LATEST APPROVED METHODS OF TREATMENT
FOR THE PRACTICING PHYSICIAN

Edited by
ROBERT E. RAKEL, M.D.

Professor and Chairman, Department of Family Medicine
Associate Dean for Academic and Clinical Affairs
Baylor College of Medicine, Houston, Texas

W.B. SAUNDERS COMPANY
A Division of Harcourt Brace & Company
Philadelphia London Toronto Montreal Sydney Tokyo

W.B. SAUNDERS COMPANY
A Division of
Harcourt Brace & Company

The Curtis Center
Independence Square West
Philadelphia, Pennsylvania 19106

Library of Congress Cataloging-in-Publication Data

Current therapy; latest approved methods of treatment for the practicing physician.

Editors: H. F. Conn and others.

v. 28 cm. annual.

ISBN 0–7216–6259–5

1. Therapeutics.　　2. Therapeutics, Surgical.　　3. Medicine—
　　Practice.　　I. Conn, Howard Franklin, 1908–1982 ed.

RM101.C87　　　616.058　　　49–8328 rev*

Conn's Current Therapy 1996　　　　　　　　　　　　　　　　　　　ISBN 0–7216–6259–5

Printed in the United States of America

Last digit is the print number:　　9　8　7　6　5　4　3　2　1

Contributors

JENNIFER M. ABIDARI, M.D.

Chief Resident, Scott Department of Urology, Baylor College of Medicine, Houston, Texas
Bacterial Infections of the Urinary Tract in Girls

JONATHAN ABRAMS, M.D.

Professor of Medicine (Cardiology), University of New Mexico School of Medicine, Albuquerque, New Mexico
Congestive Heart Failure

PAUL C. ADAMS, M.D.

Associate Professor of Medicine (Gastroenterology), University of Western Ontario; University Hospital, London, Ontario, Canada
Hemochromatosis

KEDAR K. ADOUR, M.D.

Director of Research, Senior Consultant, and Department of Head and Neck Surgery; Chairman, Cranial Nerve Research Clinic, Kaiser Permanente Medical Center, Oakland, California
Acute Facial Paralysis

H. RICHARD ALEXANDER, Jr., M.D.

Assistant Professor of Surgery, Uniformed Services University School of Medicine; Senior Investigator, Surgery Branch, National Cancer Institute, National Institutes of Health, Bethesda, Maryland
Tumors of the Stomach

DAVID ALTARAC, M.D., M.P.A.

Assistant Professor of Medicine, Albert Einstein College of Medicine of Yeshiva University; Chief, Infectious Disease Services, Methadone Maintenance Treatment Program; Assistant Attending Physician, Department of Medicine and Division of Infectious Diseases, Beth Israel Medical Center, New York, New York
Management of the Patient with Human Immunodeficiency Virus Disease

MAMMO AMARE, M.D.

Texas Oncology, PA, Dallas, Texas
Vitamin K Deficiency

JAYASEELAN AMBROSE, M.B.

Fellow, Division of Cardiology, Oregon Health Sciences University, Portland, Oregon
Infective Endocarditis

C. ALAN ANDERSON, M.D.

Instructor and Neurobehavioral Fellow, Department of Neurology, University of Colorado School of Medicine; Instructor and Fellow, Department of Neurology, University of Colorado Health Sciences Center, Denver, Colorado
Viral Meningitis and Encephalitis

KENNETH C. ANDERSON, M.D.

Associate Professor of Medicine, Harvard Medical School; Medical Director, Blood Component Laboratory, Dana-Farber Cancer Institute, Boston, Massachusetts
Adverse Reactions to Blood Transfusion

RON J. ANDERSON, M.D.

Professor of Internal Medicine, University of Texas Southwestern Medical Center; President and Chief Executive Officer, Parkland Memorial Hospital, Dallas, Texas
Disturbances Due to Heat

KATHRYN M. ANDOLSEK, M.D., M.P.H.

Clinical Associate Professor, Duke University Medical Center; Division Chief and Program Director, Family Medicine Residency Program, Duke University Medical Center, Durham, North Carolina
Antepartum Care

AŚOK C. ANTONY, M.D.

Professor of Medicine, Division of Hematology-Oncology, Department of Medicine, Indiana University School of Medicine; Attending Physician, Indiana University Hospitals, Indianapolis, Indiana
Pernicious Anemia and Other Megaloblastic Anemias

JAMES V. AQUAVELLA, M.D.

Clinical Professor of Ophthalmology and Director, Cornea Research Laboratory, University of Rochester School of Medicine and Dentistry; Surgeon, Strong Memorial Hospital, Rochester, New York
Conjunctivitis

JAMES E. ARNOLD, M.D.

Associate Professor of Otolaryngology, Head and Neck Surgery and Pediatrics, Case Western Reserve University School of Medicine; Chief, Pediatric Otolaryngology, Rainbow Babies and Children's Hospital, Cleveland, Ohio
Otitis Media

ANN M. ARVIN, M.D.

Professor, Stanford University, Stanford; Attending Physician, Packard Children's Hospital, Palo Alto, California
Chickenpox (Varicella)

DEAN G. ASSIMOS, M.D.

Associate Professor of Surgical Sciences (Urology), Bowman Gray School of Medicine; Attending Physician, The Wake Forest University Medical Center, Winston-Salem, North Carolina
Nephrolithiasis

OMAR T. ATIQ, M.D.

Assistant Clinical Professor of Medicine, University of Arkansas for Medical Sciences, Little Rock; Medical Director, Cancer Treatment Program, Jefferson Regional Medical Center, Pine Bluff, Arkansas
Tumors of the Colon and Rectum

PHYLLIS AUGUST, M.D.

Associate Professor of Medicine and Obstetrics and Gynecology, Cornell University Medical College; Associate Attending Physician, The New York Hospital, New York, New York
Hypertensive Disorders of Pregnancy

KEVIN A. AULT, M.D.

Assistant Professor, Department of Obstetrics and Gynecology, University of Kansas Medical Center, Kansas City, Kansas
Acute Pyelonephritis

ABDU F. AZAD, Ph.D.

Professor, Department of Microbiology and Immunology, University of Maryland Medical School, Baltimore, Maryland
The Typhus Fevers

DAVID A. BAKER, M.D.

Associate Professor and Director, Division of Infectious Diseases, Department of Obstetrics, Gynecology, and Reproductive Medicine, State University of New York at Stony Brook, Stony Brook, New York
Rubella and Congenital Rubella

JAMES R. BAKER, Jr., M.D.

Associate Professor and Chief, Division of Allergy, Department of Internal Medicine, University of Michigan Medical School; Attending Physician, University of Michigan Medical Center, Ann Arbor, Michigan
Thyroiditis

JAMES C. BALLENGER, M.D.

Chairman and Professor, Department of Psychiatry and Behavioral Sciences; Director, Institute of Psychiatry, Medical University of South Carolina, Charleston, South Carolina
Anxiety Disorders

ARIEL L. BARKAN, M.D.

Professor of Medicine, Division of Endocrinology and Metabolism, University of Michigan Medical School; Veterans' Affairs and University of Michigan Medical Centers, Ann Arbor, Michigan
Hypopituitarism

ERIC R. BATES, M.D.

Professor of Medicine, University of Michigan; Director, Cardiac Catheterization Laboratory, University Hospital, Ann Arbor, Michigan
Acute Myocardial Infarction

MARC J. BAYER, M.D.

Professor of Medicine and Surgery, University of Connecticut School of Medicine; University of Connecticut Health Center, Farmington, Connecticut
Drugs of Abuse

STEVEN R. BAYER, M.D.

Boston Regional Center for Reproductive Medicine, Stoneham, Massachusetts
Dysfunctional Uterine Bleeding

ANTONIO BAYÉS de LUNA, M.D., Ph.D.

Professor of Medicine (Cardiology), Universitat Autònoma de Barcelona; Director, Department of Cardiology and Cardiac Surgery, Hospital de la Santa Creu i Sant Pau, Universitat Autònoma de Barcelona, Barcelona, Spain
Pericarditis

DAVID J. BAYLINK, M.D.

Distinguished Professor of Medicine, Loma Linda University; Chief, Mineral Metabolism, Jerry L. Pettis Veterans' Administration Hospital, Loma Linda, California
Osteoporosis

JOSHUA B. BEDERSON, M.D.

Director of Cerebrovascular Surgery and Assistant Professor of Neurosurgery, Mount Sinai School of Medicine; Attending Neurosurgeon, Mount Sinai Hospital, New York, New York
Trigeminal Neuralgia

RAYMOND BÉGIN, M.D.

Professor of Medicine, University of Sherbrooke; Centre Hospitalier Universitaire de Sherbrooke, Sherbrooke, Quebec, Canada
Silicosis

WILLIAM D. BELVILLE, M.D.

Associate Professor of Surgery, Section of Urology, University of Michigan Medical Center; Associate Professor with Tenure, Department of Surgery (Urology), University of Michigan, Ann Arbor, Michigan; Clinical Professor, Department of Urology, University of Washington, Seattle, Washington; Clinical Associate Professor, Department of Surgery (Urology), Uniformed Services, University of the Health Sciences, Bethesda, Maryland
Benign Prostatic Hyperplasia

MARSHALL E. BENJAMIN, M.D.

Vascular Surgery Fellow, Department of Surgery, Bowman Gray School of Medicine, Winston-Salem, North Carolina
Acquired Diseases of the Aorta

ANN BERGIN, M.B.

Clinical Fellow, Department of Neurology, Johns Hopkins University, School of Medicine; Clinical Fellow, Johns Hopkins Hospital, Baltimore, Maryland
Gilles De La Tourette Syndrome

JUDITH A. BETTS, M.D.

Assistant Professor of Medicine, Department of Internal Medicine, College of Medicine, Division of Nephrology, The Ohio State University Medical Center; Attending Physician, Department of Internal Medicine/Division of Nephrology, The Ohio State University Medical Center, Columbus, Ohio
Primary Glomerulopathies

HENRY R. BLACK, M.D.

Charles J. and Margaret Roberts Professor of Preventive Medicine, Chairman, Department of Preventive Medicine, Professor of Internal Medicine, Senior Attending Physician, Rush-Presbyterian-St. Luke's Hospital, Chicago, Illinois
Pheochromocytoma

KIRBY I. BLAND, M.D.

J. Murray Beardsley Professor and Chairman, Department of Surgery, Brown University School of Medicine; Surgeon-in-Chief, Rhode Island Hospital, Providence, Rhode Island
Diseases of the Breast

THOMAS P. BLECK, M.D.

Associate Professor of Neurology and Neurological Surgery, and The Louise Nerancy Professor in Neurology, The University of Virginia; Director, Neurocritical Care Unit, and Chief, Division of Critical Care, Department of Neurology, University of Virginia, Charlottesville, Virginia
Tetanus

WILLIAM Z. BORER, M.D.

Associate Professor, Department of Pathology, Anatomy, and Cell Biology, Thomas Jefferson University; Director of Clinical Chemistry, Thomas Jefferson University Hospital, Philadelphia, Pennsylvania
Reference Intervals for the Interpretation of Laboratory Tests

DERALD E. BRACKMANN, M.D.

Clinical Professor of Otolaryngology, Head, and Neck Surgery; Clinical Professor of Neurosurgery, University of Southern California School of Medicine; President, House Ear Clinic; Board of Directors, House Ear Institute, Los Angeles, California
Meniere's Disease

ROBERT W. BRADSHER, Jr., M.D.

Professor and Vice-Chairman of Medicine and Director, Division of Infectious Diseases, University of Arkansas for Medical Sciences; Attending Physician, University Hospital of Arkansas, John L. McClellan Veterans' Medical Center, Little Rock, Arkansas
Blastomycosis

CHARLES BRADY, M.D.

Associate Professor of Medicine, University of Texas Health Science Center at San Antonio; Director, Endoscopy Center, University Hospital; Attending Physician, Audie L. Murphy Memorial Veterans' Hospital, San Antonio, Texas
Gastritis

DOUGLAS L. BRAND, M.D.

Associate Professor of Medicine and Associate Chair and Director of Education, Department of Medicine, State University of New York at Stony Brook, Stony Brook, New York
Dysphagia and Esophageal Obstruction

CALVIN R. BROWN, JR., M.D.

Assistant Professor of Medicine, Rush Medical College; Attending Physician, Rush-Presbyterian-St. Luke's Medical Center, Chicago, Illinois
Bursitis, Tendinitis, Myofascial Pain, and Fibromyalgia

LUCINDA S. BUESCHER, M.D.

Assistant Professor and Residency Program Director, Division of Dermatology, Southern Illinois University School of Medicine; Attending Physician, Memorial Medical Center and St. John's Hospital, Springfield, Illinois
Spider Bites and Scorpion Stings

ROBERT K. BUSH, M.D.

Professor of Medicine, University of Wisconsin-Madison; Chief of Allergy, William S. Middleton Veterans' Administration Hospital, Madison, Wisconsin
Asthma in Adults and Adolescents

WILLIAM R. BYRNE, M.D.

Assistant Professor of Medicine, Uniformed Services University of the Health Sciences, Bethesda; Chief, Genetics and Physiology Branch, Bacteriology Division, US Army Medical Research Institute of Infectious Diseases, Fort Detrick, Frederick, Maryland; Attending Physician, Walter Reed Army Medical Center, Washington, District of Columbia
Bacterial Meningitis

JOHN J. BYRNES, M.D.

Professor of Medicine, University of Miami School of Medicine; Chief of Hematology and Oncology Section, Miami Veterans' Administration Medical Center, Miami, Florida
Disseminated Intravascular Coagulation; Thrombotic Thrombocytopenic Purpura and the Hemolytic-Uremic Syndrome

THOMAS R. CARACCIO, Pharm.D.

Assistant Professor of Emergency Medicine, State University of New York at Stony Brook, Stony Brook; Assistant Professor of Pharmacology/Toxicology, New York College of Osteopathic Medicine, Old Westbury; Assistant Professor of Clinical Pharmacy, St. John's University College Pharmacy, Jamaica; Assistant Director of Long Island Regional Poison Control Center, East Meadow; Winthrop University Hospital, Mineola, New York
Acute Poisonings

DANIEL E. CASEY, M.D.

Professor of Psychiatry and Neurology, Oregon Health Sciences University; Chief of Psychiatry Research/Psychopharmacology, Veterans' Administration Medical Center, Portland, Oregon
Schizophrenia

CONNIE CELUM, M.D., M.P.H.

Assistant Professor of Medicine, University of Washington; Medical Director, Harborview STD Clinic, Seattle, Washington
Nongonococcal Urethritis in Men

WALTER CHAIM, M.D.

Senior Lecturer, Department of Obstetrics and Gynecology, Soroka Medical Center of Kupat Holim, Ben Gurion University, Beer-sheva, Israel; Visiting Professor, Department of Obstetrics and Gynecology, Grace Hospital, Detroit Medical Center, Detroit, Michigan
Postpartum Care

HELENA R. CHANG, M.D., Ph.D.

Associate Professor of Surgery and Pathobiology, Brown University School of Medicine; Director of the Hybridoma Laboratory; Surgeon, Roger Williams Hospital, Providence, Rhode Island
Diseases of the Breast

STEPHEN A. CHARTRAND, M.D.

Professor and Chairman, Department of Pediatrics, and Director, Pediatric Infectious Disease Training Program, Creighton University School of Medicine; Director of Pediatric Infectious Disease, University of Nebraska Medical Center and Children's Hospital of Omaha, Omaha, Nebraska
Pertussis (Whooping Cough)

WISSAM CHATILA, M.D.

Pulmonary Fellow, Bridgeport Hospital, Bridgeport, Connecticut
Cough

GLENN M. CHERTOW, M.D., M.P.H.

Instructor in Medicine, Harvard Medical School; Chief Medical Resident, Brigham and Women's Hospital, Boston, Massachusetts
Chronic Renal Failure

ELLIOT CHESLER, M.D.

Professor of Medicine, University of Minnesota; Chief, Cardiovascular Division, Veterans' Administration Hospital, Minneapolis, Minnesota
Mitral Valve Prolapse

P. JOAN CHESNEY, M.D.

Professor of Pediatrics, University of Tennessee; Active Staff, Le Bonheur Children's Medical Center, Memphis, Tennessee
Toxic Shock Syndrome

BRUCE D. CHESON, M.D.

Head, Medicine Section, Cancer Therapy Evaluation Program, Division of Cancer Treatment, National Cancer Institute; Senior Staff, National Cancer Institute, Bethesda, Maryland
Non-Hodgkin's Lymphomas

BARRETT H. CHILDS, M.D.

Instructor, Cornell University Medical College; Clinical Assistant, Memorial Sloan-Kettering Cancer Center, New York, New York
Aplastic Anemia

STACY J. CHILDS, M.D.

Associate Clinical Professor of Urology, University of Colorado Health Sciences Center, Denver, Colorado; Staff Urologist, United Medical Center, West Cheyenne, Wyoming
Prostatitis

MARC I. CHIMOWITZ, M.B., Ch.B.

Associate Professor of Neurology and Director of Cerebrovascular Program, Emory University School of Medicine; Attending Physician, Emory University Hospital, Atlanta, Georgia
Focal Ischemic Cerebrovascular Disease

YANEK S. Y. CHIU, M.D.

Associate Clinical Professor of Surgery, University of California at San Francisco; Active Staff, California Pacific Medical Center, San Francisco, California
Hemorrhoids, Anal Fissure, and Anorectal Abscess and Fistula

BRUNO B. CHOMEL, D.V.M., Ph.D.

Assistant Professor, School of Veterinary Medicine, University of California at Davis, Davis, California
Q Fever

G. PATRICK CLAGETT, M.D.

Professor of Surgery and Head of Vascular Surgery, Department of Surgery, University of Texas Southwestern Medical Center at Dallas; Attending Staff, Vascular and General Surgery and Head of Vascular Surgery, Parkland Memorial Hospital; Attending Staff, Vascular and General Surgery, Zale Lipshy University Hospital, Dallas, Texas
Deep Venous Thrombosis of the Lower Extremities

KEITH A. CLARK, D.V.M., PH.D.

Director, Zoonosis Control Division, Texas Department of Health, Austin, Texas
Rabies

HARRIS R. CLEARFIELD, M.D.

Professor of Medicine and Director, Division of Gastroenterology, Hahnemann University, Medical College of Pennsylvania; Attending Physician, Hahnemann University Hospital, Philadelphia, Pennsylvania
Diverticula of the Alimentary Tract

MARC S. COHEN, M.D.

Associate Professor of Surgery/Urology, The University of Florida College of Medicine; Attending Faculty, Shands Teaching Hospital and Affiliated Clinics, Gainesville Veterans' Administration Medical Center, Gainesville, Florida
Epididymitis

JONATHAN CORREN, M.D.

Clinical Assistant Professor, Department of Medicine, and Director, Allergy and Immunology Clinic, University of California at Los Angeles, Los Angeles, California
Allergic Rhinitis Caused by Inhalant Factors

CHRISTOPHER M. CORSI, M.D.

Fellow in Endocrinology, University of Virginia, Charlottesville, Virginia
Hyperprolactinemia

DAVID M. COSENTINO, M.D.

Physician, University of Connecticut Health Center, Farmington, Connecticut
Drugs of Abuse

FERNANDO G. COSIO, M.D.

Professor of Medicine, Department of Internal Medicine, College of Medicine, Division of Nephrology, The Ohio State University Medical Center; Attending Physician, Department of Internal Medicine/Division of Nephrology, The Ohio State University Medical Center, Columbus, Ohio
Primary Glomerulopathies

JOSEPH J. COTTRELL, M.D.

Assistant Professor of Medicine, University of Pittsburgh School of Medicine; Associate Chief of Staff, Veterans' Affairs Medical Center, Pittsburgh, Pennsylvania
Acute Respiratory Failure

JOHN V. COX, D.O.

Texas Oncology, PA, Dallas, Texas
Vitamin K Deficiency

MALCOLM COX, M.D.

Professor of Medicine; Vice Chairman, Department of Medicine, University of Pennsylvania School of Medicine, Philadelphia, Pennsylvania
Diabetes Insipidus

CHRISTINA M. COYLE, M.D.

Assistant Professor of Medicine, Division of Internal Medicine and Division of Infectious Diseases, Albert Einstein College of Medicine; Associate Director of Medicine, Bronx Municipal Hospital, New York, New York
Malaria

SCOTT CROW, M.D.

Assistant Professor of Psychiatry, University of Minnesota Medical School; Director, Consult Liaison Psychiatry, University of Minnesota Hospital and Clinic, Minneapolis, Minnesota
Bulimia Nervosa

JAMES P. CROWLEY, M.D.

Professor of Medicine, Brown University School of Medicine; Director of Clinical Hematology, Rhode Island Hospital, Providence, Rhode Island
Nonimmune Hemolytic Anemia

JAMES M. CRUTCHER, M.D., M.P.H.

Clinical Researcher, Naval Medical Research Institute, Bethesda, Maryland
Typhoid Fever

JOHN P. CURTIN, M.D.

Assistant Professor, Department of Obstetrics and Gynecology, Cornell University Medical School; Associate Attending Surgeon, Gynecology Service, Department of Surgery, Memorial Sloan-Kettering Cancer Center, New York, New York
Endometrial Cancer

ALBERT J. CZAJA, M.D.

Professor of Medicine, Mayo Medical School; Consultant in Gastroenterology, Mayo Clinic, Rochester, Minnesota
Bleeding Esophageal Varices

ALAN DALKIN, M.D.

Assistant Professor, Department of Internal Medicine, Division of Endocrinology, University of Virginia, Charlottesville, Virginia
Hyperprolactinemia

ARISTOTLE J. DAMIANOS, M.D.

Assistant Professor of Medicine, The Milton S. Hershey Medical Center, Pennsylvania State University, Hershey, Pennsylvania
Irritable Bowel Syndrome

ROBERT N. DAVIDSON, M.D.

Senior Lecturer, St. Mary's Hospital Medical School, London; Consultant in Infection and Tropical Medicine, Northwick Park Hospital, Harrow, Middlesex, England, United Kingdom
Leishmaniasis

KELLY D. DAVIS, M.D.

Assistant Professor of Medicine, Division of Endocrinology Diabetes and Metabolism, University of Pennsylvania School of Medicine; Medical Staff, Hospital of the University of Pennsylvania, Philadelphia, Pennsylvania
Hypothyroidism

CATHERINE L. DEAN, M.D., M.P.H.

Clinical Instructor in Obstetrics and Gynecology, Washington University School of Medicine; Attending Physician, Department of Obstetrics and Gynecology, Barnes Hospital, Jewish Hospital, Missouri Baptist Hospital, and Christian Northwest Hospital, St. Louis, Missouri
Contraception

RICHARD H. DEAN, M.D.

Chairman, Department of Surgery, Professor of Surgery, and Director of the Division of Surgical Sciences, Bowman Gray School of Medicine; Chief of Surgery, North Carolina Baptist Hospital, Winston-Salem, North Carolina
Acquired Diseases of the Aorta

ALAN H. DeCHERNEY, M.D.

Professor and Chairman of Obstetrics and Gynecology, Tufts University School of Medicine, Chief of Services, Department of Obstetrics and Gynecology, New England Medical Center, Boston, Massachusetts
Dysfunctional Uterine Bleeding

ROSS M. DECTER, M.D.

Associate Professor of Surgery (Urology) and Director of Pediatric Urology, The Milton S. Hershey Medical Center, Pennsylvania State University, Hershey, Pennsylvania
Childhood Enuresis

ALBERT A. DEL NEGRO, M.D.

Clinical Assistant Professor of Medicine, Georgetown University School of Medicine, Washington, District of Columbia; Director, Pacemaker Clinic, Fairfax Hospital, Falls Church; Director of Clinical Cardiac Electrophysiology, Alexandria Hospital, Alexandria, Virginia
Heart Block

KATHLEEN A. DELANEY, M.D.

Associate Professor of Surgery and Associate Professor of Internal Medicine, University of Texas, Southwestern Medical Center, Dallas, Texas
Disturbances Due to Heat

DAVID T. DENNIS, M.D., M.P.H.

Chief, Bacterial Zoonoses Branch, Centers for Disease Control and Prevention, National Center for Infectious Diseases, Division of Vector-Borne Infectious Diseases, Fort Collins, Colorado
Plague

ANNE E. DE PAPP, M.D.

Assistant Professor of Medicine, Thomas Jefferson Medical School, Philadelphia, Pennsylvania
Acromegaly

RICHARD D. DeSHAZO, M.D.

Professor of Medicine and Pediatrics and Director, Division of Allergy and Clinical Immunology, Departments of Medicine and Pediatrics, College of Medicine, University of South Alabama; Attending Physician, University of South Alabama Hospitals and Clinics, Mobile, Alabama
Allergic Reactions to Insect Stings

REGIS A. DeSILVA, M.B., B.S.

Assistant Professor of Medicine, Harvard Medical School; Staff Cardiologist, Cardiovascular Division, Deaconess Hospital, Boston, Massachusetts
Care After Myocardial Infarction

EDWARD A. DOMINGUEZ, M.D.

Assistant Professor, Department of Internal Medicine, University of Nebraska Medical Center; Attending Physician, University of Nebraska Medical Center, Omaha, Nebraska
Bacterial Pneumonia

FRITZ E. DREIFUSS, M.B.

Thomas E. Worrell Jr. Professor of Epileptology and Neurology, University of Virginia School of Medicine; Neurologist and Director, Comprehensive Epilepsy Program, University of Virginia Health Sciences Center, Charlottesville, Virginia
Epilepsy in Infants and Children

ANN-CHRISTINE DUHAIME, M.D.

Assistant Professor, University of Pennsylvania School of Medicine; Associate Neurosurgeon, Children's Hospital of Philadelphia, Philadelphia, Pennsylvania
Acute Head Injuries in Children

JEFFERY S. DZIECZKOWSKI, M.D.

Assistant Professor of Pathology, Wayne State University School of Medicine; Medical Director of Laboratories, Hutzel Hospital, Detroit, Michigan
Adverse Reactions to Blood Transfusion

GRETCHEN M. EAMES, M.D., M.P.H.

Fellow, Division of Pediatric Hematology/Oncology/Bone Marrow Transplant, Department of Pediatrics, University of Minnesota, Minneapolis, Minnesota
Acute Leukemia in Childhood

KEVIN O. EASLEY, J.D., M.D.

Gynecologic Oncology Fellow and Instructor, Department of Obstetrics and Gynecology, Washington University School of Medicine; Attending Physician, Barnes Hospital, St. Louis, Missouri
Neoplasms of the Vulva

JAMES S. ECONOMOU, M.D., PH.D.

Professor of Surgery, Louis D. Beaumont Chair in Surgery, Division of Surgical Oncology, Department of Surgery, University of California at Los Angeles School of Medicine; Attending Surgeon, University of California at Los Angeles Medical Center, Los Angeles, California
Malignant Melanoma

STEVEN V. EDELMAN, M.D.

Associate Professor of Medicine, Division of Endocrinology and Metabolism, University of California; Staff Physician, Veterans' Affairs Medical Center; Staff Physician, University of California, San Diego, Medical Center, San Diego, California
Diabetes Mellitus in Adults

RICHARD F. EDLICH, M.D., Ph.D.

Distinguished Professor of Plastic Surgery and Biomedical Engineering, University of Virginia School of Medicine, Charlottesville, Virginia
Bacterial Diseases of the Skin

NATHANIEL C. EDWARDS, M.D.

Clinical Fellow in Medicine, Harvard Medical School; Cardiology Fellow, Deaconess Hospital, Boston, Massachusetts
Care After Myocardial Infarction

EDWARD S. EISENBERG, M.D.

Assistant Professor of Medicine, Albert Einstein School of Medicine, Bronx, New York; Attending Physician, Mountainside Hospital, Montclair, New Jersey
Rat-Bite Fever

KENNETH A. ELLENBOGEN, M.D.

Associate Professor of Medicine, Medical College of Virginia; Director, Clinical Electrophysiology and Pacing Laboratory, Medical College of Virginia, and McGuire Veterans' Administration Medical Center, Richmond, Virginia
Atrial Fibrillation

KATHRYN J. ELLIOTT, M.D.

Assistant Attending Neurologist, Memorial Hospital for Cancer and Allied Diseases, Memorial Sloan-Kettering Cancer Center; Assistant Professor, Department of Neurology, Cornell University Medical College, New York, New York
Pain

CRAIG A. ELMETS, M.D.

Professor of Dermatology and Director, Skin Diseases Research Center, Case Western Reserve University; Attending Physician, University Hospitals of Cleveland, Cleveland Veterans' Administration Medical Center, Cleveland, Ohio
Cutaneous Vasculitis

WILLIAM L. EPSTEIN, M.D.

Professor, Department of Dermatology, University of California at San Francisco, San Francisco; Consultant, U.S. Department of Health, Education, and Welfare; Consultant in Dermatology, Oak Knoll Hospital, Oakland, California
Contact Dermatitis

JAVIER I. ESCOBAR II, M.D.

General Surgery Resident, University of Connecticut Health Center, Farmington, Connecticut
Drugs of Abuse

FUAD S. FARAH, M.D.

Professor of Medicine and Chief, Division of Dermatology, State University of New York at Syracuse, Health Science Center; Chief, Division of Dermatology, and Director, Dermatology Clinics, State University Hospital, Syracuse, New York
Parasitic Diseases of the Skin

EDWARD FELDMANN, M.D.

Associate Professor of Neurology, Brown University School of Medicine; Director, Division of Cerebrovascular Diseases and Sonography, and Director, Neurology Cerebrovascular Laboratory, Rhode Island Hospital, Providence, Rhode Island
Intracerebral Hemorrhage

BRUCE A. FERRELL, M.D.

Assistant Professor, University of California at San Francisco, School of Medicine, San Francisco, California; Associate Director for Clinical Programs of the Geriatric Research, Education, and Clinical Center, Sepulveda Veterans' Administration Medical Center, Sepulveda, California
Pressure Ulcers

JILL S. FISCHER, B.A.

Medical Student, Yale University School of Medicine, New Haven, Connecticut
Endometriosis

MARCELA FISHER-TABUENCA, M.D.

Fellow, Department of Medicine, Loma Linda University, Loma Linda, California
Osteoporosis

LORRAINE A. FITZPATRICK, M.D.

Professor Medicine, Mayo Medical School; Consultant in Endocrinology and Metabolism, Mayo Clinic and Mayo Foundation, Rochester, Minnesota
Paget's Disease of Bone

ALAN B. FLEISCHER, JR., M.D.

Assistant Professor of Dermatology, Bowman Gray School of Medicine of Wake Forest University; Liaison to the Center on Aging; Director, CTCL Clinic; Attending Physician, North Carolina Baptist Hospital, Winston Salem, North Carolina
Pruritus (Itching)

THOMAS E. FLEMING, M.D.

Resident, Department of Dermatology, University Hospitals of Cleveland, Cleveland Veterans' Administration Medical Center, Cleveland, Ohio
Cutaneous Vasculitis

SCOTT W. FOSKO, M.D.

Assistant Professor of Internal Medicine, Division of Dermatology; Director, Mohs Cutaneous Micrographic Surgery, Saint Louis University Health Sciences Center, Saint Louis, Missouri
Cancer of the Skin

AIDAN FOY, M.B., M.Sc.

Clinical Lecturer, Faculty of Medicine, University of Newcastle; Director, Alcohol and Drug Unit, Newcastle Mater Misericordiae Hospital, Newcastle, New South Wales, Australia
The Management of Alcoholism

ELLIOT FRANK, M.D.

Clinical Associate Professor, University of Medicine and Dentistry of New Jersey, Robert Wood Johnson Medical School, New Brunswick; Director, Division of Infectious Diseases, and Associate Program Director, Department of Medicine, Jersey Shore Medical Center, Neptune, New Jersey
Lyme Disease and Ehrlichiosis

J. MICHAEL FULLER, M.D.

Fellow, Pulmonary and Critical Care Medicine, University of Alabama, Birmingham, Alabama
Sarcoidosis

HOWARD J. FULLMAN, M.D.

Assistant Clinical Professor of Medicine, University of California at Los Angeles, Los Angeles; Attending Physician and Chief, Biliary Endoscopy Divison of Gastroenterology, Department of Internal Medicine, Kaiser Permanente, West Los Angeles, California
Gaseousness and Indigestion

JACK D. FULMER, M.D.

Professor of Medicine and Ben V. Branscomb Chair of Respiratory Disease, University of Alabama at Birmingham; Attending Physician, University of Alabama Hospitals and Clinics, Birmingham, Alabama
Sarcoidosis

KAREN L. FURIE, M.D.

Research Fellow in Cerebrovascular Disease, Brown University School of Medicine; Fellow in Cerebrovascular Disease, Department of Neurology, Rhode Island Hospital, Providence, Rhode Island
Intracerebral Hemorrhage

ANNE-SOPHIE J. GADENNE, M.D.

Dermatology Resident, University of Cincinnati Medical Center, Cincinnati, Ohio
Pigmentary Disorders

JOHN N. GALGIANI, M.D.

Chief, Section of Infectious Diseases, Veterans' Administration Medical Center, Tucson, Arizona
Coccidioidomycosis

RON MATTHEW GALL, B.M.R.(P.T.)

Staff Therapist, Sports Physiotherapy Centre, Pan Am Sports Medicine Centre, Winnipeg, Manitoba, Canada
Ankylosing Spondylitis

NELSON M. GANTZ, M.D.

Clinical Professor of Medicine, Pennsylvania State University College of Medicine, Hershey; Chairman of Medicine and Chief of Infectious Diseases, Polyclinic Medical Center, Harrisburg, Pennsylvania
Sinusitis

MARIA A. GEORGSSON, M.D.

Senior Fellow, Division of Gastroenterology-Hepatology, State University of New York at Stony Brook, Stony Brook, New York
Dysphagia and Esophageal Obstruction

ALFRED L. GEST, M.D.

Assistant Professor of Pediatrics, Baylor College of Medicine; Neonatologist, Texas Children's Hospital, Houston, Texas
Resuscitation of the Newborn

MUHAMMAD GHADAI, M.D.

Fellow in Geriatric Medicine, University of California, Los Angeles, School of Medicine, Los Angeles; Fellow, Sepulveda Veterans' Administration Medical Center, Sepulveda, California
Pressure Ulcers

VINCENZO F. GIANNELLI, M.D.

Assistant Clinical Professor, Department of Dermatology, Washington Hospital Center and George Washington University Medical Center, Washington, District of Columbia
Viral Diseases of the Skin

ALLAN GIBOFSKY, M.D., J.D.

Professor, Departments of Medicine and Public Health, Cornell University Medical College; Attending Rheumatologist, The Hospital for Special Surgery; Attending Physician, Department of Medicine, The New York Hospital, New York, New York
Rheumatic Fever

DONALD H. GILDEN, M.D.

Professor and Chairman, Department of Neurology, University of Colorado School of Medicine; Professor, Department of Neurology, University Hospital, University of Colorado Health Sciences Center, Denver, Colorado
Viral Meningitis and Encephalitis

DAVID M. GILLIGAN, M.D.

Assistant Professor of Medicine, Medical College of Virginia; Co-Director, Clinical Electrophysiology Laboratory, McGuire Veterans' Administration Medical Center, Richmond, Virginia
Atrial Fibrillation

SERGIO A. GIRALT, M.D.

Assistant Internist and Instructor, University of Texas M. D. Anderson Cancer Center, Houston, Texas
Chronic Leukemias

ELI GLATSTEIN, M.D.

Professor and Chairman, Radiation Oncology Department, University of Texas Southwestern Medical School, Dallas, Texas
Hodgkin's Disease: Radiation Therapy

MATTHEW BIDWELL GOETZ, M.D.

Associate Professor of Medicine, University of California, Los Angeles, School of Medicine; Associate Chief, Infectious Diseases, West Los Angeles Veterans' Administration Medical Center, Los Angeles, California
Bacteremia and Septicemia

MITCHELL GOLDMAN, M.D.

Assistant Professor, Department of Medicine, Division of Infectious Diseases, Indiana University School of Medicine; Attending Physician, Indiana University Hospital, Wishard Memorial Hospital, Indianapolis, Indiana
Histoplasmosis

JERRY GOLDSTONE, M.D.

Professor of Surgery, Division of Vascular Surgery, Department of Surgery, University of California; Director, S.T.A.M.P. Veterans' Administration Medical Center, San Francisco, California
Peripheral Arterial Disease

LOREN E. GOLITZ, M.D.

Professor of Dermatology and Pathology and Training Director for Dermatopathology, University of Colorado School of Medicine; Chief of Dermatology and Clinical Director, Ambulatory Care Center, Denver General Hospital, Denver, Colorado
Nevi

BERNARD GONIK, M.D.

Professor and Associate Chairman, Department of Obstetrics and Gynecology, Wayne State University School of Medicine; Chief, Department of Obstetrics and Gynecology, Grace Hospital/The Detroit Medical Center, Detroit, Michigan
Postpartum Care

E. ANN GORMLEY, M.D.

Assistant Professor of Surgery (Urology), Dartmouth Medical School, Hanover; Staff Urologist, Dartmouth-Hitchcock Medical Center, Lebanon, New Hampshire
Urinary Incontinence

RAFAEL GORODISCHER, M.D.

Professor of Pediatrics, Faculty of Health Sciences, Ben Gurion University of the Negev; Director, Department of Pediatrics, Soroka Medical Center, Beersheva, Israel
Fever

MARK F. GOURLEY, M.D.

Senior Staff Fellow, Clinical Investigations Section, Arthritis and Rheumatism Branch, National Institutes of Health, Bethesda, Maryland
Connective Tissue Disorders

GLEN A. GREEN, M.D.

Assistant Professor of Pediatrics, Eastern Virginia Medical School; Neonatologist, Children's Hospital of The King's Daughters, and Medical Director Intermediate Nursery, Sentara Hospitals, Norfolk, Virginia
Care of the High-Risk Neonate

ROBERT P. GREEN, M.D.

Associate Clinical Professor, Department of Otolaryngology, Mount Sinai School of Medicine; Attending Physician, Mount Sinai Hospital, New York, New York
Tinnitus

BARRY H. GREENBERG, M.D.

Professor of Medicine, University of California, San Diego; Director, Heart Failure/Cardiac Transplantation, Division of Cardiology, University of California at San Diego, Medical Center, San Diego, California
Infective Endocarditis

RICHARD N. GREENBERG, M.D.

Associate Professor of Medicine, Division of Infectious Diseases, University of Kentucky Medical School; Attending Physician, University of Kentucky Medical Center and Lexington Veterans' Administration Medical Center, Lexington, Kentucky
Osteomyelitis

JOSEPH GREENSHER, M.D.

Professor of Pediatrics, State University of New York at Stony Brook, Stony Brook; Medical Director and Associate Chairman, Department of Pediatrics, Winthrop University Hospital, Mineola; Associate Director, Long Island Regional Poison Control Center, East Meadow, New York
Acute Poisonings

JOHN A. GRISWOLD, M.D.

Associate Professor of Surgery, Texas Tech University Health Sciences Center; Director, Timothy J. Harnar Burn Center, University Medical Center, Lubbock, Texas
Burns

DIETER H. M. GRÖESCHEL, M.D., PH.D.

Professor of Pathology, University of Virginia School of Medicine; Director of Microbiology, Department of Pathology, University of Virginia School of Medicine, Charlottesville, Virginia
Bacterial Diseases of the Skin

CARLOS GUARNER, M.D.

Associate Professor of Medicine, Autonomous University of Barcelona; Attending Physician, Hospital Sant Pau, Barcelona, Spain
Cirrhosis

RICHARD L. GUERRANT, M.D.

Thomas H. Hunter Professor of International Medicine and Chief, Division of Geographic Medicine, University of Virginia School of Medicine, Charlottesville, Virginia
Food-Borne Illness

WILLIAM GRAHAM GUERRIERO, M.D.

Surgical Professor of Urology, Baylor College of Medicine; Surgical Director, Kidney Transplant Program, Texas Children's Hospital; Director of Kidney Transplantation, The Methodist Hospital, Houston, Texas
Trauma to the Genitourinary Tract

JERE D. GUIN, M.D.

Professor and Chairman, Department of Dermatology, University of Arkansas for Medical Sciences, Little Rock, Arkansas
Urticaria

JOSEP GUINDO, M.D.

Staff, Coronary Care Unit, Department of Cardiology and Cardiac Surgery, Hospital de la Santa Creu i Sant Pau, Universitat Autònoma de Barcelona, Barcelona, Spain
Pericarditis

DAVID S. GUZICK, M.D., PH.D.

Henry A. Thiede Professor and Chairman, Department of Obstetrics and Gynecology, University of Rochester Medical Center, Rochester, New York
Amenorrhea

RAYMOND G. HADDAD, M.D.

Associate Clinical Professor of Medicine, Yale University School of Medicine, New Haven; Senior Attending Physician and Chief, Pulmonary Section, Bridgeport Hospital, Bridgeport, Connecticut
Cough

TIMOTHY C. HAIN, M.D.

Associate Professor, Departments of Neurology and Otolaryngology, Northwestern University Medical School; Attending Physician, Northwestern Memorial Hospital, Chicago, Illinois
Episodic Vertigo

WILLIAM D. HAIRE, M.D.

Associate Professor, Division of Oncology and Hematology, Department of Internal Medicine, University of Nebraska Medical Center, Omaha, Nebraska
Pulmonary Embolism

EDWARD L. HALL, M.D.

Director, Trauma Center; Staff Surgeon, John D. Archbold Memorial Hospital, Thomasville, Georgia
Snake Venom Poisoning

LORI-LINELL H. HALL, M.D.

Assistant Professor of Obstetrics, Gynecology and Reproductive Sciences, Division of Reproductive Endocrinology, University of Pittsburgh; Attending Physician, Magee-Women's Hospital, Pittsburgh, Pennsylvania
Amenorrhea

BRUCE W. HALSTEAD, M.D.

Director, World Life Research Institute, Colton, California
Marine Animal Injuries

STEPHEN B. HANAUER, M.D.

Professor of Medicine and Clinical Pharmacology, University of Chicago; Attending Physician, University of Chicago Medical Center, Chicago, Illinois
Crohn's Disease

JAMES B. HANSHAW, M.D., D.SCI.(HON.)

Professor of Pediatrics, University of Massachusetts Medical School; Chair, Department of Pediatrics Medical Center of Central Massachusetts, Worcester, Massachusetts
Measles

JAMES E. HAYES, M.D.

Associate Professor of Surgery and Chairman, Division of Emergency Medicine, University of Texas Southwestern Medical Center; Medical Director, Emergency Services, Parkland Memorial Hospital, Dallas, Texas
Disturbances Due to Heat

KAREN A. HEIDELBERG, M.D.

Resident in Dermatology, Mayo Graduate School of Medicine, Rochester, Minnesota
Polyarteritis Nodosa and Cutaneous Polyarteritis Nodosa

JONATHAN D. HEILICZER, M.D.

Associate Professor of Pediatrics, The Children's Kidney Center of Illinois, University of Illinois College of Medicine; Attending Physician, University of Illinois Hospital, Chicago, Illinois
Parenteral Fluid Therapy for Infants and Children

ROBERT R. HENRY, M.D.

Associate Professor of Medicine, Division of Endocrinology and Metabolism, University of California, San Diego; Staff Physician, Veterans' Affairs Medical Center; Staff Physician, University of California, San Diego, Medical Center, San Diego, California
Diabetes Mellitus in Adults

HENRY G. HERROD, M.D.

Le Bonheur Professor of Pediatrics, University of Tennessee; Staff Physician, Le Bonheur Children's Medical Center, Memphis, Tennessee
Anaphylaxis and Serum Sickness

CHARLES B. HICKS, M.D.

Assistant Professor of Medicine, Division of Infectious Diseases, Duke University Medical Center, Durham, North Carolina
Syphilis

JAMES A. HIGGINS, PH.D.

Post-Doctoral Fellow, Department of Microbiology and Immunology, University of Maryland Medical School, Baltimore, Maryland
The Typhus Fevers

HENRY T. HOFFMAN, M.D.

Associate Professor of Otolaryngology, Director, Head and Neck Oncology, and Director, Voice Clinic, University of Iowa; Attending Physician, University of Iowa Hospitals and Clinics, Iowa City, Iowa
Hoarseness and Laryngitis

STEPHEN L. HOFFMAN, M.D., D.T.M.H.

Director, Malaria Program, Naval Medical Research Institute; Adjunct Professor, Department of Preventive Medicine and Biometrics, Uniformed Services University of the Health Sciences; Attending Staff, Department of Medicine, Division of Infectious Diseases, National Naval Medical Center, Bethesda, Maryland
Typhoid Fever

W. KEITH HOOTS, M.D.

Associate Professor of Pediatrics and Internal Medicine, The University of Texas Medical School at Houston; Associate Pediatrician and Associate Professor of Pediatrics, University of Texas, M. D. Anderson Cancer Center; Associate Professor, Hermann Hospital, Houston, Texas
Hemophilia and Related Conditions

RICHARD T. HOPPE, M.D.

Professor and Chairman, Department of Radiation Oncology and Henry S. Kaplan-Henry Lebeson Professor of Cancer Biology, Stanford University School of Medicine, Stanford, California
Mycosis Fungoides

MARK C. HOUSTON, M.D.

Associate Clinical Professor of Medicine, Vanderbilt University Medical Center; Chief, Hypertension Institute, Saint Thomas Medical Group, Saint Thomas Hospital, Nashville, Tennessee
Hypertension

JAMES F. HOWARD, Jr., M.D.

Professor of Neurology, The University of North Carolina at Chapel Hill; Professor of Neurology, The University of North Carolina Hospitals, Chapel Hill, North Carolina
Myasthenia Gravis

COLIN W. HOWDEN, M.D.

Professor of Medicine, University of South Carolina School of Medicine; Staff Gastroenterologist, Richland Memorial Hospital; Consulting Gastroenterologist, Dorn Veterans' Administration Hospital, Columbia, South Carolina
Peptic Ulcer Disease

ABDOLLAH IRAVANI, M.D.

Director, Central Florida Medical Research Center, Orlando; Clinical Faculty, College of Health Science, University of Central Florida, Orlando; Professor of Pediatric Nephrology, University of Florida, Gainesville; Attending Physician, Orlando Regional Medical Center; Florida Hospital, Orlando; and Winter Park Hospital, Winter Park, Florida
Bacterial Infections of the Urinary Tract in Women

JOHN A. JERNIGAN, M.D.

Assistant Professor of Medicine, Division of Infectious Diseases, Emory University School of Medicine; Hospital Epidemiologist, Emory University Hospital, Atlanta, Georgia
Amebiasis

JAMES R. JETT, M.D.

Professor of Medicine, University of Pittsburgh, Pittsburgh, Pennsylvania
Primary Lung Cancer

PAULA H. JOHNSON, M.B., Ch.B.

Clinical Teacher, Nottingham University; Respiratory Registrar, Nottingham City Hospital, Nottingham, England, United Kingdom
Psittacosis

SCOTT A. JOHNSON, M.D.

Staff Neonatologist, Memorial Medical Center, Candler Hospital, and St. Joseph's Hospital, Savannah, Georgia
Resuscitation of the Newborn

NIGEL I. JOWETT, M.D.

District Tutor, Royal College of Physicians (UK); Consultant Physician and Director of Clinical Medicine, Pembrokeshire Health Trust, Pembrokeshire, Wales, United Kingdom
Brucellosis

FRANKLYN N. JUDSON, M.D.

Professor, Departments of Medicine and Preventive Medicine, University of Colorado Health Sciences Center; Chief of Infectious Diseases, Denver General Hospital, Denver, Colorado
Gonorrhea

JEFFREY W. KALENAK, M.D.

Associate Professor of Clinical Ophthalmology, Medical College of Wisconsin; Attending Physician, John L. Doyne Hospital; Consultant in Glaucoma, Children's Hospital of Wisconsin and Zablocki Department of Veterans' Affairs Medical Center, Milwaukee, Wisconsin
Glaucoma

H. BENFER KALTREIDER, M.D.

Professor of Medicine, University of California at San Francisco; Chief, Pulmonary and Critical Care Medicine, Veterans' Affairs Medical Center, San Francisco, California
Hypersensitivity Pneumonitis (Allergic Alveolitis)

HAGOP M. KANTARJIAN, M.D.

Professor of Medicine, University of Texas M. D. Anderson Cancer Center, Houston, Texas
Chronic Leukemias

MICHAEL P. KARNELL, Ph.D.

Associate Professor of Otolaryngology and Speech Pathology, The University of Iowa; Speech Pathologist, The University of Iowa Hospitals and Clinics, Iowa City, Iowa
Hoarseness and Laryngitis

JUDITH E. KARP, M.D.

Assistant Director for Applied Science, National Cancer Institute, Rockville; Associate Professor of Oncology and Medicine, The Johns Hopkins University School of Medicine; Member, Clinical Center Medical Staff, National Institutes of Health; Active Staff (Part-time), The Johns Hopkins Hospital, Baltimore, Maryland
Acute Leukemia in Adults

BARRY M. KARPEL, D.O.

Fellow in Maternal-Fetal Medicine, Department of Obstetrics, Gynecology and Reproductive Medicine, State University of New York at Stony Brook, Stony Brook, New York
Rubella and Congenital Rubella

JON M. KATZ, M.D.

Staff Perinatologist, Department of Obstetrics and Gynecology, Columbia Hospital for Women Medical Center, Washington, District of Columbia
Vaginal Bleeding in Late Pregnancy

RITVA KAUPPINEN-MÄKELIN, M.D., Ph.D.

Senior Consultant in Internal Medicine, Peijas Hospital, Vantaa, Finland
Adrenocortical Insufficiency

MARTIN B. KELLER, M.D.

Mary E. Zucker Professor and Chairman, Brown University; Executive Psychiatrist-in-Chief, Butler Hospital, Emma Pendleton Bradley Hospital, Memorial Hospital, Miriam Hospital, Rhode Island Hospital, Roger Williams Hospital, Veterans' Administration Medical Center, and Women and Infants Hospital, Providence, Rhode Island; Admitting Staff, Westwood Lodge Hospital, Canton, Massachusetts
Mood Disorders

RICK KELLERMAN, M.D.

Associate Professor, University of Kansas School of Medicine, Wichita; Program Director, Smoky Hill Family Practice Residency; Attending Physician, Salina Regional Medical Center, Salina, Kansas
Immunization Practices

MICHAEL F. KELLEY, M.D., M.P.H.

Chief, Bureau of Communicable Disease Control, Texas Department of Health, Austin, Texas
Rabies

NANCY KEMENY, M.D.

Professor of Medicine, Cornell University Medical College; Attending Physician, Memorial Sloan-Kettering Cancer Center, New York, New York
Tumors of the Colon and Rectum

JAMIL H. KHAN, M.D.

Associate Professor of Pediatrics, Eastern Virginia Medical School; Medical Director, Neonatal Intensive Care Unit, Children's Hospital of The King's Daughters; Neonatologist, Sentara Hospitals, Norfolk, Virginia
Care of the High-Risk Neonate

R. PHILIP KINKEL, M.D.

Director of Medical Programs, Mellen Center for Multiple Sclerosis Treatment and Research, Cleveland Clinic Foundation, Cleveland, Ohio
Multiple Sclerosis

DONALD F. KIRBY, M.D.

Associate Professor of Medicine and Chief, Section of Nutrition, Division of Gastroenterology, Medical College of Virginia Hospitals, McGuire Veterans' Administration Medical Center, Richmond, Virginia
Obesity

LANNING B. KLINE, M.D.

Professor of Clinical Ophthalmology, Combined Program in Ophthalmology, Eye Foundation Hospital, University of Alabama School of Medicine, Birmingham, Alabama
Optic Neuritis

MARK W. KLINE, M.D.

Associate Professor of Pediatrics, Baylor College of Medicine; Attending Physician, Texas Children's Hospital, Houston, Texas
Otitis Externa

JOHN H. KLIPPEL, M.D.

Clinical Director, National Institute of Arthritis and Musculoskeletal and Skin Diseases, National Institutes of Health, Bethesda, Maryland
Connective Tissue Disorders

WILLIAM J. KLISH, M.D.

Professor of Pediatrics, Baylor College of Medicine; Head, Department of Pediatric Gastroenterology and Nutrition, Texas Children's Hospital, Houston, Texas
Normal Infant Feeding

RICHARD T. KLOOS, M.D.

Fellow in Endocrinology and Metabolism, and Nuclear Medicine, Department of Internal Medicine, The University of Michigan Medical Center, Ann Arbor, Michigan
Thyroiditis

KENNETH L. KOCH, M.D.

Professor of Medicine, The Milton S. Hershey Medical Center, Pennsylvania State University, Hershey, Pennsylvania
Irritable Bowel Syndrome

KEITH C. KOCIS, M.D.

Post-Doctoral Fellow, Department of Anesthesiology and Critical Care Medicine, The Johns Hopkins Medical Institutes, Baltimore, Maryland
Congenital Heart Disease

BRIAN S. KOLL, M.D.

Assistant Professor of Medicine, Albert Einstein College of Medicine of Yeshiva University; Assistant Hospital Epidemiologist and Assistant Attending Physician, Department of Medicine and Division of Infectious Diseases, Beth Israel Medical Center, New York, New York
Management of the Patient with Human Immunodeficiency Virus Disease

KENNETH J. KOPACZ, M.D.

Assistant Clinical Professor of Orthopaedics, New Jersey Medical School, Newark, New Jersey
Low Back Pain

NEIL J. KORMAN, Ph.D., M.D.

Assistant Professor, Department of Dermatology, Case Western Reserve University; Dermatologist, University Hospitals of Cleveland, Cleveland, Ohio
Skin Diseases of Pregnancy

THEODORE A. KOTCHEN, M.D.

Professor and Chairman, Department of Medicine, Medical College of Wisconsin, Milwaukee, Wisconsin
Primary Aldosteronism

RICHARD A. KOZAREK, M.D.

Clinical Professor of Medicine, University of Washington; Chief of Gastroenterology, Virginia Mason Medical Center, Seattle, Washington
Chronic Pancreatitis

PHYLLIS E. KOZARSKY, M.D.

Associate Professor of Medicine, Division of Infectious Diseases, Emory University School of Medicine; Director, Travel Well Clinic, Crawford Long Hospital of Emory University, Atlanta, Georgia
Amebiasis

ALFONS L. KROL, M.D.

Director, Pediatric Dermatology Clinic; Clinical Associate Professor of Dermatology, University of Alberta, Edmonton, Alberta, Canada
Atopic Dermatitis

ROBERT S. KUNKEL, M.D.

Clinical Assistant Professor of Medicine, College of Medicine of Pennsylvania State University, Hershey, Pennsylvania; Staff Physician, Cleveland Clinic Headache Center, Department of Internal Medicine, Cleveland Clinic Foundation, Cleveland, Ohio
Headache

DEMETRE LABADARIOS, MB., Ch.B., Ph.D.

Head, Department of Human Nutrition, University of Stellenbosch and Tygerberg Hospital; Chief Specialist, Tygerberg Hospital, Tygerberg, South Africa
Vitamin Deficiency

ELAINE LAMBERT, M.D.

Assistant Professor of Medicine, Stanford University School of Medicine, Stanford, California
Rheumatoid Arthritis

W. THOMAS LAWRENCE, M.P.H., M.D.

Professor and Chief, Division of Plastic and Reconstructive Surgery, University of Massachusetts Medical Center, Worcester, Massachusetts
Keloids

LAWRENCE F. LAYFER, M.D.

Associate Professor, Section of Rheumatology, Department of Medicine, and Associate Dean, Rush Medical College, Chicago; Vice President, Medical Affairs, Rush North Shore Medical Center, Skokie, Illinois
Bursitis, Tendinitis, Myofascial Pain, and Fibromyalgia

MITCHELL A. LAZAR, M.D., Ph.D.

Associate Professor of Medicine and Genetics, Division of Endocrinology, Diabetes, and Metabolism, University of Pennsylvania School of Medicine; Medical Staff, Hospital of the University of Pennsylvania, Philadelphia, Pennsylvania
Hypothyroidism

J. MICHAEL LAZARUS, M.D.

Associate Professor of Medicine, Harvard Medical School; Director of Clinical Services, Division of Nephrology, Brigham and Women's Hospital, Boston, Massachusetts
Chronic Renal Failure

CASEY K. LEE, M.D.

Professor of Orthopaedics, New Jersey Medical School, Newark, New Jersey
Low Back Pain

TONY LEMBO, M.D.

Fellow in Gastroenterology, University of California, Los Angeles, Medical Center, Los Angeles, California
Acute and Chronic Viral Hepatitis

JACK L. LESHER, JR., M.D.

Professor and Chief, Section of Dermatology, Department of Medicine, Medical College of Georgia, Augusta, Georgia
Fungal Diseases of the Skin

BARRY LESHIN, M.D.

Associate Professor of Dermatology and Otolaryngology, Bowman Gray School of Medicine of Wake Forest University; Attending Physician, North Carolina Baptist Hospital, Winston-Salem, North Carolina
Premalignant Skin Lesions

ROLAND A. LEVANDOWSKI, M.D.

Acting Chief, Laboratory of Respiratory Viruses, Center for Biologics Evaluation and Research, Rockville, Maryland
Influenza

DOUGLAS S. LEVINE, M.D.

Associate Professor of Medicine, Division of Gastroenterology, University of Washington School of Medicine; Attending Staff Physician, University of Washington Medical Center and Affiliated Hospitals, Seattle, Washington
Ulcerative Colitis

JAMES H. LEWIS, M.D.

Associate Professor of Medicine, Division of Gastroenterology, Georgetown University School of Medicine; Attending Physician, Georgetown University Hospital, Washington, District of Columbia
Hiccups

GARY R. LICHTENSTEIN, M.D.

Assistant Professor of Medicine, University of Pennsylvania School of Medicine; Director, Inflammatory Bowel Disease Center, Division of Gastroenterology, Department of Medicine, Hospital of the University of Pennsylvania, Philadelphia, Pennsylvania
Malabsorption Syndromes

CAROL B. LINDSLEY, M.D.

Professor of Pediatrics and Director of Pediatric Rheumatology, University of Kansas Medical Center, Kansas City, Kansas
Juvenile Rheumatoid Arthritis

FRANK W. LING, M.D.

Faculty Professor and Chairman, Department of Obstetrics and Gynecology, University of Tennessee, Memphis College of Medicine, Memphis, Tennessee
Ectopic Pregnancy

N. SCOTT LITOFSKY, M.D.

Assistant Professor of Surgery (Neurosurgery) University of Massachusetts Medical Center, Worcester, Massachusetts
Brain Tumors

LEO X. LIU, M.D., D.T.M.H.

Assistant Professor of Medicine, Harvard Medical School; Physician, Beth Israel Hospital, Boston, Massachusetts
Trichinosis

DIRK S. LUCAS, PHARM.D.

Assistant Professor, College of Pharmacy, University of Houston; Adjunct Assistant Professor, Department of Family Medicine, Baylor College of Medicine, Houston, Texas
Drugs Approved in 1994; Top 200 Drugs Prescribed in the United States

CHRISTINA LUEDKE, M.D., PH.D.

Clinical Fellow, Harvard Medical School; Fellow in Endocrinology, Children's Hospital, Boston, Massachusetts
Diabetes Mellitus in Children and Adolescents

BENJAMIN J. LUFT, M.D.

Acting Chairman, Department of Medicine; Chief, Division of Infectious Diseases; Associate Professor of Medicine, State University of New York at Stony Brook, Stony Brook, New York
Toxoplasmosis

DENIS P. LYNCH, D.D.S., PH.D.

Professor, Department of Biologic and Diagnostic Sciences, College of Dentistry; Professor, Department of Medicine, Division of Dermatology, College of Medicine, The University of Tennessee, Memphis, Tennessee
Diseases of the Mouth

JOHN T. MACFARLANE, D.M.

Consultant Respiratory Physician, Nottingham City Hospital; Clinical Teacher, Nottingham University, Nottingham, England, United Kingdom
Psittacosis

MALCOLM R. MacKENZIE, M.D.

Professor Emeritus, Division of Hematology and Oncology, University of California, Davis, Medical Center, Sacramento, California
Multiple Myeloma

JAMES MAJESKI, PH.D., M.D.

Assistant Clinical Professor of Surgery, Medical University of South Carolina, Charleston; Chief of Surgery, East Cooper Hospital, Mt. Pleasant, South Carolina
Necrotizing Skin and Soft Tissue Infections

LAWRENCE E. MALLETTE, M.D., PH.D.

Associate Professor of Medicine, Baylor College of Medicine; Acting Chief of Endocrinology, Veterans' Administration Medical Center, Houston, Texas
Hyperparathyroidism and Hypoparathyroidism

HEIDI C. MANGELSDORF, M.D.

Chief Resident, Department of Dermatology, Bowman Gray School of Medicine of Wake Forest University; Attending Physician, North Carolina Baptist Hospital, Winston-Salem, North Carolina
Premalignant Skin Lesions

DAVID E. MANN, M.D.

Associate Professor of Medicine, University of Colorado Health Sciences Center; Director, Cardiac Electrophysiology Laboratory, University Hospital, Denver, Colorado
Premature Beats

PETER MARIUZ, M.D.

Assistant Professor of Medicine, State University of New York at Stony Brook, Stony Brook, New York
Toxoplasmosis

SANFORD M. MARKHAM, M.D.

Assistant Professor, Georgetown University Medical Center, Washington, District of Columbia; Chairman, Department of Obstetrics and Gynecology, The Union Memorial Hospital, Baltimore, Maryland
Uterine Leiomyoma

THOMAS J. MARRIE, M.D.

Professor of Medicine, Dalhousie University; Attending Physician, Victoria General Hospital, Halifax, Nova Scotia, Canada
Legionellosis (Legionnaires' Disease and Pontiac Fever)

PAUL MARTIN, M.D.

Associate Professor of Medicine, University of California at Los Angeles; Director, Hepatology Division of Digestive Diseases, Uni-

versity of California, Los Angeles, Medical Center, Los Angeles, California
Acute and Chronic Viral Hepatitis

GLENN E. MATHISEN, M.D.

Associate Clinical Professor of Medicine, University of California, Los Angeles, School of Medicine, Los Angeles; Chief, Infectious Disease Division, Olive View Medical Center, Sylmar, California
Tularemia

MICHAEL E. MAY, PH.D., M.D.

Assistant Professor of Medicine, Vanderbilt University; Attending Physician, Vanderbilt Hospital, Nashville, Tennessee
Diabetic Ketoacidosis

JAMES M. McCARTY, M.D.

Adjunct Assistant Professor of Pediatrics, University of California, San Francisco, San Francisco; Director, Infectious Diseases Division, Valley Children's Hospital, Fresno, California
Streptococcal Pharyngitis

MARIAN L. McCORD, M.D.

Assistant Professor, Division of Gynecology, Department of Obstetrics and Gynecology, University of Tennessee, Memphis, Tennessee
Ectopic Pregnancy

MICHEL McDONALD, M.D.

Resident in Dermatology, Vanderbilt University Medical Center, Nashville, Tennessee
Papulosquamous Diseases

JAMES L. McGUIRE, M.D.

Associate Professor of Medicine and Associate Dean for Graduate Medical Education, Stanford University School of Medicine; Chief of Staff, Stanford University Hospital, Stanford, California
Rheumatoid Arthritis

JEFFRY P. McKINZIE, M.D.

Assistant Professor, Department of Emergency Medicine, Vanderbilt University Medical Center, Nashville, Tennessee
Disturbances Due to Cold

MICHAEL MELLON, M.D.

Associate Clinical Professor of Pediatrics, University of California, San Diego, School of Medicine, La Jolla; Staff Allergist, Kaiser Permanente Hospital, San Diego, California
Allergic Reactions to Drugs

MARIO F. MENDEZ, M.D., PH.D.

Associate Professor of Neurology, University of California, Los Angeles, School of Medicine; Director, Neurobehavior Unit, West Los Angeles Veterans' Affairs Medical Center, Los Angeles, California
Alzheimer's Disease

MARK L. METERSKY, M.D.

Assistant Professor of Clinical Medicine, University of Connecticut School of Medicine; Attending Physician, University of Connecticut Health Center, Farmington, Connecticut
Primary Lung Abscess

RALPH M. MEYER, M.D.

Associate Professor, Department of Medicine, McMaster University; Head, Service of Clinical Hematology, Hamilton Civic Hospitals and Hamilton Regional Cancer Centre, Hamilton, Ontario, Canada
Hodgkin's Disease: Chemotherapy

WILLIAM C. MEYERS, M.D.

Professor and Chief of Gastrointestinal Surgery, Duke University Medical Center; Chief of Hepatobiliary Surgery; Chief of Endoscopic Surgery, Duke University Medical Center; Chief of Gastro-

intestinal Surgery, Durham Veterans Administration Medical Center, Durham, North Carolina
Gallstones and Gallstone Syndromes

DANIEL B. MICHAEL, M.D., PH.D.

Assistant Professor of Neurosurgery, Wayne State University School of Medicine; Chief of Neurosurgery, Detroit Receiving Hospital, Detroit, Michigan
Acute Head Injuries in Adults

MOHAMAD MIKATI, M.D.

Professor and Chairman, Department of Pediatrics; American University of Beirut; Director, Epilepsy Program, American University of Beirut Medical Center, Beirut, Lebanon
Epilepsy in Adolescents and Adults

JAMES E. MITCHELL, M.D.

Professor of Psychiatry, University of Minnesota Medical School, Minneapolis, Minnesota
Bulimia Nervosa

ANNA JACQUELINE MITUS, M.D.

Instructor in Medicine, Harvard Medical School; Associate Physician, Brigham and Women's Hospital, Boston, Massachusetts
Platelet-Mediated Bleeding Disorders

HOWARD C. MOFENSON, M.D.

Professor of Pediatrics and Emergency Medicine, State University of New York at Stony Brook, Stony Brook; Professor of Pharmacology/Toxicology, New York College of Osteopathy, Old Westbury; Professor of Clinical Pharmacy, St. John's University, Jamaica; Medical Director, Long Island Regional Poison Control Center, East Meadow; Attending Physician, Winthrop University Hospital, Mineola, New York
Acute Poisonings

KENNETH J. MOISE, JR., M.D.

Associate Professor of Obstetrics and Gynecology and Director, Division of Maternal-Fetal Medicine, Baylor College of Medicine; Chief of Obstetrics, Ben Taub General Hospital, Houston, Texas
Hemolytic Disease of the Fetus and Newborn (Red Cell Alloimmunization)

JOHN C. MORRIS, M.D.

Assistant Professor, Mayo Medical School; Consultant, Division of Endocrinology and Metabolism, St. Mary's Hospital, Rochester, Minnesota
Thyrotoxicosis

MITCHELL MORRIS, M.D.

Associate Vice-President for Informatics and Associate Professor of Gynecologic Oncology, University of Texas M. D. Anderson Cancer Center, Houston, Texas
Carcinoma of the Uterine Cervix

JOSEPH F. MORTOLA, M.D.

Associate Professor of Obstetrics, Gynecology, and Reproductive Medicine and Associate Professor of Psychiatry, Harvard Medical School; Director, Division of Reproductive Endocrinology, Beth Israel Hospital, Boston, Massachusetts
Premenstrual Syndrome

RAJA MUDAD, M.D.

Fellow, Division of Hematology/Oncology, Department of Medicine, Duke University Medical Center, Durham, North Carolina
Autoimmune Hemolytic Anemia

J. PAUL MUIZELAAR, M.D., PH.D.

Professor of Neurosurgery and Director, Detroit Neurotrauma Institute, Wayne State University School of Medicine; Attending Physician, Detroit Receiving Hospital, Detroit, Michigan
Acute Head Injuries in Adults

WILLIAM K. MURPHY, M.D.

Internist and Professor of Medicine, University of Texas M. D. Anderson Cancer Center, Houston, Texas
Nausea and Vomiting

DENNIS L. MURRAY, M.D.

Professor and Division Chief, Infectious Diseases Department of Pediatrics and Human Development, Michigan State University, East Lansing; Attending Physician, Sparrow Hospital, Regional Children's Center; Consulting Staff, Michigan Capital Medical Center; Courtesy Staff, Saint Lawrence Hospital, Lansing, Michigan
Mumps

DIYA F. MUTASIM, M.D.

Associate Professor of Dermatology, Dermatopathology, and Immunodermatology, University of Cincinnati; Residency Program Director, University of Cincinnati Medical Center, Cincinnati, Ohio
Bullous Diseases

DAVID G. MUTCH, M.D.

Associate Professor of Obstetrics and Gynecology and Director of Division of Gynecologic Oncology, Washington University School of Medicine; Attending Physician, Barnes Hospital, St. Louis, Missouri
Neoplasms of the Vulva

KENRAD E. NELSON, M.D.

Professor of Epidemiology, Medicine, and International Health, School of Hygiene and Public Health and School of Medicine, Johns Hopkins University, Baltimore, Maryland
Leprosy (Hansen's Disease)

MARK E. NESBIT, Jr., M.D.

Professor of Pediatrics, Therapeutic Radiology and Nursing, Department of Pediatrics, University of Minnesota, Minneapolis, Minnesota
Acute Leukemia in Childhood

R. MITCHELL NEWMAN, M.D.

Chief Resident, Combined Program in Ophthalmology, Eye Foundation Hospital, University of Alabama School of Medicine, Birmingham, Alabama
Optic Neuritis

CARLETON NIBLEY, M.D.

Fellow in Cardiology, Duke University Medical Center, Durham, North Carolina
Tachycardias

STEPHEN D. NIMER, M.D.

Chief, Hematology Service, Memorial Sloan-Kettering Cancer Center, and Associate Professor of Medicine, Cornell University Medical College; Associate Attending Physician, Memorial Hospital, New York, New York
Aplastic Anemia

ERIC A. NOFZINGER, M.D.

Assistant Professor of Psychiatry, University of Pittsburgh; Chief, Sleep Evaluation Center, Highland Drive Veterans Affairs Hospital, Pittsburgh, Pennsylvania
Insomnia

JAMES J. NORDLUND, M.D.

Professor and Chairman, Department of Dermatology, University of Cincinnati College of Medicine; Attending Physician, University Hospital, and Children's Hospital Medical Center; Consultant/Attending Physician, Veterans' Administration Hospital; Consultant Physician, Jewish Hospital of Cincinnati, Good Samaritan Hospital, Providence Hospital, and Shriners Burns Institute, Cincinnati, Ohio
Pigmentary Disorders

YVES NORDMANN, M.D.

Professor of Medical Biochemistry, Faculty of Medicine Xavier Bichat, University of Paris; Executive Head of Biochemical Department, Hospital Louis Mourier, Paris, France
The Porphyrias

ANDREW J. NORTON, M.D.

Assistant Professor of Medicine, Medical College of Wisconsin, Milwaukee, Wisconsin
Primary Aldosteronism

MICHAEL O'BRIEN, M.D.†

Fellow, UCLA Multicampus Program in Infectious Diseases and Microbial Pathogenesis, Department of Medicine, University of California at Los Angeles, Los Angeles, California
Bacteremia and Septicemia

BLANCA N. OCAMPO-LIM, M.D.

Fellow, Division of Endocrinology and Metabolism, University of Michigan Medical School, Ann Arbor, Michigan
Hypopituitarism

AMY L. O'DONNELL, M.D.

Research Assistant Professor of Medicine, Division of Endocrinology and Metabolism, State University of New York at Buffalo; Attending Physician, Buffalo Veterans' Administration Medical Center, Buffalo, New York
Goiter

DAVID L. OLIVE, M.D.

Associate Professor and Chief, Reproductive Endocrinology and Infertility, Department of Obstetrics and Gynecology, Yale University School of Medicine; Attending Physician, Yale–New Haven Hospital, New Haven, Connecticut
Endometriosis

DEBORAH ORTEGA-CARR, M.D.

Allergy Fellow, Department of Medicine, University of Wisconsin, Madison, Wisconsin; Attending Physician, Riverside-Methodist Hospital, Columbus, Ohio
Asthma in Adults and Adolescents

GASTON OSTIGUY, M.D.

Associate Professor of Medicine, University of Montreal; Attending Physician, Maisonneuve-Rosemont Hospital, Montreal, Quebec, Canada
Silicosis

PAUL M. PALEVSKY, M.D.

Associate Professor of Medicine, University of Pittsburgh School of Medicine; Chief, Renal Section, Veterans' Administration Medical Center, Pittsburgh, Pennsylvania
Diabetes Insipidus

MARK S. PALLER, M.D.

Associate Professor of Medicine, University of Minnesota; Attending Physician, University of Minnesota Hospital and Clinic, Minneapolis, Minnesota
Acute Renal Failure

SUN M. PARK, M.D.

Resident in Emergency Medicine, University of Virginia School of Medicine, Charlottesville, Virginia
Bacterial Diseases of the Skin

†Deceased.

GAVRIL PASTERNAK, M.D., Ph.D.

Member, Memorial Sloan-Kettering Cancer Center; Professor, Departments of Neurology, Neuroscience and Pharmacology, Cornell University Medical College; Attending Neurologist, Memorial Hospital and New York Hospital, New York, New York
Pain

DILIP PATEL, M.D.

Assistant Professor, Albert Einstein College of Medicine of Yeshiva University, Bronx; Attending Physician, Long Island Jewish Medical Center, New Hyde Park, New York
Polycythemia Vera

ROY PATTERSON, M.D.

Professor of Medicine and Chief, Division of Allergy-Immunology, Northwestern University Medical School, Chicago, Illinois
Allergic Reactions to Drugs

H. T. PERRY, D.D.S., Ph.D.

Professor (Emeritus), Northwestern University Dental School; Dental Attending Staff, Northwestern Memorial Hospital, Chicago, Illinois
Temporomandibular Disorders

EDWARD L. PESANTI, M.D.

Professor of Medicine, University of Connecticut Health Center; Attending Physician, Veterans' Affairs Medical Center, Newington; University of Connecticut Health Center, Farmington, Connecticut
Tuberculosis and Other Mycobacterial Diseases

DONALD D. PETERSON, M.D.

Clinical Associate Professor of Medicine, Jefferson Medical College, Philadelphia; Director, Lankenau Hospital Sleep Disorders Center, Lankenau Hospital, Wynnewood, Pennsylvania
Sleep Apnea Syndrome

PATTI L. PETERSON, M.D.

Associate Professor of Neurology/Emergency Medicine, Wayne State University School of Medicine; Chief of Neurology/Neurotrauma, Detroit Receiving Hospital, Detroit, Michigan
Acute Head Injuries in Adults

JOHN M. PETTIFOR, M.B., B.Ch., Ph.D.

Chairman, Department of Paediatrics, University of the Witwatersrand, Johannesburg; Director, MRC/University Mineral Metabolism Research Unit, University of the Witwatersrand; Chief Paediatrician, Baraqwanath Hospital, Soweto, South Africa
Vitamin Deficiency

SAMANTHA M. PFEIFER, M.D.

Assistant Professor of Obstetrics and Gynecology, Division of Human Reproduction, University of Pennsylvania Medical Center, Philadelphia, Pennsylvania
Dysmenorrhea

STEPHANIE H. PINCUS, M.D.

Professor and Chair, Department of Dermatology; Professor, Department of Medicine, State University of New York at Buffalo; Chief, Department of Dermatology, Buffalo General Hospital, Buffalo, New York
Pruritus Ani and Vulvae

BIANCA MARIA PIRACCINI, M.D.

Doctor in Research, Department of Dermatology, University of Bologna, Bologna, Italy
Diseases of the Nails

ANDREW P. PITMAN, M.D.

Chief, Pulmonary and Critical Care Medicine; Director, Intensive Care Unit, Bryn Mawr Hospital, Bryn Mawr, Pennsylvania
Sleep Apnea Syndrome

SHEREE R. POITIER, M.D.

Assistant Clinical Professor of Medicine, University of California, Los Angeles, School of Medicine, Los Angeles; Director of Women's Clinic, Department of Medicine, Division of Infectious Disease, Olive View Medical Center, Sylmar, California
Tularemia

JAMES C. PUFFER, M.D.

Professor and Chief, Division of Family Medicine, University of California, Los Angeles, School of Medicine; Attending Physician, University of California at Los Angeles Medical Center, Los Angeles, California
Common Sports Injuries

GARY S. RACHELEFSKY, M.D.

Clinical Professor, Department of Pediatrics, University of California at Los Angeles; Director, Allergy Research Foundation, Los Angeles, California
Allergic Rhinitis Caused by Inhalant Factors

STEVEN E. RADEMACHER, M.D.

Fellow in Infectious Disease, University of Texas Southwestern Medical Center at Dallas; Attending Physician, Dallas Veterans' Administration, Dallas, Texas
Bacterial Infections of the Urinary Tract in Males

KANTI R. RAI, M.D.

Professor of Medicine, Albert Einstein College of Medicine; Chief, Division of Hematology-Oncology, Long Island Jewish Medical Center, New Hyde Park, New York
Polycythemia Vera

SHARON S. RAIMER, M.D.

Professor of Dermatology and Pediatrics and Director, Pediatric Dermatology, University of Texas Medical Branch, Galveston, Texas
Acne Vulgaris and Rosacea

A. KONETI RAO, M.D.

Professor of Medicine, Thrombosis Research and Pathology and Director, Thromboembolic Diseases Program, Temple University School of Medicine; Attending Physician, Temple University Hospital, Philadelphia, Pennsylvania
Venous Thromboembolism in Obstetrics and Gynecology

LAWRENCE D. RECHT, M.D.

Professor of Neurology and Neurosurgery, University of Massachusetts Medical Center, Worcester, Massachusetts
Brain Tumors

REBECCA REDMAN, M.D.

Fellow, Pediatric Infectious Diseases, Stanford University School of Medicine, Stanford, California
Chickenpox (Varicella)

BARBARA D. REED, M.D., M.S.P.H.

Associate Professor, Department of Family Practice, University of Michigan, Ann Arbor, Michigan
Vulvovaginitis

T. M. S. REID, M.B., Ch.B.

Honorary Senior Lecturer in Microbiology, University of Aberdeen; Consultant Microbiologist, Aberdeen Royal Infirmary, Aberdeen, Scotland, United Kingdom
Salmonellosis

JOSEPH G. RENNEY, D.O.

Fellow in Rheumatology, Division of Rheumatology and Immunology, Medical University of South Carolina, Charleston, South Carolina
Polymyalgia Rheumatica and Giant Cell Arteritis

CHARLES F. REYNOLDS III, M.D.

Professor of Psychiatry and Neurology, University of Pittsburgh School of Medicine; Director, Sleep and Chronobiology Center, and Director, Mental Health Clinical Research Center for the Study of Late-Life Mood Disorders, Pittsburgh, Pennsylvania
Insomnia

PETER B. RINTELS, M.D.

Assistant Professor of Medicine, Brown University School of Medicine; Associate Director of Clinical Hematology, Rhode Island Hospital, Providence, Rhode Island
Nonimmune Hemolytic Anemia

RODERICK ROBINSON, M.D.

Resident, University of Tennessee; Resident Physician, Le Bonheur Children's Medical Center, Memphis, Tennessee
Anaphylaxis and Serum Sickness

PAUL F. ROCKLEY, M.D.

Chief Resident, Department of Dermatology, Washington Hospital Center, Washington, District of Columbia
Viral Diseases of the Skin

JONATHAN E. RODNICK, M.D.

Professor and Chair, Department of Family and Community Medicine, University of California, San Francisco, California
Acute Bronchitis

ROBERT L. RODNITZKY, M.D.

Professor and Vice-Chairman, Department of Neurology, University of Iowa College of Medicine; Director, Movement Disorders Clinic, University of Iowa Hospitals and Clinics, Iowa City, Iowa
Parkinson's Disease

ROBERT M. ROGERS, M.D.

Professor of Medicine and Chief, Division of Pulmonary, Allergy, and Critical Care Medicine, University of Pittsburgh School of Medicine; Attending Physician, University of Pittsburgh Medical Center, Pittsburgh, Pennsylvania
Acute Respiratory Failure

CHERYL F. ROSEN, M.D.

Assistant Professor, Department of Medicine, University of Toronto; Staff Physician, Women's College Hospital, Toronto, Ontario, Canada
Sunburn

GERALD B. ROSEN, M.D.

Instructor and Fellow, Department of Ophthalmology, University of Rochester School of Medicine and Dentistry, Rochester, New York
Conjunctivitis

TED ROSEN, M.D.

Professor of Dermatology, Baylor College of Medicine; Chief of Dermatology, Veterans' Administration Medical Center; Deputy Chief of Dermatology, The Methodist Hospital, Houston, Texas
Granuloma Inguinale (Donovanosis); Lymphogranuloma Venereum

DAVID I. ROSENTHAL, M.D.

Assistant Professor, University of Texas Southwestern Medical Center, Dallas, Texas
Hodgkin's Disease: Radiation Therapy

NICHOLAS P. ROSSI, M.D.

Professor of Surgery, University of Iowa Hospitals and Clinics, Iowa City, Iowa
Pleural Effusion and Empyema Thoracis

DAVID R. ROTH, M.D.

Associate Professor of Urology, Scott Department of Urology, Baylor College of Medicine; Attending Urologist, Texas Children's Hospital, Houston, Texas
Bacterial Infections of the Urinary Tract in Girls

ELLIOT J. ROTH, M.D.

Professor and Chairman, Department of Physical Medicine and Rehabilitation, Northwestern University Medical School; Medical Director, Rehabilitation Institute of Chicago; Chairman, Physical Medicine and Rehabilitation, Northwestern Memorial Hospital, Chicago, Illinois
Rehabilitation of the Stroke Patient

GERALD ROTHSTEIN, M.D.

Director and Chief, Division of Human Development and Aging, University of Utah School of Medicine; Director, Geriatric Research, Education, and Clinical Center, Veterans Administration Hospital, Salt Lake City, Utah
Neutropenia

FREDERICK L. RUBEN, M.D.

Professor of Medicine, University of Pittsburgh School of Medicine; Staff Physician, University of Pittsburgh Medical Center Hospitals, Pittsburgh, Pennsylvania
Viral Respiratory Infections

RICHARD A. RUDICK, M.D.

Director, Mellen Center for Multiple Sclerosis Treatment and Research, Cleveland Clinic Foundation, Cleveland, Ohio
Multiple Sclerosis

BRUCE A. RUNYON, M.D.

Professor of Medicine, University of Louisville; Director of Liver Service and Medical Director of Liver Transplantation, University of Louisville and Jewish Hospital, Louisville, Kentucky
Cirrhosis

MARK E. RUPP, M.D.

Assistant Professor, Department of Internal Medicine, University of Nebraska Medical Center; Attending Physician, University of Nebraska Medical Center, Omaha, Nebraska
Bacterial Pneumonia

DAVID A. SACK, M.D.

Professor, Department of International Health, Johns Hopkins University School of Hygiene and Public Health; Attending Physician, Johns Hopkins Hospital, Baltimore, Maryland
Cholera

JOSE H. SALGADO, M.D., M.P.H.

Infectious Disease Specialist, St. Mary's Medical Center, Evansville, Indiana
Osteomyelitis

JAMIE D. SANTILLI, M.D.

Assistant Professor, Department of Family and Community Medicine, University of Minnesota, Minneapolis; Attending Physician, St. Joseph's Hospital, St. Paul, Minnesota
Peripheral Arterial Disease

STEVEN M. SANTILLI, M.D., Ph.D.

Assistant Professor, Department of Surgery, University of Minnesota; Attending Physician, Section of Vascular Surgery, Veterans' Administration Medical Center, Minneapolis, Minnesota
Peripheral Arterial Disease

MICHAEL SCHATZ, M.D.

Clinical Professor, Department of Medicine, University of California, San Diego, School of Medicine; Staff Allergist, Kaiser-Permanente Medical Center, San Diego, California
Allergic Reactions to Drugs

W. MICHAEL SCHELD, M.D.

Professor of Internal Medicine and Neurosurgery and Associate Chair for Residency Programs, University of Virginia School of Medicine; Attending Physician, University of Virginia Health Sciences Center, Charlottesville, Virginia
Brain Abscess

CHRISTOPHER F. SCHULTZ, M.D.

Fellow in Gastroenterology, University of Pennsylvania School of Medicine; Attending Physician, Division of Gastroenterology, Department of Medicine, Hospital of the University of Pennsylvania, Philadelphia, Pennsylvania
Malabsorption Syndromes

BEVERLY E. SHA, M.D.

Assistant Professor of Medicine, Rush Medical College, Rush-Presbyterian-St. Luke's Medical Center; Assistant Attending Physician, Rush-Presbyterian-St Luke's Medical Center, Chicago, Illinois
Infectious Mononucleosis

REZA SHAKER, M.D.

Associate Professor of Medicine, Radiology and Surgery (Otolaryngology), Medical College of Wisconsin; Senior Attending Physician, Froedtert Memorial Lutheran Hospital, Milwaukee, Wisconsin
Gastroesophageal Reflux Disease

JERRY SHAPIRO, M.D.

Clinical Associate Professor, Division of Dermatology, Faculty of Medicine, University of British Columbia; Director, University of British Columbia Hair Clinic; Research, Treatment and Transplant Centre; Consultant, Vancouver Hospital and Health Science Centre, Vancouver, British Columbia, Canada
Diseases of the Hair

NEIL H. SHEAR, M.D.

Associate Professor of Medicine (Dermatology and Clinical Pharmacology), Pharmacology, and Pediatrics, University of Toronto Medical School; University Director of Clinical Pharmacology and Head of Clinical Pharmacology Program, Sunnybrook Health Science Centre, North York, Ontario, Canada
Erythema Multiforme

SUNITA B. SHETH, M.D.

Assistant Professor of Medicine and Thrombosis Research, Temple University School of Medicine; Attending Physician, Temple University Hospital, Philadelphia, Pennsylvania
Venous Thromboembolism in Obstetrics and Gynecology

ROBERT W. SHIELDS, Jr., M.D.

Staff Neurologist, Cleveland Clinic Foundation and Director, Quantitative Peripheral Nerve Laboratory, Cleveland Clinic Foundation, Cleveland, Ohio
Peripheral Neuropathies

KAM SHOJANIA, M.D.

Rheumatology Fellow, Department of Medicine, University of British Columbia, Vancouver; Staff Physician, Richmond Hospital, Richmond, British Columbia, Canada
Hyperuricemia and Gout

RICHARD M. SILVER, M.D.

Professor of Medicine and Pediatrics, Division of Rheumatology and Immunology, Medical University of South Carolina, Charleston, South Carolina
Polymyalgia Rheumatica and Giant Cell Arteritis

HARVEY S. SINGER, M.D.

Professor, Departments of Neurology and Pediatrics, Johns Hopkins University School of Medicine; Director of Pediatric Neurology, Johns Hopkins Hospital, Baltimore, Maryland
Gilles De La Tourette Syndrome

NAV T. SINGH, M.B.B.S.

Assistant Professor, University of Connecticut Health Center; Veterans' Administration Medical Center, Newington, Connecticut; Attending Physician, University of Connecticut Health Center, Farmington, Connecticut
Tuberculosis and Other Mycobacterial Diseases

RAYMOND A. SMEGO, Jr., M.D., M.P.H.

Associate Professor of Medicine (Infectious Diseases) and Director, International Health Program, Robert C. Byrd Health Sciences Center of West Virginia University; Attending Physician, Ruby Memorial Hospital, Morgantown, West Virginia
Relapsing Fever

BRADLEY E. SMITH, M.D.

Professor of Anesthesiology, Vanderbilt University School of Medicine; Attending Physician, Vanderbilt University Hospital, Nashville, Tennessee
Obstetric Anesthesia

JAMES W. SMITH, M.D.

Professor of Internal Medicine, University of Texas Southwestern Medical School at Dallas; Staff Physician, Infectious Diseases, Dallas Department of Veterans' Affairs Medical Center, Dallas, Texas
Bacterial Infections of the Urinary Tract in Males

JOSEPH A. SMITH, Jr., M.D.

William L. Bray Professor and Chairman, Department of Urology, Vanderbilt University Medical Center; Chairman, Urology Service, Vanderbilt University Hospital, Nashville, Tennessee
Malignant Tumors of the Urogenital Tract

THOMAS F. SMITH, M.D.

Professor of Pediatrics, Washington University School of Medicine; Associate Director for Allergy and Asthma, Division of Allergy and Pulmonary Medicine, Department of Pediatrics; Attending Physician, Allergy and Pulmonary Medicine, St. Louis Children's Hospital, St. Louis, Missouri
Asthma in Children

A. REBECCA SNIDER, M.D.

Professor of Pediatrics, Division of Pediatric Cardiology, The Johns Hopkins Medical Institutes, Baltimore, Maryland
Congenital Heart Disease

PETER J. SNYDER, M.D.

Professor of Medicine, University of Pennsylvania School of Medicine, Philadelphia, Pennsylvania
Acromegaly

WILLIAM H. SNYDER III, M.D.

Professor of Surgery, University of Texas Southwestern Medical Center; Attending Physician, Zale Lipshy University Hospital and Parkland Memorial Hospital; Specialist Physician, Veterans' Administration Hospital; Visiting/Teaching Staff, St. Paul Medical Center; Courtesy Staff, Children's Medical Center and Medical Arts Hospital; Consulting Physician, Presbyterian Hospital of Dallas, Dallas, Texas
Thyroid Cancer

DAVID A. SOLOMON, M.D.

Clinical Assistant Professor of Psychiatry and Human Behavior, Brown University; Assistant Director of Mood Disorders Program, Butler Hospital, Providence, Rhode Island
Mood Disorders

MARCIO SOTERO, M.D.

Assistant Professor, Department of Neurology, University of New Mexico School of Medicine, Albuquerque, New Mexico
Epilepsy in Adolescents and Adults

SARA V. SOTIROPOULOS, M.D.

Assistant Professor of Pediatrics and Director, Pediatric Residency Program, University of Missouri School of Medicine; Attending Physician, Children's Hospital at University Hospital and Clinics, Columbia, Missouri
Otitis Externa

MARIA SOTO-AGUILAR, M.D.

Assistant Professor of Medicine and Pediatrics, Division of Allergy and Clinical Immunology, Departments of Medicine and Pediatrics, College of Medicine, University of South Alabama; Attending Physician, University of South Alabama Hospitals and Clinics, Mobile, Alabama
Allergic Reactions to Insect Stings

STEPHEN W. SPAULDING, M.D., C.M.

Professor of Medicine, State University of New York at Buffalo; Associate Chief of Staff for Research, Buffalo Veterans' Administration Medical Center, Buffalo, New York
Goiter

MURRAY B. STEIN, M.D.

Associate Professor, Department of Psychiatry; Director, Anxiety and Traumatic Stress Disorders Program, University of California, San Diego, La Jolla, California
Panic Disorder

PETER STEIN, M.D.

Chief, Section of Endocrinology and Nutrition, and Associate Professor of Medicine, Medical College of Georgia; Attending Physician, Medical College of Georgia Clinics and Hospital, Augusta, Georgia
Pheochromocytoma

EVAN A. STEINBERG, M.D.

Associate Professor of Clinical Pediatrics, University of Southern California School of Medicine; Assistant Chief of Pediatrics and Consultant in Pediatric Infectious Diseases, Kaiser Permanente Los Angeles Medical Center, Los Angeles, California
Diphtheria

SAMUEL MARK STEINFIELD, B.Sc., B.M.R.(P.T.)

Partner/Owner, Sports Physiotherapy Centre, Pan Am Sports Medicine, Orthopaedic and Rehabilitation Centre, Winnipeg, Manitoba, Canada
Ankylosing Spondylitis

JAMES H. STEWART, M.D.

Instructor in Medicine, Mayo Medical School; Director, Vascular Medicine Section, Division of Cardiovascular Diseases, Mayo Clinic, Jacksonville, Florida
Venous Stasis Ulcerations

JAMES A. STOCKMAN III, M.D.

Professor of Clinical Pediatrics, University of North Carolina School of Medicine; Consultant Professor, Duke University School of Medicine, Durham, North Carolina
Iron Deficiency Anemia

NEIL J. STONE, M.D.

Associate Professor of Medicine, Northwestern University School of Medicine; Jacques Smyth Distinguished Physician in Medicine, Northwestern Memorial Hospital, Chicago, Illinois
Hyperlipoproteinemia

LARRY JAMES STRAUSBAUGH, M.D.

Professor of Medicine, School of Medicine, Oregon Health Sciences Center; Hospital Epidemiologist and Staff Physician, Infectious Diseases, Portland Veterans' Affairs Medical Center, Portland, Oregon
Viral and Mycoplasmal Pneumonias

ROBERT C. STRUNK, M.D.

Professor of Pediatrics, Washington University School of Medicine; Director, Division of Allergy and Pulmonary Medicine, Department of Pediatrics, St. Louis Children's Hospital, St. Louis, Missouri
Asthma in Children

W. P. DANIEL SU, M.D.

Consultant, Department of Dermatology, Mayo Clinic and Mayo Foundation; Professor of Dermatology, Mayo Medical School, Rochester, Minnesota
Polyarteritis Nodosa and Cutaneous Polyarteritis Nodosa

STEPHEN B. SULAVIK, M.D.

Professor and Head, Division of Pulmonary Medicine, University of Connecticut School of Medicine; Clinical Professor of Medicine, Yale University School of Medicine, New Haven; Attending Physician, University of Connecticut Health Center, Farmington, Connecticut
Primary Lung Abscess

PAUL S. SWERDLOW, M.D.

Associate Professor of Medicine, Division of Hematology-Oncology, Wayne State University School of Medicine; Director of Red Cell Disorders, Harper Hospital, Detroit Medical Center, Detroit, Michigan
Sickle Cell Disease

IRMA O. SZYMANSKI, M.D.

Professor of Pathology and Medicine, University of Massachusetts Medical School; Medical Director, Transfusion Services, University of Massachusetts Medical Center, Worcester, Massachusetts
Therapeutic Use of Blood Components

STEPHEN R. TABET, M.D., M.P.H.

Senior Fellow, Division of Infectious Diseases, Department of Medicine, University of Washington, Seattle, Washington
Nongonococcal Urethritis in Men

JAMES S. TAYLOR, M.D.

Head, Section of Industrial Dermatology, The Cleveland Clinic Foundation, Cleveland, Ohio
Occupational Dermatoses

MARILYN J. TELEN, M.D.

Associate Professor of Medicine, Division of Hematology/Oncology, Duke University Medical Center, Durham, North Carolina
Autoimmune Hemolytic Anemia

R. THOMAS TEMES, M.D.

Assistant Professor of Surgery, Division of Thoracic and Cardiovascular Surgery, University of New Mexico School of Medicine; Faculty, University of New Mexico Health Sciences Center; Faculty, Veterans' Administration Medical Center Albuquerque; Faculty, Lovelace Medical Center, Albuquerque, New Mexico
Atelectasis

NATHAN M. THIELMAN, M.D., M.P.H.

Fellow in Infectious Diseases, University of Virginia School of Medicine, Charlottesville, Virginia
Food-Borne Illness

JOEL A. THOMPSON, M.D.

Associate Professor of Pediatrics and Neurology, University of Utah Medical Center; Attending Physician, University of Utah Medical Center and Primary Children's Medical Center, Salt Lake City, Utah
Reye's Syndrome

GLEN T. D. THOMSON, M.D.

Associate Professor, University of Manitoba; Director of Rheumatology Services, St. Boniface Hospital, Winnipeg, Manitoba, Canada
Ankylosing Spondylitis

ANTONELLA TOSTI, M.D.

Associate Professor of Dermatology, University of Bologna, Bologna, Italy
Diseases of the Nails

L. WILLIAM TRAVERSO, M.D.

Associate Clinical Professor of Surgery, University of Washington School of Medicine; Attending Surgeon, Virginia Mason Medical Center, Seattle, Washington
Chronic Pancreatitis

KENNETH F. TROFATTER, JR., M.D., PH.D.

Professor, Department of Obstetrics and Gynecology; Director, East Tennessee Regional Perinatal Program, University of Tennessee Medical Center, Knoxville, Tennessee
Condylomata Acuminata (Genital Warts)

LARRY E. TUNE, M.D.

Professor of Psychiatry and Geriatrics, Emory University; Chief of Psychiatry, Wesley Woods Geriatric Center at Emory University, Atlanta, Georgia
Delirium

MARK TYNDALL, M.D.

Assistant Professor of Medicine, Centre for International Health, Faculty of Health Sciences, Department of Internal Medicine, McMaster University; Attending Physician, St. Joseph's Hospital, Hamilton, Ontario, Canada
Chancroid

WULF H. UTIAN, M.D., PH.D.

Professor and Chairman, Department of Reproductive Biology, Case Western Reserve University School of Medicine; Director, Department of Obstetrics and Gynecology, University Hospitals of Cleveland, Cleveland, Ohio
Menopause

R. JAMES VALENTINE, M.D.

Associate Professor of Surgery, Associate Director of Graduate Medical Education, Department of Surgery, University of Texas Southwestern Medical Center; Chief of Vascular Surgery, Department of Veterans' Affairs; Chief, Vascular Surgery Section, Department of Surgery, Veterans' Administration Medical Center; Attending Physician, Department of Surgery, Parkland Memorial Hospital; Attending Physician, Department of Surgery, Zale Lipshy University Hospital, Dallas, Texas
Deep Venous Thrombosis of the Lower Extremities

MATTI VÄLIMÄKI, M.D., PH.D.

Chief Physician, Division of Endocrinology, Helsinki University Central Hospital, Helsinki, Finland
Adrenocortical Insufficiency

JOHN P. WADE, M.D.

Clinical Associate Professor, University of British Columbia; Consulting Rheumatologist, Vancouver Hospital, Vancouver, British Columbia, Canada
Hyperuricemia and Gout

ARNOLD WALD, M.D.

Professor of Medicine, University of Pittsburgh School of Medicine; Associate Chief, Division of Gastroenterology and Hepatology, University of Pittsburgh Medical Center, Pittsburgh, Pennsylvania
Constipation

MICHAEL R. WARE, M.D.

Associate Professor in Psychiatry, Department of Psychiatry and Behavioral Sciences and Institute of Psychiatry, Medical University of South Carolina, Charleston, South Carolina
Anxiety Disorders

THOMAS J. WARGOVICH, M.D.

Associate Professor of Medicine, Division of Cardiology, University of Florida, Gainesville, Florida
Angina Pectoris

CHARLES H. WATT, JR., M.D.

Private Practice, Thomasville, Georgia
Snake Venom Poisoning

ARTHUR L. WEAVER, M.D.

Medical Director, Arthritis Center of Nebraska, Lincoln; Clinical Associate Professor of Medicine, University of Nebraska Medical School, Omaha; Attending Physician, Department of Medicine, Department of Rheumatology, Bryan Memorial Hospital; Courtesy Staff, Lincoln General Hospital and St. Elizabeth's Community Health Center, Lincoln, Nebraska
Osteoarthritis

LOUIS M. WEISS, M.D., M.P.H.

Associate Professor of Medicine, Division of Infectious Diseases, and Associate Professor of Pathology, Division of Parasitology, Albert Einstein College of Medicine; Assistant Attending Physician, The Jack D. Weiler Hospital of the Albert Einstein College of Medicine, Montefiore Medical Center; Attending Physician, Bronx Municipal Hospital, Bronx, New York
Malaria

PETER F. WELLER, M.D.

Associate Professor of Medicine, Harvard Medical School; Physician, Beth Israel Hospital, Boston, Massachusetts
Trichinosis

ERIC L. WESTERMAN, M.D.

Clinical Professor, Section of Infectious Diseases, University of Oklahoma Health Science Center; Director of Epidemiology, Hillcrest Medical Center, Tulsa, Oklahoma
Rocky Mountain Spotted Fever

J. MARCUS WHARTON, M.D.

Associate Professor of Medicine and Director, Clinical Cardiac Electrophysiology, Duke University Medical Center, Durham, North Carolina
Tachycardias

L. JOSEPH WHEAT, M.D.

Professor of Medicine and Pathology, Indianapolis University School of Medicine; Staff Physician, Richard L. Roudebush Veterans' Affairs Medical Center, Indianapolis, Indiana
Histoplasmosis

ROGER D. WHITE, M.D.

Professor of Anesthesiology, Mayo Medical School; Consultant in Anesthesiology (Cardiovascular), Mayo Clinic; Medical Director, Mayo Clinic/Gold Cross Ambulance Service, Rochester, Minnesota
Cardiac Arrest: Sudden Cardiac Death

BRIAN WISPELWEY, M.S., M.D.

Associate Professor of Medicine and Director, Infectious Diseases Clinic, University of Virginia; Attending Physician, University of Virginia Health Sciences Center, Charlottesville, Virginia
Brain Abscess

ROY WITHERINGTON, M.D.

Professor of Surgery (Urology), Medical College of Georgia School of Medicine; Active Staff, Medical College of Georgia Hospital and Clinics; Consultant, Veterans' Affairs Medical Center, University Hospital, and St. Joseph Hospital, Augusta, Georgia
Urethral Stricture

MURRAY WITTNER, M.D., PH.D.

Professor of Pathology and Parasitology, Albert Einstein College of Medicine; Director of Parasitology and Tropical Medicine Clinic and Laboratory, Jacobi Medical Center, Bronx, New York
Intestinal Parasites

LAWRENCE WOLFE, M.D.

Associate Professor of Pediatrics, Tufts University School of Medicine; Chief, Division of Hematology/Oncology, Floating Hospital for Children, New England Medical Center, Boston, Massachusetts
Thalassemia

MARTIN S. WOLFE, M.D.

Clinical Professor of Medicine, George Washington University Medical School; Attending Physician, George Washington University Hospital, Washington, District of Columbia
Acute Infectious Diarrhea

JOSEPH I. WOLFSDORF, M.B., B.CH.

Associate Professor of Pediatrics, Harvard Medical School; Clinical Director of Endocrinology, Children's Hospital; Chief of Pediatrics, Joslin Diabetes Center, Boston, Massachusetts
Diabetes Mellitus in Children and Adolescents

KIMBERLY A. WORKOWSKI, M.D.

Assistant Professor of Medicine, Division of Infectious Diseases, Emory University; Attending Physician, Crawford Long Hospital of Emory University and Grady Memorial Hospital, Atlanta, Georgia
Chlamydia trachomatis *Infection*

KEITH D. WRENN, M.D.

Professor, Departments of Emergency Medicine and Medicine, Vanderbilt University Medical Center, Nashville, Tennessee
Disturbances Due to Cold

MARIAN E. WULF, M.D.

Assistant Professor of Obstetrics and Gynecology, Department of Obstetrics, Gynecology and Reproductive Sciences, University of Texas Medical School; Attending Physician, Hermann Hospital, Houston, Texas
Pelvic Inflammatory Disease

SUMNER J. YAFFE, M.D.

Director, Center for Research for Mothers and Children, National Institute of Child Health and Human Development, Bethesda, Maryland
Fever

CHARLES J. YEO, M.D.

Associate Professor, Departments of Surgery and Oncology, The Johns Hopkins University School of Medicine; Attending Surgeon, The Johns Hopkins Hospital, Baltimore, Maryland
Acute Pancreatitis

CONNIE YOUNG, R.N., M.S.N.

Adjunct Faculty, School of Nursing, Vanderbilt University; Clinical Nurse Specialist, Vanderbilt Hospital, Nashville, Tennessee
Diabetic Ketoacidosis

WILLIAM F. YOUNG, JR., M.D.

Associate Professor of Medicine, Mayo Medical School; Consultant, Divisions of Endocrinology, Hypertension, Internal Medicine; Mayo Clinic and Mayo Foundation, Rochester, Minnesota
Cushing's Syndrome

K. YUGAMBARANATHAN, M.B.

Assistant Medical Registrar, Withybush General Hospital, Pembrokeshire, Wales, United Kingdom
Brucellosis

JOHN B. ZABRISKIE, M.D.

Associate Professor, Rockefeller University; Attending Physician, Rockefeller University Hospital, New York, New York
Rheumatic Fever

KAREN E. ZANOL, M.D.

Assistant Professor of Medicine, Division of Dermatology, Department of Medicine, University of Missouri Hospital and Clinics, Columbia, Missouri
Warts (Verruca Vulgaris)

MICHAEL ZANOLLI, M.D.

Associate Professor of Medicine, Division of Dermatology, Vanderbilt University Medical Center; Director of Clinical Dermatology Services and Director of Vanderbilt Phototherapy Treatment Center, Nashville, Tennessee
Papulosquamous Diseases

SHARON ZELLIS, D.O.

Resident, Department of Dermatology, Philadelphia College of Osteopathic Medicine, Philadelphia, Pennsylvania
Pruritus Ani and Vulvae

THOMAS R. ZIEGLER, M.D.

Assistant Professor of Medicine, Emory University School of Medicine; Associate Director, Nutrition and Metabolic Support Services, Emory University Hospital, Atlanta, Georgia
Parenteral Nutrition in Adults

IRWIN ZIMENT, M.D.

Professor of Medicine, University of California, Los Angeles, School of Medicine, Los Angeles; Chief of Medicine and Medical Director, Olive View–UCLA Medical Center, Sylmar, California
Chronic Obstructive Pulmonary Disease

TONY G. ZREIK, M.D.

Postdoctoral Fellow, Reproductive Endocrinology and Infertility, Department of Obstetrics and Gynecology, Yale University School of Medicine; Attending Physician, Yale–New Haven Hospital, New Haven, Connecticut
Endometriosis

Preface

This is the 48th edition of *Current Therapy,* and as always, it is an entirely new book when compared with the 1995 edition. This year 95% of the authors are new, with the other 5% of authors updating their material from last year when the new author was not able to meet our tight deadline.

Although the great majority of our authors are from the United States, each year some of the authorities are from other countries. This year 31 authors are from other countries, including France (The Porphyrias), Spain (Pericarditis), Finland (Adrenocortical Insufficiency), and Australia (Alcoholism). Fifteen authors are from Canada.

The goal of this book remains the same as first conceived by Howard Conn in 1949: to provide up-to-date information on recent advances in medicine, focusing on the treatment of problems frequently encountered in practice. Also included are less common problems that can be serious if not diagnosed and managed appropriately. The material is presented in a concise and easy-to-read format.

An unusually large number of new topics have been added this year. One is on current immunization practices, which discusses new vaccines (such as for varicella) and includes a table showing the most recent recommended childhood immunization schedule. Also new is an excellent chapter on persistent and intractable hiccups, including the causes and varied treatments (mechanical and pharmacologic) and five useful tables. Other new topics are on the management of sleep apnea syndrome, polyarteritis nodosa, and condylomata acuminata (including a variety of treatments ranging from the old standard podophyllin to the new interferons). Finally, GERD (gastroesophageal reflux disease) is presented as a separate topic, with the discussion including diagnostic evaluation, management, and extraesophageal complications.

Another new feature this year is a list of the 200 most frequently prescribed drugs in the United States, the brand name, manufacturer, and relative cost, to serve as a quick reference when that is all that is needed.

My special thanks to Jeanne Ullian, my editorial assistant who manages the many logistic problems, which allows the book to consistently be published on time, and to Ray Kersey and the excellent editorial staff at W. B. Saunders for their commitment to quality.

ROBERT E. RAKEL, M.D.

NOTICE

Medicine is an ever-changing field. Standard safety precautions must be followed, but as new research and clinical experience broaden our knowledge, changes in treatment and drug therapy become necessary or appropriate. The editors of this work have carefully checked the generic and trade drug names and verified drug dosages to ensure that the dosage information in this work is accurate and in accord with the standards accepted at the time of publication. Readers are advised, however, to check the product information currently provided by the manufacturer of each drug to be administered to be certain that changes have not been made in the recommended dose or in the contraindications for administration. This is of particular importance in regard to new or infrequently used drugs. It is the responsibility of the treating physician, relying on experience and knowledge of the patient, to determine dosages and the best treatment for the patient. The editors cannot be responsible for misuse or misapplication of the material in this work.

THE PUBLISHER

Contents

SECTION 3. THE RESPIRATORY SYSTEM

SECTION 4. THE CARDIOVASCULAR SYSTEM

SECTION 5. THE BLOOD AND SPLEEN

SECTION 6. THE DIGESTIVE SYSTEM

SECTION 7. METABOLIC DISORDERS

SECTION 8. THE ENDOCRINE SYSTEM

SECTION 9. THE UROGENITAL TRACT

SECTION 10. THE SEXUALLY TRANSMITTED DISEASES

SECTION 11. DISEASES OF ALLERGY

SECTION 12. DISEASES OF THE SKIN

SECTION 13. THE NERVOUS SYSTEM

SECTION 14. THE LOCOMOTOR SYSTEM

SECTION 15. OBSTETRICS AND GYNECOLOGY

SECTION 16. PSYCHIATRIC DISORDERS

SECTION 17. PHYSICAL AND CHEMICAL INJURIES

SECTION 18. APPENDICES AND INDEX

Symptomatic Care Pending Diagnosis

PAIN

method of
KATHRYN J. ELLIOTT, M.D., and
GAVRIL PASTERNAK, M.D., PH.D.
Memorial Sloan-Kettering Cancer Center
New York, New York

Pain is one of the most common symptoms addressed by physicians. Drug therapies are used most frequently, but psychotherapy, relaxation therapies, biofeedback, self-hypnosis, physical therapy, stress management, psychiatric and psychosocial support, occupational retraining, cognitive therapies, and neurosurgical and anesthetic techniques also have a role (Table 1). One of the most powerful factors in the treatment of pain is establishing a close, supportive relationship with the patient.

Pain can be difficult to assess because of its subjectivity. Different stimuli can produce different levels of pain among subjects and over time for a given patient. Pain intensity is dependent on the situation in which it occurs, and its perception by the patient can be greatly enhanced by anxiety or fear about its significance. Acute pain may have autonomic signs, such as tachycardia, diaphoresis, hypertension, and pupillary dilatation, but these signs are lost in chronic pain, even when the pain is severe. Thus, the most accurate means of assessment of pain remains simply asking the patient.

PHARMACOTHERAPY

The major groups of drugs used in pain management include the nonsteroidal anti-inflammatory drugs (NSAIDs), the opioids, and a variety of adjuvants. Somatic pain and visceral pain are the most common types encountered clinically and are treated with NSAIDs or opiates, or a combination of both. Patients should be started on weaker agents

TABLE 1. **Principles of Pain Management**

Administer analgesics around the clock.
Provide rescue doses for breakthrough pain.
Titrate analgesics to effect or side effect.
Use drug combinations to maximize analgesia and minimize side effects.
Treat side effects.
Watch for opioid analgesic tolerance.
Use alternative pain therapies if there is inadequate analgesia (anesthetic, neurosurgical, psychotherapeutic techniques).
Follow patients' reports of pain intensity and relief.

first. If increasing the dose is not effective, more potent drugs should be used. Administering the drugs around the clock is more effective than giving them on an "as-needed" (prn) basis. Patients require lower daily analgesic doses using the around-the-clock approach than when given medications as needed. The patient should also be given access to "rescue" dosages for the management of breakthrough pain.

Nonsteroidal Anti-Inflammatory Drugs

A number of NSAIDs are available without prescription, including aspirin, ibuprofen, and naproxen. Acetaminophen is widely used, but it lacks much of the anti-inflammatory actions of the others. Although these drugs can be very effective, their ceiling effects for analgesia limit their use to relief of mild to moderate pain.

Acetaminophen (650 to 1000 mg every 4 hours) has a predominantly central mechanism of action and is equipotent with aspirin. The total daily adult dose should not exceed 6 grams. Side effects with acetaminophen use are uncommon. Hepatoxicity can develop, particularly in patients fasting or using alcohol. Acetaminophen overdose can result in hepatic necrosis, a medical emergency. Overdose patients require liver function tests, and acetylcysteine should be given immediately on evidence of hepatotoxicity.

Aspirin (650 to 1000 mg every 4 hours) is an effective analgesic with both peripheral and central actions. The anti-inflammatory actions of aspirin and the other NSAIDs distinguish them from acetaminophen and may offer significant benefits. Adverse effects include nausea, vomiting, and gastrointestinal bleeding. The tendency toward bleeding may be significant because of the additional inhibition of platelet aggregation by the drug. These platelet effects can last up to a week after the drug is discontinued, and aspirin should be avoided in patients undergoing surgery. Higher dosages may result in tinnitus, headache, and dizziness. Aspirin, like the other NSAIDs, should be used with caution by patients with impaired renal function.

A number of NSAIDs have similar mechanisms of action. Ibuprofen (200 to 600 mg every 4 hours) and naproxen (Naprosyn) (250 to 500 mg twice a day) have been approved for over-the-counter use, illustrating their overall safety. Longer-acting NSAIDs include diflunisal (Dolobid) (500 mg twice a day), piroxicam (Feldene) (20 to 40 mg a day), and choline magnesium trisalicylate (Trilisate), a nonacetylated salicylate (500 to 1000 mg twice a day), which has the advantage of limited gastrointestinal, renal, or platelet toxicity as there is minimal interference with prostaglandin synthesis. Ketorolac tromethamine (Toradol) is an injectable NSAID that can be useful in acute pain management. Ketorolac has an onset of analgesia similar to that of the opioids but a longer duration of action. Ketorolac 30 mg intramuscularly is equivalent in efficacy to meperidine 100 mg intramuscularly or morphine 12 mg intramuscularly in single-dose studies.

Opioid Analgesics

General Principles

Opioids can relieve pain through peripheral, spinal, and supraspinal mechanisms and through a family of related but distinct receptors. Most opioids used clinically act through mu, or morphine, receptors, but mixed agonist-antagonists, such as pentazocine (Talwin), act through a combination of mu and kappa receptors. Mixed agonist-antagonists should be used cautiously, and their use should be limited to opioid-naive patients. Their analgesic actions are mediated, in large part, through kappa receptors. However, they are typically antagonists at the mu receptors and can precipitate withdrawal in dependent persons. Other opiates, like buprenorphine (Temgesic), are partial agonists with limited analgesic potency. They too can be problematic in physically dependent patients.

Patients with moderate pain should be tried on one of the weak opioids, such as codeine, oxycodone, hydrocodone, or propoxyphene, used in combination with acetaminophen, aspirin, or another NSAID. If patients fail to obtain adequate analgesia on maximal doses, they should be switched to a stronger opioid, with the dose again titrated to effect or side effect. Patients often respond better to one medication than to another, and even side effects can be more problematic with one drug than with another. Indeed, if a side effect is experienced with one medication, it is often helpful to switch to another. Opioid responsiveness varies among the various pain syndromes, with both somatic and visceral pain relatively more responsive than neuropathic pain. With chronic use, all patients develop tolerance and dependence. Tolerance is often noted by the patient as a shorter duration of analgesic action, and it is overcome by an increase in the dose. As the dose increases, patients on weak opioids should be switched to stronger drugs. Sometimes patients switched from one medication to another regain pain relief because of the lack of complete cross-tolerance among drugs. Tolerance develops to all opiate actions, including respiratory depression and constipation. Taking dependent patients off opiates can be done relatively easily by cutting the dose every 3 to 4 days. Withdrawal signs can be prevented by giving the patient as little as 25% of the previous drug dosage. Although all patients become dependent with chronic dosing, very few become addicted, as defined by drug-seeking behavior and craving. The unfounded fear of addiction by both the patient and the physician can interfere with adequate pain control. Although pain should be adequately treated in all patients, special care should be taken with patients with a history of drug abuse.

Routes of Opioid Administration

Oral administration is the most common, and preferred, route of administration of opioids, but it may be suboptimal in patients with impaired swallowing, gastrointestinal obstruction, or the need for rapid pain control. Parenteral administration provides the fastest relief of pain, but bolus injections can be associated with alternating toxicity at the peak concentrations and breakthrough pain at the trough levels. This problem can be overcome by using either intravenous or subcutaneous infusions. Continuous subcutaneous infusion has proved effective in ambulatory patients, primarily with morphine, hydromorphone (Dilaudid), or oxymorphone (Numorphan). Fentanyl (Duragesic) is available in a transdermal patch. It has a slow onset of action and should be used only in patients with stable pain. The dosing schedule is approximately 72 hours. Intranasal butorphanol has been used for the management of acute postoperative pain. Opiates also are used epidurally and intrathecally, but these routes should be used only in refractory cases.

Adverse Effects of Opioids

Opioids have a variety of side effects. Respiratory depression is mediated through brainstem mu receptors and is always accompanied by other signs of central nervous system depression, including sedation and mental clouding. Patients tolerant to the analgesic actions of opioids are tolerant to their respiratory depressant actions. If significant respiratory depression occurs, administering naloxone (Narcan) improves ventilation if the patient cannot be aroused with stimulation or physical activity. Care must be used with naloxone. The duration of naloxone action is typically shorter than that of many analgesics, so that repeated dosing may be required. Since naloxone induces withdrawal, the naloxone dose (0.4 mg) should be diluted to 10 mL with saline and administered slowly to dependent patients. When naloxone is given carefully, it is possible to achieve reversal of respiratory depression without precipitating withdrawal. Protection of the airway with an endotracheal tube should be considered, to prevent aspiration.

Constipation is the most common adverse effect encountered during chronic opioid therapy, and only limited tolerance develops. All patients should be prescribed prophylactic laxatives. Sedation commonly occurs with the initiation of opioid therapy, and tolerance to this effect develops in days to weeks.

Patients should be warned to avoid dangerous activities. Patients with underlying central nervous system disorders or using other sedating drugs, particularly the benzodiazepines, are at increased risk for sedation, confusion, or delirium. In patients in whom sedation cannot be managed with dose titration, psychostimulants such as dextroamphetamine* (5 mg orally every 6 hours) or methylphenidate (Ritalin)* have been widely used in the cancer pain population. Both agents enhance the analgesic actions of the opioid as well as increasing alertness.

Nausea and vomiting may occur in up to 40% of patients started on opioids. Tolerance can develop rapidly, and the routine prophylactic administration of an antiemetic is not necessary. When needed, an antiemetic such as prochlorperazine (Compazine) or metoclopramide (Reglan) is often sufficient to manage opioid-induced nausea. If these symptoms are severe or persist, a change to another opioid may eliminate the problem.

Multifocal myoclonus may develop with any of the opioid analgesics and is often associated with subtle mental clouding that may progress to delirium. Its mechanism is unknown, but decreasing the drug dose usually eliminates the problem.

Opioid Drugs

Weak opioids, including codeine, hydrocodone, and oxycodone, are distinguished from the strong opioids by the intensity of the pain for which they are customarily used. Codeine alone (30 to 60 mg every 4 hours) or in combination with other drugs such as acetaminophen (Tylenol No. 3) is a commonly used opioid for mild to moderate pain. Codeine is metabolized to morphine, which is believed to be the active metabolite since codeine itself does not bind to opioid receptors. Orally, 30 mg of codeine is equivalent to 650 mg of aspirin. Oxycodone is a codeine analogue typically given with acetaminophen (Percocet) or aspirin (Percodan), as is hydrocodone (Vicodin). Anecdotal experience suggests that oxycodone may produce fewer central nervous system side effects than other strong opioids. Propoxyphene is a weak opioid that also is used in conjunction with aspirin (Darvon with A.S.A.) or acetaminophen (Darvocet).

Morphine is a potent opioid used for the management of severe pain. Dosing often starts at 30 mg every 4 hours orally, but the dose should be titrated since some patients require far greater doses. Parenterally, morphine doses are approximately one-third of the oral doses. Care must be taken with patients who have impaired renal function. In addition to being converted to inactive metabolites, morphine is converted to morphine-6β-glucuronide, which is more potent than morphine and which can accumulate and result in renal failure. Controlled-release preparations of morphine (such as MS Contin) allow dosing on an 8- or 12-hour schedule. This dosing schedule is helpful in managing patients' pain, especially during the nighttime hours. Patients should be titrated with immediate-release morphine, and when the pain is stabilized the same daily dose can then be given with the slow-release preparations. At least 24 hours is required to approach steady-state plasma concentrations after dosing is either started or changed. Hydromorphone may be an alternative to morphine, given its significant solubility and the availability of a concentrated preparation (10 mg per mL), although pharmacologically it is quite similar. It is particularly useful with continuous subcutaneous or intravenous infusions.

Although meperidine (Demerol) is widely used to manage acute or chronic pain, we rarely use it. Particular care must be taken in patients with renal disease because of the accumulation of the metabolite normeperidine, which has been associated with mood changes, multifocal myoclonus, tremor, and occasionally seizures. Naloxone does not reverse meperidine-induced seizures. In addition, meperidine interacts with monoamine oxidase (MAO) inhibitors, to produce a syndrome of malignant hyperthermia characterized by hyperpyrexia, muscle rigidity, seizures, and death.

Methadone (Dolophine) is a long-acting synthetic opioid that can be effectively used to treat pain. However, its use as an analgesic should be limited to situations in which the other opioids are not adequate. Despite its long half-life, patients still require doses every 4 to 8 hours to maintain analgesia. This can create difficulties since the plasma levels of methadone increase for days after the institution of a fixed dosing schedule, posing a risk of toxicity to the patient. Methadone therapy should initially be administered on an as-needed dosing schedule only. Levorphanol (Levo-Dromoran) is a long-acting opioid that can be given every 4 to 6 hours. As with methadone, its long plasma half-life predisposes patients to drug accumulation after changes in the dose. This drug should be used cautiously in the opioid-naive patient.

Fentanyl is a potent semisynthetic opioid. The transdermal preparation slowly releases drug and requires many hours to reach maximal effect; it should not be used in the initial dose titration in patients with severe pain. After the removal of the fentanyl patch, the drug is still released from the cutaneous depot for many hours.

Adjuvant Analgesics

Adjuvant analgesics are agents useful in specific pain syndromes or in combination with traditional pharmacologic therapies. The use of the adjuvant drugs in pain management remains largely empirical, though their use in some cases has been validated in clinical trials. Many agents are primarily used for other reasons. There is great interindividual variability in the response to all the adjuvant analgesics.

Corticosteroids

Corticosteroids are widely used as analgesics in patients with cancer. In addition, corticosteroids also

---

*Not FDA-approved for this indication.

improve appetite and mood and reduce nausea and malaise in this population. Analgesic properties of the corticosteroids may result from their actions against edema and inflammation. The use of corticosteroids in nonmalignant pain is not recommended as the long-term use of these agents has significant toxicity. They have been used empirically for the management of acute intractable migraine or cluster headache.

Antidepressants

The antidepressants are analgesic in diverse types of chronic pain syndromes, including neuropathic pain syndromes, and can be effective for prophylaxis in migraine. Amitriptyline (Elavil)* is most widely used, although imipramine (Tofranil),* doxepin (Sinequan),* and clomipramine (Anafranil)* all demonstrate analgesic effects as well. The choice of antidepressant is often empirical and is based largely on consideration of side effects. Amitriptyline is usually the first agent to be tried. It is started as a single 10-mg dose at bedtime to minimize side effects. The dose is then escalated slowly until relief is obtained or side effects intervene. Not all patients respond. If a patient has not obtained relief at a daily dose of 150 mg, it is unlikely that higher doses will be effective. At this point, another antidepressant can be tried. Serious adverse effects are uncommon, but sedation, postural hypotension, and delirium may occur, especially in the elderly population. Acute urinary retention, acute angle-closure glaucoma, constipation, and cardiac arrhythmias may also be a concern.

Local Anesthetics

Two oral lidocaine analogues show efficacy in neuropathic pain: tocainide (Tonocard)* has demonstrated analgesia in patients with trigeminal neuralgia, and mexiletine (Mexitil)* has demonstrated analgesia in patients with painful diabetic neuropathy. Subcutaneous lidocaine has also been used for refractory neuropathic pain. Topical lidocaine preparations have decreased the allodynic component of the pain in herpetic neuralgia, and regional injection and intraspinal instillation are other effective ways of delivering lidocaine for analgesia. The oral local anesthetic mexiletine produces nausea, vomiting, dizziness, unsteadiness, and tremor at higher dosages and should be avoided in patients with cardiac disease.

Anticonvulsant Drugs

The anticonvulsant drugs are active against paroxysmal pains of trigeminal neuralgia and peripheral neuropathies and other lancinating pains. The evidence is strongest for carbamazepine, but anecdotal experience suggests that phenytoin (Dilantin),* clonazepam (Klonopin),* and valproate (Depakote) also are effective. Carbamazepine (Tegretol) may produce sleepiness, dizziness, nausea and vomiting, or unsteadiness, but these effects can be minimized by a dose titration. Carbamazepine may cause leukopenia and/or thrombocytopenia and, rarely, aplastic anemia and hepatoxicity, requiring monitoring of blood counts and liver functions. Phenytoin may also show efficacy in lancinating neuropathic pain; its use is associated with sedation, dizziness, and ataxia and may lead to hepatotoxicity. Allergic reactions are particularly troublesome, and at the first indication of a rash the patient should be taken off the drug. Valproate is a third-line adjuvant anticonvulsant for use in lancinating neuropathic pain, and side effects may include sedation, tremor, nausea, hepatotoxicity, encephalopathy, dermatitis, alopecia, and a rare hyperammonia syndrome.

Baclofen

Baclofen (Lioresal)* likely acts as a gamma-aminobutyric acid (GABA) agonist. Although effective in trigeminal neuralgia, it is a second-line drug behind carbamazepine. A dose of 5 mg once a day may be gradually escalated to 30 to 90 mg per day in divided doses, with sedation as the principal side effect. Much larger dosages have been used in the spinal cord–injured population, and anecdotal experience suggests that higher dosages of baclofen, if titrated slowly, can be effective both in lancinating neuralgias and in central neuropathic pain. Discontinuation requires dose tapering to prevent a withdrawal syndrome.

Calcitonin

Calcitonin is effective against bone pain from osteoporotic vertebral collapse, against pain from metastatic tumor or Paget's disease, and in central neuropathic phantom limb pain. Its mechanism of analgesic action is unknown. Anecdotal experience suggests that side effects are minimal. Elderly patients do not develop cognitive impairment or constipation. Nausea and/or vomiting appears to be doserelated and a minor problem. A test dose beforeinduction of therapy is required if the salmon preparation is used.

NEUROSURGICAL APPROACHES

Neurosurgical approaches to pain control are limited and should be used as a last resort. Cordotomy involves the transection of the pain pathways in the spinal cord and is usually performed percutaneously. Although this is quite effective, the relief of pain is often limited to 6 months. Cordotomy can be associated with an ipsilateral paresis, and bilateral cordotomies can result in loss of sphincter control, paresis, or sleep apnea ("Ondine's curse"). Trigeminal neuralgia that is refractory to medical treatment can be treated surgically through exploration of the posterior fossa or through radiofrequency ablation.

OTHER APPROACHES

Many factors modify pain perception. Relieving anxiety through reassurance or use of an anxiolytic

---

*Not FDA-approved for this indication.

*Not FDA-approved for this indication.

agent can help control pain. Chronic pain poses special problems. First, many physicians are reluctant to use pain medications for prolonged periods of time in nonmalignant pain. Second, chronic pain is associated with significant psychological problems. Oftentimes patients are helped by psychotherapy, biofeedback, or relaxation therapy. Many patients also report positive results from transcutaneous electrical nerve stimulation (TENS).

NAUSEA AND VOMITING

method of
WILLIAM K. MURPHY, M.D.
*University of Texas M. D. Anderson Cancer
Center
Houston, Texas*

The symptom complex of nausea and vomiting and the physical manifestations thereof are encountered in all the specialties and subspecialties in the field of medicine. Each may occur without the other, but nausea usually precedes vomiting, and nausea and vomiting usually occur together and may have various other associated symptoms such as diarrhea, headaches, abdominal pain, or fever. Although the association with antineoplastic chemotherapy has been emphasized in recent literature, nausea and vomiting as manifestations in other widely varied circumstances, not infrequently life-threatening, constitute the majority of incidences.

Nausea and vomiting involve basic neural reflexes. Nausea itself is an ill-defined but universally recognized sensation mediated through unknown pathways and associated with hypersalivation, diminished gastric tone and peristalsis, and increased duodenal tone and duodenal-gastric reflux. It may be associated with retching, which is characterized by spasmodic respiratory movements against a closed glottis with contractions of the abdominal musculature without expulsion of gastrointestinal contents. Vomiting involves, in addition, sustained contracture of abdominal musculature with forceful expulsion of gastric contents. The reflexes involved in this process may be triggered by at least four different afferent pathways either simultaneously or independently and involve the chemoreceptor trigger zone (CTZ), located in the brain in the area posterior to the medulla (humoral pathway). Activation of the CTZ results in neural messages to the vomiting center located nearby in the lateral reticular formation of the medulla, which coordinates the act of vomiting. A peripheral afferent pathway involves activation of peripheral nerve endings in the gastrointestinal tract (and other peripheral sites) with transmission to the vomiting center via the vagus nerve. A cerebral afferent pathway involves nonchemical stimuli such as unpleasant sights or odors. The fourth afferent pathway is the vestibular pathway. Central and peripheral neurotransmitters important in nausea and vomiting include dopamine, acetylcholine, serotonin, histamine, and endorphins.

ASSESSMENT AND DIAGNOSIS

The cornerstone in the assessment of the cause of nausea and vomiting clinically is a thorough history accompanied by an equally thorough physical examination. As may be seen in Table 1, the causes of nausea and vomiting are myriad and this list is by no means comprehensive. In the setting of cancer chemotherapy, where the cause would seem to be evident and the solution the administration of antiemetics, complicating factors must still be considered. Protracted nausea and vomiting, associated fever and/or pain, or the development of unusual associated symptoms should prompt an investigation for unrelated medical-surgical conditions. The fact that a patient has cancer for which chemotherapy is being given does not affect the fact that other conditions, some of which may be serious or even life-threatening, may not coincidentally supervene. Thorough assessment may reveal the presence of unrelated bowel obstruction, peptic ulcer disease, infectious processes, reaction to other medications, or other emetogenic problems.

In any patient presenting with nausea and/or vomiting, history alone may identify the cause. Reaction to medication recently started, infectious processes (including gastroenteritis), food poisoning, a history of diabetes mellitus, known peptic ulcer disease, ingestion or use of various recreational drugs (including alcoholic overindulgence) are but a few of the causes in this category. History enhanced by physical examination will reveal most additional causes of nausea and vomiting, although specific confirmatory tests will often be required. Jaundice, fever, cough, abdomi-

TABLE 1. **Some Causes of Nausea and Vomiting**

Gastrointestinal Disorders

Peptic ulcer disease/gastritis
Intestinal obstruction/ileus/perforation/volvulus
Cholelithiasis/cholecystitis
Constipation/fecal impaction
Adhesions
Gastric cancer
Pancreatitis/pancreatic tumors
Motility disorders
Autonomic neuropathy
Pyloric obstruction

Central Nervous System

Cerebral edema
Migraine
Vestibular dysfunction/Meniere's disease/motion sickness
Brain tumor/carcinomatous meningitis
Brain abscess
Hydrocephalus
Cerebral/anticipatory/reactive

Iatrogenic Causes

Medications
  Antibiotics
  Antineoplastic agents
  Morphine/analgesics
  Theophylline
  Digitalis/digoxin
  Anesthetic agents
  L-dopa/bromocriptine (Parlodel)
Radiation therapy
Postoperative factors

Systemic Causes

Pregnancy
Infectious causes/food poisoning
Diabetic ketoacidosis
Uremia
Chronic hepatic disease/hepatic failure
Adrenal insufficiency
Paraneoplastic syndromes
Hypercalcemia
Drug overdose
Heavy metal poisoning

Psychogenic Causes

nal distention with or without tenderness, absent bowel sounds, hyperactive bowel sounds with or without diarrhea, hepatomegaly, fecal impaction, epigastric tenderness, fruity or alcoholic breath odor, perforated nasal septum, amenorrhea with enlarged uterus, point tenderness in the right lower quadrant, and papilledema are a few of the physical findings that point to specific causes of nausea and vomiting.

The medical history and positive physical findings more often than not suggest specific laboratory or imaging studies to pinpoint the specific cause of nausea and vomiting. Complete blood count, a chemistry battery, and urinalysis may be sufficient alone for conditions including infections, gastrointestinal bleeding (plus stool guaiac testing), or thrombocytopenia. Elevated bilirubin with or without enzyme elevations indicate probable liver problems and hematuria/pyuria indicates urinary problems at various sites in the urinary tract. Abdominal tenderness and distention with or without fever are an indication for abdominal radiologic studies including flat plate and supine and upright films. Contrast imaging studies and endoscopy may be needed for more difficult diagnoses, but a simple amylase/lipase level may suffice if pancreatitis is suspected. Headaches, papilledema, seizures, and more focal abnormalities associated with nausea and vomiting suggest brain imaging for diagnosis. Fever and cough indicate the need for chest imaging studies. Nausea and vomiting may be related to esophageal disease, cancer, hiatal hernia, and various cardiac causes. A simple pregnancy test can clarify another otherwise obscure cause of nausea and vomiting. The list is not comprehensive but indicates how ubiquitous the symptoms of nausea and vomiting are as reflections of significant medical problems. There are psychogenic causes as well.

TREATMENT

The treatment of nausea and vomiting is, first and foremost, the treatment of the underlying cause. The extent to which this cause may be corrected will control the success of other modalities of treatment. Not infrequently, ordering bed rest, temporarily stopping the patient's oral intake, and administering corrective intravenous fluids and electrolytes will either solve the problem by itself (in the most common causes—gastroenteritis and various types of overindulgence) or alleviate the patient's discomfort until the diagnosis is made and curative or corrective procedures can be applied. In this setting, antiemetic agents may be administered for palliative purposes but not to the extent that significant pathology is obscured, which would delay life-saving intervention.

Adequate and correct fluid and electrolyte therapy may be lifesaving in patients with protracted nausea and vomiting, particularly in children and elderly persons, and should be pursued aggressively at the initiation of therapy. A variety of medications may be causes of significant nausea and vomiting, and to continue any of these by switching to intravenous forms may only aggravate or perpetuate the problem. Such medications include theophylline, digoxin, antibiotics, and agents to relieve pain, particularly narcotics.

Pregnancy very often is associated with nausea and vomiting, classically as morning sickness in the first trimester. Extended nausea and vomiting throughout pregnancy (hyperemesis gravidarum) may be a complication of major consequence. These problems associated with the gravid state are beyond the scope of this treatise and should be addressed by specialists in the field of obstetrics. Suffice it to say that antiemetics administered to a pregnant woman may enter the fetal circulation, with potential adverse effects. If a female patient with nausea and vomiting is in the childbearing years and the cause of her gastrointestinal problems remain obscure, the possibility of pregnancy should be assessed and pharmacologically active antiemetic regimens avoided.

The occurrence of nausea and vomiting in the postoperative state and in motion sickness is also of consequence. Postoperative nausea and vomiting may occur as a result of anesthetic agents and of the type of surgery itself. In the former instance, much progress has been made in the development of new anesthetic agents and techniques that have lessened or eliminated nausea and vomiting as a problem. Serotonin antagonists (ondansetron [Zofran], granisetron [Kytril]) have been found effective and useful in this setting. Studies continue of their use in the postoperative situation and, as always, other correctable causes should be sought. Nasogastric suction may be particularly useful postoperatively for thoracoabdominal surgery or any persistent nausea and vomiting in the postoperative setting.

Motion sickness is a particularly vexing problem for a segment of the population. Its cause is not well understood, but mild sedation with anxiolytic agents may be helpful when used along with anticholinegics and antihistamines. Agents used for this disorder include dimenhydrinate, cyclizine and meclizine. Another interesting approach is the transdermal administration of scopolamine. Cessation of motion is curative.

Antiemetic Agents

Antiemetics are used primarily for symptom control while the cause of the nausea and vomiting is determined. Much impetus has been given to research in this field by the rapid development of anticancer chemotherapy since the mid-1960s. One of the principal side effects of these agents is nausea and vomiting, in some cases severe enough to interfere with effective therapy. The use of antiemetics, particularly the relatively new class of serotonin antagonists, has been responsible for major improvement in control of emesis, particularly when used in rational combinations.

There are eight classes of antiemetic agents, as listed in Table 2, plus some adjunctive agents. These agents may be used for varied conditions as adjuncts to primary treatment of the underlying causes of nausea and vomiting or in the setting of cancer chemotherapy.

Serotonin Antagonists

The newest class of antiemetics, and perhaps the most effective, is the specific 5-hydroxytryptamine

TABLE 2. **Antiemetic Classification and Recommended Dosage/Administration**

Drug	Trade Name	Dosage/Administration
Serotonin Antagonists		
Ondansetron	Zofran	0.15 mg/kg q 4 h IV × 3 or a single 32-mg IV dose; 8 mg q 8 h PO × 24 h
Granisetron	Kytril	10 µg/kg (or 1 mg) IV, once Not available orally
Phenothiazines		
Prochlorperazine	Compazine	5–10 mg q 4–6 h PO or IM 10 mg q 3 h IV × 4 maximum 25 mg q 4–6 h rectally
Thiethlyperazine	Torecan	10 mg q 6–8 PO or IM, rectally
Promethazine	Phenergan	25 mg q 4–6 h PO or IM, rectally 12.5 mg q 4–6 h IV
Perphenazine	Trilafon	8–16 mg q 4–6 h PO
Chlorpromazine	Thorazine	10–25 mg q 3–6 h PO or IV 50–100 mg q 6–8 h rectally
Butyrophenones		
Droperidol		
	Inapsine	1–2 mg q 6–8 h PO or IM 0.5–2 mg q 4 h IV
Haloperidol	Haldol	1–3 mg q 2–6 h IV
Substituted Benzamides		
Metoclopramide	Reglan	1–3 mg/kg q 2 h IV for three doses 10 mg 30 min a.c. PO
Steroids		
Dexamethasone		
Methylprednisolone	Decadron Solu-Medrol	10–20 mg once PO or IV (q 6 h × 24–48 h for severe nausea and vomiting) 250–500 mg q 4–6 h IV
Antihistamines		
Diphenhydramine	Benadryl	25–50 mg q 6–8 h PO, IM, or IV
Hydroxyzine	Vistaril	25–100 mg q 6–8 h PO or IV
Meclizine	Antivert	20–50 mg q 24 h PO
Dimenhydrinate	Dramamine	50 mg q 4–8 h PO or IV
Benzodiazepines		
Lorazepam	Ativan	1.0–1.5 mg IV or IM
Diazepam	Valium	5–10 mg q 6–8 h PO or IV
Cannabinoids		
Dronabinol	Marinol	5–10 mg/m² q 4–6 h PO
Anticholinergics		
Scopolamine	Transderm Scōp	1 patch q 3 days behind ear
Miscellaneous		
Trimethobenzamide	Tigan	250 mg PO or 200 mg IM 3 or 4 times daily (adults)
Benzquinamide	Emete-con	50 mg q 3–4 h IM 25 mg IV (1 mg/min)

Abbreviations: IV = intravenously; PO = orally; IM = intramuscularly; a.c. = before meals.

(5-HT$_3$) receptor antagonist or serotonin antagonists. These agents, ondansetron (Zofran) and granisetron (Kytril), in addition to being highly effective, have relatively few side effects including headaches, transient elevation of serum aspartate aminotransferase (AST) and alanine aminotransferase (ALT), and lightheadedness. Most effective for acute nausea and vomiting of chemotherapy within the first 24 hours, the value of these agents in delayed nausea and vomiting has yet to be established. Both are available in intravenous and oral form. Additional 5-HT$_3$ blockers are under development and will be marketed in the near future. The determining factor in utilization may turn out to be economic, since the agents so far appear to be relatively equivalent in efficacy.

Substituted Benzamides

The principal agent in this class is metoclopramide (Reglan), an agent that blocks both dopamine recep-

tors and, in high dose, 5-HT$_3$ receptors. An older agent that has been extensively studied, it is very effective in doses of 1 to 3 mg/kg given every 2 to 3 hours beginning before chemotherapy (see Table 2). Side effects such as akathisia, diarrhea, and acute dystonic reactions, particularly in younger patients (under 30 years old), may be controlled with diphenhydramine (Benadryl) and lorazepam (Ativan). The 5-HT$_3$ blockers for antiemetic therapy for highly emetogenic drugs or combinations have been favored because they do not cause this class of side effects and are equally effective, if not more so.

Butyrophenones

These agents used intravenously are dopamine receptor blockers. Haloperidol (Haldol) and droperidol (Inapsine) are effective antiemetics with a lower order of efficacy and are used most often in combinations or in delayed emesis. As with several antiemetics, they may cause sedation. Sedation may be a beneficial side effect but must be taken into account when treating ambulatory patients or outpatients who drive automobiles.

Corticosteroids

These agents have been recognized for many years as having significant antiemetic effects, although they are not approved by the FDA for this indication. Dexamethasone and prednisone or methylprednisolone are the agents most often used. The dosage is not well standardized and the mechanism of action is unknown but multiple studies have confirmed their efficacy, particularly in combinations as with ondanestron, granisetron, and metoclopramide. Corticosteroids are not without significant side effects and should be administered cautiously in patients with active peptic ulcer disease, insulin-dependent diabetes mellitus, history of heart failure, or known psychotic disorders. The use of these agents in refractory nausea and vomiting may afford significant benefit but the potential for side effects from more intensive and more prolonged administration must be carefully considered.

Cannabinoids

Long-touted as an ameliorative agent for nausea and vomiting of chemotherapy, marijuana remains basically unavailable and illegal per se. Research into its effectiveness has been performed, and tetrahydrocannabinol has been isolated and marketed as dronabinol (Marinol). It is a mild antiemetic that may cause drowsiness, ataxia, and dysphoria, and it is more acceptable to younger patients.

Phenothiazines

One of the oldest classes of antiemetics, phenothiazines are best used for mild-to-moderate nausea and vomiting. Available orally, intravenously, and by suppository, these agents find their widest use for continuing therapy at home and for more transient nonchemotherapy-related use. Agents and doses are partially listed in Table 2. Although less used than formerly, agents such as prochlorperazine (Compazine), and promethazine (Phenergan) are useful in management of emesis and nausea from less emetogenic antineoplastic agents and for delayed emesis. Their long-term and generic availability make them a less expensive alternative. Side effects include extrapyramidal sequelae, sedation, and anticholinergic manifestations.

Anticholinergics/Antihistamines

These agents have only low-level antiemetic properties and are useful mostly in combination therapy and for motion sickness. Doses and schedules are shown in Table 2. Scopolamine dermal patches (Transderm Scōp) may be particularly useful in motion sickness and in amelioration of side effects of pain medication.

Benzodiazepines and Miscellaneous

Benzodiazepines act on cortical pathways and possibly on the vomiting center. They have a low level of antiemetic activity but may be particularly useful in combination therapy for their sedative properties and for amnesic effects, of benefit in lessening the conditioned behavior (anticipatory nausea and vomiting) resulting from emetogenic therapy.

Miscellaneous agents used in antiemetic therapy include trimethobenzamide (Tigan) and benzquinamide (Emete-con). These agents are useful for less severe nausea and emesis and have minimal side effects.

Management of Chemotherapy-Induced Nausea and Vomiting

Nausea and vomiting induced by the administration of antineoplastic drugs is a relatively new area of medical research, although some agents used to treat cancer go back a long time. Since about 1970 (some earlier), carboplatin, cisplatin, dacarbazine, the nitrosoureas, cytarabine, daunorubicin, doxorubicin, and idarubicin have all been introduced and have become commercially available (Table 3). These agents are all considered to be moderately to severely emetogenic. Metoclopramide in high doses (see Tables 2 and 4 regarding dosing) with dexamethasone, diphenhydramine, and lorazepam has proved to be an effective agent and combination for management of the nausea and vomiting caused by most of these agents. With the introduction of the 5-HT_3 antagonists, ondansetron (Zofran) and now granisetron (Kytril), even more effective antiemetic control is possible, particularly when these are combined with

TABLE 3. **Emetic Potency of Chemotherapeutic Agents**

Severe

Cisplatin (Platinol)
Dacarbazine
Nitrogen mustard
Streptozocin (Zanosar)

Moderately Severe

Cyclophosphamide (Cytoxan)
Ifosfamide (Ifex)
Doxorubicin (Rubex)
Nitrosoureas
Actinomycin D

Moderate

Cytarabine (Cytosar-U)
Procarbazine (Matulane)
Mitomycin C (Mutamycin)
High-dose methotrexate

Mild

Etoposide (VePesid)
5-Fluorouracil
Hydroxyurea (Hydrea)
Bleomycin (Blenoxane)
Vinblastine (Velban)
Vincristine (Oncovin)
Chlorambucil (Leukeran)
Low-dose methotrexate
Vinorelbine (Navelbine)

intravenous dexamethasone in a dose of 10 mg to 20 mg, possibly combined with lorazepam (Ativan) (Table 4). For less emetogenic anticancer therapy, oral ondansetron or granisetron or any of a number of less expensive drugs of lesser potency may be effective, including (low-dose) metoclopramide, butyrophenones, corticosteroids, and phenothiazines. Combinations of these agents with anticholinergics and/or antihistamines are often useful. Benzodiazepines are particularly useful in highly anxious and overreactive patients. The combination of haloperidol (1.5 mg), diphenhydramine (25 mg), and lorazepam (0.5 mg) is very useful given orally or in suppositories. The key to successful antiemetic therapy is to premedicate patients to avoid nausea and vomiting initially rather than to wait until the problem develops and then to administer rescue medication.

"Delayed emesis" is a term that has come to mean nausea and vomiting persisting or starting 24 hours following chemotherapy. Whereas ondansetron and granisetron are highly effective in the first 24 hours, their use for delayed emesis has not been very effective, although research in this area continues. Metoclopramide (0.5 mg/kg orally four times daily), prochlorperazine (10 mg intravenously, 25 mg suppository, or oral extended release 15 to 30 mg) or dexamethasone (4 mg orally every 4 to 6 hours) may be helpful in this setting, as may other of the ancillary antiemetics. If one regimen does not work, another agent should be tried. For intense, protracted nausea and vomiting in which other more serious causes have been ruled out, intravenous corticosteroids (dexamethasone 10 mg intravenously every 6 hours around the clock for 24 to 48 hours) may be remarkedly effective. In such prolonged administration at high dose, the more serious adverse effects of corticosteroids must be kept in mind.

"Anticipatory emesis," a conditioned response characterized by sights, smells, food, and even people or places eliciting significant nausea and vomiting, has been a problem in cancer chemotherapy. Its origins generally relate to poorly controlled or uncontrolled nausea and vomiting from chemotherapy for which the patient has developed specific associations. Management lies in effective antiemetic therapy started prior to chemotherapy administration. Treatment with benzodiazepines and/or behavioral modification may be helpful in the management of this vexing problem. The introduction of more effective antiemetic agents and their combinations has lessened the incidence of this complication.

Notes and Cautions

In the management of nausea and vomiting, the assessment of underlying cause remains the key to successful and rational management. The possibility of complicating conditions should be kept in mind at all times, even when the cause, such as administration of cancer chemotherapy, seems obvious. Fluid and electrolyte therapy is of prime importance. Although significant progress has been made in antiemetic therapy, particularly in the field of cancer chemotherapy, primary treatment failures still occur and virtually all patients treated with highly emetogenic agents have some nausea and often delayed nausea and vomiting. There is need for continued research into more effective antiemetic therapy.

The economics of antiemetic therapy cannot be ignored, particularly with the advent of managed care, health maintenance organizations, and preferred provider organizations. Cost effectiveness must be considered but cost alone must not be allowed to dictate inferior or ineffective antiemetic therapy. Physicians must refrain from indiscriminate use of the more expensive agents, particularly when the indications for their use are not clearly defined. Research into the medical/economic aspects of antiemetic utilization is needed for rational prescribing practices.

GASEOUSNESS AND INDIGESTION

method of
HOWARD J. FULLMAN, M.D.
Kaiser Permanente
West Los Angeles, California

GASEOUSNESS

The phenomenon of gaseousness may be manifested as excessive belching, a sense of abdominal fullness, or excessive flatus. Often these sensations are not truly pathologic but rather are physiologic or are due to excessive sensitivity to normal function. Sometimes these symptoms are caused by reflux esophagitis, maldigestion of food substances (as in lactose intolerance), or the irritable bowel syndrome.

Aerophagia, the swallowing of air, may cause belching and distention. Patients with this condition should be advised to avoid talking while eating, chewing gum, drinking through a straw, smoking

TABLE 4. **Combination Antiemetic Regimens for Moderate-to-Severe Emetogenic Chemotherapy***

Regimen 1	
Ondansetron (Zofran)	0.15 mg/kg q 4 h for three doses IV or 32 mg IV as a single dose
Dexamethasone	10–20 mg IV once
Lorazepam (Ativan)†	1.0–1.5 mg IV once; may repeat
Regimen 2	
Granisetron (Kytril)	10 µg/kg (or 1 mg) IV once
Dexamethasone	10–20 mg IV once
Lorazepam (Ativan)†	1.0–1.5 mg IV once; may repeat
Regimen 3	
Metoclopramide (Reglan)	3 mg/kg q 2–4 h for three doses IV
Dexamethasone	10–20 mg IV once
Lorazepam (Ativan)	1.5–2.0 mg IV once; may repeat
Diphenhydramine	25–50 mg q 4–6 h IV

*Antinausea medication should begin 30 min before the start of chemotherapy.
†Lorazepam inclusion is optional.
Abbreviation: IV = intravenously.

cigarettes, and drinking carbonated beverages. This can be a neurotic condition amenable to appropriate psychotherapy.

Belching occurs when atmospheric air in the stomach overwhelms the lower esophageal sphincter, resulting in forceful eructation. It rarely reflects serious disease, although it can occasionally be a reflection of reflux esophagitis. When the presence of pyrosis or endoscopic findings suggest reflux disease, antireflux measures (small, frequent meals, elevating the head of the bed at night, and avoiding fats and chocolate) and H₂ blockers may be helpful.

Abdominal gaseousness or fullness is usually an innocent condition but can result at times from a more serious gastrointestinal ailment. Acute onset of these symptoms raises the possibilities of gastric outlet obstruction, intestinal obstruction, food poisoning, gastroenteritis, and biliary colic. Longer duration of symptoms might result from intra-abdominal neoplasia or ascites.

A gassy feeling in the abdomen usually relates to maldigestion of food or heightened sensitivity to normal amounts of gastrointestinal gas (heightened visceral nociception). When excessive flatus or diarrhea is present, maldigestion is particularly suggested. Hydrogen, carbon dioxide, and methane are produced as by-products of bacterial fermentation of carbohydrates. Lactose intolerance is common in patients of African and Asian descent and symptoms occur after the patient eats milk, ice cream, or soft cheese. Elimination of these foods or the use of lactase prior to the consumption of dairy foods (e.g., chewing several caplets of LactAid) will reduce symptoms. Gas-producing vegetables (e.g., beans, broccoli, and cauliflower) can be eliminated from the diet or eaten with alpha-D-galactosidase (commonly known as Beano). Therapy directed at the irritable bowel syndrome with anticholinergics such as dicyclomine (Bentyl) and treatment of associated constipation, if present, with fiber supplements often ameliorate this condition. Finally, the use of charcoal or simethicone may reduce gaseousness.

The evaluation of patients with gaseousness should start with a history and physical examination. A food diary directed toward the association of various foods and symptoms may yield clues about lactose intolerance. Severe acute symptoms may suggest gastroenteritis, food poisoning, and intestinal obstruction. Weight loss and change in bowel habits may suggest neoplasia. The vast majority of patients with this symptom have a more innocent cause and can be managed with dietary manipulation and medication.

INDIGESTION

Indigestion or dyspepsia is classically burning epigastric pain frequently affected by food intake. Often this pain is caused by peptic ulcer disease (PUD); however, biliary tree disease (such as gallbladder colic), gastroesophageal reflux disease, the irritable

TABLE 1. Treatments for Peptic Ulcer Disease

Agent	Dosage
H₂ Blockers	
Cimetidine (Tagamet)	800 mg hs for 8 weeks
Ranitidine (Zantac)	300 mg hs for 8 weeks
Famotidine (Pepcid)	40 mg hs for 8 weeks
Nizatidine (Axid)	300 mg hs for 8 weeks
Sucralfate (Carafate)	1 gm before meals and bedtime 4 times daily
Omeprazole (Prilosec)	40 mg daily for 4–6 weeks

bowel syndrome, and other conditions may cause similar symptoms.

Patients with PUD or nonulcer dyspepsia often show improvement with antacid therapy. Duodenal ulcers are usually relieved with food intake, with pain recurring several hours after eating, such as in the early morning. The causes of PUD include *Helicobacter pylori*, the use of nonsteroidal anti-inflammatory drugs, and tobacco use. Patients with symptoms suggestive of PUD can often be treated empirically with H₂ blockers for 10 to 14 days. If symptoms persist, upper endoscopy should be performed to document ulcer disease and to detect the presence of *H. pylori*.

Nonulcer dyspepsia is of unclear etiology. Proposed causes include dietary factors, duodenitis, *H. pylori*, gastric acid hypersecretion, gastric motor dysfunction, heightened visceral nociception, and stress. Patients having symptoms suggestive of ulcer disease but with normal endoscopic findings may be treated in a variety of manners, all with variable and somewhat unproven success. Treatments include H₂ blockers (e.g. cimetidine [Tagamet] and ranitidine [Zantac]), promotility agents (e.g., metoclopramide [Reglan] and cisapride [Propulsid]), and possibly antibiotic therapy directed at *H. pylori*, although the efficacy of eradication therapy for *H. pylori* in nonulcer dyspepsia is still unproved.

Gastroesophageal reflux disease should be suspected when pyrosis, sour brash, and burning substernal pain (particularly while reclining or after meals) occur. It should be treated with elevating the head of the bed at night; smaller, more frequent meals; and avoidance of fats and chocolates. Medical therapy includes the use of antacids, H₂ blockers,

TABLE 2. Treatments for *Helicobacter pylori* Eradication

Tetracycline 500 mg qid for 14 days, metronidazole 250 mg qid for 14 days, bismuth subsalicylate (Pepto-Bismol) 2 tablets qid for 14 days

Amoxicillin 750 mg tid for 14 days, metronidazole 500 mg tid for 14 days, bismuth subsalicylate (Pepto-Bismol) 2 tablets qid for 14 days

Omeprazole (Prilosec) 20 mg bid for 14 days, amoxicillin 500 mg qid or 1 gm bid for 14 days

Omeprazole (Prilosec) 20 mg bid for 14 days, clarithromycin (Biaxin) 500 mg tid for 14 days omeprazole, and promotility agents (metoclopramide or cisapride).

Treatment of indigestion often starts with empiric therapy with an H_2 blocker. If 10 to 14 days of therapy does not lead to substantial improvement, endoscopy should be considered. If a peptic ulcer is seen, 6 to 8 weeks of therapy should be given (Table 1). If biopsy, serologic test, or breath test indicate *H. pylori* is present, antibiotic therapy should be initiated (Table 2). Treating *H. pylori* has been shown to substantially reduce recurrences of duodenal ulcers. Finding a gastric ulcer at endoscopy warrants a follow-up examination in 8 weeks to ensure healing and to exclude the possibility of the occasional malignant gastric ulcer.

HICCUPS

method of
JAMES H. LEWIS, M.D.
Georgetown University Medical Center
Washington, District of Columbia

The term "hiccup" refers to the onomatopoietic attempt to vocalize the sound produced by sudden contraction of the inspiratory muscles terminated by abrupt closure of the glottis. The term "hiccough" has been used as an alternative spelling of hiccup, but more likely represents the previously held (but mistaken) belief that hiccups occur as a result of a respiratory reflex. The medical term for hiccups, "singultus," may have been derived from the Latin root "singult," meaning a sob or the act of catching the breath in sobbing.

Most hiccups occur as brief, self-limited episodes lasting only a few seconds or minutes. Hiccups that last more than 48 hours or recur at frequent intervals are referred to as "persistent" and often imply an underlying physical or metabolic cause. Occasionally, hiccups are intractable, occurring continuously for months or years, and may result in significant morbidity and even death.

PATHOPHYSIOLOGY

Unlike reflexes such as coughing, sneezing, vomiting, and withdrawal from heat or pain, hiccups do not appear to serve any useful or protective function. However, because other mammals can hiccup, and because hiccups may occur during fetal and neonatal life, they may represent a vestigial remnant of a primitive reflex whose functional or behavioral significance is now lost. In 1833, a relationship between hiccups and the phrenic nerve producing diaphragmatic contractions was recognized when an Edinburgh physician recommended blistering the skin over the origin and course of the phrenic nerves as a means of treating the condition. It was not until 1943, however, that a central basis for hiccuping was described. In current theory, the afferent limb of the reflex is composed of the vagus and phrenic nerves and by the sympathetic chain arising from the sixth to the twelfth thoracic segments, with the "hiccup center" located in the spinal cord between the third and the fifth cervical segments. The efferent limb remains primarily the phrenic nerve, although nerves to the glottis and accessory muscles of respiration are also

thought to be involved, since there are reports of patients who continue to hiccup even after transection of both phrenic nerves.

CONDITIONS ASSOCIATED WITH HICCUPS

More than 100 causes have been described, separated into those that are considered benign and self-limited (Table 1) and those that are associated with underlying structural, metabolic, inflammatory, neoplastic, or infectious causes (Table 2).

Overdistention of the stomach is one of the most frequent causes of self-limited hiccups. The mechanism by which gastric distention causes hiccups appears to be stimulation (stretching?) of the gastric branches of the vagus nerve or possible direct irritation of the diaphragm by the overinflated stomach. The mechanism of alcohol-induced hiccups is unclear, but may relate to the ingestion of large quantities of alcoholic beverages causing gastric distention, or possibly to the effects of alcohol on the cerebral cortex that remove inhibitions normally serving to dampen the hiccup reflex. Predisposing factors for intraoperative hiccups include hyperextension of the neck resulting in stretching of the roots of the phrenic nerve, traction on the diaphragm or viscera during surgery, the use of short-acting barbiturates, inadequate ventilation, and gastric distention or ileus in the recovery period. In addition, too light a plane of anesthesia may suppress inhibitory influences that normally function to prevent hiccups. Similarly, as the neuromuscular blocking action of certain muscle relaxants starts to wear off, return of diaphragmatic activity may be associated with hiccups.

Postoperative hiccups accounted for 25% of their occurrence in men with an established organic basis for their hiccups in a Mayo Clinic series. The hiccups usually appeared within 4 days of surgery with more than half of the episodes following intra-abdominal operations; the remainder resulted from urinary tract, central nervous system, and chest operations.

HICCUP TREATMENTS

Historical Cures

The origins of many of the better known hiccup cures can be traced back hundreds and even thousands of years. Hippocrates wrote in the fourth century B.C. that "in the case of a person afflicted with hiccough, sneezing coming on removes the hiccough."

TABLE 1. **Conditions Associated with Self-Limited Hiccups**

Gastric distention
  Overeating, eating too fast
  Drinking carbonated beverages
  Aerophagia
  Air insufflation during gastroscopy
Sudden change in temperature
  Ingesting very hot or cold food or beverages
  Taking a cold shower
  Entering or leaving a hot or cold room
Alcohol ingestion
Excess smoking
Psychogenic
  Sudden excitement
  Emotional stress

TABLE 2. **Causes of Persistent and Intractable Hiccups**

Central Nervous System

Intracranial or brain stem neoplasms
Hydrocephalus
Multiple sclerosis
Syringomyelia
Ventricular-peritoneal shunt
Glaucoma
Parkinson's disease
Skull fracture
Vascular insufficiency
Arteriovenous malformation
Intracranial hemorrhage
Temporal arteritis

Toxic-Metabolic Causes

Uremia
Diabetes mellitus
Alcohol
Gout
Hyponatremia
Hypokalemia
Hypocalcemia
Hypocapnia (hyperventilation)
Fever
Insulin shock therapy

Diaphragmatic Irritation

Diaphragmatic tumors
Eventration
Myocardial infarction
Pericarditis
Hiatus hernia
Splenomegaly (various causes)
Hepatomegaly (various causes)
Subphrenic abscess
Esophageal cancer
Aberrant cardiac pacemaker electrode

Irritation of the Vagus Nerve

Meningeal Branches

Meningitis

Pharyngeal Branches

Pharyngitis
Laryngitis

Auricular Branches

Hair, insect, or foreign body irritating tympanic membrane

Recurrent Laryngeal Nerve

Goiter
Neck cysts, tumors, or lymphadenopathy

Thoracic Branches

Pneumonia
Pleuritis
Achalasia
Sarcoidosis
Esophageal obstruction
Esophagitis
Thoracic aortic aneurysm
Tuberculosis
Mediastinitis
Cor pulmonale
Herpes zoster
Lung cancer

Abdominal Branches

Gastric atony (distention)
Gastric cancer
Gastritis
Peptic ulcer
Pancreatic cancer
Pancreatitis
Pseudocyst
Intra-abdominal abscess
Bowel obstruction
Cholelithiasis
Cholecystitis
Abdominal aortic aneurysm
Inflammatory bowel disease
Hydronephrosis
Prostatic disorders
Parasitic infestation
Appendicitis
Hepatitis

Drugs

Alpha-methyldopa
Short-acting barbiturates
Dexamethasone
Methylprednisolone
Diazepam
Chlordiazepoxide

General Anesthesia

Inadequate ventilation
Suppression of normal inhibitory influences
Intubation (stimulation of glottis)
Traction of viscera
Hyperextension of the neck (stretching of phrenic nerve roots)
Gastric distention or ileus

Postoperative Causes

Manipulation of diaphragm or adjacent organs
Prostatic and urinary tract surgery
Craniotomy (various operations)
Thoracotomy (various operations)
Laparotomy (cholecystectomy, gastrectomy, colectomy, sympathectomy)

Infectious Causes

Meningitis
Encephalitis
Typhoid fever
Cholera
Candida esophagitis
Malaria
Herpes zoster
Acute rheumatic fever
Influenza
Tuberculosis

Psychogenic Causes

Hysterical neurosis (worry, anxiety, fear)
Conversion reaction
Sudden shock
Grief reaction
Malingering
Personality disorders
Anorexia nervosa
Enuresis

Miscellaneous Causes

Familial
Idiopathic

Plato is credited with being the first to recommend sudden thump on the back as means of "scaring away" hiccups. Eryxmachus the Physician is quoted as telling Aristophanes to hold his breath, gargle with water, and if need be, tickle his nose to induce a sneeze, after which "even the most violent hiccough is sure to go." Paulus Aegineta advocated emetics (assisted by sneezing) to empty the stomach if it was distended or contained "spoiled food." Herbal remedies were prescribed by a number of other medical authorities in the Middle Ages. Plugging the ears with the fingers (in combination with breath holding) was advocated in London by Lupton in 1627. Grandmothers going back several generations have recommended swallowing granulated sugar or eating peanut butter.

Physical and Mechanical Means of Treating Hiccups (Table 3)

Measures aimed at conunterstimulating the diaphragmatic contractions that occur during hiccuping have included pulling the knees up to the chest or leaning forward to compress the diaphragm. Continuous positive airway pressure or other means to hyperinflate the lungs is thought to act by stimulating the Hering-Breuer inflation reflex, which disrupts not only the normal respiratory rhythm but the abnormal hiccup pattern as well. Other acts to reduce hiccup frequency to below a critical threshold level include sneezing, performing a Valsalva maneuver, breath holding, hyperventilating, and involuntary gasping induced by the inhalation of smelling salts or the result of being surprised by sudden fright or pain. Inhaling 5% carbon dioxide or breathing into a paper bag have also been used, which may terminate hiccups via the effect of acute respiratory acidosis on diaphragmatic contractility.

Relief of gastric distention by emetics, gastric lavage, or nasogastric aspiration has been effective when the stomach is overdistended by food, liquid, or air or is obstructed by mechanical or functional disorders. Stimulation of the soft palate, uvula, and pharynx is often able to terminate a bout of hiccups. Forcible traction of the tongue (credited to William Osler), lifting the uvula with a spoon, and manipulating the pharynx with a cathether or cotton-tipped swab have all been used successfully. Intraoperative hiccups may be stopped with a rubber or plastic catheter inserted through a nostril to a depth of 3 or 4 inches using a to-and-fro motion. The success of this method suggests that irritation of the soft palate or the pharynx inhibits afferent impulses transmitted via the vagus nerve.

Stimulation of vagal afferents may also account for the success of swallowing dry granulated sugar, sipping ice water, or eating peanut butter. Although sugar has been given to countless numbers of persons with hiccups, as with most other "cures," few published reports on the method are available, and nearly all have been anecdotal and uncontrolled.

Alcohol-related hiccups have been treated success-

TABLE 3. Common Mechanical Methods Available for Treating Hiccups

Stimulation of Uvula or Nasopharynx
Forcible traction of the tongue
Lifting the uvula with a spoon
Catheter stimulation
Gargling with water
Sipping ice water
Sucking on hard candy
Swallowing dry granulated sugar
Swallowing hard bread or peanut butter
Drinking from the far side of a glass
Noxious taste (vinegar, angostura bitters)
Instillation of noxious irritants (ammonia, ether)

Interruption of Respiratory Rhythm
Valsalva maneuver
Gasping (noxious odors or sudden fright)
Sneezing
Continuous positive airway pressure
Breath holding
Compression of the thyroid cartilage

Respiratory Center Stimulants
Breathing 5% carbon dioxide
Hyperventilation
Breath holding
Rebreathing into a paper bag or dead space tubing

Counterirritation of the Diaphragm
Pulling the knees up to the chest
Leaning forward to compress the chest
Applying pressure at points of diaphragmatic insertion

Relief of Gastric Distention
Gastric lavage
Nasogastric aspiration
Emetic-induced vomiting

Disruption of the Phrenic Nerve
Bupivacaine or alcohol injection (nerve block)
Electrical stimulation
Phrenic crush
Transection

Counterirritation of the Vagus Nerve
Supraorbital pressure
Carotid sinus message
Removal of hair or foreign body irritating tympanic membrane
Digital rectal massage

Psychiatric
Hypnosis
Behavior modification

Miscellaneous
Cardioversion
Acupuncture
Prayer

fully with a lemon wedge soaked with angostura bitters. Of 16 patients in one series, 14 responded within 1 minute and remained hiccup-free for at least 2 hours. Drinking from the far side of a glass has been proposed as a means of terminating hiccups through "cerebral concentration," although it may act simply as a pharyngeal stimulant.

Miscellaneous Nondrug Hiccup Treatments

The successful use of hypnosis for hiccups has been reported by several authors for a variety of underlying conditions, including myocardial infarction, metastatic adenocarcinoma of the colon unresponsive to phrenic nerve block, and postoperative hiccups. In some patients, hypnosis can uncover psychological problems that may be the cause of hiccups. Acupuncture has been used in Asia to treat hiccups for generations and the technique has been reported to favorably influence the course of intractable hiccups in a number of patients in the West. Its major limitation as a hiccup cure appears to be the availability of physicians skilled in its application.

DRUG THERAPY FOR HICCUPS

A variety of pharmacologic agents have been used in the treatment of intractable hiccups when mechanical or physical measures fail. As is the case with most reports dealing with physical maneuvers to stop hiccups, the results of nearly all these reports have been anecdotal. Those that are considered the most likely to be successful are summarized here, with dosages provided in Table 4. None of these agents is U.S. Food and Drug Administration (FDA)–approved for this indication.

Major Tranquilizers

Chlorpromazine (Thorazine) is the agent that has been most widely utilized since the 1950s when re-

TABLE 4. **Pharmacotherapy of Hiccups***

Major tranquilizers
    Chlorpromazine 25–50 mg IV q 6 h; if successful, switch to
      PO at the same dose
    Haloperidol† 2–12 mg/day PO
Anticonvulsants
    Phenytoin† 200 mg IV bolus, then 100 mg PO qid
    Valproic acid† 15 mg/kg/day PO or rectally
    Carbamazepine† 200 mg PO qid
    Magnesium sulfate† 5 ml of a 25% solution IM
Central nervous system stimulants
    Methylphenidate† 6–20 mg IV bolus
    Amphetamine sulfate† 10–20 mg PO bid
    Ephedrine† 5 mg IV bolus
Anesthetic stimulant
    Ketamine† 0.4–0.5 mg/kg IV during anesthesia
Antispasticity agent
    Baclofen† 5–20 mg PO q 6–12 h
Calcium channel blocker
    Nifedipine† 10 mg PO bid (escalated to 20 mg tid)
Antidepressant
    Amitriptyline† 10 mg PO tid
Serotonin antagonist
    Ondansetron† 4–32 mg IV bolus or 8 mg PO tid
Dopamine antagonist
    Metoclopramide† 10 mg PO q 6 h or 5–10 mg IM or IV
      q 8 h
Dopamine agonist
    Amantadine† 100 mg PO daily
Parasympathomimetic
    Edrophonium† 5 mg IV
Parasympatholytics
    Atropine† 1 mg IV
    Quinidine† 10 grains PO or IM q 3–4 h
Antiarrhythmic
    Lidocaine† mg/kg IV loading dose followed by 2–4 mg
      per min continuous IV infusion

*Medications and doses listed are those with reported success.
†Not FDA-approved for this indication.

ports first cited cure rates in the range of 80% among patients with intractable hiccups of various causes. If intravenous therapy proves successful, then oral chlorpromazine (at the same dosage) can be maintained for a period of 7 to 10 days. *Haloperidol* (Haldol), a butyrophenone, has also been reported to be effective, perhaps relating to its dopamine antagonist effects.

Anticonvulsants

Phenytoin (Dilantin) is given as an initial intravenous bolus followed by oral therapy, although it is not consistently effective. *Valproic acid* (Depakene), given orally or rectally, has controlled hiccups for periods up to 1 year. It is postulated to act in the central nervous system (CNS) by enhancing the inhibitory effects of gamma-aminobutyric acid (GABA). Its use in children may be complicated by hepatic injury. *Carbamazepine (Tegretol)*, given orally, has successfully stopped hiccups due to multiple sclerosis, and hiccups associated with pulmonary tuberculosis have responded to *magnesium sulfate* given intramuscularly. The *benzodiazepines* have not been useful in treating hiccups. In fact, diazepam (Valium) has been reported to worsen hiccuping episodes, a finding consistent with the observation that hiccups may be induced when the drug is given as premedication for the induction of anesthesia or endoscopy. *Chlordiazepoxide (Librium)* has also been reported to cause hiccups.

Central Nervous System Stimulants

A number of CNS stimulants have been used with variable success in treating anesthesia-related hiccups, including *methylphenidate (Ritalin)* and *ephedrine*. *Amphetamine sulfate* has arrested postoperative hiccups, possibly because of its smooth muscle relaxant effect. *Ketamine* (Ketalar), an anesthetic stimulant, has been reported to terminate hiccups in both the anesthesia and the postoperative settings, in a dose that is only about 20% of the usual anesthetic dose. In animals, ketamine has caused seizures owing to its pronounced CNS stimulant effect. In humans, it is postulated that the drug blocks the hiccup center by increasing efferent impulses and decreasing afferent stimuli.

Sedative/Hypnotics

Among the various sedative-hypnotic agents, *pentobarbital* has been effective in patients who developed hiccups after transurethral prostatectomy. However, *phenobarbital* is regarded as being unreliable in controlling hiccups, perhaps because it has also been implicated as a cause of hiccups. As mentioned under "Anticonvulsants," the *benzodiazepines* have not been useful as a class in the control of hiccups.

Antispasticity Agents

Baclofen (Lioresal), a derivative of the inhibitory neurotransmitter GABA, was initially developed for reducing the frequency and severity of spasticity caused by multiple sclerosis and other disorders of the spinal cord. It has also been reported to cure hiccups unresponsive to most other agents, including hiccups due to renal failure in patients receiving chronic peritoneal dialysis or hemodialysis, and an interesting entity referred to as "familial hiccups." In addition to baclofen's anecdotal success, it has been shown to be useful in a randomized controlled clinical trial. Baclofen is rapidly absorbed after oral administration with a half-life of 3 to 4 hours and is excreted largely unchanged by the kidneys. Side effects include drowsiness, insomnia, dizziness, weakness, ataxia, and confusion. It is said to be poorly tolerated by elderly patients, and sudden withdrawal after long-term use may cause auditory and visual hallucinations, anxiety, and tachycardia. Respiratory depression, seizures, and coma have been reported following significant overdose. Abrupt withdrawal should be avoided and the drug should be administered cautiously in patients with impaired renal function. It is not recommended for use in patients with spasticity owing to stroke or other cerebral lesions.

Tricyclic Antidepressants

Amitriptyline (Elavil) is known to synchronize electroencephalogram (EEG) activity and to act on brain amines, although its exact mechanism of action in the treatment of hiccups remains unclear. Anecdotal success has been reported.

Calcium Channel Blocking Agents

Several patients have been treated successfully with *nifedipine (Procardia)*, although its efficacy is variable. As nifedipine does not readily enter the CNS, its actions are thought to be peripheral.

Dopamine Antagonists

Agents in this class act on the autonomic nervous system, and are regularly tried in patients with chronic hiccups. *Metoclopramide (Reglan)* has terminated hiccups of diverse causes, including gastric dilatation due to diabetic gastroparesis. Unpleasant neuropsychiatric side effects are common and represent a limiting factor to its use.

Parasympathomimetics/ Parasympatholytics

Edrophonium chloride (Tensilon) has been effective in terminating hiccups, possibly by disrupting cholinergic impulse transmission. *Atropine* is said to be beneficial in preventing hiccups during anesthesia. *Quinidine sulfate* has been helpful in patients with chronic hiccups, perhaps by prolonging the refractory period of striated muscle.

Serotonin Antagonists

Ondansetron (Zofran), a specific 5-hydroxytryptamine (5-HT)–3 antagonist, is currently used in the management of chemotherapy-induced emesis and postoperative nausea and vomiting. It has been used successfully to control hiccups in patients with metastatic gastric adenocarcinoma, whose symptoms also included uncontrolled vomiting. Although the mechanism by which ondansetron stops hiccups is unclear, it may relate to the drug's effects on blocking the serotonin neurotransmitter, 5-hydroxytryptamine (5-HT-1), at its receptors in the central and peripheral nervous systems.

Antiarrhythmics

Lidocaine (Xylocaine) is an antiarrhythmic that has been reported to reduce the risk of hiccups associated with induction of anesthesia with methohexital, and more recently was successful in alleviating hiccups associated with a pneumonitis. It should be used only while monitoring for lidocaine toxicity in a hospital setting.

SPECIFIC HICCUP CURES

Table 5 lists a number of causes of hiccups that have been successfully treated by physical maneuvers or drug therapy directed specifically at the underlying cause. Although most of these treatments seem self-evident, relatively few reports chronicle the success of a specific therapy directed against a specific cause of hiccups in the literature.

TABLE 5. **Specific Hiccup Therapies***

Hiccup Cause	Successful Physical Maneuver/ Drug Treatment
Addison's disease	Steroid replacement
Alcohol	Angostura bitters–soaked lemon wedge
Candida esophagitis	Antifungal treatment
Carcinomatosis with vomiting	Ondansetron
Cardiac arrhythmia (ventricular tachycardia)	Cardioversion
Coronary artery or valvular heart disease	Nifedipine
Esophageal obstruction or achalasia	Esophageal dilatation
Foreign body in ear canal	Removal
Herpetic esophagitis	Acyclovir (Zovirax)
Hyponatremia	Correct electrolyte imbalance
Intraoperative	Catheter stimulation of pharynx; ether instillation into nostrils
Parkinson's disease	Amantadine (Symmetrel)
Postoperative	Splanchnicectomy
Reflux esophagitis	Acid suppression or antireflux surgery
Renal failure requiring dialysis	Baclofen

*As reported in the literature. Specific agents may also be useful in treating other causes of hiccups.

GUIDELINES FOR TREATING TRANSIENT HICCUPS

Hiccup episodes that last only a few minutes may be annoying or sometimes socially embarrassing, but rarely require treatment other than simple physical maneuvers. Breath holding, breathing into a paper bag, pulling on the tongue, sneezing, swallowing a teaspoonful of granulated sugar or peanut butter, sucking on hard candy, drinking from the far side of the glass, holding one's nose and ears closed while swallowing, or sudden fright, alone or in combination, are usually effective. In cases in which hiccups last longer than 30 or 60 minutes, manual stimulation of the nasopharynx with a finger, rubber catheter, or cotton-tipped applicator, lifting the uvula with a spoon or other device, or inducing a gasp with smelling salts or other noxious substances can be tried if simpler measures are ineffective. Not recommended as home measures are instilling ammonia or ether into the nasopharynx, performing carotid sinus massage, applying supraorbital pressure or digital compression to the root of the neck over the course of the phrenic nerve, compressing the thyroid cartilage, or massaging the rectum digitally. Nasogastric aspiration and manipulation or removal of an aberrant hair, insect, or other foreign object in the auditory canal should also not be employed without proper instruction or supervision.

Occasionally, women in their second or third trimester of pregnancy will note rhythmic fetal movements that can be attributed to fetal hiccuping. These hiccups can routinely be seen on sonography, and in many instances, such episodes can be terminated when the mother leans forward or turns onto her side to change position. Interestingly, fetal hiccups are said to recur in subsequent pregnancies, often occur at the same time of the day, and may persist in the infant after birth.

GUIDELINES FOR TREATING PERSISTENT HICCUPS

A thorough search for an underlying cause is thought to reveal an organic etiology in over 90% of men with persistent hiccups. Women, however, are less likely to have an identifiable organic cause, according to older reports. No studies have examined what percentage of hiccups can be expected to resolve when the underlying disorder is corrected, although it is assumed that many, if not most, hiccups will stop when the specific cause is successfully treated (see Table 5). If hiccups persist despite specific therapy, physical manipulation such as pharyngeal stimulation or gastric aspiration can be tried. Hiccups that remain refractory to these measures often require the use of pharmacologic agents as listed in Table 4. I personally favor the use of one of the more recently described therapies such as baclofen, nifedipine, amitriptyline, or ondansetron as initial therapy. Should these agents fail, chlorpromazine or intravenous lidocaine can be tried.

For hiccups unresponsive to both physical maneuvers and drug therapy, such as those due to widespread intra-abdominal carcinoma or surgical adhesions, disruption of the phrenic nerve can be considered, especially in patients in whom persistent hiccups are the cause of significant discomfort or serious morbidity. It is recommended that a fluoroscopic examination of the diaphragm be performed to determine which leaflet is contracting, or to determine if one leaflet is dominant in cases of bilateral involvement. A temporary phrenic nerve block using a long-acting agent such as bupivacaine should be attempted before a more permanent phrenic crush or transection procedure is carried out. It should be remembered that phrenic nerve block and phrenic crush procedures have not been uniformly successful in terminating bilateral hiccups, even when both sides have been treated. Moreover, impaired pulmonary function or respiratory failure have occurred as a result of bilateral diaphragmatic paralysis, and such an approach seems justified only in extreme cases and with ventilatory support services available. It is reasonable to first exhaust all conservative treatment approaches, including hypnosis, psychotherapy, behavioral modification techniques, and even acupuncture if it is available, before proceeding with a bilateral phrenic nerve crush or transection.

ACUTE INFECTIOUS DIARRHEA
method of
MARTIN S. WOLFE, M.D.
Traveler's Medical Service of Washington and
George Washington University Medical School
Washington, District of Columbia

Acute infectious diarrhea is generally defined as the passage of three or more loose stools in a 24-hour period, and continuing for less than 14 to 21 days. Associated symptoms may include nausea, vomiting, abdominal cramps, or fever. The occurrence of fever with blood or mucus in the stool indicates a more severe dysenteric syndrome related to infection with a more invasive organism.

The causative agents of acute infectious diarrhea include bacteria, viruses, parasites, and certain fungi. Incubation periods may vary from 1 to 48 hours for viruses and bacteria to 7 or more days for certain parasites. A very common bacterial agent, particularly in travelers, is enterotoxigenic *Escherichia coli,* which causes a relatively mild syndrome that is self-limited within a few days. Potentially colonic tissue-invasive bacteria include *Shigella, Campylobacter,* and *Salmonella,* which can cause a more severe debilitating and often prolonged infection if left untreated. Less common bacterial causes in travelers include *Aeromonas* spp, *Plesiomonas shigelloides,* and *Vibrio parahaemolyticus* and other *Vibrio* spp. *Clostridium difficile* must be considered when there has been a recent use of an antimicrobial agent. Food-borne bacterial infections, including such cosmopolitan organisms as *Clostridium* sp, *Staphylococcus aureus,* and *Bacillus cereus,* are more often the cause of common source diarrhea outbreaks. Most viral infections are caused by rotavirus in infants and Norwalk agent in older children and adults. The most common parasitic protozoal agents are *Cryptosporidium, Giardia lamblia,* and *Entamoeba histolytica,* with usual incubation periods of 7 to 10 days or more. Overgrowth of *Candida* spp secondary to antibiotic use can be an essential factor in the development of both acute and chronic diarrhea not due to other causes.

DIAGNOSIS

Initial evaluation should be with an immediate microscopic examination for fecal leukocytes. When many leukocytes are present, this indicates colonic inflammation and a high likelihood of the presence of an invasive bacteria (*Shigella, Campylobacter, Salmonella*). With prior antibiotic use, *C. difficile* could also be possible. Acute amebiasis may cause blood in the stool but is usually not accompanied by leukocytes. *G. lamblia* and *Cryptosporidium* are only rarely associated with blood or mucus in the stool. Enterotoxigenic *E. coli* and other less common bacteria and viruses are noninvasive pathogens of the small bowel and do not lead to leukocytes or red blood cells in the stool. Cultural identification of a particular bacterial species should be made with standard techniques and with other specialized media for *Campylobacter* and *Vibrio* spp. When indicated, stool can be tested for the presence of *C. difficile* cytotoxin. Only specialized laboratories can identify enterotoxigenic *E. coli,* and diagnosis is usually made from clinical features and exclusion of other organisms. An antigen test is available for rotavirus, but not for Norwalk agent. Standard procedures for ova and parasite detection should be performed on a series of preserved stool specimens. The most common fungal agents, *Candida* spp, can be suspected on a stool smear and confirmed by stool fungus culture.

TREATMENT

Symptomatic Treatment

An otherwise healthy individual with acute diarrhea is not likely to develop dehydration and can replace lost fluids and electrolytes with any beverage plus a source of sodium chloride (such as salted crackers). Young children, elderly people, and those individuals with certain underlying medical problems requiring diuretics, who have severe diarrhea, are more threatened by dehydration. With mild-to-moderate diarrhea, hydration can be accomplished with flavored mineral water containing glucose and a salt solution. Packets of World Health Organization formula oral rehydration salts may be used with more severe diarrhea. During the acute diarrheal episode, the diet should be modified. Milk and other dairy products should be avoided and a bland diet emphasizing such foods as bananas, clear soups, juice, gelatin, and boiled vegetables should be consumed. As stools become formed, the diet can gradually return to normal as tolerated.

Antimotility agents such as loperamide (Imodium) or diphenoxylate (Lomotil), or bismuth subsalicylate (Pepto-Bismol) can improve the symptoms of moderately severe diarrhea (Table 1). Loperamide, unlike diphenoxylate, does not contain atropine and is better tolerated by older men with prostatic hypertrophy in whom atropine could cause acute urinary retention, as well as other unpleasant anticholinergic side effects. Loperamide liquid and caplets are available as over-the-counter products. These products and diphenoxylate should not be administered to children younger than 2 years of age. If symptoms persist over 48 hours or if fever or blood or mucus in the stool develops, these medications should be discontinued. Bismuth subsalicylate liquid taken as 1 ounce every half hour for 8 doses works somewhat slower but is also effective in moderately severe diarrhea. It may produce darkening of the stools and tongue, but this is harmless. Other agents such as kaolin-pectin and aciduric bacteria such as *Lactobacillus* have been found ineffective in clinical trials.

Antimicrobial Treatment

In patients with fever and dysenteric stools, while awaiting culture results, empirical antimicrobial treatment can be directed against the most likely bacterial causes, *Shigella, Campylobacter,* or *Salmonella.* With appropriate treatment, symptoms are usually improved within the time required for culture confirmation. The only antimicrobials effective

TABLE 1. **Symptomatic Therapy for Acute Diarrhea**

Drug	Adult Dosage	Pediatric Dosage
Loperamide (Imodium) Prescription (Imodium) 2-mg capsule OTC (Imodium A-D) 2-mg caplet Liquid—5 mL contains 1 mg	4 mg, then 2 mg after each loose stool; not to exceed 16 mg/day (prescription) or 8 mg/day (OTC)	Use Imodium A-D (OTC) 24–47 lb: 1 tsp initially, then 1 tsp after each loose stool; not to exceed 3 tsp/day 48–59 lb: 2 tsp or 1 caplet initially, then 1 tsp or ½ caplet after each loose stool; not to exceed 4 tsp or 2 caplets/day 60–95 lb: Same as 48–59 kg, but not to exceed 6 tsp or 3 caplets/day
Bismuth subsalicylate (Pepto-Bismol)	30 ml every 30 min for 8 doses	3–8 yr: 5 mL 6–9 yr: 10 mL 9–12 yr: 15 mL Dose to be taken every 30 min for 8 doses

Abbreviation: OTC = over the counter.

against all three of these invasive organisms are the quinolones (Table 2). I prefer ciprofloxacin 500 to 750 mg twice daily for 3 to 5 days. Quinolones are contraindicated in children, who could alternatively receive trimethoprim/sulfamethoxazole (TMP–SMX) (Bactrim, Septra) plus erythromycin, since the former drug alone does not treat *Campylobacter*. There is some recent evidence of developing resistance of *Campylobacter* to quinolones. In travelers' diarrhea, the most common agent is noninvasive enterotoxigenic *E. coli,* which causes a self-limited illness after a few days and usually can be managed with symptomatic treatment alone. However, moderate and distressing symptoms can be more quickly and dramatically improved with a 3-day course of TMP–SMX or a quinolone, together with loperamide. *Aeromonas* spp and *Plesiomonas shigelloides* will generally respond to TMP–SMX or a quinolone. *Vibrio parahaemolyticus* is self-limited and most patients do not require antimicrobial therapy. Supportive therapy is adequate for food poisoning, which usually lasts less than 24 hours.

Acute diarrhea following antibiotic use could be due to *C. difficile* or a *Candida* sp. With a positive *C. difficile* cytotoxin test, treatment should initially be with metronidazole 250 mg four times daily for 10 to 14 days. Persistent or very severe infections would require oral vancomycin 125 mg four times daily for 10 to 14 days. In the absence of other causative agents, or with considerable yeast found on a wet stool smear or stool fungus culture, treatment for *Candida* may be given with oral mycostatin (Nystatin) 500,000 units three times daily for 7 days.

For acute invasive amebic dysentery, initial treatment is with metronidazole (Flagyl) 750 mg three times daily for 10 days. This should always be followed with a course of a poorly absorbed luminal drug, either paromomycin (Humatin) 500 mg three times a day for 7 days or iodoquinol (Yodoxin) 650 mg three times a day for 20 days. For moderate nondysenteric amebiasis, 500 mg of metronidazole three times daily for 10 days, followed by a luminal drug, should be adequate. For very mild amebiasis, a luminal drug alone is sufficient. Acute giardiasis can be treated with metronidazole 250 mg three times daily for 7 days. Quinacrine (Atabrine)* in a 5-day course of 100 mg three times daily is an even more effective treatment for giardiasis, albeit with potentially more troublesome side effects. However, this drug is currently unavailable. Furazolidone (Furoxone) is a less effective treatment, but it is available as a liquid preparation, which is better

---

*Not available in the United States.

TABLE 2. **Therapeutic Drugs for Acute Diarrhea**

Drug	Indication	Adult Dosage	Pediatric Dosage
Trimethoprim/ sulfamethoxazole (TMP–SMX) (Bactrim, Septra)	*Shigella,* invasive *Salmonella,* toxigenic *Escherichia coli, Aeromonas,* and *Plesiomonas*	160 mg TMP/800 mg SMX bid for 3–5 days	TMP 10 mg/kg/day/SMX 50 mg/kg/day in 2 divided doses for 3–5 days
Ciprofloxacin (Cipro)	*Campylobacter* (plus above bacteria)	500 or 750 mg for 3–5 days	Contraindicated in children
Erythromycin	Drug of choice for *Campylobacter* in children and alternative for adults	250 mg qid for 5 days	40 mg/kg/day in 4 divided doses for 5 days
Metronidazole (Flagyl)	Giardiasis	250 mg tid for 7 days	15 mg/kg/day in 3 divided doses for 7 days
	Clostridium difficile	250 mg qid for 10–14 days	20 mg/kg/day in 4 divided doses for 10–14 days
	Amebiasis—moderate to severe	500–750 mg tid for 10 days	30–45 mg/kg/day in 3 divided doses for 10 days
Paromomycin (Humatin)	Amebiasis—follow-up to metronidazole; alone for mild amebiasis	500 mg tid for 7 days	25–30 mg/kg/day in 3 divided doses for 7 days
Iodoquinol (Yodoxin)	Same as for paromomycin	650 mg tid for 20 days	30–40 mg/kg/day in 3 divided doses for 20 days
Furazolidone (Furoxone)	Giardiasis—liquid form for young children	100 mg qid for 7 days	6 mg/kg/day in 4 divided doses for 7 days
Quinacrine (Atabrine)	Giardiasis	100 mg tid for 5 days	6 mg/kg/day in 3 divided doses for 5 days
Nystatin (Mycostatin)	Intestinal candidiasis	500,000 units tid for 7 days	500,000 units tid for 7 days

tolerated by young children. Cryptosporidiosis in a nonimmunosuppressed individual is self-limited within 3 or 4 weeks and symptomatic treatment alone is generally sufficient, as there is currently no reliable curative treatment.

PREVENTION

Appropriate food and water hygiene are the best preventive measures against infection with the agents causing acute diarrhea. Antimicrobial drug prophylaxis is generally not recommended for travelers because of resistance and potential side effects. In particular situations where antimicrobial drug prophylaxis is indicated, quinolones are considered most effective and safe. Bismuth subsalicylate, taken as 2 tablets chewed four times a day, has given about 65% protection against diarrhea. This should not be used for more than 3 weeks, or by persons who either cannot take salicylates or are already taking salicylates for other purposes.

CONSTIPATION

method of
ARNOLD WALD, M.D.
University of Pittsburgh Medical Center
Pittsburgh, Pennsylvania

CLINICAL CONSIDERATIONS

Constipation is a symptom rather than a disease and therefore represents a subjective interpretation of a real or an imaginary disturbance of bowel function. Although it has been defined, on the basis of large population surveys in Western countries, as a frequency of defecation of twice-weekly or less, frequency alone is not a sufficient criterion. Many constipated patients complain of excessive straining or discomfort at defecation, with or without small or hard stools, although frequency of defecation is within the normal range. For clinical purposes, the physician must use a combination of subjective and objective criteria in assessing such complaints. These criteria include a frequency of defecation less than three times weekly alone, or in conjunction with other subjective complaints, especially if there has also been a distinct change in regular bowel habits. Understanding what the patient's perceptions are and attempting to correct misconceptions are critical aspects of the initial evaluation.

PATHOPHYSIOLOGY

Constipation may be conceptually regarded as disordered movement through the colon and/or anorectum, since, with few exceptions, transit through the proximal gastrointestinal tract is normal. Slowing of colonic transit occurs as a primary motor disorder, in association with many diseases, or as a side effect of many drugs. Diseases associated with constipation include neurologic, metabolic, and endocrine disorders and obstructing lesions of the gastrointestinal tract. Other abnormalities such as congenital aganglionosis (Hirschsprung's disease) and acquired functional outlet disorder (pelvic floor dyssynergia), lead to

impairment of defecation. Finally, colonic transit is normal in many patients who complain of constipation, and various factors influence colorectal function or an individual's perception that constipation exists. These factors include dietary fiber and fluid intake, physical activity, level of education, psychological makeup, and emotional factors. These should be considered when a patient is initially evaluated for chronic constipation or a recent alteration in bowel habits.

INITIAL EVALUATION

The initial evaluation incorporates a careful history with particular attention to identifying potential risk factors. This includes defining the nature and duration of the complaint and determining whether such complaints arise from patient misconceptions concerning normal bowel habits. A recent and persistent change in bowel habits, if not associated with a readily definable cause of constipation (e.g., medications), should prompt an evaluation to exclude structural bowel changes or organic diseases. This is especially important in older adults who complain of excessive straining or a sense of incomplete evacuation or who also exhibit anemia or occult gastrointestinal bleeding. Only after such diseases have been excluded should a diagnosis of functional constipation be considered.

Flexible sigmoidoscopy and colonoscopy are superior techniques to identify lesions that narrow or occlude the bowel. They will also detect melanosis coli, a brown-black discoloration of the bowel mucosa associated with chronic use of anthraquinone laxatives.

Barium radiographs complement sigmoidoscopy in detecting organic causes and are also useful to diagnose megacolon and megarectum. Barium radiographs will show the aganglionic distal bowel with proximal dilatation of the colon in classical Hirschsprung's disease and should be obtained in children or young adults if this disorder is suspected. In such patients, bowel cleansing should not be ordered so that the characteristic changes will be accentuated, and the insertion catheter should be removed to identify a short aganglionic segment. However, barium enema provides limited information about colonic transit and motor function in most patients with chronic constipation. Plain films of the abdomen can detect significant stool retention in the colon, can suggest the diagnosis of megacolon, and can be used to monitor bowel cleansing in patients with fecal retention.

Rectal biopsies are useful in patients with suspected Hirschsprung's disease. Suction biopsies should be obtained from the nondilated rectum at least 3 centimeters above the internal anal sphincter for appropriate testing.

INITIAL MANAGEMENT

The initial management of functional chronic constipation includes patient education, behavior modification, dietary changes, and judicious use of laxatives or enemas.

Patient education may include reassurance and an explanation of normal bowel habits. Efforts are made to reduce excessive use of laxatives and cathartics, to increase fluid and fiber intake, to encourage moderate exercise, and to utilize postprandial increases in colonic motility by instructing patients to defecate after meals, particularly in the morning when colonic motor activity is highest. Use of dietary fiber and bulk laxatives such as psyllium or methylcellulose together with adequate fluids is the safest and most physiologic approach in most patients with constipation. In general, the use of stimulant laxatives should be restricted to those patients who do not respond to initial measures.

Dietary fiber is that portion of plant food that escapes digestion and is composed of both insoluble and soluble components. Cereal fibers generally possess cell walls that resist digestion and retain water within their cellular structures, whereas fiber found in citrus fruits and legumes stimulates the growth of colonic flora, which increases fecal mass. Wheat bran is one of the most effective fiber laxatives, and there is a clear dose response to fiber with respect to fecal output. Particle size appears to be crucially important and the large particle size of cereal products appears to enhance fecal-bulking effects.

Patients with poor dietary habits may add raw bran (2 to 6 tablespoons with each meal) followed by a glass of water or another beverage. A significant laxative effect may not be observed for 3 to 5 days, and up to several weeks may be required to relieve chronic constipation. Raw vegetables and fruits contain soluble fiber and often are not adequate substitutes for raw bran. Patients should be warned that consuming large amounts of bran can cause abdominal bloating or flatulence. This can be modulated by starting with small amounts and slowly increasing to tolerance and efficacy.

Psyllium (Metamucil), calcium polycarbophil (FiberCon), and methylcellulose (Citrucel) are more refined and concentrated than bran, but they also are considerably more expensive. These agents should be well diluted to ensure adequate mixing with food and are generally consumed before meals or at bedtime. They increase the water content and bulk volume of the stool to decrease colonic transit time. There is some evidence that mechanical stimulation of nerves in the bowel wall also contributes to the action of dietary fiber and bulk-forming agents.

Sorbitol and lactulose (Chronulac, Cephulac) are often useful in patients with chronic constipation who do not tolerate or respond to dietary fiber or bulk-forming agents. These poorly absorbed sugars are hydrolyzed, in part, to lactic, acetic, and formic acids by coliform bacteria. Accumulation of fluid in the colon is stimulated by the osmotic effect of these acid metabolites, which usually produces soft, formed stools. In one well-controlled study in elderly patients with chronic constipation, sorbitol 70% administered at bedtime was as effective as lactulose and was well tolerated. Thus, sorbitol can be used as a low-cost alternative to lactulose. Patients should also be advised that these agents can cause abdominal bloating and flatulence.

Docusates (Colace, Surfak) soften the feces by reducing surface tension, thus permitting penetration of the fecal mass by intestinal fluids. However, the efficacy of docusates is highly questionable and they are of marginal use for chronic constipation.

Mineral oil softens stool owing to its emollient action and is particularly effective in enemas to soften fecal impactions. However, aspiration with lipoid pneumonia is a recognized hazard of oral mineral oil, especially in the elderly and in those patients with impaired swallowing, and anal seepage may also occur. It is an unattractive agent in view of the availability of effective bulk and osmotic laxatives.

When patients fail to respond to initial measures, stimulant laxatives may be considered for relatively short periods of time (weeks to months). These agents include cascara, senna (Senokot), bisacodyl (Dulcolax), phenolphthalein (Ex-Lax), and castor oil. Although the precise mechanism(s) of action for each drug is not established, all produce a net accumulation of fluid and electrolytes in the lumen.

Because stimulant laxatives are often abused, some clinicians recommend that they be taken for no longer than 1 week, but this seems unduly restrictive. The continuous use of stimulant laxatives may produce diarrhea that is severe enough to cause hyponatremia, hypokalemia, dehydration, hyperaldosteronism, protein-losing gastroenteropathy, and steatorrhea. Subtle mucosal and myenteric nerve alterations have been seen with long-term use of stimulant laxatives, as have changes in the radiologic appearance of the colon, known as the "cathartic colon."

The anthraquinone-containing laxatives (e.g., senna, cascara sagrada) are widely used and abused. Their onset of activity is within 6 to 12 hours. Cascara has the mildest action and produces a soft or formed stool with little or no colic. Senna may be particularly helpful in patients with severe constipation and is apparently safe even in large doses. When combined with psyllium or other bulk-forming agents, smaller amounts of senna may be employed. Aloe-containing preparations are the most potent of the anthraquinone-containing laxatives and are best avoided because they almost always produce colic. Although most anthraquinone-containing laxatives discolor the colonic mucosa (melanosis coli), this effect is presumed to be innocuous and is reversible.

Bisacodyl (Dulcolax) and phenolphthalein (Ex-Lax, Feen-A-Mint) both stimulate peristalsis and alter active electrolyte transport to affect fluid movement. Bisacodyl produces a soft-to-formed stool, usually with little or no colic, whereas phenolphthalein is more likely to produce a semifluid stool. Because of its enterohepatic circulation, the duration of action of phenolphthalein may be prolonged (3 to 4 days) in sensitive patients.

Patients who do not respond to oral laxatives can self-administer tap-water enemas every 3 to 4 days. The addition of other substances to an enema solution is of uncertain therapeutic value. However, the small-volume prepackaged sodium phosphate–biphosphate enema kits (Fleet's) are convenient and safe to administer.

Isotonic sodium chloride enema (1 level teaspoonful per pint of water) should be used cautiously in patients with sodium and fluid retention. Some enema solutions irritate the mucosa and can simulate early changes of ulcerative proctosigmoiditis. Hot water, peroxide, household detergents, and strong hypertonic salt solutions are most irritating and should not be used.

Weakness, shock, convulsions, and/or coma may result from water intoxication and dilutional hyponatremia in children and the elderly, and in patients with megacolon who are given a tap-water enema. Severe hypokalemia may also follow the use of a tap-water enema, especially in patients also receiving diuretics. Convulsions with hypocalcemia and hyperphosphatemia have occurred in children or adults with renal dysfunction who absorbed large amounts of the phosphate present in sodium phosphate–biphosphate enemas.

THERAPY FOR SEVERE CONSTIPATION

Ideally, therapy for patients with severe chronic constipation should be based on the nature of the complaint and presumed pathophysiologic mechanisms. More rational choices and consistent therapeutic outcomes will require further understanding of both the psychological and the physiologic characteristics of this diverse group of patients.

Behavioral Approaches

Habit training has been successfully employed in children with severe constipation. The goal of such an approach is to achieve regular evacuation to prevent build-up of stool. A modified program may also be effective in many adults with neurogenic constipation, patients with dementia, and those with physical impairments.

Initially, patients should be disimpacted and the colon evacuated effectively. This can be accomplished with twice-daily enemas for up to 3 days. An alternative approach is to drink 4 to 8 liters (occasionally more) of a balanced electrolyte solution containing polyethylene glycol (Colyte, GoLYTELY) until cleansing is complete.

After bowel cleansing, sorbitol or lactulose is given to produce one stool per day or every other day. The patient is instructed to use the bathroom after eating breakfast to take advantage of meal-stimulated increases in colonic motility (the gastrocolonic response). An enema is administered if there is no defecation after 2 days, to prevent recurrence of fecal impaction. Once defecation occurs regularly for several months, gradual weaning of laxatives may be attempted. Positive reinforcement is given for successful toileting, and punishment for failure is prohibited. Office visits should be maintained regularly.

Such behavioral approaches have achieved success rates of up to 78% in children with idiopathic constipation, although relapses are not uncommon. Treatment failures have been attributed to patient and family behavioral disturbances and noncompliance, but underlying disturbances of bowel function may also play a role in some children.

A modified program may be used in demented or bedridden patients of all ages with fecal impaction. Initially, mineral oil enemas (Fleet Mineral Oil) may be used to soften hard impactions and permit rectal evacuation. After disimpaction, bowel cleansing with enemas or polyethylene glycol–containing solutions should be performed. In demented patients or those with neurogenic bowel disorders, a fiber-restricted diet together with cleansing enemas once or twice per week will assist nursing management by decreasing build-up of stool and recurrence of fecal impaction.

Another behavioral approach is biofeedback to correct inappropriate contraction of the pelvic floor muscles and external anal sphincter during defecation in patients with pelvic floor dyssynergia. Various techniques, including anal plugs and anorectal manometers that monitor external anal sphinter pressures during attempted expulsion of the apparatus, have been used to record defecation dynamics. The patient watches the recordings of electromyographic activity or sphincter pressure responses and is asked to modify inappropriate responses through trial-and-error efforts. Clinical improvement has been reported in both children and adults who have received biofeedback for pelvic floor dyssynergia.

Pharmacologic Approaches

The use of drugs to promote colonic transit by increasing colonic motor activity has generally proved disappointing. Cholinergic agents such as bethanechol (Urecholine) and neostigmine have been tried with little success and may be associated with side effects. Prokinetic agents such as metoclopramide (Reglan) and cisapride (Propulsid) appear to be ineffective in most severely constipated patients. Some patients with severe constipation have been treated successfully with misoprostol (Cytotec), a prostaglandin used to prevent peptic ulcers associated with the use of nonsteroidal anti-inflammatory drugs. Further studies are needed to assess the possible efficacy of this agent in severely constipated individuals.

Surgical Approaches

Severe Slow Transit Constipation. Although somewhat controversial, subtotal colectomy with ileorectal anastomosis can dramatically ameliorate incapacitating constipation in carefully selected patients. If surgery is undertaken, at least three criteria should be met: (1) the patient has chronic, severe, and disabling symptoms from constipation that are unresponsive to medical therapy; (2) the patient has slow colonic transit of the inertia pattern; (3) the patient does *not* have intestinal pseudo-obstruction. as demonstrated by radiologic or manometric studies. Potential complications of surgery include persistent abdominal pain and bloating, diarrhea, small intestine obstruction, and postoperative infections. Recent studies have documented that greater than 90% of carefully studied patients have satisfactory long-term results.

Rectoceles and Rectal Intussusceptions. These conditions are common in older, nonconstipated women, and caution must be used when attributing defecatory difficulties to these entities. Indeed, surgical repairs frequently do not alleviate symptoms of difficult defecation. Optimally, the patient should demonstrate improved rectal evacuation when pressure is placed on the posterior wall of the vagina during defecation before a rectocele repair should be entertained.

Hirschsprung's Disease. Surgery is the treatment of choice for Hirschsprung's disease and varies according to the length of the aganglionic segment. In patients with short-segment or ultra-short-segment disease, anal myotomy, in which the internal sphincter and a varying length of rectal smooth muscle are incised, is often effective. With larger segments, bypassing or removing the aganglionic bowel is necessary to overcome the obstructing effect of the denervated segment. The choice of surgical technique depends on the surgeon but excellent results have been reported for all of them.

ACKNOWLEDGMENT

The author thanks Ms. Helen Gibson for the expert preparation of this manuscript.

FEVER

method of
RAFAEL GORODISCHER, M.D.
Ben-Gurion University of the Negev
Beer-Sheva, Israel

and

SUMNER J. YAFFE, M.D.
National Institute of Child Health and Human
Development
Bethesda, Maryland

Fever is often the focus of concern when treating a patient and is one of the main reasons that infants and children are brought for medical attention. It is frequently a manifestation of an infectious illness but may be due to other causes (e.g., malignancies, inflammatory conditions) (Table 1). In fever, the hypothalamic set point regulating body temperature is raised, and as a result, thermoregulatory effectors are activated and mechanisms of heat pro-

TABLE 1. Conditions Associated with Fever

Infections
Malignancies
Inflammatory conditions
Conditions due to immune mechanisms
Tissue infarction and thrombosis
Vascular inflammation
Trauma
Metabolic diseases
Miscellaneous

TABLE 2. Conditions Associated with Heat Illness

Malignant hyperthermia
Anhydrotic ectodermal dysplasia
Heat stroke
Hyperthyroidism
Drug (e.g., aspirin, atropine) overdose
Use of street drugs
Miscellaneous

duction (increased muscle tone, chills) and heat conservation (vasoconstriction) predominate over mechanisms of heat loss until the temperature of the blood bathing the hypothalamus reaches the new setting. The rise of the set point seems to be mediated by locally released prostaglandins through the action of interleukin-1 originating in polymorphonuclear leukocytes and other phagocytic cells. Exogenous pyrogens (viruses, bacteria, fungi, polynucleotides) act on those cells and promote the production and release of interleukin-1.

Generally, the accepted normal limits of rectal temperature (which measures core temperature closely) are between 36.1° and 37.8° C (97° and 100° F). Body temperature is higher in the evening than in the early morning and increases during physical exercise. It also is higher in infants than in older children and adults; it decreases in childhood and stabilizes during puberty. Rectal temperature is about 0.6° C (1° F) higher than oral temperature and about 0.8° to 1.4° C (2° to 2.5° F) higher than axillary temperature.

Both from a pathophysiologic perspective and as an approach to treatment, fever must be distinguished from heat illness (Table 2). In fever, body temperature rarely exceeds 41.1° C (106° F) and does not pose a serious risk to the patient; in contrast, in heat illness (a rare condition), body temperature may reach higher values, and the illness must be treated promptly and vigorously, as it is life-threatening. Whereas external cooling is the mode of lowering body temperature in heat illness, lowering the set point is the principal aim in the symptomatic treatment of fever.

Certain febrile patients require special attention during the initial evaluation: infants less than 2 months of age who look ill or who have a focus of infection, leukocytosis, leukocyturia, or stool leukocytes; children less than 2 years of age with temperature above 39° C (102° F) and leukocytosis; and patients with asplenia or sickle cell disease. These patients may have serious bacterial infections, and early consideration should be given to initiating antibiotic therapy.

Despite conflicting theoretical opinions about whether fever plays a significant defensive role in infection, a clinically beneficial effect of fever has not been demonstrated in infectious illnesses (except perhaps in syphilis). It has been shown that the use of antipyretics does not alter children's rate of recovery from viral illnesses. Thus, the treatment of fever should be individualized, with the focus on the patient rather than on the thermometer. The patient's comfort is the main purpose of the symptomatic treatment of fever, although the fear of febrile seizures, which affect 2 to 4% of children aged 6 months to 6 years, and the feeling of "doing something" are other reasons to use antipyretics. Febrile children who are given antipyretics may show improvement in alertness and activity, but there is no evidence that fever-control measures decrease the risk of febrile seizures. Acetaminophen given at the time of diphtheria-pertussis-tetanus immunization (one dose every 4 hours for a total of three doses) may reduce the frequency and severity of local and systemic reactions, and use of this agent should be considered in children with a family history of convulsive disorders. Because fever increases oxygen demands, antipyretic therapy may benefit patients with cardiac or pulmonary insufficiency. Febrile patients may also have a component of heat illness (due to overclothing and dehydration), and attention should be paid to proper fluid balance and external cooling.

DRUG THERAPY OF FEVER

The medications most commonly used today in the management of fever include acetaminophen and ibuprofen (Table 3). Aspirin, which was widely used in the past, has lost popularity owing to its presumptive role in the pathogenesis of Reye's syndrome in children with viral infections (in particular influenza and varicella). These drugs reduce fever by lowering the hypothalamic set point (presumably through inhibition of prostaglandin synthesis) and activating heat loss mechanisms (vasodilatation, sweating).

Acetaminophen, a *p*-aminophenol derivative and an active metabolite of phenacetin, is also known in Europe as paracetamol. Physicians have been familiar with the use of acetaminophen for half a century; it is generally well tolerated and has become a common household antipyretic and analgesic. It has antipyretic and analgesic (but not anti-inflammatory) properties. Its elimination is decreased in young infants; thus, lower doses should be given and caution exercised in such patients. When acetominophen is used in combination with external cooling, the drug's antipyretic effect is somewhat more pronounced. (Because cold water causes discomfort and shivering, only tepid water should be used for external cooling; sponging with alcohol is not recommended, as it may be absorbed.)

Ibuprofen is a nonsteroidal anti-inflammatory propionic acid derivative that has gained increasing popularity for the treatment of fever. The antipyretic effects of ibuprofen 10 mg per kg and of acetaminophen 15 mg per kg given to children every 6 hours are similar, and both drugs are equally well tolerated. Given in single doses, ibuprofen may have a longer duration of effect.

When the decision is made to use an antipyretic medication, acetaminophen is generally preferred because of its familiarity and relative safety; it is also cheaper than ibuprofen. However, when an anti-inflammatory effect is also a goal of therapy, ibuprofen or another nonsteroidal anti-inflammatory drug should be used. Acetaminophen should not be given to patients with liver disease or to chronic alcohol abusers. Massive acetaminophen overdose can cause fatal hepatic necrosis. Although ibuprofen and other nonsteroidal anti-inflammatory drugs cause less gastritis, gastrointestinal bleeding, and impaired platelet function than aspirin, they should be used with caution in patients with peptic disease. Elderly patients and those with asthma, bleeding disorders, and cardiovascular disease should be carefully monitored when receiving repeated doses of ibuprofen. Adults who often take acetaminophen or nonsteroidal anti-inflammatory drugs are at increased risk for the development of end-stage renal disease.

COUGH

method of
RAYMOND G. HADDAD, M.D., and
WISSAM CHATILA, M.D.
Bridgeport Hospital
Bridgeport, Connecticut

Cough is a normal protective mechanism and a component of lung defenses; it allows the expulsion of normally produced secretions or inhaled substances from the tracheobronchial tree. As such, cough is not considered a manifestation of disease or a pathologic process. On the other hand, cough can also be a prominent symptom in respiratory and nonrespiratory disorders. Its prevalence among nonsmokers ranges between 5 and 23% and it is the fifth most common symptom for which patients seek medical evaluation.

Cough can be voluntary or involuntary; it is stimulated by mechanical, chemical, or physical agents that act on various components of the cough reflex. These include: (1) thoracic and extrathoracic cough receptors (C fibers, rapidly adapting receptors, slowly adapting receptors), (2) afferent nerves (trigeminal, glossopharyngeal, superior laryngeal, and vagus nerves), (3) cough center located in the medulla, (4) efferent nerves (vagus, phrenic, recurrent laryngeal, and spinal motor nerves), (5) effector organs (respiratory muscles, larynx). Stimulation of the cough reflex results in a deep inspiration with subsequent glottic closure, accompanied by a significant increase in pleural and airway pressures, followed by opening of the glottis to release the pressure. This process generates high flow rates and shearing forces that aid to clear the airways from irritants and retained secretions. Various inflammatory mediators, with or without epithelial damage, can increase the sensitivity of the cough reflex by acting on the afferent limb.

DIAGNOSIS

A thorough history and physical examination will provide clues that will guide the approach to the patient with cough (Table 1; see text). The mode of onset, character, timing, and duration of the cough as well as associated

TABLE 3. **Usual Doses of Antipyretic Agents**

Drug	Child Single Dose	Child Maximum Daily Dose	Adult Single Dose	Adult Maximum Daily Dose
Acetaminophen	10–15 mg/kg every 4–6 h	65 mg/kg	0.5–1 gm every 4–6 h	4 gm
Aspirin	10–15 mg/kg every 4–6 h	65 mg/kg	0.5–1 gm every 4–6 h	4 gm
Ibuprofen	5–10 mg/kg every 6–8 h	—	0.4 gm every 4–6 h	—

TABLE 1. **Evaluation of Chronic Cough**

History and physical examination
Chest radiograph
Spirometry with or without bronchoprovocation
Upper gastrointestinal series/endoscopy/24-h esophageal
  pH monitoring
Imaging of facial sinuses
Others: Fiberoptic bronchoscopy, computed tomography,
  echocardiography

respiratory or systemic symptoms should be noted. Additional data need to include a history of cigarette smoking and allergies, exposures in the work place or with avocations, and use of medications, especially angiotensin-converting enzyme (ACE) inhibitors or beta blockers. Table 2 lists some common causes of cough and their associated clinical clues and symptoms.

A rational therapy for cough requires a diagnosis of the underlying cause and determination whether it is a component of an acute or a chronic process. A duration of less than 3 weeks is often chosen as the definition of an acute cough. Because cough related to a viral respiratory infection can last up to 8 weeks, it may be warranted to withhold a full diagnostic work-up until the end of that period if the history is not suggestive of other causes and the physical examination is unrevealing. Similarly, testing can be delayed in patients on ACE inhibitors until the response to discontinuation of the drug has been assessed. Cigarette smoking and chronic bronchitis are a common cause of chronic cough; however, it is unusual for affected individuals to complain or be aware enough of the cough to seek medical attention, since they may consider it a

TABLE 2. **Causes Associated with Various Signs and Symptoms**

Clues	Causes
Acute cough*	Upper and lower respiratory tract infections (laryngitis, pneumonia, tracheobronchitis), irritants (environmental, occupational)†
Nocturnal cough	Asthma, gastrointestinal reflux, early congestive heart failure, rhinosinusitis, bronchitis
Sputum production	Smoking, chronic bronchitis, respiratory infections
Putrid sputum	Lung abscess, bronchiectasis
Bronchorrhea	Pulmonary edema, alveolar cell cancer
Hemoptysis	Lung cancer, tuberculosis, bronchiectasis, bronchitis
Wheezing	Airway obstruction: asthma, chronic obstructive pulmonary disease, foreign body, endobronchial tumor
Crackles	Congestive heart failure, interstitial lung disease, pneumonia
Stridor	Vocal cord dysfunction, laryngeal tumor
Dry cough	Drug-related, sarcoidosis, pulmonary fibrosis, tumor, mechanical pressure (aortic aneurysm), interstitial lung disease, psychogenic
Fever	Infections (bacterial, mycobacterial, viral, fungal)
Weight loss	Malignancies (lung, mediastinal tumor, metastatic), tuberculosis

*Less than 3 weeks.
†Cause chronic cough with prolonged exposure.

normal occurrence. Therefore, when such patients ask for medical evaluation, they should undergo a thorough work-up to exclude other conditions. Several investigators have shown that postnasal drip syndrome (PND), asthma, gastroesophageal reflux disease (GERD), and chronic bronchitis acting individually or in concert are the most common causes of chronic cough. Hence the history, physical examination, and ancillary testing, if needed, should be directed at these causes, bearing in mind that a positive test does not always predict a favorable response to therapy. Some authors demonstrated up to a 95% response by following a sequential anatomic approach in all patients with chronic cough (Figure 1).

Asthma can present as a nonseasonal paroxysmal nonproductive cough with no history of dyspnea or wheezing and normal prebronchodilator and postbronchodilator spirometry. Bronchoprovocation challenge with methacholine or histamine has been found to be the most useful test to exclude cough-variant asthma. The cause of the cough will be non–asthma related in almost all patients whose bronchoprovocation test is negative; nevertheless, a positive test is not always indicative of cough resolution on asthma therapy (i.e., bronchoprovocation test is highly sensitive but moderately specific). In nonsmokers, PND is the most common cause of an *unexplained* chronic cough even in the absence of nasal/sinus congestion or throat clearing. It is related to various rhinosinus disorders such as sinusitis and allergic or nonallergic rhinitis. An allergy evaluation and computed tomography (CT) scan of the sinuses will help identify the underlying cause; however, there is no objective test for PND, hence cough resolution with an antihistamine (H_1 antagonist) and a decongestant is considered to be diagnostic. Similarly, cough may be the only manifestation of some patients with GERD. Gastroesophageal reflux–associated cough is thought to be vagally mediated through an esophageal-tracheobronchial reflex that starts with a distal esophagus hypersensitive to various stimuli. Barium study or upper endoscopy may be required when symptoms persist after appropriate therapy and when the 24-hour distal esophageal pH monitoring is nondiagnostic.

A chest radiograph (CXR) should be obtained on all patients with chronic cough in whom history and physical examination do not provide a readily plausible cause, especially if a therapeutic trial for the suspected etiology is initiated without benefit. The CXR can be considered as an extension of the physical examination and will assist to establish a differential diagnosis and direct further testing. When the evaluation for chronic cough fails to establish a diagnosis and the patient has no response to various therapies, then one may consider bronchoscopy, CT scan of the chest, or noninvasive cardiac studies. In general, bronchoscopy has a low diagnostic yield in the assessment of a chronic cough but it is a valuable tool in the presence of an abnormal CXR or a suspected endobronchial lesion.

SPECIFIC THERAPY

Specific therapy is aimed at the cause rather than at the symptom itself. Figure 1 highlights the major therapeutic strategies for the most common disorders associated with chronic cough. Every effort should be made to define the cause since specific treatment directed at the underlying pathophysiology is frequently successful. Cough related to asthma usually improves after several days of combined therapy with an inhaled beta agonist (albuterol [Proventil, Ven-

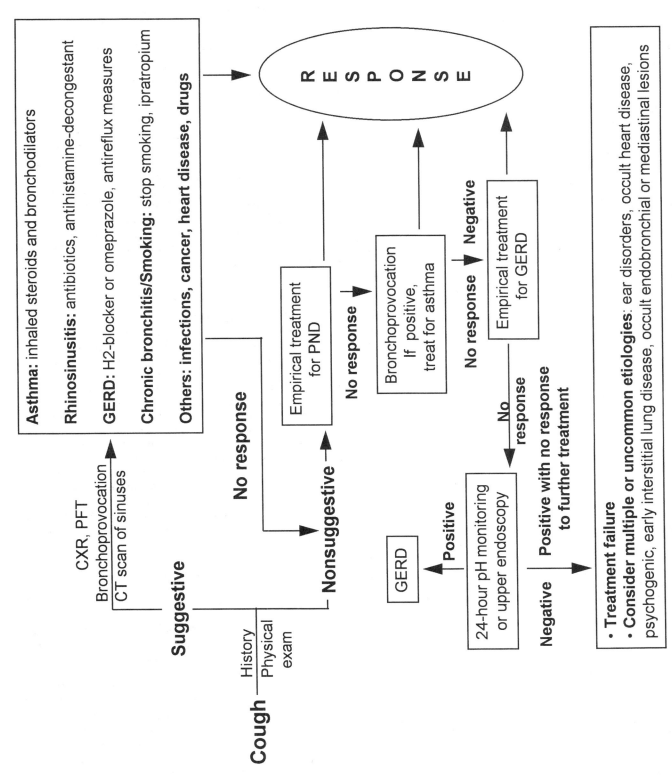

Figure 1. Algorithm for the investigation and treatment of cough based on a stepped anatomical approach. *Abbreviations:* CXR = chest x-ray; PFT = pulmonary function test; CT = computed tomography; GERD = gastroesophageal reflux disease; PND = postnasal drip.

tolin], metaproterenol [Alupent]) and an inhaled corticosteroid such as beclomethasone dipropionate (Beclovent, Vanceril) or triamcinolone acetonide (Azmacort). If cough persists, one should consider another cause.

Allergic and nonallergic rhinitis with PND often respond to a combination of intranasal corticosteroid (beclomethasone [Beconase], triamcinolone [Nasacort], budesonide [Rhinocort]) and an antihistamine-decongestant such as Trinalin (pseudoephedrine 120 mg, azatadine 1 mg), Actifed (pseudoephedrine 60 mg, triprolidine 2.5 mg), or Claritin-D (pseudoephedrine 120 mg, loratidine 5 mg) in conjunction with avoidance of precipitating factors. Sedating H_1 antagonists appear to be more effective than the newer generation antihistamines in controlling the nonallergic rhinitis because the former have a greater anticholinergic activity. When chronic sinusitis is present, the addition of oral antibiotics for 3 to 6 weeks is required. Trimethoprim-sulfamethoxazole or a second-generation cephalosporin (cefuroxime [Ceftin], cefaclor [Ceclor]) usually covers the common pathogens such as *Streptococcus pneumoniae, Moraxella catarrhalis,* and *Haemophilus influenzae.* Prior to discontinuation of the antibiotic, another clinical assessment may be prudent in patients with severe and chronic sinusitis, because of the high relapse rates. Unlike PND and asthma, the response to therapy of cough due to GERD may be delayed as long as 3 months. Since H_2 antagonists or blockers with head-of-bed elevation and dietary measures may fail, other medications will be needed if the diagnosis is strongly suspected. These include proton pump inhibitors (omeprazole [Prilosec]) or prokinetic agents (cisapride [Propulsid]).

The treatment of chronic bronchitis is smoking cessation, which may result in cough resolution and improved pulmonary function. Nicotine patches and gums have high failure rates for smoking cessation when prescribed without any attempts at behavioral modification. If patients remain symptomatic and have chronic obstructive pulmonary disease (COPD), then ipratropium bromide (Atrovent) up to three puffs (18 μg/actuation) four times per day with or without beta agonists often helps alleviate the symptoms and improve pulmonary function. The addition of inhaled corticosteroids may also prove to be beneficial, especially for patients with airway hyper-responsiveness, and their general use is currently being investigated in large international studies. Episodes of acute bronchitis may require appropriate antibiotic therapy.

NONSPECIFIC THERAPY

Nonspecific therapy (Table 3) is considered when cough causes significant morbidity, when the etiology is undetermined and specific therapy is noncurative, e.g., unresectable lung cancer, or when cough interferes with sleep. Symptomatic nonspecific cough products can be classified as antitussive or protussive agents and may include in addition H_1 antagonists,

sympathomimetic decongestants, and demulcents. While antitussive therapy attempts to eliminate the cough, protussive drugs (expectorants and mucolytics) tend to enhance the effectiveness of the antitussive agent and to improve mucus clearance. Most of these drugs are found in combination in over-the-counter products. Occasionally, these combination products should be avoided because some patients do not require the various ingredients in a given mixture. Even though the cough associated with the common cold is self-limited, the majority of patients tend to self-medicate themselves with one of the many available over-the-counter cough and cold remedies. So far there is no convincing evidence that antihistamines and expectorants provide more relief than a placebo. Under those circumstances, demulcents (e.g., cough drops, tea with honey, menthol) and simple humidification should be tried first. If those measures are not adequate to relieve the cough and nasal congestion, then an oral decongestant such as pseudoephedrine (Sudafed) may be useful.

Antitussive Therapy

Few of the nonspecific antitussive drugs have been evaluated critically or have been shown to be effective in all clinical settings. For instance, H_1 antagonists are beneficial in the management of allergic disorders but their use in viral upper respiratory tract infections (URI) remains controversial. The benefits of the first-generation antihistamines for viral infections are thought to be related to their anticholinergic effect by drying secretions. Likewise, in some studies codeine has been shown to suppress cough in chronic bronchitis but was no more effective than placebo for viral URI. Antitussive drugs are classified based on their site of action on the cough reflex. Table 3 lists some of these products, their recommended dosages, and proposed site of action. Many of these agents may also alter mucociliary function.

Protussive Therapy

The accumulation of mucus leads to airway obstruction, which in turn may exacerbate lung infection and symptoms. Antitussive measures alone are contraindicated when cough is associated with mucus production because these agents will hinder airways clearing. Expectorants increase the volume of the sputum and mucolytics liquefy the mucus, hence facilitating its clearance. Protussive therapy should be reserved for patients with chest congestion who have difficulty expectorating their copious and viscid secretions. Except for dornase alfa (recombinant human deoxyribonuclease; DNase [Pulmozyme]), the efficacy of protussive therapy has not been well demonstrated. Dornase alfa has been shown to improve pulmonary function over a period of 6 months and to maintain its effects up to 18 months in patients with cystic fibrosis. Aerosolized amiloride and hypertonic saline have been shown to improve mucus clearance

TABLE 3. **Nonspecific Therapy for Cough**

Classification	Drug	Dosage	Remarks/Precautions
Protussive			
Expectorant	Guaifenesin (Robitussin)	200–400 mg q 4 h PO	?Effective only at its maximal recommended dosage
Mucolytic	Acetylcysteine (Mucomyst))	2–3 ml 10% solution NEB	Restricted for in-hospital use
	Dornase alfa (Pulmozyme)	2.5 mg q 24 h NEB	Currently being studied for chronic bronchitis
Antitussive			
Afferent limb	Benzonatate (Tessalon Perles)	100 mg q 4–8 h PO	May cause local anesthesia and impair swallowing if chewed
	Lidocaine (Xylocaine)	3 ml of 1–2% solution NEB	Restricted for procedures
Cough center	NARCOTIC		
	Codeine	10–20 mg q 4–6 h PO	Adverse effects are uncommon with the recommended doses
	Hydrocodone (Hycodan)	5–10 mg q 4–6 h PO	Higher potency, less constipation, greater addiction potential than codeine
	NON-NARCOTIC		
	Dextromethorphan	10–30 mg q 4–8 h PO	Contraindicated in patients on MAOI; no narcotic effects
	Diphenhydramine (Benadryl)	25 mg q 4–6 h PO	The only H_1 antagonist recommended as an antitussive
	Caramiphen (Tuss-Ornade)	10–20 mg q 4–6 h PO	Found only in combination preparations; weak anticholinergic effect
Efferent limb	Ipratropium (Atrovent)	2–3 puffs q 6 h MDI	Most effective for COPD and ? GERD
Sympathomimetic Decongestant	Pseudoephedrine	60 mg q 4–6 h PO	No hypertensive response at 15–30-mg doses
	Phenylpropanolamine	25 mg q 4 h PO	Associated with a hypertensive response
	Oxymetazoline	2–3 nasal sprays q 12 h	Will cause rebound nasal congestion if used for >4 days
	Phenylephrine	2–3 nasal sprays q 3–4 h	
H_1 *Antagonist*			
First-generation	Chlorpheniramine (Chlor-Trimeton)	4 mg q 4–6 h PO	MAOIs may prolong and intensify their anticholinergic effects and may cause hypotension and extrapyramidal reactions with the phenothiazine antihistamines
	Clemastine (Tavist)	1 mg q 12 h PO	
	Brompheniramine (Dimetane)	4 mg q 4–6 h PO	
	Promethazine (Phenergan)	12.5–25 mg q 6–24 h PO	
Second-generation	Astemizole (Hismanal)	10 mg q 24 h PO	Possible serious arrhythmias when given with azole antifungals or macrolide antibiotics or to patients with liver disease
	Terfenadine (Seldane)	60 mg q 12 h PO	
	Loratadine (Claritin)	10 mg q 24 h PO	No changes in QTc on ECG; drug-drug interaction not yet completely excluded

Abbreviations: PO = orally; NEB = nebulizer; MAOI = monoamine oxidase inhibitor; MDI = metered dose inhaler; COPD = chronic obstructive pulmonary disease; GERD = gastroesophageal reflux disease; ECG = electrocardiogram; QTc = corrected QT interval.

in patients with cystic fibrosis and chronic bronchitis, respectively, but without improving lung function. Iodinated glycerol, another mucolytic agent, has been recently withdrawn from the U.S. market. Guaifenesin is the only agent approved by the Food and Drug Administration for use as an over-the-counter expectorant. Even though the effectiveness of guaifenesin has not been established, several studies have demonstrated increased sputum volume at its maximal recommended dosage (2400 mg/day).

SUMMARY

Acute cough related to a viral URI is usually self-limited and responds to demulcents and decongestants if necessary. When the cough is disruptive or nagging, the addition of a non-narcotic antitussive such as dextromethorphan may be helpful. The key to therapy of a chronic cough is to establish its cause so that specific treatment can be implemented according to the algorithm in Figure 1. A common pitfall in the management of chronic cough is the assumption that it is always related to a single cause. Finally, before labeling a patient a treatment failure and resorting to nonspecific therapy, one needs to ensure that the patient was not undertreated with a suboptimal regimen for the illness.

HOARSENESS AND LARYNGITIS

method of
HENRY T. HOFFMAN, M.D., and
MICHAEL P. KARNELL, Ph.D.
The University of Iowa Hospitals and Clinics
Iowa City, Iowa

Hoarseness as a medical complaint may appear trivial when considered in the context of many of the life-threatening diseases physicians commonly encounter. Although the vast majority of processes causing hoarseness are benign, the rough voice associated with laryngeal cancer, the breathy voice associated with laryngeal paralysis from a thyroid cancer, and the weak voice of a patient with Parkinson's disease are early tip-offs to diseases that warrant serious attention.

Even in the absence of associated systemic disease, hoarseness as an isolated problem interferes with the lives of many otherwise healthy patients. Harshness in a singer's voice resulting from vocal nodules may mark the end of a career. The negative impact of voice abnormalities on the careers of other professionals who depend on their voices, such as clergy, teachers, salespersons, physicians, and lawyers, is acknowledged, but not yet fully quantified. The difficulties President Clinton experienced with his voice during the 1992 campaign clearly demonstrate how a relatively minor disease process may interfere with the work of a voice professional.

The largest study to date addressing the impact of voice disorders consists of an evaluation of 113 patients seen for chronic voice problems at weekly voice clinics held at the Universities of Iowa and Utah. Questionnaires were administered to identify lifestyle effects of voicing abnormalities. Voice disorders in this group were primarily due to vocal nodules, laryngeal polyps, laryngitis, vocal cord paralysis, spasmodic dysphonia, and laryngeal trauma. Among these 113 patients, 52% related that their voice problem had negatively affected their past career options and 75% felt that their condition limited future career choices. Over 70% felt that social interactions were negatively affected by their voice problem, with 55% avoiding social situations when possible. Over half of the patients related that they experienced difficulty in being understood over the phone.

Whereas the social impact of chronic voice disorders has just recently become apparent, the overall importance of infections of the upper aerodigestive system (including laryngitis) has been known for many years. A yearly loss of more than 250 million days of work with over 100 million physician office visits has been estimated to result from upper respiratory tract infections in the United States.

The *glottis* is the segment of the larynx composed of the vocal folds, extending from the ventricles to 1 cm below the free surface of the vocal cords. The glottis functions as a *valve* that opens and closes in an oscillating fashion to convert the direct current of air traveling up the trachea from the lungs into an alternating current that generates the *voice*. The position, length, and tension of the vocal cords depend on contraction of the laryngeal muscles, which set the vocal folds into a position leading to passive opening and closing of the valve (vocal fold vibration) as the tracheal air column passes through. The configuration of the glottic valve and the nature of the substance of the vocal cords determine the character of the voice, including pitch and loudness. Voice should be differentiated from *speech,* which is the end result of modulation of voice (the laryngeal output) by supraglottic, oropharyngeal, and oral cavity structures including the palate, tongue, teeth, and lips.

Hoarseness or *dysphonia* describes abnormal voice production that reflects impaired vocal cord or lung function. *Aphonia* represents complete loss of voice. An abnormal voice termed "hoarse" or "dysphonic" is more specifically characterized as breathy, weak, rough, or strained. A *breathy voice* may result from *glottic incompetence* with incomplete closure of the valve if one of the vocal cords is paralyzed. A *weak (asthenic) voice* may occur as a combination of inadequate pulmonary support and general muscle wasting such as is commonly seen in debilitated, elderly patients. A *rough voice* commonly results from mass lesions of the vocal cord(s) such as the thickenings and irregularities associated with chronic smoking and excessive use of the voice. A *strained voice* may reflect abnormal motor control of the larynx resulting in excessively tight closure of the glottis. Several causes of vocal strain exist, with the most common, termed *"muscle tension dysphonia,"* thought to be functional in nature.

The vocal cords are complex structures composed of several interacting layers that permit wavelike motion of the mucosa and overlying mucosal blanket during voice production. The term *"vocal fold"* is used by some (in a pedantic fashion) to emphasize the complicated nature of what is more commonly referred to as *"vocal cord."*

Inflammation of the larynx is termed *"laryngitis"* and can be associated with pain, hoarseness, dysphagia, odynophagia, and airway obstruction. Laryngitis with associated hoarseness can be acute or chronic. Factors responsible for laryngitis are infectious (viral, bacterial, fungal), toxic (smoke, gastroesophageal reflux, caustic ingestion), traumatic, and allergic.

The following discussion is organized according to presenting signs and symptoms as would be evaluated by a physician without the capacity to visualize the vocal cords. An emphasis is placed on those processes that require urgent referral as well as those that can be treated without imaging the larynx. Most cases of chronic hoarseness warrant referral to an otolaryngologist on a nonemergency basis. The discussion of these processes is therefore truncated.

SIGNS AND SYMPTOMS
Acute Hoarseness: Traumatic

Traumatic laryngitis may be the most common cause of hoarseness, and is caused by closing the glottis with excessive muscular force. It affects large segments of the population attending sporting events and other activities associated with loud or prolonged cheering or singing. For the great majority of these people, resuming normal voice use for several days after the event permits resolution of vocal cord edema without sequela. However, repetition of such injury to the larynx may result in changes that become permanent (see "Chronic Hoarseness: Traumatic/Environmental"). Vocal cord hemorrhage may occur acutely with the development of a hematoma that does not resolve but matures to become a polyp. The larynx altered by inflammation from an active upper respiratory tract infection or esophageal reflux is more susceptible to injury from vocal abuse. Desiccation of the vocal cords from low humidity or dehydration, as well as irritation of the vocal cords from tobacco smoke, increases the likelihood of permanent injury following excessive voice use. Many medications may affect the larynx in a negative fashion primarily by systemic dehydration (as with diuretics) or diminishing surface moisture (antihistamines) (Table 1). Although continued use of some agents known to negatively affect the voice may be required to maintain health, many of these medications can be either eliminated or substituted with agents without such drying effects.

Medications including ingested emollients, inhaled steroids, and mists containing anesthetics or vasoconstrictors are popular among some voice professionals but are generally not recommended owing to the potential for irritating the larynx. Systemic mucolytics and wetting agents such as iodinated glycerol and guaifenesin may be of some benefit in thinning secretions. The placebo effect of these medications may be difficult to separate from true pharmacologic benefit. Because of their few side effects, it is reasonable to offer these medications to patients with complaints of thick secretions or frequent throat clearing in association with hoarseness. Attention to possible sinonasal disease or gastroesophageal reflux is warranted in patients complaining of secretions in their throat.

Treatment of hoarseness developing after an episode of vocal abuse consists of a period of voice rest as well as attention to adequate hydration and humidification, with consideration for referral should the hoarseness persist for more than 1 or 2 weeks. Complete voice rest entails communication by nonverbal methods, usually employing a writing pad and a bell or buzzer to gain the listener's attention. Radical voice rest to this extent is of questionable value and is a true hardship for the patient. Although complete voice rest is commonly used in the care of professional vocalists and postoperatively after surgical manipulation of the vocal cords, "relative voice rest" may be a more reasonable goal for most patients during an episode of acute hoarseness. The "arm's length rule" is easily communicated by instructing the patient to speak in an easy, soft manner only to those within arm's reach. Adequate hydration is ensured by avoidance of diuretics (including caffeine) and attention to drinking sufficient fluids "to make the urine the color of water." Humidification of the environment is best accomplished by use of a bedside vaporizer, which should be cleaned between uses to prevent aerosolizing proliferating bacteria.

External trauma to the larynx is rare owing to the protected location of the larynx between the mandible and the sternum, which limits exposure unless the neck is extended. Even a minor degree of hoarseness associated with external neck injury may herald rapid progression to airway obstruction and therefore warrants immediate referral for inspection of the larynx with mirror examination or fiberoptics. Palpation of the neck may reveal crepitus, indicating mucosal disruption that allows tracking of air into the soft tissue of the neck. Maintenance of the airway is the primary concern, with further evaluation needed via computed tomography (CT) imaging of the larynx and rigid endoscopy performed with the patient under general anesthesia. Surgical intervention by way of a tracheotomy may also be required to deal with laryngeal cartilage fracture or dislocation, hematoma, or soft tissue laceration.

Acute Hoarseness: Infectious

Infectious laryngitis is a common cause of hoarseness and is usually viral. Hoarseness arising in this setting is often associated with other symptoms that may overshadow those due to vocal cord inflammation. Several days of fever, pharyngitis, rhinitis, bronchitis, and cervical adenitis are frequently associated with hoarseness. The diagnosis of laryngitis in this setting does not require visualization of the larynx unless additional symptoms such as stridor or significant dysphagia develop.

Treatment consists of adequate hydration, humidification, vocal conservation, and symptomatic treatment of associated symptoms with, e.g., an antitussive

TABLE 1. **Medications in Common Use Affecting the Voice (Attenuated List)**

Adverse Effect	Medications
Desiccation of vocal cords	Antihistamines; diuretics; tricyclic antidepressants; others (many)
Alteration of cord substance	Birth control pills; androgens
Inflammation of cord surface	Propellants in inhalants
Development of *Candida* laryngitis	Steroid inhalants
Induction of intracordal hemorrhage	Aspirin; anticoagulants
Useful Agents	
Mucolytics	Iodinated glycerol; guaifenesin
Antitussives	Dextromethorphan; codeine
Replacement therapy	Estrogen (menopause); thyroxine (hypothyroid states)

Data from Sataloff RT, Lawrence VL, Hawkshaw MJ, Rosen DC: Medications and their effects on the voice. Reprinted with permission from Benninger MS, Jacobson BH, Johnson AF (eds): Arts Medicine—The Care and Prevention of Professional Voice Disorders, pp 216–225, 1994, copyright Thieme Medical Publishers, Inc.

for cough or nasal decongestants for rhinitis. Suppression of a cough with codeine or dextromethorphan may protect the vocal cords from repeated trauma that could lead to edema and hemorrhage.

While the vocal cords are inflamed, trauma resulting from excessive use may lead to permanent laryngeal injury (e.g., polyps or nodules). Systemic steroids (e.g., methylprednisolone [Medrol Dosepak] or burst and taper of prednisone) have been used by the voice professional to avoid cancelling a speaking or singing engagement or to diminish inflammation during an episode of laryngitis; this is controversial and should be dealt with on an individual basis. The patient with a single chance—a "once-in-a-lifetime" opportunity—to perform a significant engagement may justifiably receive this type of medical intervention. As a general rule, however, voice conservation is a better approach to take in the case of acute laryngitis regardless of whether this requires cancelling a performance. The services of speech pathologists with an interest in the vocal arts are invaluable in situations such as these. They may be helpful in suggesting technical modifications to diminish laryngeal injury with voice use as well as modifications of the speaking or singing environment (e.g., use of a microphone, avoidance of difficult songs, and lip syncing when performing with a group).

Viral laryngitis may result from infection by one of more than 200 viruses known to be responsible for upper respiratory tract infections. The supportive management of these clinically indistinguishable illnesses is the same, with the exception of influenza A infection, which can be treated with amantadine (Symmetrel) or, in high-risk individuals, prevented with vaccination.

Like viral laryngitis, *bacterial laryngitis* rarely presents in isolation and usually is associated with rhinosinusitis and/or laryngotracheal bronchitis. Purulent rhinorrhea or cough is considered sufficient evidence of a bacterial infection to treat with antibiotics supplemented by the same supportive care given for viral laryngitis. Erythromycin combined with sulfonamide, amoxicillin with clavulanic acid (Augmentin), cefuroxime (Ceftin), or clarithromycin (Biaxin) are antibiotic choices currently recommended for bacterial laryngitis.

Fungal laryngitis is still rare but becoming increasingly more common owing to its association with acquired immune deficiency syndrome as well as other forms of immune suppression. It usually represents infection with *Candida*. Although isolated laryngeal involvement in otherwise healthy newborns has been reported, involvement of the larynx generally represents a small part of a more generalized mucocutaneous candidiasis. Symptoms of hoarseness in an immunocompromised patient should raise concern about this diagnosis and warrant referral. Inspection of the larynx reveals a thick white covering to an erythematous and edematous larynx. Parenteral antifungal agents may be required for treatment, with either intubation or tracheotomy and maintenance of the airway. Endoscopic removal of the fungus under general anesthesia may permit maintenance of an adequate airway without the need for prolonged intubation or tracheotomy.

North American blastomycosis is a rare cause of fungal laryngitis that is managed with antifungal agents with attention to maintenance of an adequate airway. Concern about this process exists in a disproportionate scale to its incidence because of its similarity in appearance both grossly and microscopically to squamous cell carcinoma.

Acute Hoarseness: Toxic Exposure

Inhalation of toxic gases such as anhydrous ammonia and *ingestion of toxic solids or liquids* such as hydrochloric acid may injure the vocal cords and the adjacent upper aerodigestive tract. Depending on the type of exposure, hoarseness may be the significant presenting symptom or may be a minor consideration in the face of a life-threatening pulmonary or esophageal injury. Urgent referral should be made for visualization of the larynx, with the work-up extended according to signs and symptoms of pulmonary or esophageal injury. Pending imaging of the larynx, supportive treatment should be offered, including humidification (by face mask acutely), voice rest, and attention to signs of progressive airway compromise.

Acute Hoarseness with Aspiration: Neurogenic

Unilateral vocal cord paralysis in the adult is frequently associated with hoarseness or vocal fatigue, is occasionally asymptomatic, and is only rarely a cause of airway obstruction. Patients may complain of shortness of breath, which results from excessive air escape during speech owing to incomplete closure of the glottis. Extra effort is required to generate sufficient airflow to produce voice. Symptoms due to unilateral vocal cord paralysis may present as an acute process or more gradually. Urgent but not emergent referral is suggested if aspiration is not significant. More timely intervention through either immediate referral or maintenance of nothing-by-mouth status may be required in selected cases to diminish the risk of life-threatening aspiration pneumonia.

Reflex closure of the glottis is an important part of the swallowing reflex that is impaired in the paralyzed larynx. Aspiration of liquids is a common symptom but is frequently offered as a minor complaint such as "when I drink water rapidly, it goes down the wrong pipe and I cough." Modification of swallowing technique is generally adequate treatment. More severe forms of aspiration may occur if the paralyzed vocal cord is positioned so as to leave the glottis widely open during the swallow. Additional neurologic deficits either generalized or more focal, such as an ipsilateral superior laryngeal nerve paralysis, can result in life-threatening aspiration. Institution of nasogastric feedings generally permits a studied approach to the evaluation and treatment. More severe aspiration in those unable to tolerate their own oral secretions warrants emergent intervention to include vocal cord medialization to restore glottic competence. A tracheotomy may be required for pulmonary toilet with the understanding that the presence of a tracheotomy tube interferes with the mechanism of deglutition to further impair swallowing.

Key to the evaluation is identification of the cause of the paralysis. Although some cases ultimately are labeled "idiopathic" and ascribed to a viral infection (Table 2), cancer must be excluded. Associated history, signs, and symptoms may help to identify the cause of the paralysis and to direct evaluation. Hoarseness developing immediately after carotid endarterectomy in association with the finding of an immobile vocal cord may be assumed to be caused by surgical injury of the recurrent laryngeal nerve without need for further work-up. Laryngeal paralysis presenting along with an ipsilateral neck mass determined to be thyroid cancer with fine-needle aspiration biopsy may be considered to reflect tumor involvement of the recurrent laryngeal nerve without need for further evaluation. In the absence of such localizing signs, we currently evaluate laryngeal paralysis with a chest x-ray to rule out lung neoplasm, followed by a single tailored magnetic resonance imaging scan to track the course of the vagus and recurrent laryngeal nerves from the midbrain, base of skull, neck, and mediastinum. The absence of findings results in the diagnosis of idiopathic laryngeal paralysis with the understanding that long-term follow-up may permit identification of an occult tumor in a small percentage of patients.

The treatment of unilateral vocal cord paralysis has advanced over the past decade to the point that a near-normal voice may be restored in the great majority of cases following treatment with one of several surgical procedures that have improved on the standard technique of Teflon augmentation of the paralyzed vocal cord. When prognosis for return of function of the paralyzed vocal cord is uncertain, injection with Gelfoam may improve swallowing, cough, and voicing without inducing irreversible changes to the larynx. The Gelfoam resorbs within 3 months, at which time reinjection or a more permanent treatment may be considered.

Posterior glottic scarring, traumatic arytenoid subluxation, and *cricoarytenoid arthritis* are processes that may mimic laryngeal paralysis and present with all the symptoms associated with an immobile vocal cord. Evaluation with laryngeal electromyography and/or direct laryngoscopy including palpation of

laryngeal structures may reconcile this differential diagnosis. A trial of a burst and taper of systemic steroids may be used as a diagnostic and therapeutic trial to benefit the patient with rheumatoid arthritis with an immobile vocal cord suspected to represent cricoarytenoid arthritis.

Acute Hoarseness with Airway Obstruction

Interference with the passage of air through the larynx commonly occurs at levels other than the glottis and often occurs without hoarseness. A supraglottic lesion such as a tumor or edema of the epiglottis permits unimpaired lung and laryngeal output. The voice is therefore normal or may be muffled as a "hot-potato" voice if the mass above the vocal cords is sufficiently large. Similarly, subglottic narrowing will impair airflow but is likely to affect the voice only by decreasing the breath support without otherwise changing vocal cord function. Any process that predominantly affects an adjacent structure to cause airway obstruction may also extend to involve the glottis and cause hoarseness.

Acute Hoarseness with Airway Obstruction: Infectious

Inflammation of the larynx is common in the pediatric patient and, as in adults, is generally a self-limited viral infection without long-term sequelae once the hoarseness, cough, and symptoms related to inflammation in adjacent upper respiratory structures resolve. Because the larynx, subglottis, and trachea are smaller in children than in adults, inflammation with attendant edema is much more likely to result in airway obstruction. As a result, clinical evaluation suggesting laryngeal infection in children is more likely to warrant immediate intervention, including hospitalization.

Supraglottitis, croup, and *bacterial tracheitis* are three processes commonly seen in the emergency department that share the potential to progress to complete airway obstruction but are managed differently.

Supraglottitis, formerly termed "epiglottitis," is a rapidly progressive cellulitis of the supraglottis with marked edema that, if considered as a diagnosis in an adult, warrants admission for observation. A more aggressive approach is required for pediatric cases with emergent transfer to the operating room for either endotracheal intubation or tracheotomy. Although supraglottitis is most commonly seen between the ages of 3 and 5 years, it can present at any age. It is generally caused by *Haemophilus influenzae* type B in the pediatric age group but may be caused by *Streptococcus viridans, Staphylococcus pyogenes,* and *Pneumococcus* in the adult. The process is potentially lethal, as reported by Hawkins and associates who, in 1973,* reviewed previously published accounts totaling 62 adults with supraglottitis with a 32% mortality rate. Subsequent series have noted a

TABLE 2. **Common Causes of Laryngeal Paralysis**

Adults	Children
Surgery	Neurologic
Idiopathic	Surgery
Malignancy	Idiopathic
Trauma	Trauma
Neurologic	(Birth)

*Hawkins DB, Miller AH, Sacks GG, Benz RT: Acute epiglottitis in adults. Laryngoscope 83:1211, 1973.

much lower mortality felt to result from improved physician awareness of the need for urgent intervention.

The presentation in pediatric and adult patients is similar with the exception that airway obstruction occurs more rapidly in the child. The initial symptom is usually throat pain that may be accompanied by fever and malaise followed rapidly by the development of odynophagia and dysphagia. Odynophagia is present in all cases of supraglottitis and, as it worsens, causes drooling. At this stage, the airway is likely to be compromised somewhat by the swollen epiglottis, which the patient generally maneuvers in a way to maximally open the airway by sitting erect and leaning forward. A muffling of the voice is generally present owing to increased mass above the vocal cords. Stridor is generally a late sign that predicts the onset of complete airway obstruction, which, in the absence of acute intervention, is followed by death.

The key to successful treatment lies in making the diagnosis before airway collapse. Emergent referral to a specialist capable of difficult intubation, rigid bronchoscopy, and tracheotomy in the supportive environment of the operating room is indicated. In pediatric patients, maneuvers such as placing the patient supine, performing a phlebotomy, inserting an intravenous tube, and manipulating the oral cavity may precipitate complete airway obstruction. As a result, immediate transfer to the operating room without the need for any further intervention is indicated for the child with signs and symptoms strongly suggestive of rapidly progressing supraglottitis.

Although an adult presenting with airway obstruction may require similar treatment, the larger airway may permit a less urgent approach to the workup. Flexible fiberoptic laryngoscopy may be safely performed in most adults without inducing airway obstruction. Observation in-hospital in a closely monitored environment without intubation or tracheotomy may be possible for adults with milder cases. Radiographic imaging with anteroposterior and lateral soft tissue films of the neck may be useful in those cases not requiring urgent intervention and will demonstrate marked enlargement of the epiglottis and aryepiglottic folds with filling of the hypopharynx and obliteration of the valleculae. Blood cultures as well as a complete blood count may be useful in predicting recovery without the need for airway intervention. A white blood count greater than 15,000 with a left shift and positive blood cultures predict a more fulminant course.

Observation of adult patients without intubation may be supplemented with general measures to limit progression of supraglottic edema with cool mist by face mask, inhalations of racemic epinephrine, and intravenous dexamethasone. Antibiotic therapy should be targeted initially toward *H. influenzae* and modified according to blood culture results. Popular drugs as initial treatment include ceftriaxone (Rocephin), cefuroxime (Ceftin), or ampicillin/sulbactam combination (Unasyn), with chloramphenicol or az-

treonam (Azactam) as alternatives in the penicillin-allergic patients. Bacterial supraglottitis generally resolves rapidly following initiation of therapy, with dysphagia and odynophagia resolving within 24 hours and epiglottic swelling disappearing 2 to 3 days later.

Croup is used to describe several different clinical syndromes with the common features of respiratory obstruction along with a barking cough.

Laryngotracheobronchitis (*LTB*) and *spasmodic croup* are two separate syndromes worthy of discriminating.

LTB most commonly presents in children under 3 years of age with the dominating signs of biphasic stridor and a "croupy" cough. A mild upper respiratory tract infection generally precedes the onset of these symptoms, which generally intensify at night and improve during the day. LTB generally occurs during the winter months and is due to infection of the larynx, subglottis, and lungs with parainfluenza or respiratory syncytial viruses. Other viruses may be implicated as well, with bacterial superinfection by *Streptococcus, Staphylococcus,* or *Haemophilus* developing with more extensive involvement.

The most concerning feature of LTB is biphasic stridor resulting from edema with narrowing of the subglottis. Soft tissue radiographs of the neck will demonstrate a characteristic narrowing in this region referred to as a "steeple sign" or "pencil point sign."

Supportive therapy with cool mist inhalations and racemic epinephrine treatments as necessary are generally sufficient to permit natural resolution of the disease process. The value of systemic steroids is controversial. Repeated mild episodes or progression of a moderate episode warrants referral to an otolaryngologist to assess for possible predisposing factors such as subglottic stenosis.

Spasmodic croup generally presents as recurrent episodes of upper airway obstruction associated with a barking cough in children without other signs of toxicity. Airway intervention or even admission to the hospital for observation is rarely necessary. Symptoms generally resolve quickly when treated with exposure to high humidity (e.g., running the shower). The value of other treatment with medication such as systemic corticosteroids, antihistamines, and subcutaneous epinephrine is questionable.

Acute Hoarseness with Airway Obstruction: Foreign Body Ingestion

Owing to protective reflexes and anatomic relationships, foreign bodies rarely lodge in the larynx at the level of the glottis and therefore generally are unassociated with the onset of hoarseness. They more commonly come to rest above the glottis in the oropharynx or adjacent to the larynx in the hypopharynx or pass inferiorly into the lungs or esophagus. Depending on the size and location of the object, a patient with a laryngeal foreign body may present with dysphonia or aphonia in addition to stridor and pain. Treatment begins with emergent consultation for visualization of the larynx. In those patients without signs of airway compromise and in clinics where visualization of the larynx is not possible, a lateral neck radiograph may help in demonstrating a radiopaque structure. Endoscopic removal with the patient under general anesthesia is usually the treatment of choice. In cooperative adults, removal with the patient under local anesthesia may occasionally be attempted as an office procedure employing indirect mirror examination and specially designed instruments.

Acute Hoarseness with Airway Obstruction: Neurogenic

Bilateral vocal cord paralysis may occur after either neck injury or surgery (e.g., thyroidectomy) and therefore may present acutely. The onset of symptoms most often occurs immediately after the injury or within several days. Rarely the immobile vocal cords may be positioned such that symptoms are not noted until long after the injury. More gradual onset of airway obstruction may develop in the face of bilateral vocal cord paralysis that develops in association with a malignancy or progressive neurologic disorder.

Airway obstruction with a normal voice will occur if the vocal cords are positioned in the midline with the glottis closed. Hoarseness as breathiness will occur without airway obstruction if the vocal cords are positioned laterally with the glottis open. Dysphagia with aspiration is most likely to occur with the vocal cords in this position. In an intermediate fashion, both hoarseness and airway obstruction develop if the position of the vocal cords permits the glottis to be partially open, resulting in both breathiness and inspiratory stridor.

The treatment of bilateral vocal cord paralysis is based on a compromise to improve either the airway or the voice.

Surgery may be performed to remove or reposition part of the vocal cord or arytenoid cartilage to enlarge the glottic opening, resulting in a breathy voice.

Alternatively, the voice and swallowing may be improved at the expense of the airway with procedures to close the glottis with vocal cord medialization requiring a tracheotomy. Prognosis for the return of function, associated symptoms (aspiration), and the desires of a fully informed patient should be considered when choosing among the many treatment options. The occupation of the patient is a critical consideration as to choice of treatment. The choices of a lawyer who requires a strong voice and can hide a tracheotomy tube under a collar may be significantly different from those of a professional scuba diver who cannot work with a tracheotomy tube. Experimental surgery performed to reinnervate the larynx to restore the potential to open the glottis for inspiration and to close the glottis for speech and swallowing has been under investigation for many years but is still not widely practiced.

Chronic Hoarseness

Chronic hoarseness generally warrants referral to an otolaryngologist. The urgency with which the referral is made depends on the symptom complex. If upper airway obstruction is considered, evaluation by the otolaryngologist should be made within minutes. If cancer is a concern, the referral should be made within days. If vocal nodules are the most likely diagnosis, the referral is not urgent, unless the patient is a singer, in which case she or he may request an evaluation emergently in order to prepare for a performance.

Chronic Hoarseness: Neoplastic

Most patients with *laryngeal cancer* are smokers who, prior to the development of cancer, may have a rough voice associated with the chronic laryngeal irritation of tobacco smoke. Voice abnormalities developing with a laryngeal cancer vary according to the location of the tumor in the larynx and may consist of voice changes identified as breathy, harsh, or muffled. Additional presenting symptoms include hemoptysis, stridor, dysphagia, pain, airway obstruction, and the appearance of a neck mass.

Glottic cancers developing on the vibrating surface of the vocal cord cause a dramatic change in voicing with a harshness that may have a breathy component if interference with glottic closure occurs. Because these symptoms usually present early in the development of the cancer, many glottic cancers are identified at an early stage that makes them readily curable. Glottic cancers rarely present with neck metastases both because the draining lymphatics in the vocal cords are sparse and because treatment is generally begun early in the course of the disease.

Supraglottic tumors develop in a "silent area" that generally does not produce symptoms until the tumor has enlarged to a significant size. A change in voice develops as a result of a tumor in this location generally only after the tumor is sufficiently large to muffle the laryngeal output, resulting in a "hot-potato" voice similar to that seen with supraglottitis. Extension from the supraglottis to involve the vocal cord may occur at a later stage to cause a harsh or breathy voice. Supraglottic tumors may progress to a sufficiently large size without detection to present with acute airway obstruction. Hemoptysis and dysphagia are relatively late symptoms. Otalgia owing to referred pain involving a branch of the vagus nerve often presents along with other symptoms. Because of the late development of symptoms associated with supraglottic tumors, many tumors are identified only after regional lymphatic metastases to the neck develop.

Subglottic tumors are rare and account for 1 to 2% of all laryngeal cancers. These tumors often present with airway obstruction owing to their location within the confines of the cricoid cartilage. In this region, narrowing presents with inspiratory and expiratory stridor owing to the rigid, nondistensible nature of the cartilage cricoid ring.

Recurrent respiratory papillomatosis is a benign neoplastic process with a potential for malignant degeneration. It occurs commonly in a juvenile form, which may disappear at puberty but may also persist throughout life. Wartlike growths occur in the upper aerodigestive tract with a predisposition for accumulation at the junction between respiratory epithelium and either squamous epithelium or scar. As a result, the vocal cords are commonly involved, with symptoms developing in a fashion similar to that of glottic cancer with hoarseness and occasionally airway obstruction.

The disease is felt to be viral in nature and affects not only grossly involved tissue but also adjacent normal-appearing mucosa. As a result, treatment with endoscopic removal is usually associated with recurrence. Symptoms may develop as early as several weeks after treatment or as late as years after treatment, depending on the rate of growth. The current treatment of choice is endoscopic removal employing carbon dioxide laser ablation with microscopic control. Biopsy to rule out cancer is important to perform in adult patients because of the potential for malignant transformation. Experimental work with photodynamic therapy as well as interferon has yet to show results that make these interventions first-line therapy.

Chronic Hoarseness: Neurogenic

The voice is affected by a large number of disease processes involving both the central and the peripheral nervous systems in a fashion that may be predicted by the systemic symptoms. *Tremor,* which may compromise fine motor control by interference of digital coordination by oscillations in hand movement, may also cause rhythmic alterations in the pitch and amplitude of the voice. Successful treatment of the systemic process may result in associated voice improvement. Unfortunately, many neurologic diseases with associated voice problems cannot be cured. As a result, for many of these processes, the goal of the laryngologist and speech pathologist is not to restore normal function but to maximize potential with a clear understanding of the limitations posed by the underlying disorder.

Spasmodic dysphonia is characterized by a stress-strained voice quality with intermittent breaks that often is severe to the point that the affected patient will retire from work and withdraw socially. Distinction between this process and muscle tension dysphonia may be difficult and, in our hands, is done through our voice clinic with a trial of voice therapy. Spasmodic dysphonia is generally resistant to improvement with voice therapy alone. Spasmodic dysphonia often presents in association with vocal tremor. The cause of spasmodic dysphonia remains unclear, although it is generally felt to represent a true dystonia rather than a psychiatric abnormality. Spasmodic dysphonia may be related to a disorder localized to the midbrain that is felt to represent a dystonia that may be isolated to the larynx or exist as part of a more generalized dystonia such as a Meige syndrome.

The diagnosis of spasmodic dysphonia is supported by fiberoptic imaging of irregular and intermittent glottic closure with hyperadduction of the vocal cords

more evident during connected speech than with sustained utterances. Laryngeal electromyography is of questionable value in supporting the diagnosis but some feel that characteristic patterns of activity may be elicited from the intrinsic laryngeal muscles.

Treatment is most effective with the use of botulinum neurotoxin A (Botox)* placed within the substance of the laryngeal muscles to dampen the excessive action-induced muscle contractions causing the characteristic voicing patterns. Systemic treatment with medications used for generalized dystonias such as trihexyphenidyl (Artane) is generally not as effective as botulinum toxin.

Myasthenia gravis is a disorder of muscle activity related to the presence of antibodies reacting with the receptor site of the neuromuscular junction that may initially present with weakness associated with swallowing or speech impairment. Although specific distribution of muscle weakness may be limited, there is usually weakness noted around the orbicularis oculi and upper facial muscles that may progress to more widespread involvement. In addition to an asthenic vocal quality, hypernasal speech may be apparent because of palatal weakness.

There is an urgency in diagnosing this disease in order that treatment be instituted. Myasthenia gravis is a potentially lethal disease that may result in death from respiratory failure. The diagnosis is made by identifying a response with improved muscle strength following the administration of neostigmine (Prostigmin) or edrophonium (Tensilon). To establish the diagnosis in a patient with laryngeal complaints (which requires more time to assess than eye weakness), evaluation of the patient 30 to 40 minutes after administration of the longer-acting neostigmine is generally preferred to the use of edrophonium, which acts for only 30 seconds to 2 minutes.

Amyotrophic lateral sclerosis is a disease caused by loss of anterior horn neurons and is characterized by progressive weakness that commonly presents with involvement of the tongue, pharynx, and vocal cords. Atrophy of the sides of the tongue coupled with fasciculations as well as palatal weakness and a decreased gag reflex are tip-offs to this disease process. There is no treatment available to reverse the progression of this disease toward death, but supportive help with speech and swallowing therapy can be of significant benefit. Tracheotomy and enteral tube feedings are commonly required as the disease approaches its final stages.

The voicing pattern of patients with *Parkinson's disease* is distinctive as a monotonous breathy voice characterized as "hypophonic." The presentation of voice in an emotionless manner coupled with the masklike facies common to these patients may mistakenly identify this process as a psychiatric disorder. The additional findings of cogwheel rigidity of the limbs, pillrolling tremor, and disorders of posture and gait are distinctive of more advanced cases of Parkinson's disease. Speech disability has been re-

---

*Investigational drug in the United States.

ported as the most significant aspect of this disease process interfering with quality of life. This interference in the ability to communicate has been identified in 75% of patients with the disease. In addition to the general medical management of Parkinson's disease, speech therapy may be of benefit.

Chronic Hoarseness: Psychogenic

Functional aphonia or *psychogenic aphonia* most commonly occurs in females and is identified by the absence of voicing in a patient whose laryngeal examination is otherwise normal. The capacity to effect glottic closure may be identified through a number of mechanisms including eliciting a normal cough. Treatment is with psychiatric counseling and voice therapy. Occasionally, resistant cases may be treated with procedures to interfere with the normal laryngeal mechanisms, such as lidocaine injection to the recurrent laryngeal nerve to induce a temporary laryngeal paralysis.

Muscle tension dysphonia is a common voicing disorder most often seen in patients with stressful jobs and significant demands on use of their voice. A tight, strained voice is commonly seen that, in severe cases, may be difficult to differentiate from spasmodic dysphonia. Associated neck muscle tightness may be identified. Treatment is with speech therapy, which may include innovative techniques such as circumlaryngeal massage and biofeedback.

Chronic Hoarseness: Traumatic/Environmental

Voice misuse (voice abuse) with or without other forms of laryngeal irritation may result in chronic changes to the vocal cords resulting in nodules, polyps, cysts, scarring, and chronic edematous changes termed "polypoid chorditis." These disorders are most commonly diagnosed with laryngeal imaging with mirror examination. Disorders of the vocal cords that are not clearly apparent on mirror examination can often be identified with use of the newer videostroboscopic units that not only permit more sophisticated assessment of the motion of the vocal cord structures during phonation but also provide enhanced illumination and magnification. If cancer is suspected, a biopsy usually with the patient under general anesthesia is performed. Those patients who are surgical risks or at relatively low risk for laryngeal cancer may be followed with sequential videoendoscopies to determine whether the nature of the vocal cord lesion is stable and less likely to require biopsy.

For the majority of laryngeal lesions felt to represent benign processes, a course of voice therapy is offered before surgical treatment in order that the vocal behavior that initially induced the abnormality be modified. Surgical treatment is reserved for those who have persistence of symptoms following voice therapy, who have modified their vocal behavior sufficiently to make recurrence of the lesion unlikely, and who accept the risks of surgical intervention, which include permanent scarring of the vocal cords.

INSOMNIA

method of
ERIC A. NOFZINGER, M.D., and
CHARLES F. REYNOLDS III, M.D.
Western Psychiatric Institute and Clinic
Pittsburgh, Pennsylvania

Although insomnia has been recognized as a common experience for ages, only recently has this complaint been recognized as a significant and disabling medical condition, worthy of accurate assessment and treatment within the medical community. The most notable recent recognition came in 1993, when a congressional mandate, Section 424 of the Public Health Service Act, established a National Center on Sleep Disorders Research within the National Heart, Lung and Blood Institute. The threefold purpose of the center is to (1) conduct and support research, (2) educate and train scientists, and (3) educate the public regarding sleep disorders, of which insomnia is a major complaint. The current chapter reviews the varied causes of a clinical complaint of insomnia and outline treatment strategies that are tailored to the underlying pathophysiology of the insomnia complaint.

INSOMNIA AS A FINAL COMMON PATHWAY

In our approach to the treatment of insomnia, we tend not to view the insomnia as the focus of treatment, but rather as a final common pathway of a variety of diverse, often multifactorial causative factors. In the medical management of a fever, it would generally be considered inappropriate to try to lower the temperature of a patient without first exploring all the potential causes of a fever from which more specific treatment recommendations could be made. In this view, our approach parallels that of professionals in the fields of sleep medicine and psychiatry, who have recently revised their diagnostic criteria for the classification of sleep disorders (the International Classification of Sleep Disorders [ICSD], 1990; Diagnostic and Statistical Manual of Mental Disorders, 4th ed [DSM–IV], 1994), based on a pathophysiologically based system, in contrast to the symptom-based classification system that they replaced (the Diagnostic Classification of Sleep and Arousal Disorders [DCSAD], 1979; DSM, 3rd ed, revised [III-R], 1987).

EVALUATION OF THE INSOMNIA COMPLAINT

Given that insomnia is a symptom as opposed to a disorder, the most important aspect of treatment is the accurate diagnosis of the underlying condition that results in the insomnia complaint. In sleep disorders, especially in the evaluation of insomnia, the most important diagnostic tool is the clinical interview of the patient. The initial phase of the clinical interview should be open-ended rather than structured, allowing the patient free rein to expound on the chief complaint. It is this complaint that is subsequently the focus for all other aspects of the evaluation and it is the resolution of this complaint, the subjective suffering of the patient, that determines the ultimate success of the medical intervention. In this phase, the clinician should focus on the subjective experience of the patient, clarifying the individual meaning of the insomnia for that patient, as it is different for every patient. A common opening question might be, "If there is anything you could change about your sleep, what would that be?" If the response is, "I would simply like to sleep at night," some effort should be made to establish why sleeping at night is important to that individual. Responses to this probing give early clues as to diagnosis. Patients with psychophysiologic or conditioned insomnia (described later) do not understand this last question and express surprise that it is being asked given their automatic thought process that convinces them of the essential need to obtain their 8 hours of sleep in order to function the next day. Patients with depression say that sleep is necessary so that their minds can get some rest from the incessant ruminations and worries about their lives that plague them during the day. "If only I could sleep at night, then I know I would be fine" is a common retort. Patients with insomnia associated with the normative process of aging answer this question by saying, "Well, I'm not sure why I should get more sleep; I know I always used to," as the decreased sleep time is often not disabling for them, but more a curiosity.

The duration of the insomnia complaint should be identified. Transient insomnias (less than 1 month) and chronic insomnias (greater than 1 month) have different prognoses and treatment strategies, which are reviewed later.

After the subjective chief complaint has been clarified, the interview should take a more structured approach, clarifying aspects of the patient's usual sleep and wake habits, which may provide additional clues for diagnosis. One way of structuring this aspect of the interview is to ask the patient about 24-hour sleep and wake habits, beginning, for example, at bedtime, then gradually working through the night, and then the following day until questioning has completed a 24-hour cycle. Bedtime issues to be clarified include the following: (1) is there a regular time at which the patient goes to bed (irregular times may suggest a circadian rhythm or sleep and wake schedule disorder) and (2) are there any special habits or routines engaged in before going to bed or performed in bed before attempting sleep, e.g., brushing teeth, drinking an ounce of liquor, reading a book, or watching television? Sleep-onset symptoms to be screened include the following: (1) hypnagogic hallucinations (visual images seen before sleep onset that suggest narcolepsy or sleep deprivation secondary to sleep apnea), (2) sleep-onset paralysis (ranging from a sense of heaviness in the limbs to complete skeletal muscle paralysis occurring immediately before sleep onset in the still-conscious patient, indicative of narcolepsy), and (3) restlessness in the legs (often requiring the patient to get out of bed for relief, indicative of restless legs syndrome and/or periodic limb movement disorder).

Once bedtime issues have been addressed, intrinsic sleep disturbances should be clarified. Corroborative information from a bed partner is often helpful here. The examiner should ask about sleep onset. (1) How long does it take to fall asleep? (2) Is the patient relaxed when attempting sleep, or is sleep forced (psychophysiologic insomnia)? The patient should be asked about the general quality and duration of sleep. At this time, the patient may describe the presence or absence of specific sleep complaints, including a history of snoring or gasping for breath in the middle of the night, and parasomnias, such as sleepwalking, or sleeptalking. Patients with a sleep state misperception may claim that they do not sleep at all at night despite objective signs of sleep. Patients with psychophysiologic insomnia generally underestimate the quantity of sleep, giving more weight to the period in the night when they are lying awake frustrated at their attempts to sleep. The examiner should ask about awakening. Does the patient awaken (1) in the middle of the night, (2) at the end of the night, (3) in relation to any internal stimuli (such as a nightmare or loss of air) or external stimuli (such as a baby crying, noises in the street, or the rustling of a bed partner)? How long do the awakenings last? On awakening in the middle of the night, is the mental status (1) vigilant and angry (psychophysiologic insomnia), (2) physically exhausted yet mentally unable to return to sleep (depression), or (3) fatigued, unrefreshed, and sleepy (sleep apnea)? Is there a regular time when the patient gets out of bed? How is the patient awakened? How does the patient feel on awakening after a night's sleep?

Questions covering the daytime should focus on degrees of alertness and sleepiness, and on sleep and wake habits. How alert does the patient feel during the daytime? Patients suffering from disorders that disrupt sleep (sleep apnea, or periodic limb movement disorder) generally appear sleep-deprived the following day. Patients with depression are not able to sleep (rest) either at night or during the daytime. Patients with psychophysiologic insomnia may experience a blunting of performance yet may be vigilant, mentally stimulated, and aroused during the daytime. Patients with disturbances of sleep and wake scheduling or circadian rhythm sleep disturbances may reveal differential degrees of alertness according to the time of day. The examiner should find out if the patient drinks coffee, caffeinated beverages, or alcohol or smokes cigarettes during the day and how much. The patient's daily schedule and major work and activity times, as well as the regularity of these activities throughout the week should be determined.

Following this 24-hour review of sleep and wake habits, the interview should turn to a review of the more common medical and psychiatric disorders associated with insomnia. Since the most common cause of insomnia identified in patients who report to sleep disorders clinicians is related to a mental disorder, the major focus at this point should be the psychiatric history. As in the elicitation of the chief complaint, the attitude of the interviewer at this point should be open-ended and nonjudgmental, creating an atmosphere in which the patients feel comfortable sharing more personal aspects of their lives. Of the mental disorders that have been associated with insomnia, depression is the most frequent diagnosis, necessitating a brief review of cognitive and physiologic signs and symptoms that may suggest the presence of a depressive disorder. Anxiety disorders and substance use disorders should also be reviewed. Persons with insomnias associated with the psychoses, such as schizophrenia and acute mania, will most likely not present to a generalist with the chief complaint of an insomnia.

DIAGNOSTIC INSTRUMENTS

Sleep Diary

Either before or after the clinical interview with the patient, it is often helpful to ask the patient to fill out a sleep diary to provide more objective measures of the patient's routine sleep and wake habits. Sleep diaries range from simply asking the patients to write down the times they go to bed and wake up in the morning to more elaborate self-report forms that include information on eating habits, coffee and alcohol consumption, the timing of daytime naps, the amounts and timing of exercise, and self-ratings of mood, alertness, and the quality of sleep. The patient is instructed to fill out the diary at a regular time each day to increase compliance. Reviewing the results of the diary often becomes the focus for clarifying the diagnosis or for following responses to treatment interventions.

Activity Monitoring

A more objective longitudinal measure of sleep and wake activity can be obtained by the use of a wrist activity monitor, or actigraph. These devices are generally provided by a sleep disorder center during a consultation for a sleep complaint. They measure the frequency and patterning of daily activity, which is approximated by the activity of the nondominant wrist. Inspection of activity patterns over consecutive days in the patient's natural environment can yield clinically valuable information regarding sleep and wake scheduling, the amplitude of activity or inactivity during the day, and the degree of sleep disruption caused by active periods in the middle of the night.

Polysomnography

If the cause of the insomnia is not apparent from the initial clinical interview or if initial treatment efforts have not been successful, then referral to a sleep evaluation center is recommended. There a formal sleep study or polysomnographic assessment can be obtained under the guidance of a sleep disorders specialist. Polysomnography is the simultaneous assessment of several different psychophysiologic measure, for example, by using electroencephalography (EEG), electromyography (EMG), oximetry, and electrocardiography (ECG). Polysomnography can establish sleep staging as well as identify disturbances in respirations, or body movements that aid diagnosis when interpreted by a sleep disorders specialist.

This test is generally not recommended for routine use in all cases of insomnia but is reserved for cases that are refractory to treatment or in which the insomnia is presumed to be related to sleep apnea or periodic limb movement disorder.

DIFFERENTIAL DIAGNOSIS

Normative Alterations in Sleep Across the Life Cycle

In evaluating and treating patients with insomnia, it is essential to understand the normative changes in sleep across the life cycle so that expectations for treatment are not inflated. With aging, the ability to sleep diminishes, while the need for sleep does not. This is reflected by reductions in deeper aspects of sleep (Stages 3 and 4 sleep) and by an increase in wakefulness throughout the night, with corresponding attempts to restore some sleep deprivation during the daytime by taking naps. As a result of this decreased ability to sleep, the patterning of sleep in the elderly may become displaced when they either go to bed earlier in the night (which then leads to early morning awakenings, or "insomnia") or redistribute sleep between the nighttime and the daytime hours (which then leads to "insomnia" during the night). With aging, then, the subjective experience of "insomnia" is often simply the result of a normative change in the physiology of sleeping. Treatment of this normal insomnia of aging therefore relies heavily on educating the patient about the normative changes in sleep associated with aging. These patients should be encouraged to rely less on daytime naps to recover their sleep debt, since napping decreases nighttime sleep propensity.

In these patients, middle-of-the-night awakenings and early-morning awakenings may be relieved by sleep restriction therapy. In this technique, sleep is consolidated by restricting the total time spent in bed to the amount of time the patients actually feel they are sleeping at night. For example, if a patient feels that he or she only gets 5 hours of sleep at night and is actually in bed between 10:00 P.M. and 7:00 A.M. (9 hours), then inevitably, sometime during the night the patient is awake for at least 4 hours. Shortening the time in bed to between 12:00 midnight and 5:00 A.M. consolidates sleep to the actual period spent in bed and reduces the subjective experience of "insomnia" (time spent awake in bed) while not increasing the total sleep time. A healthy dose of education and reassurance must accompany these recommendations as these patients have been accustomed to the longer sleeping schedule without difficulties for most of their lives.

Transient Versus Chronic Insomnia

The duration of the insomnia complaint has been shown to be important in establishing the cause of the insomnia and in determining the appropriate treatment intervention. In general, transient insomnia is defined as a duration of less than 3 to 4 weeks and chronic insomnia as longer than 1 month. The transient insomnias are thought to be a normal variant of sleep and have a good prognosis. The chronic insomnias are thought to reflect a more severe pathophysiologic process. They require a more comprehensive diagnostic treatment strategy and are associated with a less favorable prognosis.

Transient insomnias in general are short-lived by definition and do not come to the attention of the clinician. Examples might include environmental sleep disruptions related to alterations in noise, light, or temperature in the sleeping environment, or to alterations in the scheduling of sleep in a 24-hour cycle related either to shift work or to travel across multiple time zones (jet lag). The most common form of transient insomnia is that related to an acute stressor, such as a personal loss or excitement about a promotion. Treatment efforts should focus on education, reassurance, and promotion of good sleep and wake hygiene (reviewed later). A brief (generally less than 3 weeks) course of a sedative medication (reviewed later) may be considered. For more chronic insomnias, which do not respond to acute therapy for transient insomnias, the clinician should seek a more specific cause on which to base more focused treatment.

CHRONIC INSOMNIAS

Insomnia Related to a Mental Disorder

Insomnia related to a mental disorder is the most common diagnosis within the chronic insomnias. A review of psychiatric symptoms is essential in any patient presenting to a clinician with insomnia complaints. An understanding of some of the more common sleep disturbances associated with the various mental disorders will help the clinician to arrive at an accurate diagnosis and to enhance the treatment specificity.

Depression

Within mental disorders, the most common cause of insomnia that may present to a general clinician is major depression. Depressed patients complain of difficulty sleeping, despite the simultaneous experience of physical fatigue. These patients appear to be in a state of heightened arousal related to the state of depression in which their brains do not allow sleep to proceed in a restorative fashion. Over 3 decades of research into the objective alterations in sleep physiology have demonstrated reliable sleep alterations associated with depression that may relate to this subjective experience of the patient. Difficulty in falling asleep, manifested in prolonged sleep latencies; difficulties in maintaining sleep, reflected by frequent arousals in the night; and early-morning awakenings are found. In general, these patients do not feel refreshed on awakening in the morning, and they would like to sleep or take naps during the daytime if only they could. Alternatively, some depressed patients describe atypical sleep complaints, including prolonged sleep periods resembling sleep drunkenness, or difficulty arising from sleep in the morning, and frequent napping in bed during the daytime.

Psychoses

A patient with schizophrenia in general would not come to the attention of a general clinician with a complaint of insomnia, although certainly insomnia is one of the cardinal manifestations of schizophrenia, especially during acute psychotic exacerbations. At those times it is not unusual for these patients to have profound reductions in the amount of time spent asleep, approximating a 50% reduction in sleep duration. The accompanying psychotic manifestations, which may include auditory hallucinations and vivid delusional thinking, are the symptoms that bring these patients to the attention of the medical system, rather than primary sleep complaints.

Anxiety Disorders

Patients with anxiety disorders (generalized anxiety disorder, panic disorder, obsessive compulsive disorder, and post-traumatic stress disorder) often present with insomnia. This may include difficulty initiating sleep at night and difficulty maintaining sleep throughout the night. The insomnia appears related to excessive worry or apprehensive expectation about one or more life circumstances. Objective sleep studies confirm that these patients have long sleep latencies, increased time spent in "lighter" stages 1 and 2 non–rapid eye movement (NREM) sleep, and decreased "deeper" stages 3 and 4 NREM sleep. Symptoms of anxiety disorders include panic attacks, anxious mood, nervousness, jitteriness, shortness of breath, palpitations, smothering feelings, dizziness, faintness, sweating and trembling, or recurrent nightmares of traumatic experiences. The presence of these symptoms should raise suspicion that an anxiety disorder is a cause of the insomnia.

Dementia

Insomnia is also a common feature of dementia. These patients may have nocturnal delirium, agitation, combativeness, wandering, and vocalization without ostensible purpose during the early evening and nighttime hours. Sleep is fragmented with frequent awakenings throughout the night. These clinical symptoms have objective correlates based on polysomnographic studies in this population and include an increase in lighter stages of sleep, reduction of delta and rapid eye movement (REM) sleep, and a tendency to redistribute the major sleeping period to fragmented periods throughout a 24-hour cycle.

Approaches to treatment in these cases are primarily behavioral and educational. Minimizing daytime naps may increase sleep propensity at night, thereby consolidating nocturnal sleep. Increasing both activity levels and light illumination during the daytime may help to entrain the sleep and wake system to separate the major active period to the daytime and the major inactive period to the nighttime. When there is a significant reduction in total sleep time over a 24-hour period, restricting the time in bed to the actual amount of time spent sleeping may be helpful. Planned activities for all other hours should be considered. Education of nursing home staff or other family members may be necessary in order to adjust their expectations that the demented patient should be sleeping longer than is possible. Low dosages of neuroleptic medications such as thiothixene (Navane)* (2 mg), haloperidol (Haldol)* (0.5 to 1.0 mg), perphenazine (Trilafon)* (2 to 4 mg), thioridazine (Mellaril) (25 to 50 mg), or risperidone (1 to 2 mg) may be useful. Sedative hypnotic medications in general should be avoided in an elderly population owing to the potential exacerbation of sleep-related breathing disturbances, which are known to occur more frequently in this population, and to the possible induction of daytime sedation.

Substance Abuse

Insomnia is a complication in acute and chronic alcohol abuse as well as a lingering clinical complaint following complete abstinence from alcohol use. Although alcohol has a short-acting central nervous system depressant effect and can facilitate sleep, these effects of alcohol generally wear off in the middle of the night as the drug is metabolized, producing withdrawal-associated bizarre nightmares and insomnia later in the night. Many patients habitually drink before bedtime to help them get to sleep but become involved in a vicious circle as the alcohol produces later insomnia. With chronic use, the ability to sleep soundly becomes physiologically more diffi-

---

*Not FDA-approved for this indication.

cult, resulting in more fragmented, lighter sleep. In short-term abstinence, or withdrawal, there are severe sleep-disrupting effects, which tend to normalize with increasing duration of abstinence; however, losses of the deeper stages of sleep have been noted years after complete cessation of alcohol use. This suggests that profound pathophysiologic disturbances of sleep may be associated with chronic alcohol use.

General Guidelines for Treating Insomnia Related to a Mental Disorder

Although there are diverse mental disorders that may contribute to insomnia complaints, there are some general guidelines for treatment. First, the proper diagnosis of the underlying mental disorder should be established. If this cannot be done in the initial evaluation, then referral to a psychiatric specialist may be warranted. Second, focus should be on treating the mental disorder as opposed to the insomnia complaint. Third, once a mental disorder has been diagnosed, medications should be chosen that are specific to the disorder and whose side-effect profile may optimize alleviation of the sleep complaint. Fourth, the patient should be educated about the expected duration to maximal clinical response. Often this time period approximates the response time to alleviation of the mental disorder. For example, in depression, the patient on an antidepressant medication may not experience significant benefit in insomnia or depression until 4 to 8 weeks after initiation of the medication trial, although sleep often is one of the first symptoms to improve.

Psychophysiologic Insomnia

Following insomnia related to a mental disorder, psychophysiologic insomnia is the most common form of insomnia that presents to sleep disorders clinicians for treatment, although the incidence in the community is unknown. This form of insomnia is also referred to as "learned" or "conditioned" insomnia. In these patients the insomnia is "primary" and not secondary to another mental or physical disorder. The insomnia in these patients is theorized to result from a vicious circle, in which recurrent unsuccessful attempts to sleep lead to frustration and physiologic tension, which in turn makes sleep less likely. Although a variety of precipitating factors may instigate the initial insomnia, subsequent sleepless nights are the result of learned associations between frustration and attempts to sleep. These patients present with exaggerated concerns regarding their difficulties sleeping and the degree of incapacitation that this sleeplessness may produce in their waking lives if it is not corrected. Paradoxically, when not trying to fall asleep—for example, during changes in environment associated with vacations or travel— these patients may sleep better than they do in their own bedrooms.

Treatment of psychophysiologic insomnia revolves around behavioral interventions and judicious transient use of sedative-hypnotic medications. General sleep and wake hygiene education should emphasize using the bed for sleeping purposes only. This prevents the learned pairing of frustration and somatized tension with the sleeping environment. Relaxation training may be considered under the supervision of a behavioral therapist and may include progressive muscle relaxation and biofeedback training. Restricting the time in bed to the total amount of time in which the patient is actually sleeping may help to consolidate sleep and decrease the amount of time spent in bed in a frustrated, angry cognitive state. Cognitive therapy, in which automatic negative thoughts are identified and tested, may be helpful to reduce the psychophysiologic arousal associated with middle-of-the-night awakenings. Finally, occasional (once or twice weekly) use of a hypnotic may help to break the cycle of sleeplessness and provide relief on nights before days in which maximal alertness is desired, e.g., an important meeting or test.

Insomnia Related to a Medical Disorder

Several medical conditions are known to be associated with insomnia. Sleep apnea, characterized by periodic cessation of respiration during sleep, is most often associated with hypersomnia at night as well as during the daytime, although occasionally patients complain of insomnia. Referral to a sleep disorders center is recommended for further evaluation and treatment of the sleep apnea.

Restless legs syndrome, experienced as a deep muscle restlessness most often in the legs, is a common cause of difficulties initiating sleep on going to bed. The restlessness often becomes apparent only on lying down in bed, and the discomfort can be severe enough to inhibit sleep onset. Periodic limb movement (PLM) disorder is a syndrome in which rhythmic extensions of the big toe and dorsiflexions of the ankle occur on a frequency of 20 to 40 seconds during sleep; this can be associated with insomnia if the movements are associated with arousals from sleep. Carbidopa-levodopa (Sinemet)* (initial dose 25-100 mg to 50-200 mg titrated upward to clinical response), as well as benzodiazepines such as clonazepam (Klonopin)* (dosage 0.25 to 2.0 mg at bedtime) have been shown to be helpful for restless legs syndrome and PLM disorder.

Several chronic medical disorders are associated with insomnia. Chronic pain often causes insomnia related to an inability to find a comfortable position in which to sleep. Chronic illnesses such as rheumatoid arthritis and fibromyositis may cause insomnia and are associated with signs of central nervous system arousal during sleep. Anti-inflammatory medications and benzodiazepines may help insomnia related to rheumatoid arthritis, and low doses of tricyclic antidepressant medications such as amitriptyline

---

*Not FDA-approved for this indication.

(Elavil)* (10 to 50 mg at bedtime) may help insomnia related to fibromyositis. Chronic fatigue syndrome is often associated with insomnia and daytime fatigue. No clear treatments for this disorder have emerged, although occasional success has been noted with tricyclic antidepressants, selective serotonin re-uptake inhibitors, nonsteroidal anti-inflammatory agents, and monoamine oxidase inhibitors.

Of neurologic disorders, parkinsonism is strikingly associated with severe loss of sleep propensity to the point where often a 50% reduction in the duration of sleep is observed. Treatment of these patients is difficult and often unsuccessful. Education regarding the decreased sleep propensity associated with the condition is indicated rather than trying to re-establish an 8-hour nighttime sleep duration. The addition of bedtime dosing of dopaminergic agonists may be helpful, as may low dosages of benzodiazepine hypnotics and tricyclic antidepressants such as amitriptyline. These medications should be monitored closely since they may cause complications in a parkinsonian patient including delirium, nightmares, and worsening insomnia.

TREATMENT TECHNIQUES

Sleep Hygiene

Patients who complain of insomnia should be educated about sleep hygiene, which can be broadly defined as healthy behaviors that promote good sleep. Outlined in Table 1, these guidelines are a combination of common sense rules and condensed guidelines that incorporate techniques used in more extensive behavioral treatments for insomnia. After reviewing these guidelines with the patient, the clinician can give them to the patient for home review and use.

Stimulus Control

Stimulus control techniques are instructions to the patient to use the bed and bedroom for sleeping and sexual purposes only. Reading or watching television in bed should be discouraged. If the patients are awake for longer than 10 to 15 minutes at any point in the middle of the night, they are instructed to get out of the bed and the bedroom, occupying themselves with waking activities, such as reading or watching television in another room, until they feel sleepy, at which time they can return to bed. The goal is to associate the stimulus of the bed with sleeping and not with frustrated attempts to try to sleep. This technique is a general guideline for overall sleep hygiene as well as a specific technique that can be used in patients with psychophysiologic insomnia. These patients often develop negative associations with the bed and bedroom through repeated frustrated, angry attempts to "force" sleep after spontaneous arousals in the night.

*Not FDA-approved for this indication.

TABLE 1. **Rules for Better Sleep**

1. Sleep only as much as you need to feel refreshed during the following day. Restricting your time in bed helps to consolidate and deepen your sleep. Excessively long times in bed lead to fragmented and shallow sleep.
2. Get up at the same time each day, 7 days a week. A regular wake time in the morning leads to regular times of sleep onset and helps to set your "biologic" clock.
3. A steady daily amount of exercise helps to deepen sleep. Exercise should not be taken too close to bedtime; plan to finish by 7:00 P.M.
4. Insulate your bedroom against sounds that disturb your sleep. Carpeting, insulated curtains, and closing the door may help.
5. Excessively warm rooms may disturb sleep; keep the room temperature moderate.
6. Hunger may disturb sleep. A light snack at bedtime may help sleep, but avoid greasy or "heavy" foods.
7. Avoid excessive liquids in the evening, in order to minimize the need for nighttime trips to the bathroom.
8. Avoid caffeinated beverages, especially in the evening.
9. Avoid alcohol, especially in the evening. Although alcohol helps tense people fall asleep more easily, the ensuing sleep is fragmented.
10. The use of tobacco disturbs sleep.
11. Do not take your problems to bed. If necessary, plan some time earlier in the evening for working on your problems or planning the next day's activities.
12. Train yourself to use the bedroom only for sleeping and sexual activity. This will help condition your brain to see the bed as the place for sleeping. Do *not* read, watch TV, or eat in bed.
13. People who feel angry and frustrated because they cannot sleep should *not* try harder and harder to fall asleep. This only makes the problem worse. Instead, turn on the light, leave the bedroom, and do something different like reading a boring book. Do not engage in stimulating activity. Return to bed only when you are sleepy. Get up at your regular time the next day, no matter how little you slept.
14. If you find yourself waking up and looking at the clock, put the clock under the bed or turn it so that you can't see it.
15. Avoid naps. Staying awake during the day helps you to fall asleep at night.

Sleep Restriction

Sleep restriction therapy is a general technique for the treatment of insomnia, especially in cases in which the patient is noted to be spending excessive time in bed trying but unable to sleep. The clinician should first estimate the actual time over a 24-hour period in which the patients think they are actually sleeping. The duration of both nighttime sleep and daytime naps should be included. Second, which sleep period in the 24-hour day the patient would most like to be sleeping should be determined, based on the duration of time estimated from Step 1. Third, the patients should be instructed to retire to bed only at the time they have specified from Step 2 and to get out of bed regularly at the ending time they have specified. They should remain out of bed for the entire rest of the day, retiring to bed on the following evening only at the specified time. These patients will gradually become sleep-deprived, increasing their sleep propensity, which will subsequently lead to improved sleep maintenance at night. As their sleep becomes more consolidated, they can gradually increase the time in bed as long as they are maintaining sleep for the majority of the time in bed. Often, a beneficial effect of the treatment is enabling the patients to develop mastery over their sleep cycles, decreasing their sense of helplessness and building their confidence that their insomnia is not a hopeless condition.

Relaxation Techniques

Relaxation before bedtime has been shown to reduce insomnia complaints in patients for whom increased muscular tension makes sleep onset difficult. This is most prominent in patients with psychophysiologic insomnia. Progressive muscle relaxation techniques train patients to relax their muscles by actively tensing and relaxing various muscle groups throughout the body. Biofeedback training uses EMG-recorded muscle activity or "tension" to produce visual or auditory "feedback" to help the patient recognize when the muscles have successfully been relaxed. This training helps the patient to learn to relax the muscles in bed before sleep onset. Guided imagery and meditation before sleep onset have also been tried in an attempt to break the vicious circle of progressive heightening of somatic tension that results from the negative focus on the inability to sleep. Although these techniques are helpful, there is significant expense in terms of time and training of the clinician and the patient that may make widespread application of these techniques difficult.

Pharmacotherapy

Some general guidelines should be followed in considering the use of pharmacotherapy for patients with insomnia complaints: (1) medications should be viewed as adjunctive treatment for most cases of transient and chronic insomnia as opposed to the primary treatment, (2) benzodiazepine hypnotics should be confined to the treatment of transient insomnia unless the specific form of insomnia, e.g., insomnia related to PLM disorder, is best treated by a long-term benzodiazepine, in this case, clonazepam, and (3) therapy, including pharmacotherapy should be directed toward the underlying etiologic agent, as opposed to alleviating the insomnia per se.

Pharmacotherapy for insomnia related to a mental disorder should, in general, follow pharmacotherapy guidelines for the individual mental disorder. Since the sleep disturbance is related to the underlying mental disorder, treatment of the mental disorder usually results in alleviation of the sleep complaint, often before alleviation of the mental disorder. Referral to a psychiatrist for further evaluation of a mental disorder and for initiation of psychotropic medications may be indicated at the discretion of the clinician. In depression, sleep consolidation has been objectively documented for most antidepressant agents including the tricyclic antidepressants and the selective serotonin re-uptake inhibitors (SSRIs), such as fluoxetine (Prozac). For anxiety disorders, the initiation of tricyclic antidepressant or SSRI medications to relieve the anxiety disorder should proceed with lower doses than typically used for the treatment of depression, because these drugs tend to have a paradoxical insomnia side effect in these patients when they begin antidepressant medications; this side effect subsides with long-term therapy.

In addition to the treatment of depression, the tricyclic antidepressants and trazodone (Desyrel)* may have broader spectrums of treatment that are appropriate in the treatment of more chronic forms of insomnia. Unlike the benzodiazepine class of hypnotics, these medications do not appear to result in tolerance to their hypnotic effects when used for longer than a month. The abuse potential for these medications is thought to be minimal, although occasionally psychological dependence may occur with more chronic forms of treatment. Patients with primary insomnia, which by definition is chronic, may benefit from low doses of more-sedating tricyclic antidepressants such as amitriptyline* (25 to 50 mg at bedtime), or from trazodone (25 to 200 mg at bedtime). Tricyclic antidepressants have also been helpful in the treatment of the specific insomnia associated with fibromyositis and may be helpful in insomnia related to chronic pain syndromes. Some caution should be observed, however, in using these medications in patients with PLM disorder, as they have been noted to exacerbate this condition.

Benzodiazepines are most appropriate in treating transient insomnias, and then only on an intermittent (every two or three nights) basis over a 2- to 3-week period. The smallest effective doses should be used to avoid the side effects of impaired daytime performance and anterograde amnesia. Short-term (less than 1 month) use is advised to minimize the development of dependence to the medication. Patients who have primarily difficulty in falling asleep may be helped by benzodiazepines that have relatively rapid to ultrarapid elimination such as temazepam (Restoril) (10 to 60 mg, or 10 to 20 mg in the elderly), triazolam (Halcion) (0.125 to 0.250 mg, 0.125 mg in the elderly), and zolpidem (Ambien) (5 to 10 mg). Rebound insomnia may occur with these rapidly eliminated hypnotics if withdrawn abruptly or if large doses are used. If the insomnia is more related to frequent arousals in the night, or if daytime anxiety is also present, then a hypnotic with more prolonged elimination such as flurazepam (Dalmane) (15 to 30 mg, 15 mg in the elderly), or clorazepate (Tranxene)* (15 to 22.5 mg, 7.5 to 15 mg in the elderly) may be considered. With these latter medications, the effects on daytime performance as well as the accumulation of dose over successive administrations are apparent. Rebound insomnia, however, is less likely to occur with the use of these medications given their longer half-lives.

---

*Not FDA-approved for this indication.

PRURITUS
(Itching)

method of
ALAN B. FLEISCHER, JR., M.D.
*The Bowman Gray School of Medicine of
Wake Forest University
Winston-Salem, North Carolina*

PRURITUS SENSATIONS

Pruritus or itching is that sensation that provokes scratching behavior. Although many patients with pruritic conditions complain of itching, others patients state that they have burning, stinging, tingling, tickling, or a crawling sensation. These symptoms appear to be closely related to pruritus and have similar pathogenic mechanisms. Pruritus is a distinct, complex sensation that may be considered a primary sensory modality.

Many cutaneous diseases, including atopic dermatitis, contact dermatitis, urticaria, scabies, and dermatitis herpetiformis, present with pruritus. These cutaneous diseases are often readily diagnosed by careful clinical examination. To aid diagnosis, the physician should attempt to distinguish primary from secondary lesions. Primary lesions may consist of scaling macules, papules, or vesicles. By contrast, secondary lesions represent the changes that patients have wrought, including excoriations (scratch marks) and lichenification (thickening due to rubbing or scratching). The location of the disease is critical for diagnosis. Atopic dermatitis commonly affects the antecubital and popliteal fossae, whereas scabies typically affects the interdigital web spaces, wrists, and anogenital areas.

There is no question that internal diseases may be associated with pruritus. Of patients who present with generalized pruritus, systemic diseases account for a small number of cases. Thus, a careful history to establish the location, duration, and history may rule out significant internal disease. Generalized pruritus may be associated with thyroid disease, renal insufficiency, liver disease, iron deficiency, diabetes mellitus, paraproteinemia, Sjögren's syndrome, and various malignancies (Table 1).

TOPICAL TREATMENT

In the best possible world, the physician would choose the single topical medication that corrects the underlying condition. Although this scenario occasionally occurs (e.g., permethrin [Elimite] for scabies infestation), symptomatic treatment is less specific. Therefore clinicians must use their diagnostic skills to provide the patient with reasonable relief.

In the presence of visible scaling, the author strongly recommends a topical emollient. Emollient creams, ointments, and lotions are widely available and are indispensable in treating atopic dermatitis, asteatotic dermatitis, hand eczema, and psoriasis. Topical emollients have been shown to decrease the irritancy of the skin and may therefore serve as an adjunct to any other therapy.

Age-old remedies such as cool compresses (application of a wet washcloth for 20 minutes), shake lotions (calamine), and menthol may prove highly efficacious. Either cooling the skin or giving the sensation of cooling may provide remarkable pruritus relief.

TABLE 1. **Systemic Conditions Reported to be Associated with Generalized Pruritus**

Organ Systems/ Etiology	Example
Autoimmune	Sjögren's syndrome
Endocrine	Hyperthyroidism
	Hypothyroidism
	Diabetes mellitus
Central nervous system	Cerebrovascular accident
	Delusions of parasitosis
	Depression
	Multiple sclerosis
	Neurodermatitis
	Psychosis
Hematopoietic	Paraproteinemia
	Iron-deficiency anemia
	Mastocytosis
Liver	Primary biliary cirrhosis
	Extrahepatic biliary obstruction
	Hepatitis
Malignancy	Polycythemia rubra vera
	Carcinoid syndrome
	Multiple myeloma
	Hodgkin's disease
	Non-Hodgkin's lymphomas
	Lung cancer
	Leukemia
	Prostatic carcinoma
	Thyroid carcinoma
	Gastrointestinal tract cancers: tongue, stomach, and colon
	Cutaneous T cell lymphoma
	Breast carcinoma
	Uterine carcinoma
Pharmacologic	Drug ingestion
Infectious	Human immunodeficiency virus
	Parasitic diseases
	Syphilis
Renal	Chronic renal insufficiency and renal failure
	Dialysis dermatosis

Oatmeal baths (Aveeno) or baths in therapeutic salts may also effect short-term symptomatic relief.

Topical corticosteroids are exceptionally useful agents for pruritus control. Their anti-inflammatory activity makes them the mainstay of topical therapy. Hydrocortisone (Hytone) 1% or 2.5% twice-daily and triamcinolone (Aristocort) 0.025% or 0.1% twice-daily are reasonably inexpensive and effective for most cases of dermatitis. Other topical corticosteroid agents have advantages and disadvantages. The author encourages the use of the least potent topical corticosteroid that works for the patient.

Compounds with pramoxine (Prax) or menthol and camphor (Sarna) may be helpful for selected patients. These agents are found either mixed in various combinations with one another or combined with topical corticosteroid agents. Table 2 reviews some of the

TABLE 2. **Topical Agents Used in Treatment of Pruritus**

Topical Agent	Examples	Advantages	Disadvantages
Emollients and moisturizers	Petrolatum Moisturizing lotions Bath oils	Inexpensive Correct xerosis and reduce irritant dermatitis	May be too greasy Not sufficient for inflammatory dermatoses
Corticosteroids	Hydrocortisone Triamcinolone Fluocinonide	Effective for inflammatory dermatoses, the mainstay of topical therapy	May cause atrophy and sensitivity May cause adrenal suppression
Anesthetics	Camphor Pramoxine Benzocaine Emla (lidocaine and prilocaine)	May provide excellent adjunctive pruritus relief Do not cause atrophy or adrenal suppression	Potentially sensitizing
Antihistamines	Diphenhydramine (Benadryl) Doxepin (Sinequan)	May provide excellent adjunctive pruritus relief Do not cause atrophy or adrenal suppression	Potentially sedating and sensitizing
Cooling agents	Calamine Menthol Alcohol	May be soothing and cooling	Calamine leaves visible film Alcohol dries the skin
Miscellaneous	Coal tar Capsaicin (Zostrix)	Coal tar has excellent anti-inflammatory activity Capsaicin works differently from other agents	Tar is not elegant and stains Capsaicin may burn

topical therapeutic agents available and their relative merits.

ORAL TREATMENT

Great care must be taken when prescribing systemic medications. Nevertheless, in patients with pruritus that interferes with sleep, oral antipruritic agents may prove important in symptomatic relief. Antihistamines such as hydroxyzine and diphenhydramine not only are antipruritic but also have important central nervous system effects. Occasionally, memory impairment or impaired psychomotor function may result from their administration. Both hydroxyzine (Atarax) and diphenhydramine (Benadryl) may be administered to adults in doses ranging from 10 mg at bedtime to 50 mg four times daily depending on patient tolerance.

Doxepin (Sinequan),* a tricyclic antidepressant, at doses ranging from 10 to 100 mg every bedtime, may also be an effective agent for the treatment of refractory pruritus. Doxepin may exacerbate glaucoma and urinary retention.

All these agents may also cause drowsiness, postural hypotension, and cardiac disturbances.

In conditions other than urticaria, the nonsedating antihistamines may have only marginal therapeutic effect. Urticaria generally responds to most of the systemic antihistamines. Because around-the-clock histamine blockade is desirable, nonsedating antihistamines including astemizole (Hismanal) and terfenadine (Seldane) are first-line agents. Because of potentially serious cardiac arrhythmias, these agents should not be used in patients also taking systemic agents, including antifungal agents and erythromycin.

Systemic corticosteroids for pruritus are often highly effective, but their use is problematic. Prednisone and methylprednisolone are well known to exacerbate hypertension, diabetes, fluid retention, and osteoporosis. Systemic corticosteroids are particularly effective for brief periods for allergic or irritant contact dermatitis. More prolonged use may induce adverse sequelae.

PHYSICAL TREATMENT MODALITIES

Ultraviolet A (UVA), ultraviolet B (UVB), and psoralen photochemotherapy (PUVA) have been successfully employed in a wide range of pruritic disorders, from psoriasis and atopic dermatitis to the pruritus of renal failure. Because of its high degree of efficacy, UVB has become the treatment of choice for uremic pruritus in some centers, including the author's own.

TINNITUS

method of
ROBERT P. GREEN, M.D.
Mount Sinai School of Medicine
New York, New York

Tinnitus is an abnormal perception of sound that is localized within the head or ears. Tinnitus can range from a

*Not FDA approved for this indication.

minor annoyance to a disabling symptom complex. Often patients are fearful of the presence of a brain tumor, and this, in fact, may not be unfounded. It is estimated that over 12 million Americans suffer from severe tinnitus that is disabling in quality. Some degree of tinnitus is common in many millions more.

Two general types of tinnitus may be defined.

1. *Objective tinnitus* may be heard by an observer, often with a stethoscope, as well as by the patient. The cause is often vascular or neuromuscular. Vascular lesions such as glomus tumors, arteriovenous malformations, and turbulent venous or arterial flow must be considered and appropriate radiographic and vascular studies performed. Besides computed tomography (CT) scanning with contrast, magnetic resonance angiography (MRA) can be very helpful in defining vascular lesions that may be a source of objective tinnitus. Traditional angiography may be appropriate when a vascular lesion appears to be present. Myoclonic contractions of the palate, stapedius, or tensor tympani muscles may also present as objective tinnitus but are easily distinguished by the lack of correlation to the arterial pulse. Therapy is often successful and is generally surgical and directed at eliminating the offending lesion.

2. *Subjective tinnitus* (that heard only by the patient) is unfortunately far more common and less amenable to treatment. Establishing the cause, however, is paramount in providing reassurance and, at times, therapeutic intervention. Conductive hearing deficits will often be associated with tinnitus. The correction of these problems, thus improving hearing, will often mask out an underlying tinnitus, making it imperceptible. Therefore, correction of a cerumen impaction, drainage of a middle ear effusion, or performance of a stapedectomy in an otosclerotic patient will often provide dramatic relief.

The most difficult cases, however, are those associated with inner ear hearing loss or no identifiable hearing loss at all. Benign, age-related hearing loss, ototoxicity, noise-induced hearing loss, and Meniere's disease must be distinguished from cerebellopontine angle tumors.

In addition to obtaining routine audiometry, it cannot be emphasized too strongly that a detailed neuro-otologic work-up is essential, including a CT scan or magnetic resonance imaging (MRI) to rule out a cerebellopontine angle tumor. At present, auditory brain stem response represents an accurate and useful screening examination, particularly if routine audiometry reveals asymmetrical hearing loss or retrocochlear signs. There should, however, be no hesitation to obtain an MRI scan with the infusion of intravenous gadolinium, as this is highly accurate in detecting even small acoustic neuromas or related lesions. A detailed blood work-up should include at least a Venereal Disease Research Laboratory–fluorescent treponemal antibody (VDRL–FTA) and serologic tests to help identify those patients with neurosyphilis or autoimmune sensorineural hearing loss, both of which can be helped with conventional medical therapy. Lyme titers, thyroid function tests, and serum glucose complete an appropriate evaluation.

TREATMENT

Most often, the tinnitus patient has an identifiable sensorineural hearing loss caused by age, noise, or ototoxicity. Tinnitus can often be relieved by amplifying environmental sounds to mask out the perception of tinnitus. A hearing aid during the day may be effective in this regard and the use of an FM radio tuned between stations may help patients fall asleep. Mixed success has been obtained using the tinnitus masker. This device, worn like a hearing aid, provides a band of noise that masks out the tinnitus without interfering with the speech frequencies. Biofeedback has proved to be a useful technique by shifting body awareness away from the tinnitus.

It is becoming increasingly clear that certain forms of tinnitus represent spontaneous neural activity probably originating at the brain stem level. With this in mind, limited success has been obtained using a variety of centrally acting medications including anticonvulsants, antidepressants, and anxiety-reducing agents. There is unquestionably a strong association of depression with severity of tinnitus. At times, therefore, the help of a psychiatrist may be in order.

Pharmacotherapy at present consists of conventional trial doses of phenobarbital,* carbamazepine (Tegretol),* amitriptyline (Elavil),* or benzodiazepines such as alprazolam (Xanax).* Carbamazepine may be given as a starting dose of 100 mg at night to a maximum of 200 mg three times a day, increasing by 100 mg each week. Complete blood counts as well as renal and hepatic function must be monitored. Alprazolam may be given as 0.5 mg at night, increasing to 0.5 mg three times a day in gradual increments.

The converse of administering centrally acting medications is the elimination of medications that may be likely causes of tinnitus. Included for consideration would be salicylates, quinine, psychoactive drugs, and any other medication whose initiation coincides with the onset of tinnitus.

When all is said and done, many patients respond to simple reassurance following a thorough investigation to rule out a serious problem. A referral to the American Tinnitus Association (503-248-9985) can provide additional support via newsletters and up-to-date literature.

LOW BACK PAIN

method of
KENNETH J. KOPACZ, M.D., and
CASEY K. LEE, M.D.
New Jersey Medical School
Newark, New Jersey

An estimated 50% of working-age people admit to back symptoms, and 1% of the U.S. population is chronically disabled because of back symptoms. Back pain is a common presenting symptom in patients seen by their primary care physician and the most common presentation to the orthopedic surgeon. The cost of back disease in both economic and psychosocial terms is tremendous. Estimates of the cost of back pain in the United States range from $20 to $50 billion annually.

The natural history of acute low back pain (LBP) has

---

*Not FDA-approved for this indication.

been documented by studies in the United Kingdom, Sweden, and Rochester, New York. The episode appears to be self-limited in the majority of patients. The mean duration for return to work is 20 to 30 days, and 44% of patients will be better in 1 week. However, a small subset of patients (approximately 8%) proceed to have chronic LBP, defined as that lasting for more than 7 to 12 weeks. This group utilizes 80 to 90% of the costs related to LBP.

Several factors have been investigated relating to back pain. Aerobic exercise seems to have a benefit in both prevention and treatment. Cigarette smoking has been shown to be a significant risk factor for LBP as well as sciatica. Occupation also has a detrimental effect on the risk for LBP, especially related to recovery. This is due not only to heavy occupation but also to factors such as dissatisfaction with work, poor interactions between employer and employee, and unpleasant and noisy work environments.

EVALUATION

Initial evaluation should include a thorough history and physical examination focusing on the presence of atypical findings such as constitutional symptoms, recent trauma, history of cancer, alcohol or drug abuse, severe back or bilateral leg pain, bowel or bladder complaints, pain at rest, neuromotor deficits, or age under 15 or over 50 years. Patients with a typical presentation do not need initial diagnostic studies for the first 4 weeks while undergoing nonoperative therapy.

Radiography, computed tomography (CT) scan, or magnetic resonance imaging (MRI) is indicated for initial failure of treatment or for atypical presentation. The results of these imaging studies reveal a high incidence of positive findings in both the symptomatic and the asymptomatic population. The radiographic results need to be correlated to the physical findings in each patient to increase diagnostic accuracy.

The Quebec Task Force Report in 1987 categorized back problems into 11 classes based on patients' signs and symptoms (Table 1). This classification allows the treating physician to easily group patients for treatment and acknowledges that most patients do not have a verifiable structural abnormality. The report also evaluates many treatment categories according to the scientific efficacy determined in the literature.

TREATMENT

Bed Rest

Rest is the treatment most frequently prescribed for back pain. Most people are symptomatically improved at rest, and studies of intradiskal pressure have shown decreases in the supine position. Bed rest for a brief period (2 days) has been shown to be as effective as longer periods. Short periods of bed rest have no effect on natural history; however, prolonged rest seems to slow return to "usual activities."

Exercise

Nonoperative therapy is the hallmark of initial treatment of LBP. Since the natural history is self-limited, therapy is directed at symptomatic relief. Scientific evaluation of these treatments is difficult owing to the problems with defining therapeutic endpoints and blinded evaluation of treatment. Several treatments—including traction, acupuncture, biofeedback, the use of corsets or braces, and trigger point injections—although widely used, do not have any scientific validation.

There is consensus that active programs with direct patient involvement play a major role in the treatment of acute LBP. However, the specific type of exercise program is controversial. The most widely known is an isometric flexion program described by Williams. The principle is to open the intervertebral foramen with flexion and also to strengthen the abdominal musculature to act as an internal corset. McKenzie emphasized an exercise regimen individualized to the patient's symptoms. This program primarily relies on extension movements; however, it can be altered depending on the patient's response. Extension exercises may exacerbate the symptoms of patients with lumbar stenosis or facet joint syndromes. Aerobic exercise has a preventive effect on LBP, but the therapeutic effect in acute situations has not been properly evaluated. Nevertheless, aerobic conditioning exercises will theoretically benefit patients with acute low back symptoms.

Medications

Narcotic analgesics such as codeine are often useful in the acute setting. Their use should be limited to a very short period because of their addictive nature and decreasing efficacy in chronic syndromes. Furthermore, the depressant effect of narcotics may create psychological maladjustment.

Nonsteroidal anti-inflammatory drugs (NSAIDs) are another class of medications useful in the treatment of LBP. Several studies document their benefit over placebo. Theoretically, they act as both analgesic

TABLE 1. **Quebec Task Force Classification for Disorders of the Lumbar Spine**

Class	Symptoms
1	Pain without radiation
2	Pain with radiation to extremity, proximally
3	Pain with radiation to extremity, distally
4	Pain with radiation to upper/lower limb, neurologic signs
5	Presumptive compression of a spinal nerve root on a simple roentgenogram
6	Compression of a spinal nerve root confirmed by special imaging techniques or other diagnostic studies
7	Spinal stenosis
8	Postsurgical status, 1–6 months after intervention
9	Postsurgical status, >6 months after intervention 9.1 Asymptomatic 9.2 Symptomatic
10	Chronic pain syndrome
11	Other diagnoses

From Report of the Quebec Task Force on Spinal Disorders. Scientific approach to the assessment and management of activity-related spinal disorders. A monograph for clinicians. Spine 12(Suppl):S1–S59, 1987.

and anti-inflammatory agents in the acute process. No NSAID has been shown to be more effective than aspirin; however, they often have fewer side effects.

Muscle relaxants have not been shown to be any more effective than NSAIDs. Also, the side effects of drowsiness and addiction limit their usefulness. Oral corticosteroids and tricyclic antidepressants have not been shown to be efficacious in the acute setting.

Epidural Injections

The use of epidural steroid injections has not been proved efficacious in rigorous scientific studies. However, they are widely used and seem to be beneficial in a subset of patients for the treatment of lumbar disk disease.

CHRONIC LOW BACK PAIN

Patients with chronic low back problems often need a team approach to evaluation and treatment. The surgeon, the rehabilitation physician, the anesthesiologist trained in pain management, and often a psychologist work together to evaluate the patient. Psychological testing may be a useful adjunct to the therapies already discussed.

PATIENT EDUCATION

Patients with LBP deserve adequate information concerning their symptoms. Discussion of natural history, methods of symptom control, activity modifi-cation, and further diagnostic avenues for persistent symptoms helps to allay patients' fears and may reduce the utilization of medical resources and encourage compliance with treatment. This may be accomplished through multiple media including printed material, audiovisual tapes, and direct patient discussion.

"Back school," a formal education program for patients with low back disorders, is useful especially in the industrial setting. This training allows patients to understand disorders of the back, proper posture and body mechanics, and protection of the low back in various activities. Although the data concerning efficacy are confusing, it appears these programs have at least a positive short-term effect on low back disorders.

SURGERY

Absolute surgical indications in lumbar disk disease are progressive neurologic deficit and a cauda equina syndrome. Patients with signs and symptoms of a disk herniation consistent with their imaging studies may also be candidates for surgical decompression after an adequate trial of nonsurgical therapy lasting at least 4 to 6 weeks. Surgical results for patients with herniated disks show short-term benefits, but after 4 years, the two groups have similar results. Spinal fusion in acute disk herniation has been shown to be unnecessary. However, spinal fusion for LBP in patients with degenerative disk disease may be beneficial.

The Infectious Diseases

MANAGEMENT OF THE PATIENT WITH HUMAN IMMUNODEFICIENCY VIRUS DISEASE

method of
DAVID ALTARAC, M.D., M.P.A., and
BRIAN S. KOLL, M.D.
*Beth Israel Medical Center in affiliation with the
Albert Einstein College of Medicine of Yeshiva
University*
New York, New York

Since the epidemic first appeared in the early 1980s, the World Health Organization (WHO) estimates that 16 million adults and 1 million children have been infected with the human immunodeficiency virus (HIV), the virus that causes acquired immune deficiency syndrome (AIDS). Estimates are that the number of full-blown cases of AIDS worldwide increased to 4 million in 1994. At the current rate, between 30 and 40 million people will have been infected with HIV by the end of the century. HIV infection, once thought to be a medical enigma affecting only a small subset of the population, has become a pandemic of global proportions with social, biologic, economic, cultural, and ethical implications for the entire world.

EPIDEMIOLOGY

The epidemiology of AIDS is changing. Sub-Saharan Africa continues to account for the highest number of cases, with 33.5% of reported cases in 1994. However, the global pandemic is now spreading in Asia faster than anywhere else in the world. Parts of Asia, particularly the more populous areas, have experienced an eightfold increase in rates in 1994. In Thailand, about one-fifth of military recruits in a northern province were HIV-infected, and in another province, 8% of women attending prenatal clinics carried the virus. Although these figures are alarming, the numbers are vastly underestimated because there is a huge discrepancy between reported and estimated cases owing to underdiagnosis and incomplete reporting, especially in developing countries.

The United States accounts for 42% of the reported cases but represents only 10% of the overall global estimates. In 1993, there were 105,990 reported cases of AIDS in the United States. AIDS still affects homosexual men more than any other risk group in the United States. However, the incidence is increasing in the heterosexual population because of unsafe sexual practices and injection drug use. The proportion of AIDS cases linked with heterosexual transmission has increased from 26% in 1986 to 36% in 1991. Approximately 34% of all cases of AIDS in adults have occurred in either injection drug users or in their sexual partners.

Curtailment of some high-risk behaviors has resulted in an initial decline and then a leveling off of new case rates among homosexual men. The risk of infection from contaminated blood products has also been reduced over the past decade. However, the epidemic is progressing in large urban areas in the United States, and a large upward trend in rates is seen disproportionately in women and ethnic minorities. Of the 105,990 cases in 1993, 58,538 (55%) were diagnosed among racial or ethnic minorities; 66% were African American, 32% Hispanic, 1% Asian or Pacific Islander, and 1% American Indian or Alaskan natives. African Americans were disproportionately affected by HIV. The AIDS rate for African American females was 15 times greater than for white females, and the rate for African American males was five times that for white males. Among children less than 13 years of age, 84% of cases were among racial or ethnic minorities.

PATHOPHYSIOLOGY

In 1984, HIV-1 was shown to be the etiologic agent of AIDS. Since then, another retrovirus, HIV-2, has also been found to infect humans and cause AIDS. HIV-2 is most frequently found in infected persons from West Africa but has been found in persons with AIDS in the United States, Europe, and South America. HIV-2 has been molecularly cloned and characterized, and shows a 40 to 50% nucleoside sequence homology to HIV-1. HIV-1 and HIV-2 are RNA viruses that have an affinity for cells expressing the CD4 lymphocyte receptor. CD4 lymphocytes (T helper cells), a key component of cell-mediated immunity, are depleted by HIV infection, leading to the profound immunologic defects that are the hallmark of AIDS.

HIV is not spread by casual contact. It is spread through intimate sexual contact or by parenteral contact with blood or body fluids infected with the virus. Incidental transmission through saliva, tears, minor bites, scratches, or insect bites has no solid scientific support. Anecdotal reports have implicated the sharing of toothbrushes or razor blades as risks for the spread of the virus. Once inoculated, HIV infects and begins to replicate in susceptible cells, predominantly CD4 lymphocytes and macrophages, but also epithelial cells of the gastrointestinal tract, uterine cervical cells, and glial cells of the nervous system.

Once HIV is within the macrophage, it remains undetected by the body's immune surveillance system and replicates freely. Thus the macrophage can serve as both a haven and a reservoir for HIV. It also appears that macrophage function is impaired. Macrophages can introduce HIV to the brain and contribute to the AIDS dementia complex. HIV also infects myeloid monocyte precursor cells in the bone marrow. This is believed to contribute to the pancytopenia seen in patients with AIDS. B cell impairment, as well as functional impairment of neutrophils, is also seen in patients infected with HIV. Poor antibody responses are apparently due to a breakdown in CD4 lymphocytes' ability to inform B cells to produce specific antibody. The reason for the functional impairment of neutrophils is not clear.

NATURAL HISTORY

Within a few weeks after infection, HIV replicates to a level at which it produces detectable viral antigens and elicits host antibody production. During this period, the patient may have an acute "flulike" syndrome known as the "acute retroviral syndrome." Patients may present with fever, sweats, malaise, myalgias, anorexia, nausea, diarrhea, and a nonexudative pharyngitis. Other symptoms may include headaches, photophobia, and meningismus associated with a truncal maculopapular rash. Aseptic meningitis, peripheral neuropathy, or an ascending polyneuropathy (Guillain-Barré syndrome) has also been described.

As the host mounts an immune response, viral antigen is neutralized and disappears or is detected at low levels. The patient is usually asymptomatic and may remain so for weeks to months to years. During this time, approximately 50 to 70% of infected individuals develop persistent generalized lymphadenopathy (PGL), which is defined as the presence of two or more extrainguinal sites of lymphadenopathy for a minimum of 3 to 6 months for which no other explanation can be found. The most frequent sites of involvement include the posterior and anterior cervical nodes; the submandibular, occipital, and axillary chains; and the epitrochlear and femoral nodes. Biopsy specimens of these sites reveal a follicular hyperplasia without specific pathogens.

In most cases, although the infected individual exists in a clinically latent state, viral replication progresses at differing rates. As viral replication continues, there is progressive destruction of CD4 lymphocytes, either directly or by syncytial formation, and macrophage dysfunction. The combination of CD4 depletion and macrophage destruction leads to abnormal activation of other immune mechanisms resulting in B cell dysfunction manifested by hypergammaglobulinemia and thrombocytopenia. There are also abnormal cytotoxic T cell responses.

As the immune system deteriorates, the host is less able to slow the progression of HIV replication, resulting in further CD4 lymphocyte depletion. Antibodies to HIV antigen become undetectable and HIV antigens reappear. The clinical syndrome observed depends on the degree of immunosuppression. Studies have shown a strong association between the development of life-threatening opportunistic illnesses and the absolute number or percentage of CD4 lymphocytes. As the CD4 lymphocyte count decreases, the risk and severity of opportunistic infections increases. An overwhelming opportunistic infection can result in death.

Classification of Disease

In 1993, the Centers for Disease Control and Prevention (CDC) revised its classification system for HIV infection in adolescents and adults to include clinical conditions associated with HIV infection and CD4 lymphocyte counts (Table 1). Infection with HIV should be considered an evolving process from asymptomatic carriage of the virus to full-blown AIDS as defined by the CDC, with a number of intermediate stages referred to as "AIDS-related complex" (ARC). The clinical approach toward managing patients infected with HIV includes the prevention of infection, the management of asymptomatic infection and ARC, and the management of AIDS-associated opportunistic infections and neoplasms and other medical conditions.

TABLE 1. Centers for Disease Control and Prevention Surveillance Criteria for the Diagnosis of Acquired Immune Deficiency Syndrome

I. Without laboratory evidence of human immunodeficiency virus (HIV) infection and with definitive evidence of
  Candidiasis of the esophagus, trachea, bronchi, or lungs
  Cryptococcosis, extrapulmonary cryptosporidiosis with diarrhea lasting >1 month
  Herpes simplex esophagitis, bronchitis, pneumonitis; or mucocutaneous disease for >1 month
  Cytomegalovirus disease of an organ other than liver, spleen, or lymph nodes in a patient >1 month of age
  Kaposi's sarcoma in a patient <60 years of age
  Primary brain lymphoma in a patient <60 years of age
  Lymphoid interstitial pneumonia in a patient <13 years of age
  Disseminated *Mycobacterium avium* complex or *M. kansasii* disease
  Pneumocystis carinii pneumonia
  Progressive multifocal leukoencephalopathy
  Toxoplasmosis of the brain in a patient >1 month of age
II. With laboratory evidence of HIV infection and
  A CD4 T lymphocyte count <200 cells per mm^3
  Pulmonary or extrapulmonary tuberculosis
  Any mycobacterial disease caused by mycobacteria other than *Mycobacterium tuberculosis* disseminated at a site other than or in addition to lungs, skin, or cervical or hilar lymph nodes
  Recurrent pneumonia within a 12-month period
  Recurrent *Salmonella* sp septicemia
  Multiple infections with encapsulated or pyogenic bacteria in a child <13 years of age
  Invasive cervical cancer
  Kaposi's sarcoma
  Lymphoma of the brain
  Other lymphomas of B cell or unknown phenotype
  Coccidioidomycosis, disseminated at a site other than or in addition to the lungs or cervical or hilar lymph nodes
  Histoplasmosis, disseminated at a site other than or in addition to the lungs or cervical or hilar lymph nodes
  HIV encephalopathy
  HIV wasting syndrome
  Isosporiasis with diarrhea persisting >1 month
  Recurrent salpingitis
III. Presumptive diagnosis of
  Esophageal candidiasis
  Cytomegalovirus retinitis with loss of vision
  P. carinii pneumonia
  Toxoplasmosis of the brain in a patient >1 month of age
  Disseminated mycobacterial disease (no culture)
  Lymphoid interstitial pneumonia in a child <13 years of age
  Kaposi's sarcoma

Surrogate Markers

Surrogate tests that are often performed in persons with HIV infection include serum beta$_2$ microglobulin, neopterin, and p24 antigen levels, as well as measures of delayed-type hypersensitivity (DTH). Such tests are of limited clinical utility, and the precise use of these markers is not yet clear.

Levels of beta$_2$ microglobulin, a low-molecular-weight immunoglobulin found on the surface of all nucleated cells, are elevated in HIV infection. Elevations are most often seen in persons with advanced HIV disease. Some studies have shown that HIV-infected persons with elevated levels of beta$_2$ microglobulin are at increased risk of progressing to AIDS.

Neopterin is excreted in high amounts from human monocytes/macrophages responding to stimulation with interferon-gamma and thus is seen in the serum of individuals infected with viral illnesses. It has been found in increased amounts in the serum and urine of patients with HIV disease.

A major structural core protein of HIV is the p24 antigen. Viremia is associated with high levels of p24 antigen. When antibodies to viral core and envelope proteins appear, p24 antigen is no longer detectable. Increasing levels of p24 antigen, with concomitant decreasing levels of p24 antibody, correlate with the progression of HIV disease and indicate a poor prognosis. The p24 antigen has been used in clinical studies to monitor the efficacy of drug treatments. Other clinical uses for p24 antigen have not been developed.

In addition to increases in levels of beta$_2$ microglobulin, neopterin, and p24 antigen, elevations in levels of acid-labile interferon-alpha and alpha$_1$-thymosine have been reported in persons with AIDS. Elevations of levels of these compounds are also of unknown clinical significance.

The absence of a response to skin test antigens (skin test anergy) purified protein derivative (PPD) of tuburculin, *Candida,* mumps, tetanus toxoid, and/or *Trichophyton* indicates an abnormality in DTH. Decreasing levels of CD4 lymphocytes have been correlated with decreased DTH. Conversely, the presence of skin test anergy may indicate low levels of CD4 lymphocytes, placing the individual at high risk of acquiring an opportunistic infection.

Idiopathic CD4 Lymphocytopenia

Recently, individuals with profound and progressive CD4 lymphocyte depletion and opportunistic infections, alone or with Kaposi's sarcoma, and with AIDS risk factors but without evidence of HIV-1 or HIV-2 by serologic tests or culture, have been reported. This syndrome is called "idiopathic CD4 lymphocytopenia" (ICL). Most cases of ICL have been reported in the United States. Initial studies show that in contrast to those with HIV infection, persons with ICL have a relatively good prognosis with stable CD4 lymphocyte counts. The case definition is as follows: (1) a CD4 lymphocyte count less than 300 cells per mm^3 or less than 20% on more than one determination; (2) no laboratory evidence of HIV infection; and (3) no defined immunodeficiency or therapy associated with CD4 lymphopenia. Individuals suspected of having ICL should be referred to the CDC for further evaluation.

MANAGEMENT OF ASYMPTOMATIC INFECTION

Individuals with known HIV infection may be completely asymptomatic on presentation. Alternatively, individuals without prior HIV testing may present with complications of HIV infection. The most common findings on initial evaluation are shown in Table 2. Any individual who demonstrates any of these clinical findings should be recommended for HIV testing.

HIV Testing

HIV testing is voluntary and should include informed consent along with appropriate pretest and post-test counseling. When HIV infection is suspected, an enzyme-linked immunosorbent assay (ELISA) should be used as a screening test for HIV antibody. If a positive test is obtained, it should be

TABLE 2. **Common Clinical Findings on Initial Evaluation**

Persistent generalized lymphadenopathy
Cytopenias including anemia, leukopenia, and/or
   thrombocytopenia
Pneumocystis carinii pneumonia
Kaposi's sarcoma
Localized candidal infections, especially of the oropharynx
   (thrush) and esophagus and recurrent or refractory vaginal
   infections
Constitutional symptoms including fevers, weight loss, night
   sweats, and persistent diarrhea
Bacterial infections, including recurrent pneumococcal
   pneumonias, *Haemophilus influenzae* infections, and
   Salmonella bacteremias
Tuberculosis
Sexually transmitted diseases, particularly those causing genital
   ulcers such as syphilis, herpes simplex, and chancroid
Neurologic syndromes, most commonly dementia and peripheral
   neuropathies

confirmed with a Western blot. False-positive and false-negative tests results for both the ELISA and the Western blot are rare. Periodic testing is recommended every 6 to 12 months for individuals who test negative but continue to practice high-risk behaviors.

Initial Screening

The usual baseline evaluation of the HIV-infected individual should include (1) a complete blood cell count (CBC) with differential and platelet count, (2) a chemistry panel (Sequential Multiple Analyzer [SMA] 12, 14, 20), (3) a CD4 lymphocyte count and percentage, (4) a PPD and anergy test using two of the skin test antigens *Candida albicans,* mumps, tetanus toxoid, and *Trichophyton,* (5) a Venereal Disease Research Laboratory (VDRL) test or rapid plasma reagin (RPR), (6) a chest x-ray examination, (7) serologic tests for anti–hepatitis B surface antigen or anti–hepatitis B core antigen if the patient is being considered for vaccination, and tests for hepatitis B surface antigen and anti–hepatitis C virus if the person has abnormal liver function tests suggesting chronic hepatitis, (8) toxoplasmosis serologic tests (immunoglobulin G [IgG]), and (9) a Pap smear for all women regardless of age.

A follow-up evaluation is recommended 1 to 2 weeks after the initial evaluation to review the laboratory findings, provide further counseling, and develop an acceptable treatment plan for the patient.

Measurements of CD4 T lymphocyte counts are pivotal in the evaluation and are used to guide clinical and therapeutic management of HIV-infected persons, particularly the initiation of antimicrobial prophylaxis and antiretroviral therapy. Antimicrobial prophylaxis and antiretroviral therapy have been shown to be most effective at certain levels of immune dysfunction. Antiretroviral therapy is usually initiated at CD4 T lymphocyte counts of less than 500 cells per mm^3. As the CD4 T lymphocyte count declines, the patient becomes more susceptible to opportunistic infections, and prophylaxis against certain microorganisms is warranted.

Antiretroviral Therapy

Antiretroviral therapy has been shown to retard HIV replication but does not kill the virus. Since 1985, several clinical trials of antiretroviral agents have demonstrated benefits for patients infected with HIV. These benefits include (1) improved short-term survival in patients with CD4 T lymphocyte counts less than 200 cells per mm³, (2) improvement in neurologic function for some patients treated with zidovudine, (3) modest and transient increases in CD4 T lymphocyte counts in some patients, (4) a decrease in viral titers in the blood, for a period of time, (5) increased energy and weight gain in some patients, and (6) a reduction in the transmission of HIV from mothers to their neonates, decreasing vertical transmission in some women treated with zidovudine.

There are presently four licensed antiretroviral agents approved for the therapy of HIV infection: zidovudine (ZDV, AZT, Retrovir), dideoxyinosine (ddI), didanosine (Videx), dideoxycytidine (ddC, zalcitabine [Hivid]), and d4T (stavudine [Zerit]). Before antiretroviral therapy is initiated, CD4 T lymphocyte counts should be determined by two separate assays, at least 1 week apart. Two assays are needed because of the substantial variation in CD4 T lymphocyte counts that can occur because of analytic variation, seasonal and diurnal fluctuations, and other causes such as intercurrent illnesses or corticosteroid therapy. If CD4 T lymphocyte counts are greater than 500 cells per mm³, the patient should not be started on antiretroviral therapy. T cell subset counts should be followed every 4 to 6 months.

There has been some controversy as to when to begin antiretroviral therapy. Several U.S. studies suggest a benefit for patients with CD4 T lymphocyte counts between 200 and 500 cells per mm³, whereas a recent European (Concorde) study did not show a similar benefit. The conclusion made from the Concorde study was that the early use of AZT offers no additional advantage over deferred use among asymptomatic patients with greater than 200 CD4 cells per mm³ in delaying the progression to AIDS, ARC, or death over 3 years. A benefit for patients with CD4 T lymphocyte counts less than 200 cells per mm³ is generally agreed on. Because of the different conclusions from these studies, a patient may be observed without therapy if the patient is asymptomatic, has CD4 T lymphocyte counts between 200 and 500 cells per mm³, is clinically well, and is stable over time. Antiretroviral therapy should be started if clinical or laboratory deterioration occurs. If a patient is symptomatic with CD4 T lymphocyte counts between 200 and 500 cells per mm³, or has a history of an opportunistic infection regardless of CD4 T lymphocyte counts, antiretroviral therapy should be started.

AZT has been the cornerstone of antiretroviral therapy and is usually the initial agent that is started. It is a thymidine analogue that inhibits the in vitro replication of HIV by blocking the viral enzyme reverse transcriptase. The suggested dose is 500 to 600 mg per day (100 mg orally every 4 hours while awake or 200 mg orally every 8 hours). CBCs should be monitored monthly for the first 3 months. If no toxicity is seen, the frequency of CBCs can be decreased to every 3 months thereafter. Higher doses may be indicated for HIV-associated thrombocytopenia or HIV-related encephalopathy. The lowest dose that has been found to have antiretroviral activity is 300 mg a day.

Early toxicities of AZT include nausea, vomiting, dyspepsia, malaise, and headaches. Symptoms usually occur during the first few weeks of therapy and tend to be self-limited. Elevations of levels of liver transaminases, alkaline phosphatase, and bilirubin have also been reported. These elevations are generally not severe and do not require dose modification.

Bone marrow suppression is seen later with therapy and is the primary dose-limiting toxicity of AZT. Bone marrow suppression is thought to occur by suppression of cellular thymidine metabolism, DNA polymerase, and DNA synthesis. Some patients with AIDS and AZT-induced anemia have a suboptimal compensatory erythropoietin level response. Controlled trials have demonstrated a benefit from exogenous recombinant erythropoietin for those persons with serum erythropoietin levels less than 500 IU per liter. Granulocyte-macrophage colony-stimulating factor (GM-CSF, sargramostim [Leukine]) and granulocyte colony-stimulating factor (G-CSF, filgrastim [Neupogen]) are being studied as adjuvant agents for patients with AZT-induced neutropenia.

Long-term (greater than 1 year) AZT use has been associated with the development of myocyte mitochondrial toxicity resulting in clinical myopathy. The use of AZT for more than 6 months in patients with advanced AIDS has led to the recovery of virus isolates resistant in vitro to AZT. Resistance develops less often in patients with fewer HIV-related symptoms and higher CD4 T lymphocyte counts. It is felt that patients with resistant isolates may have a more rapid clinical deterioration. These isolates may remain sensitive to other antiretroviral agents.

Despite the proven benefits of AZT, patients infected with HIV have disease progression over time. These patients should be evaluated for other antiretroviral therapy. The drug ddI has a mechanism of action similar to that of AZT but a different toxicity profile. The two primary toxicities associated with ddI are peripheral neuropathy and acute pancreatitis. The peripheral neuropathy seen with ddI therapy is common but usually not severe. Persons who develop this complication complain of numbness, tingling, or painful extremities. Symptoms generally improve with the discontinuation of the medicine, and some patients tolerate lower doses of the agent. Pancreatitis occurs less often and can be subclinical. A prior history of pancreatitis or excessive alcohol use should be considered a relative contraindication to ddI therapy. Therapy with ddI should also be withheld during treatment with pentamidine to minimize the development of pancreatitis. Neurologic examinations and laboratory evaluations of amylase and lipase levels should be done monthly to monitor for the development of these two toxicities.

Currently, ddI is approved for adults who have advanced AIDS and who are intolerant to or failing to respond to therapy with AZT. Therapeutic failure is considered to be the development of significant clinical or immunologic deterioration while receiving treatment with AZT. The drug ddI may also benefit patients who have received AZT for 4 months or longer and have CD4 T lymphocyte counts less than 300 cells per mm^3. Doses are based on weights in adults and are presented in Table 3. To date no data exist to guide the use of ddI in asymptomatic patients or those with CD4 T lymphocyte counts greater than 200 cells per mm^3. Further studies with ddI alone and in combination with AZT therapy are continuing. Resistant HIV isolates have been recovered after 6 months of therapy with ddI. As with AZT, patients with these resistant isolates may have a more rapid clinical deterioration.

The drug ddC is presently approved for monotherapy and combination therapy with AZT. Studies have shown that monotherapy with ddC has equal or more benefit than monotherapy with AZT. The side effects seen with ddC are similar to those seen with ddI but occur less often. Other adverse effects seen with ddC include transient aphthous mouth ulcers, skin eruptions, arthralgias, and fever. These early side effects are usually self-limited.

The drug ddC should be considered as monotherapy or combination therapy with AZT in adults with advanced HIV infection (CD4 T lymphocyte counts less than 300 cells per mm^3) who have developed significant clinical or immunologic deterioration while receiving AZT monotherapy. The dosage of ddC is 0.75 mg orally every 8 hours with AZT 200 mg orally every 8 hours (see Table 3). If side effects develop with ddC, 0.375 mg orally every 8 hours

may be used. As with the other antiretroviral agents, resistant viral isolates have been recovered.

The drug d4T is a newer nucleoside analogue reverse transcriptase inhibitor approved for use in advanced HIV infection in individuals (1) intolerant to other approved therapies, (2) who have experienced significant clinical or immunologic deterioration while receiving these therapies, or (3) for whom such therapies are contraindicated. The most common clinical toxicity associated with d4T is peripheral neuropathy, occurring in 15 to 21% of patients in controlled trials. As with the other agents, the neuropathy is reversible once the therapy is discontinued. Other adverse effects include chills, fever, nausea and vomiting, insomnia, and anorexia. For patients of greater than or equal to 60 kg, d4T is administered in doses of 40 mg orally every 12 hours; for those of less than 60 kg, 30 mgs given orally every 12 hours. Doses for all currently approved antiretrovirals are shown in Table 3.

The use of combination therapy with 2-dideoxynucleoside analogues that have differing toxicity profiles or with two agents of different classes and mechanisms of action is presently being evaluated. Preliminary data suggest that multidrug antiretroviral therapy is more effective in vitro at inhibiting replication of HIV compared with single-drug regimens. Combination therapy will likely provide the next major advancement in the treatment of HIV infection.

Vaccinations

Pneumococcal and influenza vaccines should be routinely given to patients with HIV infection. Other recommended vaccines include those against hepatitis B, *Haemophilus influenzae,* and childhood viral infections as well as vaccines recommended for travel. These vaccinations should be given early in the course of HIV infection to get optimal responses, preferably when the CD4 lymphocyte count is equal to or greater than 200 cells per mm^3.

Pneumococcal Vaccine

Pneumococcal pneumonia and pneumococcal bacteremia are increased 20 to 100 times in persons with HIV infection. Although the efficacy of pneumococcal vaccine is debated, it is considered cost-effective and is recommended for all persons with HIV infection according to the current guidelines.

Influenza Vaccine

Although there is little evidence that influenza is more frequent in HIV infection, the CDC recommends annual influenza vaccination for all HIV-infected persons. This is particularly true for HIV-infected persons who are over 65 years of age or likely to be in chronic care facilities or housed in congregate settings and for those with chronic cardiovascular or pulmonary disorders.

TABLE 3. **Recommended Dosages of Approved Antiretroviral Therapies**

Zidovudine (AZT, ZDV, Retrovir)

Adults	200 mg orally tid	

ddI (dideoxyinosine, didanosine, Videx)

	Weight (kg)	Tablets
Adults	75	300 mg bid
	50–74	200 mg bid
	35–49	125 mg bid

ddI may be given as monotherapy or with AZT 200 mg tid

ddC (dideoxycytidine, zalcitabine, Hivid)

Adults	0.75 mg orally tid

ddC may be given as monotherapy or with AZT 200 mg tid

d4T (stavudine, Zerit)

	Weight (kg)	Tablets
Adults	≥60	40 mg bid
	<60	30 mg bid

Haemophilus influenzae *Type B Vaccine*

Increased frequencies of *H. influenzae*-pneumonia and bacteremia are seen in advanced HIV disease. Although the efficacy of *H. influenzae* Type B vaccine in the adult population has not been demonstrated, some authors recommend considering it, especially in HIV-infected persons who have chronic lung disease or are otherwise predisposed to *H. influenzae* infections.

Hepatitis B

Hepatitis vaccination is advocated for persons who lack serologic evidence of hepatitis B markers and are in any of the following risk groups: active intravenous drug users, sexually active homosexual men, and sexual or household contacts of hepatitis B virus surface antigen (HBsAg) carriers. The usual serologic test to screen candidates is surface antibody. The usual regimen involves three serial vaccinations given at months 0, 1, and 6. Vaccinated patients should be tested for anti-HBsAg response 1 to 6 months after the third dose, and if no response is seen, one to three additional doses can be given.

Measles, Mumps, and Rubella Vaccinations

Live attenuated virus vaccines have not been shown to cause unusual side effects in HIV-infected persons, so the recommendation for vaccinations remains identical for patients with and without HIV infection. Measles vaccine is advocated for susceptible adults attending post–high school institutions and for medical personnel. Mumps vaccine is advocated for susceptible adults, especially men. Rubella vaccine is advocated for susceptible adults, especially nonpregnant women with childbearing potential.

Tetanus-Diphtheria

Tetanus-diphtheria (Td) vaccine can be safely given to adults according to standard practice. Booster vaccinations should be given every 10 years.

Polio

Oral polio vaccine (OPV) is a live-virus vaccine and should not be given to adults with HIV infection or their household contacts. The administration of inactivated polio vaccine (IPV) can safely be given to HIV-infected adults.

Travel

With the exception of live vaccines (yellow fever vaccine, OPV, live oral typhoid-Ty21a vaccine), recommendations are identical for patients with or without HIV infection. IPV, inactivated parenteral typhoid vaccine, and vaccines for cholera, rabies, Japanese B encephalitis, anthrax, plague, and meningococcal infection are considered safe.

OPPORTUNISTIC INFECTIONS

Opportunistic infections are the major cause of morbidity and mortality in patients infected with HIV. There should be a low threshold for obtaining a diagnosis to explain the relatively nonspecific signs and symptoms that can herald the onset of a new infection. Empirical therapy is discouraged, when possible, because of the high incidence of multiple infections, the diverse causes of various syndromes, and the toxicities that can occur with treatment. Although most infections are responsive to therapy, there is a high relapse rate, so chronic suppressive therapy and prophylaxis are important in the management of HIV-infected patients. Table 4 illustrates the common opportunistic pathogens seen in AIDS.

Parasitic Infections

Toxoplasma gondii

Neurologic disease occurs in up to 40% of patients with AIDS. Toxoplasmosis develops in 5 to 10% of patients with AIDS in the United States, and higher rates are seen in Europe, where there is a higher incidence of latent infection. *Toxoplasma gondii* is the most common cause of focal encephalitis in individuals infected with HIV, and in 99% of cases the encephalitis is due to reactivation of latent infection. The neurologic manifestations of toxoplasmosis include encephalitis, meningoencephalitis, and mass lesions, which can present as headache, fever, altered mental status, seizures, focal motor and sensory deficits, and coma. Pneumonia, pericarditis, chorioretinitis, and disseminated infection with *T. gondii* have also been reported.

Patients at risk of developing toxoplasmosis have elevated IgG titers representing past exposure to the parasite. The absence of IgG for *T. gondii* makes the diagnosis unlikely. As most patients do not mount a rising titer of IgG antibody because of defects in humoral immunity, serologic diagnosis of reactivated infection is difficult. Cerebrospinal fluid (CSF) is also often negative for antibody against *T. gondii*.

Computed tomography (CT) or magnetic resonance imaging (MRI) of the brain usually demonstrates multiple bilateral contrast-enhancing lesions in the cerebral hemispheres at the junction of the gray and white matter. Edema may or may not be present. Brain biopsy, looking for the tachyzoites of *T. gondii*, is the only certain way to make a definite diagnosis.

Empirical therapy may be required if the brain lesions are inaccessible or a brain biopsy contraindicated. In practice, empirical therapy is now the rule. Improvement with empirical therapy for a presumptive diagnosis of cerebral toxoplasmosis should be expected within 14 days of treatment. If there is no improvement or if the patient deteriorates, further attempts at making a tissue diagnosis should be reconsidered.

The standard therapy for toxoplasmosis includes pyrimethamine (Daraprim), 100 mg orally per day for 3 days, followed by 25 to 75 mg orally per day, and sulfadiazine, 4 grams orally as a loading dose followed by 6 to 8 grams in four divided doses every day. Folinic acid, 5 mg orally per day, is usually given

TABLE 4. **Opportunistic Infections in Acquired Immune Deficiency Syndrome**

Pathogen	Usual Clinical Presentation
Bacteria	
Mycobacterium tuberculosis	Pulmonary or extrapulmonary disease
M. avium complex	Dissemination
M. haemophilum	Skin or joint lesions, pneumonia
M. kansasii	Pulmonary disease
Streptococcus pneumoniae	Pneumonia, sinusitis
Haemophilus influenzae	Pneumonia, sinusitis
Staphylococcus aureus	Pneumonia
Salmonella typhimurium	Enteritis or dissemination
Treponema pallidum	Central nervous system infection
Rochalimaea spp	Skin or hepatic lesions
Rhodococcus equi	Pneumonia, central nervous system, skin lesions
Listeria monocytogenes	Disseminated disease, meningitis
Fungi	
Pneumocystis carinii	Pneumonia or dissemination
Candida albicans	Oral thrush, esophagitis
Cryptococcus neoformans	Dissemination
Histoplasma capsulatum	Dissemination
Coccidioides immitis	Dissemination
Aspergillus spp	Pneumonia
Protozoans	
Toxoplasma gondii	Brain mass lesion, encephalitis, chorioretinitis
Cryptosporidium	Chronic diarrhea
Isospora belli	Recurrent diarrhea
Microsporidia	Recurrent diarrhea
Viruses	
Cytomegalovirus	Chorioretinitis, pneumonitis, colitis, esophagitis, dissemination
Herpes simplex	Mucocutaneous ulcers, stomatitis
Varicella-zoster	Dissemination
Epstein-Barr	Lymphoma, oral hairy leukoplakia, lymphocytic interstitial pneumonitis
Papovavirus	Progressive multifocal leukoencephalopathy
Poxvirus	Molluscum contagiosum
Human immunodeficiency virus (HIV)	Acute retroviral syndrome, AIDS dementia, nephropathy, cardiomyopathy, cytopenias

to minimize bone marrow suppression from these agents. Other side effects include rash, fever, and gastrointestinal intolerance. Most reactions are due to sulfadiazine. Response rates are in the 90% range with this regimen in patients diagnosed early.

Alternatives to sulfadiazine include clindamycin (Cleocin), 900 mg orally three times daily, or dapsone, 100 mg orally per day. Pyrimethamine should be given with either agent. Other agents that may be effective include oral azithromycin (Zithromax), oral clarithromycin (Biaxin), oral atovaquone (Mepron), or intravenous trimetrexate. Oral trimethoprim-sulfamethoxazole (TMP–SMX) (Bactrim, Septra), given as prophylaxis against *Pneumocystis carinii* pneumonia, is felt to be adequate as prophylaxis against toxoplasmosis.

Lifelong maintenance therapy is required to prevent relapse of infection, as up to 80% of patients relapse after treatment is discontinued. Maintenance therapy is usually begun after 4 to 6 weeks of initial therapy and clinical and radiographic improvement is observed. Most clinicians use decreased doses of pyrimethamine, 50 mg daily, and sulfadiazine, 4 grams divided in four doses. With the exception of clindamycin, the efficacy of other agents has not been established. Pyrimethamine alone at doses of 50 mg per day and above has been successful as a maintenance dose.

Cryptosporidium

Cryptosporidiosis is caused by the protozoan *Cryptosporidium parvum*. In the normal host, it usually causes a self-limited diarrheal syndrome. AIDS patients with cryptosporidiosis may have protracted, voluminous, and watery diarrhea, profound malabsorption with electrolyte disturbances, and weight loss. Biliary tract involvement, seen in up to 10% of patients, can present with severe right upper quadrant abdominal pain, nausea, and vomiting. Laboratory studies reveal an elevated alkaline phosphatase level, gallbladder wall thickening, and dilated bile ducts. Cryptosporidiosis is seen mostly in Africa and Haiti, where 50% of AIDS patients have it; only 5% of AIDS patients in the United States have this disease. Occasionally patients have only mild diarrhea, and spontaneous remissions occur.

The diagnosis is established by the detection of acid-fast cryptosporidial oocysts in the stool or by a sucrose gradient technique. No effective therapy for cryptosporidial infections has been established. Small double-blind placebo-controlled trials comparing the aminoglycoside paromomycin (Humatin) to placebo have shown both a clinical and a parasitologic response when paromomycin is given in dosages of 25 to 35 mg per kg per day. The drug was well tolerated in most cases. Treatment regimens with the oral aminoglycoside spiramycin,* oral diclazuril,* oral azithromycin, or subcutaneous somatostatin have yielded inconsistent results. Recently albendazole has been tried as a therapeutic agent. Further clinical trials are continuing.

Isospora belli

Isospora belli is also an acid-fast parasite seen mostly in patients of Haitian origin. It can also produce watery diarrhea, but unlike *Cryptosporidium,* it can cause disseminated disease. It responds to treatment with oral TMP–SMX, one double-strength tablet four times daily for 10 to 14 days. Metronidazole (Flagyl) and pyrimethamine-sulfadoxine (Fansidar) are also effective. Recurrence is common, and chronic suppressive therapy may be required.

Microsporidia

Microsporidiosis, caused by the tiny coccidian organisms Microsporidia, is responsible for diarrhea in

---

*Not available in the United States.

some patients with AIDS. It is difficult to diagnose, so the true prevalence is unknown. In several studies in which selected AIDS patients with unexplained diarrhea were examined for microsporidians, the prevalence of the organism ranged from 7.5 to 50%. A trichrome stain of the stool is now available through the CDC, and bowel biopsies have been diagnostic. There is no proven effective therapy, but there are anecdotal reports of both success and failure using albendazole, metronidazole, and paromomycin. The most promising agent appears to be albendazole,* given orally in doses of 400 mg twice a day.

Other Parasitic Infections

Entamoeba histolytica, Giardia lamblia, and *Amoeba* are frequently implicated in acute enteritis in patients infected with HIV and often respond to standard treatment regimens. Disseminated *Strongyloides stercoralis* and severe visceral leishmaniasis has been reported in HIV-infected persons who have lived in or traveled to endemic areas.

Fungal Infections

Pneumocystis carinii

Pneumocystis carinii has been thought to be a protozoan, but based on reviews of molecular genetic data, it has been recently reclassified as a fungus. *Pneumocystis carinii* pneumonia (PCP) is the most common opportunistic infection in patients with AIDS. It is the initial manifestation of AIDS in 64% of patients. PCP is the leading cause of morbidity and mortality in patients infected with HIV and is the cause of death in 25% of patients. In the United States, 80% of patients with AIDS have had at least one episode of PCP. The onset of PCP can be insidious and prolonged, or acute. Cough, usually nonproductive, and fever are the most common presenting symptoms. Other signs and symptoms include dyspnea, tachypnea, exercise intolerance, chest tightness, and spontaneous pneumothorax. Physical examination of the chest is often unremarkable.

The chest film is the best screening test for PCP. The pneumonia can appear as diffuse interstitial infiltrates, cavities, or pneumothorax or may appear normal on a chest film. If a patient is receiving aerosol pentamidine, PCP can present as biapical disease. Gallium scanning is 100% sensitive but only 50% specific. It may be useful if PCP is strongly suspected and the patient has a normal chest film. An arterial blood gas (ABG) measurement may reveal hypoxia and an increased arterial-alveolar (A-a) gradient. The ABG may be normal with early PCP. Paired rest and exercise ABGs, however, usually show a pronounced A-a gradient (>10 mmHg) with early PCP, and this is suggestive of an interstitial process. A decreased diffusing capacity is also suggestive of an interstitial disease and can indicate early PCP. The lactate dehydrogenase level is often elevated in PCP but the elevation is nonspecific.

Since the signs and symptoms of PCP are nonspecific, additional studies are necessary to document the infection. *Pneumocystis carinii* cannot be cultured, and at the present time there are no reliable serologic tests. Therefore, to clearly establish the diagnosis of PCP, *P. carinii* must be identified in pulmonary secretions or in lung tissue. All specimens should be examined with toluidine blue and Giemsa stains and examined cytologically with Gram-Weigert stain. Direct fluorescent antibody studies have been successful in some laboratories.

Sputum induction should be the first test when PCP is strongly suspected because it is the least invasive method. Depending on the institution, *P. carinii* can be detected in 52 to 92% of cases of PCP. The use of aerosol pentamidine prophylaxis decreases the yield in detecting *P. carinii* from induced sputum samples. The diagnostic yield of bronchoscopy and bronchoalveolar lavage (BAL) has been reported to approach 100%. However the sensitivity of BAL may also be decreased with the use of aerosol pentamidine (NebuPent) prophylaxis. The sensitivity increases to 100% when a transbronchial biopsy is performed. However, many patients cannot undergo transbronchial biopsy because of thrombocytopenia or an underlying coagulation disorder. An open lung biopsy is the diagnostic procedure of last resort to determine the diagnosis.

Agents used for the treatment of PCP are presented in Table 5. Adverse reactions develop in 50 to 100% of patients receiving anti-PCP therapy. Side effects with TMP–SMX include rash, leukopenia, thrombocytopenia, fever, nausea, and vomiting. Pentamidine can induce hypoglycemia, pancreatitis, nephrotoxicity, hepatic dysfunction, neutropenia, hypotension, and cardiac arrhythmias. Corticosteroids are recommended when the presenting Po_2 is less than 70 mmHg. The dosage of prednisone as adjunctive therapy for PCP is also presented in Table 5. With early diagnosis, treatment with TMP–SMX or intravenous pentamidine should result in 90% response rates.

Atovaquone (Mepron) is a new nonsulfonamide that has been recently approved as therapy for PCP in patients with mild PCP who are intolerant to TMP–SMX. In clinical trials, oral atovaquone had similar rates of success as intravenous pentamidine for the treatment of mild to moderate PCP. There were fewer treatment limitations with atovaquone than with pentamidine. However, notable failures and early recurrences have been observed with the use of atovaquone.

Trimetrexate (Neutrexin) is an inhibitor of dihydrofolate reductase in *P. carinii*. In preliminary clinical trials, trimetrexate with leucovorin rescue was effective in treating severe cases of PCP but was less effective than TMP–SMX. Although trimetrexate was better tolerated than TMP–SMX, there was a higher rate of treatment failures and relapse with trimetrexate. Therefore, it can be an alternative for moderate to severe PCP when TMP–SMX or pentamidine cannot be used.

---

*Not available in the United States.

TABLE 5. **Recommended Regimens for *Pneumocystis carinii* Pneumonia Therapy***

Drug	Dosage	Route
Trimethoprim-sulfamethoxazole (Bactrim, Septra)	Trimethoprim, 20 mg/kg/day, and sulfamethoxazole, 100 mg/kg/day, in four divided doses	oral† or IV
Pentamidine (Pentam)	4 mg/kg in a single daily dose	IV
Dapsone-trimethoprim (Proloprim)	Dapsone 100 mg, in a single daily dose, and trimethoprim, 20 mg/kg/day, q 8 h	oral†
Atovaquone (Mepron)	750 mg q 8 h	oral†
Clindamycin-primaquine	Clindamycin 600 mg IV q 6–8 h or 450 mg orally q 6 h and Primaquine 15 mg base orally per day	oral† or IV
Trimetrexate (Neutrexin)	45 mg/m² per day	IV
Prednisone‡	40 mg bid for 5 days, 20 mg bid for 5 days, and 20 mg once a day for 5 days	oral

*All regimens given for 21 days.
†Oral therapy not recommended for moderate-to-severe disease.
‡Adjunctive therapy to antibiotics as defined in the text.

Less effective therapies for PCP include dapsone, dapsone with trimethoprim, and clindamycin with primaquine. These agents are associated with a variety of toxicities and should only be considered if a patient is failing to respond to primary therapy.

Prophylaxis against PCP is indicated when the person infected with HIV has a CD4 T lymphocyte count less than 200 cells per mm³, a rapid decline in CD4 T lymphocyte counts, thrush, or any opportunistic infection, regardless of the CD4 T lymphocyte count. TMP–SMX is the most effective agent. Aerosol pentamidine can be used when there is intolerance to TMP–SMX. Aerosol pentamidine is usually well tolerated but may induce bronchospasm during administration. Other potential prophylactic agents include (1) oral dapsone, (2) pyrimethamine-sulfadoxine, (3) intravenous or intramuscular pentamidine, (4) atovaquone, (5) clindamycin with primaquine, and (6) trimethoprim with dapsone (Table 6).

Pneumocystis carinii may disseminate. The organisms may be found in the bone marrow, lymph nodes, thyroid, liver, spleen, or retina. Aerosol pentamidine prophylaxis may predispose to disseminated infection with *P. carinii*. Therapy with TMP–SMX or intravenous pentamidine may be effective.

Candida albicans

Mucocutaneous candidiasis is often the first sign of infection with HIV. Candidal infections are common clinically, with as many as 80% of AIDS patients experiencing candidiasis at some time during their illness. However, candidal organisms are infrequent causes of major morbidity or mortality in patients with AIDS. Oropharyngeal disease occurs most often, but cutaneous, vaginal, and esophageal involvement is not unusual in the absence of invasive disease. Hematogenous candidiasis can occur but is usually associated with intravascular catheters.

The most common presentation of oral candidiasis (thrush) appears as creamy-white or yellow plaques on red mucosa, which can bleed after easy removal of the plaques. Lesions are most commonly seen on the dorsal or lateral surface of the tongue but can also appear on the palate and buccal or gingival mucosa. Diagnosis is made by wet mount with potassium hydroxide or Gram's stain of accessible lesions.

Esophagitis clinically presents with gradually progressive burning dysphagia, which can occur without oropharyngeal disease. When the clinical suspicion of esophageal candidiasis is strong, symptomatic improvement with therapy is presumptive support for the diagnosis. If improvement does not occur, endoscopy should be considered.

Topical therapy of cutaneous and vaginal disease is usually effective. Oropharyngeal disease often clears with oral preparations of nystatin (Mycostatin) or clotrimazole (Mycelex). Suspensions, suppositories,

TABLE 6. **Recommended Regimens for *Pneumocystis carinii* Pneumonia Prophylaxis**

Drug	Dose/Route
Trimethoprim-sulfamethoxazole	One double-strength tablet daily 7 days/week or two double-strength tablets bid 3 days/week
Aerosol pentamidine (NebuPent)	300 mg, once monthly via Respirgard II nebulizer or 60 mg five times over 2 weeks; then 60 mg every 2 weeks via Fisoneb nebulizer
Dapsone-pyrimethamine	50 mg/day plus 50 mg/week plus folinic acid 25 mg/week
Dapsone	50 mg/day or 100 mg twice weekly
Pentamidine (Pentam)	4 mg/kg IM or every 2 weeks

Other options include clindamycin-primaquine or atovaquone, but there are no studies at this time to support the use of these drugs and the troche forms of these medications are equally efficacious, although patients usually express preference for the troche form. Nystatin, 500,000 to 1 million U orally three to five times per day, or clotrimazole troches, 10 mg orally five times per day, are the standard therapy.

Systemic therapy with ketoconazole (Nizoral) or fluconazole (Diflucan) is indicated for candidal esophagitis. Ketoconazole, 100 to 200 mg twice daily, or fluconazole, 200 mg orally on the first day followed by 100 mg daily, is usually well tolerated. Itraconazole (Sporanox), the newest oral azole, has no clear advantages over the other agents for candidal infections. It is unknown whether candidal infections refractory to other treatment regimens will respond to therapy with this agent. Patients may develop mild gastrointestinal side effects from both drugs, and cross-reactivity with other medications can occur with either azole. Ketoconazole, unlike fluconazole, requires a normally low gastric pH to be absorbed. Recent studies have shown that fluconazole may be more beneficial than ketoconazole in the treatment of esophageal candidiasis. Refractory disease may require treatment with 0.5 mg per kg per day of intravenous amphotericin B (Fungizone). After response to systemic therapy, suppressive use of topical preparations can be employed as needed. Recurrence is common, and more severe disease is seen with progression of infection with HIV.

Cryptococcus neoformans

The spectrum of disease caused by *Cryptococcus neoformans* ranges from asymptomatic pulmonary lesions to meningoencephalitis to fungemia with disseminated infection. Cryptococcal infections occur in approximately 5% of all patients with AIDS. It is the second most common fungal infection, the most common cause of fungal meningitis, and the fourth most common opportunistic infection in patients infected with HIV.

The central nervous system (CNS) is the most frequent site of extrapulmonary involvement. Symptoms include fever, headache, and mental status changes lasting from days to weeks. Because patients have relatively minimal cerebrospinal fluid (CSF) inflammation, the meningeal findings may be subtle and the only sign may be an unexplained fever. A presumptive diagnosis is made by a positive test for cryptococcal antigen in blood and CSF. *Cryptococcus neoformans* cultured from the blood and CSF establishes the infection. The CSF should also be examined with an India ink preparation looking for budding yeasts. The India ink preparation has a 15% false-negative rate. CSF pleocytosis may or may not be evident. CSF glucose and protein levels can also be normal.

Pulmonary infection can also occur, with or without cryptococcal meningitis. It can present as lobar pneumonia, interstitial pneumonia, or pleural effusion. Other manifestations of cryptococcal disease include adenopathy, mediastinitis, chorioretinitis, sinusitis, CNS cryptococcoma, arthritis, prostatitis, pustules, and molluscum-like skin lesions. Because of the protean manifestations of cryptococcal disease, it is recommended that a serum test for cryptococcal antigen be routinely obtained in the evaluation of unexplained symptoms and fever in persons infected with HIV, although the test result is usually negative with localized disease. Once the diagnosis is established, the patient should be treated with amphotericin B.

Amphotericin B is initially given intravenously as a 1-mg test dose. If this is tolerated, the dose is escalated to 1.0 mg per kg per day within the first 24 hours. Oral 5-flucytosine (5FC) (Ancobon), 50 to 100 mg per kg per day in divided doses every 6 hours, is given with amphotericin B. Treatment of acute reactions to amphotericin B infusion such as rigors and fevers can be managed as needed with acetaminophen, diphenhydramine, and meperidine. Both amphotericin B and 5FC are nephrotoxic, requiring frequent evaluations of renal function. The use of 5FC may be limited by myelosuppression or gastrointestinal intolerance. To minimize side effects, 5FC peak and trough levels should be measured and maintained between 25 and 50 μg per mL. Therapy with high-dose fluconazole (800 mg per day) is presently being compared with therapy with amphotericin B and 5FC, and some small studies have shown it to have both clinical and microbiologic efficacy in selected patients. Itraconazole may be inferior to fluconazole for the therapy of cryptococcal disease, but it may be considered if the patient cannot receive any other therapy because drug allergy or intolerance.

Therapeutic efficacy should be monitored by serial sampling of blood, and CSF examination every 2 weeks, for culture and testing for cryptococcal antigen. The amount of cryptococcal antigen is not predictive of response to treatment, but serial titers may be useful in assessing a response to therapy. When the fungal culture has remained sterile for at least 7 days, oral fluconazole, 400 mg a day, can be given for a total of 10 weeks of induction therapy.

Although response to treatment is expected, up to 33% of patients with cryptococcal disease will succumb to their initial infection, 50 to 90% of patients will relapse, and most patients will die 5 months after their presentation with cryptococcal disease.

Cryptococcal infection is rarely if ever cured. Patients infected with HIV require chronic maintenance therapy to prevent relapse. Oral fluconazole maintenance therapy of 100 mg per day is felt to be more effective than treatment with amphotericin B one to three times weekly. Fluconazole is usually well tolerated but can cause mild elevations in transaminase levels, gastrointestinal distress, and a rash, including a Stevens-Johnson–like syndrome in a small number of individuals. Unlike ketoconazole, fluconazole is well absorbed, even in the absence of gastric acid and in patients taking antacids and H_2 blockers.

Histoplasma capsulatum *and* Coccidioides immitis

Although cryptococci are ubiquitous, certain mycotic diseases such as coccidioidomycosis and histoplasmosis are epidemic in certain regions of North America. Disease with either organism should be considered in a person with AIDS who lives in or who has traveled to an endemic area and has an unexplained fever. Pulmonary involvement is most common, but disseminated disease has been noted with increased frequency in patients infected with HIV. Symptoms are often nonspecific, with complaints of cough, fever, malaise, and weight loss often reported. Disseminated histoplasmosis can present with the previous symptoms along with respiratory complaints, hepatosplenomegaly, lymphadenopathy, anemia, leukopenia, thrombocytopenia, mucocutaneous lesions, renal insufficiency, chorioretinitis, meningitis, and/or encephalitis.

AIDS patients with coccidioidomycosis most often present with focal or diffuse pulmonary disease, meningitis, extrathoracic lymphadenopathy, hepatic disease, and/or cutaneous lesions. Radiologic studies may reveal perihilar calcification and/or splenic calcifications with histoplasmosis. Serologic tests are valuable in the diagnosis of infection with either yeast. A positive test for *Histoplasma* antigen in urine, serum, or CSF correlates with active disease. Positive cultures or demonstration of the organism by fungal stains in peripheral blood buffy coat, bone marrow, or bronchoalveolar lavage, or in biopsy specimens of lung, skin, liver, or lymph nodes, establish the diagnosis of infection with these fungi.

Treatment with amphotericin B, 1.0 mg per kg per day up to a total dose of 2 to 2.5 grams, is recommended. As with cryptococcosis, chronic suppressive therapy is required. Amphotericin B, 50 to 100 mg given once or twice weekly or biweekly, has been used successfully. Alternative therapies include ketoconazole, fluconazole, or itraconazole. Itraconazole is presently not recommended for coccidioidomycosis, but is for histoplasmosis. A 12-week induction phase of itraconazole, 200 mg orally twice a day, followed by lifelong suppressive maintenance with 100 mg orally twice a day, has been used as an alternative to amphotericin B. Alternative suppressive therapies for coccidioidomycosis include fluconazole, 200 to 400 mg orally per day, or ketoconazole, 400 mg per day.

Aspergillus *Species*

Invasive aspergillosis is an uncommon infectious complication in patients with AIDS despite the frequent recovery of *Aspergillus* spp from sputum. Risk factors associated with invasive aspergillosis include neutropenia, hematologic malignancy, and corticosteroid use. As more aggressive chemotherapy protocols are developed for Kaposi's sarcoma, lymphoma, and other malignancies that occur in patients infected with HIV, the predisposing factors for invasive aspergillosis will occur with increased frequency. Treatment with amphotericin B must be considered for the neutropenic patient with AIDS who has a pneumonia of uncertain cause and from whom *Aspergillus* spp has been isolated from a respiratory specimen. Itraconazole is also an effective agent to treat aspergillosis. Every effort should be made to establish a definitive microbial diagnosis before therapy is initiated.

Common Bacterial Infections

Mycobacteria

The mycobacteria have been a prominent part of the AIDS pandemic since its very beginning. Two species predominate, *Mycobacterium tuberculosis* (MTb) and *M. avium* complex (MAC), the latter comprising those organisms previously identified as either *M. avium* or *M. intracellulare* but now recognized as so similar as to be classified together. Recently, infections with *M. haemophilum* and *M. kansasii* have also been associated with AIDS. Other mycobacterial infections only rarely recognized until now include *M. genavense, M. malmoense, M. xenopi,* and *M. gordonae.*

Approximately 10 to 12 million people are infected with MTb in the United States; many of them are co-infected with HIV. Infection with MTb has been seen in up to 10% of patients with AIDS, and the incidence of tuberculosis among patients with HIV infection ranges from 4 to 21% depending on the geographic area. Tuberculosis is often the first manifestation of HIV infection. It can be reactivated disease or primary infection. In the mid-1990s reports suggest that over 30% of cases in two geographic areas (San Francisco and the Bronx, New York City) were due to new infection. When tuberculosis occurs early in HIV infection, its features are indistinguishable from those of tuberculosis occurring in non–HIV-infected persons. The clinical features include night sweats, fever, weight loss, and productive cough with typical chest x-ray findings. In the later stages of HIV infection, tuberculosis is more likely to present in an atypical manner with nonspecific constitutional symptoms and nonproductive cough. Pulmonary disease is often atypical on chest film, lacking cavitation, and may involve the mediastinal lymph nodes or the lower lobes or present as a diffuse interstitial infiltrate. Histopathologic examination may show poorly formed granulomas without caseation necrosis.

Up to 70% of patients with tuberculosis have extrapulmonary disease, often involving the adrenal glands. Lymphadenopathy is the most common manifestation of extrapulmonary tuberculosis and can be an unsuspected cause of lymphadenopathy in HIV-infected persons. Extrapulmonary tuberculosis also manifests itself in patients with AIDS as pericarditis, peritonitis, meningitis, brain lesions, bone and joint involvement, or disseminated tuberculosis.

The diagnosis of tuberculosis in HIV-infected patients can be difficult and is often missed because of its atypical presentation, the high frequency of extrapulmonary manifestations, the occurrence of other mycobacterial diseases, and a frequently poor delayed hypersensitivity response. Because anergy is seen in about 50% of HIV-infected persons and in over 90% of people in the later stages of AIDS, many have a negative skin test, even when the classic test response criterion is relaxed and induration of less than 5 mm is considered positive.

Patients with pulmonary tuberculosis in the later stages of AIDS produce scanty sputum that may be nondiagnostic by direct microscopic examination. A positive sputum smear can be helpful, and at least three sputum smears should be tested; if they do not contain acid-fast bacilli, other specimens should be obtained through induced sputum samples; bronchial washing and lavage; gastric lavage; pleural fluid, blood, or urine samples; and lymph node, bone marrow, or liver biopsy if indicated. A culture with complete identification of mycobacterial species and drug-susceptibility tests should be obtained. Serologic tests are still limited, and polymerase chain reaction tests are under development.

Treatment for active tuberculosis should include oral isoniazid (INH), 300 mg per day; oral rifampin (RIF) (Rifadin), 600 mg per day; oral pyrazinamide (PZA), 20 to 30 mg per kg per day; and either oral ethambutol (EMB) (Myambutol), 15 to 25 mg per kg per day, or streptomycin (STM), 1 gram intramuscularly per day, until susceptibilities are known. If the isolate is susceptible to INH and RIF, INH and RIF at the same dosages should be given for the remainder of the treatment. Acceptable intermittent therapy includes two- or three-times-a-week regimens at adjusted doses (Table 7). Therapy should continue for a minimum of 9 months or for at least 6 months after the last culture conversion. Many public health experts recommend that all therapy be directly observed to ensure adherence to the often-difficult-to-tolerate therapy. Oral EMB, 15 mg per kg per day, should be added if disseminated or CNS infection is suspected. HIV-infected patients have a similar response rate to therapy compared with uninfected patients. However, HIV-infected patients have a higher relapse rate.

HIV-infected patients are at a higher risk for developing drug-resistant tuberculosis. Factors associated with drug resistance include prior antituberculous therapy, exposure to persons with resistant tuberculosis, homelessness, injection drug use, imprisonment, and sporadic health care. Nosocomial outbreaks of multidrug-resistant tuberculosis (MDR–TB) have been described, primarily among HIV-infected persons. The risk factors for MDR–TB are similar to those for single-drug-resistant tuberculosis, with prior inadequate or inappropriate therapy and injection drug use the greatest predictors of multidrug resistance. The initial treatment regimen should take into consideration the knowledge regarding the incidence of drug-resistant isolates from a given community. If drug-resistant tuberculosis is suspected, therapy may require starting with more than four drugs, including INH, RIF, PZA, EMB, and either STM or amikacin (Amikin), and one or more other drugs, which include ethionamide (Trecator-SC), 10 to 15 mg per kg per day; cycloserine (Seromycin), 15 mg per kg per day; kanamycin (Kantrex), 0.5 gram per day; capreomycin (Capastat), 15 mg per kg per day; para-aminosalicylic acid (PAS), 10 to 12 grams per day in two to three divided doses; ciprofloxacin (Cipro), 750 mg orally twice a day; ofloxacin (Floxin), 400 mg orally twice a day; and clofazimine (Lamprene), 100 mg orally once per day. Treatment regimens for MDR–TB are outlined in Table 8.

Individuals with HIV infection who have been previously infected with MTb are more likely to develop active disease than those who are HIV-seronegative. Whereas seronegative persons have a 10% lifetime risk of developing active disease (with the greatest

TABLE 7. **Therapy for Tuberculosis**

	Doses*		
	Daily	*Three Times/Week*	*Two Times/Week*
INH	5 mg/kg (300 mg)	15 mg/kg (900 mg)	15 mg/kg (900 mg)
RIF	10 mg/kg (600 mg)	10 mg/kg (600 mg)	10 mg/kg (600 mg)
PZA	15–30 mg/kg (2 gm)	50–70 mg/kg (2.5–3 gm)	50–70 mg/kg (3–3.5 gm)
EMB	5–25 mg/kg (2.5 gm)	25–30 mg/kg (2.5 gm)	50 mg/kg (2.5 gm)
STM	15 mg/kg (1 gm)	25–30 mg/kg (1 gm)	25–30 mg/kg (1.5 gm)

*Maximal dose in parentheses.

Duration: 9 months and ≥6 months after culture conversion.

Option 1: INH, RIF, and PZA, plus STM or EMB daily for 8 weeks, then INH and RIF daily for 16 weeks if isolate is sensitive to INH and RIF. If INH resistance is likely, add EMB for 8 weeks.

Option 2: INH, RIF, and PZA, plus STM or EMB daily for 2 weeks, then DOT with same four drugs two times/week for 6 weeks, then INH and RIF for 16 weeks.

Option 3: DOT with INH, RIF, and PZA, plus STM or EMB three times/week for 6 months.

INH should be supplemented with pyridoxine (vitamin B$_6$) 25–50 mg/day.

Abbreviations: INH = isoniazid; RIF = rifampin; PZA = pyrazinamide; EMB = ethambutol; STM = streptomycin.

Directly observed therapy (DOT) two to three times a week is preferred.

TABLE 8. **Therapy for Multidrug-Resistant Tuberculosis**

Resistant To	Suggested Regimen
INH, STM, PZA	RIF, PZA, EMB, plus an aminoglycoside*
INH, EMB ± STM	RIF, PZA, ciprofloxacin (Cipro) or ofloxacin (Floxin), plus an aminoglycoside
INH, RIF	PZA, EMB, Cipro or Oflox, plus an aminoglycoside
INH, RIF, EMB	PZA, Cipro or Oflox, plus an aminoglycoside plus two other drugs†
INH, RIF, PZA	EMB, Cipro or Oflox, plus an aminoglycoside plus two other drugs
INH, RIF, PZA, EMB	Cipro or Oflox, plus an aminoglycoside plus at least two other drugs to which the organism is sensitive

*Aminoglycosides include amikacin (Amikin), STM, kanamycin (Kantrex), and capreomycin (Capastat) and should be based on in vitro susceptibilities; they can be given daily or two or three times per week IV or IM for 4–6 months.

†Ethionamide (Trecator-SC), cycloserine (Seromycin), para-aminosalicylic acid (PAS), clofazimine (Lamprene).

Abbreviations: INH = isoniazid; STM = streptomycin; PZA = pyrizinamide; RIF = rifampin; EMB = ethambutol.

risk the first 2 years after infection), the risk for an HIV-infected person is 8 to 10% per year. In addition, studies suggest that people with HIV infection are more likely to develop active disease after recent infection. This has led to the recommendation that all persons with HIV be tested for PPD and that all persons with active tuberculosis be tested for HIV.

PPD skin testing should be performed using the Mantoux method, introducing 5 TU of PPD intradermally. The current CDC guidelines recommend using 5 mm of skin induration as an indication of latent MTb infection. Because persons with HIV infection have abnormalities with delayed-type hypersensitivity, false-negative PPD skin tests are common, particularly in advanced disease. As a result, the CDC recommends PPD testing with concomitant anergy testing using two of three control antigens: *C. albicans,* mumps, or tetanus toxoid.

Individuals found to be PPD-positive or anergic should receive a chest x-ray examination. If clinically indicated, a further investigation for tuberculosis should be initiated, including examination (smear and culture) of the sputum for acid-fast bacilli. Chemoprophylaxis is recommended for asymptomatic HIV-infected persons with any of the following indications: (1) PPD indurations greater than or equal to 5 millimeters, (2) radiographic evidence of old tuberculosis, (3) household exposure, or (4) anergy in individuals from populations with a 10% or greater prevalence of tuberculosis, including injection drug users, prisoners, homeless persons, migrant laborers, and foreign-born individuals from tuberculosis-endemic areas. Prophylaxis using INH 300 mg per day or INH 15 mg per kg per day twice weekly for 9 to 12 months is recommended. Studies of shorter duration are under way, including an investigation of RIF combined with PZA for 2 months. For patients unable to take INH, RIF may be given for 6 to 12 months. Other potential prophylactic agents include the rifamycin derivative rifabutin (Mycobutin).

Some studies have found a higher frequency of side effects to drug therapy in HIV-infected patients with tuberculosis, whereas others have found no significant difference. The most frequent adverse reactions included skin rashes; some cases of hepatitis have been reported. Treatment should be adjusted in cases of severe drug toxicity. INH has been associated with a peripheral neuropathy postulated to be a result of pyridoxine (vitamin B_6) deficiency. Individuals suspected of malnutrition should receive supplemental oral pyridoxine, 25 to 50 mg per day. There appears to be no drug interaction with AZT, but RIF can increase the hepatic metabolism of fluconazole, oral contraceptives, methadone, and warfarin. Individuals maintained on any of these drugs should be informed of the possible effects. Women using oral contraceptives should be educated about other forms of contraception. Patients maintained on methadone may need to be closely monitored to prevent the onset of withdrawal symptoms. Increases in doses in increments of 5 to 10 mg per day, up to 50% of the initial methadone starting dose, may be necessary.

MAC is found antemortem in 20% of patients with AIDS and has been found in greater than 50% at autopsy. MAC usually presents as a disseminated infection in patients with far-advanced AIDS. Diffuse involvement of bone marrow and structures of the reticuloendothelial system in the spleen, liver, lymph nodes, lungs, and gastrointestinal tract with massive mycobacterial loads and poorly formed granulomas is often seen along with a continuous high-grade bacillemia.

Symptoms include persistent fevers, weight loss, and night sweats. Signs of end-organ involvement include diarrhea, anemia, an elevated alkaline phosphatase level, hypoalbuminemia, and progressive debilitation. Disseminated disease is associated with a relentlessly deteriorating clinical course and an extremely poor prognosis. It is rarely the only direct cause of death.

Diagnosis depends on culturing possible sites of involvement, including blood, lymph nodes, liver, stool, and bone marrow, for mycobacteria. The finding of acid-fast bacilli in direct smears of stool with positive cultures often correlates with disseminated disease and should prompt consideration of treatment or intensive further evaluation. In contrast, the finding of MAC in sputum or bronchoalveolar lavage specimens does not necessarily imply systemic infection because, unlike MTb, MAC seldom causes invasive pulmonary disease.

Patients who are symptomatic usually benefit from a trial of therapy. However, no consistently effective or curative therapy has been found for MAC. Regimens using four to five drugs, including rifabutin, clofazimine, RIF, ethionamide, cycloserine, ciprofloxacin, and amikacin, with either clarithromycin or azithromycin, have been used with some improvement in symptoms and often a temporary reduction in bacillemia. The adequate duration of therapy has not been determined, but most clinicians choose to continue maintenance therapy indefinitely if the patient has a clinical or mycobacteriologic response and the regimen is tolerated.

Rifabutin, 300 mg orally per day, is recommended to prevent the development of disseminated MAC infection in patients infected with HIV who have CD4 lymphocyte counts less than 100 cells per mm^3. Since rifabutin monotherapy is inadequate for disseminated MAC, a thorough investigation to rule out disease is warranted before initiation of therapy. It is also imperative that the patient be evaluated for the presence of MTb before initiation of therapy so that the selection of rifabutin- or RIF-resistant strains can be prevented. Clarithromycin also appears to be effective in MAC prophylaxis.

Recently, *M. haemophilum* has been found to infect the skin and underlying tissues of HIV-infected patients. Skin lesions begin as painful, erythematous, or violaceous nodules that can progress to form an abscess. They are often exudative and can form ulcers. The synovium of joints such as the knee, ankle, digits, and wrist, as well as tendon sheaths, can also be infected. Isolation from bronchoalveolar lavage, blood, skin ulcers, joint effusion, eye, or lymph nodes requires special culturing techniques. The optimal treatment regimen and duration of therapy are presently unclear, but four drug regimens utilizing RIF or rifabutin, ciprofloxacin, clarithromycin, amikacin, or clofazimine may be effective. Infection with this organism should be in the differential diagnosis of any HIV-infected patient who presents with cutaneous lesions, joint effusion, osteomyelitis, or unexplained pneumonia. The microbiology laboratory must be notified so that special culture conditions using hemin and room temperature incubation can be used.

Other mycobacteria, including *M. kansasii,* can present with pulmonary and extrapulmonary disease and multiorgan dissemination. The symptoms are often indistinguishable from those of MTb or MAC. The diagnosis can be made by gene probe after growth of the organism in culture. Treatment for *M. kansasii* consists of INH 300 mg per day, RIF 600 mg per day, and EMB 15 to 25 mg per kg per day for 15 to 18 months.

Other Bacterial Infections

Treponema pallidum

Syphilis is increasingly being recognized as a cause of CNS disease in patients with AIDS. Patients may be asymptomatic or have an array of signs and symptoms. Patients infected with HIV and with a history of treated primary or secondary syphilis may develop CNS infection months or years after therapy. This can include cerebral infarcts, meningitis, and polyradiculitis. The diagnosis is difficult because both the clinical course and the serologic examination may be altered in HIV infection. Nearly all patients with HIV infection and primary or secondary syphilis have a positive serum VDRL or RPR test, even after adequate treatment. As a result, fluorescent treponemal antibody absorption (FTA–ABS) test must be performed to rule out a false-positive result. Treatment for primary or secondary syphilis is identical to that for HIV-negative persons.

Serologic testing after treatment for early syphilis is important in those co-infected with HIV. Quantitative nontreponemal tests (VDRL, RPR) should be repeated at 1, 2, and 3 months and at 3-month intervals thereafter, until a satisfactory serologic response to treatment occurs. It the titer does not decrease by two dilutions within 3 months in primary syphilis or within 6 months in secondary syphilis, the patient should be re-evaluated for the possibility of treatment failure, reinfection, or neurosyphilis.

In neurosyphilis, the cerebrospinal fluid may show a pleocytosis and an elevated protein level or may be normal, including a nonreactive VDRL test. Therapy with intravenous penicillin G, 12 to 24 million U per day, is given for a minimum of 2 weeks. Alternatively, aqueous procaine penicillin 2.4 million U intramuscularly daily for 10 to 14 days along with oral probenecid 500 mg four times a day followed by three weekly doses of 2.4 million U of intramuscular benzathine penicillin can be given. Patients with neurosyphilis should have cerebrospinal fluid examinations every 6 months for 2 years, or until the VDRL is consistently negative or cell counts are normal. Failure to normalize the cerebrospinal fluid is reason to re-treat. The need for suppressive therapy in neurosyphilis is unclear.

Salmonella

Salmonella infections in patients with AIDS are common. They are distinguished by a high frequency of bacteremia and disseminated infection and a high likelihood of recurrence after treatment is discontinued. Patients often have unexplained fever and rigors, with or without associated diarrhea. Isolation of salmonella species, especially *Salmonella typhimurium,* from blood or other sterile body sites provides a diagnosis. Isolation of salmonella from stool samples should be followed by blood cultures. Treatment for bacteremia includes 10 to 14 days of intravenous antibiotics. Agents commonly used include ampicillin, 1 to 2 grams every 4 to 6 hours; TMP–SMX, 10 to 20 mg per kg per day in four divided doses; or ciprofloxacin, 750 mg twice a day. Individuals with gastroenteritis without bacteremia can be treated orally with the same drugs at adjusted doses.

Most patients with salmonella infection require chronic suppressive therapy regardless of the presentation and initial treatment. The choice of agent should be based on antimicrobial susceptibility results. Similar agents used for the acute phase can be used orally for chronic suppressive therapy.

Other Bacterial Infections

Other bacterial infections to which HIV-infected persons are predisposed because of defects in cell-mediated immunity include listeriosis, legionellosis, and nocardial infections. These organism respond well to conventional therapy. HIV-infected persons are also predisposed to infections with encapsulated organisms because of their impaired humoral immune system. Bacterial pneumonia occurs frequently in AIDS patients and may be seen concurrently with PCP. *Streptococcus pneumoniae* and *Haemophilus influenzae* pneumonia often occur in this patient population. Pneumococcal pneumonia is typically lobar and responds to conventional therapy. Pneumonia due to *H. influenzae* can have a variety of radiographic presentations and may be indistinguishable from PCP. It is therefore recommended that treatment for bacterial pneumonia be added to pentamidine when allergy to TMP–SMX precludes its use in the early empirical therapy of presumed PCP, as pentamidine has no activity against bacterial pneumonia.

Pyogenic infections with *Staphylococcus aureus* and *Pseudomonas aeruginosa* occur with increased frequency in HIV-infected patients, especially in those persons with neutropenia. The most common presentations are bronchitis, sinusitis, and pneumonia. These infections respond to conventional therapy, but relapse is common.

Campylobacter jejuni, C. fetus, and *Shigella flexneri* are also seen with increased frequency in patients with AIDS. These organisms are usually associated with chronic diarrhea, but bacteremia can occur. Conventional therapy is indicated.

Rochalimaea henselae, the causative agent of cat-scratch fever, has been shown to cause bacillary angiomatosis in patients with AIDS. It presents with multiple small hemangioma-like lesions of the skin, but the disease may involve the viscera, especially the liver and spleen. Involvement of the lymph nodes, bone, and soft tissues has been described. Because of the dermatologic manifestations, bacillary angiomatosis is often mistaken for Kaposi's sarcoma. The diagnosis is made by identification of the characteristic histologic findings, genetic amplification by means of polymerase chain reaction, or culture of the organism. Therapy with erythromycin or doxycycline is usually effective. The organism *Rochalimaea quintana* may also play a role in this infection.

Rhodococcus equi, formerly called *Corynebacterium equi,* can cause a necrotizing pneumonia resembling tuberculosis or nocardiosis in patients with AIDS. Subcutaneous nodules and brain abscesses have also been described as in nocardiosis. The organism is sensitive to vancomycin, erythromycin, aminoglycosides, and chloramphenicol, but the optimal duration of therapy is unknown. Some patients may require surgical intervention for cure.

Viral Infections

Cytomegalovirus

Cytomegalovirus (CMV) infections are among the most common in persons with AIDS. CMV is transmitted sexually, by saliva, or by exposure to blood products. Approximately 100% of homosexual men infected with HIV are seropositive for CMV. Therefore, in this population, CMV disease is believed to be due to reactivation of latent infection. CMV itself may contribute to immunosuppression. Retinitis is the major manifestation of infection with CMV, but encephalitis, polyradiculopathy, pneumonitis, esophagitis, hepatitis, and colitis are being found with increasing frequency. Adrenalitis with adrenal insufficiency may occur. Ventriculitis with pathognomonic CT scan results has also been seen.

Diagnosis of infection with CMV is not easy. Serologic testing is seldom helpful, owing to the high prevalence of seropositivity in the HIV-infected population. Positive cultures of CMV are difficult to interpret because it is difficult to distinguish between active disease due to CMV and intermittent viral shedding or even viremia with CMV.

Two clinical syndromes that may be accepted as presumptive evidence of invasive CMV disease include (1) a characteristic chorioretinitis with hemorrhages, perivascular exudates, and vascular sheathing, and (2) adrenalitis in the presence of CMV infection viremia or uremia and without another explanation. Organ system involvement such as pneumonia, colitis, esophagitis, and hepatitis must be accompanied by histopathologic evidence of pathognomonic "owl's-eye" inclusions before a diagnosis can be made. Pap smears of cells may also show the typical inclusions.

Presenting signs and symptoms of CMV infection depend upon the organ system infected. Between 5 and 10% of patients with AIDS develop CMV retinitis, which is the most common sight-threatening disease in patients with AIDS. Retinitis usually develops during the later stages of AIDS, and patients should have ophthalmologic evaluations every 3 to 4 months, even if asymptomatic. Patients may complain of floaters, a change in acuity, or a unilateral visual field defect. Pain is rare. Blindness results if therapy is not instituted. Blood and urine cultures are often positive for CMV at the time of diagnosis but can be negative.

Ganciclovir (dihydroxy propoxymethyl guanine [DHPG]) (Cytovene) is an effective therapeutic agent in 80% of patients with CMV retinitis. Treatment is intravenous and is given initially as 10 mg per kg per day in two divided doses for 2 weeks, and then maintenance therapy at 5 mg per kg per day indefinitely to prevent relapse. Close monitoring of the CBC and ophthalmic examinations is necessary. If the total granulocyte count falls below 750 cells per mm³, ganciclovir should be temporarily discontinued. The use of GM-CSF or G-CSF with ganciclovir may ameliorate the myelosuppression seen with therapy. If there is no improvement in the total granulocyte count, therapy should be changed to foscarnet. Patients may need to discontinue AZT therapy while receiving ganciclovir because of both drugs' myelosuppressive effects. With effective therapy, progression of the retinitis is aborted and vision may improve as edema and inflammation subside.

Intravenous foscarnet (Foscavir) is a broad-spectrum antiviral agent with good activity against CMV. It is effective in ganciclovir-resistant strains of CMV. The induction dose is 180 mg per kg per day in three divided doses for 2 weeks then 90 to 120 mg per kg per day in a single dose indefinitely. Foscarnet does not cause myelosuppression, but a rise in serum creatinine levels is often seen and may require dose adjustments. Other adverse effects include fever, nausea, anemia, diarrhea, vomiting, headache, hypokalemia, hypocalcemia, seizures, and granulocytopenia.

As both ganciclovir and foscarnet are usually given intravenously, most persons with CMV retinitis require indwelling vascular access devices for indefinite treatment. Patients should have frequent ophthalmologic examinations to assess the response to therapy and to monitor for recurrence of disease. Both drugs are equally effective, but an apparent 4-month survival advantage has been seen with patients receiving foscarnet, as foscarnet may have some antiretroviral activity.

A new oral formulation of ganciclovir is approved

for maintenance treatment of CMV retinitis in AIDS patients. Clinical trials have shown the drug to be effective in patients in whom retinitis is stable following appropriate induction therapy and for whom the risk of more rapid progression is balanced by the benefit associated with avoiding intravenous therapy. The recommended dose following induction therapy is 1000 mg three times a day with food or, alternatively, 500 mg taken six times a day every 3 hours with food.

Signs and symptoms of CMV pneumonitis resemble those of PCP or any interstitial pneumonitis. Patients with biopsy-proven disease and no other demonstrable pathogen to explain an interstitial pneumonia may benefit from treatment. Intravenous therapy with ganciclovir given 5 mg per kg twice daily is effective in 50% of patients. The optimal duration of therapy is not established. Some patients respond after 2 to 4 weeks of treatment, but many relapse. Chronic suppressive therapy may be necessary. Intravenous foscarnet given for 14 to 21 days, 60 mg per kg three times daily, has had promising results. The effective maintenance dose has not been determined.

CMV esophagitis is clinically indistinguishable from esophagitis due to *C. albicans* or herpes simplex virus. Endoscopy reveals erythema, submucosal hemorrhages, and diffuse ulcerations. Vasculitis, neutrophilic invasion, and destructive changes are seen at biopsy. Diagnosis is made by finding the pathognomonic inclusions seen with CMV. CMV colitis occurs in at least 5 to 10% of patients with AIDS. Findings at sigmoidoscopy are similar to the findings seen on endoscopy. Treatment with ganciclovir, 5 mg per kg twice daily, is effective in at least 75% of patients. Chronic suppressive therapy may not be required. All patients with CMV colitis should have an ophthalmologic examination to rule out retinitis.

Herpes Simplex Virus

Herpes simplex virus (HSV) infections are common and unusually severe in HIV-infected patients. Manifestations of HSV infection include large persistent perianal erosions that may lack typical vesicle formation, stomatitis, and esophagitis. Diagnosis of perianal, oral, and genital HSV infection is made by culture of swabs of the lesions. Endoscopy is required to diagnose HSV esophagitis, as it is clinically indistinguishable from esophagitis due to *C. albicans* or CMV.

Treatment with oral acyclovir (Zovirax), 200 mg five times daily, is usually effective for mild infections. Treatment should continue until all lesions are crusted. More severe disease requires intravenous therapy with acyclovir, 5 mg per kg three times daily. Ganciclovir is also effective for HSV esophagitis. Recurrence is common and may require suppressive medication. Oral acyclovir given at doses of 600 to 800 mg daily is effective as secondary prophylaxis but is associated with the emergence of thymidine-kinase-deficient, acyclovir-resistant HSV infections.

Foscarnet is the drug of choice for acyclovir-resistant HSV.

Varicella-Zoster Virus

Reactivation varicella-zoster virus (VZV) infection is common in HIV-infected persons and can be the first sign of clinically significant immunosuppression. VZV disease can be severe and chronic, and although usually dermatomal, it may disseminate. Diagnosis is usually made clinically but can include a biopsy, Tzanck's preparation, or virus isolation from an affected region. Therapy with oral acyclovir, 800 mg five times per day for dermatomal disease, or intravenous acyclovir, 10 mg per kg three times daily for disseminated disease, is usually effective. Famciclovir is a recently released antiviral agent that is approved for acute VZV infection. It is given in doses of 500 mg orally, three times per day. Intravenous foscarnet is required for resistant VZV infections. Treatment is usually continued until all lesions have crusted over. Recurrences with VZV are less frequent than with HSV, and therefore secondary prophylaxis is usually not necessary.

Epstein-Barr Virus

High titers of antibody to Epstein-Barr virus (EBV) are found in many AIDS patients but have not been clearly associated with disease. There is evidence that B cell lymphomas and lymphoid interstitial pneumonitis (LIP) seen in HIV-infected persons, especially children, are caused by EBV. EBV has also been associated with oral hairy leukoplakia (OHL). Patients may present with hypertrophy of the lateral tongue or painless white plaques anywhere on the tongue or posterior oropharynx. Unlike thrush lesions, these lesions do not scrape off. There is no known treatment, and the lesions usually do not progress. Regression of OHL has been seen with AZT therapy.

Papovavirus

The JC and SV40 papovaviruses are the most common causes of progressive multifocal leukoencephalopathy (PML) seen in patients with AIDS. Presentation depends on the area of the brain involved, ranging from a diffuse encephalopathy to focal deficits. Symptoms usually progress rapidly over several months, although some patients may have a waxing and waning clinical course. Brain-imaging studies reveal multiple nonenhancing lesions scattered throughout the white matter. MRI images are more specific than CT images. Diagnosis is made at brain biopsy, which shows focal myelin loss with abnormal astrocytes. There is no known therapy at present, but cytarabine (ara-C) may be useful and is currently being evaluated for treatment. Prognosis with PML is poor.

Pox Viruses

Molluscum contagiosum occurs as an opportunistic infection in patients with AIDS. The presentation is clinically the same as in non–HIV-infected persons except that the lesions may not resolve spontaneously but instead continue to increase in size, number, and severity. Patients should be referred to a dermatologist for cryotherapy with liquid nitrogen.

Human Immunodeficiency Virus

HIV can cause a variety of clinical syndromes on its own. It has been associated with a mononucleosis-like syndrome, acute aseptic meningitis, myocarditis, cardiomyopathy, immune thrombocytopenic purpura, progressive generalized lymphadenopathy, subacute encephalitis, spinal vacuolar myopathy, and peripheral neuropathies. Some of these syndromes respond to antiretroviral therapy. HIV-associated nephropathy is a distinct form of renal disease that is becoming increasingly important as a cause of morbidity and mortality. It is characterized by nephrotic-range proteinuria and rapid progression to end-stage renal disease. The role of antiviral agents is unclear. Dialysis therapy does not appear to prolong life substantially in most patients.

Opportunistic Tumors

Kaposi's Sarcoma

Kaposi's sarcoma (KS) is a malignancy of presumed endothelial cell origin. It occurs in approximately 10% of all cases of AIDS but in closer to 20% of male homosexuals. Recent studies have shown an association between KS and a herpesvirus. This virus is undergoing further evaluation and identification. KS is characterized by mucocutaneous lesions that can appear as erythematous to violaceous macules, plaques, and/or nodules. KS can spread to lymph nodes and cause lymphedema, or can spread to the viscera, especially the lungs or gastrointestinal tract. The diagnosis of KS is made by biopsy of the involved organ system showing typical endothelial cell proliferation with spindle cell formation.

Treatment for KS is palliative. Prospective studies have not shown a clear survival advantage for those who receive treatment. Complete responses to treatment are not common, and most responses are short-lived. The indications for initiation of therapy include (1) cosmetically disturbing lesions, (2) lymphedema, (3) visceral involvement, (4) locally symptomatic disease, and (5) rapidly progressive disease.

Patients requiring local therapy have cosmetic lesions or local symptoms, especially of the oropharynx. Local therapies that are well tolerated include (1) surgical excision, (2) cryotherapy with liquid nitrogen, (3) radiotherapy, or (4) intralesional vinblastine (Velban). Radiotherapy of the oropharynx can be complicated by severe and debilitating mucositis.

Patients who have more advanced or rapidly progressive disease, or have visceral involvement, require systemic therapy. The combination of bleomycin (Blenoxane) and vincristine (Oncovin), a relatively nonmyelosuppressive regimen, has shown good antitumor activity. Interferon-alpha has also been shown to have good antitumor activity. It is most effective in individuals who have a CD4 lymphocyte count greater than 400 cells per mm³. The major side effects of interferon-alpha include myelosuppression, fever, myalgias, a flulike syndrome, depression, and liver function abnormalities.

Non-Hodgkin's Lymphoma and Primary Central Nervous System Lymphoma

Non-Hodgkin's lymphoma is an aggressive disease in patients who are HIV-infected. These tumors are usually of B cell phenotype and are of high-grade histologic type, either small noncleaved cell lymphoma or immunoblastic lymphoma. These patients often present with disseminated disease, and there is frequently extranodal involvement, including the bone marrow, gastrointestinal tract, liver, spleen, subcutaneous and soft tissues, lungs, pleura, heart, pericardium, kidney, gingiva, parotid gland, and paranasal sinus. Non-Hodgkin's lymphoma may present with fevers, weight loss, and night sweats, or with local organ dysfunction from extranodal disease. It can also present as asymptomatic progressive lymphadenopathy.

Treatment regimens for non-Hodgkin's lymphoma include cyclophosphamide (Cytoxan), doxorubicin (Adriamycin), vincristine, and dexamethasone. Response rates approximate 50%, and the median survival ranges from 4 months to 1 year depending on other risk factors.

Primary CNS lymphoma represents a unique syndrome associated with profound immunosuppression and presents at advanced stages of HIV disease. It is the second most common cause of an enhancing CNS mass lesion in AIDS patients. Patients may present with headache, confusion, lethargy, memory loss, hemiparesis, aphasia, seizures, and cranial nerve palsies. CT scanning of the brain reveals single or multiple discrete iso- or hypodense lesions, which enhance with contrast and have associated mass effect and edema. Cytologic examination of cerebrospinal fluid provides a diagnosis in 25% of patients. A brain biopsy may be necessary for a definitive diagnosis. Treatment for CNS lymphoma is primarily radiotherapy along with corticosteroids to control cerebral edema. The average survival for AIDS patients with CNS lymphoma and previous opportunistic infections is 2 months. This is in contrast to those patients without previous opportunistic infections who have an average survival of 12 months.

Hematologic Abnormalities

The majority of patients with HIV infection develop cytopenias, either anemia, leukopenia, or thrombocytopenia. Whereas thrombocytopenia is commonly caused by immune *destruction* of the platelets, anemia and leukopenia are generally due to inadequate *production* of blood cells. Some of the more common causes of cytopenias include (1) a direct suppressive effect of HIV, (2) myelosuppressive effects of drug therapy (e.g., AZT, ganciclovir, TMP–SMX), (3) infiltration of bone marrow by malignant cells, (4) infiltration of bone marrow by infection (e.g., MAC, MTb, *Histoplasma, Cryptococcus*), (5) anemia of chronic disease, (6) malnutrition, (7) blood loss, (8) autoimmune destruction, and (9) pre-existing or coexisting diseases (e.g., hypersplenism).

Identification of the underlying cause of the cytopenia can allow specific therapy. If cytopenia is drug-induced, either discontinuing the offending agent or adjusting the dose may be appropriate. For acute blood loss, transfusions of packed red blood cells may be beneficial. Leucovorin has been recommended in doses ranging from 10 to 50 mg daily to prevent leukopenia due to therapy with pyrimethamine and sulfadiazine for toxoplasmosis, as well as trimetrexate for PCP. Recombinant erythropoietin (Epogen) has been approved for treating anemia secondary to AZT therapy in patients with HIV infection. Patients with serum erythropoietin levels less than 500 mU per mL have a greater chance of responding to exogenous erythropoietin. Myeloid colony-stimulating factors G-CSF and GM-CSF have been approved for use in the amelioration of neutropenia due to cytotoxic chemotherapy and bone marrow transplantation, not for myelosuppression in the setting of HIV infection. Their use in HIV infection could be considered when alternative regimens are not appropriate and the benefits are felt to outweigh the potential risks.

Idiopathic Thrombocytopenic Purpura

Idiopathic thrombocytopenia purpura (ITP) is seen in association with HIV infection and can occur at any stage of disease. Thrombocytopenia is due to immune destruction of the platelets, either by immune complex deposited on the surface of the platelets or through antiplatelet antibody production. Other causes of thrombocytopenia include drug-induced suppression and hypersplenism. Clinical manifestations of ITP include petechiae, ecchymosis, mucosal bleeding, menorrhagia, and most seriously, intracranial bleeding.

Thrombotic Thrombocytopenic Purpura

Thrombotic thrombocytopenic purpura (TTP) has been reported in association with HIV infection. It is marked by thrombocytopenia, microangiopathic hemolytic anemia, fever, renal dysfunction, and neurologic dysfunction. It is treated with plasma infusion or plasma exchange.

Spontaneous bleeding due to thrombocytopenia is rare. Treatment for thrombocytopenia may include platelet transfusions. In patients with ITP, platelet counts have increased in response to glucocorticoids, AZT, danazol (Danocrine), and as a last resort, splenectomy. Patients should receive pneumococcal vaccine before splenectomy.

Neurologic Complications

Neurologic complications are frequent in HIV infection, often with subtle manifestations. Neurodysfunction in patients with AIDS may be a consequence of HIV infection of the CNS, toxic-metabolic disorders, or infectious or neoplastic diseases.

The most common CNS complication is HIV encephalopathy (AIDS dementia). It eventually develops in 10 to 50% of patients with AIDS. The cause is presumed to be directly related to HIV infection. It may present as a behavioral syndrome with characteristics of depression or psychosis. The most common finding is increasing difficulties with mental and motor activity, especially cognitive impairment. Discrete lateralizing neurologic findings such as hemiparesis or visual field defects are rare and suggest another diagnosis. CT and MRI show generalized atrophy with white matter changes late in the course. Approximately 25% of patients have accompaniment of signs of spinal cord involvement, including unilateral or bilateral leg weakness, sensory loss, or sphincter dysfunction. Some studies suggest encouraging results with the use of AZT.

Noncompressive myelopathy is usually due to vacuolar degeneration. It is present in 10 to 25% of patients. It is often associated with cognitive impairment, as a part of the AIDS dementia complex. Other causes include human T cell lymphotropic virus type I (HTLV I) (tropical spastic paraparesis), HSV, CMV, MTb, and *T. pallidum*. Specific diagnosis is made by immunologic and other studies of CSF.

Peripheral Nervous System Syndromes

Distal symmetric peripheral neuropathy is common in patients with advanced AIDS. It is the most common presentation of generalized neuropathy in patients with AIDS. It typically begins with a distal sensory loss of fingers or toes that spreads proximally. Trophic changes of the skin may be seen. Small doses of tricyclic antidepressants, for example, nortriptyline,* 10 mg every evening with increasing doses up to 50 mg per day, may ameliorate the symptoms.

Cranial nerve neuropathy can occur in the setting of HIV infection. Cranial nerves V and VII are most frequently affected. Nerves III, IV, and VI may also be involved.

Chronic inflammatory demyelinating polyradiculopathy is more common in patients with symptomatic HIV than in those with AIDS. It has a presentation similar to that of the Guillain-Barré syndrome (GBS) with weakness in both proximal and distal muscles of both upper and lower extremities. It tends to be more subacute or chronic than the typical GBS. Deep tendon reflexes may be hyporeflexic or absent. Sensory loss is usually mild and, if present, affects mostly hands and feet. Some patients respond dramatically to plasmapheresis.

Mononeuritis multiplex is a syndrome in which patients develop abrupt mononeuropathies, followed by additional mononeuropathies at other sites. Symptoms commonly include facial weakness, foot drop, cranial nerve involvement, and patchy sensory abnormalities.

---

*Not FDA-approved for this indication.

Progressive polyradiculopathy is characterized by progressive sensory and motor loss of subacute onset. It involves contiguous lumbar and sacral roots and can cause impaired bladder and rectal sphincter control, and sacral sensory loss.

Autonomic neuropathies have been described in patients with AIDS. Signs and symptoms include syncope, orthostatic hypotension, diarrhea, cardiac arrhythmias, cardiopulmonary arrest, disordered sweating, and impotence. Treatment is symptomatic.

Psychiatric Complications

Psychiatric complications are common in patients with AIDS and pose an extreme problem in diagnosis and treatment. Psychiatric referrals are indicated when treatment is beyond the clinician's expertise. Conditions that may warrant psychiatric assessment include (1) chronic anxiety that interferes with daily functioning or adherence to medical treatment recommendations, (2) depression with vegetative symptoms, (3) substance dependence, (4) organic mental disorders with marked impairment in alertness, orientation, memory, and intellectual tasks not due to other causes, and (5) suicidal ideation. As psychiatric symptoms may be seen with infections, tumors, and endocrine abnormalities, a complete investigation to assess for these conditions must be performed, along with any psychiatric referral.

WOMEN AND HIV

Women, especially young women aged 15 to 25 years, are facing the fastest rate of increase in HIV infection. Projections are that the number of women infected in the United States will equal that of HIV-infected men by the year 2000. Heterosexual contact is the second most frequent exposure category and accounts for 34% of all reported cases. Most heterosexual contacts in women are related to sexual contact with an HIV-infected injection drug user. Heterosexual transmission may be linked by both drug use and sexually transmitted diseases. Genital ulcerative diseases, like chancroid and syphilis, have been noted to facilitate the acquisition and transmission of HIV.

The overall survival with HIV and AIDS appears to be similar in women and men receiving similar treatments; however, several population-based studies indicate the women are less likely to have received antiretroviral therapy than men. The current recommendations for the initiation of antiretrovirals and antimicrobial prophylaxis are similar to those for HIV-infected men. Alternative therapies may be necessary during pregnancy, as some agents may be toxic to the fetus.

Since HIV infection is often associated with other sexually transmitted diseases, women with HIV infection should be evaluated for such conditions. Screening gynecologic exams should be performed with appropriate cultures for gonorrhea and chlamydial infection, as well as serologic examination for syphilis. Pap smears should be obtained to monitor for human papillomavirus and cervical dysplasia. A normal Pap smear should be repeated in 6 months to rule out false-negative results.

The current evidence suggests that there is an increased risk of cervical dysplasia in HIV-infected women. Many of the preinvasive lesions can be expected to progress to invasive carcinoma. Data suggest that progression to cervical cancer is more rapid in HIV infection. As a result, all HIV-infected women should have Pap smears annually. Any evidence of abnormal Pap smears, including squamous intraepithelial lesions or atypical squamous cells of undetermined significance, should be investigated promptly with colposcopy. Because lesions are often undiagnosed and untreated in many HIV-positive women, results of colposcopic testing show a tendency for high-grade lesions and more extensive disease than seen in the general population. Therefore, standard therapies often yield fewer cures and more recurrences than seen in HIV-negative women. Invasive cervical carcinoma is an AIDS-defining diagnosis based on the CDC revised case definition.

Human papillomavirus is thought to be the agent responsible for most cervical cancers, cervical dysplasia, and condylomata acuminata (genital warts), all of which are more common in HIV infection. Condylomata acuminata may be profuse with frequent recurrences despite therapy.

Chronic or recurrent vaginal candidiasis has been noticed in increased frequency in HIV-infected women. It can occur in early stages of HIV infection. Treatment with standard topical agents is usually satisfactory. Rarely, systemic antifungal therapy with ketoconazole or fluconazole is needed for severely immunosuppressed individuals or those with refractory infections.

Pelvic inflammatory disease occurs more frequently in HIV infection. It often requires inpatient treatment and prolonged antibiotic therapy and has more frequent complications, especially tubo-ovarian abscesses. HIV-infected women with pelvic inflammatory disease are more likely to need surgery for complications.

Pregnancy in HIV-infected women carries a 30 to 35% risk of HIV infection in the infant. The rate is highest for women with p24 antigenemia or low CD4 lymphocyte counts. Viral transmission can occur in utero, at delivery, or with breast feeding. Recent clinical trials have shown that AZT reduces in utero viral transmission. As a result, it is recommended that all pregnant females have an HIV test.

CONCLUSIONS

Although many strides have been made in identifying the etiologic agent of HIV, determining the pathophysiology of the disease, and defining the natural history of the process, HIV/AIDS is still a formidable challenge. There appears to be no cure in sight, and a vaccine is years away. In addition, as patients are living longer, surviving opportunistic infections and maintaining their health on a multitude of antimicrobial agents, the list of new pathogens and resistant organisms is increasing. As a result, the approach toward reducing morbidity and mortality in AIDS is through three basic strategies: (1) intervening in the natural history of HIV-associated immunodeficiency, (2) preventing the acquisition of new opportunistic pathogens, and (3) suppressing or eliminating latent infections.

Intervening in the natural history is an attempt to prolong survival and improve the quality of life. Strategies to slow the immunologic decline associated with HIV include the development and investigation of antiretroviral therapies. Other strategies to boost the immune system show some promise but have not yet proved to have any clinical benefit. Identifying surrogate markers with clinical utility, including a better use of CD4 lymphocyte counts, will help guide treatment options in the future.

Preventing the acquisition of pathogens means behavior modification for individuals practicing unsafe sex or exposing themselves to potential pathogens. Educating individuals on how to limit their exposure to pathogens may have an impact on their quality of life and ultimately, their survival. Judicious use of antimicrobial agents and the early identification of potential pathogens may limit the emergence of new and resistant organisms.

Suppressing or eliminating latent infections consists of primary or secondary prophylaxis and chronic suppressive therapy. Organisms that persist latently in normal hosts and may become active and cause disease in immunosuppressed persons include *P. carinii,* CMV, HSV, VZV, *T. gondii,* and MTb. Other organisms that may recur in immunosuppressed persons include: *Candida* spp, *H. capsulatum, C. neoformans,* MAC, and *Salmonella* spp. Providing safe, convenient, and economic prophylactic agents can substantially reduce morbidity and mortality.

Research in the next decade is likely to improve on the progress that has already been made. New oral agents are being developed, and current existing agents are being investigated for other uses. Many agents may be appropriate for the prophylaxis or multiple opportunistic infections. For example, TMP–SMX may be useful in preventing PCP, toxoplasmosis, and bacteremias due to streptococci and *H. influenzae.* The macrolides may be useful for PCP and mycobacterial, *Cryptosporidium,* and *Toxoplasma* infections. Rifabutin is showing some promising activity against *Toxoplasma,* mycobacterial, and other bacterial infections. Lastly, newer antiretroviral agents are being investigated, and vaccine trials continue.

ACKNOWLEDGMENT

The authors thank Dr. Donna Mildvan for her helpful discussions and review of the manuscript.

AMEBIASIS

method of
PHYLLIS E. KOZARSKY, M.D., and
JOHN A. JERNIGAN, M.D.
*Emory University School of Medicine
Atlanta, Georgia*

Entamoeba histolytica is an enteric protozoan that causes intestinal and extraintestinal disease worldwide. An estimated 10% of the world population is infected, but the great majority of infections occur in developing countries, where amebiasis is a leading cause of morbidity and mortality. Approximately 50 million cases of invasive disease occur each year, resulting in up to 100,000 deaths.

Recent data suggest that only 10% of those infected with the parasite harbor strains having the potential to cause invasive disease. In the past, morphologically indistinguishable pathogenic and nonpathogenic strains were classified within the same species *(E. histolytica).* There is now clear evidence that pathogenic and nonpathogenic strains are genetically distinct. Accordingly, it has recently been proposed that the nonpathogenic strains be reclassified as a separate species, *Entamoeba dispar. E. dispar* is not associated with invasive disease.

The infective form of the parasite is the cyst, which is excreted in large numbers in the stool of infected patients. Transmission is by the fecal-oral route. Cysts that are ingested excyst in the small bowel, resulting in trophozoite infection of the colon. In developing countries, the prevalence of infection may be as high as 50%. Although the overall prevalence of *E. histolytica / E. dispar* is much lower in developed countries, certain groups within nonendemic areas have a much higher incidence of infection. These include male homosexuals, Native Americans, immigrants from developing countries, and institutionalized mentally challenged individuals. Such risk factors should raise the diagnostic suspicion for amebiasis.

CLINICAL MANIFESTATIONS

The major clinical syndromes produced by *E. histolytica* infection include asymptomatic infection, acute rectocolitis, chronic intestinal amebiasis, and liver abscess.

Patients with acute amebic rectocolitis usually present with subacute (over 7 to 10 days) onset of crampy lower abdominal pain, small-volume diarrhea, bloody mucus in stools, and tenesmus. About one-third of patients have fever, and virtually all patients test positive for occult blood in the stool. Rarely, patients may present with a fulminant course characterized by high fever, profuse bloody diarrhea, colonic dilatation, and/or perforation, with signs of peritoneal irritation. Individuals at risk for fulminant amebiasis include those who are immunosuppressed, particularly those taking corticosteroids.

Chronic intestinal amebiasis is characterized by chronic intermittent diarrhea (sometimes bloody), abdominal pain, and weight loss. It can be clinically mistaken for inflammatory bowel disease, which may lead to treatment with corticosteroids and result in fulminant amebic colitis. Therefore, amebiasis should always be excluded before making the diagnosis of inflammatory bowel disease. Another form of chronic intestinal amebiasis is ameboma, which presents as a colonic mass, usually in the right colon, and is often mistaken for colonic carcinoma.

The most common form of extraintestinal amebiasis is hepatic abscess. Patients generally present acutely with fever and right upper quadrant pain; however, infrequently the presentation can be more chronic in nature with generalized abdominal pain and weight loss in the absence of fever. Other rare forms of extraintestinal amebiasis include extension of a liver abscess to involve the lung, pericardium, or peritoneum. Hematogenous dissemination rarely results in the formation of abscesses of the lung, brain, skin, and other organs.

DIAGNOSIS

The cornerstone of diagnosis of intestinal amebiasis remains the detection of *E. histolytica* cysts or trophozoites in stool by light microscopy. However, errors are frequent, and multiple stool samples are required. Numerous factors can interfere with the correct identification of the organism, including the experience of the microscopist, prior administration of hypertonic enemas (e.g., barium), and medications such as bismuth, laxatives, antacids, tetracyclines, and erythromycin. Stool antigen detection assays are now being studied, and the emerging data suggest that the assays not only are sensitive and specific but also distinguish pathogenic *E. histolytica* from nonpathogenic *E. dispar*. The precise clinical role for such assays in the diagnosis of amebiasis has not yet been fully established.

Other observations during stool examination are of importance in evaluating patients with suspected invasive amebiasis. Occult blood is present in the stools of virtually all patients with invasive intestinal amebiasis; a negative test for occult blood in the stool therefore argues against the disease. In addition, the presence of large numbers of polymorphonuclear leukocytes in the stool is not typical; *E. histolytica* lyses neutrophils, resulting in few, if any, fecal leukocytes on stool examination. The presence of hematophagous trophozoites is diagnostic of invasive disease.

Serologic testing is very helpful in the diagnosis of pathogenic *E. histolytica* infection. Ninety percent of patients infected with a pathogenic strain, including those with asymptomatic infection, will be seropositive by the seventh day of infection. Those infected with *E. dispar* have negative results using standard serology tests. Negative amebic serology is therefore useful in ruling out the presence of an invasive strain. In endemic areas where infection is very common, the presence of antibodies is less helpful in the diagnosis because patients may remain seropositive for years following treatment. The presence of antibodies, therefore, may not reflect active disease.

The diagnosis of amebic liver abscess can usually be established by the presence of a space-occupying liver lesion (e.g., by computed tomography or ultrasound), combined with epidemiologic risk factors and a positive amebic serology. Occasionally a fine-needle aspiration may be necessary to rule out a pyogenic abscess or a necrotic hepatoma. Amebic liver abscesses do not contain pus but rather proteinaceous "anchovy paste–like" fluid with necrotic cellular debris. Trophozoites are usually not found in this fluid. In addition, typically no trophozoites are detectable in the stool at the time of presentation in patients with amebic liver abscess.

TREATMENT

In general, the successful treatment of amebiasis involves a dual approach: (1) the use of agents directed toward trophozoites that have invaded tissue (if invasive disease is present), and (2) the use of agents directed toward intraluminal organisms. Luminal agents are required because the tissue amebicides fail to reach sufficiently high luminal levels to kill luminal trophozoites. If there is no evidence of invasive disease, luminal agents alone are sufficient.

Intestinal Infections

Asymptomatic Passage of Cysts and Trophozoites

The optimal management of the asymptomatic patient with cysts or red cell–free trophozoites in the stool is a matter of some controversy. Many of these patients are infected with nonpathogenic *E. dispar*. There is no evidence that infection with *E. dispar* poses any health risk to the infected individual or others, and therefore these individuals probably require no treatment. However, pathogenic and nonpathogenic strains are morphologically identical, and antigenic tests capable of distinguishing *E. dispar* from *E. histolytica* are not yet widely available. In nonendemic areas, we therefore favor presumptive treatment of asymptomatic excreters of cysts and/or red cell–free trophozoites with luminal agents only (Table 1). In endemic areas where the prevalence of infection may be as high as 50% and the risk of reinfection is great, the decision to treat asymptomatic persons is more complex. In this setting clinicians might opt to seek additional evidence for pathogenic infection by testing for antiamebic antibodies. A positive serologic test should be considered an indication for presumptive therapy in asymptomatic cyst or trophozoite excreters, even in an endemic area. However, we would not recommend therapy for a seronegative resident of an endemic area who is an asymptomatic cyst or trophozoite excreter.

Individuals who asymptomatically pass cysts or trophozoites and who require treatment should be given one of the following luminal agents: diloxanide furoate, paromomycin, or iodoquinol. Diloxanide furoate (Furamide)* is the preferred agent owing to its high efficacy and relative lack of toxicity. Unfortunately, the drug is only available in the United States from the Centers for Disease Control and Prevention

---

*Investigational drug in the United States.

TABLE 1. **Treatment of the Asymptomatic Cyst-Passer**

Drug	Adult Dosage (Oral)	Pediatric Dosage (Oral)
Diloxanide furoate (Furamide)*	500 mg tid × 10 days	20 mg/kg/day in 3 doses × 10 days
Paromomycin (Humatin)	25–30 mg/kg/day in 3 doses × 7 days	25–30 mg/kg/day in 3 doses × 7 days
Iodoquinol (Yodoxin)	650 mg tid × 20 days	30–40 mg/kg/day in 3 doses × 20 days

*In the United States, available only through the Centers for Disease Control and Prevention: 404-639-3670 (evenings, weekends, and holidays: 404-639-2888). In Canada, Bureau of Drugs, Health Protection Branch, Otttawa.

(CDC) in Atlanta, Georgia, and in Canada with the authorization of the Bureau of Drugs, Health Protection Branch, Ottawa. It is highly efficacious: a 10-day course results in an 85% eradication rate. The most common side effects are flatulence and, much less frequently, nausea, vomiting, and diarrhea. Paromomycin (Humatin), a poorly absorbed aminoglycoside, is also effective and is safe in pregnancy. Its major side effects are gastrointestinal disturbances. It is, however, very expensive. Iodoquinol (Yodoxin) is as effective as diloxanide furoate, but because it requires a prolonged (20 days) course, it is less convenient and makes full compliance less likely. Its side effects include nausea, diarrhea, cramping, and rarely neurotoxicity, including optic nerve damage and peripheral neuropathy (usually after prolonged use or high doses). In addition, iodoquinol has a high iodine content and therefore should be avoided in patients with iodine hypersensitivity or thyroid disease.

Asymptomatic persons who are excreting hematophagous trophozoites should be treated as though they have invasive amebic colitis (see next section).

Amebic Colitis

Nitroimidazoles (metronidazole [Flagyl], tinidazole* [Fasigyn]) are the mainstays of therapy for all invasive *E. histolytica* infections (Table 2). They penetrate well into all tissues and are highly amebicidal. However, they usually fail to eliminate intestinal carriage and should therefore be given in conjunction with a lumen-active agent. Although the lumen-active agent can be given concomitantly, it is usually withheld until metronidazole (or tinidazole) is completed in order to avoid additive side effects. The most common side effects of nitroimidazoles include nausea, abdominal discomfort, headache, metallic taste, and dark-colored urine. Other less common side effects include ataxia, confusion, insomnia, and paresthesias. Tinidazole is associated with fewer gastrointestinal complaints. Ethanol should be avoided during metronidazole therapy because of a disulfiram-like effect. Teratogenesis has been a concern with nitroimidazole use. However, in one uncontrolled study, over 200 women received metronidazole during the third trimester of pregnancy without any adverse effects to the fetus. Many authorities feel that the risk of fulminant disease in pregnancy outweighs the risk of drug-induced adverse fetal effects and therefore advise the use of metronidazole in pregnant patients with documented invasive *E. histolytica* infection.

Tetracyclines and erythromycins have amebicidal activity and, when followed by luminal agents, can be used as second-line therapy for mild intestinal disease in patients who do not tolerate metronidazole. They are, however, ineffective in treating liver abscess.

Dehydroemetine (Mebadin)† is an alternative

---

*Not available in the United States.
†Investigational drug in the United States.

TABLE 2. **Treatment of Amebic Colitis***

Drug	Adult Dosage	Pediatric Dosage
Metronidazole (Flagyl)	750 PO or IV tid × 10 days	35–50 mg/kg/day in 3 doses × 10 days
Tinidazole (Fasigyn)†	2 gm q day × 3 days	50 mg/kg (maximum, 2 gm) q day × 3 days
Alternative: Dehydroemetine (Mebadin)‡	1–1.5 mg/kg/day IM (maximum, 90 mg/day) for up to 5 days	1–1.5 mg/kg/day IM in 2 doses (maximum, 90 mg/day) for up to 5 days

*All regimens should be followed by a complete course of a luminal agent to eradicate intestinal colonization (see Table 1).
†Not available in the United States or Canada.
‡In the United States, available only through the Centers for Disease Control and Prevention: 404-639-3670 (evenings, weekends, and holidays: 404-639-2888). In Canada, Bureau of Drugs, Health Protection Branch, Ottawa.

agent that is rapidly amebicidal. Because of significant cardiovascular and neuromuscular toxicity, however, the drug is rarely recommended. It is available only through the CDC in the United States or with the authorization of the Bureau of Drugs, Health Protection Branch, Canada.

Regardless of the therapeutic regimen used, relapses can occur. All patients treated for amebic colitis should have eradication of the parasite documented by examination of at least two separate stool specimens collected 2 weeks following completion of therapy.

Liver Abscess

The therapy of choice for an amebic liver abscess is metronidazole followed by a luminal agent (Table 3). Although the traditional regimen calls for a 7- to 10-day course of therapy, patients with uncomplicated mild-to-moderate disease can be treated effec-

TABLE 3. **Treatment of Amebic Liver Abscess***

Drug of Choice	Adult Dosage	Pediatric Dosage
Metronidazole	750 mg PO or IV tid × 10 days **OR** 2.5 gm PO × 1 dose (mild-to-moderate disease only)	35–50 mg/kg/day in 3 doses × 10 days
Tinidazole†	800 mg PO tid × 5 days	60 mg/kg (maximum, 2 gm) q day × 3 days
Alternative: Dehydroemetine‡	1–1.5 mg/kg/day IM (maximum, 90 mg/day) for up to 5 days	1–1.5 mg/kg/day IM in 2 doses (maximum, 90 mg/day) for up to 5 days

*All regimens should be followed by a complete course of a luminal agent to eradicate intestinal colonization (see Table 1).
†Not available in the United States or Canada.
‡In the United States, available only through the Centers for Disease Control and Prevention: 404-639-3670 (evenings, weekends, and holidays: 404-639-2888). In Canada, Bureau of Drugs, Health Protection Branch, Ottawa.

tively with a single dose of 2.5 gm of metronidazole. Dehydroemetine is an alternative agent for critically ill patients but is not recommended because of its toxicity.

Patients usually respond within 48 to 72 hours with gradual improvement in fever and abdominal pain. Fine-needle aspiration of the abscess on presentation is usually unnecessary except when the abscess is very large, if there is impending rupture or a high suspicion of primary or secondary bacterial infection, or if the patient is moribund. Needle aspiration should also be considered if the patient is not responding to metronidazole.

Radiographic or sonographic evidence of hepatic abscess resolution takes months, and some patients will have a permanent hepatic cyst following completion of curative therapy. Repeated imaging studies are not necessary if the patient clinically responds to therapy. A recurrence of symptoms, however, merits investigation.

Patients with peritonitis due to rupture of an abscess have traditionally been managed by open surgical drainage, but some patients have now been managed nonoperatively. Similarly, lung abscesses can be managed without drainage. Amebic empyema and pericardial effusion, however, should be drained. All patients treated with surgical drainage still require a full course of antiamebic therapy.

NONPATHOGENIC AMEBAS

A variety of amebas are found in the intestine that are at present considered nonpathogenic and for which treatment is not indicated. These include *Entamoeba hartmanni, Entamoeba coli, Endolimax nana,* and *Iodamoeba bütschlii. Dientamoeba fragilis,* a flagellate (and not an ameba, but often confused with one because of its name), has been associated with bowel symptoms and can be treated with iodoquinol, paromomycin, or tetracycline.

BACTEREMIA AND SEPTICEMIA

method of
MICHAEL O'BRIEN, M.D., and
MATTHEW BIDWELL GOETZ, M.D.
UCLA School of Medicine
Los Angeles, California

The signs and symptoms of bacteremia are variegated, reflecting the interaction between bacterial toxins and the host immunologic response. The mere presence of bacteria in the bloodstream does not assure disease. During toothbrushing and defecation, the bloodstream is transiently seeded by small numbers of low-virulence bacteria, which are quickly cleared by the reticuloendothelial system. No symptoms usually attend such events.

A range of nomenclature is used to define the many possible consequences of bacterial bloodstream invasion. The term "bacteremia" refers only to the presence of bacteria within the bloodstream; clinical illness may or may not accompany this condition. In contrast, septicemia implies *systemic* disease caused by the presence of microorganisms and their toxins in the circulating blood. Because of the overlapping clinical manifestations, many physicians use the term "sepsis" to describe seriously ill infected patients, regardless of the presence or absence of bacteremia. Infected patients with otherwise unexplained evidence of organ hypoperfusion, e.g., hypoxemia, elevated lactate levels, or oliguria, are said to have "sepsis syndrome"; "septic shock" is defined by a fall in the systolic blood pressure to less than 90 mm Hg or by more than 40 mm Hg from baseline. Finally, since the inflammatory reaction that accompanies the sepsis syndrome may resemble that found in noninfectious ailments, such as severe pancreatitis, multiple trauma, or thermal injury, some investigators use the phrase "systemic inflammatory response syndrome" (SIRS) to describe the common features of these critically ill patients. It is important to recognize that even in the absence of detectable bacteremia, local bacterial infections may provoke the severe, systemic metabolic derangements of sepsis syndrome.

PATHOPHYSIOLOGY

Although gram-negative bacteria are the most notorious and common etiologic agents, sepsis syndrome often accompanies serious infection by gram-positive bacteria such as *Staphylococcus aureus* and is occasionally due to bloodstream infections by *Candida* species. More rarely, sepsis syndrome is caused by overwhelming infection by other fungi, as well as by mycobacteria, rickettsiae, viruses, and parasites. A common pathway by which virulent microorganisms and noninfectious ailments trigger this syndrome is through the provocation of cytokine release by macrophages. The best-described microbial trigger of sepsis syndrome is the lipopolysaccharide component of the outer cell membrane of gram-negative bacteria (otherwise known as endotoxin). The conserved lipid A moiety of endotoxin directly activates macrophages, causing the release of various cytokines. Similarly, the peptidoglycan component of the cell wall of gram-positive bacteria and various bacterial toxins (e.g., the toxic shock toxins of *S. aureus* and the exotoxins of *Streptococcus*) also activate macrophages. The relative importance of the uncontrolled activation of various cytokines and of other humoral and cellular mediators of the inflammatory response remains to be determined fully. Nevertheless, administration of tumor necrosis factor (TNF) and interleukin-1 (IL-1) to various animals results in the full-blown sepsis syndrome; in animal models, the administration of monoclonal antibodies that bind these cytokines blocks the septic response to subsequent microbial challenges.

The systemic release and activation of cytokines and other humoral and cellular inflammatory mediators result in the widespread loss of endothelial integrity, with subsequent capillary leak and intravascular volume depletion. Blood flow is further compromised by the activation of the fibrinolytic system early in sepsis, followed by the subsequent development of disseminated intravascular coagulation (DIC) and the attendant depletion of coagulation factors and the formation of microclots and microinfarcts. These events lead to the development of common complications of sepsis, including the adult respiratory distress syndrome, renal failure, and failure of other major organs. Hence sepsis syndrome is a systemic, inflammatory host response to pathogenic microorganisms, their components (e.g., endotoxin, peptidoglycans), or their toxins (e.g., the toxic shock syndrome toxins) in the blood or tissues. This state is largely provoked via a complicated cascade of cytokines and results in diffuse endothelial damage, which in turn injures adjacent tissues and compromises organ function. The severity of this reaction is related to the interplay of the number of infecting organisms, the quantity and type of microbial toxin released, and the intensity of the host's response.

CLINICAL PRESENTATION

Clinically detectable bacteremia is most often secondary to spillage into the blood of microorganisms from an extravascular site of infection, such as "pus under pressure" (e.g., abscesses; obstructed bowel or biliary or urinary tract), or to necrotizing infections (e.g., necrotizing fasciitis or gram-negative pneumonia) rather than to the sustained multiplication of bacteria within the vascular compartment (so-called primary bacteremia). Thus the manifestations of a local infection usually underlie the clinical presentation of sepsis (a systemic pathologic condition). Early symptoms and signs suggesting that the sepsis syndrome is developing include hyper- or hypothermia, tachypnea, tachycardia, chills and rigors, encephalopathy, diarrhea, oliguria, hypo- or hyperglycemia, and leukocytosis or leukopenia. Given the heterogeneity of infecting microorganisms and the varying fury of the consequent host response, it is not surprising that the signs and symptoms of bacteremia are highly variable. The late manifestations of sepsis, such as hypotension, the adult respiratory distress syndrome, renal insufficiency, dysglycemias, DIC, and lactic acidosis, reflect the consequences of the generalized activation of the host's inflammatory response.

The probability that the aforementioned nonspecific symptoms and signs are related to an underlying bacteremia increases with the presence of epidemiologic features, such as injection drug use or increasing age, co-morbidities such as organ transplantation, multiple trauma, severe burns, or diabetes mellitus, clinical features including fever, rigors, or an acute abdomen, and laboratory tests demonstrating an elevated sedimentation rate (more than 30 mm per hour), white blood cell count (more than 15,000 per mm^3), or immature granulocyte count (more than 1500 per mm^3). Nevertheless, it is still difficult to predict with any great accuracy the presence of sepsis in any single patient. For example, only one-third of all patients entered into clinical studies of agents to treat gram-negative bacteremia were subsequently found to have such an infection. Another third of the patients had nonbacteremic gram-negative infections, and 10% had gram-positive infections, but no infection was ultimately documented in nearly 20% of such patients. The immunologically compromised host offers other challenges. When bacteremia coexists with neutropenia (i.e., 500 neutrophils per mm^3 or less), a paucity of signs and symptoms is the rule, as the lack of neutrophils obviates pus formation or inflammation. For this reason, fever and minimal inflammation at any site must be taken seriously in the neutropenic patient.

DIAGNOSIS OF BACTEREMIA

Whereas the presence in blood cultures of organisms such as *S. aureus*, group A streptococci, *Streptococcus pneumoniae*, and *Escherichia coli* is a highly specific marker of serious infection, virtually all blood isolates of *Corynebacterium* or *Bacillus* species represent false positives. Similarly, most isolates of coagulase-negative staphylococci (e.g., *Staphylococcus epidermidis*) or *Propionibacterium acnes*, especially if found in only a single set of blood cultures or after greater than 2 days of blood culture incubation, represent false positives, except perhaps in patients with prosthetic cardiac valves or other prosthetic intravascular devices.

Most false-positive blood cultures arise because of poor technique. In obtaining blood cultures, the skin should be prepared as in a surgical scrub, being first cleansed with antiseptic soap and water and followed by the vigorous application of 70% isopropyl alcohol and then by an iodine solution that should be allowed to dry. Most authorities recommend the use of sterile gloves before insertion of the needle. Each venipuncture must be repeated with a new needle set, although needles need not be changed between the blood draw and the bottle inoculation. Increasing the volume of blood inoculated per blood culture set (up to the maximum recommended for a given system) increases the likelihood of a positive culture. Three sets of blood cultures, from three different blood draw sites, are nearly always adequate to obtain a positive culture when continuous bacteremia exists. Because of sampling error and difficulties in properly interpreting the finding of coagulase-negative staphylococci, a minimum of two sets of blood cultures should always be obtained. Unfortunately, the fevers and rigors of intermittent bacteremia often *follow* a bacteremic episode by 1 to 2 hours. When the patient is receiving antibiotics, attempts should be made at the nadir of the antibiotic blood levels; in such patients, blood culture systems equipped with antibiotic removal devices appear to increase bacterial yield modestly.

TREATMENT

Often antimicrobial therapy must be started in the septic patient before the identity of the infecting pathogen, let alone its antimicrobial susceptibility, is known (Tables 1 and 2). Nonetheless, haphazard, empirical antimicrobial therapy must be avoided. Although broad, empirical antimicrobial therapy is often necessary, the use of targeted antimicrobial therapy will better preserve a patient's endogenous microbial flora than will ultrabroad-spectrum regimens. The benefits of maintaining the endogenous flora are significant. The risk of superinfection, and especially of fungemia, increases with the use of broad-spectrum antimicrobial regimens.

It is difficult to institute appropriate empirical antimicrobial therapy in the absence of a scrupulous epidemiologic evaluation, careful attention to a patient's co-morbidities, a meticulous physical examination, recognition of the hallmarks of infection by specific pathogens, careful review of the Gram stain of infected materials, and knowledge of the patterns of antimicrobial resistance within the local community. Specific antimicrobial therapy directed at the susceptibility of the pathogen actually causing the septic state is, of course, superior to empirical therapy. Therefore, not only must the blood be cultured but cultures also should be made of all other infected sites so that therapy can be rapidly tailored to attack the microorganisms present in the specific patient.

Appreciation of the epidemiology of a given patient will provide clues as to the identity of the probable infecting pathogen. Fever in a patient who has recently returned from a trip to India may suggest the presence of *Salmonella typhi*. *S. aureus* sepsis is

TABLE 1. **Parenteral Antibiotics and Their Appropriate Dosage in Bacteremic Adults with Normal Renal Function**

Antimicrobial Agent	Dosage
Penicillins	
Beta-lactamase–susceptible (not active against *S. aureus*)	
Penicillin*	2–4 million U q 4 h
Ampicillin*	1–2 gm q 4–6 h
Beta-lactamase–resistant (not active against methicillin-resistant *S. aureus*)	
Oxacillin (Prostaphilin),† nafcillin (Unipen)†	1–2 gm q 4–6 h
Antipseudomonal penicillins	
Mezlocillin (Mezlin),* piperacillin (Pipracil)*	3–4 gm q 4–6 h
Ticarcillin (Ticar)*	3 gm q 4 h
Penicillins and beta-lactamase inhibitor combinations	
Ampicillin/sulbactam (Unasyn)*	1.5–3.0 gm q 6 h
Ticarcillin/clavulanate (Timentin)*	3.1 gm q 4 h
Piperacillin/tazobactam (Zosyn)*	3.375 gm q 6 h
Cephalosporins	
First-generation	
Cefazolin (Ancef)*	1–2 gm q 8 h
Cephradine (Velosef),* cephalothin (Keflin),* cephapirin (Cefadyl)*	1–2 gm q 4 h
Second-generation	
Cefoxitin (Mefoxin)*	1–2 gm q 4–6 h
Cefotetan (Cefotan)*	1–2 gm q 12 h
Cefuroxime (Zinacef)*	0.75–1.5 gm q 8 h
Third-generation (not active against *P. aeruginosa*)	
Cefotaxime (Claforan)*	2 gm q 4–12 h
Ceftriaxone (Rocephin)†	1–2 gm q 12–24 h
Ceftizoxime (Cefizox)*	2–4 gm q 8–12 h
Third-generation (active against *P. aeruginosa*)	
Ceftazidime (Fortax)*	1–2 gm q 8–12 h
Cefoperazone (Cefobid)†	2–4 gm q 8–12 h
Aminoglycosides	
Gentamicin,* tobramycin (Nebcin)*	3–5 mg/kg/day in three daily doses, with 1.7–2.0 mg/kg load
Amikacin (Amikin)*	15 mg/kg/day in two daily doses with 7.5 mg/kg load
Monobactam	
Aztreonam (Azactam)*	1–2 gm q 6 h
Carbapenem	
Imipenem plus cilastatin (Primaxin)*‡	0.5–1.0 gm q 6 h
Fluoroquinolones	
Ciprofloxacin (Cipro)*	200–400 mg q 12 h
Ofloxacin (Floxin)*	200–400 mg q 12 h
Other Antimicrobials	
Vancomycin (Vancocin)*	15 mg/kg q 12 h
Metronidazole (Flagyl)†	500 mg q 6–8 h
Erythromycin†	500 mg–1 gm q 6 h
Clindamycin (Cleocin)†	600–900 mg q 8 h
Chloramphenicol†	0.75–1.0 gm q 6 h
Trimethoprim/sulfamethoxazole (Bactrim, Septra)*	8/40–15/75 mg/kg/day in three to four daily doses
Tetracycline*§	0.5–1.0 gm q 12 h
Doxycycline (Vibramycin)†	100 mg q 12 h

*May require dosage adjustment in patients with renal insufficiency.
†Does not require dosage adjustment in patients with renal insufficiency.
‡Reserve high dose for patients with normal renal function and serious *P. aeruginosa* infections.
§Avoid in patients with renal insufficiency.

especially common among injection drug users and diabetic patients. HIV-infected patients are predisposed to sepsis due to *S. pneumoniae*, as well as to *S. aureus*. Hospitalized patients are likely to develop sepsis as a complication of an infected vascular catheter, surgical wound, or other medical or surgical intervention. These nosocomial infections tend to be more often caused by antimicrobe-resistant pathogens such as methicillin-resistant *S. aureus* or *S. epidermidis*, *Pseudomonas aeruginosa*, or other resis-

TABLE 2. Initial, Empirical Therapy for Suspected Septicemia by Clinical Syndrome

Clinical Syndrome	Likely Pathogens	Empirical Therapy*
Suspected sepsis in neutropenic patient (≤500 PMN/mm³)	Enterobacteriaceae, *P. aeruginosa*, *S. aureus*, *Streptococcus* spp (*S. epidermidis* if catheter infection suspected)	1. PS† + PSAG‡ 2. Ceftriaxone (or pip/tazo or ticar/clav§) + PSAG (limit to settings where infection by *P. aeruginosa* is unlikely). *Note: Add vancomycin to these regimens if catheter infection suspected*
Primary Bacteremia, Without Obvious Source		
Adult, neither recently hospitalized nor immunocompromised	*E. coli*, *K. pneumoniae*, *Enterobacter*, *S. aureus*, *S. pneumoniae*, and other *Streptococcus* spp	1. Non-PS3G cephalosporin‖ 2. Ampicillin/sulbactam 3. 1 gm ceph¶ + aminoglycoside
Adult with recent hospitalization and/or antimicrobial therapy	Enterobacteriaceae, *P. aeruginosa*, *S. aureus*, *S. pneumoniae*, and other *Streptococcus* spp	1. PS + PSAG 2. Pip/tazo (or ticar/clav)† + PSAG 3. Imipenem/cilastatin
Adult with illicit parenteral drug use	*S. aureus*	1. β-lactamase–resistant penicillin (or 1 gm ceph) + aminoglycoside 2. Vancomycin + aminoglycoside (if methicillin-resistant *S. aureus* strains are prevalent)
Contaminated intravascular device suspected	*S. aureus*, *S. epidermidis*, enterococci; rarely gram-negative bacteria	Vancomycin
Secondary Bacteremias		
Complicated soft tissue infections (e.g., necrotizing fasciitis, decubitus ulcers)	*S. aureus*, *Streptococcus* spp, Enterobacteriaceae, *P. aeruginosa*, anaerobes	1. 1 gm ceph¶ + aminoglycoside + metronidazole 2. Ampicillin/sulbactam or cefoxitin 3. Pip/tazo or ticar/clav†
*Acute Cellulitis**	*S. pyogenes*, occasionally *S. aureus*	1. β-lactamase–resistant penicillin (or 1 gm cephalosporin) + aminoglycoside 2. Vancomycin
Pulmonary Infections		
Community-acquired pneumonia	*S. pneumoniae*, *H. influenzae*, *S. aureus* (after influenza), *K. pneumoniae* (rare)	Ampicillin/sulbactam, cefuroxime, or non-PSAG cephalosporin
Hospital-acquired pneumonia	*P. aeruginosa*, *S. aureus*, Enterobacteriaceae, *Streptococcus* spp	1. PS + PSAG 2. Pip/tazo (or ticar/clav)† + PSAG 3. Imipenem/cilastatin
Urinary Tract Infections	*E. coli* and other Enterobacteriaceae (enterococci and *P. aeruginosa* are unusual)	1. Ampicillin + aminoglycoside 2. Non-PS3G cephalosporin 3. PS
Intra-Abdominal Infections: e.g., Intra-Abdominal Abscesses, Peritonitis, Biliary Tract Disease		
Community-acquired infection	Enterobacteriaceae, *Enterococcus*, *Bacteroides* spp	1. Ampicillin + aminoglycoside + metronidazole 2. Clindamycin + aminoglycoside 3. Cefoxitin or ampicillin/sulbactam
Hospital-acquired infection	As above, and consider *P. aeruginosa*	1. PS + PSAG + metronidazole 2. Pip/tazo (or ticar/clav)† + PSAG 3. Imipenem/cilastatin
Gynecologic Infections (Nonsexually Transmitted)		
Community-acquired infection	Enterobacteriaceae, *Enterococcus*, *Bacteroides* spp	1. Ampicillin + aminoglycoside + metronidazole 2. Clindamycin + aminoglycoside 3. Cefoxitin or ampicillin/sulbactam
Hospital-acquired infection	As above, and consider *P. aeruginosa*	1. PS + PSAG + metronidazole 2. Pip/tazo (or ticar/clav)† + PSAG 3. Imipenem/cilastatin
Central Nervous System Infections		
Community-acquired meningitis	*S. pneumoniae*, *N. meningitidis*	1. Cefotaxime (or ceftriaxone) 2. Chloramphenicol 3. Vancomycin (if ceftriaxone-resistant pneumococci suspected)
Meningitis during pregnancy or in patients with impaired cell-mediated immunity	*S. pneumoniae*, *N. meningitidis*, *Listeria monocytogenes*	1. Cefotaxime or ceftriaxone + ampicillin 2. Chloramphenicol + trimethoprim/sulfamethoxazole
Postneurosurgical meningitis	*S. epidermidis*, *S. aureus*, Enterobacteriaceae, *P. aeruginosa*, *S. pneumoniae*	Vancomycin + ceftazidime

*Strongly consider adding an aminoglycoside for all clinical syndromes accompanied by evidence of septic shock.

†Beta-lactam with activity against *P. aeruginosa*—e.g., ceftazidime, mezlocillin, piperacillin, or ticarcillin. Note that piperacillin/tazobactam and ticarcillin/clavulanic acid have a lower maximal dose and are no more active against *P. aeruginosa* than are piperacillin and ticarcillin. Therefore, piperacillin/tazobactam and ticarcillin/clavulanic acid should not be used to treat potentially life-threatening infections by *P. aeruginosa*.

‡Aminoglycoside with activity against *P. aeruginosa* (check local antimicrobial susceptibilities).

§Piperacillin/tazobactam or ticarcillin/clavulanic acid.

‖Third-generation cephalosporin without activity against *P. aeruginosa*.

¶First-generation cephalosporin.

**In the setting of chronic liver disease and cellulitis, especially when there is a history of seawater/oyster exposure, consider *Vibrio vulnificus* infection (to be treated with tetracycline, doxycycline, or cefotaxime).

Abbreviations: PS = antipseudomonal β-lactam; PSAG = antipseudomonal aminoglycoside; PS3G = antipseudomonal third-generation cephalosporin.

tant gram-negative rods, and thus differ from community-acquired infections.

Some microorganisms such as *S. pneumoniae* are highly virulent and rapidly invade the bloodstream in nonimmune hosts. Other pathogens are more likely in septic, immunocompromised patients. For example, *P. aeruginosa* and other gram-negative rods such as *E. coli* and *Klebsiella pneumoniae* are common pathogens in neutropenic patients (especially in persons with less than 100 polymorphonuclear neutrophils per mm^3). Similarly, *Salmonella* and *Listeria monocytogenes* are over-represented in patients with impaired cell-mediated immunity (e.g., patients receiving high doses of corticosteroids), as is *Vibrio vulnificus* in patients with hepatic cirrhosis. Encapsulated bacteria such as *S. pneumoniae, Neisseria meningitidis*, and *Haemophilus influenzae* often cause acute, fulminant septic shock in asplenic patients and are common causes of sepsis syndrome in other patients who have abnormalities in humoral immunity (e.g., patients with hypogammaglobulinemia or complement defects). The risk of gram-negative sepsis increases in patients with disruption of mucosal barriers (e.g., by ischemia, trauma, malignancy), an obstructed viscus (biliary, bowel, or urinary), cirrhosis, nosocomial factors, or extensive tissue necrosis (e.g., burns or decubiti). Thus, a neutropenic patient with acute leukemia who was recently in the hospital for a long course of antibiotics and who now presents with a urinary tract infection deserves consideration of *P. aeruginosa* infection; this pathogen is extremely uncommon in an otherwise healthy, not recently hospitalized, young, sexually active female who presents with a urinary tract infection, no matter its severity.

Patients with infections by certain organisms present with distinctive clinical features. Meningococcemia, for example, classically manifests as a petechial rash. In neutropenic patients, gram-negative infections, especially with *P. aeruginosa*, can lead to ecthyma gangrenosum. *V. vulnificus* is frequently the pathogen in a patient, often with liver disease, recently exposed to seawater and presenting with a rapidly progressive cellulitis.

Bacterial endocarditis should be considered in any patient with a fever of unknown origin (FUO). Although embolic manifestations are present in over half of all patients, nearly 30% of patients with endocarditis present primarily with musculoskeletal symptoms, and 15% have a primary neurologic event. Fever is initially absent in nearly 25% of patients with bacterial endocarditis, whereas up to 10% lack a cardiac murmur at presentation, and up to 35% have no history of prior valvular disease. Osler's nodes, Janeway's lesions, petechiae, and retinal lesions are each present in less than a third of patients with bacterial endocarditis.

Subacute bacterial endocarditis is generally due to infection by low-virulence organisms such as the viridans group of streptococci, the so-called HACEK bacteria (*Haemophilus, Actinobacillus, Cardiobacter, Eikenella, Kingella*), and occasionally enterococci.

Acute endocarditis is generally due to *S. aureus*; enterococci, enteric gram-negative rods, *S. pneumoniae*, and *Neisseria gonorrhoeae* are less common causes. In patients with prosthetic valve endocarditis, *S. aureus*, coagulase-negative staphylococci, enteric gram-negative rods, *P. aeruginosa*, corynebacteria, and fungi are of greatest concern during the first 60 days after surgery, after which streptococci and staphylococci predominate.

In summary, the patient is well served if an exhaustive physical examination reveals the nidus of infection, and Gram's stain of material from that region supports the targeted use of antimicrobials. If the bacteremia is secondary, for example, when a urinary tract infection coexists with sepsis, a list of likely pathogens can generally be formulated, so antibiotic coverage need not be haphazard or overly broad. Furthermore, removal, débridement, decompression, or drainage of infected prosthetic devices, abscesses, or obstructed viscera is a critical therapeutic adjunct.

The principle that the prompt administration of appropriate antimicrobial agents in the correct dose improves the outcome of infected patients holds doubly true for septic patients. Thus for potentially toxic agents, such as aminoglycosides, serum drug levels should be obtained to assure that adequate serum concentrations are achieved. Bactericidal agents are strongly recommended; their use is mandatory in the treatment of endocarditis and meningitis and in the neutropenic patient. Treatment of streptococcal endocarditis also is highly dependent on the minimal inhibitory concentration (MIC) of penicillin needed to inhibit growth of the infecting microorganism.

Once the pathogen is known, from either a positive blood culture or the culture of a local site, the antimicrobial regimen should be simplified to reflect that pathogen's antimicrobial susceptibility. In so doing, attention needs to be paid to antimicrobial toxicity and to the penetration of the antimicrobial into the infected site. Intuitive as this concept may be, too often practitioners continue empirical broad-spectrum therapy, apparently concerned that altering what has been a successful course of action may be harmful. The real concern should be for the integrity of the patient's endogenous flora, which is eroded daily by the use of antibiotics—the broader the spectrum, the more dangerous in this regard. The duration of antimicrobial therapy is highly dependent on the site of infection and the clinical course of the patient. Specific guidelines for the treatment of endocarditis are shown in Table 3. In regard to the treatment of the septic neutropenic patient who has responded to therapy, antimicrobials may be discontinued 5 to 7 days after resolution of signs of infection or after the absolute neutrophil count has increased to more than 500 per mm^3. In patients who are not clinically well, antimicrobial therapy should be continued at least until the absolute neutrophil count has increased to more than 500 per mm^3. In persistently febrile neutropenic patients for whom no cause of continued fever has been found, empirical vanco-

TABLE 3. **Treatment of Endocarditis**

Empirical Therapy

Subacute bacterial endocarditis   Penicillin G + gentamicin
Acute bacterial endocarditis   Penicillin G, gentamicin, + oxacillin
Early prosthetic valve endocarditis   Ceftazidime, amikacin, + vancomycin
Late prosthetic valve endocarditis   Vancomycin, gentamicin, + rifampin

***Streptococci* with Penicillin, MIC <0.5 μg/mL**

Native Valve Endocarditis
Penicillin, MIC ≤0.1 μg/mL
    Penicillin G (10–20 million U/day × 4 weeks) + gentamicin (3 mg/kg/day × 2 weeks)* **or**
    Penicillin G (10–20 million U/day × 2 weeks) + gentamicin (3 mg/kg/day × 2 weeks)
Penicillin, MIC 0.2–<0.5 μg/mL
    Penicillin G (10–20 million U/day × 4 weeks) + gentamicin (3 mg/kg/day × 2 weeks)
Prosthetic Valve Endocarditis
Penicillin, MIC <0.5 μg/mL
    Penicillin G (10–20 million U/day × 4–6 weeks) + gentamicin (3 mg/kg/day × 2 weeks)

***Enterococci* or *Streptococci* with Penicillin, MIC >0.5 μg/mL**

Native Valve
    Penicillin G (20–24 million U/day) + gentamicin (3 mg/kg/day), both for 4–6 weeks†
Prosthetic Valve
    Penicillin G (20–24 million U/day) + gentamicin (3 mg/kg/day), both for 6–8 weeks†

Staphylococci

Native Valve
    Oxacillin (12 gm/day) for 4–6 weeks **or**
    Vancomycin (30 mg/kg/day) for 4–6 weeks if methicillin-resistant
Prosthetic Valve
    Oxacillin (12 gm/day) for 6–8 weeks **or**
    Vancomycin (30 mg/kg/day) for 6–8 weeks

    All the above must be combined with

    Rifampin (900 mg/day) for 6–8 weeks **plus**
    Gentamicin (3 mg/kg/day) for 2 weeks

Penicillin-Allergic Patients

Streptococci with MIC <0.5 μg/mL: Substitute cephalothin (12 gm/day) or ceftriaxone (4 gm/day)

Enterococci or *streptococci* with MIC ≥0.5 μg/mL: Substitute vancomycin (30 mg/kg/day); consider penicillin desensitization

Staphylococci: Substitute cephalothin. Vancomycin must be used if the isolate is resistant to methicillin

---

*Add gentamicin for prolonged (>12 weeks) symptoms. Avoid gentamicin with old age or renal disease. Two weeks' therapy with penicillin plus gentamicin is adequate only for uncomplicated cases. Aim for peak levels of 3–5 μg/mL of gentamicin (or 20 μg/mL of streptomycin).

†Isolates with high-level gentamicin resistance (MIC > 2000 μg/mL) may be sensitive to streptomycin. If no synergy can be demonstrated, consider 8–12 weeks of therapy; valve replacement may be required for cure. Rare isolates produce β-lactamase or, less commonly, are vancomycin-resistant.

---

mycin is added after 4 to 5 days of therapy if a long-term vascular catheter is present. After 5 to 7 days of persistent fever, amphotericin is added.

In treating septic shock, antibiotics alone do not suffice. Aggressive intravascular volume repletion is critical, and the use of pressors can be lifesaving, although their use should await normalization of pulmonary capillary wedge pressure. If hypotension persists after the pulmonary capillary wedge pressure is greater than 14 mm Hg, dopamine should be considered in order to support major organ perfusion while not unduly vasoconstricting the renal vascular bed. Once the dose of dopamine exceeds about 15 μg per kg per minute, norepinephrine should be begun, with dopamine dosing lowered to below 5 μg per kg per minute, to maintain renal vascular flow.

Aside from antibiotics, fluid, and pressors, there are no other universally accepted treatments for septic shock. Corticosteroids *do* benefit experimental animals with sepsis but only if given *before* the animal becomes septic. Recent clinical studies have shown clearly that steroids have no benefit in the treatment

of septicemia. Similarly, although acidemia is a common complication of sepsis, the administration of bicarbonate may actually be harmful to patients with sepsis and low blood pH. Most experts emphasize the need for treating the underlying causes of septic acidosis (infection, poor perfusion) and completely shun the use of bicarbonate; a few recommend it as a last-ditch effort when the blood pH falls below 7.10.

Millions of dollars have been spent recently on clinical trials of antiendotoxin and anticytokine therapies. Monoclonal antibodies (HA-1A and E5) directed against the lipid A moiety of endotoxin have not been shown to offer overall significant clinical benefit in the treatment of patients with suspected gram-negative septicemia. More recently, a trial of a receptor antagonist to IL-1 was halted before completion of the study because of lack of benefit. These failures suggest that by the time sepsis is recognized, using the currently available, insensitive, and imprecise diagnostic tools, the inflammatory cascade cannot be consistently reversed merely by blocking the activation and activity of TNF and IL-1.

PREVENTION

It is estimated that there are 400,000 episodes of sepsis yearly in the United States, 50% of which are associated with shock and 25% of which are fatal. About one-half of septic episodes occur in hospitals. Prevention of many of these tragedies is a realistic goal. Minimizing the duration of use of intravenous and intra-arterial catheters and indwelling Foley catheters, keeping neutropenic episodes as short as possible, and not overusing corticosteroids would reduce much of the risk. Pneumococcal vaccine should be administered to asplenic patients, and prophylactic antibiotics should be used in accordance with published recommendations in patients with prosthetic heart valves or other cardiac indications who are about to undergo an invasive procedure.

BRUCELLOSIS

method of
NIGEL I. JOWETT, M.D., and
K. YUGAMBARANATHAN, M.B.
Withybush General Hospital
Pembrokeshire, Wales, United Kingdom

Brucellosis in humans is acquired from infected domestic animals, and although animal brucellosis occurs worldwide, human brucellosis is now uncommon in developed countries, where bovine eradication programs and pasteurization of dairy products have contributed to its decline.

Most human cases occur in those people occupationally exposed to animals, following inhalation or inoculation of the organism when in close contact with infected animals (e.g., farmers, shepherds, veterinary surgeons), or via the animal carcass, where the organism can survive for several weeks, placing butchers and abattoir workers at risk. The remainder of cases usually occur following ingestion of contaminated meat or dairy products, particularly milk and goat cheese.

The *Brucella* organism is a gram-negative, aerobic, nonmotile, nonsporing coccobacillus, which grows very slowly in vitro. Four *Brucella* species are known to infect humans:

Most common: B. melitensis—from sheep, goats, and camels; B. abortus—from cattle.
Less common: B. suis—from pigs.
Very uncommon: B. canis—from dogs.

Brucellae are rapidly phagocytosed by neutrophils at the portal of entry and carried to the regional lymph nodes, where they may be eradicated without consequence or they may replicate. Subsequent dissemination leads to localization in reticuloendothelial cells of the liver, spleen, kidneys, and lymph nodes, where granulomata, similar to those found in sarcoidosis and tuberculosis, may form. Other sites of localization are the endocardium, bone, testes, central nervous system, and peripheral nerves. This intracellular localization helps to protect the organism from host defenses (and antibiotics), providing the potential for chronic infection. It is not clear whether clinical symptoms are related to destruction of the organism with endotoxin release or are due to periodic release of bacteria into the bloodstream.

Following an incubation period of 1 to 3 weeks (although occasionally several months), acute brucellosis presents with nonspecific symptoms, so early diagnosis requires a high index of suspicion. The clinical features depend largely on the virulence of the infecting organism and are usually those of an influenza-like illness with fever, myalgia, headache, fatigue, and sore throat. There may be an acute epididymo-orchitis, arthritis, or cholecystitis.

The term "chronic brucellosis" is applied when symptoms continue or recur 6 months or more after an acute attack or occur insidiously. There is a low-grade undulant fever, sweats, fatigue, headache, musculoskeletal pains, and marked depression. Low back pain and hepatosplenomegaly may be other features.

Confirming the diagnosis is usually serologic, where a tube agglutination titer of 1:160 or over or evidence of seroconversion suggests active infection. Isolation of the microorganism from the blood is possible in about two-thirds of cases, and marrow or other tissue culture may be of value.

TREATMENT

The most effective, least toxic chemotherapy for brucellosis has not been established. In vitro susceptibility is not always possible to determine in the absence of a bacterial isolate, and it is more usual for empirical therapy to be administered. No single drug will reliably eradicate the organism and prolonged combination antibiotic therapy is recommended. The drugs chosen must have good tissue penetration and intracellular activity because of the intracellular localization of the *Brucella* organism. Despite many different antibiotics being tried, the synergistic combination of a tetracycline and an aminoglycoside remains the most effective therapy. Even this fails to prevent relapse in up to 10% of cases, despite persisting organisms retaining their antibiotic sensitivities.

Doxycycline, 100 mg twice daily orally, is the tetracycline of choice because of its excellent absorption, tissue penetration, and long half-life (18 to 24 hours).

The most used aminoglycoside is intramuscular streptomycin, at a dose of 1 gram per day in patients under 40 years old and 0.5 to 0.75 gram per day in older patients or those weighing less than 50 kg. Alternatives are intramuscular gentamicin and netilmicin. Gentamicin (Garamycin),* 2 to 5 mg per kg, needs to be given every 8 hours, but netilmicin (Netromycin), 4 to 6 mg per kg, may be given once daily. Plasma levels should always be monitored.

Combination therapy is continued for 14 to 21 days, followed by doxycycline alone for a total duration of 6 weeks. In severe cases, combination therapy is extended to 4 weeks, followed by oral doxycycline and trimethoprim 80 mg and sulfamethoxazole 400 mg (Bactrim, Septra) twice daily for a further 4 to 8 weeks.

Although rifampin (Rifadin),* 15 mg per kg per day, is currently recommended by the World Health Organization in preference to the aminoglycosides in combination with doxycycline for 6 weeks, a recent

---

*Not FDA-approved for this indication.

meta-analysis of treatment trials suggests reduced efficacy. This needs to be balanced against the more complex arrangements required for intramuscular administration of aminoglycosides, the need to assay drug levels, and the greater potential for toxicity. The authors initially use the rifampin/doxycycline regimen for reasons of improved safety, compliance, convenience, and cost. Oral ofloxacin (Floxin),* 200 mg twice daily, is used instead of doxycycline if gastric side effects are severe.

Treating Patients with Renal Impairment

Aminoglycosides should be used with great caution in those patients with renal impairment, and frequent plasma drug concentrations with renal function tests should be performed. Doxycycline (although not tetracycline) is safe, and may be used with rifampin or trimethoprim and sulfamethoxazole at reduced doses.

Brucellosis in Pregnancy

Untreated pregnant women may suffer fetal death. Chemotherapy is difficult because of the risk of fetal harm, and the aminoglycosides and tetracyclines are particularly toxic. Treatment strategies depend on the severity of the illness and the stage of pregnancy at diagnosis. Discussion among patient, physician, and obstetrician is recommended to assess the risks and benefits of treatment. The use of rifampin alone for 2 months is suitable, but seldom effects a cure. More definitive therapy in the first trimester involves 6-week combination therapy of doxycycline and rifampin. In the second and third trimesters, rifampin with trimethoprim and sulfamethoxazole for 2 to 3 months appears to be relatively safe.

Childhood Brucellosis

Childhood brucellosis is often a mild, self-limiting disease. Treatment is therefore controversial, particularly with the potential adverse effects of the aminoglycosides and tetracyclines in the young. Children under the age of 8 years should not be treated with these drugs, but the combination of trimethoprim and sulfamethoxazole with rifampin is both effective and safe.

For those over the age of 8 years, doxycycline, 3 mg per kg orally in divided doses for 6 weeks, and streptomycin, 15 to 20 mg per kg per day for 2 weeks, has been the usual first-line therapy. Most physicians now prefer to avoid aminoglycosides and use oral doxycycline with trimethoprim 40 mg and sulfamethoxazole 200 mg, twice daily for 6 weeks, or doxycy-

*Not FDA-approved for this indication.

cline and rifampin, 15 mg per kg once daily for 6 weeks.

Treatment of Complications

Skeletal Brucellosis

Weight-bearing joints are most affected, and become hot, swollen, and tender. Vertebral osteomyelitis is particularly common, sometimes associated with paraspinal or psoas abscesses. Relapse is common following treatment of osteoarticular brucellosis, and prolonged therapy (minimum, 12 weeks) is recommended, combined with surgery if indicated.

Brucella *Endocarditis*

Endocarditis is an uncommon, but often lethal, complication of brucellosis, mostly occurring on previously damaged valves (usually the aortic). Triple therapy with a combination of tetracycline, aminoglycoside, and rifampin or trimethoprim and sulfamethoxazole is recommended to increase serum bactericidal activity. Treatment is needed for at least 2 months, but virtually all patients require surgical intervention. Early transfer to a cardiothoracic unit is therefore recommended before fulminating cardiac failure develops. Antibiotic therapy should be continued for several weeks after valve replacement.

Neurobrucellosis

Neurobrucellosis usually manifests as meningitis, although encephalitis, stroke, cranial nerve lesions, or bleeding from mycotic aneurysms may occur. Central manifestations are often serious, and drugs that cross the blood-brain barrier should be used. Aminoglycosides are particularly poor in this respect. The authors therefore use doxycycline with rifampin for 3 to 6 months. Trimethoprim and sulfamethoxazole or chloramphenicol may be added in severe cases.

Response to Treatment

Patients should be warned that there is often an initial transient deterioration of symptoms soon after the start of therapy (the Spink effect), particularly if tetracyclines are used. This Jarisch-Herxheimer reaction should not necessitate discontinuation of treatment. Clinical improvement can be expected within 14 days of starting antibiotics. Relapses usually occur within 2 months of completing therapy, and may be difficult to distinguish from other causes of the chronic fatigue syndrome or depression. Expert interpretation of appropriate serology helps identify persistent infection. Splenomegaly or positive blood cultures occur in a minority of patients, but these are major clues of relapse.

The authors follow up patients for 3 years with clinical examination, blood cultures, and serologic tests performed quarterly in the first year, and then every 6 months for 2 years.

CONJUNCTIVITIS

method of
GERALD B. ROSEN, M.D., and
JAMES V. AQUAVELLA, M.D.

University of Rochester
Rochester, New York

The conjunctiva, along with the corneal epithelium and tear film, constitutes the ocular surface. Conjunctival inflammation may result from infectious, allergic, mechanical, or immunologic processes or from contiguous inflammation from an adjacent tissue. In the normal eye, the tear film provides an effective barrier to infection by virtue of a mechanical lavaging effect and its antimicrobial constituents, such as lysozyme, lactoferrin, betalysin, and immunoglobulins. Nevertheless, conjunctival infection may result from dysfunctional tear film, abnormal conjunctival anatomy caused by trauma or disease, and exposure to virulent or opportunistic pathogens.

The clinical presentation of infectious conjunctivitis varies, depending on the offending organism and its disease-producing capabilities. Common symptoms include burning, itching, tearing, and foreign-body sensation. Examination usually reveals varying degrees of conjunctival hyperemia, chemosis (edema), discharge, and lid edema. The predominant symptoms and signs, including the characteristics of the discharge, help determine the underlying cause of the conjunctivitis (Table 1). When present, conjunctival follicles, subconjunctival hemorrhage, or ipsilateral preauricular adenopathy helps limit the differential diagnosis.

Although unnecessary for most primary episodes of conjunctivitis, conjunctival swabbing for culture and sensitivity should be performed for any case of persistent, recurrent, or hyperacute conjunctivitis. Other ancillary laboratory studies occasionally used in the work-up of conjunctivitis include conjunctival scraping for cytology, swabbing for direct fluorescent antibody or enzyme-linked immunoassay tests, and conjunctival biopsy. Indications for these procedures are discussed later.

OPHTHALMIA NEONATORUM

Neonatal conjunctivitis (ophthalmia neonatorum) refers to the occurrence of conjunctivitis in the first month of life. In addition to its significant ophthalmic morbidity, ophthalmia neonatorum can represent a manifestation of potentially serious systemic infection. Historically, this was an important cause of blindness prior to the introduction of silver nitrate prophylaxis by Credé in 1881. Although the widespread use of chemoprophylaxis has dramatically reduced the incidence of neonatal blindness, the potentially devastating consequences of ophthalmia neonatorum require that this entity be given special consideration in any discussion of infectious conjunctivitis.

The normal conjunctival flora of the neonate reflects the normal bacterial flora of the vagina. Likewise, conjunctival pathogens in the first month of life are usually neonatal extensions of venereal diseases. The most devastating of these pathogens is *Neisseria gonorrhoeae*. This aerobic gram-negative diplococcus elicits a fierce inflammatory response leading to a copious purulent discharge that typically begins 12 to 24 hours after birth. Neisserial organisms are capable of penetrating intact epithelial cells, and, consequently, conjunctival infection may progress rapidly to corneal ulceration and perforation. Gram's stain of the discharge reveals the characteristic microorganisms along with an abundance of polymorphonuclear leukocytes. *N. gonorrhoeae* is most easily cultured on chocolate agar or Thayer-Martin medium with 5 to 10% carbon dioxide.

Infants must be treated both systemically and topically. Topical therapy consists of penicillin G drops, 20,000 U per mL every 30 minutes. Alternatively, bacitracin, erythromycin, or gentamicin ointment may be used. Frequent lavage is also recommended. Because disseminated infection may occur, systemic treatment is mandatory. Ceftriaxone (Rocephin), 25 to 40 mg per kg intravenously every 8 hours, is recommended for at least 3 days. Alternatively, penicillin G (if sensitivity is documented), 25,000 U per kg intravenously four times a day, or gentamicin, 2 to 2.5 mg per kg intravenously every 8 hours, may be used. Because chlamydial co-infection often exists, oral erythromycin, 50 mg per kg per day in four divided doses for 14 days, is also recommended.

Chlamydia trachomatis is the most common cause of infectious neonatal conjunctivitis in the United States, occurring in up to 40% of infants born through chlamydia-infected birth canals. Typically, a mucopurulent conjunctivitis becomes apparent 5 to 14 days after birth, although an earlier presentation may occur if the amniotic membranes rupture prematurely. The condition is usually mild; however, conjunctival scarring and corneal opacification have been reported. Diagnosing *C. trachomatis* as the etiologic agent in a neonate with conjunctivitis may aid the diagnosis of concurrent chlamydial pneumonitis, which occurs in up to 20% of infants with conjunctivitis. Giemsa staining of conjunctival scrapings may reveal intracytoplasmic inclusion bodies within epithelial cells. A monoclonal antibody test (Micro-Trak) and an enzyme-linked immunoassay are also available for rapid and accurate diagnosis. The treatment strategy for neonatal chlamydial conjunctivitis includes consideration of the need to treat not only the conjunctivitis, but the often-associated respiratory colonization, the mother's genital tract, and that of her sexual partner.

TABLE 1. **Discharge Characteristics of Different Types of Conjunctivitis**

	Watery	Mucoid	Mucopurulent	Purulent
Viral*	+	+		
Chlamydial*†		+	+	
Bacterial			+	+
Allergic‡	+	+		

*Conjunctival follicles common.
†Giemsa stain of conjunctival scrapings may reveal intracytoplasmic inclusions.
‡Giemsa stain of conjunctival scrapings may reveal eosinophils.

The neonate must be treated systemically with erythromycin, 50 mg per kg per day in four divided doses for 2 weeks. Although probably of minimal benefit, erythromycin ointment may also be applied topically. The mother and her partner can be treated most easily by a single oral dose of azithromycin (Zithromax), 1 gram. Alternatively, they may be treated with oral tetracycline, 500 mg four times a day for 1 week. The breast-feeding mother should be given oral erythromycin instead of tetracycline.

Herpes simplex virus (HSV) type 2 is a rare but important pathogen to consider in the differential diagnosis of ophthalmia neonatorum. Should disseminated disease occur, the mortality may be as high as 50 to 80%. Onset is in the first 2 weeks postpartum as a unilateral or bilateral conjunctivitis. Ophthalmic manifestations may include lid vesicles, serosanguineous conjunctival discharge, corneal epithelial dendrites, cataract, and uveitis. In the absence of skin vesicles and keratitis, the diagnosis may be difficult to make. Multinucleated giant cells or eosinophilic intranuclear inclusions may be seen on Papanicolaou stain of infected conjunctival or corneal epithelium. Viral cultures should be performed. Monoclonal antibody tests are now also available. Topical trifluridine (Viroptic) every 2 hours while the patient is awake is the drug of choice for conjunctivitis or dendritic keratitis. Uveitis or disseminated disease should be treated with systemic acyclovir.

Other commonly encountered causes of neonatal conjunctivitis are staphylococcal and chemical conjunctivitis. Chemical conjunctivitis, caused most often by the prophylactic application of topical 1% silver nitrate solution, occurs in 50 to 100% of treated neonates and is the most common overall cause of neonatal conjunctivitis. The typical picture is one of mild hyperemia and tearing, which usually resolves after 1 to 2 days. Concern over induced ocular toxicity and ineffectiveness has led to the substitution of erythromycin or tetracycline ointment in many hospital centers.

In summary, management of ophthalmia neonatorum should be prompt and thorough. Stains and cultures should be performed routinely, and systemic treatment is mandatory.

ADULT CONJUNCTIVITIS

Viral Conjunctivitis

Viral conjunctivitis is one of the most common conditions presenting to an acute care setting. Onset is usually unilateral at first, with involvement of the second eye within 1 week. Itching and tearing are the predominant symptoms. Examination reveals a watery discharge, often with a follicular conjunctival reaction and a preauricular node. Most viral conjunctivitides resolve without sequelae within 2 weeks. For these uncomplicated cases, treatment is directed toward relief of symptoms with cold compresses and artificial tears. Patients must also be instructed to practice meticulous hygiene to decrease the risk of transmission to others. Adenovirus, which is responsible for pharyngoconjunctival fever (PCF) and the highly contagious epidemic keratoconjunctivitis (EKC), is probably the most common viral cause of conjunctivitis; however, many different viruses have been implicated.

Primary HSV conjunctivitis (usually caused by HSV type 1) may be diagnosed by its association with typical eyelid vesicles; a follicular conjunctivitis; and punctate, dendritic, or geographic keratitis. Recurrent ocular HSV infection in an adult is usually a corneal process with the conjunctivitis secondary. Topical application of trifluridine is effective in reducing viral replication and decreasing the risk of corneal scarring. Topical steroids, which potentiate viral replication, are contraindicated unless given under the supervision of an ophthalmologist. Advanced herpetic keratitis is the leading infectious cause of corneal blindness in the United States. In general, any conjunctivitis that is complicated by keratitis or the formation of conjunctival membranes that may lead to scarring should be managed by an ophthalmologist.

Chlamydial Conjunctivitis

Adult inclusion conjunctivitis is a chronic, remittent conjunctivitis caused by C. trachomatis serotypes D to K and transmitted via sexual exposure. Although the organism is the same that causes neonatal inclusion conjunctivitis, the mature immune system of the adult accounts for the different clinical expression of the disease. In adults, inclusion conjunctivitis has an insidious onset with a scant mucopurulent discharge and a follicular reaction. Multiple corneal infiltrates may persist for up to 18 months. One oral dose of azithromycin, 1 gram, is effective in treating both the conjunctivitis and the genital infection. Oral tetracycline or erythromycin for 3 weeks is an alternative. Sexual partners must be treated as well.

Bacterial Conjunctivitis

Adult bacterial conjunctivitis may be classified as acute purulent, acute mucopurulent, chronic catarrhal, and the conjunctivitis associated with Parinaud's oculoglandular syndrome. Acute purulent (hyperacute) conjunctivitis, as the name implies, refers to the very rapid development of copious purulent exudate. The organism most frequently responsible is N. gonorrhoeae, which is found primarily in young, sexually active adults. The profuse discharge, lid edema, hyperemia, and chemosis can be quite impressive. An enlarged, tender, preauricular node may also be present. Because Neisseria exhibits epithelial parasitism, the integrity of the corneal epithelial layer is in jeopardy, and corneal ulceration and perforation may occur. N. meningitidis infection is less common and tends to cause a less severe conjunctivitis, but it may be complicated by disseminated meningococcemia. Prompt diagnostic procedures and systemic treatment are required for suspected neisserial conjunctivitis (ceftriaxone, 1 gram intramuscularly daily for 5 days). Still less common causes of hyperacute conjunctivitis include *Staphylococcus aureus*, streptococcal species, *Haemophilus aegyptius*, and enteric gram-negative bacilli.

Acute mucopurulent conjunctivitis is commonly known as "pink eye." *Streptococcus pneumoniae* and *H. aegyptius* are the most common bacteria responsible, although infections caused by *Staphylococcus* and *H. influenzae* are not unusual. The typical irritation, tearing, and discharge may involve the second eye 12 to 24 hours after the first. Usually, this is a self-limiting condition, lasting 7 to 12 days, with no sequelae. Despite this, topical therapy is advocated to shorten the course of infection, reduce patient discomfort, prevent chronic conjunctivitis (from *Staphylococcus*), and limit spread to adjacent tissues. A broad-spectrum antibiotic such as a polymixin B/trimethoprim combination (Polytrim) is usually appropriate. Conjunctivitis caused by *H. influenzae* tends to afflict young children and may be associated with a systemic complex of fever, upper respiratory tract infection, and leukocytosis. Suspected *H. influenzae* conjunctivitis should be cultured on chocolate agar and treated systemically.

S. aureus, the most common worldwide cause of bacterial conjunctivitis, accounts for most cases of chronic conjunctivitis. Its pathogenicity results not only from its direct contact with conjunctival tissue but also from its elaboration of toxins, which may result in keratitis and phlyctenulosis. *Moraxella* also produces a chronic conjunctivitis, which typically causes a follicular reaction.

Parinaud's oculoglandular syndrome refers to a unilateral granulomatous conjunctivitis associated with a visibly enlarged and tender ipsilateral preauricular or submandibular lymph node. By far, the most common etiology is cat-scratch disease, which is now thought to be caused by *Rochalimaea*, a member of the family Rickettsiaceae. A history of a cat scratch is helpful but not essential to the diagnosis. Conjunctival biopsy often shows a granulomatous inflammation. Recently, *Rochalimaea* infection has been documented by performing polymerase chain reaction on DNA extracted from a conjunctival swab. A cat-scratch skin test is also available. Systemic treatment with either doxycycline (if the patient is over 8 years of age) or ciprofloxacin (Cipro) for at least 2 weeks is recommended. Other antibiotics have also been advocated. The prognosis for cat-scratch disease is excellent. In the appropriate clinical setting, other etiologic agents for Parinaud's syndrome should be suspected, such as tuberculosis, tularemia, and sporotrichosis.

Allergic Conjunctivitis

The hallmark of allergic conjunctivitis is itching. Bilateral involvement is typical and usually consists of nonspecific hyperemia and chemosis, with a watery discharge. Conjunctival scrapings reveal eosinophils. Attempts should be made to identify the agent responsible for inciting the allergic response. Topical therapy may include a vasoconstrictor, a mast cell stabilizer such as lodoxamide (Alomide), an antihistamine such as levocabastine (Livostin), a nonsteroidal agent, or topical steroids. Chronic use of vasoconstrictors may lead to a rebound effect, and they should be used with caution. Topical steroids may lead to development of cataract and glaucoma, and they should be reserved for refractory cases.

DIFFERENTIAL DIAGNOSIS

When patients present with a red eye, the clinician must consider alternative diagnostic possibilities to conjunctivitis. Dacryostenosis, which is more common in elderly people, may cause a unilateral purulent discharge. In these cases, palpation of the lacrimal sac may express pus from the lacrimal puncta. Primary blepharitis, keratitis, scleritis, and iritis can all cause secondary conjunctival injection. Patients with angle-closure glaucoma characteristically present with blurred vision, periocular pain, and nausea. Examination reveals corneal edema, a fixed midposition pupil, and elevated intraocular pressure. In general, any patient with decreased visual acuity should be evaluated for conditions other than conjunctivitis.

CHICKENPOX
(Varicella)

method of
REBECCA REDMAN, M.D., and
ANN M. ARVIN, M.D.
Stanford University School of Medicine
Stanford, California

Varicella is a generalized vesicular exanthem caused by varicella-zoster virus (VZV), a DNA virus that belongs to the herpesvirus group. The scattered cutaneous lesions seen during the primary infection with the virus result from a viremia associated with peripheral blood mononuclear cells. After primary infection, the virus produces latent infection of neuronal cells in the dorsal root ganglia that may reactivate to cause herpes zoster (shingles).

EPIDEMIOLOGY

Varicella is transmitted to a susceptible individual by contact with another person who has varicella or herpes zoster. Airborne transmission occurs via respiratory droplets from patients with varicella but not from those with herpes zoster; transmission from individuals with herpes zoster requires direct contact with the noncrusted lesions. The incubation period of varicella is 10 to 21 days in the immunocompetent host; it may be shorter in the immunodeficient host or as long as 28 days in recipients of varicella-zoster immune globulin (VZIG). Transmission can occur from patients 24 to 48 hours before the appearance of the exanthem. Varicella should be considered contagious until no new lesions have appeared for 24 to 48 hours and crusting of old lesions is noted. Children with varicella need not be isolated from other healthy children. Exposure of adults and pregnant women who are susceptible and of immunocompromised patients should be avoided. More than 90% of adults who are natives of the United States have had varicella, but only about 50% have a clinical history of past infection; the percentage of immune adults is significantly lower among individuals from tropical areas.

DIAGNOSIS AND MANAGEMENT IN THE NORMAL HOST

The diagnosis of varicella is usually made based on the characteristic vesicular exanthem and does not require laboratory documentation. The initial lesions appear on the face, scalp, and trunk and are followed by new lesions for up to 7 days in the healthy host. The period of new lesion formation may be longer in immunocompromised patients. Mucous membrane lesions are common. Later lesions usually appear on the extremities and may be maculopapular rather than vesicular.

The management of varicella in healthy individuals is supportive. Discomfort caused by the rash can be decreased by application of calamine lotions or cool compresses and by bathing with tepid water. Oral antihistamines may be helpful during the first few days if pruritus is severe and interferes with sleep, but care should be taken that their administration does not mask neurologic symptoms. Daily bathing is indicated to minimize risk of secondary bacterial infection of the lesions; use of medicated soaps is not necessary. Trimming fingernails may also help prevent secondary bacterial infection. Fever and malaise can be treated with acetaminophen; salicylates are contraindicated because of the association with Reye's syndrome. Activity should be allowed as tolerated. Scabbed lesions may take several weeks to resolve. Areas of increased or decreased skin pigmentation may be prominent but gradually resolve. A few of the larger lesions may produce scarring, but these scars become less obvious with time.

The routine use of oral acyclovir (Zovirax) in otherwise healthy children with uncomplicated varicella is not recommended. Oral acyclovir should be considered in populations who are at an increased risk of moderate-to-severe varicella disease. These populations include: children greater than 11 years of age and otherwise healthy adults; patients with a history of chronic cutaneous disorders; patients with a history of chronic pulmonary disorders; patients who have received therapy with parenteral, oral, or aerosol corticosteroids; or patients with a history of chronic salicylate use. The physician may also consider initiating oral acyclovir within 24 hours of the development of exanthem in secondary household contacts in whom the disease is often more severe. The dose of acyclovir in the immunocompetent host with varicella is 20 mg per kg per dose, four times a day (with a maximum of 800 mg per dose) for 5 days. The use of oral acyclovir in infants cannot be extrapolated from the recommendations regarding older children because the safety and efficacy of oral acyclovir in infants under 12 months old has not been established.

COMPLICATIONS OF VARICELLA IN THE NORMAL HOST

The most common complication in normal individuals with varicella is secondary bacterial infection of the skin lesions, but significant pyoderma or cellulitis occurs in fewer than 5% of patients. The usual organisms causing secondary infections are *Staphylococcus aureus* and group A beta-hemolytic *Streptococcus.* Manifestations include rapidly progressive enlargement of skin lesions, impetigo, and cellulitis surrounding involved lesions; rarely, staphylococcal scalded skin syndrome or scarlet fever may develop. Bacteremia is rare, even in patients with infected skin lesions. After the lesions have been cultured, a first-generation cephalosporin or amoxicillin with clavulanate potassium (Augmentin) should be given. If the organism is a streptococcus or penicillin-sensitive *S. aureus,* penicillin may be used. Invasive bacterial superinfection requires parenteral antibiotic therapy.

Vesicular lesions of the conjunctivae can occur. These lesions usually resolve without residua, but ophthalmic evaluation for keratitis and possible topical antiviral therapy is indicated if ocular infection is extensive.

The most common neurologic complications of varicella are cerebellar ataxia and encephalitis. Cerebellar ataxia is a self-limited syndrome that may occur in the acute phase of the illness or within 2 or 3 weeks after the exanthem appears. It resolves without treatment in 1 to 3 weeks and leaves no sequelae. Encephalitis in the normal host usually begins with symptoms of personality change, confusion, drowsiness, irritability, or seizures 5 to 7 days after the appearance of the rash. Symptoms may progress rapidly to obtundation and coma. Encephalitis is estimated to occur in 1 per 1000 cases of varicella. Lumbar puncture is indicated to rule out bacterial infection; the cerebrospinal fluid usually shows a moderate increase in white blood cells, predominantly lymphocytes, with a normal glucose level and a normal or moderately elevated protein level. Lumbar puncture should be performed only after careful assessment for signs of increased intracranial pressure. These patients should be treated with intravenous acyclovir, 500 mg per m² per kg per dose, given every 8 hours. Supportive care with attention to maintaining the airway, restricting fluids, and monitoring vital signs is essential. Seizures are treated with anticonvulsants. Patients who have increased intracranial pressure should be treated with dexamethasone, 1.5 mg per kg initially, with a maintenance dose of 1.5 mg per kg per day, with a maximal dose of 16 mg per day, divided every 4 to 6 hours. Mannitol, 20% solution, can be given at a dose of 0.25 gram per kg by intravenous push and increased to 1 gram per kg per dose if necessary. Mannitol should not be given if the serum osmolality is above 320 mOsm per liter. Steroid therapy for increased intracranial pressure should be tapered as soon as the problem has resolved. Symptoms of varicella encephalitis often reverse rapidly after 24 to 48 hours, and sequelae are unusual. The fatalities that occur, estimated at 10%, are attributed to increased intracranial pressure. The pathogenesis in healthy children is considered to be demyelination rather than viral infection of brain tissue.

Other neurologic manifestations that have been associated with varicella include Guillain-Barré syndrome, cranial nerve palsies, optic neuritis with transient blindness, and transverse myelitis. Reye's syndrome may follow varicella infection. Children with persistent vomiting should be evaluated for this complication because repeated vomiting is unusual with varicella.

Varicella pneumonia is estimated to occur in about 15% of healthy adults who acquire varicella. Its severity may range from asymptomatic pulmonary infiltrates on chest films to life-threatening pneumonia. Respiratory symptoms develop within 2 to 5 days after the onset of the rash and are usually accompanied by continued formation of new skin lesions. Tachypnea is the initial sign; other findings on physical examination may be minimal. The chest film shows diffuse infiltrates with multiple nodular densities, often in the hilar and perihilar regions. This pattern is quite distinct from pneumonia caused by secondary bacterial infection, which produces a unilateral lobar infiltrate with effusion in most cases. Arterial Po_2 should be measured in patients with extensive pneumonia demonstrated by chest film, even if respiratory symptoms appear mild. In severe cases, there is rapid progression with increased dyspnea, cyanosis, pleuritic pain, and tachycardia. Assisted high-pressure ventilation with 100% oxygen may be required. Antiviral therapy is indicated because varicella pneumonia is caused by replication of the virus in lung tissue. Intravenous acyclovir, 500 mg per m² per dose, every 8 hours, should be given. Clinical recovery generally parallels the cessation of formation of new skin lesions. Antibiotics are not indicated unless there is evidence of secondary bacterial infection. Steroids are of no known benefit in this complication of varicella.

Although the virus appears to infect the liver (normal children with varicella have moderately abnormal liver function tests), severe hepatitis with varicella is rare.

Thrombocytopenia may occur during acute varicella as part of a generalized intravascular coagulopathy associated with purpura fulminans and hemorrhage into the skin lesions. Patients with these symptoms should be treated with broad-spectrum antibiotics until bacterial sepsis can be ruled out. Intensive supportive care is required, including platelet and blood transfusions. Some patients have transient thrombocytopenic purpura as a postinfectious complication of varicella. These patients may require platelet support and steroid therapy.

Varicella can cause arthritis during or immediately after the acute infection. Patients with bone or joint symptoms should be evaluated carefully because osteomyelitis caused by S. aureus may follow varicella. Varicella arthritis is self-limited and does not require surgical management other than aspiration if necessary.

Other rare but important complications of varicella include glomerulonephritis, which may be caused by the virus or by intercurrent group A streptococcal infection, and myocarditis.

DIAGNOSIS AND MANAGEMENT IN SPECIAL RISK POPULATIONS

Pregnant Women and Newborn Infants

Varicella during pregnancy is unusual because most women of childbearing age are immune. Varicella is more likely to cause pneumonia in pregnant women, but whether the risk is age-related or associated with pregnancy is uncertain. VZV can cause embryopathy, but the risk is estimated to be less than 5% even after maternal varicella during the first trimester. Clinical findings reported with intrauterine varicella include microcephaly, cerebral atrophy, mental retardation, seizures, chorioretinitis, limb atrophy, and cicatricial skin scars. Spontaneous abortion may also occur. If an exposed pregnant woman is proved to be susceptible by a sensitive serologic assay for antibodies to VZV, such as enzyme immunoassay or the fluorescent antibody membrane antigen method, VZIG prophylaxis should be given within 96 hours, and preferably within 48 hours of exposure, to modify the severity of varicella. There is no evidence that its administration prevents infection of the fetus or decreases the risk of sequelae. VZIG is available through the American Red Cross Blood Services and the dose for pregnant women is 125 IU for each 10 kg (22 pounds) of body weight with the maximal dose being 625 IU (five vials). VZIG is not indicated once a patient develops varicella. The use of oral acyclovir is not recommended in pregnant woman with uncomplicated varicella because the risks to the fetus and mother are not well documented. Parenteral acyclovir should be considered for the pregnant patient with serious complications of VZV because the potential benefits to the pregnant woman with complicated VZV outweigh the known risks of acyclovir to the fetus.

If the mother develops varicella within 5 days before to 2 days after delivery, the infant is at risk for severe disseminated varicella, which may be fatal. These infants should be given VZIG, 125 IU intramuscularly, as soon as possible after delivery. Infants who receive VZIG may develop varicella and should be treated with intravenous acyclovir if progression occurs. If varicella occurs in an infant born under these circumstances who was not given VZIG, antiviral therapy should be given. Varicella in infants born to mothers who develop the rash more than 5 days before delivery will be modified by transplacentally acquired antibody. Some of these infants have skin lesions at birth, but their prognosis for uncomplicated infection is good. In general, infants who are exposed to siblings or other contacts with varicella are usually protected from severe disease by transplacentally acquired maternal antibody. Although there is no definite evidence that varicella is more severe during the first few months of life, if an infant under 2 months of age whose mother is not immune to varicella has a close exposure, it seems prudent to give VZIG.

Immunocompromised Children

Risk of visceral dissemination of varicella is increased in patients with congenital immunodeficiency, such as Wiskott-Aldrich syndrome and thymic dysplasia, or immunodeficiency related to treatment with immunosuppressive agents. Corticosteroids, cytotoxic chemotherapy, antithymocyte globulin, and radiation diminish the immune response to varicella. Children with human immunodeficiency virus infection are also at risk because severe varicella is associated with impaired cellular immunity. Severe varicella may develop in children who are receiving more than 2 mg per kg per day of prednisone. Children with malignancies who are most likely to have life-threatening varicella are those whose absolute lymphocyte count is 500 cells per mm^3 or less and whose disease is in relapse. Bone marrow and organ transplant recipients are likely to develop progressive varicella.

Parents of high-risk children should immediately report any exposure to varicella or herpes zoster. Prophylaxis with VZIG, 125 IU per 10 kg of body weight with the minimal dose of 125 IU (one vial) and the maximal dose of 625 IU (five vials), should be given for household contact or other close indoor exposure. Modification of varicella is optimal if passive antibody prophylaxis is administered within 2 days after the exposure and is not likely to modify the disease if given after 4 to 5 days. Parents should also be educated to recognize possible varicella lesions. The diagnosis of suspicious lesions should be pursued by scraping cells from the base of the lesion and staining with immunofluorescent reagents that detect VZV-infected cells. If possible, children who are receiving high-dose steroids or chemotherapy should have the steroid dose decreased and chemotherapy interrupted for the duration of the incubation period. Although varicella is modified in most children who receive prophylaxis shortly after exposure, some children develop severe varicella despite its administration and may require intravenous acyclovir therapy.

Immunocompromised children who develop varicella may have fulminant infection with pneumonia, hepatic failure, and disseminated intravascular coagulation during the first few days of the illness. However, most children appear to do well initially but develop progressive varicella with new lesion formation for more than 5 to 6 days after the appearance of the exanthem. Progressive cutaneous infection may be accompanied by pneumonia, hepatitis, thrombocytopenia, encephalitis, and glomerulonephritis with severe hypertension. Severe abdominal or back pain is an ominous prognostic sign. Bacterial sepsis may also occur. To be effective, antiviral therapy should be initiated early in the clinical course, preferably within 3 days after the appearance of the rash. Acyclovir is the drug of choice; the dosage is 500 mg per m^2 per dose, every 8 hours. The drug must be given as a 1-hour infusion, and the patient should be kept well hydrated. The dose must be decreased in patients with impaired renal function if the creatinine clearance is less than one-half of normal. Some children develop severe varicella despite antiviral therapy, and intensive support is essential for the management of these patients. There is no evidence that passive antibody administration after the appearance of clinically apparent varicella modifies the severity of the disease. Immunosuppressive therapy can be resumed 1 week after skin lesions have crusted.

A live attenuated varicella vaccine is now available for administration to healthy children and adults; its use in immunocompromised patients, however, remains investigational.

NOSOCOMIAL TRANSMISSION OF VARICELLA

Nosocomial varicella can be a serious problem in pediatric wards. All patients being admitted to the hospital should be questioned about recent exposure to varicella and herpes zoster; if an exposure has occurred, elective admissions should be delayed. If hospital exposure occurs, high-risk susceptible patients with close exposure should be given prophylaxis. Susceptible patients should be discharged during the incubation period if possible, and those who must remain in the hospital should be placed in strict isolation at the end of the incubation period. Hospital personnel who are susceptible to varicella should not care for these children. Isolation rooms for children with varicella should have negative airflow relative to the corridor and should be vented to the outside. In implementing these measures, it is helpful to screen high-risk susceptible patients for antibody to varicella at the time the underlying disease is diagnosed.

Infants with nosocomial exposure to varicella or herpes zoster are rarely at risk because most infants have maternally acquired antibodies to varicella. The maternal history should be determined; if there is doubt about the mother's immunity, the maternal varicella antibody titer should be measured. Infants with close exposure whose mothers have no antibodies to varicella should receive VZIG. Hospitalized infants born before 28 weeks of gestational age and/or who weigh less than 1000 gm and remain in the hospital for reasons of prematurity should receive VZIG regardless of maternal varicella history because these infants are not protected by the transfer of maternal antibodies that occurs during the third trimester.

CHOLERA

method of
DAVID A. SACK, M.D.
Johns Hopkins University School of Hygiene and Public Health
Baltimore, Maryland

Cholera is an acute diarrheal disease that tends to occur in epidemics and is caused by intestinal infection with *Vibrio cholerae*. The spectrum of illness is wide; some individuals infected with this bacterium experience no symptoms, some have mild diarrhea, and others develop severe, dehydrating diarrhea. The latter syndrome, often called cholera gravis, is a life-threatening condition in which perfectly healthy persons can become moribund and die within a few hours. These severely affected patients generally have associated symptoms of nausea, vomiting, and muscle cramps and signs of shock. As the fluid loss continues, dehydration progresses, the radial pulse becomes weak, the blood pressure drops to undetectable levels, the mental status becomes depressed, and coma ensues. Hyperventilation (Kussmaul breathing) frequently occurs because of metabolic acidosis. If left untreated, about 50% of patients with cholera gravis will die, yet almost all these patients will survive if given effective rehydration therapy.

Vibrio cholerae, a gram-negative, comma-shaped rod (formerly called *Vibrio comma*), is a member of the Vibrionaceae family. It has a single polar flagellum, which gives it a characteristic motility when viewed under a dark-field microscope. Although other members of the family can cause diarrhea, only toxigenic *V. cholerae,* belonging to serogroup O 1 or O 139, has been associated with epidemic cholera. Other serogroups of *V. cholerae,* as well as nontoxigenic *V. cholerae* O 1 or O 139, do not cause epidemic cholera, although they may cause individual cases of diarrhea.

Toxigenic *V. cholerae* serogroup O 1 can be subdivided into El Tor and classical biotypes and Ogawa and Inaba serotypes. Through history, the known epidemics have been caused by classical strains until the current (seventh) pandemic, which is caused by the El Tor biotype. The El Tor pandemic spread from Indonesia in 1961 has now affected most of the countries of Asia, Africa, and the Americas. The introduction of cholera to South America occurred in 1991, with an outbreak in Peru; this was followed by spread to nearly all the other countries in the region. Although the Latin American epidemic was remarkable for its rapid spread from country to country, treatment was generally well managed, and fatality rates were low (about 1%). By contrast, cholera in Africa has been sporadic, and fatality rates have been about 10%. In the Rwandan refugee camps in western Zaire in 1994, an estimated 50,000 persons died during the explosive cholera epidemic. The contrast between fatality rates in Latin America and Africa illustrates the importance of the availability of health facilities where adequate rehydration can be administered quickly.

As the seventh pandemic due to El Tor cholera continued, a new serotype, O 139 (synonym Bengal), appeared in India and Bangladesh during 1992. This was the first epidemic caused by a serogroup other than O 1. Although cholera caused by the Bengal strain is clinically identical to that caused by other strains, persons who are partially immune to O 1 cholera through natural exposure are not immune to the new strain. The Bengal strain has now spread to areas throughout India and Bangladesh and to the neighboring countries of Pakistan, Afghanistan, Nepal, southern China, Myanmar, Thailand, and Malaysia. Imported cases have also been seen in the United States, Western Europe, and Hong Kong. Whether this strain will continue its spread around the world and become the eighth pandemic strain cannot be predicted at this point.

Epidemic cholera is spread by the fecal-oral route; thus, those at highest risk are poor people with inadequate sanitation and contaminated water. Surface and estuarine waters serve as a frequent vehicle of transmission, but they also serve as a reservoir for the bacterium. Thus, primary cases can occur when undercooked shellfish contaminated with *V. cholerae* is eaten, even in the absence of fecal contamination. Such an exposure does not progress to a cholera epidemic, however, unless poor sanitation leads to multiple secondary cases. Epidemic transmission of cholera has occurred through contaminated municipal water systems, contaminated commercial ice used by street vendors, and contaminated food that has come in contact with contaminated water. When food becomes contaminated, the vibrio may multiply in the food, resulting in a large inoculum when ingested. As an epidemic progresses, more contaminated feces enter the environment, and the chance of spread becomes even greater.

The pathogenesis of cholera involves several steps. The ingested bacteria must first be swallowed in sufficient numbers. A high inoculum is more likely to cause severe illness than a low inoculum. Because vibrios are acid sensitive, they must survive the gastric acid barrier. Persons who have had gastric surgery or who take antacids or acid-suppressing medications (e.g., cimetidine) are thus at higher risk. Once the surviving vibrios enter the small intestine, they colonize the mucosa with the help of specific colonization factors and begin secreting the potent cholera toxin. The cholera toxin, a protein made of an active (A) subunit and five binding (B) subunits, binds to the GM_1 ganglioside of the surface of the mucosal cells and stimulates adenylate cyclase, leading to an increase in intracellular cyclic adenosine monophosphate (AMP). Because of the toxin's effects, the mucosal crypt cells secrete so much isotonic fluid into the small intestine that the absorptive villus small intestinal cells and the colon cannot reabsorb it. The excess fluid is thus excreted as diarrhea. The volumes of fluid lost can be massive; some adult patients lose more than a liter per hour, and some children lose more than 10 mL per kg per hour. The fluid lost in the stool comes primarily from the circulating blood volume and extracellular spaces, resulting in a lowered blood volume, hemoconcentration (increased hematocrit), lowered blood pressure, and shock.

Knowledge of the composition of cholera stool is important, because treatment is designed to replace the volume and the electrolytes that are lost. The stool is generally isotonic and has electrolyte concentrations that are similar to those of serum, as shown in Table 1. The electrolytes in highest concentration are sodium and chloride. Although the concentration of potassium is less, a large amount of potassium is lost, and cholera patients are always depleted of potassium. The loss of bicarbonate leads to metabolic acidosis. Thus, all the symptoms of cholera can be attributed to the loss of fluids and electrolytes from the gut.

Not all people are equally susceptible to cholera. Sub-

TABLE 1. **Electrolyte Composition of Cholera Stool in Adults and Children and of Rehydration Solutions (Concentration in mmol/L)**

Cholera Stool	Na$^+$	K$^+$	Cl$^-$	HCO$_3$	Carbohydrate
Adults	135	15	100	45	—
Children	105	25	90	30	—
Rehydration Fluid	**Na$^+$**	**K$^+$**	**Cl$^-$**	**Citrate**	**Carbohydrate**
Cereal ORS (for oral use)*	90	20	80	10†	20–50
Glucose ORS (for oral use)*	90	20	80	10	111
Ringer's lactate (for IV use)	131	4	111	29	—
Dhaka solution (for IV use)	133	13	98	48	—
Normal saline (for IV use)‡	154	—	154	—	—

*Glucose oral rehydration solution (ORS) contains (per L) NaCl 3.5 gm, KCl 1.5 gm, trisodium citrate 2.9 gm, and glucose 20 gm. This has a total osmolality of 311. The electrolytes in cereal ORS are the same, but the glucose is replaced by a cereal (e.g., rice) 40–80 gm/L. Cereal ORS has a total osmolality of about 220–250. Cereal ORS is available as CeraLyte from Cera Products, Inc., Columbia, MD.

†Either sodium bicarbonate 2.5 gm (which provides 30 mmol of bicarbonate) or trisodium citrate 2.9 gm (which provides 10 mmol of citrate) can be used as the base. The World Health Organization prefers citrate.

‡Use normal saline only for patients in shock when Ringer's solution or another polyelectrolyte solution is not available. Start ORS immediately to replace potassium and base, which are not included in saline.

stantial immunity follows previous infection, as seen by the lower rates of cholera in older children and adults living in cholera endemic areas compared with the rates in young children. Breast-feeding provides important protection to infants because of protective breast milk antibodies and less exposure to contaminated food and water. Persons with hypochlorhydria have a substantially increased risk because of the loss of the gastric acid barrier. Finally, persons with blood group O have a higher risk for El Tor cholera than do persons with blood group A, B, or AB.

DIAGNOSIS

Cholera should be considered in a patient with severe, acute (less than 48 hours' duration), watery diarrhea in which the stool looks like "rice water." The index of suspicion increases if the patient is an adult, if there are other cases of cholera in the area, if there is severe vomiting, if the patient is from an area of poor sanitation or has recently traveled to a cholera endemic area, and if the patient is severely dehydrated or in shock. Cholera does not generally cause fever (although a low-grade fever is sometimes seen); it does not cause blood in the stool and does not cause subacute or chronic diarrhea. The diagnosis is confirmed by identifying *V. cholerae* from a stool culture, but the laboratory must be informed that cholera is suspected so that special media (thiosulfate citrate bile salts sucrose [TCBS] agar) can be used to identify it. Only a sample of specimens needs to be cultured during epidemics in developing countries, because the clinical diagnosis is highly accurate in these circumstances, and the culture results do not alter treatment for individual cases. All new cases of cholera in other areas (including all cases in the United States) should be confirmed with culture and reported to the national health authorities. Highly sensitive and specific rapid diagnostic tests are now available to detect the organism directly from stool, but cultures should be used to confirm new cases in an area.

TREATMENT

Rehydration saves the lives of patients with cholera, and antibiotics shorten the illness. Therefore, appropriate rehydration is the key to successful management of cholera patients. Rehydration involves determining how much fluid to give, what route to use (intravenous or oral), the rate of administration, and the composition of fluid to use. The choice of antibiotics depends on the sensitivity pattern of the epidemic strains, the proven efficacy of the antibiotic for cholera, and the logistics and economics of using a particular antibiotic regimen.

Assessment of Dehydration. When determining how much fluid to give, an assessment of the fluid deficit is needed. This is accomplished by examining the patient for signs and symptoms of dehydration and then categorizing the patient as one who has no signs of dehydration (<5% deficit), some dehydration (5 to 7% deficit), or severe dehydration (10% deficit). Important symptoms of dehydration include lack of urination, lack of tears, dry mouth, and thirst. Signs of dehydration include poor skin turgor, weak or absent radial pulse, low blood pressure, depressed mental status, sunken eyes, and wrinkled skin of the fingers (washerwoman's fingers). Muscle cramps in the extremities are frequent symptoms but are not indicative of the degree of dehydration.

Patients with symptoms of cholera and who have poor skin turgor, a weak or absent radial pulse, and other signs of dehydration should be categorized as being severely dehydrated. These patients are estimated to have lost about 10% of their body weight. If patients have less severe signs and symptoms but still have evidence of dehydration (e.g., some loss of skin turgor, dry mucous membranes, thirst), they are categorized as having some dehydration and are estimated to have lost about 5 to 7% of their body weight. It should be remembered that some patients will have no objective signs of dehydration yet be somewhat dehydrated, because clinical signs generally appear after about 5% of the body weight has been lost.

Rehydration. Severely dehydrated patients are at high risk of death within a very short time, and rehydration is urgent. These patients should be given intravenous fluids to fully replace their fluid deficit, and the fluids should be given rapidly to accomplish full rehydration in less than 4 hours. This means that a 50-kg patient should receive 10% of his or her body weight (5 liters) of fluid during the rehydration phase. The optimal intravenous fluid is an isotonic, polyelectrolyte solution containing a base and potassium. Of the commonly available intravenous fluids, Ringer's lactate (Hartman's solution) is the best, although other intravenous polyelectrolyte fluids, such as Dhaka solution, are better formulated for replacing the electrolytes that have been lost. With rapid rehydration, the dehydrated patient will quickly show evidence of improvement: skin turgor will improve, the pulse will return, breathing will become normal, and mental abilities will return. Providing rapid rehydration requires a large-bore intravenous needle and sometimes requires more than one infusion. Failure to provide this rapid rehydration is the most common cause of death and complication in cholera. Measuring the patient's body weight periodically helps to monitor the state of hydration. Subcutaneous and intraperitoneal parenteral fluids should not be used, because absorption from these sites is not sufficiently rapid to restore circulation.

If cholera occurs in a remote setting where intravenous fluids cannot be given, rehydration should be given with oral rehydration solution (ORS) by mouth or by nasogastric tube, using the same volumes of fluid as described for intravenous fluid. Such patients should then be evacuated to a more adequate treatment facility while oral or nasogastric rehydration continues.

Patients who have some dehydration but are not severely dehydrated can generally be rehydrated using ORS. ORS equivalent to 5 to 7% of the patient's body weight should be provided during the rehydration phase to restore circulating volume; thus, a 50-kg patient should drink 2.5 to 3 liters of ORS within about 4 hours. Vomiting may sometimes complicate oral rehydration, but if the ORS is given in frequent small amounts, it is generally possible to adequately rehydrate these patients.

Maintenance Hydration. Hydration needs to continue after the patient has been rehydrated to replace the ongoing stool losses. This maintenance phase blends with the rehydration phase. Patients who were originally rehydrated with intravenous fluids should begin ORS as soon as they are able to drink, because it is expected that they will continue to have diarrhea. Likewise, patients who were rehydrated orally need to continue to drink ORS until the diarrhea stops. "Cholera cots" are frequently used to assist in measuring the stool output and to help prevent soiling. These simple cots have a hole cut into them where the buttocks lay, and a plastic sheet funnels the liquid stool into a plastic bucket beneath. The rate at which liquid stool is being lost can easily be estimated so that the same volume of ORS can be given to the patient to make up for fecal losses. ORS is intended to replace only the stool losses; it is not intended to provide all fluid needs. Therefore, patients should drink normal amounts of water or other fluids in addition to the ORS. Infants should continue to drink normal amounts of breast milk or formula, and all patients should continue to eat normal foods as soon as they are able—generally within a few hours.

Oral Rehydration Solution. The standard ORS promoted by UNICEF and the World Health Organization and that is commonly available in packets throughout the world uses glucose as the carbohydrate substrate. The carbohydrate substrate is critical to the absorption of salt and water, due to the fact that without the substrate, "oral saline" would simply pass through without being absorbed. Because of the glucose-mediated transport of sodium, the water and electrolytes are absorbed and rehydra-

tion is accomplished. Excessively high concentrations of glucose are less effective, however, since the high osmolality results in osmotic diarrhea. Thus, for these critically ill cholera patients, a complete formula ORS, with proper amounts of salts and substrate, is critical.

Recently, cereal ORS, which uses cereal starches rather than glucose as the substrate, have been found to be more effective for cholera patients, in that purging rates are lowered by about 30 to 40% and the duration of illness is shortened relative to treatment with glucose ORS. Because of logistic difficulties in preparing cereal ORS, only a few cholera treatment centers are using it, but, when feasible, cereal ORS should be used.

Antibiotics. Antibiotics are not needed to save the lives of cholera patients, but they should be given to shorten the illness. In epidemic areas where resources are scarce, shortening the illness also saves rehydration supplies and is therefore very cost effective. The antibiotic of choice is doxycycline or tetracycline if the strain causing the illness is sensitive to the drug. Depending on the logistic requirements, single-dose doxycycline 300 mg can be used. Alternatively, 3 days of the antibiotic may be used, as shown in Table 2. When antibiotic-resistant strains occur, alternative antibiotics that can be given include trimethoprim-sulfamethoxazole (Bactrim, Septra), furazolidone (Furoxone), chloramphenicol, and the new quinolones (e.g., ciprofloxacin [Cipro]). The tetracyclines and quinolones are generally not recommended during pregnancy or for children, so furazolidone or trimethoprim-sulfamethoxazole is used in these circumstances. During an epidemic, the choice of antibiotic depends on the sensitivity of a sample of strains. Occasionally, the antibiotic pattern changes, and an ongoing sampling surveillance is needed to detect this change. If the strains become resistant to all practical antibiotics, patients will still recover in about 5 to 7 days if proper hydration is maintained.

Other Drugs. Drugs that should not be used in

TABLE 2. **Antimicrobial Agents Used in the Treatment of Cholera**

Antibiotic	Adult Dose	Pediatric Dose
Doxycycline*	300 mg single dose† or 100 mg bid for 3 days	—
Tetracycline†	500 mg qid for 3 days	12.5 mg/kg qid for 3 days
Furazolidone (Furoxone)‡	100 mg qid for 3 days	1.25 mg/kg qid for 3 days
TMP–SMX (Bactrim, Septra)§	TMP 160 mg + SMX 800 mg bid for 3 days	TMP 5 mg/kg + SMX 25 mg/kg bid for 3 days
Ciprofloxacin (Cipro)‖	500 mg bid for 3 days	—

*The drug of choice for most situations, since a single dose can be used.
†Be aware of policies against using tetracycline in children in whom teeth staining can occur.
‡The drug of choice in pregnant women.
§The preferred drug for children.
‖Reserve for strains resistant to all other antibiotics.
Abbreviation: TMP–SMX = trimethoprim-sulfamethoxazole.

cholera include nonspecific intestinal drugs (e.g., activated charcoal, kaolin, loperamide [Imodium], diphenoxylate [Lomotil]), drugs to treat shock (e.g., dopamine, norepinephrine, high-dose steroids), and colloid or crystalloid intravenous fluids.

Prophylactic Antibiotics. During epidemics of cholera, prophylactic antibiotics will prevent other cases in the households of cholera patients who come to the hospital for treatment. These should be used only if they can be limited to immediate family members and to a single treatment dose (e.g., single-dose doxycycline 300 mg). The rationale for using prophylactic antibiotics is to prevent illness in persons who were exposed at the same time as the patient. Prophylactic antibiotics should not be given to whole neighborhoods or communities, because this wide-scale use leads to antibiotic resistance.

COMPLICATIONS

Complications from cholera are largely related to inadequate or slow rehydration or to the use of the wrong rehydration fluid. Acute tubular necrosis with renal failure can result if the patient remains hypotensive for a prolonged period; this complication is especially common if the volume of fluids given is barely sufficient to prevent death but not sufficient to restore circulating volume, or if the rehydration fluid used was 5% dextrose in water rather than a salt-containing fluid. Pulmonary edema is rarely seen but is more common if normal saline rather than Ringer's lactate is used, because this does not correct metabolic acidosis. Overhydration and generalized edema can occur if excessive intravenous fluids are given. Ileus, paralytic bladder, and cardiac arrhythmias occasionally occur, and these are usually related to hypokalemia when the rehydration fluids do not contain sufficient potassium. Cardiac arrhythmias can also result from hyperkalemia if renal failure is not recognized. Shock from cholera can precipitate abortion in pregnant women, although this is less likely to occur if rehydration is prompt. Finally, hypoglycemia, manifested by generalized seizures, occurs rarely in children. Rapid intravenous glucose is needed for this complication.

PREVENTION

Having established that contaminated water and food are the primary vehicles of transmission for cholera, the primary interventions should include providing clean food and water, communication programs on disinfecting water and on safe food preparation, and communication programs on when and where to seek medical care for diarrhea.

In recent years, vaccination has been discouraged because the injectable vaccine that is available provides only limited, short-term protection and has many side effects. New oral inactivated as well as oral live vaccines have recently been developed and are available in some countries (but not the United States). These oral vaccines have no significant side effects and provide better and more long-lasting protection than the injectable vaccine. As these oral vaccines become available, high-risk travelers to cholera-endemic areas will benefit from them, although the development of public health vaccination programs for developing countries will require further evaluation of their cost effectiveness.

DIPHTHERIA

method of
EVAN A. STEINBERG, M.D.
Southern California Permanente Medical Group
Los Angeles, California

Diphtheria is an acute infection caused by *Corynebacterium diphtheriae*. Symptoms include those localized to the site of infection, including pain, adenopathy, and possibly airway obstruction, as well as life-threatening complications from diphtheria toxin, such as cardiac, renal, and neurologic damage. The toxin is an extracellular protein. Only strains infected by a bacteriophage are able to elaborate diphtheria toxin. Humans are the only reservoir, and infection is acquired by contact with carriers or people with active disease. The bacteria may be transmitted via droplets or contact with infected skin lesions. The period of communicability in untreated individuals is usually 2 weeks but may last up to 2 months. The mean incubation period is 2 to 3 days but may be as long as 1 week. The organism remains localized to mucosal or cutaneous surfaces. A localized inflammatory response results in tissue necrosis with formation of the characteristic diphtheritic pseudomembrane in the upper respiratory tract. Toxin produced and absorbed at the local site of infection is distributed via the blood, causing potential damage to the heart, nervous system, or kidneys. The severity of disease and resultant symptoms depend on the site of the primary infection (e.g., nasopharynx, larynx, or trachea) and immune status of the infected individual. The diagnosis is made clinically. To minimize the risk of toxin-mediated complications, the decision to treat with antitoxin should be made rapidly, without cultural confirmation, which may take several days. Definitive diagnosis requires the isolation of *C. diphtheriae* on culture with selective media and the subsequent demonstration of toxin production.

TREATMENT

Treatment is directed toward (1) neutralization of free toxin, (2) elimination of further toxin production by eradication of the toxigenic organism, and (3) supportive therapy. The only specific treatment available is antitoxin of equine origin (diphtheria equine antitoxin).

Antitoxin Administration

Antitoxin is preferably delivered intravenously. It should be given in a single dose to avoid the risk of sensitization from repeated doses. A syringe containing aqueous epinephrine (1:1000) should be available whenever antitoxin is being injected. The epinephrine dose for an anaphylactic reaction is 0.01 mL per kg, up to 0.3 mL. Resuscitative and monitoring equipment should also be available.

Testing for sensitivity to horse serum should always be done. The patient should be questioned for prior exposure to horse serum and for a history of asthma or allergic symptoms on exposure to horses or horse serum. If the history is positive, testing should first be performed with either a scratch test or intracutaneous injection of dilute antitoxin. The scratch test is performed by application of one drop of 1:100 saline dilution of serum to the site of a superficial scratch, prick, or puncture on the volar aspect of the forearm. A positive test response is indicated by a wheal with surrounding erythema at least 3 mm larger than that seen with a control test with normal saline (at 15 to 20 minutes after application). Alternatively, for patients with a history of possible hypersensitivity, intracutaneous injection of 0.02 mL of a 1:1000 saline dilution of antitoxin may be administered. An erythematous region greater than 10 mm across or occurrence of a wheal within 20 minutes is considered a positive reaction. For patients with a negative history and for those whose first test is negative, intracutaneous injection should be performed or repeated, respectively, by injection of 0.02 mL of a 1:100 dilution. If the patient is sensitive to horse serum, then desensitization is necessary. All desensitization regimens should be done by personnel familiar with the treatment of anaphylaxis and with appropriate drugs and equipment available and thus are optimally performed in an intensive care unit. The American Academy of Pediatrics Committee on Infectious Diseases recommends a regimen employing increasing intravenous doses administered at 15-minute intervals as shown in Table 1. Administration of serum under the protection of a desensitization procedure must be continuous. If administration is interrupted, protection from desensitization is lost. If signs of anaphylaxis occur, epinephrine should be administered immediately. If no reaction to antitoxin occurs, the remaining dose of antitoxin is given by slow intravenous infusion.

Patients may benefit from premedication with antihistamines, with or without the addition of hydrocortisone or methylprednisolone. Intravenous administration of antitoxin results in higher levels of antibodies in saliva and presumptively more rapid neutralization of toxin and subsequent detoxification of horse serum products.

The dose of equine antitoxin is empirical (Table 2) and is dependent on the site and duration of infection and degree of toxicity, rather than the age or size of the patient. The degree of lymph node involvement in the neck increases with the degree of toxin absorption.

In the United States, antitoxin is available from the National Immunization Program of the Centers for Disease Control and Prevention, 404–639–8200, Atlanta, Georgia. An immediate reaction, including a variety of rashes, fever, and anaphylaxis, may be seen in up to 16% of patients, whereas a delayed reaction of serum sickness (rash, urticaria, fever, and arthralgia or arthritis) may occur in 10 to 30% of children or adults. Serum sickness characteristically occurs at 5 to 21 days after infusion and may be treated symptomatically with acetaminophen, aspirin, or ibuprofen, or with corticosteroids in severe cases.

Antibiotic Therapy

Antibiotics are important to eradicate the organism, prevent further toxin production, and decrease the likelihood of disease transmission. Both erythromycin and penicillin are effective. Erythromycin may be given orally or intravenously at a dosage of 40 to 50 mg per kg per day in four divided doses (maximum 2.0 grams per day). Penicillin may be given as aqueous penicillin, 100,000 to 150,000 U per kg per day in four divided doses (maximum 10 mU), or procaine penicillin G, 25,000 to 50,000 U per kg per day, intramuscularly in two divided doses (maximum 1.2 mU per dose). Erythromycin-resistant strains have been identified. All regimens of penicillin or erythromycin should be given for a total of 14 days. These antibiotic regimens eliminate group A streptococci, which commonly co-infect diphtheria patients. Elimination of the organism should be documented by consecutive negative cultures after completion of therapy.

In cutaneous diphtheria, lesions should be cleaned vigorously with soap and water. Either oral erythromycin or penicillin V should be administered for 10 days. Antitoxin therapy is of unproven value for this

TABLE 1. **Suggested Dosage Schedule of Diphtheria Equine Antitoxin for Desensitization**

Dose	Amount (mL)	Dilution	Preferred Route*	Alternative Route
1	0.10	1:1000	Intravenous	Intradermal
2	0.30	1:1000	Intravenous	Intradermal
3	0.60	1:1000	Intravenous	Subcutaneous
4	0.10	1:100	Intravenous	Subcutaneous
5	0.30	1:100	Intravenous	Subcutaneous
6	0.60	1:100	Intravenous	Subcutaneous
7	0.10	1:10	Intravenous	Subcutaneous
8	0.30	1:10	Intravenous	Subcutaneous
9	0.60	1:10	Intravenous	Subcutaneous
10	0.10	undiluted	Intravenous	Subcutaneous
11	0.20	undiluted	Intravenous	Subcutaneous
12	0.60	undiluted	Intravenous	Intramuscular
13	1.0	undiluted	Intravenous	Intramuscular

*Intravenous is the preferred route because of better control.

TABLE 2. **Dosage of Diphtheria Antitoxin**

Clinical Indication	Antitoxin Dose (U)
Pharyngeal or laryngeal disease of 48 hours' duration or less	40,000
Nasopharyngeal lesions	40,000–60,000
Extensive disease of more than 3 days' duration or brawny neck swelling	80,000–120,000

form of diphtheria, but some authorities recommend the administration of 20,000 to 40,000 U of antitoxin. Because of its uncertain value in this situation, antitoxin should not be given to patients who are sensitive to horse serum by history or skin testing.

Supportive Therapy

Patients with diphtheria should be hospitalized for horse serum therapy and careful monitoring. Most deaths from diphtheria are due to myocarditis or mechanical airway obstruction.

Myocarditis may present suddenly, with congestive heart failure or circulatory collapse, or indolently. Continuous cardiac monitoring should be employed during hospitalization; thereafter, serial electrocardiographic or echocardiographic studies, or both, should be performed two to three times per week to assess for cardiac arrhythmias and to monitor myocardial function, for up to 6 weeks. Patients with diphtheria may be given digitalis carefully if congestive heart failure develops. In severe cases prednisone, 1 to 1.5 mg per kg for up to 2 weeks, has been employed, but its therapeutic efficacy is unknown. Serial urinalyses and renal function studies should also be obtained to detect renal damage. Similarly, serial neurologic examinations should be carefully performed to detect any evidence of neurologic toxicity. Maintenance of adequate hydration and nutrition, including parenteral nutrition if necessary, should be provided because palatal paralysis may complicate oral hydration or alimentation. Careful attention should be directed to signs of airway obstruction. Patients with laryngeal disease may require diagnostic or therapeutic bronchoscopy with intubation in order to provide an unobstructed airway. A section of necrotic membrane in nasal or throat locations may dislodge and obstruct the airway. Tracheostomy may be required early for severely ill patients. Corticosteroids may be helpful in acute laryngeal diphtheria.

Bed rest is important. Isolation of the patient with measures to prevent airborne spread is necessary and should continue until two cultures from both the nasopharynx and throat are negative for *C. diphtheriae*. Cultures should be obtained 24 hours apart after completion of therapy.

Since diphtheria does not necessarily confer immunity, patients should be actively immunized with diphtheria toxoid during convalescence.

Treatment of Contacts

When the diagnosis of diphtheria is made, the local public health department should be notified promptly. A history of symptoms and immunization status should be sought in all contacts. Close contacts, regardless of immunization status, should have pharyngeal cultures for *C. diphtheriae* performed and receive antimicrobial prophylaxis with either oral erythromycin or phenoxymethylpenicillin for 7 days, or a single intramuscular dose of penicillin G benzathine* (600,000 U for those weighing less than 30 kg and 1.2 million units for those weighing greater than 30 kg). Since the efficacy of prophylaxis is unproven, contacts who are carriers should have cultures repeated at least 2 weeks after completion of therapy. Asymptomatic, previously immunized close contacts should receive a booster dose of diphtheria toxoid appropriate for age. Asymptomatic close contacts who are unimmunized or who are not fully immunized, or whose immunization status is unknown, should be actively immunized with diphtheria-pertussis-tetanus (DPT), diphtheria-tetanus (DT), or adult diphtheria-tetanus (dT) vaccine, as appropriate for age. A close contact who cannot be kept under close surveillance should be given penicillin G benzathine* and a dose of an appropriate immunizing agent, depending on age and immunization status.

PREVENTION

Universal immunization with diphtheria toxoid is the only effective control measure. Children up to their seventh birthday should receive DPT vaccine (or DT vaccine in those in whom pertussis immunization is contraindicated) according to the currently approved schedule at 2, 4, 6, and 15 to 18 months, repeated at 4 to 6 years. After the age of 7 years, booster immunization with dT toxoid is recommended at 10-year intervals or with the administration of tetanus prophylaxis for wounds. An alternative strategy, proposed by the Task Force on Adult Immunization,† which includes the American College of Physicians, the Infectious Diseases Society of America, and the Centers for Disease Control and Prevention, is to administer a single, midlife (50 years of age) dT booster to persons who have received the full pediatric series, as well as a booster dose during adolescence. The recommendation for dT boosters for wound management has not changed. Childhood preparations of diphtheria toxoid (DPT or DT) contain 7 to 25 flocculating units (Lf) of diphtheria toxoid per dose, compared with the preparation of vaccine for older children and adults (dT), which contains no more than 2 Lf per dose. A primary series of immunizations for older children and adults who have not previously been immunized is two doses given at a 2-month interval and a booster dose at 6 to 12 months. It is important to verify that all individuals have completed the primary series during routine or urgent care visits. People over 60 years of age warrant special attention, since they may never have been immunized during childhood or adolescence.

---

*Not FDA-approved for this indication.
†Task Force on Adult Immunization: Adult immunizations 1994. Ann Intern Med *121*:540–541, 1994.

FOOD–BORNE ILLNESS

method of
NATHAN M. THIELMAN, M.D., M.P.H., and
RICHARD L. GUERRANT, M.D.
University of Virginia School of Medicine
Charlottesville, Virginia

Diverse pathogenic microorganisms, toxins, and chemicals ingested with food may lead to varied gastrointestinal, neurologic, and systemic syndromes. Evaluation of the patient with a suspected food-borne illness should include careful attention not only to presenting symptoms and signs but also to a detailed food history and timing of symptoms in relation to food ingestion, recent travel, season, and the presence of similar symptoms among those who have shared similar meals (Figure 1). Although a food-specific attack rate is important for those who ate the suspected food, the most important additional figure is the attack rate among those who did not eat the suspected food to help implicate that food. Laboratory testing for suspected microorganisms or their toxins may help to establish the definitive etiology and enable directed therapy.

For many food-borne illnesses, appropriate treatment is primarily supportive because the toxic insult is generally short-lived and reversible. Patients with food-borne gastroenteritis caused by certain bacterial pathogens may, however, benefit from additional antimicrobial therapy (Table 1 and see text later). The cornerstone of therapy for patients with diarrheal illnesses is replacement of lost fluid and electrolytes. In most cases this is best accomplished with the simple and inexpensive oral rehydration therapy (ORT) recommended by the World Health Organization (WHO). This lifesaving, simple, and cost-effective formulation can be reconstituted from packets (Jianas Brothers Packaging Co., Kansas City, Missouri), or approximations of this formulation can be made at home (Table 2). In addition, food or cereal-based ORT can be prepared as noted in Table 2; rice powder–based ORT packets can also be purchased inexpensively (Cera Products, Inc., Columbia, Maryland). A number of more expensive commercially available products (such as Pedialyte and Lytren) vary from the WHO formulation but remain safe and effective alternatives. Regardless of which solution is used, therapy should be prompt and aimed at replacing both the existing fluid deficit and the continuing fluid losses resulting from diarrhea and basal metabolism. Uncontrolled vomiting, ileus, severe fluid deficit with obtundation or toxicity, or severe monosaccharide malabsorption are contraindications to ORT and mandate intravenous fluid resuscitation.

Most food-borne diarrheal illnesses are self-limited and brief. With more prolonged illnesses not associated with inflammatory colitis, symptomatic therapy with loperamide (Imodium) for adults, 4 mg initially, followed by 2 mg after each loose stool, not to exceed 16 mg per day, usually provides significant relief. Bismuth subsalicylate (Pepto-Bismol), although in general not as effective as loperamide, has shown modest efficacy in treating traveler's diarrhea.

Protracted nausea and vomiting associated with food-borne illnesses may be controlled with an antiemetic agent. Prochlorperazine (Compazine), 5 to 10 mg orally, 25 mg per rectal suppository, or 10 mg intramuscularly; promethazine (Phenergan), 12.5 to 25 mg orally, intramuscularly, or per rectum; or trimethobenzamide (Tigan), 250 mg orally, or 200 mg intramuscularly or per rectum, may help to control nausea and vomiting in adults. Trimethobenzamide can be used in children over 2 years of age.

MICROBIAL FOOD POISONING SYNDROMES

Early-Onset Nausea and Vomiting

Food poisoning characterized primarily by nausea and vomiting within 1 to 6 hours of ingestion is typically caused by preformed enterotoxins of *Staphylococcus aureus* or *Bacillus cereus*. If symptoms occur within 5 to 60 minutes of ingestion, and are associated with a metallic taste, heavy metal poisoning should also be considered (see later).

Staphylococcal food poisoning typically follows ingestion of foods such as ham, cream-filled cakes, poultry, and egg salads—all of which favor the growth of staphylococci following contamination by an infected or colonized food handler and improper storage at room temperature. About 75% of patients present with nausea and vomiting, and a slightly lower percentage of patients will subsequently develop diarrhea. Fever and other systemic symptoms are rare. Definitive diagnosis can be established by culturing the stool or vomitus of a patient or the implicated food itself.

Ingestion of a preformed emetic toxin produced by *B. cereus* causes an acute emetic syndrome similar to that seen with staphylococcal food poisoning. The strong association of *B. cereus* emetic syndrome with consumption of fried rice has been attributed to germination of heat-resistant spores on cooling boiled rice to room temperature; flash-frying does not produce sufficient heat to inactivate the heat-stable emetic toxin.

Because the duration of both staphylococcal and *B. cereus* emetic illnesses is usually less than 12 to 24 hours, therapy aimed at correcting fluid and electrolyte abnormalities is generally sufficient. Antibiotic therapy is not indicated.

Noninflammatory Diarrhea

Early Onset (6–24 Hours)

Profuse watery diarrhea and abdominal cramping occurring 6 to 24 hours after ingestion of contaminated food is frequently caused by the in vivo production of either a heat-labile toxin from *Clostridium perfringens* or by the diarrheogenic toxin of *B. cereus*. Although nausea may occur, vomiting is usually not seen, and fever is rare. In most patients symptoms

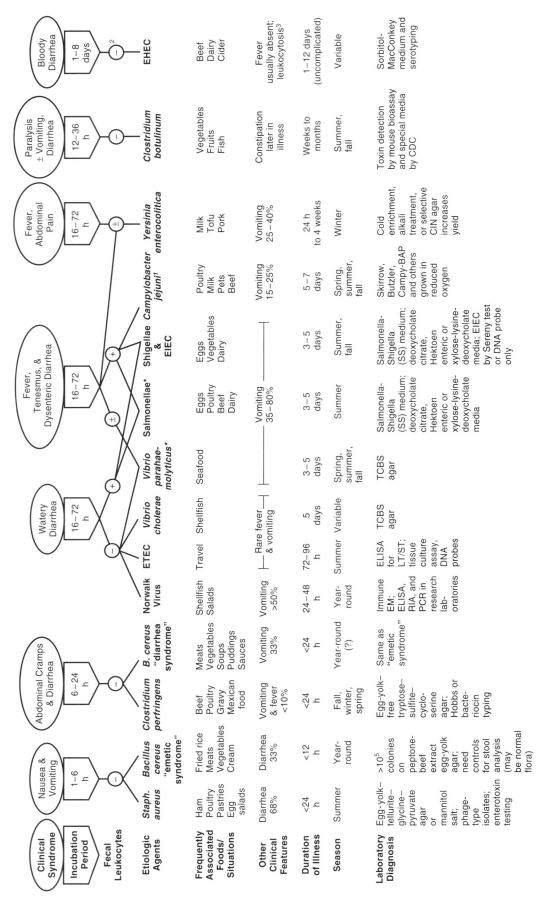

Figure 1. Characteristics of infectious food poisoning syndromes. *Abbreviations:* ETEC = enterotoxic *Escherichia coli;* EIEC = enteroinvasive *E. coli;* EHEC = enterohemorrhagic *E. coli;* EM = electron microscopy; ELISA = enzyme-linked immunosorbent assay; RIA = radioimmunoassay; PCR = polymerase chain reaction; LT/ST = labile toxin/stable toxin; TCBS = thiosulfate citrate bile salts sucrose; BAP = blood agar plate; CIN = cefsulodine-irgasan-novobiocin; CDC = Centers for Disease Control and Prevention.

$\cdot$Incubation periods for *V. parahaemolyticus* and Salmonellae may rarely be as short as 5 h.

[1]Incubation periods for *C. jejuni* may be as long as 7 days.

[2]Fecal leukocytes are present in approximately 30% of patients with EHEC.

[3]Systemic leukocytosis may herald the onset of hemolytic uremic syndrome.

90

TABLE 1. **Antibiotics for Acute Bacterial Food-Borne Illnesses***

Pathogen	Drug	Usual Adult Dosage	Notes
Shigella	**Ciprofloxacin** (Cipro)†	500 mg PO bid × 3–5 days	A single 1-gram dose of ciprofloxacin may be as effective as a 5-day/10-dose course in patients with *Shigella* other than *S. dysenteriae* type 1
	Norfloxacin (Noroxin)†	400 mg PO bid × 3–5 days	
	TMP–SMX (Bactrim, Septra)	1 DS PO bid × 3–5 days	Increasingly resistant strains are reported in many developing regions
	Ampicillin	500 mg PO or 1 gm IV q 6 h × 3–5 days	Increasingly resistant strains are noted in many developing regions
	Nalidixic acid (NegGram)	1 gm q 6 h × 3–5 days	Like 4-fluoroquinolones, causes arthropathy when given in high doses to immature animals
Nontyphoid *Salmonella*‡	**Ciprofloxacin**†	500 mg PO bid or 400 mg IV q 12 h until patient is free of fever for at least 24 h	Antimicrobial therapy may prolong intestinal shedding of *Salmonella* spp
	TMP–SMX	1 DS PO bid	
	Amoxicillin	500 mg PO tid	
	Ampicillin	1–2 gm IV q 4–6 h	
	Cefoperazone (Cefobid)	2 gm IV q 12 h	
	Ceftriaxone (Rocephin)	1 gm IV q 12 h	
Campylobacter jejuni§	**Erythromycin**	250–500 mg PO qid × 5–7 days	Increased rates of resistance reported in Thailand
	Ciprofloxacin†	500 mg PO bid × 7 days	Rarely resistance and associated clinical relapse has developed during therapy
	Tetracycline‖	500 mg PO qid × 7 days	Higher resistance rates (~30%)
Travelers' diarrhea¶	**TMP–SMX**	2 DS once or 1 DS PO bid × 3–5 days	Loading dose regimen followed by standard doses for 3 days may be more effective
	Ciprofloxacin†	1 gm once or 500 mg PO bid × 3–5 days	
	Norfloxacin†	800 mg once or 400 mg PO bid × 3–5 days	
	Ofloxacin (Floxin)	600 mg once or 300 mg PO bid × 3–5 days	
	Furazolidone (Furoxone)	100 mg PO qid × 7 days	
*Vibrio cholerae***	**Tetracycline**‖	500 mg qid or 2 gm q day × 2 days	Tetracycline-resistant outbreaks have been reported in Africa and Asia
	Doxycycline‖	300 mg PO × 1 day	
	TMP–SMX	1 DS PO bid × 3 days	
	Furazolidone	100 mg PO qid × 3 days	Alternative for treatment of children and pregnant women

*Preferred antibiotics are listed in **bold;** directed antibiotic therapy should also take into account local sensitivity patterns if available.

†Quinolones in immature animals can cause arthropathy, and their safety and efficacy has not been established in persons <18 years of age, pregnant women, and nursing mothers.

‡Treatment is particularly recommended for bacteremia prophylaxis in patients at extremes of age, with prosthetic material(s) present, or immunocompromised hosts (see text).

§Studies in which antibiotic treatment is initiated early in the course of illness (≤4 days) demonstrate clinical benefit.

‖Should not be used in children <7 years of age.

¶Most common bacterial enteropathogens include enterotoxigenic, enteroadherent, and enteroinvasive *Escherichia coli* as well as *Shigella, C. jejuni,* and *Salmonella.*

**Although the mainstay of therapy should be volume replacement, antibiotics diminish volume and duration of diarrhea and volume replacement requirements.

Abbreviations: TMP–SMX = trimethoprim-sulfamethoxazole; DS = double strength.

Modified from Thielman NM, Guerrant RL: Acute infectious diarrhea. *In* Rakel RE (ed): Conn's Current Therapy 1995. Philadelphia, WB Saunders Co, 1995.

resolve within 24 hours. Typically *C. perfringens* food poisoning occurs when meat products are allowed to sit at temperatures between 15° and 60° C for 2 to 3 hours or more, thereby allowing clostridial spores (commonly present in raw meats and vegetables) to germinate and multiply. In outbreaks of *C. perfringens* food poisoning, around 50% of individuals consuming the contaminated food will develop symptoms. The diarrheal syndrome of *B. cereus* has been associated with ingestion of proteinaceous foods, sauces, puddings, and vegetables.

Later Onset (16–72 Hours)

Norwalk virus and other small, round, structured viruses (SRSVs) cause diarrhea after a longer incubation period of 24 to 48 hours. Poorly cooked or raw shellfish, salads, and contaminated drinking water have all been implicated in point-source outbreaks caused by this organism. Secondary cases among close contacts not initially exposed to the contaminated food suggests Norwalk virus as a possible cause. Clinically, infection is usually manifest first

TABLE 2. **Oral Rehydration Formula**

WHO Formula		Home Recipe	
Ingredient	Amount*	Ingredient	Amount*
NaCl	3.5 gm	Table salt	¾ tbsp
NaHCO₃	2.5 gm	Baking soda	1 tsp
KCl	1.5 gm	Orange juice	1 cup
Glucose	20 gm	Table sugar†	4 level tbsp

*Per 1 liter (1.05 quarts) of clean water.
†Food-based oral rehydration formulations, prepared by replacing table sugar with 50–60 gm of cereal flour or 200 gm of mashed boiled potato, may help to reduce fluid output.
Abbreviation: WHO = World Health Organization.

by abdominal cramping and nausea, followed by myalgias with diarrhea and/or vomiting. Malaise and headaches are not uncommon; low-grade fevers occur in close to 50% of patients. Various tests are available to definitively diagnose Norwalk infection (see Figure 1), but these are not practical in most clinical situations. Treatment with bismuth subsalicylate has been shown to decrease gastrointestinal symptoms in Norwalk-induced disease in human volunteers.

Enterotoxigenic *Escherichia coli* (ETEC) is the leading identifiable cause of diarrhea among travelers from industrialized regions to the developing world and has been rarely associated with food-borne outbreaks in the United States. Like cholera, ETEC causes a profuse watery diarrhea unaccompanied by fevers or vomiting. The incubation period for each of these illnesses is between 16 and 72 hours. Although symptoms rarely last longer than 5 days, the severe dehydration caused by ETEC may be life-threatening. ORT is the mainstay of therapy in mild-to-moderate disease; in severely dehydrated patients, intravenous therapy may be necessary. Early antimicrobial therapy further reduces fluid losses and the duration of diarrhea. ETEC infections typically respond to ciprofloxacin (Cipro), norfloxacin (Noroxin), or trimethoprim-sulfamethoxazole (TMP–SMX) (Bactrim, Septra), although resistance to all of these agents is increasing globally. Occasionally food-borne diarrhea associated with *Vibrio cholerae* has been reported in the United States. Tetracycline is the drug of choice for most patients with cholera; doxycycline, TMP–SMX, and furazolidone (Furoxone) are also effective.

Inflammatory Diarrhea

Food-borne diarrheal illnesses associated with fever, tenesmus, mucoid stools, severe dehydration, or prolonged duration should prompt examination for fecal leukocytes or fecal lactoferrin (a sensitive and specific surrogate marker for leukocytes in adults). Such syndromes usually occur within 16 to 72 hours of ingesting contaminated food (or water) and are characteristically caused by invasive pathogens including *Salmonella, Shigella*, and *Campylobacter*.

Salmonellosis is the single leading identified cause of food-borne disease in the United States, with ap-

proximately 40,000 cases reported annually. Improperly prepared poultry, eggs, beef, pork, and dairy products are the most common sources for food-borne salmonella infections. In most patients, the illness is usually self-limited with resolution of fever within 2 days and resolution of diarrhea after 3 to 5 days. Among human immunodeficiency virus (HIV)–infected patients the disease is frequently more severe, and bacteremia more common. The diagnosis is readily made by culturing the organism from freshly passed stools onto a variety of standard enteric laboratory media. Although some antibiotics (particularly ciprofloxacin) may reduce the duration of symptoms in *Salmonella* gastroenteritis, they may prolong the intestinal carriage state and have been associated with clinical relapse. Thus, the routine use of antibiotics in the uncomplicated patient is controversial. However, patients with *Salmonella* gastroenteritis who are younger than 12 weeks of age or older than 50 years; those with lymphoproliferative disorders, malignancies, hemoglobinopathies (including sickle cell disease), or acquired immune deficiency disease (AIDS); transplant recipients; those with vascular grafts, artificial joints, marked degenerative joint disease, valvular heart disease; and those on steroids should receive antibiotics until afebrile for at least 24 hours. All bacteremic patients should be treated for 7 to 14 days (longer if a metastatic focus is present). Fluoroquinolones or a third-generation cephalosporin are reasonable initial antibiotic choices until culture sensitivity results become available.

Recent estimates suggest that the annual incidence of food-borne *Campylobacter* gastroenteritis in the United States may rival that of *Salmonella*-induced disorders. Common food sources include poultry, milk, and beef, and infection usually occurs in nonwinter months. The gastrointestinal symptoms associated with inflammatory diarrhea are often preceded by a 12- to 24-hour prodrome of headache, fever, and malaise; diarrhea generally lasts for 5 to 7 days. Routine stool cultures often do not detect campylobacter organisms; thus, selective media (such as Skirrow, Butzler, Campy-Bap) should be used when this organism is suspected. Because the illness is short-lived and self-limited, antibiotics generally do not alter the course of disease unless administered early. Erythromycin has been shown to eradicate *Campylobacter* from stool but does not alter the natural course of the disease when initiated 4 days or longer after the onset of symptoms. Ciprofloxacin is also usually effective, although resistant organisms and clinical relapses occasionally occur. In general, if the patient presents soon after the onset of symptoms, appears toxic, or is immunocompromised, antimicrobial therapy is indicated.

Shigellosis, also a relatively common cause of food-borne disease, occurs most frequently in the summer and fall. As ingestion of fewer than 200 *Shigella* organisms readily causes disease, transmission of shigellosis is very efficient, rendering direct person-to-person contact a common means of infection. Food-borne transmission, when it occurs, tends to be associated with large outbreaks coupled with cases of secondary transmission. Fever is documented in 33% of cases and grossly bloody stools are seen in 40%; tenesmus and abdominal pain is frequent. As with *Salmonella*, *Shigella* can be cultured on routine enteric media. Microbiologic recovery of the organism is best accomplished early in the illness when higher concentrations of viable organisms are present. For shigellosis acquired in the United States, either TMP–SMX or a fluoroquinolone is a reasonable initial antimicrobial choice; shigellosis acquired in developing regions (where trimethoprim resistance is common) should be treated with a fluoroquinolone (the newer agents are not approved for use in children; see Table 1), pending susceptibility testing.

Rarely in the United States, but more frequently in Japan, *Vibrio parahaemolyticus* has been implicated in food-borne infections. Illness is characterized by the sudden onset of watery diarrhea associated with ingestion of seafood. In some patients the disease appears to be more inflammatory and is characterized by fever, chills, and bloody dysentery. Because of the short duration of illness, treatment beyond supportive measures generally is not necessary.

Yersinia enterocolitica is also a relatively rare cause of food-borne disease in the United States; it is more prevalent in Europe. Children under 5 years of age are particularly susceptible to *Yersinia* food poisoning, which occurs primarily during the winter months and is associated with improperly prepared meat or dairy products. In addition to causing diarrhea, *Y. enterocolitica* infection may be complicated by mesenteric adenitis or a reactive polyarthritis, the latter particularly in adults. There are no data to support the use of antibiotics in uncomplicated *Y. enterocolitica* gastroenteritis; in complicated illnesses, treatment should be guided by in vitro susceptibility data.

Hemorrhagic Diarrhea

Enterohemorrhagic *E. coli* (EHEC) (particularly *E. coli* serotype O157:H7) and *Shigella* are the most common food-borne causes of bloody diarrhea and colitis. EHEC infections have been linked to the consumption of rare hamburgers, unpasteurized dairy products, fresh-pressed apple cider, and contaminated water—usually 72 to 120 hours prior to the onset of symptoms. Most patients with hemorrhagic colitis remain afebrile, and fecal leukocytes are seen in only 30 to 40% of cases. The potentially devastating complication, hemolytic uremic syndrome (HUS), a constellation of microangiopathic hemolytic anemia, thrombocytopenia, and acute renal failure, occurs most frequently in children between 1 and 4 years of age and in elderly people; it may be heralded by the onset of fever and leukocytosis during the acute illness. When EHEC is suspected, stool should be plated on sorbitol-MacConkey medium, and any sorbitol-negative *E. coli* isolates should be serotyped. In addition, serologic testing for *E. coli* O157 infections is a potentially useful clinical diagnostic tool.

The role of antibiotics in treating EHEC infections has not been clearly established. Some potentially biased epidemiologic data have associated TMP–SMX administration with the development of HUS in some patients, and clinical EHEC isolates in vitro have been found to actually secrete more toxin in response to TMP–SMX and other antibiotics. Other studies, however, have found that prolonged antibiotic therapy either had no effect on or decreased the incidence of progression to HUS. Currently, supportive care with particular attention toward maintaining euvolemia and monitoring for signs of HUS (by following platelet counts, blood smears, and renal function) remains the mainstay of management of EHEC infections.

NEUROLOGIC SYMPTOMS (FOOD–BORNE BOTULISM)

A rare but serious food-borne disease manifested primarily as a symmetrical descending paralysis is caused by toxins produced by *Clostridium botulinum*. Among adults, the disease usually occurs after ingestion of improperly canned foods or fish contaminated with botulinum toxin, whereas among infants under 1 year of age disease has been associated with in vivo toxin production after ingesting honey contaminated with *C. botulinum* spores. Early symptoms include blurred vision and photophobia, dry mouth, dysphagia, dysphonia, nausea and vomiting, and generalized weakness. This may be followed by constipation, postural hypotension, and paralysis with respiratory compromise. Major considerations in the differential diagnosis of botulism includes Guillain-Barré syndrome, myasthenia gravis, poliomyelitis, stroke, and drug reaction. The diagnosis may be supported by specific electromyographic findings; definitive diagnosis may be established by a mouse bioassay for the toxin in the patient's stool or serum or in the suspected food. Intensive monitoring and aggressive respiratory support are mandatory in any patient with suspected botulism. Patients with suspected botulism should be reported immediately to state health department officials and to the Centers for Disease Control and Prevention (404-329-3753 or 404-329-3644 after 5 P.M.) from whom trivalent equine antitoxin may be obtained. Antitoxin therapy does not reverse pre-existing paralysis, but it does prevent its progression. It is associated with hypersensitivity reactions in nearly 10% of patients.

Syndromes Associated with Seafood Ingestion

Ciguatera Fish Poisoning

Ciguatera fish poisoning results from ingestion of fish contaminated with ciguatoxin, a neurotoxin originating from dinoflagellates and propagated through the aquatic food chain. More than 400 species of fish (restricted to oceans within a 30-degree latitude on either side of the equator) have been noted to harbor ciguatoxin; grouper, red snapper, and barracuda have been most frequently implicated. Nausea, vomiting, and diarrhea may be followed by pruritus, paresthesias, dry mouth, photophobia, and blurred vision. In severe cases, cranial nerve palsies, bradycardia, hypotension, and respiratory paralysis may occur.

If the patient presents within 4 hours of ingestion, emesis induction or gastric lavage may prevent further toxin absorption, and in severe cases, atropine may be useful to control symptomatic bradycardia. Mechanical ventilation may be necessary if the patient develops respiratory failure secondary to paralysis.

Scombroid Fish Poisoning

Ingestion of spoiled fish, most commonly from the families Scombridae and Scomberesocidae (which include tuna, mackerel, skipjack, mahi-mahi, and bonito) may lead to scombrotoxicosis, a syndrome resembling a histamine reaction. Typically within 10 minutes to 3 hours after ingesting the contaminated fish, patients will develop symptoms including sudden onset flushing, headache, nausea, vomiting, diarrhea, and in severe cases, respiratory distress. The diagnosis is confirmed by demonstrating greater than 100 mg of histamine per gram in the suspected fish. Antihistamines and bronchodilators may provide symptomatic relief, although most symptoms usually resolve within 6 hours.

Puffer Fish Poisoning

Ingestion of improperly prepared puffer fish may lead to tetrodotoxin intoxication. Such poisoning is characterized by the rapid onset of weakness, paresthesias, and abdominal pain, which may be followed by a general flaccid ascending paralysis with respiratory failure and death. In Japan, where most cases are described, mortality rates as high as 60% have been reported.

Paralytic Shellfish Poisoning

Paralytic shellfish poisoning is caused by eating mussels, clams, or oysters containing concentrated saxitoxin, a potent neurotoxin that cause nausea, vomiting, diarrhea, and facial paresthesias. In severe cases, dysphonia, dysphagia, paralysis, and respiratory compromise may occur. Most illnesses occur in the summer and early fall and may be associated with a red tide event that reflects high concentrations of potentially toxin-producing dinoflagellates. The incubation period is probably inversely related to the amount of toxin ingested, ranging from 30 minutes to 10 hours; symptoms last from a few hours to a few days. If not contraindicated by the presence of an ileus, enemas or cathartics may be used in an attempt to remove unabsorbed toxin from the intestinal tract.

Neurotoxic Shellfish Poisoning

Neurotoxic shellfish poisoning usually occurs within 4 hours of eating shellfish harvested during the spring or fall from the Gulf Coast or Florida's Atlantic coast. Much like paralytic shellfish poisoning, illness is characterized by nausea, vomiting, and paresthesias; however, paralysis does not occur, and symptoms are usually milder in neurotoxic shellfish poisoning.

Amnesic Shellfish Poisoning

Described in a 1987 outbreak in Canada, amnesic shellfish poisoning (also called "toxic encephalopathic shellfish poisoning") was associated with ingesting mussels contaminated with domoic acid. Clinical features of amnesic shellfish poisoning include initial nausea, vomiting, and diarrhea, often followed by confusion, anterograde amnesia, coma, and cardiovascular instability in severe cases.

Mushroom Poisoning

Toxic mushroom ingestion may lead to a variety of clinical syndromes, depending on the type of mushroom ingested (Table 3). Although many mushroom intoxication syndromes are self-limited and require only supportive therapy, others may be fatal. If mushroom poisoning is suspected, a local poison control center should be contacted promptly. Thirty minutes to 2 hours after ingestion of the muscarine-containing mushrooms *Clitocybe* spp and *Inocybe* spp, patients develop an anticholinergic syndrome of sweating, salivation, lacrimation, and bradycardia, among other indications of parasympathetic hyperactivity. Although symptoms usually resolve within 24 hours, severe cases may be fatal and thus should be treated with parenteral atropine sulfate, 1 to 2 mg every 2 to 6 hours as warranted for bradycardia.

Most fatal mushroom poisonings occur with ingestion of *Amanita phalloides* and several other species that produce amatoxins and phallotoxins. The resultant illness is characteristically biphasic with abdominal pain, vomiting, and diarrhea occurring 6 to 12 hours after ingestion and usually resolving within 24 hours. After appearing well for 1 to 2 days, the patient develops both renal and hepatic failure. Despite intensive supportive care, the mortality rate may be as high as 30 to 50%. Hemoperfusion may be useful to help remove circulating toxin. A similar syndrome without renal failure may occur after ingestion of mushrooms of the genus *Gyromitra* containing gyromitrin, an inhibitor of pyridoxal phosphate. In addition to hepatic failure, hemolysis and methemoglobinuria are seen in the later phases of the illness. Intravenous pyridoxine hydrochloride may be useful for treatment of neurologic symptoms.

Other Food-Related Illnesses

Acute food-related syndromes rarely result from ingestion of various plant-derived foods that contain high levels of endogenous toxicants. Consumption of fava beans (*Vicia faba*), particularly by individuals who are glucose-6-phosphate dehydrogenase–deficient, may lead to an acute hemolytic crisis within 5 to 24 hours after ingestion. The acute illness typi-

TABLE 3. **Seafood, Mushroom, and Plant Poisoning Syndromes**

Food	Toxic Compound	Incubation Period	Syndrome
Seafood			
Ciguatera fish poisoning (grouper, red snapper, barracuda)	Ciguatoxin	1–6 h	Nausea, vomiting, diarrhea, pruritus, paresthesias
Scombroid poisoning (tuna, mackerel, bonito, skipjack, mahi-mahi)	Scombrotoxin	Within 30 min	"Histamine-like" reactions: headache, flushing, pruritus, urticaria, nausea, vomiting
Puffer fish poisoning	Tetrodotoxin	5–30 min	Paralysis, respiratory failure
Paralytic shellfish poisoning	Saxitoxin and others	1–10 h	Paresthesias (face, extremities), nausea, vomiting, diarrhea, paralysis in severe cases
Neurotoxic shellfish poisoning	Several neurotoxins	Within 3 h	Paresthesias, nausea, vomiting, diarrhea
Amnesic shellfish poisoning	Domoic acid	15 min–6 h	Vomiting, cramps, diarrhea—sometimes followed by confusion, amnesia, coma, cardiovascular instability
Mushrooms			
Clitocybe and *Inocybe* groups	Muscarinic compounds	30 min–2 h	Anticholinergic syndrome: sweating, salivation, lacrimation, bradycardia, vomiting
Amanita spp	Ibotenic acid and isoxazole derivatives	20–90 min	Confusion, restlessness, visual disturbances
Psilocybe or *Panaeolus* spp	Psilocybin, psilocin, and related indoles	30–60 min	Mood elevation, hallucination, hyperkinetic activity, and muscle weakness
Coprinus spp	Coprine	Up to 5 days	Disulfiram-like reaction within 30 min after alcohol ingestion
Amanita phalloides	Amatoxins and phallotoxins	6–24 h	Initially: abdominal pain, vomiting, diarrhea 2–3 days later: renal failure, hepatic failure
Gyromitra spp	Gyromitrin	2–12 h	Nausea, vomiting, hemolysis, methemoglobinemia, hepatic failure
Corinarius spp	Orellanine	3–5 days	Thirst, nausea, headache, abdominal pain, visual disturbance
Plants			
Favism (fava bean)	Vincine and convincine	5–24 h	Acute hemolytic crisis in patients with G6PD deficiency
Lathyrism (chickling vetch, sweet peas)	Possibly neurolathyrogen	Prolonged; insidious	Muscle spasm, cramps, leg weakness, signs of degeneration in posterolateral tract of spinal cord
Solanine poisoning (potato tubers, vines, leaves, new sprouts; tomato plant stems, leaves)	Solanine	8–12 h	Headache, abdominal pain, diarrhea, confusion
Acute cyanide poisoning (lima beans, manioc, unripe sorghum, bitter almonds, apricot kernels, apple seeds)	Cyanogenetic glycosides	Within 1 h	Hyperventilation, headache, paralysis, seizures, respiratory arrest
Chronic cyanide poisoning (cassava)	Cyanogenetic glycosides	Prolonged; insidious	Ataxic neuropathy, goiter, possibly amblyopia

Abbreviation: G6PD = glucose-6-phosphate dehydrogenase.

cally lasts for 24 to 48 hours, although support with blood transfusions may be necessary. Solanine poisoning, primarily associated with potato tubers, causes abdominal pain, diarrhea, and confusion typically 8 to 12 hours after ingestion. Rarely, acute cyanide poisoning may result from ingestion of a number of different plant-derived foodstuffs. Chronic cyanide poisoning from high consumption of cassava, particularly in some African cultures, may lead to tropical ataxic neuropathy, tropical amblyopia, and possibly goiters. Lathyrism, an insidious neurologic illness progressing from muscle spasm and cramps to weakness and paralysis, and associated with degeneration of the posterolateral tracts of the spinal cord, results from chronic ingestion of large quantities of legumes of the genus *Lathyrus*. Lathyrism is generally confined to Africa and Asia and is particularly associated with increased consumption of *L. sativus* (sweet peas).

Monosodium glutamate (MSG) ingestion, particularly on an empty stomach, may cause nausea, headache, flushing, and a burning sensation in the skin. Symptoms typically occur soon after beginning the meal and resolve within 4 hours. Because MSG is commonly used in Chinese foods (particularly won ton soup) the syndrome associated with its ingestion has been called the "Chinese restaurant syndrome."

Heavy metal poisoning with copper, zinc, iron, tin, or cadmium is known to cause nausea, vomiting, diarrhea, and a metallic taste within 5 to 60 minutes after ingestion. In addition, cadmium may be associated with increased salivation and cadmium and zinc may cause myalgias. Heavy metal contamination often occurs when acidic (especially citric or carbonated) beverages are allowed to come in contact with metal containers or tubing for prolonged periods of time.

NECROTIZING SKIN AND SOFT TISSUE INFECTIONS

method of
JAMES MAJESKI, PH.D., M.D.
Charleston, South Carolina

The necrotizing lesions of the skin and soft tissues are severe, progressive, often lethal, usually mixed synergistic gangrenous infections. The infectious gangrenes are occasionally seen in clinical practice. They have been classified into several categories: (1) necrotizing fasciitis, (2) bacterial synergistic gangrene, (3) streptococcal gangrene, and (4) clostridial myonecrosis. All these necrotizing soft tissue infectious conditions have been recognized as variations of the same disease process. They are now collectively termed the "infectious gangrenes" and should be initially managed by a unified approach. Further classification based on the organism or tissue level involved will add to the initial diagnostic confusion, as this information is usually not available preoperatively. These necrotizing soft tissue infections should be treated as potentially life-threatening emergencies. They are often associated with severe disability and frequent mortality.

The bacteriology is complex. The majority of these infections consist of a mixture of beta-hemolytic streptococcus (90%), anaerobic gram-positive cocci, aerobic gram-negative bacilli, and bacteroides. These infections have very rarely been caused by a single organism. Frequently the actual bacterial cultures are contaminated with secondary infecting organisms. Also, many laboratories are not able to correctly identify the organisms and false-negative reports may also be encountered. Most frequently the infection is caused by a mixed and rich variety of organisms, aerobic and anaerobic, in a synergistic type of association that inflicts massive damage to the subcutaneous tissue, fascia, and occasionally muscle.

These infectious gangrenes tend to occur in compromised elderly and debilitated patients, especially patients with atherosclerotic vascular disease, malignancy, or diabetes. These infections are now being recognized in increasing frequency in younger patients who sustain wounds and traumatic injuries or undergo surgical procedures of the gastrointestinal tract. Postpartum women and intravenous drug abusers are also at increased risk. These gangrenous infections may also occur in healthy patients after minor trauma and lacerations, after clean operations, and after blunt, nonpenetrating trauma. They can also occur spontaneously, especially in obese, alcoholic, and diabetic patients. They have been noted to occur in patients with autoimmune diseases and acquired immune deficiency syndrome (AIDS), and in transplant patients.

Clostridial and mycotic infections must always be considered in the initial evaluation of a necrotizing skin and soft tissue infection. Mucormycosis can produce an extremely aggressive gangrenous infection. Clostridial infections should always be suspected when necrotic muscle is found during débridement of an infectious gangrene.

CLINICAL PRESENTATION

The disease process is a bacterial synergistic infection produced by a combination of gram-positive cocci and gram-negative bacilli. Modern bacteriology laboratories will frequently isolate both aerobes and anaerobes. The actual organisms and specific conditions needed for these necrotic processes to develop are unknown. Much of the bacteriology data in the literature are invalid owing to frequent secondary infection by opportunistic organisms. Most current reports, however, speculate that synergism between aerobic and anaerobic organisms is responsible for the necrotizing skin and soft tissue infectious process.

The clinical history and manifestations are very helpful to establish an early diagnosis of infectious necrotizing soft tissue infection. The patient generally appears ill and has a rapid pulse and a mild-to-high temperature elevation. A characteristic occasional finding is numbness of the infected area, although most patients present with localized pain of the involved site, and the overlying skin is red, hot, and swollen. Skin anesthesia is probably due to infarction of cutaneous nerves located in necrotic subcutaneous fascia. An apparent cellulitis that fails to respond to standard therapy must raise suspicion of more extensive underlying subcutaneous infection. Necrotic tissue and a muddy, brown serous fluid exudate are very diagnostic.

Tissue biopsies, tissue cultures, exudate cultures, and blood cultures are made early in the evaluation of the patient with an infectious gangrene. The exact site of entry of the bacteria occasionally cannot be determined with certainty. The extremities are the most common site of involvement, followed in frequency by the perineum. Ultrasound or computed tomography may be helpful in the diagnosis of some deep necrotic infections when they identify air or extensive soft tissue edema. Nuclear medicine scans, such as indium or gallium scans, require too much time for results to be of any significant value.

Anemia, possibly due to a bacterial hemolysin, is a consistent finding. Hemoglobin levels below 10 grams per dL are found in most patients. Hypocalcemia is noted but very infrequently are there any accompanying symptoms of muscle twitching, Chvostek's sign, or carpopedal spasms. All patients have a leukocytosis with a left shift in the white cell differential count. Frequently, the presence of gas in the subcutaneous and soft tissue is noted radiographically. The clinical sign of crepitus is found in only 25% of patients. Most patients have hypoproteinemia and hypoalbuminemia. Electrolyte and fluid deficits are frequently severe, even though no external losses of fluid occur.

When a gangrenous or necrotizing infection is suspected, the rapid performance of a frozen-section biopsy helps establish the diagnosis on the basis of the typical histologic changes of subcutaneous necrosis, polymorphonuclear cell infiltration, fibrinous vascular thrombosis with necrosis and microorganisms within the destroyed fascia and dermis, and sparing of muscle. Early tissue biopsy also permits the identification of fungus in the tissues, with characteristic invasion and occlusion of blood vessels. Tissue biopsy or Gram's stain of the exudate may also reveal the characteristic finding of clostridia, which are gram-positive rods with blunt ends resembling boxcars.

The clinical course of necrotizing infections is characterized by moderate pain, moderate fever, and marked edema of the skin, which is initially spared from necrosis, a feature that often causes errors and delays in the diagnosis. Local signs that suggest a deep tissue infection may include cyanosis or bronzing of the skin. The destruction of subcutaneous fat, under the erythematous skin, typically exhibits minimal pain or tenderness. The easy and painless diagnostic introduction of a probing instrument into the necrotic subcutaneous space is an accurate bedside clinical test. Progression of the occlusive vascular process brings about delayed cutaneous gangrene. As the disease process advances, systemic toxicity develops. If prompt and radical treatment is not established, the condition advances rapidly into severe systemic sepsis and fatal multiple organ system failure. A seroma and partial or complete dehiscence of a recent operative incision are suggestive of a possible necrotizing infection. If a necrotizing process is suspected in a recent operative incision, the patient should be returned to the operative suite for tissue biopsy and absolute examination of all layers of the skin, subcutaneous tissue, fascia, muscle, and peritoneum. Partial examination in the patient's bed of postoperative wounds under local anesthesia with a gloved hand is frequently associated with an incorrect assessment of the type or extent of the infectious process and a delay in treatment.

TREATMENT

The cornerstone of treatment of necrotizing skin and soft tissue infection is early diagnosis and prompt initiation of treatment. As the period of time increases from onset of the necrotizing process to its diagnosis and treatment, the morbidity and mortality increase.

The physician must keep a high index of suspicion, viewing any area of spreading cellulitis with extreme caution and close monitoring, performing immediate needle aspiration for specimens for bacterial examination and culture and biopsies of the affected tissue and the advancing edge. Emergency radical resection of all necrotic tissue until healthy and unaffected tissue is reached, accompanied by broad-spectrum antibiotic coverage and full hemodynamic and physiologic monitoring for vigorous organ and metabolic support, is required.

At the outset, under the preliminary guidance of Gram-stained smears while aerobic and anaerobic tissue and blood cultures are under way, a triple regimen of antibiotic coverage is favored to cover the diverse and varied causative bacteria:

Penicillin for clostridia, enterococci, and peptostreptococci;

Clindamycin (Cleocin) or metronidazole (Flagyl) for anaerobes, *Bacteroides fragilis*, and peptostreptococci;

Gentamicin (Garamycin) (or another aminoglycoside) for Enterobacteriaceae and various gram-negative organisms.

Imipenem (Primaxin), by virtue of its very high beta-lactamase resistance and wide-spectrum efficacy, may be the initial agent of choice if only one antibiotic is to be used. The antibiotic coverage is subsequently tailored to the results of the meticulous microbiology-monitoring tissue biopsy cultures that are mandatory for these patients.

Patients with mucormycosis and progressive necrotizing lesions are at high risk of death. Once invasive mucormycosis has been demonstrated, treatment with amphotericin B (Fungizone), currently the agent of choice, must be promptly started.

Clostridial infections may be initially recognized at the time of surgery on identification of necrotic muscle. Radical débridement should be performed in clostridial infections, but amputation of an extremity should be considered early in the treatment as it may be lifesaving. High-dose penicillin should be administered; clindamycin or metronidazole is substituted for patients with penicillin allergy. Hyperbaric oxygenation can also be given to the patient as it is bacteriostatic to the organism and appears to hinder the production of some exotoxins. It is important to emphasize that primary treatment is radical surgical débridement, as both in vitro and in vivo studies reveal an insignificant effect by hyperbaric oxygenation in the presence of residual necrotic tissue.

Tetanus prophylaxis with absorbed tetanus toxoid and passive immune coverage with tetanus hyperimmune globulin are indicated in the management of all high-risk wounds because tetanus is an occasional complication of severe lesions of this nature.

Once the diagnosis of necrotizing skin and soft tissue infection is made or highly suspected, aggressive fluid resuscitation and stabilization are absolutely necessary prior to surgery. Occasionally, this will require placement of a Swan-Ganz catheter and preoperative preparation in a surgical intensive care unit. Broad-spectrum antibiotics are always administered preoperatively.

The management of these entities constitutes a major surgical emergency. As soon as the patient's condition will permit a general anesthetic, an aggressive radical débridement of the area is undertaken in the operating room. Occasionally a patient may remain in septic shock after resuscitation and antibiotics are begun. Surgical débridement should not be delayed, as correction of the septic state does not occur until the infectious process is radically excised. All necrotic tissue should be removed at the initial operative procedure.

Minor drainages and débridements are attended by prohibitive mortality rates, and the surgeon must always undertake a radical resection of all affected tissues. This débridement may occasionally require several teams of surgeons. Whenever possible, the affected limb should not be amputated nor any viable tissue removed.

Amputation is rarely needed in cases of infectious gangrene. During all operative procedures, the infected areas are frequently copiously irrigated with saline containing antibiotics. Kanamycin* or neomycin* is an effective agent in a concentration of 1 gram per 1 liter of normal saline. Despite reports of aminoglycoside-induced myoneural blockade and its resultant respiratory arrest, these complications are rare when the drugs are used judiciously in surgical wounds. Another irrigation solution that has been effective consists of 1 gram of a cephalosporin* in 1 liter of normal saline. The use of topical irrigation has been a factor in reducing intraoperative bacteria and reducing the actual bacterial count in the affected tissue. The operative areas are always packed open with gauzes soaked in povidone-iodine (Betadine) or antibiotics.

Patients are taken back to the operating room daily for anesthesia with dressing changes and for additional débridement if necessary. Dressing changes are all initially performed in the operating room on a daily basis. This provides a second and third look at the affected tissues and underlying tissue, muscle, and overlying skin. Its purpose is for the careful reexploration of the wound and the identification of residual necrotic foci and any advancing edge of the necrotizing infection. A daily regimen of exploration and dressings with the patient under general anesthesia in the operating room is continued until the patient's condition allows the dressings to be changed in the intensive care unit or the ward without anesthesia.

The wound is best covered with saline-soaked dressings. In areas of loss of the abdominal wall, a plastic sheet is used rather than a mesh, which occasionally will produce an enterocutaneous fistula. I recommend repeated culturing of the wounds, because a secondary infection of Pseudomonas, Serratia, or Candida occasionally develops. The wound and all flaps should be packed open. When the wound is ready (less than 10^5 organisms per gram of tissue or when healthy granulation tissue appears), the large skin flaps are replaced. When the flaps have healed in place, the residual open area is then covered with split-thickness skin grafts. Mafenide acetate (Sulfamylon) or silver sulfadiazine (Silvadene) is applied to all open areas, as in the treatment of burns, to retard secondary infection.

Hyperbaric oxygen has not been demonstrated to be of any consistent value in the treatment of necrotizing infections. Its true value is confirmed only in the treatment of gas gangrene.

Most patients with necrotizing infections will have or will rapidly develop malnutrition. Consequently, the last point in the postoperative and perioperative treatment of these necrotizing processes is aggressive nutritional support with either oral or intravenous hyperalimentation. I recommend nutritional support at a rate of one and one-half to two times the patient's basal requirement for energy intake, with a high-protein dietary supplement. The oral route of hyperalimentation is preferred. Serial serum transferrin levels are a good reflection of protein nutritional status.

INFLUENZA

method of
ROLAND A. LEVANDOWSKI, M.D.
Center for Biologics Evaluation and Research
Rockville, Maryland

Influenza viruses, which are lipid-enveloped viruses and contain a segmented RNA genome, are classified as myxoviruses. Influenza viruses have two major surface glycoproteins: hemagglutinin (HA) and neuraminidase (NA). HA binds to sialic acid on cells and permits fusion with cells to internalize the viral nucleocapsid. NA enzymatically cleaves sialic acids on the surface of the infected cells to permit dispersion of new virions during viral morphogenesis. Antibodies to HA block receptor binding and prevent infection, and those to NA limit the extent of spread. Cytolytic T lymphocytes develop in response to other structural and nonstructural viral proteins and lyse infected cells to facilitate elimination of virus from infected individuals.

Since HA and NA undergo continuous antigenic alterations because of natural and immunologic selection, repeated illnesses of varying severity are possible during each person's lifetime. The alterations occurring in HA and NA are detected readily by antibodies in the sera of immune animals and people. Infrequently, a major antigenic change occurs in HA or NA as the result of natural exchange of viral gene segments between human strains and other animal strains (termed "antigenic shift"), and a pandemic occurs in a large segment of the world population. More often, minor but detectable changes in HA and NA occur as a result of point mutations in the viral genome (termed "antigenic drift"). Under either condition, the susceptible population increases and excess mortality occurs, particularly in those patients with conditions that interfere with proper function of host defense mechanisms. The goals of prevention and treatment are, therefore, similar for pandemics and interpandemic periods, but the intensity of public health activities increases in the face of a pandemic threat when essentially all people are susceptible, as happened most recently during the 1958 shift from H1N1 to H2N2 influenza A viruses and during the 1968 shift from H2N2 to H3N2 influenza A viruses.

DISEASE

Although "intestinal flu" is a term used frequently, it should not be inferred that influenza viruses are a major cause of this syndrome. Gastrointestinal symptoms are minor in infections caused by influenza viruses that replicate in the epithelium of the nasal and pulmonary airways. In severe instances, the respiratory epithelium of the pulmonary airways may be completely denuded by infection with an influenza virus. In milder forms, little or only

---

*Not FDA-approved for this indication.

patchy involvement may be evident. Consequently, the disease caused by influenza viruses ranges from mild upper respiratory illness to viral pneumonia and death.

Fever, chills, headache, myalgia, sore throat, coryza, and cough occur after an incubation period of 24 to 48 hours and resolve gradually in a few days in uncomplicated cases, but even uncomplicated illness is associated with alterations in lung function that may be subtle but can persist for weeks to months in otherwise healthy persons. Impairment of mucociliary clearance mechanisms and alterations in epithelial cells contribute to the colonization of the airways and contiguous spaces by pathogenic bacteria including *Streptococcus pneumoniae, Haemophilus influenzae,* and *Staphylococcus aureus*. Productive bronchitis, sinusitis, and otitis media are all increased in frequency by acute influenza virus infections. Although viral pneumonia is infrequently identified, secondary bacterial pneumonia is an all too common event. Complications of influenza such as bronchitis and pneumonia are generally more frequent and potentially more debilitating in persons with underlying cardiopulmonary diseases that affect oxygenation, particularly in those conditions that compromise oxygen exchange or increase interstitial lung fluid.

The extremes of age are also associated with increased risk of complications. Children under 12 months of age are more frequently hospitalized and have a higher mortality rate during influenza epidemics than any age group other than the elderly. Although death complicating acute influenza infection begins to accelerate after age 40 years, mortality is highest after 65 years of age, which is used as a convenient but arbitrary division point for defining population risk. Immaturity of the immune system, premature birth with bronchopulmonary dysplasia, and initial exposures to influenza in the absence of protective immunologic mechanisms contribute to the morbidity and mortality of the very young. Impairments of the immune response of the elderly may reflect a sort of immunologic distraction caused by inflammatory and other immune-modulating (and possibly immune-suppressing) events that accumulate with age. It has been noted during pandemics that the risk of mortality is increased for women during pregnancy. The mild immune suppression and the increase in vascular and interstitial fluids inherent to normal pregnancy are potentially contributory to the risk.

DIAGNOSIS

In epidemic situations, febrile nonpneumonic respiratory illness should be considered to be influenza, although symptoms are by no means specific and many other respiratory viruses including respiratory syncytial virus, parainfluenza viruses, and sometimes even rhinoviruses can cause influenza-like illnesses. Usually, however, the isolation of an influenza virus in a well-defined population sufficiently reduces the probability of any other cause to warrant a presumptive diagnosis for subsequent contemporary cases. The relative ease of transmission of influenza viruses by aerosol and contact and the rapidity of onset of illness make it unlikely that other respiratory viruses will co-circulate in the same household or closed population such as a school or a nursing home.

A specific diagnosis in an individual patient is best made from the isolation and identification of virus by inoculating respiratory secretions onto appropriate tissue cultures or embryonated eggs. Although virologic procedures typically require several days to complete, the finding of a hemadsorbing agent after 48 hours' incubation is provisionally diagnostic. Rapid immunologic and molecular techniques

are also available and, when carefully controlled, are valuable in making a presumptive diagnosis when urgency exists. The probability of success for diagnostic procedures depends on the quality of the specimens collected. Usually, nasal secretions obtained by saline washing are the most reliable source of virus, but throat gargles and swabs may also be of value. Samples taken during the first few days of the illness are more likely to yield virus than a sample taken at the end of illness. Serologic procedures help to confirm the diagnosis retrospectively and may be useful in dealing with subsequent cases, but generally 2 to 3 weeks must elapse before a definitive rise in antibody titer occurs.

Information and guidance on influenza activity in specific areas of the United States and elsewhere are available from a number of sources. Local, state, and territorial health departments track activity and report to the Centers for Disease Control and Prevention (CDC), which confirm and place the data on their Voice Information System (404-332-4555), incorporating weekly surveillance updates on the Influenza Hotline as to the level of activity of influenza and the types of viruses being encountered.

PREVENTION AND TREATMENT

Vaccine

Although restriction and isolation of ill persons may serve as adjunct measures to prevent transmission of influenza viruses in certain populations and effective drugs specific for influenza viruses exist, the unpredictable and explosive appearance of influenza in a given community makes the use of inactivated influenza virus vaccines the major focus of public health measures. The ease and speed of modern travel greatly facilitate the spread of influenza. It is not uncommon to hear of influenza occurring in travelers, and there have been notable outbreaks on cruise ships returning to the United States from Asia. Therefore, a continuing effort is made to provide vaccines that reflect the strains currently circulating in humans. Critical surveillance and epidemiologic efforts begin with individual physicians who recognize disease and take appropriate cultures in order to report to and alert public health authorities. Without the information from surveillance, accurate predictions of changes in strains are impossible, and knowledge of the beginning and end of the influenza season cannot be provided with geographic specificity.

Currently available vaccines are produced in eggs, contain chemically inactivated viruses, and are standardized for HA content. Whole-virus vaccines are now a minority of the product made. The majority of inactivated vaccines currently available are produced by disrupting viruses and partially purifying the viral proteins to minimize the presence of extraneous materials derived from the egg or additives used in purification. The immune response to inactivated vaccines is predominantly in the form of antibodies to HA, although antibodies to NA may also be produced. Compared with natural infection, inactivated vaccines are poor at stimulating cytotoxic T lymphocytes.

Although a single dose (0.25 ml for children less than 3 years old and 0.5 ml for older children and adults) of inactivated vaccine containing 30 μg/ml of HA for each vaccine component is adequate for the majority of the population, two doses are needed by the immunologically naive (generally children), who because of age have not been exposed to specific types or subtypes of virus. However, multiple or larger doses of vaccine in a single season do not necessarily increase immunogenicity for primed adults or elderly persons. In addition, although the effects of immunologic immaturity on the response of the infant are not entirely determined, premature birth and age under 6 months may also adversely affect the immunogenicity of inactivated influenza virus vaccines.

In temperate climates, influenza occurs predominantly during the winter months, but in tropical areas, transmission of influenza viruses occurs sporadically and in outbreaks throughout the year. In the United States, vaccine is best given in the fall to maximize antibody titers at the time of exposure to influenza. The newest vaccine formulation is usually available by September, and often during the summer. Although the fall months of October and November are appropriate for organized immunization activities, it is difficult to reach all persons in that period of time, and many individuals appear at hospitals, clinics, and physicians' offices at other times. As a practical matter to improve convenience for patients and to avoid missed opportunities, vaccine can and should be offered to all high-risk patients whenever they present for medical care from the time the new vaccine is available up to and even after influenza appears in the community, as long as vaccine is available. Since travel is one mechanism of transmission, the most current vaccine should also be offered to these patients as preparation for travel to areas where influenza may be active.

An obstacle to vaccine use is the perception of potential adverse effects, but most adverse events are minor and of less than 2 days' duration, including local inflammation at the injection site and systemic complaints such as fever, myalgias, and malaise. The benefits of protection greatly outweigh the short-lived discomfort, and patients generally respond positively when they are fully informed of the rationale for use of vaccine. Guillain-Barré syndrome (GBS), a usually reversible, immunologically mediated paralysis, requires special comment. GBS is not specifically related to influenza virus infection or vaccine. It has been associated with many other infectious causes. GBS is rare enough that risk is difficult to quantify precisely. Most authorities agree that it was increased in frequency for persons who received the swine flue vaccine in 1976. However, subsequent studies have shown no increased risk of GBS associated with vaccine or have not been definitive because of the extreme rarity of GBS. The best estimate is that the risks of complications of influenza virus infection outweigh any risk of GBS.

The current supplies of vaccine have increased to approximately 70 million doses for the United States. Since this amount is insufficient to immunize the majority of the population, efforts currently emphasize persons who are more likely to suffer morbidity and mortality from acute infection by influenza viruses. Persons who should be targeted for special attention include those with chronic pulmonary or cardiovascular disorders including asthma; those who may be at increased risk of morbidity and mortality because of age alone; residents of chronic care facilities, particularly those with chronic medical conditions; and those who have required regular medical follow-up or hospitalization for chronic metabolic diseases, renal dysfunction, hemoglobinopathy, or immune suppression. Persons providing medical and nursing care to these individuals and the household contacts of these individuals are also strong candidates for immunization to reduce the risk of transmission of influenza virus infection. Children who need aspirin therapy on a regular basis are also candidates for immunization to reduce the potential for Reye's syndrome, which has been associated with influenza infections. Since excess mortality has been documented for women pregnant during previous pandemics, consideration should be given to providing vaccine to women who will be in the third trimester of pregnancy during the influenza season, especially those who have any other indication for immunization. Even though the quantity of vaccine available in the United States is relatively limited, no one wishing to receive vaccine to prevent influenza should be refused while supplies exist.

Persons who should not be immunized are those who have experienced a severe adverse reaction that might be related to influenza vaccine such as anaphylaxis or GBS. The very few patients who do have IgE-mediated allergy to influenza vaccine (usually because of antibodies to egg proteins) may be considered for desensitization procedures if the risk from influenza and its complications is sufficient to warrant. Otherwise, measures such as antiviral agents may be more prudent for use in these patients.

Antiviral Agents

Drugs licensed in the United States for the treatment and prevention of acute influenza A virus infections include amantadine (Symmetrel) and rimantadine (Flumadine). These drugs prevent viral infection by interfering with a viral protein that probably functions as an ion channel required for the packaging of new viruses and the uncoating of virus particles on entry into cells. These drugs are not effective against influenza B virus strains, and they do have adverse consequences that would discourage their use if no effect were likely. Therefore, knowledge of the influenza viruses in circulation is invaluable for a logical decision on whether to institute antiviral chemotherapy.

Antiviral agents have been shown to shorten the duration of symptoms, and they can help to speed recovery when used early in the course of illness. For maximal effect, treatment should begin as soon as possible after onset of symptoms (within 24 to 48 hours) and continued for 24 to 48 hours after the acute symptoms subside. Resistant strains of influenza A virus have developed during treatment with both amantadine and rimantadine. Even if resistant strains develop during treatment, therapy is effective in reducing the acute symptoms. However, drug resistance as a result of treatment may render prophylaxis ineffective in the same household or treatment unit.

The use of amantadine and rimantadine for prophylaxis in persons who cannot be immunized or who are not yet immunized can also be recommended. Antiviral chemotherapy may be particularly helpful in institutional outbreaks for residents who have not yet been immunized. For patients who cannot be immunized, the drug must be continued for as long as the threat of infection exists (usually several weeks), which can be determined by knowing the status of spread of viruses as tracked by public health authorities. For those persons who can be immunized, administration for the weeks needed until antibodies develop in response to vaccine (2 to 3 weeks after the single dose in immunologically primed and 2 to 3 weeks after the second dose of vaccine in immunologically unprimed) is sufficient.

The adverse events associated with amantadine and rimantadine are similar, although the incidence of adverse events is considerably less with rimantadine. The adverse events are readily reversible on discontinuation of medication and are predominantly related to central nervous system excitement or depression including such symptoms as nausea, dizziness, insomnia, anxiety, irritability, hallucinations, confusion, anorexia, and ataxia. In order to minimize adverse events and maintain effective concentrations, both drugs must be adjusted for renal function. Rimantadine, which is also metabolized, requires adjustment for hepatic function as well. In addition, dosage reduction is indicated for children under 10 years of age (to accommodate smaller body mass and volume of distribution) and for persons over 65 years (who are more likely to have reduced renal function and to experience adverse events).

Recommendations for control of influenza virus infections are made by the Advisory Committee on Immunization Practices at CDC and are published and updated yearly in *Morbidity and Mortality Weekly Reports*. These recommendations provide a coherent approach to preventing influenza virus infection, and are widely accepted by practitioners in infection control. The recommendations are now being made available via Internet, and are also reprinted in the fall in several medical journals including the *Journal of the American Medical Association* and the *Annals of Internal Medicine*.

Other Measures

Symptomatic relief can be very important during the acute illness caused by influenza viruses. Rest is usually self-initiated and is highly recommended during the occurrence of systemic symptoms of fever, chills, headache, and myalgia. Maintenance of hydra-

tion is important particularly when respiratory secretions increase and become mucopurulent, since water is needed for the proper function of mucous transport mechanisms, for reducing the viscosity of the secretions, and for easing their removal. When mucociliary transport mechanisms are impaired by acute infection, cough serves as an important and possibly the only lung clearance mechanism for gross removal of secretions and cellular debris from the airways. Therefore, cough is probably better left alone unless it threatens to exhaust the patient or is otherwise undesirable. Analgesia with aspirin has been associated with development of Reye's syndrome during influenza virus infections, particularly influenza B in children. If treatment is required for fever, headache, or myalgia during an influenza-like illness, aspirin should not be given. However, acetaminophen is acceptable when dose is adjusted for age.

The bacteria associated with pneumonia, bronchitis, sinusitis, and otitis media complicating influenza virus infection are most predictably those inhabiting the respiratory tract for which empirical therapy can be begun based on local patterns of antimicrobial susceptibility. However, a specific diagnosis is an indispensable guide to antimicrobial therapy. Materials for microscopic examination and microbial cultures should be collected early, and these may take advantage of drainage procedures for fluid collections in the pleural space, sinuses, or middle ear.

S. pneumoniae (pneumococcus), *H. influenzae,* and *S. aureus* are the most common causes for secondary bacterial pneumonia complicating influenza virus infection. Until specific results of cultures of sputum and blood are available, the gram-stained sputum can be a valuable diagnostic tool to narrow the spectrum of empirical therapy for bacterial pneumonia. Consideration of the emergence of resistant strains has increasing importance, and consultation with local hospital microbiologists, epidemiologists, and infectious diseases physicians can be helpful in determining the most appropriate antimicrobial agents for use, particularly if treatment failures or unexpected microflora arise.

A vaccine exists for preventing infection by the majority of the most prevalent human serotypes of pneumococci (Pneumovax 23), and is strongly recommended for any patient at risk of complications of influenza. Both pneumococcal and influenza vaccines can be given at the same visit for patient convenience. Although influenza vaccine must be given yearly for changing strains of virus, the need for additional doses of pneumococcal vaccine after the first is not established.

LEISHMANIASIS

method of
ROBERT N. DAVIDSON, M.D.
Northwick Park Hospital
Harrow, Middlesex, England, United Kingdom

BIOLOGY AND ECOLOGY

The leishmaniases are visceral, cutaneous, and mucocutaneous infections caused by *Leishmania* protozoans. Female sandflies of the genus *Phlebotomus* (in Africa, Asia, and Europe) and *Lutzomyia* (in the Americas) infect humans by injecting promastigotes in their saliva into the human skin as the flies feed. Host dendritic cells and macrophages take up the promastigotes (flagellate stage) of *Leishmania,* which become rounded forms, called amastigotes. Amastigotes are able to survive and reproduce within the parasitophorous vacuoles of macrophages. The clinical outcome of the infection is determined both by the host cellular immune responses and by the species of *Leishmania*: some are dermotropic, others viscerotropic. Most species are capable of producing more than one clinical syndrome, although there are typical patterns of disease. The parasite species can be determined by zymodeme (isoenzyme) typing of cultured promastigotes and by polymerase chain reaction using small numbers of parasites. Host cellular immunity determines whether clinical or subclinical infection occurs; whether the disease is visceral, cutaneous, or mucocutaneous; whether lesions are few or diffuse; and whether response to treatment is complete or partial.

The diagnosis of leishmaniasis is suggested by the clinical features and supported by serologic or skin tests but should wherever possible be confirmed by finding or culturing the parasite. Amastigotes (Leishman-Donovan bodies) are 2 to 3 μm long and are found within macrophages in tissue sections. Amastigotes lie free in smears, because infected macrophages burst while being smeared. Nuclei and kinetoplasts of amastigotes stain blue with hematoxylin and eosin, and red with Giemsa stain. *Histoplasma* are the main source of mistaken identification: however, *Histoplasma* lack these structures.

About 10 million cases of cutaneous leishmaniasis (CL) occur annually, and 400,000 cases of visceral leishmaniasis (kala-azar, VL). Both VL and CL are increasing in many areas because of environmental changes. In Brazil, the increase in VL and CL is due to deforestation, which brings humans into close contact with sylvatic reservoirs and forest vectors of *L. braziliensis* and other species. In North Africa and the Middle East, irrigation projects have increased the numbers of gerbils, and the construction of new townships in these areas has led to marked increases in endemic CL caused by *L. major.* Breakdown of the infrastructure in Afghanistan has caused outbreaks of urban CL due to *L. tropica.* Reduction of DDT spraying against malaria vectors in India and Bangladesh has been blamed for the present epidemic of VL caused by *L. donovani,* which affects hundreds of thousands annually. Since 1988 there has been a major epidemic of VL in south Sudan brought on by famine, civil war, and ecologic change. In Europe, VL caused by *L. infantum* is increasing, and half the new patients are co-infected with human immunodeficiency virus (HIV). HIV co-infection has also begun to be reported among VL patients from Africa, and also among CL, VL, and mucocutaneous leishmaniasis (MCL) patients from South America.

VISCERAL LEISHMANIASIS

L. infantum is the cause of VL in Europe in the countries bordering the Mediterranean, and in north Africa; the animal host is the domestic dog. *L. donovani* causes VL in Africa (Sudan and Kenya are most affected, with sporadic cases as far south as Malawi and Angola) and in India; no animal host has been positively identified, and person-to-person transmission is thought to be important. VL is endemic in Bangladesh; Pakistan; the south of the former Soviet Union; Nepal; and China. VL occurs commonly in Brazil, where it is caused by *L. chagasi,* which is identical to *L. infantum*; the animal host is the domestic dog.

Clinical Features of Visceral Leishmaniasis

In VL, the amastigotes disseminate throughout the reticuloendothelial system. After an incubation period of weeks to months (range: 10 days to over 2 years), the patient develops pyrexia, wasting, and hepatosplenomegaly, which may become massive. Lymphadenopathy is common in Sudan. Males and females are equally affected, with a predominance of children and infants in Europe. Patients report fever, malaise, abdominal distention or discomfort, diarrhea, cough, and epistaxis. Laboratory tests reveal pancytopenia, polyclonal hypergammaglobulinemia, and hypoalbuminemia. The erythrocyte sedimentation rate (ESR) and C-reactive protein level are elevated. In 95% of cases, serologic examination for *Leishmania* is positive at high titers, using the direct agglutination test (DAT), immunofluorescent antibody test (IFAT), or enzyme-linked immunosorbent assay (ELISA). The leishmanin skin test is invariably negative, indicating antigen-specific anergy and an absence of Th1 cell–mediated immunity. After several weeks to months of illness, most patients with VL succumb, often with uncontrolled bleeding or secondary bacterial pneumonia, tuberculosis, or dysentery. Serologic and leishmanin skin test surveys of endemic populations indicate that subclinical self-healing infection occurs more frequently than clinical cases. For example, in the Mediterranean countries, about 30% of adults living in rural areas typically have a positive leishmanin skin test, indicating good cellular immunity against *Leishmania,* and presumptive evidence of prior subclinical infection with *L. infantum.* In the same areas, typically about 30% of dogs are actively and chronically infected with *Leishmania.* In epidemics with *L. donovani,* however, most infections are symptomatic and the mortality rate is high.

VL occurs as an opportunistic infection among immunosuppressed individuals: those co-infected with HIV (typically in an advanced stage of immunosuppression), those on corticosteroid treatment, and those who have undergone organ transplantation or thymectomy. Travel to an endemic area may have been years previously. Clinical features in HIV-positive patients are often atypical: symptoms may be vague, laboratory abnormalities may be less severe, and hepatosplenomegaly may be absent or unimpressive. Amastigotes may be found unexpectedly in bone marrow aspirates of oligosymptomatic HIV-positive patients, or in unusual cells, such as circulating neutrophils or gut mucosa. *Leishmania* serologic findings are negative in one-third of immunosuppressed patients. Such patients may respond well to antileishmanial treatment, only to relapse 2 to 12 months later; alternatively, response to treatment may be incomplete, or the patient may be totally nonresponsive or suffer exaggerated drug toxicity.

A few U.S. soldiers who served in the Persian Gulf area in 1990 to 1991 were found to have systemic infection caused by viscerotropic *L. tropica,* normally the cause of urban CL in the Middle East. The manifestations among these soldiers included an acute-to-subacute febrile illness with fatigue, arthralgia, and diarrhea. Some soldiers recovered spontaneously, whereas others progressed to a more chronic condition, associated with adenopathy or splenomegaly. Most responded to treatment with sodium stibogluconate.

After successful treatment for VL due to *L. donovani,* a minority of patients develop a rash called post–kala-azar dermal leishmaniasis (PKDL). This occurs within a few weeks or months of stopping apparently successful treatment in Africa, or months to years later in India. PKDL is occasionally acute and severe, with desquamation of skin and mucosas. More commonly, there are hypopigmented patches, nodules, and plaques. Parasites are scanty or absent from the biopsies. PKDL patients may be a continuing reservoir of *L. donovani* between outbreaks.

CUTANEOUS LEISHMANIASIS

In CL, amastigotes multiply in macrophages near the site of inoculation, typically on the arms, legs, face, or ears. Lesions may be nodular or ulcerative; they may be single, or there may be multiple satellite nodules or lymphangitic spread. The most typical lesion of CL is a chronic 2- to 5-cm-diameter ulcer with raised, indurated margins. The ulcer may be covered by a dry fibrinous crust or have a serous or purulent exudate. The ulcers are painful if large or secondarily infected. The histologic picture is of intense lymphoid and monocytic infiltrate, with granulomas. The diagnosis of CL is confirmed by finding amastigotes in a biopsy or on tissue touch impression smears made on slides from the biopsy material. An alternative is to perform a slit-skin smear. Amastigotes are most abundant in the dermis near the raised ulcer edge and may be scanty in old lesions. The base of the ulcer or secondarily infected lesions are avoided because the parasite yield is low. In CL, *Leishmania* serologic findings may be weakly positive, but the leishmanin skin test is usually positive. A "tissue paper" scar remains after healing, whether this occurs spontaneously or with treatment. The spontaneous healing rate is different for each species.

In the Middle East, zoonotic CL is caused by *L. major* and is linked to living or working near gerbil burrows. In towns in the same areas, person-to-person transmission of *L. tropica* CL occurs commonly. In the Americas (South and Central America, the Caribbean, Mexico, and as far north as Texas), CL is caused mainly by *L. mexicana* and *L. braziliensis,* both of which have many subspecies. Determination of the species that caused the CL in Central and South America is important, because MCL can occur after *L. braziliensis* subsp *braziliensis* CL.

Leishmania infantum causes occasional CL in Europe, often in the elderly. *Leishmania aethiopica* causes CL in Ethiopia and parts of Kenya.

Two chronic forms of CL occur. Diffuse cutaneous leishmaniasis (DCL) is rare but disfiguring. Widespread dermal plaques containing huge numbers of amastigotes persist for decades. DCL patients are anergic to *Leishmania* antigen but do not have visceral dissemination or any systemic symptoms. DCL is caused mainly by *L. aethiopica* in Africa and *L. mexicana amazonensis* in South and Central America. Leishmaniasis recidivans (LR) is a chronic non-healing or relapsing cutaneous infection, seen mainly in the Middle East. LR patients are hypersensitive to parasite antigens, and organisms are few.

MUCOCUTANEOUS LEISHMANIASIS

Mucocutaneous leishmaniasis (MCL; espundia) occurs in about 3 to 10% of cases of CL due to *L. braziliensis braziliensis;* it is commonest in Peru and Bolivia. The mucosal lesions usually become apparent months to years after the cutaneous sores have healed, but cases of simultaneous CL and MCL occur, as do cases in those who have no history of CL. Usually the tip of the nose, nasal cartilage, or upper lip is involved first, with a painless induration or ulceration. MCL may remain static, or there may be gradual extension into the nasopharynx, palate, uvula, larynx, and upper airways. Mutilating destruction of the nose may occur. Biopsies of the lesions show a chronic inflammatory and granulomatous infiltrate with very scanty amastigotes. Cultures of biopsies are usually positive for *L. braziliensis,* but this may require repeated attempts. *Leishmania* serologic findings and the leishmanin skin test are both usually positive. A less severe degree of oral or nasal mucosal involvement rarely occurs with other species causing CL, such as *L. infantum;* this often indicates an underlying defect of host immunity.

TREATMENT

Since the 1940s, the first-line drugs for all forms of leishmaniasis have been the pentavalent antimonials (Sb^v). In English-speaking countries the drug most used is sodium stibogluconate (Pentostam);* in India, the identical compound is known as sodium antimony gluconate† (Albert David Ltd, Calcutta); in most other parts of the world, meglumine antimonate (Glucantime, Rhone, Spain, and Specia, France; Glucantim, Farmitalia Carlo Erba, Milan)† is used. It is assumed that these drugs are identical in activity and toxicity, but they have never been directly compared in patients. Meglumine antimonate solution contains 85 mg of Sb^v per mL; sodium stibogluconate solution contains 100 mg of Sb^v per mL. In the United States, virtually all cases of leishmaniasis are treated with sodium stibogluconate, which is available only through the Drug Services of the Centers for Disease Control and Prevention in Atlanta, Georgia.‡

The drug is given by intravenous infusion or intramuscular injection at a daily dose of 20 mg of Sb^v per kg. The upper limit of 850 mg of Sb^v per day, proposed by the World Health Organization (WHO), should be ignored. Undertreatment is often a cause of relapse, and the practice of giving VL patients 10 mg of Sb^v per kg daily, short courses, or intermittent treatment often leads to relapse. Parasites from relapsed cases are 10- to 17-fold less sensitive to Sb^v than primary isolates.

Toxicity relates to the cumulative dose of Sb^v and may be due to the slow accumulation of trivalent antimony. Children tolerate Sb^v better than adults and may be given higher doses according to body surface area. Before therapy is initiated, patients should be thoroughly evaluated by a history and physical examination, and a baseline full blood count,

---

*Investigational drug in the United States.
†Not available in the United States.
‡Telephone: 1-404-639-3670.

biochemistry profile, and electrocardiogram (ECG) should be obtained. If no significant cardiac, renal, or hepatic abnormalities are found, therapy can begin.

Patients should be hospitalized during systemic Sb^v therapy, and blood tests and ECGs should be performed twice weekly. Hospital-based Sb^v treatment is expensive, inconvenient, and often impossible in rural settings. In poor countries, a nurse usually administers Sb^v to outpatients, without the facilities for monitoring toxicity. Serious adverse events are rare, and deaths due to Sb^v very rare, even in VL patients who have severe disease. Toxicity is reversible and includes elevation of liver enzyme and serum amylase levels; arthralgia and myalgia; thrombocytopenia; leukopenia; anorexia, and thrombophlebitis. Patients may complain of lethargy, headache, nausea, vomiting, metallic taste, or pruritus. The most common ECG changes are ST segment and T wave changes and prolongation of the QT interval. A corrected QT interval greater than 0.50 second is an indication to interrupt therapy, because sudden death from arrhythmia has occurred after prolonged, high-dose intravenous Sb^v therapy. Acute renal failure, acute pancreatitis, severe thrombocytopenia, renal failure, arthritis, and exfoliative dermatitis occur occasionally.

Second-line drugs are amphotericin B desoxycholate (Fungizone) and pentamidine isethionate (Pentam 300). Amphotericin B is used at daily doses of 0.5 mg per kg, or every-other-day doses of 1 mg per kg. Pentamidine is used intravenously at 4 mg per kg two or three times weekly.

Under investigation are liposomal amphotericin B (AmBisome, Vestar, San Dimas, CA) and amphotericin B lipid complex (Amphocil, Liposome Technology, Menlo Park, CA). Also undergoing trials is an aminoglycoside, aminosidine (Gabbriomycin, Farmacia, Milan, Italy),* also called paromomycin.

Visceral Leishmaniasis

Standard treatment of VL is with Sb^v 20 mg per kg intravenously or intramuscularly for 30 days, or longer in India.

Amphotericin B is a good alternative to Sb^v; it is given to a total dose of 7 mg per kg in India but 20 mg per kg elsewhere. Liposomal amphotericin B is highly effective in VL. It achieves very high drug levels in liver and spleen, where liposomes are taken up by macrophages (the infected cells in leishmaniasis), thus targeting the drug to the site of infection. In addition, the toxicity of liposomal amphotericin B is much less than that of conventional amphotericin B. Liposomal amphotericin B* has been used in Mediterranean VL at a dosage of 3 mg per kg daily for 10 days, with a very rapid response and a lack of toxicity.

Aminosidine (paromomycin) may be synergistic with Sb^v, and the most widely studied regimen in VL is aminosidine, 15 mg per kg daily, plus Sb^v, 20 mg per kg daily, given together for 17 days.

The combination of interferon-gamma (IFN-γ) (Actimmune) and Sb^v may improve cure rates in relapsed cases. Of eight Brazilian patients with VL in relapse after multiple courses of meglumine antimonate, six responded to combination therapy of Sb^v plus IFN-γ for 10 to 40 days. In previously untreated VL patients in Kenya, the addition of IFN-γ did not markedly improve the response to Sb^v.

Successful treatment of VL results in defervescence by the end of a week, and by 14 days the clinical and laboratory abnormalities should improve. Parasites are present in greatest numbers in the spleen, and estimates of the parasite burden can be made by doing weekly splenic aspirates, particularly if the clinical response is in doubt. Wherever possible, parasite clearance should be established before treatment is stopped. After successful treatment, amastigotes are absent from aspirates and negative on culture. Although scanty parasites may yet be cleared immunologically, this should not be relied on, and treatment should be continued for 1 to 2 weeks after parasitologic testing becomes negative.

Clinical improvement should be sustained after treatment, although slight splenomegaly may persist for a year or more. Cellular immunity to *Leishmania* returns after successful treatment of VL, with a fall in the *Leishmania* IFAT titer and a positive leishmanin test by 6 to 12 months. The patient should be reviewed 1, 3, 6, and 12 months after treatment. The patient's body weight, spleen size, full blood count, serum albumin level, and ESR are all sensitive markers of recurrent VL.

A relapse rate of less than 5% is expected in VL in immunocompetent patients, but more than 80% of HIV–co-infected patients relapse. Almost all relapses occur within 6 months. To prevent or delay relapse in HIV–co-infected patients, maintenance with intravenous pentamidine isethionate 4 mg per kg for 2 to 4 weeks has been used, but its prophylactic efficacy has not been carefully evaluated. A second course of Sb^v in high dose may succeed in treating relapses of VL, but a second-line drug such as amphotericin B is probably more effective. In HIV–co-infected cases, relapses may be milder than the first attack and accompanied by vague, minor, or atypical clinical features. In such patients, the benefit to be gained must be carefully weighed against the adverse effects of prolonged or repeated courses of toxic drugs.

PKDL, if mild, may settle spontaneously over several months. More severe PKDL may require 3 to 4 months of Sb^v therapy.

Cutaneous Leishmaniasis

Most simple sores heal in months, and treatment is only necessary if the lesions are large, multiple, disfiguring, or over a joint. CL due to *L. braziliensis* must be treated with systemic drug therapy to eradicate metastatic organisms and reduce the risk of subsequent MCL. Heat and cold treatments, laser

---

*Investigational drug in the United States.

and diathermy, and careful curettage have all been advocated to accelerate natural healing. Removing the crusts is of no benefit. Intralesional injections of Sb^v are usually effective: to induce blanching of the infected tissue, the ulcer base and edges are infiltrated with sodium stibogluconate (Pentostam) or meglumine antimonate (Glucantime) from a syringe that has a fine needle. Usually 1 mL suffices for a lesion measuring 2 by 3 cm; injections should be repeated twice weekly for 3 weeks. Systemic treatment, if required, is with Sb^v 20 mg per kg daily by intravenous infusion or intramuscular injection for 20 days, or longer if healing is slow. Epithelialization may occur during treatment or may be delayed, but in *L. braziliensis* infections, treatment should continue for 1 to 2 weeks after parasites are negative in biopsies or smears. Most relapses of CL occur within 12 months.

Because CL is self-healing, the numerous published reports of cures with a wide range of topical and oral medications must be evaluated carefully; placebo-controlled trials and randomized comparative studies are few. Topical treatment with aminosidine* 15% and methylbenzethonium chloride (P-ointment, Teva Pharmaceuticals, Jerusalem) is available in Israel. In a study of 67 patients with CL due to *L. major,* most were cured after twice-daily application for 10 to 30 days.

Ketoconazole (Nizoral), 600 mg daily for 28 days, is effective in CL caused by *L. major;* it is ineffective against *L. tropica* or *L. aethiopica.* In Guatemala, ketoconazole was more effective than Sb^v in CL caused by *L. mexicana* but less effective in CL caused by *L. braziliensis.* In Colombia, ketoconazole and Sb^v were similarly effective in CL caused by *L. braziliensis.* In another Colombian study, a short course of pentamidine was highly effective in CL. Itraconazole (Sporanox), 200 mg daily for 28 days, has had variable success rates in the treatment of CL in different countries. Allopurinol (Zyloprim) has excellent in vitro activity against *Leishmania,* but clinical efficacy in CL is variable. The best results are from a study in Colombia, where allopurinol at a dosage of 20 mg per kg daily in four divided doses combined with Sb^v cured 76% of CL patients and allopurinol alone cured 80%. Immunotherapy with a vaccine consisting of live bacille Calmette-Guérin (BCG) plus heat-killed *Leishmania* promastigotes, three doses injected intradermally into CL patients at 6- to 8-week intervals, has been used in Venezuela. The cure rate was greater than 90%, equivalent to that of Sb^v therapy in the control group.

DCL requires very prolonged treatment; Sb^v is usually effective in South and Central America, and aminosidine may succeed in Ethiopia. LR usually responds to a prolonged course of Sb^v.

Mucocutaneous Leishmaniasis

Because untreated MCL usually progresses and causes extensive, mutilating lesions, early treatment

*Not available in the United States.

is important. MCL responds slowly to treatment, and relapses are common. Sb^v 20 mg per kg daily for 28 days cures most cases with MCL confined to the nose and lip. Patients with extensive MCL such as laryngeal involvement should receive amphotericin B to a total dose of 30 mg per kg.

Corticosteroids should be used if the larynx or airways are involved, because edema often occurs at the start of therapy with an effective drug. Relapse may occur many months to several years after treatment, and clinical follow-up with repeated biopsies may be necessary. Falling *Leishmania* IFAT titers over 6 to 12 months are encouraging evidence of cure in MCL.

Note: The use of ketaconazole, itraconazole, pentamidine, amphotericin B, IFN-γ, and allopurinol for leishmaniasis is not listed in the manufacturers' official directives. AmBisome has a product license for VL in the United Kingdom and some other European countries, but not in the United States.

LEPROSY
(Hansen's Disease)

method of
KENRAD E. NELSON, M.D.
Johns Hopkins University
Baltimore, Maryland

Leprosy is a chronic infectious disease involving primarily the peripheral nervous system, skin, and mucous membranes. It is endemic in many countries in Asia, Africa, the Pacific Islands, Latin America, Southern Europe, and the Middle East. There are endemic areas of infection in the United States as well, particularly in Louisiana, Texas, and California. The major sequelae of leprosy are physical deformities involving the extremities, face, and eyes due primarily to damage to the sensory nerves from *Mycobacterium leprae* infection and the immune reaction. The resultant deformities often lead to stigmatization that continues after the infection becomes inactive and the patient is noninfectious.

The disease is caused by *M. leprae*, an acid-fast organism that, despite its identification in 1873 by Gerhard Henrik Armauer Hansen, has not been reproducibly cultivated in vitro. It is a very slow growing organism that divides only every 12 days when it is in the log phase of growth. This slow growth coincides with the indolent, slowly progressive clinical course of the disease. The human being is the only epidemiologically significant reservoir of the disease. However, several other animals are infected naturally, including the nine-banded armadillo, the sooty mangabey, and possibly other primates. The disease is probably transmitted by infection of the upper respiratory tract through inhalation or contact with infectious cases. Skin-to-skin contact has been shown to be another less important route of transmission. The incubation period is quite long; it may vary from 2 to 10 years in paucibacillary (tuberculoid) disease and 5 to 20 years or more in multibacillary (lepromatous) disease.

CLINICAL MANIFESTATIONS

The clinical manifestations of leprosy are quite variable. The clinical presentation and course depend on the interaction between the bacterial load and the host immune system, especially the cellular immune system. The most widely utilized system for clinical-immunologic classification of leprosy is that developed by Ridley and Jopling, which subdivides leprosy into five general classes: polar lepromatous leprosy (LL), borderline lepromatous (BL) leprosy, mid-borderline (BB) leprosy, borderline tuberculoid (BT) leprosy, and polar tuberculoid (TT) leprosy. In addition, a very early form of leprosy, which is not readily classified into any of the above groups, is called indeterminate (I) leprosy. Indeterminate leprosy often resolves spontaneously without specific therapy. Leprosy is often divided into only two groups: multibacillary leprosy, consisting of LL, BL, and BB leprosy, and paucibacillary leprosy. These groupings are useful for purposes of therapy.

There is a good correlation between the clinical appearance, the number and distribution of organisms, and the patient's classification according to the Ridley-Jopling criteria. Patients with paucibacillary leprosy have well-defined macular skin lesions that are few in number but increase and become more ill defined if the disease moves toward the lepromatous end of the spectrum. In contrast, patients with BL or LL leprosy have more ill defined, even diffuse or nodular, skin lesions without clear borders. Loss of eyebrows or hair is quite common in patients with lepromatous disease. Also characteristic of leprosy is anesthesia of the skin lesions. The skin lesions of leprosy generally spare the warmer intertriginous areas of the body. Enlargement and nodularity of the peripheral nerves, especially the ulnar, posterior tibial, and great auricular nerves, are characteristic. Patients may have corneal anesthesia and keratitis or lagophthalmos due to involvement of the facial nerve. Damage to the hands, feet, and eyes is characteristic of lepromatous disease. Trophic ulcers and resorption of digits may result from the sensory nerve damage and repeated trauma that these patients undergo.

DIAGNOSIS

The diagnosis of leprosy is usually made clinically. Skin lesions that are anesthetic, enlarged nerves to palpation, lagophthalmos, and distal stocking-glove anesthesia are characteristic of leprosy. The diagnosis should be confirmed by skin biopsy and slit-skin smears if possible. When taking a punch biopsy, it is important to include specimens of the entire dermis at the active border of a lesion, because the organisms are often deeply located in the skin. The histopathologic features of leprosy correlate well with the clinical picture of the disease. Patients with lepromatous disease have many organisms in their lesions and lack a well-developed granulomatous response due to their ineffective cellular immunity to the organism. In contrast, tuberculoid patients have few organisms with a granulomatous infiltrate. Consultation for the interpretation and classification of skin biopsies can be obtained from Dr. David Scollard at the National Hansen's Disease Center at Baton Rouge, Louisiana (Phone: 504-642-4740) or Dr. Wayne Meyers at the Armed Forces Institute of Pathology, Washington, D.C.

An important clinical feature of leprosy that often complicates treatment is leprosy reaction, of which there are two basic types. A reversal reaction, or Type 1 reaction, is seen most often in tuberculoid and borderline leprosy. It consists of a relatively abrupt increase in the size and erythema of the skin lesions and often neurologic dysfunction. It is believed to be due to an increase in cell-mediated immunity. It is important to recognize and treat reversal reactions, usually with corticosteroids, when they include

neuritis, in order to preserve neurologic function. Reactions associated with decreased cellular immunity are called downgrading reactions. The second type of reaction, erythema nodosum leprosum (ENL), or Type 2 reaction, is seen most commonly in patients with LL or BL leprosy. ENL reactions are believed to be due to a humoral immune mechanism that involves immune complexes. However, shifts in cellular immunity may also play some role in Type 2 reactions. Type 2 reactions are characterized by tender erythematous nodules involving the skin, fever, and sometimes joint pain, iridocyclitis, or orchitis. Another type of reaction, which is thought by some experts to be a distinct subtype of the Type 2 reaction, is the Lucio phenomenon. Lucio reactions are seen primarily among leprosy patients in Central America and Mexico. These reactions, which can be life-threatening, are characterized by vasculitis and punched-out skin ulcers due to small infarcts.

TREATMENT

Antileprosy Drugs

At present, three drugs are commonly used for the treatment of leprosy: dapsone (Avlosulfon), rifampin (Rifadin), and clofazimine (Lamprene). The use of ethionamide-prothionamide (Trecator) has been abandoned due to its hepatotoxicity and the availability of better alternative drugs. Dapsone and clofazimine have weak bactericidal activity against M. leprae, and rifampin has potent bactericidal activity against nearly all strains of the organism. Other drugs have recently been shown to have good antibacterial activity against M. leprae. Included are ofloxacin (Floxin),* minocycline (Minocin),* and clarithromycin (Biaxin).* Isoniazid (INH), which is an important first-line drug for the treatment of tuberculosis, is ineffective for treating leprosy.

Dapsone

Dapsone is available as 25- and 100-mg tablets. The usual dose is 100 mg daily for adults and 1.0 mg per kg for children. It is a safe, cheap, and effective drug for treating all types of leprosy. Strains of M. leprae that are fully sensitive to dapsone have a minimal inhibitory concentration (MIC) of about 0.003 mg per mL as determined in the mouse footpad assay. Although doses of 100 mg per day of dapsone exceed the MIC by a factor of nearly 500-fold, the increasing prevalence of mild, moderate, or complete resistance to dapsone among M. leprae organisms—either primary resistance in untreated leprosy or secondary resistance that emerges during treatment—and the relatively weak bactericidal action of the drug have dictated the current recommendation of the 100-mg daily dosage.

The most common side effect of dapsone therapy is anemia. However, this is usually mild and well tolerated, unless the patient has a complete glucose-6-phosphate dehydrogenase (G6PD) deficiency, in which case the anemia may be more severe. Therefore, it is useful to screen patients to detect G6PD

---

*Not FDA-approved for this indication.

deficiency prior to instituting dapsone therapy. Occasionally, patients may develop gastrointestinal complaints while on dapsone. More serious but, fortunately, rare side effects include agranulocytosis, exfoliative dermatitis, hepatitis, and the "dapsone syndrome," which includes hepatitis and a generalized rash that can progress to exfoliation. Since these more serious toxic effects generally occur soon after the initiation of therapy, patients should be seen periodically, and complete blood counts and liver enzymes should be measured after therapy is begun. If serious toxicity occurs, dapsone should be stopped immediately and the patient treated with steroids and alternative antileprosy therapy.

Rifampin*

Because of its excellent bactericidal activity against *M. leprae*, rifampin is usually included in the therapy of leprosy patients. Patients with lepromatous leprosy who are treated with a drug regimen that includes rifampin become noncontagious after only 2 to 3 weeks of treatment. The usual adult dose is 600 mg daily; children should be treated with 10 to 20 mg per kg, not to exceed 600 mg per day. The cost of daily administration is prohibitive for leprosy control programs in the developing world. Therefore, an alternative regimen recommended by the World Health Organization (WHO) for leprosy control programs includes administration of 600 mg of rifampin at monthly intervals. This regimen of once monthly administration of rifampin (directly observed therapy) has been shown to be equivalent to daily doses of the drug. The major toxic side effect of rifampin is hepatotoxicity, especially if the drug is used in combination with ethionamide. Generally, rifampin should be discontinued if the alanine aminotransferase or aspartate aminotransferase levels increase to more than 2.5 to 3.0 times the upper limit of normal. Other complications of rifampin therapy include thrombocytopenia, skin rashes, headache, and gastrointestinal symptoms (epigastric distress, nausea, vomiting, and diarrhea). The "flulike" syndrome, which has been reported in tuberculosis patients receiving intermittent rifampin, is not common in leprosy patients given intermittent therapy at 1-month intervals. Rifabutin, a drug licensed for therapy of *M. avium* complex infections, also has bactericidal activity against *M. leprae*.

Clofazimine

Clofazimine is a substituted iminophenazine dye with an antimycobacterial activity roughly equivalent to that of dapsone. It is useful in the treatment of leprosy because it also has some anti-inflammatory activity, which helps control leprosy reactions. The usual adult dose is 50 to 100 mg daily. Higher doses of 200 to 300 mg daily have more pronounced anti-inflammatory activity but are more likely to lead to gastrointestinal toxicity with chronic use. Also, clofazimine has been used in doses of 100 mg three times weekly for the chronic treatment of leprosy. The drug is deposited in the skin and slowly released, thus providing a repository effect in chronic therapy.

The most frequent side effect of therapy with clofazimine is a reddish-black pigmentation of the skin. The degree of pigmentation is dose related. However, the pigmentation tends not to be uniform and is concentrated in the areas of the lesions, producing a blotchy pigmentation that many patients consider unsightly. Since virtually all fair-skinned patients will have some pigmentation with clofazimine therapy, it also serves as a useful marker of drug compliance. The pigmentation is slowly cleared 6 to 12 months or more after therapy is discontinued.

Aside from pigmentation, the major side effects of clofazimine therapy involve the gastrointestinal tract. Patients may develop crampy abdominal pain, which is sometimes associated with nausea, vomiting, and diarrhea. On high doses of clofazimine (over 100 mg daily), these symptoms are common after more than 3 to 6 months of therapy. Studies of the small bowel may show a pattern compatible with malabsorption. Fortunately, these symptoms are usually reversible upon discontinuation of the drug.

Other side effects include anticholinergic activity, which may result in diminished sweating and tearing. Since patients with lepromatous leprosy may have autonomic nerve involvement, they commonly have ichthyosis from decreased sweating, and this problem may be intensified by clofazimine.

Ethionamide-Prothionamide

Although ethionamide-prothionamide has been used in multidrug therapy for patients who are intolerant to one of the main drugs, its use has been discontinued due to the frequency of drug toxicity.

Ofloxacin*

A number of fluoroquinolones have been developed; some, such as ciprofloxacin, are not active against *M. leprae*. Among those that are active against *M. leprae*, most attention has focused on ofloxacin. It interferes with bacterial DNA replication by inhibiting the A subunit of the enzyme DNA gyrase. It has been shown in animal and short-term human experiments to have good bactericidal activity, though somewhat less than that of rifampin. It is well absorbed orally and generally given in a dose of 400 mg once daily. A large-scale trial is currently under way to determine whether a combination of rifampin and ofloxacin can reduce the treatment period of multibacillary leprosy to just 1 month. Side effects include nausea, diarrhea, and other gastrointestinal complaints and a variety of central nervous system symptoms, including insomnia, headaches, dizziness, nervousness, and hallucinations. Serious problems are infrequent, however, and usually do not require the drug to be discontinued.

*Not FDA-approved for this indication.

*Not FDA-approved for this indication.

Minocycline*

Minocycline is the only member of the tetracycline group of antibiotics that has significant bactericidal activity against *M. leprae*. The standard dose is 100 mg daily, which gives a peak serum level that exceeds the MIC of minocycline against *M. leprae* by a factor of 10 to 20. Clinical trials are under way to determine optimal usage of the drug. The drug is relatively well tolerated, although vestibular toxicity has been reported in some patients. It has been used chronically for the treatment of severe acne.

Clarithromycin*

Among the macrolide antibiotics, clarithromycin is the only drug shown to have significant bactericidal activity against *M. leprae*. When given in a dose of 500 mg once daily to patients with lepromatous leprosy, 99% of bacilli were killed within 28 days and 99.9% by 56 days. The drug is relatively nontoxic, but gastrointestinal irritation, nausea, vomiting, and diarrhea are the most common side effects.

Treatment Regimens

The standard treatment for leprosy should include multidrug therapy for all forms of the disease. Prior to the early 1980s, patients were often treated with dapsone alone. This led to the emergence of dapsone resistance and rendered further dapsone therapy ineffective in many areas. In 1981, a WHO study group met to develop new treatment regimens for leprosy control programs (WHO Technical Report Series No. 675, 1982). The WHO group reviewed the data on the resistance of *M. leprae* to dapsone and their sensitivity to rifampin and clofazimine and recommended that multidrug therapy be used to treat all active cases of leprosy (Table 1). The group recommended that patients with paucibacillary disease be treated with 100 mg (1 to 2 mg per kg) of dapsone daily, unsupervised, and 600 mg of rifampin once a month as directly observed therapy. Therapy should be continued for 6 months and then stopped. Patients with multibacillary leprosy are to be treated with dapsone 100 mg daily and clofazimine 50 mg daily, both self-administered, and with rifampin 600 mg once monthly and clofazimine 300 mg once monthly, both supervised. This regimen is continued for at least 2 years or until the disease becomes inactive. Patients in whom acid-fast organisms are identified on their slit-skin smears or skin biopsies should be treated with the regimen for multibacillary disease. Also, patients with currently "inactive" leprosy who have had only monotherapy with dapsone should be given multidrug therapy to prevent relapse. The results of these regimens of multidrug therapy were evaluated recently by a WHO study group (WHO Technical Report Series No. 847, 1994) and found to be satisfactory. Relapse rates of 1.0% or less have occurred in the 5 to 9 years after completion of these regimens in patients who were successfully treated.

*Not FDA-approved for this indication.

TABLE 1. **World Health Organization Recommendations for Multidrug Therapy for Leprosy**

Multibacillary Leprosy*	
Drug	*Dose*
Rifampin (Rifadin)	600 mg once a month, supervised
Dapsone	100 mg/day, self-administered
Clofazimine (Lamprene)	300 mg once a month, supervised, and 50 mg/day, self-administered
Paucibacillary Leprosy	
Drug	*Dose*
Rifampin	600 mg once a month, supervised
Dapsone	100 mg/day, self-administered

*Therapy should be continued for 2 years or until leprosy is inactive. Any of the following three drugs can be substituted for one of the above drugs in case of drug intolerance: ofloxacin (Floxin) 400 mg/day, minocycline (Minocin) 100 mg/day, or clarithromycin (Biaxin) 500 mg/day.

Patients should be followed at frequent intervals after treatment is started. Follow-up should include examination for new skin lesions, new areas of anesthesia, new motor deficits, enlargement or tenderness of nerves, and clinical evidence of reactions. In addition, annual skin biopsies are useful in documenting changes in disease status. Also, slit-skin smears are helpful in estimating bacillary load and probable viability of acid-fast organisms remaining in the skin. These are done by pinching the skin to reduce bleeding, cleaning with alcohol, and making a slit about 5 mm long through the epidermis and superficial dermis. The tissue fluid is scraped from the slit skin with a scalpel blade and transferred to a circular area 5 to 6 mm in diameter on a clean glass slide. Slit-skin smears are taken from six or more sites (e.g., earlobe, eyebrow, trunk, elbow, thigh, and knee) at 6- to 12-month intervals and stained using the Fite-Fataco acid-fast stain. The bacteriologic index (BI) is a semiquantitative logarithmic estimate of the number of organisms in the skin (Table 2). The morphologic index (MI) is the percentage of organisms that are solid staining and therefore viable. With effective therapy of lepromatous patients, the MI generally falls to zero within 3 to 4 months, and the average BI should decrease at a rate of about $\frac{1}{2}$ to 1 each year. Failure of the MI or BI to fall suggests poor compliance with therapy or infection with drug-resistant organisms. The National Hansen's Disease Center at Carville, Louisiana, will stain

TABLE 2. **Bacterial Index**

Bacteriologic Index	Number of Organisms
0	No bacilli in 100 OIFs
1+	1–10 bacilli per 100 OIFs
2+	1–10 bacilli per 10 OIFs
3+	1–10 bacilli per OIF
4+	10–100 bacilli per OIF
5+	100–1000 bacilli per OIF
6+	Over 1000 bacilli per OIF

Abbreviation: OIF = oil immersion field.

and examine slides prepared by the slit-skin smear technique. Inactivity of leprosy is defined as a BI of zero on slit-skin smear, no active lesions on skin biopsy, and no clinical evidence of disease activity for at least 1 year. In cases of intolerance to one of the primary drugs (i.e., dapsone, clofazimine, or rifampin) one of the other antileprosy drugs can be substituted (i.e., ofloxacin, minocycline, or clarithromycin). The patient is then given a full course of multidrug therapy.

Treatment of Reactions

Reactions are common during leprosy treatment and complicate the outcome of therapy. Educating patients to recognize reactions and seek prompt treatment is essential for a successful therapeutic outcome. Such reactions, especially those involving neuritis, can cause permanent incapacitation if they are not promptly recognized and properly treated.

Type 1 Reactions

The most important goals in the treatment of Type 1 reactions (reversal reactions) are to prevent nerve damage, control severe inflammation, and prevent necrosis of skin lesions. Antileprosy chemotherapy should not be interrupted during the reaction. In mild reactions, especially those without neuritis or facial lesions, treatment with analgesics and close observation may suffice. However, any reaction in which there is evidence of acute neuritis with pain, tenderness, and loss of nerve function should be treated with steroids, starting with prednisone in doses of 40 to 60 mg per day. The patient may need hospitalization and should be closely observed with frequent voluntary muscle tests (VMT) to evaluate nerve weakness. The dose of prednisone may be reduced by 5 to 10 mg every 1 to 2 weeks until a maintenance dose of 20 to 25 mg is reached. It can then be reduced slowly over the course of 6 months or more while repeating VMT and observing for recurrence of the reaction. Careful management of Type 1 reactions is essential to prevent long-term sequelae.

Type 2 Reactions

Although Type 2 (ENL) reactions are less important from the standpoint of causing nerve damage, they are nonetheless important because of their frequency and the potential for organ damage. Mild ENL reactions can be managed with anti-inflammatory agents, such as salicylates or nonsteroidal anti-inflammatory drugs. However, severe or persistent ENL often requires therapy with corticosteroids, thalidomide,* or clofazimine. Commonly, prednisone 40 to 60 mg is given, and the patient is started on 400 mg per day of thalidomide. Although thalidomide is quite effective in controlling ENL reactions, it cannot be given to women of childbearing age unless they are following a foolproof method of contraception, since the drug is highly teratogenic. Clofazimine in doses of 100 to 300 mg per day has anti-inflammatory effects, but gastrointestinal toxicity is common when the drug is continued at this dose for more than 2 to 3 months.

Iridocyclitis

Iridocyclitis commonly accompanies Type 2 reactions and is a common cause of blindness in leprosy, along with keratitis secondary to the nerve damage that causes lagophthalmos. Acute iridocyclitis should be treated with mydriatics, such as 1% atropine or 0.25% scopolamine, and anti-inflammatory drugs, such as 1% hydrocortisone.

Other Complications

Important complications of leprosy, such as neuritis, iridocyclitis, orchitis, and glomerulonephritis, often occur during reactions. However, these manifestations sometimes occur independent of an obvious reactive episode. Therefore, it is important that leprosy patients be carefully monitored at frequent intervals, especially during the first year or two of therapy.

Patients should be trained to avoid injuries to anesthetic areas and to report injuries promptly, even in the absence of pain. Frequent inspection of the feet and hands and construction of special footwear to prevent permanent damage to anesthetic feet are important aspects of the care of leprosy patients. Reconstructive surgery, such as tibialis posterior muscle transfer to correct footdrop, may be important in treating some patients. Many leprosy patients who have ocular problems should be seen by an ophthalmologist.

CONTROL AND PREVENTION

It is critical that the patient and the patient's family understand the natural history of the disease and what to expect from therapy. Compliance with therapy and patient cooperation in preventing deformities are essential to successful treatment.

The patient's household contacts should be evaluated for signs and symptoms of disease at 6- to 12-month intervals for several years. These examinations should include inspection to detect skin lesions, biopsy of suspicious lesions, palpation for enlarged or tender nerves, and evaluation of motor and sensory nerve function. Infants and children (under age 16 years) who are household contacts of untreated lepromatous patients should receive prophylactic dapsone treatment for 3 years. Adults may be less susceptible to infection; therefore, most authorities do not recommend routine prophylaxis.

---

*Investigational drug in the United States.

MALARIA

method of
CHRISTINA M. COYLE, M.D., and
LOUIS M. WEISS, M.D., M.P.H.
Albert Einstein College of Medicine
Bronx, New York

Malaria infects more than 250 million people worldwide and results in at least 5 million deaths annually. The majority of infections occur in the developing world, where malaria is a leading cause of morbidity and mortality; however, imported malaria is a common problem in nonendemic countries. Malaria is severe in nonimmune individuals, including children, pregnant women, travelers, and immigrants. In the United States, about 1000 cases of malaria per year are reported to the Centers for Disease Control and Prevention (CDC). This is probably a significant underestimate, even though malaria remains a reportable disease. The vast majority of infections seen in North America occur in travelers or immigrants arriving from Africa. Other sources of infection in patients without a travel history include blood transfusion, the use of contaminated needles, and rarely imported infected insects (transmission at international airports). Focal malarial transmission via insect vectors has been reported in California, New York City, Florida, and New Jersey.

ETIOLOGY

Malaria is caused by obligate intracellular protozoans of the genus *Plasmodium*. The four species of protozoans that infect humans are, in order of decreasing worldwide prevalence, *P. falciparum, P. vivax, P. malariae,* and *P. ovale.* Transmission occurs when plasmodial sporozoites are inoculated into humans from the salivary glands of an *Anopheles* mosquito during a blood meal. Within 30 minutes, the sporozoites are cleared from the blood and enter hepatocytes, where they multiply asexually in a process known as "exoerythrocytic schizogony." The sporozoite nucleus undergoes repeated divisions, resulting in the formation of thousands of uninucleate merozoites. Within 7 to 10 days this tissue schizont ruptures and the merozoites enter the circulation, where they infect red blood cells, in which they undergo further division and development (erythrocytic phase). Newly formed merozoites are released from erythrocytes and reinvade and multiply in red blood cells or mature to sexual forms (gametes), which can be transmitted to a feeding female *Anopheles* mosquito to complete the cycle.

In infections with *P. falciparum* and *P. malariae,* the tissue schizonts rupture at about the same time, and none persists in the liver. In contrast, *P. vivax* and *P. ovale* develop latent tissue schizonts in the liver called hypnozoites that are capable of causing relapses of infection up to 5 years later. Such tissue-resident schizonts do not develop if blood exposure is the mechanism of transmission.

CLINICAL MANIFESTATIONS

Depending on the species involved, the incubation period for malaria usually ranges from 9 to 30 days but may be as long as 9 months. It may be prolonged in patients taking chemoprophylaxis and in those who have developed partial immunity from repeated malarial infections. In its early stages, malaria typically manifests as a flulike prodrome that includes headache, malaise, and myalgias, then fever.

In a traveler with these symptoms the differential diagnosis should include typhoid fever, early meningococcal disease, and rickettsial and arboviral infections. Malaria paroxysms usually develop within a few days of the prodromal period and correspond to the release of newly formed merozoites from red blood cells at the completion of a developmental cycle. When the majority of parasites within red blood cells undergo maturation (schizogony) at the same time, episodes of symptoms recur at 48-hour intervals except for *P. malariae* infections, which have a 72-hour erythrocytic cycle. In most patients with *P. falciparum,* development is asynchronous, and consequently fever occurs at varying intervals. During a paroxysm, the temperature rises to 104° to 105° F, and the patient experiences rigors, severe headaches, abdominal pain, and nausea and may vomit. Splenomegaly and hepatomegaly may be present without the presence of peripheral lymphadenopathy. Blood tests are likely to reveal anemia, thrombocytopenia, neutropenia, hyponatremia, and mildly elevated transaminase levels.

In the early stages, falciparum malaria is clinically indistinguishable from infection due to other species. However, life-threatening complications, which are not seen with infection by the other plasmodial species, can develop rapidly. This is probably due in part to the ability of *P. falciparum* to infect erythrocytes of all ages, unlike *P. vivax* and *P. ovale,* which develop in young erythrocytes, and *P. malariae,* which is restricted to a subpopulation of erythrocytes, probably older ones. In addition, high levels of parasitemia occur in association with cytoadherence of infected erythrocytes to postcapillary venules and to uninfected erythrocytes. Cytoadherence of infected erythrocytes protects the parasite from clearance mechanisms operating in the spleen and may lead to cerebral anoxia. The combination of severe anemia and microvascular congestion that results from deep vascular schizogony gives rise to tissue hypoxia and subsequently to organ dysfunction. As a result, symmetrical encephalopathy (termed "cerebral malaria"), acute tubular necrosis, and the adult respiratory distress syndrome (ARDS) can occur and necessitate therapeutic intervention.

TRANSMISSION AND RESISTANCE

Malarial transmission occurs in Africa, parts of Asia, many countries in Latin America, and small foci in Greece, Turkey, and the Middle East. The risk of acquiring malaria varies greatly from one region of a country to another; variables such as altitude, season, and the amount of rural travel done by the potential victim influence the density of the vector mosquito population. Since mosquito vectors only feed from dusk to dawn, evening and nighttime exposure is also a major determinant of risk. In North America, approximately 80% of cases of imported malaria are acquired in Africa.

The development of resistance to antimalarial drugs has complicated malarial therapy and prophylaxis. Chloroquine-resistant strains of *P. falciparum* have spread throughout most malarious areas of the world, leaving only west of the Panama Canal in Central America, Haiti, the Dominican Republic, Egypt, and parts of the Middle East unaffected. Resistance to the combination of pyrimethamine and sulfadoxine (Fansidar) is prevalent in some areas of Southeast Asia, the Amazon Basin of South America, and many foci in sub-Saharan Africa. In areas of Southeast Asia, *P. falciparum* malaria has shown a reduced susceptibility to the standard 3-day course of quinine. Mefloquine and halofantrine resistance is clinically important along the Thai-Kampuchean (Cambodian) and Myanmar (Burmese) borders as well as in parts of Vietnam. The results of in vitro studies from several countries in West Africa and South America, where mefloquine had not yet been used, suggest that some strains of *P. falciparum* may have an inherently decreased sensitivity to mefloquine.

Recently, chloroquine-resistant *P. vivax* malaria has been reported from Brazil, New Guinea, and Indonesia. Although the extent and frequency of this problem is unclear, recent studies suggest that *P. vivax* malaria from these geographic areas should be assumed to be chloroquine-resistant and treated with quinine. Primaquine resistance is well established in Southeast Asia and Oceania, where up to one-third of patients with *P. vivax* malaria suffer relapse after a standard 14-day course of therapy. Resistance to primaquine is uncommon in other *P. vivax* endemic areas of the world.

DIAGNOSIS

For diagnosis, it is imperative to examine several sequential blood smears (finger stick or capillary blood) for the presence of parasitized erythrocytes. The initial smear may be negative since symptoms of malaria in the nonimmune individual may occur a few days before the appearance of parasitized erythrocytes at detectable levels. Therefore, blood smears must be obtained on multiple occasions (such as every 6 hours) over a 72-hour period before a diagnosis of malaria can be excluded. Although a serologic test for malaria exists, it is not useful for diagnosis except in the diagnosis of cases of chronic malaria due to *P. malariae*. Polymerase chain reaction (PCR) techniques are available in specialized research laboratories. The QBC tube method may be useful in the diagnosis of cases with a low parasitemia when there are undetected parasites on the blood smear. This is a relatively easy technique that takes advantage of acridine orange's ability to stain nucleic acid, including that of malarial parasites. A commercially available capillary tube precoated with acridine orange and containing a float with a buoyant density midway between plasma and packed red cells is used to separate and stain parasitized erythrocytes. This technique requires microcentrifugation and an ultraviolet microscope.

Thick blood smears are prepared with Giemsa stain in a manner that optimizes the chances of detecting the presence of parasites, but the smears are unreliable for species identification. Thin blood smears are examined for the latter purpose and are prepared in the same manner as routine hematologic smears. In addition to species identification, the degree of parasitemia should be estimated, because it has prognostic value for severe *P. falciparum* infections. At low levels of parasitemia, it is helpful to estimate the number in thick smears. At higher levels of parasitemia, the percentage of infected erythrocytes can be estimated directly from thin smears by examination of several oil immersion fields. During treatment the examination and quantification of parasitemia in sequential smears is useful for monitoring the effectiveness of antibiotic therapy and for detecting resistance to therapy.

ANTIMALARIAL DRUGS

Chloroquine phosphate (Aralen) and *chloroquine sulfate* (Nivaquine) are 4-aminoquinolines that act on the erythrocytic stage of all species of *Plasmodium*. Chloroquine is still the drug of choice for the treatment of susceptible strains of *P. falciparum* and the other three malarial species; however, chloroquine-resistant *P. vivax* malaria has recently been reported. Chloroquine does not affect liver schizonts and thus does not prevent relapse with *P. vivax* or *P. ovale*. Side effects of chloroquine, which affect approximately 25% of users, include gastrointestinal upset, visual disturbances, headache, and nonallergic pruritus. With intravenous therapy, hypotension and heart block may occur, especially if the drug is administered too rapidly.

Mefloquine (Lariam) is a 4-quinolinemethanol that has blood schizonticidal activity against all four species of human *Plasmodium*, including chloroquine-resistant isolates. In North America, mefloquine is generally recommended only as prophylaxis for drug-resistant *P. falciparum* malaria, as in the higher doses required for treatment it causes unacceptable central nervous system (CNS) effects. It is also effective as a prophylactic against malaria caused by *P. vivax*, *P. ovale*, and *P. malariae*. Subsequent treatment with primaquine is recommended in *P. vivax* or *P. ovale* infections to avoid relapses, since mefloquine (or chloroquine) does not eliminate the exoerythrocytic stage of infection.

Neurologic side effects, mainly seizures and psychosis, occur with the use of mefloquine. It is estimated that serious side effects, which include seizures, occur in 1 per 10,000 to 20,000 travelers who use 250 mg weekly for prophylaxis. Mefloquine is more effective than chloroquine plus proguanil for malarial prophylaxis in short- and long-term visits to chloroquine-resistant regions and has a tolerance similar to that of chloroquine used alone. When higher doses (1250 mg once) of mefloquine are used for the treatment of active malaria, the rate of serious side effects is 0.5 to 1.0% (this rate may be decreased by dividing the dose).

Mefloquine dosage is not standardized for children weighing less than 15 kg. Because of CNS effects it is contraindicated in patients with epilepsy or psychiatric disorders. It should be avoided in patients who are known to have cardiac conduction disturbances as it prolongs the QT_C interval. In theory, quinine or quinidine may exacerbate the cardiodepressant effects of mefloquine. It should be used with caution in patients on beta blockers. Although teratogenic in rats, mefloquine taken during the second and third trimester in humans has not been associated with fetal malformations. It is unknown whether first-trimester exposure is harmful. In general mefloquine should *not* be taken during pregnancy. Because of mefloquine's long half-life, pregnancy should probably be avoided for at least 3 months after taking mefloquine.

Cinchona alkaloids such as quinine sulfate (oral) or quinine dihydrochloride (intravenous) have been used for centuries for the treatment of malaria. Parenteral quinidine gluconate or sulfate is used in the United States, as intravenous quinine is not immediately available. Both quinine and quinidine are active against asexual erythrocytic stages of all four malarial species and are also active against gameto-cytes other than those of *P. falciparum*. Quinine (650 mg three times daily for 3 to 7 days) combined with pyrimethamine-sulfadoxine, tetracycline, or clinda-mycin (Cleocin) is the first-line drug for the oral treatment of chloroquine-resistant malaria; quini-dine is reserved for ill patients requiring parenteral therapy.

Quinine has a bitter taste and is associated with the well-recognized syndrome of cinchonism: head-ache, nausea, abdominal pain, tinnitus, and tran-sient loss of hearing. These symptoms usually begin 48 hours after the initiation of therapy and subside quickly when the drug is stopped. Both quinine and quinidine cause insulin release from the pancreas and have been associated with hypoglycemia when parenteral forms have been used. Potential cardio-vascular effects include QRS widening and arrhyth-mias. Because of potential toxicity, parenteral quini-dine should be administered only with constant electrocardiographic monitoring.

Primaquine (primaquine phosphate 26.3 mg per day for 14 days) is an 8-aminoquinoline active against tissue-resident schizonts and gametocytes and used to prevent relapses of *P. vivax* and *P. ovale* malaria. Because primaquine can cause hemolysis in glucose-6-phosphate dehydrogenase (G6PD) defi-ciency, a G6PD level should be obtained before the drug is administered. Primaquine is contraindicated during pregnancy because the G6PD status of the fetus cannot be ascertained.

Pyrimethamine-sulfadoxine (Fansidar) is used for the treatment of chloroquine-resistant falciparum malaria. It was previously recommended for travel-ers to areas with chloroquine-resistant *P. falciparum*. Pyrimethamine-sulfadoxine is no longer used for pro-phylaxis because of the occurrence of life-threatening allergic reactions to the long-acting sulfa component. Fatalities with prophylactic pyrimethamine-sulfa-doxine have occurred in 1 in 11,000 to 1 in 26,000 users. Most of the severe cutaneous adverse reac-tions, including toxic epidermal necrolysis, erythema multiforme, and the Stevens-Johnson syndrome, have occurred soon after the start of prophylaxis, usually within the first 5 weeks. In addition, drug resistance has emerged in many areas. No fatal reac-tions have yet been reported when pyrimethamine-sulfadoxine (three tablets in a single dose) has been used for the treatment of chloroquine-resistant falci-parum malaria. It is still prescribed as empirical treatment for persons who develop symptoms of ma-laria in areas where they cannot obtain medical eval-uation promptly. Pyrimethamine-sulfadoxine should not be used by patients with a history of sulfa allergy. Patients with G6PD deficiency can develop hemolytic anemia when they use this drug.

Tetracyclines are active against erythrocytic schiz-onts of all four species of malaria including chlo-roquine-resistant isolates. They possess some activity against extraerythrocytic schizonts but are not active enough to be used to prevent relapses. Doxycycline (Vibramycin) (100 mg per day) is useful for prophy-laxis in patients unable to take mefloquine. Side ef-fects of importance include gastrointestinal intoler-ance, photosensitivity reactions (patients should be advised to wear SPF-15 sun screen), and vaginal candidiasis (women can take fluconazole, 150-mg tablet once, for this complication).

Macrolides and *lincomycins* are also used to treat malaria. Clindamycin is used in combination with quinine for the treatment of malaria due to chlo-roquine-resistant *P. falciparum*. *Clostridium difficile* enterocolitis is the main side effect. A single small study has shown that azithromycin can be used suc-cessfully for the prophylaxis of malaria. The macro-lides have been used mainly in pregnant patients.

Halofantrine (Halfan) (8 mg per kg orally at 0, 6, and 12 hours repeated in 7 days), a phenan-threnemethanol derivative of an amine alcohol, is one of the most recently available drugs that are effective against multidrug-resistant *P. falciparum*. A few cases of recrudescence, however, have been reported, especially after a single-dose treatment with halofantrine. The primary cause of these treat-ment failures has generally been ascribed to a vari-able and low absorption of the drug in some patients, rather than to resistance. Side effects include cough, pruritus, hemolytic anemia, and consistent dose-re-lated lengthening of the PR and QT_C intervals. The likelihood of significant QT_C prolongation was greater after halofantrine was used as a retreatment following mefloquine failure than after it was used as primary treatment. Torsades de pointes ventricular arrhythmia developed in two patients with congeni-tal prolonged QT syndrome, and three sudden deaths have been reported in patients taking halofantrine.

*Artemisinin,** derived from the Chinese medicinal plant qinghao (*Artemisia annua*), is a rapidly acting antimalarial that has already established a role in the treatment of multidrug-resistant falciparum ma-laria. It is the only reliable treatment (artesunate 10 mg then 50 mg, or artemether 200 mg intramuscu-larly, 100 mg in 6 hours and then 100 mg every day for 4 days) for some highly drug resistant strains of *P. falciparum* found in the Thai-Kampuchean and Thai-Myanmar borders and should be followed with a course of mefloquine. The compound can be given parenterally, orally, or by suppository and is schiz-onticidal and active against the asexual blood stages of *P. falciparum*. The drug is well tolerated.

Fluoroquinolones such as ciprofloxacin and nor-floxacin (Noroxin) do have antimalarial activity, but clinical trials have demonstrated a high rate of re-lapse. They are not currently used for treatment or prophylaxis.

THERAPY (Table 1)

During the initial evaluation of a patient suspected of having malaria, certain factors must be consid-ered. These include the species of malaria, the para-site density, the geographic area of potential acquisi-

---

*Not available in the United States.

TABLE 1. **Drugs Used to Treat Malaria**

Drugs	Adult Dosage	Pediatric Dosage
All Plasmodium *Species Except Chloroquine-resistant* P. falciparum		
ORAL		
Chloroquine phosphate	600 mg base (1 gm), then 300 mg base (500 mg) 6 h later, then 300 mg (500 mg) 6, 24, and 48 h	10 mg base/kg (max 600 mg base), then 5 mg base/kg 6, 24, and 48 h (maximum 300 mg base)
PARENTERAL		
Quinidine gluconate	10 mg/kg loading dose (max 600 mg) in normal saline slowly over 1 h, followed by continuous infusion of 0.02 mg/kg/min × 3 days maximum	Same as adult dose
Chloroquine-resistant P. falciparum		
ORAL		
Quinine sulfate	650 mg tid × 3 days (7 days if acquired in SE Asia or Oceania)	25 mg/kg/day in 3 doses for 3 days (7 days if acquired in SE Asia or Oceania)
plus		
Tetracycline	250 mg qid × 7 days (doxycycline 100 mg bid × 7 days)	For children ≥7 years of age, 20 mg/kg/day divided into 4 doses daily × 7 days
or		
Clindamycin	900 mg tid or 450 mg qid × 3 days	20–40 mg/kg/day in 3 doses × 3 days
or		
Pyrimethamine-sulfadiazine	Pyrimethamine 25 mg qd and sulfadiazine 1 gm qid × 5 days	>12 use adult dose
or		
Pyrimethamine-sulfadoxine (Fansidar)	Three tablets once on last day of quinine	<1 year old: ¼ tablet 1–3 year old: ½ tablet 4–8 year old: one tablet 9–14 year old: two tablets >14 year old: three tablets once on last day of quinine
PARENTERAL		
Quinidine gluconate	10 mg/kg loading dose (max 600 mg) in normal saline slowly over 1 h, followed by continuous infusion of 0.02 mg/kg/min × 3 days maximum (followed by oral quinine to complete a 7-day course of treatment in disease acquired in SE Asia or Oceania)	Same as adult
plus		
Clindamycin	10 mg/kg first dose followed by 5 mg/kg tid	Same as adult
plus		
Exchange transfusion	In patients with >10% parasitemia	
Prevention of Relapses (P. vivax *and* P. ovale)		
Primaquine phosphate	15 mg base (26.3 mg)/day × 14 days	0.3 mg base/kg/day × 14 days

tion of infection, coexisting medical complications, and the patient's ability to take oral medication. The geographic area of acquisition must be considered when the possibility of drug-resistant *P. falciparum* and *P. vivax* malaria is assessed. Patients with *P. falciparum* malaria, with mixed infections due to organisms that could include *P. falciparum,* or for whom the infecting species cannot immediately be identified should be hospitalized.

Patients with nonfalciparum malaria should receive a course of chloroquine phosphate by mouth. When this treatment is completed, primaquine phosphate should always be administered to patients with *P. vivax* or *P. ovale* infections after screening for G6PD deficiency. Patients who acquired falciparum malaria in regions of Central America west of the Panama Canal, in Haiti, or in the Middle East can be treated with chloroquine unless they are unable to take medications by mouth or have complications

that require parenteral antimalarial therapy. *P. falciparum* from all other regions of the world should be considered resistant to chloroquine. For patients with presumed chloroquine-resistant malaria, quinine is the drug of choice. If the patient is able to tolerate oral medication, quinine sulfate should be given by mouth for 3 or 7 days. This regimen should always be supplemented with sulfadiazine-pyrimethamine, tetracycline, or clindamycin to avoid recrudescence. In areas where there are strains of *P. falciparum* that exhibit reduced sensitivity to quinine (such as Southeast Asia and Oceania), the duration of oral quinine therapy should be 7 days.

Patients with falciparum malaria who are unable to take oral medication because of depressed sensorium, vomiting, or other reasons, in whom more than 5% of erythrocytes are parasitized, or who have organ dysfunction due to infection (renal failure, cerebral malaria, ARDS), should be treated with parenteral antimalarial agents, such as quinidine gluco-nate. Quinidine gluconate (10 mg per kg loading dose, to a maximum dose of 600 mg, followed by 0.02 mg per kg per minute for 3 days) is administered slowly in a large volume of 5% glucose solution (D5W) while monitoring vital signs and the QT_C interval with an electrocardiogram. When stable, the patient can be switched to oral treatment to finish the course of treatment. Chemotherapy should be initiated as soon as possible in patients with severe *P. falciparum* malaria as there is a significant association between delayed chemotherapy and increased mortality.

Adjuncts to antimicrobial therapy are often necessary in cases of complicated falciparum malaria. Hypoglycemia is a relatively common complication, particularly in pregnant women, patients receiving quinidine, patients with severe malaria, and young children. Careful monitoring of the blood glucose concentration in all patients with *P. falciparum* malaria and efforts to correct hypoglycemia by intravenous glucose administration should be initiated promptly. Severe anemia requires transfusion with packed erythrocytes; exchange transfusion may be necessary if the patient is volume-overloaded. In nonimmune patients with falciparum malaria, the mortality rises above 60% with parasitemia above 10%. These patients should probably receive exchange transfusions. Renal failure associated with severe malaria is usually secondary to hydration status and is reversible. Peritoneal dialysis can be lifesaving for patients with acute renal failure. Severe malaria can be complicated by ARDS and is associated with a poor prognosis.

Cerebral malaria is a life-threatening complication of *P. falciparum* infection. Coma or impairment in mental status resulting from malaria should be distinguished from other causes of neurologic symptoms such as hyperpyrexia, hypoglycemia, and concurrent infection. Seizures are common in the early stages, followed by coma or a decreased level of consciousness and are frequently associated with hyperpyrexia. This must be differentiated from febrile seizures in the pediatric patient. Neck rigidity and photophobia do not occur, but patients can develop neck retraction, opisthotonos, gaze disorders, and posturing. Corticosteroids are no longer recommended as adjunctive therapy in cases of cerebral malaria. Steroids have been proved to have no benefit in this setting and may be deleterious, increasing the risk of complications such as infection and gastrointestinal bleeding. Antipyretics, antiemetics, and anticonvulsants can all be used as adjunctive therapy.

Malaria (especially falciparum malaria) in pregnant women may compromise fetal development (low birthweights) or induce premature labor or spontaneous abortion. Chloroquine therapy is considered safe for the fetus. Despite the concern regarding an oxytocic effect, quinine and quinidine have been used successfully and safely in severe malaria during pregnancy. The risks of malaria to mother and child far outweigh any concerns about the use of these drugs. There is a theoretical risk of inducing hyperbilirubinemia and subsequent kernicterus with the use of sulfonamides in late pregnancy, but this has not been observed to be a problem in treatment series. Nonetheless, we routinely use quinine and clindamycin in late pregnancy and avoid the use of sulfonamides. Tetracycline and primaquine are contraindicated in pregnancy. Relapses of *P. vivax* and *P. ovale* disease should be treated with chloroquine; primaquine should be administered after delivery. Congenital transmission has been reported, and babies born to mothers with active malaria should be followed closely.

PREVENTION (Table 2)

The combination of personal protection measures and prophylaxis can be highly effective in preventing malaria, but no chemoprophylactic regimen guarantees protection against malaria. Because the *Anopheles* mosquito bites from dusk to dawn, during this time, people should wear clothing that minimizes the amount of exposed skin and remain in well-screened areas. Those in areas of high exposure should sleep in air-conditioned or screened rooms and use permethrin-impregnated bed nets. Pyrethrum insect

TABLE 2. **Malaria Prophylaxis**

Drugs	Adult Dosage	Pediatric Dosage
Chloroquine-Sensitive Areas		
Chloroquine phosphate	300 mg base (500 mg salt) PO once weekly starting 1 week before departure and for 4 weeks after leaving an endemic area	5 mg base/kg (8.3 mg salt/kg) once/week up to the adult dose of 300 mg base starting 1 week before departure for and for 4 weeks after leaving the endemic area
Chloroquine-Resistant Areas		
Mefloquine (Lariam)	250 mg PO once/week starting 1 week before departure for and for 4 weeks after leaving an endemic area	15–19 kg: ¼ tablet 20–30 kg: ½ tablet 31–45 kg: ¾ tablet >45 kg: 1 tablet weekly as described for adults
Doxycycline (Vibramycin)	100 mg/day starting 1 day before departure for and for 4 weeks after leaving an endemic area	If over 7 years of age: 2 mg/kg/day (max 100 mg/day) as described for adults
For terminal Prophylaxis		
Primaquine phosphate	15 mg base (26.3 mg salt)/day for 14 days	0.3 mg base/kg (0.5 mg salt/kg)/day for 14 days

sprays may also be useful. Insect repellant containing no more than 35% N,N-diethyl-m-toluamide (DEET) should be applied sparingly to the exposed skin when a person is outdoors during times of malarial transmission. Exposure to high concentrations (>35%) of DEET for long periods of time can be neurotoxic, especially to children, in whom DEET-induced seizures have been reported. Recent formulations of DEET that decrease evaporation and have low absorption allow the effective use of low concentrations of DEET and have been safe in children.

Chloroquine phosphate, taken once weekly by mouth, is appropriate for travelers to areas where there is no transmission of P. falciparum or to the few remaining areas where P. falciparum remains predictably sensitive to chloroquine. Travelers to areas where chloroquine-resistant P. falciparum is found should receive mefloquine. The exception to this is travel to certain regions along the Thai-Myanmar and Thai-Kampuchean borders and some parts of Vietnam, where mefloquine-resistant strains are present and doxycycline should be used. Doxycycline can also be used daily by travelers who cannot take mefloquine and are traveling to chloroquine-resistant endemic areas. In Africa, chloroquine phosphate (500 mg per week) plus proguanil (200 mg per day) has also been effective prophylaxis. In these cases a dose of pyrimethamine-sulfadoxine (three tablets) is taken along for self-treatment of malarial symptoms if medical attention cannot be obtained immediately. This regimen is less effective than mefloquine.

Women should be discouraged from traveling to malarious areas while pregnant. Mefloquine and doxycycline are both contraindicated in pregnancy. If travel is necessary chloroquine plus proguanil must be employed, and a standby dose of pyrimethamine-sulfadoxine can be provided.

Prophylactic drugs should be started before departure to optimize blood levels and ensure tolerance. Antimalarials do not prevent the exoerythrocytic life cycle and thus must be continued for 4 weeks after leaving an endemic area. All patients should be tested for G6PD deficiency before departure. After prolonged exposure in endemic regions, all patients who are not G6PD deficient should be given primaquine phosphate [15 mg base (26.3 mg salt) daily] for 14 days on leaving an endemic region to eradicate exoerythrocytic stages. Regardless of the prophylaxis taken, travelers should be advised that malaria can occur after prophylaxis and that malaria can be responsible for unexplained febrile illness within the first year after visiting an endemic region.

Despite considerable efforts in the last 2 decades to develop a malaria vaccine, none is commercially available.

Recent changes in malaria resistance, treatment, and prophylaxis can be obtained from the CDC Malaria Hotline at 1-404-332-4555.

BACTERIAL MENINGITIS*

method of
WILLIAM R. BYRNE, M.D.
U.S. Army Medical Research Institute of
Infectious Diseases
Fort Detrick, Frederick, Maryland

Acute bacterial meningitis is a medical emergency requiring rapid initial evaluation followed immediately by initiation of therapy. In adults, the disease should be considered whenever fever and mental status changes (e.g., lethargy, confusion, delirium, stupor) are encountered, particularly if associated with neck stiffness or headache. In elderly patients, a change in mental status, such as confusion, may be the only clinical indication of meningitis. In children, the diagnosis of bacterial meningitis should be considered in the presence of fever associated with mental status changes, neck stiffness or headache, focal neurologic signs, or seizures. In neonates, clinical manifestations may be limited to poor feeding, listlessness, or irritability.

The incidence of bacterial meningitis is estimated to be approximately 3 per 100,000 population per year in the United States. It is predominantly a disease of children; the highest attack rates occur in infants younger than 1 month old, followed by young children, and then adults over 60 years of age.

Initial evaluation and administration of the first dose of antibiotic therapy should be completed within 30 to 60 minutes of presentation. Diagnostic procedures, such as lumbar puncture and blood cultures, should also be completed within this interval, if at all possible. If focal neurologic signs or evidence of increased intracranial pressure is present, a computed tomographic scan of the head should be done before the lumbar puncture is performed to exclude the possibility of an expanding mass lesion, but this procedure should not delay blood cultures or the first dose of antibiotic.

Cerebrospinal fluid specimens should be processed for Gram's stain and bacterial culture promptly. In the absence of a positive Gram stain, or when prior antibiotic therapy has caused bacterial cultures to be sterile, rapid diagnostic tests for detecting bacterial antigens by latex particle agglutination (available for Haemophilus influenzae type b, Neisseria meningitidis, Streptococcus pneumoniae, group B Streptococcus, and Escherichia coli [K1]) may provide valuable information.

A chest radiograph should also be obtained, along with radiographic evaluation of the paranasal sinuses, to evaluate these sites as potential sources of infection, but these procedures need not be performed immediately.

ANTIBIOTIC THERAPY

Empirical therapy should be selected according to the patient's age (Table 1) or special clinical situation (Table 2). Appropriate antibiotic dosages are of critical importance (Table 3). Shortly after the first dose of antibiotic therapy, the coverage may be altered based on the results of Gram's stain of the cerebrospinal fluid, which will reveal a pathogen in 50 to 75% of patients with bacterial meningitis. Further adjustments in antimicrobial coverage may be indicated

*The view, opinions, and/or findings contained in this manuscript are those of the author and should not be construed as an official Department of the Army position, policy, or decision unless so designated by other documentation.

TABLE 1. **Presumptive Initial Therapy for Bacterial Meningitis by Age Group**

Age Group	Likely Pathogens	Recommended Therapy
Less than 1 month	Group B *Streptococcus* *Escherichia coli* (K1)* *Listeria monocytogenes* *Klebsiella-Enterobacter* spp.	Ampicillin plus cefotaxime (Claforan)
1–3 months	*H. influenzae*† *N. meningitidis* *S. pneumoniae* Group B *Streptococcus*	Ampicillin plus cefotaxime
3 months–9 years	*H. influenzae*† *S. pneumoniae* *N. meningitidis*	Cefotaxime *or* ceftriaxone (Rocephin)
9–59 years	*N. meningitidis* *S. pneumoniae* *H. influenzae*† ‡	Ceftriaxone *or* cefotaxime
60+ years	*S. pneumoniae* Gram-negative enteric bacilli§ *N. meningitidis* *L. monocytogenes* *H. influenzae*† ‡ Group B *Streptococcus* *S. aureus*‖	Ampicillin *plus* cefotaxime or ceftriaxone

*Approximately 75% of strains possess the K1 capsular antigen.
†Approximately 20–30% of *H. influenzae* isolated from the cerebrospinal fluid from patients in the United States produce beta-lactamase, indicating resistance to ampicillin.
‡*H. influenzae* meningitis in adults is seen in the setting of head trauma (either recent or remote), cerebrospinal fluid rhinorrhea, paranasal sinusitis, otitis media, pneumonia (particularly when associated with asthma or chronic obstructive pulmonary disease), or diabetes mellitus.
§Meningitis secondary to infection with gram-negative enteric bacilli is also seen in association with gram-negative bacillary septicemia from infection at a remote site, ruptured brain abscess, and disseminated strongyloidiasis.
‖When *S. aureus* is suspected, this organism should be treated with nafcillin (Unipen), vancomycin, or other specific therapy (see Table 4). Meningitis secondary to infection with *S. aureus* is also seen in association with paraspinal infection, staphylococcal septicemia from infection at distant sites (e.g., infective endocarditis, infected vascular graft, soft tissue abscess, cellulitis, osteomyelitis), diabetes mellitus, chronic renal failure, alcoholism, and injection drug use.

when the results of cerebrospinal fluid culture and antimicrobial susceptibility testing are available (Table 4). In general, treatment should be continued until the patient has been afebrile for at least 5 days.

In neonates and infants 1 to 3 months old, a combination of ampicillin and cefotaxime (Claforan) provides broad coverage against the most likely pathogens (see Table 1). For children older than 3 months, cefotaxime or ceftriaxone (Rocephin) is recommended; ampicillin plus chloramphenicol is also acceptable. Ampicillin may be substituted for chloramphenicol, ceftriaxone, or cefotaxime for treating beta-lactamase–negative *H. influenzae*.

Ceftriaxone or cefotaxime should be used as initial presumptive therapy in adults less than 60 years old, except in the special situations listed in Table 2.

TABLE 2. **Presumptive Therapy for Bacterial Meningitis in Special Clinical Situations**

Situation	Likely Pathogens	Recommended Presumptive Therapy
Meningitis associated with cerebrospinal fluid shunt, neurosurgery, penetrating head trauma, cerebrospinal fluid rhinorrhea, skull fracture	Gram-negative enteric bacilli Coagulase-negative staphylococci *S. aureus* *Propionibacterium acnes* *Streptococcus pneumoniae*	Vancomycin *plus* ceftazidime,* ceftriaxone, or cefotaxime
Immunocompromised patient	*Listeria monocytogenes* Gram-negative enteric bacilli *S. aureus*†	Ampicillin *plus* ceftriaxone (Rocephin), cefotaxime (Claforan), or ceftazidime (Fortaz)*
Recurrent meningitis Community-acquired	*S. pneumoniae* *H. influenzae* *N. meningitidis*	Ceftriaxone or cefotaxime
Nosocomial	Enteric gram-negative bacilli *S. aureus*† Coagulase-negative staphylococci	Vancomycin *plus* ceftazidime,* cefotaxime, or ceftriaxone

*Ceftazidime should be used if *P. aeruginosa* is suspected.
†When *S. aureus* is suspected, this organism should be treated with nafcillin, vancomycin, or other specific therapy (see Table 4). Meningitis secondary to infection with *S. aureus* is also seen in association with paraspinal infection, staphylococcal septicemia from infection at distant sites (e.g., infective endocarditis, infected vascular graft, soft tissue abscess, cellulitis, osteomyelitis), diabetes mellitus, chronic renal failure, alcoholism, and injection drug use.

TABLE 3. **Antibiotic Dosages for Bacterial Meningitis**

Antibiotic (All Intravenous)	Daily Adult Dose		Daily Child's Dose*†	
	Total	Interval	Total	Interval
Ampicillin	12/gm/day	4 h	200–300 mg/kg/day‡	4–6 h
Nafcillin (Unipen)	12/gm/day§	4 h	150–200 mg/kg/day	4–6 h
Oxacillin (Prostaphlin)	12 gm/day	4 h	150–200 mg/kg/day	4–6 h
Penicillin G	20–24 million U/day	2–4 h	200,000 to 300,000, U/kg/day	4–6 h
Cefotaxime (Claforan)	12/gm/day	4 h	150–200 mg/kg/day	4–6 h
Ceftriaxone (Rocephin)	4/gm/day	12 h	80–100 mg/kg/day‖	12 h
Ceftazidime (Fortaz)	6 gm/day	8 h	125–150 mg/kg/day	8 h
Chloramphenicol	4 gm/day** ††	6 h	75–100 mg/kg/day	6 h
Vancomycin	2 gm/day	6–12 h	40–60 mg/kg/day	6 h
Amikacin (Amikin)¶	15 mg/kg/day** ††	8–12 h**	20–30 mg/kg/day** ††	8–12 h**
Gentamicin¶	5 mg/kg/day** ‡‡	8 h	7.5 mg/kg/day** ‡‡	8 h††
Tobramycin (Nebcin)¶	5 mg/kg/day** ‡‡	8 h**	5–6 mg/kg/day** ‡‡	8 h**
Trimethoprim-sulfamethoxazole (TMP–SMX) (Bactrim, Septra)	10 mg/kg/day TMP	6 h	15–20 mg/kg/day TMP	6 h

*Doses listed are for patients aged more than 30 days. Different doses are required for infants during the first week after birth and the remainder of the first 30 days of life than for older children. Antibiotic therapy for newborn infants needs appropriate consultation.

†Doses in children should not exceed the adult dose.

‡After an initial dose of 100 mg/kg.

§After 5–7 days of nafcillin therapy, the dose should be reduced to 9 gm/day to avoid the development of neutropenia.

‖After an initial dose of 75 mg/kg.

¶Peak and trough serum drug levels should be measured at least twice weekly, along with tests of renal function.

**Adjustments to total daily dose and interval in the presence of abnormal renal function should be made with reference to standard nomograms and manufacturer's recommendations.

††After a loading dose of 7.5 mg/kg.

‡‡After a loading dose of 2 mg/kg.

Initial presumptive therapy in the elderly should consist of ampicillin plus either cefotaxime or ceftriaxone, as patients in this age group have an increased incidence of meningitis secondary to *Listeria monocytogenes*, enteric gram-negative bacilli, and group B *Streptococcus*. The incidence of meningitis secondary to *Staphylococcus aureus* and *Pseudomonas aeruginosa* is also increased in elderly people but usually in association with head trauma or neurosurgical procedures. Therapy specific for these pathogens should be initiated if they are suspected.

Follow-Up Procedures

In routine cases of bacterial meningitis in which the patient responds to therapy, a follow-up lumbar puncture is not required after the diagnosis has been established by a positive cerebrospinal fluid culture. Repeat lumbar puncture is indicated when a patient with meningitis is not responding clinically to antibiotic therapy or when the patient has a bacterial pathogen known to be difficult to treat (e.g., enteric gram-negative bacilli, *Staphylococcus aureus, L. monocytogenes*). Audiometric testing should be considered after completion of treatment, to assess whether hearing has been affected. Meningococcal disease should prompt consideration of complement deficiency.

ADJUNCTIVE THERAPY

The routine use of dexamethasone is recommended for the treatment of bacterial meningitis in children 2 months of age and older to decrease neurologic complications, such as hearing loss. Dexamethasone should be started as soon as possible after the diagnosis of bacterial meningitis is made. The dose of dexamethasone for children is 0.15 mg per kg every 6 hours for 4 days. In adults, the use of dexamethasone therapy in bacterial meningitis should be seriously considered in the presence of focal neurologic findings or a depressed level of consciousness, or if there is evidence of increased intracranial pressure. Dexamethasone may also provide benefit when treating pneumococcal meningitis, or when large numbers of bacteria are present in the cerebrospinal fluid (manifested by a positive Gram stain).

Intravenous fluids should be administered with care to prevent fluid overload during the first 24 to 48 hours of therapy to avoid the complication of hyponatremia resulting from the syndrome of inappropriate antidiuretic hormone secretion (SIADH). Seizures occur in up to 33% of children and usually respond to therapy with diazepam, phenytoin, or phenobarbital. In children, treatment for nonfocal seizures can be safely discontinued after the second hospital day in the absence of recurrence or status epilepticus.

The presence of persistent or recurrent fever, vomiting, seizures, focal neurologic findings, or signs of meningeal irritation should prompt consideration of subdural empyema or complicated subdural effusion, particularly in children. This diagnosis is established by computed tomographic scan or magnetic resonance imaging of the head in conjunction with subdural paracentesis. Daily measurement of head cir-

TABLE 4. **Specific Antibiotic Coverage Based on Results of Cerebrospinal Fluid Culture**

Bacteria (Appearance on Gram's Stain)	Antibiotics		Duration of Therapy
	First Choices	*Alternates*	
Gram-negative enteric bacilli* (gram-negative rods)			At least 21 days: 10–14 days after CSF culture has become negative
Escherichia coli, Klebsiella-Enterobacter-Serratia	Cefotaxime†, ceftriaxone†	Trimethoprim-sulfamethoxazole	Same
Pseudomonas aeruginosa	Ceftazidime plus IV aminoglycoside‡		Same
Group B *Streptococcus* (gram-positive cocci in chains)	Ampicillin or penicillin G plus gentamicin	Vancomycin, ceftriaxone, cefotaxime	14–21 days
Haemophilus influenzae (short gram-positive rods or coccobacilli, which may demonstrate bipolar staining resembling over-decolorized pneumococci)			7–10 days
Beta-lactamase–negative	Ampicillin	Chloramphenicol, cefotaxime, ceftriaxone	Same
Beta-lactamase–positive	Cefotaxime, ceftriaxone	Chloramphenicol	Same
Listeria monocytogenes (gram-positive rods resembling diphtheroids; may appear coccoid or in pairs resembling pneumococci)	Ampicillin or penicillin G plus gentamicin	Trimethoprim-sulfamethoxazole	Usually 14–21 days (4–6 weeks may be required if clinical response is slow)
Neisseria meningitidis (gram-negative diplococci, biscuit- or kidney bean-shaped, with flattened adjacent sides)	Penicillin G, ampicillin	Ceftriaxone, cefotaxime, chloramphenicol	7–10 days
Propionibacterium acnes (plemorphic gram-positive bacilli; "diphtheroids")	Penicillin G	Vancomycin, chloramphenicol	14–21 days (4–6 weeks if osteomyelitis is present)
Staphylococcus aureus§ and coagulase-negative Staphylococci‖ (gram-positive cocci as singles, pairs, clusters, and short chains of up to five cocci)			21 days
Beta-lactamase–negative	Penicillin G	Vancomycin	Same
Beta-lactamase–positive			
Methicillin-sensitive	Nafcillin, oxacillin	Vancomycin	Same
Methicillin-resistant	Vancomycin	Trimethoprim-sulfamethoxazole	Same
Streptococcus pneumoniae (gram-positive cocci in singles and pairs; cocci are spherical, oval, or lancet-shaped)			
Penicillin-sensitive	Penicillin G¶	Ceftriaxone, cefotaxime, chloramphenicol	10–14 days
Penicillin-resistant** ††			
Moderate (MIC 0.1–1.0 μg/mL)	Cefotaxime††, ceftriaxone††	Vancomycin	10–14 days
High level (MIC > 1.0 μg/mL)	Vancomycin		

*Chloramphenicol should not be considered an acceptable antibiotic for treatment of gram-negative bacillary meningitis, in spite of apparent in vitro activity, because it is bacteriostatic for most of these organisms at concentrations achievable in the cerebrospinal fluid.

†Plus intravenous and intraventricular aminoglycoside for difficult cases.

‡Plus intraventricular aminoglycoside in difficult cases until cerebrospinal fluid cultures are negative. This usually occurs within 5–7 days.

§The addition of rifampin, 600 mg twice daily, may improve outcome in difficult cases.

‖About 60–90% of coagulase-negative staphylococci are methicillin-resistant, and initial presumptive therapy when this organism is suspected should be with vancomycin.

¶Ampicillin is also effective.

**Reports of penicillin-resistant pneumococci are unusual in the United States as of this writing.

††Because of the possibility of resistance to multiple antibiotics, susceptibility of the patient's organisms to chloramphenicol and cephalosporins should be checked.

TABLE 5. **Chemoprophylaxis for Bacterial Meningitis**[*][†]

Bacterial Species	Indications for Prophylaxis	Dose	
		Adult	*Child*[‡]
Haemophilus influenzae type b[§]	All household and day care center contacts, when at least one of the contacts is 4 years old or less. Index patient should also receive prophylaxis, since antibiotic therapy for meningitis may not eradicate the carrier state	Rifampin (Rifadin), 600 mg/day as a single daily dose for 4 days	20 mg/kg/day as a single daily dose for 4 days[‖]
Neisseria meningitidis[¶]	Close daily personal contacts of index patient (household, day care, nursery school, roommates, girlfriend, or boyfriend), particularly infants. Health care workers who have had intimate contact with an infected person should receive prophylaxis[**]	Rifampin, 600 mg q 12 h for four doses Ceftriaxone (Rocephin) intramuscularly, 250 mg once Ciprofloxacin (Cipro) orally, 500–750 mg once	10 mg/kg 12 h for four doses[††] 125 mg once

[*]Pregnant women should not receive rifampin.
[†]Patients taking rifampin should be advised that this antibiotic is likely to cause a reddish-orange discoloration of urine, sweat, and tears.
[‡]Dose for children should not exceed the adult dose.
[§]Contacts should be treated within 1 week of exposure, if possible, but there may be some benefit to prophylaxis administered as late as 2–4 weeks after exposure to the index case.
[‖]Dose should not exceed a maximum of 600 mg. The dose for neonates (less than 1 month old) is 10 mg/kg/day.
[¶]Prophylaxis should be initiated as soon as possible after the index case is identified, preferably within 24 h.
[**]Intimate contact refers to such circumstances as mucosal contact with respiratory secretions, intubation, or mouth-to-mouth resuscitation. Prophylaxis in the absence of intimate contact is not routinely indicated for medical personnel, classmates, or fellow office workers.
[††]Infants 3–12 months old should receive 5 mg/kg every 12 h for four doses.

cumference should be performed in probable cases in children.

Chemoprophylaxis

Rifampin (Rifadin)[*] is the recommended drug for chemoprophylaxis of contacts of patients with *H. influenzae* meningitis (Table 5). Rifampin is also recommended for chemoprophylaxis of contacts of patients with meningococcal meningitis, although ceftriaxone and ciprofloxacin (Cipro) are also effective (Table 5). Rifampin prophylaxis should be administered to index cases.

Immunoprophylaxis

One of the *H. influenzae* type b conjugate vaccines is recommended for all infants and children. Pneumococcal vaccine is recommended for persons with chronic cardiac or pulmonary disease, illnesses that predispose to pneumococcal infection (sickle cell disease, nephrotic syndrome, Hodgkin's disease, asplenia, multiple myeloma, cirrhosis of the liver, alcoholism, renal failure, cerebrospinal fluid leaks), and conditions associated with compromised immune systems. The use of pneumococcal vaccine (Pneumovax 23) in all persons older than 65 years has been recommended but remains controversial. Meningococcal vaccine is available for serogroups A, C, Y, and W-135 (Menomune-A/C/Y/W-135). Its use is recommended in epidemics of serogroups A and C disease, in military

recruits, and in travelers to areas where disease is endemic or epidemic.

Isolation

All patients with suspected bacterial meningitis, particularly community-acquired cases, should be placed initially in respiratory isolation. After a diagnosis has been established, continued isolation is necessary only for meningococcal meningitis, for the first 24 hours after initiation of effective therapy. Rifampin chemoprophylaxis, when indicated, should be administered early to cases of *H. influenzae* or meningococcal meningitis.

Recurrent Meningitis

Recurrent attacks of bacterial meningitis usually result from a congenital defect or traumatic event that causes a communication between the subarachnoid space and the paranasal sinuses, nasopharynx, middle ear, or skin. The occurrence of recurrent bacterial meningitis should prompt a search for such a defect. Noninfectious causes of recurrent meningitis include Mollaret's meningitis, sarcoidosis, systemic lupus erythematosus, Behçet's disease, and Vogt-Koyanagi-Harada syndrome. The most common offending pathogen of community-acquired recurrent meningitis is *S. pneumoniae*, and the clinical course is usually more benign than that of meningitis resulting from other causes. Nosocomial recurrent meningitis is most commonly secondary to gram-negative bacilli, followed by *S. aureus*.

[*]This use of rifampin is not listed in the manufacturer's official directive.

INFECTIOUS MONONUCLEOSIS

method of
BEVERLY E. SHA, M.D.
Rush–Presbyterian–St. Luke's Medical Center
Chicago, Illinois

Infectious mononucleosis is a well-characterized clinical syndrome resulting from symptomatic infection with Epstein-Barr virus (EBV). The syndrome is characterized by a triad of sore throat, fever, and lymphadenopathy. Additional symptoms may include headache, malaise, anorexia, myalgias, and arthralgias. Pharyngitis, hepatosplenomegaly, and rash may be apparent on physical examination. Infectious mononucleosis typically occurs in late adolescence or early adulthood as EBV generally causes subclinical infection in early childhood. Although infection with other microorganisms including cytomegalovirus, *Toxoplasma gondii*, human immunodeficiency virus (HIV), and hepatitis A, B, and C viruses can cause similar symptoms, infectious mononucleosis has historically been used to describe the syndrome associated with acute EBV infection.

EBV is a member of the herpesvirus family. Infection is transmitted through intimate contact between susceptible persons and symptomatic or asymptomatic shedders of EBV. The average incubation period is 4 to 6 weeks. Fever generally resolves after 1 to 2 weeks. Around 10% of patients experience profound persistent fatigue for weeks to months. Further study has refuted initial reports that suggested that EBV was a cause of the chronic fatigue syndrome. Rash is present in 5% of patients and a maculopapular rash is inducible in almost all patients with the administration of ampicillin.

Laboratory findings include atypical lymphocytosis, hepatitis, and a positive heterophil test. Hematologic complications include thrombocytopenia, anemia, and neutropenia, and although these complications are generally mild, in rare circumstances they can be life-threatening. Splenomegaly predisposes to splenic rupture in less than 0.5% of patients. Encephalitis, meningitis, Guillain-Barré syndrome, transverse myelitis, and Bell's palsy are rare neurologic complications occurring in less than 1% of cases overall. Rarer complications include pleuritis, pulmonary infiltrates, pericarditis, or liver failure. Individuals with X-linked Duncan's immunodeficiency may develop overwhelming infection and death with acute EBV infection.

TREATMENT

Although there is no effective antiviral treatment for infectious mononucleosis, spontaneous recovery in 2 to 3 weeks is the rule. Supportive care with acetaminophen 650 to 1000 mg every 4 to 6 hours (maximum, 4 grams per 24 hours) for relief of fever, sore throat, and myalgias and arthralgias can be recommended. Bed rest is helpful for patients with fatigue. Because of the potential complication of splenic rupture, patients with splenomegaly should refrain from contact sports or heavy lifting for 2 to 4 weeks or until the spleen is no longer palpable.

Corticosteroids are not recommended for routine use in EBV infection and should be reserved for the treatment of tonsillar lymphadenopathy resulting in impending airway obstruction. Individuals with life-threatening airway obstruction should receive intravenous methylprednisolone (Solu-Medrol), 60 mg every 6 hours followed by rapid taper over 1 to 2 weeks. Tracheal intubation or tracheostomy may be indicated to protect the airway. Some investigators also recommend the use of corticosteroids for the treatment of severe autoimmune hemolytic anemia or thrombocytopenia; initial prednisone doses of 60 to 80 mg per day in divided doses tapered over 1 to 2 weeks is recommended. For patients who suffer severe or prolonged prostration, anecdotal reports have suggested that a short course of prednisone 80 mg per day in divided doses for 2 to 3 days and tapered over 1 week may be helpful. Support for the use of corticosteroids in treating neurologic complications, hepatitis, pericarditis, or myocarditis due to EBV is minimal, and this practice cannot be routinely recommended until more data are available.

For individuals who suffer the rare complication of traumatic or spontaneous splenic rupture, splenectomy is generally recommended. Plasmapheresis should be initiated for those with Guillain-Barré syndrome. There are no data to indicate that high doses of acyclovir, vidarabine (adenine arabinoside), or interferon-alfa are effective against EBV infection.

PREVENTION

Like other herpesviruses, EBV is associated with latency in infected individuals. The virus has been cultured from oropharyngeal washings for 12 to 18 months after acute EBV infection. Oral secretions should be considered infectious in acutely ill individuals. Virus has also been identified in exfoliated cervical cells, suggesting that EBV may also be sexually transmitted. Rarely EBV has been transmitted through blood transfusion or transplantation. Patients recovering from infectious mononucleosis should avoid blood donation for 6 months. Unfortunately, both previously infected immune-suppressed and healthy individuals may continue to shed EBV in oral secretions intermittently over years and join the pool of asymptomatic shedders capable of infecting susceptible persons.

MUMPS

method of
DENNIS L. MURRAY, M.D.
Michigan State University
East Lansing, Michigan

Mumps is a communicable, systemic illness caused by a paramyxovirus affecting primarily children and young adults. Manifestations of this viral illness were described by Hippocrates in the fifth century B.C., and the etiologic agent was first identified in 1934. A live attenuated mumps virus vaccine was licensed in the United States in 1967.

Humans are the only known natural hosts of mumps virus, and although asymptomatic infected persons may transmit the virus, no carrier state is known to exist. The virus is spread through airborne transmission or direct contact with respiratory secretions. Illness predominates in the winter and spring, but cases may occur at any time of the year. The communicability of the virus is less than that of measles or varicella-zoster virus; however, 20% or more cases of mumps may be asymptomatic. Before vaccine licensure, over 200,000 estimated cases of mumps occurred in the United States annually. After recommendation for the routine use of mumps vaccine in 1977, the annual reported incidence of mumps declined rapidly, with approximately 3000 cases reported each year from 1983 to 1985. A resurgence in disease incidence, accompanied by a change in the age of disease occurrence, began in 1986 and lasted through 1989. In 1987, approximately 13,000 cases of mumps were reported in the United States. Both before and for several years after vaccine licensure, the majority of reported mumps cases occurred in children 5 to 9 years of age. In the late 1980s, however, a dramatic increase in reported cases occurred in children 10 to 19 years of age, predominantly those not vaccinated in infancy. The number of reported mumps cases declined substantially during the early 1990s. In 1993, a total of 1692 mumps cases were reported, the lowest number ever reported in the United States.

Clinically, after an incubation period of 16 to 18 days (range 12 to 25 days), the disease typically begins with nonspecific symptoms that include myalgia, anorexia, malaise, headache, and low-grade fever. Prodromal symptoms last from 1 to several days, but may not occur in all patients. Parotitis, the most common manifestation of mumps, occurs in 30 to 40% of cases and is usually accompanied by fever. Parotid involvement may be unilateral or bilateral and occurs with or without involvement of the other salivary glands. Parotid swelling associated with pain on chewing or swallowing acidic foods or liquids may be the first and only sign of infection. Patients complain of tenderness on palpation of the angle of the jaw, and the earlobe may be pushed outward. Symptoms intensify over 1 to 3 days and take 7 to 10 days to clear.

Involvement of the central nervous system in the form of asymptomatic aseptic meningitis is common. Where studied, 50% or more of patients with clinical manifestations of mumps have inflammatory cells identified on evaluation of the cerebrospinal fluid. Meningeal signs occur in over 10% of patients, more commonly adults, and resolve without sequelae. Encephalitis is a rare complication of mumps illness, occurring in approximately 1 in 6000 cases, with a fatality rate of 1.4%.

Orchitis is the most common symptomatic nonsalivary manifestation of mumps. Orchitis occurs in 20 to 50% of postpubertal males with mumps but only rarely in prepubertal males. Testicular involvement can occur at any time in the course of mumps disease, is usually unilateral, and has been reported in the absence of parotitis. Testicular atrophy may occur after mumps involvement, but sterility is rare.

Mumps is one of the leading causes of sensorineural deafness. Hearing loss is unilateral in approximately 80% of cases and may be associated with vestibular reactions. The frequency of this complication is difficult to ascertain, but it is probably more common in adults.

Other complications of mumps include oophoritis (approximately 5% of mumps cases in postpubertal females), pancreatitis, arthritis, myocarditis, mastitis, thyroiditis, and renal dysfunction. Viruria is common in mumps infection; patients may develop nephritis, which has rarely been fatal.

Primary infection with mumps virus in the first trimester of pregnancy has been associated with an increase in fetal deaths. Based on findings of Siegal (1973),* fetal mortality, however, is not increased when maternal infection occurs in the last two trimesters. There is no evidence that mumps infection produces congenital malformations.

When confronted with a patient with unilateral or bilateral parotid swelling, the differential diagnosis, in addition to mumps, should include drug effects, metabolic diseases, systemic lupus erythematosus, parotid duct obstruction (stone, tumor, etc.), bacterial infection, and other viruses (cytomegalovirus, enterovirus, influenza A, and parainfluenza types 1 and 3). On rare occasions, enlargement of lymph nodes in proximity to the parotid gland or bony lesions of the mandible have been confused with parotid swelling.

Mumps virus can be isolated from cerebrospinal fluid, saliva, throat washings, and urine. Virus has also been recovered from biopsy specimens. For best results, culture specimens should be obtained on or before the fifth day of illness. Infection can also be confirmed serologically.

Enzyme immunoassay (EIA) is more reliable than complement fixation (CF) or hemagglutination inhibition (HI) tests. EIA testing is available to detect both IgM and IgG antibodies to mumps. Only EIA or neutralization testing should be used to assess immunity to mumps. Mumps skin tests are unreliable, difficult to interpret from an immunologic perspective, and should not be used to determine immune status.

THERAPY

There is no specific therapy for mumps. Supportive measures such as adequate hydration and alimentation as well as analgesia for parotitis, orchitis, and headache are helpful. Parenteral fluids may be required in patients with persistent vomiting from meningoencephalitis or pancreatitis.

Unless a secondary bacterial infection occurs, antibiotics are unnecessary. No antiviral therapy is indicated. There is no role for gamma-globulin administration.

ISOLATION AND OUTBREAK CONTROL

Respiratory isolation is employed for hospitalized patients with mumps. Patients should be isolated for 9 days after the onset of parotid swelling. In closed populations such as schools, the exclusion of susceptible pupils should be considered. Pupils exempted from mumps vaccination because of medical, religious, or other reasons should be excluded until at least 26 days after the onset of parotitis in the last person with mumps in the affected school. Excluded students can be readmitted immediately after vaccination.

PREVENTION

The principal strategy for the prevention of mumps is vaccination. An inactivated viral vaccine was developed in 1948, but it produced only short-term immunity and was discontinued in 1976. A live-virus vaccine, attenuated in chick embryo culture, was licensed in 1967 and continues to be used routinely in the immunization of children. This vaccine, which

---

*Siegel M: Congenital malformations following chickenpox, measles, mumps, and hepatitis: Results of a cohort study. JAMA 226:1521–1524, 1973.

does contain neomycin, elicits antibody in over 90% of vaccinees and produces presumably lifelong immunity. The clinical efficacy in preventing infection is estimated to be 95% (range 90 to 97%).

The current recommendation is for mumps vaccine to be administered in combination with measles and rubella vaccines (MMR) to all infants without contraindications at 12 to 15 months of age. A second dose of mumps vaccine, administered as MMR, is advised; the timing of the second dose is determined by the measles vaccine schedule employed (usually at either 4 to 6 or 11 to 12 years of age). Revaccination is important, because like measles, mumps can occur in highly vaccinated populations. Data from a 12-year study in Finland using a two-dose schedule of MMR vaccine have demonstrated the elimination of indigenous measles, mumps, and rubella cases in that country.

Mumps vaccine is not routinely advised for persons born before 1957 unless they are proved to be susceptible. All those born in or after 1957 should be considered susceptible unless they have documentation of (1) physician-diagnosed mumps, (2) adequate immunization with live-virus vaccine on or after 12 months of age, or (3) serologic evidence of immunity. Susceptibility testing before vaccination is not necessary since vaccination of immune (by disease or vaccination) persons is safe.

Mumps vaccine has not been demonstrated to be effective in preventing infection in exposed susceptibles. However, vaccine may be given after an exposure because immunization provides protection against any subsequent exposures. There is no increased risk of reactions after vaccination in persons found to be incubating mumps virus.

Adverse reactions to mumps vaccine are uncommon. Parotitis and fever have been reported rarely. Orchitis has been reported very rarely, and the relationship to vaccine in these few cases is questionable. Cases of nerve deafness and encephalitis, within 2 months of vaccination, have been reported. The Institute of Medicine concluded in 1993 that evidence is inadequate to accept or reject a causal relationship between the current mumps vaccine and aseptic meningitis, encephalitis, sensorineural deafness, or orchitis.

Live attenuated mumps vaccine is contraindicated in persons known to be pregnant; in those who have experienced an anaphylactic reaction to neomycin; in patients with altered immunity related to primary or secondary immunodeficiency except human immunodeficiency virus (HIV) or immunosuppressive therapy, or those receiving large systemic doses of corticosteroids or radiation; and in persons with a moderate to severe acute illness until that illness has resolved. Patients with asymptomatic or symptomatic HIV infection are advised to be vaccinated against measles using MMR vaccine. Mumps vaccine may be given to individuals with history of anaphylaxis to egg only with extreme caution using established protocols. Unlike live attenuated polio vaccine, mumps vaccine can be given to contacts of persons with altered immunity (discussed earlier) because vaccinated persons do not transmit mumps vaccine virus.

Immune response to mumps vaccine may be inhibited by receipt of blood products containing antibody (immune serum globulin, whole blood, packed red blood cells, or intravenous gamma globulin). Mumps vaccine should be given 2 weeks before or from 3 to 11 months after receiving any of the aforementioned products. High doses of intravenous gamma globulin, such as treatment for Kawasaki disease, may, in particular, necessitate deferral of vaccination for a very prolonged period (11 months).

Unless contraindicated, all persons thought to be susceptible to mumps should be vaccinated. Vaccination of adolescents and young adults, given a shift in risk of disease to these groups, should be considered a priority along with the routine immunization of infants and children.

OTITIS EXTERNA

method of
SARA V. SOTIROPOULOS, M.D.
University of Missouri School of Medicine
Columbia, Missouri

and

MARK W. KLINE, M.D.
Baylor College of Medicine
Houston, Texas

Inflammation of the external auditory canal is a common problem, particularly during warm months. Factors that may render the thin layer of skin in the external canal susceptible to infection or inflammation include excessive moisture (swimming, bathing, or increased humidity), excessive dryness (insufficient cerumen, or dermatoses), and trauma (use of cotton swabs; foreign body; or iatrogenic abrasions). Although in 30% of individuals the external canal is sterile, the normal flora of the external auditory canal includes *Staphylococcus epidermidis, Corynebacterium* spp, *Staphylococcus aureus, Micrococcus* spp, and viridans streptococci. Fungi, including *Aspergillus niger* and *Candida albicans,* are found in up to one-third of normal individuals. Any of these indigenous organisms, as well as others, may become pathogens when normal host protective mechanisms have been disrupted.

Otitis externa may be localized, diffuse, or invasive. Localized disease occurs when hair follicles or sebaceous glands, located in the outer one-half of the canal, become infected. *S. aureus* and *Streptococcus pyogenes* are common pathogens. Patients usually present with acute pain. On examination, a localized area of erythema, a furuncle, or pustules are seen. Local heat, analgesics, and occasionally incision and drainage are usually sufficient for management. Depending on the severity, local or systemic antibiotics may be necessary.

Diffuse otitis externa may be infectious (wet), dermatitic (dry), or a combination. Pathogens show geographic variation, with *Pseudomonas aeruginosa* more commonly isolated in regions with hot humid climates, and *S. aureus* more commonly isolated elsewhere. Cultures of the exudate reveal polymicrobial infection in 30% and anaerobic bacteria in 25% of cases. Gram-negative bacteria tend to be found in severe infections. On examination, the canal may be edematous and erythematous with copious exudate. The patient usually complains of pain with manipulation of the tragus, a cartilaginous structure contiguous with the cartilage of the external canal. Otitis media with perforation of the tympanic membrane should be excluded before initiating therapy. In general, otitis media is not associated with pain on manipulation of the tragus, or severe inflammation of the ear canal. If a culture of the exudate is desired, it is best obtained using a sterile calcium alginate urethral swab.

Treatment of diffuse otitis externa begins with removal of debris. This can be accomplished by suction, gentle wiping, or irrigation. When the canal is extremely narrow secondary to severe inflammation, an ear wick should be carefully inserted. A suspension containing neomycin, polymyxin, and hydrocortisone (Cortisporin) should be dripped onto the wick until it expands to fill the canal. The solution of the same medications is more irritating to the canal and is not well absorbed by the wick; therefore, the suspension is preferable for the treatment of otitis externa. The wick should be removed in 24 hours. Subsequently, an antibiotic-steroid suspension can be used four times daily in the external canal, usually for 7 to 10 days. Drops of acetic acid otic solution (Vō-Sol) or a mixture of half vinegar and half alcohol solution may be applied topically after swimming or bathing for prevention of recurrent infection.

Otomycosis, or acute fungal external otitis, accounts for up to 10% of cases of external otitis. *Aspergillus* is the most common etiologic organism. Diagnosed most commonly in subtropical areas, it can be identified during otoscopic examination, when a fungal mass may be seen. The mass may appear white or black at the time of the examination. The causative agent often can be identified microscopically from scrapings or aspirated material on a 20% potassium hydroxide preparation. A culture may clarify the diagnosis. Treatment consists of thorough cleansing of the external auditory canal and restoring the proper pH level with 2% acetic acid drops. Topical nystatin powder or tolnaftate drops may be helpful.

Dermatitis of the skin of the external canal is associated most commonly with seborrheic dermatitis present elsewhere. It also can be associated with psoriasis, systemic lupus erythematosus, neurodermatitis, contact dermatitis, sensitivities to products (including topical neomycin), purulent otitis media, and infantile eczema. The pinna may be involved with fissuring and weeping of the overlying skin. Often pruritic, these conditions are associated with excoriations and secondary bacterial infections. Treating the underlying condition is indicated. Topical steroids with 2% acetic acid may be helpful.

Invasive otitis externa, also called "malignant external otitis" (MEO), is an infection of the external auditory canal and deep periauricular tissues. This invasive infection typically begins at the bone-cartilage junction of the canal and spreads in any number of directions. It commonly involves adjacent cartilaginous and bony structures leading to chondritis of the external ear or life-threatening osteomyelitis of the base of the skull. *Pseudomonas aeruginosa* is the etiologic agent in nearly all cases.

Typically, MEO is a disease of elderly diabetic patients. They present with a history of prolonged otitis externa refractory to topical treatment. Persistent otalgia and otorrhea may be accompanied by hearing loss. Fever usually is absent. Cranial nerve palsies (usually cranial nerve VII) occur in 20 to 30% of patients. On examination, granulation tissue can be visualized at the floor of the external canal overlying the junction of the bone and cartilage. Tenderness of the temporomandibular joint or erythema and tenderness overlying the mastoid process are often present. Laboratory studies are usually unimpressive. The white blood cell count may be normal, but the erythrocyte sedimentation rate is usually elevated. Granulation tissue, when present in the external auditory canal, should be biopsied to exclude carcinoma.

Two groups of children may be affected by MEO: adolescents with diabetes and children with immune dysfunction. In contrast to adults, who have a more insidious onset of otalgia and drainage, children commonly have an acute onset of symptoms. Erythema and swelling of the preauricular area and pinna develop rapidly. Severe, relentless pain is distinctive. The tympanic membrane, usually normal in adults, is necrotic in most children with MEO. Facial nerve dysfunction, a rare finding but poor prognostic feature in adults, occurs more frequently in children. Though the facial nerve dysfunction seen with MEO in children usually is complete and permanent, it does not appear to herald a lower survival rate. Deforming chondritis, not often seen in adults, has been reported frequently in children. Recurrence, a common problem in adults, is unusual in children.

MEO must be differentiated from chronic external otitis in the child. Cultures of the exudate in both conditions may yield *P. aeruginosa*. Children with MEO usually have no recent history of aural infection, whereas children with chronic external otitis tend to have a history of ear disease.

Plain radiographs are of limited use in confirming the diagnosis of MEO. Technetium scintigraphy is more sensitive than computed tomography (CT) for diagnostic purposes. Once the diagnosis has been confirmed, serial CT or magnetic resonance imaging (MRI) scans may further delineate the extra- and intracranial extent of disease.

Historically, radical surgical excision was the treatment of choice for MEO. Treatment now has evolved to the use of systemic antibiotics with adjunctive surgical intervention reserved for the most severe cases. There are many reports in the literature of successful therapy of adults with oral ciprofloxacin (Cipro), but intravenous antibiotic therapy usually is preferred for initial management. Combination antimicrobial therapy with an aminoglycoside and an antipseudomonal penicillin should be initiated when the diagnosis of MEO is suspected. The duration of therapy depends on the severity and extent of disease and the clinical response. Generally, therapy of 4 to 8 weeks in adults and 3 to 4 weeks in children is necessary.

PLAGUE*

method of
DAVID T. DENNIS, M.D., M.P.H.
Centers for Disease Control and Prevention
Fort Collins, Colorado

Plague is an acute, sometimes fulminating, zoonotic disease caused by infection with *Yersinia pestis*, a gram-negative, bipolar-staining, nonmotile pleomorphic coccobacillus of the Enterobacteriaceae family. The latest plague pandemic spread from central Asia at the turn of the century and established itself first in port cities and later in rural foci involving indigenous rodent populations on all continents other than Australia and Antarctica. San Francisco was the city most affected in the United States, and outbreaks of human plague occurred there until about 1920; the last instance of human-to-human transmission occurred in Los Angeles in 1925. Since the early part of the century, plague has spread and established itself among wild rodent populations in all states of the western United States, and associated human cases have been mostly sporadic and geographically widely distributed. In the 50-year period 1944 through 1993, 362 cases of human plague were reported by 13 states, and approximately 90% of these occurred in Arizona, California, Colorado, and New Mexico. Plague elsewhere in the world has also moved from urban to rural settings. In its natural rural foci, enzootic *Y. pestis* transmission is "silently" maintained in flea-rodent cycles involving relatively resistant rodent species that show little or no obvious disease. Explosive epizootics that kill large numbers of animals do, however, occur intermittently among susceptible wild rodent populations, during which infection with *Y. pestis* is most likely to spill over into commensal rodents and their fleas and place humans at risk in their usual living and working environments. Humans most often acquire plague from the bites of infected rodent fleas, to a lesser extent through direct contact with fluids or tissues of infected animals, and rarely by inhaling infective respiratory droplets from an animal or human with plague pneumonia. In the period 1978 to 1992, nearly 15,000 human plague cases with 1451 deaths were reported to the World Health Organization by 21 countries, 6 of them (Brazil, Madagascar, Myanmar (Burma), Tanzania, the United States, and Vietnam) reporting cases practically every year.

---

*This article is in the public domain.

CLINICAL MANIFESTATIONS

The principal clinical forms of plague are bubonic, septicemic, and pneumonic. Bubonic plague is the most common form (accounting for about 90% of cases in the United States) and develops as a regional lymphadenopathy secondary to a flea bite or to a percutaneous or mucous membrane introduction of *Y. pestis* from direct contact with infective material. The incubation period for bubonic plague is usually 2 to 6 days. The onset of symptoms can be insidious, but the illness most often progresses rapidly with increasing pain and swelling, and exquisite tenderness of the affected regional lymph nodes accompanied by fever, chills, headache, prostration, and agitation, and sometimes by gastrointestinal symptoms of nausea, vomiting, abdominal pain, and diarrhea. Bloodstream infection occurs frequently in bubonic plague and can result in septic shock and secondary plague pneumonia, and rarely in plague meningitis and pericarditis. Plague pneumonia is rapidly progressive and fatal if not treated early and aggressively—it also poses the potential risk of direct spread via respiratory droplet from the patient to close contacts. Apparent primary septicemia occurs in nearly 10% of plague cases in the United States and usually arises from direct inoculation of *Y. pestis* when infected animal tissues are handled or ingested. In recent years, primary plague pneumonia in humans, although rare, has increasingly occurred in the United States as a result of intimate contact of pet owners and veterinary staff with cats that have infectious oropharyngeal or pneumonic plague. Cats, which are relatively susceptible to *Y. pestis* infection, acquire the infection by ingesting plague-infected rodents.

DIAGNOSIS

All patients suspected of having plague should be placed in the hospital in isolation; specimens should be obtained for laboratory diagnosis, chest roentgenography performed, and antibiotic treatment started without delay. For all patients appropriate diagnostic specimens include blood for culture and serum antibody tests; for suspected pneumonic cases, sputum samples; and for suspected bubonic cases, aspirates from affected lymph nodes. A *suspect case* is an illness with clinical and epidemiologic features compatible with plague with or without gram-negative bipolar coccobacilli in clinical material (e.g., bubo aspirate, sputum, tissue, blood). A *presumptive case* is a compatible illness in which there is either direct fluorescent antibody staining of organisms presumed to be *Y. pestis* in clinical materials or in culture, or there is a passive hemagglutination serum antibody titer of greater than or equal to 1:10. A *confirmed case* is one in which a cultural isolate of *Y. pestis* is confirmed by lysis with bacteriophage and by a diagnostic biochemical profile, or in which passive hemagglutination serum antibodies demonstrate a fourfold difference in titer between specimens taken at appropriate intervals. Specificity of the antibody reaction is validated by hemagglutination inhibition testing.

TREATMENT

Untreated plague is fatal in more than 50% of patients with the bubonic form of the disease, and in nearly all persons with septicemic, pneumonic, or meningeal plague. The recent overall mortality in plague cases in the United States is nearly 15%, and fatalities almost always arise from delays in seeking treatment and delays in making the proper diagnosis. Rapid diagnosis and appropriate antibiotic therapy are therefore essential (Table 1).

Streptomycin is the drug of choice for treating plague. Gentamicin is more readily available than streptomycin and has, therefore, increasingly been substituted for treating plague in the United States. Gentamicin has not, however, been systematically evaluated for this use. Tetracycline and chloramphenicol are excellent alternative antimicrobials; they are usually given orally with initial loading doses, but they may also be given intravenously in seriously ill patients. Penicillins, cephalosporins, and macrolide antimicrobials have a suboptimal effect and should not be used to treat plague. Although doxycycline is considered to have antimicrobial equivalence with tetracycline, its efficacy in treating plague has not been studied. In general, antimicrobial therapy should be continued for 10 days, or for at least 3 days after the patient has become afebrile and has made an apparent clinical recovery. Patients started on intravenous antimicrobials may, when warranted by clinical improvement, be switched to oral regimens. Clinical improvement is usually evident 2 to 3 days after the start of antimicrobial treatment even though the body temperature often remains elevated for several days. Buboes frequently continue to enlarge for several days after the start of treatment, and the affected nodes sometimes remain swollen and tender for weeks after successful treatment. Chloramphenicol is recommended for treating plague meningitis, endophthalmitis, myocarditis, and pleuritis because of its high tissue penetration, and it may be used for these indications in combination with streptomycin.

COMPLICATIONS

Complications that sometimes arise early in the course of illness include sepsis with shock, secondary pneumonia, disseminated intravascular coagulation (DIC) and bleeding, and adult respiratory distress syndrome (ARDS). These complications are most likely to occur in patients whose treatment has been delayed. Life-threatening complications such as septic shock, DIC, and ARDS require highly intensive monitoring and close physiologic supportive care as outlined elsewhere. Case fatality rates for these conditions are high.

Delayed complications are unusual; they include abscess formation in affected nodes, which in some instances may be intra-abdominal or intrathoracic, and rarely in other tissues, such as lung, liver, spleen, and kidney. Abscesses can be a cause of recurrent fever in patients who have had an apparent full recovery. Viable plague organisms have been cultured from affected nodes 1 to 2 weeks after clinical recovery from the acute disease. Antimicrobial treatment of lymph node abscess is guided by microbiologic examination for *Y. pestis* and possible superinfecting bacteria. Buboes may be drained surgically; occasionally, they drain spontaneously. Purulent material should be considered to be potentially infective. Streptomycin-resistant *Y. pestis* has not been identified, and *Y. pestis* appears to be genetically stable.

Diseases that can mimic (or be confused with) plague include lymphogranuloma venereum; staphylococcal, streptococcal, and various gram-negative bacterial causes of adenitis, such as tularemia, melioidosis, and cat scratch disease; sepsis and shock from causes other than *Y. pestis*; pneumococcal and other acute bacterial pneumonias; viral pneumonia, including Hantavirus infection; and ARDS. Plague presenting with gastrointestinal symptoms can be confused with shigellosis, food poisoning, viral gastroenteritis syndromes, mesenteric adenitis, and appendicitis.

PREVENTION

Plague is a disease of place. In the United States, endemic disease is found only in the western states. The Centers for Disease Control and Prevention, state and local health departments, Native American health services, and park and wildlife services maintain information on sites where enzootic and epizootic plague occur and conduct surveillance for plague outbreaks among wild animal populations. Avoiding known epizootic sites during the peak transmission season of May through October, taking precautions as directed by posted warnings, and avoiding contact with sick or dead wild animals, especially rodents, rabbits, and wild carnivores, can do much to prevent exposure to infection among persons who use natural areas for recreational and occupational purposes. Increasingly, however, as suburbanization encroaches on natural areas, people are at risk of exposure in periresidential settings and in undeveloped areas near their homes. Rock squirrels, tree squirrels, and wood rats sometimes act as infective sources in yards and outbuildings. Pet dogs and cats can bring infective fleas from wild rodents into the home environment; diseased cats can directly transmit infection to persons caring for them. Since dogs and cats acquire infection by direct contact with tissues of infected wild animals and from the bites of infected rodent fleas, persons living in endemic areas should prevent

TABLE 1. **Plague Treatment Guidelines**

Drug	Dosage	Hourly Interval	Route of Administration
Streptomycin			
Adults	2 gm/day	12	IM
Children	30 mg/kg/day	8 or 12	IM
Gentamicin			
Adults	3 mg/kg/day	8	IM or IV
Children	6.0–7.5 mg/kg/day	8	IM or IV
Infants or neonates	7.5 mg/kg/day	8	IM or IV
Tetracycline			
Adults	2 gm/day	6	PO
Children ≥9 years	25–50 mg/kg/day	6	PO
Chloramphenicol			
Adults	50 mg/kg/day	6	PO or IV
Children ≥1 year	50 mg/kg/day	6	PO or IV

TABLE 2. **Plague Prophylaxis Guidelines**

Drug	Dosage	Hourly Interval	Route of Administration
Tetracycline			
Adults	1–2 gm/day	6 or 12	PO
Children ≥9 years	25–50 mg/kg/day	6 or 12	PO
Doxycycline (Vibramycin)			
Adults	100–200 mg/day	12	PO
Children ≥9 years	0.5–1 mg/kg/day	12	PO
Trimethoprim-sulfamethoxazole (Bactrim, Septra)	40 mg/kg/day	12	PO

these pets from roaming freely and take steps to control their fleas. A plague vaccine for humans prepared from formalin-killed *Y. pestis* is available; it is given as a primary series of three intramuscular doses, followed by booster doses depending upon circumstances of continuing exposure. Outside the military, the vaccine has a restricted use for laboratory personnel regularly working with *Y. pestis* or *Y. pestis*–infected animals, and for persons whose vocation brings them into regular direct contact with wild rodents or rabbits in enzootic plague areas. The vaccine is variably immunogenic and moderately reactogenic; field trials of its efficacy have not been performed. The vaccine is unsuitable for near-term protection of health workers and other persons in close contact with cases of plague, and it is not indicated for use as a control measure during plague outbreaks.

Prophylactic antibiotic treatment should be administered within 6 days of exposure to persons who have had close (respiratory droplet) contact with a person or a cat with suspected respiratory plague, and to persons who have handled plague-infected animals. Household contacts of bubonic plague patients should also receive prophylactic antibiotic treatment if there is thought to be a peridomestic risk of exposure to infected rodent fleas. In selected circumstances, short-term antimicrobial prophylaxis may be appropriate for travelers to and health workers in known plague outbreak foci. Guidelines for prophylactic antimicrobial administration are provided in Table 2.

PSITTACOSIS

method of
PAULA H. JOHNSON, M.B., CH.B., and
JOHN T. MACFARLANE, D.M.
City Hospital
Nottingham, England, United Kingdom

Psittacosis is caused by *Chlamydia psittaci*, a gram-negative obligate intracellular organism. It is a zoonosis classically transmitted to humans via psittacine birds (e.g., parrots, parakeets, cockatoos, and budgerigars), but if it is transmitted via another species, the term "ornithosis" is used. Human-to-human transmission is well documented but rare.

The reported incidence is rising worldwide: in England and Wales about 300 chlamydial pneumonias are reported annually, 75% of which are due to *C. psittaci*. Besides psittacine birds, infection is well documented via other species: poultry, pigeons, canaries, finches, and seagulls among them. There are also case reports of transmission via sheep, cattle, rodents, and domestic cats. Those most at risk are owners of pet birds, workers in poultry-processing plants, veterinarians, and zoo or pet shop workers. Asymptomatic birds carrying *C. psittaci* can excrete organisms if stressed, such as during overcrowded transport conditions.

Contact with birds is reported by as few as 62% of patients in some series. Exposure need only be brief, and contact with infected birds need not be close. Urine, feces and feathers may be heavily contaminated, and an "aerosol" of chlamydial organisms can form. Chlamydiae may remain viable for months in the dust of bird houses. The incubation period is usually 7 to 10 days but may extend to 4 weeks.

Symptoms are often nonspecific, but the most prominent are fever, cough, headache, nausea and vomiting, and myalgia. Less common presentations include diarrhea, abdominal pain, chest pain, dyspnea, sore throat, and meningism.

Chest signs are present in 80% of patients—commonly crackles and consolidation and occasionally pleural rubs. Less common signs include relative bradycardia, confusion, lymphadenopathy, and splenomegaly.

Investigations yield an abnormal chest x-ray film in up to 85% of cases, usually consolidation, which is multilobar in 10%. Liver and/or renal function is deranged in 50% and the erythrocyte sedimentation rate is nearly always raised to a mean level of about 50 mm per hour. The white cell count is normal in 70 to 90% of patients.

Establishing the diagnosis is most commonly done using the complement fixation test, although this cannot distinguish between chlamydial species. A fourfold rise in antibody titer is most helpful, but a single titer of 1:128 or more suffices. Microimmunofluorescence usually distinguishes between chlamydial species, but *C. psittaci* has more than 11 different serotypes, and not all are routinely tested for. Diagnosis can also be established via cell culture of blood, sputum, pleural fluid, or throat swabs, but this is hazardous to laboratory workers. Other techniques include antigen detection via enzyme-linked immunosorbent assay (ELISA) and the polymerase chain reaction.

TREATMENT

The treatment of choice is tetracycline 1 to 2 grams daily or doxycycline 200 mg daily for 14 days. Erythromycin can also be used: 500 mg four times daily for 14 days is probably as effective as tetracycline, but a 21-day course of 250 mg four times daily is associated with a higher relapse rate. Chloramphenicol and rifampin (Rifadin) are effective, but more relapses are reported. There have been no formal trials comparing different treatments.

Complications of psittacosis are uncommon but include endocarditis, pericarditis, myocarditis, disseminated intravascular coagulation, meningitis, arthralgias, and spontaneous abortion.

Measures to prevent psittacosis include antibiotic administration to birds in breeding aviaries before they are distributed to pet shops, and to birds in poultry plants, although the latter is less successful in controlling carriage. Controls on the import of exotic birds are in force but are frequently flouted by illegal importers. Ill birds should be quarantined and treated with tetracycline and stringent infection control measures applied.

There is no vaccine, and lasting immunity is *not* conferred by acute infection.

Q FEVER

method of
BRUNO B. CHOMEL, D.V.M., PH.D.
University of California, Davis
Davis, California

Q fever was described for the first time in 1937 in Australia and since then, has been recognized as a zoonosis worldwide. The causative bacterium, *Coxiella burnetii*, a Rickettsiaceae, is transmitted to humans most often by the inhalation of contaminated aerosols. Human infections result from contact with infected animals, especially sheep, goats, or cattle, or from infected placentas. Cats can also be a source of human infection. In sheep, goats, and cattle, Q fever is usually subclinical. Heavy concentrations of the bacterium are shed in milk, urine, feces, and especially parturient products of infected pregnant animals. The ingestion of contaminated animal milk or meat can be another source of human infection. *C. burnetii* can survive several months in the environment, long after the infective animals are not shedding any more.

PRESENTATION AND DIAGNOSIS

After an incubation period of 2 to 6 weeks (average 20 days), typical patients have acute onset of high fever, chills with rigors, severe headaches, retrobulbar pain, general malaise, and myalgia. Chest pain, cough, nausea, vomiting, and diarrhea can also be observed. Q fever is usually describe as an atypical pneumonia, although the actual incidence of respiratory illness ranges widely, from few affected patients to more than 90%. Acute Q fever may also present as hepatitis with features suggestive of viral hepatitis, including elevated serum transaminase levels and right upper quadrant tenderness. Most cases of Q fever are self-limited, with symptoms resolving in 1 to 2 weeks. Endocarditis develops in a small proportion of patients (less than 1%) years after the acute infection and follows a chronic course. Unlike other causes of endocarditis and characteristic of this infection, routine blood cultures are negative.

Diagnosis of acute Q fever is based on serologic examination, since culturing the organism is hazardous and requires specially equipped laboratories. Antibodies to both Phase I and Phase II antigens can be detected by various methods, including indirect immunofluorescent antibody (IFA) test and enzyme-linked immunosorbent assay (ELISA). Anti–Phase I antibodies are present at higher titers only during the chronic form of the illness, whereas anti-Phase II antibodies are largely predominant in primary acute Q fever.

TREATMENT

A number of antimicrobial agents have been used to treat infections caused by *C. burnetii*, but the results have been variable, as several antibiotics have only rickettsiostatic properties. Most acute Q fever infection resolves without treatment, but uncertainty regarding the development of chronic infection makes treatment advisable. The choice of antimicrobial agent for treating the disease in human cases is based more on tradition than on scientific study, since controlled clinical trials with different agents have not been performed. In a randomized study, tetracycline reduced the duration of fever by 50% when the drug was administered within the first 3 days of the illness. Therefore, tetracycline and its analogues have been considered the treatment of choice for acute Q fever. In adults and children aged 8 years and older, 500 mg four times a day for 14 days is recommended. Children may be treated with trimethoprim (Proloprim)* or chloramphenicol.* However, more recent data suggest that the most effective antibiotic is doxycycline (Vibramycin), 100 mg twice daily for 14 days. Alternative antibiotics are ofloxacin (Floxin)* 300 mg twice daily and pefloxacin† 400 mg twice daily, for 2 weeks. The combination of pefloxacin† 800 mg per day and rifampin (Rifadin)* 1200 mg per day for 21 days successfully treated patients with prolonged Q fever.

The treatment of Q fever endocarditis has not been the subject of controlled studies. A combination of antibiotics in conjunction with periodic evaluations of the hemodynamic status of the patient are generally required. Tetracycline in combination with trimethoprim-sulfamethoxazole (Bactrim, Septra)* or lincomycin (Lincocin)* for a prolonged period has been advocated as a successful treatment for Q fever endocarditis, and an alternative is rifampin combined with doxycycline. Valve replacement should be reserved for hemodynamic failure.

PREVENTION

Strategies for the prevention of Q fever in humans should aim at high-risk occupational groups (abattoir workers, veterinarians, and medical researchers, especially those engaged in research on pregnant ewes). A reduction of shedding rather than a reduction of infection in domestic animals has been observed after vaccination of dairy cattle and sheep with an inactivated Phase I vaccine. Because Q fever is generally subclinical in animals, there is little economic incentive to eradicate the infection in livestock by widespread vaccination programs. Ewes used for medical research should be serologically tested and come from flocks regularly monitored. However, since most animals are asymptomatic and some may shed the organism despite being seronegative, it is difficult to screen for or eradicate infection in all animals. In medical facilities, surveillance of the serologic status

---

*Not FDA-approved for this indication.
†Not available in the United States.

of the workers should be performed on a regular basis, and any worker with congenital or acquired heart disease, pregnant females, and any immuno-suppressed person should be restricted from high-risk jobs. No human vaccine against *C. burnetii* is commercially available, but a number of experimental vaccines are under study.

RABIES

method of
MICHAEL F. KELLEY, M.D., M.P.H., and
KEITH A. CLARK, D.V.M., Ph.D.
Texas Department of Health
Austin, Texas

Rabies is an almost invariably fatal viral zoonosis characterized by encephalitis, typically following an animal bite. Carnivorous mammals and bats are the usual reservoirs; worldwide, dogs are the animals most often responsible for human infection. In the United States, bats have been incriminated in 9 of the last 11 indigenously acquired cases of rabies in humans.

Although rare in humans, rabies remains a dread disease because of the near certainty of death and the terrifying aspects of death due to rabies. From a public health viewpoint, the most significant problem in the United States is the large number of postexposure antirabies treatments resulting from actual or suspected exposure to rabid animals. Approximately 20,000 such treatments are administered annually. Undoubtedly, many are unnecessary, but difficulty arises when one must attempt to determine promptly, on a case-by-case basis, exactly which ones are unnecessary. Understandably, both medical personnel and bite victims usually opt to err on the conservative side.

Striped skunks, raccoons, foxes, coyotes, and various species of bats are the most commonly infected species. Specialized laboratory studies, including monoclonal antibody analysis and nucleotide sequencing after amplification by polymerase chain reaction (PCR), have demonstrated that different variants or ecotypes (approximately equivalent to strains) of rabies virus can be identified. These variants are somewhat host-specific, and rabies tends to be confined principally to a single reservoir species in a particular locality ("compartmentalization"), but two species with distinctly different strains of rabies may occupy the same locality at the same time. The reservoir species maintains the infection in nature, and fluctuations of the animal population are integrally related to characteristic enzootic-epizootic cycles.

The incubation period in humans reportedly may be as short as 4 days or as long as several years. A case occurring in Texas in 1984 is reliably reported to have had an incubation period of almost 7 years. Such latency is poorly understood, but several factors known to influence the incubation period include the site of inoculation, the quantity of virus in the inoculum, the virulence of the viral strain, and the age of the victim.

The usual mode of transmission is through the contamination of a bite wound by the biting animal's virus-laden saliva. Mucosal contact with the virus may also result in infection. Aerosol transmission of rabies has been reported, but only under specialized conditions in which the air contains a high concentration of suspended particles or drop-lets carrying viral particles. Such conditions are unusual, but have occurred in laboratory settings, in caves with extremely high populations of colonial bats, and possibly in one instance in which rabid wild animals were housed indoors near uninfected ones. There is no danger of aerosol transmission under most circumstances, and rabies virus has not been isolated from skunk musk (spray).

CLINICAL SIGNS IN ANIMALS

Rabid animals of all species exhibit typical signs of central nervous system disturbance, with minor variations between species. The most commonly reported signs of rabies in animals are behavioral changes and/or unexplained paralysis. Behavioral changes may consist of such aberrations as loss of fear of humans by wild animals, shyness on the part of a usually friendly pet, restlessness, excitability, sudden mood changes, or pica. Ataxia, incoordination, altered phonation, seeking solitude, and uncharacteristic aggressiveness may develop; a normally docile animal may suddenly become vicious. Commonly, rabid wild animals lose their fear of humans, and normally nocturnal species may be seen wandering about during the daytime. The term "furious rabies" refers to animals in which aggression (the excitative phase) is pronounced, and "dumb," or paralytic, rabies refers to those in which the behavioral changes are minimal or absent and the disease is manifested principally by paralysis. Paralysis associated with rabies may involve any part of the animal's body but is most often ascending.

Rabid foxes and coyotes frequently invade yards or even houses, attacking dogs and people. Rabid raccoons and skunks typically show no fear of humans, are ataxic and uncoordinated, frequently are aggressive, and are active during the day, despite their nocturnal nature. In urban areas, they often attack domestic pets.

In general, rabies should be suspected in terrestrial wildlife acting abnormally. The same is true of bats that are observed flying in the daytime, resting on the ground, attacking people and animals, or fighting.

Rodents and lagomorphs rarely constitute a risk for rabies exposure, but each incident must be evaluated individually. Several reports of laboratory-confirmed rabies in woodchucks have been associated with the raccoon rabies epizootic in the eastern United States.

A presumptive clinical diagnosis of rabies in an animal may be based on behavioral changes and/or paralysis, especially when rabies has been recently reported from the same species in that geographic area. Confirmation must be performed in a competent laboratory by direct immuno-fluorescence on central nervous tissue. The preferred sampling areas are hippocampus, brain stem, and cerebellum. Intracerebral inoculation of a suspension of suspect nervous tissue into suckling mice is sometimes used as an adjunct but is less sensitive and cannot be pronounced negative for 28 days postinoculation. Inoculation of in vitro cultured mouse neuroblastoma cells may eventually supplant mouse inoculation, principally because results are available as soon as 8 days postinoculation.

CLINICAL MANIFESTATIONS IN HUMANS

Although incubation periods from 4 days to 19 years have been reported, 95% are less than 1 year and two-thirds are less than 90 days, with an average of 4 to 8 weeks. Clinical rabies begins with a prodromal phase of nonspecific symptoms that may include cough, sore throat, abdominal pain, and anxiety. Frequently there are paresthesias or pain at the site of the original exposure. After 2 to 10 days of prodromal symptoms, rapid progression of clinical disease usually ensues. Agitation worsens, with periods of hyperactivity, hallucination, and delirium alternating with relatively normal behavior. Hydrophobia or aerophobia occurs during this phase in about 60% of patients. These symptoms are pathognomonic and consist of painless diaphragmatic, neck, and facial muscle spasms in response to attempts at swallowing or stimulation of the face by air currents, and may manifest themselves as avoidance of fluids and air movement. Seizures may occur, and deterioration of mental status progressing to coma is accompanied by autonomic instability, with wild fluctuations in body temperature, pulse, and blood pressure. The patient has marked diaphoresis and salivation and frequently has severe difficulty handling respiratory secretions, requiring intubation. Cardiac or respiratory arrest can be expected within a few days of the onset of clinical symptoms. Survival is typically less than a week without medical care and somewhat longer with aggressive intensive care. Only three survivors of suspected rabies have been reported. The last was in 1972, with none since, in spite of advances in critical care medicine.

There is also a human counterpart of "dumb," or paralytic, rabies, with a progression from the prodrome to an ascending paralytic phase and coma, without the excitement characterizing "furious rabies." This clinical picture is less common than furious rabies but has been observed in association with rabies acquired from vampire bats.

DIAGNOSIS

Antemortem diagnosis of rabies is difficult. False-negative results are common with all diagnostic tests available. Although a history of a bite exposure is helpful, it is frequently not obtained. Rabies should be included in the differential diagnosis of any progressive encephalopathic condition. The presence of hydrophobia or aerophobia should greatly increase clinical suspicion. Routine laboratory tests are not helpful for diagnosis. Computed tomography of the brain is typically normal, and electroencephalographic changes are not diagnostic.

Neutralizing antibody in serum or cerebrospinal fluid is diagnostic if the patient has not received rabies vaccine, but death often occurs before a rise in antibody titer can occur. Virus may be demonstrated in saliva or in a full-thickness skin biopsy from the nape of the neck before neutralizing antibodies are formed. Because these tests are insensitive, they should be repeated every few days until a diagnosis is established. Corneal impressions have also been used for antemortem diagnosis, but the yield on this test is low. Brain biopsy may be helpful, but it is not unusual for all the tests to remain negative and the diagnosis only to be confirmed at autopsy.

Other causes of encephalopathy must be excluded, including viral and toxic encephalitis and delirium tremens. Hydrophobia has caused confusion with tetanus, but the contractions of tetanus are painful and last longer than the contractions of hydrophobia. The paralytic form of rabies must be differentiated from Guillain-Barré syndrome and poliomyelitis.

TREATMENT

Treatment of human rabies is supportive. Early intubation helps control respiratory secretions and reduces the risk of exposing medical personnel to infectious secretions. There is no advantage in administering rabies immune globulin or vaccine after symptoms begin, and doing so reduces the value of some diagnostic tests. There is no evidence that antiviral agents or immunomodulators are beneficial. Steroids should be avoided.

Infection control is important, both to prevent nosocomial infection in the patient and to protect the medical staff. The use of a mask, goggles, gown, and gloves when caring for an unintubated patient, and when performing intubation or respiratory care, should adequately protect staff. Virus is not found in the blood, and universal body fluid precautions are sufficient, except that saliva and respiratory secretions should also be treated as potentially infectious fluids. Although there is no evidence that human-to-human transmission of rabies can occur, except after corneal transplantation, there is usually considerable anxiety among medical staff caring for a rabies patient. This should be addressed early by providing reassurance and factual information.

PREVENTION AND CONTROL

Immunization of dogs and cats is the cornerstone of rabies control but must be accompanied by effective stray animal control and community education.

Animal bite or nonbite exposures may place a person at risk of rabies. Although bite exposures are usually obvious, nonbite exposures can be more difficult to assess. Saliva is the infectious fluid in either case. Nonbite exposures occur when mucous membranes or broken skin comes into contact with saliva. Healing of wounds is rapid enough that exposure of broken skin that has not had serous or bloody drainage within the preceding 24 hours generally does not pose a risk of rabies transmission. Likewise, direct saliva contact is required for transmission. Handling a toy that was in a pet's mouth, or petting a pet that had been grooming itself generally does not constitute an exposure, unless there is gross contamination with undried saliva at the time of contact.

If an exposure has occurred, an assessment of the probability that the exposing animal has rabies is essential for deciding appropriate treatment. In any case, proper wound care, including prompt, thorough cleansing of the wound with *soap* and water is essential. Evaluation of the need for tetanus immunization is also important. After first aid is administered, the process of deciding on appropriate subsequent action must begin. The decision whether to initiate postexposure prophylaxis with rabies immune globulin and/or rabies vaccine must be made immediately, not awaiting results of testing or observation, on the basis of the risk of rabies transmission. This decision is based on the species of the animal, its immunization status and behavior, and the prevalence of rabies in the area. Generally, carnivores and bats should be considered higher rabies risks. Although it varies regionally, skunks, raccoons, foxes, and bats are likely to carry rabies. Lagomorphs and rodents are unlikely to have rabies. If the animal exhibits unusual behavior, as described above, rabies is more likely. Properly immunized pets are less likely to be rabid, though vaccine failures in animals do occur. If subsequent testing or observation indicates an incorrect decision, the appropriate corrective action should be taken. Asymptomatic biting domestic dogs and cats, if owned and wanted, may be observed for 10 days to determine their capability of transmitting rabies at the time of the bite. Other animals, including unwanted dogs and cats, should be humanely killed and tested for rabies as soon as possible. If the animal is capable of transmitting rabies at the time of the bite, testing of the brain yields positive results. A period of observation for animals other than cats or dogs is not appropriate.

Once the decision has been made that a potential rabies exposure has occurred, postexposure prophylaxis should be started. Because some rabies cases have followed very long incubation periods, it is appropriate to begin treatment at any point after exposure if symptoms have not begun and the exposure is deemed significant, even if weeks or months have passed.

For people who were previously unimmunized, treatment consists of a single dose of human rabies immune globulin (HRIG) (Hyperab, Imogam), 20 IU per kg, at the beginning of treatment (Day 0), plus a series of five doses of rabies vaccine administered intramuscularly on Days 0, 3, 7, 14, and 28. Up to half the HRIG should be administered at the site of the exposure, if anatomically feasible. The remainder should be given as a deep intramuscular injection into the gluteal muscle. HRIG is available in 2-mL and 10-mL vials containing 150 IU per mL of immune globulin.

Two rabies vaccines are available in the United States, human diploid cell vaccine (HDCV) (Imovax) and rabies vaccine, adsorbed (RVA). The dose for each is 1 mL given intramuscularly. Vaccine should not be given in the gluteal region, since failures have been reported with this route of administration. It is usually given in the deltoid muscle. Both vaccines have very low incidence of adverse reactions and are highly immunogenic. They may be used interchangeably. RVA may have a slightly lower incidence of Type III hypersensitivity after the administration of repeated doses. Both vaccines are prepared in cell cultures and do not contain nerve-derived tissue.

In Texas, patients are sometimes seen who were started on purified Vero cell rabies vaccine (PVRV)* in another country but have not yet completed postexposure treatment. PVRV is a third-generation rabies vaccine that appears to be as free from side effects and as immunogenic as the second-generation vaccine, HDCV. Our practice has been to complete

the series with HRIG or RVA rather than restart treatment.

If treatment is interrupted, the series should be resumed where it left off. When HRIG is not given on Day 0, it may be administered up to Day 8 of treatment. After that it is more likely to interfere with antibody formation than to give additional protection.

There is no need to measure antibody titers after a properly administered postexposure series, unless the patient is immunocompromised by illness or immunosuppressive therapy. A titer of 0.5 IU or neutralization at a serum dilution of 1:5 is considered protective.

If an exposed patient has previously been adequately immunized, the postexposure treatment is considerably simpler. For these patients, HRIG should not be administered. Two doses of HDCV or RVA should be given on Days 0 and 3. Previous adequate immunization is defined as properly administered pre- or postexposure prophylaxis with HDCV or RVA, or pre- or postexposure prophylaxis using another vaccine with documented antibody response after the series was completed.

Pre-exposure prophylaxis is given to persons with high risk of inapparent exposure to rabies. This includes laboratory workers who handle rabies specimens, veterinarians and animal handlers, and persons who regularly enter bat caves. Pre-exposure prophylaxis is given as a series of three 1.0-mL doses of HDCV or RVA, on Days 0, 7, and 21 or 28. Either vaccine may be given intramuscularly; an intradermal preparation of HDCV is also available, with a dose of 0.1 mL, and is slightly more economical. This intradermal preparation is only intended for pre-exposure use and should not be used for postexposure prophylaxis.

When the ongoing risk of exposure continues, booster doses of vaccine should be given periodically. Since the risk of allergic reaction increases with subsequent doses, antibody titers should be obtained and boosters given only when the titer falls below a protective level. Titers should be obtained every 6 months on rabies laboratory workers, and every 2 years on others. If titers are not obtained, booster doses should be given according to this same schedule.

Pre-exposure prophylaxis is also recommended for travelers who will spend extended periods in areas where adequate postexposure treatment will not be readily available or who will be working in areas with a high prevalence of animal rabies. For travelers who are also receiving chloroquine (Aralen), only the intramuscular preparations of vaccines should be used. Failure of intradermal pre-exposure prophylaxis has been reported in persons who are taking chloroquine phosphate during the time they are being immunized. It is also prudent to use the intramuscular vaccine if any live-virus vaccines are to be administered at the same time or within 30 days before the rabies immunization.

*Not available in the United States.

RAT–BITE FEVER

method of
EDWARD S. EISENBERG, M.D.
Albert Einstein College of Medicine
Bronx, New York

Rat-bite fever is an acute febrile illness that is usually acquired through the bite or scratch of a rat, mouse, other rodent, or animal that recently killed a rodent. The term "rat-bite fever" refers to two similar yet distinct disease syndromes caused by two different organisms that are part of the normal oral flora of the rat. *Streptobacillus moniliformis,* the cause of the great majority of cases in North America, is a pleomorphic gram-negative bacillus that forms beadlike chains and forms typical "puffballs" in liquid media. It occasionally can be isolated from routine blood cultures. *Spirillum minus* is a gram-negative, short, thick tightly coiled spiral rod that does not grow on standard culture media. Identification requires Giemsa- or Wright-stained or dark-field microscopic examination or intraperitoneal inoculation of infected material from patients into mice or guinea pigs.

CLINICAL MANIFESTATIONS

Both illnesses are characterized by initial healing of the bite wound, followed by the acute onset of fever, malaise, chills, headache, and rash. Untreated, both illnesses usually resolve spontaneously, over weeks, though both may lead to chronic complications of arthritis, relapsing fever, anemia, myocarditis, endocarditis, meningitis, hepatitis, and localized abscess. Both cause a leukocytosis and may be associated with a false-positive syphilis serologic test. The features that distinguish these illnesses are summarized in Table 1.

Infection caused by *S. moniliformis* usually occurs within a few days of a rat bite wound that is healing. It is characterized by the abrupt onset of fever, chills, headache, vomiting, and severe migratory arthralgias and myalgias. Regional lymphadenopathy is minimal. Within 2 to 4 days of fever, a nonpruritic maculapapular, morbilliform or petechial rash erupts over the palms, soles, and extremities. Skin lesions may become purpuric or confluent, and they may eventually desquamate. Approximately 50% of patients develop asymmetric polyarthritis or true septic ar-

thritis, most often involving the ankles, elbows, wrist, shoulders, or hips. Epidemics of disease (Haverhill fever) due to *S. bacilliformis* and associated with the ingestion of milk products contaminated with rat feces have occurred.

Bite wounds infected with *S. minus* usually heal promptly but then become painful, swollen, and purple approximately 1 to 4 weeks later, associated with regional lymphangitis and lymphadenitis and systemic illness characterized by fever, chills, headache, and malaise. The wound commonly progresses to chancre-like ulceration and induration with eschar formation. During the first week of fever a blotchy violaceous or reddish-brown macular rash erupts over the extremities, face, scalp, and trunk.

DIAGNOSIS

The diagnosis of rat-bite fever should be considered in individuals with fever, rash, a history of animal exposure (especially rodents), and leukocytosis. Direct visualization of pleomorphic bacillary organisms of *S. moniliformis* in Giemsa-stained smears of blood, joint fluid, or pus may provide an early clue to the diagnosis. Culture of the organism on enriched media occasionally yields the diagnosis. Specific agglutinins appear within 10 days of the onset of illness and reach a maximum within 1 to 3 months. An initial titer greater than 1:80 or a fourfold rise in titer is considered diagnostic. Since *S. minus* cannot be grown on synthetic media, diagnosis relies on direct visualization of characteristic spirochetes in blood, exudate, or lymph node tissue. The differential diagnosis may include leptospirosis, meningococcal sepsis, Rocky Mountain spotted fever, Lyme disease, brucellosis, viral infections, septic arthritis, endocarditis, and collagen vascular disease.

TREATMENT

The treatment of any bite begins with meticulous local wound care including cleansing, débridement, and tetanus prophylaxis. The drug of choice for rat-bite fever caused by either pathogen is penicillin. Traditional therapy is procaine penicillin, 600,000 U intramuscularly every 12 hours for 10 to 14 days. Patients who are quite ill may do better with intravenous penicillin, 600,000 U every 6 hours. Those with mild symptoms may respond to oral penicillin or ampicillin, 500 mg four times daily. For penicillin-allergic patients, tetracycline, 500 mg four times daily, or streptomycin, 15 mg per kg daily in divided doses, is recommended. Other drugs with in vitro evidence of activity but for which there is little clinical information include erythromycin, ciprofloxacin (Cipro), cefuroxime (Ceftin), and cefotaxime (Claforan).

TABLE 1. Distinguishing Features of Rat-Bite Fever Syndromes

	Streptobacillus moniliformis	*Spirillum minus*
Mode of transmission	Bite or ingestion	Bite
Incubation period	A few days	>1 week
Bite wound	Heals promptly	Heals, then ulcerates
Lymphadenopathy	Uncommon, mild	Prominent, usually regional
Arthritis	Common	Rare
Rash	Morbilliform, purpuric	Maculopapular
False-positive syphilis serologic test	25%	50%

Modified from Eisenberg ES: Rat Bite Fever. *In* Rakel R (ed): Conn's Current Therapy. Philadelphia, WB Saunders Co, 1990, p 106.

RELAPSING FEVER

method of
RAYMOND A. SMEGO, JR., M.D., M.P.H.
Robert C. Byrd Health Sciences Center of West Virginia University
Morgantown, West Virginia

Relapsing fever is an acute infectious disease caused by arthropod-borne spirochetes belonging to the genus *Bor-*

relia. It is clinically characterized by recurrent episodes of fever. Two forms of the disease exist: louse-borne and tick-borne relapsing fever. Epidemic or louse-borne relapsing fever occurs primarily in developing countries of the world. It is transmitted by the body louse *Pediculus humanus humanus* and is caused by *B. recurrentis*. The disease affects only humans. Epidemics may occur during war, famine, or other situations in which the prevalence of pediculosis is enhanced, such as among overcrowded, malnourished populations with poor personal hygiene. Endemic tick-borne relapsing fever is a less severe illness caused by several species of *Borrelia*. It is transmitted by soft body ticks of the genus *Ornithodoros*, has a worldwide distribution, and has associated rodent and small animal reservoirs of infection. Like other spirochetal infections, including syphilis, leptospirosis, and Lyme disease, relapsing fever is associated with the Jarisch-Herxheimer reaction, a complication that follows antimicrobial treatment of the infection.

CLINICAL AND LABORATORY MANIFESTATIONS

The classic clinical presentation of relapsing fever is a sudden onset of fever lasting 3 to 6 days, followed by an afebrile period of about 7 to 9 days, then followed by a sudden return of fever. Without treatment, three to five relapses of fever typically occur, with each febrile episode terminating by crisis. The severity of illness generally decreases with each recurrence. Relapses of fever correlate with spontaneous antigen variation in the abundant surface lipoproteins of the spirochete, in response to the host's antibody challenge. Apart from the recurrent nature of the illness, the clinical manifestations of relapsing fever are typically nonspecific. The spectrum of illness from relapsing fever ranges from mild self-limited febrile illness to severe systemic disease with death resulting from end-organ failure.

The initial attack usually starts abruptly with high fever and chills due to spirochetemia. Common associated symptoms include headache, myalgias, arthralgias, anorexia, dry cough, and abdominal pain. Hepatosplenomegaly, transient petechial rash, and jaundice are the most frequently encountered physical findings. Other cutaneous features may include macular or papular rashes, or a pruritic eschar at the inoculation site in tick-borne relapsing fever. Leukocytosis, thrombocytopenia, an elevated sedimentation rate, and abnormal liver function tests are common laboratory results. A notable feature of relapsing fever is the involvement of the central nervous system as a result of spirochete neurotropism. This predilection for invasion and persistence in the brain leads to complications of encephalitis, meningitis, peripheral and cranial neuritis, myelitis, and neuropsychiatric disturbances. Other end-organ complications of relapsing fever include hepatic failure, myocarditis, abortion in pregnant women, pneumonia, uveitis, iridocyclitis, and hemorrhagic phenomena.

DIAGNOSIS

The diagnosis of relapsing fever is generally made by demonstrating the presence of spirochetes in stained peripheral blood smears. During febrile episodes, *Borrelia* may be seen in approximately 70% of thin or thick Wright- or Giemsa-stained blood smears. Sensitivity can be enhanced by staining fixed smears with fluorescent acridine orange and by using dark-field or phase contrast microscopy. Serologic tests such as enzyme immunoassay or immunofluorescent assays are limited in their diagnostic util-

ity by cross-reactivity with other spirochetes and by antigenic variation of *Borrelia*. Patients with low levels of spirochetemia may be diagnosed only by intraperitoneal animal inoculation and observing for spirochetemia. In vitro cultivation of *Borrelia* from blood using Kelly's growth medium or BSK 11 medium is a specific diagnostic approach, but it is tedious and not widely performed.

TREATMENT

Tetracyclines, erythromycin, and penicillin have been standard therapies for relapsing fever for many years. Due to their rapid clearing of spirochetemia and cumulative clinical experience, tetracyclines are considered the drugs of choice. The recommended duration of treatment differs between the two clinical forms of disease: for epidemic louse-borne relapsing fever, single-dose regimens (doxycycline [Vibramycin] 100 mg, tetracycline [Achromycin, Sumycin] or erythromycin 500 mg) are generally effective, with relapse rates of less than 1%. Intramuscular penicillin aluminum monostearate 1.2 million U,* but not procaine penicillin G, is also effective single-dose therapy. For tick-borne disease, 5 to 10 days of therapy (doxycycline 100 mg twice daily; tetracycline, erythromycin, ampicillin, or penicillin V 500 mg four times a day) is recommended, and most patients can be treated orally as outpatients. Hospitalization and intravenously administered antimicrobial agents may be indicated for severely ill patients. Treatment failures with all agents may be due to an inability to eradicate organisms from the central nervous system.

In pregnant women and children, penicillin or erythromycin should be used. For patients with neurologic involvement, aqueous penicillin G should be considered the agent of choice. Ceftriaxone (Rocephin), the drug of choice in Lyme neuroborreliosis, has been successful in one patient with relapsing fever and central nervous system involvement refractory to penicillin.

JARISCH–HERXHEIMER REACTION

The Jarisch-Herxheimer reaction is a serious and frequent consequence of antimicrobial therapy for relapsing fever, more often seen in louse-borne than tick-borne disease. This clinical syndrome occurs within 1 to 3 hours after the first adequate dose of antibiotic and consists of fever, chills, tachycardia, and a transient rise in blood pressure followed by hypotension and decreased systemic vascular resistance. Blood leukocyte and platelet counts fall, and disseminated intravascular coagulation is accelerated. It is during this crisis that patients are at greatest risk of dying.

The pathophysiologic mechanisms of the Jarisch-Herxheimer reaction have not been precisely elucidated, but the interaction of antibiotics with spirochetes may trigger the release of cytokine intermediates or endogenous opioids. Treatment with penicillin may elicit a milder Jarisch-Herxheimer reaction but is associated

---

*Not available in the United States.

with a longer period of spirochetemia and hypotension than in patients treated with tetracycline. Treatment is generally supportive, emphasizing aggressive intravenous fluid support to maintain adequate intravascular volume; pressor agents may be needed. Attempts to modify or prevent the reaction with various pretreatments such as acetaminophen, hydrocortisone, or meptazinol (an opioid agonist-antagonist) have not shown consistent benefit. Similarly, waiting for an afebrile period before starting therapy or using lower initial doses of antibiotic does not appear to substantially alter the course of the reaction.

PREVENTION

Prevention of relapsing fever focuses on detection and treatment of human cases, avoidance of vector exposure (e.g., personal protection measures, including repellants on clothing and bedding, and antibiotic chemoprophylaxis), vector control (e.g., insecticides to reduce tick and lice populations), and public health education. For tick-borne relapsing fever, preventing rodents from nesting in human shelters reduces human contact with the ticks that transmit the disease. For lice-infected persons, delousing can be accomplished effectively using gamma benzene hexachloride or lindane (Kwell), permethrin (Elimite, Nix), malathion (Prioderm lotion), or pyrethrins–piperonyl butoxide (RID). Clothing and bedding should be washed and ironed to prevent reinfection. Household and close contacts must be examined and deloused if infested.

RHEUMATIC FEVER

method of
ALLAN GIBOFSKY, M.D., J.D.,
*Cornell University Medical College–The Hospital
for Special Surgery
New York, New York*

and

JOHN B. ZABRISKIE, M.D.
*The Rockefeller University
New York, New York*

Acute rheumatic fever (ARF) is a delayed, nonsuppurative outcome of a pharyngeal infection with group A streptococcus. After the initial streptococcal pharyngitis, there is a latent period of 2 to 3 weeks. The onset of disease is usually characterized by an acute febrile illness, which may manifest itself in one of three classic ways:

1. The patient may present with migratory arthritis predominantly involving the large joints of the body.
2. There may be concomitant clinical and laboratory signs of carditis and valvulitis.
3. There may be involvement of the central nervous system, manifesting itself as Sydenham's chorea.

The clinical episodes are self-limiting, but damage to the valves may be chronic and progressive, resulting in cardiac decompensation and death. Although there has been a dramatic decline in both the severity and the mortality of the disease since the early twentieth century, there have been reports of its resurgence in the United States and in many military installations around the world, reminding us that the disease is still present, even in developed countries. In addition, the disease continues unabated in many of the developing countries, with estimates of from 10 to 20 million new cases per year in those countries where two-thirds of the world's population lives.

CLINICAL FEATURES OF ACUTE RHEUMATIC FEVER

The clinical presentation of ARF is quite variable, and the lack of a single pathognomonic feature has resulted in the development of the revised Jones Criteria, as illustrated in Table 1 (Jones Criteria update, 1992), which are used to establish a diagnosis. It should be noted that these criteria were established only as *guidelines* for the diagnosis and were never intended to be "etched in stone." Thus, depending on the age of the patient, geographic location, and ethnic population, emphasis on one or the other criteria for the diagnosis of ARF may be more important than others. Manifestations of rheumatic fever that are not clearly expressed pose a dilemma because of the importance of identifying a first rheumatic attack clearly in order to establish the need for prophylaxis of recurrences (see later). Some of the isolated manifestations, particularly polyarthritis, may be difficult or impossible to distinguish from other diseases, especially at their onset. The diagnosis can be made, however, when "pure" chorea is the sole manifestation because of the rarity with which this syndrome is associated with any other cause.

Arthritis

In the classic, untreated case, the arthritis of rheumatic fever affects several joints in quick succession, each for a short time. The legs are usually affected first and later the arms. The terms "migrating" or "migratory" are often used to describe the polyarthritis of rheumatic fever, but these designations are not meant to signify that the inflammation necessarily disappears in one joint when it appears in another. Rather, the various localizations usually overlap in time, and the onset, as opposed to the full course of the arthritis, "migrates" from joint to joint.

TABLE 1. **Revised Jones Criteria for Diagnosis of Acute Rheumatic Fever**

Major Manifestations	Minor Manifestations
Carditis	Fever
Polyarthritis	Arthralgia
Chorea	Previous rheumatic fever or
Erythema marginatum	rheumatic heart disease
Subcutaneous nodules	
plus	
Supporting evidence of preceding streptococcal infection	
Increased levels of antistreptolysin O or other streptococcal antibodies	
Positive throat culture for group A beta-hemolytic streptococci	
Recent scarlet fever	

From Special Writing Group of the Committee on Rheumatic Fever, Endocarditis, and Kawasaki Disease of the Council on Cardiovascular Disease in the Young of the American Heart Association: Guidelines for the diagnosis of rheumatic fever. JAMA *268*:2069–2070, 1992. Copyright 1992, American Medical Association.

Involvement of the joints is more common, and also more severe, in teenagers and young adults than in children. This involvement occurs early in the rheumatic illness and is usually the earliest symptomatic manifestation of the disease, although asymptomatic carditis may precede it. Rheumatic polyarthritis may be excruciatingly painful but is almost always transient. The pain is usually more prominent than the objective signs of inflammation. Classically, each joint is maximally inflamed for only a few days, or a week at the most, and inflammation may be present in from 6 to 16 joints. The inflammation decreases, perhaps lingering for another week or so, and then disappears completely. Radiographs taken at this point may show a slight effusion but most likely will be unremarkable.

In routine practice, however, many patients with arthritis and/or arthralgias are treated empirically with salicylates or other nonsteroidal anti-inflammatory drugs. Accordingly, arthritis subsides quickly in the joint(s) already affected and does not "migrate" to new joints. Thus, therapy may deprive the diagnostician of a useful sign. In a large series of patients with rheumatic fever and associated arthritis, most of whom had been treated, involvement of only a single large joint was common.

Analysis of the synovial fluid in well-documented cases of rheumatic fever with arthritis generally reveals a sterile inflammatory fluid. There may be a decrease in the level of the complement components C1q, C3, and C4, indicating their consumption by immune complexes in the joint fluid.

Carditis

Cardiac valvular and muscular damage can be manifested in a variety of signs or symptoms. These include organic heart murmurs, cardiomegaly, congestive heart failure, or pericarditis. Mild to moderate chest discomfort, pleuritic chest pain, or a pericardial friction rub is an indication of pericarditis. On clinical examination, the patient can have new or changing organic murmurs. If the valvular damage is severe enough, along with concurrent cardiac dysfunction, congestive heart failure can ensue; this is the most life-threatening clinical syndrome of acute rheumatic fever. Congestive heart failure needs to be treated intensively and quickly with a combination of anti-inflammatory drugs, diuretics, and, occasionally, steroids to acutely decrease cardiac inflammation. Electrocardiographic abnormalities include all degrees of heart block including atrioventricular dissociation. The most common manifestation of carditis is cardiomegaly as seen on radiographs. Studies using echocardiographic techniques suggest that when these more sensitive measurements of cardiac dysfunction are used, nearly all patients with acute rheumatic fever have signs of acute carditis.

Rheumatic Heart Disease

Rheumatic heart disease is the most severe sequela of acute rheumatic fever. Usually occurring 10 to 20 years after the original attack, it is the major cause of acquired valvular disease in the world. The mitral valve is mainly involved, and aortic valve involvement occurs less often. Mitral stenosis is a classified finding in rheumatic heart disease and can manifest itself as a combination of mitral insufficiency and stenosis secondary to severe calcification of the mitral valve. Mitral stenosis needs to be treated surgically, especially when symptoms of left atrial enlargement are seen. However, younger patients with mitral stenosis but no valvular calcification may now be spared valve replacement for some time by the use of percutane-

ous (balloon) mitral valvuloplasty. This may have especially great potential in countries where cardiac surgery is less likely to be available.

In various studies, the incidence of rheumatic heart disease in patients with a history of acute rheumatic fever has varied. In our experience, valvular damage manifesting as organic murmur later in life is still likely to occur in half the patients if they had evidence of carditis at initial diagnosis.

Chorea

Sydenham's chorea, chorea minor, or "St. Vitus' dance" is a neurologic disorder consisting of abrupt, purposeless, nonrhythmic involuntary movements, muscular weakness, and emotional disturbances. The movements disappear during sleep but may occur at rest and may interfere with voluntary activity. Grimaces and inappropriate smiles are common. Handwriting usually becomes clumsy and provides a convenient way of following the patient's course. Speech is often slurred. The movements are commonly more marked on one side and are occasionally completely unilateral (hemichorea).

The muscular weakness is best revealed by asking the patient to squeeze the examiner's hands: the pressure of the patient's grip increases and decreases continuously and capriciously, a phenomenon known as relapsing grip, or milking sign.

The emotional changes manifest themselves in outbursts of inappropriate behavior, including crying and restlessness. In rare cases, the psychological manifestations may be severe and may result in transient psychosis.

The neurologic examination fails to reveal sensory losses or involvement of the pyramidal tract. Diffuse hypotonia may be present. Chorea may follow streptococcal infections after a latent period that is longer, on the average, than the latent period of other rheumatic manifestations. Some patients with chorea have no other symptoms, but other patients develop chorea weeks or months after arthritis. In both cases, examination of the heart may reveal murmurs.

Subcutaneous Nodules

The subcutaneous nodules of rheumatic fever are firm and painless. The overlying skin is not inflamed and can usually be moved over the nodules. The diameter of these round lesions varies from a few millimeters to 1 or even 2 cm. They are located over bony surfaces or prominences, or near tendons, and their number varies from a single nodule to a few dozen and averages three or four; when numerous, they are usually symmetrical. These nodules are present for 1 or more weeks, rarely for more than a month. They are smaller and more short-lived than the nodules of rheumatoid arthritis. Although in both diseases the elbows are most frequently involved, the rheumatic nodules are more common on the olecranon, and the rheumatoid nodules are usually found 3 or 4 cm distal to it. Rheumatic subcutaneous nodules generally appear only after the first weeks of illness, usually only in patients with carditis.

Erythema Marginatum

Erythema marginatum is an evanescent, nonpruritic skin rash, pink or faintly red, affecting usually the trunk and sometimes the proximal parts or the limbs, but not the face. This lesion extends centrifugally while the skin in the center returns to normal; hence the name "erythema marginatum." The outer edge of the lesion is sharp, whereas the inner edge is diffuse. Because the margin of the lesion is usually continuous, making a ring, it is also known as "erythema annulare."

The individual lesions may appear and disappear in a matter of hours, usually to return. A hot bath or shower may make them more evident or may even reveal them for the first time.

Erythema marginatum usually occurs in the early phase of the disease. It often persists or recurs, even when all other manifestations of disease have disappeared. Occasionally, the lesions appear for the first time, or, more likely, are noticed for the first time, late in the course of the illness or even during convalescence. This disorder usually occurs only in patients with carditis.

LABORATORY FINDINGS

The diagnosis of rheumatic fever cannot readily be established by laboratory tests. Serial chest radiographs may be helpful in following the course of carditis, and the electrocardiogram may reflect the inflammatory process on the conduction system.

Throat cultures are usually negative by the time rheumatic fever appears, but an attempt should be made to isolate the organism. It is our practice to take three throat cultures during the first 24 hours of admission before giving antibiotics. Antistreptococcal antibodies are more useful because (1) they reach a peak titer at about the time of onset of rheumatic fever, (2) they indicate true infection rather than transient carriage, and (3) by making several tests of different antibodies, any significant recent streptococcal infection can be detected. It is useful to take one serum specimen upon admission and another one 2 weeks later for comparison. The antibody usually tested for is the antistreptolysin O titer. If the test is negative, one should also test for anti-DNAse B, anti-DNAse, and antihyaluronidase antibodies.

Titers of antistreptolysin do vary with age, season, and geography. Titers of 200 to 300 Todd units per mL are common in healthy children of elementary school age. After a streptococcal pharyngitis, the antibody response peaks at about 4 to 5 weeks, which is usually during the second or third week of rheumatic fever (depending on how early it is detected). Thereafter, antibody titers fall off rapidly in the next several months, and after 6 months they decline more slowly. As only 80% of documented rheumatic fever patients show a rise in the titer of antistreptolysin, it is recommended that other antistreptococcal antibody tests be made in the absence of a positive test for antistreptolysin. Streptococcal antibodies, when their levels are increased, support but do not prove the diagnosis of acute rheumatic fever, nor are they a measure of rheumatic activity.

Acute Phase Reactants

Levels of acute phase reactants are increased during acute rheumatic fever, just as they are during other inflammatory conditions. Both the C-reactive protein and the erythrocyte sedimentation rate (ESR) are almost invariably abnormal during the active rheumatic process if the process is not suppressed by antirheumatic drugs. Pure chorea and persistent erythema marginatum are exceptions. Particularly when treatment has been discontinued or is being tapered off, the C-reactive protein or ESR is useful in monitoring "rebounds" of rheumatic inflammation, which indicate that the rheumatic process is still active. If either the C-reactive protein or ESR remains normal a few weeks after antirheumatic therapy is discontinued, the attack may be considered ended unless chorea appears. Even then, usually, there is no exacerbation of the systemic inflammation and chorea is present as an isolated manifestation.

Anemia

A mild normochromic normocytic anemia of chronic inflammation may be seen during acute rheumatic fever. Suppressing the inflammation usually improves the anemia; thus iron therapy is usually not indicated.

TREATMENT

The mainstay of treatment for acute rheumatic fever has always been anti-inflammatory agents, most commonly aspirin. Dramatic improvement in symptoms is usually seen after the start of therapy. Usually 80 to 100 mg per day in children and 4 to 8 grams per day in adults are required for an effect to be seen. Concentrations of aspirin in serum can be measured, and 20 to 30 mg per dL is the therapeutic range. The duration of anti-inflammatory therapy can vary, but it needs to be maintained until all symptoms are absent and laboratory values are normal. If severe carditis is also present, as indicated by significant cardiomegaly, congestive heart failure, or third-degree heart block, steroid therapy can be instituted. The usual dosage is 2 mg per kg per day of oral prednisone during the first 1 to 2 weeks. Depending on clinical and laboratory improvement, the dosage is then tapered off over the next 2 weeks, and during the last week aspirin may be added, in the dosage recommended above, sufficient to achieve the concentration of 20 to 30 mg per dL.

Whether or not signs of pharyngitis are present at the time of diagnosis, antibiotic therapy with penicillin should be started and maintained for at least 10 days, given in doses recommended for the eradication of a streptococcal pharyngitis. In addition, samples from all family contacts should be cultured and, if the cultures are positive, the contacts should be treated for streptococcal infection. If compliance is an issue, depot penicillins, i.e., benzathine penicillin G 600,000 U in children, 1.2 million U in adults, should be given. Recurrences of acute rheumatic fever are most common within 2 years of the original attack but can happen at any time. The risk of recurrence decreases with age. Recurrence rates have been decreasing, from 20 to between 2 and 4% in recent outbreaks. This may be due to better surveillance and treatment.

PROPHYLAXIS

Antibiotic prophylaxis with penicillin should be started immediately after the resolution of the acute episode. The optimal regimen consists of oral penicillin VK, 250,000 U twice a day, or intramuscularly injected depot penicillin (1.2 million U of penicillin G benzathine) every 4 weeks. Recent data suggest, however, that injections every 3 weeks are more effective in preventing recurrences of acute rheumatic fever than those every 4 weeks. If the patient is allergic to penicillin, erythromycin, 250 mg twice daily, can be substituted.

The end point of prophylaxis is unclear; most believe it should continue at least until the patient is a young adult, which is usually 10 years from an acute attack with no recurrence. In our opinion, individuals with documented evidence of rheumatic heart disease should be on continuous prophylaxis indefinitely, as our experience has been that rheumatic fever can recur even in the fifth or sixth decade. Another potential problem for these recurrences is in those who have young children in the household, who could transmit new group A streptococcal infections to the rheumatic fever–susceptible individual.

Obviously, the alternative to long-term prophylaxis in a person with rheumatic fever will be the introduction of streptococcal vaccines designed not only to prevent recurrent infections in rheumatic-susceptible persons but also to prevent streptococcal disease in general.

LYME DISEASE AND EHRLICHIOSIS

method of
ELLIOT FRANK, M.D.
Jersey Shore Medical Center
Neptune, New Jersey

LYME DISEASE

Lyme disease is a multisystem inflammatory illness caused by infection with the spirochete *Borrelia burgdorferi*. In Europe, skin lesions now associated with Lyme disease were described as far back as 1883 and various neurologic manifestations were documented during the first half of the twentieth century. However, not until 1976 was Lyme disease recognized as a single clinical entity, as a result of the landmark observations of Steere, then at the Yale University School of Medicine. Lyme disease has been reported from much of the world, but tends to occur in geographically defined areas. In the United States, over 90% of cases originate in eight states: New York, New Jersey, Connecticut, Rhode Island, Massachusetts, Pennsylvania, Wisconsin, and Minnesota, although cases have been reported from at least 46 states.

The principal vectors for Lyme disease in the United States are the deer ticks *Ixodes dammini* and *I. pacificus*. Other ticks and insects are unlikely to harbor or transmit *B. burgdorferi*. Ixodid nymphs (the size of a sesame seed) are responsible for 70 to 80% of Lyme disease transmission. Larvae (the size of a poppy seed) are rarely infected. Adult ticks, although frequently infected, are less likely to transmit *B. burgdorferi* to humans because there are fewer of them, they are more easily seen and re-

moved, and they appear in colder months, when fewer people venture into tick habitats and if they do are protected by layers of clothing.

Clinical Manifestations

Early Localized Lyme Disease

Erythema migrans (EM), the only pathognomonic feature of Lyme disease, occurs between 3 and 32 days after the tick bite, which is recalled by only about 30% of patients. EM begins as an erythematous macule or papule at the site of the bite, often in the groin, thigh, or axilla. The skin lesion is painless and rarely burns or itches as it expands over days. Central clearing is common, and multiple concentric circles (targets) are seen frequently; induration, vesiculation, and necrosis are rare. Many patients with EM have no symptoms. In others, a nonspecific constellation of symptoms (fatigue, malaise, headache, myalgias, arthralgias, lymphadenopathy) may precede, accompany, or follow the rash. Since only 50 to 70% of patients with early Lyme disease develop EM, it follows that early Lyme disease may manifest as a nonspecific febrile illness or may be clinically silent. Respiratory symptoms—cough, coryza, and exudative pharyngitis—are not features of Lyme disease and argue against the diagnosis.

Early Disseminated Lyme Disease

About 50% of patients with untreated EM develop multiple skin lesions due to hematogenous dissemination of the spirochete. Of greater concern, however, are cardiac and neurologic manifestations that occur in the first few months following infection. Atrioventricular conduction delay is seen in 8% of untreated patients with Lyme disease, whereas neurologic involvement occurs in 15%. Early neurologic symptoms characteristically involve cranial neuropathy (most often unilateral or bilateral seventh nerve palsy), lymphocytic meningitis or meningoencephalitis, and painful radiculopathies.

Late Lyme Disease

Lyme disease is associated with a variety of musculoskeletal manifestations, including polyarthralgias, true arthritis, tendinitis, bursitis, and fibromyalgia. The arthritis of Lyme disease is an asymmetrical, intermittent, mono- or oligoarticular disease, most often involving the knee. About 10% of patients go on to have chronic, persistent synovitis with or without erosive changes. Fibromyalgia may occur during or after Lyme disease and is not felt to be related to active infection and, therefore, not responsive to antibiotic therapy.

The greatest difficulty and confusion surround the issue of late neurologic manifestations of Lyme disease. Often termed "tertiary neuroborreliosis," this syndrome of progressive encephalomyelopathy, polyneuritis, and mental or psychiatric change is due to chronic central nervous system infection with *B. burgdorferi*. It may be the first manifestation of latent Lyme disease or occasionally occur in a patient previously treated for an earlier manifestation of Lyme disease.

Diagnosis

Lyme disease is a clinical diagnosis confirmed by serologic testing utilizing enzyme-linked immunosorbent assay (ELISA) and Western blot (WB) technologies (Figure 1). It is crucial that results of antibody detection tests be interpreted carefully. A negative serology result most often means the patient has not been infected with *B. burgdorferi*. In early disease, however, even IgM antibodies may not have had a chance to develop, and a negative result should not deter treatment when the clinical picture is suggestive. Antibiotic treatment very early in the course of Lyme disease may abrogate the antibody response; thus occasional patients given antibiotics for other diagnoses (but inadequate to treat Lyme disease) may develop progressive illness with negative serologic tests.

A positive serologic test is useful in confirming a diagnosis of Lyme disease. When the clinical picture is nonspecific, however, a positive antibody test may be misleading, reflecting either a false-positive result from cross-reacting antibodies or a true-positive result related to prior exposure to the organism but *unrelated* to the patient's current complaints. Western blotting is useful in distinguishing false-positive from true-positive results but cannot substitute for clinical judgment in the latter situation.

Comparing antibody concentrations in cerebrospinal fluid and synovial fluid with serum levels, using techniques that control for total protein synthesis, may be useful in some circumstances.

TABLE 1. Antibiotic Treatment of Lyme Disease*

Early localized Lyme disease Isolated facial palsy (with normal CSF)	Doxycycline, 100 mg PO bid Amoxicillin, 500 mg PO tid Cefuroxime axetil (Ceftin), 500 mg PO bid
All other manifestations	Ceftriaxone (Rocephin), 2 gm IV q day Cefotaxime (Claforan), 3 gm IV bid Penicillin G, 4 million U IV q 4 h

*All regimens should be administered for 21 to 28 days.
Abbreviation: CSF = cerebrospinal fluid.

B. burgdorferi is difficult to grow in the laboratory, so that culture is thus far an impractical diagnostic modality. Polymerase chain reaction, antigen detection assays, and serum borreliacidal assays are currently being investigated as possible adjuncts to diagnosis.

Treatment

Our approach to managing patients with Lyme disease is outlined in Table 1. Unfortunately, a paucity of data exists on which to base some of these recommendations, and thus controversy abounds. There certainly are anecdotal data to support the use of oral antibiotics in early, disseminated infection: cardiac disease with mild first-degree heart block (PR less than 0.28), EM with multiple lesions, early arthritis, and even mild neurologic disease. However, because early dissemination may be associated with central nervous system infection, we prefer intravenous therapy to help obviate a re-emergence of Lyme disease at a later date.

Figure 1. Diagnostic algorithm for Lyme disease (LD). *Abbreviations*: ELISA = enzyme-linked immunosorbent assay; WB = Western blot.

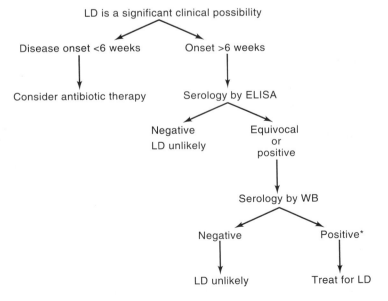

*An IgG WB is considered positive if 5 of 10 bands (18, 21, 28, 30, 39, 41, 45, 58, 66, 93) are reactive. An IgM WB is considered positive if 2 of 4 bands (21/24, 37, 39, 41) are reactive

Patients with heart block, especially with PR greater than 0.28, should be admitted and monitored; temporary pacing may be needed. Some patients with arthritis who do not respond to antibiotics have been successfully treated with hydroxychloroquine (Plaquenil) or synovectomy. Fibromyalgia—as opposed to Lyme arthritis—will not respond to antibiotics but often will improve with aerobic exercise and tricyclic antidepressants, given in small doses at bedtime.

Pregnancy

Although we know that *B. burgdorferi* can cross the placenta and several case reports have documented fetal damage in association with Lyme disease, prospective studies of pregnant women with Lyme disease have not documented the presence of a "congenital Lyme syndrome" and cord blood surveys have failed to demonstrate a link between poor fetal outcome and in utero exposure. The evidence thus suggests that if in utero exposure is associated with adverse outcomes, this is extremely uncommon. Therefore, there is currently *no* justification for screening serology studies in pregnant women; women with Lyme disease should be treated as would be appropriate for their clinical manifestations.

Tick Bites

The management of tick bites is another area of controversy. It is clear from several prospective studies that the risk of acquiring Lyme disease following a tick bite, even in highly endemic areas, is less than 1%. It should be noted that transmission of disease requires tick attachment for at least 24 hours. In general, most patients can be reassured and educated about the signs and symptoms of early Lyme disease. For patients who find fully engorged ticks in highly endemic areas or who are particularly anxious, re-evaluation with follow-up serology studies can be done 6 to 8 weeks after the tick bite and the rare, silent seroconverter then treated.

Persistent Symptoms

In our experience, the most common reasons for persistent symptoms following treatment of Lyme disease reflect either the natural history of Lyme disease, misdiagnosis, or fibromyalgia. Facial palsy, chronic neurologic symptoms, and musculoskeletal symptoms of Lyme disease may take months to resolve. Chronic fatigue syndrome (CFS) may have been mistaken for Lyme disease and both CFS and fibromyalgia have been reported following Lyme disease. In some patients with chronic neurologic disease, some residual deficit, unresponsive to antibiotics, may persist. To be sure, as in any infection, occasional patients may relapse and require retreatment. This is a clinical judgment that should be made carefully, as there is currently no test that can distinguish between adequately treated Lyme disease and active infection. In any event, there is no scientific evidence to support the use of prolonged oral or intravenous therapy, and there are very definite and occasionally life-threatening risks associated with this approach (neutropenia, biliary sludging, pseudomembranous colitis, and catheter sepsis).

EHRLICHIOSIS

Since the original report of human ehrlichiosis in 1987, more than 250 cases have been described in the United States, with most cases occurring in the South Central and South Atlantic states. Infection with the human pathogen *Ehrlichia chaffeensis* generally results in a nonspecific illness that resembles Rocky Mountain spotted fever. Fever and headache are characteristic; malaise, myalgias, nausea, vomiting, and anorexia are common. A maculopapular or petechial rash occurs in 20% of patients and only occasionally involves the palms or soles. The course may be complicated by renal failure, respiratory failure, or encephalopathy. Death due to ehrlichiosis has been documented but is rare.

Laboratory abnormalities are variable and mainly nonspecific: leukopenia, lymphopenia, thrombocytopenia, abnormal liver function tests, and cerebrospinal fluid (CSF) pleocytosis. Morulae, mulberry-like inclusion bodies representing clumps of the small, gram-negative, pleomorphic, coccobacillary causative agent, can be seen in blood leukocytes or CSF mononuclear cells and will greatly aid diagnosis in occasional patients. Treatment with a tetracycline or chloramphenicol should be initiated when the diagnosis is suspected, since confirmation of diagnosis will most often require convalescent serology as much as 4 weeks from the onset of illness.

ROCKY MOUNTAIN SPOTTED FEVER

method of
ERIC L. WESTERMAN, M.D.
Tulsa Infectious Disease Clinic, Inc.
Tulsa, Oklahoma

Rocky Mountain Spotted fever (RMSF) is the most commonly reported tick-related infection occurring in humans in the United States. It was first described by Howard Ricketts from his observations in the Bitterroot Valley of Montana. The name is a misnomer because the disease is now rarely found in the Rocky Mountain region. Rashless disease, or "spotless fever," is not uncommon, occurring in 10 to 15% of cases. The causative organism is *Rickettsia rickettsii*, an obligate intracellular parasite closely related to other arthropod-borne rickettsial organisms causing disease in the continental United States.

Ticks serve as both vectors and hosts for the organism. They become infected by feeding on infected animals. Female ticks pass the organism to their male and female offspring (transovarial passage). Thus a single infected female tick may produce thousands of infected progeny without the intervention of another host. Dogs and rodents are important reservoirs for the organism. The dog tick (*Dermacentor variabilis*), the wood tick (*Dermacentor andersoni*), and the Lone Star tick (*Amblyomma americanum*) are the major tick vectors. Humans usually acquire the infection from the attachment of an infected tick; however, infection may occur from the handling or crushing of ticks with the fingers.

The disease occurs most often in the southern and southeastern United States. Oklahoma, North Carolina, South Carolina, and Tennessee report approximately 50% of all cases annually, but few states are devoid of this illness. The history of exposure to ticks or wooded areas is obtained from 60 to 70% of infected persons. Conversely at least 30% of patients report no such risk factor. Illness occurs most often in warmer months, when ticks are active, with most cases reported between April and November. Disease occurs occasionally in urban areas (e.g., New York City), where the risk would appear to be small. Death occurs in 30 to 40% of those with untreated illness, but in only 5% of those treated before the first week of illness.

CLINICAL MANIFESTATIONS

The rickettsiae parasitize endothelial cells, leading to a diffuse vasculitis that is responsible for the clinical manifestations of the disease. All organ systems may be involved, but the skin is the most commonly recognized organ. Clinical disease usually occurs 2 to 14 days after the bite of an infected tick. The onset is usually abrupt with the classic triad of fever, chills, and the eventual development of a rash. Although the symptoms may occasionally present gradually, asymptomatic disease or disease without fever does not occur. Headache and myalgias are the next most common symptoms, and disease without at least one of these complaints is rare.

The characteristic rash occurring on the third to fifth day of the illness is one of the most common clues leading one to suspect the disease. Typically, the rash occurs on the extremities and then spreads toward the trunk. This is distinguished from the rash of murine typhus, which typically begins on the trunk and spreads outward (centrifugal). The classic involvement of the palms and soles in RMSF is present in only 10 to 15% of cases, and the absence of this finding should not be relied upon to exclude suspicion of the disease. The rash is variable, consisting of macules, papules, and petechiae, with one or more predominating. It does not itch, and the presence of pruritus should suggest another disease. Vesicles and pustules are likewise rare.

Nausea, vomiting, abdominal pain, confusion, cough, and other nonspecific symptoms illustrate the widespread organ involvement that occurs. Mild lymphadenopathy and hepatosplenomegaly are not uncommon physical findings. The most common laboratory findings include hyponatremia (95%), leukopenia, thrombocytopenia, elevated blood urea nitrogen (BUN) and creatinine levels, cerebrospinal fluid (CSF) pleocytosis, elevated (rarely above 100) transaminase and alkaline phosphatase levels, and a prolonged prothrombin time. Occasionally a single organ system finding such as the central nervous system (meningoencephalitis), gallbladder (cholecystitis), or lungs (pneumonitis) predominates. Viscerotropic disease may cause abdominal findings that lead to exploratory laparotomy. Occasionally fulminant RMSF can occur with rapid onset of shock, renal failure, and disseminated intravascular coagulation mimicking other forms of septic shock. Spotless fever may occur more often in fulminant disease.

Clinical manifestations of RMSF are similar to those of several other acute febrile illnesses that may occur after arthropod exposure, and these should be included in the differential diagnosis (Table 1). *Ehrlichia chaffeensis*, a rickettsia-like gram-negative coccobacillary organism that parasitizes mononuclear phagocytes, causes acute febrile illness after tick bite. Rash is less common (30%), but leukopenia, thrombocytopenia, transaminase level elevation, and aseptic meningitis are more prominent than in RMSF. Murine typhus caused by *Rickettsia typhi* is transmitted by the rat flea, occurring mostly in the southeastern and Gulf Coast states. Symptoms are identical to those of RMSF, but the rash distribution is different and laboratory abnormalities are mild. Tularemia may occur either after tick bite or after contact with infected animal hosts. Leukopenia is milder than with RMSF, rash is unusual, and onset is more gradual. Local organ involvement such as regional lymphadenopathy (ulceroglandular), oculoglandular disease, or pneumonitis is more common. A recently described disease, human granulocytic ehrlichiosis, is caused by an organism similar to *Ehrlichia phagocytophila* or *E. equi*. It typically presents with more profound leukopenia and thrombocytopenia, and intracytoplasmic inclusions may be found within neutrophils. Colorado tick fever, caused by an RNA virus, usually presents as a biphasic febrile illness with thrombocytopenia after tick bite.

Other diseases unrelated to tick exposure that may present with similar clinical presentations as RMSF include atypical measles, dengue fever, enteroviral infections, Stevens-Johnson syndrome, drug eruptions, hemolytic uremia syndrome, and thrombotic thrombocytopenic purpura (TTP)

DIAGNOSIS

The diagnosis of acute RMSF must be made on clinical grounds. Laboratory confirmation can only rarely be made during acute clinical illness. Immunofluorescent staining of a skin biopsy specimen is the only reliable way of confirming the diagnosis on initial presentation of illness, but this technique is not widely available. Specific serologic tests on acute and convalescent sera should be used to confirm the diagnosis. The indirect fluorescent antibody test (IFAT) is the most commonly used serologic test followed by latex agglutination (LA), complement fixation (CF), or indirect hemagglutination (IHA). A case is considered probable if a convalescent serum sample shows a titer of at least 1:128 by LA or IHA, 1:64 by IFAT, 1:16 by CF, or a fourfold rise in titer by either of these methods. The interval from the onset of illness to the initial detection of antibody for the various tests is 6 to 14 days for IFAT, IHA, and LA and 14 to 28 days for CF. The Weil-Felix test using *Proteus* OX-19 and *Proteus* OX-2 (so-called febrile agglutinins) is insensitive and nonspecific. This test is obsolete and should not be used. The failure to diagnose or suspect RMSF may result in severe disease or death. The presumptive diagnosis should be made in the proper clinical setting before laboratory confirmation can be obtained, and appropriate therapy should be instituted. In the setting of acute febrile illness during warm months of the year with headache or myalgias, leukopenia, or thrombocytopenia, with or without rash, and with potential tick exposure, the diagnosis should be strongly entertained.

TREATMENT

Tetracyclines and chloramphenicol are the only antibiotics proved to be effective for the treatment of RMSF. Treatment with one of these agents should be started as early as possible to prevent complications or death. Doxycycline (Vibramycin, Doryx) is the preferred tetracycline and has been reported to be effective with as short a course as 3 days in mild cases.

TABLE 1. **Common Characteristics of Rocky Mountain Spotted Fever and Similar Illnesses**

	RMSF	Colorado Tick Fever	Ehrlichiosis	Murine Typhus	Tularemia	Dengue
Vector	Tick	Tick	Tick	Flea	Tick, mammals	Mosquito
Fever, headache	+++	+++	+++	+++	+++	+++
Rash	+++	−	+	++	−	+++
Leukopenia	++	++	+++	−	−	−
Thrombocytopenia	+	++	+++	+	−	++
Hyponatremia	+++	−	+	+	+	−
↑ Creatinine	+	−	++	−	−	+
↑ ALT (SGPT)	+	−	+++	+	+	+

Abbreviations and symbols: ALT = alanine aminotransferase, formerly known as SGPT (serum glutamic-pyruvic transaminase); − = <10%; + = 10–25%; ++ = 25–50%; +++ = >50%

In nonpregnant adults and children over the age of 8 years it is the treatment of choice, particularly since it is also effective against ehrlichiosis, which is often included in the differential diagnosis of RMSF. The usual dose is 100 mg orally or intravenously every 12 hours. The intravenous route is recommended initially for severe disease. No dosage adjustment is necessary for renal disease. Tetracycline hydrochloride may be used, but the dosage must be adjusted for renal dysfunction. Chloramphenicol (Chloromycetin) should be used for the treatment of infants, children less than 9 years of age, and pregnant patients and when there is a suspicion of meningococcal disease. It may be given either orally or intravenously with a loading dose of 100 mg per kg and subsequently at 50 to 100 mg per kg per day in four divided doses. Therapy with either agent should be given until the patient has been afebrile for 3 to 5 days.

The mortality from the disease is considerably lower in children than in adults, and controversy exists over which drug is safest to administer in children when the diagnosis is suspected but unclear. Tetracyclines are known to stain teeth, but rarely if given for less than 5 days. There is concern about the rare complication of fatal agranulocytosis occurring after chloramphenicol therapy. Both drugs are effective, but chloramphenicol is less effective for *Ehrlichia* infections. A short course of doxycycline for children is safe. Quinolones such as ciprofloxacin (Cipro) and ofloxacin (Floxin) have been shown to be effective against rickettsiae in vitro and in other rickettsial illness, but there is no proven clinical benefit in RMSF, and they cannot be recommended at this time. Erythromycin, clindamycin (Cleocin), penicillins, cephalosporins, aminoglycosides, and sulfonamides are all ineffective.

Supportive therapy with intravenous fluid should be used, especially when azotemia or dehydration is present. Corticosteroids have not been proved to be useful but should be considered in severe disease with shock or meningoencephalitis.

PREVENTION

Prevention of tick attachment is the only effective preventive measure. The use of tick or insect repellents may be helpful. The body should be promptly inspected after travel to wooded areas so that ticks can be removed before attachment. Ticks should be removed with forceps or tissue rather than the bare hands, and they should never be crushed with the fingers. No effective vaccine exists for RMSF. Treatment of tick infestation in pet dogs is encouraged. Prophylactic treatment with antibiotics after a tick bite is ineffective, since antibiotics are bacteriostatic and they only delay but do not prevent the development of clinical disease. Infection with RMSF probably confers lifelong immunity but does not offer protection against other rickettsial infections.

RUBELLA AND CONGENITAL RUBELLA

method of
BARRY M. KARPEL, D.O., and
DAVID A. BAKER, M.D.
University Medical Center at Stony Brook
Stony Brook, New York

Rubella is a single-stranded RNA togavirus, genus *Rubivirus*. The virus is 50 to 70 nm in diameter. There is only one naturally occurring immunologically distinct type. Humans are the only known host for the rubella virus.

EPIDEMIOLOGY

Prior to the widespread availability and use of the rubella vaccine in the 1970s, rubella in the United States was episodic, with epidemics occurring at 6- to 9-year intervals. In the winter and spring of 1964–1965, it is estimated that more than 12.5 million cases of rubella occurred. During this period, congenital rubella infection occurred in an estimated 30,000 pregnancies. Fetal death occurred or therapeutic abortion was performed in 10,000 cases, and approximately 20,000 infants were born with congenital rubella syndrome. Since the initiation of rubella immunization in 1969, there have been no rubella epidemics in the United States. Only 225 cases of rubella were reported to the Centers for Disease Control and Prevention (CDC) in 1988, and in 1989 there were two cases of congenital rubella syndrome reported. However, outbreaks of rubella continue to occur. From January 1, 1990, through January 8, 1991, 23 infants with congenital rubella syndrome and two infants with congenital rubella infection were born in four southern California counties. This represents the largest cluster of congenital rubella syndrome reported in the last decade. Rubella susceptibility has shifted toward older age groups since the implementation of universal immunization of infants with the measles-mumps-rubella (MMR) vaccine. Sporadic outbreaks are now occurring on college campuses.

PATHOGENESIS

Rubella is an exanthematous viral infection usually associated with little mortality. Mild disease occurs in children, with a peak incidence between 5 and 9 years of age. The virus is spread by inhalation of aerosolized droplets or through direct contact with contaminated material or infected individuals. Rubella enters the host through the upper respiratory tract and then spreads to regional lymph nodes, where viral replication takes place. Viremia occurs 7 to 9 days after exposure, and multiple tissue sites can be affected. By 9 to 11 days after exposure, viral shedding occurs from various sites such as the upper respiratory tract, kidneys, cervix, placenta, and gastrointestinal tract. Nasopharyngeal shedding of the virus lasts 2 weeks. Rubella is thought to be most infectious from 5 days before to 6 days after the appearance of the rash. The rash typically appears 16 to 18 days after exposure.

CLINICAL MANIFESTATIONS

Rubella infection can be overlooked or misdiagnosed because its signs and symptoms are usually mild and variable. In children, approximately 50% of cases are subclinical. With increasing age, the proportion of subclinical infection falls, and in adults, the majority of infections are symptomatic. Similar exanthematous illnesses are caused by adenovirus, enterovirus, parvovirus, and other common respiratory viruses.

Symptoms of rubella occur after a 14- to 21-day incubation period. The typical macular rash is preceded by a prodrome of malaise, fever, headache, conjunctivitis, and lymphadenopathy (posterior auricular, posterior cervical, and suboccipital). The prodrome lasts from 1 to 5 days. The rash appears 16 to 18 days after exposure. It begins on the face and thorax and progresses caudally and distally over 1 to 2 days. The rash usually disappears in 3 days in the order in which it appeared. Rubella in children is usually mild, with little or no systemic upset. They may have mild or absent fever and only a fleeting rash. Infection in immunocompromised patients is not remarkably severe, nor does it have an unusual presentation. Pregnancy does not alter the clinical course of rubella infection.

COMPLICATIONS

The major complication of rubella is the potential for congenital rubella syndrome when infection occurs early in pregnancy. The rash may be accompanied by transient arthralgias in up to one-third of adults. The small joints of the hands and wrists are most frequently involved. Symptoms usually resolve within a month, but in some individuals, they can persist for much longer. Thrombocytopenic purpura, neuritis, heart block, and encephalitis are rare complications, with the latter occurring in 1 per 10,000 cases.

DIAGNOSIS

The clinical diagnosis of rubella is often difficult, since it resembles a number of other exanthemas. Diagnosis should not be based solely on clinical criteria. A number of antibody tests are available to confirm infection, including latex agglutination, fluorescence immunoassay, passive hemagglutination, and enzyme immunoassay.

In the past, the hemagglutinating inhibition antibody test was the most commonly used screening method. This method screens for IgG class antibody, which, after wild virus infection, usually remains positive for life. A titer of greater than 1:8 is conclusive evidence of immunity. A titer of 1:8 should be repeated. If the second titer is equal to or greater than 1:8, the patient probably has long-lasting immunity. If the second titer shows a fourfold rise, the patient has acute rubella infection.

Most laboratories now use the enzyme-linked immunosorbent assay (ELISA) for screening. Antibody serum is detected by an antihuman globulin conjugated to an enzyme. The amount of enzyme conjugate is proportional to the amount of serum antibody; the amount of enzyme is determined colormetrically and read in absorbance units at a given wavelength. An absorbance reading is selected as a breakpoint to correlate with the reference hemagglutinating inhibition antibody titer of 1:8. Values below this are reported as rubella nonimmune, whereas values above this are reported as rubella immune. The ELISA cannot quantitate antibody titer, so if acute infection is suspected, another method must be utilized. Complement-fixing antibody is also an IgG class antibody. Because it appears later than hemagglutinating inhibition antibody, it may be useful in patients first seen 1 to 5 weeks after exposure, when a significant rise in complement-fixing antibody may be seen but it is too late to demonstrate this change in hemagglutinating antibody.

IgM antibodies appear early and last for only a few weeks. The presence of rubella-specific IgM is indicative of recent primary infection. In some patients, IgM may disappear in less than 4 weeks, so the absence of IgM does not exclude recent infection.

TREATMENT

Treatment of rubella illness is directed at the relief of symptoms. Currently, no antiviral therapy is effective at attenuating viremia or decreasing transplacental transmission of the virus. Immune globulin is not recommended for routine use as a postexposure prophylaxis. In 1981, the advisory committee of the CDC noted that immune globulin given after exposure did not prevent infection or viremia and was therefore of no benefit.

IMMUNIZATION

Universal immunization, instituted in 1969, was aimed at eliminating maternal rubella infection and congenital rubella syndrome. Live rubella virus vaccine is recommended for all children and susceptible people older than 12 months of age. The vaccine should not be given to infants, since persisting maternal antibodies may interfere with seroconversion.

Live rubella virus vaccine distributed in the United States is prepared in human diploid cell culture. In January 1979, this vaccine (RA 27/3) replaced the HPV-77 DE-5 vaccine, which was grown in duck embryo cell culture. The newer vaccine offers a higher seroresponse, greater resistance to reinfection, and fewer side reactions. The RA 27/3 strand is included in the MMR vaccine and confers long-lasting immunity in 95% of individuals. Clinical efficacy and challenge studies have shown that the vaccine protects against both viremia and clinical rubella for at least 15 years and, based on follow-up studies, vaccine-induced protection is probably lifelong. Thus, immunity can be inferred if a patient has had one dose of rubella vaccine after age 1 year or if he or she has documented laboratory evidence of immunity.

After receiving the rubella vaccine, an individual can expect to experience mild rubella-like symptoms such as low-grade fever, rash, and lymphadenopathy. Reports of significant adverse reactions are rare. Severe joint pain and transient arthritis with visible joint swelling have been reported, but these adverse reactions are self-limited. To date, passive surveillance systems in the United States have failed to show an association between chronic joint problems and rubella vaccine.

Absolute contraindications to rubella vaccine include immunologic compromise and pregnancy. Recent blood transfusion and the administration of anti-Rh$_O$ (D) immune globulin (RhoGAM) are not contraindications to rubella vaccine. However, they represent the only cases in which routine postvaccination (6 to 8 weeks) serologic testing is recommended to confirm that seroconversion has occurred. It is recommended that rubella vaccine be given at least 3 weeks after the administration of another live virus vaccine and at least 3 months after the administration of human immune globulin.

CONGENITAL RUBELLA INFECTION

Congenital rubella syndrome was described in 1941 by N. McAlister Gregg after he found congenital defects in infants born to mothers who had had antepartum rubella infection. After this finding, rubella became a serious obstetric and public health problem.

The risk of intrauterine infection after maternal rubella at successive stages of pregnancy has been assessed. The reported risk of congenital rubella syndrome is as follows: 90% at less than 11 weeks gestation, 33% at 11 to 12 weeks gestation, 11% at 13 to 14 weeks gestation, and 24% at 15 to 16 weeks gestation. At greater than 16 weeks gestation, occasional cases of deafness may be attributable to intrauterine infection. After 24 weeks gestation, the risk to the fetus is close to zero.

The classic triad of congenital rubella syndrome consists of deformities of the eye (cataracts, microphthalmos, chorioretinitis), deformities of the heart (patent ductus arteriosus and pulmonary artery stenosis), and sensorineural deafness. Hearing loss is the most common manifestation. In utero, microencephaly, intrauterine growth restriction, and hepatosplenomegaly may develop. Mental retardation, purpura, immune-mediated pneumonitis, progressive panencephalitis, and diabetes mellitus may occur after birth.

In women with confirmed rubella infection during pregnancy, management consists of counseling about the risks and types of congenital anomalies. Fetal diagnosis is difficult because amniotic fluid culture does not distinguish an infected fetus from an uninfected one. Rubella-specific IgM has been detected in fetal blood through the use of percutaneous umbilical blood sampling (PUBS) performed at midpregnancy. PUBS must be performed more than 2 weeks after the onset of clinical infection and after 22 weeks gestation because the human fetus cannot produce detectable IgM until 19 to 20 weeks gestation. The information gained may be used to counsel patients, but there are serious limitations to the procedure, including risk of fetal loss and the possibility of false-negative or false-positive results.

Postpartum immunization can prevent 33 to 50% of all congenital rubella syndrome cases. Women who have had both negative and positive rubella titers should be vaccinated if there is no documentation of vaccination after a negative result. Women with equivocal results should be vaccinated. The CDC reported data on 324 infants born to mothers who had received rubella vaccine up to 3 months before conception or during the first trimester. None of the infants in the report had defects indicative of congenital rubella syndrome. Although the observed risk of congenital malformations after the vaccine is zero, the theoretical risk may be as high as 1 to 6%. This information must be used to counsel patients who inadvertently received vaccine during the 3 months prior to conception and during the first trimester. Rubella vaccine may be given during breast-feeding. Some infants become infected through breast milk and develop a mild rash. Most remain asymptomatic, and no serious effects have been reported.

MEASLES

method of
JAMES B. HANSHAW, M.D.
Medical Center of Central Massachusetts
Worcester, Massachusetts

Measles is an acute disease caused by an RNA virus with one antigenic type. It is classified as a morbillivirus of the Paramyxoviridae family. The illness is characterized by a course of approximately 7 days with high fever, coryza, conjunctivitis, and cough. There is a characteristic enanthem (Koplik spots) and exanthem (maculopapular rash). Death from measles in the United States declined before the use of the measles vaccine presumably because of antibiotics and improved nutrition. In developing countries, measles is still a life-threatening disease with a case fatality rate of 3 to 5% in countries with high infant mortality rates. Major factors in this mortality rate are thought to be poor nutritional status with a relatively high prevalence of vitamin A deficiency, a heavy disease burden from other infectious diseases, crowding and intensity of exposure, and lack of access to appropriate care.

EPIDEMIOLOGY

The wide use of measles vaccine in the United States since 1963 resulted in a 99% decrease in the incidence of the disease by 1981. Before the introduction of the vaccine, approximately 500,000 cases were reported annually. In 1989 and 1990, outbreaks of measles occurred among poor, inner-city preschool children. These outbreaks represented a public health failure rather than a failure of the vaccine to protect. Most cases reported in recent years have not received one dose of vaccine.

Measles remains one of the most contagious of infectious diseases. More than 90% of susceptible household contacts contract the disease. Exposure in a school, on a bus, or in a hospital results in disease in 25% of susceptible contacts. An infected person is contagious 3 to 5 days before the onset of the rash and for 5 days thereafter. The incubation period is 8 to 12 days after exposure, with the rash usually appearing an average of 14 days after exposure.

Measles is endemic over most of the world. Epidemics occur every 2 to 3 years in developing countries with peak incidence in the winter and spring.

PASSIVE IMMUNIZATION

Immune globulin (IG) (Gamastan, Gammar), if given within 6 days of exposure to measles, prevents or modifies the disease. Passive immunization with IG is indicated for susceptible household contacts of measles patients, immunocompromised contacts, and pregnant women in whom the risk of complications is high. The usual dose is 0.25 mL per kg of body weight given intramuscularly. Immunocompromised persons should receive 0.5 mL per kg. (The maximum amount of either dose is 15 mL.) Once the child is over 12 months of age, measles vaccination can begin 5 to 6 months after IG is administered.

Patients receiving intravenous IG (Gamimune N, Polygam, Sandoglobulin), at the usual dose of 100 to 400 mL per kg are protected from measles for 3 weeks or more. If 300 to 400 mL per kg is used, active immunization with measles vaccine should not be undertaken for 8 months. Larger intravenous IG doses of 1000 mL per kg or more require an interval of 10 to 11 months before vaccination should be attempted.

Passive immunization should not be used to control measles outbreaks in schools or communities. Available data suggest that live-virus measle vaccine should be the intervention of choice for the control of school or community measles outbreaks. If given within 72 hours after exposure, the vaccine provides protection in some susceptible persons exposed to the virus. Prevention of subsequent measles infection occurs in almost all cases.

ACTIVE IMMUNIZATION

Measles vaccine is prepared from a live, further-attenuated measles virus prepared in chick embryo cell culture. It is available as a monovalent vaccine (Attenuvax), or in combination with rubella (MR) and mumps vaccines (MMR). The MMR is the vaccine of choice for routine vaccination of children. When one dose is administered at 15 months or older, approximately 95% develop serum measles antibody following a mild or inapparent noncommunicable infection. Waning immunity following vaccination does occur but only in a small percentage of individuals.

At the present time, it is recommended that measles vaccine be given at 15 months (12 months in high-risk areas), and at entry to middle or junior high school unless two doses were given after the first birthday. College students should have either serologic evidence of immunity or receipt of two doses of measles-containing vaccine after 12 months of age and at least 1 month apart. Physician-diagnosed disease is no longer accepted in some states presumably because there is now a generation of physicians with little or no experience with measles.

CONTRAINDICATIONS AND PRECAUTIONS

Pregnancy, compromised immunity, and a history of anaphylactic reactions to egg or neomycin are contraindications to the receipt of measles vaccine. Women who are given the vaccine should not become pregnant for at least 30 days. There is a theoretical risk that the live vaccine virus could be transmitted to the fetus.

The Committee on Infectious Diseases of the American Academy of Pediatrics recommends testing the child with egg anaphylaxis with a scratch test followed by an intradermal skin test with measles vaccine before immunization. They recommend that children with positive skin tests undergo desensitization under careful supervision. Recent studies indicate that such children can be safely vaccinated without prior skin testing or desensitization. The vaccine should be given, however, in a setting where a rare serious reaction can be treated. The child who has had an anaphylactic reaction to topical neomycin should not be vaccinated.

Live measles vaccine can be administered to individuals who received a killed measles vaccine between 1963 and 1967. Such persons may develop atypical measles, which ranges from a mild illness to an uncommon severe form characterized by fever, pulmonary infiltrates, polyserositis, and a vesicular and/or hemorrhagic rash. Since natural measles is more likely to result in a more severe type of atypical measles than measles vaccine, most authorities advise giving the live virus vaccine to such patients with adequate warning.

IMMUNOCOMPROMISED PATIENTS

Fatal measles virus infection has occurred after live measles vaccination of children with acquired or congenital disorders of immune function. The former include children with leukemia or lymphoma and those receiving high-dose steroid, radiation, and antimetabolite therapy. Immunocompromised children may not be able to respond to live vaccines, and some may be receiving regular doses of immunoglobulin that tend to inactivate the vaccine virus. Since the transmission of measles vaccine virus does not occur, the siblings and household contacts of immunocompromised children can be vaccinated with MMR. Measles vaccine is recommended for patients with human immunodeficiency virus (HIV) infection at the recommended ages. HIV-infected patients tolerate the vaccine well and may have severe or fatal infections from natural measles.

Mild acute illness with low-grade fever, mild diarrheal illness, a family history of convulsions, breast feeding, or pregnancy in the mother are *not* contraindications to measles vaccination.

MANAGEMENT OF MEASLES

Although no specific antiviral therapy is available, measles virus is susceptible to ribavirin (Virazole) in vitro. The drug has been given intravenously and by aerosol to severely affected or immunocompromised patients. Since controlled studies have not yet been done, the Food and Drug Administration has not approved ribavirin for the treatment of measles.

In many countries of the world where vitamin A deficiency is present, the administration of this vitamin has reduced the mortality and morbidity from measles. In the United States, the American Academy of Pediatrics Committee on Infectious Diseases recommends that vitamin A supplementation be considered for

1. Infants 6 to 24 months of age hospitalized with measles and its complications (e.g., croup, pneumonia, diarrhea)
2. Patients 6 months of age or older with
   a. Immunodeficiency
   b. Ophthalmic evidence of vitamin A deficiency
   c. Impaired intestinal absorption
   d. Malnutrition
   e. A history of recent immigration from a country with a high measles mortality rate (1% or greater)

The dose of vitamin A is 200,000 IU, given orally as a single dose for children 1 year and older and half that dose for infants under 1 year. The dose should be repeated the next day and at 4 weeks if there is ophthalmic evidence of vitamin A deficiency.

Acetaminophen 5 mL per kg should be given every 4 hours for symptomatic relief of fever, headache, and general discomfort.

COMPLICATIONS

If fever continues after the full development of a rash, complications such as bacterial otitis media or pneumonia should be suspected and appropriate antibiotics employed.

Acute measles encephalitis occurs in about 1 per 1000 cases and usually appears in the early convalescent phase of the disease. Neurologic consultation is advisable when this complication is suspected.

An epidemic of measles occurred in southern California in 1990 involving 440 cases at one hospital. Forty-four percent required hospitalization. Complications included pneumonia (36%), croup (18%), dehydration, diarrhea, and vomiting. Seven percent required intensive care, and 5% required assisted ventilation. This outbreak, with higher-than-expected complication rates, presents a compelling example of the consequences of failure to vaccinate against measles.

FUTURE CONTROL OF MEASLES

Although it may be feasible to eliminate measles with current vaccines, a panel of the world's measles experts have recommended a new strategy for global control of measles. This would involve the development of a safe and effective oral vaccine that is heat-stable and able to bypass maternal antibody.

TETANUS

method of
THOMAS P. BLECK, M.D.
The University of Virginia
Charlottesville, Virginia

Tetanus begins with the invasion of a susceptible host by spores of the anaerobic gram-positive rod *Clostridium tetani*. In the majority of cases, this results from a wound, although the portal of entry is unknown in up to 20% of cases. The ubiquitous nature and hardiness of the spores ensure that virtually any wound can become infected; only appropriate wound care and active immunity stand between an injured patient and this disease.

As the spores germinate, the developing organisms produce *tetanospasmin*, or tetanus toxin. This toxin acts by inhibiting the release of neurotransmitters from presynaptic terminals. Its most apparent action is on the inhibitory neurons (gamma-aminobutyric acid [GABA]–ergic and glycinergic) of the spinal cord and brain stem, resulting in the spasms and muscular hypertonia that dominate the clinical picture. The toxin gains access to these cells by fast retrograde transport within motor neurons. This has important therapeutic implications, since the toxin can be neutralized only by systemic antibody before it enters the motor neuron. The clinical disease will therefore progress for several days after antitoxin administration.

DIAGNOSIS AND DIFFERENTIAL DIAGNOSIS

Four varieties of tetanus are recognized, which differ somewhat in their clinical manifestations but share the same basic pathophysiology. They are described in Table 1.

Although the differential diagnosis of tetanus includes many entities, the only real mimic of tetanus is strychnine poisoning. Since the emergency treatment of the two conditions is similar, such therapy need not depend on a definite diagnosis. The common condition that may resemble tetanus is a dystonic reaction to a centrally acting dopamine-blocking agent (e.g., neuroleptics, most antiemetics, metoclopramide). The patient experiencing such a reaction typically has the head turned to one side and the eyes forcefully and painfully elevated and directed to one side

TABLE 1. **Clinical Varieties of Tetanus**

Type	Description	Typical Host and Portal of Entry
Neonatal tetanus	Hypertonus, spasms, feeding difficulties, airway obstruction in the first weeks of life	Umbilical stump of the infant of a nonimmune mother
Local tetanus	Increased muscle tone in the vicinity of an injury, sometimes with flaccidity of the muscle closest to the wound	Puncture wound, laceration, or burn affecting a patient with partial immunity to tetanospasmin
Cephalic tetanus	Specialized form of local tetanus primarily affecting the cranial nerve musculature	Patient with a facial or scalp laceration, otitis media, or a foreign body in the ear canal; peripheral facial nerve paresis is common
Generalized tetanus	Hypertonus, spasms (including opisthotonic posturing), airway obstruction, autonomic dysfunction (usually a hypersympathetic state)	Patient with a puncture wound presenting days to weeks later with neck and back stiffness, abdominal rigidity, trismus (inability to open the jaw fully), and *risus sardonicus* (a facial expression involving straightening of the upper lip); often occurs in a progression from local or cephalic tetanus

(the "oculogyric crisis"); these findings are distinctly unusual in tetanus. A therapeutic trial of an anticholinergic (e.g., benztropine [Cogentin], 1 to 2 mg, or diphenhydramine [Benadryl], 50 mg intravenously) will usually abort the oculogyric crisis but have little or no effect in tetanus. The sedation produced by diphenhydramine may briefly ease spasms, however.

Trismus without the other manifestations of tetanus may be seen with oral infections, especially abscesses of the alveolar ridge. Generalized convulsive status epilepticus may involve postures similar to those of generalized tetanus, although the arms are extended in seizures and flexed in tetanic spasms. The major distinction between the two, however, is the preservation of consciousness in tetanic spasms, which as a consequence are very painful.

Local tetanus is more difficult to recognize but should be considered whenever focal neurologic findings arise in the area of a recent wound. Cephalic tetanus may occasionally present as Bell's palsy, but the development of trismus and generalized spasms quickly clarifies the diagnosis.

The patient's immunization history is crucial in the diagnosis of tetanus. Almost all patients who have undergone an initial series of immunizations with alum-adsorbed tetanus toxoid (included in diphtheria-pertussis-tetanus [DPT] and tetanus-diphtheria [Td] vaccines) and who have received booster injections at least every 10 years will be immune to tetanus. There are rare case reports of patients who have failed immunization, or who appear to have developed antibodies that are not protective despite their presence in presumably adequate concentrations (0.01 IU/mL). Most of these patients presented with local tetanus, although some have had the generalized form. Strychnine and neuroleptic drug levels should also be obtained, but no laboratory studies are diagnostically useful with sufficient rapidity to influence management in the first several hours, which are often crucial for the patient's survival.

Recognized poor prognostic features include an incubation period of less than 1 week, a period of onset (from the first symptom to the first generalized spasm) of less than 48 hours, a core temperature above 40° C, tachycardia (more than 120 beats per minute in adults), and a "high-risk" portal of entry (including burns, the umbilical stump, surgical procedures, intramuscular injections, compound fractures, or septic abortions). Elderly patients are particularly at risk for tetanus, as their immunity has often waned. They are also least able to tolerate the tremendous cardiovascular, respiratory, and psychologic demands of the illness.

TREATMENT

Once the diagnosis of tetanus is considered, the patient should be carefully moved to a quiet examination area. Both tetanus and strychnine poisoning involve stimulus-sensitive spasms, so any unnecessary lights, noises, or tactile stimuli should be avoided. The patient should be moved to an intensive care unit quickly, but only after adequate ventilation is ensured. The patient and family should be prepared for a period of critical illness lasting 2 to 4 weeks, which may be extended by complications, and recognize that the disease is still fatal in over 25% of cases.

Control of Spasms and Rigidity

The first object of treatment is to control the spasms, since they pose the most immediate risk to the patient's survival by compromising respiration. Benzodiazepines are the agents of choice; either diazepam (Valium) or lorazepam (Ativan) may be used. The doses required to control the spasms are often very large (as much as 500 mg of diazepam, or equivalent, per day); the patient usually remains awake despite these large doses, but provisions for neuromuscular junction blockade and immediate endotracheal intubation must be available in case the patient fails to maintain an adequate airway. The water-soluble benzodiazepine midazolam (Versed) is an alternative, but it must be given by continuous infusion. It is useful if the volume of vehicle necessary to administer the other benzodiazepines intravenously is sufficient to produce a metabolic acidosis. In addition to controlling spasms, these drugs also decrease the muscular hypertonicity of tetanus and will provide some useful sedation and anamnesis in the balance. Barbiturates have no advantages over the benzodiazepines in this setting, and they have more side effects. Chlorpromazine (Thorazine) no longer has a role in the management of this disorder.

Although all the benzodiazepines produce some tachyphylaxis, midazolam displays this effect most prominently. If the patient can accept enteral feedings, changing to diazepam or lorazepam administered via a feeding tube will obviate the metabolic problem of the parenteral forms.

Propofol (Diprivan)* has also been successfully employed for sedation in tetanus, but it has no apparent advantage over the benzodiazepines.

Airway and Ventilatory Management

The decision to intubate a tetanus patient depends on one's ability to control the airway with benzodiazepines; if there is any doubt in this regard, the patient should be intubated. Because the act of intubation involves many potent stimuli for spasm production, the patient should be sedated to unconsciousness and undergo neuromuscular junction blockade (e.g., with vecuronium [Norcuron], 0.1 mg per kg) prior to insertion of the laryngoscope. I favor "elective" tracheostomy at the earliest convenient moment in order to remove the oropharyngeal stimulation of the endotracheal tube, but this point is debated. It does allow some patients to breathe spontaneously who would otherwise be committed to mechanical ventilation because of the larger doses of sedatives required to tolerate the endotracheal tube.

Some severely afflicted patients will require ongoing neuromuscular junction blockade for many days or weeks. Pancuronium bromide (Pavulon) has commonly been used; vecuronium (Norcuron) has the potential advantage of fewer autonomic adverse effects. The dose must be titrated as needed; I start with 0.05 mg per kg of pancuronium or 0.1 mg per kg of vecuronium intravenously. Subsequent doses of pancuronium are given as needed to control movement; vecuronium is given by constant infusion at a dose to produce the same effect. Whichever drug is chosen, it should be stopped daily to assess the continuing need for its use, and the patient *must* be adequately sedated while under the influence of these agents. Since the goal is to prevent spasms and facilitate ventilation, complete paralysis is not necessary. For this reason, routine muscle twitch monitoring (e.g., utilizing the train-of-four test) is not necessary if the patient is making small spontaneous movements, but this should be available for patients who are making no movements to ensure that they are not receiving too much of the blocking agent.

Immunotherapy

Specific immunotherapy with human tetanus immune globulin (Hyper-Tet) should be given once the airway is safe. An adult dose of 500 U appears as effective as the older recommended dose of 5000 U, and it can be given as one or two intramuscular injections instead of ten. The formulation available in the United States is not licensed for intravenous use. The commercially available human immunoglobulin preparations for intravenous use contain varying amounts of antitetanus antibody and should not be

routinely used for the treatment of tetanus. There is no apparent advantage to the much larger doses previously recommended. Since the amount of tetanospasmin produced in the course of a natural infection is not adequate to produce an immune response, active immunization with tetanus toxoid should be initiated at the same time at a different site from the antitoxin injection. The potential role of intrathecal antitoxin remains uncertain; the tetanus immune globulin available in the United States contains a preservative (thiomersal) that should not be injected into the subarachnoid space.

Autonomic Dysfunction

During the second and third weeks of the disease, autonomic dysfunction becomes prominent in a large proportion of patients. This is primarily manifested as sympathetic overactivity and should initially be managed with combined alpha- and beta-adrenergic blockade (e.g., labetalol [Normodyne, Trandatec], 0.25 to 1.0 mg per minute). Should this drug be insufficient, constant infusion of morphine (0.5 to 1.0 mg per kg per hour) may be effective. Epidural blockade at the level of the renal nerves, to inhibit adrenal catecholamine release, may also be effective.

Other Aspects of Treatment

Wound care should be provided as would be appropriate in the absence of tetanus; such care does not affect the course of the disease.

The use of antibiotics to eradicate the toxin-forming bacteria remains debated. If one chooses to use them, then metronidazole (Flagyl), 500 mg four times daily, is probably preferable to penicillin. The latter agent, a GABA-antagonist, was associated with less favorable outcomes in the one comparison published to date.*

Nutrition should be started as soon as possible, preferably via the enteric route. Total parenteral nutrition is required if intestinal atony prevents adequate absorption. The daily caloric requirements are often very high and should be measured to calculate the appropriate replacement. If the parenteral route is chosen, an H_2 blocker or sucralfate (Carafate) should be considered in order to decrease the risk of gastrointestinal bleeding.

Patients who are sedated or paralyzed should receive prophylaxis against thromboembolic disease, with either sequential compression boots or prophylactic doses of heparin.

The psychological strain of an episode of generalized tetanus (and its therapy) is tremendous. Although adequate sedation will lessen this (and the benzodiazepines will facilitate amnesia for much of the acute period), attention to the patient's psychological needs as these drugs are slowly withdrawn is important.

---

*Not FDA-approved for this indication.

*See Ahmadsyah I, Salim A: Treatment of tetanus: An open study to compare the efficacy of procaine penicillin and metronidazole. Br Med J *291*:648–650, 1985.

PROPHYLAXIS

Tetanus should be an almost completely preventable disease. The combination of active immunization for most patients and passive immunization for the rare person who is intolerant to tetanus toxoid would eliminate most cases. Unfortunately, once the period of mandated school vaccinations has passed, only the rare physician attends to routine issues of immunization.

For the average patient, a booster injection of tetanus toxoid (always in the form of Td, unless the patient is hypersensitive to diphtheria toxoid) should be given every 10 years. Patients who have never completed a full series of immunizations should receive three monthly injections. The rare patient with a history of a true adverse reaction to this vaccine, or in whom intramuscular injections are contraindicated, should receive passive immunotherapy as outlined next. Patients who experience the common side effects of local tenderness and edema should be treated symptomatically and should not be considered hypersensitive to tetanus toxoid.

Patients who present to medical attention after any injury that breaks the skin or mucous membranes should receive tetanus toxoid if their last injection was received 10 or more years before. Patients with clean, minor wounds are not usually given passive immunotherapy. Those with tetanus-prone wounds (see earlier) are usually given tetanus toxoid if more than 5 years have elapsed. A patient with a tetanus-prone wound who has an incomplete or uncertain immunization history should also receive human tetanus immune globulin, 250 U intramuscularly. Patients with humoral immunodeficiencies should also be given human tetanus immune globulin.

PERTUSSIS
(Whooping Cough)

method of
STEPHEN A. CHARTRAND, M.D.
Creighton University
Omaha, Nebraska

Pertussis is an acute and highly contagious respiratory infection caused by the gram-negative bacterium *Bordetella pertussis*, which is a strictly human pathogen. The lay term "whooping cough" is less appropriate because not all patients develop the characteristic post-tussive whoop. Infection with *B. parapertussis*, *B. bronchiseptica*, or adenovirus occasionally may produce a clinically indistinguishable "pertussis syndrome." *B. pertussis* is transmitted by large airborne droplets deposited on ciliated respiratory epithelial cells in susceptible individuals. The organism is rather labile outside the respiratory tract, making fomite spread unlikely, although theoretically possible. Secondary attack rates approach 90 to 100% among susceptible close contacts, such as families of an index case. Transient asymptomatic nasopharyngeal colonization has been documented during epidemics, but the role of such individuals with this condition in the spread of disease is questionable. There is no evidence for a true carrier state.

EPIDEMIOLOGY

Pertussis remains a significant pediatric health problem worldwide with over 60 million cases and 500,000 deaths annually. In the United States 5500 confirmed cases of pertussis were reported to the Centers for Disease Control and Prevention during 1993, an 82% increase over 1992 and the highest annual number of cases reported since 1967. Pertussis incidence is usually characterized by a cyclical pattern with peaks occurring at 3- to 4-year intervals. The total number of reported cases has increased in each peak year since 1977.

In the prevaccine era, pertussis was most common among preschool and school-age children, but since 1980 there has been an epidemiologic shift to higher attack rates among young infants, adolescents, and adults. In the United States, for example, 44% of all confirmed cases during 1993 occurred in children less than 1 year of age, in whom morbidity and mortality are highest. Twenty-seven percent of cases occurred in individuals older than 10 years, who are now the most common vector for transmission of pertussis to children. This increase in adult pertussis cases is likely due to waning vaccine-induced immunity and a failure by physicians to recognize the nonclassic symptoms of pertussis in this age group. Contrary to most childhood infectious diseases, pertussis is consistently more common and more severe in females. Seasonal patterns of disease are not clearly marked and differ in different geographic areas. There are no racial differences in attack rates of pertussis.

SYMPTOMS

Following a 7- to 10-day incubation period, the classic symptoms of pertussis progress through three stages: (1) catarrhal (7 to 10 days), (2) paroxysmal (1 to 4 weeks), and (3) convalescent (1 to 4 weeks). The onset of illness is subtle, characterized by nonspecific symptoms of rhinorrhea, conjunctival injection, tearing, and perhaps a mild but nondistinctive cough. The nasopharyngeal secretions are most infectious during this period, but pertussis is rarely suspected unless an exposure history is elicited. Cough symptoms increase in number and severity, finally manifesting in multiple, repetitive, staccato paroxysms. The patient may strangle on the thick secretions, the eyes bulge, the tongue protrudes, and inspiratory efforts are impossible during such bouts. This is followed by a massive inspiratory effort, and the characteristic whoop may be heard as air is inhaled forcefully against a closed glottis. This distinctive whooping sound, however, is frequently absent in young infants and adults, who make up most of the pertussis cases in the 1990s. Such paroxysms may be accompanied by life-threatening apnea and hypoxemia in young infants. In partially immune adolescents and adults, the only symptom may be a lingering paroxysmal or staccato cough. Most such cases are misdiagnosed as bronchitis. During the convalescent stage there is gradual lessening of symptoms, although recurrent cough may persist for several months.

COMPLICATIONS

Respiratory. The most common complication of pertussis is secondary bacterial pneumonia, usually due to *Strep-*

tococcus pneumoniae, Haemophilus influenzae, Strep. pyogenes, or *Staphylococcus aureus*. Secondary pneumonia occurs in 20 to 25% of infants hospitalized with pertussis and is responsible for over 90% of pertussis-related deaths in children less than 3 years of age. For empirical therapy of secondary pneumonia, a third-generation cephalosporin such as ceftriaxone (Rocephin) or cefotaxime (Claforan) is appropriate. Cefuroxime (Ceftin) is another option, especially if *Staph. aureus* is suspected. If *Staph. aureus* is isolated, however, nafcillin (Unipen) or oxacillin (Prostaphlin) is preferred. Other pulmonary complications may include atelectasis, pulmonary hemorrhage, and alveolar rupture.

Central Nervous System. Overall, central nervous system complications of pertussis occur in 4 to 5 patients per 1000 cases, but they are tenfold more common in hospitalized infants. These include seizures, hemiplegia, paraplegia, hemiparesis, aphasia, ataxia, and encephalopathy. The pathogenesis of such complications is unclear; the cerebrospinal fluid is typically normal or may show only a mild pleocytosis or modest protein elevation.

DIAGNOSIS

The optimal specimen for culture of *B. pertussis* is a deep nasopharyngeal Dacron or calcium alginate swab held in place for at least 30 seconds and plated at the bedside onto selective media such as Regan-Lowe or Bordet-Gengou agar. Highest recovery rates occur during the catarrhal or early paroxysmal stage; false-negative cultures are common, especially later in the course of disease or in patients receiving antibiotics. The direct fluorescent antibody test can be performed on the same specimen, but this requires experienced personnel to avoid problems with poor sensitivity and specificity. Although absolute lymphocytosis is common in pertussis, it is a nonspecific finding and may be absent in adolescents and adults. Commercially available serologic tests for pertussis are generally inadequate for accurate diagnostic purposes. Specific assays for IgG antibody against lymphocytosis-promoting factor or IgA against filamentous hemagglutinin appear promising for the future.

MANAGEMENT

General Supportive Care. It is important to maintain adequate hydration and nutrition, especially in young infants. This may necessitate hospitalization for intravenous fluids or hyperalimentation if the paroxysmal stage is prolonged. If paroxysms are severe or if apneic/cyanotic episodes occur, young infants should be hospitalized for transcutaneous oximetry and electronic apnea monitoring. General supportive care and periodic gentle suctioning by experienced pediatric nursing personnel are critically important. Because paroxysms may be induced by pain, excitement, temperature fluctuations, and even feeding, interventions—including unnecessary blood tests—should be kept to a minimum.

Isolation. Untreated patients should be placed in respiratory isolation for 3 weeks after the onset of paroxysms. Patients treated with erythromycin should be isolated for 5 days after initiation of therapy. Children with pertussis, if their medical condition allows, may return to school or child care 5 days after initiation of appropriate antibiotics.

Treatment (Table 1). Antimicrobial therapy dur-

TABLE 1. **Antimicrobial Therapy of Pertussis**

Clinical Indication	Regimen
Prophylaxis or therapy	Erythromycin estolate (Ilosone),* 40 mg/kg/day q 8 h for 14 days *or* Clarithromycin (Biaxin),† 15 mg/kg/day q 12 h for 14 days *or* Azithromycin (Zithromax),† 10 mg/kg once, then 5 mg/kg once daily for 7 days *or* Trimethoprim-sulfamethoxazole (Bactrim, Septra), 10 mg/kg (of trimethoprim)/day q 12 h for 14 days
Secondary pneumonia	Ceftriaxone (Rocephin), 75–100 mg/kg/day q 12–24 h *or* Cefotaxime (Claforan), 200 mg/kg/day q 6 h *or* Cefuroxime (Ceftin), 200 mg/kg/day q 8 h

*Alternative: Erythromycin ethylsuccinate, 60–70 mg/kg/day q 6 h, but microbiologic and clinical cure rates are lower.

†Not approved for this indication, but its in vitro activity is similar to that of erythromycin. May be useful in patients unable to tolerate erythromycin.

ing the catarrhal or early paroxysmal stage ameliorates the course of disease in most patients. Once paroxysms have become established, however, treatment has no discernible effect, and antibiotics are prescribed primarily to prevent spread of the illness. Erythromycin estolate, 40 mg per kg per day for 14 days, is the preferred regimen due to higher microbiologic eradication rates and a lower incidence of relapse, compared with the ethylsuccinate preparation. Treatment for less than 14 days is associated with higher rates of clinical and microbiologic relapse. Recently, two macrolide derivatives of erythromycin, clarithromycin (Biaxin) and azithromycin (Zithromax), have been licensed for use in the United States. Both drugs possess in vitro activity comparable to that of erythromycin against *B. pertussis*, with fewer gastrointestinal side effects. They both have longer half-lives than erythromycin, which allows twice- or even once-daily dosing. With azithromycin, the half-life increases with an increasing number of doses, which may eventually lead to shorter courses of therapy. As of early 1995, only clarithromycin was available, in a suspension form that unfortunately has a somewhat bitter aftertaste. Neither drug has been prospectively evaluated for treatment or prophylaxis of pertussis, but they may represent reasonable alternatives for patients unable to tolerate erythromycin. Finally, trimethoprim-sulfamethoxazole (Bactrim, Septra) (10/50 mg per kg per day) has been recommended as another alternative regimen, but its efficacy remains unproved.

Pertussis immune globulin was at one time widely prescribed as both prophylaxis and treatment of pertussis. Controlled studies, however, failed to show a benefit and it is not recommended. Some experts recommend corticosteroids and the beta₂-adrenergic stimulant albuterol to reduce the paroxysms of coughing, but controlled clinical trials to document efficacy are lacking.

PREVENTION

Care of Exposed Persons. Close contacts under 7 years of age who have received fewer than four doses of pertussis vaccine should have pertussis immunization initiated or continued. Children who received their third dose 6 or more months before exposure should receive the fourth dose at this time. Those who have received their fourth dose should also receive a booster dose unless the last dose was within the last 3 years or they are more than 6 years of age. Chemoprophylaxis with erythromycin estolate (40 mg per kg per day orally, maximum 2 grams per day) for 14 days is recommended for all contacts, *irrespective of vaccine status.* Pertussis immunity is not complete and wanes with time, and patients with mild illness may not be recognized but may transmit the infection. Clarithromycin, azithromycin and trimethoprim-sulfamethoxazole are alternative but unproven regimens for those unable to tolerate erythromycin.

Immunization. Universal immunization with pertussis vaccine is recommended for all children younger than 7 years of age. Whole-cell pertussis vaccine (DTP) is usually administered, along with diphtheria and tetanus toxoids, at 2, 4, 6, 12 to 15, and 48 to 60 months of age. The whole-cell preparation is a suspension of killed bacteria that contains multiple antigens, many of which play no role in development of immunity and may contribute to adverse effects following vaccination. These adverse effects increase in frequency and severity with the increasing number of DTP doses. They can be lessened by routine administration of acetaminophen, 15 mg per kg per dose at the time of immunization and again 4 and 8 hours later. Whole-cell pertussis vaccine is 80 to 90% protective against clinical disease, depending on the severity of illness used as an end point. Acellular pertussis vaccines (DTaP) contain one to four purified antigens (lymphocytosis-promoting factor, agglutinogens, hemagglutinins, and an outer membrane protein, pertactin) in various ratios and concentrations. On the basis of similar antibody responses to DTP, two of these preparations (Acel-Imune and Tripedia) are currently licensed in the United States for the fourth and fifth booster doses for children 15 months of age or older. The incidence of local and systemic side effects with DTaP is significantly less than with DTP in all ages, including infants. Preliminary efficacy data suggest that acellular vaccines are as protective as whole-cell preparations for older children. Comparative efficacy studies in young infants are currently in progress and appear quite promising. When used for the fourth or fifth dose, these two acellular vaccines are interchangeable.

IMMUNIZATION PRACTICES

method of
RICK KELLERMAN, M.D.
*University of Kansas School of
    Medicine—Wichita
Wichita, Kansas*

The immunization of children and adults against infectious diseases is a cornerstone of health maintenance and disease prevention. Unfortunately, nearly half of all children in the United States have not received their recommended immunizations on schedule. Less than a third of high-risk adults receive appropriate influenza vaccination yearly.

There are multiple barriers that hinder appropriate immunization of children and adults. The cost of vaccines, inadequate access to medical care, inadequate public health delivery systems, and a lack of awareness on the part of the public and parents all contribute to low immunization rates. The majority of unimmunized and underimmunized children do not have health insurance that covers immunizations.

Many private physicians have discontinued giving immunizations in their offices because of perceived liability risks and the hassles involved in providing informed consent. A recent proliferation of new immunizations and immunization schedules has confused many practitioners. Although multiple vaccines can be administered simultaneously without impairment of the immunologic response and without increased risk of adverse reactions, some practitioners are unwilling to give more than two vaccines during the same visit.

This article provides an update on immunization schedules, reviews indications and contraindications to vaccination, examines the immunization of special populations such as those who are human immunodeficiency virus (HIV) positive, and clarifies commonly held misconceptions about immunizations.

Table 1 outlines a recommended childhood immunization schedule accepted by the American Academy of Family Physicians, American Academy of Pediatrics, and the Advisory Committee on Immunization Practices in 1995.

DIPHTHERIA-PERTUSSIS-TETANUS

Childhood Immunizations

Diphtheria, tetanus, and pertussis are usually administered as a combined (DTP) vaccine in children younger than 7 years of age. A combined vaccine with an acellular pertussis component (DTaP) may be used for the fourth and fifth doses of vaccine in children who have previously received three doses of whole-cell DTP vaccine. Future updated immunization schedules may allow DTaP for the first, second, and third doses. Because of the increased incidence of side effects owing to age, the pertussis component is not used at all in children over the age of 6 years, and the combined adult vaccine (dT) is used instead.

TABLE 1. **Recommended Childhood Immunization Schedule, United States— January 1995**

Vaccine	At Birth	2 Months	4 Months	6 Months	12 Months*	15 Months	18 Months	4–6 Years	11–12 Years	14–16 Years
Hepatitis B (Hep B)†	Hep B 1									
		Hep B 2		Hep B 3						
Diphtheria, tetanus, pertussis (DTP)‡		DTP	DTP	DTP	DTP or DTaP at 15+ months			DTP or DTaP	dT	
Haemophilus influenzae Type B (Hib)§		HbCV	HbCV	HbCV	HbCV					
Polio, live oral (OPV)		OPV	OPV	OPV				OPV		
Measles, mumps, rubella (MMR)‖					MMR			MMR or MMR		

This schedule is provided by AAFP only as assistance for physicians making clinical decisions regarding care of their patients. As such, it cannot substitute for individual judgment brought to each clinical situation by patient's family physician. As with all clinical reference resources, they reflect best understanding of science of medicine at time of publication but should be used with clear understanding that continued research may result in new knowledge and recommendations.

Vaccines are listed under routinely recommended ages. Boxes indicate range of acceptable ages for vaccine administration. This schedule has been approved by Advisory Committee on Immunization Practices (ACIP) of Centers for Disease Control and Prevention, American Academy of Pediatrics (AAP), and American Academy of Family Physicians (AAFP).

*Vaccines recommended in second year of life (12 to 15 months of age) may be given at either one or two visits.

†Infants born to hepatitis B surface antigen (HBsAg) negative mothers should receive second dose of hepatitis B vaccine between 1 and 4 months of age, provided at least 1 month has elapsed since receipt of first dose. Third dose is recommended between 6 and 18 months of age. Infants born to HBsAg-positive mothers should receive immunoprophylaxis for hepatitis B with 0.5 mL of hepatitis B immune globulin within 12 hours of birth, and 0.5 mL of either Recombivax HB or Engerix-B at separate site. In these infants, second dose of vaccine is recommended at 1 month of age and third dose at 6 months of age. All pregnant women should be screened for HBsAg in early prenatal visit.

‡Fourth dose of DTP may be administered as early as 12 months of age, provided at least 6 months have elapsed since third dose of DTP. Combined DTP-Hib products may be used when these two vaccines are to be administered simultaneously. DTaP is licensed for use for fourth and/or fifth dose of DTP vaccine in children 15 months of age or older and may be preferred for these doses in children in this age group.

§Three Hib conjugate vaccines are available for use in infants: HbOC; PRP-T (ActHib, Omni Hib), and PRP-OMP (Pedvax Hib). Children who have received PRP-OMP at 2 and 4 months of age do not require dose at 6 months of age. After primary infant Hib conjugate vaccine series is completed, any licensed Hib conjugate vaccine may be used as booster dose at 12 to 15 months of age.

‖Second dose of MMR vaccine should be administered at either 4 to 6 years or 11 to 12 years of age.

From AAFP, AAP, and ACIP collaborate in the development of a simplified childhood immunization schedule. Am Fam Physician 50:1826, 1994.

The diphtheria and tetanus components of DTP immunization induce very few side effects. On the other hand, the safety of the pertussis component has engendered considerable debate, controversy, and media attention. An interim report of the British National Childhood Encephalopathy Study (NCES) published in 1981 concluded that the risk of permanent brain damage after pertussis vaccination was 1 in 330,000 immunizations. Subsequent inspection of the NCES data revealed that some case reports were misclassified and that alternate causes such as meningitis explained the permanent brain damage originally attributed to the pertussis vaccine. A British legal opinion has concluded that the NCES overstated the risk of the pertussis vaccine and said that there is no specific clinical syndrome of pertussis vaccine–induced brain damage. There are no animal experiments that show permanent brain damage from pertussis vaccination.

Currently there is no consistent evidence to support allegations that the pertussis vaccine causes permanent brain damage in the previously normal child. In 1991, the Institute of Medicine concluded that although there was weak but consistent evidence that the pertussis vaccine may cause acute encephalopathy, there was insufficient evidence to indicate either the presence or absence of a causal relationship between the pertussis vaccine and chronic neurologic damage. Pertussis vaccine does appear to induce febrile seizures, and antipyretics are indicated when it is administered.

Concern about the side effects of the whole-cell pertussis vaccine led to the development of the acellular pertussis DTaP vaccines that are currently licensed in the United States. Whereas half of children vaccinated with whole-cell DTP vaccine develop fever, irritability, and fretfulness, considerably less than 20% of children receiving DTaP vaccine develop these symptoms. Three-fourths of children receiving DTP vaccine develop red, tender, swollen injection sites compared with fewer than one-third who receive DTaP vaccine. Both DTP and DTaP vaccines may induce hypotonic-hyporesponsive episodes, the cause of which is undetermined.

The absolute contraindications to the whole-cell and acellular pertussis components are identical. Contraindications include age over 6 years, acute febrile illness, neurologic disorder with progressive developmental delay or changing neurologic findings, and immediate anaphylactic reaction or encephalopathy within 7 days of administration of a previous dose. If encephalopathy from a previous dose is a contraindication, the DT vaccine may be used for the next vaccination.

Precautions include the following if they occur within 48 hours after a previous dose: fever greater than or equal to 40.5° C (104.9° F), hypotonic-hyporesponsive episode, and persistent, inconsolable crying lasting more than 3 hours. A convulsion with or without fever within 3 days of previous vaccination is also a precaution.

The CDC recommends that the risk/benefit ratio of administering the DTP or DTaP vaccine be considered when deciding to vaccinate a child who fits into a precaution category. For example, if there is a high background rate of pertussis or a serious epidemic in a community, the individual practitioner may recommend the vaccine for children who fit into the precaution categories. In other cases in which the community or individual risk of pertussis is low, the practitioner may elect to forego the pertussis component of the DTP or DTaP vaccine.

In a child who has an uncertain or uncharacterized neurologic disorder, the pertussis vaccine should not be administered until the neurologic status can be clarified. A child with a seizure disorder or positive family history of seizures without other neurologic abnormality may receive the pertussis vaccine, although the child is at increased risk of having a seizure. Children with stable cerebral palsy or nonprogressive developmental delay without seizures are not at increased risk for seizures. The pertussis immunization is not a cause of sudden infant death syndrome (SIDS).

The diphtheria and tetanus components rarely cause systemic reactions but may cause local injection site soreness. Reactions are more common if immunization with these components occurs too frequently. Contraindications to the diphtheria and tetanus components include previous anaphylactic reactions and acute febrile illness.

Adult Diphtheria-Tetanus

Although tetanus is a rare disease in the United States, most cases in the United States now occur in individuals over the age of 50. It is not sufficient to ask adult patients for the date of their last tetanus immunization. Rather, an inquiry should be made about completion of their primary vaccination series. The CDC suggests that adults receive dT boosters every 10 years after completion of their primary series.

The tetanus immunization of adults should always be done along with diphtheria immunization, as combined dT vaccination. The little "d" signifies the adult dosage, which contains 2 flocculating units of diphtheria toxoid; the big "D" signifies the children's dosage, containing 7 to 25 flocculating units of diphtheria. The dT vaccine should be used after the age of 6 years.

Table 2 outlines administration guidelines for tetanus prophylaxis in the management of wounds. An individual with a contaminated, dirty wound who has received fewer than three tetanus immunizations should receive both tetanus immune globulin (TIG) and dT vaccine and be appropriately rescheduled for

Table 2. Tetanus Prophylaxis in Wound Management

History of Adsorbed Tetanus Toxoid (Doses)	Clean, Minor Wounds		All Other Wounds*	
	Td†	TIG	Td†	TIG
Unknown or < 3	Yes	No	Yes	Yes
≥3‡	No§	No	No¶	No

*Such as, but not limited to, wounds contaminated with dirt, feces, soil and saliva; puncture wounds; avulsions; and wounds resulting from missiles, crushing, burns and frostbite.

†For children <7 years old, DTP (DT, if pertussis vaccine is contraindicated) is preferred to tetanus toxoid alone. For persons ≥7 years of age, Td is preferred to tetanus toxoid alone.

‡If only three doses of *fluid* toxoid have been received, then a fourth dose of toxoid, preferably an adsorbed toxoid, should be given.

§Yes, if >10 years since last dose.

¶Yes, if >5 years since last dose. (Most frequent boosters are not needed and can accentuate side effects.)

Reprinted from Centers for Disease Control and Prevention: Summary guide to tetanus prophylaxis in wound management: MMWR *40* (No. RR-10), August 8, 1991, p 16.

follow-up to complete the primary immunization series.

POLIO

Since 1980, approximately eight people have acquired poliomyelitis in the United States each year. Virtually all of these cases are vaccine-related. The risk of vaccine-associated poliomyelitis is 1 in 2.5 million doses of oral polio vaccine (OPV) distributed. The risk of polio infection is greatest in the immunodeficient. Because the attenuated wild poliovirus vaccine is excreted in the stool, immune-suppressed contacts of vaccinated children are also at risk. Intramuscular injections administered within 30 days of OPV administration may increase the risk of paralytic disease, a phenomenon known as "provocation" poliomyelitis.

OPV is contraindicated if the patient or a household contact is immunocompromised (cancer, leukemia, chemotherapy, radiation therapy, high-dose steroids, etc.) or is HIV-positive. The enhanced inactivated poliovirus vaccine (eIPV), administered subcutaneously, should be substituted in these instances. Because it is difficult to identify with certainty all household members who may be HIV-positive or who are immune suppressed, there has been discussion that the polio vaccination schedule should utilize eIPV.

Contraindications specific to eIPV include anaphylaxis to neomycin, polymyxin B, or streptomycin.

Contraindications common to OPV and eIPV include anaphylaxis and moderate to severe illness with or without fever. Pregnancy is a precaution. Low- to moderate-dose steroid use is not a contraindication to OPV administration.

Primary vaccination and booster doses are unnecessary for adults incompletely vaccinated against polio in the United States unless there is a risk due to foreign travel or occupation. If vaccination is required in an adult over the age of 17, eIPV is recommended, unless the patient is pregnant. If polio vaccination is required during pregnancy, OPV is recommended.

If a child spits out or regurgitates an OPV dose within 10 minutes of vaccination, another dose should be administered at the same visit.

MEASLES-MUMPS-RUBELLA

Measles-mumps-rubella (MMR) vaccine is a live-virus combination vaccine administered subcutaneously. The first dose of MMR vaccine should be administered at 12 to 15 months of age, the second dose at the age of 4 to 6 or 11 to 12 years. MMR vaccine may be administered to infants younger than 12 months of age if there is a community epidemic of measles. However, this dose does not count as the child's first MMR immunization, and the child should be revaccinated at 15 months of age and again at the age of 4 to 6 or 11 to 12 years.

Special consideration should be given to ensuring appropriate immunization of health care workers, college students, and international travelers born after 1956. Those born before 1957 are considered immune.

Contraindications to MMR immunization include anaphylaxis to egg ingestion or neomycin, moderate or severe illness with or without fever, pregnancy, and immunodeficiency. HIV positivity and low to moderate steroid use are not contraindications. Because the vaccine is not transmitted from vaccinee to susceptible contacts, children with pregnant mothers may be vaccinated.

MMR immunization precautions include the administration of immune globulin in the 3 months before scheduled vaccination. MMR vaccine may temporarily suppress tuberculin skin test reactivity; therefore, the tuberculin skin test should be administered on the same day as or 6 weeks after MMR immunization.

Women of childbearing age should be screened for rubella immunity and vaccinated unless there is a contraindication. Arthralgias may develop 1 to 3 months after MMR immunization, especially in adult women.

HAEMOPHILUS INFLUENZAE TYPE B CONJUGATE VACCINE

Single Vaccines. The *Haemophilus influenzae* Type B (Hib) polysaccharide vaccines are conjugated to protein carriers that help improve vaccine immunogenicity.

Immunization with the Hib conjugate vaccines (HbCVs) is safe. Recent epidemiologic studies show that the incidence of Hib meningitis has dropped considerably with the advent of these vaccines. Most practitioners become familiar with and consistently use one of the HbCV vaccines that can be administered to children less than 1 year of age (see Table 1).

Physicians should identify on the patient's personal immunization record and in the office chart the specific type of HbCV administered. When possible, the same HbCV should be used throughout the primary series. If different HbCVs must be administered, a total of three doses of vaccine, regardless of manufacturer, should be administered to complete the primary vaccination of children less than 15 months of age.

HbCV contraindications include anaphylaxis to a previous dose and moderate or severe systemic illness with or without fever.

The HbCV does not have to be given to a child over the age of 5 years unless there are special circumstances such as asplenia or sickle cell disease. Consideration should be given to administering the HbCV to HIV-positive or immunocompromised adults and children over the age of 5 years.

Because children younger than 24 months of age may fail to develop adequate immunity after natural disease caused by Hib, children of this age group should be immunized even if they have had invasive Hib disease. Special attention should be given to immunization of all children in day care centers.

Combination Vaccines. Recent efforts to simplify childhood dosing schedules and eliminate as many individual injections as possible have led to the development of new combination vaccines. Tetramune consists of diphtheria, whole-cell pertussis, tetanus, and Hib components. It may be administered at 2, 4, and 6 months. It may also be used as a 12- to 15-month booster, although separate DTaP and HbCV vaccines may be preferable because of the decreased incidence of reactions with the acellular pertussis component.

OmniHIB and ActHIB may be reconstituted with Connaught whole-cell DTP, allowing simultaneous vaccination with DTP and HbCV.

MENINGOCOCCAL POLYSACCHARIDE VACCINE

The meningococcal polysaccharide vaccine (Menomune-A/C/Y/W-135) includes serogroups A, C, Y, and W-135. It does not include serogroup B and in children younger than 2 years old is not effective against serogroup C; these are the serogroups most likely to cause disease in U.S. children. The vaccine is not routinely recommended but should be administered to those with asplenia, sickle cell disease, and terminal complement component deficiencies and to travelers to epidemic areas.

Contraindications include anaphylaxis and moderate illness, with or without fever. Pregnancy is considered a precaution.

HEPATITIS B VACCINE

There are two licensed hepatitis B vaccines: Recombivax HB (Merck & Company) and Engerix-B (SmithKline Beecham). The two vaccines are equally immunogenic and may be used interchangeably in their respective, recommended intramuscular doses. Both are routinely administered in a three-dose infant series at 0, 1 to 4, and 6 to 18 months. There is no consensus as to whether periodic revaccination is necessary. Because of their differing formulations, the package insert should be consulted for dosing information.

All pregnant women should be routinely tested for hepatitis B surface antigen (HBsAg), and all infants should receive hepatitis B vaccination. Infants born to HBsAg-positive mothers should receive both hepatitis B vaccination and hepatitis B immune globulin.

Hepatitis B vaccination is also recommended for the following high-risk groups: health care and public safety workers, clients and staff of institutions for the developmentally disabled, inmates of correctional facilities, hemodialysis patients, recipients of certain blood products, injecting drug users, individuals with multiple sex partners, sexually active homosexual and bisexual men, prostitutes, household contacts and sex partners of hepatitis B carriers, travelers to endemic areas, and adoptees from countries where hepatitis B is endemic.

The hepatitis B vaccine is considered safe with a minimum of side effects, and the individual practitioner may liberally recommend the vaccine to individuals or age groups considered at high risk because of their behaviors, for example, sexually active teenagers. Patients with sexually transmitted diseases and pregnancy in teenagers may be considered "red flags" for vaccination.

The only contraindication to hepatitis B vaccination is anaphylaxis to previous vaccination or to common baker's yeast. Serious active illness and pregnancy are considered precautions.

There is no consensus as to whether serologic testing should occur after administration of the hepatitis B vaccine. Many physicians test for the serologic response of health care workers, dialysis patients, infants born to HBsAg-positive mothers, and those who they anticipate may have a suboptimal response, such as immune-suppressed or HIV-positive patients. Individuals who are elderly, are obese, or smoke are also less likely to develop immunity. A patient who does not respond to the initial three-dose regimen should be revaccinated with one or more doses.

SIMULTANEOUS VACCINATION OF CHILDREN

DTP or DTaP, OPV or eIPV, MMR, HbCV, and hepatitis B vaccines may be administered simultaneously at the same office visit. The future introduction of additional combined vaccines and technological innovations such as multichambered syringes may help simplify immunization dosage schedules.

SPECIAL POPULATIONS

Recommendations for Routine Immunization of Children Infected with Human Immunodeficiency Virus

With the exception of the OPV immunization, the child with HIV infection should follow the usual im-

munization schedule for children. The eIPV vaccine should be substituted for OPV in the HIV-positive child. The HIV-positive child should receive influenza and pneumococcal vaccines. The safety of the varicella virus vaccine has not been demonstrated in asymptomatic children infected with HIV; it is contraindicated in children with AIDS.

Immunization of the Pregnant Patient

The pregnant patient may receive dT immunization if she is not up to date during pregnancy. Unless otherwise contraindicated, if an unvaccinated pregnant patient is at substantial risk for infection with poliovirus or requires immediate protection in order to travel to an endemic area, OPV is preferred over eIPV. MMR vaccination is not recommended during pregnancy, although there have been no adverse effects reported when administered during pregnancy. The rubella-negative pregnant patient should have an MMR vaccine administered shortly after delivery. All pregnant patients should be screened for hepatitis B, but the vaccine is not routinely recommended during pregnancy.

PNEUMOCOCCAL VACCINE

The pneumococcal vaccine (Pneumovax 23) contains the capsular polysaccharides of the 23 most prevalent pneumococcal types. The current high-risk groups for whom the vaccine is recommended include those aged 65 or older, those with chronic disease (cardiovascular, respiratory, hepatic, or renal disease, diabetes, immune suppression, cancer, lymphoma, multiple myeloma, leukemia, organ transplantation), those who are HIV-positive, Native Americans, those with asplenia (anatomic or sickle cell disease), those who chronically abuse alcohol, those with chronic cerebrospinal fluid leakage, those who live in closed groups such as nursing homes, and patients at high risk for influenza complications.

Children who have reached the age of 2 years who have a chronic disease such as asthma or diabetes should receive the pneumococcal vaccine. The vaccine is specifically indicated for children who are HIV-positive, immunosuppressed, or Native American or who have nephrotic syndrome, sickle cell disease, or asplenia. The vaccine is not effective in children younger than 2 years of age or for otitis media prophylaxis.

The current CDC recommendation is to administer the vaccine once a lifetime except in certain high-risk groups. There are no current studies to guide firm recommendations for revaccination of most individuals.

Current indications for revaccination of adults include those who previously received the 14-valent pneumococcal vaccine more than 3 years previously and are at highest risk because of conditions such as asplenia and those who received the 23-valent vaccine more than 5 years previously and have nephrotic syndrome, renal failure, or transplants. Children at high risk due to asplenia, sickle cell disease, and nephrotic syndrome should be revaccinated in 3 to 5 years especially if younger than 10 years of age.

Systemic reactions to the pneumococcal vaccine are rare, although severe local Arthus-like reactions may occur when booster doses are administered less than 6 years after the initial dose. Contraindications include hypersensitivity or anaphylaxis to previous pneumococcal vaccination. Precautions include febrile illness, active infection, and pregnancy.

INFLUENZA VACCINE

The influenza vaccine has relatively few side effects. The vaccine is a killed virus, so it is impossible to contract influenza from the vaccine.

In the United States, the influenza vaccine should be administered in the fall and early winter. Though the influenza vaccine is available in both whole-virus and "split" virus vaccines, most practitioners stock only the split virus in their offices since it can be administered to both children and adults. Because the influenza virus demonstrates antigenic variation from year to year, the vaccine must be administered yearly.

The influenza vaccination should be targeted to high-risk individuals who fit the following criteria: those aged 65 or older; those with chronic lung or heart disease, chronic illness such as diabetes, renal failure, hemoglobinopathy, or immune suppression including acquired immune deficiency disease (AIDS); and residents of nursing homes and other chronic care facilities.

Those who are capable of transmitting influenza to high-risk patients, including health care workers, home care volunteers, and household members, should also be vaccinated.

Although generally considered an immunization for the high-risk elderly, the influenza vaccine should also be administered to children with high-risk conditions such as asthma and diabetes. Children and teenagers receiving long-term aspirin therapy for conditions such as juvenile rheumatoid arthritis and who may be at risk for Reye's syndrome after influenza infection should be immunized. Children and adolescents capable of transmitting influenza to high-risk family members should also be immunized.

Children aged 6 months to 9 years who have not previously been vaccinated should receive two doses of split influenza virus vaccine, 4 weeks apart. The influenza vaccine has not been approved for use in children younger than 6 months.

Because of its relative safety, physicians may also administer the vaccine to individuals who request immunization against influenza even if they are not in a high-risk group.

Contraindications to influenza vaccine include acute febrile illness, anaphylaxis to chicken eggs or aminoglycosides, anaphylaxis to a previous influenza vaccination, and a past history of Guillain-Barré syndrome. Except for the 1976–1977 swine influenza vaccine, the vaccine has not been clearly associated with Guillain-Barré syndrome. Pregnancy is a precaution. Immunosuppression may decrease the immunogenic response.

If the vaccination cannot be administered to a high-risk patient, amantadine or rimantadine may be used for influenza prophylaxis.

RABIES

Pre-exposure rabies prophylaxis with human diploid cell vaccine (HDCV) should be recommended to veterinarians, animal handlers, spelunkers, certain laboratory workers, and persons visiting or living in countries where rabies risks are high.

Postexposure immunization with both HDCV and rabies immune globulin (RIG) is recommended for all bites of skunks, bats, raccoons, foxes, coyotes, bobcats, woodchucks, and other carnivores. Postexposure immunization is also recommended for bites or other wounds contaminated by saliva of dogs and cats suspected of being rabid or those that have escaped.

Postexposure vaccination of the previously unimmunized bite victim requires HDCV administered into the deltoid muscle on a 0-, 3-, 7-, 14-, 28-day schedule. One-half of the RIG, calculated on the basis of the weight of the victim, is administered into the wound after it is thoroughly cleaned. The other half of the RIG is injected intramuscularly at a site distant from the HDCV injection site.

Bites by domestic dogs and cats, unless suspected of being rabid, may be treated expectantly by close observation of the animal for 10 days. Bites by livestock, rodents, rats, mice, squirrels, hamsters, guinea pigs, gerbils, chipmunks, and rabbits should be selectively treated after consulting with the state or local health department since transmission of rabies by these animal groups is rare.

There are no clear-cut contraindications to postexposure vaccination, although previous anaphylactic reaction is a definite precaution. Contraindications to pre-exposure prophylaxis include anaphylaxis and acute illness with or without fever.

Immune suppression may interfere with immunity and may require that the rabies antibody titer be monitored.

VACCINES INDICATED FOR SELECTED INDIVIDUALS, PATIENT POPULATIONS, AND TRAVELERS

Active immunizing agents are available against anthrax (Bacillus anthracis), cholera (Vibrio cholerae), plague (Yersinia pestis), typhoid (Salmonella typhi), yellow fever, and Japanese encephalitis. Hepatitis A vaccine for travelers has recently been approved by the Food and Drug Administration (FDA). The CDC, state, or local health department may be consulted to obtain recommendations for travelers.

VARICELLA VACCINE

The varicella vaccine, approved by the FDA for use in the United States in 1995, is a live attenuated vaccine. The vaccine is indicated for individuals 12 months of age and older. Children aged 12 months to 12 years who have not had chickenpox should receive a single 0.5-mL dose. Adolescents and adults 13 years of age or older should receive two doses, administered 4 to 8 weeks apart.

Contraindications to the varicella vaccine include hypersensitivity to any component including gelatin, a history of anaphylaxis to neomycin, active untreated tuberculosis, acute febrile illness, and pregnancy. Pregnancy should be avoided for a minimum of 3 months after immunization. With the exception of children with acute lymphoblastic leukemia in remission, the vaccine should not be given to individuals with blood dyscrasias, lymphomas, leukemia, or other malignant neoplasms affecting the bone marrow or lymphatic system. In addition, individuals on immune suppressants or those with primary or acquired immunodeficiencies including AIDS should not receive the vaccine. If a patient has a family history of congenital or hereditary immunodeficiency, the vaccination should be deferred until immune competence is clearly demonstrated.

The most common side effect of the varicella vaccination is pain, redness, and swelling at the injection site. Fever occurs in less than 15% of children receiving the vaccination, and febrile seizures are associated only rarely. In clinical trials, occasionally children developed respiratory illness, cough, irritability, joint pain, or diarrhea after vaccination. A mild chickenpox-like rash that may be generalized (median of five vesicles) or a localized rash near the site of injection may occur within 3 weeks after less than 5% of injections.

Within 3 years after vaccination, less than 1% of children who are immunized develop chickenpox, a 93% decrease from the expected attack rate. The majority of these cases are milder than would be expected.

A cost-benefit analysis has suggested that for every dollar invested in varicella vaccination, a societal savings of $5.40 would accrue based on medical and parental work-loss costs. The analysis assumed a vaccine cost of $35 per dose.

FUTURE PROSPECTS

Work continues on the development of HIV vaccines, new acellular vaccines, and combination vaccinations.

TOXOPLASMOSIS

method of
PETER MARIUZ, M.D., and
BENJAMIN J. LUFT, M.D.
State University of New York at Stony Brook
Stony Brook, New York

Toxoplasmosis, the disease caused by the obligate intracellular protozoan *Toxoplasma gondii*, is a worldwide zoonosis responsible for significant morbidity and mortality in both animals and humans. With the advent of acquired immune deficiency syndrome (AIDS), toxoplasmic encephalitis is occurring in epidemic proportions. *T. gondii* is a coccidian, currently classified among the Sporozoa in the suborder Eimeria. It exists in three morphologic forms: oocyst, tachyzoite, and tissue cyst. Oocysts are produced by gametogony only within the gut of felines, the definitive host. Unsporulated, noninfectious oocysts are shed in the feces. Sporogony takes place outside the body of the host and requires 2 to 21 days to occur. Once sporulated, oocysts are infectious and may remain so for up to one year under ideal conditions. The ingestion of food or beverages contaminated with oocysts is a primary route of human infection. Exposure to boiling water for at least 5 minutes or dry heat ($>60°$ C) renders the oocysts noninfectious.

Tachyzoites are obligate intracellular parasites capable of infecting every kind of mammalian cell. They are released from ingested oocysts or tissue cysts. After invading the intestinal mucosa, they disseminate widely throughout the body. The infected host cell lyses, and contiguous cells become infected and then destroyed. The organism spreads throughout the body hematogenously and through the lymphatics. Host cell destruction continues until an adequate immune response is elicited. Subsequently, tissue cysts are formed in various tissues and a chronic, or latent, infection ensues. The clinical corollary of this is that toxoplasmosis ranges from an asymptomatic disease to a life-threatening encephalitis, depending to a large extent on the immunologic status of the host.

The chronic infection is asymptomatic but can be detected serologically. Tachyzoites play a role in the transmission of *T. gondii* in congenital disease or, rarely, during transfusions of blood or leukocytes and in laboratory accidents. The ingestion of tissue cysts contained in raw or undercooked meats, particularly lamb and pork, is an important source of human infection. Tissue cysts in meat can be rendered noninfectious by heating ($>60°$ C), smoking, curing, or freezing ($< -20°$ C for at least 24 hours). However, most home freezers are not capable of reaching and maintaining such temperatures. Tissue cysts that are present in donor organs play a prominent role in transplantation-related toxoplasmosis. When a chronically infected host becomes immunocompromised (particularly cell-mediated immunity), reactivation of the latent infection may occur, with devastating consequences. This represents the predominant mechanism of disease in patients with AIDS. In the United States, the prevalence of toxoplasmosis in adults, determined by serologic studies, varies from 10 to 30%. In Africa, Haiti, Europe, and Latin America, the incidence of latent infection is much higher. In France, for example, the incidence of toxoplasmosis in adults over 35 years of age approaches 98%. It is estimated that 30% of AIDS patients latently infected with *T. gondii* will develop active disease.

TREATMENT

Most episodes of toxoplasmosis in immunocompetent hosts are asymptomatic and do not require therapy. There are, however, specific instances—based on the location of the infection, its severity, the mode of transmission (e.g., congenital disease), and the host's immune status—when treatment is necessary (Table 1). Therapeutic regimens are based on data from in vitro and in vivo experimental animal models (mostly murine) as well as a few large, well-controlled clinical

TABLE 1. *Toxoplasma gondii* Infections Requiring Treatment

Infection in Immunocompetent Hosts
Ocular disease
Infections during pregnancy
Congenital infection
Disseminated disease (e.g., encephalitis, pneumonitis, myocarditis, or hepatitis)
Unusually prolonged or severe adenopathy

Infection in Immunocompromised Hosts
AIDS
Transplantation
Chronic steroid use
Hematologic malignancies, particularly Hodgkin's disease

Other
Transfusion-related infection
Accidental infection of laboratory personnel

trials and the practice of physicians experienced in the treatment of toxoplasmosis (Tables 2 to 5). However, the ideal dosage, combination of drugs, and length of therapy are not known.

Toxoplasmosis in Immunocompetent Hosts

The majority of infections in immunocompetent hosts are asymptomatic and do not require therapy. Lymphadenopathy, the most common manifestation, is self-limited and usually resolves within 1 to 3 weeks. Treatment in this setting should be considered only if systemic symptoms are severe or prolonged or in the rare event that there is visceral involvement (encephalitis, myocarditis, or pneumoni-

tis). Acute infection as a result of laboratory accidents or transfusions may be severe and should be treated. The treatment regimen of choice consists of a combination of pyrimethamine (Daraprim) and sulfadiazine or trisulfapyrimidine (a mixture of equal parts of sulfamethazine, sulfamerazine, and sulfadiazine) given for 2 to 4 weeks with folinic acid (leucovorin). Oral pyrimethamine is administered at a loading dose of 2 mg per kg per day, up to a maximum of 100 to 200 mg for 2 days, followed by 25 to 50 mg daily, along with 10 mg of folinic acid. Sulfadiazine or trisulfapyrimidine, 100 mg per kg per day (maximum daily dose of 4 to 8 gm) in four divided doses, is given by mouth. In the event of pyrimethamine-induced hematologic toxicity (cytopenia), the dose of folinic acid can be increased to 20 mg per day. As of August 1994, sulfadiazine is available in the United States through Eon Labs Manufacturing, Inc., 227-15 North Conduit Avenue, Laurelton, New York 11413; telephone 800-336-1595 or 718-276-8607.

Ocular Toxoplasmosis

Toxoplasmosis most frequently causes a retinochoroiditis that is usually a manifestation of congenital infection but is also seen occasionally in acute acquired disease and in patients with AIDS. Signs and symptoms include decreased visual acuity, eye pain, scotomas, photophobia, nystagmus, and strabismus. Signs of systemic involvement are uncommon except in patients with AIDS, in whom ocular toxoplasmosis can be a harbinger of central nervous system (CNS) infection. Diagnosis is based on the ophthalmic ex-

TABLE 2. **Overview of Drugs Currently Used to Treat Toxoplasmosis**

Antimicrobial	Mode of Action	Metabolism	Adverse Effects	Recommended Dose	
				Immunocompromised	*Immunocompetent*
Pyrimethamine (Daraprim) oral	Inhibits folic acid synthesis	Readily absorbed by gut; hepatic metabolism, lipid soluble	Cytopenias, rash, GI intolerance	Acute: loading dose, 100–200 mg; 50–75 mg daily for 3–6 weeks, with oral folinic acid 10–20 mg/day. Maintenance: 25–50 mg per day, with oral folinic acid 10–20 mg/day	Loading dose, 2 mg/kg per day (max 100–200 mg); then 25–50 mg daily for 2–4 weeks, with oral folinic acid 10–20 mg/day
Sulfadiazine* or trisulfapyrimidine oral	Inhibits folic acid synthesis; acts synergistically and sequentially with pyrimethamine	Readily absorbed by gut; penetrates blood-brain barrier; some hepatic metabolism	GI intolerance, rash (Stevens-Johnson syndrome), cytopenias, nephrolithiasis, crystalluria, interstitial nephritis, encephalopathy	Acute: 4–6 gm/day for 3–6 weeks. Maintenance: 2–4 gm/day in four equally divided doses	100 mg/kg/day (max 4–8 gm/day) in four equally divided doses for 2–4 weeks
Clindamycin* (Cleocin) oral and IV	Unknown; possibly inhibition of protein synthesis	Readily absorbed by gut; excellent tissue penetration	GI intolerance, rash, pseudomembranous colitis	Acute: 600 mg every 6 h for 3–6 weeks. Maintenance: same	300 mg every 6 h for 4 weeks; repeat as needed

*Most effective when used with pyrimethamine.
Abbreviation: GI = gastrointestinal.

TABLE 3. **Drugs Used to Treat Toxoplasmosis in Pregnant Women and for Congenital Toxoplasmosis**

Antimicrobial	Adverse Effects	Recommended Dose		
		(Pregnancy—1st Trimester)	Pregnancy—2nd & 3rd Trimesters	Congenital
Spiramycin* oral	Nausea, vomiting	30–50 mg/kg per day, in three divided doses	30–50 mg/kg per day, in three divided doses; if fetal infection confirmed or suspected, then pyrimethamine and sulfadiazine may be superior for treatment of fetus	50–100 mg/kg per day in two equally divided doses; 4- to 6-week course alternating with a 3-week course of pyrimethamine and sulfadiazine
Pyrimethamine (Daraprim) oral	Cytopenias, rash, GI intolerance	Not recommended— teratogenic	Loading dose, 100 mg/ day for 2 days, then 50 mg/day with folinic acid, 10 mg orally (with sulfadiazine or trisulfapyrimidine)	Loading dose 2 mg/kg for 2 days, then 1 mg/kg with folinic acid, 10 mg orally, three times per week for up to 1 year (with sulfadiazine or trisulfapyrimidine)
Sulfadiazine or trisulfapyrimidine oral	GI intolerance, rash (Stevens-Johnson syndrome), cytopenias, nephrolithiasis, crystalluria, interstitial nephritis, encephalopathy	50–100 mg/kg per day in two equally divided doses (alone)	50–100 mg/kg/day in two equally divided doses (with pyrimethamine)	50–100 mg/kg/day in two equally divided doses for up to 1 year

*Spiramycin is available on request from the U.S. Food and Drug Administration (telephone 301-443-9553).
Abbreviation: GI = gastrointestinal.
From Remington JS, McLeod R, Desmonts G: Toxoplasmosis. *In* Remington JS, Klein JO (eds): Infectious Diseases of the Fetus & Newborn Infant, 4th ed. Philadelphia, WB Saunders Co, 1995, pp 140–267.

amination combined with serologic evidence of toxoplasmosis. Treatment is required in order to prevent relapse and the risk of progressive visual loss and other complications, such as glaucoma.

The drugs of choice are oral pyrimethamine and sulfadiazine or trisulfapyrimidine with folinic acid, in the same dosages as described in the previous section. For sulfa-allergic nonimmunocompromised patients, clindamycin (Cleocin) 300 mg orally every 6 hours in combination with pyrimethamine and folinic acid has been used successfully; 600 mg every 6 hours is used for patients with AIDS. Therapy is given for 4 weeks and repeated as needed. Adjunctive therapy with systemic corticosteroids (prednisone 80 to 120 mg per day or an equivalent) is indicated if the macula, optic nerve, or papillomacular bundle is

TABLE 4. **Alternative or Investigational Drugs Used to Treat Toxoplasmosis in Immunocompromised Patients**

Antimicrobial	Mode of Action	Metabolism	Adverse Effects	Recommended Dose
Atovaquone* (Mepron) oral	Uncoupling electron biosynthesis; inhibition of de novo pyrimidine biosynthesis	Suspension has better bioavailability than old tablet formulation; improved absorption if taken with food, particularly fatty foods	Rash, elevated liver function tests	Acute: suspension—1500 mg two times/day for 3–6 weeks Maintenance: same
Azithromycin* (Zithromax) oral	Unknown; possibly inhibition of protein synthesis	Readily absorbed by gut; high intracellular levels	GI intolerance	Acute: 1250–1500 mg/day for 3–6 weeks Maintenance: same
Clarithromycin* (Biaxin) oral	Unknown; possibly inhibition of protein synthesis	Readily absorbed by gut; high tissue levels	GI intolerance, hearing loss, elevated liver function tests	Acute: 1 gm/day in two equally divided doses for 3–6 weeks Maintenance: same

*Most effective when used in combination with pyrimethamine.
Abbreviation: GI = gastrointestinal.

TABLE 5. Drugs Used for Primary Prophylaxis of Toxoplasmic Encephalitis in HIV-Positive Patients

Antimicrobial	Recommended Dose
Trimethoprim-sulfamethoxazole (Bactrim) oral	1 double-strength tablet per day
Dapsone* oral	100 mg two times/week (with pyrimethamine)
Pyrimethamine* (Daraprim) oral	25 mg/week (with dapsone)

*Most effective when used in combination.

involved. In particular cases, photocoagulation and vitrectomy may be necessary.

Toxoplasmosis in Immunocompromised Hosts

Toxoplasmic encephalitis (TE) is the most frequent manifestation of toxoplasmosis in patients with AIDS and is the most common cause of focal CNS infection in this clinical setting. The incidence of TE is directly proportional to the prevalence of antibodies to *T. gondii* in any given population. In the United States, 10 to 30% of adults with AIDS are latently infected, and it is estimated that 30% of these patients will develop TE. Over 80% of cases of TE occur when the absolute number of CD4 lymphocytes falls to less than 100 per mm^3, although the risk of developing overt infection begins when CD4 counts fall below 200 per mm^3. The large majority of patients who develop TE have serologic evidence of past infection, and this disease process is thought to be caused by reactivation of latent toxoplasmosis.

Clinical manifestations include signs and symptoms of focal or generalized neurologic dysfunction (Table 6). Neuroimaging studies typically show multiple contrast-enhancing mass lesions. The clinical manifestations and radiographic findings are not specific for toxoplasmosis. The differential diagnosis includes other infections that cause space-occupying CNS lesions, such as tuberculoma, cryptococcoma, and, most frequently in the United States, CNS lymphoma. A definitive diagnosis requires a brain biopsy. Regardless, therapy is generally started empirically, based on the clinical and neuroradiographic evidence in a patient with a CD4 lymphocyte count less than 200 mm^3 and who is seropositive for anti–*T. gondii* antibodies. Using these criteria, the predictive value according to one study was 80%. Seventy percent of patients with TE will have a quantifiable clinical improvement by Day 7 of therapy. Conversely, patients not responding to empiric therapy usually have evidence of progressive disease within the first 10 days. Ninety percent of patients will show improvement on neuroradiographic studies within 6 weeks of starting therapy.

The combination of pyrimethamine (an initial 200-mg loading dose in two divided doses followed by 50 to 75 mg per day orally) and sulfadiazine (4 to 6 gm per day by mouth in four divided doses) remains the mainstay of treatment. Oral folinic acid 10 to 20 mg per day is added to preclude the hematologic toxicities associated with antifolate agents. Acute therapy is given for at least 3 weeks; 6 weeks or more is indicated in severely ill patients and when a complete clinical or radiographic response has not been achieved. Sulfa-intolerant patients can be given clindamycin 600 mg orally or intravenously every 6 hours in combination with pyrimethamine, as described earlier. Chronic suppressive therapy (described later) is indicated in all immunocompromised patients until an adequate cell-mediated immune response is restored. Prophylactic use of anticonvulsants is not recommended. Corticosteroids should not be used routinely but are indicated if there is evidence of increased intracranial pressure. The use of corticosteroids may complicate the interpretation of the response to empiric therapy, because clinical and radiographic improvements may be related to reduced cerebral edema or the size of a steroid-sensitive CNS lymphoma. The same chemotherapeutic regimens are used for extraneural toxoplasmosis, but there are limited data available on the optimal

TABLE 6. Clinical Manifestations of Toxoplasmic Encephalitis in Patients with AIDS

Focal Neurologic Deficits	Generalized Cerebral Dysfunction	Neuropsychiatric Abnormalities
Hemiparesis	Lethargy	Dementia
Hemiplegia	Confusion	Anxiety
Dysphasia	Coma	Personality changes
Aphasia	Decreased recent memory	Psychosis
Movement disorders: hemichorea, hemiballismus	Global cognitive impairment, like AIDS dementia	
Seizures	Decreased attention	
Ataxia	Slowed motor responses	
Diplopia	Slowed verbal responses	
Visual field deficits		
Cranial nerve palsies		
Cerebellar tremor		
Parkinsonian symptoms		
Thalamic syndrome		
Hemisensory loss		
Headache (severe localized)		

length and outcome of treatment. As a rule, ocular toxoplasmosis responds favorably to therapy, and treatment of pulmonary infection has been reported to be successful in 50 to 77% of patients. Intravenous trimethoprim-sulfamethoxazole (Bactrim, Septra) 5 mg per kg of trimethoprim component every 6 hours has been used in small numbers of patients when oral therapy is contraindicated. Although available for oral use, trimethoprim-sulfamethoxazole has achieved lower response rates than those seen with standard regimens.

The drugs described thus far are active against only the tachyzoite form of *T. gondii*. Surviving tissue cysts can reinitiate TE and other manifestations of reactivated latent disease if treatment is discontinued. Therefore, it is necessary to give chronic suppressive therapy. Pyrimethamine 25 mg per day and sulfadiazine 2 to 4 gm per day orally in four equally divided doses, with 10 mg per day of oral folinic acid are recommended, based on the low relapse rate associated with this combination. In sulfa-allergic patients, clindamycin is used; a daily dose of at least 2400 mg in four divided doses by mouth is recommended. The combination of clindamycin and pyrimethamine has a higher relapse rate than pyrimethamine and sulfadiazine. Other possible prophylactic agents under investigation include pyrimethamine and sulfadoxine (Fansidar) and the combination of pyrimethamine and dapsone given two to three times per week. These agents have been used successfully in small numbers of patients.

Primary chemoprophylaxis is an attractive therapeutic option for patients known to be at risk of developing toxoplasmosis, such as HIV-infected patients with CD4 counts less than 100 per mm^3 and who are seropositive for anti–*T. gondii* antibodies. Based on retrospective data, oral trimethoprim-sulfamethoxazole (one double-strength tablet per day) may be efficacious in this regard. When used as single agents, dapsone and pyrimethamine may not be effective. However, the combination of these drugs—pyrimethamine 25 mg per week and dapsone 100 mg two times per week—may be useful in this regard. In sulfa-allergic patients, desensitization is also an option.

Drug regimens currently being studied for their usefulness as initial and maintenance therapy include atovaquone (Mepron),* which is being investigated in combination with pyrimethamine, sulfadiazine, or clarithromycin (Biaxin) because of the high relapse rate when atovaquone is used alone. The newest formulation of atovaquone is administered as an oral suspension (1500 mg twice per day) with food (preferably fatty foods) to increase the bioavailability of the drug. The new macrolide antibiotic azithromycin (Zithromax), at a daily oral dose of 1250 to 1500 mg in combination with 50 to 75 mg per day of pyrimethamine, has limited utility as an alternative regimen.

---

*Not FDA-approved for this indication.

Toxoplasmosis in Pregnant Women

Women who acquire toxoplasmosis during pregnancy expose their fetuses to risk of infection. Overall, transplacental transmission occurs in greater than 50% of untreated and approximately 20% of treated women who are pregnant at the time of infection. Infection of the fetus may result in stillbirth, spontaneous abortion, or birth of a symptomatic or asymptomatic infant. The incidence of fetal infection and the severity of infection are correlated to the trimester during which maternal infection occurs. If infection occurs at 22 to 24 weeks of gestation and the infection goes untreated, the infant has approximately a 25% chance of becoming infected transplacentally, and the infection tends to be severe. During the second and third trimesters, transplacental infection is more likely, 54 and 65%, respectively, but the disease tends to be less severe or asymptomatic during the neonatal period. However, these infants are subject to significant morbidity later in life.

Pyrimethamine plus a sulfonamide or spiramycin (a macrolide antibiotic available in Western Europe, Mexico, and Canada but only through the Food and Drug Administration in the United States: telephone number 301-443-9553) appears to decrease the incidence of congenital toxoplasmic infection when given to women who acquire *T. gondii* during pregnancy. Pyrimethamine is teratogenic and should not be used until after the first trimester, however. There is no optimal medical therapy in the United States for women who become infected during the first trimester. However, sulfadiazine or trisulfapyrimidines should be used during the first trimester, because sulfonamides alone have been shown to be effective in acute toxoplasmosis in animal models. Most experience of maternal treatment to prevent transmission is with spiramycin. If spiramycin can be obtained, pregnant women who are acutely infected in the first trimester may be treated until term with 30 to 50 mg per kg per day orally, in two equal doses every 12 hours, in 3-week courses alternating with 2-week drug-free intervals. Treatment with spiramycin alone decreases the incidence of transmission but not the severity of established congenital infection. Maternal treatment with pyrimethamine plus sulfadiazine appears to attenuate the clinical manifestations in the fetus. If fetal infection is suspected after the first trimester, pyrimethamine, sulfadiazine, and folinic acid should be used to treat the maternal infection.

Congenital Toxoplasmosis

Acute infection with *T. gondii* can be clinically manifest, usually as lymphadenopathy, in 10 to 20% of pregnant women. The fetus is at risk of transplacental infection whether or not the mother is symptomatic. Infants with clinically apparent disease at birth may have a combination of the signs and symptoms (Table 7); 8% have severe impairment of the CNS or eyes. Seventy-five percent are asymptomatic. The incidence of untoward sequelae in the asymp-

TABLE 7. **Clinical Manifestations of Toxoplasmosis in Newborns and Prominent Sequelae in Asymptomatic Newborns**

Toxoplasmosis in Newborns	Prominent Sequelae in Asymptomatic Newborns
Hydrocephalus	Sensorineural hearing loss
Microcephalus	Retinochoroiditis
Cerebral calcification	Hydrocephalus
Seizure disorders	Seizures
Psychomotor retardation	Blindness
Micro-ophthalmia	Mental retardation
Strabismus	Delayed psychomotor development
Cataracts	
Glaucoma	
Retinochoroiditis	
Optic atrophy	
Lymphadenopathy	
Myocarditis	
Pneumonitis	
Hepatosplenomegaly	
Fever	
Hypothermia	
Vomiting	
Diarrhea	
Jaundice	
Rash	
Deafness	

tomatic population has been studied prospectively and has been found to be greater than 85%. Prominent manifestations are listed in Table 7.

Optimal treatment for congenital toxoplasmosis is not yet established. A national collaborative, prospective study is being performed by a Chicago group to evaluate the outcome in infants treated with a combination of pyrimethamine, sulfadiazine, and folinic acid. Two different doses of pyrimethamine are being compared. Medications are begun when the child is 2.5 months old and continue for 1 year. Preliminary results indicate that this therapeutic regimen can be administered safely to children. The most significant adverse effect has been transient neutropenia, which responded to increased doses of folinic acid or withholding of pyrimethamine. The current guidelines for treatment of congenital toxoplasmosis are pyrimethamine 2 mg per kg for 2 days as a loading dose, then 1 mg per kg with folinic acid 10 mg orally, and sulfadiazine or trisulfapyrimidine 50 to 100 mg, three times per week up to 1 year. If spiramycin is available, the dose is 50 to 100 mg per kg per day orally, in two equal portions every 12 hours. If a patient has evidence of an inflammatory process (chorioretinitis, high cerebrospinal fluid protein content, generalized infection, jaundice), glucocorticosteroids (prednisone or methylprednisolone 1 to 2 mg per kg per day orally, as two equal portions every 12 hours) should be prescribed until the inflammatory process has subsided.

PREVENTION

As long as humans continue to eat meat and associate with domestic and wild cats, they will continue to serve as incidental hosts to the parasite *T. gondii*. One can help prevent infection by eating only meat that has been well cooked (>60° C) or that has been frozen (< −20° C for at least 24 hours) and thawed. Consistent handwashing after handling cats or their feces should decrease the ingestion of oocysts. Also, cat litter boxes should be emptied daily, before the oocysts can become infectious. Cat owners should keep their cats indoors, if possible, and feed them commercial cat food or well-cooked table food only. Specifically, pregnant women and immunocompromised hosts (particularly HIV-positive patients) should observe these prevention strategies.

TRICHINOSIS

method of
PETER F. WELLER, M.D., and
LEO X. LIU, M.D., D.T.M.H.
Harvard Medical School
Boston, Massachusetts

Trichinosis is caused by the nematode *Trichinella spiralis*. The disease is acquired by the ingestion of meat that contains encysted larvae of the parasite. Most commonly the infected meat is pork, but it may also be horse meat or that of wild animals, including bears, walruses, and boars. The severity of the infection increases with the numbers of ingested larvae. After the ingestion of infected meat, two phases of infection develop.

INTESTINAL PHASE

The digestion of meat liberates encysted larvae that develop into adult worms that burrow into the villi of the small intestine. Within 5 to 7 days after ingestion, the adult worms produce larvae that enter the circulation. During this early enteric phase of trichinosis, patients may experience nausea, vomiting, constipation, diarrhea, abdominal aches, or no symptoms at all. These intestinal symptoms may subside before or overlap with the subsequent muscle-invasion phase of the infection. Larval production continues for 2 to 5 weeks, rarely longer. Intestinal symptoms are usually short-lived over a couple of weeks, although previously infected patients can experience prolonged diarrhea.

MUSCLE PHASE

Patients may develop periorbital and facial edema, subconjunctival and retinal hemorrhages, and subungual splinter hemorrhages as a result of the hematogenous spread of larvae. About 3 weeks after infection, the larvae begin to encyst in skeletal muscle, and patients may experience myalgias, muscle edema and weakness, fever, and eosinophilia. Headache, cough, dyspnea, dysphagia, and macular or urticarial skin lesions may occur. Although larvae encyst only in skeletal muscle, in serious infections inflammatory lesions may develop in the heart, central nervous system (CNS), and lungs. Most infections are mild, and symptoms subside and disappear within a couple of weeks. In heavier infections, resolution may be prolonged and fatalities can occur, especially from myocarditis.

DIAGNOSIS

The triad of periorbital edema, myalgias, and eosinophilia is strongly suggestive of the diagnosis of trichinosis. Usually, but not always, a history of consuming potentially infected meat can be elicited from the patient, and others who ate the same meat may also have symptoms due to trichinosis. Serologic tests are available, but a diagnostic rise in specific antibody titer often does not develop until a couple of weeks after the onset of the muscle phase. Muscle biopsy can provide a definitive diagnosis by demonstrating encysting larvae.

TREATMENT AND PREVENTION

Specific anthelminthic treatment of trichinosis is not very satisfactory. The infection is self-limited and not life-threatening in most patients. Therefore, bed rest, analgesics, and antipyretics are sufficient. For those with serious infections, including myocarditis or CNS involvement, prednisone (40 to 60 mg per day) is given with mebendazole (Vermox),* 200 to 400 mg three times daily for 3 days then 400 to 500 mg three times daily for 10 days. Prednisone suppresses the eosinophil-rich inflammatory reactions within affected tissues. Whether mebendazole promotes killing of muscle-stage larvae is not certain, but this medication terminates any continuing infection from intestinal-phase parasites. Mebendazole should be avoided during pregnancy but otherwise is safe and well tolerated.

Larvae in pork can be killed by heating meat to 77° C. Alternatively, freezing meat at −15° C for 3 weeks kills larvae, except those of arctic strains of the parasite that might be present in bear or walrus meat from arctic areas.

TULAREMIA

method of
SHEREE R. POITIER, M.D., and
GLENN E. MATHISEN, M.D.
Los Angeles County/Olive View Medical Center
Sylmar, California

Tularemia is an acute febrile illness caused by the small, pleomorphic gram-negative coccobacilli *Francisella tularensis*. It is a zoonotic disease that is found throughout the Northern hemisphere between the latitudes of 30 and 71 degrees, particularly in rural areas where there are infected animal reservoirs. The disease is traditionally classified into six clinical syndromes: ulceroglandular, glandular, oculoglandular, pharyngeal, typhoidal, and pneumonic. However, this distinction is for convenience only and does not indicate any fundamental difference in the source of infection, the course of illness, or the prognosis of the disease.

Francisella tularensis is primarily a pathogen of animals, and occasionally of humans. It has been associated with over 100 species of wild animals (e.g., hares, rabbits, deer, beavers), 9 species of domestic animals such as cats,

---
*Not FDA-approved for this indication.

sheep, and cattle, and 25 species of birds, fish, and amphibians. The transmission of *F. tularensis* to humans has been associated with the direct handling of animal tissues or direct contact with animal body fluids. In addition, the disease can be transmitted by insect bites (deer flies, ticks, mosquitoes), animal bites, aerosol inhalation, and ingestion of contaminated water or undercooked meat. Blood-sucking arthropods and flies are the most important vectors for tularemia in the United States. The dog tick *(Dermacentor variabilis)*, the wood tick *(D. andersoni)*, and the Lone Star tick *(Amblyomma americanum)* are commonly involved in the transmission of disease in North America. Human-to-human transmission of tularemia has been reported only rarely, and most authorities believe this route to be of no clinical importance.

In the United States, tularemia has been reported in all 50 states, with the majority of cases in Missouri, Arkansas, Texas, Tennessee, and Oklahoma. The disease has a seasonal occurrence, being most frequent in the summer and winter months. Cases acquired in the summer months are usually tick-associated, whereas transmission in the winter months is generally associated with hunting and direct contact with infected animals. The disease is more common in the male sex and occurs in all age groups. The preponderance of males is thought to be related to greater exposure risks related to occupation as well as to outdoor recreational activities. Occupations that have been associated with tularemia include laboratory workers, farmers, veterinarians, sheep workers, hunters or trappers, and cooks or meat handlers.

The diagnosis of tularemia should be suspected in patients with a compatible clinical presentation and a potential exposure to infected animals or tick bites. The clinical manifestations of tularemia depend on several factors: the virulence of the infecting organism, the portal of entry, the extent of systemic disease, and the immune status of the host. The spectrum of disease can range from asymptomatic disease to acute sepsis and death.

The most common presentation of tularemia is ulceroglandular disease (70 to 85%), which is characterized by a painful ulcer at the site of the initial inoculation (usually on the lower extremities or trunk in patients with tick-associated disease) and painful regional lymphadenopathy. Typhoidal tularemia (5 to 15%) may be difficult to diagnose since patients usually lack lymphadenopathy and present with a nonspecific syndrome characterized by fever, chills, and weight loss. Tularemia pneumonia may be seen with any form of tularemia and occasionally results in acute respiratory distress syndrome (ARDS). Other clinical categories of infection include oculoglandular, oropharyngeal, and rarely, meningitis, osteomyelitis, and pericarditis.

All forms of tularemia have been associated with systemic symptoms such as fever, chills, headache, malaise, hepatitis, rash, anorexia, and fatigue. Fever is usually greater than 101° F and a pulse-temperature deficit has been noted in up to 42% of patients. Less virulent strains cause a milder, self-limited illness that may resolve without therapy. Other prominent symptoms may include cough, myalgia, chest discomfort, vomiting, sore throat, diarrhea, and abdominal pain. The incubation period averages from 3 to 5 days but ranges from less than 1 day to 21 days. Following inoculation, a papule develops at the site; rapid ulceration of the lesion occurs, followed by lymphadenopathy and systemic symptoms.

The definitive diagnosis of tularemia is made by recovery of the organism from blood or lymph nodes. However, because laboratory confirmation often lags by several days to weeks, strong clinical suspicion of the presence of disease generally mandates early empirical antimicrobial therapy. *Francisella tularensis* does not grow well on ordinary laboratory media, and growth must be supplemented with cysteine. The isolation and cultivation of *F. tularensis* represents a definite danger to laboratory personnel; the laboratory should be informed if tularemia is suspected so that proper precautions can be taken to prevent transmission to laboratory workers. Other methods are useful in the diagnosis of tularemia, including the use of serologic testing; a single positive titer of agglutinating antibody of 160 or greater in the appropriate clinical setting is strong evidence for the disease, although a fourfold rise in titer is required for confirmation. Serologies are usually negative during the first week but become positive in 50 to 70% of patients by the third week of illness. Diagnosis of tularemia may be made by direct immunofluorescence of infected tissues and secretions; this test is available through most state public health laboratories and serves to provide a rapid diagnosis as well as rule out other pathogens (e.g., plague) that may mimic tularemia.

TREATMENT

The antibiotic of first choice for virtually all forms of tularemia remains streptomycin. Only meningitis requires the use of a drug with greater central nervous system penetration, such as chloramphenicol. The minimal dosage of streptomycin that is effective in tularemia is 7.5 to 10 mg per kg intramuscularly every 12 hours for 7 to 10 days; treatment regimens of shorter duration are associated with a greater frequency of relapse. Higher doses of streptomycin (15 mg per kg per day in divided doses) may be more appropriate for more severely ill patients; however, doses greater than 2 grams per day do not increase the clinical efficacy of the drug and are associated with increased toxicity (renal insufficiency, ototoxicity).

Because streptomycin was unavailable in the United States for a period of time prior to its remarketing in 1993, practitioners have turned to other antibiotics as possible alternatives. Gentamicin is considered to be an effective alternative to streptomycin, although fewer studies are available to document clinical efficacy. Gentamicin should be considered in patients who are allergic to streptomycin, who are pregnant, or when the diagnosis is in doubt. Gentamicin is given intravenously at a dose of 3 to 5 mg per kg per day in divided doses for 7 to 10 days; desired peak serum levels of at least 5.0 μg per mL should be obtained. Other aminoglycosides such as kanamycin (Kantrex) and tobramycin (Nebcin) have also been reported to be active against *F. tularensis*; however, experience with these drugs is limited.

Chloramphenicol and tetracycline have both been used in tularemia. Both drugs are bacteriostatic for *F. tularensis*, and this may account for the higher relapse rates seen when these drugs are used for therapy. With the exception of meningitis, use of chloramphenicol alone should be avoided because of the potential toxicity of the drug as well as reports of high relapse rates. Chloramphenicol is administered as an oral loading dose (30 mg per kg orally), followed by 30 to 50 mg per kg per day in divided

doses for 14 days. Higher intravenous doses (50 to 100 mg per kg per day in divided doses) are more appropriate for critically ill patients. Tetracycline should be reserved for the ambulatory patient whose illness is of greater than a week's duration and who is tolerating the illness well. Tetracycline is most effective for adults if given as 2 grams per day in divided doses for at least 14 days. It should not be given to children under 9 years of age or to pregnant or lactating females. Care should also be exercised when administering the drug to patients with liver disease.

Erythromycin has been used successfully in a few patients, and some strains appear susceptible to the drug. Nevertheless, increasing in vitro resistance to erythromycin has been demonstrated (particularly in strains from outside North America), and the drug should not be relied upon in seriously ill patients with suspected tularemia. Other antibiotics reported to have in vitro activity against *F. tularensis* include ciprofloxacin, norfloxacin, and imipenem/cilastatin; however, little clinical experience has been reported aside from several favorable anecdotal case reports. Third-generation cephalosporins have been used, but a recent report documented several outpatient failures with ceftriaxone despite previously reported in vitro susceptibility to the drug. Antibiotics shown to be ineffective include penicillins, cephalexin (Keflex), cefuroxime (Zinacef), ceftazidime (Fortaz), and meropenem.*

PREVENTION

Chemoprophylaxis for persons exposed to those with tularemia is not recommended. Individuals with a high occupational risk are advised to take measures to prevent direct skin contact. Insect repellents should also be used to prevent arthropod bites. A vaccine made from live attenuated *F. tularensis* is useful for partial protection of laboratory workers but not practical for the prevention of tick-borne tularemia.

SALMONELLOSIS

method of
T. M. S. REID, M.B., C.L.B.
Aberdeen Royal Infirmary
Aberdeen, Scotland, United Kingdom

Nontyphoidal *Salmonella* infection, with its significant morbidity and mortality, presents a major therapeutic challenge worldwide. The increasing rates of antibiotic resistance in *Salmonella* spp further complicate clinical management.

ACUTE GASTROENTERITIS

Ingestion of nontyphoidal *Salmonella* results in acute gastroenteritis after an incubation period of 12

---

*Not available in the United States.

to 36 hours during which the salmonellae colonize and damage the intestinal mucosa, producing increased fluid secretion and intestinal motility. The illness is usually self-limiting, with nausea, vomiting, abdominal cramps, and diarrhea lasting for 3 to 4 days but in some more than 1 week. Fever is present in 50% of patients and persists for 1 to 2 days. Treatment is based on rehydration and correction of electrolyte abnormalities orally in mild cases or intravenously in the more severe. Symptomatic relief can be achieved with antipyretics and antiemetics, but antiperistaltic-antispasmodic agents such as loperamide and diphenoxylate are contraindicated as they can exacerbate the illness. Before the advent of the 4-fluoroquinolone group of antimicrobial agents, antibiotic therapy was not recommended in acute uncomplicated salmonella gastroenteritis since treatment frequently failed to influence the clinical course of the illness and there was concern that such treatment might prolong carriage and promote the spread of antibiotic resistance. However, despite some conflicting data, it would appear that oral treatment with ciprofloxacin (Cipro), 500 mg twice daily for 5 days; ofloxacin (Floxin), 100 mg twice daily for 6 to 10 days; or norfloxacin (Noroxin),* 400 mg twice daily for 5 days, can shorten the duration of fever, diarrhea, and fecal excretion, although relapse and persistent long-term carriage may be a problem in some patients. Antimicrobial therapy is indicated for high-risk patients such as the elderly; the immunosuppressed, including those with lymphoproliferative disorders, sickle cell disease, and acquired immune deficiency disease (AIDS); and neonates and young infants (less than 3 months of age). Nonessential use of quinolones should be avoided in children, as animal studies have suggested there may be a potential risk of cartilage dysplasia.

CONVALESCENT CARRIAGE

Convalescent carriage of nontyphoidal salmonellae is common, the mean duration of excretion being approximately 4 weeks in adults and older children and 7 weeks in children under 5 years. Oral quinolone therapy (e.g., ciprofloxacin 500 mg or 750 mg twice daily for 5 to 14 days) can be used effectively as an infection control measure when outbreaks of salmonella infection involve individuals who work in high-risk areas, for example, health care workers and food handlers. Prompt treatment can ensure that they can return to work without undue delay, and the risk of transmission to susceptible individuals is eliminated. Similarly, high-risk geriatric and psychiatric patients who are a potential source of infection to other patients and staff alike can be cleared and the need for prolonged isolation removed.

CHRONIC CARRIAGE

Approximately 1% of patients are still excreting nontyphoidal salmonellae 1 year after infection, i.e.,

*Not FDA-approved for this indication.

they are chronic carriers. Factors predisposing to chronic carriage are age (over 50 years) and biliary tract disease. In the past, attempts to eradicate chronic carriage consisted of giving ampicillin or amoxicillin (4 to 6 grams per day) in four divided doses with or without probenecid (Benemid) 2 grams per day in divided doses for 5 to 6 weeks. Such regimens are 50 to 90% successful, but failures and relapses are common, particularly in patients with biliary tract disease. The use of such high dosage results in correspondingly high rates of side effects, notably diarrhea, rashes, and eosinophilia, and the broad-spectrum suppression of the normal bowel flora predisposes to overgrowth with antibiotic-resistant species. Antibiotic treatment or surgery (cholecystectomy) alone may not be sufficient; the combination may ultimately prove to be effective.

Quinolone antimicrobial agents are of proven value in treating chronic salmonella carriers although the optimal dose and duration of therapy are open to debate. Various oral regimens have proved effective: ciprofloxacin 500 mg twice daily for 28 days or 750 mg twice daily for 14 or 21 days or ofloxacin 400 mg once a day for 7 days.

Prolonged gastrointestinal carriage of nontyphoidal salmonellae in infants (5.4% still excreting after 1 year) is a potential source of infection for close family contacts, other infants, and nursing staff. Treatment of such chronic carriage remains somewhat problematic as the quinolones may be contraindicated in view of their potential for adverse effects on growing cartilage (see later discussion). The high biliary and gall bladder wall concentrations achievable with some of the newer intravenous cephalosporins, such as ceftriaxone (Rocephin), suggest that these agents might be effective despite relatively poor intracellular penetration.

INVASIVE SALMONELLOSIS

Severe invasive infection occurs in a small proportion of patients (approximately 5%) when the salmonellae pass through the intestinal mucosa with resulting bacteremia. However, rates of 40 to 80% are not uncommon in immunosuppressed patients and immunocompromised patients with cancer or human immunodeficiency virus (HIV) infection, all of whom are prone to develop local and metastatic extraintestinal suppurative complications and frequently relapse despite appropriate antibiotic therapy, probably because of their impaired cell-mediated immunity. Recognized host factors that predispose to severe invasive salmonellosis include extremes of age (neonates and infants less than 1 year of age, and the elderly), hypochlorhydria, previous gastrectomy, chronic hemodialysis, sickle cell disease, systemic lupus erythematosus, uremia, AIDS, and neomycin therapy. Diarrhea is itself a defense mechanism designed to minimize contact time between gut pathogens and the intestinal mucosa, and consequently drugs that reduce intestinal motility such as diphenoxylate (Lomotil), loperamide (Imodium), domperidone (Motilium),* and codeine phosphate may also promote the development of toxic megacolon and bacteremia with its complications and should be avoided.

Invasive salmonella infection requires prompt antibiotic treatment to produce a rapid resolution of clinical symptoms, prevent relapse, and ideally eradicate the organism from the gastrointestinal tract. Systemic salmonellosis can be successfully treated with intravenous ampicillin, 150 to 200 mg per kg per day in 4 to 6 doses; chloramphenicol (Chloromycetin), 50 mg per kg every 6 hours for 14 days; or trimethoprim-sulfamethoxazole (TMP–SMX) (Septra, Bactrim), 5 to 25 mg per kg twice daily for 14 days, clinical improvement and defervescence in 2 to 5 days being the norm. However, resistance to all three agents is increasing in nontyphoidal salmonellae, greatly restricting the therapeutic options. Ampicillin is frequently contraindicated by a history of known or perceived beta-lactam allergy. Chloramphenicol, like TMP–SMX, lacks bactericidal activity against *Salmonella* spp at clinically achievable levels and is consequently slow to eradicate the organism from the bloodstream and has a very limited effect on the relapse or recurrence rate and the development of the chronic carrier state. Chloramphenicol and TMP–SMX are in addition associated with significant well-established toxicity: bone marrow suppression and, in the case of TMP–SMX, rashes and the development of Stevens-Johnson syndrome.

The third-generation cephalosporins such as cefotaxime (Claforan), ceftazidime (Fortaz), and ceftriaxone and the quinolones are up to 400 times more active in vitro than ampicillin or chloramphenicol. However, there is not necessarily a good correlation between the in vitro sensitivity and the clinical response, the degree of tissue and cellular penetration being of major importance. Cephalosporins show poor intracellular penetration, and thus the older cephalosporins, either alone or in combination with an aminoglycoside, are ineffective in the treatment of salmonella septicemia. Even the response to ceftazidime is variable, prolonged high-dose therapy (2 to 3 grams twice daily for 2 to 3 weeks) being required for a successful outcome. There is evidence of antagonism between chloramphenicol and the cephalosporins, and thus such combination therapy is not recommended. In view of their high activity and long serum half-lives, the newest cephalosporins are candidates for high-dose, short-course treatment, e.g., ceftriaxone, 3 to 4 grams daily intravenously for 5 to 7 days. These agents may be particularly useful in treating systemic salmonellosis in children, in whom the therapeutic choice is limited. In general, these antimicrobials with their high specific activity rapidly eliminate the salmonellae from the bloodstream but are slower to produce defervescence, probably a reflection of their limitations in cellular penetration. Low relapse rates appear to correlate with high levels of biliary excretion (ceftriaxone more than cefotaxime).

The quinolones have a profile that commends them for treating salmonella infection—high rapid bactericidal activity against *Salmonella* spp including multiresistant strains; rapid oral absorption resulting in wide tissue distribution with high concentrations achieved in bile, gall bladder wall, and feces; and excellent intracellular penetration and concentration within neutrophils and macrophages. An excellent pharmacokinetic profile is obtained after oral dosing, and consequently oral ciprofloxacin, 500 or 750 mg twice daily for 7 to 10 days; intravenous ciprofloxacin, 400 mg twice daily; or sequential intravenous and oral ciprofloxacin are all effective in treating salmonella septicemia, and prolonged high-dose therapy (1 to 2 weeks intravenously plus 3 to 4 weeks orally) has been used with some success in immunocompromised patients such as AIDS patients, in whom post-treatment relapse is a recurring problem. Long-term antibiotic suppressive treatment, oral ciprofloxacin 750 mg twice daily for up to 8 months, has been suggested for intractable cases. In patients with AIDS, zidovudine (AZT) (Retrovir),* 400 mg per day, may be beneficial by improving immune function or by direct antibacterial activity (zidovudine has in vitro activity against gram-negative organisms including salmonellae).

Salmonella septicemia can result—particularly in debilitated or immunocompromised patients—in a range of extraintestinal complications such as mycotic aneurysms; endocarditis; meningitis; septic arthritis; osteomyelitis, a well-recognized complication of sickle cell disease; and focal abscesses. Surgical excision and drainage may be required coupled with prolonged (more than 3 weeks) antibiotic treatment with a third-generation cephalosporin such as ceftriaxone or a quinolone. Both agents produce therapeutic concentrations in cerebrospinal fluid even when there is no inflammation of the meninges and are recommended for the treatment of salmonella meningitis brain abscess or subdural empyema in adults and young children. A minimum of 4 to 6 weeks of treatment may be required to prevent relapse.

Although the quinolones are not licensed (not Food and Drug Administration–approved) for use in children because of concerns regarding the finding of cartilage dysplasia in animal models, the steadily accumulating experience of use in treating severe childhood infection such as cystic fibrosis over a period of months has shown no evidence of arthropathogenicity and few if any adverse effects. Consequently, with a severe systemic salmonella infection in a child, the use of a quinolone with informed parental consent would be appropriate and potentially lifesaving. Ciprofloxacin, 10 mg per kg per day, can be given in two divided doses by intravenous infusion over 10 minutes pending a switch to oral therapy, 15 mg per kg per day. The alternative for children, including neonates, would be to use ceftriaxone intravenously,

---

*Not available in the United States.

*Not FDA-approved for this indication.

75 mg per kg per day. In pregnancy, in which chloramphenicol, TMP–SMX, and quinolones are all contraindicated, ceftriaxone would again be the preferred option.

TYPHOID FEVER*

method of
STEPHEN L. HOFFMAN, M.D., D.T.M.H.,
and JAMES M. CRUTCHER, M.D., M.P.H.
Malaria Program, Naval Medical Research Institute
Rockville, Maryland

DEFINITION

Typhoid fever is an acute illness caused by infection with *Salmonella typhi*, characterized by (1) prolonged fever, (2) sustained bacteremia without endothelial or endocardial involvement, and (3) bacterial multiplication within the mononuclear cells of the liver, spleen, lymph nodes, and Peyer's patches. Paratyphoid fever is a pathologically and clinically similar, but generally milder, illness caused most commonly by *S. paratyphi A, S. schottmülleri,* or *S. hirschfeldii.* "Enteric fever" refers to either typhoid or paratyphoid fever. Unless otherwise stated, "typhoid fever" is used to refer to either typhoid or paratyphoid fever.

EPIDEMIOLOGY

The prevalence of typhoid fever is strongly associated with the level of sanitation, and it is therefore a common infection in countries of the developing world where sanitary conditions are poor. The disease is relatively uncommon in the developed world, where cases are either imported or can be traced to contact with a chronic carrier. In the United States, 440 cases were reported in 1993, and the number of cases from 1984 to 1993 ranged from 400 to 550.

The infection is generally acquired by the ingestion of contaminated food or water but may rarely be transmitted by direct finger-to-mouth contact with the feces, urine, respiratory secretions, vomitus, or pus from an infected individual. Since humans are the only host, all cases of typhoid fever can theoretically be traced to another infected human. The stool of those with or recovering from acute infections is most commonly the source. It is generally believed that 3% of patients with acute typhoid fever become carriers. The carrier rate increases with age and the prevalence of gallbladder disease.

DIAGNOSIS

Typhoid fever can mimic most acute febrile infectious diseases. Virtually all patients have fever and a disturbance of bowel function (either constipation or diarrhea), and most have a headache. Malaise, sore throat, anorexia, nausea, abdominal pain, and myalgias are common. Rose

*The opinions or assertions herein are those of the authors and are not to be construed as official or as reflecting the views of the U.S. Navy or the naval service at large.

This work was supported by Naval Medical and Development Command work for work unit numbers 612787A.870.00101.EFX and 62300A.810.00101.HFX.1433.

spots are often difficult to detect. The incubation period is generally 7 to 14 days but may be longer. Because of its variable presentation, typhoid should be suspected in any patient with a febrile illness who lives in or has visited a typhoid endemic area in the last 2 months, particularly if ill for more than a week.

Definitive diagnosis of typhoid fever requires isolation of the organism from blood, bone marrow, duodenal secretions, or stool. Bone marrow aspirate (BMA) culture is the most sensitive diagnostic method. BMA cultures are positive in 80 to 95% of patients, even if patients have been taking antibiotics for several days, and regardless of how long they have been ill. The blood culture is positive in 40 to 80% of patients. The sensitivity of blood culture is greatest during the first week of illness, is reduced by prior ingestion of antibiotics, and is directly related to the quantity of blood cultured. The culture of intestinal secretions collected by duodenal string test has a sensitivity of 60 to 80%. The stool culture sensitivity is 30 to 40%; the sensitivity increases with the length of illness. Because of irregular shedding, several stool cultures may be necessary to identify carriers.

The Widal reaction is a serologic test that measures agglutinating antibodies to the O and H antigens of *S. typhi*. The test is highly variable among laboratories and is useful for the diagnosis of acute typhoid fever only if the sensitivity, specificity, and predictive value of the test are known for the local population. A number of new techniques have been developed for detecting *S. typhi* antibodies in serum; *S. typhi* antigen in blood, serum, and urine; and *S. typhi* DNA in blood and stool. Despite excellent results, none are currently in widespread use.

PREVENTION

Sanitation

Salmonella typhi is killed by heating water to 57° C, iodination, and chlorination. *Salmonella typhi* in food is killed at the same temperature, but the food must be heated for several minutes. When in endemic areas, individuals can decrease their risk of contracting typhoid by drinking boiled, bottled, or chlorinated water and only eating foods that are well cooked and served hot. Uncooked vegetables and unpeeled fruit should be washed in iodinated or chlorinated water.

Vaccines

The standard parenteral inactivated typhoid vaccine is only partially (50 to 90%) protective and is associated with local and systemic side effects in 25 to 50% of recipients. Newer vaccines include an oral live attenuated *S. typhi* vaccine (Ty21A Vivotif Berna) and a capsular polysaccharide vaccine for parenteral use (Typhim Vi, Pasteur Merieux). Both Ty21A and the Vi antigen vaccine appear at least as effective as the standard typhoid vaccine and cause far fewer side effects. Therefore, either of these vaccines is preferable to the standard vaccine. Typhoid vaccination should be considered for those traveling to or living in areas where typhoid is endemic. This includes most countries of the developing world.

Immunization Schedules

Ty21A. Four enteric-coated capsules are given at 2-day intervals. For continued exposure the entire four-dose series is recommended every 5 years. The vaccine is not recommended for children less than 6 years of age.

Vi Antigen Vaccine. A single 0.5-mL dose is administered intramuscularly with a similar booster dose every 2 years for continued exposure. The vaccine is not recommended for children younger than 2 years of age, although a recent study from Indonesia indicates that it is safe and immunogenic in children 6 to 13 months of age.

Standard Parenteral Vaccine. Adults and children aged 10 years and older are given 0.5 mL subcutaneously on two occasions 4 or more weeks apart. Children less than 10 years of age receive half the dose on the same schedule. If there is insufficient time for two doses at the interval specified, one dose a week for 3 weeks may be given. A single booster dose every 3 years is recommended. The manufacturer does not recommend the vaccine for children younger than 6 months of age.

TREATMENT

Optimal treatment of typhoid fever requires rapid diagnosis, the use of antibiotics, the recognition and treatment of life-threatening complications, and the treatment of relapse and the carrier state.

Antibiotic Resistance

In the 1970s there were large epidemics of typhoid fever in Mexico and Southeast Asia caused by *S. typhi* that exhibited R-plasmid-mediated resistance to chloramphenicol. Fortunately this resistance subsided. In the past 10 years isolates of *S. typhi* resistant to chloramphenicol, ampicillin, amoxicillin, and trimethoprim-sulfamethoxazole (TMP–SMX) have been reported. Multidrug resistance is most prevalent on the Indian subcontinent (with rates of 50% or higher in some series), China, and the Middle East. Multidrug resistance is also reported from South and Central America, Southeast Asia, Europe, Africa, and Saudi Arabia, but the prevalence is generally low. The prevalence of drug resistance can increase dramatically during epidemics, which occur periodically in endemic areas.

Antibiotic Recommendations

Patients with uncomplicated typhoid fever are generally treated with antibiotics, as outpatients. The choice of antibiotics is dependent on the expected antimicrobial drug sensitivities. For adults in the United States, a fluorinated quinolone, such as ciprofloxacin (Cipro), is the initial drug of choice. Alternatives include third-generation cephalosporins, TMP–SMX (Bactrim, Septra), amoxicillin, ampicillin, and chloramphenicol. Since quinolones are not rec-ommended for children, the choice of antibiotics for children is less clear-cut. In most areas with multidrug-resistant *S. typhi* the majority of organisms are sensitive to most antibiotics. In children we therefore recommend TMP–SMX for uncomplicated typhoid fever acquired everywhere in the world except the Indian subcontinent, China, the Middle East, and other areas with a reported high prevalence of multidrug resistance. Children who acquire the infections in these areas may be treated with TMP–SMX under close observation, or with intramuscular or intravenous ceftriaxone (Rocephin). Initial studies also suggest that cefixime (Suprax), an oral third-generation cephalosporin, is as effective and safe as intravenous ceftriaxone for treatment of patients with multidrug resistant *S. typhi*. Children who are seriously ill, develop complications, or fail to respond to an adequate trial of a conventional antibiotic should be treated with a parenteral third-generation cephalosporin. Fluoroquinolones are currently not recommended in children because they cause damage to growing cartilage in animals. However, no such association has been shown in humans, and many experts consider their use justified when no alternative exists. Future safety data may justify the routine use of fluoroquinolones in children.

Chloramphenicol-Sensitive Infections. Globally, chloramphenicol is still the most widely used antibiotic for the treatment of typhoid fever. The drug is inexpensive, well tolerated, and in most areas of the world remains highly effective, with a clinical cure rate of about 90%. It is not the drug of choice in the United States, however, because of drug resistance, a 5 to 10% relapse rate, and association with aplastic anemia (estimated at 1 in every 10,000 to 50,000 patients). Most studies have shown that in acute chloramphenicol-sensitive *S. typhi* infections, chloramphenicol produces more rapid defervescence (generally within 3 to 4 days) than do ampicillin, amoxicillin, and TMP–SMX, and a higher rate of clinical cure than ampicillin. The use of amoxicillin or TMP–SMX has generally been associated with clinical cure rates comparable to those of chloramphenicol, and with lower relapse and convalescent excreter rates than those of chloramphenicol. Treatment with fluoroquinolones is associated with high cure rates and low relapse rates. The use of third-generation cephalosporins like cefoperazone and ceftriaxone has been associated with cure and relapse rates at least comparable to those of chloramphenicol.

Chloramphenicol-Resistant Infections. Ampicillin, amoxicillin, TMP–SMX, fluoroquinolones, and third-generation cephalosporins are all effective against *S. typhi* with R-factor-mediated resistance to chloramphenicol.

Multidrug-Resistant Infections. Fluoroquinolones and third-generation cephalosporins are the drugs of choice for *S. typhi* resistant to chloramphenicol, ampicillin, amoxicillin, and TMP–SMX.

Drug Regimens

Fluoroquinolones. Ciprofloxacin (Cipro) 500 mg twice daily, norfloxacin (Noroxin) 400 mg twice daily, and ofloxacin (Floxin) 400 mg twice daily have all proved highly efficacious. Generally, 14 days is recommended, although ciprofloxacin for 7 days has achieved clinical cures. Relapse rates, however, may be greater with shorter therapy. Fluoroquinolones can only be used in adults (see the section "Antibiotic Recommendations").

Third-Generation Cephalosporins. Ceftriaxone (Rocephin), cefotaxime (Claforan), and cefoperazone (Cefobid) are effective for the therapy of multidrug-resistant *S. typhi*, although generally somewhat less so than the fluoroquinolones. Clinical cure rates range from 75 to 100%, depending on the dose and length of therapy. The drugs can only be administered parenterally. Ceftriaxone has a long serum half-life (6 to 9 hours) and can be given once daily. For adults, ceftriaxone in doses of 2 to 4 grams intravenously once daily (or in two divided doses) and for children 75 mg per kg per day have been effective. Regimens as short as 3 to 5 days have resulted in cure rates of 70 to 80% although best results are seen with 7 to 14 days of therapy. Intravenous cefoperazone, 100 mg per kg per day in two doses until defervescence, and then 50 mg per kg per day for a total of 14 days, is also effective. The oral drug cefixime (Suprax) has been shown to be effective in children at a dose of 10 mg per kg per day (in two divided doses) for 14 days.

Chloramphenicol. Chloramphenicol (Chloromycetin) is administered to adults and children in a dose of 50 mg per kg per day in four divided doses for 14 days, or 5 to 7 days after resolution of fever. It may be given orally, intramuscularly, or intravenously; bioavailability is greatest when it is administered orally.

TMP–SMX. For adults the dose of TMP–SMX (Bactrim, Septra) is 160 mg of TMP and 800 mg of SMX (equivalent to one double-strength tablet) administered orally or intravenously twice daily for 14 days. The children's dosage is 8 mg of TMP and 40 mg of SMX per kg per day in two divided doses for 14 days.

Recognition and Treatment of Life-Threatening Complications

Uncomplicated typhoid fever is quite easy to treat with a variety of antibiotics. However, patients with typhoid fever with abnormal levels of consciousness, intestinal perforation, or severe gastrointestinal bleeding are at high risk of dying if their condition is not rapidly recognized and treated. Patients with complicated typhoid fever have poor oral intake and high insensible water losses and tend to become dehydrated with resulting hyponatremia and hypokalemia.

Abnormal Level of Consciousness

Disturbances in the level of consciousness range from disorientation to coma. Delirium, stupor, and coma are grave prognostic signs associated with case-fatality rates that have exceeded 40%. High-dose dexamethasone has been shown to reduce mortality in patients with severe typhoid fever without increasing the incidence of complications, carriers, or relapse among survivors. Patients with suspected typhoid fever who are delirious, obtunded, stuporous, comatose, or in shock should immediately receive dexamethasone or an equivalent corticosteroid. After antibiotic therapy has been started, dexamethasone 3 mg per kg should be administered by intravenous infusion over 30 minutes. This is followed by dexamethasone 1 mg per kg given at the same rate every 6 hours for eight additional doses, the total duration of corticosteroid therapy being 48 hours. It has recently been reported from Pakistan that intravenous ciprofloxacin (5 mg per kg twice daily) was curative in 17 of 18 children with typhoid fever and abnormal levels of consciousness.

Intestinal Perforation

Intestinal perforation occurs in about 3% of hospitalized patients. It is most common during the third week of illness. The patient should be treated with antibiotics effective against *S. typhi* and the enteric organisms expected after intestinal perforation and should be given corticosteroids if severely toxic. Surgery should not be delayed for more than several hours after diagnosis.

Intestinal Hemorrhage

Intestinal hemorrhage occurs in up to 15% of cases, and bleeding is sometimes heavy enough to cause shock. The bowel usually does not perforate. In most cases, intestinal hemorrhage, even when massive, can be managed with general supportive care and blood replacement. Occasionally the use of platelets, fresh-frozen plasma to replace clotting factors, or intestinal resection is necessary, but this is uncommon.

Treatment of Relapse

Relapse may occur in 5 to 10% of patients treated with chloramphenicol and other antibiotics. Fluoroquinolones are associated with extremely low relapse rates. Relapse generally occurs about 2 weeks after the cessation of antibiotic therapy or in untreated patients about 2 weeks after defervescence. However, it can occur during therapy and has been reported several months after the initial illness. Relapse is usually, but not always, milder than the initial syndrome. Relapse is treated the same way as the primary attack.

Treatment of Carriers

A person who excretes the organism in the stool 1 year after the initial illness is considered to be a carrier. Although 10% of typhoid patients excrete the organism for 3 months after the initial illness, only 3% of patients go on to become carriers. In the absence of cholelithiasis, the majority of carriers can be cured by a 6-week course of oral ampicillin or amoxicillin, 100 mg per kg per day, plus probenecid,

30 mg per kg per day, or TMP–SMX, one double-strength tablet twice daily. Cure rates of approximately 80% have been reported with 28 days of ciprofloxacin, 750 mg twice daily, and with 28 days of norfloxacin, 400 mg twice daily. In the presence of cholelithiasis the above regimens should be tried before surgical intervention, but most fail, and in such cases cholecystectomy as well as the same antimicrobial regimen is required. A cure rate of 80 to 90% can be effected by combined surgical and antimicrobial treatment.

THE TYPHUS FEVERS

method of
JAMES A. HIGGINS, Ph.D., and
ABDU F. AZAD, Ph.D.

University of Maryland School of Medicine
Baltimore, Maryland

Rickettsial diseases of humans and animals are distributed throughout the tropical and temperate regions of the world. They are caused by obligate intracellular parasites, small gram-negative bacteria of the family Rickettsiaceae, and consist of several clinical entities, characterized by acute onset and self-limiting fever. Only pathogenic members of the typhus group *Rickettsia* are discussed in this chapter (Table 1) because of their public health importance, their presence in urban habitats, and their association with household pets.

The "classic" typhus fevers comprise related infectious diseases that occur in different parts of the world. Two species of the genus *Rickettsia* that belong to this group are pathogenic to humans; these are *R. prowazekii*, transmitted by human body lice and causing epidemic typhus, and *R. typhi* (= *R. mooseri*), transmitted by fleas and causing murine or flea-borne typhus (see Table 1).

MURINE TYPHUS

"Murine typhus is a good example of a disease whose importance is not adequately appreciated—except by the patient, and, even today, in most parts of the world, he will never know what ails him because the diagnosis will not be made." This statement, made over 15 years ago,* is as valid today as it was then. Murine typhus remains one of the most prevalent rickettsial infections throughout the world today. This is a disease so widely distributed that it occurs on every continent except Antarctica. During the period 1931 to 1946, human cases occurred by the thousands annually in the United States. In recent years the incidence has declined to fewer than 60 cases per year; however, outbreaks have been reported in Australia, China, Kuwait, and Thailand. In the United States, murine typhus is most prevalent in south Texas and southern California, with sporadic cases reported from other states. Murine typhus is a moderately severe febrile illness resulting from infection with *Rickettsia typhi*, a small (0.4 × 1.3 µm), gram-negative, obligate intracellular bacterium. It is usually transmitted to humans by the contamination of the bite site or skin abrasions with rickettsiae-containing flea feces. After an incubation period of 6 to 14 days, the disease is clinically characterized by high fever, headache, generalized pain, weakness, and a rash, which, if present, is often centrally distributed on the trunk. Important signs and symptoms of murine typhus include fever (almost all the patients), headache (75%), chills (66%), rash (about 50%), myalgias (46%), nausea (48%), vomiting (40%), anorexia (35%), and diarrhea (26%). Complications are rare, and the case fatality rate is less than 2% in untreated patients. Since this group of symptoms is shared with an array of other infectious diseases, including sev-

---

*See Traub R, Wisseman CL: The ecology of murine typhus—A critical review. Trop Dis Bull 75:237–317, 1978.

TABLE 1. **The Principal Vectors, Reservoirs, and Distribution of Human Rickettsial Diseases**

| Disease | Organism | Natural Cycle | | Mode of Transmission | Geographic Distribution |
		Arthropod Vector	Mammalian Host		
Murine typhus	*Rickettsia typhi*	*Xenopsylla cheopis* *Ctenocephalides felis*	Rodents	Contact with flea feces Flea bite	Worldwide
Epidemic typhus Epidemic	*R. prowazekii*	*Pediculus humanus*	Humans	Contact with louse feces	Worldwide
Sylvatic		Squirrel fleas	Flying squirrel	Unknown	Eastern United States
Rocky Mountain spotted fever	*R. rickettsii*	*Dermacentor variabilis* *D. andersoni*	Small mammals	Tick bite	Western Hemisphere
Rickettsialpox	*R. akari*	Mouse mites	House mice	Mite bite	Worldwide
Q fever	*Coxiella burnetii*	Ticks and other arthropods	Domestic and wild animals	Aerosols Contact with infected tissues	Worldwide
Ehrlichiosis	*Ehrlichia chaffeensis*	*Amblyomma Dermacentor*	Rodents or deer	Tick bite	United States
	Ehrlichia spp closely related to *E. phagocytophila*	Ticks	Unknown	Tick bite	North central and northeastern United States

Data from various sources.

eral bacterial and viral infections, without laboratory-confirmed diagnosis, many cases of murine typhus are overlooked. Indeed, it has been reported that undiagnosed cases of murine typhus surpassed reported cases by a factor of 4:1.

As for other vasculotropic rickettsioses, the chief target of the rickettsiae is the endothelial cells lining small blood vessels. Infection with *R. typhi* leads to massive rickettsial replication within target cells, subsequent endothelial injury, recruitment of inflammatory cells, and concomitant release of cytokines, resulting in the characteristic vasculitis. Unabated vascular damage can result in hypovolemic shock, with deleterious effects on renal function. Rickettsial dissemination from the portal of entry occurs via neighboring blood vessels and lymph nodes to vital organs such as the heart, lung, and brain. Involvement of these organs may lead to noncardiogenic pulmonary edema, respiratory failure, and multiorgan failure, requiring intensive clinical intervention.

Murine typhus is unique among the major arthropod-borne infections in that it can be a household infection because of its intimate association with commensal rats and their fleas. The natural history of murine typhus is complex; in addition to rats, a large spectrum of rodents, and even shrews, skunks, opossums, and cats, can serve as hosts for both *R. typhi* and various arthropod vectors. Even today the identity of all the vectors and reservoirs of murine typhus, as well as the precise mode(s) of transmission, is not known; the disease has also been reported in areas where either the flea or the rat was absent.

The Oriental rat flea *Xenopsylla cheopis* and the cat flea *Ctenocephalides felis* (see Table 1) are considered the major vectors of murine typhus on the basis of epidemiologic data. In general, there has been a strong correlation between the seasonal abundance of *X. cheopis* and the incidence of human murine typhus cases. In the United States, 94% of all reported cases of murine typhus have occurred in eight southern states (including coastal Texas), where warm and humid climates prevail for most of the year. The majority of cases occurred during late spring and early autumn, when the fleas were very abundant. Moreover, a marked decline in the reported cases of murine typhus in the United States occurred when *X. cheopis* populations were effectively brought under control by sustained DDT dusting campaigns. Interestingly, the approximately 200 cases reported in southern California and the Gulf Coast regions of Texas during the last 10 years have occurred in the absence of the classic transmission cycle (the flea vector *X. cheopis* and the rodent host *Rattus norvegicus*). Instead, opossums (*Didelphis marsupialis*), domestic cats, and the cat flea *C. felis* are likely to be involved in the transmission of murine typhus to humans in these cases. In addition to their abundance on household pets, cat fleas readily bite humans and are capable of maintaining and transmitting *R. typhi* to nonimmune hosts. Furthermore, the presence of an as-yet-undescribed rickettsia-like bacterium (the ELB agent) in the fleas collected from murine typhus–endemic areas of California and Texas further complicates the existing situation. Serologic studies of opossums and domestic cats have demonstrated the widespread presence of antibodies against this rickettsia throughout the murine typhus–endemic areas.

EPIDEMIC, RECRUDESCENT, AND SYLVATIC TYPHUS

Epidemic typhus fever is caused by the transmission of *R. prowazekii* to humans via the inoculation of rickettsia-laden feces of the human body louse, *Pediculus humanus humanus,* into bite wounds, abrasions, and other superficial skin lesions. Lice are extremely host-specific and spend their entire life cycle on the same host; they have poor mobility and require close physical contact between humans in order to transfer from one host to another. The clinical manifestations are similar to, but usually more severe than, those of murine typhus, including fever, intense headache, prostration, macular skin rash, malaise, myalgia, and vascular and neurologic disturbances. Case fatality rates vary from 4 to 20% if untreated. The incubation period is usually less than 14 days.

Historically, louse-borne epidemic typhus has occurred in major epidemics associated with wars and other social upheavals, when environmental conditions are conducive to louse infestation. In recent years, however, its distribution has been limited to mountainous regions of South America, the Himalayas, and highlands of North Africa. Both epidemic and recrudescent (Brill-Zinsser disease) forms are practically nonexistent in the United States. However, the presence of a sylvatic typhus in the eastern United States involving flying squirrels, *Glaucomys volans,* and their ectoparasites, was documented via isolation of *R. prowazekii* from the squirrels and their lice and fleas. Additionally, 35 serologically confirmed cases of human infection with *R. prowazekii* have been associated with contact with flying squirrels and the squirrel flea, *Orchopeas howardi.* Consequently, the prudent clinician should consider sylvatic typhus fever in the differential diagnosis of febrile illness in individuals whose occupations and/or hobbies bring them into proximity with these mammals.

LABORATORY DIAGNOSIS

Current surveys of rickettsial infections use both serologic and genetic analyses. Serologic assays test patients' sera against a complex of whole cell rickettsial antigens using immunofluorescent antibody assays. Because of the antigenic cross-reactivity between the members of typhus (*R. typhi* and *R. prowazekii*) and spotted fever group (*R. rickettsii*) rickettsiae, this is not a species-specific assay without further modification (e.g., antigenic absorption, titrations). Tests based on detecting and measuring antirickettsial antibodies are not available in most hospital laboratories. Alternative methods include latex agglutination and enzyme-linked immunosorbent assay (ELISA), which are highly sensitive and species-specific and capable of distinguishing murine typhus infection from Rocky Mountain spotted fever. However, these serologic tests are unable to distinguish between *R. prowazekii* and *R. typhi*.

Since these methods are useful only for confirmation in convalescence, antigen-based detection assays should be used, e.g., detection of rickettsiae in skin biopsies from rash lesions, and recovery of rickettsiae via tissue culture plaque assays for diagnosis in the acute phase of infection. Obviously, skin biopsies can be of diagnostic value only in those 50% of typhus patients who develop this physical finding. Cultivation of rickettsiae is very expensive and time-consuming, requiring cell culture facilities and laboratories that have authorization to maintain hazardous organisms. Newer techniques such as nucleic acid–based diagnostic procedures (e.g., DNA probes, polymerase chain reaction [PCR]) can greatly facilitate diagnosis; unfortunately, few hospital laboratories are currently equipped to use these methods routinely. PCR based on the amplification of several independent gene sequences (e.g., genes encoding the 17-kDa protein antigen, 16-S ribosomal RNA [rRNA], and citrate synthase) with *Rickettsia* genus-

TABLE 2. **Drug Treatment of the Typhus Fevers**

Drug	Oral Therapy	Intravenous Therapy	Maximum Total Daily Dose
Tetracycline	25–50 mg/kg/day, in four divided doses q 6 h	(Tetracycline hydrochloride) 10–20 mg/kg/day, in four divided doses q 6 h	2 gm/day
Doxycycline	4–5 mg/kg/day, in two divided doses q 12 h	(Doxycycline hyclate) 4–5 mg/kg/day, in two divided doses q 12 h	200 mg/day
Chloramphenicol	50–75 mg/kg/day, in four divided doses q 6 h	(Chloramphenicol sodium succinate) 50 mg/kg/day, in four divided doses q 6 h	3 gm/day

specific primers, and subsequent analysis of PCR products by specific restriction endonuclease patterns, can be used to distinguish rickettsial species. Unlike standard serologic confirmation, which is retrospective, PCR and restriction enzyme analysis allow the species of the rickettsial infection to be identified within 48 hours; this early diagnosis can be used for proper therapeutic decision making. Additionally, the utility of PCR-based diagnosis can be further exploited to discriminate between *R. typhi* and the recently described ELB agent. These rickettsiae are not distinguishable with currently available serologic reagents.

TREATMENT

The patient suspected of suffering from typhus fever should be treated promptly with antirickettsial therapy. It is recommended that therapy for rickettsial infections be initiated on the basis of clinical suspicion, in the absence of a definitive serologic diagnosis, since delayed therapy may contribute to the development of more severe infection. In murine typhus–endemic areas, several factors (season; the presence of rats or opossums; flea bites; intense headache and high fever; rash) should be considered before initiating antirickettsial therapy. Because of the sensitivity of the rickettsial organisms to tetracycline agents, including doxycycline, tetracycline, and minocycline (Minocin), these antibiotics have been extensively used as the treatment of choice for adults. Chloramphenicol remains the preferred therapy for children younger than 8 years of age. However, since these antibiotics are rickettsistatic rather than rickettsicidal, it is crucial that they be used long enough to allow the development of a strong host immune response to control further rickettsial replication and facilitate their clearance. Therapy is advocated for 6 to 10 days (minimum of 5 days) or for 2 to 3 days after defervescence, whichever is longer, to prevent relapse. These drugs are usually highly effective, and clinical improvement (e.g., defervescence) within 48 to 72 hours is commonly noted if they are given early and in adequate dosage. In patients with severe central nervous system disease, corticosteroids should be used to reduce inflammation and the po-

tential for life-threatening cerebral edema. Chloramphenicol or doxycycline therapy should be used in patients with diminished renal function. Additionally, a reduced chloramphenicol dosage is recommended for infants and young children and for patients with liver and renal dysfunction. All warnings and recommendations on drug labeling should be followed. Recommended dosages are presented in Table 2.

PREVENTION

Prevention of typhus fever transmission can be accomplished by educating at-risk populations about the diseases, their reservoirs, and their vectors. Reduction of exposure to fleas is the most important preventive measure. This can be achieved by the use of insecticides to control flea infestations, and by limiting outdoor activities for household pets, if these bring them into contact with potential reservoirs and/or vectors. Control should be aimed at the immature stages of fleas, using applications of dust formulations of residual insecticides (2% concentrations of dimpylate [diazinon], fenitrothion, and primiphos) to heavily flea-infested areas, and regular vacuum cleaning of the house, with particular attention given to nooks and corners where debris can accumulate. The application of nontoxic insecticides such as pyrethrum dust to dogs and cats, their bedding, and kennel areas is also recommended. In murine typhus–endemic areas, flea control should precede rodent control in rat-infested premises, in order to minimize the opportunistic movement of rickettsia-infected fleas from dead animals to humans and household pets. Measures to control rodents and opossums should be taken within the neighborhood, including reduction of garbage deposits, elimination of harborage sites, and the use of rodenticides. Vector control measures such as delousing of patients and clothing should be considered for the suppression of outbreaks of epidemic typhus. Suspect or documented cases of epidemic typhus should be immediately reported to local, state, or federal health officials.

The Respiratory System

ACUTE RESPIRATORY FAILURE

method of
JOSEPH J. COTTRELL, M.D., and
ROBERT M. ROGERS, M.D.
University of Pittsburgh
Pittsburgh, Pennsylvania

The expression "acute respiratory failure" is often used to describe any rapid change in the processes of respiration. Such changes result in either an elevated partial pressure of carbon dioxide (hypercarbia) or a decreased partial pressure of oxygen (hypoxemia) in arterial blood, or both. Although this common usage encompasses almost every patient who is ventilated in an intensive care unit, it does not well describe the many different illnesses that can cause respiratory failure. Successful treatment of acute respiratory failure (ARF) requires a systematic approach to the patient.

Conceptually, it is worthwhile to separate ARF into two major categories: hypoventilation (elevated partial pressure of carbon dioxide) and hypoxemia (decreased arterial partial pressure of oxygen). Frequently they occur together, for an increase in alveolar carbon dioxide tension (PA_{CO_2}) always results in a decrease in alveolar oxygen tension (PA_{O_2}). However, severe hypoxemia may occur without carbon dioxide retention in acute parenchymal lung disease. Although oxygen administration remains the key therapy for ARF, further interventions to treat defects in ventilation are different from those used for the hypoxemia of parenchymal lung disease.

A second distinction, which needs to be appreciated for proper therapy, is the distinction between ARF in a previously healthy individual and ARF occurring in an individual with prior chronic obstructive lung disease (COPD). The latter, also known as "acute on chronic" respiratory failure (AOCRF), requires a slightly different therapeutic strategy (discussed later).

VENTILATION

The process of moving air into and out of the respiratory tract is complex, involving central and peripheral nervous systems, peripheral chemoreceptors, airways, muscles, and chest and abdominal walls. Despite the complexity of the system, arterial blood gas (ABG) values are maintained within narrow limits. In health, alveolar ventilation is closely regulated to maintain the partial pressure of carbon dioxide in arterial blood ($PaPA_{O_2}$) at 40 mmHg, with a range no greater than 35 to 45 mmHg. Since $PaPA_{O_2}$ is inversely proportional to alveolar ventilation, in order for the $PaPA_{O_2}$ to rise, alveolar ventilation must decrease. Table 1 lists some of the more common causes of hypoventilation.

OXYGENATION

Healthy lung parenchyma does an excellent job of passing oxygen from the alveolar space into the arterial blood. A "normal" partial pressure of oxygen in arterial blood (Pa_{O_2}) exceeds 90 mmHg in the young but may be as low as 70 mmHg in the oldest patients. More accurate Pa_{O_2} predictions may be obtained using equations (Table 2). In illness, an excellent tool for assessing the efficiency of oxygen transfer across the alveolus is the calculated "A-a gradient." The A-a gradient is the difference between the calculated alveolar oxygen tension (PA_{O_2}) and the arterial oxygen tension (Pa_{O_2}) measured from a sample of arterial blood. Table 3 provides the alveolar gas equation, a simplified version for use on room air, and a sample calculation. Since the calculation takes into account the effect of an increased carbon dioxide level on the oxygen level, an elevation of the A-a gradient indicates the presence of parenchymal lung disease. It must be appreciated that the A-a gradient increases with the administration of oxygen. Therefore, this tool is best reserved for evaluations of patients breathing room air.

SIGNS AND SYMPTOMS

Respiratory failure should be a clinical diagnosis confirmed by laboratory studies. Although the signs (Table 4) are frequently nonspecific, their presence in any individual should lead one to consider this diagnosis. Signs are more useful than symptoms. The most common symptom, dyspnea, is so nonspecific that it is of little value.

Assessment of the respiratory rate is of great importance. Rates less than 8 per minute are abnormal and generally result in alveolar hypoventilation. Rates greater than 35 per minute are nonsustainable over time and indicate respiratory failure. A word of warning in the interpretation of cyanosis: local circulatory factors such as shock,

TABLE 1. **Common Causes of Hypoventilation**

System Component	Examples
Brain	Head trauma Drug overdose Cerebral vascular accident
Spinal cord	Cervical fracture Myasthenia gravis Guillain-Barré syndrome
Chest wall	Flail chest (trauma)
Upper airways	Neoplasms Laryngospasm Foreign body (pediatrics)
Lower airways and lungs	Asthma Bronchitis Emphysema Pneumonia

TABLE 2. **Arterial Oxygen Prediction Equations**

$$Pa_{O_2} = 104.2 - (0.27 \times age)$$
$$Pa_{O_2} = 109 - (0.43 \times age)$$
$$Pa_{O_2} = (0.279 \times age) + (0.1134 \times P_{bar}) + 14.63$$

Age is in years.
P_{bar} is barometric pressure in mmHg.

severely decreased cardiac output, and right-to-left shunts may be solely responsible for the development of this sign. In addition, since at least 5 grams of unoxygenated hemoglobin is required for clinical cyanosis to be detected, some polycythemic individuals may always be cyanotic and severely anemic individuals may never be cyanotic.

BEDSIDE TESTING

Several bedside respiratory parameters are available that can be useful in the assessment of ARF. These include maximal inspiratory force (MIF), tidal volume (TV), and vital capacity (VC). Their normal values, as well as critical values consistent with ARF, are listed in Table 5. The greatest utility for these measurements is in the repeated assessment of patients with changing neuromuscular dysfunction, including spinal cord trauma and myasthenia gravis.

ARTERIAL BLOOD GASES

In view of the nonspecificity of the signs and symptoms of respiratory failure, one cannot adequately assess the patient's condition without ABG measurements. Indeed, all decisions in caring for the patient must be made in the light of a recent measurement of pH, partial pressure of CO_2 (Pa_{CO_2}), and partial pressure of O_2 (Pa_{O_2}). Since rapid changes occur in the blood gases when the patient is unstable or when therapeutic measures are altered, there should be no hesitancy in obtaining frequent measurement of ABGs. Noninvasive monitoring, including pulse oximetry and end-tidal carbon dioxide measurements, are at best supplements to ABG determinations and not replacements for them.

OXYGEN THERAPY IN RESPIRATORY FAILURE

The basic problems for a patient with respiratory failure are hypoxemia and hypercarbia. One might

TABLE 3. **Alveolar Gas Equation**

$$PA_{O_2} = Fi_{O_2} \times (P_{bar} - P_{H2O}) - [Fi_{O_2} + (1 - Fi_{O_2}/R)] \times Pa_{CO_2}$$

Where
Fi_{O_2} is the fractional inspired concentration of oxygen.
P_{bar} is the barometric pressure. Normal sea level value is 760 mmHg.
P_{H2O} is the partial pressure of water vapor, 47 mmHg.
R is the respiratory quotient.

Solved for room air at sea level, this reduces to
$$PA_{O_2} = 149 - (1.2 \times Pa_{CO_2})$$

Example:
Calculate A–a gradient for patient with following room air arterial blood gas values:
pH 7.30, Pa_{O_2} 49, Pa_{CO_2} 60

$PA_{O_2} = 149 - (1.2 \times 60) = 149 - 72 = 77$
A–a gradient $= PA_{O_2} - Pa_{O_2} = 77 - 49$
A–a gradient $= 28$

TABLE 4. **Signs of Acute Respiratory Failure**

Respiratory rate >35 or <8 breaths/min
Paradoxical diaphragmatic movement
Use of accessory muscles for respiration
Cyanosis
Tachycardia or bradycardia
Conjunctival injection or chemosis
Altered mental status

presumably direct equal efforts toward correcting both these defects. However, *hypoxia can cause brain death within minutes*. Hypercarbia is well tolerated, even at high levels, if hypoxia is not present. Therefore, the initial therapeutic actions must be to treat hypoxia. We first discuss the use of controlled oxygen therapy in the treatment of respiratory failure and then discuss mechanical ventilation.

Conceptually, oxygen should be considered a drug, just like gentamicin (Garamycin) or dopamine (Intropin). Oxygen has a therapeutic range and known side effects. For this reason, the correct dosage of oxygen must always be used. The amount required varies with the individual patient.

Patients with hypoxemia may be divided into three categories: (1) Patients in whom Pa_{O_2} is 30 mmHg or less. This is the very critical range in which the patient can die rapidly if the hypoxemia is not corrected. (2) Patients in whom the Pa_{O_2} is between 40 and 60 mmHg. In this range, small increases in the percentage of inspired oxygen rapidly shift the patient away from the dangerous levels of hypoxemia. (3) Patients in whom the Pa_{O_2} is 60 mmHg or greater. In this setting, hemoglobin saturation is 90% or more. A Pa_{O_2} of 60 mmHg is a good "end point" for which to strive.

Table 6 demonstrates the effect of Pa_{O_2} on the oxygen content of the blood. With a Pa_{O_2} of 20 mmHg, there is 7.06 mL of oxygen combined with the hemoglobin in 100 mL of blood and 0.06 mL of dissolved oxygen, for a total of 7.12 mL. The saturation is only 35%. However, with a Pa_{O_2} of 60 mmHg, there is an increase of oxygen content to 18.16 mL of oxygen per 100 mL of blood. The saturation is 89%. Increasing the Pa_{O_2} above 60 mmHg results in very little further improvement in oxygen content.

METHODS OF CONTROLLING INSPIRED OXYGEN

In a breathing patient with suspected hypoxemia not yet confirmed by ABG measurements and without a history of COPD, we recommend the use of 100% oxygen by face mask. If there is a history of COPD, careful titration of "low-dose" oxygen is strongly suggested. Although careful control of flow rates through a nasal cannula can provide varying levels of oxygen, it is not possible to specify oxygen levels precisely using this technique. We prefer to use one of the many masks in which the Venturi principle is used to control oxygen concentration. Such masks, available from several manufacturers,

TABLE 5. **Bedside Respiratory Function Parameters**

Parameter	Normal Value	Respiratory Failure Value
Maximum inspiratory force	-80 to -100 cmH$_2$O	0 to -25 cmH$_2$O
Vital capacity	>60 mL/kg	<15 mL/kg
Tidal volume	>10 mL/kg	<5 mL/kg

are able to provide precise oxygen delivery. Masks may be of "fixed" design, able to provide inspired oxygen at a single concentration (generally 24, 28, 31, or 35%), or "variable," able to be adjusted over the same range. Initial therapy begins at 24% and is titrated upward based upon ABG analysis.

COMPLICATIONS OF OXYGEN THERAPY

Severe hypoxemia rapidly leads to irreversible brain damage. It is therefore imperative to correct the hypoxia. The fear of some physicians that oxygen administration will cause large increases in Pa$_{CO_2}$ and worsening acidosis is not well founded. Indeed, it rarely occurs. The modest rises in the Pa$_{CO_2}$ that do frequently occur with oxygen therapy can generally be tolerated and rarely cause further central nervous system depression. If an acceptable Pa$_{O_2}$ and a tolerable Pa$_{CO_2}$ cannot be achieved, then intubation and mechanical ventilation are necessary. The number of patients requiring mechanical ventilation has decreased, owing to avoidance of certain errors in management. These errors are uncontrolled or injudicious use of oxygen, causing hypercapnia and acidosis; the use of any medication that might lead to respiratory or cough depression; and discontinuance of oxygen therapy once it has commenced. If a patient develops marked worsening of hypercapnia in response to oxygen therapy, a slight lowering of the inspired oxygen concentration may be appropriate. However, too great a reduction or a complete cessation of oxygen leads to a drop of the alveolar and arterial oxygen tensions to values below pretreatment levels (PA$_{CO_2}$ is now higher; therefore PA$_{O_2}$ must be lower). We recommend intubation and ventilation as the safest course to follow if progressive hypercapnia and acidosis occur in response to oxygen therapy.

High concentrations of inspired oxygen can be injurious to the lung, causing an acute inflammatory process and leading to pulmonary fibrosis. It is unclear whether this condition can ever be caused by a loose-fitting face mask, which generally allows the entrainment of significant amounts of ambient air. However, oxygen toxicity can clearly result from pro-

longed mechanical ventilation with high levels of oxygen. Our current practice would be to use 90% oxygen for no more than 24 hours and restrict all subsequent oxygen therapy to 60% or less. Although there is very little human data, animal data suggest a wide variability in lung sensitivity to oxygen toxicity. We prefer to err on the side of caution and advocate decreasing the inspired concentration to 50% or less as quickly as possible.

INTUBATION

Although a complete discussion of intubation is beyond the scope of this chapter, it is important to note that placement of an endotracheal tube is critical to successful mechanical ventilation. We prefer true "high volume–low pressure" cuffs, rather than the intermediate-volume balloons offered by some manufacturers. To minimize complications, we advise regularly scheduled manometer checks of inflation pressure. Inflation pressure should be the lowest consistent with adequate ventilation. Many patients achieve a good seal at less than 10 cmH$_2$O. Cuff pressures should never exceed 25 cmH$_2$O. Properly cared for, most endotracheal tubes can be used for at least 2 weeks before a tracheostomy tube must be placed.

VENTILATOR MANAGEMENT

Most individuals with ARF and many of those with AOCRF require mechanical ventilation. To successfully manage ARF we must have a good working knowledge of mechanical ventilation. It is imperative that whenever we place a patient on a ventilator, we address all six items in Table 7.

Tidal Volume and Respiratory Rate

The TV and respiratory rate (RR), when multiplied together, provide the patient's minute ventilation (MV). The higher the MV, the lower the patient's

TABLE 6. **Relationship of Oxygen Content to Arterial Oxygen Tension**

Pa$_{O_2}$ (mmHg)	20	40	60	80
Saturation (%)	35	75	89	94.5
O$_2$ content (mL O$_2$/100 mL blood)	7.12	15.24	18.16	19.4

TABLE 7. **The "Big 6" of Ventilator Management**

Respiratory rate
Tidal volume
Inspired oxygen concentration
Mode
Positive end-expiratory pressure (PEEP)
Inspiratory/expiratory ratio

Whenever patient is placed on mechanical ventilator, orders for these six parameters must be written.

Pa_{CO_2}. As a general rule of thumb for ARF, a rate of 10 breaths per minute, with a TV of 10 mL per kg, provides near normalization of the Pa_{CO_2}. For initial ventilator settings in AOCRF, we decrease the rate to 6 or 7. These individuals have previously compensated for their chronic respiratory acidosis with a metabolic alkalosis. Sudden normalization of their Pa_{CO_2} can therefore lead to a severe combined alkalosis.

Oxygen

In a patient with ARF, we generally recommend starting with an inspired oxygen concentration of 90%; 100% oxygen can result in washing out all nitrogen from the lung, and this can result in atelectasis. Lesser amounts, particularly in individuals with large shunts, can result in unnecessary hypoxemia. In patients with AOCRF, we generally add 5 to 10% to their previous supplemental oxygen requirement.

Positive End-Expiratory Pressure

It has been demonstrated that if one measures functional residual capacity (FRC) before and after intubation, FRC falls after intubation. Intubation, by unclear mechanisms, causes atelectasis. It has also been shown that small amounts of positive end-expiratory pressure (PEEP) (2.5 to 5 cmH_2O) prevent this fall in FRC. We therefore routinely use PEEP with "malice aforethought." Although PEEP is beneficial for most individuals with ARF, there are several categories of patients for whom PEEP may be harmful. In individuals with asthma or COPD, in whom FRC is generally increased, PEEP can lead to further hyperinflation, and cause barotrauma. PEEP can also be problematic in young, previously healthy persons (trauma victims) who are hypovolemic. Even small increases in intrathoracic pressure can markedly decrease venous return, resulting in hypotension.

Inspiratory/Expiratory Ratio

Most of the "art" of ventilator management comes from an understanding of the proper management of inspiratory and expiratory times. Indeed, most of our nighttime telephone calls result from problems with this aspect of ventilator management. The goal of mechanical ventilation is to deliver a breath to the patient, provide fresh air to the alveolar space, and allow exhalation. This entire process must occur within the time constraints of the respiratory rate. At a respiratory rate of 10, this entire process must occur within 6 seconds. At a respiratory rate of 20, only 3 seconds are available. If the ventilator needed 1 second to deliver the breath, 2 seconds would be available for exhalation. The inspiratory/expiratory ratio (IER) would be 1:2. If all the air did not escape in those 2 seconds, the ventilator would still deliver the next breath, but now to a slightly more expanded lung. If this continued, hyperinflation and barotrauma would be the likely outcome. Exhalation is a totally passive process. In general, the longer the time available for exhalation, the better. In ARF we like IERs of at least 1:2.5. In patients with obstructive lung disease, we like IERs of at least 1:4. Having said that, we will be the first to admit that achieving such ratios may be difficult. Although some ventilators let you choose IER directly, for most ventilators, one controls IER indirectly. Inspiratory flow rate control determines inspiratory time, allowing expiration to occur in whatever time is left in the breathing cycle. At a ventilator rate of 20, in a patient with COPD and a TV of 750 mL, is an inspiratory flow of 60 liters per minute adequate? No. The inspiratory flow rate is 1 liter per second. The ventilator would require at least 0.75 second to deliver the breath, leaving 2.25 seconds for exhalation and resulting in an IER of 1:3. A more rapid inspiratory flow would improve the IER. Increasing inspiratory flow may have untoward effects, however. Peak airway pressure tends to increase with increasing flows. Therefore, particularly in patients with obstruction, management of the ventilator may require careful fine tuning and acceptance of compromise.

Ventilator Mode

We have deliberately left this decision for last. Over the past 2 decades perhaps more has been written championing "new" ventilator modes than any other topic in critical care. We believe that it is much ado about nothing. Despite the thousands of articles and the individual crusades of physicians and companies, there is little to suggest that differing modes of ventilation affect outcomes. Table 8 lists the major selections offered. "Assist/control" (A/C) is the oldest ventilator mode. In A/C, anytime the patient makes a respiratory effort, that individual receives a full ventilator TV. If the patient's spontaneous RR falls below the rate set on the ventilator, the patient receives a ventilator breath. "Synchronized intermittent mandatory ventilation" (SIMV) is probably the most widely used mode of ventilation. Originally described primarily for the safe, rapid weaning of postsurgical cases, it has found widespread use in the intensive care unit setting. In SIMV, the ventilator

TABLE 8. **Commonly Used Ventilator Modes**

Ventilator Mode	Prominent Feature
Assist/control (A/C)	Every breath is assisted. Ventilator rate setting only provides backup rate.
Intermittent mandatory ventilation (IMV)	Ventilator only gives number of breaths set on machine. Patient may make unassisted breaths.
Synchronized intermittent mandatory ventilation (SIMV)	Synchronizes machine breaths with those of patient.
Pressure support (PS)	Maintains positive pressure during inspiration. Potentially unsafe.

does not assist every patient breath. Only the number of breaths set on the ventilator are supported each minute. In essence, the patient receives two different TVs, those of his spontaneous breaths and those that are machine-assisted. The newest modality to enter widespread use is "pressure support" (PS). In PS a selected pressure is maintained in the respiratory circuit during inspiration. Although this may be helpful in decreasing the resistance in the ventilator circuit and decreasing the extra work of breathing, it cannot guarantee a TV or MV. We do not recommend the use of this mode for initial ventilation. Although we prefer A/C for AOCRF, and SIMV for simple ARF, we think that the best treatment for your patients is the mode with which you and your staff are most familiar. In the initial stages of total ventilator support, there are few real differences between any of the commonly used modalities. Their major differences only become apparent during weaning.

MANAGING THE VENTILATOR

Assessment of ABGs is critical for modifying ventilator settings. Knowing that the P_{CO_2} is inversely proportional to the MV, it is easy to calculate ventilation changes. If a patient with a TV of 700 mL and an RR of 10 had a Pa_{CO_2} of 50, what could we do to normalize the Pa_{CO_2}? To effect a 20% reduction in Pa_{CO_2} we would prescribe a 20% increase in MV. Raising the TV to 840 mL should accomplish our goal.

Control of oxygenation is not quite as simple. It is imperative that long-term levels of inspired oxygen be kept at or below 60%. If a patient does not maintain the Pa_{O_2} above 60 mmHg, despite high inspired oxygen concentrations, we add PEEP. We generally increment by 5 cmH$_2$0, as needed. The use of PEEP is empirical, and the response to any given level of PEEP is not predictable. It should be noted that the vast majority of patients, even those suffering from adult respiratory distress syndrome (ARDS), require 15 cmH$_2$0 or less of PEEP. Although we will insert a flow-directed pulmonary artery catheter (Swan-Ganz) at any sign of hemodynamic instability, it is distinctly unusual not to require one at 15 cmH$_2$0 or more of PEEP.

COMPLICATIONS OF VENTILATION

There are many known complications and therapeutic misadventures associated with mechanical ventilation. It is important to be aware of the more common ones, both to minimize their occurrence and to respond appropriately when they do occur.

The effects of mechanical ventilation on the architecture of the lung are controversial. It is quite possible that high airway pressures or local hyperinflation, in and of themselves, may cause further injury to the lung. Although it is accepted that peak airway pressures are most closely associated with the incidence of pneumothorax, the relationship is not defined as cause and effect. Peak airway pressures, as currently measured proximal to the endotracheal tube, are a reflection of lung compliance, lung volume, lung and endotracheal tube resistance, and ventilator setting and design. To attribute barotrauma to peak pressure alone is clearly incorrect. At the present time, minimization of airway pressures should be considered a secondary treatment goal. It is important for the physician to be aware of both peak and plateau airway pressures in any patient receiving mechanical ventilation. Using these pressures and the known TV, one should calculate the dynamic and static compliance of the lung. The difference between these two values is a function of the resistance of the ventilator-patient system. Any change in compliance should be addressed immediately, for it may reflect worsening of the lung injury or a pneumothorax. Similarly, a change in resistance may provide the first indication of worsening bronchospasm or a kinked endotracheal tube.

Mechanical ventilation may be uncomfortable to a patient, and sedation is generally recommended. We prefer narcotics as the sedative-anxiolytic of choice. They are titratable and reversible. Their most common side effect, hypotension, responds to fluid replacement. We generally avoid benzodiazepines because of inconsistent metabolism and less reversibility. We recognize that there are rare patients who require paralysis for successful ventilation. In general, we avoid this for all but the most serious situations. It is extremely difficult to monitor the paralyzed patient. Neurologic markers are lost as well as most protective reflexes. A perforated viscus or a ventilator disconnect, easily recognized in a nonparalyzed patient, is frequently fatal in a paralyzed one.

Displacement of the endotracheal tube should be an uncommon occurrence. All tubes should be firmly secured, and the nursing staff should be aware of the depth of insertion. A useful radiologic marker is that the tip of the endotracheal tube should be at the level of the top of the aortic knob. This is a relatively fixed marker and is resistant to the inadvertent lordotic or kyphotic angulation that frequently occurs during bedside radiography. A daily chest radiograph to confirm tube position is not unreasonable. We believe that patient restraints to prevent inadvertent tube displacement are indicated. In light of recent changes to the Joint Commission on Accreditation of Healthcare Organization standards, we suggest that you verify that your policies are consistent with their standards on this issue.

WEANING

Before consideration is given to weaning a patient from ventilator support, it is important to correct the underlying pathophysiology that led to the initial decompensation. All treatment modalities discussed to this point have been supportive rather than therapeutic. Unless the underlying conditions have been addressed and treated, the patient simply deteriorates as support is removed.

In addition to specific treatment of the primary illness, certain general therapies are important. The number one cause of mortality in intensive care remains infection. It is very important that strict infection control precautions be followed both for the use of the ventilator and for all invasive lines. There is growing recognition that nutritional support is important for respiratory muscle function. We advocate early nutritional support. Attention should be paid to calorie needs, for overfeeding can result in excess carbon dioxide production.

Once the patient has improved, consideration of withdrawing ventilator support can begin in earnest. If the patient is on more than 5 cmH$_2$O of PEEP, we generally reduce PEEP by 2.5 cmH$_2$O every 6 hours as tolerated. It is important that the patient's oxygen requirement be less than 60% on no more than 5 cmH$_2$O of PEEP or the patient is not ready for weaning.

The bedside parameters, discussed previously, are useful in assessing the ability of a patient to be weaned. The ideal weaning candidate would have a maximal inspiratory pressure (MIP) greater than 25 cmH$_2$O, a TV greater than 10 mL per kg, and a vital capacity greater than 15 mL per kg. In addition the spontaneous MV should be less than 10 liters per minute. Many patients who are successfully weaned do not meet one or more of these parameters. Nonetheless, the parameters provide useful information concerning a patient's ability to maintain spontaneous respiration.

The three commonly used ventilator modalities discussed previously are quite different in their weaning methodology. For A/C weaning, the patients are taken off the ventilator for short periods of time, initially 5 minutes or more, as tolerated, and placed on a T tube. When they show signs of fatigue, they are placed back on the "full support" that A/C provides. We favor this technique in patients with AOCRF for two reasons: (1) it mimics typical muscle training: rest, exercise, rest, exercise, and (2) it has been effectively used in several studies of "weaning the unweanable." The major disadvantage with T tube weaning is that it is very labor-intensive. When the patients are placed on the T tube, they need to be carefully observed. There is no mechanical backup to the system, so skilled practitioners need to be in immediate attendance. SIMV weaning is much less people-intensive. One simply decreases the number of breaths per minute provided by the ventilator. It is simple and, by making small decremental changes, safe even if the patient is not as well observed. The disadvantage is that if the patient develops respiratory muscle fatigue, it may continue indefinitely, for the patient does not receive the "rest" available on A/C. In addition, depending upon the model of ventilator and breathing circuit, the work of breathing may be high. Low levels of PS (2 to 5 cmH$_2$O) can be used as an adjunct to SIMV to help overcome the resistance of the breathing circuit, or high levels of PS (10 cmH$_2$O or more) may be used in a method similar to pressure-cycled ventilation. Initially, pressure support is increased to provide the patient a TV similar to what he or she was receiving with the volume-cycled settings. PS is then gradually decreased as tolerated. We discourage the use of PS in all but the most controlled circumstances. At the present time we know of no advantages to PS weaning and have great concerns about its safety. The lack of adequate "backup" mechanisms if compliance changes or spontaneous ventilation ceases is a very serious limitation.

EXPERIMENTAL MODALITIES

There are several treatments for ARF that are in use but that must be considered experimental at this time. Chief among these are noninvasive ventilation with bilevel positive airway pressure (Bi-PAP) and extracorporeal membrane oxygenation (ECMO). Bi-PAP is the technique of using positive airway pressure delivered through either a face or a nasal mask without intubation of the airway. It is essentially a PS modality without intubation. It can augment ventilation and has been reported to result in decreased need for intubation in individuals with AOCRF. Although currently used in some centers, its ultimate role remains to be determined. We do not advocate using this technique until the results of several ongoing clinical research protocols are available. ECMO has been widely used for the neonatal respiratory distress syndrome for several years. Based upon this experience, and some uncontrolled studies in adults, its efficacy was recently re-evaluated in a well-designed clinical trial. No benefit over conventional therapy was demonstrated, and any further use should be strictly limited to clinical trials.

ATELECTASIS

method of
R. THOMAS TEMES, M.D.
University of New Mexico School of Medicine
Albuquerque, New Mexico

Atelectasis is collapse of lung tissue. This may involve an entire lung, a lobe, a segment, or a subsegmental region. Atelectasis develops most frequently as a complication of surgery but may have other causes as well. These include trauma, endobronchial tumor, airway compression from mediastinal adenopathy, bronchial stricture or rupture, pneumothorax, pleural effusion, aspirated foreign body, main-stem intubation, and pulmonary parenchymal disease. In patients with atelectasis and no obvious cause, an evaluation including bronchoscopy and computed tomography of the chest must be performed to exclude an underlying disorder.

After surgery or trauma, atelectasis develops from impaired respiratory mechanics, pain, abnormal mucociliary clearance, and retained secretions. Collapse of alveoli produces shunt with mismatched ventilation and perfusion, resulting in hypoxia that may be severe. Retained secretions promote bacterial growth, which can progress to pneumonia.

TREATMENT

The treatment of atelectasis requires identification of the cause. When mechanical causes are identified, these are treated. In routine atelectasis without predisposing factors, treatment goals are increased pulmonary volumes and mobilization of secretions.

In surgical patients, treatment begins preoperatively with cessation of bronchial irritants (most commonly cigarette smoke), an exercise program to improve respiratory mechanics and lung reserve, and education. Patients learn the expected postoperative activities and their rationale, are taught incentive spirometry, and are treated for underlying lung disease with bronchodilators and antibiotics as indicated.

Intraoperatively, pulmonary trauma is minimized. Care is taken to aspirate secretions from the airway during the procedure and upon completion using suction catheters or bronchoscopy. Fluids are administered judiciously to prevent pulmonary edema. Early extubation restores near-normal pulmonary physiology and cough.

Postoperatively (or following trauma) adequate pain control is important to allow deep breathing and effective coughing. This can be provided by epidural narcotics, patient-controlled analgesia, or rib blocks. Parenteral or oral pain medications, although useful, are less effective.

Patients are kept in a chair or ambulated during daylight hours. Incentive spirometry is performed every half to 1 hour. Coughing and deep breathing are encouraged. Postural and percussion physiotherapy are given a minimum of twice daily. Bronchodilators and humidified oxygen are administered routinely. Antibiotics are given as indicated by fever, leukocytosis, worsening pulmonary function, purulent sputum, and infiltrate on a chest radiograph.

In refractory cases of atelectasis due to secretions, more aggressive measures may be required. Frequent bronchoscopy is often useful. A venous catheter inserted through the cricothyroid membrane may be used to instill saline within the airway and promote coughing. Intubation, minitracheostomy, or formal tracheostomy allow access to the airway for suctioning.

Atelectasis that fails to resolve rapidly with treatment or recurs must be aggressively evaluated. Underlying disorders, including malignancy, may present as atelectasis and be curable if diagnosed in a timely fashion.

CHRONIC OBSTRUCTIVE PULMONARY DISEASE

method of
IRWIN ZIMENT, M.D.
Olive View–UCLA Medical Center
Sylmar, California

Characteristically, chronic obstructive pulmonary disease (COPD) is a progressive disorder, and eventually chronic respiratory failure is diagnosed; exacerbations can result in acute respiratory failure that necessitates temporary ventilatory support. In the final stages, the patient has severe exercise limitation and requires chronic oxygen therapy; in selected cases, a permanent tracheostomy and maintenance on a respirator are needed. Severe COPD places a strain on the right ventricle, and in such patients cor pulmonale usually results. However, this late stage is not always recognized since coincidental ischemic heart disease may become the predominant problem in these elderly patients. The patient with COPD is susceptible to pulmonary infections, thromboembolic complications, arrhythmias, heart failure, and drug toxicity from the adverse interactions both with medications and with concomitant organ dysfunction.

PROPHYLACTIC MEASURES

Once COPD is recognized, it is important to institute measures to decrease the liability to further deterioration and to prevent common complications.

Prevention

Chronic exposure to airway irritants and toxic chemicals is associated with the risk of developing COPD. Measures to reduce the hazards of smoking are thus prophylactic as well as therapeutic; counseling and exhortations by the physician are the main requirement to help smokers quit the habit. Local support groups organized by hospitals, churches, health clubs, lung associations, and cancer societies can be of value. The various nicotine substitutes are of help if used correctly; in some patients combinations of nicotine gum and patches, perhaps with clonidine (Catapres)* as an adjuvant, are of great value, but their use should always be accompanied by counseling and behavior modification.

Diet

The exact role of diet in COPD is ill defined, but general malnourishment appears to exacerbate the condition, whereas obesity necessitates an increase in ventilatory effort. The debility associated with symptomatic COPD may interfere with food intake, thus contributing to the impaired nutritional state of the patient. Increased protein intake is probably not beneficial, whereas a predominantly carbohydrate diet, which may acutely lead to increased carbon dioxide production and thereby increase respiratory demands, is probably not harmful in long-term management. Smaller and more frequent meals, with appropriate dietary regulation to optimize weight, should be advised for symptomatic patients. Antioxidant foods and vitamins may be beneficial, and their use should be encouraged. The use of expectorant spicy foods, if tolerated, may be helpful.

Infection

Lung infection should be prevented if possible. Influenza vaccine should be given each year to suscepti-

---

*Not FDA-approved for this indication.

ble patients, and pneumococcal vaccine may be of value if given every 5 to 10 years. Sinus problems should be addressed in subjects with nasal allergy, polyps, or postnasal drip; topical steroids or decongestant drugs should be given periodically to relieve symptoms and decrease the liability to infection.

Enzyme Deficiency

Neutrophil invasion and breakdown in the alveoli occurs as a response to irritants, toxins, and infections. The resulting release of proteases is normally modulated by the presence of antiproteases such as alpha$_1$-antitrypsin (αAT). Persons with homozygous αAT deficiency are susceptible to the early development of progressive emphysema; this accounts for only 1 to 2% of patients with emphysema. A serum level of less than 180 mg per dL in a stable individual may be an indication for periodic replacement of the enzyme using a commercially available preparation. This prophylactic drug is extremely expensive and can only be justified in carefully selected persons.

PHARMACOLOGIC THERAPY

Unlike the situation with asthma, guidelines for the management of COPD have not been issued by major professional organizations. The inflammatory nature of COPD has not been perceived as offering a basis for therapy, and stepwise escalation of drug introduction may not be so relevant. In asthma, therapy is based on aerosol medications, but older subjects with COPD often find it difficult to use a metered-dose inhaler (MDI) correctly, whereas appropriate use of orally administered preparations is readily ensured. If possible, therapy should be initiated with MDIs since the usual doses of these topical drugs cause minimal side effects. Stepped-care principles should prove helpful (Table 1).

Beta-Agonist Drugs

For occasional relief of symptoms in early COPD, a beta$_2$-agonist MDI can be used as needed. In established disease, routine dosing helps to relieve symptoms, although the increase achieved in forced expiratory volume (FEV) may be less than 10 to 15%. The appropriate dosage may need to be determined by increasing from a baseline of two to three puffs three to four times a day up to four to eight puffs every 4 to 6 hours.* In many patients, the combination of a beta$_2$ agonist, such as albuterol (Ventolin, Proventil), with ipratropium (Atrovent) results in an improved outcome; this combination in a single preparation will offer an optimal regimen for patients with moderate or severe COPD.

Patients who do not achieve the desired response can try alternative formulations of beta agonists. The use of a spacer, a powder preparation, or a breath-activated device may offer advantages. Exacerbation may require the prescribing of an inhalant preparation with a jet nebulizer: the standard dose of albuterol is 2.5 mg, which is equivalent to 27 puffs from an MDI. Such nebulizer dosing may be required two to three times an hour in severe exacerbations, and continuous nebulization may be required if the patient needs ventilator support. In some patients, oral slow-release albuterol 4 to 8 mg twice a day appears to be useful. In emergencies, subcutaneous injections of epinephrine or terbutaline (Brethine) may be indicated. The combination of moderate doses of inhaled beta-agonist solution or beta agonist from an MDI with moderately large doses of ipratropium may be safer than the use of a proportionately large dose of an inhaled beta agonist alone.

Anticholinergic Drugs

Over the course of the twentieth century, stramonium cigarettes gave way to atropine by nebuliza-

---

*Dosage should not exceed 12 puffs in 24 hours.

TABLE 1. **Stepped Care for Chronic Obstructive Pulmonary Disease**

General		Correct causal or exacerbating factors, e.g., smoking
		Optimize nutrition, exercise, weight, and rest
		Anticipate problems, e.g., give influenza vaccination
Step 1	For episodic symptoms, e.g., dyspnea on effort	Beta$_2$-agonist MDI 2–3 puffs q 6–8 h prn
Step 2	For persistent symptoms due to reversible bronchospasm	Ipratropium (Atrovent) MDI 2–8 puffs bid–tid* and Beta$_2$-agonist MDI 2–6 puffs q 4–12 h prn
Step 3	For symptoms that limit exercise, add	Theophylline (slow-release) 400–1000 mg/day in 1–2 divided doses; follow dosing guidelines or Albuterol (Proventil) (slow-release oral) 4–8 mg bid
Step 4	For persistent symptoms or nocturnal wheezing, consider use of	Salmeterol (Serevent) MDI 1–2 puffs 1–2 times/day
Step 5	For asthmatic symptoms or rapid deterioration, add	Prednisone: dose varies from 5–10 mg qod to 15–60 mg/day; reduce to minimal dose, then use Aerosol steroid MDI 8–24 puffs per day*
Step 6	For exacerbations or cardiopulmonary disease, add	Antibiotic courses if needed, e.g., trimethoprim-sulfamethoxazole (Bactrim, Septra) 1–2 tabs q 12 h, tetracycline 250–500 mg qid, amoxicillin 500 mg q 8 h and Mucokinetic agents for sputum clearance problems and Cardiac drugs and diuretic for primary or secondary cardiac complications

*Exceeds dosage recommended by the manufacturer.
Abbreviation: MDI = metered dose inhaler.

tion, which has been succeeded by ipratropium. This topical preparation has minimal side effects when given in the basic dosage of two MDI inhalations three or four times a day. For moderate to severe symptomatic COPD, the regular use of ipratropium MDI is required. Although two to three puffs three to four times a day (up to a maximum of 12 puffs in 24 hours) are usually advised, four to eight puffs may be needed every 6 to 8 hours, and with such dosages side effects or complications are rare. A spacer is useful, both to improve drug delivery to the lung and to reduce the risk of precipitating glaucoma by accidental spraying of the eyes. In exacerbations, the 1% inhalant solution allows larger doses to be delivered every 3 to 4 hours by means of a nebulizer, with 0.25 to 0.5 mL providing the equivalent of 14 to 28 puffs from the MDI.

Theophylline

A major advantage of theophylline is that it can easily be given once or twice a day using one of several long-acting preparations. Theophylline is a weak bronchodilator and improves mucus clearance. There is some evidence that it improves the contractility and decreases the fatiguability of the respiratory muscles, and it may stimulate the respiratory center. In addition, theophylline can reduce pulmonary vascular resistance, increase coronary artery perfusion, and improve both left and right ventricular ejection fractions. Thus, theophylline can be a valuable drug in severe COPD, particularly if there is cor pulmonale. In exacerbations, it can be administered intravenously as aminophylline.

The main disadvantage of theophylline is its increased toxicity in the presence of various drugs, impaired liver function, or hypoxia. The precautions listed in manufacturers' brochures must be taken into account, and a lower dose should be given if there is a danger of impaired drug clearance. Measuring the serum level can help optimize it at 8 to 14 μg per mL and thereby avoid toxicity. It is essential that patients be warned that nausea, nervousness, and palpitations are indications of toxicity and that precautions must be taken to avoid overdosing by careless or unknowing administration of one or more theophylline preparations.

Corticosteroids

Although aerosol steroids have a central role in the management of asthma, they have not been shown to be useful in the management of most cases of COPD. Oral steroids may help in patients with an asthmatic component, particularly if they fail to respond adequately to other established drug treatment. Whenever oral steroids are introduced, great care is needed to demonstrate objective pulmonary benefit, since most COPD patients are at an age that makes them very susceptible to steroid complications. Low daily maintenance dosage or alternate-day dosing may be needed. Steroid-responsive patients may benefit from an aerosol. In general, exacerbations of COPD are treated with large doses of intravenous or oral steroids; however, it is uncertain that adequate benefit can be demonstrated in most patients.

Mucokinetic Drugs

Although abnormal mucus is a defining characteristic of bronchitis, most drugs that appear to affect mucus qualities have not been demonstrated to confer definite benefits in COPD. Water and traditional expectorants such as iodides and guaifenesin (Robitussin) may help. Currently, there is some evidence that aerosolized recombinant human DNase (rhDNase) may prolong life if given to patients with an exacerbation of COPD. Physical therapy and devices that use oscillatory wave applications are of limited value. Established techniques such as intubation, suctioning, or bronchoscopy may be required if excessive, abnormal production of secretions causes progressive respiratory failure.

Antibiotics

Most clinicians give a course of sulfamethoxazole-trimethoprim or derivatives of either tetracycline, ampicillin, or erythromycin to treat exacerbations characterized by increased purulence of sputum. There is little proof of antibiotic efficacy in patients unless there is clinical deterioration in respiratory function and evidence of pulmonary tissue invasion such as fever, leukocytosis, and a radiologic infiltrate. In nursing home patients, infection requires more potent antibiotics such as a cephalosporin or a broad-spectrum penicillin. Amantadine (Symmetrel) or rimantadine (Flumadine) may be useful in patients who are thought to be infected by influenza A virus.

ADDITIONAL MEASURES

Several complications that occur commonly in COPD may need attention.

Hypoxia

Once a patient is significantly hypoxic during normal activities, supplementary oxygen may be needed for symptomatic relief and to enhance mobility. If the Pa_{O_2} is persistently below 60 mmHg, oxygen delivered at about 2 to 3 liters per minute for 16 to 24 hours a day can decrease pulmonary hypertension and reduce the progress of cor pulmonale, thereby prolonging life. Oxygen can be given by tank or from a liquid oxygen supply, or by means of an electrically operated concentrator; the choice depends on individual circumstances, local practices, and the availability of a suitable service company. Patients must be prepared to cooperate in using the drug appropriately and to avoid inappropriate activities such as smoking.

Hypercarbia

In chronic progressive disease, the Pa_{CO_2} increases, but as long as the body compensates by maintaining a pH above 7.30 and oxygen is supplied, compensated respiratory acidosis can be tolerated for years. Effective therapy may stabilize the Pa_{CO_2}; excessive efforts to reduce carbon dioxide retention by the intermittent use of respirators is not necessary. A respiratory center stimulant, almitrine, is available in Europe, but in the United States the only recommended drug for selected patients is methylphenidate.

Heart Failure

Heart failure is a common complication, with left heart failure occurring in subjects with ischemic or hypertensive cardiomyopathy and right heart failure occurring in COPD as a consequence of pulmonary hypertension. Left heart failure may require diuretic, cardiotonic, vasodilator, and antiarrhythmia therapy. Right heart failure may also improve with oxygen, and in some patients theophylline is beneficial. Pulmonary artery vasodilators have not been proved to be of practical value. A hematocrit over 55% is thought to present rheologic disadvantages, and phlebotomy is advisable to reduce the level to 48 to 50%; it is unusual for more than two phlebotomies to be needed over the lifetime of a patient with polycythemia secondary to COPD.

Surgery

In some patients, surgical procedures can help in COPD. Thus, it is generally recognized that removal of large bullae may improve lung mechanics. Lung transplantation is an option for suitable patients. Chronic lung disease need not preclude major surgery for extrapulmonary problems.

Psychological Problems

Dyspnea may persist in spite of adequate bronchodilator therapy, and this symptom may be difficult to alleviate. In general, sedatives and hypnotics or narcotics do not help and may suppress the respiratory center; however, in terminal patients, or those with severe pain, such palliative therapy is humane and appropriate. Antidepressants are indicated for selected patients, particularly when there is troublesome insomnia. Patients may be candidates for polysomnography to help define and treat sleep disorders. Antitussive drugs may be required for patients who suffer from frequent painful or discomforting nonproductive coughing.

Rehabilitation

High-quality rehabilitation programs are very valuable; they offer psychosocial support, motivation, and reconditioning. Patients can learn how to conserve energy and improve exercise capacity, while gaining valuable insights into appropriate use of their medications and supplementary oxygen. Finally, patients can learn about their options when their disease enters its terminal stages; they require appropriate education about living wills, nursing homes or hospices, home care, palliative care, and other measures designed to help them avoid the indignity of a prolonged final illness on a ventilator in an ICU.

SLEEP APNEA SYNDROME

method of
DONALD D. PETERSON, M.D.
The Lankenau Hospital
Wynnewood, Pennsylvania

and

ANDREW P. PITMAN, M.D.
The Bryn Mawr Hospital
Bryn Mawr, Pennsylvania

Sleep apnea is a common disorder characterized by frequent apneas (cessation of breathing for at least 10 seconds) during sleep. Most patients with this syndrome have obstructive apnea, with intermittent blockage of the upper airway during sleep, whereas a much smaller number have central sleep apnea, with fluctuations in respiratory effort. Current estimates are that 8% of American men have symptomatic obstructive sleep apnea syndrome, compared with 4% of postmenopausal women.

PATHOPHYSIOLOGY

There appears to be a continuum between snoring and obstructive sleep apnea. The sites of the partial upper airway obstruction causing snoring and complete obstruction causing apnea are generally the hypopharynx and/or oropharynx. The cause of the repetitive obstructions is the normal sleep state–related decrease in the tone of the genioglossus and other muscles that function to open the upper airway during inspiration. The function of these muscles is particularly impaired during rapid eye movement sleep. Predisposing factors that adversely affect upper airway patency include nasal septal deformity, nasal polyps, adenotonsillar hypertrophy, retrognathia, obesity, and an inherited tendency for a structurally small pharyngeal airway (the latter two factors are by far the most common). Many of the clinical consequences of the syndrome are mediated by arousals of the central nervous system (CNS) that briefly return the CNS to the awake state in order to terminate each apnea, causing fragmentation of sleep and activation of the sympathetic nervous system. However, at the end of a few breaths, sleep resumes and the pharyngeal muscles again relax, so that the whole process repeats itself, often several hundred times in a single night. The repetitive sympathetic stimulation causes systemic hypertension, whereas repetitive hypoxia causes pulmonary hypertension, mediated by pulmonary vasoconstrictive reflexes. The term "upper airway resistance syndrome" has been used to describe patients with labored breathing due to partial upper airway obstruction (usually heavy snoring) punctuated by frequent arousals, causing the same sequelae despite the lack of actual apneas or measurable hypopneas.

Central sleep apnea syndrome is most often seen in patients with Cheyne-Stokes breathing owing to congestive heart failure, CNS disorders, chronic renal failure, and the like. Although Cheynes-Stokes breathing during sleep frequently causes no sequelae and may even be considered a normal aspect of sleep in elderly men, the sleep apnea syndrome can result if sleep architecture is disturbed.

The term "sleep-disordered breathing" is now generally used to describe any of the entities previously described, particularly since many patients have a mixture of the various types of events during a night of sleep.

CLINICAL FEATURES

The most frequent signs of obstructive sleep apnea prompting evaluation are excessive daytime sleepiness and unusually loud snoring. Obtaining a history from other observers in the bedroom or elsewhere in the household is extremely helpful, since many patients deny sleepiness and snoring, even when these are quite obvious to others. Often observers note actual apneas or periods of loud snoring punctuated by several "resuscitative" gasps of deep breathing or snorts. The brief arousals from sleep terminating these apneas or hypopneas may not be recognizable as awakenings from sleep to others; in fact patients are usually completely unaware of the frequency of sleep disruption. Daytime sleepiness is often ignored by patients, until job performance is compromised or traffic accidents occur (one of the many potentially life-threatening consequences of sleep apnea). The incidence and severity of obstructive sleep apnea is correlated with increasing obesity, but an important subset (approximately 25%) of patients are not obese; this fact often contributes to delayed recognition of the syndrome. Hypertension is found in approximately 50% of patients with sleep apnea; conversely, as many as 30% of patients with "essential" hypertension will be found to have sleep apnea, if they are appropriately tested. Whether sleep apnea is the cause of the hypertension or whether both exist because of common predisposing factors is being vigorously investigated at present. Similar efforts focus on the epidemiologic associations of snoring and sleep apnea with coronary artery disease and stroke. Other signs of sleep apnea include headaches on awakening, probably due to sleep-related elevations in arterial carbon dioxide pressure (Pa_{CO_2}), and unexplained edema of the legs, secondary to right ventricular dysfunction and pulmonary hypertension. The term "Pickwickian syndrome" (also referred to as "obesity-hypoventilation syndrome") is frequently used to describe patients with extreme obesity, sleepiness, hypoxia, and hypercapnia while awake, and cor pulmonale; this level of severity is seen in fewer than 5% of patients with sleep apnea.

Laboratory findings occasionally prompting evaluation for sleep apnea include unexplained polycythemia or CO_2 retention, pulmonary hypertension (often diagnosed incidentally during cardiac catheterization for other reasons), and nocturnal cardiac arrhythmias noted on continuous ambulatory or inpatient monitoring. Conversely, hypothyroidism can cause sleep apnea by an alteration of upper airway anatomy and a decrease in ventilatory drive, so that thyroid function testing should be performed on most patients with sleep apnea, albeit with a relatively low yield.

Diagnosis of presence and severity of suspected sleep apnea requires polysomnography, preferably an overnight study with continuous measurements of sleep stage, airflow, respiratory effort, oxygen saturation, electrocardiographic data, and so on. Results are scored as events per hour of sleep (i.e., apnea index) or more recently, the respiratory disturbance index (RDI) incorporating both apneas and hypopneas. An index of up to 5 is often accepted as normal, with 5 to 20 per hour considered mild sleep apnea, 20 to 40 per hour considered moderate, and over 40 per hour considered severe sleep apnea. Obviously other features, including hypoxemia, arrhythmias, and other possible sequelae must be taken into account when the severity of the overall clinical syndrome is judged.

TREATMENT

The most widely accepted current therapy for obstructive sleep apnea is nasal continuous positive airway pressure (NCPAP), usually at a pressure of 5 to 15 cmH_2O. Pressures are titrated during a full night of sleep with polysomnographic monitoring until apneas and snoring are eliminated in all stages of sleep. Although this therapy is frequently remarkably effective on the initial night in the laboratory, approximately one-third of patients consider NCPAP treatment too uncomfortable initially or soon after the home prescription to continue therapy. Some of the remaining groups of patients with significant symptomatic improvement only use the NCPAP apparatus for part of the night. Despite these limitations, NCPAP continues to be the most effective treatment strategy, particularly for patients with moderate or severe obstructive apnea. For patients with persistent hypoxemia despite NCPAP or patients who cannot tolerate NCPAP, bilevel positive airway pressure may be effective. At the other end of the spectrum, patients with severe snoring and/or mild sleep apnea may respond to a variety of surgical approaches, including correction of nasal septal deviation and laser-assisted uvulopalatoplasty. More aggressive measures, such as uvulopalatopharyngoplasty, hyoid resuspension, mandibular advancement, and tracheostomy (usually recommended only for patients with life-threatening arrhythmias), may be employed for patients with more severe disease. Although individual anatomic considerations and preferences may favor one approach over the other, increasing severity of sleep apnea predicts lower success rates of all but the most aggressive approaches described.

Weight loss is of potentially great benefit in the treatment of sleep apnea in the majority of patients who are obese; however, it is infrequently achieved, and then often only temporarily. Enhancing nasal patency with intranasal steroids, antihistamines, and decongestants can provide treatment for patients with mild disturbances, in addition to increasing the likelihood of success with other measures.

Pharmacotherapy has been of limited benefit, with conflicting results regarding possible modest benefits from medroxyprogesterone (Provera),* protriptyline (Vivactil),* and fluoxetine (Prozac).* Since alcohol and benzodiazepines have been shown to produce

---

*Not FDA-approved for this indication.

snoring and obstructive apneas in normal individuals, abstinence from alcohol, hypnotics, and other CNS depressants before bed is important for patients with sleep apnea.

In the current setting of rapidly evolving treatment strategies, the high incidence of sleep apnea syndrome and its many serious consequences mandate increased efforts to identify and test patients at risk.

PRIMARY LUNG CANCER

method of
JAMES R. JETT, M.D.
University of Pittsburgh
Pittsburgh, Pennsylvania

We are caught up in a lung cancer epidemic in the United States. It was estimated that in 1995, there would be 170,000 new cases of lung cancer and 157,000 lung cancer deaths. Lung cancer is now the most common cause of death from cancer in both males and females. Women account for 40% of all new lung cancers. The 5-year survival rate for lung cancer has increased from 8% in the early 1960s to 13% in the late 1980s for whites and from 5% to 11% for African Americans. Although this improvement in survival is statistically significant, it is far from acceptable. Progress in prevention and treatment is mandatory. As is the case for many diseases, lung cancer is easier to prevent than to cure.

The presenting manifestations of lung cancer are myriad. Occasionally, a lesion is discovered while the patient is still asymptomatic because a chest x-ray is obtained for other reasons. The survival in asymptomatic lung cancer patients is superior to those who present with symptoms. Symptoms are related to local tumor growth, invasion of mediastinal or thoracic structures, distant metastasis or remote tumor effects due to paraneoplastic syndromes, or constitutional symptoms. The most common symptoms are cough (new or changed), dyspnea, chest pain, and hemoptysis, which occur in 35 to 75% of individuals. Many of these symptoms indicate advanced or unresectable disease. There is a large variety of other signs and symptoms due to local disease, metastatic disease, or paraneoplastic syndromes.*

PATHOLOGY

The pathology of lung cancer is important for both diagnostic and therapeutic reasons. Pathologic proof of malignancy is usually needed prior to definitive treatment. An exception to this rule would be an enlarging pulmonary mass in an individual without signs or symptoms suggesting an infectious etiology. In this situation, it might be justifiable to resect the enlarging mass without prior confirmation of malignancy. In almost all other situations, histologic or cytologic proof of malignancy is needed before definitive treatment is begun, including patients who present with superior vena cava syndrome.

The major histologic types of lung cancer are squamous cell, large cell, adeno, and small cell. Bronchioloalveolar cell is generally considered to be a subtype of adenocarcinoma. Many cancers have mixed histology. Treatment varies, depending on the cell type, with the most important differentiation being between small cell and non–small cell (squamous, large, adeno) histology. Blinded studies of interobserver variability have shown variation between pathologists for non–small cell histology (i.e., squamous vs. large cell or adenocarcinoma vs. large cell) in one-fourth to one-third of cases. However, a majority of pathologists agreed on the designation of non–small cell carcinoma 94% of the time. Additionally, only 34% of lung cancer cases are homogeneous according to the majority of five pathologists on one review panel. Forty-five percent of cases showed a major histologic type difference on at least one slide. There was very little ($\leq 2\%$) interobserver disagreement on small cell carcinoma. Other reports have confirmed this agreement among pathologists for cases of small cell lung cancer.

STAGING

In addition to histologic type, a determination of stage is important in deciding on the most appropriate treatment. In 1986, a new international staging system for lung cancer was adopted based on tumor (T) size and location, lymph node (N) involvement, and presence or absence of distant metastasis (M). Staging is based on the letters T, N, M, with appropriate suffixes that describe the extent of the cancer (Table 1).

Lung cancer is divided into four stages (Table 2). Stage 0 is uncommon and refers specifically to carcinoma in situ. In these patients, the chest x-ray is normal and the malignancy is discovered by an abnormal sputum cytology or bronchoscopically obtained cytology or biopsy. Stage 0, I, II,

TABLE 1. **TNM Method of Tumor Staging**

Primary Tumor (T)

T0 No evidence of primary tumor
TX Cancer cell in bronchopulmonary secretions; no tumor seen on chest film or at bronchoscopy
Tis Carcinoma in situ
T1 Tumor ≤ 3 cm in greatest dimension, surrounded by lung tissue; no bronchoscopic evidence of tumor proximal to lobar bronchus
T2 Tumor >3 cm in diameter, or a tumor of any size that involves visceral pleura or associated with atelectasis extending to hilum (but not involving entire lung); must be ≥ 2 cm from carina
T3 Tumor involves chest wall, diaphragm, mediastinal pleura, or pericardium or is ≤ 2 cm from carina (but does not involve it)
T4 Tumor involves carina or trachea or invades mediastinum, heart, great vessels, esophagus, or vertebrae; or there is malignant pleural effusion

Nodal Involvement (N)

N0 No demonstrable lymph node involvement
N1 Ipsilateral peribronchial or hilar nodes involved (includes direct extension)
N2 Metastasis to ipsilateral mediastinal nodes or to subcarinal nodes
N3 Metastasis to contralateral mediastinal or hilar nodes or to scalene or supraclavicular nodes

Distant Metastasis (M)

M0 No (known) distant metastasis
M1 Distant metastasis present—specify site(s)

Adapted from Mountain CF: A new international staging system for lung cancer. Chest *89*(Suppl):225S–233S, 1986. By permission of the American College of Chest Physicians.

---

*See Patel AM, Peters SG: Symposium on intrathoracic neoplasms. Mayo Clin Proc *68*:273–287, 1993.

TABLE 2. **TNM Subsets for the Staging of Lung Cancer**

Stage	TNM Subsets
0	Tis (in situ)
I	T1, N0, M0
	T2, N0, M0
II	T1, N1, M0
	T2, N1, M0
IIIA	T3, N0, M0
	T3, N1, M0
	T1–3, N2, M0
IIIB	Any T, N3, M0
	T4, any N, M0
IV	Any T, any N, M1

Adapted from Mountain CF: A new international staging system for lung cancer. Chest *89*(Suppl):225S–233S, 1986. By permission of American College of Chest Physicians.

and some IIIA lung cancers are considered to be resectable. Stages IIIB and IV are generally not considered to be surgical diseases and are best treated with other modalities.

It is possible to use the TNM staging system for small cell lung cancer (SCLC), but there is less differentiation of survival for the various stages than has been observed with non–small cell lung cancer (NSCLC). Accordingly, most physicians use the old Veterans Administration staging system of limited and extensive disease for this cell type. Limited-stage disease is defined as disease confined to one hemithorax and the ipsilateral supraclavicular nodes. This stage of disease can usually be encompassed within one radiation port. Extensive-stage disease is defined as disease beyond the confines just stated. Contralateral hilar lymph nodes, cervical lymph nodes, or distant organ disease is extensive-stage disease. A cytologically positive or bloody effusion should be considered extensive-stage disease.

All patients should have clinical staging before undergoing definitive treatment. This should include a complete history and physical examination, complete blood count, chemistry panel, chest radiograph, and computed tomography (CT) scan of the chest and upper abdomen through the liver and adrenal glands. The CT scan is cost effective because it helps avoid unnecessary thoracotomies. Prior to operation or radiotherapy, pulmonary function evaluation is useful. A CT scan of the head or magnetic resonance imaging (MRI) is indicated for individuals with any central nervous system (CNS) complaint, no matter how vague, because of the high propensity for CNS metastasis with lung cancer. Other tests should be individualized based on specific signs and symptoms. To date, there are no tumor markers in the blood that have been proved to be of prognostic or diagnostic benefit for individual patients. The role of oncogene or tumor suppressor gene, DNA ploidy, and cytogenetic analysis of the tumor is undergoing extensive evaluation but cannot be recommended for routine clinical use at this time.

TREATMENT FOR STAGES I AND II NON–SMALL CELL LUNG CANCER

Only 20 to 25% of patients with lung cancer have resectable disease at the time of initial presentation. The treatment of choice for Stage 0, I, or II NSCLC is surgical resection, provided the patient is medi-

cally fit. The Lung Cancer Study Group reviewed the 30-day operative mortality of 2200 resections of NSCLC from 1979 to 1981.* The overall operative mortality for all patients was 3.7%. They observed a 6.2% and 2.9% mortality for patients undergoing pneumonectomy and lobectomy, respectively. The major causes of postoperative death included pneumonia, respiratory failure, bronchopleural fistula and empyema, myocardial infarction, and pulmonary emboli. The operation of choice is a lobectomy with sampling of multiple mediastinal lymph nodes from different stations. The lymph node biopsies are necessary for adequate staging and to determine the need for further therapy. Failure to biopsy mediastinal nodes is less than optimal surgery. Lobectomy is the usual and most common resection unless it results in incomplete excision. Pneumonectomy is required in 15 to 25% of patients in most series. Limited resections (less than lobectomy) may be indicated in patients with compromised pulmonary function. Several studies have demonstrated a higher rate of local recurrence in patients undergoing limited resection. Accordingly, lobectomy is the operation of choice in patients with adequate pulmonary reserve. There have been recent reports of lobectomy via video-assisted thoracoscopic surgery (VATS). The exact role of VATS lobectomy is currently being debated, but at least one report has documented dissemination of tumor in 20 cases of VATS for various malignant diseases.

The 5-year survival for resected Stage I NSCLC ranges from 60 to 80% in different series. For Stage II disease, the survival at 5 years is 33 to 50%. In patients with resected lung cancer, there is a 2 to 3% risk per year of developing a second primary lung cancer. Accordingly, patients should be followed every 3 to 4 months during the first 2 years for recurrent disease and every 6 to 12 months thereafter for the development of a new cancer.

TREATMENT FOR STAGES IIIA AND IIIB NON–SMALL CELL LUNG CANCER

Surgery is indicated for some patients with Stage IIIA NSCLC, but exactly which patients are best treated with resection is moot. There is general agreement that those with T3, N0, M0 because of chest wall invasion by direct extension are surgical candidates. Several surgical series have reported an approximate 50% survival at 5 years. It is uncertain whether postresection radiotherapy to the resected tumor bed results in increased survival. Pancoast tumors (superior sulcus tumors) are usually Stage IIIA or IIIB disease. These lesions have traditionally been treated with preoperative radiotherapy with or without chemotherapy and followed by surgery if they are deemed to be resectable by the surgeon. The preoperative radiotherapy is generally 3000 to 4500

*See Ginsberg RJ, Hill LD, Eagan RT, et al: Modern thirty-day operative mortality for surgical resections in lung cancer. J Thorac Cardiovasc Surg *86*:654–658, 1983.

cGy rather than the traditional 6000-cGy dose for "curative radiotherapy." The abbreviated dose of radiotherapy is to diminish the risk of postoperative complications. Additional radiotherapy may be given postoperatively. Some reports advocate radiotherapy alone or in combination with chemotherapy for Pancoast lesions. No randomized trials have been conducted to compare the two treatment approaches (i.e., radiotherapy with and without surgery).

Operations for patients with N2 disease (ipsilateral mediastinal nodes) is much more controversial. Pearson and associates, from Toronto, carefully selected 79 patients with NSCLC and positive mediastinoscopy (biopsy-proven mediastinal lymph node metastasis) in whom a "curative resection" was judged to be possible.* These 79 patients represented only 20% of all of their patients with a positive mediastinoscopy. The 5-year survival, after attempted curative resection, was 9%. Based on this study by Pearson and others, Stage III NSCLC with mediastinal lymph node involvement has been considered to be inoperable.

In the past 10 years, there have been numerous reports of using neoadjuvant therapy (preoperative therapy) in these patients to shrink the tumor and then proceed with surgical resection. The principle goal of neoadjuvant therapy is to convert unresectable disease into resectable disease. Preoperative radiotherapy alone was tested previously and proved to be of no benefit. The more recent trials have employed chemotherapy, usually with a cisplatin-based regimen, or combined chemotherapy and thoracic radiotherapy. In general, the response rates to neoadjuvant chemotherapy have been high (50 to 75% experience significant tumor shrinkage). Approximately 50% are subsequently resectable, and 10 to 25% of resected cases are histologically free of malignancy. The potential negative aspect of this approach is the higher rate of postoperative morbidity and mortality.

In 1994, there were two reports of small randomized trials treating carefully selected patients with Stage IIIA disease with surgery alone or preoperative chemotherapy for two cycles followed by surgery. In both studies, patients on the chemotherapy plus surgery regimen did much better than those receiving surgery only, and the difference was highly statistically significant. Both of these studies were single-institution studies with only 30 patients in each treatment arm. Accompanying editorials with each of these articles cautioned against adopting preoperative chemotherapy followed by attempted surgical resection as the standard approach to Stage IIIA disease.

A number of multi-institutional trials by cooperative oncology groups using neoadjuvant therapy have been reported. The results of two of those trials are summarized in Table 3. Patients with Stage IIIA and occasionally Stage IIIB disease have been included and treated preoperatively with chemotherapy with or without thoracic radiotherapy. The results have been enticing. In general, the 3- to 5-year survival rates have been 25 to 35%. The potential drawback to this approach is a high rate of pneumonectomy (approximately 35%) and a treatment-related mortality of 10 to 15%. Presently, it is unproved whether chemotherapy plus radiotherapy followed by surgery is superior to chemoradiotherapy alone. A large phase III trial with survival as the end point has been initiated to try to answer this question. Until completion of this phase III trial, neoadjuvant therapy followed by surgery for Stage IIIA or IIIB NSCLC should not be adopted as standard therapy. Surgery has not been proved to add to survival in patients with Stage IIIA disease (N2 disease), or Stage IIIB disease.

In the 1970s, the standard treatment for Stage IIIA and IIIB NSCLC was thoracic radiotherapy alone. The 5-year survival with radiotherapy alone was 3 to 5%, with a 70% rate of local failure (within the field of radiation) and a 50 to 70% rate of distant metastasis within 2 years. Because of these poor results, investigators have used combination chemotherapy and radiotherapy for this stage disease. Table 4 summarizes the results of four large randomized trials comparing chemotherapy plus radiotherapy versus radiotherapy alone. The chemotherapy in each trial was a cisplatin-based (Platinol) regimen. Each of these trials confirmed that combined modality therapy was superior to radiotherapy alone. There was an 8 to 14% difference in the 3-year survival. In the United States alone, this improvement in survival could translate into the saving of 4000 to 6000 lives per year. The currently recommended treatment for patients with Stage IIIA or IIIB disease is a combination of chemotherapy and thoracic radiotherapy, if their overall physical status allows it.

TABLE 3. **Results of Multi-Institutional Trials of Neoadjuvant Therapy***

	Neoadjuvant Treatment and Surgery		Chemotherapy and Thoracic Radiotherapy	
	TCG	SWOG	ECOG/RTOG	CALGB
Number of patients	55	127	150	78
Median survival (mo)	21	13/16†	13.8	13.7
2-year survival (%)	47	34/38†	32	26
3-year survival (%)	34	26/24†	15	24

*Survival of Stage III non–small cell lung cancer patients treated on neoadjuvant trials followed by surgery (TCG and SWOG trial) or treated with combined chemotherapy and thoracic radiotherapy, but no surgery (ECOG/RTOG and CALGB trial).

†Survival is reported separately for patients with Stage IIIA and Stage IIIB disease.

Abbreviations: TCG = Toronto Cooperative Group; SWOG = Southwest Oncology Group; ECOG/RTOG = Eastern Cooperative Oncology Group/Radiation Therapy Oncology Group; CALGB = Cancer and Acute Leukemia Group B.

*See Pearson FG, DeLarue NC, Ilves R, et al: Significance of positive superior mediastinal nodes identified at mediastinoscopy in patients with resectable cancer of the lung. J Thorac Cardiovasc Surg 83:1–11, 1982.

TABLE 4. **Results of Trials of Chemotherapy and Radiotherapy***

Trial	Arm	Number of Patients	Median Survival (Mo)	3-Year Survival (%)
CALGB	RT	77	9.6	10
	RT + CT	78	13.7	24
FCOG	RT	95	10.0	4
	RT + CT	99	12.0	12
ECOG/RTOG	RT	150	11.4	6
	RT + CT	150	13.8	15
		1-Year Survival (%)		
EORTC	RT	108	46	2
	RT + CT	102	54	16

*Survival of patients with Stage III non–small cell lung cancer treated in randomized trials comparing thoracic radiotherapy only versus combined chemotherapy and radiotherapy. Chemotherapeutic agents, schedule, and dose varied in the different trials.

Abbreviations: CALGB = Cancer and Acute Leukemia Group B Cooperative Group; FCOG = French Cooperative Oncology Group; ECOG/RTOG = Eastern Cooperative Oncology Group/Radiation Therapy Oncology Group; EORTC = European Organization for Research and Treatment of Cancer; RT = radiotherapy; CT = chemotherapy.

Radiotherapy alone may be given to more debilitated patients. The most commonly employed treatment schedule of radiotherapy (when it is being used with curative intent) is 6000 cGy in 30 fractions. No specific chemotherapy regimen has been shown to be superior, but it should be a cisplatin-based regimen with a dose of 75 to 100 mg per m² per treatment cycle (one cycle equals 3 to 4 weeks). Commonly utilized regimens have been vinblastine (Velban)–cisplatin and etoposide (VePesid)–cisplatin.

TREATMENT FOR STAGE IV NON–SMALL CELL LUNG CANCER

Approximately 40 to 50% of all patients with lung cancer have distant metastasis (Stage IV) at the time of initial diagnosis. For these individuals, there is no curative treatment currently available. The goal of therapy is to try to control their disease and palliate symptoms. Response rates of 10 to 30% have been noted with single-agent or combination chemotherapy. Almost all responses to treatment are partial. Complete clinical remissions occur in less than 5% of cases. Patients who respond to chemotherapy may gain an additional 3 to 9 months of life, but eventually all will relapse. A multitude of randomized trials have compared various combinations of chemotherapy drugs. Generally, the median survival time is 5 to 7 months, and the response rates range from 10 to 30%. No combination has been shown to be superior. Accordingly, there is no standard therapy for Stage IV NSCLC.

Because no therapy is curative, a large number of randomized trials have been performed to compare the best supportive care versus combination chemotherapy. One of the most frequently cited studies was carried out by the National Cancer Institute of

Canada Cooperative Group,* with patients randomized to supportive care or chemotherapy with either vindesine† and cisplatin or cyclophosphamide (Cytoxan), doxorubicin (Adriamycin), and cisplatin (Platinol) (CAP). The median survival time of the supportive care group was 17 weeks versus 33 weeks for patients on vindesine–cisplatin and 25 weeks for those on the CAP regimen. The difference in survival was statistically significant in favor of the chemotherapy treated patients.

The Canadian investigators analyzed the cost of treatment for each of the treatment arms. Treatment with CAP was the least expensive. The best supportive care was more expensive than CAP therapy because more patients in the supportive care group required radiotherapy for palliation of symptoms and had more days in the hospital. Chemotherapy with CAP was associated with a savings of $6172 per year of life gained. The major cost in all three arms of the study was related to hospitalization and not to the use of chemotherapy. Thus, chemotherapy should be given in an outpatient setting whenever possible.

A recent meta-analysis reviewed seven studies of polychemotherapy versus supportive care for patients with advanced NSCLC.‡ These studies included over 700 patients. The numbers of deaths at 3, 6, 9, 12, and 18 months were used as the study end points. The relative risk reduction of death was 0.65 at 3 months and 0.73 at 6 months in patients receiving chemotherapy. The reduction in mortality associated with systemic chemotherapy during the first 6 months was statistically significant. The benefit of chemotherapy diminished with time.

Quality of life (QOL) data are not available from any of the previously cited trials. Obviously, the QOL of lung cancer patients declines as the disease progresses, with or without treatment. A question of paramount importance is whether systemic chemotherapy increases or decreases the QOL in patients with advanced disease. There is evidence that polychemotherapy can reduce pain, cough, or dyspnea in some cases, and reduction of symptoms should improve the QOL. Additionally, spending fewer days in the hospital is likely to translate into better QOL. As stated earlier, the treated patients in the Canadian trial had fewer days of hospitalization compared with the best supportive care group. QOL issues in lung cancer patients are currently under investigation in clinical trials. To date, there are no data to support the belief that chemotherapy decreases the QOL of individuals compared with those receiving supportive care only.

Due to the current status of modest treatment benefits, lack of curative treatment, and no standard

---

*See Rapp E, Pater JL, Willan A, et al: Chemotherapy can prolong survival in patients with advanced non–small-cell lung cancer: Report of a Canadian multicenter randomized trial. J Clin Oncol 6:633–641, 1988.

†Not available in the United States.

‡See Souquet PJ, Chauvin F, Boisse JP, et al: Polychemotherapy in advanced non–small-cell lung cancer: A meta-analysis. Lancet 342:19–21, 1993.

therapy, many medical oncologists offer previously untreated patients experimental therapies. This approach is justifiable, given the need to identify new active agents against this disease. In the past few years, a number of new chemotherapeutic agents with good activity (>15% response rate) against NSCLC have been identified. These agents are paclitaxel (Taxol), docetaxel (Taxotere),* CPT-11,* vinorelbine (Navelbine), and gemcitabine.* Presently, phase II and phase III trials are under way to evaluate these agents in combination with other agents, usually cisplatin. For the first time in many years, improved treatment for Stage IV NSCLC may be forthcoming.

SMALL CELL LUNG CANCER

SCLC accounts for 20 to 25% of all lung cancers, or 34,000 to 42,000 cases per year in the United States. This cell type has the strongest association with cigarette smoking and is rarely observed in someone who has never smoked. If SCLC is diagnosed in an individual who has never smoked, an alternative diagnosis should be considered, such as bronchial carcinoid tumor or lymphoma. SCLC has a more rapid doubling time than NSCLC and a tendency for early metastasis. These cancers have neuroendocrine granules that are identified by electron microscopy and are associated with peptide hormone secretions, such as neuron-specific enolase, gastrin-releasing peptide (bombesin), and chromogranin A. SCLC is the cell type most commonly associated with ectopic production of hormones, such as arginine vasopressin (antidiuretic hormone) and adrenocorticotropic hormone (corticotropin). Treatment is based on the extent of disease. As previously stated, most physicians stage this disease as either "limited" or "extensive" disease.

Role of Surgery in Small Cell Lung Cancer

In the 1950s and 1960s, surgical resection was the preferred treatment for SCLC. Long-term survival was uncommon following surgery alone (1 to 2%). In the 1960s, the British Medical Research Council conducted a randomized trial of surgery only versus thoracic radiotherapy for limited stage patients.† The median survival time was 199 days for the surgical treatment versus 300 days for radiotherapy (p = .04). These results and the discovery of active systemic chemotherapy agents resulted in the abandonment of surgical therapy for SCLC.

More recently, surgeons have re-examined the issue of surgical treatment in patients with limited-stage disease. In highly selected nonrandomized series, 5-year survival rates of 25 to 35% have been reported. In the only other surgical randomized trial, the Lung Cancer Study Group evaluated the role of

surgery in limited-stage SCLC.* Patients received five cycles of cyclophosphamide (Cytoxan), doxorubicin (Adriamycin), and vincristine (Oncovin). Patients with at least a partial response who were medically able to tolerate resection were randomized to either thoracotomy and resection or no surgery. Subsequently, all patients received identical thoracic radiotherapy. Of the 340 patients initially enrolled, only 144 were ultimately randomized. The survival for patients in the two arms of the study was identical (p = .91). Thus, no randomized trial has shown a survival advantage in patients who received surgical treatment. The survival advantage of resected patients that has been suggested by retrospective series could be due to selection bias or to inaccuracy of the pathologic diagnosis (for example, mistaking atypical carcinoid tumors for SCLC). Most pundits would agree that the most favorable lesion for surgical treatment is the small cell cancer that is a solitary pulmonary nodule. These peripheral cancers should be resected if there is no evidence of distant metastasis, even if a preoperative biopsy suggests small cell histology. If the pathologic review of the resected specimen confirms the diagnosis of SCLC, then these patients should receive four cycles of adjuvant chemotherapy and thoracic radiotherapy. The most commonly employed chemotherapy is either cisplatin and etoposide or cyclophosphamide, doxorubicin, and vincristine.

Limited-Stage Small Cell Lung Cancer

It is estimated that one-third of patients with SCLC have limited-stage disease at initial diagnosis. These individuals are exquisitely responsive to initial chemotherapy and have major response rates of 80 to 90%. Fifty percent or more will achieve a complete remission of all clinically detectable disease (Table 5). The median survival time varies from 15 to 18 months in recent trials. Despite the high response rates, the 2-year survival is 20 to 40%, with 5-year survival rates of 10 to 15%.

SCLC is responsive to a large number of chemotherapeutic agents. In the late 1960s and early 1970s, the combination of cyclophosphamide (Cy-

---

*See Lad T, Piantadosi S, Thomas P, et al: Chest 106(Suppl): 320S–323S, 1994.

TABLE 5. **Response Rates and Survival of Patients with Small Cell Lung Cancer***

	Limited Stage	Extensive Stage
Total number	770	845
Complete response (%)	59	24
Median survival (mo)	15.1	9.3
2-year survival (%)	29	8
5-year survival (%)	12	2

*All patients were treated with Mayo Clinic or North Central Cancer Treatment Group phase II or Phase III protocols from 1975 to 1990.
Data from Shaw EG, Su JQ, Eagan RT, et al: Prophylactic cranial irradiation in complete responders with small cell lung cancer. J Clin Oncol 12:2327–2332, 1994.

---

*Investigational drug in the United States.
†See Fox W, Scadding JG: Medical research council comparative trial of surgery and radiotherapy for primary treatment of small-celled or oat-celled carcinoma of bronchus. Lancet 2:63–65, 1973.

toxan), doxorubcin (Adriamycin), and vincristine (Oncovin) (CAV) was established as effective and was generally adopted as the treatment of choice. In the early 1980s, patients who failed initial therapy with CAV were shown to be responsive to cisplatin (Platinol) and etoposide (VePesid) (PE). Subsequent studies comparing CAV versus CAV alternating with PE have shown the alternating regimen to be slightly superior. Gradually, PE gained acceptance as initial therapy and is now the most common initial therapy for this disease.

During the 1980s, randomized trials in limited-stage disease compared combination chemotherapy with and without thoracic radiotherapy. Because of conflicting reports, a meta-analysis was recently conducted. The authors reviewed data from 13 randomized trials of chemotherapy plus thoracic radiotherapy versus chemotherapy alone. These trials included over 2100 patients. The relative risk of death with combined modality therapy was 0.86, or a 14% decrease in the risk of death. The benefit in terms of overall survival at 3 years was 5.4%. Accordingly, combined modality therapy with chemotherapy and thoracic radiotherapy is recommended for limited-stage disease.

Historically, the thoracic radiotherapy has been given in between cycles of chemotherapy or after completion of chemotherapy. A randomized trial in Canada evaluated the timing of thoracic radiotherapy and concluded that early radiotherapy along with chemotherapy results in better survival than late thoracic radiotherapy. Several recent trials employed concomitant chemotherapy and thoracic radiotherapy, with both beginning on day one of treatment. These reports are very encouraging, median survival times of 17 to 20 months were observed, with 2-year survivals of 40% (Table 6). Based on these reports, one approach to limited-stage SCLC is to combine chemotherapy and concurrent radiotherapy and to administer the radiotherapy early in the treatment program. Concurrent therapy is likely to be associated with greater toxicity, but it is hoped

that this will be offset by better long-term survival. Data concerning survival benefit, if there is one, should be available in the near future.

In the 1970s, therapy for SCLC was usually continued for 1 or 2 years. Several trials in the 1980s demonstrated that six cycles of therapy are as effective as 12 cycles, with one cycle equal to 3 to 4 weeks. Additionally, multiple randomized trials have shown that maintenance therapy beyond six cycles does not increase survival. Two recent trials, one in limited-stage disease and one in extensive-stage disease, employed four cycles of cisplatin and etoposide. The limited-stage trial also utilized concurrent thoracic radiotherapy. The response rates, median survival, and long-term survival of patients in these two trials were at least as good as survival in trials with similar stage patients who were treated with six cycles.

As previously stated, approximately 50 to 60% of limited-stage patients will achieve a complete remission. Unfortunately, about 70% of the complete remissions will relapse within 2 years. If individuals were treated with cyclophosphamide, doxorubicin, and vincristine initially, then it would be advisable to treat with cisplatin and etoposide for four cycles. If patients were initially treated with cisplatin and etoposide, then the best option for second-line therapy is probably oral etoposide at a dose of 50 mg twice a day for 14 days and repeated every 28 days for six cycles, unless they develop progressive disease sooner. The response rates to cyclophosphamide, doxorubicin, and vincristine as second-line therapy following cisplatin and etoposide are poor (usually < 25%).

Extensive-Stage Small Cell Lung Cancer

Almost two-thirds of all patients with SCLC have extensive-stage disease at the time of diagnosis. The median survival time for these patients is 9 to 10 months, with 2-year survival of 10% or less and virtually no 5-year survivors (0 to 2%) (see Table 5). Extensive-stage SCLC has a 60 to 80% initial response rate, and 20 to 30% of patients will achieve a complete remission. The chemotherapeutic agents employed are identical to those for limited-stage disease. For elderly patients, some investigators have used oral etoposide as the initial therapy. The major responses are similar to those reported for combination chemotherapy. It is uncertain whether the long-term results are equivalent to those from combination chemotherapy. However, toxicity with oral etoposide appears to be less than with alternative therapies. At this time, a large phase III trial is under way to compare oral etoposide versus conventional chemotherapy with cisplatin and etoposide. In addition to response rate and survival, this trial will compare toxicity and QOL of the two regimens.

Despite the high initial response rates, the dismal 2-year survival of patients with extensive-stage SCLC emphasizes the need for new agents with activity against this disease. Recently, investigators have conducted phase II trials (the major end point of a phase II trial is response) with new single

TABLE 6. **Response Rates and Survival of Patients with Limited-Stage Small Cell Lung Cancer Treated with Concurrent Chemotherapy and Thoracic Radiotherapy***

| | ECOG/RTOG | | SWOG |
	CT + TRT	CT + HFxTRT	CT + TRT
Total number	176	182	154
Complete response (%)	46	53	56
Median survival (mo)	18.6	20.3	17.5
2-year survival (%)	42	44	40
3-year survival (%)	NA	NA	35†
4-year survival (%)	NA	NA	30

*Chemotherapeutic agents, dose, and schedule varied between the two trials.

†Approximate.

Abbreviations: ECOG/RTOG = Eastern Cooperative Oncology Group/Radiation Therapy Oncology Group; SWOG = Southwestern Oncology Group; CT = chemotherapy; TRT = thoracic radiotherapy; HFxTRT = hyperfractionated TRT (given twice daily); NA = not available.

agents. These studies are designed so that there is rapid crossover to conventional therapy for those patients with progressive or stable disease. Based on the results of phase II trials in previously untreated patients, two new agents have shown promising activity against SCLC: paclitaxel (Taxol) and topotecan.* Currently, these agents are being used in combination with other agents in ongoing clinical trials.

CONCLUSION

No major breakthroughs in the treatment of lung cancer have occurred over the past decade. However, the overall understanding of the biology of lung cancer has increased exponentially. In certain areas, small but significant improvements in therapy and survival have ensued. The methods and quality of clinical trials against this disease have been refined. Several new chemotherapeutic agents, with novel mechanisms of action, have been shown to be active against lung cancer. Exciting new clinical trials are under way, examining the most pressing clinical questions.

In an effort to improve standard therapy, primary care physicians should encourage patients to consider participating in approved prospective clinical trials at reputable medical centers. Currently, only 1% of newly diagnosed lung cancer patients in the United States are enrolled in prospective clinical trials. Information about approved clinical trials is available through the Physician Desk Query or the cancer hotline at the National Cancer Institute (1-800-4-CANCER). Progress cannot be made without the enrollment of patients in clinical trials.

COCCIDIOIDOMYCOSIS

method of
JOHN N. GALGIANI, M.D.
VA Medical Center
Tucson, Arizona

Coccidioidomycosis is a systemic infection caused by the dimorphic fungus *Coccidioides immitis*. It grows in the soil of the lower Sonoran deserts of California, Arizona, New Mexico, west Texas, and scattered parts of Central and South America. When the climate is dry, single-cell mycelial elements (arthroconidia) are inhaled and convert to spherules within tissue. Of the approximately 100,000 infections per year, only one-third come to medical attention, usually as a subacute respiratory syndrome, and most resolve without specific therapy. However, a small proportion of the patients are left with residual pulmonary lesions (nodules, cavities), others experience chronic pulmonary symptoms, and some develop lesions outside the lungs (extrapulmonary dissemination), most typically in the skin, joints, bones, or meninges. These complications require a variety of management decisions involving diagnostic evaluation, selection of antifungal treatments, and adjunctive surgery.

---

*Investigational drug in the United States.

Coccidioidomycosis is diagnosed by one of four ways: (1) identifying the organism in tissue or secretions, (2) recovering it in culture, (3) detecting antibodies against the fungus in serum or other patient fluid, and (4) evoking delayed-type dermal hypersensitivity to coccidioidal antigens. Tests for coccidioidomycosis are not routinely performed, and thus clinical suspicion is a critical first step for prompt diagnosis. Outside the endemic regions, a detailed travel history may afford the only hint that coccidioidomycosis should be considered. Since the spherule is a morphologic structure unique to *C. immitis,* the identification of a spherical structure ranging in size between 15 and 75 μm in diameter with a doubly refractile wall and containing multiple internal spherical structures (endospores) establishes the diagnosis. Spherules can be seen microscopically in potassium hydroxide preparations, cytology smears, and tissue stained with hematoxylin and eosin or other special stains. Cultures of *C. immitis* grow on nearly all laboratory media, often within the first week. Since mycelia of *C. immitis* pose a biohazard to laboratory personnel, it is helpful to indicate that this organism is being sought and any growth should be handled with Biohazard Level 3 containment procedures. Anticoccidioidal antibodies are detected in a variety of ways. Tube precipitin (TP) antibodies are characteristically IgM early responses, and complement-fixing (CF) antibodies are IgG that develops later to a different fungal antigen and are often reported quantitatively. Both TP and CF antibodies can be detected by double agar diffusion techniques sold commercially as kits. A commercial enzyme-linked immunosorbent assay (ELISA) kit that measures undefined coccidioidal antibodies is also available from Meridian Diagnostics (Cincinnati, Ohio). This ELISA is more sensitive to early infections, but its specificity is not fully defined. Delayed-type dermal hypersensitivity to coccidioidal skin-testing antigens develops in most patients after infection, although it may be absent when infection is widely disseminated. Because skin-test reactivity is lifelong, its presence may not be related to a specific current illness and therefore is not usually helpful in diagnosis.

WHO REQUIRES TREATMENT?

The vast majority of initial infections resolve without treatment, and it is not known whether treatment of early infections with any currently available therapy either speeds recovery or prevents future complications. Thus, for patients with uncomplicated primary coccidioidal pneumonia, treatment should be reserved for selected patients in whom underlying disease or severity of the clinical manifestations makes therapy advisable. The most critical predisposing factors are T cell deficiencies such as occur with acquired immune deficiency disease (AIDS), organ transplantation, Hodgkin's disease, or chronic corticosteroid therapy. Such patients should always be treated once a coccidioidal illness is manifest. Coccidioidal infection during the third trimester of pregnancy is also likely to progress and should be treated with amphotericin B because of its lack of teratogenicity. Pulmonary infections that have not resolved after 2 or more months or which recur months or years after their initial infection should be treated. Similarly, patients with extrapulmonary dissemination should also receive therapy.

USEFUL ANTIFUNGAL DRUGS

Amphotericin B

Amphotericin B (Fungizone) has been in clinical use for the longest time and may be the agent with the most rapid onset of action. It is therefore the first-line choice in patients with rapidly progressive infections. Amphotericin B is administered intravenously for all infections except coccidioidal meningitis, in which it is delivered directly into the cerebrospinal fluid by intracisternal, intralumbar, or intraventricular routes. Treatment is initiated with once-daily dosing with rapidly increasing doses to 0.4 to 0.6 mg per kg per dose. After several days, dosing can be continued on an alternate-day schedule. Amphotericin B is a very toxic drug. Common reactions include phlebitis at the injection site, nausea, and high fever. If any of these side effects occur, premedication with analgesics, antiemetics, or antipyretics may ameliorate the symptoms (Table 1). Blood pressure should be monitored during infusion. If hypotension is noted, treatment should be discontinued that day, although this does not preclude reinstitution of amphotericin B at a later time. Transient azotemia is frequent during therapy. Serum creatinine concentrations should be measured weekly or more frequently if the dose of amphotericin B has been changed recently. Permanent renal impairment has been reported in some patients who have received a total of 3 grams or more. Hemograms should be obtained at least weekly during therapy to monitor leukocyte, erythrocyte, and platelet counts. Although anemia is common, it often stabilizes at a level that does not require transfusion. Potassium, magnesium, and other electrolytes should also be monitored weekly, and deficiencies resulting from renal wasting should be replaced.

Azole Antifungal Agents

Ketoconazole (Nizoral) has Food and Drug Administration approval for the treatment of coccidioidomycosis. Although fluconazole (Diflucan)* and itraconazole (Sporanox)* have not been approved for this indication, published reports have demonstrated their efficacy. All drugs are currently available for oral administration. A parenteral form is available only for fluconazole. Ketoconazole is used at a dosage of 400 mg per day. Higher dosages have only a mar-

---

*Not FDA-approved for this indication.

TABLE 1. **Amphotericin B Premedication**

30–45 min before infusion:
Aspirin (600 mg) or acetaminophen (650 mg) *plus*
Diphenhydramine (Benadryl) (50 mg PO) *or*
Promethazine (Phenergan) (50 mg PO or IM)
If ineffective, add:
Meperidine (Demerol) (25 to 50 mg IV) for fever
Hydrocortisone (25 mg added to infusion or given IV just
before starting infusion)

ginally increased efficacy and incur a greater chance of side effects. Itraconazole is used at a dosage of 200 mg twice daily after initiating therapy with 200 mg three times daily for the first 3 days. Dose-limiting toxicity, including hyperkalemia and water retention, is often encountered at 600 mg per day. Fluconazole is used at a dosage of 400 mg per day after initiating treatment with 400 mg twice daily for 2 days. Dosages greater than 800 mg per day have been used in some patients for prolonged periods without serious consequences. However, it is not known if higher doses of fluconazole improve response for most patients. Gastric acidity is important to promote the absorption of ketoconazole and itraconazole but not fluconazole. Significant drug interactions at the level of the P-450 pathways occur between the azoles (especially ketoconazole or itraconazole) and several other drugs. For examples, all three azoles decrease the metabolism of cyclosporin (Sandimmune) and warfarin (Coumadin), whereas rifampin (Rifadin) increases the metabolism of itraconazole. Since such interactions are possible, a careful review of all concurrent medications should be made before treatment with these drugs is initiated. The most common side effect of all agents is nausea, which is dose-related. Nausea occurs in 5% of patients receiving 400 mg of ketoconazole per day and is less frequent with fluconazole or itraconazole therapy. Gynecomastia and azoospermia occur with increasing doses of ketoconazole and can be treated with testosterone replacement. Hair loss and dry skin are frequently reported by patients receiving fluconazole. Hepatitis has been reported with ketoconazole at a frequency of approximately 1 in 10,000 treated patients. It may be less frequent with itraconazole or fluconazole. Stevens-Johnson syndrome has been reported with fluconazole therapy.

TREATMENT OF SPECIFIC CLINICAL SYNDROMES

Pulmonary Nodules

Nodules, usually single, 1 to 4 cm, are common residua of the initial pneumonia. They typically cause no symptoms but may be impossible to distinguish from malignancy without a bronchoscopic or percutaneous aspirate or surgical specimen for examination and culture. If the nodule is resected for the purposes of diagnosis, antifungal therapy is not recommended either before or after the procedure.

Pulmonary Cavities and Chronic Pneumonia

Coccidioidal cavities usually measure 2 to 4 cm on chest radiographs; 75% are in the upper lung fields. They are often thin-walled, and the majority close spontaneously within 2 years of their detection. In patients with small cavities and no symptoms, no intervention is required. Patients whose cavities are associated with symptoms such as cough, sputum production, or mild hemoptysis may be treated with 400 mg of an azole per day. Fibrocavitary infections associated with more extensive infiltrates are often a source of symptoms and should be treated similarly. If symptoms abate, therapy should be continued for many months or even years. If symptoms recur on discontinuation of therapy, restarting the same therapy is often effective, and the therapy may need to be continued indefinitely. If response is not obtained, a trial of amphotericin B is warranted, and after 0.5 gram, consideration should be given to surgical resection if a well-demarcated lesion is identified. However, it may recur after this approach as well. If a cavity ruptures into the pleural space, the primary therapy is surgical resection.

Diffuse Reticular-Nodular Pneumonia

Bilateral multiple infiltrates are most frequently the result of hematogenous spread in immunosuppressed patients or occasionally multicentric primary foci that can result from exposure to high densities of arthroconidia. Amphotericin B should be used as initial therapy. Once pneumonia stabilizes (several weeks to a few months of treatment), continuation therapy can be switched to an oral azole.

Extrapulmonary Dissemination

Even when many lesions are present, patients often follow a subacute or chronic course. In such patients, the safety and convenience of oral azole therapy makes the azoles preferable for initial therapy, with amphotericin B reserved for more fulminant presentations or for those who do not respond to an azole. In responding patients, azole therapy should be continued until all pretreatment abnormalities such as symptoms, lesion size, and serum CF antibody concentrations stabilize and show no further improve. This may require many months or years of treatment but increases the chances that disease does not relapse after therapy is stopped. Coccidioidal meningitis is a special case of disseminated infection. Fluconazole at 400 mg per day may produce a clinical response in approximately 70% of new infections, and patients in whom therapy fails at this dosage may still respond if the dosage is increased. Itraconazole has also been effective in a few patients. Treatment appears to be lifelong since 75% of patients who have discontinued azole therapy have relapsed. Intrathecal amphotericin B is also effective and in some patients has been curative. However, such therapy is technically difficult, is prone to serious complications, and commonly produces side-effects. These limitations currently make intrathecal amphotericin B second-line therapy for most patients with coccidioidal meningitis.

HISTOPLASMOSIS

method of
MITCHELL GOLDMAN, M.D., and
L. JOSEPH WHEAT, M.D.
Indiana University School of Medicine
Indianapolis, Indiana

Histoplasmosis is the most common of the endemic mycoses in the United States with estimates as high as 500,000 individuals infected yearly. Although *Histoplasma capsulatum* has a near worldwide distribution, endemic areas with the highest rates of infection include the Ohio and Mississippi River valleys of the United States and areas of Central and South America. *Histoplasma capsulatum*, a dimorphic fungus, is present as a mold found sporadically throughout soil and other material rich in organic matter. Localized areas, containing heavy growth of *H. capsulatum*, or so-called microfoci, have included bird roosts, caves, and chicken coops. Documented cases of histoplasmosis have occurred as a consequence of disturbances at such sites and are believed to occur after inhalation of airborne *H. capsulatum* microconidia. The majority of infected individuals, however, do not recall direct contact with such sites. Presumably most acquire infection during daily activities from exposure to wind-borne microconidia released by activities disturbing microfoci located some distance away.

After inhalation, the microconidia of *H. capsulatum* convert into yeast forms in the lungs. The outcome of such an infection is influenced by the immunologic state of the individual and the magnitude of the exposure. In immunocompetent individuals, T cell immunity develops 10 to 14 days after infection, and activated macrophages assume fungicidal properties that are generally sufficient to control the infection. After a low-level exposure in a normal host the resultant infection is most often asymptomatic because of the success of this immune response. After high-level exposure, however, the majority of exposed individuals develop symptomatic infections. Those with impaired T cell immunity often fail to control *H. capsulatum* infection and may develop disseminated disease.

Symptomatic infection occurs in about 1% of infected individuals. The clinical manifestations of histoplasmosis are quite varied, though the majority of those with symptoms present with self-limited syndromes. These syndromes include "influenza-like" pulmonary illnesses, pericarditis, arthritis or arthralgias, and erythema nodosum. Common symptoms include fever, chills, headache, myalgia, cough, and chest pain. Examination is usually normal, though pericardial friction rubs or erythema nodosum may be identified. Chest roentgenograms typically reveal enlarged hilar or mediastinal nodes with patchy infiltrates but may be normal. The majority of these patients begin to improve within a few weeks, and the illness generally resolves spontaneously.

Acute granulomatous mediastinitis (mediastinal granuloma) is thought to occur as a result of active *H. capsulatum* infection and may be accompanied by obstructive symptoms when enlarged mediastinal lymph nodes compress the esophagus, superior vena cava, large airways, or pulmonary vessels. Rupture of necrotizing lymph nodes into the esophagus, airways, or other mediastinal structures can also occur. Chronic pulmonary infection occurs in about 1 in 2000 exposed individuals and most often affects those with pre-existing chronic obstructive lung disease. Such individuals may develop chronic cavitary infections that can be difficult to distinguish from tuberculosis on clinical grounds. Disseminated infection occurs in about 1 in 2000 exposed individuals. In those at the extremes of ages or those with impaired T cell immunity due to the acquired immune deficiency syndrome (AIDS), lymphoreticular malignancies, or immune-suppressant medications, disseminated infections are more common. These infections are characterized by involvement of the reticuloendothelial system as well as mucosal, cutaneous, adrenal gland, and central nervous system involvement. Mediastinal fibrosis is a rare complication of histoplasmosis, attributed to an immunologic-mediated response to prior *H. capsulatum* infection and occurs in about 1 in 5000 persons. This condition may present with symptoms due to mechanical obstruction of mediastinal structures.

Cultures; special stains of histologic specimens which may be complemented by specific molecular probes; serum antibody detection; and detection of *H. capsulatum* polysaccharide antigen have all been used to assist in the diagnosis of histoplasmosis. Cultures are positive in 10% of self-limited, 67% of chronic pulmonary (after multiple sputum samples), and 80% of disseminated infections. For patients with disseminated histoplasmosis, bone marrow cultures are positive in over 75%, whereas blood cultures are positive in 50 to 70% using lysis-centrifugation. Delayed culture growth (can be as long as 2 to 4 weeks) may limit the reliance on culture for diagnosis in severe cases.

Immunodiagnostic tests for histoplasmosis include serologic tests and skin testing. Skin testing is useful for determining infection rates for epidemiologic surveys but generally has no role in the diagnosis of symptomatic histoplasmosis and can interfere with the interpretation of subsequent serologic testing. The measurement of serum antibodies against yeast or mycelial antigens of *H. capsulatum* by complement fixation or the detection of M and or H precipitins by immunodiffusion techniques is useful for diagnosis of histoplasmosis. These serologic tests are positive in 90% of those with symptomatic histoplasmosis but may be falsely negative in early infection and in patients with immune-suppressive conditions. False-positive results may be seen with other fungal infections and tuberculosis. Finally, because such antibodies clear slowly, weak positive test results may be seen in patients with a past history of histoplasmosis who present with another illness.

Antigen detection of a polysaccharide antigen of *H. capsulatum* by enzyme immunoassay provides another rapid and specific method for the diagnosis of histoplasmosis, particularly in patients with severe infections who require prompt administration of antifungal therapy. This antigen may be detected in the blood or urine in 80 to 98% of those with disseminated infection and at least 50% of those with severe acute pulmonary histoplasmosis. Antigen can also be detected in cerebrospinal fluid and bronchial washings. The measurement of *H. capsulatum* antigen is not only useful for diagnosis but is also useful for following treatment, particularly in AIDS patients with disseminated infections.

TREATMENT OF HISTOPLASMOSIS

Acute Self-Limited Syndromes

Most patients with acute self-limited pulmonary, rheumatologic, or pericardial manifestations of histoplasmosis recover spontaneously and do not require antifungal therapy. Arthritis, arthralgias, and pericarditis are the results of immune-mediated responses and are rarely associated with positive cultures from the affected tissues. For patients with these self-limited conditions, restriction of activities and symptomatic treatment with anti-inflammatory agents are recommended. Although the majority of these infections are uncomplicated, pericarditis may occasionally be complicated by tamponade and require pericardiocentesis. The role of antifungal treatment in patients with self-limited syndromes other than severe acute pulmonary infection has not been adequately evaluated, though antifungals should be considered for those with moderate symptoms who have not shown improvement after a 1- to 3-week period of follow-up and for those who require hospitalization (Table 1). A trial of 2 to 6 weeks of antifungal therapy using itraconazole (Sporanox) or ketoconazole (Nizoral) is appropriate for those with less severe illnesses, reserving amphotericin B (Fungizone) for more severe illnesses. Similarly, a trial of antifungal therapy may be useful for patients with mediastinal granuloma complicated by symptoms due to obstruction or fistula formation.

Typically, after a heavy exposure to *H. capsulatum*, patients can develop a severe acute pulmonary disease characterized by severe hypoxemia, which may be accompanied by diffuse pulmonary infiltrates and adult respiratory distress syndrome. Treatment with amphotericin B intravenously at a dose of approximately 0.7 mg per kg per day for 10 to 14 days along with corticosteroid therapy at a dose equivalent to 40 to 60 mg of prednisone per day is appropriate for these patients. The corticosteroid component of this therapy is intended to treat the inflammatory response to *H. capsulatum*. The use of any of the presently available oral azole agents as initial therapy for severe acute pulmonary histoplasmosis should be avoided, as the response to these agents is slower than that with amphotericin B; however, if improvement occurs after 3 to 7 days of amphotericin B therapy, oral itraconazole or ketoconazole can be used to complete the course of therapy.

Chronic Pulmonary Histoplasmosis

Although some patients with chronic pulmonary histoplasmosis may improve without treatment, most patients experience a chronic, slowly progressive course with a gradual loss of pulmonary function. Before the development of amphotericin B, chronic pulmonary histoplasmosis was associated with considerable morbidity and mortality. Initial studies using amphotericin B showed response rates of approximately 75% and a reduction in relapse rates to less than 25% in those treated with prolonged courses. Amphotericin B given intravenously for a total course of 35 mg per kg, over 10 to 16 weeks, has been used in severely ill patients with chronic pulmonary histoplasmosis. The majority of patients with severe infections should be able to be successfully switched to oral azole therapy after initial improvement using a shorter course of amphotericin B. As most patients with chronic pulmonary histoplasmosis are not so severely ill, one can use azole therapy alone in these

TABLE 1. **Recommendations for Antifungal Treatment of Histoplasmosis**

Condition	Antifungal Agent	Dosage Used	Duration	Comments
Prolonged self-limited syndromes	Oral itraconazole (Sporanox) Oral ketoconazole (Nizoral)	200 mg/day 400 mg/day	2–6 weeks? 2–6 weeks?	Not studied Not studied
Severe acute pulmonary	Amphotericin B (Fungizone) with oral prednisone	0.7 mg/kg/day 40–60 mg/day	14 days	
Chronic pulmonary Severe	Amphotericin B	50 mg/day	Until improvement, then change to oral itraconazole or ketoconazole as described under "chronic pulmonary, mild to moderate"	
Mild to moderate	Oral itraconazole Oral ketoconazole	200–400 mg/day 400 mg/day	6–24 months 6–24 months	
Disseminated non-AIDS Severe	Amphotericin B	50 mg/day	Until improvement, then change to oral itraconazole or ketoconazole as described under "Disseminated non-AIDS, mild to moderate"	
Mild to moderate	Oral itraconazole Oral ketoconazole	200–400 mg/day 400 mg/day	6–12 months 6–12 months	
Disseminated in AIDS Induction treatment Severe	Amphotericin B followed by oral itraconazole	50 mg/day 400 mg/day	7–14 days 10 weeks	Monitor blood levels
Moderately severe	Amphotericin B followed by Oral itraconazole	50 mg/day 400 mg/day	3–7 days 12 weeks	Monitor blood levels
Mild	Oral itraconazole Oral fluconazole (Diflucan)	400 mg/day 800 mg/day	3 months 3 months	Monitor blood levels Use only in those unable to take itraconazole
Maintenance treatment	Oral itraconazole	200–400 mg/day	Life	If serum itraconazole level ≥4 μg on 400-mg dose, 200 mg/day can be used
	Oral fluconazole	400 mg/day	Life	Use in those unable to take itraconazole
	Amphotericin B	50–100 mg once or twice weekly	Life	May be poorly tolerated

patients, reserving amphotericin B for those in whom oral therapy fails.

For those with non–life-threatening chronic cavitary histoplasmosis, ketoconazole is associated with response rates of approximately 80 to 85%. Ketoconazole orally at a dose of 400 mg per day for 6 to 12 months is a reasonable choice for initial therapy in patients with less severe chronic pulmonary histoplasmosis, though poor patient tolerance because of gastrointestinal complaints, and inadequate absorption, remain potential problems. Itraconazole represents a better-tolerated oral azole agent with increased activity against *H. capsulatum*, though inadequate absorption is also a concern with itraconazole. When used in the treatment of non–life-threatening chronic cavitary histoplasmosis, itraconazole appears to have similar efficacy to that of ketoconazole. Itraconazole taken orally at a dose of 200 to 400 mg per day for at least 6 months also represents an effective therapy for patients with chronic pulmonary histoplasmosis. It should be noted that 15% of patients may relapse, and response to therapy can be slow. Because of these observations, therapy with ketoconazole or itraconazole for at least 12 months is recommended. Consideration should be given to treatment courses as long as 24 months in those still improving at 12 months, or to continue therapy for at least 3 months after chest roentgenograms are stable. Though itraconazole is better tolerated than ketoconazole, it is more expensive. With limited experience using fluconazole (Diflucan)* for the treatment of chronic pulmonary histoplasmosis, oral fluconazole used at a dose of 200 to 800 mg per day for at least 6 months appears to have less efficacy than either ketoconazole or itraconazole and should not be considered a first-line therapy for this condition.

---

*Not FDA-approved for this indication.

Although medical therapy is often successful for chronic pulmonary histoplasmosis, all patients should be followed for evidence of relapse. Additionally, surgical resection of lung tissue should be considered for uncontrolled hemoptysis or in those who fail to respond to medical therapy.

Fibrosing Mediastinitis

Fibrosing mediastinitis is a progressive, often fatal, manifestation of histoplasmosis that most often has not responded to therapy with antifungal or anti-inflammatory agents. Limited experience suggests that some patients with symptomatic superior vena caval obstruction, tracheal or esophageal compression, or other conditions affecting mediastinal structures have benefited from surgical procedures. In one report a small number of patients with high sedimentation rates and *H. capsulatum* complement fixation titers, antifungal treatment given before as well as after such surgery was thought to improve the success rate. Additionally, the use of ketoconazole in one patient with symptoms attributed to recurrent fibrotic complications was associated with a reduction in symptoms, allowing the avoidance of additional surgery.

Disseminated Histoplasmosis in Patients Without Acquired Immune Deficiency Syndrome

In nearly all AIDS patients with disseminated disease, without antifungal treatment, the disease is progressive and ultimately fatal. Treatment with amphotericin B is associated with cure rates of at least 75%. After an initial response to therapy, relapsing infection may occur in 5 to 23% of treated patients and occurs more often in those receiving less than 30 mg per kg of amphotericin B. Other conditions associated with relapse include intravascular infections, meningitis, adrenal insufficiency, or underlying immune suppression. As amphotericin B is associated with a more rapid response and because azole agents have not been studied in the treatment of severe disseminated infections, initial treatment with intravenous amphotericin B at a dose of 50 mg per day is preferred for patients with life-threatening infections or underlying immune suppression. On clinical improvement, usually within 5 to 14 days, therapy can be changed to ketoconazole or itraconazole. The total duration of therapy should be at least 6 months in those without underlying immune suppression. Longer courses may be needed in patients with persistent clinical or laboratory abnormalities after 6 months of therapy. If the *Histoplasma* antigen test is positive, treatment should be continued until the antigen clears from the urine. For those expected to have continued immune suppression, longer courses of antifungal therapy should be given with consideration for therapy continued indefinitely for those who are not expected to have immune recovery.

In patients without AIDS who have nonmeningeal non–life-threatening disseminated histoplasmosis, treatment with ketoconazole at a dose of 400 mg orally per day for 6 to 12 months has been associated with response rates from 70 to 100%. More recent studies using itraconazole for treatment of disseminated histoplasmosis in similar populations have shown oral itraconazole at a dose of 200 to 400 mg per day for 6 months to be associated with success rates as high as 100%. Either itraconazole or ketoconazole used for at least 6 months represents effective therapy for disseminated nonmeningeal, non–life-threatening histoplasmosis in patients without severe underlying immune suppression. Again, itraconazole is the better-tolerated compound, though it is more expensive. Both these agents require a low gastric pH for adequate absorption and should not be used in the presence of achlorhydria or medications known to raise gastric pH. The use of itraconazole and ketoconazole should also be avoided in patients requiring rifampin, rifabutin, isoniazid, or anticonvulsant medications that reduce the achievable levels of these azoles. Fluconazole has been the least well studied of the azole agents in the treatment of disseminated histoplasmosis. At doses of 200 to 800 mg per day, fluconazole* has been associated with response rates of about 75% in patients with non–life-threatening disseminated infections. Fluconazole at a dose of 400 mg per day for a minimum of 6 months could be considered an alternative therapy for non-AIDS patients with mild or moderate disseminated histoplasmosis who are unable to tolerate itraconazole or ketoconazole.

Central nervous system manifestations may complicate disseminated histoplasmosis in 10 to 20% of cases. An initial response to amphotericin B can be seen in up to 75 to 80%, though relapse occurs in as many as 50% of these cases. Although the optimum treatment for this condition is unknown, an initial course of at least 35 mg per kg of amphotericin B using doses of at least 50 mg per kg daily is recommended with close follow-up for relapse of infection.

Disseminated Histoplasmosis in Acquired Immune Deficiency Syndrome

Because of a relapse rate of 80% after acute treatment of disseminated histoplasmosis in AIDS patients, the goal of therapy is lifelong suppression as opposed to cure. Treatment courses are separated into induction therapy and maintenance therapy.

Successful induction therapy for disseminated histoplasmosis in patients with AIDS has been achieved in approximately 80% by the administration of amphotericin B at a dose of 50 mg per day for a 14-day course. This regimen is considered the treatment of choice in those who are severely ill, inducing a response in about half of these cases. Shorter courses (3 to 7 days) of amphotericin B may produce clinical remission in those with moderately severe illness. Before the availability of itraconazole or fluconazole,

---

*Not FDA-approved for this indication.

ketoconazole used as induction therapy for patients with disseminated histoplasmosis was associated with an unacceptably high percentage of failures and should not be used in this population. Itraconazole has been evaluated as induction treatment for disseminated histoplasmosis in AIDS patients, although those with severe infections or central nervous system involvement were excluded from these studies. Itraconazole administered orally at a dose of 200 mg three times daily for 3 days followed by 200 mg twice daily for 12 weeks was associated with response rates of 85%. Patients with moderately severe disease as indicated by a fever greater than 39.5° C (103.1° F), a Karnofsky score less than 60, an alkaline phosphatase level more than five times normal, or an albumin level less than 3 grams per dL tended to respond more poorly. Treatment failures may have resulted from an inability to achieve therapeutic itraconazole plasma concentrations ($\geq$1 μg per mL) as well. These findings suggest that itraconazole, when adequately absorbed, represents an effective convenient alternative to amphotericin B induction therapy in AIDS patients with mild to moderate disseminated histoplasmosis. Fluconazole has been studied as induction therapy for nonsevere disseminated histoplasmosis in patients with AIDS using a dose of 1600 mg on day 1, followed by 800 mg per day for 12 weeks. Fluconazole* used in this manner was less effective (approximately 75% response) than itraconazole induction therapy and should be considered as an alternative therapy only for those unable to take itraconazole.

After successful induction therapy, amphotericin B has been used as maintenance therapy to prevent relapse of infection. Amphotericin B given intravenously at a dose of 50 to 100 mg weekly or biweekly for life has been associated with relapse rates of approximately 5 to 20%. Long-term amphotericin B therapy used in this manner is an acceptable albeit inconvenient and sometimes toxic therapy for maintenance treatment of disseminated infections in this population. Oral ketoconazole use for this purpose was associated with an unacceptably high rate of relapse (approximately 50%) and should not be used in this patient group. Recently, oral itraconazole at doses of 200 to 400 mg daily has been shown to prevent relapse in as many as 95% of patients when used as chronic maintenance therapy. The dose of itraconazole chosen for maintenance therapy should depend on the plasma level of the drug achievable in any individual patient (for those with an itraconazole plasma concentration of $\geq$4 μg per mL obtained while receiving itraconazole 400 mg daily, the maintenance dose of itraconazole can be reduced to 200 mg per day). For patients with disseminated histoplasmosis and AIDS, oral itraconazole is very well tolerated and highly efficacious and at 200 to 400 mg daily should be the treatment of choice for those able to absorb this drug. For prevention of relapse of histoplasmosis in patients with AIDS, oral fluconazole should be considered significantly less effective

(approximately 30% relapse) than itraconazole. Fluconazole* given orally at a dose of 400 mg per day should only be considered as an alternative maintenance treatment in those unable to absorb or tolerate itraconazole.

Measurement of *H. capsulatum* antigen has been useful for following the response to therapy in patients with AIDS. The levels of antigen fall with successful therapy and increase with relapse. Antigen increases of more than 2 U suggest relapsed infection and support further laboratory evaluation and consideration for resumption of induction therapy. Antigen levels should be followed at 3- to 4-month intervals and require direct comparison to the last prior specimen. Antigen testing is available at the Histoplasmosis Reference Laboratory in Indianapolis, Indiana.

Areas of active or planned research at this time include the evaluation of itraconazole for prophylaxis of histoplasmosis in patients with AIDS residing in highly endemic areas and an evaluation of lipid formulations of amphotericin B for severe disseminated histoplasmosis in AIDS.

BLASTOMYCOSIS

method of
ROBERT W. BRADSHER, JR., M.D.
University of Arkansas for Medical Sciences
Little Rock, Arkansas

Blastomycosis is a systemic infection identified by round, thick-walled yeast in tissue or sputum specimens or after culture of the organisms in the mycelial phase at room temperature. The organisms are initially inhaled while in the mycelial form as found in nature, and the infection begins after conversion to the yeast phase. Organisms proliferate locally in the lung and may be spread by lymphohematogenous routes to other organs. These metastatic foci of infection due to *Blastomyces dermatitidis* are most commonly located in skin, bone, or prostate, but many other organs have been reported to be infected. Spontaneous remission of blastomycosis pneumonia may occur, but relapse of infection at a later date, either with or without previous antifungal therapy, has been reported. Very rarely, cutaneous inoculation of the yeast organisms, for example, by a pathologist at autopsy, has resulted in primary cutaneous blastomycosis.

INDICATIONS FOR THERAPY

The first consideration for the patient with blastomycosis is whether or not to treat with an antifungal agent. Because of the toxicity of amphotericin B, some patients in the past were simply observed. Spontaneous resolution of infection without therapy is most likely in patients involved with a blastomycosis epidemic; if pneumonia is acquired in this setting, observation for 1 to 2 weeks is reasonable. If deterio-

---

*Not FDA-approved for this indication.

*Not FDA-approved for this indication.

ration or progression is noted, antifungal therapy should be started. Observation only could also be considered in the patient with acute pneumonia that resolves before *B. dermatitidis* is identified by culture. The presence of pleural disease or any extrapulmonary infection during the course of illness necessitates antifungal treatment. With the development of oral agents with substantially less toxicity than amphotericin B, the option of observation alone in blastomycosis is chosen much less often than when amphotericin B was the only agent available.

TREATMENT

The blastomycosis therapy to be considered initially is listed in Table 1. If deterioration occurs in a patient being observed or if disease manifestations persist, treatment should be with an oral agent such as itraconazole. If a patient treated orally has progression of symptoms or signs of involvement, a switch to amphotericin B is indicated. In blastomycosis there appears to be no advantage to the combination of amphotericin B plus an imidazole.

POLYENE ANTIFUNGAL AGENT

Amphotericin B

Since the introduction of amphotericin B (Fungizone) in 1956, it has become well recognized that this polyene antifungal drug is effective in the treatment of blastomycosis (Table 2). In one study, when a cumulative dose of 2 grams was given, a cure rate of 97% was reported. However, in those patients, 71% had a decline in renal function with other significant toxicities, including anemia (53%), anorexia and nausea (53%), fever (49%), hypokalemia (37%), and thrombophlebitis (19%). These side effects resulted in interruption of therapy in 41% and early cessation of amphotericin B therapy in 14% of the patients.

Amphotericin B must be given intravenously, beginning with a test dose of 1.0 mg in 100 mL of 5% dextrose in water (D5W) over 2 hours. If that dosage is tolerated without fever, chills, or hypotension, the dosage is increased by 10 to 15 mg per day to reach

TABLE 1. **Therapy for Blastomycosis**

Type of Disease	Mode of Therapy
Pulmonary	
Epidemic exposure and pneumonia	Observation
Culture positive, symptoms resolved	Observation
Symptomatic, not life-threatening	Itraconazole
Overwhelming, life-threatening (e.g., ARDS)	Amphotericin B
Extrapulmonary	
Culture positive, symptoms resolved	Itraconazole
Symptomatic, not life-threatening	Itraconazole
Relapse after ketoconazole	Itraconazole
Meningitis or intracerebral infection	Amphotericin B
Overwhelming, life-threatening (e.g., ARDS)	Amphotericin B

Abbreviations: ARDS = acute respiratory distress syndrome.

a daily dosage of 40 to 45 mg per day (approximately 0.4 to 0.6 mg per kg per day) in a sufficient volume of D5W to be infused in 4 to 6 hours. In critically ill patients, a full dose of 40 to 45 mg can be given immediately after the test dose. A total of 2.0 grams should be given to adults unless toxicity is a limiting factor. There is no need to protect amphotericin B solution from light, but the agent must be mixed in dextrose in water rather than saline.

The toxicity of amphotericin B should be monitored by measuring creatinine concentrations in serum biweekly. If the serum creatinine level goes above 3.0 mg per dL, the drug should be withheld for 48 hours and adequate hydration must be ensured. When amphotericin B therapy is reinstituted, a lower dosage is used before returning to the usual daily dose. Because dehydration and amphotericin B are synergistically nephrotoxic, 500 mL of intravenous saline given daily before and after the amphotericin B dose is recommended unless the patient is unable to tolerate such fluid challenges. Hypokalemia is fairly frequent, so electrolyte assessment must be performed biweekly. Blood counts should be monitored at least weekly. Phlebitis is best avoided by frequent changing of peripheral intravenous sites or by the use of larger central veins such as subclavian catheters. The addition of 25 to 50 mg of hydrocortisone to the infusion to reduce phlebitis is thereby avoided. Premedication with aspirin or diphenhydramine is useful to decrease the fever and chills that may occur with amphotericin B; if rigors do occur, an intravenous dose of 15 to 25 mg of meperidine is often effective in stopping the chill.

AZOLE ANTIFUNGAL AGENTS

Ketoconazole

Ketoconazole (Nizoral), an imidazole antifungal agent, has in vitro activity against *B. dermatitidis* comparable with that of amphotericin B. The drug is absorbed from the gastrointestinal tract and has generally been well tolerated in the treatment of fungal infections. Adverse effects include rare hepatocellular toxicity and antitestosterone-like effects (gynecomastia, oligospermia) at high dosages (greater than 400 mg per day). More common but less severe adverse effects include nausea and vomiting when taken without a meal, dizziness, pruritus, or headache. Clinical cures are achieved with ketoconazole (Table 3). Over a 2-year period, we used ketoconazole to treat 44 patients with blastomycosis. Cure without relapse was obtained in 37. Three patients relapsed after therapy was complete, and in two the lesions did not completely resolve, causing them to be considered failures. The remaining two patients had persistent infection but were noncompliant with the therapy. Side effects were minimal.

Ketoconazole is given orally with a meal early in the day at a dose of 400 mg (two tablets). If no response is noted within 4 weeks, it was previously my practice to increase the dose by 200-mg incre-

TABLE 2. **Amphotericin B Therapy of Blastomycosis**

	Witorsch and Utz*	Lockwood et al†	Parker et al‡	Seabury and Dascomb§	Busey‖	Abernathy¶
Intent to treat	n = 20	n = 27	n = 49	n = 15	n = 41	n = 50
Cure	12/20	21/27	34/49	11/15	37/41	39/50
Relapse	5	NA	7	1	0	2
Failure	1	6	4	4	4	9
Indeterminate	4	NA	4	NA	NA	NA
Full dose: cure	11/15	NA	21/28	11/12	37/41	28/31

*Witorsch P, Utz JP: North American blastomycosis: A study of 40 patients. Medicine 47:169, 1968.
†Lockwood WR, Allison F Jr, Batson BE, et al: The treatment of North American blastomycosis. Ten years' experience. Am Rev Respir Dis 100:314, 1969.
‡Parker JD, Doto IL, Tosh FE: A decade of experience with blastomycosis and its treatment with amphotericin B. Am Rev Respir Dis 99:895, 1969.
§Seabury JH, Dascomb HE: Results of the treatment of systemic mycoses. JAMA 188:509, 1964.
‖Busey JF: Blastomycosis. 3. A comparative study of 2-hydroxystilbamidine and amphotericin B therapy. Am Rev Respir Dis 105:812, 1972.
¶Abernathy RS: Amphotericin treatment of blastomycosis. Antimicrob Agents Chemother 3:298, 1966.
Abbreviations: NA = not available.

ments to a maximum of 800 mg per day (800 mg per day exceeds manufacturer's recommended dosage). However, because of greater toxicity with high doses of ketoconazole, I now switch to another oral agent. Nausea and vomiting with ketoconazole are reduced and greater absorption is achieved by administering the drug with a meal. Liver transaminase levels should be monitored once a month. It has been my practice to continue ketoconazole therapy for at least 6 months. In those with more extensive disease, a total of 1 year of therapy has been given. Relapse rates with ketoconazole are greater than with amphotericin B, so subsequent infection in a patient treated with ketoconazole should be carefully examined for evidence of blastomycosis. Ketoconazole is less expensive than the other azole agents.

Itraconazole

Itraconazole (Sporanox) is another oral agent with activity in blastomycosis. The major theoretical advantage of itraconazole compared with ketoconazole has been a lower rate of toxicity in investigational trials, particularly with regard to endocrine abnormalities associated with ketoconazole (Table 4). The drug was used at a dosage of 200 to 400 mg per day in the Mycoses Study Group of the National Institutes of Health (NIH) beginning in 1985. Of the 40 patients with blastomycosis treated with itraconazole, only two patients were not considered to be cured. We have used itraconazole at a dosage of 200 mg per day to treat an additional 42 patients with blastomycosis, including 16 who had relapse or progressive disease while on ketoconazole or fluconazole. All the patients had a rapid initial response with itraconazole, and only 5 of the 42 patients had a less-than-satisfactory response with a follow-up period of up to 5 years. A patient with malabsorption had rapid clearing of the pulmonary infiltrate but had a relapse 9 months later; this was cured with a second course of itraconazole. A myeloma patient likewise had a relapse and was successfully retreated with the agent. One patient was found by computed tomographic scans to have intracerebral lesions after being on itraconazole for only 4 days; amphotericin B was used since itraconazole has no better penetration into spinal fluid than ketoconazole. Three patients had a relapse after itraconazole; one was receiving immunosuppressive therapy for a renal transplant, but the other patients had no obvious reason for the relapse. All three were cured with amphotericin B.

Despite the added expense of itraconazole over ketoconazole, the greater efficacy rate and the lower toxicity rate has caused me to consider itraconazole as the drug of choice in treatment of blastomycosis.

Newer imidazole and triazole antifungal agents are being developed. There has been some experience with fluconazole (Diflucan) in *B. dermatitidis* infections. With a low dosage of 50 mg per day in an NIH Mycoses Study Group trial, in a small number of blastomycosis patients fluconazole was not associated with the same cure rates as ketoconazole or itraconazole. This failure was considered to be more an inadequacy of the dosage that was given than a

TABLE 3. **Ketoconazole Therapy of Blastomycosis**

	Dismukes et al*	NIAID†	Bradsher et al‡	McManus and Jones§
Intent to treat	n = 16	n = 80	n = 46	n = 8
Cure	7/16	62/80	35/46	6/8
Relapse	5	4	35	0
Failure	4	14	6	2
Full course: cure	NA	58/65	35/40	6/6

*Dismukes WE, Stamm AM, Graybill JR, et al: Treatment of systemic mycoses with ketoconazole. Ann Intern Med 98:13, 1983.
†National Institute of Allergy and Infectious Diseases (NIAID) Mycoses Study Group: Treatment of blastomycosis and histoplasmosis with ketoconazole. Results of a prospective randomized clinical trial. Ann Intern Med 103:861, 1985.
‡Bradsher RW, Rice DC, Abernathy RS: Ketoconazole therapy for endemic blastomycosis. Ann Intern Med 103:872, 1985.
§McManus EJ, Jones JM: The use of ketoconazole in the treatment of blastomycosis. Am Rev Respir Dis 133:141, 1986.
Abbreviations: NA = not available.

TABLE 4. **Itraconazole Therapy of Blastomycosis**

	Dismukes et al*	Bradsher†
Intent to treat	(9 after other treatment failure)	(16 after other treatment failure)
Cure	43/48	38/42
Relapse	1	4
Failure	4	1
Full course: cure	38/40	36/39

*Dismukes WE, Bradsher RW, Cloud GC, et al: Intraconazole therapy of blastomycosis and histoplasmosis. Am J Med 93:489, 1992.
†Bradsher RW: Clinical considerations in blastomycosis. Infect Dis Clin Practice 1:97, 1992.

deficiency of the agent itself, but in trials with 200 to 400 mg per day of fluconazole, a lower response rate was noted. At higher dosages of 400 to 800 mg per day, higher cure rates have been achieved. However, the cost of fluconazole at such high dosages becomes prohibitive. Fluconazole is approved by the Food and Drug Administration (FDA) only for treatment of cryptococcal infection in acquired immune deficiency syndrome (AIDS) patients and for *Candida* infections; for blastomycosis I do not consider it to be equivalent in efficacy to itraconazole. Other agents are in early investigations as well.

The results of oral therapy of blastomycosis are encouraging. However, in the very ill patient, amphotericin B remains the treatment of choice. In such a patient, after improvement with 500 mg or so of amphotericin B, a switch to itraconazole for the remainder of the treatment may be appropriate. One major disadvantage of oral therapy is the potential for noncompliance. Most ketoconazole treatment failures were documented in patients who had not taken the drug as they were instructed, a problem that is usually not encountered with intravenous therapy with amphotericin B. In addition, central nervous system infection with blastomycosis may occur while a patient is on itraconazole or ketoconazole since penetration into the brain is minimal. Cases have been reported in which there is clearing of the cutaneous or pulmonary infection with ketoconazole but subsequent diagnosis of central nervous system infection. Fluconazole* has been successful in the treatment of a few patients with central nervous system blastomycosis, but amphotericin B would be my preference for this site of infection.

SUMMARY

On the basis of available information, itraconazole, at a dosage of 200 mg per day for 6 months, should replace amphotericin B as therapy in compliant patients who do not have overwhelming or life-threatening blastomycosis. Because of less toxicity and a lower apparent relapse rate, itraconazole is considered to be superior to ketoconazole for first-line therapy, despite a higher cost. However, for the person with life-threatening manifestation of infection, such as the appearance of adult respiratory distress syndrome (ARDS), or the person with central nervous

*Not FDA-approved for this indication.

system involvement with blastomycosis, amphotericin B remains the treatment of choice.

PLEURAL EFFUSION AND EMPYEMA THORACIS

method of
NICHOLAS P. ROSSI, M.D.
The University of Iowa Hospitals and Clinics
Iowa City, Iowa

The presence of a pleural effusion always indicates significant systemic or local disease and demands immediate diagnosis and appropriate treatment. Important systemic diseases such as congestive heart failure, cirrhosis, and superior vena caval obstruction provide the driving force moving fluid into the pleural space with characteristics of transudates, in contrast to exudates usually due to intrathoracic disease processes such as bacterial or viral pneumonia, tuberculosis, or malignancy. The chest x-ray film, anamnesis, and physical examination many times offer strong initial hints about which type of process is occurring, but in either event thoracentesis is the next required step that results in an early diagnosis in a majority of the patients. The gross appearance of the fluid is extremely important, as 90% of malignant effusions are bloody, while infected fluids may be characterized by odor, consistency, and purulence; chyle is usually easily identified but may be distinguished from purulent exudates by the fact that the latter produce a clear supernatant on settling. If the fluid contains amylase, then suspicion is immediately raised toward pancreatitis or esophageal perforation. Exudates produce a pleural fluid with protein values greater than 3 grams per dL, a pleural fluid protein/serum protein ratio greater than 0.5, and a lactate dehydrogenase (LD) level greater than 1000 IU per mL. Exudates are also cloudy and have a high white cell count, usually greater than 1000 cells per mm³, while transudates are clear, straw-colored fluids. If a concomitant pulmonary process is going on, then determination of the pleural fluid pH and glucose level may be helpful in deciding whether an immediate drainage procedure is required.

MALIGNANT EFFUSIONS

When malignancy is suspected, cytologic examination of the fluid may provide the diagnosis, but experience has shown that cytologic examination of the fluid sediment is more efficacious than diagnosis of a smear of the fluid itself or of a percutaneous needle biopsy of the parietal pleura. Both failures are caused not by the inability to recognize malignant cells but by the lack of shed cells in the fluid at the time of the sampling or to a fault in the procedure used to convey the cells to the slides. Multiple smears of this type may be required. If such measures fail to establish a diagnosis, then thoracoscopic examination of the pleura itself yields a very high positive rate of diagnosis as well as providing the opportunity for therapeutic treatment of the malignant effusion; 75% of malignant effusions are caused by three primary malignancies: lung, breast, and lymphoma. When recurrence of effusions is frequent and bothersome, the placement of an intrathoracic Hickman line allows ready withdrawal of the fluid in the home environment without further intervention.

PARAPNEUMONIC EFFUSIONS AND EMPYEMA

The high prevalence of bacterial pneumonia in the general population and the fact that as many as 40% of such patients have an accompanying pleural effusion presents challenging problems not only in the treatment but also in the timing of the treatment of pleural effusions. Most of these effusions can be managed by measures directed at the underlying process in the lung, but a certain percentage become empyemas, which if not drained early obviate the employment of extensive procedures (open thoracotomy or decortication) to eradicate the underlying problem. Light's criteria for the drainage of such effusions have been widely accepted and are valid to use. However, a significant number of these effusions can still be managed without tube drainage, although draining is better than lingering in doubt. Gross pus and a positive Gram stain (visible organism) are definite indications for tube drainage. A pleural fluid glucose level less than 40 mg per dL and a pH below 7 should also indicate tube drainage. Perhaps 20 to 30% of patients with the last two criteria could escape tube drainage, but they cannot be selected a priori. Early drainage saves a greater number of patients from further major interventions. When parapneumonic effusions become infected, they often pass quickly from the initial exudative stage into one in which the infectious process produces heavy loculations within a very short time. The essential point in treatment is to intervene between the first and the second stages before the loculations form or become too thick. Judgment is required; if the underlying process is well controlled, the effusion seems to be the sympathetic collection of fluid that frequently accompanies these pneumonias, there are no bacteria on Gram stain, and the treatment has been initiated early, then the effusion can be watched. Since the window of opportunity is very small and the production of loculated empyema can occur within hours, surgical drainage should be the first and immediate therapeutic intervention. Fluid should be tested for bacteria before the institution of antibiotic therapy. There are no specific guidelines specifying when drainage is essential or contraindicated. If there has been a delay in diagnosis or if there is any hint of beginning bacterial contamination, such as thickening or cloudiness of the fluid

with a slight odor, then tube thoracostomy is required. Drainage is more likely required if the organism is staphylococcal or anaerobic, the effusion large, the contamination heavy, or the patient immunocompromised. All too frequently, the window of opportunity is lost and the second (fibroproliferative) stage produces such thick loculations that simple tube drainage is not sufficient to drain the infection and open tube thoracostomy is required. Intrapleural streptokinase (Streptase)* has been used in conjunction with open drainage to break up loculations, and its use alone to obviate the need for a tube thoracostomy is only successful if it is used before the second stage is established. The recommended dose is 250,000 U diluted in 100 mL of normal saline. The solution is injected into the chest, the tube is clamped for 4 hours, and the treatment is repeated daily for up to 2 weeks. The prolonged period of treatment is a big disadvantage to the use of this modality as a primary procedure. Such prolonged treatment is not often cost-effective for many patients, as has been noted in several countries. Early surgical intervention (in the second stage) has been advocated as the most cost-effective method of treatment. I have personally seen this method applied in Argentina at the Hospital de Clinicas José de San Martin, Universidad de Buenos Aires under the direction of Doctor Hugo Esteva, who found that the hospital stay and the need for subsequent procedures were both decreased by half when early limited thoracotomy was employed. An extension of this treatment is early intervention not by open thoracotomy but video thoracoscopic débridement, irrigation, and drainage. This procedure can many times prevent the need for a larger surgical operation, but at this point it has not succeeded 30% of the time, and the procedure has had to be converted into a limited open thoracotomy. One must remember that 10% of established empyemas that result from pulmonic processes have some underlying condition initiating the pneumonia such as bronchogenic carcinoma, pulmonary infarction, esophageal rupture, or chronic pulmonary abscess.

Surgical treatment must ensure (1) control of the underlying process, which may require pulmonary resection for an underlying carcinoma or unhealed abscess, (2) removal of all infected exudate, and (3) obliteration of any potential space. If the empyema has entered the stage of organization (third stage), decortication of the "peel" is required to prevent restriction of the lung or its incomplete expansion.

Pleural effusion is seen in significant numbers in patients with acquired immune deficiency syndrome (AIDS). The principles of treatment are the same. The most common cause is a parapneumonic infection, but unexpectedly, *Pneumocystis* is not a common cause of the effusion despite being the most common opportunistic infection. Bacterial pneumonia is the most common underlying problem. Tuberculous effusions are more likely to be seen in this group, and

---

*Not FDA-approved for this indication.

many small lymphocytes in the fluid help make the diagnosis. Large effusions accompany Kaposi's sarcoma. In noninfectious effusions, hypoalbuminemia is the most common cause.

PRIMARY LUNG ABSCESS

method of
MARK L. METERSKY, M.D., and
STEPHEN B. SULAVIK, M.D.
University of Connecticut Health Center
Farmington, Connecticut

Primary lung abscess may best be defined as a solitary area of pulmonary parenchymal necrosis resulting in the formation of a single cavity, with or without an air-fluid level due to pyogenic infection. Thus primary lung abscess must be differentiated from necrotizing pneumonia, in which multiple, contiguous small cavities may develop, most commonly in the setting of pneumonia caused by aerobic gram-negative rods and *Staphylococcus aureus*. The designation "primary" refers to abscesses not due to hematogenous spread or secondary infection of a previously existing cavity.

PATHOGENESIS

Aspiration of oral secretions into the lung during sleep is frequent. A lung abscess results when sufficient organisms are aspirated into the lung to overwhelm the protective mechanisms such as ciliary action, cough, and alveolar macrophage activity. Factors that predispose patients to large-volume aspiration include those associated with altered levels of consciousness, such as seizure disorders and abuse of alcohol or narcotics. Patients with impaired swallowing due to cerebrovascular accidents or esophageal disorders are also at risk. Factors that augment the number of pathogenic bacteria in oral secretions increase the risk of infections developing once aspiration has occurred. The most notable of these is periodontal disease, in the setting of which the normal population of bacteria that reside in the gingival crevices is tremendously increased in number. The most important of these organisms are the anaerobic *Fusobacterium* spp, *Peptostreptococcus,* and *Bacteroides* spp; and aerobic species such as microaerophilic streptococci. Consequently, these are the most common causes of solitary lung abscesses. Conversely, lung abscesses are unusual in edentulous patients and when they do occur are often associated with endobronchial obstruction from bronchogenic carcinoma. Enteric gram-negative bacilli frequently colonize the oropharynx of debilitated persons and may play a role in the development of lung abscess. Pus from lung abscesses most commonly grows two or more anaerobic species, often with an aerobic species. Early studies documented that synergy between these organisms plays a role in the development of infection. Occasionally, pure cultures of enteric gram-negative bacilli, *S. aureus,* or *Haemophilus influenzae* are obtained from solitary lung abscesses.

Many lung abscesses can be traced to a specific episode of aspiration or period of altered consciousness. Observation of such patients has revealed that lung abscess occurs because of a local area of necrosis in the setting of an aspiration pneumonitis. After aspiration, as long as 3 weeks elapse before a cavity develops. The area of aspiration is dependent upon the position that the patient is in. Because aspiration occurs into the gravity-dependent areas of the lung and occurs most commonly in the supine position, lung abscesses are most commonly found in the posterior segment of the upper lobes and the superior segments of the lower lobes, with the basilar segments of the lower lobes the next most common areas. The right lung is involved more frequently than the left because of the straighter takeoff of the right main-stem bronchus.

DIAGNOSIS AND EVALUATION

Usually, the diagnosis of lung abscess is not difficult. In over 90% of patients, a risk factor for aspiration is evident. The clinical presentation can be identical to that of a typical community-acquired pneumonia but usually is more indolent, with fevers, cough, and putrid (foul-smelling and -tasting) sputum present for over 2 weeks. Thus, the presence of symptoms long enough to cause weight loss is an important clue to the presence of a lung abscess. The presence of putrid sputum is particularly important, as this finding is seen in over 60% of lung abscesses and is unusual even in anaerobic pneumonia. The chest roentgenogram, of course, is the most important diagnostic aid and usually shows a single cavity with an air-fluid level and a surrounding infiltrate, often in the pulmonary segments described above. Occasionally a lung abscess can develop without effective communication with the bronchial tree. In such cases, sputum production is less prominent and because of the lack of drainage, the patient may appear more acutely ill. The diagnosis can be more difficult, as no air-fluid level is visible and the abscess may appear as a well-circumscribed oval or circular mass or may be completely hidden within a pneumonia. Computed tomography can be helpful in identifying the presence of an abscess in this situation. The presence of a lung abscess can also be missed if the chest roentgenogram is obtained with the patient in the supine position, as an air-fluid level will not be seen. Consequently, when the presence of a lung abscess is suspected, it is important to attempt to obtain a chest roentgenogram with the patient in the upright position. If the patient is too debilitated to allow this, a decubitus view may reveal the presence of an air-fluid level.

The examination of expectorated sputum may be helpful in diagnosing anaerobic lung abscess if purulent material with mixed flora is identified. Anaerobic culture of expectorated sputum is generally not helpful because of contamination with oral flora (i.e., the same organisms that cause lung abscess). Rarely, the sputum culture may be helpful by revealing an alternative diagnosis such as tuberculosis or fungal infection.

Because of the usual presence of risk factors, the typical clinical presentation, and the distinctive roentgenographic findings, most lung abscesses can be treated without a definitive bacteriologic diagnosis. Occasionally, it is important to obtain abscess material for culture because of diagnostic uncertainty or lack of response to empirical treatment. In such settings, transthoracic needle aspiration and transtracheal aspiration are often successful. Bronchoscopy with protected specimen brush sampling has also been used successfully but is probably less specific. Parapneumonic pleural effusions are commonly seen in the setting of anaerobic lung infection and when noted, should be evaluated with standard studies and anaerobic cultures to assess for the presence of empyema.

MANAGEMENT

As with any abscess, the mainstays of therapy of anaerobic lung abscess include effective drainage and antimicrobial therapy. In the 1960s, penicillin was almost always effective, even when penicillin-resistant organisms were cultured, again illustrating the polymicrobial and synergistic nature of this infection. However, with the increasing development of penicillin resistance, more recent studies have shown a significant rate of failure using penicillin alone. When compared with penicillin, clindamycin (Cleocin) results in a shorter duration of fever and putrid sputum production, as well as a lower treatment failure rate. Consequently, penicillin is not recommended as a single agent for the treatment of anaerobic lung abscess. Clindamycin given intravenously at a dosage of 600 to 900 mg every 8 hours is a very effective initial therapy for anaerobic lung abscess and is generally the treatment of choice. Disadvantages include its relatively high cost and the side effects of diarrhea and pseudomembranous colitis. Metronidazole (Flagyl) has been shown to have an unacceptably high failure rate and should not be used as a single agent for anaerobic lung abscess. Metronidazole with penicillin has been used with success. In patients who develop nosocomial lung abscess, it is more important to obtain accurate culture results because of the frequent oral colonization with gram-negative bacilli and *S. aureus*. In such patients, antibiotic therapy should be directed by the culture and sensitivity results. Patients can be switched to oral therapy once they defervesce, usually within a week of starting therapy. Initial radiographic improvement is a decrease in the size of the cavity or in the diameter of the pericavitary infiltrate. Oral antibiotic therapy should be continued until serial chest roentgenographic examinations reveal that the abscess cavity has completely closed or a stable cavity remains, with no surrounding infiltrate. This usually requires 6 to 10 weeks of therapy and not uncommonly takes longer. While drainage of any abscess is integral, the presence of an air-fluid level signifies that some communication with the bronchial tree is occurring. Postural drainage and chest physiotherapy are usually employed to facilitate drainage.

Patients with large fluid-filled abscess cavities need to be considered separately for two reasons. First, sudden emptying of the cavity into the bronchial tree can result in rapid death by asphyxiation. Second, these patients often respond very slowly to antibiotic treatment alone. We avoid the use of postural drainage in patients with large cavities because of the risk of rapid emptying. Indeed, such patients should be instructed to avoid lying with the uninvolved lung in a dependent position. Transthoracic catheter drainage has been shown to be effective in achieving rapid clinical improvement in patients with large volumes of abscess fluid and those with poor response to conservative therapy. The feared complications of empyema or bronchopleural fistula are unusual; however, hemorrhage is occasionally seen. While older reports note a requirement for resectional surgery in 10 to 15% of patients with lung abscess because of a poor response to conservative management, this number is likely to diminish with the more frequent use of transthoracic catheter drainage. Severe pulmonary hemorrhage can occasionally occur secondary to lung abscesses, and in this setting, resectional surgery or bronchial artery embolization may be required.

Fiberoptic bronchoscopy is frequently indicated for patients with a solitary lung abscess. Patients without obvious risk factors for lung abscess should undergo bronchoscopy to rule out the presence of tumor or foreign bodies resulting in bronchial obstruction. Likewise, patients at high risk for bronchogenic carcinoma should be considered for bronchoscopy. Bronchoscopy should also be performed in any patient who does not appear to be draining the abscess cavity appropriately, i.e., no air-fluid level at presentation, minimal sputum production, lack of clinical improvement, and no decrease in the amount of fluid despite appropriate antibiotic treatment, as these may be clues to the presence of bronchial obstruction.

If possible, risk factors for the development of the lung abscess should be addressed. Periodontal disease should receive dental attention. Gastrostomy tube placement should be considered for patients found to have a swallowing disorder that is not reversible.

OTITIS MEDIA

method of
JAMES E. ARNOLD, M.D.
Rainbow Babies & Childrens Hospital,
University Hospitals of Cleveland
Cleveland, Ohio

Acute otitis media is second only to upper respiratory viral infections in terms of the number of diagnoses made yearly by pediatricians. Up to 85% of children have at least one episode of otitis media by 3 years of age, and approximately one-third of them have at least three infections during that time. Some children have multiple recurrent episodes of otitis media. Risk factors for these otitis-prone children include onset of otitis at less than 1 year of age, with the younger the age of onset, the greater the likelihood of recurrent infections; a sibling with a history of recurrent ear infections; secondhand exposure to cigarette smoke; and attendance at day care centers. Children with head and neck malformations, such as those with Down's syndrome or cleft palate, as well as immunosuppressed patients are more likely to have recurrent otitis media. Being breast-fed appears to decrease the likelihood of a patient developing otitis media. Although otitis media is primarily a disease of childhood, it does occur in adolescents and adults, with a similar microbiologic pattern.

Acute otitis media is commonly recognized as being an acute inflammation of the middle ear space. Adults and older children usually complain of otalgia, ear fullness, hearing loss, and sometimes unsteadiness. Younger children may be seemingly asymptomatic or slightly fussy, with irregular feeding. Noninfected middle ear effusion that is present following acute otitis or that is associated with upper respiratory tract infections or eustachian tube dysfunction is otitis media with effusion. This fluid may be thin and serous in nature or thick and mucoid. Patients may be asymptomatic due to the indolent nature of this condition, or they may experience fullness, pressure, and a plugging sensation, along with conductive hearing loss and occasional unsteadiness. Since the mastoid air cells are contiguous with the middle ear space, any episode of otitis media also causes inflammation of the mastoid. However, clinical mastoiditis involves focal infection within the mastoid air cell system, causing postauricular pain, tenderness, and swelling, along with edema of the posterior ear canal. Extension of otitis media and mastoiditis may occur to the intracranial cavity by direct extension, through the valveless veins, or through hematogenous spread. The sternocleidomastoid muscle and the posterior belly of the digastric muscle are attached to the mastoid tip. If an infection spreads deep to these muscles, it presents in the neck, forming a Bezold abscess.

MICROBIOLOGY

A bacterial pathogen is isolated in approximately two-thirds of children with acute otitis media. The bacteriology of otitis media has been established through multiple studies. *Streptococcus pneumoniae* is the leading bacterial pathogen, accounting for 25 to 50% of cases. The second most common bacterium is nontypeable *Haemophilus influenzae*, accounting for approximately 20% of infections, followed by *Moraxella cattarhalis*, causing approximately 15% of infections. Group A streptococcus and *Staphylococcus aureus* each account for approximately 2% of the episodes of acute otitis media. Evidence of respiratory viral infection is found in approximately 20% of infected middle ears, either alone or in combination with bacterial pathogens. *Mycoplasma pneumoniae* and *Chlamydia trachomatis* rarely cause otitis media. The bacteriology of adult and pediatric otitis media is similar.

Most strains of *S. pneumoniae* are sensitive to penicillin and amoxicillin; however, there has been a recent increase in penicillin-resistant strains, as well as in strains that are resistant to multiple antibiotics. These have most often been identified in children in group settings, such as day care centers. The resistance is due to a change in the penicillin-binding proteins within the bacterial cell wall and is not caused by penicillinase activity.

EXAMINATION

Visualization of the tympanic membrane must be part of the evaluation of any child or adult with complaints related to the ear and adjacent structures. An uncooperative child should be gently restrained by having the parent hold the child in his or her lap with one arm around the child's arms and one hand steadying the child's forehead against the parent's shoulder. Since visualization of the eardrum is mandatory, forceful restraint is sometimes needed. The lateral portion of the external auditory canal contains skin with adnexal structures, as well as extra cushioning of soft tissue and cartilage. The medial half of the ear canal is covered with thin skin over periosteum and bone and is very sensitive. Obstructing cerumen may be bypassed or gently removed with a wire loop using an open-head otoscope. Gentle irrigation, using body-temperature water, may be helpful; sometimes, commercial drops are needed.

On rare occasions, examination requires sedation or anesthesia. The color, thickness, and contour of the eardrum should be noted. Is it bulging or retracted? The tympanic membrane is often translucent, and an effort should be made to determine whether there is air or fluid in the middle ear space. If fluid is present, it must be determined whether it is infected. Infected fluid is generally present in a painful ear with a full or bulging red tympanic membrane. Noninfected fluid is usually present with a retracted eardrum. In a crying child, the tympanic membrane, even if not infected, may turn red just as his or her cheeks turn red. The mobility of the tympanic membrane should be determined by pneumatic otoscopy. A gentle seal with the speculum is needed in the external auditory canal. A normal eardrum should move easily with both light positive and negative pressure. A retracted eardrum will move better with negative pressure on the bulb. A complete examination also requires noting any redness, fullness, or tenderness of the mastoid, as well as a neck examination.

TREATMENT

Treatment of an episode of acute otitis media is based on the known bacteriology. In general, amoxicillin is still considered the drug of choice because of its long record of effectiveness, safety, low cost, and palatability. If a child has received other recent antibiotics, the possibility of a resistant strain is more likely and an alternative drug should be chosen. Table 1 lists the currently used antibiotics and their relative effectiveness for the major bacterial pathogens, as well as dosage schedule, palatability, and estimated cost for both adults and children. In general, unless a child is not responding clinically to a course of antibiotics, he or she should be examined within 2 to 3 weeks of the institution of therapy. If the child has not responded clinically or if the follow-up examination indicates evidence of active, ongoing infection, a different class of antibiotics should be used, and the patient should be rechecked in several days. If there is still no response, the patient has become obviously ill, there is evidence of spread of infection, or the patient is immunocompromised, a diagnostic tympanocentesis should be performed to identify the infecting organism to better determine antibiotic therapy. A needle is inserted through the tympanic membrane (the needle in an 18-gauge intravenous catheter that has been bent at the hub works well) and fluid is aspirated and sent for culture and sensitivity. The posterior superior portion of the quadrant of the eardrum should be avoided due to the location of the ossicles.

In patients with recurrent otitis media, loosely defined as three or more infections within a 6-month period or four infections within a year, prophylactic antibiotics with amoxicillin 20 mg per kg per day or sulfisoxazole (Gantrisin) 500 mg per day in one or two doses is effective in reducing the number of recurrent ear infections in many children. Prophylaxis is generally carried through the wintertime and midspring. If prophylactic antibiotics are ineffective, the child should be referred for consideration of ventilation tube placement. Adenoidectomy may be beneficial in children who become reinfected despite pre-

TABLE 1. **Features of Commonly Used Oral Antibiotics for Acute Otitis Media**

Drug	Susceptibility			Frequency	Palat-ability‡	Adult		Pediatric	
	*Streptococcus pneumoniae**	*Haemophilus influenzae†*	*Moraxella cattarhalis†*			*Dosage*	*Cost§*	*Dosage*	*Cost§, ‖*
Amoxicillin	+ + +	—	—	tid	+ + + +	250 mg	$ 8	20 mg/kg/day	$ 6
Amoxicillin-clavulanate (Augmentin)	+ + +	+ + +	+ + +	tid	+ +	250 mg	$ 56	20 mg/kg/day	$30
Cefaclor (Ceclor)	+ + +	+	+ + +	bid/tid	+ + +	250 mg	$ 58 $ 50	20 mg/kg/day	$30 $25¶
Cefuroxime axetil (Ceftin)	+ +	+ + +	+ + +	bid	+	250 mg	$ 64	30 mg/kg/day	$54
Cefixime (Suprax)	+	+ + +	+ + +	qd/bid	+ + + +	400 mg	$ 66	8 mg/kg/day	$48
Cefpodoxime proxetil (Vantin)	+ +	+ + +	+	bid	+ +	200 mg	$ 74	10 mg/kg/day	$58
Cefprozil (Cefzil)	+ + +	+ + +	+ + +	bid	+ + +	500 mg	$105	30 mg/kg/day	$30
Loracarbef (Lorabid)	+ +	+ +	+ + +	bid	+ + + +	400 mg	$ 78	30 mg/kg/day	$36
Trimethoprim-sulfamethoxazole (Bactrim, Septra)	+ +	+ + +	+ + +	bid	+ +	1 double-strength tablet	$ 9	5 mL/10 kg bid	$ 7
Clarithromycin (Biaxin)**	+ +	+ +	+ +	bid	+	250 mg	$ 63	15 mg/kg/day	$26
Azithromycin (Zithromax)††	+ +	+ +	+ +	qd × 5 days	—††	500 mg × 1 day, then 250 mg/day × 4 days	$ 36	—††	—††

*Does not include penicillin-resistant strains.
†For penicillinase-producing strains (*H. influenzae* 25%; *M. cattarhalis* > 80%).
‡Personal reports from patients and parents for liquid.
§Average charge to patient, four pharmacies in metropolitan Cleveland, March 1995.
¶Generic cefaclor.
‖For an approximately 15-kg child.
**The primary metabolite is most effective against *H. influenzae*.
††Pediatric approval pending for liquid preparation.

vious ventilation tube placement or in whom there is evidence of significant nasopharyngeal obstruction. Tonsillectomy does not prevent otitis media.

Acute otitis media in the presence of a perforated tympanic membrane or a ventilation tube is accompanied by purulent drainage, unless the tube is blocked or the discharge is unusually thick. These cases should be treated with oral antibiotics as previously described. Topical antibiotic suspension drops are helpful in mechanically cleaning the drainage as well as in providing antibiotic therapy. Eye drops used in the ear are mild but provide effective antibiotic treatment. Treatment is continued for 10 days, after which a follow-up examination is done. In cases of persistent drainage, suctioning may be helpful, and in rare cases, intravenous antibiotics are needed. In the unusual case in which an infection does not clear, a computed tomography scan of the middle ear and mastoid should be considered to rule out significant underlying pathology.

Middle ear effusion follows nearly all cases of acute otitis media and is more common in children than adults. It may also be associated with the congestion of an upper respiratory infection and is most often related to abnormal eustachian tube function. The natural history of middle ear effusion is one of spontaneous resolution. If its presence is detected after an ear infection, the ear can be observed for clearance. If there is no evidence of clearance after a month, a 20-day therapeutic course of antibiotics effective against organisms producing beta-lactamase is warranted, since bacteria with a distribution similar to those causing acute otitis media have been identified in this clinically noninfected fluid. The antibiotics may also function by decreasing adenoid and nasopharyngeal inflammation, thereby improving eustachian tube function. The presence of middle ear effusion causes a conductive hearing loss, and if it is present bilaterally, earlier treatment is warranted. If there is no resolution with observation or medical treatment after 3 months and both ears are involved, if one ear is still involved after 6 months, or if there is evidence of structural damage to the eardrum, such as severe retraction, referral for pressure equalizing (PE) tube placement for middle ear ventilation and possible adenoidectomy is indicated. Patients with learning or developmental disabilities in whom a conductive hearing loss is more of a handicap may require earlier, more aggressive treatment of middle ear effusion.

ACUTE BRONCHITIS

method of
JONATHAN E. RODNICK, M.D.
University of California, San Francisco
San Francisco, California

Acute bronchitis divides into two syndromes—an acute lower respiratory infection in those patients who have no significant underlying lung disease and an exacerbation of symptoms in those with chronic bronchitis and/or asthma. The cause and treatment of each differs.

The defining characteristic of acute bronchitis is cough. In acute infectious bronchitis it is associated with other symptoms of upper and/or lower respiratory tract infection, but there is no evidence for pneumonia. The cough often develops after a few days of predominantly upper respiratory symptoms such as coryza or sore throat. Initially the cough is dry, but usually becomes productive of mucopurulent phlegm. Other signs and symptoms may include low-grade fever, malaise, pleuritic chest pain, wheezing, and occasionally hemoptysis. The lung examination is usually clear, but rales, rhonchi, and wheezes may be heard on auscultation. Acute bronchitis is self-limited, but one-third of patients will cough for more than 1 month.

Laboratory tests are usually not necessary. Sputum cultures, if done, typically show normal flora. A chest x-ray is occasionally helpful to differentiate bronchitis from pneumonia, for example, in an elderly patient with fever and abnormal chest findings. In the absence of auscultatory findings, a chest x-ray is very likely to be normal.

Recently it has been appreciated that bronchospasm and bronchial edema are part of the syndrome of acute bronchitis. Pulmonary function tests, if done, often show a decreased peak expiratory flow. An association exists between recurrent episodes of acute bronchitis and asthma, and occasionally persistent new asthmatic symptoms will follow an episode of bronchitis.

The cause of acute infectious bronchitis is usually viral; indeed, over 180 viruses can cause respiratory infections. Most common are the rhinoviruses, followed by the adenoviruses; influenza, parainfluenza, and respiratory syncytial viruses, although less common, cause more severe symptoms. In children and young adults, both *Mycoplasma pneumoniae* and *Chlamydia pneumonia* are relatively common causes. It is not possible to differentiate viral from other respiratory pathogens, although a more prolonged course of illness may be associated with *Mycoplasma* and *Chlamydia* infections. Viral infections are more common in the winter months. *Mycoplasma* and *Chlamydia* are more sporadic.

Other bacterial causes of acute bronchitis are uncommon. *Bordetella pertussis* should always be kept in mind. *Haemophilus influenzae, Streptococcus pneumoniae,* and *Moraxella catarrhalis* are more likely causes of flare-ups of chronic bronchitis.

TREATMENT

Because acute infectious bronchitis is a self-limited disease, antibiotics are usually not indicated. Symp-tomatic treatment includes double-dose dextromethorphan (30 to 60 mg) or 15 to 30 mg codeine to suppress nocturnal cough. Guaifenesin (Humibid), 300 to 600 mg four times daily, may be used as a mucolytic.

The most effective way to relieve cough is with a metered-dose inhaler (MDI) with a spacer containing either a beta$_2$ agonist such as albuterol (Proventil, Ventolin) or ipratropium (Atrovent). MDIs work whether or not one hears wheezes or whether the patient smokes or is on antibiotics. Obviously, in a smoker an episode of bronchitis is an ideal time to assess or reinforce the patient's motivation for quitting.

If a productive cough is prolonged (more than 2 weeks) or constitutional symptoms are prominent, it is reasonable to treat with antibiotics on the premise one is dealing with a mycoplasmal or chlamydial infection. In this case, appropriate choices are erythromycin 250 mg four times daily, clarithromycin (Biaxin), 250 mg twice daily, tetracycline, 250 mg four times daily, doxycycline (Vibramycin), 100 mg twice daily—all for 7 to 14 days—or azithromycin (Zithromax), 500 mg, then 250 mg daily for 5 days.

ACUTE EXACERBATIONS OF CHRONIC BRONCHITIS

Chronic bronchitis is defined as the production of sputum on most days for at least 3 months per year for at least 2 years. The majority of patients are men and smokers (relative risk of smokers vs. nonsmokers is 8.8 for men and 5.9 for women). An acute exacerbation of chronic bronchitis is a clinical syndrome characterized by an increase in cough, an increase in phlegm (usually with altered color or tenacity), and an increase in breathlessness. Most patients do not have findings suggestive of a systemic infection, such as fever or leukocytosis. A chest x-ray, if ordered, reflects the underlying chronic obstructive pulmonary disease and/or bronchiectasis with hyperaeration, bullae, atelectasis, or peribronchial cuffing.

The cause of these acute exacerbations is not clear. Besides environmental factors, viruses, mycoplasma, and bacteria may be involved. Bacterial colonization of the normally sterile tracheobronchial tree is common in chronic bronchitis. *H. influenzae* (nontypeable), *S. pneumoniae,* and *M. (Branhamella) catar-*

TABLE 1. **Oral Antibiotics with Broad Activity Against Bacteria Associated with Acute Exacerbations of Chronic Bronchitis**

Generic	Trade Name	Dosage	Comments	Cost
Amoxicillin/clavulanic acid	Augmentin	250–500 mg tid	Good spectrum of activity	High
Azithromycin	Zithromax	500 mg, then 250 mg qd	Few *Streptococcus pneumoniae* are resistant	High
Cefixime	Suprax	400 mg qd	Less active against *S. pneumoniae*	High
Cefpodoxime	Vantin	200 mg bid	Good spectrum	High
Cefprozil	Cefzil	500 mg bid	Less active against *Haemophilus influenzae* and *Moraxella catarrhalis*	High
Cefuroxime axetil	Ceftin	250–500 mg bid	Good spectrum	High
Loracarbef	Lorabid	400 mg bid	Less active against *H. influenzae*	High

TABLE 2. **Oral Antibiotics with More Limited Activity Against Bacteria Associated with Acute Exacerbations of Chronic Bronchitis**

Generic	Trade Name	Dosage	Comments	Cost
Ampicillin		250–500 mg qid	Many *Haemophilus influenzae* and most *Moraxella catarrhalis* are resistant	Low
Amoxicillin		250–500 mg tid	Many *H. influenzae* and most *M. catarrhalis* are resistant	Low
Erythromycin		250–500 mg qid	Most *H. influenzae* and a few *S. pneumoniae* resistant	Low
Clarithromycin	Biaxin	500 mg bid	Some *H. influenzae* and a few *Streptococcus pneumoniae* are resistant	High
Cefaclor	Ceclor	250 mg tid	Less active against *H. influenzae* and *M. catarrhalis*	High
Doxycycline		100 mg bid	Some *S. pneumoniae* and *H. influenzae* are resistant	Low
Ciprofloxacin	Cipro	500 mg bid	Less active against *S. pneumoniae*	High
Trimethoprim-sulfamethoxazole	Bactrim, Septra	160/800 mg bid	Less active against *S. pneumoniae*	Low

rhalis may be frequently cultured. Although not proved, it is thought that infection with these organisms is responsible for most exacerbations. *H. parainfluenzae* and species of *Neisseria, Klebsiella, Pseudomonas,* and *Staphylococci* may also occasionally be causative agents.

Laboratory tests are usually not indicated, unless hospitalization is contemplated. However, sputum Gram's stain may be helpful in determining therapy. If there are more than 25 neutrophils and fewer than 10 epithelial cells per low-power field, infection is more likely. The presence of bacteria on high-power examination (in a field with white blood cells) is further presumptive evidence of infection. Sputum culture and sensitivity are generally not necessary and are not reliable, as they do not differentiate between colonization and infection. Oximetry and/or peak air flow tests may be helpful in determining the degree of respiratory compromise.

TREATMENT

Because a bacterial cause is more likely for an exacerbation of chronic bronchitis than it is for acute bronchitis in an otherwise healthy individual, antibiotics are frequently given in an effort to shorten the duration of the exacerbation and prevent deterioration of pulmonary function in patients with minimal respiratory reserve. A benefit is more likely in those with more severe and frequent exacerbations or who have more severe underlying lung disease. The oral antibiotics of choice are listed in Table 1. Because all are high cost, less expensive and other commonly used antibiotics are listed in Table 2. A good Gram stain can help guide the decision of which antibiotic to use, particularly noting the presence or absence of *M. catarrhalis,* an intracellular and extracellular gram-negative diplococci. The usual length of treatment is 7 to 14 days (except for 5 days for azithromycin). Prophylactic low-dose antibiotics should be considered in those who get frequent (more than 4 times per year) exacerbations and have significant underlying lung diseases.

Ancillary treatments such as chest physiotherapy,

humidification, and expectorants (iodinated glycerol and guaifenesin) may be helpful, but are unproved. Bronchodilators (beta₂ agonists, ipratropium, or theophylline), anti-inflammatory agents (oral or inhaled steroids), supplemental oxygen, and maintenance of hydration may be necessary in those with more severe underlying disease. Pneumococcal vaccine and yearly influenza vaccine are important preventive measures. Because strains of *H. influenzae* that are associated with bronchitis are nontypeable, Hib vaccine has no benefit. Amantidine or rimantidine (Flumadine) 200 mg daily (100 mg in the elderly) will decrease the incidence of influenza A in high-risk patients in epidemic situations and will shorten the duration of illness when administered within 48 hours of onset of symptoms. Smoking cessation is the most important step that can be taken to decrease morbidity.

BACTERIAL PNEUMONIA

method of
EDWARD A. DOMINGUEZ, M.D., and
MARK E. RUPP, M.D.
University of Nebraska Medical Center
Omaha, Nebraska

Bacterial pneumonia may be of two types, community-acquired or hospital-acquired (i.e., nosocomial). Both are significant causes of morbidity and mortality. In the United States, community-acquired pneumonia afflicts almost 3 million adults per year and accounts for 800,000 hospital admissions. Annually, there are 50,000 deaths attributable to community-acquired pneumonia, making this infection the sixth leading cause of death in the United States. Despite the availability of broad-spectrum antibiotics, the mortality rate remains 6 to 13%. The economic impact is enormous, with cost estimates exceeding $4 billion per year (1984 U.S. dollars). The high-risk groups for both types of bacterial pneumonias include the elderly, the immunocompromised (e.g., those with malignancies or human immunodeficiency virus [HIV] infection), and the chronically ill, particularly those with cardiac or pulmonary diseases. Nosocomial bacterial pneumonia occurs in approximately 300,000 patients per year and is the second most common hospital-acquired infection in the United States. The mortality rate of this infection is 20 to 50%. Although the same risk factors for community-acquired pneumonia are applicable in this disease, the major risk factor is mechanical ventilation.

ETIOLOGY

The human body has an elaborate defense mechanism against the invasion of the lower respiratory tract by bacterial pathogens. This includes (1) epiglottic and cough reflexes, (2) mucociliary transport and tracheobronchial secretions, (3) cell-mediated immunity (CMI), (4) humoral immunity, and (5) phagocytosis (particularly by polymorphonuclear neutrophils). Aberrations in one or more of these components increase the risk of developing pneumonia. The pathophysiology of bacterial pneumonia is now well understood. The first step involves colonization of the upper respiratory tract with pathogenic bacteria. This process is important in nosocomial pneumonia, as the likelihood of colonization with bacteria such as *Pseudomonas aeruginosa* increases with the days of hospitalization. Colonization is followed by aspiration into the lower tract. Certain iatrogenic factors, such as sedation or endotracheal intubation, can enhance aspiration. Once the infection is in the lower tract, inflammation ensues. If the infection cannot be contained, bacteremia may occur. Pneumonia with bacteremia is usually associated with a worse outcome.

Organisms causing bacterial pneumonia vary with the type of pneumonia (Table 1). Most surveys of patients with community-acquired pneumonia have found *Streptococcus pneumoniae* as the most frequently isolated bacterium, responsible for about one-third of cases. Importantly, these studies involved patients treated as both outpatients and inpatients. In patients requiring admission, bacteria like *Haemophilus pneumoniae*, *Staphylococcus aureus*, *Legionella* species, and aerobic gram-negative bacilli (e.g., *Klebsiella pneumoniae*) are more likely to be involved. In outpatients, *Mycoplasma pneumoniae* and *Chlamydia pneumoniae* are commonly found. However, about one-third of all patients do not have an identifiable pathogen. There are often clues in a patient's history that suggest a particular pathogen. A preceding influenza infection increases the likelihood of *Staph. aureus* pneumonia. Smokers and patients with underlying pulmonary disease often develop infections with *H. pneumoniae* and *Moraxella catarrhalis*. Patients with severe underlying diseases (e.g., alcoholic cirrhosis) are prone to infection with *Strep. pneumoniae* and aerobic gram-negative bacilli. Those with poor dentition or altered mentation may aspirate and develop

TABLE 1. **Causes of Community-Acquired and Nosocomial Pneumonias**

Agent	Community (%)	Nosocomial (%)
Streptococcus pneumoniae	33	6
Mycoplasma pneumoniae	9	—
Haemophilus influenzae	7	5
Virus	7	—
Legionella spp	6	—
Chlamydia spp	6	—
Staphylococcus aureus	3	8
Aerobic gram-negative bacteria	5	80

anaerobic or polymicrobial pneumonias. Finally, specific environmental or geographic exposures may suggest diseases like tularemia, psittacosis, Q fever, or pneumonic plague.

The etiologic agents of nosocomial pneumonia are diverse but consist primarily of aerobic gram-negative bacilli, especially *P. aeruginosa* and *Staph. aureus*. However, a recent study from a community hospital reported that bacteria causing nosocomial pneumonia were similar to those causing community-acquired pneumonia. Thus, the patient mix of a hospital is an important factor in the spectrum of bacteria causing nosocomial pneumonia. It is not uncommon to find more than one species in specimens from the lower respiratory tract, making treatment of nosocomial pneumonia more complicated. The role of anaerobic bacteria remains unclear, but they may be involved in up to one-third of cases.

DIAGNOSIS

The typical patient with bacterial pneumonia complains of acute onset of fever, cough with purulent sputum, pleuritic chest pain, and dyspnea. Physical examination typically reveals fever, tachypnea, and lung consolidation. A chest x-ray film is usually confirmatory. This clinical presentation, however, is highly dependent on the status of the host's defense mechanisms. The elderly are more likely to present with worsening of underlying diseases or with altered mental status. They may also have hypothermia and a normal white cell count. Patients on corticosteroids may not have the local signs of inflammation, such as pleurisy. Importantly, there are no signs or symptoms that are pathognomonic for pneumonia with a particular organism.

Despite occasional reports to the contrary, the sputum Gram stain remains an important part of the evaluation. When performed and interpreted carefully, it helps direct empirical therapy. An adequate specimen has fewer than 10 epithelial cells and more than 25 polymorphonuclear leukocytes per high-powered field. For pneumonia with *Strep. pneumoniae*, the sensitivity and specificity of the sputum Gram stain exceeds that of sputum culture. Thus, sputum cultures are probably less reliable for the diagnosis of community-acquired pneumonia than generally thought. An array of specialized tests, based on antigen-detection techniques such as immunofluorescence, electrophoresis, and nucleic acid amplification and hybridization, have been developed to overcome this problem. *Legionella pneumophila* pneumonia, for example, may be diagnosed by urinary antigen detection. *Strep. pneumoniae* infections can frequently be diagnosed with sputum counterimmunoelectrophoresis. Some of these methods are not standardized or are not readily available, however.

Although the chest x-ray film is important in clinical decision making, the distinction of typical versus atypical patterns may not be as useful as previously thought. Lobar or segmental infiltrates are most often found in pneumococcal pneumonia but may be seen in pneumonia caused by "atypical" agents like *Mycoplasma* and *Legionella* as well. Parapneumonic effusions are more common, in staphylococcal and pneumococcal pneumonias, and are rare with legionellosis. Cavitary lesions are frequently found in anaerobic, staphylococcal, and mycobacterial pneumonias. So, although the chest x-ray film pattern may be suggestive of certain pathogens, it does not preclude Gram's stain and culture of respiratory secretions. In fact, for patients with an acute cough, the sensitivity of a chest x-ray film is less than 3%. Thus, chest x-ray examinations should probably be limited to patients with fever, tachycardia, abnormal lung examinations, and absence of asthma, all factors that are predictive of bacterial pneumonia.

In the diagnosis of nosocomial pneumonia, clinical parameters (fever, purulent sputum, and new pulmonary infiltrates on chest x-ray films) are woefully inadequate. Recent studies using protected-brush bronchoscopic techniques demonstrate that bacterial pneumonia occurs in only about 50% of mechanically ventilated patients with these findings. Consequently, protected-brush bronchoscopy with quantitative bacteriologic culture is currently the best method for diagnosing nosocomial pneumonia.

TREATMENT

Community-Acquired Pneumonia

Before a decision on antimicrobial therapy is made, the clinician must decide whether or not to admit a patient with community-acquired pneumonia. Recent prospective studies suggest the following criteria as relative indications for hospitalization:

1. Age greater than 65 years
2. Immunosuppression
3. Symptom duration greater than 4 weeks or less than 1 week
4. Temperature greater than 38.3° C
5. Co-morbid illness (e.g., pulmonary disease)
6. Multilobar involvement
7. Disease associated with worse outcome (staphylococci; gram-negative bacilli; aspiration; or postobstructive pneumonia)
8. Altered mental status
9. Hypoxemia, or severe renal, hematologic, or electrolyte abnormalities
10. Hypotension, or other severe vital sign abnormalities

Even without any of these findings, social factors may occasionally be compelling enough to warrant admission. Thus, issues like compliance and independence in activities of daily living should be included in the decision process, particularly in the elderly and in those with suspected mycobacterial infections.

Therapy should be guided by the most likely pathogen in a clinical setting. Table 2 includes recommendations for specific situations from several published reviews. In general, it is important to base initial therapy on a suitable sputum Gram stain. For example, if gram-positive diplococci are seen, then pneumococcal pneumonia should be suspected and penicillin should be started (a macrolide, like erythromycin, can be substituted in penicillin-allergic patients). However, if the patient recently had influenza, then a penicillinase-resistant antistaphylococcal penicillin (e.g., nafcillin [Unipen] or dicloxacillin [Dynapen]) would be appropriate until cultures were finalized. When the Gram stain in a previously untreated patient shows numerous inflammatory cells without bacteria, a macrolide would be an excellent broad-spectrum choice. Such a Gram stain would be likely when *Mycoplasma*, *Legionella*, or *Chlamydia* is the causative agent. The newer macrolides, clarithromycin (Biaxin) and azithromycin (Zithromax), provide broader coverage than erythromycin and cause less gastrointestinal upset.

Patients with pre-existing lung disease, particularly chronic bronchitis, are more likely to harbor *H. influenzae* or *M. catarrhalis*. A second-generation cephalosporin like cefuroxime (Zinacef) would be appropriate. A reasonable and cost-effective alternative, however, is trimethoprim-sulfamethoxazole (Septra or Bactrim). Immunocompromised patients are more likely to develop gram-negative bacillary pneumonia, and thus extended-spectrum penicillins (piperacillin [Pipracil]) or third-generation cephalosporins (cefotaxime [Claforan]) are suitable for initial therapy. Once an organism has been identified, therapy should be individualized based on in vitro sensitivity data.

For most patients, 5 to 7 days of therapy is adequate. Hospitalized patients may complete their course as outpatients on either parenteral or oral antibiotics. However, bacteremic patients should receive a minimum of 7 days of parenteral therapy. After completion, consideration should be given to appropriate vaccinations (e.g., influenza or pneumococcal).

TABLE 2. **Guidelines for Outpatient Treatment of Community-Acquired Pneumonia**

Sputum Gram's Stain	Primary Treatment	Alternative
If sputum available:		
Gram-positive diplococci	Penicillin	Macrolide
Small gram-negative bacilli	Trimethoprim-sulfamethoxazole	Doxycycline
Large gram-negative diplococci	Trimethoprim-sulfamethoxazole	2° Cephalosporin Doxycycline
Polymorphonuclear cells without organisms	Macrolide	2° Cephalosporin Doxycycline

Clinical Situation	Initial Therapy	Alternative
If sputum unavailable:		
Nonelderly	Erythromycin	Doxycycline Macrolide
Chronic lung disease/elderly	Trimethoprim-sulfamethoxazole	Macrolide 2° Cephalosporin
Aspiration pneumonia	Clindamycin	Penicillin

TABLE 3. **Empirical Therapy of Nosocomial Pneumonia**

Class of Antibiotic	Example
3 Ceph + APAG	Ceftazidime 2 gm IV q 8 h & IV gentamicin 5 mg/kg/day
AP PCN–BLAINH + APAG	PIP–TZ 3.375 gm IV q 6 h & IV gentamicin 5 mg/kg/day
AP PCN + APAG	Pipercillin 3 gm IV q 4 h & IV gentamicin 5 mg/kg/day
Carbapenem	Imipenem-cilastatin 500 mg IV q 6 h
FQ + Clind	Ofloxacin 400 mg IV q 12 h & clindamycin 900 mg IV q 8 h

Abbreviations: 3 Ceph = third-generation cephalosporin (e,g., cefotaxime [Claforan], ceftriaxone [Rocephin], ceftazidime [Fortaz, Tazidime]); APAG = antipseudomonal aminoglycoside (e.g., gentamicin [Garamycin], amikacin [Amikin], tobramycin [Nebcin]); AP PCN = antipseudomonal penicillin (e.g., piperacillin [Pipracil], ticarcillin [Ticar], mezlocillin [Mezlin]); AP PCN–BLAINH = antipseudomonal penicillin–beta-lactamase inhibitor (piperacillin-tazobactam (PIP– TZ [Zosyn]), ticarcillin-clavulanate [Timentin]); FQ = fluoroquinolone (e.g., ciprofloxacin [Cipro], ofloxacin [Floxin]); Clind = clindamycin.

Nosocomial Pneumonia

Therapy for nosocomial pneumonia is often empirical and generally utilizes combinations of broad-spectrum antibiotics (Table 3). No single antibiotic regimen has been conclusively demonstrated to be superior, and the regimen chosen must be based on the local antimicrobial susceptibility pattern (i.e., antibiogram). Many authorities recommend therapy with a third-generation cephalosporin or an antipseudomonal penicillin–beta-lactamase inhibitor combined with an aminoglycoside.

Alternative regimens could include imipenemcilastatin (Primaxin) as single-agent therapy. A fluoroquinolone such as ofloxacin (Floxin) or ciprofloxacin (Cipro) may be used instead of a beta-lactam. Often a fluoroquinolone is used in combination with clindamycin (Cleocin), to coverage of gram-positive cocci and anaerobic organisms. Aztreonam (Azactam) may be used in patients with compromised renal function to avoid the nephrotoxicity associated with aminoglycosides. The above regimens do not cover methicillin-resistant *S. aureus* (MRSA), which should be treated with vancomycin. Despite the development of excellent antibiotics, the mortality rate of nosocomial pneumonia remains significant and emphasizes the need for improvements in preventive strategies.

VIRAL RESPIRATORY INFECTIONS

method of
FREDERICK L. RUBEN, M.D.
University of Pittsburgh Medical Center
Pittsburgh, Pennsylvania

Viral respiratory infections affect all age groups and are the most common type of acute illness seen by physicians in the United States. The principal virus families responsible for these illnesses are rhinovirus, coronavirus, respiratory syncytial virus, adenovirus, parainfluenza virus, and influenza virus. Other less common virus groups are herpes simplex virus Type 1, coxsackievirus, Epstein-Barr virus, echovirus, and poliovirus. Syndromes caused by these agents range from the common cold to severe pneumonia. Different viruses can cause the same clinical picture. Cultures or viral serologic studies can identify the specific virus responsible, but until these diagnostic tests are more widely available, management is usually empirical. In many instances it is necessary to exclude the group A hemolytic streptococci, which can mimic a viral respiratory infection and should be treated with antibiotics.

SYMPTOMATIC TREATMENT

Rhinorrhea and Nasal Stuffiness

Nasal congestion can be adequately treated with topically applied sympathomimetic amines. Drops of sprays of 0.05% oxymetazoline or 0.1% xylometazoline (each marketed under a variety of brand names) are available, with half-strength preparations also available for use in children. Prolonged or excessive use should be avoided to prevent rebound congestion with chronic swelling of nasal mucosa. These medications should not be used in patients who are taking monoamine oxidase (MAO) inhibitors or tricyclic antidepressants.

Oral sympathomimetic amines are generally less effective than the topical ones and may cause systemic side effects such as excessive nervousness or transient increases in blood pressure.

Antihistamines, although widely used for symptomatic relief of nasal congestion, are not conclusively effective.

Sore Throat

As indicated above, infection with group A streptococci can mimic viral respiratory disease. Sore throat is a symptom that is common with these bacteria. Although sore throat associated with viruses may be milder than that with the streptococci, it may require therapy. Either aspirin or acetaminophen is effective with viral sore throat; however, aspirin should not be used in children 16 years of age or younger because of the danger of inducing Reye's syndrome. If the sore throat is unusually severe, some relief may be obtained with lidocaine (Xylocaine Viscous), usually 2%. For adults 15 mL is a single dose; as a gargle it may, if necessary, be swallowed. The pediatric dose must be individualized by the physician. Dosages should not exceed eight doses in 14 hours.

Cough

Cough suppression is generally not needed in patients with uncomplicated viral respiratory infection. Moderate to severe cough can be treated with either codeine or dextromethorphan hydrobromide. Codeine can be given orally every 4 hours at a dose of 10 mg in adults and 0.25 mg per kg in children. Dextromethorphan is given orally every 6 to 8 hours, 15 to 30 mg in adults and 0.25 mg per kg in children. Neither medication should be used in patients taking MAO inhibitors.

Headache and Myalgia

Headache and myalgia are not prominent except in patients with influenza, for which specific antiviral therapy is available. Mild analgesics as described above for sore throat are usually effective.

Croup

In managing croup it is essential to rule out the presence of epiglottitis. The latter usually has a sudden onset and rapid progression in conjunction with high fever and dysphagia.

Most viral croup can be managed in the outpatient setting without therapeutic intervention. Signs of significant respiratory compromise such as restlessness, severe retractions, or cyanosis require that the patient be hospitalized for observation and for any necessary intervention to ensure adequate ventilation.

Symptomatic treatment of viral croup is directed at reducing airway edema. The most effective medication is racemic epinephrine as an aerosol. The aerosol solution is made by mixing 0.5 mL of racemic epinephrine with 3.5 mL of saline, and the mixture is given via aerosolization in a face mask. The use of intermittent positive-pressure breathing (IPPB), although more effective, makes it more difficult to give the aerosol. The effect of therapy may last from 1 to 3 hours, and aerosols are usually given every 3 to 4 hours or more frequently if needed. Tachycardia is the most common side effect. These aerosols provide only temporary relief and do not alter the natural course of the disease. In general they should only be used in the hospitalized patient.

Croup tents and corticosteroids are probably not helpful. Cool mist does seem to be beneficial for acute spasmodic croup.

SPECIFIC ANTIVIRAL THERAPY

Respiratory Syncytial Virus

Ribavirin (Virazole) as an aerosol has been approved for the treatment of respiratory syncytial virus (RSV) infection. Previously healthy patients with uncomplicated disease are not candidates for ribavirin aerosol. Patient populations with high morbidity and mortality from RSV disease such as patients with underlying cardiac or pulmonary disease, neonates, and immunocompromised patients may benefit from therapy. The drug is given as an aerosol via tent, head box, or face mask for 12 to 18 hours daily for 3 to 7 days. A small-particle aerosolizer is available from ICN Pharmaceuticals. Ribavirin is not administered through a ventilator.

Influenza Virus, Type A

Amantadine hydrochloride (Symmetrel) is effective for both the prophylaxis and the treatment of influenza A infections in adults and children. The use of amantadine in children less than 1 year of age has not been adequately evaluated. Amantadine dosage for prophylaxis and treatment should be based on age and renal function. For children 1 to 9 years of age, 4.4 to 8.8 mg per kg per day, not to exceed 150 mg per day, is recommended, with the lower range of doses preferable to avoid toxicity. For adults, 200 mg per day is suggested, but studies have shown efficacy at 100 mg per day, and this author prefers the lower dosage. For patients with reduced renal function the package insert gives the reduced dosages. Prophylaxis is generally needed for up to 6 weeks after the influenza outbreak is noted. Therapy with amantadine should begin within 24 to 48 hours of the onset of symptoms for maximal benefit and should continue for 5 to 7 days. A derivative of amantadine, rimantadine (Flumadine), is also available for use. It has the advantage of not needing dosage adjustments for reduced renal function, making it useful for elderly patients. Neither drug is effective against Type B influenza viruses.

The toxicity and side effects of amantadine and rimantadine mainly affect the central nervous system (e.g., insomnia, drowsiness) or the gastrointestinal tract. Lower dosages reduce the likelihood of side effects. Both drugs have been more efficacious against influenza A than aspirin or placebo in controlled trials.

VIRAL AND MYCOPLASMAL PNEUMONIAS

method of
LARRY JAMES STRAUSBAUGH, M.D.
Portland Veterans Affairs Medical Center
Portland, Oregon

VIRAL PNEUMONIAS

Viruses commonly cause pneumonia in children and adults. In published series of pediatric cases viruses account for 15 to 20% of pneumonias in outpatients and for up to 50% of pneumonias in inpatients. In series of adult cases the percentage of pneumonias caused by viruses has ranged from 4 to 39%, averaging about 15%. The most frequently encountered viral causes of pneumonia in the general population are listed in Table 1. These agents may account for sporadic cases of pneumonia throughout the year, but cases caused by respiratory syncytial virus (RSV), parainfluenza viruses, and influenza viruses are recognized most frequently in seasonal epidemics. Outbreaks of respiratory disease caused by all of these viruses with associated cases of pneumonia occasionally occur in hospitals, nursing homes,

TABLE 1. **Viruses That Commonly Cause Pneumonia and Associated Epidemiologic Features**

Virus (Types)	Epidemiologic Features
Respiratory syncytial virus (RSV)	All ages; most common cause in children <5 years; winter and spring
Influenza virus (A & B)	All ages; most common cause in adults; winter
Parainfluenza virus (I–III)	All ages but most frequent in children <5 years; Types I and II in fall; Type III year round
Adenovirus (1–5, 7, 14, 21, 35)	All ages; generally uncommon; Types 4 & 7 in military recruits; spring and summer
Varicella-zoster virus (VZV)	All ages; especially immuno-compromised children, young men, and pregnant women; winter and spring
Measles virus	Uncommon in vaccine era

and other closed populations. Case reports indicate that other viruses, e.g., enteroviruses and rhinoviruses, may rarely cause pneumonia; and new viral agents are still being described, e.g., the hantavirus recovered in 1993 from patients dying with the adult respiratory distress syndrome in the four corners region of the southwestern United States. Additional viral causes of pneumonia need to be considered in immunocompromised patients (Table 2). Of these, cytomegalovirus (CMV) is encountered most frequently, especially in seronegative recipients of bone marrow, kidney, or liver transplants from seropositive donors.

Clinical Features

The clinical manifestations of viral pneumonias are quite diverse, seldom permitting a specific viral diagnosis and often mimicking features of bacterial pneumonia. In general, viral pneumonias present with a more gradual onset of symptoms than is characteristic in patients with bacterial pneumonia. Cough with or without sputum production, respiratory distress, rales and rhonchi on physical examination, and pulmonary infiltrates on chest x-ray films are the most common presenting features of viral pneumonias. Radiographic features run the gamut from small patchy infiltrates to diffuse bilateral disease. Air trapping and hyperinflation may also be noted in RSV disease. Leukocytosis is unusual in patients with viral pneumonia unless bacterial superinfection has supervened. Patients infected with RSV or parainfluenza virus frequently report antecedent upper respiratory symptoms, and they are less likely to be febrile. Prostration and myalgias are

TABLE 2. **Viruses That Cause Pneumonia Primarily in Immunocompromised Patients**

Cytomegalovirus (CMV)
Herpes simplex virus (HSV)
Human herpesvirus 6 (HHV6)

often noteworthy in patients infected with influenza virus. Pneumonia caused by varicella-zoster virus (VZV) or measles virus is accompanied by the characteristic exanthem. Fever and systemic toxicity often overshadow pulmonary symptoms in immunocompromised patients with viral pneumonia.

Diagnosis

Clinical features are usually sufficient to make a diagnosis of pneumonia, but establishing a viral cause is difficult. The diagnostic process is confounded by the overlapping features of viral and bacterial respiratory infections as well as by the frequency of bacterial superinfections in patients who start out with viral respiratory diseases. Nevertheless, negative bacteriologic studies, epidemiologic considerations (age, season, clinical setting, knowledge of other illness in the family or community), and the presence of generalized vesicular or morbilliform rashes frequently permit a reasonable guess about viral causes. Confirmation, however, requires either isolation of the virus in tissue culture or documentation of an antibody response—procedures that are not readily available and require a week or more for completion. An RSV diagnosis, however, can be confirmed more rapidly: commercially available fluorescent antibody reagents and enzyme-linked immunosorbent assay (ELISA) systems allow the rapid detection of RSV antigens in respiratory secretions with sensitivities exceeding 80% and specificities of 95%. In transplantation centers, shell vial tissue culture methods are often available to identify CMV in buffy coat and respiratory tract specimens within a day or two of collection.

Treatment

In recent years the armamentarium of agents for possible use in patients with viral pneumonia has expanded considerably (Table 3), but controversy and uncertainty about efficacy persist. At the present time three generalization can be made. Ribavirin (Virazole) warrants a trial in pediatric patients with severe RSV pneumonia, impending respiratory failure, significant risk factors for a bad outcome (prematurity, age less than 1 year, neuromuscular disorders, and underlying cardiac or pulmonary disease), and no response to supportive therapy within 24 hours of admission. Acyclovir (Zovirax) is of definite value in herpes simplex virus (HSV) and VZV* pneumonia, especially when started within a day or two of disease onset. Ganciclovir (Cytovene)* in combination with CMV immune globulin has proven efficacy in transplant patients with CMV pneumonia. Other considerations listed in Table 3 must be regarded as speculative.

Supportive therapy remains the mainstay for most patients with viral pneumonia. Supplemented oxygen administration, the humidification of inspired

---

*Not FDA-approved for this indication.

TABLE 3. **Antiviral Agents for Possible Use in Viral Pneumonia**

Agents	Indications	Dose	Comments
Ribavirin (Virazole)	RSV	1.1 gm/day by aerosol (delivery by oxygen mask, hood, mist tent, or endotracheal tube, depending on severity of illness); treatment for 3–7 days; pregnant caregivers should avoid contact with aerosol because of possible teratogenecity and toxicity to fetus	Severe cases only (see text); activity against influenza A & B and parainfluenza viruses but not FDA-approved for infections caused by these viruses; being tried on investigational basis in hantavirus pulmonary syndrome (by IV route)
Amantadine (Symmetrel) and Rimantdine (Flumadine)	Influenza A	100 mg PO bid; treatment for 5 days	Benefit in uncomplicated influenza A if administered within 48 h of disease onset; efficacy in patients with pneumonia unproved
Acyclovir (Zovirax)*	HSV VZV	5 mg/kg IV q 8 h 10–12 mg/kg IV q 12 h, treatment for 7–14 days	Dosage adjustments necessary for patients with renal insufficiency; neurologic and renal side effects of concern with higher dose
Ganciclovir (Cytovene)*	CMV	5 mg/kg IV q 12 h initially	Usually combined with IV immune globulin
Foscarnet (Foscavir)*	CMV Acyclovir-resistant HSV VZV	Undetermined at present	Efficacy in patients with pneumonia unproved

*Not FDA-approved for this indication.
Abbreviations: RSV = respiratory syncytial virus; HSV = herpes simplex virus; VZV = varicella-zoster virus; CMV = cytomegalovirus.

air, and the parenteral or oral administration of sufficient fluids to maintain adequate volume status are key considerations for patients that are sick enough to be hospitalized. Fever suppression is indicated for markedly febrile patients. Bronchodilators are indicated for patients with evident bronchospasm. Some patients require periodic suctioning of the airway to manage secretions, and a small percentage require intubation and mechanical ventilation. Early recognition and treatment of bacterial superinfection is also important.

MYCOPLASMAL PNEUMONIA

Mycoplasma pneumoniae—the so-called Eaton agent, a cell wall–deficient bacterium—is a common cause of pneumonia. It accounts for approximately 15 to 20% of pneumonias in the population at large, and in closed populations such as military barracks it may account for 50% of pneumonias. Since 95% of cases are not severe enough to warrant hospitalization, it accounts for only a small percentage of cases in hospital series. Human infections caused by *M. pneumoniae* include not only pneumonia but also rhinitis, pharyngitis, and tracheobronchitis. These infection occur throughout the year without apparent seasonality, and some data suggest that epidemics occur every 4 to 8 years. Epidemics begin gradually and may endure for as long as 2 years. Cumulative attack rates in families approach 90%, but only 5 to 10% of those infected develop pneumonia. Pneumonia can develop in persons of any age, but it is most common in persons between the ages of 5 and 20; in fact, *M. pneumoniae* is the leading cause of pneumonia in this age group.

Clinical Features

Mycoplasmal pneumonia generally has a gradual onset with headache, malaise, and low-grade fever. Within a few days a nagging cough becomes a prominent symptom. It is usually nonproductice. Upper respiratory tract symptoms may also be present, and a small percentage of patients may exhibit bullous myringitis. Pleuritic pain, purulent sputum production, and hemoptysis are uncommon. Physical examination usually discloses fever, but chest findings are highly variable, ranging from no abnormalities to evidence of lobar consolidation. About 15% of patients exhibit a maculopapular rash. Laboratory findings are rarely distinctive. About 25% of patients have leukocyte counts exceeding 10,000 cells per μL, and about 5% have counts greater than 15,000. Chest x-ray films most frequently reveal a unilateral, segmental bronchopneumonia, but multiple-lobe involvement and lobar involvement also occur. Pleural effusions when present are usually small.

Extrapulmonary manifestations are uncommon and for the most part involve less than 5% of infected patients. Hematologic complications include hemolytic anemia with immunoglobulin M (IgM) antibody directed against I antigens on erythrocytes. Neurologic manifestations include meningoencephalitis, aseptic meningitis, transverse myelitis, and various neuropathies. Cardiac manifestations include pericarditis, myocarditis, congestive heart failure, hemopericardium, and heart block. Case reports of rare complications, e.g., Stevens-Johnson syndrome, glomerulonephritis, pancreatitis, are also encountered.

Diagnosis

Diagnosis currently rests largely on clinical grounds and remains imprecise, but the occurrence of a mild pneumonia in a young person is certainly suggestive. Although cold agglutinins have often been sought as a diagnostic aid, the low sensitivity and specificity of this test argue against its use. Confirmation of the diagnosis requires either isolation of the bacterium on special media, which is not generally available and requires 2 to 3 weeks to detect growth, or demonstration of seroconversion or four-fold rises in antibody titers using complement fixation or other serologic tests on acute and convalescent serum specimens. Polymerase chain reaction (PCR) techniques, now in development and not yet commercially available, appear to offer the best hope for early diagnosis. These techniques can detect minute quantities of *M. pneumoniae* DNA sequences in respiratory secretions with a high degree of specificity.

Treatment

Mycoplasma pneumoniae infections are usually treated with either erythromycin or tetracycline antibiotics. Both agents have demonstrable activity in susceptibility tests, and both have been demonstrated to reduce the duration of respiratory symptoms and pulmonary infiltrates. The clinical response, however, is rarely dramatic, and neither drug eradicates the carrier state. In adults 2.0 grams of erythromycin base (Ilotycin) or tetracycline hydrochloride (Achromycin) are administered daily in four divided doses. In children the equivalent dose of erythromycin would be 40 mg per kg per day in four divided doses. Tetracyclines should be avoided in children under 9 years of age. Although newer antimicrobial agents, e.g., clarithromycin (Biaxin) and azithromycin (Zithromax), are active in vitro against *M. pneumoniae*, there is insufficient clinical experience at present to recommend their use.

LEGIONELLOSIS
(Legionnaires' Disease and Pontiac Fever)

method of
THOMAS J. MARRIE, M.D.
Dalhousie University
Halifax, Nova Scotia, Canada

Legionellosis refers to two clinical syndromes caused by bacteria from the family Legionellaceae. These two syndromes are pneumonia (legionnaires' disease) and a self-limited, flulike illness (Pontiac fever).

The family Legionellaceae now includes 29 species and more than 49 serogroups. At least 17 members of this family have been implicated in pneumonia; however, *Legionella pneumophila* serogroup 1 accounts for 70 to 90% of these cases. *L. micdadei* (also known as "Pittsburgh pneumonia agent") is the most common of the non-*pneumophila* species of Legionellaceae to cause pneumonia.

L. pneumophila is an aerobic, gram-negative rod that is widely distributed in natural and manufactured water systems. In these systems, *Legionella* is amplified by growth in amebae and ciliated protozoa.

EPIDEMIOLOGY

Legionnaires' disease can be both community- and hospital-acquired and can occur in sporadic, endemic, and epidemic forms.

Exposure to *Legionella pneumophila*–contaminated aerosols (showers, tap-water faucets, cooling towers and evaporative condensers, whirlpool baths, decorative fountains, ultrasonic mist machines) is the prime mode of acquisition for cases of epidemic legionnaires' disease. The disease accounts for about 2% of the cases of community-acquired pneumonia in adults. Risk factors for legionnaires' disease include older age, tobacco smoking, diabetes, cancer, acquired immune deficiency syndrome (AIDS), and end-stage renal disease. There is a markedly elevated risk for persons with AIDS developing legionnaires' disease. The periods of highest risk are the summer months. The rate of nosocomial legionnaires' disease varies considerably, but outbreaks occur from time to time.

Domestic hot water heaters are frequently contaminated with Legionellaceae. The importance of this contamination as a source of sporadic community-acquired legionnaires' disease is currently undergoing investigation.

Risk factors for death from legionnaires' disease include older age, male gender, nosocomial acquisition of disease, immunosuppression, end-stage renal disease, cancer, and infection with *L. pneumophila* serogroup 6.

CLINICAL MANIFESTATIONS

Legionnaires' disease presents as pneumonia that may range from mild to severe overwhelming pneumonia requiring ventilator support. Fever is present in 75% of patients. Contrary to initial descriptions, the cough may be productive, especially in elderly people. Pleuritic chest pain, anorexia, nausea, and vomiting occur in one-third to one-half of patients. Myalgia, chills, and confusion are found in about one-third. Headache or abdominal pain and diarrhea occur in 7 to 20%. Hemoptysis is unusual but occasionally can be present, and the clinical picture of legionnaires' disease in this setting may mimic that of pulmonary infarction. Almost half the patients have the physical findings of consolidation. On occasion, extrapulmonary manifestations may dominate the clinical picture. These include encephalitis, cerebellar ataxia, fulminant diarrhea, hepatitis, rapidly progressive glomerulonephritis, myoglobinuria, myocarditis, pericarditis, prosthetic valve endocarditis, hemodialysis shunt infection, and erythema multiforme.

DIAGNOSIS

Knowledge of the local epidemiology and a high index of suspicion are necessary for diagnosis of legionnaires' disease. This entity should be suspected in all cases of rapidly progressive, community-acquired pneumonia, defined as any two of the following: most of two or more lobes involved by the pneumonia; increase in extent of the opacity by 50% or greater within 48 hours; a respiratory rate of greater than 32 per minute; or shock state due to the pneumonia. Cigarette smoking, chronic lung disease, immunosuppression, and chronic illness are risk factors for this infection. Corticosteroids are the most important immunosuppressive agents predisposing patients to legionnaires' disease.

Onset of pneumonia following travel (exposure to contaminated air conditioning) also suggests legionnaires' disease. However, even a trip to the local grocery store (exposure to a contaminated ultrasonic mist machine) can be the source.

Despite the foregoing clues, the diagnosis cannot be made on clinical grounds and has to be confirmed by the laboratory. The organism can be grown from sputum; however, this takes 3 to 5 days. The direct fluorescent antibody test for detecting the organism in sputum has a sensitivity of 25 to 75% and a specificity of 95 to 99%. A radioimmunoassay is available for detecting *L. pneumophila* serogroup 1 antigen in urine. This test is 80 to 99% sensitive and 99% specific. The antigen may persist in the urine for days to weeks, even after initiation of specific therapy. The major drawback to this test is that it detects only disease caused by *L. pneumophila* serogroup 1.

Diagnosis also may be confirmed by testing acute serum samples and 6- to 9-week convalescent serum samples for a four-fold rise in antibodies to *Legionella*.

TREATMENT

Choice and route of therapy depend on the severity of illness of the patient. For patients seriously ill with confirmed or suspected legionnaires' disease, I start treatment with erythromycin, 1 gm intravenously every 6 hours. In addition, I add rifampin (Rifadin), 300 mg orally every 12 hours. Once there has been definite clinical improvement, the rifampin can be discontinued and the erythromycin given orally in a dose of 500 mg every 6 hours. Total duration of therapy should be at least 21 days, since relapses occur with durations shorter than this. High-dose erythromycin can result in temporary hearing loss.

If erythromycin and rifampin cannot be given, my second choice is doxycycline (Vibramycin), 200 mg every 12 hours for two doses, then 200 mg once daily intravenously. Other options for therapy include ciprofloxacin (Cipro), 400 mg every 12 hours intravenously or 750 mg every 12 hours orally. Trimethoprim-sulfamethoxazole (Bactrim, Septra), 5 mg of the trimethoprim component per kg every 8 hours also has been used, usually in conjunction with rifampin; however, there have been reports of failure of therapy with trimethoprim-sulfamethoxazole alone for legionnaires' disease in patients with AIDS.

A newer macrolide, clarithromycin (Biaxin), at a dose of 500 to 1000 mg every 12 hours orally, also has been effective in the treatment of legionnaires' disease.

PREVENTION

If nosocomial legionnaires' disease is identified, the hospital's water distribution should be cultured for *Legionella*. If *Legionella* is found, a variety of methods are used for eliminating it from the distribution system. These include (1) heating the water to about 70°C (160°F) for several days and then flushing the hot water through all the outlets, (2) hyperchlorinating the water, or (3) adding copper and silver ions to the water supply. If Legionellaceae cannot be eradicated from the water supply, all organ transplant recipients and all patients who are receiving corticosteroids should not drink the water or shower with it.

PULMONARY EMBOLISM

method of
WILLIAM D. HAIRE, M.D.
University of Nebraska Medical Center
Omaha, Nebraska

Pulmonary embolism (PE) is a major public health problem for two basic reasons: (1) it is a common occurrence, affecting 300,000 patients annually in North America alone, and (2) once it occurs it is often fatal. Untreated, the mortality rate of PE is estimated at 30%. With current standard treatment the mortality rate is approximately 8% and is significantly higher in the subgroup of patients with major co-morbidities, especially underlying cardiopulmonary disease. In addition to these difficulties, PE poses another major problem to the clinician: the difficulty of diagnosis. Presenting signs and symptoms are nonspecific, and diagnostic tests either have limited specificity or are invasive, expensive, and not readily available. Because of its high frequency, difficulty in detection, and high mortality, the best way to deal with PE is to prevent it.

PROPHYLAXIS

PE is a one component of a larger group of disorders termed "venous thromboembolism" (VT). VT generally begins with thrombosis of one or more veins, usually the deep veins of the legs. Consequently, methods of preventing PE are directed at preventing deep vein thrombosis (DVT) in the legs. A key component of prophylaxis of VT is the ability to predict its occurrence. This is accomplished by understanding the factors that put a patient at risk for VT (Table 1). In addition to those listed in Table 1, perhaps the strongest risk factor for future VT is a past history of VT. These risk factors are felt to be

TABLE 1. **Risk Factors for Venous Thromboembolism**

Exogenous Risk Factors

Inflammation, due to the effects of
  Surgery
  Trauma
  Infection
  Malignancy
  Diseases such as Crohn's disease, ulcerative colitis, or systemic
    lupus erythematosus
Medications, such as
  Estrogens
  Cancer chemotherapy
Direct venous trauma, such as encountered in hip and knee
  arthroplasty

Endogenous Risk Factors

Advanced age
Obesity
Pregnancy
Immobility or vascular stasis
Abnormalities of the natural anticoagulant or fibrinolytic
  systems—both congenital and acquired

additive in individual patients, i.e., patients with several of these abnormalities are at higher risk of VT than those with only a few.

Many of the risk factors for VT are transient (see Table 1). Consequently, thromboprophylactic maneuvers often are required for the limited periods of time during which the patient is at unusually high risk of VT. There are two basic methods of prophylaxis: (1) pharmacologic, usually with heparin or warfarin, and (2) mechanical, usually accomplished with external pneumatic compression of the calves. Standard heparin at a dose of 5000 U given subcutaneously every 12 hours is effective prophylaxis in low-risk medical and surgical patients (those with one or two risk factors). For patients with intermediate risk of VT, such as knee or hip arthroplasty in older patients, standard heparin given in doses adjusted to prolong the partial thromboplastin time (PTT); warfarin in doses adjusted to prolong the prothrombin time to an international normalized ratio (INR) of 2.0 to 3.0; or low-molecular-weight heparin in fixed doses (in the United States, enoxaparin 30 mg subcutaneously every 12 hours) are required. For knee arthroplasty, low-molecular-weight heparin is preferred. For patients falling into either the low- or the intermediate-risk group, external pneumatic compression can be effectively substituted. This is especially helpful in patients with a significant risk of bleeding, such as neurosurgical patients or those with multisystem trauma. For patients at high risk of VT (those with four or more risk factors *or* a history of VT plus one other risk factor), it is generally felt that a single mode of thromboprophylaxis is inadequate. In these patients combining external pneumatic compression with a pharmacologic agent (often low-molecular-weight heparin) is recommended during the postoperative period (7 to 10 days).

DIAGNOSIS

The presenting signs and symptoms of PE are manifold and nonspecific. PE can mimic a variety of cardiac, pulmonary, and other disorders (Table 2). Consequently, *a high degree of clinical suspicion cannot be overestimated* as a prerequisite for making the diagnosis. The clinician who does not think of PE rarely diagnoses PE! This diagnosis should be suspected in any patient with new cardiopulmonary symptoms or signs, regardless of their underlying disease process.

Once the diagnosis of PE has been considered, other tests must be done to confirm the diagnosis and/or exclude other diagnostic possibilities. Chest x-ray and electrocardiographic examination are done initially to eliminate the possibilities of pneumothorax, pericarditis, and acute myocardial ischemia. After that, ventilation/perfusion lung scans have classically been the first diagnostic test ordered to specifically evaluate for the presence of PE. Unfortunately, although a normal lung scan virtually eliminates any possibility of PE, abnormalities are generally not specific. Scans read as "high probability"

TABLE 2. **Disorders That Can Mimic Acute Pulmonary Embolism**

Cardiac Disease

Acute myocardial infarction
Acute pericarditis
Aortic dissection
Papillary muscle rupture

Pulmonary Disease

Pneumothorax
Pleuritis, infectious or sterile
Lung cancer
Pneumonia
Bronchitis
Exacerbation of chronic obstructive pulmonary disease
Acute asthma

Other

Sepsis
Varicella-zoster infection of a chest dermatome
Esophageal spasm or rupture
Chest wall pain
Acute anxiety or psychosis
Hyperventilation syndrome

represent PE almost 90% of the time. However, "high probability" scans are rare—seen in less than 15% of all patients with PE. Scans falling between "normal" and "high probability" have a 15 to 50% probability of representing a PE and are not particularly helpful in making or excluding the diagnosis. In addition to the relatively low sensitivity and specificity, lung scans are relatively expensive. Despite these drawbacks, lung scans are widely available and are occasionally helpful in either making or excluding the diagnosis of PE. Consequently, they remain the first test used to evaluate for PE.

The approach to the patients who might have a PE but whose scan is neither "normal" nor "high probability" is not standardized. A recommended approach is outlined in Figure 1. This algorithm is based on two observations. The first is that most PEs are fragments of thrombi that have formed in the deep veins of the legs. Consequently, patients with evidence of DVT in the leg who have symptoms of PE are highly likely to really have PE. In patients with suspected PE who have non–high-probability scans, ultrasound examination of the leg veins looking for DVT is recommended. If evidence of DVT is found, therapy for both DVT *and* PE can begin. The second observation is based on the fact that D dimer is the end product of cross-linked fibrin dissolution. Patients who have formed a significant amount of fibrin ultimately have fibrin dissolution and, consequently, have elevated levels of D dimer. Therefore, high levels of D dimer suggest the formation of significant amounts of fibrin-based thrombus. The converse of this observation is relevant to the diagnosis of PE: patients with *normal* levels of D dimer have *not* formed abnormal amounts of fibrin-based thrombi and, consequently, cannot be suffering from pulmonary thromboemboli. This premise has been supported by clinical research showing that approximately 90% of patients suspected of having PE but whose D dimer levels were normal were found not to

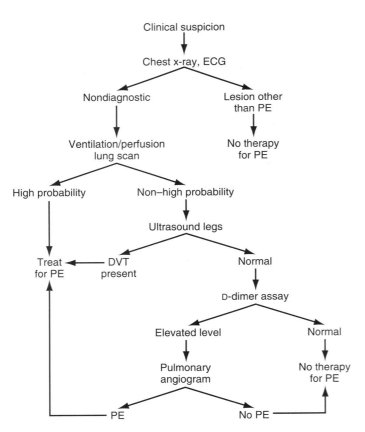

Figure 1. Diagnostic algorithm for pulmonary embolism (PE). *Abbreviations*: ECG = electrocardiogram; DVT = deep vein thrombosis.

have PE on subsequent pulmonary angiograms. For patients with indeterminate lung scans in whom ultrasound shows no evidence of DVT, normal levels of D dimer strongly suggest that the patient does not have PE. Consequently, withholding therapy for PE is reasonable. A variety of simple D dimer assays are commercially available for clinical use, and many, though not all, are appropriate for use in this setting. In patients with suspected PE with indeterminate lung scans, no ultrasound evidence of DVT and elevated levels of D dimer, a pulmonary angiogram is the only way to reliably make or exclude the diagnosis. Recent studies have suggested, however, that treatment of these patients can be withheld without proceeding to angiography *if* they do not have impaired cardiopulmonary reserve (no hypotension, tachycardia, hypoxia) *and* they are willing to be followed with serial noninvasive venous studies for the subsequent 2 weeks. For patients with impaired cardiopulmonary function at time of presentation, proceeding to angiography and providing definitive therapy for PE if found is strongly recommended.

THERAPY

Acute therapy for PE falls into three basic types: (1) anticoagulant, (2) fibrinolytic, and (3) mechanical. These therapies all have different mechanisms of action and differing outcome goals. The degree to which each of these treatments' goals are required in any given patient determines which is the most appropriate therapy for that patient (Figure 2).

Anticoagulation is the most common form of therapy. It is intended to improve patient outcomes by limiting the growth of the embolized thrombus and prevent re-embolization by inhibiting coagulation and preventing new clot deposition. This form of therapy allows the naturally occurring fibrinolytic system to eventually remove the thrombus and is generally accomplished with standard heparin. Heparin is most likely to be effective if given as an initial intravenous bolus followed by a continuous intravenous infusion, though it can be given subcutaneously in patients with limited venous access. The goal is to achieve a level of heparin in the blood that causes a significant prolongation of the PTT very soon after hospitalization. This is best accomplished if heparin dosage and PTT monitoring are done by adhering to a protocol designed with this goal in mind (Table 3). The dose of heparin is escalated to a maximum of approximately 25 U per kg per hour. If given subcutaneously, the starting dose of heparin is 17,500 U given every 12 hours. The dose is adjusted to keep the PTT in the 45- to 70-second range when tested 6 hours after the morning dose of heparin. Once the patient is clinically stable, warfarin at a dose of 5 to 10 mg daily is begun. In many patients, warfarin can be started shortly after an adequate dose of heparin has been achieved. The heparin is continued until the patient's prothrombin time has been prolonged to an INR of 2.0 to 3.0 for two consecutive days or the heparin and warfarin have been given concurrently for 5 days, *whichever is longer*. A therapeutic degree of anticoagulation cannot be

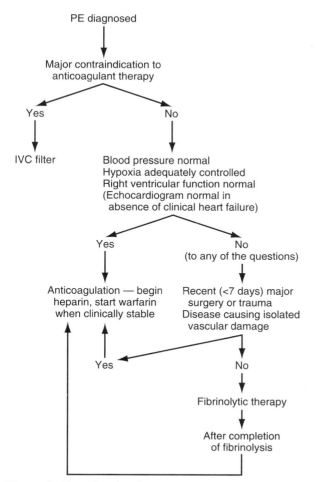

Figure 2. Algorithm for choosing treatment for PE. *Abbreviation*: IVC = inferior vena cava.

achieved with less than 5 days of warfarin therapy, *independent of the degree of prolongation of the prothrombin time.*

The two major complications of heparin anticoagulation are bleeding and thrombocytopenia with thrombosis. The greatest determinants of bleeding are the number of co-morbid conditions and the total daily dose of heparin. The first can be estimated

TABLE 3. Intravenous Heparin Dose Titration Nomogram

PTT	Dose	Repeat PTT
Baseline	80 U/kg bolus, then 18 U/kg/h	4–6 h
<35 s	80 U/kg bolus, then increase by 4 U/kg/h	4–6 h
35–45 s	40 U/kg bolus, then increase by 2 U/kg/h	4–6 h
36–70 s	No change	Next morning
71–90 s	Decrease by 2 U/kg/h	Next morning
>90 s	Stop for 1 h, decrease by 3 U/kg/h	6 h

Abbreviation: PTT = partial thromboplastin time.
Adapted from Raschke RA, Reilly BM, Guidry JR, et al: The weight-based heparin dosing nomogram compared with a "standard care" nomogram. Ann Intern Med *119*:874, 1993.

by the patient's functional status. Patients who are sufficiently ill to be confined to bed are at significantly higher risk of bleeding than those with a normal functional status. Heparin dose escalation should be done more cautiously in patients with numerous concomitant medical problems, and they should be monitored more closely for bleeding complications. Heparin-induced thrombocytopenia is an idiosyncratic reaction occurring in approximately 3% of patients. The thrombocytopenia is caused by the development of antibodies that react with platelets in the presence of heparin, causing the platelets to aggregate in the vascular space. These aggregates serve as a nidus for the growth of larger thrombi. These thrombi often grow sufficiently large to occlude major arteries and veins, with disastrous consequences (stroke, myocardial infarction, acute limb ischemia). This complication is heralded by a rapid drop in the platelet count and the occurrence of symptoms of thrombosis while the patient is on heparin. If this occurs, the *heparin therapy must be stopped* and alternative therapy for PE instituted.

The goal of fibrinolytic therapy is different from that of anticoagulant therapy. Although anticoagulation prevents thrombi from enlarging and embolizing, it does nothing to remove the thrombi causing the patient's symptoms. Fibrinolytic therapy is directed at removing the thrombus and rapidly improving the patient's cardiopulmonary function by minimizing the degree of obstruction of the pulmonary vasculature. Fibrinolytic therapy is reserved for patients with significant clinical problems caused by obstruction to right ventricular outflow such as hypotension, right ventricular failure (manifesting clinically or as hypokinesis on echocardiography), or hypoxia not readily reversed with supplemental oxygen. These patients can be treated with either streptokinase, urokinase, or recombinant tissue plasminogen activator (Table 4). For rapid restoration of cardiopulmonary function, the 2-hour infusions of either urokinase or recombinant tissue plasminogen activator are recommended. Bleeding complications are likely to occur in patients with incompletely healed vascular injury. Consequently, fibrinolytic therapy is relatively contraindicated in patients for approximately 7 days after trauma or surgery or in patients with diseases such as cancer or gastrointestinal ulcer-

TABLE 4. Drugs Available for Fibrinolytic Therapy of Pulmonary Embolism

Drug	Dose
Streptokinase (Kabikinase, Streptase)	250,000 U over 30 min followed by 100,000 U/h for 12–24 h*
Urokinase (Abbokinase)	4400 U/kg over 30 min followed by 4400 U/kg hourly for 12 h*, *or* 3 million U over 2 h
Recombinant tissue plasminogen activator (Activase)	100 mg over 2 h*

*FDA-approved.

ation, who have injured vessels in isolated anatomic areas. Fibrinolytic therapy does not take the place of anticoagulation. After the thrombus has been removed with the fibrinolytic agent, heparin and warfarin therapy must be used to prevent it from recurring. Heparin therapy can be started shortly after fibrinolysis is completed, but without the use of a bolus dose.

PE is treated mechanically by placing a filter in the inferior vena cava (IVC). The goal of this type of therapy is to prevent large, possibly fatal, thromboemboli from reaching the pulmonary circulation. This treatment is *not* designed to prevent extension of the DVT from which the original embolus came or to prevent small emboli from occurring. Worsening symptoms of DVT owing to its enlargement caused by lack of anticoagulant therapy often occurs if IVC filter placement is the only treatment given. Consequently, IVC filters are recommended as sole treatment only in patients with *major* contraindications to anticoagulation, such as active bleeding, recent major surgery or trauma, or an intracranial lesion that is likely to bleed during anticoagulant therapy. If the contraindication to anticoagulation resolves (the patient recovers 7 to 10 days from surgery or trauma, the hemorrhagic gastritis heals) adding anticoagulation to the IVC filter is recommended.

Chronic therapy for PE is generally directed at preventing recurrent VT by limiting the rate of activation of the hemostatic system with warfarin. Warfarin should be given in doses sufficient to prolong the prothrombin time to an INR of 2.0 to 3.0 until the risk of recurrence of VT is minimal. In patients whose risk of VT was due to transient abnormalities, such as the postoperative state, pregnancy, or immobilization, 3 to 6 months of treatment is generally adequate. For patients with more persistent risk factors for VT, such as protein C deficiency, anticardiolipin antibody syndrome, or cancer, more prolonged anticoagulation (often indefinite) is reasonable.

SARCOIDOSIS

method of
J. MICHAEL FULLER, M.D., and
JACK D. FULMER, M.D.
University of Alabama at Birmingham
Birmingham, Alabama

Sarcoidosis is a multisystem disease of unknown etiology, most commonly affecting young adults and presenting most frequently with bilateral hilar adenopathy, pulmonary infiltration, and skin or eye lesions. This disease is diagnosed by typical clinical and roentgenographic features, as well as the histologic presence of noncaseating granulomas in multiple organs. Sarcoidosis has a worldwide distribution but appears to be more prevalent in certain geographic areas and certain races. In America, there is a predilection for female African Americans.

Current concepts of the pathogenesis of sarcoidosis are that there is some type of unidentified stimulus that in a susceptible individual activates and recruits macrophages and lymphocytes into target organs. Macrophages differentiate into epithelioid and giant cells, and there is a clonal proliferation of T helper lymphocytes (CD4+). Primitive mesenchymal cells are recruited and differentiate into collagen-producing fibroblasts, forming typical granulomas. If this granulomatous process is unchecked, there is tissue destruction, revision of organ architecture, and ultimately fibrosis and loss of organ function.

CLINICAL MANIFESTATIONS

Intrathoracic Involvement

The most common presentation of sarcoidosis is intrathoracic involvement. Whereas lung parenchyma and lymph nodes are major sites of intrathoracic disease, endobronchial involvement is common, ranging from submucosal granulomas to total airway obstruction. The chest roentgenograms of patients with sarcoidosis are, by convention, grouped according to the following scheme: Stage 0, normal; Stage I, bilateral hilar adenopathy; Stage II, hilar adenopathy with diffuse parenchymal involvement; and Stage III, diffuse parenchymal involvement without hilar adenopathy. Some clinicians use another grouping, Stage IV, which is characterized by diffuse infiltration, fibrosis, and upper lobe cystic and bullous disease. These bullous or cystic lesions are sometimes colonized by *Aspergillus fumigatus,* which forms mycetomas. There are roentgenographic patterns that do not fit this grouping. Nodular sarcoidosis is characterized by large nodular lesions simulating metastatic disease. In comparison, alveolar sarcoidosis is characterized by diffuse airspace disease. These two latter roentgenographic patterns are uncommon.

Extrapulmonary Involvement

Extrapulmonary sarcoidosis may present as isolated disease but more often is associated with thoracic disease. Virtually every organ can be involved. Cutaneous involvement is common and offers an acceptable site for biopsy. Several common forms of cutaneous sarcoidosis are erythema nodosum, lupus pernio, and granulomatous infiltration of old scars.

Ophthalmic sarcoidosis may include involvement of conjunctiva, lacrimal glands, uveal tracts, and retina or retinal vessels. An early diagnosis is mandatory to prevent blindness, and the ophthalmologist is uniquely positioned to obtain tissue for diagnosis and to treat the disease.

Cardiac sarcoidosis, previously thought to be rare, is common. Heart failure, heart block, arrhythmias, and sudden death are some of the modes of presentation. However, many patients have asymptomatic, transient, electrocardiographic abnormalities. Early diagnosis and treatment is critical to prevent complications.

Neurosarcoidosis is an uncommon, but potentially devastating, form of sarcoidosis. While any part of the nervous system can be affected, cranial and peripheral nerve involvement is the most common. Facial paresis from involvement of cranial nerve VII can be unilateral or bilateral. The pattern of peripheral nerve involvement is that of a mononeuritis multiplex. Central nervous system lesions can range from masses to meningeal involvement; the hypothalamus and pituitary gland may also be involved. Granulomatous involvement of vasculature can result in vascular insufficiency and cerebral vascular accidents.

SPECIAL SITUATIONS

Pregnancy in Sarcoidosis

Sarcoidosis has no apparent effect on the course of pregnancy. In contrast, pregnancy improves the clinical manifestations of sarcoidosis in some patients. On delivery, however, the disease may worsen.

Sarcoidosis and Autoimmunity

Sarcoidosis has been considered an autoimmune disease. However, data to support this concept are weak. There are recent reports of antibody-mediated thrombocytopenia, which responds to treatment.

Sarcoidosis and Human Immunodeficiency Virus Infection

There are isolated reports of sarcoidosis in cases of human immunodeficiency virus (HIV) infection. This is of great interest since the alveolitis of sarcoidosis is characterized by excessive T helper lymphocytes (CD4+). Limited data are available on lung lavage cellular analysis in these cases, but there appear to be low numbers of T helper lymphocytes, causing confusion on the role of these cells in the pathogenesis of sarcoidosis. Reported cases of sarcoidosis in HIV-positive patients appear to have responded to treatment.

Sarcoidosis and Transplantation

Transplantation is a viable alternative for patients with end-stage lung, cardiac, or renal disease. There have, however, been reported cases of recurrent sarcoidosis in the allograft of both heart and lung recipients. The incidence of recurrence is unknown, but cases have responded to treatment.

DIAGNOSIS AND TREATMENT OF SARCOIDOSIS

Sarcoidosis can be easily diagnosed in patients who have the typical clinical presentation and tissue showing noncaseating granulomas, with negative special stains and cultures for fungi, bacteria, and protozoa. The clinician should be aware of local microbes that can mimic sarcoidosis and exclude these. Clinicians must also be aware that lymphatic tissue draining gastrointestinal malignancies, and malignancies of other organ systems, may develop noncaseating granulomas. Adjunctive laboratory studies that may add supporting evidence to the clinical diagnosis of sarcoidosis include an elevation of the serum angiotensin-converting enzyme (ACE) level, a positive gallium 67 scan, and bronchoalveolar lavage lymphocytosis. Abnormalities in these studies may also be present in diseases that mimic sarcoidosis. Hypercalcemia is present in 30% of patients.

Sarcoidosis has a protean course; some cases are progressive while others remit spontaneously. For this reason, it would be helpful to find an indicator of the stage or activity of the disease. Serum ACE levels, gallium 67 scanning, and analysis of bronchoalveolar lavage lymphocyte counts have all been studied, but none reliably stage or predict the natural history or treatment response of sarcoidosis. Currently, clinical assessment and examination and the use of appropriate imaging and functional studies, such as routine chest roentgenograms and pulmonary function tests, are the best means to assess and monitor sarcoidosis. Studies of the use of high-resolution computerized chest tomography in pulmonary sarcoidosis are under way, but further investigation must be done before this technology can be accepted.

Corticosteroids are the mainstay for the treatment of sarcoidosis. Virtually every organ can be involved and at some point may require treatment. In general, however, patients with Stage I sarcoidosis and nodular sarcoidosis do not require treatment, unless there is endobronchial sarcoidosis with obstruction. Often these patients have chest pain, arthralgias, and fever that respond well to nonsteroidal anti-inflammatory drugs. Stages II and III disease should be treated if there is evidence of progression. Prednisone at a dosage of 30 to 40 mg daily in a single dose is usually adequate. After a period of 6 to 8 weeks, the dosage is reduced to a maintenance level of 10 to 15 mg daily over a period of 6 months. If the disease stabilizes or improves, then prednisone is gradually stopped. Relapses are common, however, and repeat treatment may be needed. Recently, inhaled steroids have been used with some success. Patients with extensive pulmonary fibrosis with bullous or cystic disease should not ordinarily be treated with corticosteroids. Hemoptysis, a major complication of those who have mycetomas, can be managed with bronchial artery embolization. However, if ventilatory reserve is adequate, surgery is indicated for massive hemoptysis. Itraconazole has been used, but its efficacy is not established. The management of airway distortion is empirical; bronchodilators may help with excessive secretions, and broad-spectrum antibiotics may improve bronchitis.

Uncommonly, pulmonary sarcoidosis may be aggressive, not responding to conventional doses of corticosteroids. The initial approach is to augment the prednisone dosage to 60 to 100 mg per day. If it is clear that the patient's disease is steroid-resistant, then immunosuppressive or cytotoxic agents are used. Methotrexate at a dosage of 5 to 10 mg weekly is a reasonable second-line drug. The white blood cell count should be monitored and not allowed to go below 3000 to 3500. Other drugs that have been used include cyclophosphamide (Cytoxan),* azathioprine (Imuran),* and cyclosporin A (Sandimmune).* Chloroquine (Aralen)* appears to be the drug of choice for refractory skin disease but has also been used successfully in steroid-resistant pulmonary sarcoidosis.

Eye examinations should be part of the routine care of sarcoidosis patients. If ophthalmic involvement is present, a qualified ophthalmologist should direct the treatment.

Myocardial sarcoidosis must be contemplated

---

*Not FDA-approved for this indication.

when considering cardiac disease with appropriate symptoms, sex, and race. Confirmation may, however, be difficult. The combination of thallium 201 and gallium 67 radionuclide cardiac scans with normal coronary artery arteriography provides the best diagnostic approach. Cardiac biopsy is desirable but has a low yield. Treatment is best accomplished with high-dose prednisone, 60 to 80 mg per day. Cases unresponsive to corticosteroids may benefit from methotrexate or the combination of methotrexate and corticosteroids. Heart block should be treated with a pacemaker.

Neurosarcoidosis is often difficult to diagnose and manage. Multisystem sarcoidosis allows early entertainment of the diagnosis, which may be supported by data from lumbar puncture and magnetic resonance imaging or computerized tomography. However, the diagnosis of isolated central nervous system sarcoidosis may be far more challenging and may require biopsy. Central nervous system or cord sarcoidosis is treated with high-dose corticosteroids (60 to 80 mg daily) but may be quite refractory. Cerebral or cord irradiation has been used with some success. Cranial nerve involvement is, by contrast, much easier to diagnose. The prognosis for cranial nerve sarcoidosis is good; often no treatment is needed.

Preventive and palliative measures are important in managing pulmonary sarcoidosis. The structural changes constitute a significant host defense problem, and bacterial pneumonias may be a cause of death. Influenza and pneumococcal vaccines are recommended, and acute bacterial bronchitis should be treated. Some patients develop reversible airway obstruction, which should also be treated with bronchodilators. Supplemental oxygen is recommended for patients who have an arterial oxygen tension less than 55 mmHg at rest or during exercise. Advanced sarcoidosis can develop recurrent pneumothoraces, which may require chemical pleurodesis. Finally, transplantation may be the only alternative treatment for some with end-stage organ involvement. Successful transplantation for myocardial disease, pulmonary disease, and renal disease has been reported. Limited data are available, but most of these patients do well.

SILICOSIS

method of
RAYMOND BÉGIN, M.D.
CHU de Sherbrooke
Sherbrooke, Québec, Canada

and

GASTON OSTIGUY, M.D.
Hôpital Maisonneuve-Rosemont
Montréal, Québec, Canada

Silicosis is a mineral dust pneumoconiosis caused by inhalation and excessive retention of free or crystalline silica generating a pathologic tissue reaction. In spite of vastly improved industrial hygiene regulations, the incidence is still approximately 10 cases per 1 million males in developed countries. In North America, 2 to 3% of the male population is occupationally exposed to silica, but the exact prevalence of silicosis is unknown.

The earth's crust is composed mainly of silicon and silicate. They constitute the bulk of most kinds of rocks, soils, clays, and sands. Silicon occurs as silica (SiO_2), also known as free silica, and as combined silica or silicates. The three forms of free silica are crystalline, amorphous, and cryptocrystalline. The main forms of crystalline silica are quartz, tridymite, and crystobalite, which are responsible for the pathogenesis of silicosis. The silica content of various rocks such as sandstone, granite, or slate varies. Occupational exposure to silica particles of respirable size (0.5 to 5 μm in diameter) is associated with various types of work such as mining; quarrying and tunneling; stonecutting; engraving and polishing; glass and ceramic manufacturing; the use of silica-containing abrasives and fillers; foundry work; manufacturing of ceramics and refractories; sandblasting; grinding; and pottery manufacturing.

The pathogenesis of silicosis is as follows: the surface of quartz particles is hydrated to form silanol groups, and these react with phospholipids of cell membranes and produce free radicals (particularly at the surface of freshly fractured particles), inducing peroxidative changes in the cell membranes. (These surface properties of silica can be altered by surface coating, rendering the particles inactive.) Silica is initially rapidly ingested by alveolar macrophages, which are activated to release cytokines that have chemotactic activity for macrophages, lymphocytes, and neutrophils and activate these cells at the site of tissue injury. (Affected macrophages may be impaired in their ability to defend against *Mycobacterium tuberculosis* and *Nocardia asteroides* infection.) Hypertrophy, hyperplasia, and activation of Type II pneumocytes also occur, producing excessive amounts of surfactant-related substances found in the silicotic nodules (see later). Fibroblast growth factors are also released to sustain a chronic fibrosing activity. Following these events, the lung initiates an alveolitis, which if sustained—and depending on the amount of dust retained, its constituents, the duration of exposure, and individual susceptibility—can evolve into the fundamental lesion of silicosis, the silicotic nodule.

The silicotic nodule is pathologically a hyaline nodule containing a central acellular zone incorporating free silica, surrounded by whorls of collagen, fibronectin, lipids, and fibroblasts, and an active outer zone of macrophages, fibroblasts, plasma cells, and free silica. The silicotic nodule is initially well separated from the surrounding lung tissue. The nodules are located predominantly in the subpleural areas of the lungs and are associated with variable amounts of fibrosis, hypertrophy, and hyperplasia of the Type II pneumocytes. With progression of the disease, confluence of the disease process, dense fibrosis, and associated paracicatricial emphysema appear.

CLINICAL FORMS OF DISEASE

Simple (Chronic) Silicosis

The most common presentation of silicosis is in its simple form. This is seen in workers with long-term (15 to 20 years) and relatively low intensity exposure to silica dust. Simple silicosis is recognized on routine chest radiographs. It is characterized by small (less than 10 mm) round nonconfluent opacities seen either predominantly in the upper lung fields or more diffusely. At this simple stage of disease, the worker is usually asymptomatic and the pulmonary function tests are normal, although mild reduction in diffusion capacity and airflow limitation may be seen. The disease may remain in its simple form in 70 to 80% of cases but progresses to confluent silicosis in others. The intensity and duration of exposure appear to influence the outcome.

Confluent Silicosis

In confluent silicosis (also called "complicated silicosis" or "progressive massive fibrosis"), confluence is the result of progression of the interstitial fibrosis; fusion or coalescence of adjacent silicotic nodules; and fibrosis to form large masses of disease, surrounded by adjacent paracicatricial emphysema in the most severe form. Progression is almost the rule in this form of silicosis. The patient often has exercise dyspnea and nonproductive cough. Radiographically, the nodular opacities may be more than 10 mm. More specifically, the opacities become confluent, and larger masses of dense opacity are seen, with reduced amounts of nodules and rarefaction of the vascular markings around these large opacities. The lung function is now altered, reflecting a reduction in lung volumes, diffusion capacity, and airflow and giving a mixed pattern of restrictive and obstructive change. Distortion of the bronchial tree can be seen at bronchoscopy. Although cough is usually nonproductive, productive cough is often present and signals chronic bronchitis, recurrent bacterial infection, and occasionally bronchiectasis. Weight loss and cavitation of the large masses may prompt consideration of avascular necrosis or tuberculosis. Pneumothorax due to difficult expansion of fibrotic lung tissues can be a life-threatening complication. Hypoxia and pulmonary hypertension lead to end-stage cor pulmonale and respiratory failure, a common terminal event.

Acute Silicoproteinosis

Acute silicoproteinosis, an uncommon form of silicosis, is a rapidly progressive and fatal disease developing after massive high-intensity silica exposure of short duration. This occurs in unprotected and/or confined sandblasting work, silica flour work, or ceramic work. The disease becomes manifest as severe dyspnea, generalized weakness, and weight loss. The radiograph shows diffuse ground glass–like infiltrates, reflecting the alveolar fillings by acellular surfactant-like materials; some sparse poorly demarcated silicotic nodules; interstitial fibrosing pneumonitis; and occasionally poorly formed loose granulomas, resembling those of sarcoidosis. In this form of silicosis, extrapulmonary manifestations can be seen in the liver and kidneys. Rapid progression to respiratory failure is the course.

Accelerated Silicosis

Accelerated silicosis has an intermediate rate of progression between that of simple silicosis and that of acute silicoproteinosis. It usually appears after 5 to 10 years of silica exposure of high intensity, with inappropriate protection, often in sandblasters. Dyspnea and cough usually bring the worker to the physician. The nodular infiltrates are dense with some confluence at initial radiography. Lung functions are altered as in the complicated form. Pathologically, the disease has features of simple and confluent silicosis. Progression is the rule, autoimmune associated diseases are frequent, and tuberculosis is seen in

up to 25% of cases. The disease is usually fatal within 10 years.

End-Stage Silicosis

In end-stage silicosis, patients have advanced lung infiltrations, confluence, airway distortion and emphysematous changes, severe deterioration of lung functions, and cor pulmonale. Medical interventions are most needed. Problems of shortness of breath; productive or dry cough; hemoptysis secondary to avascular necrosis of confluent silicosis or rheumatoid nodules; active tuberculosis; acute bronchitis; pneumonia, often anaerobic; lung cancer; and chronic cor pulmonale call for careful investigation and appropriate therapy.

Silicosis and Autoimmune Diseases

SEROLOGIC FACTORS. Exposure to silica is associated with immunologic phenomena such as an increased incidence of positive rheumatoid factor in up to 25% of patients, increased incidence of antinuclear factor, and increased levels of immunoglobulins.

SCLERODERMA. In the absence of radiographic silicosis, a definitely increased incidence of scleroderma has been reported in persons with more than 3 years of exposure, high intensity of exposure being a contributor. In case reports the incidence of other autoimmune disorders has been reported to have been increased in the absence of silicosis, but without convincing studies.

RHEUMATOID SILICOTIC NODULES AND ARTHRITIS. The rheumatoid nodules in silicosis are not as frequent as in coal workers' pneumoconiosis but have been seen pathologically in up to 2% of cases. These are recognized as one or a few irregularly located nodules larger than the usual silicotic nodules and with a paler or necrotic center, associated with overt rheumatoid arthritis and/or a positive rheumatoid factor. Systemic rheumatoid arthritis is of variable severity and is definitely associated with silicosis. Rheumatoid arthritis, but not a positive rheumatoid factor alone, is associated with faster progression of silicosis.

SILICOSIS AND TUBERCULOSIS

Patients with silicosis are at greater risk of tuberculosis, particularly those with any but the simple form, which has been associated with a macrophage dysfunction in the lower respiratory tract. Atypical mycobacteria are at times recovered from sputum of silicotic patients. If these nontuberculous mycobacteria (*M. avium-intracellularis* or *M. kansasii*) are causing symptoms, loss of function, and radiographic changes, multiple drug treatment is indicated.

SILICOSIS AND LUNG CANCER

Silicosis is likely associated with an increased incidence of lung cancer, which may not be true for silica exposure alone. According to the International Agency for Research on Cancer (IARC), there is limited evidence for the carcinogenicity of crystalline silica to humans. In the absence of silicosis, the standard mortality ratio (SMR) for lung cancer is not increased, but in the presence of silicosis, SMRs of two to six times normal have been reported. These findings are not fully accepted, given that it is difficult to dissociate the effects of smoking and chronic obstructive lung disease and that several studies are based on Workers' Compensation Board data.

COMPLICATIONS

Tuberculosis remains today the most prevalent, difficult, and serious complication of silicosis. Fungal colonization of a cavity, an aspergilloma with positive, circulating precipitating antibody to *Aspergillus,* may be the cause of recurrent hemoptysis. Acute and chronic bronchitis, and segmental atelectasis, are associated with confluent silicosis in distorting the airways or with airway compression by adjacent nodes (middle lobe collapse). Enlarged silicotic lymph nodes may cause irreversible paralysis of the left recurrent laryngeal nerve and dysphagia associated with esophageal compression. An acute glomerulonephritis similar to that from heavy metal exposure has been associated with acute silicosis.

MEDICAL INTERVENTIONS

Prevention

Prevention remains the cornerstone of eliminating silicosis. This is done through legislative regulation of hygiene at work places; education of workers on the risks of their jobs; and control of the silica dust level by ventilation and exhaust systems, process enclosures, and personal protection with appropriate respirators. The recognition of new cases of silicosis should be reported to state or federal agencies (the National Institute of Occupational Safety and Health, for instance, at 1-800-35-NIOSH) to obtain work place evaluation and thus help other workers at risk.

Treatments

For silicosis prevention, the inhalation of aerosolized aluminum or other silica surface–coating compounds has been successful in experimental animal settings before but not after radiographic silicosis. In human situations, such practices are unacceptable. To date, the search for a specific therapy has been unrewarding.

In bronchial complications of silicosis, treatments to relieve bronchospasm, cough, and infection are similar to those of other chronic airway diseases. For bronchospasm, oral theophylline therapy to blood levels between 10 and 20 μg per mL and inhaled bronchodilators at the usual dosages of two puffs four times daily are recommended. The additional use of inhaled steroids is of unproven value in such cases. Cough medicine may be of temporary help. For treating acute bronchitis or acute exacerbation of chronic bronchitis, we recommend the use of broad-spectrum antibiotics such as ampicillin 250 to 500 mg three or four times a day for 7 to 10 days. Alternative antibiotics would be tetracycline, erythromycin, or trimethoprim-sulfamethoxazole (Bactrim, Septra). In rare cases of beta-lactamase–producing bacterial infection, alternative antibiotics would be amoxicillin-clavulanate (Augmentin) 250 to 500 mg three times a day, or cefuroxime (Ceftin) or the newer clarithromycin (Biaxin) at 250-mg doses twice daily.

In acute or accelerated silicosis, one may consider the use of high-dose prednisone (1 mg per kg per day) for a few months tapered gradually over 12 months, which may result in short-term reduction of the alveolitis and provide some clinical improvement but may accelerate infections such as tuberculosis. Its benefits are still unproven. Such steroid treatment should only follow rigorous elimination of tuberculosis by the usual methods, including bronchoscopy, and be associated with isoniazid therapy, 300 mg per day. Alternatively, one may consider massive whole-lung lavage under general anesthesia to improve gas exchange and remove alveolar materials, although its efficacy has not been proven. Hypoxemia should be treated with supplemental oxygen to improve the Pa_{O_2} to 60 torr, improve exercise tolerance, and prevent the development of polycythemia, pulmonary hypertension, and cor pulmonale. Ventilatory support should be considered when respiratory failure is precipitated by a reversible condition such as pneumonia. Pneumothorax should be drained, preferably with a small chest tube and a Heimlich valve, and surgical intervention in cases of failure. A bronchopleural fistula can be precipitated by high negative suction pressure. In acute or accelerated silicosis rapidly progressing to end-stage silicosis, lung transplantation should be considered in younger patients.

In patients with silicosis, a positive tuberculin skin test with a negative sputum smear and culture for tuberculosis is an indication for the prophylactic administration of isoniazid (300 mg per day). Active tuberculosis in silicotic patients should be treated initially for 2 months with three mycobactericidal drugs (isoniazid, 300 mg per day; rifampin (Rifadin), 400 to 600 mg per day; and pyrazinamide, 500 to 1000 mg per day) for 2 months followed by two-drug therapy (isoniazid and rifampin) for at least 12 months. Additional details on drug therapy regimens for tuberculosis and atypical mycobacterial infections can be found in the article "Tuberculosis and Other Mycobacterial Diseases."

Finally, in advanced end-stage silicosis, anaerobic lung infections may be symptomatic and cause additional tissue damage if not treated properly with antibiotics.

HYPERSENSITIVITY PNEUMONITIS
(Allergic Alveolitis)

method of
H. BENFER KALTREIDER, M.D.
School of Medicine, University of California at San Francisco
San Francisco, California

The syndromes of hypersensitivity pneumonitis, or allergic alveolitis, constitute a group of related inflammatory interstitial lung diseases that result from hypersensitivity immune reactions to the repeated inhalation or ingestion of a variety of antigens derived from fungal, bacterial, animal protein, or reactive chemical sources. Table 1 lists the major etiologic agents responsible for hypersensitivity

TABLE 1. **Representative Syndromes of Hypersensitivity Pneumonitis**

Clinical Syndromes by Etiologic Category	Major Causative Agents	Environmental Source
Thermophilic Actinomycetes		
Farmer's lung	*Faeni rectivirgula** *Thermoactinomyces vulgaris*	Moldy hay
Bagassosis	*T. sacchari, T. vulgaris*	Moldy pressed sugar cane
Humidifier lung	*T. vulgaris, T. candidus*	Contaminated humidifiers, air conditioners
Avian Proteins		
Bird fancier's lung	Avian proteins	Bird droppings, feathers
Fungi		
Malt worker's lung	*Aspergillus clavatus*	Moldy malt
Cheese worker's lung	*Penicillium caseii*	Cheese mold
Suberosis	*Penicillium frequentans*	Moldy cork
Reactive Chemicals and Drugs		
Hypersensitivity pneumonitis	Toluene diisocyanate Trimellitic anhydride	Plastics industry
	Amiodarone, gold, minocycline	Medications

*Formerly *Micropolyspora faeni.*

pneumonitis. The most important groups of etiologic agents are (1) the thermophilic actinomycetes, which are responsible for farmer's lung, bagassosis, and humidifier lung, (2) avian serum proteins, which induce bird fancier's lung, (3) fungi such as *Aspergillus* and *Penicillium* spp, which cause maltworker's and cheeseworker's lung, and (4) reactive chemical compounds such as toluene diisocyanate and certain drugs. A large number of additional environmental agents have been associated with the development of hypersensitivity pneumonitis in case reports and small series. Regardless of the precise etiologic agent or the environmental setting in which the disease is encountered, the pathogenesis and clinical manifestations of the syndromes of hypersensitivity pneumonitis are all identical.

The syndromes of hypersensitivity pneumonitis are inflammatory and granulomatous interstitial lung diseases for which the offending antigens are generally known and the immune and inflammatory mechanisms causing lung injury have been identified. The pathogenicity of an environmental agent is dictated by its chemical composition (usually an organic particle or a reactive chemical), its particle size, and the dose and duration of exposure. The susceptibility of the host to immune lung injury is also of critical importance, since only a minority of equally exposed individuals develop pneumonitis. The pathogenesis of hypersensitivity pneumonitis requires ongoing or repeated exposure to the offending antigen. During the initial sensitizing exposures, the host generates appropriate immune responses to the antigen, which result in the generation of specific antibody and sensitized T lymphocytes. Subsequent antigen exposure of sensitized individuals produces lung injury in those who are predisposed to develop hypersensitivity immune responses.

Two distinct clinical syndromes, with differing presentations and manifestations, are recognizable: *acute* and *subacute* or *chronic* hypersensitivity pneumonitis. The different manifestations are primarily determined by the intensity and frequency of antigen exposure. Episodes of *acute hypersensitivity pneumonitis* result from intermittent intense exposure and are reversible. Symptoms of a flulike illness characterized systemically by fever, chills, malaise, and myalgias occur 4 to 6 hours after inhalation of antigen. Pulmonary symptoms consist of severe dyspnea, chest

tightness, and a nonproductive cough. There are physical signs of fever, tachypnea, cyanosis, and bibasilar crackles in the lungs. The diagnosis is readily apparent when the onset of illness occurs 4 to 6 hours after exposure to an identifiable environmental antigen and the symptoms resolve with the cessation of exposure. The clinical syndrome is otherwise nonspecific and indistinguishable from an acute respiratory infection. *Subacute* or *chronic hypersensitivity pneumonitis* results from chronic, low-level exposure to antigen. The onset is insidious, with few if any symptoms during the early stages of the disease. In the later stages, after interstitial inflammation and fibrosis have been established, symptoms of increasing dyspnea on exertion, fatigue, anorexia, cough, and weight loss appear. Physical signs include restriction of ventilation, bibasilar crackles, and eventually, signs of right ventricular failure. The clinical findings frequently do not bear an obvious temporal relationship to antigen exposure and are characteristic of interstitial lung disease of any cause. Only a detailed occupational, environmental, and drug-ingestion history coupled with a high index of suspicion will suggest a possible cause of the lung disease.

The chest radiograph in acute disease reveals interstitial reticulonodular infiltrates of variable intensity at the lung bases. When the x-ray film is normal, high-resolution computed tomography (CT) scanning of the chest is a remarkably sensitive tool for detecting early interstitial changes. In subacute or chronic disease, the chest radiograph shows reduced lung volumes, diffuse interstitial fibrosis, and honeycombing. Pulmonary physiologic abnormalities are characterized by a restrictive ventilatory defect. There are reductions in the vital capacity, the total lung capacity, and the diffusing capacity for carbon monoxide. Airway obstruction is absent or mild. Moderate hypoxemia and mild hypocapnia may be present. In acute disease, physiologic abnormalities parallel the acute episodes; between episodes they revert to normal. In chronic disease, functional abnormalities are progressive and may be irreversible.

Routine laboratory studies are nonspecific. During acute disease, there is a neutrophilic leukocytosis; the white blood cell count is normal in subacute or chronic disease. Eosinophilia is distinctly unusual. Serum protein electrophoresis demonstrates a polyclonal increase in immunoglobulin levels, but the serum concentration of immunoglobulin E (IgE) is normal. Immunologic studies of serum reveal precipitating antibodies against the suspect antigen in greater than 90% of cases. The presence of precipitins indicates intense exposure to antigen but does not necessarily establish a causal relationship between antigen exposure and lung disease. Bronchoalveolar lavage reveals a marked increase in the percentages of lymphocytes (up to 80% total cells), the majority of which are T cells with a predominance of CD8$^+$ T cells (cytotoxic or suppressor cells). In the absence of a characteristic clinical syndrome, such as frequently occurs in subacute or chronic disease, a lung biopsy may be necessary to suggest the diagnosis of hypersensitivity pneumonitis. Inhalation provocation with highly purified antigen preparations under controlled laboratory conditions elicits the reproduction of the acute clinical syndrome and, while investigational, can definitively establish the causal role of an environmental antigen.

TREATMENT

The mainstays of treatment are early and accurate diagnosis, avoidance of continued exposure to antigen, and corticosteroid therapy. Accurate diagnosis is the essential first step, since the maneuvers used to establish the diagnosis consequently suggest the appropriate therapy. An accurate diagnosis of acute hypersensitivity pneumonitis is established clinically based on a high index of suspicion, a thorough environmental and drug history, and the onset of the typical clinical syndrome several hours after antigen exposure. Amelioration of symptoms after the patient leaves the suspect environment and exacerbation of symptoms after the patient reenters that environment establish a presumptive diagnosis and provide strong evidence for the correct cause. When available, confirmation of the offending antigen can be obtained from serum precipitin analysis. A positive test indicates intense exposure to the antigen and, in the proper clinical setting, indicates a causal relation between exposure and disease. Open lung biopsy occasionally may be required when the diagnosis is not apparent on clinical grounds. Inhalation provocation is definitive but investigational and should be reserved for selected cases in which the causal relationship between antigen and lung disease must be established.

Having established an accurate diagnosis and having identified the offending agent and environment, one can design and institute measures to avoid exposure. The patient may avoid antigen exposure by eliminating the offending antigen or its source from the work place or domestic environment, discontinuing suspect drugs, avoiding the offending environment, using a respiratory protective device, avoiding specific areas of the work place, changing the nature of employment in the work place, or, when all else fails, changing occupations altogether. When avoidance is successful, the syndrome of acute hypersensitivity pneumonitis resolves completely and spontaneously. Subacute disease relentlessly progresses unless exposure to the offending antigen is completely eliminated. Subacute or chronic disease may not resolve spontaneously and usually requires additional therapy with corticosteroids.

Mild episodes of acute pneumonitis resolve spontaneously upon removal of the patient from the offending environment. Resolution of severe episodes of acute hypersensitivity pneumonitis can be hastened by a brief course of oral or parenteral corticosteroid therapy, in addition to oxygen and other supportive measures. Such patients can safely be treated with the equivalent of prednisone, 0.5 to 1.0 mg per kg per day for 7 to 14 days, depending on the severity of illness. Subacute or chronic hypersensitivity pneumonitis, like other inflammatory interstitial lung diseases, requires moderate doses of prednisone (1.0 mg per kg per day) for weeks to months. The effectiveness of therapy is monitored by measuring clinical, radiographic, and physiologic parameters. An objective response should be evident after 4 to 6 weeks, in which case therapy should be continued until no further improvement occurs, followed by a gradual reduction to a low dose or to discontinuation. Current practice dictates prompt and aggressive treatment of both the acute and the subacute or chronic forms of hypersensitivity pneumonitis to prevent progression to fibrosis. However, the long-term beneficial effects of corticosteroids on arresting disease progression remain to be definitively established.

SINUSITIS

method of
NELSON M. GANTZ, M.D.
Pennsylvania State University College of Medicine
Hershey, Pennsylvania

Sinusitis or inflammation of the paranasal sinuses is an extremely common problem. Adults have about three to four upper respiratory infections each year, and it is estimated that 0.5 to 1% of these disorders is complicated by a sinus infection. Sinusitis may be classified by duration as acute (present for less than 1 month), subacute (disease present for more than 1 month but less than 3 months), and chronic (disease of more than 3 months). The illness can be classified also by the type of inflammation as either infectious or not infectious. The diagnosis of sinusitis is problematic for both patients and physicians. The self-diagnosis of sinusitis made by patients is frequently incorrect. For the clinician, recognition of the illness is also difficult because the classic symptoms of headache, facial pain, and fever may be absent. It is often difficult to differentiate a viral upper respiratory infection from bacterial sinusitis. No simple, inexpensive diagnostic methods are available. Conventional radiographs may be misleading and lack the sensitivity of a computed tomography (CT) scan or magnetic resonance imaging (MRI) study. Finally, confirmation of the cause requires an invasive procedure.

The pathogenesis of sinusitis results from one of three mechanisms—obstruction of the sinus ostia, abnormal local host defenses, and factors that damage the mucociliary sinus lining. Obstruction of the sinus ostia results from mucosal swelling usually due to a viral upper respiratory infection or allergic disease. At times, obstruction is a result of anatomic causes such as a foreign body. Examples of abnormal host defenses include patients with cystic fi-

TABLE 1. **Predisposing Factors in Sinusitis**

Seasonal

Allergy
Viral upper respiratory infection
Swimming, flying
Low humidity

Obstruction

Foreign body—nasogastric or nasotracheal tube
Adenoidal hyperplasia
Nasal polyps
Neoplasms
Septal deviation

Other

Dental infection
Immunodeficiency
Conditions impairing ciliary clearance (e.g., smoke, air pollution)
Facial trauma

brosis or IgA or IgG antibody deficiency. Finally, a normal mucociliary mechanism is critical for preventing the accumulation of fluid within the sinus. Agents that interfere with ciliary function include viruses, smoke, air pollution, and low ambient humidity. Fluid within a sinus cavity can lead to sinusitis by providing a culture medium that permits bacteria to multiply. Patients with acquired immune deficiency syndrome (AIDS) have both an increased frequency of sinusitis and an infection that is less responsive to therapy.

Patients with recurrent sinusitis should be evaluated for the presence of predisposing factors (Table 1). The use of allergy and immunologic testing, CT scan or MRI, and/or endoscopy may uncover a cause for the recurrent disease.

ACUTE SINUSITIS

Acute sinusitis is usually a result of allergic rhinitis or secondary to a viral upper respiratory infection. Allergic disease is usually seasonal and often associated with itching of the eyes and throat. The diagnosis of sinusitis should be considered in an adult with an upper respiratory infection that persists for more than 10 days. Although the triad of headache, facial pain, and fever suggests the diagnosis, fever is present in only 25 to 50% of patients with acute maxillary sinusitis. Patients usually complain of nasal discharge that is often purulent. Cough, which is a feature of bronchitis and pneumonia, occurs in 70% of patients with sinusitis. Percussion tenderness over the involved sinus and periorbital edema may be present. Diagnostic methods include transillumination, conventional sinus x-rays, CT scan, MRI study, and fiberoptic rhinoscopy. Conventional sinus x-rays lack the sensitivity of a CT scan or MRI study. For most patients, the diagnosis is made clinically without radiographic studies. If a patient fails to respond to therapy, is seriously ill, or has a possible complication of sinusitis such as an intracranial abscess, then radiographic studies are indicated. The organisms most often involved in patients with acute sinusitis include *Streptococcus pneumoniae*, *Haemophilus influenzae*, *Moraxella catarrhalis*, *Staphylococcus aureus*, and *Strep. pyogenes*. Over 50% of cases are caused by *Strep. pneumoniae* or *H. influenzae*. The

yield from either a throat or a nasopharyngeal culture correlates poorly with sinus aspirate results. Since sinus aspirates are not usually obtained, microbiologic data are unavailable in the majority of patients with sinusitis. *Mycoplasma pneumoniae* and *Chlamydia pneumoniae* are not important pathogens in acute sinusitis. In patients with cystic fibrosis, *Pseudomonas aeruginosa* is the most frequent organism isolated.

In recent years, about 15 to 20% of isolates of *H. influenzae* and 75% of strains of *Moraxella catarrhalis* produce beta-lactamase and are resistant to ampicillin. Penicillin- and cephalosporin-resistant *Strep. pneumoniae* is another organism that poses problems. The frequency of resistant pneumococci in patients with acute sinusitis is unknown. Vancomycin is the drug of choice to treat infections caused by resistant pneumococci.

Antibiotic therapy in acute maxillary sinusitis is usually empirical. In patients without a penicillin allergy, amoxicillin (Amoxil), is still recommended. Those who have a history of a penicillin allergy such as a delayed skin rash can be given a cephalosporin such as cefaclor (Ceclor), loracarbef (Lorabid) or cefuroxime axetil (Ceftin). Patients who report an immediate type hypersensitivity reaction to penicillin may be given doxycycline (Vibramycin), clarithromycin (Biaxin), azithromycin (Zithromax), or trimethoprim-sulfamethoxazole (Bactrim, Septra) but not a cephalosporin. If a patient fails to improve after 5 days, consideration should be given to changing the antimicrobial agent (Table 2). Drugs such as loracarbef, cefaclor, cefuroxime axetil, or amoxicillin-clavulanate (Augmentin) may be used in patients who fail to respond to amoxicillin. Antibiotic therapy is usually given for 10 to 14 days.

Measures to improve drainage such as steam from a shower or saline nasal spray may be helpful. Systemic decongestants and mucolytic agents such as guaifenesin are of limited value. Topical decongestants such as phenylephrine or oxymetazoline (Afrin) may be tried for 3 days. The older antihistamines such as chlorpheniramine tend to thicken the sinus secretions and are best avoided during an acute infection. In patients with allergic rhinitis, topical ste-

TABLE 2. **Antimicrobial Therapy of Acute Sinusitis**

Drug	Oral Dose in Adults
Amoxicillin (Amoxil)	500 mg tid*
Loracarbef (Lorabid)	200–400 mg bid*
Amoxicillin-clavulanate (Augmentin)	500 mg tid*
Cefaclor (Ceclor)	500 mg tid*
Cefuroxime (Zinacef)	250 mg bid*
Doxycycline (Vibramycin)	100 mg bid*
Trimethoprim-sulfamethoxazole 160 mg/800 mg (Bactrim DS, Septra DS)	1 tablet bid*
Clarithromycin (Biaxin)	500 mg bid*
Azithromycin (Zithromax)	500 mg then 250 mg qd†

*Course of therapy: 10–14 days.
†5-day course.

roid nasal sprays such as beclomethasone can be useful in decreasing mucosal swelling.

Consideration should be given to hospitalization of patients who are ill with infection limited to the sphenoid sinus or frontal sinuses. Infection of these sinuses often requires parenteral therapy because of the risk of developing an intracranial complication or osteomyelitis.

CHRONIC SINUSITIS

Chronic sinusitis refers to disease that is present for more than 3 months. Symptoms include nasal discharge that is often foul-smelling, and facial pain at times. Fever is often absent. The infection is often polymicrobial with anaerobes present in most cases. Amoxicillin-clavulanate, in a dose of 500 mg three times a day orally, or clindamycin 300 mg four times a day orally, may be useful. Antimicrobial therapy is usually given for 2 to 3 weeks but controlled studies are lacking. In addition to antimicrobial agents, therapy of chronic sinusitis often requires fiberoptic rhinoscopy to relieve obstruction in the area of the osteomeatal complex. In addition, patients may benefit from an allergy and immunologic evaluation.

COMPLICATIONS OF SINUSITIS

Complications of sinusitis, although rare, can be life-threatening. Because of the proximity of the orbit, intracranial structures, and bone to the sinus cavities, infection may involve these areas by direct extension (Table 3). Patients will present with a complication and then, using a CT scan, the clinician must determine that the source of the infection is sinusitis. Therapy consists of drainage and an appropriate antimicrobial agent based on the results of data from aspiration of the pus. Since it is impossible to predict the occurrence of a complication, it is important to ensure that adequate follow-up is present when treating a patient for sinusitis.

IMMUNOCOMPROMISED HOST

Patients with impaired host defenses—such as those with diabetes mellitus, AIDS, or a malignancy—who are receiving chemotherapy or corticosteroids may develop sinusitis with the usual pathogens such as *Strep. pneumoniae* or unusual organisms such as *Aspergillus*. For example, the patient with diabetes mellitus with ketoacidosis or leukemia with prolonged neutropenia is at risk for an invasive sinus infection with *Aspergillus* or *Mucor*. Rhinocerebral mucormycosis is a life-threatening infection with involvement of *Mucor* in the nose, sinuses, eyes, and brain. In the compromised host who fails to respond to therapy with drugs effective against the common bacterial pathogens, sinus aspiration is needed to diagnose the unusual opportunistic organisms. Patients with AIDS have an increased frequency of sinusitis. Infection has been reported with the common sinus pathogens or unusual organisms. Patients generally respond poorly to appropriate therapy and chronic sinusitis often occurs.

Fungal sinusitis occurs in both the immunocompetent and the immunocompromised host. In the normal host, fungal sinusitis can be categorized as (1) chronic indolent disease, which responds to surgical resection, (2) mycetoma ("fungus ball of the sinus"), which responds to surgical resection, and (3) allergic fungal sinusitis, which can be treated with surgery and steroids. Antifungal therapy is not needed to manage fungal disease in the immunocompetent patient. Invasive fungal sinusitis can occur in the immunocompromised patient. The disease is characterized histologically by tissue necrosis and mycelial invasion of blood vessels. Prognosis is poor even with surgical resection and antifungal therapy.

STREPTOCOCCAL PHARYNGITIS

method of
JAMES M. McCARTY, M.D.
Valley Children's Hospital
Fresno, California

Pharyngitis is one of the most common reasons for patient visits to primary health care providers. Although most cases are of viral etiology, the bacterium most frequently isolated is *Streptococcus pyogenes* (group A beta-hemolytic streptococci [GABHS]), occurring in up to 30% of patients with acute sore throat. Other bacteria implicated less frequently include group C and G streptococci, *Neisseria gonorrhoeae* and possibly *Mycoplasma pneumoniae* and *Chlamydia pneumoniae*, although the role of the latter two organisms is less clear. Many cases of acute pharyngitis are idiopathic in nature but of presumed viral origin.

GABHS pharyngitis is spread via person-to-person contact with infectious nasal or oral secretions and is more common in situations of crowding, as occur in schools, and during the colder months of the year. It may occur at any age but is most common in school-age children and is uncommon in those younger than 3 years. There is no evidence that the incidence of streptococcal pharyngitis has increased in the past decade. However, there have been a disturbing number of outbreaks of acute rheumatic fever and an increase in the incidence of invasive group A

TABLE 3. **Complications of Acute Sinusitis**

Orbital Complications
Preseptal or periorbital cellulitis
Orbital cellulitis
Subperiosteal abscess
Orbital abscess
Optic neuritis
Osteomyelitis of the Frontal or Maxillary Bone
Intracranial Complications
Epidural abscess
Subdural abscess
Cavernous or sagittal sinus thrombosis
Meningitis
Brain abscess

streptococcal infections recently. A streptococcal toxic shock syndrome very much like that caused by *Staphylococcus aureus*, with fever, rash, hypotension, and multisystem organ failure, has also been recognized.

CLINICAL PRESENTATION

The "classic" patient with GABHS pharyngitis presents acutely with fever, dysphagia, tonsillopharyngeal erythema/exudate, cervical lymphadenopathy, and an elevated white blood cell count. The majority of GABHS pharyngitis patients do not present with these classic findings; in addition, many will also have abdominal pain, nausea, or headache. Patients presenting with rhinorrhea, cough, or hoarseness are more likely to have infection of viral etiology. Unfortunately, there is significant clinical overlap between viral and streptococcal pharyngitis and experienced physicians are able to make a specific diagnosis on the basis of clinical findings only 50 to 75% of the time. Of note is that young children 1 to 3 years of age with GABHS upper respiratory infection may sometimes present with fever and serous rhinitis.

Suppurative complications of GABHS pharyngitis include peritonsillar and retropharyngeal abscess, otitis media, sinusitis, suppurative cervical lymphadenitis, and possibly bacteremia or GABHS toxic shock syndrome. Nonsuppurative complications include acute rheumatic fever and acute glomerulonephritis and are associated with certain M-protein serotypes of GABHS.

DIAGNOSIS

Since the clinical diagnosis of streptococcal pharyngitis is so inaccurate and since most patients presenting to a physician with pharyngitis do not need antimicrobial therapy, more reliable techniques of diagnosis are needed. The throat culture, a vigorous swab of the tonsillopharyngeal area plated on blood agar and incubated overnight, is considered the most reliable method of identifying the presence of GABHS. Unfortunately, up to 20% of school-age children will be carriers of GABHS during the winter, and a positive throat culture does not differentiate patients with streptococcal infection from those who are streptococcal carriers and have pharyngitis of viral etiology. False-negative throat cultures are infrequent in patients with true streptococcal infection.

More recently, a number of rapid diagnostic techniques have become available, allowing the diagnosis of infection due to GABHS within minutes. In research settings these tests are highly sensitive and specific and will detect GABHS in most patients. However, studies done in "real-life" situations have demonstrated false-negative rates as high as 50%. Therefore, the recommended practice for the patient presenting to the clinician's office with acute pharyngitis is to obtain two swabs of the throat. If the rapid "strep" test is positive, treatment is initiated and the second specimen discarded; if it is negative, the second specimen is submitted for conventional culture.

THERAPY

Antibiotic treatment is effective in shortening the duration of signs and symptoms of streptococcal pharyngitis and in preventing suppurative complications such as peritonsillar abscess. Ten-day antibiotic therapy has also been demonstrated effective in preventing the nonsuppurative complication of acute rheumatic fever if given within 9 days of the onset of pharyngitis.

Penicillin has traditionally been the drug of choice for streptococcal pharyngitis. There have been no reports of resistance of group A streptococcus to this antibiotic; also, there has been some association of penicillin "tolerance" with treatment failures. Tolerance is an in vitro phenomenon that occurs when the minimal bactericidal concentration (MBC; the concentration of antibiotic needed to kill the organism) is significantly greater than the minimal inhibitory concentration (MIC; the concentration of antibiotic necessary to inhibit growth of the organism). The clinical significance, if any, of penicillin tolerance remains controversial.

Penicillin V may be given orally at a dose of 400,000 U (250 mg) three times per day or 800,000 U (500 mg) twice per day. It is important to complete 10 days, despite clinical improvement, to prevent acute rheumatic fever. However, compliance with 10-day treatment regimens is often poor, and this may lead to treatment failures. Intramuscular benzathine penicillin G as a single injection is just as effective as oral penicillin and eliminates any problems with compliance, but it is painful. The usual dosage is 600,000 U for children who weigh less than 60 pounds and 1,200,000 U for larger children and adults. Some of the pain associated with intramuscular administration of benzathine penicillin G can be diminished by adding procaine penicillin to the previously mentioned dosages of benzathine penicillin.

Recent studies have suggested a decreased efficacy of penicillin in the treatment of streptococcal pharyngitis, with failure rates as high as 38%. A number of possible explanations for this have been proposed, including decreased sensitivity of GABHS to penicillin, bacterial tolerance, and the interference of normal upper respiratory tract flora with GABHS colonization. The available evidence does not consistently support any of these ideas. Another suggested explanation for decreased penicillin efficacy is the concept of "copathogenicity." Although not universally accepted, some studies have suggested that beta-lactamase–producing organisms in the throat, such as *S. aureus*, *Haemophilus influenzae*, *Moraxella catarrhalis*, and oral anaerobes inactivate penicillin. A recent meta-analysis of 19 clinical trials comparing beta-lactamase–stable cephalosporins with penicillin for the treatment of GABHS pharyngitis demonstrated significantly better clinical and bacteriologic cure rates with cephalosporins and led the author to consider replacing penicillin with cephalosporins as the treatment of choice of GABHS pharyngitis. However, a number of investigators have criticized this meta-analysis, citing incomplete compliance data, lack of serotyping of GABHS isolates in cases of bacteriologic failure, lack of consistent bacteriologic end-points, and study designs that encouraged the inclusion of GABHS carriers in the trials. These workers concluded that, because of its lower cost and more narrow spectrum of activity, penicillin remains the drug of choice for GABHS pharyngitis.

Early penicillin therapy within 24 hours of symptoms seems to result in a higher relapse rate than therapy instituted after a waiting period of 3 to 4 days. This may be secondary to a diminished antibody response seen with early treatment. Some have advocated waiting 2 to 3 days before beginning antibiotic therapy of streptococcal pharyngitis to allow an antibody response to develop. However, this will no doubt prolong the pain and suffering associated with pharyngitis and may increase the incidence of serious complications, such as retropharyngeal abscess or other invasive complications. At this time, the American Academy of Pediatrics recommends penicillin V as the drug of choice for GABHS pharyngitis. Oral erythromycin for 10 days is indicated for penicillin-allergic patients, either erythromycin estolate at 20 to 40 mg per kg per day in two to four divided doses or erythromycin ethyl succinate at 40 to 50 mg per kg per day, with a maximal dose of 1 gram per day. The newer macrolides clarithromycin (Biaxin) and azithromycin (Zithromax) have also been demonstrated effective in the treatment of GABHS pharyngitis. Narrow-spectrum oral cephalosporins for 10 days may be an acceptable alternative in penicillin-allergic patients, particularly those intolerant of macrolides, although up to 15% of these patients will also be allergic to cephalosporins. Tetracyclines and sulfonamides should not be used for the treatment of streptococcal pharyngitis.

Azithromycin given orally for 5 days has been shown to be as effective as a 10-day course of oral penicillin for GABHS pharyngitis. A number of studies have been recently completed or are in progress comparing 5-day courses of oral cephalosporins with conventional therapy for this illness.

CHRONIC CARRIERS

GABHS can be cultured from the throats of 5 to 15% of healthy, asymptomatic school-age children. Most of these individuals represent streptococcal carriers and pose no risk to themselves or others. Therefore, routine throat cultures are not recommended in asymptomatic patients after completion of antibiotic therapy of streptococcal pharyngitis. Chronic carriers of GABHS should be treated only under certain circumstances, such as in families where siblings are having recurrent episodes of streptococcal pharyngitis and in those with a history of rheumatic fever. GABHS is difficult to eradicate from the pharynx in these patients, but clindamycin (Cleocin), amoxicillin-clavulanate (Augmentin), dicloxacillin (Dynapen), and a combination of penicillin and rifampin (Rifadin) have all been shown to be effective. Unfortunately, many chronic carriers of GABHS will demonstrate streptococci on rapid test or culture when presenting with viral upper respiratory infections and will receive antibiotic therapy when it is not needed.

RECURRENT PHARYNGITIS

Patients with recurrent symptomatic streptococcal pharyngitis may represent chronic carriers with re-

current viral infections or may indeed represent true reinfections. When evaluating the patient with recurrent GABHS pharyngitis, it is important to make sure that compliance with a complete treatment regimen is adequate. If compliance is uncertain, then intramuscular therapy with penicillin G should be considered. In compliant patients with recurrent streptococcal pharyngitis, alternative therapy with cephalosporins, macrolides, amoxicillin-clavulanate, or clindamycin may be necessary. Some clinicians will culture other members of the family and treat all who are positive for GABHS. Finally, tonsillectomy may be considered for some individuals.

TUBERCULOSIS AND OTHER MYCOBACTERIAL DISEASES

method of
NAV T. SINGH, M.B.B.S., and
EDWARD L. PESANTI, M.D.
University of Connecticut Health Center
Farmington, Connecticut

During this century, tuberculosis therapy has evolved from essentially lengthy observation in sanatoria (with rest, nutritious diets, fresh air) to "collapse therapy," with pneumothorax, pneumoperitoneum, thoracoplasty, and extrapleural plombage or resection of the diseased lung. Streptomycin was discovered in 1943, followed by para-aminosalicylic acid (PAS) (1944), isoniazid (1952), and later rifampin (1965). During this period, the incidence, morbidity, and mortality steadily declined in the United States. A tuberculosis mortality of about 50% dramatically changed to an almost 100% cure rate in patients with previously untreated pulmonary tuberculosis.

Two pivotal changes in this trend with major public health consequences have occurred in the last 10 years. First, since 1985, the steady decline in incidence was reversed; and second, there appeared an accelerated emergence of multiple-drug–resistant strains of *Mycobacterium tuberculosis*. Among the critical elements in the effort to reverse these trends is a careful, rational, and determined approach to therapy in individual cases.

FIRST-LINE DRUGS (Table 1)

Isoniazid

Isoniazid (INH) is the mainstay of therapy of tuberculosis. The drug is inexpensive and well tolerated and causes relatively few side effects. It is administered in a single daily dose of 10 mg per kg up to a maximum of 300 mg per day. Use of larger doses causes a higher incidence of side effects without, in most situations, increasing therapeutic activity.

The most commonly encountered serious adverse effects of INH are hepatotoxicity and neurotoxicity; the incidence of the latter is dose related whereas that of the former is not. Deaths have resulted from INH-induced hepatotoxicity, most commonly in patients who continued to take the medication despite

TABLE 1. **Common Antituberculous Drugs**

Drug	Usual Dose	Common Side Effects
Isoniazid	300 mg	Hepatitis, neurotoxicity
Rifampin (Rifadin)	600 mg	Hepatitis, red-orange secretions, flulike syndrome, thrombocytopenia
Pyrazinamide	30 mg/kg	Hepatitis, hyperuricemia
Ethambutol (Myambutol)	15 mg/kg	Optic neuritis
Streptomycin	15 mg/kg	Auditory or vestibular toxicity, nephrotoxicity

the onset of symptomatic hepatitis. Periodic screening of asymptomatic patients for abnormalities of hepatic function may identify a group of patients at high risk of developing serious toxicity. However, interpretation of the results of such routine screening is difficult. During the first few months of INH administration, elevated liver enzyme levels can be seen in about 25% of patients followed with serial determinations; in the great majority, the changes are clinically insignificant. In addition, many patients who develop hepatitis have normal liver enzyme levels in the routine screening prior to their illness.

Patients prescribed INH should be advised to contact their physician if they develop fever, malaise, nausea, or vomiting. Serum transaminase and bilirubin levels should be measured in such patients. If the results are consistent with hepatitis, INH and any other potentially hepatotoxic drugs should be discontinued. Prophylactic administration of INH probably should not be resumed on improvement of liver function tests, but gradual reintroduction of INH may be attempted in patients being treated for active disease. A substantial number of these patients will not experience further difficulty with the drug.

Neurotoxicity from INH is rare in healthy individuals treated with no more than 300 mg per day. It usually causes peripheral neuropathy but in some cases may cause drowsiness, seizures, and rarely, coma. Neurotoxicity may be a particular problem in malnourished patients, alcoholics, and diabetics. These patients may also develop neuropathy from their underlying disease. Clinical distinction between alcoholic or diabetic neuropathy and INH-induced neuropathy is virtually impossible. For such high-risk patients, use of pyridoxine (10 mg per day) is warranted. The routine use of pyridoxine is unnecessary and does not contribute to improved therapy of tuberculosis.

In addition to these direct effects of INH, serious side effects can result from its interaction with other drugs. INH diminishes hepatic elimination of phenytoin and carbamazepine, causing toxic reactions to these agents with doses that would otherwise be well tolerated; those drugs also retard INH elimination.

Rare adverse effects of INH include typical drug rashes, systemic lupus erythematosus, and pellagra, among those affecting the skin, as well as a number of apparently rare biochemical interactions.

INH is inactivated by hepatic enzyme–mediated acetylation. The speed of inactivation of the drug is a genetically determined trait. Slow inactivators are more susceptible to neurotoxicity than are rapid inactivators; rapid inactivators have responded poorly to therapy with experimental regimens utilizing once-weekly INH. Patients with renal impairment may be treated with 300 mg of INH daily, as may most patients with pre-existing liver disease. Active hepatitis is a relative contraindication. Prophylactic INH probably should not be administered until liver enzyme levels stabilize (not necessarily at normal values). Patients with acute hepatitis can be treated with other agents until the disease subsides. INH can be added subsequently. Patients with chronic active hepatitis can be treated with INH as long as liver function tests are periodically monitored. There is no evidence that such patients are particularly prone to worsening liver function as a result of having received INH.

Rifampin (Rifadin)

Unlike INH, which has an extremely narrow spectrum, rifampin is effective against a variety of bacteria and has a role in therapy of many infections other than tuberculosis. The usual daily dosage for adults is 600 mg taken at one time.

The drug causes few side effects. To allay anxiety, patients should be warned that their urine may become brick-red. Typical hepatitis indistinguishable from that due to INH is the most common serious adverse effect. It is possible that the combination of INH and rifampin is slightly more hepatotoxic than is either agent alone. Rifampin also may cause isolated hyperbilirubinemia. The development of symptomatic hepatitis or of very high transaminase levels is an indication for stopping the drug, at least temporarily. Isolated hyperbilirubinemia may simply be observed if the elevation is minor, or it may respond to a slight reduction in rifampin dosage.

The most serious side effect of rifampin is the rare reaction causing thrombocytopenia, renal insufficiency, fever, and myalgias. The reaction was reported to occur most often during intermittent therapy using high doses of rifampin, but it has also occurred in patients receiving daily rifampin, possibly related to irregular ingestion of the drug by poorly compliant patients. Newly devised intermittent regimens using no more than 600 mg of rifampin per dose have not been complicated by this side effect with any greater frequency than is seen with daily administration.

Since rifampin is eliminated by hepatic excretion, its clearance is not diminished by renal failure, but high levels can accumulate in hepatic disease. In that situation, drug toxicity will be clinically and biochemically indistinguishable from progression of the underlying hepatic disease, a clinical dilemma that will require discontinuation of rifampin to resolve.

Like INH, rifampin may alter the elimination of other therapeutic agents. However, although the common interactions of INH reflect inhibition of the elimination, rifampin accelerates clearance of a variety of agents that are detoxified in the liver. Rifampin enhances clearance of estrogens (birth control pills are unreliable contraceptives in patients on rifampin), warfarin (high doses of warfarin are often required in patients on rifampin, and the requirement rapidly decreases when rifampin is discontinued), quinidine, methadone, and several others.

Ethambutol (Myambutol)

Ethambutol is a valuable companion drug to be used in conjunction with INH and rifampin, especially when there is a high risk of INH resistance, pending the results of cultures and sensitivity reports. The drug does not appear to cause fetal anomalies and, in combination with INH, is a drug of choice in pregnant women with active tuberculosis. Ethambutol is well tolerated and relatively inexpensive. Although dosages of up to 25 mg per kg are sometimes recommended, we generally never exceed a daily dosage of 15 mg per kg, in an effort to limit side effects.

The only serious side effect of ethambutol is optic (retrobulbar) neuritis, and this is rare when no more than 15 mg per kg per day of ethambutol is administered. Typically, it presents first as a loss of color vision, followed by decrements in visual acuity. These alterations are usually reversible when ethambutol is discontinued, but permanent blindness has occurred. Since the most common early sign of visual toxicity—loss of red-green color discrimination—is also the most spontaneous anomaly of color vision, pretreatment screening is particularly important. Although formal ophthalmic consultation is not required to initiate therapy or to follow patients on the drug, it is essential that patients' color vision and visual acuity be tested, both prior to initiation of therapy and at monthly intervals during therapy. Patients should also be advised to report any suspected alterations in visual acuity that they notice between visits. Patients whose vision cannot be reliably tested, for example, small children, should not receive the drug if other effective agents are available.

Clearance of ethambutol is mediated entirely by renal excretion. Unless accurate serum levels of the drug can be obtained, other agents should be used in patients with markedly depressed renal function (creatinine levels greater than 3 mg per dL). The ethambutol-induced visual toxicity is usually observed in patients with pre-existing renal impairment who nonetheless were treated with 15 mg per kg per day of the drug.

Pyrazinamide

This is one of the most intrinsically active of the drugs available for use against *M. tuberculosis*, especially within the acidic environment of macrophages. It is inactive against other species of mycobacteria. It is very well absorbed and penetrates the blood-brain barrier with good cerebrospinal fluid levels. The most important side effect is hepatic injury, which is handled in a manner similar to that with INH and rifampin. Although gout is an uncommon reaction, serum hyperuricemia is frequent, sometimes with arthralgias responding to salicylates or nonsteroidal anti-inflammatory drugs (NSAIDs). Occasionally gastrointestinal intolerance and rash are seen.

Streptomycin

The first major antituberculosis drug has long been reliable for therapy of active tuberculosis and is an obvious choice when an injectable agent is desired. The usual dosage is 15 mg per kg intramuscularly or 12 mg per kg intravenously as a single daily dose for 5 days a week. It is excreted almost exclusively through the kidney and has generally good tissue penetration (except into the cerebrospinal fluid). Its principal side effects are drug fever, seen in up to 15% of patients, and vestibular neurotoxicity. The latter reaction is particularly common and troublesome in elderly people, in whom it should be used with caution, if at all. Administration of streptomycin to pregnant women has resulted in fetal deafness; the drug is not recommended for use in pregnancy. It is less often nephrotoxic compared with other aminoglycosides, but caution is appropriate in the settings of renal insufficiency and simultaneous use of other nephrotoxic agents.

SECOND-LINE DRUGS
Cycloserine (Seromycin)

Because of an unacceptable risk of serious neurotoxicity when used at doses that produce therapeutic levels in serum and tissues, this drug is seldom utilized in therapy of tuberculosis when other drugs are available. Adverse reactions include abnormal behavior, convulsions, and peripheral neuropathy (especially with INH). Like the penicillins, the drug reaches very high concentrations in the kidneys and urine and is sometimes useful in treating renal tuberculosis. It is given orally in doses of 15 to 20 mg per kg per day in divided doses.

Capreomycin (Capastat) and Kanamycin (Kantrex)*

These are also aminoglycosides, used mainly for drug-resistant tuberculosis, and although probably less effective than streptomycin, they do not demon-

---

*Not FDA-approved for this indication.

strate cross-microbial resistance. They are given in dosages like those of streptomycin. They are also ototoxic (especially kanamycin), but hearing loss can occur before vestibular dysfunction. Therefore, audiograms should be obtained initially and then monthly, in addition to clinical examinations for vestibular dysfunction. Renal toxicity consists of elevated creatinine levels and occasionally electrolyte disturbances. Elderly people are especially susceptible to these toxicities. Combined use is usually avoided.

Para-Aminosalicylic Acid

This drug was an integral part of primary therapy regimens 20 years ago. Its use has been curtailed, not because it lacks efficacy but because of its high incidence of gastrointestinal side effects (nausea, vomiting, and diarrhea) at the necessary doses. Hypersensitivity reactions, sodium overload, and hepatitis occur. The usual therapeutic dose is 10 to 20 grams per day in divided doses.

Ethionamide (Tretacor SC)

This second-line drug is often included in lists of agents useful in treating drug-resistant tuberculosis and disease due to *M. avium-intracellulare*. The usual daily dose is 15 mg per kg per day to a maximum of 1 gram. The drug causes nausea, vomiting, anorexia, and abdominal discomfort in most patients, making it necessary to gradually increase the dose to the full amount. Giving it at night with an antiemetic and a sedative is sometimes useful. Hepatitis, arthralgias, gynecomastia, impotence, menstrual irregularities, hair loss, photosensitivity, and hypothyroidism are other side effects, making this a difficult drug to tolerate.

Other Agents

Drugs utilized experimentally and in multiple-drug–resistant disease that show promise include the quinolones ciprofloxacin (Cipro) and ofloxacin (Floxin), amikacin (Amikin), rifabutin (Mycobutin), clofazimine (Lamprene), and amoxicillin-clavulanate (Augmentin). Inexpensive thiacetazone is used in many developing countries but is not available in the United States. It is contraindicated in HIV-infected patients because of frequent and severe side effects.

PRINCIPLES OF ANTITUBERCULOSIS THERAPY

The general aims of therapy include prevention of disease (either soon after infection or later through reactivation); treatment of active cases promptly with various combinations of multiple drugs (to avoid the development of drug-resistant strains), which are to be taken regularly and for a sufficient period (Table 2); and finally, limiting transmission to other persons.

At the outset, it is important to establish and record patient characteristics that may influence therapy. These include age; weight; details of prior therapy (including exact drugs, dates, efficacy, adverse reactions); travel and ethnic background; possible exposure to drug-resistant strains; the level of understanding and ability to communicate effectively; presence of other medical conditions—hepatic, ocular, renal, neurologic abnormalities, and so on; other medications; the patient's economic and social circumstances, from the ability to afford medications, tests, and visits, to family and other contacts and stability of abode. Risk factors (and better still, laboratory evaluation) for HIV infection need to be evaluated. Public health officials must be informed of the case, these details, and results of susceptibility tests.

Noncompliance has long been recognized as a significant problem in therapeutics. The many factors predisposing to, and suggested remedies for, noncompliance have been extensively discussed in the literature. Its adverse implications in antituberculous therapy, however, not only affect the noncompliant patient but also put others in the community at significant and possibly life-threatening risk. As a response to this and because of the relatively easy transmissibility of the disease and problems associated with largely avoidable multiple-drug–resistance, some have advocated consideration of directly observed drug therapy for the duration of treatment in all active cases.

Antituberculous drugs are administered in three situations: prophylaxis, prevention, or active disease.

1. *Prophylactic treatment* may be given to previously uninfected persons shortly after exposure to an active case, with the intent to kill all the infecting organisms even before an immune response develops (i.e., before a positive tuberculin skin test reaction), especially in highly susceptible hosts such as young children and the immunocompromised.

2. *Preventive treatment* is considered in individuals who have already mounted an initial immune response strong enough to control but not eradicate the infecting tubercle bacilli. They have a positive tuberculin test without evidence of active disease (i.e., asymptomatic and culture-negative [if done]).

TABLE 2. **A Standard 6-Month Regimen**

Initial Therapy for 2 Months

Isoniazid, 300 mg/day PO
Rifampin (Rifadin), 600 mg/day PO
Pyrazinamide, 30 mg/kg/day PO
and either: Ethambutol (Myambutol), 15 mg/kg/day PO
    or: Streptomycin, 15 mg/kg/day IM (5 days/week)

Continuation Therapy for Another 4 Months

Isoniazid, 300 mg, and rifampin, 600 mg, either daily or twice-weekly, preferably with directly observed therapy

Although it is indisputable that preventive therapy with INH is effective in decreasing the subsequent risk of developing active tuberculosis, there is considerable debate over who should receive preventive therapy, mainly centering on cost efficacy and safety issues in patients at low risk of reactivation.

There is less controversy, however, about therapy for high-risk individuals, such as persons with abnormal chest radiographs indicating prior disease and therefore a greater bacillary burden (e.g., apical scarring), close contacts of recently diagnosed active cases, and the immunocompromised.

INH, 3 to 5 mg per kg per day (maximum, 300 mg), usually for 9 months, has been the mainstay of therapy because of its proven efficacy, good safety profile, and low cost.

Close contacts or converters suspected of having been exposed to strains resistant to INH can be treated with rifampin. The Centers for Disease Control and Prevention has recommended a combination of pyrazinamide and a quinolone in patients known to be exposed to strains resistant to both INH and rifampin.

Therapy is monitored monthly for symptomatic adverse reactions and compliance. Baseline liver function tests are repeated if patients have symptoms suggestive of hepatitis that may represent an adverse drug reaction.

3. *Active tuberculosis* is present when, despite host defenses, the tubercle bacilli have replicated to an extent sufficient to result in tissue damage and illness. This must be treated both to improve the health of the afflicted patient and to decrease the spread of the disease to others in the community. Therapy is often begun empirically before a positive culture is available, on the basis of clinical or radiologic signs compatible with tuberculosis (e.g., upper lobe cavitary pulmonary infiltration with fever, night sweats) after obtaining secretions or tissue samples from the affected organs.

Therapy for active tuberculosis can be divided into two phases: Phase I: Initial Therapy. This is directed against rapidly growing intra- and extracellular (i.e., host macrophage) bacilli and consists generally of four or more drugs given simultaneously for 2 months on a daily basis. Phase II: Continuation Therapy. This is aimed at killing the initially dormant intramacrophage bacilli not destroyed during the initial phase. This phase lasts a minimum of 4 months. The number of drugs used during this phase should be dictated by the antibiotic susceptibility patterns of the individual strain (by now identified by culture and sensitivity testing). These should include a minimum of two first-line drugs to which the strain is susceptible, and more if the resistance pattern requires usage of second-line drugs.

Medications during this phase can be given on an intermittent high-dose basis twice- or thrice-weekly. This allows for monitoring by medical or public health personnel; it probably improves compliance and reduces the likelihood of toxic reactions.

Therapy is monitored at least monthly. Symptomatic improvement usually occurs within the first few weeks of therapy, although fever can persist for up to 3 months in successfully treated cases. In pulmonary tuberculosis, sputum culture samples are usually obtained every 2 weeks until the smears are negative, and then monthly. Antibiotic susceptibility testing must be performed on *all* initial cultures and repeated if there is evidence of treatment failure (i.e., inability to produce negative cultures after 4 months of therapy). The sputum cultures become negative in greater than 90% of cases 3 months after initiating therapy. Relapse (i.e., recurrence of disease after completion of a regimen) usually occurs in less than 5% of cases. Routine radiologic monitoring is usually not necessary in most cases, although a radiologic examination at the end of a treatment period is useful to record the "new baseline."

DRUG-RESISTANT DISEASE

Drug resistance in mycobacteria is spontaneous, predictable, and mediated by unlinked random chromosomal mutations. The likelihood of spontaneous mutation conferring resistance to INH is roughly 1 in 10^6, whereas that to rifampin is roughly 1 in 10^8. Therefore, the likelihood of an organism developing resistance to both these drugs is the product of probabilities—i.e., 10^{14}—many logfold more than is the usual mycobacterial burden. This is the underlying principle for modern combination antimycobacterial drug therapy. Appropriate therapy, therefore, consists of two or more effective drugs given simultaneously throughout treatment. Drug-resistant strains emerge when only one effective drug is given or taken, allowing the spontaneously resistant organisms to multiply while the susceptible ones are being killed. This is clinically translated into an initial response with later recurrence of symptoms when the mycobacterial burden is re-established, now with the resistant strain. This error has often been compounded by the addition of another single drug to this failing regimen. This selects out another strain, now resistant to both the first two drugs. **Never add a single drug to a failing regimen**.

Drug resistance is more likely in previously treated cases, patients from developing nations, large cities, patients with HIV infection, and patients with cavitary lesions. Whereas acquisition of drug-resistant strains in the past was primarily through multiple treatments with ineffective regimens, recent outbreaks in hospitals and correctional institutions provide evidence for a second mechanism: transmission of multiple-drug–resistant strains to contacts. Although most of those affected by this mechanism have been HIV-infected, non–HIV-infected hospital and prison workers have developed at least tuberculin skin reactivity if not active disease after exposure to the index case.

The treatment success rate in non–HIV-infected patients with drug-resistant mycobacteria is considerably lower than in those with susceptible organisms (as much as 83-fold in large trials). The relapse rate was doubled. The success rate falls farther when the number of first-line drugs the organism is resistant to increases.

The outcome is considerably worse in HIV-infected patients with multiple-drug–resistant tuberculosis. Some studies show that despite aggressive therapy, 70 to 90% died within 1 to 5 months. Apart from obvious defects in immunity, there is evidence that HIV-infected patients have impaired absorption of antituberculous medications.

Because the prevalence of drug resistance is rising, initial therapy should now be with four first-line drugs: INH, rifampin, pyrazinamide, and either ethambutol or streptomycin. Therapy with solely the first three drugs should be considered only when the likelihood of single-drug resistance is less than 2%. Conversely, in New York City, the prevalence of multiple-drug–resistant strains is so high that initial therapy with five drugs is recommended.

Directly observed therapy, as either an outpatient or preferably an inpatient, should be prescribed for cases with multiple-drug–resistant organisms, many of which have occurred because of incomplete compliance with prior self-administered regimens.

Retreatment after failed therapy should be started with at least four, if not more, drugs, depending on the extent of disease and the strength of available medications. Therapy will have to be individualized, and monitoring for side effects and changing susceptibility has to be more stringent. Early and continued consultation with specialists in the therapy of multiple-drug–resistant tuberculosis is strongly recommended. Treatment often has to be prolonged by as much as 12 to 24 months, depending on the response to and strength of the regimen.

Lung surgery has been used at specialized centers with some success as a last-ditch attempt to reduce the multiple-drug–resistant mycobacterial burden and therefore tip the balance in favor of the host.

EXTRAPULMONARY TUBERCULOSIS

Extrapulmonary sites of tuberculosis have generally been shown to respond as effectively to standard regimens as do the lungs. Skeletal tuberculosis may require longer periods of treatment. Response to therapy is more often monitored by clinical and radiologic parameters than microbiologic studies because of the relative inaccessibility of these tissues. Surgery is sometimes employed both to obtain diagnostic specimens and to treat complications of spinal tuberculosis (Pott's disease) and constrictive pericarditis. Corticosteroids may be beneficial in reducing the sequelae and symptoms from pericarditis, menin-

gitis, and postprimary pleural effusions when given as adjunctive therapy with effective antituberculous drugs. Prednisone, 40 to 60 mg per day for 4 to 6 weeks, is usually added in the initial phases.

Corticosteroids also often relieve marked constitutional symptoms and fever; improve serious hypoxemia, anemia, anorexia, and inanition in debilitated patients; and have been used successfully, again as adjunctive therapy, with effective antituberculous medications.

PREGNANCY AND LACTATION

Pregnant women with tuberculosis must be treated promptly. The disease presents much more of a hazard to both mother and fetus than does the therapy. Therapeutic abortion is not usually indicated. The initial therapy should consist of INH (with pyridoxine supplements), rifampin, and ethambutol. All three drugs cross the placenta without teratogenic effects. Streptomycin is contraindicated, with demonstrated harmful effects on the ear of the developing fetus. There is insufficient information about the routine addition of pyrazinamide during pregnancy. Other drugs should also be avoided if possible.

Drug concentrations appearing in breast milk are neither sufficient to be therapeutic or even preventive for the fetus nor are they obviously toxic.

THERAPY OF OTHER MYCOBACTERIAL DISEASES

Therapeutic data on nontuberculous (atypical) mycobacterial diseases is based on much smaller studies. A good understanding of the natural history of these infections is as important as in tuberculosis: some resolve spontaneously, some respond very well (often despite apparent in vitro resistance), some require prolonged therapy, whereas in others drug therapy is often futile. In general, *M. kansasii*, *M. xenopi*, *M. szulgai*, *M. marinum*, and *M. ulcerans* are easier to treat than *M. avium-intracellulare*, *M. scrofulaceum*, *M. simiae*, *M. chelonae*, and *M. fortuitum*.

M. kansasii. This photochromogenic species most commonly causes pulmonary disease that responds well to drug therapy. Rifampin, ethambutol, and INH for 12 to 24 months is generally successful. The INH dose is often doubled because of relative in vitro insensitivity.

M. marinum. This causes indolent cutaneous infections that may heal spontaneously. If the superficial skin infection spreads or there is deeper involvement, many drugs are often successfully used. Antituberculous drugs (especially rifampin, trimethoprim-sulfamethoxazole, and minocycline) are given singly until the lesions have completely subsided (usually within a few months).

M. fortuitum and ***M. chelonae.*** These rapidly growing species cause disease in a variety of sites and are invariably resistant to the usual antimycobacterial drugs. Cutaneous infections sometimes resolve spontaneously or require surgical removal (including any associated foreign body). Pulmonary disease and disseminated disease are also seen. Serious disease is treated with parenteral amikacin and either cefoxitin or imipenem for 4 to 6 weeks, followed by oral monotherapy with drugs such as sulfamethoxazole, quinolones, and clarithromycin, to which the organism may be susceptible. *M. chelonae* is often resistant to oral medications, and surgery is often used for local disease.

M. avium-intracellulare **Complex.** Therapy is far from adequate for these organisms, which cause various manifestations from slowly progressive pulmonary disease in patients with other chronic parenchymal abnormalities to disseminated infections in HIV-infected patients. They are often resistant to INH and pyrazinamide, but responses have been obtained with four or more drugs given simultaneously after susceptibilities are known. Combinations have included rifampin, INH, ethambutol, and streptomycin and more recently rifampin, ethambutol, clarithromycin, and ciprofloxacin. Surgical excision of localized disease is often recommended in younger patients with good lung function. Consultation with specialists is recommended. Although the duration of mycobacteremia in AIDS patients has been shortened with rifabutin, there is little evidence that the overall outcome is beneficially affected.

The Cardiovascular System

ACQUIRED DISEASES OF THE AORTA

method of
MARSHALL E. BENJAMIN, M.D., and
RICHARD H. DEAN, M.D.
*Bowman Gray School of Medicine, Wake Forest
University
Winston-Salem, North Carolina*

Complications of atherosclerosis play an integral role in the pathogenesis of greater than 95% of all acquired diseases of the aorta. Even the acquired manifestations of atherosclerosis may have some genetic predetermination, since the rate of development of occlusive disease, as well as the prevalence of aneurysmal degeneration, appears to have familial predisposition. Nevertheless these lesions are assumed to be acquired and will be the main focus of this chapter. Other rarely encountered acquired lesions of the aorta that include embolic, inflammatory, and infectious causes are discussed here only briefly.

AORTIC OCCLUSIVE DISEASE

With respect to occlusive disease, the abdominal aorta is involved to a much greater extent than the thoracic segment, although stenosis and occlusion of the branches of the thoracic aorta have been well described. Atherosclerosis accounts for the majority of thoracic disease, but occlusive lesions resulting from fibromuscular disease, Buerger's disease, and giant cell, Takayasu's, and irradiation arteritis are all well recognized.

In the abdominal aorta, the atherosclerotic process usually begins in the terminal aorta or, more commonly, the iliac vessels. An occlusive lesion at these sites allows the thrombotic process to progress proximally to the level of the renal vessels, making the site of origin difficult to identify. The thrombotic process rarely extends proximal to the renal arteries. Important collateral pathways, such as the internal mammary to inferior mesenteric, superior mesenteric to inferior mesenteric and internal iliac, and intercostal and lumbars to circumflex iliac and internal iliac, usually enlarge to compensate for such occlusive lesions of the terminal aorta.

Clinical Diagnosis

Typically the patients are middle-aged male smokers who present with buttock, thigh, and calf claudication. They may have some degree of sexual dysfunction secondary to hypoperfusion to the pelvis, but their lower extremities are usually warm and well perfused from the collateral circulation. A bruit may be noted low in the abdomen or groin region, and femoral pulses are characteristically weak or absent. The patient commonly has signs and symptoms of other systemic atherosclerotic disease. The differential diagnosis most commonly includes complaints of low-back, buttock, and/or thigh pain that is neurogenic rather than muscular in origin. When the symptoms are neurogenic, the onset of pain is usually secondary to positional changes, and relief is generally provided by flexing the spine, lying, or sitting. An uncommon presentation of aortic occlusive disease may be the "blue toe syndrome," in which an ulcerative plaque in the aortic flow stream acts as the embolic source to the distal extremity. This will be discussed in greater depth later in the chapter.

Objective Diagnosis

Although the diagnosis can usually be established by history and physical examination alone, noninvasive tests such as ankle-brachial indexes (ABIs), segmental limb pressures, Doppler waveforms, or pulse volume recordings can document the severity of limb ischemia. Treadmill testing may be particularly helpful in establishing the diagnosis. Although computed tomography (CT) scans usually demonstrate the heavily diseased or occluded distal aorta, they rarely add information. Duplex ultrasound scanning may help establish the hemodynamic significance of some stenotic iliac lesions, but because of the depth in the pelvis and overlying bowel gas, imaging of the more proximal iliac segments and distal aorta may be difficult.

An arteriogram is considered a preoperative test and is only obtained when the patient is considered for intervention, either noninvasive or surgical. With aortic occlusion, either an axillary or a translumbar approach usually gives a clear image of the extent of disease, with particular interest to the juxtarenal segment, as well as the runoff vessels. In the case of aortic or iliac stenoses, direct pressure measurements across the lesions should be obtained. A gradient of greater than 10 to 15 mmHg is considered to indicate a hemodynamically significant lesion.

Treatment

Mild nondisabling claudication from aortoiliac stenosis may remain stable for many years; however, symptomatic improvement is unlikely without treatment. Intervention is usually reserved for patients with significant disability. Efforts to modify risk factors such as smoking, obesity, hypertension, and diabetes should be undertaken. Structured exercise programs have been shown to significantly increase walking distance. Patients should be informed that the pain they experience with ambulation is in fact causing no damage, and they should be encouraged to "walk through the pain." Because of its progressive nature, with its tendency to encroach on the renal arteries, patients with significant disease or aortic occlusion are nearly always considered for operative repair, if their other medical conditions allow.

In the iliac segments, percutaneous transluminal balloon angioplasty (PTA) has a success rate of about 70% at 1 year, and about 50% at 5 years. Slightly better results are reported for lesions of the common iliac artery. These results may be even better when intraluminal stents are employed. PTA of the aortic segment has only been attempted at a few specialized centers, with results that are less satisfactory than surgical repair. Surgical repair of aortoiliac occlusive disease can be accomplished by several means including endarterectomy for relatively localized disease, as well as anatomic or extra-anatomic bypass grafting.

In experienced hands, the perioperative mortality for aortic surgery is between 2 and 3%. Myocardial infarction accounts for the majority of deaths, with stroke and pulmonary or renal failure accounting for a large portion of the rest. Many reports have established the excellent long-term patency of anatomic aortic bypass surgery, with expected patency rates of 85% at 5 years and 70% at 10 years. Because of the generalized nature of the atherosclerotic process, a reported 25% of patients will be dead 5 years after surgery, and 50% after 10 years. Thus, 10 years after aortic surgery, patients have a 50% chance of being alive and a 70% chance that the bypass graft will be patent.

Complications of aortic replacement surgery can include the systemic problems of myocardial infarction, stroke, pulmonary or renal failure, and bleeding or graft thrombosis. By far the most devastating complication is prosthetic graft infection, which, with the use of routine perioperative antibiotics, seems to occur about 1% of the time. This, however, can occur many months or years from operation, and if the entire graft is involved, complete removal and extra-anatomic reconstruction is usually required.

ANEURYSMAL DISEASE

Aneurysms of Ascending Aorta and Transverse Aortic Arch

Although syphilis was at one time a leading cause of aneurysmal disease in the ascending and arch aorta, today the majority of aneurysms of this location are from atherosclerosis. Aneurysm formation secondary to chronic aortic dissection accounts for a significant number of cases, while cystic medial necrosis and congenital causes account for a smaller

fraction. The majority of patients are asymptomatic, with symptoms arising when there is pressure on, or obstruction of, adjacent structures. In general, aneurysms larger than 5 cm in diameter should be considered for resection. Repair can be complex, with concomitant procedures on the aortic valve or coronary arteries often required. With arch disease, the arch vessel may need to be reimplanted onto the graft, requiring temporary interruption of the cerebral circulation. These procedures obviously require cardiopulmonary bypass, usually with some combination of profound hypothermia and circulatory arrest.

Acute Thoracic Dissection

In contradistinction to chronic dissection, which is a common cause of aneurysmal dilatation, acute aortic dissection represents a catastrophic emergency. Characterized by a transverse intimal tear with, most commonly, separation of the medial layer of the arterial wall, it can occur anywhere along the course of the thoracic aorta. The condition usually occurs between the ages of 40 and 70 years, with hypertension an important predisposing factor. It is three times more common in men. In younger women, it has been reported during the third trimester of pregnancy. The most common location of the tear (66% of the cases) is in the ascending aorta, within 2 cm of the aortic valve. In contrast to the commonly held belief, the majority of the patients are sleeping or lying down at the onset of symptoms. Syncope is a common presenting symptom. The dissection of blood between the layers of the arterial wall, manifests as a "tearing or ripping" type of chest or back pain, which can migrate distally as abdominal or lower extremity discomfort as the process involves more of the arterial tree.

Clinical Diagnosis

These patients are usually in shock, pale, and sweating, with severe hypertension. When the dissection involves the aortic valve, a crescendo diastolic murmur may be heard. A pericardial friction rub may be noted if the dissection has made its way to the pericardium. The dissecting column of blood usually involves the greater curvature of the thoracic aorta, and the visceral and renal vessels can become sheared off or occluded as it makes its way distally. This manifests with signs and symptoms of acute mesenteric ischemia, severe hypertension, oliguria, or anuria.

DeBakey proposed the first classification based on the location of the tear and its subsequent extension. In Types I and II, the dissection starts in the ascending aorta. Type I dissections extend to involve portions beyond the ascending aorta, whereas Type II dissections are confined to the ascending portion. Type III dissections originate in the proximal descending aorta and continue distally for a variable degree. They may also dissect in a retrograde fashion, although still originating from the proximal descending aorta. Another commonly used classification is based on the anatomic site of origin of the dissection, with Type A dissections originating in the ascending aorta and Type B originating beyond the aortic arch.

Objective Diagnosis and Treatment

Although aortography remains the mainstay of diagnosis, CT and magnetic resonance imaging (MRI) scans and transesophageal echocardiograms are increasingly accurate at establishing the diagnosis, as well as aiding in follow-up. Chronic dissections are defined as occurring more than 2 weeks before presentation and carry a much better prognosis, since these patients have already survived the most critical period and can be treated conservatively. The catastrophic series of events set in motion by acute dissection, however, results in free rupture and death in greater than 75% of the cases. These patients require a combination of medical and surgical therapy. The goal of medical management is to expediently reduce the blood pressure to normotensive levels and, with the use of a beta blocker, decrease myocardial contractility and therefore the steepness of the pulse wave (dP/dt). This is usually carried out with a combination of nitroprusside and propranolol (Inderal) or labetalol (Normodyne, Trandate).

Most surgeons feel that all acute dissections involving the ascending aorta (Stanford Type A) be treated with surgery. Type B dissections are usually approached with a combination of initial medical therapy followed by surgery. The timing of operation, however, remains controversial. For those patients treated with medical therapy alone, the 3-year survival is about 30%, while survival is increased to 60% at 3 years with the combination of medical and surgical therapy.

Thoracoabdominal Aortic Aneurysms

Thoracoabdominal aneurysms are classified into three groups: Type I involves the descending thoracic and the upper abdominal aorta, Type II involves the entire descending thoracic and entire abdominal segments, and Type III involves the distal descending thoracic aorta and the entire abdominal aorta. Type IV, although not a true thoracoabdominal aneurysm, has been described when the upper abdominal aorta is involved. Atherosclerosis and cystic medial degeneration account for nearly 85% of thoracoabdominal aneurysms. The presentation is similar to that of other forms of aneurysmal disease, with back and abdominal pain or a pulsatile abdominal mass being frequent complaints. The diagnosis may be suggested by routine chest x-ray examination and then confirmed with CT scan, MRI scan, or arteriography.

Without treatment, the natural history of the disease leads to a 2-year survival rate of only 24%, with half of these deaths due to rupture. Treatment is surgical and involves graft replacement based on the endoaneurysmal techniques devised by E. Stanley Crawford. If a patient's general medical condition does not contraindicate it, surgical repair allows a 2-

year survival of 61% for patients between 67 and 70, and 46% for those 71 years and over.

Abdominal Aortic Aneurysms

The prevalence of abdominal aortic aneurysm is reported to be increasing. In western countries, approximately 10% of a vascular surgeon's practice is made up of patients suffering from abdominal aortic aneurysms, and the majority are men. At 67 years, the mean age of patients with aneurysmal disease is about a decade older than that of patients with occlusive disease of the same area. Of major concern is that abdominal aortic aneurysms have a propensity for sudden rupture and death, with nearly 15,000 deaths reported per year, making it the thirteenth leading cause of death. In the 1950s, Estes reported the classic study of untreated abdominal aortic aneurysms, showing that the 1-year survival rate for patients with abdominal aortic aneurysm was 60%, and at 5 years, 19%. The survival of aged-matched controls *without* aneurysmal disease was 80% at 5 years. Therefore, it seems intuitive that the only way to affect the natural history is to identify and treat the disease before rupture occurs.

The relationship between size and risk of rupture was described by Szilagyi. He demonstrated that the 5-year risk of rupture for 4-cm aneurysms is less than 15%, but for one aneurysm 8 cm in diameter, it was 75%. The risk of rupture increases dramatically once the aneurysm has reached 5 cm. An aneurysm growing in excess of approximately 0.5 cm per year (the average) is also at increased risk of rupture and should be repaired electively.

Clinical Diagnosis

Nearly 75% of infrarenal aortic aneurysms are asymptomatic at diagnosis and found with routine studies or on physical examination. Most symptoms are from expansion or rupture, but embolization or thrombosis may also occur. Pressure on adjacent structures is the cause of the most common symptoms, and nearly any type of back, hip, flank, or abdominal pain can be secondary to an abdominal aortic aneurysm. The sudden onset of severe pain is characteristic of expansion or rupture and heralds an urgent or emergent situation. Small tears in the aneurysm wall may result in a transient leak, which quickly seals and then is followed by a massive, usually lethal, uncontrolled hemorrhage. Leaks in the posterior or posterolateral location may be contained by the spine or paraspinal muscles, allowing chronic contained ruptures. Any patient who presents with abdominal or back pain, shock, syncope, and a pulsatile abdominal mass should be taken directly from the emergency room to the operating room without further diagnostic studies. Hypotension and shock normally do not occur in the absence of rupture, and in this setting of a symptomatic but nonruptured aneurysm, a CT scan is usually warranted to establish the diagnosis. This patient's operation is then handled on an urgent basis. Nearly all symptomatic aneurysms, regardless of size, should be considered for surgery. As a general rule, small (less than 5 cm) asymptomatic aneurysms can be followed with serial CT scans or ultrasound. Although the 5-year risk of rupture is only 15% for aneurysms in the 4- to 4.5-cm range, because of the very high mortality associated with rupture, surgical repair of these smaller aneurysms may be considered in an otherwise healthy patient.

Objective Diagnosis

Arteriography is generally not used to diagnose an abdominal aortic aneurysm, since only the normal caliber of the luminal flow stream is opacified. In fact, aortography may not be required for most routine repairs. Certainly, as occurs frequently in our practice, if the patient has hypertension, renal insufficiency, signs and symptoms suggestive of mesenteric involvement, or a CT scan suggestive of renal or iliac involvement, an arteriogram should be obtained preoperatively. MRI scanning can provide information similar to that of the CT scan; however, in addition it can also provide information on the arteries and veins (magnetic resonance angiographic scanning) without the use of contrast agents. As the technology advances, these advantages may allow it to become the preoperative test of choice.

Treatment

Coronary artery disease is responsible for nearly 50 to 60% of the early and late deaths after surgery on the aorta, and therefore preoperative screening and optimization are critical. High-risk patients can be identified by clinical assessment, exercise stress testing, or more commonly a dipyridamole-thallium scan or stress echocardiogram. Patients with positive screening tests or prior coronary artery bypass grafting (CABG) surgery, or those requiring thoracic aortic clamping, should have coronary angiography. Preliminary myocardial revascularization seems to be required in approximately 10% of abdominal aortic aneurysm repairs. Similarly, carotid duplex ultrasound scanning identifies those patients at risk for perioperative neurologic events originating from extracranial cerebrovascular disease. Repair is usually performed with in situ prosthetic replacement, with either a straight or a bifurcated Dacron or polytetrafluoroethylene (ePTFE) graft. The mortality in most centers active in this type of surgery is less than 5% for elective repair. For ruptured aneurysms, nearly 50% of patients die before reaching the hospital. Of those who have free intraperitoneal ruptures and do make it to the hospital, less than 10% survive.

Complications are similar to those of aortic replacement for occlusive disease, with graft infection the most feared. Ischemic colitis is reported to occur in about 2% and is usually manifest with prolonged hypotension, acidemia, oliguria, or early postoperative diarrhea. Paraplegia secondary to spinal cord ischemia, although well recognized as a complication of thoracic aortic surgery, is exceedingly rare for infrarenal replacement, with a reported incidence of 0.2%. Interestingly, it is reported 10-fold more frequently in cases of ruptured aneurysms.

ATHEROEMBOLIC DISEASE

Occasionally patients with abdominal aortic aneurysm or atherosclerotic disease of the aorta present with lower extremity ischemia secondary to embolization. Atheroma dislodges from an ulcerative plaque within the high-flow circuit of the diseased aorta, or thrombus may embolize from the sac of an aneurysm. Although it may be true that "aneurysms within the abdomen tend to rupture while peripheral aneurysms tend to embolize," atheroembolic disease from any proximal location must always be considered as a cause of acute limb ischemia.

Clinical and Objective Diagnosis

There are two general types of atheroembolic pathologic lesion. Macroemboli generally are large clumps of white thrombus or atherosclerotic plaque and usually result in major vessel obstruction, such as popliteal or tibial occlusion. Microemboli are much smaller and are made up of fibrinoplatelet aggregates or cholesterol crystals. These tend to migrate to the distal aspects of the arterial tree, resulting in digital occlusion, with pedal pulse typically being spared ("blue toe syndrome"). Regardless of the cause, several studies have demonstrated that the natural history of untreated disease is that of recurrent embolic episodes, with eventual limb loss in up to 60% of the patients. We prefer a CT scan as an initial study. An abdominal aortic aneurysm with laminated thrombus within the sac, and a heavily diseased and atherosclerotic aorta, are both easily demonstrated. If this is not diagnostic and embolic disease is still suspected, an arteriogram may help demonstrate an ulcerative lesion upstream in the arterial circuit, acting as the site of embolization.

Treatment

The treatment depends on the cause of the embolic process. Embolization from an abdominal aortic aneurysm or a heavily diseased aorta should be treated with prompt surgery. In major axial vessel occlusion, embolectomy or bypass may be employed. Treatment of microembolic disease is more difficult, with heparin, dextran, or thrombolytic therapy playing a controversial but sometimes helpful role.

AORTIC INFLAMMATORY DISEASES

The vast majority of patients with aortic disease have atherosclerosis as the cause; however, numerous conditions have inflammation or vascular necrosis as their pathologic feature and are collectively termed "vasculitis." Most of these syndromes affect small to medium-sized vessels with immunologic factors thought to play a central role in the pathogenesis. A few syndromes, however, most notably Takayasu's and temporal arteritis, typically affect the aorta and its major branches.

Takayasu's arteritis is now known to occur in all races and nationalities, in addition to all age groups, but it most commonly affects young to middle-aged women. Presentation may vary, but ideally three stages of the disease can be recognized. The first phase of the disease manifests with malaise, fever, weight loss, arthralgia, and myalgias. The second phase involves vague discomfort about the involved arteries, and the final stage involves symptoms of ischemia from arterial involvement of the disease. The subclavian, carotid, renal, and mesenteric arteries, in addition to the aorta, are most commonly involved, leading to upper extremity or cerebral ischemia, as well as renovascular hypertension or mesenteric ischemia. In addition to this branch vessel disease, aortic involvement may lead to aneurysm formation anywhere along the length, as well as occlusive manifestations. Elective vascular surgical bypass during the inactive phase of the disease remains the mainstay of treatment.

Similarly, temporal arteritis has a 1- to 3-week phase of flulike symptoms with fever and headache. Later, abnormally enlarged and tender temporal arteries may appear. An erythrocyte sedimentation rate (ESR) of 40 to 140 mm per hour is usual, and ocular symptoms occur in about 50% of the patients sometime in the second or third month. Diagnosis is made with biopsy. In view of the danger of permanent visual loss or morbidity from extracranial involvement, high-dose corticosteroids are the initial therapy. The need for surgical intervention is rare in temporal arteritis, unlike that in Takayasu's arteritis, with prompt steroid therapy typically reversing most symptoms in addition to preventing involvement of the contralateral eye.

ANGINA PECTORIS

method of
THOMAS J. WARGOVICH, M.D.
University of Florida College of Medicine
Gainesville, Florida

Angina pectoris, defined in the most basic terms, is the result of an imbalance between myocardial oxygen supply and demand. Angina pectoris results from ischemia, a state of oxygen deprivation caused by decreased perfusion of the myocardium. Myocardial ischemia is relative, however, and varies for each individual, depending not only on absolute blood flow but also on systolic wall tension, contractility, and heart rate—the three major determinants of myocardial oxygen consumption. The reduction of myocardial oxygen consumption is the primary mechanism by which antianginal agents relieve symptoms.

The diagnosis of angina pectoris is a clinical one but should be based on typical symptoms and corroborated by results of objective testing. A detailed discussion of noninvasive and invasive testing in the diagnosis of ischemic heart disease is beyond the scope of this article. Silent myocardial ischemia will also not be addressed in this article.

PROFILE OF PATIENTS

Our perception that the typical patient with chronic stable angina is a middle-aged man needs correction. As the American population ages, the characteristics of this group of patients are also changing. In a retrospective analysis of 5125 patients enrolled in a large multicenter study, the mean age of patients was 69 years, and 53% were women. The mean age for women, as one might expect, was higher, at 71 years. More than one cardiovascular-related illness was present in the majority of patients (hypertension, 58%; previous myocardial infarction [MI], 44%; hypercholesterolemia, 34%; congestive heart failure [CHF], 25%; diabetes, 23%; and conduction disease, 6%). The majority of patients take more than one cardiovascular-active medication. These findings demonstrate that the management, particularly the drug therapy, of chronic stable angina is becoming more complex. Patients are very likely to have multiple medical problems. There are also more concerns regarding drug efficacies and drug interactions in an elderly population.

TREATMENT

The medical management of chronic stable angina includes modification of ongoing risk factors, pharmacologic treatment, and the appropriate selection of patients for revascularization procedures. General measures include counseling patients about diet and weight loss, as obesity increases myocardial oxygen requirements. Hyperlipidemia should be investigated and treated. Daily exercise should be encouraged, but the level of intensity may need to be modified. Chronic stable angina clearly follows a circadian pattern related to circulating plasma catecholamines. Patients should plan their daily activities to avoid attacks when the anginal threshold is lower.

Aggressive treatment of hypertension is always warranted. Secondary causes of hypertension should be considered; atherosclerotic renal artery stenosis is a relatively frequent finding in patients with coronary artery disease and hypertension. Patients should discontinue cigarette smoking. Smokers have a higher incidence of MI and cardiovascular mortality. Cigarette smoking has been shown to cause endothelial dysfunction, precipitating angina as a result of inappropriate vasoconstrictor responses to physiologic stimuli, such as exercise or cold weather.

Finally, management of patients with chronic stable angina includes the timely identification of coexistent illnesses (e.g., anemia, hyperthyroidism, tachyarrhythmias, infection) or drugs (sympathomimetics or other stimulants) that may exacerbate anginal episodes.

Pharmacotherapy

There are three general classes of antianginal medications: nitrates, beta blockers, and calcium antagonists. A number of newer medications, including metabolic agents and potassium channel openers, are still under investigation but show benefit in a limited number of clinical studies. Anticoagulants, such as aspirin and warfarin, are discussed separately later.

Nitrates

Mechanism of Action. Nitroglycerin is a time-honored treatment for chronic stable angina, and nitrates remain the most commonly used antianginal medication. Organic nitrates have numerous effects: they increase coronary blood flow by a direct vasodilator effect on epicardial (conductance) arteries of the heart, even in the most severely diseased vessels, as well as resistance vessels (arterioles). The vasodilator effect is even more potent in the venous system. Changes in venous conductance markedly reduce preload, shrinking cardiac chamber size, resulting in a decrease in systolic wall tension. It is safe to assume, then, that nitrates act to reduce or prevent symptoms of angina by a combination of increasing oxygen delivery to ischemic myocardium and also by reducing oxygen demand.

In healthy blood vessels with normally functioning endothelium, endothelium-derived relaxing factor (EDRF), since identified as nitric oxide is responsible for maintaining vascular tone and permeability. In patients with coronary artery disease, EDRF release is impaired secondary to endothelial dysfunction. This may result in enhanced vascular tone and paradoxical vasoconstriction in response to normal stimuli. Nitroglycerin is an exogenous nitric oxide donor. Nitrates act by activating intracellular guanylate cyclase to produce cyclic guanosine monophospate (GMP), which initiates vascular smooth muscle cell relaxation. Thus nitrates exert their effects independent of the state of health of the endothelium.

Dosing and Administration. Nitrates are available in a number of formulations (Table 1). Nitroglycerin by the sublingual, buccal, or lingual spray route enters the systemic circulation rapidly because it bypasses the effects of first-pass hepatic metabolism. Isosorbide dinitrate has low bioavailability owing to first-pass hepatic metabolism, and it is available in oral, sustained-release oral, and sublingual forms. Isosorbide mononitrate is the active metabolite of

dinitrate and does not undergo a significant first-pass effect. Topical and transdermal nitrate formulations are also available.

Short-acting nitrates are the treatment of choice for acute episodes of myocardial ischemia. Long-acting nitrates have been shown to be clinically effective during chronic administration, decreasing symptoms and increasing exercise ability; however, tolerance is a major limitation of long-acting nitrate therapy. Nitrate tolerance is a well-known but not completely understood phenomenon. Tolerance is thought secondary to depletion of sulfhydryl co-factors within the vascular smooth muscle cell since treatment with N-acetylcysteine partially reverses it. When selecting long-acting nitrate therapy for patients, the clinician must balance the restraints of efficacy with the development of tolerance. Tolerance only occurs when therapy is prescribed that results in consistently high levels of drug maintained over time. Tolerance can be decreased with designation of a nitrate-free interval, lasting 6 to 10 hours. On occasion, aggravation of angina may occur during the nitrate-free interval. This is known as rebound angina. There is some evidence to suggest that the controlled release form of 5-isosorbide mononitrate (Imdur), given once daily, may result in a nitrate-poor interval that would prevent the rebound phenomenon but not diminish its antianginal efficacy. Tolerance can also be avoided by administering the lowest clinically effective dose.

Headache is still the most common side effect occurring with all nitrates. Dizziness results from nitrates' hypotensive effect secondary to vasodilatation and typically occurs after acute administration of the short-acting preparation. Hypotension is exacerbated by hypovolemia.

Beta-Adrenergic Blockers

Mechanism of Action. Beta blockers represent a very important class of drugs in the treatment of chronic stable angina. A number of drugs have been extensively studied and approved (Table 2). Beta blockers have been convincingly shown to decrease symptoms and to improve the exercise anginal threshold. They act by competitively inhibiting $beta_1$- and $beta_2$-adrenergic receptor sites in cardiac and vascular tissue, respectively. Their major effect is likely due solely to reduction of myocardial oxygen consumption, both at rest and during stress, because of their negative chronotropic and inotropic effects, as well as by decreasing systemic arterial pressure. Beta blockers do not cause coronary vasodilatation; in fact, in certain situations such as coronary vasospasm, they have been reported to induce vasoconstriction.

Classification. Beta blockers are classified according to the predominance of $beta_1$ versus $beta_2$ effects (cardioselectivity). Cardioselectivity is a useful feature in attempting to avoid effects on $beta_2$ receptors that might aggravate reactive airway disease and claudication or mask symptoms of diabetes. However, cardioselectivity is relative and disappears

TABLE 1. **Common Formulations of Nitrates**

Medication	Dose	Duration of Action
Nitroglycerin		
Sublingual	0.3–0.8 mg	10–30 min
Buccal	1–3 mg	30–300 min
Spray	0.4 mg	10–30 min
Oral (SR)	2.5–17.5 mg	2–8 h
Ointment (2%)	0.5–2 inches	3–8 h
Transdermal	5–20 mg	8–18 h
Isosorbide dinitrate (Isordil)		
Sublingual	2.5–10 mg	1–2 h
Oral	5–60 mg	2–6 h
Oral (sustained release)	60–180 mg	6–10 h
Isosorbide mononitrate (IsMO)		
Oral	10–40 mg	6–8 h
Oral (sustained release)	40–100 mg	6–10 h

Adapted from Abrams J: Nitrates. *In* Parmley W, Chatterjee K (eds): Cardiology. Philadelphia, JB Lippincott, 1994, pp 1–21.

TABLE 2. **Common Formulations of Beta Blockers**

	Daily Dose (mg)	Beta₁-Selectivity	Intrinsic Sympathomimetic Activity	Alpha₁-Receptor Antagonism	Lipid Solubility
Propranolol (Inderal)	80–480	0	0	0	+ +
Metoprolol (Lopressor)	50–300	+ +	0	0	+
Atenolol (Tenormin)	25–200	+ +	0	0	0
Nadolol (Corgard)	40–240	0	0	0	0
Timolol (Blocadren)	10–45	0	0	0	0
Acebutolol (Sectral)	100–400	+	+	0	+
Labetalol (Normodyne)	200–2000	0	+	+ +	0
Pindolol (Visken)	10–40	0	+ +	0	0
Betaxolol (Kerlone)	5–40	+ +	0	0	+
Carteolol (Cartrol)	2.5–10	0	+	0	0
Penbutolol (Levatol)	20–40	0	+	0	+ +

Adapted from Frishman W, Charlap S: The alpha and beta-adrenergic blocking drugs. *In* Parmley W, Chatterjee K (eds): Cardiology. Philadelphia, JB Lippincott, 1994, pp 1–18.

as the dose is increased. In addition, there is no advantage to selectivity in regard to angina efficacy. Some beta blockers have potent peripheral vasodilator effects owing to partial alpha-adrenergic antagonism and beta₂ agonism. Labetalol (Normodyne, Trandate) is a very useful agent in patients with hypertension. Studies with carvedilol show a possible cardioprotective role in patients with poor left ventricular function, because of the beneficial effects of modulation of peripheral resistance. Potency, a measure of the dosage needed to inhibit tachycardia during exercise, is clinically important only when changing the patient from one beta-blocking agent to another.

Some beta blockers have intrinsic sympathomimetic activity (ISA), i.e., less reduction of resting heart rate while retaining the ability to block beta receptors during exercise or stress. Again, there is little evidence from results of controlled studies that partial agonism in beta blockers is superior clinically to full antagonists.

Beta blockers are also classified according to lipid solubility. This is relevant to deciding dosing schedules and minimizing side effects. Lipophilic beta blockers have shorter half-lives (that is, dosed more often), and because they are more likely to cross the blood-brain barrier, they may be prone to cause more central nervous system side effects, particularly depression and sleep disturbance. Beta blockers may affect serum lipids, most commonly causing elevation of serum triglycerides while decreasing high-density lipoproteins (HDL), with no major effect on low-density lipoproteins (LDL). There is no evidence that this effect on lipid levels translates to a mortality disadvantage.

Dosing and Administration. A wide array of beta blockers are available, with varying properties (see Table 2). The clinician is encouraged to become familiar and comfortable with at least one agent from each classification (that is, hydrophilic, lipophilic, ISA, alpha₁ antagonism), since therapy should be tailored to the individual. Beta blockers are dosed to effect or titrated until the resting heart rate is consistently within 50 to 70 beats per minute, in the absence of symptoms. This class of antianginals should be used with caution in patients with chronic obstructive lung disease, CHF, and conduction disease. It is likely that the range of limiting side effects and contraindications lead to decreasing use as the patient age increases.

Calcium Channel Antagonists

Mechanism of Action. Intracellular calcium concentration within vascular smooth muscle cells, as well as myocardial cells, regulates contractile function. Calcium antagonists interfere with entry of extracellular calcium across cellular membranes and facilitate vascular smooth muscle relaxation. Vasodilatation occurs primarily as an arteriolar effect in both systemic and coronary vascular beds, with little effect on the venous system. Calcium antagonists have different selectivity for vascular tissues, thus some have greater peripheral effects than cardiac effects. Several, however, have important negative inotropic (depress contractility), negative chronotropic (depress conduction within sinoatrial node), and negative dromotropic (depress conduction within atrioventricular node) effects. Calcium antagonists increase coronary blood flow but act primarily to reduce myocardial oxygen consumption. The antianginal effect of bepridil (Vascor) is attributed mainly to improved or redistributed coronary blood flow, but it may also decrease myocardial workload by afterload reduction.

Classification. Calcium antagonists are categorized into three main classes: the phenylalkylamines (verapamil), the benzothiazepines (diltiazem), and the dihydropyridines (nifedipine, nicardipine, isradipine, amlodipine, felodipine) (Table 3). Bepridil is a diarylaminopropylamine with additional sodium channel effects.

Dosing and Administration. Calcium antagonists are effective monotherapy in patients with chronic stable angina and are the treatment of choice in managing patients with vasospastic angina. The pharmacokinetic properties of calcium antagonists are similar. Absorption by oral administration is rapid, but bioavailability is low due to hepatic first-

TABLE 3. **Common Formulations of Calcium Antagonists**

	Daily Dose (mg)	Lower Peripheral Resistance	Negative Inotropic Effects	Effect on Atrioventricular Nodal Conduction
Verapamil (Calan)	120–480	+	+ +	+ +
Diltiazem (Cardizem)	90–480	+	+	+ +
(Cardizem CD)	120–360	+	+	+ +
Nifedipine (Procardia)	30–120	+ +	0	0
(Procardia-XL)	30–90	+ +	0	0
Nicardipine (Cardene)	60–120	+ +	0	0
Amlodipine (Norvasc)	2.5–10	+ +	0	0
Bepridil (Vascor)	200–400	0	+	+

pass effect. Older forms have short half-lives and require dosing at three or four times daily. Controlled-release formulations provide 24-hour efficacy for most patients. Newer agents, such as amlodipine, have long half-lives and can also be administered once daily. Currently, verapamil, diltiazem, nifedipine, nicardipine, amlodipine, and bepridil are all U.S. Food and Drug Administration (FDA)–approved for angina pectoris. Approved long-acting, sustained-release forms include only Cardizem CD and Procardia-XL, although there is no reason to suspect that the newer as yet unapproved formulations would not be equally efficacious.

When selecting a calcium antagonist for a patient with chronic stable angina, one must consider the characteristics of each individual patient, such as the presence of hypertension, left ventricular dysfunction, conduction disease, or cerebrovascular disease. Dihydropyridines have the greatest selectivity for vascular smooth muscle and are the most potent peripheral vasodilators; they are very effective antihypertensive agents. They lower both systolic and diastolic blood pressure to such a degree that reflex tachycardia might precipitate angina in a subgroup of patients with severe coronary disease. Combination therapy with beta blockers is often effective in the treatment of these patients. Because of their negative chronotropic effects, verapamil and diltiazem cause little change in heart rate and may actually decrease resting pulse.

The net clinical effects of calcium antagonists vary in patients with heart failure. The newer dihydropyridines reportedly have fewer negative inotropic effects and may be better tolerated in patients with left ventricular dysfunction. Verapamil and to a lesser extent diltiazem are contraindicated in patients with clinically significant bradyarrhythmias, whether due to sinus node dysfunction or heart block, and they should be used with caution in patients with CHF.

Clinically important drug interactions occur mainly due to the effect of calcium antagonists on hepatic blood flow or metabolism. Verapamil may increase plasma digoxin levels up to 75%. Increased digoxin levels have also been reported with bepridil. Patients taking digoxin concomitantly with these agents should be monitored for signs and symptoms of digoxin toxicity and the dosage adjusted as necessary. Verapamil, diltiazem, and nicardipine can cause elevations in plasma cyclosporine levels and can increase the risk of cyclosporine-induced nephrotoxicity. In these patients, careful monitoring of plasma cyclosporine levels and renal function is warranted. Bepridil may cause significant prolongation of the QT interval and may precipitate torsades de pointes.

Antithrombotics

Mechanism of Action. Aspirin and other antiplatelet agents inhibit platelet activation by irreversible inhibition of cyclooxygenase, which regulates production of the vasoactive prostanoids thromboxane A_2 and prostacyclin. Inhibition of function lasts the length of the platelet's life, approximately 10 days. Warfarin and other coumarin derivatives inhibit vitamin K–dependent circulating clotting factors. The putative mechanism of action of antithrombotic agents is inhibition of progression of stable coronary plaques to unstable ones, prone to acute thrombosis.

Dosage and Administration. A number of studies indicate a role for aspirin in both the primary and the secondary prevention of coronary artery disease. In the Physicians Health Study, use of low-dose aspirin reduced the incidence of first MI by 87%; however, total deaths were not different in the aspirin group. There are similar data indicating a beneficial effect of aspirin in patients with stable angina. The daily dose of aspirin can be individualized. The usual dose is 324 mg per day, but benefits are also likely at doses as low as 80 mg per day. Results of meta-analyses found no difference between high- or low-dose aspirin, sulfinpyrazone, or dipyridamole.

There have been conflicting results pertaining to the use of oral anticoagulants in the prevention of ischemic events or mortality in patients with ischemic heart disease. The majority of studies have included mainly survivors of MI, with little information available in the subgroup of patients with chronic stable angina. Until further data are available, routine long-term use of oral anticoagulants cannot be recommended at this time.

GUIDELINES FOR SELECTION OF ANTIANGINAL AGENTS IN PATIENTS WITH CHRONIC STABLE ANGINA

Selection of antianginal medication for the patient with chronic stable angina should be individualized, taking into account the patient's frequency of symptoms, activity level, and concurrent illnesses and medications. It is important to remember that patients judge their quality of life and overall health based on the frequency and severity of the symptoms they experience. In general, once-daily treatment regimens are associated with a higher compliance rate; however, newer formulations also tend to be more expensive, which also has an impact on compliance.

In the absence of contraindications, all patients should receive aspirin or other antiplatelet therapy. There is presently no consensus as to whether calcium antagonists or beta blockers should be first-line monotherapy for patients with chronic stable angina. As outlined earlier, advantages and disadvantages exist for both agents, and therapy should be individualized for each patient. The clinically important phenomenon of nitrate tolerance limits the use of this agent as monotherapy. Nitrates might be used as monotherapy in the group of patients with predictable angina, occurring only with strenuous activity, without rest or nocturnal symptoms.

As yet there are no firm data to determine whether drug therapy improves prognosis in the group of patients with chronic, stable angina. Much more is known about patients with unstable angina and MI. It is well known, however, that patients with chronic angina are much more likely to experience ischemic episodes and events in the morning, with a secondary peak in the evening related to circadian catecholamine and neurohumoral activity. Beta blockers are more effective in reducing these episodes than calcium antagonists, although it is not yet shown that this would influence prognosis. Compiled studies have shown that calcium antagonists clearly do not improve prognosis in patients with chronic, stable angina, whereas enough evidence exists regarding beta blocker use in related groups of patients with ischemic heart disease to infer a possible favorable prognostic effect. Therefore, it is my personal approach to try beta-blocker therapy in all patients with effort angina in the absence of contraindications.

In patients with severe hypertension, the use of potent systemic vasodilators is frequently necessary, and calcium antagonists may be started as initial therapy. As previously mentioned, however, reflex tachycardia, particularly with use of dihydropyridines, may require the addition of low-dose beta blockers. When used concomitantly with verapamil or diltiazem, be aware of additive effects on sinus and atrioventricular nodal conduction, especially in the presence of digitalis.

In patients with ischemic heart disease and a history of intermittent or chronic supraventricular tachyarrhythmia, both beta blockers and calcium antagonists (verapamil or diltiazem) are useful in suppressing or controlling symptoms.

Patients with symptoms of heart failure with objective evidence (by echocardiogram or catheterization) of primarily diastolic dysfunction may benefit more from the use of calcium antagonists than beta blockade. Caution is necessary when using either agent in patients with systolic left ventricular dysfunction, as exacerbation of symptoms of heart failure may occur. Nevertheless, there is mounting evidence for the routine use of beta blockers in CHF. Physiologically, beta blockade may ameliorate or prevent the down-regulation and loss of beta-adrenergic cardiac receptors that occur from chronic sympathetic activation accompanying uncompensated heart failure. This may in turn prevent further myocardial contractile deterioration or prevent life-threatening arrhythmias, resulting in a favorable prognostic effect in this group of high-risk patients. It is important that beta-blocker therapy (with cardioselective properties) be initiated at subclinical doses and then titrated upward as tolerated.

Patients with chronic obstructive lung disease, frequently seen in our aging population, often will not tolerate beta blockers, and calcium antagonists may be the drug of choice.

In patients with bradyarrhythmias, whether due to sinus node dysfunction or atrioventricular nodal conduction abnormalities, it is prudent to avoid the use of beta blockers and the calcium antagonists verapamil and diltiazem. The dihydropyridine group of antagonists—nifedipine, nicardipine, and so on—can be safely used.

In patients with stable angina with recent MI, there is evidence to suggest that beta blockers exert a cardioprotective effect in reducing mortality and the occurrence of ischemic events. It has been reported that verapamil and diltiazem reduce the incidence of reinfarction following MI.

Although caution is necessary, it has not been my experience that adverse effects occur with judicial use of beta blockers in patients with claudication or diabetes.

CARDIAC ARREST: SUDDEN CARDIAC DEATH

method of
ROGER D. WHITE, M.D.
Mayo Medical School and Mayo Clinic
Rochester, Minnesota

"Sudden cardiac death" (SCD) is the term used to denote unexpected cardiovascular collapse culminating in pulselessness and apnea (cardiorespiratory arrest). Although it may follow the onset of ischemic signs and/or symptoms, it not infrequently occurs without preceding warning signs of impending collapse and without a prior history of ischemic cardiac disease. The majority of these events occur outside the hospital, and therefore are out-of-hospital cardiac arrests (OHCAs). Although there are many possible causes of OHCA, coronary artery disease (CAD), with or without acute myocardial infarction, is the most frequent cause. Ventricular fibrillation (VF) is the presenting electrical derangement in 60 to 65% of these episodes, preceded in many instances by ventricular tachycardia (VT) that then degenerates into VF. Other presenting conditions are pulseless VT, pulseless electrical activity (PEA), and asystole. Fortunately the most frequent presenting SCD arrhythmia (VF) is also the most treatable, and therefore an aggressive effort is warranted in treating patients experiencing SCD. In well-organized emergency medical service (EMS) systems, as many as 30 to 35% of patients in OHCA and VF can be resuscitated and discharged without neurologic impairment. The likelihood of survival is directly dependent upon rapid and sequential implementation of the American Heart Association (AHA) chain of survival; its critical links are rapid EMS access via calling for help (911 telephone call), prompt bystander cardiopulmonary resuscitation (CPR), early defibrillation, and follow-up advanced cardiac life support (ACLS) care (Figure 1). Early defibrillation has emerged as the most critical lifesaving intervention that has the potential for substantially increasing survival from SCD caused by VF. A major national initiative is needed to educate health care professionals on the benefits of early defibrillation in order to improve survival from cardiac arrest. However, because the benefit of rapid defibrillation is frequently dependent upon the integration of the other components of the chain of survival, these components need to be understood as well.

The victim who is most likely to survive cardiac arrest is one whose arrest is caused by VF and is witnessed, for whom EMS is called immediately (early access), who receives prompt CPR by bystanders (early CPR), who is defibrillated within 6 to 8 minutes of collapse (early defibrillation), and finally who receives follow-up stabilizing ACLS treatment (early advanced care) as needed. The latter might include the administration of antiarrhythmic drugs, endotracheal intubation, or other definitive interventions. Each of these components will now be discussed.

EARLY ACCESS

As soon as a victim is observed to be unresponsive, the EMS system should be called, ideally via the universal emergency number 911. If this number is not yet established in a community, then all citizens should have posted by their telephones the number to call to access the EMS system.

EARLY CPR

Preservation of cerebral viability during the arrested state is totally dependent upon delivery of oxygenated blood to the brain by ventilation and external chest compression. Surely it is reasonable to assume that all physicians will be knowledgeable and skillful in the performance of CPR (basic life support). It is a regrettable experience for an arrested patient to have spontaneous circulation restored by defibrillation, only to die or vegetate from irreversible ischemic brain injury. While it is acknowledged that CPR is only a "holding" function, awaiting more definitive interventions, it can be the major determinant of whether or not a patient awakens without neurologic deficit after cardiac arrest. All physicians should avail themselves of the opportunity to learn this skill and periodically (every 1 or 2 years) be updated in the performance of CPR. New CPR techniques that have the potential of increasing survival are being investigated clinically. One of the most promising of these is active compression-decompression (ACD) CPR carried out by means of a simple plunger device applied to the chest wall. Physicians should be aware of these new developments, which may increase the likelihood of survival of their own patients.

EARLY DEFIBRILLATION

The most significant advance in improving the chances for survival from VF cardiac arrest has been

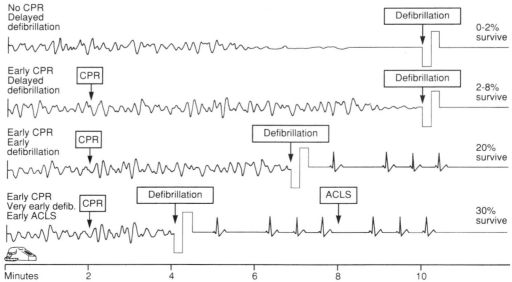

Figure 1. Dependency of survival from cardiac arrest in ventricular fibrillation (VF) on integration of the links in the chain of survival: early access to care, early cardiopulmonary resuscitation (CPR), early defibrillation, and early definitive (advanced cardiac life support [ACLS]) care. (Reproduced with permission. © *Textbook of Basic Life Support for Healthcare Providers,* 1994. Copyright American Heart Association.)

the implementation of early defibrillation programs in out-of-hospital settings. Automated external defibrillators (AEDs) make possible the delivery of defibrillatory shocks rapidly, effectively, and safely. AEDs are attached to the chest wall by means of cables connected to adhesive conductive electrode pads, which are used to both monitor the rhythm and deliver shocks (Figure 2). The rhythm is automatically analyzed by a microprocessor-based algorithm program. If a treatable rhythm (VF or pulseless VT with a rate beyond the cutoff, typically 180 beats per minute ± 10%) is detected, the AED capacitor is automatically charged and visually (screen display) and audibly (voice synthesizer) the operator is requested to deliver a shock. After the shock, most devices are programmed to automatically reanalyze the rhythm to determine if a shockable rhythm is still present. If so, the cycle is repeated, and again a third time if needed. Thus a total of three shocks can be delivered rapidly if needed. Following a third shock, or after any shock that terminates VF, the device calls for a pulse check. If none is present, CPR is performed for 1 minute, and then the analyze-shock cycle can be repeated. The microprocessor-based algorithms that analyze the rhythm have a high degree of both specificity (98%) and sensitivity (greater than 90%). Sensitivity could approach 100% if low-amplitude VF (less than 200 μV) were included in the "treat" category. AEDs are battery-powered and therefore portable, relatively lightweight (13 pounds or less), and easy to operate. The next generation of AEDs will be even more portable and lightweight, extending still further their portability and more widespread use. AEDs are available with event

documentation systems such as dual-channel (voice and electrocardiogram [ECG]) cassette-tape recorders and memory modules or event cards (PCMCIA cards), which store times and ECG data for subsequent printout and review (Figure 3; see also Figure 2).

Improved survival from VF cardiac arrest is very dependent upon early defibrillation. All patient care areas should be equipped with AEDs, including physicians' offices. In out-of-hospital settings, AEDs are carried in basic life support ambulances and by many first-responder EMS personnel, such as firefighters and police officers. It is evident that physicians seeing patients in their offices or in outpatient clinics would be well-advised to consider the placement of AEDs in those settings, and to have office or clinic staff, as well as themselves, trained in their proper operation and maintenance. AEDs can be purchased for $4000 to $4500, including accessories such as spare batteries and extra sets of electrodes.

The AHA algorithm for interventions in VF and pulseless VT is shown in Figure 4. There is a form of VT that can lead to cardiac arrest and necessitates an awareness of modes of presentation, cause, and intervention. This is torsades de pointes, a form of pleomorphic ventricular tachycardia (PVT) caused by prolonged repolarization, manifest electrocardiographically as QT-interval prolongation. It is characterized by the typical twisting of the points QRS complexes on the ECG (Figure 5). The patient may have paroxysms of this tachycardia, between which the QT interval prolongation is evident. When the disorder is suspected a search should be made for a cause (Table 1). Sustained episodes of torsades can

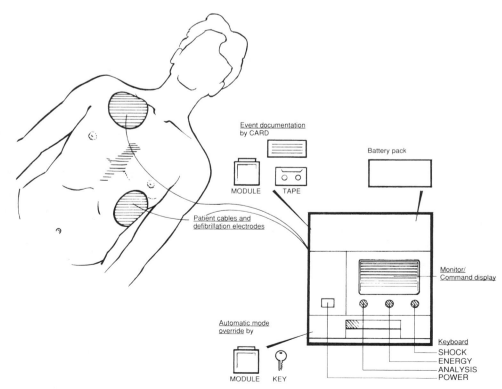

Figure 2. Schematic depiction of the components of an automated external defibrillator (AED). See text for description of the function of these components. Some AEDs have a module or key override that permits the device to be operated as a manual defibrillator if desired. (Reproduced with permission. © *Textbook of Basic Life Support for Healthcare Providers*, 1994. Copyright American Heart Association.)

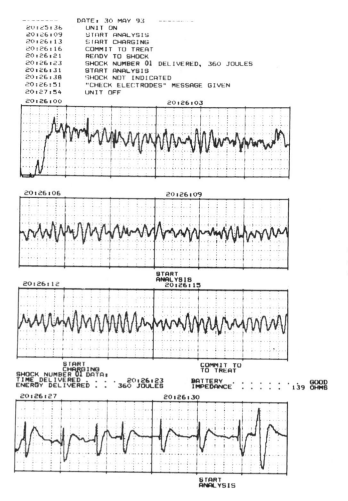

Figure 3. Example of a printout of a defibrillation event in an out-of-hospital cardiac arrest (OHCA) caused by VF. These data are obtained from the device's internal memory, such as memory modules or event cards. (Courtesy of Mayo Foundation.)

Figure 4. American Heart Association (AHA) algorithm for treatment of VF and pulseless ventricular tachycardia (VT). *Abbreviations:* ABC = airway, breathing, and circulation; PEA = pulseless electrical activity. (From Emergency Cardiac Care Committee and Subcommittees, American Heart Association: Guidelines for cardiopulmonary resuscitation and emergency cardiac care. Part III. Adult advanced cardiac life support. JAMA 268:2199–2241, 1992. Copyright 1992, American Medical Association.)

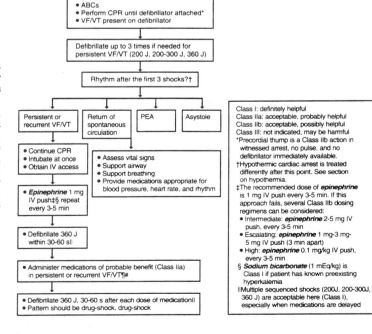

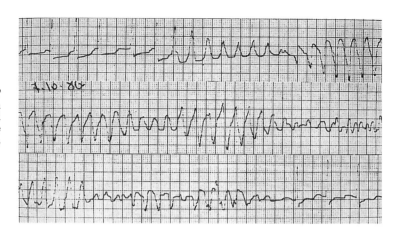

Figure 5. Torsades de pointes. Prolongation of the QT interval is evident both before and following the paroxysm of tachycardia. (Reproduced with permission. From Tzivoni D, Banai S, Schuger C, et al: Treatment of torsade de pointes with magnesium sulfate. Circulation 77:392–397, 1988. Copyright 1988 American Heart Association.)

cause cardiac arrest and should be treated with defibrillation using the same doses of energy as specified for VF and pulseless VT. Magnesium sulfate (1 to 2 grams intravenously) can be injected to control the episodes of torsades, or, if available, overdrive atrial or ventricular pacing can suppress the tachycardia. It is important to appreciate that PVT can occur without QT prolongation, e.g., after acute myocardial infarction, in which case standard antiarrhythmic therapy with lidocaine, procainamide, or bretylium is used. The primary care physician must therefore be alert not only to the ECG appearance of PVT, but also to the etiologic mechanisms that define the PVT

as torsades and thus lead to treatment with magnesium sulfate and/or overdrive pacing.

EARLY ADVANCED CARDIAC LIFE SUPPORT CARE

In many patients experiencing VF cardiac arrest, prompt defibrillation is all that is required to restore spontaneous circulation. After this an intravenous line can be initiated and lidocaine injected to reduce the risk of recurrent VF. In some patients more definitive and aggressive interventions will be required, such as additional drugs, and airway control and ventilation. Pharmacologic and additional electrical therapy is outlined in Figure 4. While endotracheal intubation is the intervention of choice for airway protection and for both oxygenation and ventilation, it should not be attempted by persons who are not trained in this skill. Instead a mask with a one-way valve can be used to ventilate the patient, using a mouth-to-mask technique. Bag-valve mask devices are very difficult for one person to use effectively, and their use in this manner is discouraged. Flow-restricted (peak flow rate 40 liters per minute), oxygen-powered, manually cycled ventilation devices can be used by one person more effectively than bag-valve masks. These devices also have the advantage of delivering 100% oxygen. They are an alternative to masks with one-way valves if the caregiver is trained in their use. Also, a multilumen airway such as the esophageal-tracheal tube (Combitube) can be inserted by trained persons in order to protect the airway if endotracheal intubation cannot be accomplished. All these skills are incorporated in the AHA ACLS training program. Primary care physicians are strongly encouraged to avail themselves of this training opportunity to become thoroughly acquainted with all these ACLS procedures and devices.

TABLE 1. **Causes of Torsades de Pointes**

Congenital prolonged QT syndromes
  Romano-Ward
  Jervell and Lange-Nielsen
Acquired prolonged QT
  Drug-induced
    Quinidine
    Procainamide (Pronestyl)
    Disopyramide (Norpace)
    Sotalol (Betapace)
    Bepridil (Vascor)
    Amiodarone (Cordarone)
    Phenothiazines
      Thioridazine (Mellaril)
      Chlorpromazine (Thorazine)
    Tricyclic antidepressants
      Amitriptyline (Elavil)
      Imipramine (Tofranil)
    Lithium
    Terfenadine (Seldane) and astemizole (Hismanal) in
      combination with ketoconazole (Nizoral), itraconazole
      (Sporanox), erythromycin, or hepatic disease
  Electrolyte derangements
    Hypokalemia
    Hypomagnesemia
    Hypocalcemia
  Neurologic
    Subarachnoid hemorrhage
    Cerebrovascular accident
  Bradycardia of any cause
    Sinus or junctional
    AV block
  Any combination of above, e.g., subarachnoid hemorrhage
    with bradycardia and hypokalemia

OTHER FORMS OF CARDIAC ARREST (PULSELESS ELECTRICAL ACTIVITY AND ASYSTOLE)

As discussed above, VF is the most common and treatable presenting rhythm in SCD and cardiac ar-

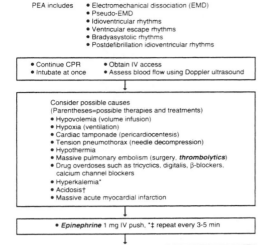

PEA includes
- Electromechanical dissociation (EMD)
- Pseudo-EMD
- Idioventricular rhythms
- Ventricular escape rhythms
- Bradyasystolic rhythms
- Postdefibrillation idioventricular rhythms

• Continue CPR	• Obtain IV access
• Intubate at once	• Assess blood flow using Doppler ultrasound

Consider possible causes
(Parentheses=possible therapies and treatments)
- Hypovolemia (volume infusion)
- Hypoxia (ventilation)
- Cardiac tamponade (pericardiocentesis)
- Tension pneumothorax (needle decompression)
- Hypothermia
- Massive pulmonary embolism (surgery, *thrombolytics*)
- Drug overdoses such as tricyclics, digitalis, β-blockers, calcium channel blockers
- Hyperkalemia*
- Acidosis†
- Massive acute myocardial infarction

- *Epinephrine* 1 mg IV push, *‡ repeat every 3-5 min

- If absolute bradycardia (<60 beats/min) or relative bradycardia, give *atropine* 1 mg IV
- Repeat every 3-5 min up to a total of 0.04 mg/kg§

Figure 6. AHA algorithm for interventions in PEA. (From Emergency Cardiac Care Committee and Subcommittees, American Heart Association: Guidelines for cardiopulmonary resuscitation and emergency cardiac care. Part III. Adult advanced cardiac life support. JAMA 268:2199–2241, 1992. Copyright 1992, American Medical Association.)

Class I: definitely helpful
Class IIa: acceptable, probably helpful
Class IIb: acceptable, possibly helpful
Class III: not indicated, may be harmful
Sodium bicarbonate 1 mEq/kg is Class I if patient has known preexisting hyperkalemia.
†*Sodium bicarbonate* 1 mEq/kg:
  Class IIa
- if known preexisting bicarbonate-responsive acidosis
- if overdose with tricyclic antidepressants
- to alkalinize the urine in drug overdoses
  Class IIb
- if intubated and long arrest interval
- upon return of spontaneous circulation after long arrest interval
  Class III
- hypoxic lactic acidosis
‡The recommended dose of *epinephrine* is 1 mg IV push every 3-5 min. If this approach fails, several Class IIb dosing regimens can be considered.
- Intermediate: *epinephrine* 2-5 mg IV push. every 3-5 min
- Escalating: *epinephrine* 1 mg-3 mg-5 mg IV push (3 min apart)
- High: *epinephrine* 0.1 mg/kg IV push, every 3-5 min
§ Shorter *atropine* dosing intervals are possibly helpful in cardiac arrest (Class IIb).

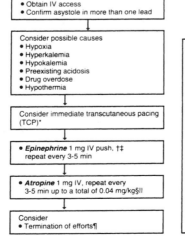

Figure 7. AHA asystole algorithm. (From Emergency Cardiac Care Committee and Subcommittees, American Heart Association: Guidelines for cardiopulmonary resuscitation and emergency cardiac care. Part III. Adult advanced cardiac life support. JAMA 268:2199–2241, 1992. Copyright 1992, American Medical Association.)

- Continue CPR
- Intubate at once
- Obtain IV access
- Confirm asystole in more than one lead

Consider possible causes
- Hypoxia
- Hyperkalemia
- Hypokalemia
- Preexisting acidosis
- Drug overdose
- Hypothermia

Consider immediate transcutaneous pacing (TCP)*

- *Epinephrine* 1 mg IV push, †‡ repeat every 3-5 min

- *Atropine* 1 mg IV, repeat every 3-5 min up to a total of 0.04 mg/kg§‖

Consider
- Termination of efforts¶

Class I: definitely helpful
Class IIa: acceptable, probably helpful
Class IIb: acceptable, possibly helpful
Class III: not indicated, may be harmful
*TCP is a Class IIb intervention. Lack of success may be due to delays in pacing. To be effective TCP must be performed early, simultaneously with drugs. Evidence does not support routine use of TCP for asystole.
†The recommended dose of *epinephrine* is 1 mg IV push every 3-5 min. If this approach fails, several Class IIb dosing regimens can be considered:
- Intermediate: *epinephrine* 2-5 mg IV push, every 3-5 min
- Escalating: *epinephrine* 1 mg-3 mg-5 mg IV push (3 min apart)
- High: *epinephrine* 0.1 mg/kg IV push, every 3-5 min
‡*Sodium bicarbonate* 1 mEq/kg is Class I if patient has known preexisting hyperkalemia.

§Shorter *atropine* dosing intervals are Class IIb in asystolic arrest.
‖*Sodium bicarbonate* 1 mEq/kg:
  Class IIa
- if known preexisting bicarbonate-responsive acidosis
- if overdose with tricyclic antidepressants
- to alkalinize the urine in drug overdoses
  Class IIb
- if intubated and continued long arrest interval
- upon return of spontaneous circulation after long arrest interval
  Class III
- hypoxic lactic acidosis
¶If patient remains in asystole or other agonal rhythms after successful intubation and initial medications and no reversible causes are identified, consider termination of resuscitative efforts by a physician. Consider interval since arrest.

rest. However, in approximately 30 to 35% of arrests the presenting rhythm is either PEA or asystole. Neither of these, of course, is treatable with defibrillation. In PEA, which by definition is some form of electrical activity on the ECG without palpable pulses, a concerted effort must be made to identify a potentially correctable cause, such as hypovolemia (e.g., exsanguination from concealed or evident hemorrhage), cardiac tamponade from trauma or secondary to ventricular rupture with acute myocardial infarction, tension pneumothorax after trauma or after attempted subclavian venous puncture, or acute pulmonary thromboembolism. The approach to PEA is depicted in the AHA PEA algorithm (Figure 6).

Asystole is most commonly an irreversible derangement secondary to long-standing hypoxia. However, even here, a rapid search should be initiated for a treatable cause, as outlined in Figure 7. For example, successful resuscitation has been described after prolonged asystolic cardiac arrest associated with hyperkalemia. External pacing can be tried, but it has not been shown to alter outcome from this form of arrest.

SUMMARY

SCD and cardiac arrest are most commonly the consequence of CAD. VF is the most frequent presenting rhythm and is often correctable with rapid interventions centered on early defibrillation. AEDs provide a means for rapid delivery of defibrillatory shocks to persons in VF cardiac arrest and constitute the single most important means for improving survival from VF arrest. All patient care areas, including physicians' offices and outpatient clinics, should be equipped with AEDs. In PEA or asystolic arrest a rapid assessment should be made to determine if a potentially correctable cause of arrest is present.

ATRIAL FIBRILLATION

method of
DAVID M. GILLIGAN, M.D., and
KENNETH A. ELLENBOGEN, M.D.
Medical College of Virginia
Richmond, Virginia

Atrial fibrillation is the most common cardiac arrhythmia requiring intervention, with an estimated 1 million persons affected in the United States. The prevalence of atrial fibrillation increases with age, affecting up to approximately 5% of the population older than 65 years. With an increasingly elderly population, atrial fibrillation is becoming more common. Also, with improving therapy for various forms of structural heart disease, more patients are surviving into later life at increased risk for atrial fibrillation. The management of atrial fibrillation has evolved in recent years. Large randomized trials have shown that anticoagulation markedly reduces the risk of stroke in atrial fibrillation. The number of antiarrhythmic agents has increased such that clinicians find themselves

TABLE 1. **The Five Aspects of Management of Atrial Fibrillation**

1. Identification of underlying cause(s) and precipitating factor(s)
2. Control of ventricular rate
3. Restoration of sinus rhythm
4. Maintenance of sinus rhythm
5. Anticoagulation or antiplatelet therapy

with a bewildering array of choices for treating this common arrhythmia. Clinicians are also more aware of the potential proarrhythmic side effects of these drugs. Finally, new procedures, such as atrioventricular junction ablation and permanent ventricular pacing, have an increasing role in the management of atrial fibrillation.

The diagnosis of atrial fibrillation can usually be made on the basis of an irregularly irregular pulse. However, electrocardiographic confirmation should be obtained, ideally a 12-lead electrocardiogram. Irregularly irregular QRS complexes with absent P waves and a variable degree of baseline fibrillatory activity confirm the diagnosis. Once atrial fibrillation has been diagnosed, five aspects of management need to be addressed in every case (Table 1); each aspect will be discussed in detail.

IDENTIFICATION OF UNDERLYING CAUSE

In every patient presenting with atrial fibrillation, it is important to ask: What are the underlying cause(s) and precipitating factor(s) for atrial fibrillation in this patient? Answering this question requires a careful history, physical examination, and ancillary investigation as necessary. All patients presenting with new atrial fibrillation should probably undergo transthoracic echocardiography and measurement of thyroid function. It is valuable to have a measure of left ventricular function in every case as this affects both the hemodynamic and symptomatic consequences of atrial fibrillation and its management. The causes and precipitating factors of atrial fibrillation are shown in Table 2. Every effort should be made to identify the underlying cause or precipitating factor, as this aids in controlling the ventricular rate and in restoring and maintaining the sinus rhythm. It is also important to assess whether the presentation with atrial fibrillation is a

TABLE 2. **Causes and/or Precipitating Factors for Atrial Fibrillation**

Structural heart disease
Hypertensive heart disease
Coronary artery disease—acute infarction, chronic ventricular dysfunction
Valvular heart disease, especially mitral valve disease (rheumatic)
Cardiomyopathies: dilated, hypertrophic, and restrictive
Postcardiac surgery
Pericarditis
Congenital heart disease, e.g., atrial septal defect
Systemic conditions
Major noncardiac surgery
Major infection
Thyrotoxicosis
Electrolyte disturbance
Malignancy, especially lung and mediastinal
Ethanol excess
Miscellaneous: sarcoidosis, pheochromocytoma, amyloidosis

"marker" for an underlying cardiac or systemic disease, the management of which may be the most important aspect of patient care.

CONTROL OF VENTRICULAR RATE

In every patient in atrial fibrillation the following questions need to be addressed: Is control of the ventricular rate needed? If so, how rapidly does the rate need to be controlled? What is likely to be the optimum rate-controlling drug(s) in this specific clinical setting? How will the efficacy of rate control be assessed? In individuals with normal atrioventricular (AV) node conduction, the ventricular response will be greater than 70 and often greater than 120 beats per minute, and therefore rate control will be necessary. The ventricular response is increased by high sympathetic tone, e.g., postoperatively, and by sympathomimetic agents. In Wolff-Parkinson-White syndrome, antegrade conduction of atrial fibrillation over an accessory pathway produces broad complex tachycardia and may conduct very rapidly with a risk of ventricular fibrillation. On the other hand, patients with inherent conduction system disease may have a slow ventricular response to atrial fibrillation, less than 70 beats per minute at rest without drug therapy. Such patients do not require AV-nodal-blocking agents.

Urgent Direct-Current Cardioversion

Initial management should follow the guidelines for advanced cardiac life support of the American Heart Association. Patients who are unstable hemodynamically because of rapid ventricular rate require urgent synchronized direct-current cardioversion. In such patients the administration of rate-slowing drugs may exacerbate hypotension and delay definitive therapy. Patients with rapid atrial fibrillation are usually conscious, and brief sedation is required. The need for emergency cardioversion is relatively unusual in atrial fibrillation, and more commonly there is an opportunity to administer rate-slowing medication and plan for elective cardioversion.

Initial Rate Control

In the patient with stable hemodynamics, the rapidity of the ventricular rate and the associated symptoms dictate the urgency of ventricular rate control. Table 3 provides an overview of the drug therapy available to control the ventricular response in atrial fibrillation. All these drugs act by slowing conduction in the AV node but achieve this in different ways: calcium channel blockers directly impair AV node conduction, beta blockers reduce sympathetic enhancement of AV node conduction, and digoxin increases vagal inhibition of AV node conduction.

Intravenous Therapy

Rapid ventricular rates that are symptomatic require intravenous therapy. We use intravenous diltia-

zem (Cardizem); an initial average bolus of 20 mg (0.25 mg per kg) is given over 2 minutes, if necessary a second additional 25 mg (0.35 mg per kg) bolus is given 15 minutes later, and a continuous infusion is begun at 5 to 10 mg per hour, increasing to a maximum of 15 mg per hour. The slowing of AV conduction with intravenous diltiazem is rapid, within 5 to 10 minutes. The drug is well tolerated and can be used in patients who have mild left ventricular dysfunction and even evidence of congestive heart failure, but it should be avoided in patients who have marked hypotension and known severe left ventricular dysfunction.

Other choices for immediate rate control include intravenous verapamil (Isoptin), which can be given in boluses of 5 to 10 mg intravenously, approximately 1 mg per minute. Like diltiazem, verapamil has an immediate heart rate–slowing effect, but it has a more marked hypotensive effect. The bolus dose may be repeated to obtain sustained heart rate control. Intravenous beta blockers may also be used to control rate acutely, especially in situations of high sympathetic drive, e.g., postoperatively. We use metoprolol (Lopressor) in 5-mg boluses every 5 minutes to a total of 15 mg. Intravenous digoxin (Lanoxin) does not provide immediate heart rate control; the onset of digoxin effect occurs around 3 hours, and the maximum effect may not be seen for 24 to 48 hours. In addition, digoxin is typically ineffective in settings of high sympathetic tone.

Oral Therapy

In less acute situations, when the ventricular rate is not rapid and there are mild or minimal symptoms, oral therapy is appropriate. The same drug choices exist for the initiation of oral therapy as for intravenous therapy. Again, calcium channel blockers such as diltiazem and verapamil or beta blockers have a more rapid onset of action compared with digoxin. Patient features and the clinical setting usually point to a preferred class to use.

Importantly, if atrial fibrillation occurs in Wolff-Parkinson-White syndrome and there is rapid conduction over the accessory pathway, some AV-node-slowing drugs are ineffective and may increase the ventricular rate. Direct-current cardioversion or intravenous procainamide should be used to terminate the arrhythmia. Subsequently, electrophysiologic study and ablation of the accessory pathway should be performed because of the risk of sudden death in this syndrome.

Long-Term Rate Control

In chronic sustained or intermittent atrial fibrillation, ventricular rate control is important in order to minimize symptoms and reduce the risk of tachycardia-induced ventricular dysfunction. In the past, digoxin has been the mainstay of therapy. Its dosing, therapeutic range, side effects, and interactions are well known. However, because digoxin's effect is primarily to increase vagal tone on the AV node, it may

TABLE 3. **Control of the Ventricular Rate in Atrial Fibrillation**

Clinical Setting	Drug	Dosing	Efficacy	Comments
Acute Atrial Fibrillation				
Rapid rate, hypotensive	None			Urgent direct current cardioversion.
Rapid rate, symptomatic	Diltiazem (Cardizem)	IV bolus 20 mg over 2 min, at 15 min 25 mg over 2 min, infusion 5–15 mg/h	Rapid rate control	Well tolerated.
	Verapamil (Isoptin)	5–10 mg IV; repeat after 10–30 min	Rapid rate control	Hypotension may occur. May be difficult to titrate.
	Metoprolol (Lopressor)	5 mg IV q 5 min; total 15 mg	Rapid rate control	Useful in postoperative setting.
	Esmolol (Brevibloc)	0.5 mg/kg over 1 min, 0.05 mg/kg/min infusion	Short-acting	Hypotension is common.
	Digoxin (Lanoxin)	IV 0.25–0.5 mg; total 1 mg/24 h	Moderately low efficacy	Delayed onset of atrioventricular slowing (h).
Slow ventricular rate	None			No therapy.
Chronic Atrial Fibrillation				
Rapid rest and/or exercise ventricular rate	Verapamil (Isoptin SR)	PO 120–480 mg daily	Reduce resting, and exercise rate	
	Diltiazem (Cardizem CD)	PO 90–360 mg daily	Reduces resting and exercise rate	
	Atenolol (Tenormin)	PO 25–100 mg daily	Reduces exercise rate	Any beta blocker may be used.
	Digoxin (Lanoxin)	PO 0.1–0.75 mg daily	Reduces resting rate	Often exercise tachycardia persists.
Rapid symptomatic ventricular rate despite medical therapy				His ablation and permanent pacemaker.

control resting ventricular rate well but have little effect on the exercise heart rate. Monotherapy with digoxin may be effective in sedentary patients or in those in need of inotropic support. Other agents, either used alone or in combination with digoxin, provide better overall control of the ventricular response in chronic atrial fibrillation, and these should be first-line therapy. The calcium channel blockers, diltiazem or verapamil (given in a slow-release, once-daily preparation for convenience), reduce both rest and exercise heart rates. Beta blockers also have an excellent effect in controlling the ventricular response, especially during exercise. To achieve optimum rate control, drugs may need to be combined. Digoxin can be added to a calcium channel blocker or a beta blocker to improve control of the resting rate. Caution should be exercised if combining a calcium channel blocker with a beta blocker because of the risk of bradycardia. Clonidine has also recently been reported to be effective in the control of the ventricular response in atrial fibrillation.

Finally, it is important to objectively assess heart rate control and the effect of therapy in patients with continuing symptoms. Thus, formal and informal exercise testing and/or Holter monitoring can guide therapy in an objective fashion.

Nonpharmacologic Methods of Rate Control

Some patients, 5 to 10%, with chronic or intermittent atrial fibrillation are persistently symptomatic with rapid ventricular rates despite maximum drug therapy with AV-blocking agents. Such patients should be referred for consideration of AV junction ablation and implantation of a ventricular, rate-responsive, permanent pacemaker. With this procedure, complete heart block is induced by radiofrequency catheter ablation of the AV junction area. A permanent pacemaker with an activity sensor allows a programmable heart rate response to physical activities such as walking and stair climbing. Patients with paroxysmal atrial fibrillation can receive a dual chamber mode-switching pacemaker to avoid tracking of atrial fibrillation. Patients with chronic atrial fibrillation who undergo AV junction ablation do require continued anticoagulation because the atria are still in fibrillation. A variation on this procedure has recently been described in which radiofrequency ablation modifies rather than ablates the AV junction; rapid ventricular rates are prevented, but permanent pacing is not required.

RESTORATION OF SINUS RHYTHM

In every patient presenting with atrial fibrillation, one must decide whether an attempt should be made to restore sinus rhythm. In patients with rapid atrial fibrillation who are hypotensive, direct-current cardioversion should be performed urgently as discussed earlier. In patients with stable hemodynamics, elective cardioversion should be considered. In up to 50% of cases of recent onset, atrial fibrillation reverts spontaneously to sinus rhythm within 48 hours, especially if precipitating factors can be reversed. The AV-nodal-blocking agents (including digoxin) do not have any specific effect in restoring sinus rhythm, although the improvement in hemodynamics resulting from rate control may facilitate return to sinus rhythm. The indications for an approach to cardioversion are summarized in Table 4.

Indications and Contraindications to Cardioversion

First Presentation of Atrial Fibrillation

We believe that elective cardioversion is indicated for all patients who first present with atrial fibrillation unless relative contraindications exist such that the benefits of restoring and/or the chances of maintaining sinus rhythm are minimal. Relative contraindications include conditions with a poor prognosis such as an advanced malignancy; high-risk anesthesia such as in severe respiratory disease; very advanced age; severe functional limitation; or long-standing (years) atrial fibrillation.

In addition to relative contraindications, there is a large group of patients whose ventricular rate is controlled with medication and who have few or no symptoms. In this situation, the advantages of leaving the patient in chronic atrial fibrillation are the avoidance of further procedures and possibly the avoidance of antiarrhythmic agents (see later). The disadvantages of not restoring sinus rhythm are that long-term anticoagulation is usually required, atrial fibrillation may cause ventricular dysfunction, and effort limitation may go unrecognized (such patients may feel a substantial benefit when sinus rhythm is restored). Therefore, the decision to proceed with cardioversion involves a discussion between the patient and the physician of the advantages of maintaining sinus rhythm.

Recurrent Atrial Fibrillation

Consideration of cardioversion in recurrent atrial fibrillation should address not only the issues described for first presentation, i.e., relative contraindications and symptomatic status, but also the ability to maintain sinus rhythm. This decision is made on an individual basis, balancing the severity of symptoms associated with episodes of atrial fibrillation against the side-effect profile of the antiarrhythmic agents available (see later).

Anticoagulation Before Cardioversion

Once the decision has been made to attempt cardioversion of atrial fibrillation, the next issue that must be addressed is the need for anticoagulation. In an emergency situation of rapid atrial fibrillation requiring urgent therapy, cardioversion should proceed immediately. In elective cardioversion, the need for anticoagulation depends primarily on the duration of atrial fibrillation.

Duration Less Than 48 Hours

Current practice is that in atrial fibrillation of less than 48 hours' duration, the risk of thromboembolism is very low and cardioversion can be performed safely without anticoagulation. Thus in episodes of atrial fibrillation occurring in hospital or episodes with a clear symptomatic onset in patients presenting from the community when the duration of the arrhythmia can be accurately determined, cardioversion can be scheduled within the 48-hour window. In these situations we do begin intravenous heparin anticoagulation when atrial fibrillation has been documented and continue this until cardioversion is performed.

Duration More Than 48 Hours

When atrial fibrillation is more than 48 hours in duration, or when the onset of the arrhythmia is unclear, we begin anticoagulation with warfarin. For patients presenting at or near the 48-hour limit, the presence of risk factors for thromboembolism may influence decisions to anticoagulate or not. A therapeutic international normalized ratio (INR) is

TABLE 4. **Restoration of Sinus Rhythm in Atrial Fibrillation**

Clinical Presentation	Duration	Anticoagulation	Cardioversion
Unstable hemodynamics: (hypotension)	Usually recent onset	No	Urgent direct-current cardioversion
	<24–48 h	No	Pharmacologic cardioversion: Quinidine (Quinaglute) Procainamide (Procan SR) Disopyramide (Norpace) Flecainide (Tambocor) Propafenone (Rhythmol) Sotalol (Betapace) Amiodarone (Cordarone)
Stable hemodynamics: cardioversion indicated (see text)	TEE negative	Short-term	
	>48 h	Yes: 4 weeks before and 3 weeks after cardioversion	Direct-current cardioversion

Abbreviation: TEE = transesophageal echocardiography.

achieved (2.0 to 3.0) and maintained for 4 weeks, at which time the patient returns for elective cardioversion. In the interim, drug therapy is used to control heart rate and minimize symptoms as necessary. The hypothesis behind a period of anticoagulation before cardioversion is that 4 weeks of therapy allows any pre-existing atrial thrombus to either resolve or fibrose and prevents the formation of new thrombus in that time. It is fresh thrombus that carries a risk of embolism. In patients who are anticoagulated before cardioversion because the duration of the arrhythmia was greater than 48 hours, it is important to continue anticoagulation for approximately 3 weeks after cardioversion. The hypothesis behind this practice is that although sinus rhythm is restored, left atrial mechanical function does not recover immediately. Thus, stasis may persist in the atrium with the risk of thromboembolism in the days after conversion from atrial fibrillation.

If there is urgency to proceed with cardioversion because of marked symptoms or heart failure despite good rate control or there is a contraindication to anticoagulation, we perform transesophageal echocardiography to exclude thrombus in the left atrium. If thrombus is excluded and there is no spontaneous echo contrast, then recent studies suggest that cardioversion can proceed with minimal risk of thromboembolism. It is important to note that transthoracic echocardiography is inadequate for this purpose.

Method of Cardioversion

Once the decision has been made to attempt cardioversion and the issue of anticoagulation has been addressed, there are two methods by which cardioversion can be achieved: pharmacologic or electrical.

Pharmacologic Cardioversion

Antiarrhythmic agents of Class IA, IC, and III all have some effect in restoring and maintaining sinus rhythm in atrial fibrillation. For all agents, the likelihood of success is closely related to the duration of atrial fibrillation. Sinus rhythm may be restored in up to 80% of recent-onset (less than 24 hours) atrial fibrillation with antiarrhythmic drug therapy (compared with a 40% spontaneous reversion rate), whereas long-standing atrial fibrillation is much less likely to convert with pharmacologic therapy. All these antiarrhythmic agents have proarrhythmic potential; therefore, we initiate therapy in the hospital during continuous cardiac monitoring. It is best to become familiar with the use of one or two drugs. Quinidine has traditionally been used, formerly in high doses until conversion or side effects occurred, but now we use quinidine sulfate in typical doses of 200 mg every 4 to 6 hours. Procainamide (Procan SR) is our most commonly used agent for pharmacologic cardioversion. The oral dosage varies from 500 to 1500 mg every 6 hours. Procainamide may be given by intravenous infusions of 15 mg per kg at 50 mg per minute. Disopyramide (Norpace) is the other Class IA agent that has some effectiveness given as 150 mg every 6 to 8 hours. Sotalol (Betapace) and amiodarone (Cordarone) are Class III agents, and flecainide (Tambocor) and propafenone (Rhythmol) are Class IC agents that also have an effect in restoring sinus rhythm in recent-onset atrial fibrillation. Intravenous preparations of these agents are available in many countries.

Usually 24 hours is allowed for pharmacologic conversion to occur. If pharmacologic cardioversion has not occurred by this time, direct-current countershock proceeds. This allows cardioversion of recent-onset atrial fibrillation to proceed within the 48-hour time window of low thromboembolic risk. Patients should be monitored for proarrhythmia for 24 hours after restoration of sinus rhythm.

Direct-Current Cardioversion

Direct-current cardioversion may be the first-line therapy to restore sinus rhythm or may be used when drug therapy fails. Direct-current cardioversion should be performed in an environment in which full resuscitation equipment is available. Patients should be fasting for at least 6 hours. The procedure should be carried out either with the assistance of an anesthesiologist or by a cardiologist experienced in airway management and ventilation during sedation and anesthesia. Usually anesthesia is achieved with rapid short-acting intravenous agents such as methohexital (Brevital) or short-acting benzodiazepines such as midazolam (Versed). We use adhesive chest patches placed in an anteroposterior position. Synchronized shocks are delivered, initially at 200 joules and if unsuccessful, followed by up to three shocks at 360 joules, usually with different patch positions. If these shocks are unsuccessful, the procedure is terminated, but direct-current cardioversion of atrial fibrillation is successful in over 90% of cases. Following cardioversion, sinus bradycardia and junctional rhythm are frequent. Sinus node function usually recovers rapidly, but in those patients with sinus node dysfunction (often associated with a slow untreated ventricular response to atrial fibrillation), recovery may be slower and equipment for transcutaneous or transvenous temporary pacing should be available. Postcardioversion ventricular arrhythmias are rare but are associated with digoxin toxicity, and therefore digoxin-toxic patients should not undergo direct-current cardioversion.

MAINTENANCE OF SINUS RHYTHM IN ATRIAL FIBRILLATION

Once atrial fibrillation reverts spontaneously or is cardioverted to sinus rhythm, the question of maintaining sinus rhythm is addressed. If there is a clear underlying cause or precipitating factor that can be reversed, this may be adequate to prevent further episodes. Infrequent episodes (fewer than one per year) can be managed as they arise with repeated cardioversions, if acceptable to the patient and the physician. If more frequent recurrences occur, consid-

TABLE 5. **Maintenance of Sinus Rhythm in Intermittent Atrial Fibrillation and After Cardioversion**

Drug	Dose	Useful in	Avoid in
Class IA			
Quinidine gluconate (Quinaglute Dura)	324–648 mg q 8–12 h	Chronic renal failure	CHF Liver failure
Procainamide (Procan SR)	0.5–1.5 g q 6 h	Men, short-term therapy	Renal failure CHF
Disopyramide (Norpace CR)	200–400 mg q 12 h	Women	Older men—risk of urinary retention Glaucoma Renal failure, CHF
Class IC			
Flecainide (Tambocor)	75–150 mg q 12 h	Failure of Class IA agents	Any LV dysfunction, CAD
Propafenone (Rhythmol)	150–300 mg q 8 h	Failure of Class IA agents	Any LV dysfunction
Class III			
Sotalol (Betapace)	180–360 mg q 12 h	Failure of IA, IC agents; may be used with mild–moderate LV dysfunction	Where beta-blocker contraindicated
Amiodarone (Cordarone)	1200 mg daily for 5 days followed by 400 mg daily for 1 month; long-term 200–400 mg daily	Severe LV dysfunction failure of other drugs CHF patients	Young patients Severe pulmonary disease

Abbreviations: LV = left ventricular; CHF = congestive heart failure; CAD = coronary artery disease.

eration is given to long-term antiarrhythmic drug therapy.

In general, because of the hemodynamic deterioration associated with the onset of atrial fibrillation (due to a loss of atrial contraction plus the irregular and rapid ventricular rate), patients experience significant symptoms with this arrhythmia. Thus, maintenance of sinus rhythm is an important goal of therapy when possible. In addition, maintenance of sinus rhythm may obviate the need for anticoagulation. It is also possible that long-standing atrial fibrillation, especially with rapid ventricular rates, may cause deterioration of left ventricular function with time. On the other hand, antiarrhythmic agents have only moderate efficacy in maintaining sinus rhythm, some have three- and even four-times-daily dosing, and all carry the risk of side effects. Proarrhythmic effects are of greatest concern. A meta-analysis of trials of quinidine for atrial fibrillation found a threefold increased mortality in patients on quinidine, although the absolute number of events was small and occurred especially in patients with congestive heart failure. Class IC agents, flecainide and encainide, increased mortality in patients with asymptomatic ventricular arrhythmia in the Cardiac Arrhythmia Suppression Trial, again an effect seen in patients with ischemia and/or left ventricular dysfunction. Only the Class III agents, such as amiodarone, currently appear to offer a survival benefit in patients treated for ventricular arrhythmias. There are no survival studies of these agents in atrial fibrillation. Therefore, the decision to begin antiarrhythmic drug therapy depends on a discussion between the patient and the physician of the risks and benefits involved and may depend largely on the severity of symptoms associated with atrial fibrillation.

If one decides to proceed with drug therapy, several options are available. All drugs have only moderate efficacy in maintaining sinus rhythm, approximately 50% at 1 year versus 25% with no therapy. In Table 5 each drug is listed with its typical dose, the general categories of patients in whom the drug is best used, and the particular situations in which the drug should be avoided. All Class IA and III agents should be started in the hospital under continuous cardiac monitoring (Class 1C agents can be begun as outpatient therapy in patients with structurally normal hearts). Daily electrocardiograms should be performed, and it is wise to avoid a greater than 25 to 30% increase in the QRS or QT duration with the initiation of these medications.

Quinidine is the most commonly used drug for the maintenance of sinus rhythm and has been most thoroughly studied. However, quinidine often causes gastrointestinal side effects (nausea, vomiting, diarrhea) and has been associated with increased mortality. Procainamide has the disadvantage of four-times-a-day dosing and in the long term, the risk of a lupus-like syndrome, thrombocytopenia, and other autoimmune phenomena. Disopyramide may be taken twice daily in the sustained-release preparation; however, it has prominent anticholinergic side effects, and in older men, this may lead to urinary retention. Disopyramide is a reasonable choice in women for long-term treatment, whereas procainamide may be more appropriate in men. All class IA agents should be used with care in patients with left ventricular ejection fraction less than 40% or with New York Heart Association Class II to IV heart failure given the potential of these agents to cause increased mortality.

There is less experience with the Class IC agents.

TABLE 6. **Randomized Trials of Anticoagulation in Atrial Fibrillation**

| Trial | Sample Size | INR | ASA | Embolic Event (% year) | | Percentage Risk Reduction |
				Control	Warfarin	
BAATAF	420	1.5–2.7	No	3.0	0.4	87
CAFA	383	2.0–3.0	No	4.5	2.5	45
SPINAF	536	1.5–2.5	No	4.4	1.1	76
AFASAK	1007	1.8–4.2	75 mg	5.5	2.0	59
SPAF	1330	2.0–4.5	325 mg	7.4	2.3	67

Abbreviations: BAATAF = Boston Area Anticoagulation Trial for Atrial Fibrillation; CAFA = Canadian Atrial Fibrillation Anticoagulation; SPINAF = Stroke Prevention in Nonrheumatic Atrial Fibrillation; AFASAK = The Copenhagen AFASAK Study; SPAF = Stroke Prevention in Atrial Fibrillation; INR = international normalized ratios; ASA = aspirin.

It is clear that drugs such as flecainide should only be used in patients with preserved left ventricular function and no structural heart disease. In this setting these agents appear efficacious and reasonably well tolerated. Class III agents are also effective in maintaining sinus rhythm. Sotalol therapy, reserved for those with normal or mildly depressed left ventricular function, should be started, again in the hospital with daily monitoring of the QT interval. Progressive prolongation of the QT interval is directly correlated with the risk of torsade using sotalol. At corrected QT intervals greater than 500 ms, the drug dose should be reduced. Amiodarone is considered the most effective medication to maintain sinus rhythm in atrial fibrillation and is the drug of choice in patients who have severe left ventricular dysfunction. In small trials, amiodarone has been associated with improved survival over that with placebo in patients with nonsustained ventricular arrhythmias. However, amiodarone does have potentially serious side effects—thyroid, pulmonary, skin, and neurologic—with long-term use. We reserve its use for older patients and in younger patients after multiple other drugs have failed.

Any patient committed to long-term antiarrhythmic therapy for the maintenance of sinus rhythm should be examined regularly, with 12-lead electrocardiography, measurement of drug levels, and monitoring for side effects. With Class IA agents, it is important to remember that these agents do not slow AV conduction and can accelerate it. Therefore, these agents should be combined with an AV-nodal-blocking drug. By contrast, Class III agents have independent AV-node-slowing properties; when these drugs are introduced, it is usually necessary to re-

duce or even stop therapy with drugs such as digoxin and calcium channel blockers.

Novel methods to maintain sinus rhythm are being explored. Two types of open heart surgery have been shown to maintain sinus rhythm in chronic atrial fibrillation: the "corridor" procedure and the "maze" procedure. Both operations depend on breaking up macro-reentry circuits for atrial fibrillation by making a series of incisions in the right and left atria. These operations are currently in clinical trial for patients with intractable symptoms or embolic events despite anticoagulation therapy.

ANTICOAGULATION AND ANTIPLATELET THERAPY

The final yet most important consideration regarding the long-term management of the patient with atrial fibrillation is the need for anticoagulation. The most serious complication of atrial fibrillation is thromboembolism, which is frequently cerebral (more than 90%) and may result in a large cerebrovascular accident. Importantly, five large, recent, multicenter randomized trials have demonstrated the ability of anticoagulation, and to a lesser extent aspirin, to reduce the risk of thromboembolism in patients with atrial fibrillation (Table 6). The average risk of ischemic stroke in these studies was 4.5% per year, and this was reduced, on average, to less than 1% per year with warfarin. In these studies, the risk reduction ranged from 45 to 87% and far outweighed the slightly increased risk of serious bleeding. Two of these studies incorporated the use of aspirin, and although aspirin also reduced the risk of stroke, the effects were more modest. These studies also identi-

TABLE 7. **Anticoagulation and Antiplatelet Therapy in Atrial Fibrillation**

	Age	Structural Heart Disease*		Systemic Risk Factors†
Anticoagulation benefit clear (warfarin)	<75	Present	or	Present
Risk/benefit of warfarin vs. aspirin must be individualized	>75	Present or absent	or	Present or absent
Aspirin adequate	<60–75	Absent		Absent
	<60–65	Absent		Absent

*Structural heart disease = depressed left ventricular systolic function, left atrial enlargement, congestive heart failure, valvular disease, or coronary artery disease.
†Systemic risk factors = prior thromboembolic event, hypertension, or diabetes.

TABLE 8. **Contraindications to Anticoagulation in Atrial Fibrillation**

Prior bleeding events—gastrointestinal or intracranial
    hemorrhage
Systemic malignancy
Uncontrolled hypertension
Diabetic retinopathy
Dementia
Noncompliance
Difficult-to-control international normalized ratio (INR)
Unsteady or gait disturbance
Chronic alcoholism
Hemostasis disorder

fied subsets of patients who were at greatest risk for systemic embolism in atrial fibrillation. From these data, an approach to anticoagulation in atrial fibrillation can be drawn up as illustrated in Table 7. Contraindications to anticoagulation therapy are listed in Table 8. Each decision to anticoagulate must be individualized.

In patients under 75 years of age who have structural disease or systemic risk factors, we recommend anticoagulation with warfarin (Coumadin) achieving an INR of 2.0 to 3.0. Future studies may demonstrate that lower INRs are adequate. High INRs increase the risk of bleeding. In patients under 60 years of age with no structural heart disease and no systemic risk factors, the risk of thromboembolism is low, and aspirin alone or no therapy appears adequate in these patients. Patients aged 60 to 75 have a slightly increased risk of thromboembolism simply as a result of their increased age. In these patients, even in the absence of structural heart disease or systemic risk factors, there may be benefit from anticoagulation over aspirin, particularly if this can be achieved with good control of the INR. In patients over 75 years of age, there may be an increased risk of bleeding complications with anticoagulation. Thus, even if these patients have structural heart disease or systemic risk factors for stroke, the risk benefit ratio of anticoagulation with warfarin over aspirin is still present, but decisions must be individualized.

Patients with one episode of atrial fibrillation who are converted to sinus rhythm and in whom it can be shown that this is maintained long term, e.g., at 6 months to 1 year, may not require long-term anticoagulation. Similarly, very infrequent and short episodes of atrial fibrillation may not require anticoagulation. In each of these groups, aspirin, 325 mg daily, is advisable. More frequent episodes of intermittent atrial fibrillation or episodes of atrial fibrillation that last longer than 48 hours should be treated in the same way as described in Table 7 for chronic atrial fibrillation.

PREMATURE BEATS

method of
DAVID E. MANN, M.D.
University of Colorado Health Sciences Center
Denver, Colorado

Premature supraventricular or ventricular beats occur in most if not all persons from time to time. They are the most common "abnormal" heart rhythm. Usually premature beats result in no symptoms and are of little consequence. However, occasionally premature beats can be markers of occult heart disease, metabolic disturbance, or drug toxicity and may call attention to an underlying problem that might otherwise have been overlooked. On the other hand, the search for the cause of premature beats often reveals no other abnormalities, which emphasizes the widespread prevalence and nonspecific nature of these beats.

Premature beats can cause symptoms, which include palpitations, fatigue, shortness of breath, chest pain, and light-headedness. These symptoms may be worse at night, when the patient is lying quietly before sleeping. It is striking that often there is little correlation between the severity of symptoms and the frequency of premature beats. Some people with only rare premature beats are highly symptomatic, whereas others, with very frequent premature beats, complain of no symptoms whatsoever. Most often, symptoms are mild and not life-threatening. This is because by their nature, premature beats cause a disturbance in cardiac output that is too brief to affect consciousness to any degree. Obviously I am excluding from this discussion patients with more sustained arrhythmias, such as ventricular tachycardia, who may be very symptomatic. The approach to those patients is different, and is discussed in the article "Tachycardias." Patients who complain of more serious symptoms, such as presyncope or syncope, should be suspected of having more sustained arrhythmias, and a search for such arrhythmias, either by Holter monitoring, event recorders, or electrophysiologic testing may be justified. When severe symptoms do correlate only with premature beats, there is usually an element of psychological overlay present that magnifies the symptoms. In most cases, the typically minor nature of the symptoms produced by premature beats justifies a conservative treatment approach that avoids potentially dangerous antiarrhythmic drugs.

Premature beats, like most cardiac arrhythmias, can be ascribed to three mechanisms: reentry, triggered activity, or automaticity. In most cases, the exact mechanism is neither apparent nor important. In some situations, certain mechanisms are likely to be present. Exercise- or catecholamine-induced premature beats or tachycardias are likely to be due to triggered activity from delayed afterdepolarizations. Premature beats from digitalis toxicity are due to the same mechanism. Premature beats and tachycardia associated with QT-interval prolongation (drug-induced or congenital) are most likely due to triggered activity associated with early after-depolarizations. Ventricular arrhythmias associated with chronic coronary artery disease are most likely reentrant. Knowledge of the likely mechanism of these arrhythmias is occasionally useful. For example, catecholamine- or exercise-induced arrhythmias are often sensitive to drugs that inhibit delayed afterdepolarizations, such as beta blockers or calcium channel blockers. Arrhythmias due to early after-depolarizations may be exacerbated by bradycardia and hypokalemia and treated by correction of these factors.

DIAGNOSIS

Usually the origin of premature beats is evident from the electrocardiogram (ECG). Supraventricular beats are preceded by P waves, whereas ventricular beats are not. Although ventricular beats invariably have a wide QRS complex (120 msec or more), supraventricular beats may also be wide because of aberrant conduction. Supraventricular beats of junctional origin may not be preceded by P waves. They are recognized as junctional by a QRS configuration identical to that of sinus beats.

Because P waves preceding premature beats may be relatively isoelectric in any one ECG lead, it is easier to determine the origin of premature beats if multiple simultaneous ECG channels are available. The P waves may be buried in the T wave of the preceding beat and thus easy to miss. Careful inspection of the T wave of the beat preceding a suspected premature supraventricular beat and comparison of this T wave with that of another beat not followed by a premature beat can be very useful in determining if a superimposed P wave is present.

Besides the 12-lead ECG and in-hospital telemetry, other tools are available to diagnose the presence of premature beats. Typically these tools are used in patients who have symptoms potentially caused by sporadic arrhythmias, but sometimes these techniques are used for other purposes and asymptomatic premature beats are detected incidentally. For symptoms that occur daily, 24-hour Holter monitoring is useful. For less frequent symptoms, transtelephonic event recorders, which can be used for periods of up to months, are more cost-effective and useful than repeated 24-hour Holter monitors. With any kind of long-term ECG monitoring it is essential that the patient fill out a diary, so that symptoms can be accurately correlated with the presence or absence of arrhythmias. If a patient's symptoms occur with exercise, exercise stress testing may be useful to replicate these symptoms and document a possible arrhythmic cause.

TREATMENT

Although premature beats occur in normal individuals, they can be an indication that underlying heart disease is present. Thus a good history, including risk factors, a family history, a physical examination, an ECG, measurement of serum electrolyte levels, and a chest x-ray examination are usually in order. Depending on the patient's age, risk factors, and other symptoms or physical signs, further evaluation may be in order, including stress testing, echocardiography, or cardiac catheterization. If cardiac abnormalities are present, their identification and treatment become the overriding concern.

Besides cardiac disease, premature beats may indicate the presence of noncardiac abnormalities. Electrolyte abnormalities, especially hypokalemia and hypomagnesemia, and proarrhythmic effects from antiarrhythmic drugs (including digoxin) or other drugs (e.g., tricyclic antidepressants, antihistamines, both of which may be associated with QT prolongation and torsades de pointes) should be considered as causes of premature beats and may lead to more serious arrhythmias if not identified and corrected.

Drug-induced proarrhythmia usually requires hospitalization for monitoring because of the danger of this condition. Other metabolic disturbances, such as hypoxia or hyperthyroidism, can cause premature beats. Premature beats documented during sleep may indicate the presence of sleep apnea. Cocaine use can result in premature beats as well as more serious arrhythmias.

Besides identification and treatment of underlying heart disease or noncardiac causes of premature beats, there are certain general measures that are useful in dealing with symptomatic premature beats. The mainstays of therapy are

1. The elimination of precipitating factors (including caffeine, nicotine, stress)
2. Reassurance

In my experience, the first option, eliminating precipitating factors, often involves lifestyle changes that the patient is unable or unwilling to make but can be helpful in some cases. Reassurance is very important. Patients are frightened by irregularities of their heartbeat, which in their minds translate into unreliability of the heartbeat and the possibility of the heart's stopping. This belief may be heightened in some cases because of a family member who had a heart attack or died suddenly (of course, the physician should always be alert to the possible presence of familial heart disease in such situations). Health care personnel may add to this anxiety, by focusing the patient's attention on these beats. If the patient has at some point been hospitalized on a telemetry ward, the medical staff sometimes contributes to this kind of anxiety, usually by offhand comments in the presence of the patient about his or her premature beat frequency, or by awakening the patient from sleep after an episode of bigeminy, couplets, or triplets, to see if the patient is "all right." Anxious medical staff transfer their anxiety to patients, and it can be very difficult to undo the damage. It is important to emphasize to patients with symptomatic premature beats and normal cardiac function that the presence of these beats is benign and will not cause sudden death. Such reassurance is often enough to relieve symptoms and avoid other therapy. In addition, providing the patient accurate information about the risks of proarrhythmia from antiarrhythmic drugs is usually enough to convince him or her that it is better to live with these symptoms. This reassurance that the treatment may be worse than the disease is especially useful for patients with premature ventricular beats (PVBs) and left ventricular dysfunction, in whom premature ventricular beats are a constant reminder of the presence of heart disease, and in whom the fear of a premature and sudden death may to some degree be justified.

Premature Atrial Beats

Premature atrial beats in themselves are benign, though they might form the trigger for atrial fibrillation, atrial flutter, or other more sustained supraventricular arrhythmias. Nevertheless, there is no evidence that antiarrhythmic drug suppression of these beats helps prevent sustained supraventricular arrhythmias. On the other hand, prophylactic treatment of atrial tachyarrhythmias with antiarrhythmic drugs (e.g., prevention of atrial fibrillation with quinidine or sotalol) may at least in part be successful because of the effect of these drugs on suppressing premature supraventricular beats. Regardless of this, treatment should be aimed at prevention of sustained supraventricular tachyarrhythmias, and not at suppression of premature supraventricular beats, and there is no role for antiarrhythmic drug therapy in patients with only premature supraventricular beats.

Premature Ventricular Beats: The Asymptomatic Patient

In patients without underlying heart disease and with normal ventricular function, the presence of PVBs has no adverse effect on survival. In patients with reduced left ventricular function, several studies promote the idea that the presence of PVBs has an independent, adverse effect on survival. However, it should be emphasized that PVBs are not the most important predictor of prognosis. Nearly all natural history studies indicate that the most important determinant of survival is left ventricular function, measured by ejection fraction or by functional heart failure class. Signal-averaged electrocardiography probably assesses arrhythmia risk better than quantification of PVBs by Holter monitoring.

Several studies have addressed the issue of the use of suppression of PVBs in the primary prevention of sudden death. The most publicized and best of these studies are the two Cardiac Arrhythmia Suppression Trials (CAST I and II). CAST examined the hypothesis that Holter monitor–guided suppression of PVBs in patients after myocardial infarction would decrease the incidence of sudden death. The drugs used were flecainide (Tambocor), encainide (Enkaid), and moricizine (Ethmozine). These drugs all best fit in the Vaughn-Williams Class Ic (slow conduction markedly without prolonging repolarization). They were selected because they were found to be the most effective Class I drugs in suppressing PVB frequency in the pilot study before CAST. After PVB reduction by one of these drugs was documented, patients were randomized to drug therapy versus placebo. Patients treated with antiarrhythmic drugs had increased mortality compared with those given placebo. This result confirmed smaller studies of other Class I antiarrhythmic drugs, which showed similar trends toward increased mortality with these drugs. Similarly, meta-analysis of studies of the Class I drug lidocaine, used prophylactically during acute myocardial infarction, showed increased mortality in the treated group, and analyses of Class I antiarrhythmic drug use for the treatment of atrial fibrillation show similar results. Thus there is no evidence that suppression of PVBs with Class I antiarrhythmic drugs prevents sudden death; in fact, all evidence points to the opposite result.

Class II drugs (beta blockers) are well documented to improve survival when used after myocardial infarction, though it is not clear if this beneficial effect relates to their antiarrhythmic or their anti-ischemic properties. Thus all post–myocardial infarction patients who can tolerate it should be treated with beta-blocking drugs for a period of at least 2 years after the infarction, regardless of the presence or absence of PVBs.

Class III drugs (e.g., amiodarone [Cordarone] and sotalol [Betapace]) have been studied in the post–myocardial infarction setting. Data thus far are insufficient to support their routine use in this setting.

Premature Ventricular Beats: The Symptomatic Patient

Although the risks of proarrhythmia are probably low in persons with normal ventricular function and symptomatic PVBs, I feel it is difficult to justify the use of Class I or III antiarrhythmic drugs in these patients. Most patients with symptomatic PVBs are satisfied with the results of elimination of precipitating factors and reassurance. If the patient still insists on further treatment and if it appears that anxiety is a problem, psychiatric evaluation and/or treatment with antianxiety agents might be helpful. If this is not appropriate, beta blockers should be tried. Although this may not reduce PVB frequency, it may alter to force of contraction so that palpitations are not as much of a problem. In addition, PVBs in persons with normal hearts frequently seem to arise in the right ventricular outflow tract (left bundle branch block morphology, vertical QRS axis) and are catecholamine-sensitive. Beta blockers or calcium channel blockers may reduce PVB frequency in this situation and may sometimes reduce PVB frequency in other settings as well. In the post–myocardial infarction patient, beta blockers are the ideal choice for the treatment of symptomatic PVBs, as these drugs have been demonstrated to reduce the risk of sudden death and reinfarction after myocardial infarction. In these patients and other patients with structural heart disease, Class I antiarrhythmic drugs must be strictly avoided.

HEART BLOCK

method of
ALBERT A. DEL NEGRO, M.D.
Fairfax Hospital
Fairfax, Virginia

"Heart block" is a general term referring to a spectrum of atrioventricular (AV) conduction abnormalities. An understanding of the anatomy and physiology of the AV conduction system is integral to the proper diagnosis and treatment of the several forms of AV block.

NORMAL CONDUCTION

Sinus node impulses travel from the high right atrium to the AV node in less than 0.045 second. Contiguous spread of excitation occurs to the left atrium. Conduction through the AV node occurs in a relatively slow 0.110 second at a maximum. The spread of excitation thereafter rapidly proceeds through the bundle of His to the right and left bundle branches and to the Purkinje system in no more than 0.055 second. These conduction times account for the usual normal PR interval of less than 0.21 second.

AUTONOMIC INFLUENCES

The sinus node and the AV node depolarizations depend on the flow of a calcium current, and both halves of the autonomic nervous system richly enervate and influence conduction and automaticity in these two areas. Thus, an excess of parasympathetic influences over sympathetic influences slows sinus node automaticity and prolongs the AV nodal portion of the AV conduction time. Increases in sympathetic influences over parasympathetic influences have the reverse effect.

Thus, for patients with inferior wall myocardial infarction complicated by heart block that resides at the AV node level, pharmacologic manipulation of the autonomic nervous system with the use of the parasympathetic blocker atropine may be all that is required to restore conduction or at least to speed the automaticity of the junctional rhythm that results.

Below the mid bundle of His, conduction depends on the flow of a sodium current, and parasympathetic influences on conduction and automaticity are negligible. Heart block at or below this level, as seen in anterior myocardial infarction or idiopathic conduction system disease (Lev's disease), therefore cannot be treated by parasympathetic withdrawal. Furthermore, increasing sympathetic influences pharmacologically by the use of sympathomimetic agents (i.e., isoproterenol) runs the risk of inducing dangerous tachyarrhythmias. Patients with block below the bundle of His require pacemaker therapy because of the failure of pharmacologic therapy as well as because of the generally profoundly slow ventricular escape rhythms upon which they must rely.

An understanding of the clinical and therapeutic differences between these loci of potential heart block leads to the classification of heart block as *proximal* (AV nodal, usually reversible and often asymptomatic) or *distal* (intra- or infra-Hisian, never reversible, and usually symptomatic). Careful electrocardiographic analysis usually can make the distinction between these two varieties of block, but on occasion, proper diagnosis requires invasive electrophysiologic study before the prescription of definitive therapy.

MANAGEMENT

First-Degree AV Block

First-degree AV block exists when there is intact AV conduction with a PR interval greater than 0.21 second. This finding implies delay in conduction from atrium to ventricle, but it is not specific for the site of delay. No therapy is required for this finding, but one should search for reversible causes. Common settings are excessive pharmacologic therapy with drugs that prolong AV conduction such as digitalis, beta blockers, or calcium channel blockers either alone or in combination. Other drugs such as sotalol and amiodarone may also prolong AV conduction in the susceptible patient. Most of these agents exert their effect at the AV nodal level, and the prolongation is reversible with withdrawal of the drug. Bilateral bundle branch delay is another cause of first-degree AV block and is indistinguishable from delay due to AV nodal delay on the surface electrocardiogram (ECG). Progression to higher forms of AV block may occur with drugs that block the sodium fast channel such as quinidine, procainamide, disopyramide (Norpace), and flecainide (Tambocor). No therapy for first-degree AV block is necessary, but if syncope or presyncope is present, one should pursue a thorough cardiac electrophysiologic diagnostic evaluation.

Second-Degree AV Block

Second-degree AV block exists when there is a failure of any of the normal atrial events to conduct to the ventricle. This form of heart block is usually benign when the locus of the block is within the AV node, since it commonly disappears with exercise or with lysis of parasympathetic influences. Noninvasive maneuvers such as exercise and the use of intravenous atropine 0.5 to 1.0 mg can cause the disappearance of block. The abolition of second-degree AV block by these measures indicates that the AV node is the site of block. No pacemaker treatment is indicated since the block is usually asymptomatic and self-limited if it is due to reversible factors such as drug effects. If, however, the site of the AV block is within the bundle of His or within the bundle branches, eventual progression to complete heart block with inappropriately slow ventricular escape rhythm and syncope or presyncope is the rule. Since both proximal and distal second-degree AV block may be initially asymptomatic, the differentiation between the two is fairly important in order to make the correct therapeutic choice.

Clues to the distinction between these two forms of second-degree AV block lie in careful electrocardiographic analysis. Wenckebach or Mobitz I block associated with a narrow QRS is classically due to AV nodal block. This is usually benign and self-limited and requires therapy only if there is extreme bradycardia or hemodynamic compromise. Wenckebach patterns with a QRS duration of 0.12 second or greater also are usually due to AV nodal block, but up to 30% may result from distal conduction disease and thus require therapy. Patients with this finding are candidates for cardiac electrophysiologic study to define the site of block with certainty.

Mobitz II AV block refers to 3:2 or lower ratios of AV conduction in which there is no change in the PR interval before or after the dropped beat. Intracardiac electrophysiologic studies universally demonstrate distal conduction system block in this circumstance. Even if the patient is asymptomatic, permanent pacemaker therapy is indicated since progression to complete heart block resulting in extreme bradycardia and Stokes-Adams attacks is the rule for this form of AV block.

Finally, any form of AV block associated with symptoms clearly due to bradycardia warrants permanent pacing therapy. This is the case irrespective of the anatomic site of block.

Third-Degree AV Block

In complete AV block without demonstrable AV relationships to judge the site of heart block, it is more difficult to arrive at therapeutic decisions in the asymptomatic patient. Even the patient with a wide QRS interval (>120 msec) may have AV nodal block rather than the more malignant distal block, and pacing for these patients may not be mandatory. Without intracardiac recordings, certain therapeutic judgments may still be easily made. A profoundly slow heart rate (<35 per minute) while awake even in the absence of symptoms of presyncope and syncope is grounds for permanent pacing. Heart block resulting in pauses of greater than 3 seconds while awake is also an indication for permanent pacing. Any patient with a slow pulse resulting from third-degree heart block in association with symptoms attributable to bradycardia should receive pacing therapy.

The heart rates of patients with third-degree AV block who are asymptomatic are usually not profoundly slow, and no therapy may be necessary especially if appropriate increases in heart rate occur after the administration of atropine or with exercise. This response suggests that the AV node is the site of block and pacing is not mandated. Conversely, the lack of increase in heart rate with exercise or after the administration of atropine suggests distal complete heart block. For these patients, pacing is highly recommended. When symptoms are absent in third-degree AV block and there is indecision about therapy, intracardiac electrophysiologic study can resolve the question (Table 1).

Heart Block in Acute Myocardial Infarction

Heart block is a known complication of anterior as well as inferior wall myocardial infarction. This is much more common for inferior myocardial infarction, in which some degree of AV block may be a complication in up to 30% of cases. Heart block in this setting is due to increased vagal effects or to direct ischemic effects on the AV node. Since the AV node is virtually always the site of block in inferior myocardial infarction, vagolysis with atropine 0.5 to 1.0 mg either restores conduction or speeds the escape of the vagally responsive AV junctional pacemakers to which the rhythm defaults. This situation warrants temporary pacing only if vagolysis does not restore heart rate and hemodynamics satisfactorily or if persistent bradycardia encourages the appearance of ventricular ectopy. The need for permanent pacing in this circumstance is exceedingly rare since complete recovery of AV nodal conduction is the rule.

When AV block accompanies anterior myocardial infarction, the block is due to injury to the proximal interventricular septum in the vicinity of the bundle branches affecting conduction below the bundle of His and proximal bundle branches. Lower-order pacemakers to which the rhythm defaults reside in the Purkinje system and are profoundly slow and unreliable. Moreover, since parasympathetic influences on automaticity and conduction in this region are negligible, vagolysis with atropine has no salutary effect on speeding the escape rhythm or on improving conduction. Finally, the extreme bradycardia encourages ventricular ectopy and magnifies the medical emergency. Temporary pacing should be initiated immediately in this setting. Even if conduction recovers, eventual permanent pacing should receive strong consideration since recovery is never complete and recurrence of heart block is likely.

One may lessen the catastrophic occurrence of AV block in acute anterior infarction by anticipating its possibility. Clues to impending AV block lie in the careful observation of the monitored electrocardiogram. An episode of at least transient complete heart block complicates acute anterior myocardial infarction in up to 40% of cases when a new right bundle branch block accompanies the infarction. Often, new right bundle branch block insidiously develops after admission to the hospital for anterior infarction, and monitoring lead V_1 is the most useful for its identification. When identified, new right bundle branch block is grounds for a prophylactic temporary pacemaker.

Positive chronotropic agents should never be used in the setting of heart block and acute myocardial infarction except as a last resort because of their tachyarrhythmia potential. If necessary, isoproterenol in a starting dose of 0.5 to 1.0 mg per minute intravenously is the usual initial drug of choice for hemodynamically unstable bradycardia due to AV block, but this therapy should be discontinued once temporary pacing is in place. Lidocaine and procainamide, commonly used in myocardial infarction, may suppress escape pacemakers in heart block with acute infarction and should be used only after establishing rate control with temporary pacing.

TABLE 1. **Clinical and Anatomic Correlations in Heart Block**

Locus	AV Node (Proximal)	Bundle Branches (Distal)
Escape mechanism	Junctional	Idioventricular
Exacerbating drugs	Digitalis	Sodium channel
	Beta blockers	blockers
	Calcium channel	
	blockers	
Myocardial infarction	Inferior	Anterior
Clinical course	Reversible	Progressive
Therapy	Atropine, rarely	Pacemaker
	pacemaker	

PACING MODALITIES

Temporary Pacing

For sudden heart block in the patient under observation in the hospital, one may use temporary transcutaneous pacing. This modality uses electrodes cutaneously applied to the chest so that the heart is in the line of a current passing between them. This is an effective therapy, but careful electrode placement is essential to ensure cardiac capture. Sedation will comfort the conscious patient, who will nonetheless be disturbed by the vigorous intercostal muscle and diaphragmatic stimulation accompanying this form of temporary cardiac pacing.

Percutaneous transthoracic pacing is a temporary pacing modality little used today. This technique involves the passage of a needle through the chest either from the subxiphoid area aiming for the left shoulder or from the fourth left intercostal space aiming directly posteriorly until right ventricular chamber blood is aspirated. A J-shaped pacing wire introduced through the needle then passes into the right ventricle and is used for pacing. Pitfalls of this technique include entry into the right atrium instead of the right ventricle. This method of temporary pacing results in a low success rate, usually because it is not attempted until quite late in the course of a resuscitative effort.

The preferred form of temporary cardiac pacing for heart block is transvenous pacing. One may pass a temporary bipolar pacing electrode by the percutaneous internal jugular, subclavian, or femoral venous routes. This requires fluoroscopy to ensure proper electrode placement at the apex of the right ventricle. When the subclavian or internal jugular venous routes are used, it is common to position the lead erroneously into the mouth of the coronary sinus and down the posterior interventricular vein. One cannot ensure adequate pacing and sensing from this position, which is, after all, extracardiac. Pacing from this site produces a right ventricular conduction delay instead of the expected left ventricular conduction delay. This error is easily avoided if the passage of the electrode is first into the right ventricle and into the pulmonary artery before its withdrawal and placement at the right ventricular apex.

Once the electrode is properly positioned, one should ensure adequate parameters for sensing and pacing. Carefully securing the lead to the skin around the entry point helps prevent inadvertent dislodgment. Once the pacing electrode is connected to a temporary pacemaker, careful insulation of electrode connectors is important to avoid conduction of stray currents to the heart capable of inducing ventricular fibrillation. Some go as far as to place the temporary pacer and its connections with the electrode into a rubber glove sealed with adhesive tape. Proper grounding of all electric appliances in the vicinity of the patient also ensures protection from the risk of stray electrical currents.

Most heart block patients do well with temporary right ventricular pacing, with few problems, but many patients may actually deteriorate hemodynamically with single-chamber pacing because of the loss of the atrial contribution to ventricular filling. Despite an increase in heart rate, the stroke volume may remain quite low and congestive symptoms may be present. Patients most vulnerable to this syndrome are those with a lack of left ventricular compliance noted in any form of left ventricular hypertrophy. These patients benefit from the restoration of AV synchrony by means of temporary dual chamber pacing. Special leads are available for temporary atrial appendage pacing or coronary sinus atrial pacing. Special temporary AV sequential pacemakers are generally available for this pacing modality.

Spontaneous temporary pacing lead dislodgment occurs in as many as 20% of patients. This requires a daily assessment of all aspects of the pacing system including threshold measurement and sensing evaluation. A rising threshold may be the first clue to impending lead dislodgment. Repositioning of dislodged temporary pacing leads should be prompt to ensure continued pacing support as well as to prevent the induction of arrhythmias from the mechanical stimulation of an improperly positioned lead. Finally, daily wound care can ensure freedom from infection, and carefully maintained systems need not be changed for several days.

Permanent Pacing

Permanent transvenous cardiac pacing most commonly uses leads passed by the percutaneous subclavian route. Cephalic vein cutdown and internal jugular cutdown surgery for lead placement is more time-consuming but still widely used. Of these approaches, the internal jugular approach is least desirable since it requires an acute bend in the lead within the subcutaneous tissues of the neck. This bend is a common site of lead fracture and constitutes a major cause of pacing system failure. After satisfactorily placing the leads, the operator creates a subcutaneous pocket of adequate size to accommodate the pacemaker subadjacent to the entry point of the leads and verifies parameters for sensing and pacing. Pacing at a high output for a brief time verifies that diaphragmatic or intercostal stimulation does not occur, which would necessitate lead repositioning. Depending on the implantation parameters and the needs of the patient, one determines the programming of the pacemaker including the rate ranges, AV interval, voltage outputs, pulse widths, and sensing. For dual-chamber pacing, an assessment of the potential for retrograde conduction assists in programming the pacer to avoid pacemaker-mediated tachycardia. Such a procedure obviously requires skill and considerable expertise as well as intimate knowledge of the engineering aspects of the pacemaker used.

Permanent dual-chamber pacing, using a rate-responsive pacemaker, is the contemporary pacing mode of choice for heart block patients in sinus rhythm. Rate responsiveness adds little to the cost of the pacemaker and permits great flexibility in the management of patients with heart block. Furthermore, for patients with atrial fibrillation and heart block, rate-responsive single-chamber pacing is the mode of choice.

After implantation, observation in a monitored setting for at least 24 hours ensures normal postimplantation function. Commonest among postimplantation problems are lack of sensing, mechanically induced ventricular ectopy, and failure of pacing to capture the heart. These are most commonly related to lead dislodgment, which may necessitate reoperation if reprogramming does not correct the problem. Long-term follow-up includes periodic office visits at least biannually for pacing threshold and sensing determinations. This permits the programming of outputs for pacing to ensure cardiac capture without using greater-than-required energies for pacing. Such careful programming of pacing output lengthens battery life and leads to fewer pacemaker replacements in the course of the patient's life. Transtelephonic monitoring with and without a magnet in place over the pacer reveals the time of impending battery exhaustion by a gradual drop in magnet rate and permits safe outpatient observation until the time of needed pacemaker replacement. After 4 years, monthly transtelephonic monitoring ensures adequate time to permit pacemaker replacement after reaching the battery exhaustion indicator.

TACHYCARDIAS

method of
CARLETON NIBLEY, M.D., and
J. MARCUS WHARTON, M.D.
Duke University Medical Center
Durham, North Carolina

In adults, the term "tachycardia" is used to describe any cardiac rhythm with a rate greater than or equal to 100 beats per minute. With the exception of sinus tachycardia, which usually occurs in response to physiologic stress, tachycardias are the result of abnormal impulse formation due to reentry, automaticity, or triggered activity. The tachycardias are broadly classified as either supraventricular or ventricular, depending on the tissues involved. Supraventricular tachycardias are critically dependent on atrial and/or atrioventricular (AV) junctional tissue for maintenance, whereas ventricular tachycardias arise in the ventricles, independent of the atrium or AV junction. Patients with tachycardias have varied clinical presentations, ranging from an absence of symptoms to full cardiorespiratory arrest. The clinical status of the patient, rather than the site of origin of the tachycardia, determines the urgency of diagnostic and therapeutic interventions.

ACUTE MANAGEMENT

Conscious asymptomatic or minimally symptomatic patients with sustained tachycardia should undergo a problem-focused history and physical examination concurrent with the establishment of continuous electrocardiographic monitoring and intravenous access. A standard 12-lead electrocardiogram should be obtained whenever possible, since electrocardiographic documentation of the presenting tachyarrhythmia will facilitate accurate diagnosis and planning of subsequent diagnostic and therapeutic steps. In clinically stable patients, vagal maneuvers such as Valsalva or carotid sinus massage may be performed for diagnostic purposes or as therapy for tachycardias that are sensitive to enhanced vagal tone. Increasingly, adenosine (Adenocard) administered at a starting dose of 6 mg as a rapid intravenous injection has supplanted the use of vagal maneuvers to produce transient complete AV nodal blockade for diagnostic purposes or for termination of tachyarrhythmias that are dependent on the AV node for maintenance. In addition, many atrial tachycardias and ventricular tachyarrhythmias due to triggered activity may be terminated by adenosine. If no effects are observed, a second dose of 12 mg may be used. When properly administered, adenosine may result in profound bradycardia or asystole lasting several seconds, followed by spontaneous restoration of baseline sinoatrial and AV nodal function. Treatment of the bradycardia or asystole associated with adenosine administration is rarely necessary, although patients receiving dipyridamole may experience potentiation of these effects. In most cases in which ventricular tachycardia is suspected, the failure of intravenous adenosine to terminate the tachycardia lends indirect support to this diagnosis.

The approach to unconscious or hemodynamically unstable patients with sustained tachycardia differs substantially. Following initiation of emergency resuscitation measures, including airway management and intravenous access, electrocardiographic documentation of the tachycardia should be obtained, followed by direct current cardioversion. Specific treatment guidelines have been established by the American Heart Association, and approved courses in advanced cardiac life support (ACLS) are recommended for physicians and allied professionals responding to clinical emergencies. Although 12-lead electrocardiographic documentation is not feasible prior to emergent direct current cardioversion or defibrillation, the importance of even single-lead electrocardiographic documentation of the presenting tachycardia cannot be overemphasized. Conscious patients in severe distress associated with a sustained tachyarrhythmia should have rapid establishment of intravenous access and electrocardiographic monitoring, followed by administration of antiarrhythmic medications or direct current cardioversion. Trained airway management personnel should be available to assist with intubation and mechanical ventilation if necessary. Commonly used sedating agents such as midazolam (Versed), diazepam (Valium), methohexital (Brevital), fentanyl (Innovar), meperidine (Demerol), or morphine sulfate should be given prior to direct current cardioversion in awake patients whenever possible.

ELECTROCARDIOGRAPHIC DIAGNOSIS

Tachycardias are broadly classified electrocardiographically as having either narrow (<0.12 second) or wide (≥0.12 second) QRS complexes, generally reflecting the manner in which ventricular activation or depolarization occurs. During sinus rhythm, orderly ventricular activation normally occurs within 0.08 to 0.10 second via the His bundle, bundle branches, and Purkinje network, generating a narrow QRS complex. All narrow complex tachycardias may, therefore, be accurately classified as supraventricular, although narrow complex ventricular tachycardia has been described. In contrast, if conduction within the bundle branches is abnormal, atrial activation of the ventricles occurs via an accessory pathway, or ventricular tachycardia is present, then ventricular activation is slowed by intraventricular impulse propagation, and a QRS complex width greater than 0.12 second results. Proper classification of wide complex tachycardias is, therefore, inherently more difficult, since supraventricular tachycardias occurring in the setting of bundle branch block or an accessory AV pathway capable of antegrade conduction can resemble ventricular tachycardia.

Once the tachycardia is classified as having a narrow or wide QRS complex, the arrhythmia may be further subclassified as regular or irregular, as shown in Table 1. Although most tachycardias show minor variation in the measured R-R intervals or rate, irregularity in this context refers to changes in R-R intervals that are readily seen upon examination of the electrocardiogram. Among narrow complex tachycardias, atrial fibrillation and multifocal atrial tachycardia are the only irregular tachycardias. The regular, narrow complex tachycardias are often more difficult to distinguish from one another, and identification of the P wave association to the QRS com-

TABLE 1. Classification of Tachycardias

Narrow Complex Tachycardias

Regular
Sinus tachycardia
Sinoatrial nodal reentrant tachycardia
Inappropriate sinus tachycardia
Atrioventricular nodal reentrant tachycardia
Atrioventricular reciprocating tachycardia (WPW)
Atrial flutter
Atrial tachycardia

Irregular
Atrial fibrillation
Multifocal atrial tachycardia

Wide Complex Tachycardias

Regular
Ventricular tachycardia
Supraventricular tachycardia with bundle branch block or ventricular pre-excitation (WPW)

Irregular
Polymorphic ventricular tachycardia (torsades de pointes)
Atrial fibrillation with bundle branch block or ventricular pre-excitation (WPW)

Abbreviation: WPW = Wolff-Parkinson-White syndrome.

TABLE 2. Electrocardiographic Criteria Used to Differentiate Ventricular Tachycardia from Supraventricular Tachycardia with Bundle Branch Block

ECG Features of Ventricular Tachycardia

Diagnostic
Atrioventricular dissociation
Fusion complexes

Suggestive
QRS duration >0.14 s
Superior frontal QRS axis
Precordial QRS concordance or absence of precordial RS complex
R to nadir of S interval >0.10 s in precordial lead

If RBBB pattern present:
Lead V1: monophasic R complex; QR or RS complex
Lead V6: R:S ratio <1; QS or QR complex
If LBBB pattern present:
Lead V1 or V2: notching of downstroke of S wave
Lead V6: QR or QS complex

Abbreviations: ECG = electrocardiogram; RBBB = right bundle branch block; LBBB = left bundle branch block.

plexes is necessary, as will be discussed (Figure 1). Among wide complex, irregular tachycardias, polymorphic ventricular tachycardia and ventricular fibrillation are considered in addition to the irregular supraventricular tachycardias with a widened QRS complex due to bundle branch block or conduction via an accessory AV pathway.

Accurate classification of wide complex tachycardias as supraventricular or ventricular requires careful evaluation of the standard 12-lead electrocardiogram in the context of clinical variables. Patients with known cardiac disease, particularly previous myocardial infarction or dilated cardiomyopathy, presenting with a wide complex tachycardia are much more likely to have ventricular tachycardia than supraventricular tachycardia with bundle branch block. The opposite is true for young, otherwise healthy patients, although a diagnosis of ventricular tachycardia should be considered in any patient with a wide complex tachycardia.

Common electrocardiographic criteria used to differentiate ventricular tachycardia from supraventricular tachycardia with bundle branch block are summarized in Table 2. AV dissociation or fusion beats are diagnostic of ventricular tachycardia. However, ventricular tachycardia is not excluded by a 1:1 P-to-QRS ratio, since up to 25% of cases of ventricular tachycardia can exhibit retrograde atrial activation. A QRS duration greater than 0.14 second, superior frontal plane QRS axis, absence of an RS complex or QRS concordance in all precordial leads, and an R to nadir of S interval that exceeds 0.10 second (Figure 2) suggest ventricular tachycardia. Other morphologic criteria supporting the diagnosis of ventricular tachycardia include a monophasic R wave in lead V1, notching of the downstroke of the S wave in lead V1 or V2, or a QS or QR complex in lead V6; however, exceptions to all the QRS morphology criteria exist. As previously discussed, vagal maneuvers or adeno-

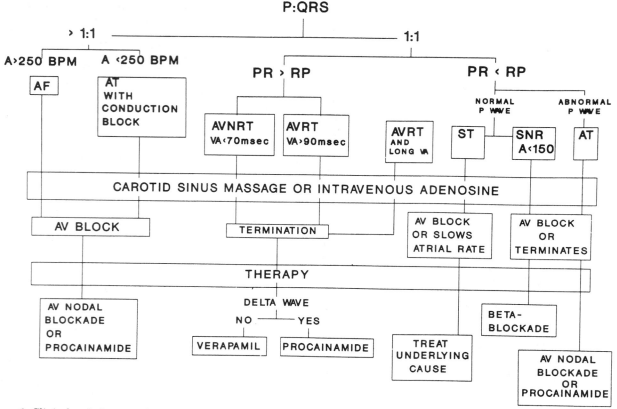

Figure 1. Clinical and electrocardiographic algorithm used to differentiate among the various regular, narrow QRS complex tachycardias. See text for discussion. *Abbreviations:* A = arrhythmia; BPM = beats per minute; AF = atrial flutter; AT = atrial tachycardia; AV = atrioventricular; AVNRT = AV nodal reentry tachycardia; AVRT = AV reciprocating tachycardia; ST = sinus tachycardia; SNR = sinus node reentry; VA = ventriculoatrial. (From Greenfield RA, Vitullo RN, Bacon ME, Wharton JM: Diagnosis and treatment of arrhythmias. *In* Schwartz GR, Cayten CG, Mangelsen MA, et al. [eds]: Principles and Practice of Emergency Medicine. Malvern, PA, Lea & Febiger, 1992.)

sine can improve diagnostic accuracy, since abrupt termination of a wide complex tachycardia in this manner supports a diagnosis of supraventricular tachycardia dependent on AV nodal function. Adeno-

sine administered during ventricular tachycardia usually has no effect, although ventricular tachycardia that is sensitive to adenosine may occur in patients with structurally normal hearts. Adenosine

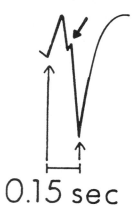

0.15 sec

RS complex lead V2

Figure 2. Characteristic RS complex during ventricular tachycardia recorded from precordial lead V_2. The interval from the onset of R to the nadir of S exceeds 0.10 s, favoring the correct diagnosis of ventricular tachycardia (VT). In addition, there is notching of the downstroke of the S wave (*dark arrow*) also consistent with VT.

is also used to demonstrate AV dissociation during ventricular tachycardia in patients with 1:1 ventriculoatrial conduction at baseline.

SINUS TACHYCARDIA

Sinus tachycardia occurs normally in patients in response to physiologic stress, usually in association with increased sympathetic tone. Therefore, treatment is usually directed at the underlying cause rather than control of the tachycardia. Among nonexercising patients, sinus tachycardia rarely exceeds 180 beats per minute, and the onset and resolution of tachycardia are gradual, not abrupt. Identification of upright P waves similar to sinus rhythm is expected. When P waves are not visible due to overlap of the preceding T wave, vagal maneuvers or adenosine used to transiently slow the sinus rate will reveal the characteristic P waves followed by rapid reestablishment of the pretreatment tachycardia. Other than for diagnostic purposes, attempts to slow sinus tachycardia with medications that depress sinus node function may be harmful by reducing cardiac output in settings where the opposite is needed by the patient.

There are abnormal tachycardias that share a sinus node origin. Inappropriate sinus tachycardia is characterized by the persistence of sinus tachycardia in the absence of an identifiable precipitant. The mechanism of inappropriate sinus tachycardia is unknown, but abnormally low resting vagal tone, elevated resting sympathetic tone, or both may play a role in some patients. Afflicted patients are often young and otherwise healthy, although frequently deconditioned. Following a complete diagnostic evaluation for occult sources of elevated sympathetic tone, treatment with beta-adrenergic blocking agents is occasionally effective. In contrast, sinus nodal reentry is a rare, paroxysmal form of atrial tachycardia, arising solely or partially from sinus node tissue. As expected, the P wave morphology during tachycardia is identical to that found in sinus rhythm, but the tachycardia has an abrupt onset and offset and is abruptly terminated by vagal maneuvers and adenosine. Beta-adrenergic blockers, calcium channel blockers, and Class IA, IC, and III antiarrhythmic agents are usually effective. Radiofrequency current catheter ablation of the tachycardia focus is also very effective therapy for medically refractory patients.

ATRIAL FIBRILLATION

Atrial fibrillation is the most common arrhythmia encountered in clinical practice, afflicting an estimated 2 million Americans. The prevalence increases as the population ages, so that 5% of individuals over 65 years of age have atrial fibrillation. Initially, most patients experience paroxysmal episodes that may progress to chronic atrial fibrillation. Several medical conditions in addition to advanced age contribute to the development of atrial fibrillation, including

ischemic and nonischemic cardiomyopathies, hypertension, diabetes mellitus, and valvular heart disease. Atrial fibrillation may also result from acute illness or injury, including recent cardiac surgery, acute myocardial infarction, hyperthyroidism, pulmonary embolism, alcohol withdrawal, or sepsis. In these instances, treatment of the underlying medical problem usually results in resolution of atrial fibrillation. When atrial fibrillation occurs in the absence of identifiable heart disease or predisposing medical conditions, the arrhythmia is called lone atrial fibrillation. The loss of atrial function and the usually rapid, irregular ventricular response during atrial fibrillation account for symptoms of lethargy, dyspnea, palpitations, and lightheadedness.

Electrocardiographically, atrial fibrillation is recognized by the absence of clearly recognizable P waves and the irregular ventricular rate. Atrial activity consists of continuous, low-amplitude electrical activity. Ventricular rates in the absence of medical therapy vary from fast to slow; at faster ventricular rates, the degree of irregularity may be diminished, leading to misdiagnosis. A slow, regular ventricular rate during atrial fibrillation suggests underlying complete heart block. Transient bundle branch block often occurs with a closely coupled ventricular response that follows a relative pause (the Ashman phenomenon). These aberrantly conducted ventricular beats may be misclassified as premature ventricular complexes or, if bundle branch block persists, nonsustained ventricular tachycardia, creating the potential for inappropriate treatment.

In patients presenting with atrial fibrillation and ventricular rates greater than 100 beats per minute and with associated hemodynamic compromise, uncontrolled angina, or unstable clinical conditions, synchronized direct current cardioversion following adequate patient sedation is appropriate. However, pharmacologic slowing of the ventricular response can be performed in most cases. Intravenous beta-adrenergic blockers, verapamil (Calan) and diltiazem (Cardizem), can provide immediate slowing of the ventricular rate, but these agents may result in hemodynamic deterioration. Digoxin (Lanoxin) is less effective in slowing the ventricular rate in clinically unstable patients, since its principal action on AV nodal tissue is mediated by vagal tone, which is usually diminished in these situations.

The loss of atrial contraction during atrial fibrillation may result in stasis of blood flow in the atria and atrial mural thrombus formation. Atrial fibrillation, whether paroxysmal or chronic, has been associated with a thromboembolic event rate of approximately 5% per year. The risk is highest in patients with mitral valvular disease, depressed left ventricular function, left atrial enlargement, and previous thromboembolic events. In several recent studies, warfarin (Coumadin) has been shown to reduce the risk of thromboembolic events in patients with atrial fibrillation. Data are conflicting as to whether aspirin is as effective as low-dose warfarin, although aspirin has been demonstrated to be superior to placebo.

Long-term therapy for atrial fibrillation is controversial. Control of the ventricular rate is essential, but the use of antiarrhythmic drugs to maintain sinus rhythm may be associated with an increased mortality, particularly among patients with depressed left ventricular function (Table 3). The restoration of sinus rhythm in patients with atrial fibrillation can be performed with antiarrhythmic agents alone or in combination with electrical conversion. When atrial fibrillation has been present for an indeterminate length of time or for longer than 72 hours, anticoagulation is generally recommended prior to cardioversion. Warfarin administered for 4 weeks prior to planned cardioversion is an accepted clinical practice, and continuation of either aspirin or warfarin indefinitely is indicated in light of the high risk of recurrence and the associated thromboembolic risks. Although transeosphageal echocardiography may be helpful prior to elective cardioversion in an attempt to exclude left atrial thrombi, this approach cannot be recommended in lieu of anticoagulation at the present time. Ideally, patients deemed eligible to receive antiarrhythmic drugs should be hospitalized and monitored for 48 to 72 hours when therapy is initiated, since roughly half of all cases of drug proarrhythmia occur within this time frame. Despite the use of antiarrhythmic drugs, at least 50% of patients experience a recurrence of atrial fibrillation within 1 year. Since there are no prospectively acquired data that treatment with antiarrhythmic drugs is associated with a decreased risk of thromboembolic events, antithrombotic therapy should be continued with antiarrhythmic drug therapy. Given the expense, numerous side effects, and potential for life-threatening proarrhythmia associated with antiarrhythmic drugs, only symptomatic patients with atrial fibrillation should be treated with these agents.

Alternative treatment strategies have been devised for symptomatic patients with medically refractory atrial fibrillation. Surgical treatment of atrial fibrillation using a series of atrial incisions, known as the maze procedure, is effective in maintaining sinus rhythm; however, the substantial morbidity, mortality, and cost associated with this procedure make it difficult to recommend for most patients. In patients for whom adequate ventricular rate control has not been possible, ablation of the AV junction to create heart block effectively improves symptoms related to the rapid ventricular rates and may improve overall quality of life; however, a permanent pacemaker is required after the procedure. Radiofrequency current catheter modification of AV nodal function has recently been shown to slow AV nodal conduction without producing the need for a permanent cardiac pacemaker in most patients. With either AV junction ablation or modification, the thromboembolic and hemodynamic consequences of loss of atrial function are not altered. Not infrequently, poor control of the ventricular response rate during chronic atrial fibrillation has resulted in a tachycardia-induced cardiomyopathy, and AV junction ablation followed by placement of a permanent pacemaker may result in improvement in left ventricular function.

ATRIAL FLUTTER

Atrial flutter occurs in patients similar to those who develop atrial fibrillation. In contrast to atrial fibrillation, atrial activation is organized, and mechanical atrial contraction is usually maintained during atrial flutter. This may account for the lower frequency of thromboembolic events with atrial flutter when compared with atrial fibrillation. Atrial flutter is often subdivided into typical and atypical varieties. The electrocardiogram during typical atrial flutter produces characteristic sawtooth waves, with a corresponding atrial rate of 250 to 350 beats per minute (Figure 3A). Atypical atrial flutter waves lack the classic sawtooth appearance, often having a more sinusoidal appearance with even faster atrial rates. For both types of atrial flutter, the corresponding ventricular rate is dependent on AV nodal function. A 2:1 ratio of AV conduction is commonly seen and should be considered in the differential diagnosis of any tachycardia with a ventricular rate of 150 beats per minute (see Figure 1). Characteristic flutter

TABLE 3. **Comparative Efficacy and Risk for Proarrhythmia and Noncardiac Organ Toxicity Among Antiarrhythmic Agents by Vaughan Williams Classification**

Class	Drug	Efficacy*			Proarrhythmia	Toxicity
		VT	SVT	AF		
IA	Quinidine	+	+ +	+ +	+	+ +
	Procainamide	+	+ +	+ +	+	+ +
	Disopyramide (Norpace)	+	+ +	+ +	+	+ +
IB	Lidocaine	+	−	−	±	±
	Mexiletine (Mexitil)	+	−	−	±	+
IC	Flecainide (Tambocor)	+	+ +	+ +	+ +	+
	Propafenone (Rythmol)	+	+ +	+ +	+ +	+
II	Beta blockers	±	+	+	−	−
III	Sotalol (Betapace)	+ +	+ +	+ +	+	±
	Amiodarone (Cordarone)	+ + +	+ + +	+ + +	±	+ + +
IV	Calcium blockers	−	+	±	−	−

*Efficacy is defined as the ability of the medication to prevent arrhythmia recurrences.
Abbreviations: VT = ventricular tachycardia; SVT = supraventricular tachycardia; AF = atrial fibrillation.

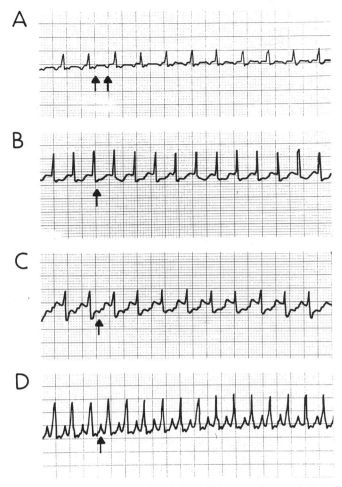

Figure 3. Comparison of limb lead II among four varieties of regular narrow complex tachycardia, demonstrating the P (*arrows*) to QRS relationship for each. *Panel A*, Typical atrial flutter with 2:1 atrioventricular (AV) conduction and negative, "saw-tooth" flutter waves. *Panel B*, AV nodal reentrant tachycardia (AVNRT) with retrograde P waves occurring at the terminal portion of the QRS complex. *Panel C*, AV reciprocating tachycardia (Wolff-Parkinson-White [WPW] syndrome) and retrograde P waves occurring later than with AVNRT. *Panel D*, Atrial tachycardia with tall, peaked P waves. See text for further discussion.

waves are often not visible in patients with 2:1 AV conduction, but either vagal maneuvers or adenosine can produce transient AV block to unmask the flutter waves.

The mechanism of typical and atypical atrial flutter is macroreentry. The macroreentrant circuit in typical atrial flutter occurs in the same right atrial site in all patients, accounting for the uniform appearance of the flutter waves in these patients. The reentrant circuit of atypical flutter is more variable. Treatment of atrial flutter is similar to that used for atrial fibrillation, although anticoagulation prior to elective cardioversion is often not performed. Since many patients with atrial flutter have episodes of atrial fibrillation, some form of antithrombotic therapy, whether aspirin or warfarin, may be useful for the prevention of thromboembolic events. Attempts to control the ventricular rate during atrial flutter

may be more difficult than during atrial fibrillation, because the constant rate of AV nodal stimulation in atrial flutter is slower and the antiarrhythmic drugs that slow the atrial flutter rate increase the probability of 1:1 or more rapid AV nodal conduction. The efficacy of antiarrhythmic drugs in preventing recurrence of atrial flutter is similar to that for atrial fibrillation. Increasingly, patients with isolated, medically refractory typical atrial flutter are treated with radiofrequency current catheter ablation of the flutter circuit, providing a curative approach to the treatment of this arrhythmia without necessitating permanent pacemaker implantation. Catheter ablation of the AV junction and placement of a permanent pacemaker may be necessary in some patients with medically refractory atrial flutter, especially if there is coexistent atrial fibrillation, when medical control of the ventricular rate has been unsuccessful.

ATRIOVENTRICULAR NODAL REENTRANT TACHYCARDIA

Atrioventricular nodal reentrant tachycardia (AVNRT) is the most common form of paroxysmal supraventricular tachycardia encountered in clinical practice. Individuals prone to the development of AVNRT may present with symptomatic paroxysmal tachycardia in adolescence or early adulthood, but later presentations are also common. Tachycardia is usually associated with symptoms of palpitations, frequently with pulsations in the neck or throbbing in the head due to the nearly simultaneous activation of the atria and ventricles during tachycardia and the retropulsion of atrial blood. Near syncope or syncope may occur rarely. Termination of the tachycardia with vagal maneuvers is often successful, although refractory episodes are promptly terminated with intravenous adenosine.

The mechanism of AVNRT is believed to be reentry in which two functionally (but not anatomically) distinct AV nodal pathways participate in the reentry circuit. The slow (posterior) pathway provides the antegrade limb, and the fast (anterior) pathway provides the retrograde limb of the circuit in typical AVNRT. In most cases, tachycardia is initiated by a premature atrial complex that finds the fast anterior pathway refractory. The impulse then conducts over the slow posterior pathway, reaching the distal AV node after a sufficient amount of time has elapsed for recovery of the fast pathway in the retrograde direction. Retrograde atrial activation occurs almost simultaneously with ventricular activation, and the 12-lead electrocardiogram during AVNRT generally reveals an absence of identifiable atrial activity, since the retrograde P waves are eclipsed by the QRS complexes during tachycardia. Sometimes, a slight negative deflection on the terminal portion of the QRS in the inferior limb leads or a pseudo-R′ in V1 are present and represent retrograde atrial activation (see Figure 3B).

Control of AVNRT has historically consisted of treatment with AV nodal blocking agents such as beta-adrenergic blockers, calcium channel blockers (verapamil or diltiazem), or digoxin (see Table 3). Medically refractory cases often respond to conventional Class IA, IC, or III antiarrhythmic drugs, although the considerable expense, frequent side effects, and proarrhythmic risks make this option less appealing. Radiofrequency current catheter ablation is an effective curative treatment of this arrhythmia. The region of the slow posterior pathway of the AV node is ablated, preventing further reentry from occurring. The risk for inadvertent complete heart block with this procedure when performed by experienced electrophysiologists is less than 1%.

ATRIOVENTRICULAR RECIPROCATING TACHYCARDIA

Reentrant tachycardia due to a circuit involving an accessory AV pathway in one direction and the AV node in the other direction is known as atrioventricular reciprocating tachycardia. If the accessory pathway is capable of antegrade conduction, then premature ventricular activation (i.e., ventricular pre-excitation) can occur during sinus rhythm, producing characteristic PR interval shortening (<0.12 second) and slurring of the initial QRS complex to form a delta wave. These patients have the Wolff-Parkinson-White (WPW) syndrome. When the accessory AV pathway functions only in the retrograde direction (no delta wave), the patient is said to have concealed WPW syndrome. Collectively, these tachycardias are responsible for approximately 20% of cases of paroxysmal supraventricular tachycardias.

An accessory AV pathway is an anomalous band of electrically active myocardium that joins the atrium and ventricle at a site remote from the AV node. When ventricular pre-excitation is present during sinus rhythm, the resultant electrocardiogram can resemble other conditions, including myocardial infarction, hypertrophy, or bundle branch block. Since not all accessory AV pathways are capable of antegrade conduction, a normal resting 12-lead electrocardiogram does not exclude the possibility of a concealed accessory AV pathway that participates in reciprocating tachycardia.

The macro-reentrant circuit responsible for over 90% of reciprocating tachycardias is referred to as orthodromic, and this involves antegrade conduction via the AV node, His bundle, and bundle branches, followed by retrograde conduction in the accessory pathway. This results in a regular, narrow complex tachycardia in which the retrograde atrial activation may be visible as inverted P waves occurring 0.04 to 0.08 second after the preceding QRS complex (see Figure 3C). The tachycardia is classically initiated by a premature atrial or ventricular complex. In fewer than 10% of reciprocating tachycardias, the circuit is reversed, or antidromic, with antegrade conduction over the accessory pathway, producing a fully pre-excited, wide QRS complex tachycardia that may be difficult to distinguish from ventricular tachycardia. During other forms of supraventricular tachycardia, the accessory pathway can function as an innocent bystander in which impulses from the tachycardia are transmitted to the ventricles via the accessory pathway, but the accessory pathway is not essential for tachycardia formation. This also produces a pre-excited, wide QRS complex tachycardia.

Patients with the WPW pattern and recurrent paroxysmal supraventricular tachycardia usually present in adolescence or young adulthood with recurrent tachypalpitations. Pharmacologic therapy with AV nodal blocking agents or conventional antiarrhythmic medications is often effective in decreasing the frequency and severity of recurrent tachycardia episodes. For medically refractory cases, radiofrequency current catheter ablation can be successfully performed in over 95% of cases. Surgical ablation is also highly effective but seldom necessary since the advent of catheter ablation.

Atrial fibrillation has been found in up to 20 to 30% of patients with the WPW syndrome. Accessory pathways capable of antegrade conduction can function in a bystander capacity, resulting in very rapid ventricular rates and a characteristic irregular wide complex tachycardia (Figure 4). In rare instances, atrial fibrillation with rapid ventricular response can degenerate into ventricular fibrillation, accounting for the increased risk of sudden cardiac death in patients with the WPW syndrome. By slowing AV node conduction and shortening accessory pathway refractoriness, digoxin may cause a paradoxical increase in ventricular rate during atrial fibrillation and increase the risk for developing ventricular fibrillation in patients with WPW (see Figure 4). Verapamil may also have a similar effect; therefore, these drugs are contraindicated in patients with WPW syndrome capable of rapid antegrade conduction. Radiofrequency current catheter ablation of the accessory pathway is generally recommended for WPW patients with atrial fibrillation, syncope, or aborted sudden cardiac death to eliminate the risk of recurrent atrial fibrillation.

ATRIAL TACHYCARDIA

The atrial tachycardias are a relatively uncommon and heterogeneous group of supraventricular tachycardias that arise from various atrial sites. Atrial tachycardias are not dependent on the sinoatrial or AV nodes for maintenance, distinguishing them from sinoatrial nodal and AV nodal reentrant tachycardias. The atrial rates are usually from 150 to 250 beats per minute with an isoelectric baseline between P waves, distinguishing atrial tachycardia from atrial flutter. However, at faster rates, atrial tachycardia may be difficult to distinguish from atrial flutter. The P wave morphology during atrial tachycardia, when visible, is different from that of sinus rhythm and is determined by the atrial site of origin of the tachycardia (see Figure 3D). The corresponding ventricular rate is determined by AV nodal function and the atrial rate. If the atrial rate is fast or AV nodal function is depressed by disease or medica-

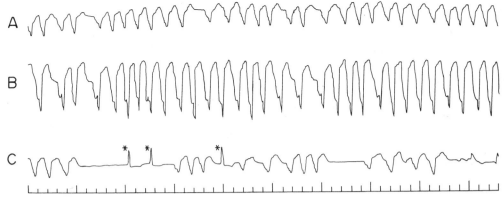

Figure 4. Single-lead electrocardiogram during atrial fibrillation in a patient with an accessory AV pathway (WPW syndrome). *Panel A*, Baseline recording demonstrating rapid ventricular response. *Panel B*, Acceleration of ventricular rate associated with administration of digoxin. *Panel C*, Slowing of ventricular rate associated with administration of magnesium sulfate to antagonize the effects of digoxin. Most of the QRS complexes are wide owing to conduction across the accessory pathway. Normally conducted (narrow) QRS complexes *(asterisk)* are seen only after magnesium was administered. (From Merrill JJ, Deweese G, Wharton JM: Magnesium therapy for digoxin-facilitated atrioventricular conduction during atrial fibrillation in the Wolff-Parkinson-White syndrome. Am J Med 97:25–28, 1994. Reprinted with permission from American Journal of Medicine.)

tions, 2:1 or higher ratios of AV conduction are often observed. In patients with atrial tachycardia rates less than 200 beats per minute and normal AV nodal function, 1:1 AV conduction may occur. Distinguishing atrial tachycardia from AVNRT and AV reciprocating tachycardia may be accomplished by vagal maneuvers or adenosine to cause transient AV nodal block.

The mechanisms responsible for the various atrial tachycardias determine the clinical response to drugs. In general, atrial tachycardias due to intra-atrial reentry occur in patients with structural heart disease and are usually paroxysmal. Intravenous adenosine does not result in termination of reentrant atrial tachycardia, although high-grade AV nodal block will occur and confirm the diagnosis. Reentrant atrial tachycardias may respond to Class I or III antiarrhythmic agents, and radiofrequency current catheter ablation has been successful in eliminating the tachycardia in medically refractory cases. Atrial tachycardias due to enhanced or abnormal automaticity also occur in patients with heart disease; however, they are often incessant. Automatic atrial tachycardias may cause a tachycardia-induced cardiomyopathy and congestive heart failure. Control or elimination of the tachycardia can result in reversal of the cardiomyopathy and restoration of normal ventricular function. Intravenous adenosine may transiently slow or suppress automatic atrial tachycardias, but the focus quickly recovers and the tachycardia resumes. Conventional antiarrhythmic agents are usually ineffective in controlling automatic atrial tachycardia, although amiodarone may have some efficacy. Therefore, surgical or radiofrequency current catheter ablation is often recommended. Finally, atrial tachycardias can result from triggered activity, usually in patients with structurally normal hearts. In these cases, adenosine can be expected to abruptly terminate the atrial tachycardia, and treatment with verapamil, beta-adrenergic blockers, or Class I or III antiarrhythmic drugs may

be effective. As with the other forms of atrial tachycardia, those due to triggered activity are also cured with catheter ablation.

NONPAROXYSMAL JUNCTIONAL TACHYCARDIA

Nonparoxysmal junctional tachycardia is an uncommon source of supraventricular tachycardia characterized by enhanced or abnormal AV nodal automaticity, with typical rates from 100 to 130 beats per minute. The electrocardiogram in most cases reveals a narrow QRS complex tachycardia with ventriculoatrial dissociation, although cases with 1:1 retrograde atrial activation are sometimes encountered. Nonparoxysmal junctional tachycardia classically occurs in the setting of digitalis toxicity. Other precipitating factors include recent cardiac surgery, acute myocardial infarction, myocarditis, chronic pulmonary disease, and states of severe sympathetic stimulation. Patients are usually asymptomatic with this arrhythmia, but hemodynamic deterioration may occur. Treatment should be directed at identification and correction of the underlying cause, although medical therapy with beta-adrenergic blockers, verapamil, or Class I or III antiarrhythmic drugs is also effective.

MULTIFOCAL ATRIAL TACHYCARDIA

Multifocal atrial tachycardia is a chaotic atrial tachyarrhythmia in which at least three different P wave morphologies are present, producing atrial rates from 100 to 150 beats per minute. The ventricular response during multifocal atrial tachycardia is irregular and rapid, and the arrhythmia may be confused with atrial fibrillation. Afflicted patients typically suffer from chronic pulmonary disease with hypoxemia, and the arrhythmia may be aggravated by superimposed acute illnesses such as infection, acute respiratory decompensation, pulmonary embolism, theophylline toxicity, or poorly controlled diabetes mellitus.

Treatment of multifocal atrial tachycardia should be directed at the underlying cause. In cases in which the ventricular rate is rapid, the administration of agents to slow AV nodal conduction is warranted. Beta-adrenergic blockers have been shown to be effective therapy for multifocal atrial tachycardia, both as primary treatment of the arrhythmia and in slowing the ventricular response, but these agents are contraindicated in patients with underlying chronic pulmonary disease due to potential worsening of bronchoconstriction. Verapamil and Class I or III antiarrhythmic drugs may also be effective for this arrhythmia; digoxin, however, is generally ineffective in slowing the ventricular rate, given the increased sympathetic stimulation in patients with this arrhythmia.

VENTRICULAR TACHYCARDIA

Ventricular tachycardia is a potentially life-threatening arrhythmia that accounts for at least 50% of sudden cardiac deaths. Ventricular tachycardia occurs most commonly in the setting of acquired structural heart disease, particularly previous myocardial infarction or dilated cardiomyopathy, where differences in conduction and refractoriness in damaged myocardium presumably provide an environment for the development of reentrant tachycardia. The heart rate during ventricular tachycardia is usually between 150 and 250 beats per minute, although both slower and faster forms are encountered clinically. The 12-lead electrocardiogram can provide important clues for the correct diagnosis (Figure 5; also see Table 2). Patient stability during an episode of sustained ventricular tachycardia is generally determined by a combination of the tachycardia rate and the severity of the underlying ventricular dysfunction; therefore, hemodynamic stability during a wide complex tachycardia does not exclude ventricular tachycardia. Very rapid rates are tolerated by some patients for hours, whereas slower rates can result in cardiac arrest in patients with depressed left ventricular function. Since ventricular muscle is minimally affected by vagal maneuvers or adenosine, ventricular tachycardia is rarely affected by these interventions. The absence of termination of slowing with vagal maneuvers or adenosine suggests ventricular tachycardia in cases in which supraventricular tachycardia with bundle branch block or ventricular pre-excitation is suspected.

Ventricular tachycardia is considered nonsustained when the arrhythmia persists for less than 30 seconds. Patients with asymptomatic nonsustained ventricular tachycardia that occurs in the absence of underlying heart disease have the same prognosis as patients without the arrhythmia. In contrast, patients with nonsustained ventricular tachycardia in the setting of underlying heart disease are at increased risk for sudden cardiac death. Despite this increased risk, attempts to treat these patients with

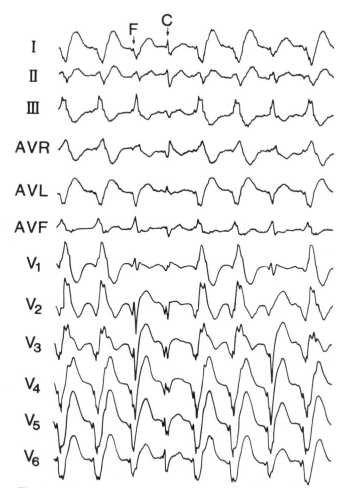

Figure 5. Twelve-lead electrocardiogram recorded during monomorphic ventricular tachycardia with right bundle branch block (RBBB)–rightward axis morphology demonstrating fusion (F) and capture (C) complexes, features diagnostic of VT. The QRS duration >0.14 s, monophasic R wave in lead V_1, and notching of the downstroke of the S wave in the precordial leads further support the diagnosis of VT. (From Greenfield RA, Vitullo RN, Bacon ME, Wharton JM: Diagnosis and treatment of arrhythmias. *In* Schwartz GR, Cayten CG, Mangelsen MA, et al. [eds]: Principles and Practice of Emergency Medicine. Malvern, PA, Lea & Febiger, 1992.)

Class I antiarrhythmic agents have been associated with an increased mortality; therefore, these patients should generally not receive Class I antiarrhythmic drugs. The Class III agents sotalol (Betapace) and amiodarone (Cordarone) may be helpful, but the results from limited studies have been conflicting. The beta-adrenergic blockers have been repeatedly shown to increase survival in these patients, and their use is therefore recommended in all patients who are able to tolerate them.

Conventional antiarrhythmic drug therapy for patients with symptomatic nonsustained or sustained ventricular tachycardia should optimally be guided by serial electrophysiologic testing to assess drug efficacy (see Table 3). Quantitative suppression of premature ventricular complexes as shown by electrocardiographic monitoring has been associated with a 30 to 40% recurrence rate at 1 year, a rate that is generally unacceptable for this population of patients. Amiodarone, an implantable cardioverter-defibrillator (ICD), and surgical or catheter ablation are appropriate options for selected medically refractory cases.

POLYMORPHIC VENTRICULAR TACHYCARDIA AND TORSADES DE POINTES

When the QRS complexes during ventricular tachycardia are constantly changing, this is known as polymorphic ventricular tachycardia (Figure 6). Polymorphic ventricular tachycardia that occurs in the setting of an electrocardiographically prolonged QT interval is called torsades de pointes, or "twisting of the points." There are numerous clinical conditions and medications that can result in torsades de pointes (Table 4). In rare instances, the condition is inherited, sometimes in association with congenital sensorineural deafness. A careful review of the patient's family history often reveals cases of unexplained sudden death in other family members. Patients with congenital or acquired long QT syndromes experience a range of symptoms, from absence of arrhythmia to cardiac arrest associated with sustained torsades de pointes. Recurrent near syncope or syncope is an ominous finding in patients with QT interval prolongation. Polymorphic ventricular tachycardia can also occur in patients with normal QT intervals, especially in association with acute myocardial infarction or severe underlying ischemia or left ventricular dysfunction. Determining whether polymorphic ventricular tachycardia occurs in the setting of a normal or prolonged QT interval is important, since therapeutic strategies are different.

Patients with sustained polymorphic ventricular tachycardia require prompt defibrillation. In cases in which QT interval prolongation is observed, conventional antiarrhythmic agents, especially Classes IA and III, are contraindicated, since they usually aggravate the arrhythmia. In cases of acquired long QT

TABLE 4. **Common Causes of Electrocardiographic QT Interval Prolongation and Associated Polymorphic Ventricular Tachycardia (Torsades de Pointes)**

Acquired Syndromes (*Bradycardia or Pause Dependent*)
  Antiarrhythmic drugs
    Class IA (quinidine, procainamide, disopyramide)
    Class III (sotalol, amiodarone)
    Class IV (bepridil)
  Electrolyte imbalances (hypokalemia, hypomagnesemia)
  Psychotropic drugs (neuroleptics, tricyclic antidepressants, lithium)
  Other medications
    Pentamidine (IV or aerosol) (Pentam)
    Terfenedine (Seldane)
    Erythromycin
    Trimethoprim-sulfamethoxazole (Bactrim, Septra)
    Amantadine (Symmetrel)
    Cisapride (Propulsid)
    Chloroquine (Aralen)
  Organophosphate insecticide poisoning
  Bradycardia (sinus node dysfunction or high-grade AV node block)
  Intracerebral hemorrhage
  Starvation (liquid protein diets, anorexia nervosa)
  Acute myocardial ischemia or infarction; myocarditis
  Mitral valve prolapse

Congenital Syndromes (*Adrenergic Dependent*)
  Jervell and Lange-Nielsen syndrome (autosomal recessive, congenital deafness)
  Romano and Ward syndrome (autosomal dominant, normal hearing)
  Sporadic form (inheritance not established)

syndrome, correction of electrolyte imbalances and elimination of offending medications can prevent recurrences. Acute management includes intravenous isoproterenol (Isuprel) at 1 to 5 μg per minute to produce acceleration of the sinus rate and overdrive suppression of the torsades de pointes. However, isoproterenol may be contraindicated in patients with non-revascularized coronary artery disease. Overdrive atrial or ventricular pacing is preferred in patients who are unable to tolerate isoproterenol. For the congenital long QT syndromes, treatment with

Lead MCL₁

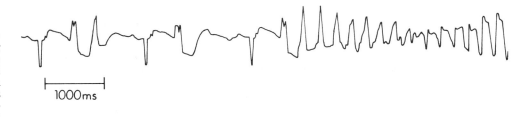

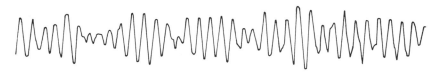

Figure 6. Single-lead electrocardiographic recording showing typical initiation of torsades de pointes, in this case associated with quinidine administration. A prolonged QT interval is apparent even during the ventricular bigeminy that precedes tachycardia initiation.

1000ms

beta-adrenergic blockers can be used acutely or as long-term therapy to prevent recurrences of polymorphic ventricular tachycardia. Class IA and III agents or other drugs that cause QT interval prolongation should be avoided. An ICD is increasingly used in patients with congenital long QT syndromes who have survived an episode of sudden cardiac death.

Treatment is considerably different in cases of polymorphic ventricular tachycardia without QT interval prolongation. These cases are most commonly associated with severe myocardial ischemia and sympathetic overstimulation; therefore, the use of isoproterenol or overdrive pacing may actually exacerbate the tachyarrhythmia. In these instances, antiarrhythmic agents, particularly amiodarone, may be effective therapy. Finally, emergent coronary revascularization may be highly effective therapy for patients with recurrent polymorphic ventricular tachycardia due to myocardial ischemia.

VENTRICULAR FIBRILLATION

Ventricular fibrillation is defined by rapid, nonuniform ventricular activation that produces characteristic fine or coarse undulations on the electrocardiogram. Prompt direct current defibrillation is required; otherwise, death results within minutes. Many cases of ventricular fibrillation occur secondary to untreated episodes of ventricular tachycardia. In cases in which ventricular fibrillation is the primary arrhythmia, acute myocardial ischemia or infarction is usually responsible, and further treatment of the ventricular fibrillation after treatment of the acute coronary syndrome is seldom necessary. All patients who have been resuscitated following an episode of ventricular fibrillation should be evaluated for acute myocardial infarction and underlying coronary artery disease.

Patients who are resuscitated from ventricular fibrillation should also be evaluated for other potentially reversible etiologies, including disturbances in electrolytes and proper or improper use of prescribed medications. The standard 12-lead electrocardiogram should be carefully evaluated during sinus rhythm for the presence of acute myocardial ischemia or infarction, QT interval prolongation, ventricular preexcitation (WPW syndrome), pulmonary hypertension, or hypertrophic obstructive cardiomyopathy. A formal assessment of ventricular function is also necessary, although a prolonged resuscitation can often result in transient depression of ventricular function.

Most cases of ventricular fibrillation occur in patients with underlying structural heart disease. When this heart disease is left untreated, the risk for recurrent lethal ventricular tachyarrhythmias approaches 30% per year. In addition to therapy for underlying heart disease, long-term treatment strategies parallel those used for sustained ventricular tachycardia, including antiarrhythmic drug therapy guided by serial electrophysiologic testing, empiric amiodarone therapy, or placement of an ICD. Prospective trials are presently under way to compare the effectiveness of each of these approaches. The use of beta-adrenergic blockers is also encouraged for this population.

CONGENITAL HEART DISEASE

method of
KEITH C. KOCIS, M.D., and
A. REBECCA SNIDER, M.D.
The Johns Hopkins University
Baltimore, Maryland

The prevalence of congenital heart disease (CHD) is approximately 5 cases per 1000 live births excluding cases of mitral valve prolapse and bicuspid aortic valve. Approximately one-third of newborns with CHD present with cyanosis. We will describe a method for evaluating, categorizing, and diagnosing the more typical forms of CHD.

Most forms of CHD can be categorized into (1) *acyanotic CHD* with subdivision into groups with (a) increased pulmonary vascularity or (b) ventricular outflow obstruction, or (2) *cyanotic CHD* with subdivision into groups with (a) decreased pulmonary vascularity or (b) increased pulmonary vascularity. Patients can be appropriately categorized into the above groups and a presumptive diagnosis made by integrating information obtained from the physical examination, chest radiograph, and pulse oximeter.

The initial evaluation of any infant or child with suspected CHD should include a comprehensive history and physical examination, posteroanterior and lateral chest radiographs, 12-lead electrocardiogram, and pulse oximetry. During the physical examination, particular attention must be given to the child's vital signs (including four-limb blood pressure measurements and height and weight plotted for age), general appearance (cyanotic vs. acyanotic; well-nourished vs. wasted), state (comfortable, distressed, shock), cardiac findings (see later), pulmonary signs (depth and rate of breathing, use of accessory respiratory muscles, presence of rales), abdominal examination (location and size of liver and location of stomach), femoral pulses (intensity and presence of radial-femoral delay), and distal extremities (temperature, cyanosis, clubbing, edema).

The cardiac examination should proceed serially and methodically with (1) *inspection* of the chest for detection of precordial bulging and visualization of the cardiac impulse, (2) *palpation* of thrills and the apical impulse, noting both the location and the intensity, (3) *percussion* of the cardiac dimensions, and, finally, (4) *auscultation*. When auscultating the pediatric heart, the examiner should note the quality of the first and second heart sounds and the presence of the third or fourth heart sounds. The second heart sound should be analyzed closely and its variation with respiration noted. Systolic murmurs are quantified on a scale of 1 to 6 with murmurs of Grade 4 or above associated with the presence of a thrill.

Regurgitant (holosystolic) murmurs begin with the first heart sound and therefore obscure it; whereas *ejection murmurs* begin after the first heart sound. Diastolic murmurs are quantified on a scale of 1 to 4, with Grade 4 murmurs associated with the presence of a thrill. Continuous murmurs extend through both systole and diastole. Localization of the murmurs to the classic mitral, tricuspid, aortic, and pulmonic areas is helpful. Additionally, auscultation over the posterior thorax bilaterally and over the supraclavicular regions is necessary.

Cyanosis is detected clinically when 3 grams per dL of desaturated hemoglobin is present. Central cyanosis, best seen in the tongue and buccal mucosa, must be differentiated from acrocyanosis (peripheral), which is usually a normal finding in infants and children. Noninvasive pulse oximetry is easily performed and most useful for diagnosing and quantifying cyanosis. Typically, oxygen saturations should be greater than 90% in neonates and 95% in infants and children. If cyanosis is present in the neonate, then the hyperoxia test should be performed to help differentiate pulmonary from cardiac disease. Classically, this test is performed by obtaining preductal (right radial) arterial blood gas measurements both before and after the neonate is placed in 100% oxygen. Infants with pulmonary disease usually can increase their partial oxygen pressures in arterial blood to greater than 150 mmHg, whereas infants with cardiac disease cannot.

ACYANOTIC CONGENITAL HEART DISEASE WITH INCREASED PULMONARY VASCULARITY

Several congenital heart defects present with acyanosis and increased pulmonary vascularity. The most common defects in this category are (1) ventricular septal defect, (2) atrial septal defect, (3) patent ductus arteriosus, and (4) atrioventricular septal defect. In total these four lesions account for the majority of CHD cases.

Ventricular Septal Defect

Ventricular septal defect (VSD) is the most common form of CHD, occurring in 32% of children with heart disease.

The ventricular septum is a complex structure that can be described embryologically as having four major regions: (1) *inlet* septum located posteriorly and superiorly between the tricuspid and mitral valves, (2) *outlet* septum located anteriorly beneath the aortic and pulmonary valves, (3) *trabecular* septum located inferiorly, and (4) *membranous* septum located in the subaortic region and beneath the septal leaflet of the tricuspid valve. The largest part of the ventricular septum is the trabecular region, and fusion of the inlet, outlet, and trabecular septa occurs in the membranous region.

Patients with a VSD have a dependent left-to-right shunt, meaning that the relative pressures and resistances of both the systemic and the pulmonary circulation determine the amount and direction of ventricular level shunting. At birth, when the pulmonary vascular pressures and resistances are high, little left-to-right ventricular shunting occurs. During the first 2 to 6 weeks of life, pulmonary pressures and vascular resistances drop, creating a pressure difference between the left and right ventricles and therefore allowing shunting from left to right. The amount of ventricular shunting is also dependent on the size of the VSD, with larger defects allowing more blood to shunt. Lastly, other associated cardiac lesions may alter the amount and direction of shunting.

The clinical signs and symptoms of children with VSD are the result of the amount of left-to-right ventricular shunting. Neonates are often without symptoms, and only as pulmonary pressures and vascular resistances drop do clinical symptoms develop. Beyond the neonatal period, children with a VSD can be categorized into four physiologic groups: (1) small VSD, (2) moderate VSD, (3) large VSD, and (4) VSD with pulmonary vascular obstructive disease (Eisenmenger's syndrome).

Children with a small VSD are asymptomatic. On physical examination, they are normal with the exception of a loud Grade 3 to 6 systolic regurgitant murmur. The vast majority of these defects close completely with time, most within the first few years of life. Their only risk is the development of subacute bacterial endocarditis (SBE), for which they require prophylaxis.

Children with a moderate VSD are often symptomatic. Infants often take longer to feed, and they may have inadequate weight gain in relation to their linear growth. These children also have a higher incidence of pulmonary infections. On physical examination, mild tachypnea may be present. A hyperdynamic impulse is usually present in the midaxillary line. A loud Grade 3 to 4 systolic regurgitant murmur is present. Mild hepatomegaly is found. Most of these defects diminish in size, and some close completely as late as young adulthood. As these defects become smaller, the patients' symptoms often disappear. A small percentage of children require surgical closure. For symptomatic children, the use of digoxin and/or diuretics is helpful. Caloric intake must be recorded frequently along with weight gain, and in children with poor growth, hypercaloric formula (24 to 30 calories per ounce) should be given with a goal of approximately 130 to 150 calories per kg per day. These children are at risk for SBE and require prophylaxis.

Children with a large VSD are all symptomatic. These infants typically are failing to thrive, and pulmonary infections are common. On physical examination, a hyperdynamic impulse is found in the axillary line. A loud Grade 3 to 4 systolic regurgitant murmur is present with a prominent (Grade 2 to 4) diastolic rumble at the apex. These children are tachypneic with retractions and rales present on auscultation. Marked hepatomegaly is found. These defects often diminish in size, but surgical closure is often required to prevent pulmonary vascular obstructive disease. Maximum medical therapy should be initiated. This includes using digoxin, diuretics, and hypercaloric formula (30 calories per ounce) with a goal of approximately 140 to 150 calories per kg per day. These children are at risk for SBE and require prophylaxis.

Eisenmenger's syndrome develops when a large VSD is left unrepaired and pulmonary hypertension and irreversible pulmonary vascular obstructive disease develop with resultant right-to-left ventricular shunting and cyanosis. Death follows as a result of pulmonary hemorrhage, infections, and/or paradoxical emboli. Fortunately, only rarely do children under 3 years of age develop this disease. In those who do, large defects are identified by echocardiography, but few symptoms exist because of the pulmonary hypertension and therefore lesser amount of left-to-right shunting. This entity is more often seen in previously undiagnosed adolescents and adults with large VSDs.

The diagnosis of VSD is often made clinically. An electrocardiogram (ECG) often reveals left atrial and left ventricular volume overload. Chest radiography reveals cardiomegaly with increased pulmonary vascularity if the left-to-right shunt is significant. Confirmation of the diagnosis is made using echocardiography. Recent technologic advances in equipment and image processing have allowed excellent visualization of the entire ventricular septum. Color Doppler ultrasonography has improved the detection of even tiny VSDs, and pulsed Doppler ultrasonography allows the estimation of right ventricular and pulmonary artery systolic pressures. Cardiac catheterization is often not required in the management of children with VSD. This procedure is reserved for those in whom multiple defects may exist or in whom the question of pulmonary vascular obstructive disease exists and the measurement of pulmonary artery pressures, resistances, and flow is desired.

With advances in the medical and surgical care of children with CHD, cardiothoracic surgery is now being performed safely, even in small infants. Indications for surgical closure of a VSD include (1) uncontrolled congestive heart failure, (2) increased pulmonary vascular resistance with a risk for the development of pulmonary vascular obstructive disease, (3) failure to thrive despite maximal medical therapy, (4) recurrent pulmonary infections, (5) endocarditis, and (6) paradoxical emboli. Lifelong follow-up with a pediatric cardiologist is required. Right ventricular infundibular stenosis (including double-chambered right ventricle) develops in approximately 20% of patients, even after spontaneous or surgical closure of the VSD. In addition, a subaortic membrane can develop in association with a VSD. SBE prophylaxis can be discontinued 6 months after surgical closure of a VSD assuming no residual defects are present. Typically, no restriction to the child's activity is necessary in the asymptomatic child or in children after closure (spontaneous or surgical).

Atrial Septal Defect

Atrial septal defect (ASD) is the third most common form of CHD, occurring in 8% of children with heart disease. ASD is found more frequently in girls than in boys (2:1).

ASDs occur in three separate locations in the atrial septum. *Ostium primum* defects are located in the lower third of the atrial septum near the atrioventricular valves. *Ostium secundum* defects are found in the midportion of the septum. *Sinus venosus* defects occur in the posterior portion of the septum adjacent to the venae cavae. Ostium secundum defects are the most common type found.

The direction and amount of atrial level shunting is determined by the relative compliances of the right and left ventricles and the size of the defect. Typically, the right ventricle is more compliant, and therefore predominantly left-to-right shunting occurs.

Most children with an ASD are asymptomatic. They typically present to the primary care physician with a heart murmur. Atrial arrhythmias are present more frequently in older children and adults. In about 6% of patients with large, unrepaired ASDs, irreversible pulmonary vascular obstructive disease develops, typically in adulthood.

On physical examination, these children have a hyperdynamic subxiphoid impulse. There is a normal first heart sound, but a fixed and widely split second heart sound is present. Often a Grade 2 to 3 systolic ejection murmur is heard in the pulmonic region because of the increased blood flow that must traverse the normal pulmonary valve, creating a "relative pulmonary stenosis." An ECG reveals right atrial and right ventricular enlargement (rSR' pattern in lead V1). A chest radiograph often reveals cardiomegaly with increased pulmonary vascularity and a prominent main pulmonary artery shadow. Confirmation of the diagnosis is made using echocardiography, during which the location and size of the defect and the degree of right ventricular volume overload are assessed.

Indications for closure of an ASD are (1) right ventricular volume overload, (2) arrhythmias, (3) paradoxical emboli, (4) elevated pulmonary vascular resistance. Closure is typically performed surgically with very little morbidity or mortality. SBE prophylaxis is not recommended for an isolated ASD. No restriction to the child's activity is necessary. In children who are repaired, atrial arrhythmias may occur and monitoring for this should be performed periodically.

Patent Ductus Arteriosus

Approximately 2% of children with CHD have an isolated patent ductus arteriosus (PDA). Premature infants have a high incidence of PDA that is inversely proportional to their gestational age. The ductus arteriosus is a normal embryologic structure connecting the main pulmonary artery to the descending aorta. In normal term infants this structure closes within the first few days of life. Patients with a PDA have left-to-right shunting dependent on the size of the PDA and pressures in the descending aorta and pulmonary artery.

Most infants with a large PDA are symptomatic with signs of congestive heart failure. Many infants and children with smaller PDAs are asymptomatic and present to the physician with only a heart murmur. Patients with large PDAs left untreated develop irreversible pulmonary vascular obstructive disease in young adulthood.

On physical examination, these children have a hyperdynamic apical impulse. The heart sounds are normal. Often a Grade 3 to 4 continuous murmur is heard best in the pulmonic region. The pulses are bounding. In patients with congestive heart failure, tachypnea, pulmonary edema, and hepatomegaly are present.

An ECG often reveals left atrial and left ventricular enlargement. A chest radiograph reveals cardiomegaly with increased pulmonary blood flow. Confirmation of the diagnosis is made using echocardiography. All patients with a PDA require closure either with medications, surgery, or interventional cardiac catheterization. Indomethacin (Indocin) is successful in closing most PDAs in premature infants, and surgical closure is only occasionally necessary. Surgical ligation is extremely effective with essentially no morbidity or mortality. Newer interventional catheterization techniques using either PDA closure devices or coils are being used at select centers with reasonable success. The risk for SBE is high and is the rationale for recommending closure of all PDAs. Until closure is accomplished, these patients require SBE prophylaxis. Asymptomatic children require no restriction to activity.

Atrioventricular Septal Defect

Atrioventricular septal defect (AVSD) occurs in 7% of children with CHD. It is commonly found in children with Down's syndrome. The defect consists of a large defect in the atrioventricular septum along with a common atrioventricular valve. The clinical presentation, physical examination, and medical treatment are similar to those of children with a large VSD. The ECG demonstrates a superior axis. Echocardiography is used to confirm the diagnosis and assess the surgical anatomy of the defect. Cardiac catheterization is rarely necessary but may be needed to measure the pulmonary artery pressure and resistance or calculate the amount of systemic-to-pulmonary shunting. Surgical repair is required in infancy, ideally at 3 to 6 months of age. SBE prophylaxis is necessary preoperatively but may be discontinued if no residual lesions exist 6 months postoperatively.

ACYANOTIC CONGENITAL HEART DISEASE WITH VENTRICULAR OUTFLOW TRACT OBSTRUCTION

Ventricular outflow tract obstruction occurs in both the left and the right ventricle. Obstruction to either ventricle can occur in isolation or in combination with other defects at the (1) subvalvar, (2) valvar, or (3) supravalvar levels.

Aortic Stenosis

Aortic stenosis (AS) occurs in 3% of children with CHD. The commissures of the aortic valve are fused, resulting in a thickened, domed, stenotic orifice. The presenting symptoms and findings on physical examination are variable and relate roughly to the degree of narrowing of the valve. In infants with mild AS, an ejection click and a systolic ejection murmur are present at the right upper sternal border. The intensity of the murmur increases with the severity of the disease, and thrills can be felt in the suprasternal notch in patients with moderate or severe AS. Infants with critical AS present in shock at birth. Often, a murmur is difficult to appreciate because of little forward flow across the valve. Patients with severe AS may complain of substernal chest pain, typically with exercise, and are at risk for sudden death. An ECG often reveals left ventricular hypertrophy with ST-T wave changes. Echocardiography is used to confirm the diagnosis, assess the severity of the lesion, and calculate pressure gradients from the left ventricle to the aorta using Doppler techniques. Cardiac catheterization is usually reserved for intervention rather than diagnosis since the treatment of choice for these patients is balloon valvuloplasty. This procedure is very effective with good initial and long-term results. Surgery is recommended for those in whom the annulus and valve are very small and require valve replacement or in whom interventional catheterization was unsuccessful. Exercise is restricted in patients with moderate or severe disease, and SBE prophylaxis is required.

Coarctation of the Aorta

Coarctation of the aorta (CoA) occurs in 5% of children with CHD. CoA is a constriction of the descending aorta that usually occurs opposite the ductus arteriosus–ligamentum arteriosum. The symptoms in these patients are variable. Typically, children with mild disease have no symptoms, whereas infants with critical CoA present with shock in the first week of life after spontaneous closure of the ductus arteriosus. The classic physical findings are right upper extremity hypertension with diminished or absent femoral pulses. The heart sounds are normal. In the left supraclavicular region, a variable Grade 2 to 4 systolic ejection murmur that spills into diastole is usually present. An ECG reveals left ventricular hypertrophy. A chest radiograph in older patients may reveal cardiac enlargement, rib notching, and the posterior indention of the descending aorta (so-called 3 sign). The diagnosis is confirmed by echocardiography or magnetic resonance imaging techniques. Pressure gradients across the CoA are calculated using Doppler techniques. Cardiac catheterization is usually reserved for patients undergoing intervention. Prostaglandin E$_1$ infusion is lifesaving for neonates with critical CoA in shock, because of its ability to open and maintain the patency of the ductus arteriosus and, therefore, allow blood flow into the descending aorta. Treatment of hypertension is frequently necessary and usually responsive to beta-receptor blockade. Hypertension may persist even after successful repair. Most children with CoA undergo surgical repair. Increasingly, interventional cardiologists have been successful in treating this lesion with balloon dilatation. Early and long-term results for balloon angioplasty are good except in neonates and young infants (under 6 months). Long term, a significant number of repaired patients develop restenosis requiring balloon angioplasty and/or surgery. Isometric exercises and contact sports are prohibited for these patients. SBE prophylaxis is required lifelong.

Pulmonic Stenosis (PS)

Pulmonary stenosis (PS) is the second most common form of CHD, occurring in 9% of children with heart disease. The pulmonary valve is abnormal, with fusion of the commissures resulting in a thickened, domed, stenotic orifice. Except for newborns with critical PS, most children with PS are asymptomatic. A prominent subxiphoid impulse is palpated. On auscultation, an ejection click and a Grade 3 to 5 systolic ejection murmur are present at the left upper sternal border. The intensity and duration of the murmur increase with the severity of the disease. Neonates with critical PS present with cyanosis due to right-to-left atrial shunting through the patent foramen ovale at birth. A murmur is often difficult to appreciate because of the lack of blood flow across the severely obstructed valve. An ECG reveals right atrial and right ventricular hypertrophy. The diagnosis of PS is made using echocardiography, and Doppler techniques can be used to assess the severity of the lesion by calculating pressure gradients across the valve. Balloon valvuloplasty is the treatment of choice for these patients. This procedure is usually curative with excellent long-term results. SBE prophylaxis is required for all except those with mild PS.

CYANOTIC CONGENITAL HEART DISEASE WITH DECREASED PULMONARY VASCULARITY

Patients with cyanotic CHD and decreased pulmonary vascularity have obstructed pulmonary blood flow and right-to-left shunting of blood at either the atrial or the ventricular level. In the neonatal period, children with this category of defects are usually intensely cyanotic with hyperpnea but not dyspnea. This presentation is due to the decrease in pulmonary blood flow and absence of congestive heart failure.

Tetralogy of Fallot

Tetralogy of Fallot (TOF) is the most common form of cyanotic CHD, occurring in 7% of children with CHD. The tetralogy consists of (1) pulmonary stenosis (subvalvar, valvar, supravalvar), (2) VSD, (3) aorta overriding the ventricular septum, and (4) right ventricular hypertrophy. Patients present with different degrees of cyanosis dependent on the severity of the pulmonary stenosis. A hypercyanotic spell, or "tetralogy spell," is a characteristic sequence of clinical events that begins with irritability and hyperpnea followed by a prolonged period of intense cyanosis leading to syncope.

On physical examination, the patient may appear cyanotic if the degree of pulmonary stenosis is more than mild. A prominent subxiphoid impulse is palpated. The first heart sound is normal, whereas the second is single. A systolic ejection click and a Grade 2 to 4 (depending on the degree of pulmonary stenosis) systolic ejection murmur is heard at the left upper sternal border. Clubbing of the distal extremities is present in older children with long-standing cyanosis.

Pulse oximetry documents the degree of cyanosis, whereas the chest radiograph often reveals a boot-shaped heart with absent main pulmonary artery shadow and decreased pulmonary vascularity. A right aortic arch is found in 25% of children with TOF. An ECG demonstrates right atrial and right ventricular enlargement. Echocardiography is used to diagnose the defect and to assess the severity of the individual components of the lesion. Cardiac catheterization and angiography are still being performed frequently in these children to assess and/or confirm the severity of the individual components of the defect.

Medical treatment is lifesaving in children with a hypercyanotic spell. Initially, the child should be calmed and comforted and placed in a knee-to-chest position. Maximal supplemental oxygen by face mask is then given. If the spell continues, morphine is given intramuscularly at a dose of 0.1 mg per kg. If the spell persists, then more aggressive therapy is initiated. This includes rapid placement of an intravenous catheter by the most experienced personnel followed by intravenous fluid administration (10 to 20 mL per kg of 0.9% saline) and sodium bicarbonate administration (1 mEq per kg). Anemia (hemoglobin less than 10 grams per dL), when present, often precipitates a hypercyanotic spell, and blood transfusion may be required.

Surgical repair of this defect is indicated for any child with hypercyanotic spells or increasing cyanosis (typically oxygen saturations less than 75%). Until recently, the approach to these patients had been a palliative operation involving placement of a modified Blalock-Taussig shunt (Gore-Tex tube connection between the innominate artery and the pulmonary artery) in infancy followed by definitive repair (pulmonary valvotomy with resection of right ventricular infundibular muscle bundles and VSD closure) in older childhood (3 to 4 years of age). With advancements in the combined medical and surgical management of younger infants, definitive repair is now usually being performed in infancy as the only surgical procedure. Immediate and long-term results for these children are excellent. SBE prophylaxis is required lifelong, and these children are prohibited from participating in strenuous sports.

Tricuspid Atresia

Tricuspid atresia (TA) is a rare form of CHD in which the tricuspid valve orifice is not patent. A patent foramen ovale or ASD is present to allow systemic venous blood to shunt from right to left. The right ventricle and pulmonary outflow tract are typically hypoplastic unless a large VSD is present. These patients present in the immediate neonatal period with marked cyanosis. The cardiac examination is variable and nonspecific. An ECG reveals leftward axis deviation and left ventricular hypertrophy. The diagnosis is made using echocardiography. Catheterization is required infrequently and is reserved for infants who require balloon atrial septostomy because of restriction of blood flow across the atrial septum. Initial medical therapy includes the initiation of prostaglandin E_1 (Prostin VR Pediatric) infusion (0.05 μg per kg per minute) to maintain the PDA. Palliative surgery is performed in the first week of life and consists of placement of a modified Blalock-Taussig shunt. A modified Fontan operation is performed in children at approximately 2 years of age. The modified Fontan operation allows complete bypass of the right side of the heart by directing inferior and superior venae cavae flow into the pulmonary arteries. These children require lifelong SBE prophylaxis and are restricted from strenuous activities.

CYANOTIC CONGENITAL HEART DISEASE WITH INCREASED PULMONARY VASCULARITY

Cardiac lesions with cyanosis and increased pulmonary vascularity can be divided further into those with increased pulmonary (1) *arterial* (transposition of the great arteries and truncus arteriosus) or (2) *venous* vascularity (total anomalous pulmonary venous connection and hypoplastic left heart syndrome). Along with cyanosis, children in this category are usually dyspneic because of congestive heart failure associated with pulmonary congestion.

Transposition of the Great Arteries

In transposition of the great arteries (TGA), the aorta arises from the right ventricle, whereas the pulmonary artery arises from the left ventricle. Under these circumstances, the pulmonary and systemic circulations are configured in parallel rather than in series, resulting in cyanotic blood's being recirculated back to the systemic circulation rather than passing through the pulmonary circulation and becoming oxygenated. These neonates present immediately after birth with deep cyanosis. The cardiac examination and ECG are often nonspecific. The classic chest radiograph reveals an "egg on a string" appearance consisting of a globular heart with a narrow mediastinum. The diagnosis is made with echocardiography. Catheterization is undertaken to perform a balloon atrial septostomy. Medical management involves stabilization of the neonate and the initiation of prostaglandin E_1 infusion (0.05 μg per kg per minute) while awaiting balloon septostomy. The infants are typically stabilized after balloon septostomy and undergo surgical repair of the defect in the first week of life. The arterial switch operation in which the aorta is connected to the left ventricle and the pulmonary artery to the right ventricle is now the surgical procedure of choice. Immediate and intermediate-term outcome are good. These children require SBE prophylaxis for their lifetime and are restricted from strenuous activities.

Truncus Arteriosus

Truncus arteriosus (TA) is a rare form of CHD whereby a single-valved vessel is located above both right and left ventricles via a VSD allowing common egress of blood from both ventricles. This common vessel, the truncus arteriosus, gives rise to the aorta, coronary arteries, and pulmonary arteries. A significant percentage of these patients have DiGeorge's syndrome (thymic hypoplasia, third and fourth pharyngeal pouch defects) and should be evaluated immediately for hypocalcemia secondary to hypoparathyroidism and T cell immune deficiency. These children should only receive irradiated blood cell transfusions so as to prevent the development of graft-versus-host disease. Cyanosis in these patients is often mild, and most infants present with symptoms of congestive heart failure and a heart murmur. A prominent right ventricular impulse is palpable, and the first and second heart sounds are single. An ejection click and continuous Grade 3 murmur are often heard. The murmur is appreciated well into the back bilaterally. An ECG shows biventricular hypertrophy, and the chest radiograph demonstrates a right aortic arch in one-third of patients. Echocardiography is diagnostic. Cardiac catheterization is frequently not required. Initial medical management involves control of the congestive heart failure with digoxin and/or diuretics. Definitive surgical repair can usually be performed soon after diagnosis and involves placement of a valved homograft conduit from the right ventricle to the main pulmonary artery, which has been separated from the truncus arteriosus. The VSD is closed so as to direct the left ventricular blood into the truncus arteriosus. Long-term outcome is good in patients without immune deficiency. Subsequent surgical procedures are necessary to change the size of the conduit as the children grow. These patients all require SBE prophylaxis for a lifetime and are restricted from strenuous activity.

Total Anomalous Pulmonary Venous Connection

Patients with total anomalous pulmonary venous connection (TAPVC), a rare form of CHD, have their entire supply of oxygenated pulmonary venous blood returning to the systemic venous circulation. This admixture of oxygenated and desaturated blood produces cyanosis. The severity of the cyanosis increases if there is an obstruction to the return of the pulmonary venous blood, as commonly occurs. Neonates with TAPVC frequently present in extremis with severe cyanosis. Physical examination is variable. The ECG is nonspecific, often showing right atrial and right ventricular enlargement. The chest radiograph in patients with obstruction of the pulmonary veins reveals a small heart with diffuse bilateral pulmonary edema. Echocardiography when performed meticulously is diagnostic. Cardiac catheterization is performed only when the pulmonary venous drainage cannot be determined with certainty. Surgical repair is done immediately upon presentation with very good long-term results. Following complete recovery, no SBE prophylaxis or restriction of activity is required.

Hypoplastic Left Heart Syndrome

Hypoplastic left heart syndrome (HLHS) occurs in 4% of children with CHD and comprises stenosis or atresia of the mitral and/or aortic valves, CoA, and hypoplasia of the left ventricle. Neonates present within the first few days of life, typically with mild cyanosis and a shocklike state after the PDA begins to close. Physical examination reveals a prominent right ventricular impulse, single first and second heart sounds, a gallop rhythm, and a systolic ejection murmur in the pulmonary region. All pulses are diminished, and hepatomegaly is frequent. The ECG reveals right ventricular hypertrophy with a paucity of left ventricular forces and occasionally ischemic changes. The chest radiograph usually shows signs of pulmonary venous congestion. Echocardiography is diagnostic and is used to evaluate the severity of the individual components of the syndrome. Cardiac catheterization is rarely required. Initial medical management is lifesaving. Control of the airway and mechanical ventilation are commonly needed. Prostaglandin E_1 infusion (0.05 μg per kg per minute) is begun and the state of shock treated with fluid administration (bolus 10 to 20 mL per kg of 0.9% saline) and inotropic support (dopamine infusion of 3 to 10 μg per kg per minute). Surgical treatment for this disease is variable and controversial. In some centers, no therapy is offered and the neonates die after intensive support is withdrawn. Cardiac transplantation at a few centers has had some success, but the limited number of donor organs and lifelong immune suppression are of major concern. In select quaternary care centers, a staged surgical approach similar to that for children with TA has been undertaken. With this approach, neonates undergo the palliative Norwood operation (anastomosis of the divided main pulmonary artery to the aorta, aortic arch reconstruction, atrial septectomy, modified Blalock-Taussig shunt). This procedure transforms the right ventricle into the single pumping chamber for both the

systemic circulation and, via the shunt, the pulmonary circulation. At 3 to 6 months of life, the infant proceeds to the bidirectional Glenn operation (anastomosis of the superior vena cava to the pulmonary arteries) with takedown of the Blalock-Taussig shunt followed by the modified Fontan operation at 2 years of age. In a few select centers, the results have been promising. SBE prophylaxis and restriction of strenuous exercise is lifelong.

MITRAL VALVE PROLAPSE

method of
ELLIOT CHESLER, M.D.
Veterans Administration Medical Center
Minneapolis, Minnesota

Names such as "floppy," "prolapsing," "systolic click-murmur syndrome," "anatomic MVP," "MVP syndrome," and "billowing mitral leaflet syndrome" refer to some anatomic or functional abnormality associated with myxomatous degeneration and prolapse of mitral valve leaflets. Prolapse detected by echocardiography, however, does not necessarily mean that the mitral valve is abnormal. For example, prolapse of normal thin leaflets may be found with left ventricular or papillary muscle dysfunction because of failure of chordal restraint in systole. Because the term "mitral valve prolapse" (MVP) is now widely accepted, it seems reasonable to restrict its use to the condition in which the clinical and echocardiographic features are compatible with those of a myxomatous mitral valve.

PATHOLOGY OF THE MYXOMATOUS VALVE

Myxomatous infiltration of the fibrous supporting layer weakens the mitral leaflets, leading to prolapse into the left atrium superior to the plane of the annulus. Usually the posterior leaflet is involved alone or at least more prominently than the anterior leaflet. The criterion for making a gross anatomic diagnosis is interchordal hooding of 4 mm or more, involving at least one-half of the anterior leaflet or two-thirds of the posterior leaflet. Fibrosis of the free aspect of the leaflets is a response to contact with an opposite prolapsing element or adjacent segment of the valve, and fibrosis of the left ventricular surface of the leaflets develops in response to stretching and tension. The chordae tendineae may be elongated and thickened, simulating rheumatic disease, but commissural fusion is absent.

Contact thrombosis may be found in two sites; one is on the atrial aspect of prolapsed units, and the other is situated between the posterior mitral leaflet and the left atrial wall (so-called angle lesion). Both are potential sources for systemic embolism.

Left ventricular endocardial friction lesions are formed as chordae make contact with subjacent left ventricular mural endocardium when the posterior leaflet prolapses. These lesions may coalesce, so that considerable portions of the base of the left ventricle become thickened and even calcified.

GENETICS AND EPIDEMIOLOGY

The myxomatous mitral valve is inherited as an autosomal dominant disorder. Most studies of the prevalence of

MVP are based on findings of echocardiography. These studies have disadvantages, however, because some interchordal "hooding" is present in the normal mitral valve, and criteria for diagnosis of prolapse are variable. There is also considerable variation in interobserver and intraobserver interpretation. Epidemiologic studies based on loose echocardiographic criteria have reported the incidence of MVP in as much as 21% of the general population. The "true" incidence is probably in the vicinity of 4% of the general population. The prevalence is lower in childhood and adolescence but increases with advancing years. There is a higher frequency among elderly men, who also tend to have more severe mitral regurgitation and left ventricular dysfunction. The myxomatous valve is now a leading cause of mitral regurgitation in the United States. This is because of a decline in the incidence of rheumatic fever and a greater awareness of the condition by clinicians and pathologists. Some instances of "rheumatic" mitral regurgitation were actually myxomatous valves associated with secondary fibrosis, erroneously diagnosed as healed rheumatic or infective endocarditis.

ASSOCIATED ABNORMALITIES

An association with Marfan's and Ehlers-Danlos syndromes, pectus excavatum, straight back, scoliosis, and high-arched palate is established. MVP has also been described in association with many other cardiac and general medical conditions, but this is almost certainly fortuitous. Because MVP is identified in approximately 4% of the general population, coincidental association occurs when there is a high background prevalence of some other cardiac or noncardiac condition, such as mitral annular calcification or migraine.

CLINICAL FINDINGS

Symptoms

Most subjects are asymptomatic, and the condition is often diagnosed by detection of a nonejection click during routine physical examination of a young person. Exertional dyspnea, leading to symptoms of frank congestive heart failure, occurs in patients with a holosystolic murmur and significant mitral regurgitation, particularly when the chordae rupture.

Physical Examination

Occasionally there are some features of Marfan's syndrome or formes frustes thereof, such as, high-arched palate, pectus excavatum, or scoliosis.

Auscultation

A high-pitched click in mid-systole is the keystone finding. It is heard in the region between the apex and the left sternal border and coincides with maximal excursion and tension on the posterior leaflet. Depending on volume changes in the left ventricle, the click may occur quite early in systole (Figure 1). The murmur is late systolic and follows the click and also responds to maneuvers that change left ventricular volume. The intensity and character are variable, but it is best heard at the apex or left mid-precordium when mitral regurgitation is mild.

When myxomatous degeneration is severe and particularly when chordae rupture, the murmur becomes holosystolic and may have a loud vibratory "honking" quality, simulating the murmur of aortic stenosis. The murmur is usually crescendo-decrescendo in shape and ends before the aortic component of S_2. S_3 is common, S_1 is of normal or increased intensity, and a mid-diastolic murmur is absent. These findings are quite different from rheumatic mitral regurgitation, in which S_1 is soft, the holosystolic murmur ends after S_2, and there is a significant mid-diastolic murmur.

Electrocardiography

The electrocardiogram is usually normal. The most commonly reported abnormality is flattening or inversion of the T waves in leads II and III and arteriovenous fistula. T wave inversion may occur spontaneously and independent of effort or may follow the patient's assumption of the erect position. The exact prevalence of these findings is unknown because of different selection criteria in various series. The Framingham study of the general population showed that persons with and without echocardiographic MVP were equally likely to have repolarization abnormalities. Left ventricular hypertrophy and left atrial enlargement are found when mitral regurgitation is significant.

Echocardiography

Invasive procedures are rarely indicated now because clinical and echocardiographic findings are so accurate. Both M-mode and two-dimensional techniques play a pivotal role in the diagnosis and assessment of patients with MVP.

M-Mode Echocardiography

MID-SYSTOLIC OR LATE SYSTOLIC BUCKLING. The sudden posterior displacement of the leaflets in mid-systole—is quite characteristic of MVP, and there are few false-positive results.

HOLOSYSTOLIC "HAMMOCKING." Holosystolic posterior displacement is not absolutely specific for MVP. False-positive results may occur when there is excessive cardiac movement in systole (e.g., pericardial effusion).

Two-Dimensional Echocardiography

The important changes are thickening of the leaflets and chordae, with systolic displacement of segments of the valve into the left atrium above the plane of the saddle-shaped mitral annulus, which has high points anteriorly and posteriorly. Because of this configuration of the mitral annulus, the mitral leaflets frequently appear to prolapse when viewed in the apical four-chamber view. Therefore, false diagnosis can be avoided by insisting that prolapse be visible in the long axis parasternal view. A calcified left atrial angle lesion above and calcified left ventricular endocardial friction lesion below the mitral annulus assist in diagnosis. When chordae rupture, there is (1) failure of leaflet coaptation, with the edges frequently observed in several views; (2) a whipping motion of the leaflet and attached chordae when a sizable portion of leaflet is detached; and (3) an eccentric jet demonstrated on color-flow Doppler imaging, depending on which chordae have ruptured. The transesophageal technique is particularly useful for defining anatomy more precisely.

COMPLICATIONS AND PROGNOSIS

The risk factors are infective endocarditis, mitral regurgitation, stroke, and sudden death. Infective endocarditis is a definite but infrequent hazard in patients with a late or holosystolic murmur. Progressive mitral regurgitation and congestive cardiac failure may supervene when

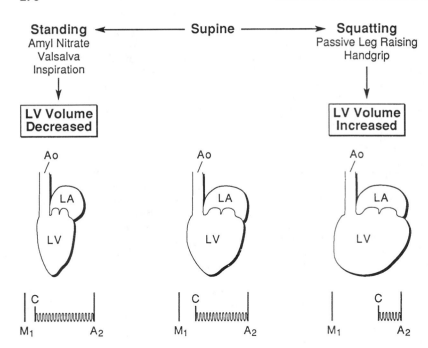

Figure 1. Effect of changes in left ventricular volume on timing of mid-systolic click (C) and late systolic murmur. *Abbreviations*: LV = left ventricle; LA = left atrium; Ao = aorta.

chordae rupture. Elderly men are particularly prone to this complication and also to severe left ventricular dysfunction and its attendant risk of sudden dysrhythmic death as a result of long-standing mitral regurgitation. The incidence of systemic embolism is low, and the risk for sudden death among young people with mild mitral regurgitation and normal left ventricular function is minuscule. The prognosis is excellent, and few patients suffer complications. Pathologic studies comparing the age at death of patients with myxomatous valves with control autopsy material showed that patients with myxomatous valves lived longer.

MANAGEMENT

Effective management of patients with MVP requires a careful assessment of the clinical, electrocardiographic, and echocardiographic findings so that triage is appropriate.

Mitral Valve Prolapse Without Mitral Regurgitation

When MVP is discovered in asymptomatic subjects without clinical evidence of mitral regurgitation, even after provocative maneuvers (see Figure 1), it should be strongly emphasized to patients that their prognosis is excellent, and every effort should be made to avoid engendering cardiac neurosis. Antibiotic prophylaxis is not necessary, but the physician should recognize that this does not completely solve the problem, because patients who have intermittent murmurs may be at increased risk. Doppler evidence of mild mitral regurgitation is not a reason for prophylaxis because the technique is too sensitive. The majority of subjects remain asymptomatic for their lifetimes without complications.

Mitral Valve Prolapse with Mitral Regurgitation

Infective Endocarditis

Infective endocarditis is a hazard for patients with MVP and a late systolic or holosystolic murmur. Thickened redundant leaflets identified by echocardiography and a predisposition to bacteremia through drug addiction or immune suppression are additional strong reasons for meticulous antibiotic prophylaxis even when mitral regurgitation is mild.

PROCEDURES NECESSITATING ANTIBIOTIC PROPHYLAXIS

Dental Procedures. Patients should be educated to maintain the best possible dental hygiene. All dental procedures likely to result in gingival damage with bleeding, including routine cleaning by a dentist, should be preceded by antibiotic treatment. Flossing, brushing, rinsing with chlorhexidine gluconate (Peridex) mouthwash, and professional cleaning help reduce bacteremia before routine dental procedures. Dentures should be regularly checked for the presence of gingival ulceration. Shedding of primary teeth and adjustment of orthodontic appliances are not usually accompanied by *Streptococcus viridans* bacteremia, and prophylaxis is therefore unnecessary.

Upper Respiratory Tract Procedures. *S. viridans* bacteremia may follow bronchoscopy, tonsillectomy, and adenoidectomy, and prophylaxis is therefore recommended.

Genitourinary and Gastrointestinal Procedures. These are important portals of infection in elderly men, and the organism is usually *Streptococcus faecalis*. Procedures include cystoscopy, urethral dilatation, prostatic massage, genitourinary and gall-

TABLE 1. Recommended Standard Prophylactic Regimen for Dental, Oral, or Upper Respiratory Tract Procedures in Patients Who Are at Risk

Drug	Dosing Regimen
	Standard Regimen
Amoxicillin	3.0 gm PO 1 h before procedure, then 1.5 gm 6 h after initial dose
	Amoxcillin/Penicillin–Allergic Patients
Erythromycin	Erythromycin ethylsuccinate, 800 mg, or erythromycin stearate, 1.0 gm PO 2 h
or	before procedure, then half the dose 6 h after initial dose
Clindamycin	300 mg PO 1 h before procedure and 150 mg 6 h after initial dose

Abbreviation: PO = orally.
From Dajani AS, Bisno AL, Kyung JC, et al.: Prevention of bacterial endocarditis. JAMA 264:2919–2922, 1990. Copyright 1990. American Medical Association.

bladder surgery, and sclerotherapy for esophageal varices. Vaginal childbirth and hysterectomy also require prophylaxis.

ANTIBIOTIC REGIMENS

These follow the recommendations of the American Heart Association and are given in Tables 1 through 3.

TABLE 2. Alternative Prophylactic Regimens for Dental, Oral, or Upper Respiratory Tract Procedures in Patients Who Are at Risk

Drug	Dosing Regimen
	Patients Unable to Take Oral Medications
Ampicillin	IV or IM administration of ampicillin, 2.0 gm, 30 min before procedure, then IV or IM administration of ampicillin, 1.0 gm, or PO administration of amoxicillin, 1.5 gm, 6 h after initial dose
	Ampicillin/Amoxicillin/Penicillin–Allergic Patients Unable to Take Oral Medications
Clindamycin	IV administration of 300 mg 30 min before procedure and an IV or PO administration of 150 mg 6 h after initial dose
	Patients Considered High Risk and Not Candidates for Standard Regimen
Ampicillin, gentamicin, and amoxicillin	IV or IM administration of ampicillin, 2.0 gm, plus gentamicin, 1.5 mg/kg (not to exceed 80 mg), 30 min before procedure, followed by amoxicillin, 1.5 gm, PO 6 h after initial dose; alternatively, the parenteral regimen may be repeated 8 h after initial dose
	Ampicillin/Amoxicillin/Penicillin–Allergic Patients Considered High Risk
Vancomycin	IV administration of 1.0 gm over 1 h, starting 1 h, before procedure; no repeated dose necessary

Abbreviations: IV = intravenous; IM = intramuscular; PO = orally.
From Dajani AS, Bisno AL, Kyung JC, et al.: Prevention of bacterial endocarditis. JAMA 264:2919–2922, 1990. Copyright 1990. American Medical Association.

TABLE 3. Regimens for Genitourinary and Gastrointestinal Procedures

Drug	Dosage Regimen
	Standard Regimen
Ampicillin, gentamicin, and amoxicillin	IV or IM administration of ampicillin, 2.0 gm, plus gentamicin, 1.5 mg/kg (not to exceed 80 mg), 30 min before procedure, followed by amoxicillin, 1.5 gm, PO 6 h after initial dose; alternatively, the parenteral regimen may be repeated once, 8 h after initial dose
	Ampicillin/Amoxicillin/Penicillin–Allergic Patient Regimen
Vancomycin and gentamicin	IV administration of vancomycin, 1.0 gm, over 1 h plus IV or IM administration of gentamicin, 1.5 mg/kg (not to exceed 80 mg), 1 h before procedure; may be repeated once, 8 h after initial dose
	Alternative Low-Risk Patient Regimen
Amoxicillin	3.0 gm, PO 1 h before procedure, then 1.5 gm 6 h after initial dose

Abbreviations: IV = intravenous; IM = intramuscular; PO = orally.
From Dajani AS, Bisno AL, Kyung JC, et al.: Prevention of bacterial endocarditis. JAMA 264:2919–2922, 1990. Copyright 1990, American Medical Association.

Progressive Mitral Regurgitation

Signs of severe mitral regurgitation and heart failure supervene in a small proportion of patients with MVP, and men older than age 45 years are particularly prone to this complication. The average age of patients having mitral repair at our institution is 61 ± 2 years, and in most cases, the underlying pathology is myxomatous mitral valve, with or without rupture of chordae. Similar findings have been noted in larger surgical centers. Mechanisms for increasing mitral regurgitation include (1) increasing prolapse because progressive myxomatous degeneration weakens the leaflets; (2) dilatation of the annulus, which goes along with and may aggravate, in a vicious circle, increasing degrees of regurgitation; and (3) rupture of the chordae tendineae.

Patients with a holosystolic murmur and significant mitral regurgitation should be examined annually, particularly when there is echocardiographic evidence of marked leaflet redundancy and lengthening of chordae. Left ventricular function and internal dimensions should be carefully assessed at each visit. Afterload reduction with angiotensin-converting enzyme (ACE) inhibitors such as enalapril (Vasotec) in a dose of 2.5 to 10 mg twice a day may be useful in diminishing mitral regurgitation and preserving left ventricular function.

SURGICAL TREATMENT

Operation is indicated when the left ventricular end-systolic dimension exceeds 5.6 cm as measured by echocardiography. Although mitral anatomy, left atrial size, and functional status are important in predicting the outcome of operation, age and left ventricular ejection fraction are the crucial prognostic factors.

Repair is accomplished by excision of excess leaflet

tissue (valvuloplasty) and annuloplasty or insertion of an annular ring. When monitored by transesophageal echocardiography, the results are excellent. Conservative repair has the obvious advantage of avoiding long-term anticoagulation, which is frequently risky in the elderly. In cases in which the valve anatomy is unsuitable for repair, replacement should be with a metallic or porcine valve.

Systemic Embolism

There is considerable evidence in the neurologic literature showing that MVP is associated with transient ischemic attacks or stroke in young patients. Although the exact mechanism for systemic embolism has not been documented, there are at least two sources for platelet, fibrin, and even calcific emboli: (1) contact thrombosis on surfaces of redundant leaflets and (2) angle lesion within the left atrium.

Antiplatelet treatment is recommended in patients who have had systemic embolism. Aspirin (160 to 320 mg) daily is effective. When embolism is recurrent, large, and associated with atrial fibrillation, warfarin (Coumadin) should be added.

Dysrhythmias

Atrial Dysrhythmias

Supraventricular tachycardia, atrial fibrillation, atrial flutter, and atrial ectopic beats are not specific for MVP but are a result of left atrial distention. They may complicate significant mitral regurgitation of any cause and should be treated in the same way: Pharmacologic cardioversion with Type Ia agents such as quinidine sulfate (Quinidex) or procainamide (Pronestyl) should be attempted and followed by synchronized DC cardioversion if the former fails. When atrial fibrillation persists, the ventricular response should be controlled with beta-blocking agents, such as atenolol (Tenormin) or metoprolol (Lopressor), or calcium channel blockers, such as verapamil (Isoptin) or diltiazem (Cardizem).

Ventricular Dysrhythmias

It is the ventricular dysrhythmias, particularly high-grade ventricular ectopy and ventricular tachycardia, that have attracted so much attention and have been correlated with the risk of sudden death. It should be strongly emphasized, however, that sudden unexpected death resulting from dysrhythmia among young people with MVP is rare. Many cases of sudden death attributed to MVP were actually a result of drug toxicity, left ventricular dysfunction associated with long-standing mitral regurgitation, or an independent cardiomyopathy. In a recent review from the Pathology Branch of the National Institutes of Health, there were records of only 15 patients studied at necropsy who had died suddenly with MVP as the only explanation for death, and in their review of the literature, only an additional 39 cases had been reported elsewhere. Most victims were young women with little or no mitral regurgitation.

TREATMENT

The rare, small subset of patients who complain of dizziness, presyncope, or syncope and have high-grade ventricular ectopy should be fully evaluated. Left ventricular ejection fraction should be measured by two-dimensional echocardiography or radionuclide angiography because impaired left ventricular function of any cause carries a poor prognosis and a risk of sudden dysrhythmic death. Holter monitoring for 24 or 48 hours is useful for assessing the severity of ventricular dysrhythmias when these are manifest on the resting electrocardiogram. When the resting electrocardiogram is normal and symptoms are infrequent, however, patient-activated event recorders are much more informative. Exercise electrocardiography is cost effective only when symptoms are clearly related to exertion.

If ventricular dysrhythmia is excluded as a cause of syncope, vagal stimulation (carotid massage) and orthostatic tilt testing should be employed to exclude neurally mediated hypotension and bradycardia. The sensitivity of orthostatic tilt may be enhanced by isoprenaline infusion, which stimulates the mechanoreceptors in the left ventricle thought to be responsible for reflex, vagal-induced bradycardia and hypotension.

When serious symptomatic ventricular dysrhythmias such as nonsustained and sustained ventricular tachycardia are demonstrated, provocative electrophysiologic study to select an appropriate antidysrhythmic drug is indicated. Favorable experience has been reported with the use of sotalol (Betapace) a beta-blocking agent with antidysrhythmic activity. Sotalol, as with all antidysrhythmic agents, must be used with caution in the presence of hypokalemia because it may lead to QT prolongation and torsades de pointes. The usual dose is 80 to 320 mg daily. Amiodarone (Cordarone) is highly efficacious in suppressing serious ventricular dysrhythmias, but because of its serious side effects, it should not be used in long-term treatment of young patients. The maintenance dose is 200 to 400 mg daily.

Patients with disease refractory to or who suffer serious side effects from antidysrhythmic drugs should be considered for mitral valvuloplasty, which has proved effective in treating a few patients with intractable ventricular dysrhythmias. The mechanism may be relief of mechanical stimulation of the endocardium by elongated chordae of the posterior mitral leaflet, a notion supported by experiments showing that traction on papillary muscles may induce ventricular ectopy.

When carotid massage or orthostatic tilt reproduces syncope as a result of neurally mediated hypotension and bradycardia, left ventricular mechanoreceptor activity should be blocked with the use of a beta-blocking agent. Disopyramide (Norpace) is also effective because it has not only an anticholinergic effect that blocks vagal transmission but also a negative inotropic action that diminishes activity of the ventricular mechanoreceptors. The usual dose is 150 mg every 6 hours. The drug should be used with caution in elderly men because it frequently causes urinary retention.

Mitral Valve Prolapse Syndrome, Autonomic Dysfunction, and Somatization Disorder

A group of patients described as having "MVP syndrome" present with nonspecific symptoms such as palpitation, fatigue, stabbing left inframammary pain, dizziness, and lightheadedness. These symptoms are indistinguishable from those occurring in "panic disorder with somatization," which affects 2 to 5% of the general population, 10 to 14% of patients in cardiologic practice, and 6 to 10% of patients in primary care clinics. The nature and severity of symptoms are unrelated to the degree of prolapse or mitral regurgitation. An association between anxiety state, panic disorder, agoraphobia, and autonomic dysfunction with a hyperadrenergic state and MVP has been described, but controlled studies have not supported these findings.

It is more likely that co-morbidity among highly symptomatic individuals is responsible and that many of the symptoms are a result of superimposed, or iatrogenic-induced anxiety in individuals who have been subjected to excessive medical attention. Many such patients respond to reassurance, and in some, a beta-blocking agent such as propranolol (Inderal) or metoprolol (Lopressor) has a useful anxiolytic effect by breaking up the vicious circle of tachycardia aggravating anxiety. Patients presenting with anxiety neurosis or panic attacks and found to have coexisting MVP should receive appropriate professional psychotherapy.

CONGESTIVE HEART FAILURE

method of
JONATHAN ABRAMS, M.D.
University of New Mexico, School of Medicine
Albuquerque, New Mexico

Congestive heart failure (CHF) is an extremely common condition, and it is increasing in incidence in the United States. As treatment targeted at cardiovascular disorders becomes more effective and individuals live longer, heart failure is more likely to complicate the course of many with underlying cardiovascular disorders. Although the classic definition of heart failure relates to an inadequate ability of the heart to distribute blood to vital organs, this is a somewhat simplistic and old-fashioned view. CHF is a syndrome, typically characterized by pulmonary or systemic congestion, or both, and often, but not always, accompanied by easy fatigability, lassitude, and decreased exercise tolerance. Pulmonary congestion is one of the hallmarks of CHF. Most, but not all, individuals with heart failure are short of breath because of elevated left ventricular (LV) filling pressure, which is transmitted to the pulmonary capillary bed; this results in pulmonary interstitial

fluid retention at rest or during exercise and, in severe cases, free alveolar fluid. When right ventricular or right-sided heart failure ensues, systemic venous pressure is elevated, and peripheral edema occurs. In severe cases, ascites may be present as well as marked jugular venous distention.

It is important to recognize that LV failure may be present or intermittently may be manifest, in the absence of signs and symptoms of right-sided heart failure. Conversely, the most common cause of right ventricular (RV) failure is abnormal left-sided heart hemodynamics resulting from LV failure. Dominant LV failure, characterized by decreased forward cardiac output and pulmonary congestion, is relatively common. LV failure may be transient, particularly in ischemic or hypertensive heart disease. On the other hand, isolated RV failure is uncommon and is typically associated with serious pulmonary disease, such as severe chronic obstructive pulmonary disease (COPD), long-standing pulmonary hypertension, or extensive parenchymal lung disease.

Certain categorizations of heart failure are common and worth reviewing. These include *systolic versus diastolic heart failure*. Most patients with clinical heart failure have systolic or contractile dysfunction of the left ventricle. The term "diastolic failure" generally relates to individuals with preserved LV systolic function and a relatively normal LV ejection fraction who manifest the CHF syndrome because of decreased compliance and distensibility of the left ventricle, accompanied by increased LV filling pressure and relative restriction to mitral diastolic inflow. *Forward versus backward failure* relates to specific signs and symptoms; forward failure is a result of decreased stroke output and is manifested by easy fatigue, renal dysfunction, and a small LV stroke volume. Backward failure reflects the more typical pulmonary congestive component of CHF and is characterized by rales, pleural effusions, elevated jugular venous pressure, peripheral edema, hepatomegaly, and in late stages, overt ascites. Certainly, not all patients manifest all of these signs and symptoms. Most patients with backward failure are short of breath, either with effort or, in severe cases, at rest. Orthopnea, or the inability to lay flat, is common in such cases, as is paroxysmal nocturnal dyspnea. *Left-sided versus right-sided failure* refers to whether there is clear-cut LV dysfunction or dominant RV dysfunction.

ASYMPTOMATIC LEFT DYSFUNCTION AND LEFT VENTRICULAR REMODELING ("PRE-CHF")

Contemporary treatment of CHF has expanded into therapeutic interventions in patients who have deranged LV contractile function but no overt clinical evidence of the heart failure syndrome. Such patients are typically detected by an echocardiogram or LV radionuclear angiogram demonstrating regional or global LV dysfunction with an ejection fraction of less than 40%; this represents significant subclinical LV dysfunction. Many data indicate that LV dysfunction is progressive. Treatment with angiotensin-converting enzyme (ACE) inhibitors helps slow the rate of subsequent deterioration and the likelihood of new CHF. In two large studies (SAVE and SOLVD), ACE inhibition has been shown to increase long-term survival. The natural history of LV dysfunction is one of progressive LV dilatation and decreasing ejection fraction. The late increase in LV cavity size, with or without compensatory hypertrophy, is known as "left ventricular remodeling." This is usually associated with increased LV compliance and an expansion in both end-systolic and end-diastolic volumes. Ejection fraction typically declines over time. Most individuals with substantial LV damage will undergo LV remodeling. The classic substrate for such events is a large anterior-apical myocardial infarction (MI), particularly when it results in a depressed ejection LV fraction (less than 35 to 40%). Inferior wall, small, or non-Q MIs in general do not remodel significantly.

DIASTOLIC DYSFUNCTION OR DIASTOLIC HEART FAILURE

LV function should be assessed in patients who have a clinical diagnosis or suspicion of heart failure. Subjects with relatively isolated diastolic heart failure represent a small proportion of individuals with CHF; such individuals have a better prognosis, and treatment is quite different, focusing mostly on symptomatic relief. Furthermore, definite diastolic failure should prompt a search for specific myocardial infiltrative processes, marked left ventricular hypertrophy (LVH), or hypertrophic cardiomyopathy. *It is essential that all patients suspected of or diagnosed as having heart failure have an assessment of LV function (echo, radionuclear study, cardiac catheterization) to document the degree of systolic dysfunction, if any, as well as the presence or absence of diastolic heart failure.*

THE PATHOPHYSIOLOGY OF CHF AS IT RELATES TO THERAPY

It is useful to address some of the important derangements in CHF and see how these might relate to choosing therapeutic agents. Table 1 lists specific features of heart failure and corresponding potential or actual therapeutic interventions. There may be overlap among various categories.

SYMPTOMATIC HEART FAILURE

This discussion focuses on chronic heart failure. Because treatment of asymptomatic LV dysfunction

TABLE 1. **Pathophysiologic Aspects of Congestive Heart Failure—Correlation with Treatment Strategies**

Pathophysiologic Aspect	Treatment
Depressed myocardial contractility	Digitalis
	Inotropes (nonglycoside)
	Afterload reduction (vasodilators)
Salt and water retention	Diuretics
	ACE inhibitors—mild action
Neurohormonal activation (↑ catecholamines, renin, angiotensin II, vasopressin, ANP, endothelin)	ACE inhibitors
	Beta blockers (use with extreme caution)
Chronic LV remodeling (chamber enlargement, ↓ compliance, ↑ sphericity, decreasing ejection fraction)	ACE inhibitors
	Nitrates (limited data)
Pulmonary venous congestion (high LV filling pressure) —can be primary problem in isolated diastolic dysfunction	Diuretics
	Nitrates
	ACE inhibitors

Abbreviations: ACE = angiotensin-converting enzyme; LV = left ventricular; ANP = atrial natriuretic peptide.

is indicated in many instances, this new concept is also reviewed.

Asymptomatic LV Dysfunction

A large database has accumulated regarding post-MI subjects followed serially with LV function testing. LV remodeling, i.e., LV chamber dilatation, usually with inadequate LV hypertrophy and a progressive decline in ejection fraction, commonly occurs following a large MI, particularly anterior-apical in location. This process begins very early after the infarct and appears to continue for months and years. Adverse consequences include the development of heart failure and decreased survival. Numerous studies have confirmed that ACE inhibitor therapy will attenuate the remodeling process and decrease morbidity and mortality in such populations. The U.S. Food and Drug Administration has recently approved captopril for post-MI LV dysfunction. It is important to stress that such individuals deserve therapy even though they have not had an episode of clinical heart failure. The SOLVD database confirms that the use of another ACE inhibitor, enalapril, limits LV remodeling and the subsequent development of heart failure; the SOLVD patients were not all post-MI and included a substantial number of individuals with dilated cardiomyopathy. *All individuals with depressed LV function and an ejection fraction of less than 35 to 40%, not associated with an acute event and not felt to be reversible, should be given an ACE inhibitor, even in the absence of any suggestion of heart failure or exercise limitation.*

Therapy of Symptomatic Heart Failure

General Measures. Salt restriction, adequate rest, weight loss in overweight individuals, control of hypertension, control of supraventricular arrhythmias, treatment of infections, and other general hygienic measures are obligatory in the management of heart failure patients. In advanced CHF, fluid restriction is often necessary to prevent or improve hyponatremia. Precarious volume status is typical of end-stage heart failure; excessive salt and water restriction and diuresis may produce symptomatic hypovolemia and prerenal azotemia, whereas excess salt and water retention results in a worsening of heart failure. On occasion, revascularization is indicated for individuals with coronary artery disease who have evidence of significant myocardial ischemia and who have coronary artery obstructions amenable to angioplasty or bypass surgery.

Diuretics. Patients with overt CHF usually require diuretic therapy. Although it is true that many such individuals who are maintained on diuretics do not need these drugs, a recent study confirms that withdrawal of diuretics in many patients with heart failure is detrimental. For mild-to-moderate CHF, a thiazide diuretic is satisfactory. The long duration of action of these agents makes them particularly desirable. However, with increasing severity of heart

TABLE 2. **Diuretics for Congestive Heart Failure**

Diuretic	Initial Dose (mg)	Maximal Dose (mg)
Furosemide (Lasix)	10–40 q day	240 bid
Metolazone (Zaroxolyn)	2.5 q day	10 q day
Hydrochlorothiazide (Oretic)	25 q day	50 q day
Chlorthalidone (Hygroton)	25 q day	50 q day
Bumetanide (Bumex)	0.5–1.0 q day	10 q day
Ethacrynic acid (Edecrin)	50 q day	200 bid
Spironolactone (Aldactone)	25 q day	100 bid
Triamterene (Dyrenium)	50 q day	100 bid
Amiloride (Midamor)	5 q day	40 q day

failure, particularly as renal dysfunction ensues, a loop diuretic is necessary. For refractory subjects, combinations of a loop diuretic and a thiazide can be extremely effective. Table 2 lists recommended diuretics and doses.

Digitalis. The digitalis glycosides have been the subject of considerable discussion and controversy over the past decade or more, but most recent evidence underscores the effectiveness of these relatively weak inotropic drugs for patients with depressed LV function. Although no longer first-line therapy, digitalis is needed for severe CHF, an enlarged left ventricle, or the presence of pulmonary congestion and a third heart sound. Conversely, patients with mild heart failure, minimally depressed LV function, or those who are easily maintained on diuretics do not benefit from digitalis. Remember that patients with atrial fibrillation may require and tolerate substantially higher digoxin doses than those in sinus rhythm.

Vasodilators. The advent of vasodilator therapy for heart failure 2 decades ago has had an enormously beneficial impact on the management of such patients. In essence, vasodilator drugs "unload" the heart by decreasing LV work by lowering afterload; drugs that relax the venous circulation also decrease cardiac preload. Afterload reduction results from decreases in LV wall stress related to a lowering of systolic blood pressure and systemic vascular resistance. These actions improve LV stroke work and ejection fraction and, therefore, should decrease the signs and symptoms of forward heart failure. Drugs with venodilating capacity lower LV and RV filling pressures and therefore reduce the signs and symptoms of pulmonary and systemic congestion.

It is not necessary to hospitalize patients to institute vasodilator therapy, although caution is necessary when beginning such therapy, particularly in individuals with borderline blood pressure, low potassium, or azotemia. Only three groups of vasodilators have been shown to be beneficial in CHF: ACE inhibitors, nitrates,* and hydralazine* (in combination with isosorbide dinitrate). The latter combination has been demonstrated to improve mortality in CHF; no studies are available to confirm that nitrates or hydralazine alone imparts a survival advan-

tage. On the other hand, numerous data attest to survival benefits of ACE inhibitors in CHF subjects with depressed LV function, who also achieve a decrease in morbidity. *ACE inhibitor therapy is mandatory for all patients with the heart failure syndrome and decreased LV function (ejection fraction less than 35 to 40%).* Nitrates can be used when ACE inhibitors are not tolerated, or in addition to ACE inhibitors in patients who remain symptomatic on diuretics, digitalis, and an ACE inhibitor. Table 3 indicates the recommended doses for commonly used ACE inhibitors, nitrates, and hydralazine.

One class of vasodilators that has been controversial in CHF therapy is the calcium channel blockers. Until recently, such drugs were relatively proscribed in patients with major depression of LV function because of their intrinsic negative inotropic properties and propensity to exacerbate heart failure. However, amlodipine (Norvasc) and felodipine (Plendil), two third-generation dihydropyridines, appear to be beneficial in heart failure and, at the very least, are safe. These drugs have very few negative inotropic properties, and their arterial vasodilating effects effectively unload the LV. Although these agents cannot be recommended as primary vasodilator drugs of choice, amlodipine or felodipine is clearly the calcium antagonist of choice for individuals with depressed LV function and ischemic heart disease and angina or those with hypertension, who otherwise might benefit from a calcium channel blocker. Ongoing clinical trials may subsequently demonstrate that these agents are safe and efficacious in CHF and should be used as first-line vasodilators. However, such a recommendation cannot be made at this time.

Other Pharmacologic Therapies. Considerable basic and clinical research efforts have gone into the development of inotropic drugs for heart failure patients. Adverse experience with amrinone, milrinone, flosequinan, and other such drugs has resulted in strong negative opinions about inotropes. In any event, such agents are not available in oral

TABLE 3. **Vasodilators for Congestive Heart Failure**

Vasodilator	Dose
ACE Inhibitors	
Captopril (Capoten)	12.5 to 100 mg tid
Enalapril (Vasotec)	2.5–20 mg q day, or bid
Lisinopril (Zestril, Prinivil)	5–20 mg q day
Ramipril (Altace)	2.5–20 mg q day
Benazepril (Lotensin)	10–20 mg q day, or bid
Fosinopril (Monopril)	10–40 mg q day
Quinapril (Accupril)	5–20 mg bid
*Nitrates**	
Nitroglycerin	0.6–2.4 mg/h for 12–14 h q
Patch	day
Isosorbide dinitrate (Isordil)	40–80 mg tid
Sustained release	120–240 mg q day
Isosorbide mononitrate (ISMO)	20–40 mg bid taken 7–8 h apart
Sustained release	120–180 mg q day
*Hydralazine**	50–100 mg q 6 h

*Not FDA-approved for this indication.

*Not FDA-approved for this indication.

formulation. The future of oral inotropic therapy is very limited as of this writing. Dobutamine infusions for 1 or more days are used by some in end-stage heart failure. In general, such an approach should be limited to cardiovascular specialists.

Beta-blocker therapy continues to receive attention as a potentially effective approach to patients with severe heart failure and depressed LV function, particularly dilated or ischemic cardiomyopathies. There is considerable evidence that extremely low doses of beta blockers can be instituted relatively safely, with dosage carefully increased. Some patients have had dramatic benefits from this approach. Treatment with beta blockers is not recommended except under the supervision of a cardiologist who has a special interest in heart failure or cardiac transplantation.

INFECTIVE ENDOCARDITIS

method of
JAYASEELAN AMBROSE, M.B., and
BARRY H. GREENBERG, M.D.
Oregon Health Sciences University
Portland, Oregon

"Acute and subacute bacterial endocarditis" are classic clinical syndromes of infected heart valves, and these distinctions remain useful in making empirical management decisions. However, most authorities use the broader term "infective endocarditis" (IE). IE often presents with protean symptoms and signs that may result in a missed or delayed diagnosis. Before the antibiotic era, IE was a uniformly fatal disease. This outcome suggests that host defense mechanisms play a relatively minor role in the eradication of this infectious process and highlights the importance of effective antimicrobial therapy and/or timely surgical intervention. Despite significant advances, the overall mortality remains significant at approximately 10 to 20%. Basic principles of management remain important in all forms of IE; they include recognition of the clinical syndrome, isolation of the organisms from blood or tissue samples, appropriate antimicrobial therapy, prompt recognition and treatment of complications, and antibiotic prophylaxis for individuals at risk.

PATHOGENESIS

Animal models have been used to study the mechanisms leading to the formation of bacterial vegetations, the pathologic hallmark of IE. This process is thought to begin with endothelial damage resulting from immune complex deposition or hemodynamic changes such as regurgitant blood flow, high pressure gradients, or turbulent flow through narrow orifices. This results in the accumulation of platelets, red blood cells, and fibrin strands, termed "nonbacterial thrombotic endocarditis," which adhere to the endothelial surface of the valve. These microthrombi appear to be a prerequisite for IE and form the nidus for bacterial growth as a result of seeding during transient bacteremia. Bacterial adherence is an important component of this process, and it appears that elaboration of dextran by the organisms and binding to fibronectin are important pathogenic mechanisms. Subsequently, additional platelet and fibrin deposition and further bacterial deposition occur, creating a series of layers that ultimately forms a vegetation. This allows both rapid unrestricted growth of bacterial colonies within the vegetation and protection from normal host defense mechanisms. Depending on the host factors and the virulence of the microorganism, the presentation may be acute, subacute, or chronic. The understanding of the pathogenic mechanisms leading to IE has established the principle of using high-dose bactericidal antimicrobials for effective treatment.

EPIDEMIOLOGY

With the caveat that published data reflect the referral bias of tertiary care institutions, the estimated incidence of IE is approximately 1 per 1000 hospital admissions, or 3 to 4 cases per 100,000 person-years. Although the incidence has remained relatively unchanged, there has been an evolution in the epidemiology as well as in the clinical and microbiologic spectrum. As in other illnesses, the mean age of affected individuals has increased.

Previously, chronic rheumatic valvular heart disease was the most common predisposing cardiac lesion. This has been supplanted by mitral valve prolapse, along with degenerative aortic and mitral valve disease and hypertrophic cardiomyopathy. There is also an increasing proportion of patients over the age of 65 with IE who have minimal or no identifiable underlying structural heart disease. A relatively new group of affected individuals is the intravenous drug users. Another population that continues to grow is individuals with prosthetic valve endocarditis. Among children, congenital heart disease is the most common predisposing cause, with cyanotic heart disease associated with shunts and stenotic valves being particularly high risk.

The microbiologic spectrum has been altered by the aging population, the increase in the number of intravenous drug users, and the aggressive use of medical interventions, in particular intravascular prostheses and monitoring equipment. Further apparent microbiologic diversity has been brought about by improved microbiologic techniques that have demonstrated a slightly increased prevalence of nutritionally variant streptococci, *Chlamydia*, *Legionella*, *Coxiella burnetii* (Q fever), and other fastidious organisms.

ETIOLOGY

Streptococci and staphylococci continue to be the most prevalent isolates, affecting at least 75% of patients who are not intravenous drug users (Table 1). Intravenous drug use (IVDU) associated IE is most often caused by *Staphylococcus aureus*, *Staph. epidermidis*, gram-negative bacilli, or *Candida*. Prosthetic valve endocarditis (PVE) can be divided into "early-onset," less than 60 days postoperatively, or "late-onset," greater than 60 days postoperatively. Early PVE is most commonly due to *Staph. epidermidis* and *Staph. aureus*. Other organisms include aerobic gram-negative bacilli and fungi (usually *Candida* or *Aspergillus*). On the other hand, the organisms responsible for late PVE are similar to those that cause "native valve endocarditis."

"Culture-negative endocarditis" occurs in less than 5% of cases of IE and is usually due to the effects of prior antibiotic therapy. Other causes include failure to grow fastidious organisms, such as the HACEK group (*Haemophilus* spp, *Actinobacillus actinomycetemcomitans*, *Cardiobacterium hominus*, *Eikenella* spp, and *Kingella kingae*), nutri-

TABLE 1. **Etiologic Agents of Infective Endocarditis**

Organism	Approximate Percentage	
	Native Valve	Prosthetic Valve
Streptococci		
Alpha-hemolytic	60	10–30
Enterococci	10	5–10
Pneumococci	1–2	<1
Beta-hemolytic	<1	<1
Others	<1	<1
Staphylococci		
Staphylococcus aureus	25	15–20
Coagulase-negative	<1	25–30
Gram-Negative Organisms		
Enterics	<5	<5
Pseudomonas spp	<5	<5
HACEK	<5	<1
Neisseria spp	<1	<1
Fungi		
Candida spp	<1	5–10
Others	<1	<1

Abbreviations: HACEK = *Haemophilus* spp, *Actinobacillus actinomycetemcomitans*, *Cardiobacterium hominis*, *Eikenella* spp, and *Kingella kingae*.

From Dajani AS: Infective endocarditis. *In* Rakel RE (ed): Conn's Current Therapy 1994. Philadelphia, WB Saunders, 1994.

tionally variant streptococci, *Corynebacterium*, *Legionella*, and fungi, such as *Aspergillus*. These organisms may require specialized culture techniques for isolation. Rare causes of sterile blood cultures include IE with *Coxiella burnetii* (Q fever) and *Chlamydia*. Systemic illnesses such as systemic lupus erythematosus and malignancies may also give rise to a syndrome of noninfective endocarditis.

Polymicrobial IE is a relatively recent problem that has predominantly affected intravenous drug users and patients with indwelling central venous catheters. These patients have an overall mortality of 30%, and prognosis is worse with infections involving *Candida*, *Pseudomonas*, and enterococci.

CLINICAL FEATURES

The presentation of IE is quite variable. The virulence of the organism and the host response in large part determine the presentation of the illness. Previously used diagnostic criteria were too strict, and therefore IE was uniformly underdiagnosed. Recently D. T. Durack and colleagues of the Duke University Endocarditis Service have proposed new diagnostic criteria that more closely reflect the changing epidemiology of IE and also take into account advances in echocardiographic diagnosis. These are modeled after the Jones criteria for rheumatic fever (Tables 2 and 3). Several different investigators have demonstrated the validity of these criteria when compared with the "gold standard" of IE diagnosis, namely, pathologic confirmation of valvular vegetations at surgery or autopsy. However, further evaluation of these criteria are required, especially in situations such as PVE and IE in children.

Clinical features of IE are a reflection of systemic toxicity, localized intracardiac infection and their related complications, bland or septic embolic phenomena, and immune complex disease.

Systemic features almost always include fever, and in subacute forms there may be complaints of malaise, weight loss, myalgias, and arthralgias.

Intracardiac infection primarily involves the valvular apparatus and usually results in a regurgitant murmur. The sensitivity of this finding in defining the presence of endocarditis increases significantly if the murmur is new-onset or has changed in character. Rupture of chordae tendineae or papillary muscle and perforation of the valve leaflet usually results in hemodynamically significant regurgitation and can lead to the abrupt onset of congestive heart failure (CHF).

The presentation of acute aortic insufficiency (AI) differs from chronic AI in that the diastolic murmur tends to be short, and it may decrease in intensity as the degree of regurgitation worsens. This is explained by rapid elevation in left ventricular (LV) end-diastolic pressure with consequent reduction in the gradient between the aortic root and the left ventricle. LV dilatation is also not marked since there has been insufficient time for the ventricle to adapt to the acute volume load. However, a drop in the diastolic blood pressure, a soft S1 and loud S3 along with pulmonary congestion remain consistent findings in hemodynamically significant acute AI.

Acute mitral insufficiency may result from destruction of the chordae, the papillary muscle, or the valve leaflet itself. Examination reveals a hyperdynamic precordium with evidence of pulmonary congestion and a systolic murmur of variable quality.

Tricuspid valve endocarditis with regurgitation is almost entirely a disease associated with IVDU. Quite often there is no discernible murmur. However, the peripheral manifestations of tricuspid regurgitation are usually obvious. These include a large V wave in the jugular venous pulse, an enlarged pulsatile liver, and peripheral edema in the absence of pulmonary congestion.

Prosthetic valve dysfunction may manifest with a new regurgitant murmur and/or loss of appropriate opening and closing sounds.

Occasionally intramyocardial abscesses may form and rupture, resulting in a variety of intracardiac shunts. Rarely, valvular stenosis may result from an obstructing vegetation or thrombus.

Clinically evident emboli occur in approximately 25% of

TABLE 2. **Proposed New Criteria for Diagnosis of Infective Endocarditis**

Definite Infective Endocarditis

Pathologic Criteria

  Microorganisms: Demonstrated by culture or histologic appearance in a vegetation, *or* in a vegetation that has embolized, *or* in an intracardiac abscess, *or*

  Pathologic Lesions: Vegetation or intracardiac abscess present, confirmed by histologic examination showing active endocarditis

Clinical Criteria, Using Specific Definitions Listed in Table 3

  2 major criteria, *or*

  1 major and 3 minor criteria, *or*

  5 minor criteria

Possible Infective Endocarditis

  Findings consistent with infective endocarditis that fall short of "definite," but not "rejected"

Rejected

  Firm alternative diagnosis for manifestations of endocarditis, *or*

  Resolution of manifestations of endocarditis, with antibiotic therapy for ≤ 4 days, *or*

  No pathologic evidence of infective endocarditis at surgery or autopsy, after antibiotic therapy for ≤ 4 days

From Durack DT, Lukes AS, Bright DK: New criteria for diagnosis of infective endocarditis: Utilization of specific echocardiographic findings. Reprinted from American Journal of Medicine: Vol. 96; 1994 (pp 200–209).

TABLE 3. **Definitions of Terminology Used in the Proposed New Criteria**

Major Criteria

1. *Positive blood culture for infective endocarditis*

   Typical microorganism for infective endocarditis from two separate blood cultures

   Viridans streptococci,* *Streptococcus bovis,* HACEK group, *or*

   Community-acquired *Staphylococcus aureus* or enterococci, in absence of primary focus, *or*

   Persistently positive blood culture, defined as recovery of microorganism consistent with infective endocarditis from

   (a) Blood cultures drawn more than 12 h apart, *or*

   (b) All of three sets, or majority of four or more separate sets of blood cultures, with first and last drawn at least 1 h apart

2. *Evidence of endocardial involvement*

   Positive echocardiogram for infective endocarditis

   (a) Oscillating intracardiac mass, on valve or supporting structures, *or* in path of regurgitant jets, *or* on implanted material, in absence of alternative anatomic explanation, *or*

   (b) Abscess, *or*

   (c) New partial dehiscence of prosthetic valve, *or*

   New valvular regurgitation (increase or change in pre-existing murmur not sufficient)

Minor Criteria

1. *Predisposition:* Predisposing heart condition *or* intravenous drug use

2. *Fever:* ≥38.0° C (100.4° F)

3. *Vascular phenomena:* Major arterial emboli, septic pulmonary infarcts, mycotic aneurysm, intracranial hemorrhage, conjunctival hemorrhages, Janeway lesions

4. *Immunologic phenomena:* Glomerulonephritis, Osler's nodes, Roth's spots, rheumatoid factor

5. *Microbiologic evidence:* Positive blood culture but not meeting major criteria as noted previously† *or* serologic evidence of active infection with organism consistent with infective endocarditis

6. *Echocardiogram:* Consistent with infective endocarditis but not meeting major criteria as noted previously

---

*Including nutritional variant strains.

†Excluding single positive cultures for coagulase-negative staphylococci and organisms that do not cause endocarditis.

From Durack DT, Lukes AS, Bright DK: New criteria for diagnosis of infective endocarditis: Utilization of specific echocardiographic findings. Reprinted from American Journal of Medicine: Vol. 96; 1994 (pp 200–209).

patients. The classic embolic findings consist of Osler's nodes (painful nodules on the pads of the fingers and toes), Janeway's lesions (nontender hemorrhagic lesions on the palms and soles), Roth's spots (white-centered hemorrhages in the fundus), splinter hemorrhages (linear red streaks in the nail beds), and petechiae (conjunctiva, palate, buccal mucosa, and skin above the clavicle). These classic findings are more often seen in the subacute form of IE. It should be noted that although these are considered classic "embolic phenomena," they may in fact be related to immune complex formation. In addition, emboli may occur to the cerebral circulation, resulting in stroke or mycotic aneurysm formation. Mycotic aneurysms may form in any part of the arterial tree and are due to bacterial seeding of the endothelial surface, which results in structural damage to the arterial wall with subsequent aneurysm formation. These aneurysms can rupture and bleed and cause clinical syndromes based on their location. Other organs such as the spleen and rarely the kidney may be sites for systemic emboli. A common feature among IVDU-associated IE is septic pulmonary emboli that appear as

nodules, infiltrates, and cavitary lesions on chest x-ray films.

The immune system is activated in IE with the formation of circulating immune complexes, which may be responsible for Osler's nodes and also for the glomerulonephritis that sometimes accompanies IE.

Splenomegaly is present in approximately 30% of affected individuals and may be related to activation of the immune system or as a result of splenic infarcts. Clubbing is a chronic manifestation of IE and is seen typically in illnesses lasting greater than 6 weeks.

Acute IE may present rapidly with fever, metastatic abscesses, valvular destruction, and CHF.

LABORATORY EVALUATION

The presence of continuous bacteremia with an organism known to cause endocarditis in the appropriate clinical setting confirms the diagnosis of IE. Therefore, the most important diagnostic test is properly obtained blood cultures.

Since the number of cfu per mL of blood is relatively low, it has been shown that at least 10 mL of blood is necessary per culture. In order to demonstrate continuous bacteremia, three sets should be collected at 1-hour intervals or longer. At least two of the three sets should be positive. If antibiotics have been used previously, it may be more beneficial to wait 48 hours before drawing blood in order to improve the chances of isolating the infecting organism. However, if the clinical course is fulminant, three blood samples for culture should be obtained at 30-minute intervals and empirical antibiotic therapy initiated.

It is extremely important to alert the microbiology laboratory that the diagnosis of IE is being considered. This enables the laboratory to hold cultures for longer periods of time and also to initiate any specialized techniques that may be necessary to isolate fastidious organisms.

Other laboratory parameters may be abnormal but are not diagnostic. Normochromic, normocytic anemia is usually present, and the white blood cell count may be normal or elevated depending on the acuity of the illness. Thrombocytopenia may occur, and the erythrocyte sedimentation rate is usually elevated. Up to 50% of patients with IE develop a positive rheumatoid factor. The urinalysis may be abnormal, with the presence of microscopic hematuria and/or proteinuria. This may indicate immune complex–mediated glomerulonephritis or renal emboli. A reduction in serum complement levels usually parallels abnormal renal function.

An electrocardiogram (ECG) is an important tool in the assessment of conduction system disease that may result from extension of the infection into the septum, particularly from the aortic valve. Abnormalities in conduction typically manifest as atrioventricular (AV) block, hemiblock, or bundle branch block. Conduction system disease may be transient or permanent, reflecting either edema or complete destruction of the conduction system, respectively. Higher degrees of AV block and bundle branch block are more specific for the detection of septal extension of the infective process. The sensitivity of ECG abnormalities for this condition, however, remains low and should not be relied on to rule out intramyocardial involvement secondary to IE.

The chest roentgenogram is valuable in the assessment of the hemodynamic status and complements the physical examination findings of left heart CHF. In tricuspid valve endocarditis, the x-ray film is an extremely important diagnostic tool and usually demonstrates the presence of infiltrates and cavitatory lesions consistent with septic emboli.

ECHOCARDIOGRAPHY

Because of significant advances in echocardiographic technology and the relative ease and noninvasiveness of this technique, it has become a frequently used test in the evaluation of patients with suspected IE. The recent introduction of the Duke University criteria for IE (see Table 2) recognizes the diagnostic importance of echocardiographically defined abnormalities; however, the definitive diagnosis of IE must be made in conjunction with clinical and microbiologic findings. The existing echocardiographic technology includes two-dimensional color flow and Doppler evaluation. Imaging can be performed using either transthoracic echocardiography (TTE) or transesophageal echocardiography (TEE).

The issue of vegetation size and its prognostic significance has been the subject of much debate. The overall consensus suggests that larger vegetations (particularly greater than 10 mm) are associated with a higher embolic rate. However, whether this embolic potential predicts progression to heart failure, the development of perivalvular extension of infection, the need for valve surgery, or death remains controversial. What remains clear is that the decision to proceed with valve surgery should not be based exclusively on vegetation size. Furthermore, follow-up studies to document the resolution of vegetations have not provided any greater prognostic information than can be obtained clinically.

In cases of CHF, echocardiography becomes an indispensable tool that can evaluate the degree of valvular abnormality, define underlying structural heart disease, and assess left ventricular function. With the addition of color mapping and Doppler flow techniques, it is possible to define in a semiquantitative fashion the degree and nature of the valvular regurgitation. In addition, these modalities can be helpful in the diagnosis of fistulous tracts and intracardiac shunts, which can develop as complications of IE. An absolute indication for either TEE or TTE would be persistent bacteremia despite adequate antibiotic therapy, suggesting perivalvular extension of infection.

Some debate still exists in the choice of TTE versus TEE. In general, TTE and TEE are complementary in the assessment of LV function. Furthermore, the relative ease of performing a TTE tends to favor this technique as the initial approach followed by the TEE if there is inadequate visualization or further information is required.

Screening for IE by echocardiography remains a complex issue, and several factors need to be considered. Since a missed diagnosis and delayed therapy can be fatal, echocardiography by itself, even by the transesophageal approach, cannot entirely rule out the diagnosis of IE. This is true for several reasons, which include the inability to resolve structures less than 2 mm and impaired visualization in the presence of heavily calcified leaflets or prosthetic valves. On one hand, in the specific case of nosocomial *S. aureus* bacteremia, it appears fairly clear that screening for IE is not cost-effective unless there is a new regurgitant murmur, underlying structural heart disease, or persistent bacteremia despite removal of the presumed primary focus. On the other hand, community-acquired *S. aureus* bacteremias with no clinical stigmata of IE are associated with a 20% likelihood of having occult vegetations or predisposing structural heart disease. Finally, not all cases of endocarditis are associated with vegetations, particularly early in the course of the disease. For all these

reasons, echocardiography is a tool that should be used thoughtfully, and, more importantly, the findings must be integrated with the existing clinical and microbiologic information.

CARDIAC CATHETERIZATION

The primary role of cardiac catherization is the preoperative evaluation of patients who require surgery for complications related to IE. Most clinical cardiologists would agree that preoperative catheterization is a useful step to assess hemodynamics, assess LV function, define aortic root anatomy, and evaluate for the presence or absence of coronary artery disease. In addition, when there are uncertainties regarding the echocardiographic assessment of valvular insufficiency and LV function, cardiac catheterization remains a useful tool for clarifying the diagnosis and severity of disease. Prosthetic valves can also be evaluated visually under fluoroscopy, and if the characteristic rocking motion is seen, this suggests valve dehiscence.

TREATMENT

The cornerstones of the management of IE are identification of the organism, initiation of appropriate antimicrobial therapy (Table 4), recognition of complications, and prompt surgical intervention when indicated. The principles of antimicrobial therapy are to use bactericidal agents, ensure adequate blood levels of these agents, utilize synergistic combinations when possible, and maintain therapy for an appropriate duration. In general, all forms of IE should be treated for a period of not less than 4 weeks. The two notable exceptions are IE caused by "pencillin-susceptible" *Streptococcus viridans* and selected cases of right-sided endocarditis due to *Staph. aureus.*

Acute IE is usually quite fulminant and is accompanied by some degree of sepsis syndrome, and therefore therapy should not be delayed. In the subacute form, therapy may be initiated after identification of the organism. In the case of previous antibiotic therapy, organism recovery is extremely low for approximately 2 weeks, and therefore the risk of delayed therapy must be weighed against the benefit of organism isolation. Despite these uncertainties in diagnosis, fairly reliable empirical judgments can be made based on the acuity of the clinical presentation and also the site and type of valvular involvement. The major categories of IE are native valve endocarditis (NVE), PVE, and right-sided endocarditis, which is usually associated with IVDU.

The vast majority of NVE cases are caused by viridans streptococci, enterococci, and staphylococci. A combination of penicillin G, gentamicin (Garamycin), and nafcillin (Unipen) is a reasonable choice if one cannot wait for the results of microbiologic cultures. In the setting of early PVE, there is a greater concern for *Staph. epidermidis* infections, and therefore vancomycin should be used in place of nafcillin. Late-onset PVE has organisms similar to those of NVE, and therefore a similar empirical regimen may be used. Infective endocarditis related to IVDU is predominantly *Staph. aureus* infection, and

TABLE 4. **Antimicrobial Therapy for Endocarditis***

Microorganism	Regimen	Duration (Weeks)
Penicillin-Susceptible Streptococci (Viridans streptococci)		
Native valve (Relatively resistant viridans streptococci and *Streptococcus bovis* should be treated with 4 weeks of penicillin G and 2 weeks of gentamicin.)	Aqueous penicillin G 10–20 × 10⁶ U IV q 24 h + Gentamicin 1 mg/kg IM or IV q 8 h *or*	2 2
	Aqueous penicillin G 10–20 × 10⁶ U IV q 24 h *or*	4
	Ceftriaxone (Rocephin) 2 g IV or IM single daily dose *or*	4
	Vancomycin 15 mg/kg IV q 12 h	4
Prosthetic valve	Aqueous penicillin G *or* vancomycin in same dose as above +	4–6
	Gentamicin 1 mg/kg IM or IV q 8 h	2
Enterococci (Streptococcus faecalis, Strep. faecium, Strep. durans) *and resistant viridans streptococci*		
Native valve and infections of <3 months' duration (For prosthetic valves and infections of >3 months' duration, 6 weeks of therapy is recommended.)	Aqueous penicillin 20–30 × 10⁶ U IV q 24 h + Gentamicin 1 mg/kg IV q 8 h *or*	4 4
	Vancomycin 15 mg/kg IV q 12 h + Gentamicin 1 mg/kg IV or IM q 8 h	4 4
Coagulase-Positive Staphylococci		
Native valve		
Staphylococus aureus, methicillin-susceptible	Nafcillin (Unipen) *or* oxacillin (Bactocill) 2 g IV q 4 h *or*	6
	Cefazolin (Ancef) 2 g IV q 8 h *or*	6
	Vancomycin 15 mg/kg IV q 12 h	6
Staph. aureus, right-sided, methicillin-susceptible (If extrapulmonary infection exists, nafcillin should be continued for 4–6 weeks.)	Nafcillin *or* oxacillin 2 g Iv q 4 h + Tobramycin (Nebcin) *or* gentamicin 1 mg/kg IV q 12 h	2 2
Staph. aureus, methicillin resistant	Vancomycin 15 mg/kg IV q 12 h	6
Prosthetic valve		
Staph. aureus, methicillin-susceptible (The use of rifampin in this setting is controversial.)	Vancomycin 15 mg/kg IV q 12 h +	≥6
	Rifampin (Rifadin) 300 mg PO q 8 h +	≥6
	Gentamicin 1 mg/kg IV or IM q 8 h	2
Coagulase-Negative Staphylococci (*Staph. epidermidis,* methicillin-resistant)†		
Native valve	Vancomycin 15 mg/kg IV q 12 h	6
Prosthetic valve	Vancomycin 15 mg/kg IV q 12 h +	≥6
	Rifampin 300 mg PO q 8 h +	≥6
	Gentamicin 1 mg/kg IV or IM q 8 h	2
Diptheroids	Vancomycin 15 mg/kg IV q 12 h	6
HACEK organisms	Ampicillin 2 g IV q 4 h + Gentamicin 1.0 mg/kg IV q 8 h *or*	4 4
	Ceftriaxone 2 g IV *or* IM q 24 h single dose	3
Gram-Negative Organisms (Should be treated according to antibiotic susceptibility; suggested regimes are listed.)		
Pseudomonas aeruginosa	Piperacillin (Pipracil) 3 g IV q 4 h *or* ceftazidime (Fortaz, Tazicef) 2 g IV q 8 h *or* Aztreonam (Azactam) 2 g IV q 6 h *or* imipenem 0.5–1 g IV q 6 h +	6
	Tobramycin 1.7 mg/kg IV q 6 h	6
Enterobacteriaceae	Cefotaxime 2 g IV q 6 h *or* imipenem 0.5–1 g q 6 h *or* aztreonam 2 g IV q 6 h +	4–6
	Tobramycin 1.7 mg/kg IV q 8 h	6

TABLE 4. **Antimicrobial Therapy for Endocarditis*** *Continued*

Microorganism	Regimen	Duration (Weeks)
Q-Fever Bacteria and Chlamydia	Doxycycline 100 mg PO q 12 h *or* Tetracycline 500 mg PO q 6 h + Co-trimoxazole (160 mg trimethoprim and 800 mg sulfamethoxazole) PO q 8 h	1–2 years or longer
Fungi	Amphotericin B (Fungizone) IV 1 mg/kg/24 h + Flucytosine (Ancobon) 37.5 mg/kg PO q 6 h	6–8
Culture-Negative (empirical therapy)	Vancomycin 15 mg/kg IV q 12 h	6
	+	
	Gentamicin 1 mg/kg IV or IM q 8 h	6

*Dosages recommended are for patients with normal renal and hepatic function.
†Antimicrobial therapy for methicillin-susceptible strains is identical to that for methicillin-susceptible *Staph. aureus.*
From Wilson WR, Thandroyen FT: Infective endocarditis. *In* Willerson JT, Cohn JN (eds): Cardiovascular Medicine. Churchill Livingstone, New York, 1995.

a combination of nafcillin and gentamicin would be a reasonable choice. It should be emphasized that these are short-term empirical regimens that should be modified as soon as culture and susceptibility testing are available.

"Susceptible" viridans streptococci are defined by the minimal inhibitory concentration (MIC), which is the minimal concentration of antibiotic that inhibits the growth of the organism in a test tube. Organisms with MICs of 0.1 µg per mL or less can be effectively treated with a 2-week course of penicillin G and gentamicin. The concentrations of gentamicin required to act synergistically with penicillin G are quite low (peak of 3 µg per mL or less; trough of 1 µg per mL or less) and minimize the risk of nephrotoxicity and eighth cranial nerve damage. Recent studies have demonstrated efficacy with a 4-week regime of ceftriaxone (Rocephin) two grams per day intravenously or intramuscularly. This antibiotic course offers the possibility of a home-based form of therapy that could significantly reduce health care costs and at the same time be safe, effective, and convenient. However, only patients with uncomplicated IE who are hemodynamically stable and have documented clearance of bacteremia would qualify for this treatment option. For relatively resistant strains of viridans streptococci (MIC 0.1 to 0.5 µg per mL), e.g., nutritionally variant streptococci, *Strep. bovis,* a 4-week course of penicillin G along with gentamicin in the first 2 weeks is recommended. Resistant viridans streptococci (MIC of 0.5 µg per mL or more) are treated with a 4- to 6-week course of penicillin G and gentamicin.

Enterococci (*Strep. faecalis, Strep. faecium, Strep. durans*) are the third most common cause of NVE and occur more commonly in elderly men. Such NVE is best treated with a 4-week course of both penicillin G and gentamicin, or ampicillin and gentamicin. The likelihood of cure using antibiotics alone improves if the infection has been less than 3 months in duration. Highly gentamicin-resistant strains may require surgical removal of the infected valve for a complete cure. Enterococci causing PVE should be

treated with the same regime as above for a period of 6 weeks.

Staphylococcal IE is treated on the basis of methicillin susceptibility or resistance, left- versus right-sided valvular involvement, and the presence or absence of prosthetic material. Methicillin-susceptible staphylococcal left-sided NVE or PVE (right- or left-sided) can be treated with 6 weeks of nafcillin alone or it can be combined with low-dose gentamicin for 3 to 5 days. The addition of gentamicin decreases the duration of bacteremia but does not improve survival or reduce complications. Methicillin-susceptible right-sided staphylococcus NVE (typically IVDU-related) not associated with an extrapulmonary foci of infection can be treated successfully with a 2-week course of nafcillin and tobramycin, or nafcillin and gentamicin. Those with extrapulmonary involvement should receive a 4- to 6-week course of nafcillin, combined in the initial 2 weeks with tobramycin or gentamicin. *Staphylococcus aureus* (methicillin-resistant) NVE should be treated with vancomycin for 6 weeks. Methicillin-resistant strains of *Staph. epidermidis* are typically associated with early-onset PVE and are best treated with a combination of vancomycin and rifampin for 6 weeks with gentamicin added in the first 2 weeks.

Endocarditis associated with the HACEK group of organisms accounts for approximately 9% of non-IVDU-associated cases. These can be effectively treated with 3 weeks of ampicillin. In penicillinase-producing strains, ceftriaxone may be substituted.

Gram-negative infections with other than the HACEK group account for 5% of NVE, 13% of PVE, and 30% of IVDU-associated IE. According to their in vitro susceptibility, these infections should be treated for 4 to 6 weeks utilizing cefotaxime, imipenem, or aztreonam in combination with high-dose gentamicin. There is some evidence to suggest that intravenous ciprofloxacin may now be the preferred therapy in Enterobacteriaceae and *Pseudomonas aeruginosa* infections. A combination of an extended-spectrum penicillin (piperacillin or azlocillin) combined with high-dose tobramycin also appears to be an effective regime for *P. aeruginosa* IE. This combination therapy may be effective in right-sided NVE; however, the cure rate for left-sided infections is quite dismal, and early valve replacement is recommended.

COMPLICATIONS

The vast majority of deaths related to IE result from congestive heart failure. The major complications can be broadly divided into (1) local valvular destruction, (2) perivalvular extension of infection, (3) embolic complications, (4) systemic sepsis, and (5) intractable infection (Table 5).

Local valvular destruction caused by bacterial vegetations constitutes the most common cause of valvular regurgitation; however, infection of the chordal apparatus or perivalvular abscesses formation may also give rise to insufficiency of the affected valve. In the case of acute aortic insufficiency or mitral regurgitation, rapid evaluation of the hemodynamic status and prompt intervention form the basis for effective therapy. Right heart catheterization can be invaluable in making this important assessment. If CHF is suspected by clinical examination, the patient should be transferred to the coronary care unit and a pulmonary artery (PA) catheter placed. If normal pulmonary capillary wedge pressures (PCWPs) are found, the PA catheter can be removed and medical therapy for IE may be continued. In the case of mild elevations in the PCWP, medical treatment for CHF should be initiated with diuretics and aggressive intravenous vasodilator therapy. We prefer using intravenous nitroprusside as a first-line agent. If the CHF can be easily controlled, continued medical management would be appropriate and the patient may be followed sequentially to determine the need for valve

TABLE 5. **Complications of Infective Endocarditis**

Local valvular destruction, which often accounts for congestive heart failure
    Aortic insufficiency
    Mitral regurgitation
    Tricuspid regurgitation (right-sided heart failure, particularly in the presence of pulmonary hypertension)
Perivalvular extension of infection, may be associated with
    Persistent, uncontrolled infection
    Valvular insufficiency
    Cardiac conduction defects
    Left-to-right shunts
    Arrhythmias
Embolic phenomena
    Systemic: cerebrovascular accidents, splenic or renal infarcts, myocardial infarction, mesenteric/limb ischemia, or metastatic abscesses
    Pulmonary: cavitary lesions or pneumonia
Other
    Systemic sepsis (usually secondary to staphylococcal or gram-negative infections)
    Mycotic aneurysms
    Valve obstruction by vegetation (rare, but may occur with exuberant growth of large, bulky vegetations, particularly on prosthetic valves)

From Larsen G, Greenberg B: Infective endocarditis. *In* Rakel RE (ed): Conn's Current Therapy 1988. Philadelphia, WB Saunders, 1988.

replacement. If, however, there is a failure of medical therapy for CHF or initial catheterization reveals severe elevation in the PCWP, urgent surgical evaluation should be planned with concomitant aggressive treatment of CHF. Failure to proceed with surgical therapy within 24 to 48 hours after the diagnosis of severe unresponsive heart failure usually results in cardiogenic shock and death.

Right-sided endocarditis differs in that the effects of tricuspid valvular regurgitation with right ventricular volume overload can often be controlled with diuretic therapy. However, if right-sided heart failure becomes intractable, a number of surgical procedures may be considered. These include replacement with a prosthetic valve and valvuloplasty. Since most cases of right-sided IE are found in intravenous drug users, there are significant implications when considering the placement of prosthetic valves in these patients. Unfortunately, a large percentage of these individuals continue to use intravenous drugs and therefore put themselves at significant risk for PVE, which carries a higher mortality and almost always requires surgical intervention. This has led several groups to consider valvuloplasty as a possible alternative. Initial reports have been encouraging; however, these were at fairly specialized centers and therefore their wider application must await larger clinical experience.

The incidence of perivalvular extension of infection (PVEI) varies considerably depending on the series that is studied. The incidence among NVE patients is in the order of 10%, and the incidence among PVE patients is approximately 50 to 60%. Aortic valve infections are the most common source of PVEI. Typically, PVEI comes to the attention of the clinician as persistent bacteremia despite adequate antibiotic therapy, or as worsening CHF. In both these situations TTE and TEE become invaluable for appropriate management. The manifestations of PVEI may reflect both its extent and its location. PVEI secondary to prosthetic valve endocarditis may result in paravalvular regurgitation as well as valve dehiscence. From 5 to 10% of patients may develop arrhythmias and heart block as a result of PVEI, and therefore the ECG remains a valuable although somewhat insensitive tool for diagnosis. Occasionally, infection may spread outside into the pericardium, resulting in purulent pericarditis, which requires prompt surgical drainage. Infection may also involve the papillary muscles, causing disruption of the subvalvular apparatus and resulting in mitral regurgitation. Destruction of intracardiac septae may result in shunt formation with consequent volume overload. All these conditions may be associated with myocardial abscess formation. Usually surgery is indicated; however, with the increasing use of TEE earlier in the course of IE, smaller myocardial abscesses are likely to be detected and may not necessarily require immediate surgical intervention.

Clinically evident embolic phenomena occur in 22 to 43% of patients with IE. There are also likely to be a large number of clinically silent events, particu-

TABLE 6. **Indications for Surgery in Infective Endocarditis**

Generally Accepted Indications
Congestive heart failure refractory to routine management
Uncontrolled infection despite appropriate antimicrobial
  therapy
Fungal endocarditis
Suppurative pericarditis
Unstable prosthetic valve
Recurrent disabling systemic emboli after 1–2 weeks of
  adequate antimicrobial therapy
Mycotic aneurysms

Relative Indications
Infection with gram-negative organism
Staphylococcus aureus infection of left-sided valve (particularly
  aortic)
Recurrent relapse after apparent cure
Evidence of perivalvular extension of infection
Rupture of sinus of Valsalva or of ventricular septum
Early prosthetic valve endocarditis
New periprosthetic leak
Metastatic abscesses not responding to antimicrobial therapy

From Larsen G, Greenberg B: Infective endocarditis. *In* Rakel RE (ed): Conn's Current Therapy 1988. Philadelphia, WB Saunders, 1988.

larly to the spleen or kidney. They may also present dramatically with an acute arterial occlusion in the limb or mesentery. Rarely, vegetations may embolize to the coronary arteries, resulting in myocardial infarction. However, cerebral emboli remain the most profound embolic complication because of their potential for death and long-term disability. The embolic risks appear to be related to the size of the vegetation, the duration of antimicrobial therapy, and the type of organism. Despite the advances in echocardiographic technique, valvular surgery cannot be recommended strictly on the basis of vegetation size. If, however, there are recurrent embolic events despite adequate antimicrobial therapy, especially in the presence of organisms such as group B streptococci, nutritionally variant streptococci, HACEK organisms, or fungi, a stronger consideration could be given for surgical intervention. Currently the most effective treatment for reduction of embolic risk is prompt antimicrobial therapy, which results in a significant reduction in embolic rates in the second and third week of treatment.

Septic embolization can result in metastatic abscesses and also mycotic aneurysms. Metastatic abscesses are most often caused by *Staph. aureus* and in general require surgical drainage. There are, however, clinical situations in which they may resolve with antibiotic therapy, in particular septic emboli to the lung from right-sided IE. Mycotic aneurysms are caused by weakening of the vascular wall as a result of local endovascular bacterial seeding. They can occur in any vascular structure and in most cases result in catastrophic hemorrhage. They are relatively rare complications and are usually diagnosed by their pressure effects. Cerebral mycotic aneurysms typically present with unremitting headache and homonymous hemianopsia, and this symptom complex should alert the physician to the possibility of a

serious intracranial complication. In general, if mycotic aneurysms are detected, the therapy of choice is surgical excision.

Systemic complications include systemic inflammatory response syndrome (SIRS), particularly with *Staph. aureus* and aerobic gram-negative infections. These complications may not reverse immediately with prompt antibiotic therapy and may therefore require supportive care in an intensive care setting. In addition, meningitis and encephalopathy may result secondary to the bacteremia and systemic sepsis.

Intractable infection may occur in the setting of fungal, gram-negative, or staphylococcal infection of prosthetic valves. Consequently these infections are associated with a greater incidence of complications including valve dysfunction and PVEI. In addition native valve infections due to aminoglycoside-resistant enterococcus and *P. aeruginosa* have a very poor response to antimicrobial therapy, and therefore early valve replacement may be the only viable option.

In general most IE relapses occur between 4 and 8 weeks of stopping antimicrobial therapy. Though there are no clear guidelines, most authorities agree that IE relapse caused by antibiotic-sensitive viridans streptococci and enterococci can be successfully treated with a repeat course of antibiotics. In cases of recurrent relapses and in first-time infections involving Q-fever or other resistant organisms, cardiac valve replacement is the appropriate approach.

A summary of the absolute and relative indications for surgery are listed in Table 6. However, the decision to proceed to surgical intervention and valve replacement must be made carefully after assessing all the available clinical, laboratory, echocardiographic, and hemodyamic information.

TABLE 7. **Cardiac Conditions**

Endocarditis Prophylaxis Recommended
Prosthetic cardiac valves, including bioprosthetic and
  homograft valves
Previous bacterial endocarditis, even in absence of heart
  disease
Most congenital cardiac malformations
Rheumatic and other acquired valvular dysfunction, even after
  valvular surgery
Hypertrophic cardiomyopathy
Mitral valve prolapse with valvular regurgitation

Endocarditis Prophylaxis Not Recommended
Isolated secundum atrial septal defect
Surgical repair without residua beyond 6 months of secundum
  atrial defect, ventricular septal defect, or patent ductus
  arteriosus
Previous coronary artery bypass graft surgery
Mitral valve prolapse without valvular regurgitation*
Physiologic, functional, or innocent heart murmurs
Previous Kawasaki disease without valvular dysfunction
Previous rheumatic fever without valvular dysfunction
Cardiac pacemakers and implanted defibrillators

*Individuals who have mitral valve prolapse associated with thickening and/or redundancy of the valve leaflets may be at increased risk for bacterial endocarditis, particularly men 45 years of age or older.
From Dajani AS, Bisno AL, Chung KJ, et al: Prevention of bacterial endocarditis. Recommendations by the American Heart Association. JAMA *264*:2919–2922, 1990. Copyright 1990, American Medical Association.

TABLE 8. **Endocarditis Prophylaxis**

Procedures for Which Endocarditis Prophylaxis Is Recommended

Dental Procedures
　Dental extraction
　Professional dental cleaning
　Periodontal surgery
Oropharyngeal and Respiratory Tract Procedures
　Tonsillectomy
　Adenoidectomy
　Surgical procedures involving respiratory mucosa
　Bronchoscopy with a rigid bronchoscope
Genitourinary Procedures
　Cystoscopy
　Prostatic surgery
　Urethral dilation
　Urethral catheterization if urinary tract infection is present*
　Urinary tract surgery if urinary tract infection is present*
Gastrointestinal Procedures
　Gallbladder surgery
　Esophageal dilation
　Sclerotherapy for esophageal varices
　Intestinal surgery
Gynecologic and Obstetric Procedures
　Vaginal hysterectomy
　Vaginal delivery in the presence of infection*
Incision and Drainage of Infected Tissue

Procedures for Which Endocarditis Prophylaxis Is Not Recommended†

Dental or Oral Procedures
　Filling of cavities above the gum line
　Simple adjustment of orthodontic appliances
　Shedding of primary teeth
　Injection of local intraoral anesthetic (except intraligamentary injections)
Lower Respiratory Tract Procedures‡
　Endotracheal intubation
　Bronchoscopy with a flexible bronchoscope, with or without biopsy
Genitourinary Procedures‡
　Gastrointestinal endoscopy with or without biopsy
Gynecologic and Obstetric Procedures (in the absence of infection)‡
　Cesarean section
　Uncomplicated vaginal delivery
　Dilation and curettage
　Therapeutic abortion
　Sterilization procedures
　Insertion or removal of intrauterine devices
Cardiac Catheterization

---

　*In addition to prophylaxis for genitourinary procedures, antibiotic therapy should be directed against the most likely pathogen.
　†Not intended to be all-inclusive.
　‡In patients who have prosthetic heart valves, a previous history of endocarditis, or surgically constructed systemic-pulmonary shunts or conduits, physicians may choose to administer prophylactic antibiotics.
　From Dajani AS, Bisno AL, Chung KJ, et al: Prevention of bacterial endocarditis. Recommendations by the American Heart Association. JAMA *264:*2919–2922, 1990. Copyright 1990, American Medical Association.

PREVENTION

　Despite the lack of data from controlled trials, there does seem to be a strong association between medical and surgical instrumentation and IE in individuals with underlying structural heart disease. Antibiotic prophylaxis has assumed an important role in the prevention of IE in such individuals. These guidelines were last revised by the American Heart Association (AHA) in 1990 and are summarized in Tables 7, 8, and 9. They represent an attempt to simplify the antibiotic regimen previously used before dental procedures. Specifically, patients with prosthetic valves no longer require parenteral prophylaxis. It is important to remember that general measures are also important. These include the maintenance of excellent oral hygiene and also the use of chlorhexidine (Peridex) mouthwash before dental procedures. These general measures can significantly decrease the amount of subsequent bacteremia. As a corollary to these preventive measures, there is a need to improve awareness among physicians, dentists, and patients regarding the need for

TABLE 9. **Recommended Regimens for Various Procedures**

Recommended Prophylactic Regimen for Dental, Oral, or Upper Respiratory Tract Procedures in Patients Who Are at Risk

Standard Regimen

PATIENTS NOT ALLERGIC TO PENICILLINS
　Amoxicillin 3.0 g PO 1 h before procedure, then 1.5 g 6 h after initial dose
PENICILLIN-ALLERGIC PATIENTS
　Erythromycin ethylsuccinate 800 mg or *erythromycin stearate* 1.0 g PO 2 h before procedure, then half the dose 6 h after initial dose
or
　Clindamycin 300 mg PO 1 h before procedure, then 150 mg 6 h after initial dose
Parenteral Regimen for Patients Unable to Take Oral Medications
PATIENTS NOT ALLERGIC TO PENICILLINS
　Ampicillin 2.0 g IV or IM 30 min before procedure, followed by ampicillin, 1.0 g IV or IM, or amoxicillin 1.5 g PO, 6 h after initial dose
PENICILLIN-ALLERGIC PATIENTS
　Clindamycin 300 mg IV 30 min before procedure, followed by 150 mg IV or PO 6 h after initial dose

Regimens for Genitourinary or Gastrointestinal Procedures

Standard Regimen

PATIENTS NOT ALLERGIC TO PENICILLIN
　Ampicillin 2 g IM or IV plus *gentamicin* 1.5 mg/kg (not to exceed 80 mg) IM or IV 30 min before procedure; followed by *amoxicillin* 1.5 g orally 6 h after initial dose; alternatively, parenteral regimen may be repeated once, 8 h after initial dose
PENICILLIN-ALLERGIC PATIENTS
　Vancomycin 1.0 g IV slowly over 1 h plus *gentamicin* 1.5 mg/kg (not to exceed 80 mg) IM or IV, 1 h before procedure, may be repeated once, 8 h after initial dose
Alternate Low-Risk Patient Regimen
　Amoxicillin 3.0 g orally 1 h before procedure; then 1.5 g 6 h after initial dose

Pediatric Doses
　Initial pediatric doses are as follows: amoxicillin, 50 mg/kg; erythromycin ethylsuccinate or erythromycin stearate, 20 mg/kg; clindamycin, 10 mg/kg; gentamicin 2 mg/kg; and vancomycin 20 mg/kg. Follow-up doses should be half the initial dose. *Total pediatric dose should not exceed total adult dose.* Following weight ranges also may be used for initial pediatric dose of amoxicillin; <15 kg, 750 mg; 15–30 kg, 1500 mg; and >30 kg, 3000 mg (full adult dose).

　From Dajani AS, Bisno AL, Chung KJ, et al: Prevention of bacterial endocarditis. Recommendations by the American Heart Association. JAMA *264:*2919–2922, 1990. Copyright 1990, American Medical Association.

antibiotic prophylaxis and the maintenance of good oral health. The AHA has IE-prevention patient cards that can alert both physicians and dentists to the need for antimicrobial prophylaxis. Using this type of system can significantly improve patient and doctor compliance with the AHA guidelines.

HYPERTENSION

method of
MARK C. HOUSTON, M.D.
Vanderbilt University Medical Center
Nashville, Tennessee

The primary short- and long-term goal in the management of essential hypertension should be the reduction of target organ damage. This includes cerebrovascular, cardiac, cardiovascular, and renal effects, the predominant events leading to the excess morbidity and mortality in hypertensive patients (Table 1). The preoccupation to reduce blood pressure (BP) *only* and ignore the metabolic, biochemical, and structural issues inherent in the hypertensive patient is to pursue a misguided approach.

Essential hypertension is a *syndrome* of metabolic and structural abnormalities, both genetic and acquired, that includes at least the following:

1. Elevated BP
2. Dyslipidemia
3. Insulin resistance and/or hyperinsulinemia
4. Carbohydrate intolerance
5. Central obesity
6. Structural abnormalities of cardiac and vascular smooth muscle (hypertrophy, hyperplasia, and abnormal vascular remodeling)
7. Membranopathy or abnormal cation transport

TABLE 1. Hypertension-Related End-Organ Damage

Cerebrovascular: cerebrovascular accidents
  Cerebral infarctions: thrombotic or lacunar infarcts
  Intracranial hemorrhage: hemorrhagic cerebrovascular
    accidents
  Hypertensive encephalopathy
Cardiac
  Coronary heart disease
    Angina pectoris
    Myocardial infarction
Congestive heart failure
  Systolic congestive heart failure
  Diastolic congestive heart failure (diastolic failure and
    dysfunction)
  Left ventricular hypertrophy
  Sudden death
Renal
  Chronic renal insufficiency
  Chronic renal failure
Large artery disease
  Carotid artery stenosis and obstruction
  Lower extremity arterial disease or peripheral vascular disease
    and claudication
  Aortic aneurysms and dissections
Progression of hypertension: accelerated and malignant
  hypertension
Retinopathy

TABLE 2. Treatment of Hypertension: Risks Versus Benefits

Pharmacologic treatment of mild to moderate hypertension (DBP $\leq$ 110 mmHg) has reduced only some of end-organ damage
Blood pressure reduction has reduced consequences of pressure-related arteriolar disease:
  Intracranial hemorrhage
  Congestive heart failure (CHF), systolic CHF
  Progression of hypertension: accelerated and malignant
  Retinopathy
  Aortic aneurysms and dissection
  Hypertensive encephalopathy
Blood pressure reduction has not achieved expected reduction in
  Cerebral infarction
  Left ventricular hypertrophy
  Diastolic CHF
  Renal insufficiency and failure
Blood pressure reduction has not reduced consequences of
  atherosclerotic-related diseases:
  Coronary heart disease
  Angina pectoris
  Myocardial infarction
  Sudden death
  Large artery disease: carotid lower extremities

Abbreviation: DBP = diastolic blood pressure.

This constellation of abnormalities results in accelerated vascular disease. Antihypertensive therapy must be directed toward correction of *all* the components of this syndrome in order to achieve an optimal decrease in target organ damage.

The pharmacologic treatment of diastolic BP (DBP) $\leq$110 mmHg has reduced cerebrovascular accidents (CVAs) and systolic congestive heart failure (CHF), but the reduction in coronary heart disease (CHD), angina, and myocardial infarction (MI) has been less than predicted and somewhat disappointing. Recently, studies have even suggested that traditional antihypertensive therapy does not prevent many cases of hypertention-related renal insufficiency despite BP control (Table 2). Obviously we have learned much but have much more to learn about the best methods to treat the hypertensive patient. Effective lifestyle modifications (nonpharmacologic therapy) and numerous antihypertensive drugs are presently available. A logical approach to the selection of these treatment modalities must be based on a comprehensive understanding of the hypertension syndrome and the effects of the treatment not only on BP but on the numerous other components that coexist. This is the challenge.

INCIDENCE AND PREVALENCE

Approximately 50 million adults in the United States (one in four) have hypertension (BP $\geq$ 140/90 mmHg) according to the National Health and Nutrition Examination Survey (NHANES III, 1988–1991). Hypertension remains the most frequent medical problem seen by physicians in the United States. Black, male, and elderly persons have the greatest incidence. Blacks have the highest morbidity and mortality compared with whites at equivalent BP levels. Most of the excess mortality occurs in patients with DBP $\leq$ 105 mmHg (60% of hypertensive-related deaths). In the United States, BP tends to increase with age: the average life expectancy of a 35-year-old white man with a blood pressure of 120/80 mmHg is 74 years, but at a BP of 150/100 mmHg, the life expectancy falls to 55 years.

CLASSIFICATION

The fifth report of the Joint National Committee on the Detection, Evaluation and Treatment of Hypertension (JNC-V) published in 1993 has established a new classification of BP based on both systolic BP (SBP) and DBP (Table 3). This classification recognizes the importance of SBPs having a greater risk for CVA and CHD than DBP. Although this classification is better than previous ones, it is important to remember that coexisting risk factors or diseases (hyperlipidemia, smoking, diabetes mellitus, CHF, CHD, left ventricular hypertrophy [LVH], etc.) compound the morbidity and mortality for all target organ events.

DETECTION AND EVALUATION

Accurate measurement of BP is obviously the most important initial step in the evaluation of the hypertensive patient (Table 4). Repeated BP measurements on several visits days to weeks apart should be done before making a diagnosis of sustained hypertension, unless the level of BP requires more immediate attention (i.e., ≥210/115 mmHg and/or target organ damage exists). Home BP measurements and 24-hour ambulatory BP monitors (ABPM) may provide more accurate BP measurements and correlate better with target organ damage than casual in-office BP readings. It is estimated that 25 to 30% of patients exhibit "white coat hypertension" in the physician's office and their BP is normal when measured by these other means. In addition, the white coat hypertensive patient is more often female, elderly, or overweight and has lower cardiovascular risk, a lower incidence of LVH, and fewer metabolic disturbances (carbohydrate intolerance, hyperinsulinemia, hyperlipidemia) compared with the chronically hypertensive patient.

Evaluation of a patient with confirmed hypertension should include assessment of these questions:

1. Is the hypertension primary (essential) or secondary (reversible)?
2. Does target organ damage exist?
3. What coexisting diseases and risk factors are present?
4. What is the most appropriate classification of the patient's hypertension and the urgency to treat based on the BP level and the above considerations?

A complete medical history should be obtained with a family history and patient history including symptoms of hypertension and cardiovascular, cerebrovascular, and renal disease as well as risk factors such as dyslipidemia and diabetes mellitus. Questions regarding tobacco, alcohol, prescription and over-the-counter (OTC) drug use, ex-

TABLE 4. Indirect Measurement of Blood Pressure

Equipment
Sphygmomanometer (aneroid or mercury manometer)
Methodology
1. Patient is seated with back supported for 5 min in quiet, comfortable environment, with arm free of restrictive clothing or other materials and supported at heart level. Patient should avoid exertion, temperature extremes, caffeine, eating, or smoking for 30 min before measurement.
2. Observer (clinician) is at eye level of meniscus of mercury column or centered in front of gauge; avoiding strained posture.
3. Appropriate cuff size is selected. Cuff bladder should be 20% wider than diameter of extremity. Bladder length should be approximately twice recommended width.
4. Deflated cuff is placed at least 2.5 cm above antecubital space. Cuff should fit smoothly and snugly around arm, with bladder centered directly over brachial artery.
5. Clinician palpates for brachial pulse. To estimate systolic blood pressure (SBP), cuff is rapidly inflated until brachial pulse can no longer be felt.
6. Bell of stethoscope is placed over previously palpated brachial artery. Cuff is rapidly deflated to 30 mmHg above point at which radial pulse disappears; cuff is deflated at rate of 2–3 mmHg/s.
7. SBP is recorded as first Korotkoff sound and diastolic blood pressure (DBP) as fifth Korotkoff sound.
8. Two minutes are allowed between blood pressure determinations.
9. Blood pressure is determined with patient in upright posture after patient has been standing for 2 min. Arm is positioned at heart level, with forearm at horizontal level of fourth intercostal space.
10. On initial visit, BP readings are performed in both arms. Subsequent BP determinations are performed in arm with higher reading if there is more than 10-mmHg discrepancy in BP reading. A leg BP should be measured at least once.

ercise, weight changes, dietary habits, stress, and symptoms of secondary hypertension are all important.

The physical examination should be directed at signs of target organ damage, coexisting diseases, and potential secondary causes of hypertension. This should include at least a funduscopic examination; evaluation of all pulses and the presence of bruits over all arteries and the abdomen; a cardiac examination; and neurologic assessment.

Selected and specific laboratory tests help identify target organ damage, coexisting diseases, and risk factors and clues to secondary causes of hypertension, if present. These should include a fresh urinalysis, possibly measuring microalbumin levels; a complete blood cell count; a fasting glucose and lipid profile; renal function tests; measurements of electrolyte, uric acid, and calcium levels; an electrocardiogram; and possibly a limited echocardiogram to detect LVH and diastolic dysfunction. Additional testing may be appropriate if secondary causes of hypertension are suspected, including 24-hour urine studies; measurements of plasma cortisol levels; and renal artery Doppler and radionucleotide renal scans.

TREATMENT: LIFESTYLE MODIFICATIONS, OR NONPHARMACOLOGIC THERAPY

The treatment of hypertension should be effective and safe, have minimal side effects, and if possible improve coexisting risk factors or diseases. Many

TABLE 3. Classification of Blood Pressure for Adults Aged 18 Years and Older

Category	Systolic (mmHg)	Diastolic (mmHg)
Normal	<130	<85
High normal	130–139	85–89
Hypertension		
Stage I (mild)	140–159	90–99
Stage II (moderate)	160–179	100–109
Stage III (severe)	180–209	110–119
Stage IV (very severe)	≥210	≥120

From National Heart, Lung, and Blood Institute I, Publication No 93–1088, US Department of Health and Human Services, January, 1993.

TABLE 5. **Lifestyle Modifications: Nonpharmacologic Treatment of Hypertension**

Weight reduction to ideal body weight
Tobacco and smoking cessation
Caffeine cessation or restriction
Alcohol reduction
Aerobic exercise implementation (avoidance of isometric exercise)
Behavior modification—relaxation and biofeedback
Drug interactions—avoidance of the following:
    Oral contraceptives
    Nonsteroidal anti-inflammatory drugs
    Sympathomimetics (decongestants, diet pills)
    Steroids
Sodium restriction
Potassium supplementation
Polyunsatured/saturated fat ratio increase
Calcium supplementation
Magnesium supplementation
Carbohydrate restriction
Crude fiber consumption increase
Dietary amino acids consumption (leucine)
Trace mineral consumption
Omega-3 fatty acid consumption (fish oil supplement)
Garlic consumption

hypertensive patients with Stage I and II hypertension can be treated with lifestyle modifications or nonpharmacologic therapy (Table 5). A number of studies, including the NHANES III, INTERSALT, Therapy of Hypertension Program (TOHP), Trial of Antihypertensive Intervention and Management (TAIM), Therapy of Mild Hypertension Study (TOMHS), Multiple Risk Factor Intervention Trial (MRFIT), and Hypertension Control Program (HCP), have demonstrated the antihypertensive efficacy of many of the items listed in Table 5 as sole and as adjunctive therapy to antihypertensive drugs.

Weight Reduction. Weight reduction has consistently been the most effective method of reducing BP (TOMHS, TOHP, INTERSALT). Central obesity has the strongest correlation with BP. Those with elevated plasma renin activity (PRA) have the greatest reduction in BP with weight loss. A waist/hip ratio (truncal or abdominal obesity) above 0.85 in women and 0.95 in men is correlated with dyslipidemia, diabetes, insulin resistance, increased CHD, and hypertension.

Tobacco and Smoking Cessation. Although tobacco use may not increase BP, it is a risk factor for CVA and CHD and should be stopped. Nicotine gum, patches, clonidine, and smoking cessation programs can be effective means of discontinuing tobacco use.

Caffeine Restriction and Cessation. Although the role of caffeine in hypertension is controversial and perhaps minor, there are some patients in whom restriction or discontinuation of caffeine may lower BP. It is, therefore, reasonable to limit caffeine use even though tolerance to its effects is common.

Alcohol Reduction. Excessive alcohol use can elevate BP and reduce the effectiveness of antihypertensive drug therapy through its vasoconstrictive effects. Alcohol should be limited to 1 ounce of ethanol per day or less.

Aerobic Exercise. Regular aerobic exercise (three times per week or more) at a level of 80% of maximal aerobic capacity (80% of maximal heart rate for age) reduces BP an average of 10 to 15 mmHg systolic and 5 to 10 mmHg diastolic. Isometric exercise (weight lifting), however, may acutely and chronically elevate BP and should be used with caution or avoided.

Behavior Modification. Stress and anxiety can contribute to BP elevation, but relaxation techniques have not been demonstrated to have a significant effect on BP in short- or long-term controlled clinical trials.

Drug Interactions. Many prescription and OTC drugs may induce hypertension directly or interfere with antihypertensive drug therapy. Nonsteroidal anti-inflammatory drugs (NSAIDs) may counterbalance the antihypertensive effects of diuretics, beta blockers, and angiotensin-converting enzyme inhibitors (ACEIs). Oral contraceptives, sympathomimetics, and steroids may also exacerbate hypertension.

Sodium Restriction. Many epidemiologic and clinical studies have demonstrated that a reduction in sodium chloride intake lowers BP and is a useful adjunct to most antihypertensive medications. In TAIM, sodium restriction to below 70 mEq per day significantly lowered BP, especially when combined with high potassium and reduced caloric intake. Similar BP reductions of 5 to 7 mm Hg systolic and 2 to 3 mm Hg diastolic have been documented in NHANES III, TOMHS, INTERSALT, and others. Patients with high-volume low-renin hypertension, blacks, and the elderly have the most dramatic BP reduction with sodium chloride restriction. Sodium should be reduced to 2 to 3 grams per day.

Potassium Supplementation. High potassium intake of 100 to 150 mEq per day lowers BP, reduces the risk of CVAs, and may provide vascular protection. Hypokalemia may predispose to cardiac arrhythmias, especially ventricular ectopy.

Other. Magnesium supplements, crude fiber, micronutrients, calcium, and fish oil may be effective, but their use is controversial. In recent studies garlic intake produces consistent reductions in BP. Low-fat diets are important to reduce CHD risk and may lower BP.

If the hypertensive patient is compliant with these various lifestyle modifications for 4 to 6 months and BP remains elevated, then antihypertensive drug therapy should be started.

PHARMACOLOGIC THERAPY

Numerous effective antihypertensive drugs are available, but the appropriate selection of a drug for an individual patient may present a dilemma. The most logical approach is individualized therapy, or the *subsets of hypertension approach*. This approach is based on the following parameters:

1. Pathophysiology
   a) Membranopathy, ion transport defects
   b) Structural abnormalities of cardiac and vascular smooth muscle
   c) Functional abnormalities

TABLE 6. **Hemodynamics: Logical and Preferred Method to Reduce Blood Pressure**

Reduce systemic vascular resistance (SVR)
Preserve cardiac output (CO)
Improve arterial compliance
Maintain organ perfusion
Achieve all the above by
  avoiding compensatory neurohumoral reflexes such as reflux tachycardia, salt and water overload, and reflex vasoconstrictors (norepinephrine, angiotensin II, antidiuretic hormone)
  controlling 24-h blood pressure
  controlling blood pressure with all activities: rest, exercise, stress, mental function, and diurnal variation

2. Hemodynamics
   a) Systemic vascular resistance (SVR)
   b) Cardiac output (CO)
   c) Arterial compliance (AC)
   d) Organ perfusion
   e) SBP, DBP, mean arterial pressure (MAP)
3. Target organ damage and risk factor reduction
4. Concomitant medical diseases or problems
5. Demographics based on race, gender, and age
6. Quality of life and adverse effects of treatment
7. Compliance with treatment
8. Total health care cost (direct and indirect)

These parameters allow for an approach that is

TABLE 7. **Antihypertensive Drugs: Hemodynamic Effects**

Reduce SVR + preserve CO + improve arterial compliance and perfusion.
  Calcium channel blockers
  Angiotensin-converting enzyme inhibitors
Reduce SVR + preserve CO + improve perfusion. Effects on arterial compliance unknown.
  Central alpha agonists
  Alpha blocker
Reduce SVR + preserve CO and perfusion, but worsen arterial compliance.
  Direct vasodilators
  Beta blockers with ISA
  Alpha-beta blocker combination
Reduce SVR + reduce CO, perfusion, and arterial compliance.
  Diuretics
  Neuronal inhibiting drugs
Increase SVR + reduce CO, perfusion, and arterial compliance.
  Beta blockers without ISA

Abbreviations: SVR = systemic vascular resistance; CO = cardiac output; ISA = intrinsic sympathomimetic activity.

logical, rational, and simple to use and avoids the cookbook treatment to every hypertensive patient. Generalizations that suggest that initial drug therapy should always be the same and prescribed in a stepwise fashion ignore many basic and newer concepts in the management of hypertension. JNC-V continues to emphasize diuretics and beta blockers as primary antihypertensive drugs despite their neg-

TABLE 8. **Effects of Antihypertensive Drugs on Coronary Heart Disease Risk Factors**

Risk Factors	Diuretics	Indapamide (Lozol)	Beta Blockers without ISA	Beta Blockers with ISA	Labetalol (Normodyne, Trandate)	Guanethidine (Ismelin) Guanadrel (Hylorel)
Hypertension	Reduced	Reduced	Reduced	Reduced	Decreased	Decreased
Dyslipidemia	Increased	Neutral	Increased	No change	No change	No change
Glucose intolerance	Increased	Neutral or Increased	Increased	Increased	Increased	No change
Insulin resistance	Increased	No change	Increased	Increased	Unknown	Unknown
Left ventricular hypertrophy	No change or Increased	Reduced	No change	Increased	Decreased	Decreased
Exercise	No change or Decreased	No change	Decreased	Decreased	No change or Decreased	Decreased
Potassium level	Decreased	Decreased	No change or Increased	No change	No change	No change
Magnesium level	Decreased	Decreased	No change	No change	No change	No change
Uric acid level	Increased	Increased	Increased	Increased	Increased	No change
Blood viscosity	Increased	No change	No change	No change	No change	No change
Blood velocity	No change or Increased	No change	Decreased	No change	No change	No change
Catecholamine levels	Increased	Decreased	Increased	Increased	No change	Decreased
Angiotensin II level	Increased	No change or Decreased	Decreased	No change	Decreased	Increased
Arrhythmia potential	Increased	No change	Decreased	No change or Increased	No change	Increased
Fibrinogen level	Increased	No change	Unknown	Unknown	Unknown	Unknown
Platelet function	Increased	Decreased	No change or Decreased	Unknown	Unknown	Unknown
Thombogenic potential	Increased	Decreased	Unknown	Unknown	Unknown	Unknown
Antiatherogenic potential	No	Neutral	Yes (animal studies)	Unknown	Unknown	Yes
CHD relative risk ratio Unfavorable Total	$\frac{16}{18}$	$\frac{3-4}{18}$	$\frac{6}{18}$	$\frac{7}{18}$	$\frac{3}{18}$	$\frac{3}{18}$

Abbreviation: ISA = intrinsic sympathomimetic activity; CHD = coronary heart disease; ACE = angiotensin-converting enzyme.

ative impact on many of the parameters mentioned in the subsets of hypertension approach.

Pathophysiology

Essential hypertension is a genetic disorder that comprises abnormalities in membrane ion transport (Na^+, K^+, Ca^{2+}, Mg^{2+}), metabolic and biochemical function, and trophic and structural changes in vascular and cardiac smooth muscle. The calcium channel blockers (CCBs) and ACEIs, in particular, as well as the central alpha agonists (CAAs) and alpha blockers (ABs) correct many of these metabolic and structural abnormalities. However, beta blockers (BBs), diuretics, and vasodilators may worsen many of these factors.

Hemodynamics

BP is elevated in essential hypertensive patients because of an elevated SVR, not an elevated CO. Arterial compliance is also decreased, and organ perfusion may be compromised. Drug therapy should decrease the SVR, maintain or improve the CO and perfusion, and increase the AC (Table 6). The CCBs, ACEIs, CAAs, and ABs achieve these hemodynamic goals better than diuretics and BBs. Table 7 divides the drugs into five classes based on hemodynamic profiles.

Target Organ Damage and Risk Factor Reduction

All modifiable risk factors should be reduced in order to achieve an optimal decrease in target organ damage such as CHD, CVA, and renal insufficiency. There are 18 CHD risk factors that can be altered by antihypertensive therapy. Diuretics induce 16 adverse effects, and BBs with or without intrinsic sympathomimetic activity (ISA) induce six or seven adverse effects, whereas CCBs, ACEIs, CAAs, and ABs have *no* adverse effects on CHD risk factors (Table 8).

Concomitant Medical Diseases or Problems

Antihypertensive drugs should reduce BP effectively without producing adverse effects on coexisting medical diseases or problems such as diabetes mellitus, dyslipidemia, angina, renal insufficiency, etc. The drugs of choice, alternatives, and those which are contraindicated for various diseases that occur with hypertension are listed in Table 9. Specific selected examples are discussed below.

TABLE 8. **Effects of Antihypertensive Drugs on Coronary Heart Disease Risk Factors** *Continued*

Central Alpha Agonists	Methyldopa	Direct Vasodilators	Alpha Blockers	ACE Inhibitors	Calcium Channel Blockers	Reserpine
Decreased	Decreased	Decreased	Decreased	Decreased	Decreased	Decreased
Decreased	Increased	No change	Decreased	No change	Decreased	Increased
No change	No change	No change	Decreased	Decreased	No change	No change
No change	No change	No change	Decreased	Decreased	No change or Decreased	Unknown
Decreased	Decreased	Increased	Decreased	Decreased	Decreased	Decreased
No change	No change	No change	No change	No change	No change	Decreased
No change	No change	No change	No change	Increased	No change	No change
No change	No change	No change	No change	No change or Increased	No change	No change
No change or Decreased	No change or Decreased	No change	No change	Decreased	No change or Decreased	No change
No change	No change	Decreased	Decreased	No change	Unknown	Unknown
Decreased	Increased	Increased	Decreased	Decreased	Decreased	Decreased
Decreased	Decreased	Increased	No change or Decreased	Decreased	Decreased	Decreased
Decreased	Decreased	Increased	No change	Decreased	Decreased	Decreased
Decreased	Decreased	Increased	No change	Decreased	Decreased	Increased
Unknown	Unknown	Unknown	Unknown	Unknown	Unknown	Unknown
Decreased	No change	Unknown	Unknown	Decreased	Decreased	Unknown
Unknown	Unknown	Unknown	Unknown	Unknown	Decreased	Unknown
Unknown	Unknown	Unknown	Unknown	Yes but decreased (animals)	Yes but decreased (animals, humans)	Yes (animals)
$\frac{0}{18}$	$\frac{2}{18}$	$\frac{5}{18}$	$\frac{0}{18}$	$\frac{0}{18}$	$\frac{0}{18}$	$\frac{3}{18}$

TABLE 9. **Concomitant Diseases and Problems: Antihypertensive Drugs**

Concomitant Disease or Problems	Drug(s) of Choice	Alternatives	Relative or Absolute Contraindications
Diabetes mellitus	ACEI AB CAA CCB	BB with SA DV Indapamide (Lozol) Labetalol	BB without ISA Diuretic Methyldopa NI Reserpine
Dyslipidemia	AB CAA CCB	ACEI BB with ISA DV Indapamide Labetalol	BB without ISA Diuretic Methyldopa NI Reserpine
Hyperuricemia	ACEI AB CAA CCB	DV Labetalol NI Reserpine	BB without ISA BB with ISA Diuretic
Renal insufficiency	ACEI* AB CAA CCB	Diuretic⁺ DV Labetalol	BB without ISA BB with ISA NI Reserpine
Exercise	ACEI AB CAA CCB	BB with ISA Diuretic DV Labetalol Methyldopa	BB without ISA NI Reserpine
Congestive heart failure (systolic failure)	ACEI Amlodipine (Norvasc) Diuretic DV Isradipine (DynaCirc) Nicardipine (Cardene) Nifedipine	AB CAA Diltiazem	BB without ISA BB with ISA Labetalol NI Reserpine Verapamil
Diastolic dysfunction or failure	CCB	ACEI AB BB without ISA CAA Labetalol	BB with ISA Diuretic DV NI Reserpine
Left ventricular hypertrophy	ACEI AB CAA CCB Indapamide Labetalol	BB without ISA Reserpine	BB with ISA Diuretic DV NI
Angina Obstructive	BB without ISA CCB	ACEI AB CAA Diuretic Labetalol	BB with ISA DV NI Reserpine
Mixed	BB without ISA CCB	ACEI AB CAA Diuretic Labetalol	BB with ISA DV NI Reserpine
Vasospastic angina	CCB	ACEI AB CAA Diuretic	BB without ISA BB with ISA DV Labetalol NI Reserpine
Arrhythmias SVT	BB CAA Diltiazem Verapamil	ACEI AB Amlodipine Diuretic Felodipine (Plendil) Labetalol Nicardipine Nifedipine Reserpine	BB with ISA DV NI

TABLE 9. **Concomitant Diseases and Problems: Antihypertensive Drugs** *Continued*

Concomitant Disease or Problems	Drug(s) of Choice	Alternatives	Relative or Absolute Contraindications
PVCs	BB without ISA CCB	ACEI AB CAA Labetalol	BB with ISA Diuretic DV NI Reserpine
Chronic liver disease	AB CAA CCB	ACEI Diuretic DV Labetalol	BB Methyldopa NI Reserpine
Migraine headache (prophylaxis)	BB without ISA CAA CCB	AB ACEI BB with ISA Diuretic Labetalol	DV NI Reserpine
Cerebrovascular disease	ACEI CCB	AB CAA DV Labetalol	BB without ISA BB with ISA Diuretic NI Reserpine
Depression	ACEI AB CCB	CAA Diuretic DV	BB without ISA BB with ISA Labetalol Methyldopa NI Reserpine
Obstructive airway disease	AB CAA CCB	ACEI Diuretic DV	BB without ISA BB with ISA Labetalol NI Reserpine
Pregnancy (first and second trimester)	Hydralazine Methyldopa	AB (?)‡ CAA (?)‡ CCB (?)‡	ACEI BB without ISA BB with ISA Diuretic Labetalol NI Reserpine
Toxemia of pregnancy (eclampsia)	CAA CCB Hydralazine	AB (?)‡	BB without ISA BB with ISA Diuretic Labetalol NI Reserpine
Glaucoma	BB CAA Diuretic		
Sinusitis or rhinitis	CAA	ACEI AB CCB Diuretic DV	BB Labetalol NI Reserpine
Peripheral vascular disease	CCB	ACEI AB CAA Diuretic DV	BB without ISA BB with ISA Labetalol NI Reserpine
Microvascular angina	CCB	ACEI AB CAA	BB without ISA BB with ISA Diuretic DV Labetalol NI Reserpine

Table continued on following page

TABLE 9. **Concomitant Diseases and Problems: Antihypertensive Drugs** *Continued*

Concomitant Disease or Problems	Drug(s) of Choice	Alternatives	Relative or Absolute Contraindications
Young patient	ACEI AB CAA CCB	BB with ISA DV Labetalol	BB without ISA Diuretic NI Reserpine
Elderly patient	AB CAA CCB	ACEI BB without ISA BB with ISA Diuretic Labetalol	DV NI Reserpine
Black patient	AB CAA CCB	ACEI Diuretic ↔ DV	BB without ISA BB with ISA Diuretic Labetalol NI Reserpine
White patient	ACEI AB CAA CCB	DV Labetalol	BB without ISA BB with ISA NI Reserpine

Sick sinus syndrome or atrioventricular block	ACEI
	AB
		CCB
		  Amlodipine
		  Felodipine
		  Isradipine
		  Nifedipine
		  Nicardipine
		Diuretic
		DV
			BB without ISA
			BB with ISA
			CAA
			CCB
			  Verapamil
			  Diltiazem
			Labetalol
			NI
			Reserpine

Nonsteroidal anti-inflammatory drugs	CCB CAA	AB	ACEI BB with ISA BB without ISA Diuretic DV Labetalol NI Reserpine
Postmyocardial infarction Q wave	BB without ISA	ACEI CAA CCB Labetalol	BB with ISA Diuretic DV NI Reserpine

Non–Q wave	Diltiazem
	Verapamil
		ACEI
		AB
		BB without ISA
		CAA
		CCB
		  Amlodipine
		  Felodipine
		  Isradipine
		  Nifedipine
		  Nicardipine
		Labetalol
			BB with ISA
			Diuretic
			DV
			NI
			Reserpine

Essential tremor	CAA BB without ISA		
Anxiety or stress	CAA BB without ISA		
Raynaud's phenomenon	CCB	ACEI AB CAA DV NI Reserpine	BB without ISA BB with ISA Labetalol

TABLE 9. **Concomitant Diseases and Problems: Antihypertensive Drugs** *Continued*

Concomitant Disease or Problems	Drug(s) of Choice	Alternatives	Relative or Absolute Contraindications
Menopausal symptoms	CAA		DV
Peptic ulcer disease	CAA CCB	ACEI AB BB Diuretic DV Labetalol	NI Reserpine
Volume overload	ACEI CCB Diuretic	AB CAA Labetalol	BB DV NI Reserpine
Obesity	ACEI AB CAA	Diuretic DV	BB without ISA BB with ISA NI
Pulmonary hypertension	CCB DV	ACEI AB CAA Diuretic	BB
Sexual dysfunction	ACEI AB CCB	CAA DV	BB without ISA BB with ISA Diuretic Labetalol Methyldopa NI Reserpine
Mitral valve prolapse	BB without ISA CAA CCB	AB ACEI Labetalol	BB with ISA Diuretic DV NI Reserpine
Diabetic diarrhea and gustatory sweating	CAA		
Addictive syndromes: withdrawal from tobacco, alcohol, opiates, etc.	CAA		

*Caution in renal artery stenosis (bilateral).
†Caution (see text). Volume overload states.
‡Unconfirmed.
Abbreviations: ACEI = angiotensin-converting enzyme inhibitor; AB = alpha blocker; CAA = central alpha agonist; CCB = calcium channel blocker; BB = beta blocker; ISA = intrinsic sympathomimetic activity;DV = direct vasodilator; NI = neuronal inhibitor, SVT = supraventricular tachycardia; PVC = premature ventricular contraction.

Diabetes Mellitus. In a Joslin Clinic study, CHD and total mortality were increased two- to fourfold in diabetic hypertensive patients with or without proteinuria who were treated with diuretics compared with untreated hypertensive patients or those receiving alternative antihypertensive therapy (Figure 1). Diuretics should be avoided or used with extreme caution in diabetic hypertensive patients.

Renal Insufficiency. Hypertensive patients receiving diuretics and/or BBs have a 16 to 30% chance of developing progressive renal insufficiency despite normal BP. However, CCBs and ACEIs used as monotherapy or in combination preserve renal function better than diuretics or BBs at equal BP levels in hypertensive patients with or without renal insufficiency, and in normotensive or hypertensive diabetic patients with or without proteinuria. In the Melbourne Study, ACEIs and CCBs reduced BP and proteinuria and preserved renal function after 1 year of therapy. In an Italian study, nifedipine (Procardia) or captopril (Capoten) therapy resulted in similar BP control and renal function at the end of 3 years. ACEIs have consistently reduced proteinuria and stabilized renal function in these patients.

Cardiac Arrhythmias. A recent article in the *New England Journal of Medicine* has confirmed that there is a dose-related effect of thiazide diuretics on ventricular ectopy and sudden death by inducing hypokalemia and hypomagnesemia, and prolonging the QT interval on the electrocardiogram (ECG). Patients with diabetes mellitus, LVH, CHD, abnormal ECGs, and hypertension are at high risk of a cardiovascular event on higher-dose diuretics.

Coronary Heart Disease. Several human as well as animal studies have demonstrated an antiatherogenic effect of CCBs in the coronary circulation that

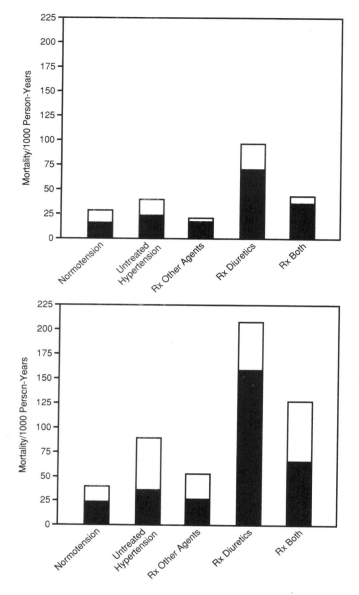

Figure 1. Mortality per 1000 person-years in diabetic patients without proteinuria (*top*) and with proteinuria (*bottom*) according to hypertension status and type of antihypertensive treatment (Rx) during each year of follow-up. *Shaded areas of bars* indicate cardiovascular mortality; *open areas*, other mortality. Mortality during diuretic treatment was significantly higher than with untreated hypertension (p < .025 for cardiovascular mortality; p < .025 for total mortality) with or without proteinuria. In patients with proteinuria, cardiovascular mortality during treatment with both diuretics and other agents was significantly lower than during treatment with diuretics alone (p < .025). Mortality was adjusted by the direct method (see Rothman KJ: Modern Epidemiology. Boston, Little, Brown & Co, 1986) to the age distribution of all patients receiving antihypertensive treatment. (From Warram JH, Laffel LMB, Valsania P, et al: Excess mortality associated with diuretic therapy in diabetes mellitus. Arch Intern Med 151:1350–1356, 1991. Copyright 1991, American Medical Association.)

is independent of BP control and traditional CHD risk factors. This may offer an additional means to prevent CHD.

Cerebrovascular Disease. Recent animal studies have suggested that CCBs and ACEIs have a cerebro-protective effect through neuroprotection and anti-ischemic effects that is independent of BP control. CCBs and ACEIs prevent CVA and improve neurologic symptoms after a CVA better than diuretics, BBs, and hydralazine (Apresoline).

TABLE 10. **Mean Costs Per Drug Per Cost Category for 1 Year of Use**

	Acquisition Cost ($)	Supplemental Drug Cost ($)	Laboratory Cost ($)	Clinic Visit Cost ($)	Side Effect Cost ($)	Total Cost ($)
Diuretics	133	232	117	298	263	1043
Beta bockers	334	115	56	187	203	895
Alpha₁ blockers	401	290	114	227	256	1288
Centrally acting alpha₂ agonists	285	295	125	267	193	1165
Angiotensin-converting enzyme inhibitors	444	291	95	218	195	1243
Calcium channel blockers	540	278	87	214	306	1425

Adapted from Hilleman DE, Mohiuddin SM, Lucas BD, Jr, et al: Cost-minimization analysis of initial antihypertensive therapy in patients with mild-to-moderate essential diastolic hypertension. Clin Ther 16:88–102, 1994.

TABLE 11. Maximal Recommended Doses of Antihypertensive Drugs with Best Treatment Characteristics*

Antihypertensive Drugs	Dose/Day (mg)
Calcium channel blockers	
Nifedipine (Procardia XL, Adalat CC)	120
Verapamil (Calan SR, Isoptin SR, Verelan)	360
Diltiazem (Cardizem CD)	360
Nicardipine (Cardene SR)	120
Isradipine (DynaCirc)	10
Amlodipine (Norvasc)	10
Felodipine (Plendil)	10
Angiotensin-converting enzyme inhibitors	
Captopril (Capoten)	50
Enalapril (Vasotec)	20
Lisinopril (Prinivil, Zestril)	20
Fosinopril (Monopril)	40
Ramipril (Altace)	20
Benazepril (Lotensin)	40
Quinapril (Accupril)	40
Central alpha-agonists	
Clonidine (Catapres and Catapres-TTS)	0.4 mg/TTS-3
Guanabenz (Wytensin)	16
Guanfacine (Tenex)	2
Alpha blockers	
Prazosin (Minipress)	10
Terazosin (Hytrin)	10
Doxazosin (Cardura)	10
Indapamide (Lozol)	2.5

*Doses represent approximately 80 to 90% of total antihypertensive effect achieved in most patients.
Abbreviations: TTS = transdermal delivery system.

CCBs and ACEIs may have cardioprotective, cerebroprotective, and renoprotective properties that are superior to those of older traditional diuretic and BB therapy.

Other Factors

Demographics. Black and elderly hypertensive patients and those with low-renin hypertension have a suboptimal BP response to BBs and ACEIs compared with other antihypertensive drugs, especially CCBs. Monotherapy with an ACEI or BB reduces BP significantly in only 40 to 50% of these patients, but CCBs achieve a 60 to 80% response.

Adverse Effects and Quality of Life. In well-controlled studies that have evaluated the effects of various antihypertensive drugs on the quality of life (QOL) by using patient interviews, spouse interviews, and independent questionnaires, the CCB and ACEI patients have a better QOL than those on diuretics and BBs.

Compliance with Treatment. Compliance with any antihypertensive drug regimen is primarily dependent on the frequency of dosing, side effects, QOL, and cost. Once-a-day doses achieve 84% compliance, but three-times-a-day doses drop compliance to 59%. Once-a-week treatment with the clonidine transdermal patch (Catapres-TTS) may improve compliance over the 84% level.

Total Health Care Costs. The total cost of a drug regimen depends not only on the acquisition cost but also the requirement to prescribe secondary drugs to combat side effects of initial therapy (i.e., KCl with diuretics), office visits, ancillary laboratory tests, costs to the patient's lifestyle, and the potential cost of increasing risk factors, complications, and end-organ damage (i.e., CHD, renal insufficiency, diabetes). In a study by Hilleman (Table 10) some of these issues are addressed. If the cost of morbidity and mortality is included, then diuretics and BBs may be more expensive than CCBs, ACEIs, CAAs, and ABs.

PRACTICAL DOSING CONSIDERATIONS

A single antihypertensive drug should be selected based on the subsets of hypertension approach and titrated to one-half to three-fourths of the maximal recommended dose (Table 11) or to side effects (Table 12). Depending on the initial BP level and response to treatment, the patient should return within 1 week for adjustment of the dose. The relative efficacy as monotherapy is shown in Table 13. At this point, if the BP has responded to a safe level, then it is reasonable to wait 4 to 8 weeks before increasing the dose or adding a second or third drug. Many drugs demonstrate improved efficacy over time because of alteration in functional or structural vasoconstriction or other hemodynamic changes. If the BP is not satisfactory, then a second drug should be added. A good rule of thumb is to titrate slowly and give low doses of combination therapy (Table 14) in order to enhance BP control and optimize the effects on the metabolic and structural components of the hypertensive syndrome. The characteristics of the best drugs and combinations are summarized in Table 15. Available antihypertensive drugs are listed in Table 16.

If the patient is resistant to the antihypertensive drugs, then causes should be identified, such as noncompliance, excessive alcohol or NaCl intake, secondary forms of hypertension, drug interactions, volume overload, or pseudohypertension.

Once BP has been controlled for a prolonged time period, it is often possible to reduce the number or dosage of antihypertensive drugs and still maintain good BP control.

HYPERTENSIVE URGENCIES AND EMERGENCIES

Accurate diagnosis, assessment, and treatment of hypertensive urgencies and emergencies can prevent imminent catastrophic target organ damage. A hypertensive urgency is defined as a DBP $\geq$120 mmHg without significant target organ damage. These patients may be treated safely as outpatients with oral or sublingual medications in most circumstances. A hypertensive emergency is defined as a DBP $\geq$120 mmHg with significant end-organ damage (CVA, angina, CHF, acute renal failure [ARF], etc.). These patients should be admitted to an intensive care unit, have an arterial line placed to monitor BP, and be given parenteral medication to promote a controlled

TABLE 12. **Adverse Drug Effects**

Drugs	Selected Side Effects
Diuretics	
Thiazides and related diuretics	Hypokalemia, hypomagnesemia, hyponatremia, hyperuricemia, hypercalcemia, hyperglycemia, hypercholesterolemia, hypertriglyceridemia, sexual dysfunction, weakness, gout
Loop diuretics	Same as for thiazides except loop diuretics do not cause hypercalcemia; volume depletion
Potassium-sparing agents	Hyperkalemia
Amiloride	
Spironolactone	Gynecomastia, mastodynia, menstrual irregularities, diminished libido in males
Triamterene	Hyperkalemia
Adrenergic inhibitors	
Beta blockers	Bronchospasm, claudication, fatigue, insomnia, exacerbation of congestive heart failure, masking of symptoms of hypoglycemia, hypertriglyceridemia, decreased high-density lipoprotein cholesterol (except for those drugs with ISA); reduces exercise tolerance and causes bradycardia, hyperglycemia, insomnia, depression
Alpha-beta blocker	
Labetalol	Bronchospasm, claudication, orthostatic hypotension
Alpha-receptor blockers	Orthostatic hypotension, syncope, weakness, palpitations, headache
Angiotension-converting enzyme inhibitors	Cough, rash, angioedema, hyperkalemia, dyspepsia, renal insufficiency
Calcium antagonists	
Dihydropyridines	Headache, dizziness, peripheral edema, tachycardia, gingival hyperplasia, flushing
Amlodipine	
Felodipine	
Isradipine	
Nicardipine	
Nifedipine	
Diltiazem	Headache, dizziness, peripheral edema, gingival hyperplasia, constipation (especially verapamil), atrioventricular block, bradycardia
Verapamil	
Centrally acting alpha agonists	
Clonidine	Drowsiness, sedation, dry mouth, fatigue, orthostatic dizziness, reduced hypertension
Guanabenz	
Guanfacine hydrohcloride	
Clonidine TTS (patch)	Same as for clonidine but less frequent skin reaction to the patch in 15–20%
Methyldopa	Hemolytic anemia, drug-induced hepatitis
Peripheral acting adrenergic antagonists	
Guanadrel sulfate	Diarrhea, orthostatic and exercise hypotension
Guanethidine monosulfate	
Rauwolfia alkaloids	Lethargy, nasal congestion, depression
Reserpine	
Direct vasodilators	Headache, tachycardia, fluid retention, angina
Hydralazine	Positive antinuclear antibody test
Minoxidil	Hypertrichosis

Abbreviations: ISA = intrinsic sympathomimetic activity.

TABLE 13. **Efficacy: Monotherapy of Antihypertensive Therapy**

Drug Class	White (%)	Black (%)	Elderly (%)
Diuretic	50	60	50
Beta blocker	50	30–40	30–40
Calcium blocker	60–75	75–80	75–80
Angiotensin-converting enzyme inhibitor	50–60	40	40
Alpha blocker	40–50	40–50	40–50
Central alpha agonist	50–60	50–60	50–60

BP reduction to no more than 25 to 30% of initial baseline MAP the first 48 to 72 hours. Blood pressure can then be slowly reduced to normal over the next few days. In most instances, diuretics should be avoided as initial therapy since volume depletion is common except in obvious cases of CHF or ARF. BBs are less effective and should be used cautiously or avoided except in dissecting aortic aneurysms, acute MI, or BB withdrawal states as they may increase the SVR, decrease the CO, and produce other undesirable effects. Table 17 lists the suitable drugs for hypertensive urgencies and emergencies.

PREGNANCY

Pregnancy-induced hypertension and preeclampsia is best treated with aspirin, bed rest, calcium supplements, ad lib NaCl intake, and antihypertensives such as methyldopa (Aldomet), clonidine (Catapres), hydralazine (Apresoline), CCBs, or ABs. Diuretics, ACEIs and BBs are associated with fetal abnormalities, growth retardation, reduced placental or fetal blood flow, volume depletion, or premature delivery and should be avoided.

SUMMARY AND CONCLUSION

1. Establish a firm diagnosis of hypertension and do a complete history, physical examination, and selected laboratory tests to identify target organ damage, coexisting metabolic problems, risk factors, and other diseases, and to exclude secondary causes of hypertension.

2. Initiate lifestyle modifications and patient education for 4 to 6 months if BP levels are not excessive, target organ damage is not significant, or early treatment is not mandatory. Continue as an adjunct to drug therapy if that therapy is started. Select the best antihypertensive agent based on the eight parameters of the *subsets of hypertension* approach: pathophysiology; hemodynamics; target organ damage and risk factor reduction; concomitant diseases; demographics; adverse effects and quality-of-life; compliance, and total cost.

3. Initiate *monotherapy* to one-half to three-quarters maximal recommended dose or to side effects, and moniter BP at frequent intervals (1 to 2 weeks).

4. Use *combination* low-dose treatment with those agents that have additive or syngeristic BP reduction *and* improve the components of the hypertensive syndrome.

TABLE 14. **Combination Antihypertensive Therapy with Selected Drugs**

Calcium channel blocker plus
  Alpha blocker, *or*
  ACE inhibitor, *or*
  Central alpha agonist
Alpha blocker plus either
  Calcium channel blocker *or*
  ACE inhibitor
  (Not with central alpha agonist [reduced response rate])
Central alpha agonist plus either
  Calcium channel blocker *or*
  ACE inhibitor
  (Not with alpha blocker [reduced response rate])
ACE inhibitor plus
  Calcium channel blocker, *or*
  Alpha blocker, *or*
  Central alpha agonist
Diuretic plus any other antihypertensive class except possibly calcium channel blockers (does not usually enhance effects)
Beta blocker plus
  Calcium channel blocker (use caution if systolic dysfunction or conducting problems exist, particularly with verapamil or diltiazem)
  ACE inhibitor
  Diuretic
  Central alpha agonist (avoid when there is possible central antagonism and potential for severe withdrawal syndrome)
  Alpha blocker

Abbreviation: ACE = angiotension-converting enzyme.

TABLE 15. **Characteristics of Ideal Antihypertensive Drugs**

Is efficacious as monotherapy in more than 50% of all patients (demographics)
Gives 24-h blood pressure control during all activities
Requires once-daily dosing
Is hemodynamically logical and effective; reduces systemic vascular resistance, improves arterial compliance, preserves cardiac output, and maintains perfusion to all vital organs
Has lack of tolerance or pseudotolerance: no reflex volume retention or stimulation of neurohumoral mechanisms
Has favorable biochemical and metabolic effects
Reverses structural, vascular smooth muscle, cardiac and left ventricular hypertrophy; improves systemic and diastolic compliance, left ventricular contractility, and function; and reduces ventricular ectopy if present
Reduces all end-organ damage: cardiac, cerebrovascular, renal, retinal, and large artery
Maintains normal hemodynamic response to aerobic and anerobic exercise
Has low incidence of side effects and gives good quality of life
Has record of good compliance with drug regimen
Has good profile in concomitant diseases or problems

TABLE 16. **Chronic Antihypertensive Therapy**

	Starting Dose (mg)	Maximum Dose (mg)	Dosing Frequency (Doses/Day)
Diuretics			
Thiazides and related diuretics			
Hydrochlorothiazide	12.5–25	25–50	1–2
Chlorthalidone (Hygroton)	12.5–25	25	1
Indapamide (Lozol)	2.5	5	1
Loop-active diuretics			
Furosemide (Lasix)	20	320–480	2
Potassium-sparing diuretics			
Amiloride (Midamor)	5	20	1
Triamterene (Dyrenium)	37.5	150	1–2
Sympatholytics			
Beta-adrenoreceptor blockers without intrinsic sympathomimetic activity			
Timolol (Blocadren)	10	60	1–2
Atenolol (Tenormin)	25–50	100	1–2
Metoprolol (Lopressor)	50	200	1–2
Nadolol (Corgard)	20	240	1
Propranolol (Inderal)	40	240–480	2
Betaxolol (Kerlone)	10	20	1
Beta-adrenoreceptor blockers with intrinsic sympathomimetic activity			
Acebutolol	200	1200	1–2
Pindolol (Visken)	10	60	2
Penbutolol (Levatol)	10	80	1–2
Peripheral alpha$_1$-adrenoreceptor blockers			
Doxazosin (Cardura)	1	16	1
Prazosin (Minipress)	1	20	2
Terazosin (Hytrin)	1	20	1 or 2
Alpha- and beta-adrenoreceptor blocker			
Labetalol (Normodyne, Trandate)	200	1200	2
Centrally acting alpha$_2$ agonists			
Alphamethyldopa	500	2000	2
Clonidine (oral) (Catapres)	0.1	0.8	2
Clonidine TTS	TTS-1	TTS-3	weekly
Guanabenz (Wytensin)	4	24–32	2
Guanfacine (Tenex)	1	3	1
Peripherally acting			
Reserpine	0.1	0.25	1
Guanethidine (Ismelin)	10	100	1
Angiotensin-converting enzyme inhibitors			
Benazepril (Lotensin)	10	40	1
Captopril (Capoten)	25	150	2
Enalapril (Vasotec)	2.5–5	40	1–2
Fosinopril (Monopril)	10	40	1
Lisinopril (Zestril)	5–10	40	1–2
Quinapril (Accupril)	10	40–80	1
Ramipril (Altace)	1.25	20	1
Nondihydropyridines			
Diltiazem (Cardizem)	30	360–480	3–4
Verapamil (Isoptin, Calan)	40	480	2–3
Dihydropyridines			
Amlodipine (Norvasc)	5	10	1
Felodipine (Pendil)	5	20	1
Isradipine (DynaCirc)	2.5	10	2
Nicardipine (Cardene)	20	120	3
Nifedipine (Procardia, Adalat)	10	120	3
Direct vasodilators			
Hydralazine (Apresoline)	10	300	2–4
Minoxidil (Loniten)	5	40	2–3

TABLE 17. **Management of Hypertensive Urgencies and Emergencies**

Parenteral Agent	Dose
Sodium nitroprusside (Nipride)	0.25–10 µg/kg/min as IV infusion
Nicardipine (Cardene)	Maximal dose for 10 min only 5 mg/h IV infusion initially Maximal dose 15 mg/h
Nitroglycerin	50–100 µg/min as IV infusion
Diazoxide (Hyperstat IV)	5–100 mg IV bolus, repeated, *or* 15–30 mg/min by IV infusion Avoid or use with caution
Hydralazine	10–20 mg IV bolus 10–40 mg IM Avoid drug or use with caution
Enalaprilat (Vasotec IV)	0.625–1.25 mg q 6 h IV
Phentolamine (Regitine)	5–15 mg IV bolus
Trimethaphan camsylate (Arfonad)	1–4 mg/min as IV infusion
Labetalol (Normodyne, Trandate)	20–80 mg IV bolus every 10 min 2 mg/min IV infusion
Methyldopa	250–500 mg IV infusion q 6 h
Oral agents	
Nifedipine (not extended release) (Procardia)	10–20 mg PO, repeat after 30 min
Captopril (Capoten)	25 mg PO, repeat as required
Clonidine (Catapres)	0.1–0.2 mg PO, repeated every hour as required to total dose of 0.6 mg
Labetalol (Normodyne)	200–400 mg PO, repeat every 2–3 h

5. Allow time between dose changes or adding medications for the antihypertensive agent to have its full effect (4 to 8 weeks, on average).

6. Identify causes for resistant hypertension.

7. After a period of time, if BP is controlled (6 to 12 months) it may be possible to reduce the number of medications or dose and still maintain BP control.

The ultimate goal in the management of hypertensive patients is to reduce target organ damage, which will decrease hypertensive-related morbidity and mortality—cardiovascular, cerebrovascular, and renal. Newer concepts and newer medications coupled with long-term prospective clinical trials comparing various drug regimens will continue to enhance our chances to achieve these goals.

ACUTE MYOCARDIAL INFARCTION

method of
ERIC R. BATES, M.D.
University of Michigan
Ann Arbor, Michigan

Acute myocardial infarction (MI) is the leading cause of death in Western society. As many as 1.5 million people per year develop MI in the United States, with 800,000 receiving in-hospital treatment. Approximately 500,000 deaths per year, or 25% of all deaths in this country, are a result of MI. Over half of these occur within 1 hour of symptom onset, usually secondary to ventricular fibrillation. Cardiogenic shock, not arrhythmia, is the most common cause of in-hospital death. Additionally, the morbidity due to MI alters the quality and quantity of life in many survivors.

Although angina pectoris was described as early as 1772 by Heberden, it was not until 1912 that Herrick suggested that postmortem coronary thrombi are related to the clinical events that precipitate myocardial necrosis. A longer life expectancy due to other medical advances, a more sedentary lifestyle, and an atherogenic diet have made MI a disease of the twentieth century.

For decades, therapeutic interventions for MI were limited to prolonged bed rest for several weeks and drug treatment for congestive failure. Hospital mortality rates were greater than 30%. The major treatment breakthrough for MI occurred in the 1960s, when the electric defibrillator became clinically available and coronary care units were established for the purpose of detecting life-threatening ventricular arrhythmias. Hospital mortality rates were halved. Beta-adrenergic blockers were introduced in the 1970s in an attempt to limit infarct size by decreasing oxygen demand, but the second most important treatment breakthrough occurred in the 1980s. Based on angiographic proof by DeWood that coronary thrombosis initiates MI and the description by Rentrop that intracoronary streptokinase lyses thrombus and restores blood supply to the ischemic myocardium, the reperfusion era was initiated. Several international clinical trials subsequently demonstrated mortality reduction, proving infarct artery patency and myocardial salvage as the mechanism. Hospital mortality rates for thrombolytic candidates have subsequently dropped to 6 to 10% but remain in double digits despite improved adjunctive therapy for certain subsets and in patients not eligible for thrombolysis. Current research is directed toward decreasing triggering of MI, stabilizing the vulnerable plaque, and ultimately preventing atherogenesis.

ATHEROGENESIS

Atherosclerosis begins as a fatty streak, evolves to a fibrous plaque, and can progress to a complex plaque at risk for thrombosis. The "response to injury" hypothesis best explains this progression. Endothelial denudation due to smoking, hypertension, elevated low-density lipoprotein cholesterol levels, diabetes mellitus, or other insult exposes collagen and other vascular wall constituents. Platelet adhesion and aggregation are stimulated. Thromboxane A_2, serotonin, growth factors, and other substances are released, promoting vasoconstriction and thrombus formation. The healing process involves smooth muscle cell proliferation and/or incorporation of thrombus into the lesion, both of which can cause plaque enlargement. Intraplaque hemorrhage or lipid accumulation can also cause lesion progression.

PLAQUE RUPTURE

Plaque rupture is the cause of more than 90% of MIs. Rare nonatherosclerotic causes include vasculitis, anomalous origin of a coronary artery, coronary artery spasm, coronary artery embolus, or hypercoagulable states. Chronic, fibrotic plaques that severely obstruct the vascular lumen are involved in only a minority of clinically significant infarctions. These lesions more commonly cause myocardial ischemia and angina pectoris. Slow progression often results in collateral circulation recruitment, such that progression to coronary artery occlusion may be clinically silent and not cause myocardial necrosis. The most common substrate for plaque rupture, coronary artery thrombosis, and MI is the hemodynamically insignificant plaque. The "vulnerable plaque" has a large lipid core and a thin fibrous cap. Infiltration of lipid-filled macrophages results in release of proteolytic enzymes that cause focal loss of collagen in the cap. Rupture occurs when there is an imbalance between systolic stress on the cap and the innate mechanical strength of the cap. Thus, treatment options that could decrease either lipid content or macrophage infiltration or reduce macrophage activation should decrease clinical events and decrease the development of high-grade stenoses.

Plaque rupture is mostly a spontaneous event. However, approximately one of six MIs is triggered by activation of the sympathetic nervous system due to heavy exertion, anger, or awakening. Interestingly, platelet activation, coagulability, ischemic sudden death, transient ischemic attacks, MI, and stroke all follow the same circadian pattern that peaks 2 hours after awakening. Aspirin and beta blockers blunt the morning increase in these events.

HEMOSTATIC AND FIBRINOLYTIC SYSTEMS

Life can be viewed as a delicate balance between bleeding and thrombosis. Vascular damage or bleeding activates the hemostatic system, which consists of platelets and the coagulation cascade. While platelet adhesion and aggregation are occurring, the coagulation system is generating thrombin, which converts fibrinogen to fibrin. Strands of fibrin stabilize the platelet thrombus. Physiologic thrombus produces hemostasis and promotes vascular healing, although vascular lumen narrowing may result. Pathologic thrombus formation produces ischemia or tissue necrosis by interfering with nutrient blood flow. The duration of ischemia in patients with unstable angina pectoris is not long enough to produce significant cell death. Myocardial necrosis requires at least 20 minutes of arterial occlusion and proceeds from the endocardium toward the epicardium as a wavefront, requiring hours to complete transmural infarction. Interruption of this process by reperfusion results in nontransmural MI.

The fibrinolytic system exists as a balance to the hemostatic system and normally prevents pathologic thrombus formation by maintaining a dynamic equilibrium between thrombosis and thrombolysis. Tissue plasminogen activator, released by endothelial cells, converts plasminogen within the thrombus to plasmin, which degrades fibrin to degradation products, lysing thrombus. Only when this system is overwhelmed does thrombotic vascular occlusion develop.

DIAGNOSIS

History

Many patients with MI have risk factors for coronary artery disease. These include a family history of atherosclerosis; hypertension; cigarette smoking; diabetes mellitus; and hypercholesterolemia. Other factors that increase the likelihood of chest pain being ischemic are male gender, older age, estrogen deficiency in women, type A personality, and cocaine use. Unfortunately, none of these descriptors predict MI, which can occur in the absence of risk factors. Often, the initial clinical manifestation of coronary artery disease is ischemic sudden death.

Very frustrating, especially to the emergency department physician, is the challenge of diagnosing MI by chest pain description. However, most of the important decisions including whether to admit the patient to the hospital are based on the history. An accurate description of pain onset, duration, severity, nature, and location; aggravating or alleviating factors; and prior episodes needs to be obtained quickly. Only a minority of patients with MI describe retrosternal pressure radiating to the neck or arm, associated with nausea, diaphoresis, or dyspnea. Conversely, chest pain complaints in most patients have noncardiac causes. These include esophageal, stomach, and gallbladder disease; pulmonary disease; aortic dissection; pericarditis; musculoskeletal complaints; and anxiety.

Physical Examination

Patients often appear anxious or restless. The most important part of the physical examination is the assessment of vital signs. Tachycardia, bradycardia, or hypotension predict higher risk, whereas hypertension may make a patient thrombolytic-ineligible. Interestingly, low body weight and short stature have also been associated with greater mortality risk, perhaps because the diameter of the coronary arteries is smaller in these people. Acute mitral regurgitation or ventricular septal defect needs to be considered in patients with systolic murmurs. The absence of pulmonary rales or jugular venous distention in a hypotensive patient suggests hypovolemia. The presence of pulmonary rales and a ventricular gallop suggests congestive heart failure from left ventricular dysfunction, whereas the triad of clear lung fields, hypotension, and jugular venous distention is found in the syndrome of right ventricular infarction. Deceased mentation, oliguria, peripheral cyanosis, clammy skin temperature, and hypotension are found in patients with cardiogenic shock. A normal neurologic examination and the absence of active bleeding should be documented before the administration of thrombolytic therapy.

Alternative diagnoses can also be suggested by the physical examination. Fever may indicate the presence of pneumonia. Chest wall tenderness can occur with musculoskeletal abnormalities but cannot be used to exclude MI. Asymmetry of breath sounds is seen with spontaneous pneumothorax. Unilateral leg swelling increases the odds for pulmonary embolism as the cause of chest pain. Pericardial friction rubs are associated with pericarditis. Differential blood pressures in the arms, absent femoral pulses, or the murmur of aortic insufficiency is suggestive of aortic dissection.

Laboratory Tests

The standard 12-lead electrocardiogram (ECG) needs to be obtained in all patients in whom the diagnosis of MI is being entertained. This should include all patients who complain of chest pain in the emergency department. The presence of new left bundle branch block or ≥ 1 mm of ST segment elevation in two contiguous leads should immediately activate the screening protocol for thrombolytic therapy. Patients with equivocal ST segment elevation, ST segment depression, or ischemic T wave changes should be monitored very carefully with repeat ECGs every 30 minutes since they may develop ST segment elevation and qualify for thrombolysis. Repeat ECGs are also indicated in patients with convincing symptoms but nondiagnostic tracings, or when symptoms increase in severity. Right-sided precordial leads should be recorded in all patients with inferior MI in an attempt to diagnose right ventricular infarction. The failure of Q waves to develop despite cardiac enzyme release may indicate nontransmural necrosis. The ECG may be normal in as many as 20% of patients who present with MI.

Elevation of ST segments in both anterior and inferior leads with PR segment depression is seen in acute pericarditis. Early repolarization, left ventricular hypertrophy, previous infarction in the same distribution, and chronic left bundle branch block can also cause ST segment elevation not related to MI. Left ventricular hypertrophy, digitalis therapy, hypokalemia, and hyperventilation can cause ST segment depression or T wave changes not related to MI. Bypass tracts, hypertrophic and dilated cardiomyopathies, chronic lung disease, and neuromuscular disorders can cause Q waves not related to MI.

The only blood tests needed to confirm the diagnosis of MI are the creatinine kinase (CK) and creatinine kinase–MB (CK–MB) isoenzyme tests. The lactic dehydrogenase (LD) and aspartate aminotransferase (AST; formerly SGOT) enzyme tests seldom add useful information. Initial levels are normal in patients presenting soon after symptom onset; the levels peak more than 15 hours later if infarct artery patency is not restored, and they return toward normal in the next 2 to 3 days. Peak levels within 15 hours suggest reperfusion. Serial enzyme patterns are necessary to confirm the diagnosis of MI if ECG changes are nondiagnostic. Occasionally enzyme levels may be normal if patients present late. Hypothyroidism, defibrillation, strenuous exercise, chronic renal failure, and myositis can produce falsely abnormal CK–MB levels. The diagnosis of MI usually requires at least two out of three descriptors: history of ischemic chest pain of more than 20 minutes' duration; new persistent ECG changes consistent with ischemia, injury, or infarction; and the rise and fall of the CK–MB isoenzyme.

The chest roentgenogram should be obtained in all patients. It may show pneumothorax, pneumomediastinum, pleural effusions, infiltrates, congestive heart failure, or widening of the mediastinum. Radionuclide studies in the acute setting are neither useful nor practical but are used in postinfarct risk stratification. Alternatively, echocardiography can be of considerable value in defining regional wall motion abnormalities, global left ventricular function, and right ventricular function. Echocardiography is essential in diagnosing mitral valve dysfunction, ventricular septal rupture, aneurysm formation, mural thrombus, or pericardial effusion.

PREHOSPITAL TREATMENT

With the knowledge that treatment delays increase the morbidity and mortality of MI, at least 20 studies have evaluated the feasibility and efficacy of prehospital treatment. Early studies demonstrated that thrombolytic therapy could be given and that approximately 45 minutes could be saved in time to treatment. The Myocardial Infarction Triage and Intervention Project (MITI), the European Myocardial Infarct Project (EMIP), and three other randomized studies showed a 17% reduction in mortality as well. Importantly, 96% of chest pain patients screened for the MITI study were considered ineligible for prehospital treatment because of contraindications to thrombolytic therapy, atypical or noncardiac chest pain, etc. That only 4% of patients were considered eligible for prehospital treatment highlights the logistic problem of committing resources to this approach. Moreover, in the United States, physicians

are not part of the emergency response team. Thus, there are logistic, medical, and legal barriers to widespread implementation. A more practical approach is prehospital diagnosis of MI with facsimile transmission of an ECG to the emergency department and rapid transfer of the patient.

EMERGENCY DEPARTMENT TREATMENT

Several studies have demonstrated an emergency department delay of 60 to 90 minutes before thrombolytic therapy is started in appropriate candidates. This deficiency has recently been addressed by the National Heart Attack Alert Program Coordinating Committee, which has set 30 minutes as the target time from hospital arrival to thrombolytic treatment initiation in obvious candidates. That committee divided the treatment delay period into four time points ("the four Ds"): arrival and triage in the emergency department (door), obtaining an ECG (data), deciding to administer thrombolytic therapy (decision), and initiating the thrombolytic infusion (drug).

Door. Registration and triage account for the initial delay. Time can be saved for walk-in patients if the triage nurse, rather than the registration clerk, immediately evaluates patients who complain of chest pain or an equivalent syndrome. Valuable time can also be saved for those transported by ambulance if the initial health care provider can telephone a history or Fax an ECG to the emergency department before the patient arrives.

Data. It takes time to order, obtain, and interpret an ECG. The emergency department nurse responsible for treating potential MI patients should immediately initiate cardiac monitoring and have a standing order to obtain a 12-lead ECG. Moreover, an ECG machine should be located in the emergency department and the nurses or emergency technicians trained to record a 12-lead ECG in case the ECG technician is not readily available. Although a computerized preliminary interpretation may help with diagnosis, a physician should be available to interpret the ECG within 5 minutes of its being ordered.

Decision. When the diagnosis is clear, the emergency physician should be empowered to initiate thrombolytic therapy in appropriate candidates. A checklist of inclusion and exclusion criteria should be used to assist in the decision (Table 1). Complicated presentations, relative contraindications to thrombolytic therapy, or unclear diagnosis may require consultation with a cardiologist. This should be done by telephone and facsimile transfer of the ECG, if possible. Echocardiography, continuous ST segment monitoring, or serial 12-lead ECGs may be necessary to confirm the diagnosis.

Drug. Once it has been determined that the patient is a candidate for thrombolysis, the patient and family should be informed of the benefits and risks of thrombolytic therapy, including the risk of stroke. Acceptance or refusal of this therapy should be documented in the medical record; standard consent

TABLE 1. **Indications and Contraindications for Thrombolytic Therapy**

Indications
1. Ischemic chest pain <12 h
2. ST segment elevation in two contiguous leads or left bundle branch block
3. Low bleeding risk

Absolute Contraindications
1. Altered consciousness
2. Known bleeding disorder
3. Active internal bleeding
4. Trauma or surgery less than 2 weeks previously
5. Suspected aortic dissection
6. Prolonged or traumatic cardiopulmonary resuscitation
7. Recent head trauma or known intracranial neoplasm
8. Diabetic hemorrhagic retinopathy or other hemorrhagic ophthalmic condition
9. Pregnancy
10. Previous allergic reaction to the thrombolytic agent (streptokinase or APSAC)
11. Recorded blood pressure higher than 200/120 mmHg
12. History of cerebrovascular accident known to be hemorrhagic

Relative Contraindications
1. Major trauma or surgery less than 2 months previously
2. History of chronic severe hypertension with or without drug therapy
3. Active peptic ulcer disease
4. History of ischemic or embolic cerebrovascular accident
5. Known bleeding diathesis or current use of anticoagulants
6. Subclavian or internal jugular venous cannulation

Abbreviation: APSAC = anisoylated plasminogen streptokinase activator complex.

forms are not recommended. To decrease treatment delay, the thrombolytic drug should be stored, mixed, and administered in the emergency department. Patients who are not candidates for thrombolysis should be started on aspirin and heparin therapy and considered for beta blocker therapy and emergency percutaneous transluminal coronary angioplasty (PTCA) before transfer to the coronary care unit. A worksheet documenting the precise timing of these events should be completed and used as part of the quality assurance program to improve efficiency.

REPERFUSION THERAPY

Of all the therapeutic interventions to consider in patients with MI, the most time-dependent is reperfusion therapy. Thrombolytic therapy is the most widely available reperfusion mode, but emergency coronary angioplasty is a reasonable option in a tertiary care hospital, especially for patients with anterior MI, history of previous MI, hemodynamic instability, or age greater than 70 years.

Thrombolytic Therapy

Four large, multicenter, placebo-controlled trials demonstrated the survival benefit associated with alteplase (tPA) (Activase), anistreplase (anisoylated plasminogen streptokinase activator complex, or APSAC (Eminase), and streptokinase (Streptase) (Table 2). These agents are now considered the most important acute treatment that can be given to eligi-

ble patients. The greatest survival benefit is seen in patients treated within 1 hour of symptom onset.

Indications

Patients with ischemic chest pain of less than 12 hours' duration, ST segment elevation or new left bundle branch block on their ECG, and low bleeding risk must be considered for thrombolytic therapy (see Table 1). Note that the treatment window has been expanded from 6 to 12 hours because of the results from four trials showing a survival benefit within this time frame. Left bundle branch block has been included because these patients have a 50% reduction in mortality when treated. A survival advantage has also been shown for patients with inferior MI, prior MI, prior coronary artery bypass graft surgery, and age greater than 70 years. No data support using these drugs, however, in patients with unstable angina pectoris or MI without ST segment elevation.

Contraindications

The contraindications for thrombolytic therapy are listed in Table 1. They are meant to exclude patients who are at increased risk of bleeding. Defibrillation is recommended before cardiopulmonary resuscitation (CPR) for witnessed cardiac arrests to avoid chest trauma, but patients who have short periods of nontraumatic CPR are still candidates. Central line placement is strongly discouraged and is considered by many to constitute a contraindication for thrombolytic therapy.

Thrombolytic Drug

Great controversy has raged over which thrombolytic drug to use (Table 2). Two trials (Gruppo Italiano per lo Studio della Sopravvivenza nell' Infarto Miocardico [GISSIM-2] and Third International Study of Infarct Survival [ISIS-3]) showed no differ-

TABLE 2. **Randomized Thrombolytic Trial Mortality Data**

Placebo-Control Trials

	Placebo (%)	Treatment (%)
GISSI-1 (SK)	13.0	10.7*
AIMS	12.2	6.4*
ASSET (tPA)	9.8	7.2*
ISIS-2 (SK)	12.0	9.2*

Comparative Trials

	Streptokinase (%)	tPA (%)
GISSI-2/International	8.6	9.0†
ISIS-3	10.6	10.3‡
GUSTO-1	7.3	6.3§

*Statistically significant.
†3-h Activase administration.
‡4-h Duteplase administration.
§1.5-h Activase administration.

Abbreviations: APSAC = anisoylated plasminogen streptokinase activator complex; AIMS = APSAC Intervention Mortality Study; ASSET = Anglo-Scandinavian Study of Early Thrombolysis; GISSI = Gruppo Italiano per lo Studio della sopravvivenza nell' Infarto Miocardico; GUSTO = Global Utilization of Streptokinase and Tissue Plasminogen Activator for Occluded Coronary Arteries; ISIS = International Study of Infarct Survival; SK = streptokinase; tPA = tissue plasminogen activator.

ence in outcome between tPA (3 to 4-hour infusion), APSAC, or streptokinase and no advantage from subcutaneous heparin administration. However, the Global Utilization of Streptokinase and Tissue Plasminogen Activator for Occluded Coronary Arteries (GUSTO-1) trial showed lower mortality with a 90-minute infusion of tPA combined with a monitored intravenous heparin infusion, compared with streptokinase. Thus, from a biologic and clinical trials standpoint, accelerated tPA plus intravenous heparin infusion appears to have an advantage. Unfortunately, tPA is approximately $2000 more expensive than streptokinase per dose, so from a clinical practice and economic standpoint, streptokinase is still a viable treatment option (Table 3). Many hospitals use only one agent. Others use tPA only for patients who present early or have anterior MI, in which the best advantage for tPA was demonstrated. Patients who present later or have smaller predicted infarct size or who cannot receive heparin may reasonably be given streptokinase. APSAC is the easiest drug to administer, but bleeding complications are more difficult to control because of its prolonged duration of action, and it is more expensive than is streptokinase without offering any advantage.

Complications

Bleeding is the major complication of thrombolytic therapy. Any recent vascular puncture can bleed, so pressure dressings should be aggressively applied and additional vascular punctures avoided if possible. Antacids or H_2 blockers should also be considered as prophylaxis against gastrointestinal bleeding. The most serious complication of thrombolytic therapy is intracerebral hemorrhage. It occurs in 0.5 to 1.0% of patients. Risk factors include low body weight, severe hypertension, age greater than 70 years, and partial thromboplastin time greater than 100 seconds. One additional stroke per 1000 patients treated occurs with tPA therapy. Conversely, anaphylaxis occurs in 1 per 1000 patients treated with streptokinase or APSAC, and hypotension or allergic reactions occur in 5%. Because streptokinase and APSAC produce antibodies that can neutralize repeat doses after 5 days from the initial exposure, tPA should be used for subsequent therapy. Packed red blood cell transfusions need not be given in stable patients until the hematocrit falls below 24% to decrease the risk of

TABLE 3. **Thrombolytic Therapy for Acute Myocardial Infarction**

Agent	Dose
Alteplase (tPA) (Activase)	15-mg bolus, 0.75 mg/kg up to 50 mg over 30 min, 0.5 mg/kg up to 35 mg over 60 min
Anistreplase (APSAC) (Eminase)	30 U over 5 min
Streptokinase (Streptase)	1.5 million U over 60 min

Abbreviations: APSAC = anisoylated plasminogen streptokinase activator complex; tPA = tissue plasminogen activator.

viral infection. Serious bleeding may require protamine to reverse the effect of heparin, fresh-frozen plasma to replace coagulation factors, cryoprecipitate to replace fibrinogen, or platelet transfusions to provide functional platelets.

Coronary Angioplasty

Four small trials randomizing patients to thrombolytic therapy or coronary angioplasty were recently reported (Table 4). With PTCA, two suggested a survival advantage, three demonstrated less recurrent ischemia, and two showed fewer strokes. The sample sizes are too small, however, to reach definitive conclusions, and the pooled results were greatly influenced by the Primary Angioplasty in Myocardial Infarction (PAMI) trial. Moreover, only the Dutch trial showed improvement in left ventricular function. There is no doubt that an experienced interventional cardiologist working in a hospital that performs several hundred PTCAs per year can achieve excellent results, perhaps superior to those of thrombolytic therapy, with this technique. Less clear is whether this strategy is reasonable if low-volume operators are performing PTCA or if time to reperfusion is delayed by patient transfer or cardiac catheterization laboratory mobilization. Two groups of patients should strongly be considered for emergency PTCA, even if interhospital transfer is required. First, patients with cardiogenic shock, in which no other treatment has been shown to reduce the 80% mortality risk, have a 50% mortality rate after PTCA. Second, patients with moderate to large infarct size (anterior MI, inferior MI with precordial ST segment depression) and contraindications for thrombolytic therapy can receive the benefits of reperfusion therapy by undergoing PTCA, without the same bleeding risk. Additionally, some physicians refer patients with anterior MI for emergency PTCA if symptoms and ST segment elevation do not resolve by the conclusion of the thrombolytic infusion.

CONJUNCTIVE THERAPY
General Measures

Every patient, whether receiving reperfusion therapy or not, is a candidate for other therapies. Oxygen should be provided in the first few hours of MI (Table 5). Modest hypoxia can be present even in patients with uncomplicated MI, partly secondary to ventilation-perfusion mismatch. Tracheal intubation and mechanical ventilation are needed when supplemental oxygen does not correct hypoxemia.

When the pain of myocardial ischemia is not quickly relieved by sublingual nitroglycerin tablets, morphine can be administered. Peripheral venous and arterial dilation also result, decreasing myocardial oxygen demand, and catecholamine levels may be reduced when pain and anxiety are relieved. Naloxone can reverse the effects of morphine if hypotension, bradycardia, or respiratory depression complicates treatment.

TABLE 4. **Randomized Percutaneous Transluminal Coronary Angioplasty**

Study	N	Lytic	Mortality*		Recurrent Ischemia and MI*		CVA*	
			PTCA	Lytic	PTCA	Lytic	PTCA	Lytic
PAMI	395	tPA	5 (2.6)	13 (6.5)	20 (10.3)	56 (28.0)	0 (0)	7 (3.5)
Dutch	142	SK	0 (0)	4 (5.6)	6 (8.6)	27 (37.5)	0 (0)	2 (2.8)
Mayo Clinic	103	tPA	2 (4.3)	2 (3.6)	7 (14.9)	20 (35.7)	0 (0)	0 (0)
Brazil	100	SK	3 (6.0)	1 (2.0)	4 (8)	5 (10)	0 (0)	0 (0)
Pooled	740		10 (2.8)	20 (5.3)	37 (10.2)	108 (28.6)	0 (0)	9 (2.4)

*Numbers in parentheses represent percent.
Abbreviations: CVA = cerebral vascular accident; MI = myocardial infarction; PAMI = Primary Angioplasty in Myocardial Infarction; PTCA = percutaneous transluminal coronary angioplasty; SK = streptokinase; tPA = tissue plasminogen activator.

Drug Therapy

Aspirin. Whereas only 20 to 30% of patients with MI receive thrombolytic therapy, only aspirin sensitivity should preclude patients from receiving aspirin as antiplatelet therapy. Aspirin costs very little, has almost no side effects, and decreases mortality. In the ISIS-2 trial, 35-day mortality was reduced by 23% with aspirin compared with 25% with streptokinase. Importantly, the benefit appears to be additive: there was a 42% reduction when both were administered together. The reinfarction rates were also halved with this treatment. Aspirin therapy should be continued indefinitely, because of its proven ability to reduce subsequent risk of death, reinfarction, and stroke. Ticlopidine (Ticlid) 250 mg twice daily can be used in patients allergic to aspirin, but complete blood counts need to be performed every 2 weeks for 3 months to monitor for neutropenia.

Heparin. The utility of thrombin inhibition with heparin is controversial. In the prethrombolytic era, heparin therapy was shown to reduce mortality, reinfarction, stroke, deep venous thrombosis, and pulmonary embolism. The benefit is much less clear in patients already receiving aspirin and thrombolytic therapy. The present data suggest that neither subcutaneous nor intravenous heparin additionally re-

duce mortality when streptokinase or APSAC are administered, so heparin is not necessary during the first hospital day. Conversely, therapeutic intravenous heparin is strongly recommended to prevent infarct artery reocclusion with tPA, because of tPA's short half-life, and with PTCA, because of the additional vascular trauma that occurs. In patients receiving intravenous heparin, it is very important to frequently monitor the activated partial thromboplastin time (APTT) in the first 24 to 48 hours and to prolong it 2.0 to 2.5 times normal. Prophylactic heparin (5000 U subcutaneously twice a day to prevent venous thrombosis or 12,500 U twice a day in patients with anterior MI at risk for mural thrombus formation) is recommended for the remainder of the hospital stay in patients not receiving intravenous heparin.

Beta-Adrenergic Blockers. Beta blockers decrease heart rate, blood pressure, and left ventricular contractility, the major determinants of oxygen demand. Like heparin, beta blockers were shown to reduce mortality in the prethrombolytic era but have not been shown to additionally reduce acute mortality in patients treated with thrombolytic therapy. There is a reduction in recurrent ischemia and reinfarction, however, and some studies have suggested that the risk of both myocardial rupture and cerebral

TABLE 5. **Conjunctive Pharmacologic Treatment for Acute Myocardial Infarction**

Oxygen	2–4 L/min by nasal cannula
Sublingual nitroglycerin	0.4 mg every 2–5 min × 3
Morphine	2–5 mg IV every 5–30 min
Aspirin	160 mg PO every day
Heparin	5000 or 12,500 U subcutaneously bid; or 5000 U IV followed by 1000 U/h IV, adjusted to keep aPTT 2.0–2.5 × control
Beta-adrenergic blockers	
Atenolol (Tenormin)	5 mg IV × 2 over 10 min; 50 mg PO 10 min later; then 100 mg PO every day
Metoprolol (Lopressor)	5 mg IV × 3 over 15 min; 50 mg PO 10 min later; then 100 mg PO twice daily
Intravenous nitroglycerin	10–200 mcg/min infusion
ACE inhibitor	
Captopril (Capoten)	12.5–50 mg PO tid
Enalapril (Vasotec)	2.5–10 mg PO bid
Lisinopril (Prinivil, Zestril)	5–20 mg PO daily
Ramipril (Altace)	2.5–5 mg PO bid
Warfarin (Coumadin)	2–10 mg PO daily adjusted to INR

Abbreviations: ACE = angiotensin-converting enzyme; aPTT = activated partial thromboplastin time; INR = International Normalized Ratio.

hemorrhage is reduced with adjunctive beta blocker therapy. Excellent candidates for therapy include patients with reflex tachycardia, systolic hypertension, continuing ischemic pain, or atrial fibrillation with fast ventricular response. Contraindications exist in 50% of patients and include bradycardia, hypotension, congestive heart failure, atrioventricular conduction abnormalities, and bronchospastic lung disease. Long-term therapy saves approximately 2 lives per 100 treated patients.

Nitroglycerin. Nitrates reduce preload and afterload and increase myocardial perfusion. Limitation of left ventricular dilatation, a major independent predictor of a poor outcome after MI, has been documented. Although several small early trials from the prethrombolytic era suggested a mortality benefit with nitroglycerin, two recent large trials (GISSI-3, ISIS-4) did not show a statistically significant advantage. Nevertheless, intravenous nitroglycerin is easily administered, has advantageous physiologic properties, and relieves ischemic chest pain, so it is a good drug for the coronary care unit phase of the hospitalization. The infusion can be initiated at 10 μg per minute and increased quickly by 10 μg per minute increments until systolic blood pressure is reduced 10 to 15 mmHg or headache or tachycardia develop. Long-term nitrate therapy has not reduced subsequent mortality.

Angiotensin-Converting Enzyme Inhibition. Converting enzyme inhibitors, like nitrates, inhibit infarct expansion and ventricular dilatation. In contrast to nitrates, however, excellent reduction in mortality has consistently been seen in treated patients with left ventricular ejection fraction less than 40% or clinical evidence of congestive heart failure. Despite statistically significant mortality reductions with early therapy in two recent trials, the absolute early advantage of converting enzyme inhibition versus nitrate therapy is similar. Therefore, nitroglycerin can be used in the coronary care unit because it is easier to titrate against blood pressure and relieves ischemic chest pain. In patients with moderate left ventricular dysfunction or clinical evidence of congestive heart failure, converting enzyme inhibitor therapy can be substituted for nitrates in the step-down unit phase of the hospitalization. Subsequent mortality, congestive heart failure, recurrent MI, and hospitalization rates are all reduced by approximately 20%.

Calcium Channel Blockers. It was initially hoped that the improvement in coronary blood flow that can be achieved with calcium channel blockers would complement the reduction in demand obtained with beta blockers and lead to a further reduction of mortality in MI. Unfortunately, this hypothesis has been disproved, and nifedipine may actually increase mortality. Whereas calcium channel blockers are useful agents to treat systemic hypertension and stable angina pectoris, they are not recommended for patients with MI.

Magnesium. Magnesium infusions have been shown to limit infarct size, increase coronary blood flow, decrease afterload, and prevent serious ventricular arrhythmias. Seven small trials and one larger trial (Leicester Intravenous Magnesium Intervention Trial [LIMIT-2]) initially suggested a large mortality reduction with early magnesium administration when patients were not treated with thrombolytic therapy. The ISIS-4 megatrial (58,000 patients) showed an excess mortality with magnesium therapy when given late and usually after aspirin and thrombolytic therapy. Therefore, magnesium infusions should not be routinely used in MI but may be beneficial in patients with high mortality risk who are not reperfusion candidates.

Lidocaine. Prophylactic lidocaine administration has been a frequently studied topic. Pooled data suggest that lidocaine does decrease the incidence of ventricular tachycardia, but mortality rates are paradoxically increased, probably because of an increased incidence of asystole. Thus, lidocaine should only be given for therapeutic indications including more than six ventricular premature beats (VPBs) per minute, closely coupled VPBs (R-on-T phenomenon), multiform VPBs, nonsustained ventricular tachycardia, and sustained ventricular tachycardia or fibrillation.

Warfarin. Warfarin (Coumadin) has shown similar benefit to aspirin in preventing reinfarction, thromboembolic events, and death after MI, but the bleeding risk and the need to monitor the prothrombin time with warfarin make aspirin a superior therapy. However, warfarin should be given for 3 months to patients with left ventricular thrombus or large anterior MI and may be beneficial with severe left ventricular dysfunction. The efficacy of low-dose aspirin and low-dose warfarin combination therapy is being investigated.

ACUTE VENTRICULAR DYSFUNCTION

General Measures

Frequent nursing assessments for hemodynamic instability or signs of recurrent ischemia in a Coronary Care Unit (CCU) setting for 48 to 72 hours are recommended. Invasive hemodynamic monitoring and pharmacologic treatment are required in patients with significant pulmonary congestion, arterial hypotension not responding rapidly to fluid administration, or both. A pulmonary artery capillary wedge pressure of less than 12 mmHg supports the diagnosis of hypovolemia. Disproportionately high right-sided filling pressures, low or normal left-sided filling pressures, and low cardiac output are seen in severe right ventricular MI. Hypotension, a left ventricular filling pressure of greater than 18 mmHg, and a cardiac index of less than 1.8 confirm the diagnosis of cardiogenic shock. A large V wave in the pulmonary artery capillary wedge pressure tracing suggests mitral regurgitation, whereas an oxygen saturation step-up in the right ventricle proves ventricular septal rupture.

Hypovolemic patients should receive intravenous fluid to maintain a pulmonary capillary wedge pressure of 15 to 18 mmHg to optimize left ventricular function. Blood gas, serum electrolyte, and acid-base abnormalities should be corrected promptly. Hemoglobin levels may need to be maintained with packed red blood cell transfusions. Therapy with negative inotropic agents, including beta blockers, calcium channel blockers, and unnecessary antiarrhythmics, should be discontinued. Nitroglycerin, morphine, and diuretics are contraindicated in hemodynamically significant right ventricular MI because they decrease preload. Bradyarrhythmias and tachyarrhythmias need to be promptly controlled pharmacologically or with electric countershock. Normal atrioventricular (AV) conduction is especially important in right ventricular infarction and cardiogenic shock to maintain cardiac output and can be restored with AV sequential pacing when AV block is present. Two-dimensional echocardiography can provide important serial information about left ventricular regional and global function. It is also very useful in diagnosing ventricular septal or free wall rupture, valvular heart disease, pericardial effusion, or right ventricular MI.

Diuretics

Intravenous furosemide (Lasix) can be used to induce diuresis in patients with pulmonary congestion and preserved arterial pressure (Table 6). Bumetanide (Bumex) can be used if there is no response to furosemide. Attention to electrolyte balance is important because hypokalemia or hypomagnesemia facilitates ventricular arrhythmias.

Vasodilating Agents

Nitroglycerin in low doses decreases preload and improves myocardial perfusion by dilating epicardial coronary arteries and improving collateral flow. It may decrease infarct expansion and has an afterload-reducing effect at higher doses. It is therefore a good agent to use in the early hours after MI when ischemia is present, and in patients with pulmonary congestion and normal systemic vascular resistance. The dosing is the same as described earlier for acute

ischemia. In situations in which ischemia is no longer present or when systemic vascular resistance is increased, nitroprusside becomes the agent of choice. Nitroprusside is a direct-acting balanced arteriodilator and venodilator. Prolonged use can result in cyanide toxicity.

Positive Inotropic Agents

Dobutamine (Dobutrex) is an effective agent for right or left ventricular pump failure when arterial pressure is greater than 90 mmHg. If arterial pressure is 70 to 90 mmHg, dopamine may be the best initial agent. Low-dose dopamine can be used in combination with dobutamine therapy to achieve desired hemodynamic effects. Higher doses of dopamine may worsen ischemia by increasing the heart rate and decreasing the alveolar-capillary gas exchange because of a rise in the pulmonary capillary wedge pressure. Also, high-dose dopamine therapy can be arrhythmogenic. When the arterial pressure is below 70 mmHg, norepinephrine, which has less chronotropic effect, is the agent of choice until the pressure can be increased to at least 80 mmHg.

Phosphodiesterase inhibitors (amrinone [Inocor], milrinone [Primacor]) are a new class of noncatecholamine inotropic drugs that have both inotropic and arterial vasodilating properties but little effect on myocardial oxygen demand or arrhythmogenesis. They can be given to patients with stable arterial pressure when both effects are needed.

Support Devices

Several support devices are available for patients in cardiogenic shock who do not respond to pharmacologic therapy. Intra-aortic balloon counterpulsation decreases the afterload without changing the mean arterial pressure and augments diastolic perfusion pressure. Although some patients survive without further therapy, most gain only temporary benefit unless myocardial revascularization or correction of mechanical defects is undertaken. Contraindications for use include aortic dissection, aortic regurgitation, severe peripheral vascular disease, thrombocyto-

TABLE 6. **Pharmacologic Treatment for Acute Ventricular Dysfunction**

Drug	Dose	Side Effects
Furosemide (Lasix)	20–160 mg IV	Hypokalemia, hypomagnesemia
Bumetanide (Bumex)	1–3 mg IV	Nausea, cramps
Nitroglycerin	10 mcg/min increased by 10 mcg every 10 min	Headache, hypotension, tolerance
Nitroprusside (Nipride)	10 mcg/min IV increased by 5 mcg every 10 min	Hypotension, cyanide toxicity
Dobutamine (Dobutrex)	5–15 mcg/kg/min IV	Tolerance
Dopamine (Intropin)	2–20 mcg/kg/min IV	Increased oxygen demand
Norepinephrine (Levophed)	2–16 mcg/min IV	Peripheral and visceral vasoconstriction
Amrinone (Inocor)	0.75 mg/kg over 2 min IV, then 5–10 mcg/kg/min	Thrombocytopenia
Milrinone (Primacor)	50 mcg/kg over 10 min IV, then 0.375–0.75 mcg/kg/min	Ventricular arrhythmia

penia, and marked arrhythmias that interfere with the QRS complex triggering of the inflation-deflation sequence.

Percutaneous cardiopulmonary bypass can be used to initiate extracorporeal membrane oxygenation. Experimental devices include the Hemopump, a catheter-mounted transvalvular left ventricular assist device, and retrograde coronary sinus counterpulsation. Left ventricular assist devices or the total artificial heart can also be used, usually as a bridge to cardiac transplantation, but complication rates are high.

Angioplasty

Coronary angioplasty is the treatment of choice for patients with cardiogenic shock. Mortality rates of 80% despite pharmacologic therapy and intra-aortic balloon counterpulsation are reduced to about 50% when angioplasty is employed. No other interventions have been shown to be lifesaving. The role of angioplasty in patients with congestive heart failure and pulmonary edema needs to be defined, because thrombolytic therapy appears relatively ineffective.

Surgery

Surgery is the primary therapy for ventricular septal defect, free wall rupture, or papillary muscle rupture. These complications typically occur in the first week after MI, often are associated with abrupt onset of heart failure, and can quickly be diagnosed by echocardiography. Mortality rates with medical therapy exceed 80%. Coronary revascularization or heart transplantation is also an option for treating cardiogenic shock.

ARRHYTHMIAS AND CONDUCTION ABNORMALITIES

General Measures

Continuous ECG monitoring for 48 to 72 hours in a CCU setting and then for 3 to 7 days in a step-down unit is performed to detect any arrhythmia or conduction abnormality. Persistent sinus tachycardia is the most ominous early arrhythmia, because it suggests low cardiac output, most ominous unless it is due to hypovolemia, pain, anxiety, hypoxia, or infection. Sinus bradycardia occurs in 25% of patients and is usually benign.

Ventricular premature beats (VPBs), couplets, triplets, multiform VPBs, and short runs of nonsustained ventricular tachycardia are common and generally do not require treatment, although lidocaine can be used to suppress them. Attempts at long-term suppression of these arrhythmias with antiarrhythmics has increased mortality. Sustained ventricular tachycardia with adequate systemic pressure can be treated pharmacologically, but direct current (DC) cardioversion is required when hypotension develops. Prompt DC defibrillation is indicated for ventricular fibrillation.

Atrial fibrillation, atrial flutter, and supraventricular tachycardia occur in approximately 10% of patients. The heart rate should be controlled pharmacologically to decrease myocardial oxygen demand if the arrhythmia cannot be pharmacologically converted. Patients with hemodynamic compromise should be treated with DC cardioversion.

Second- or third-degree atrioventricular block develops in 10 to 15% of patients. Mobitz Type I (Wenckebach) second-degree block is characterized by progressive PR interval prolongation, followed by a nonconducted P wave, then a normally conducted P wave with a short PR interval. Mobitz Type II second-degree block is present when nonconducted P waves follow a constant PR interval. Mobitz Type II block or bundle branch block (10 to 20% incidence) suggests larger infarct size and increased in-hospital and 1-year mortality.

Countershock

Two-thirds of the deaths due to MI occur within 1 hour of symptom onset and are usually due to ventricular fibrillation. As many as 40% of patients can survive to hospital discharge if basic life support is initiated within 4 minutes and defibrillation occurs within 8 minutes. More realistically, less than 10% of patients with cardiac arrest outside of the hospital survive because of delayed treatment. In contrast, defibrillation in a monitored situation should always be initiated as quickly as possible without intervening basic life support and is successful in the great majority of patients. A shock of 200 joules is usually sufficient. If not, subsequent shocks at 300 and 360 joules should follow. When ventricular tachycardia or supraventricular tachyarrhythmias are being treated by countershock, the defibrillator must first be placed in the synchronized mode. Tachyarrhythmias associated with hemodynamic compromise should always be treated with countershock instead of pharmacologic agents. Because fine ventricular fibrillation may be difficult to distinguish from asystole, countershock should always be attempted in a pulseless, unconscious patient.

Drug Therapy

Atropine. Atropine (Table 7) enhances the rate of discharge of the sinus node and facilitates AV conduction by reducing vagal tone. Sinus bradycardia or Mobitz I second-degree AV block need not be treated when patients are stable. However, atropine should be used in patients with associated hypotension, frequent ventricular ectopy, or heart failure. Atropine should not be used for Mobitz II second-degree AV block, because it may enhance the block, and is rarely useful in third-degree AV block. Doses of less than 0.5 mg may paradoxically result in bradycardia and depressed AV conduction secondary to central reflex stimulation of the vagus nerve or to a parasympathomimetic effect on the heart. Sinus tachycardia may increase ischemia, and rarely ven-

TABLE 7. **Pharmacologic Treatment for Bradycardia and Atrioventricular Block**

Drug	Dose	Side Effects
Atropine	0.5 mg IV q 5 min to maximum of 2.0 mg	Hallucinations, fever, VT-VF, urinary retention, acute angle glaucoma
Isoproterenol	2–10 mcg/min IV titrated to HR	Tachycardia, hypotension, increased O_2 demand, arrhythmia
Aminophylline	300–400 mg IV over 15–30 min	Tachycardia, atrial arrhythmia, CNS toxicity

Abbreviations: VT-VF = ventricular tachycardia and ventricular fibrillation; HR = heart rate; CNS = central nervous system.

tricular tachycardia and fibrillation are stimulated, so patients should be closely monitored.

Isoproterenol. Isoproterenol (Isuprel) can be used temporarily to stabilize patients with bradycardia resistant to atropine, or patients with torsades de pointes ventricular tachycardia while preparations are being made to insert a temporary pacemaker for overdrive pacing. Long-term infusions are not recommended because isoproterenol increases the metabolic demands of the heart, may increase infarct size, and is arrhythmogenic.

Aminophylline. Whereas Mobitz I second-degree AV block within 6 hours of symptom onset occurs secondary to increased vagal tone, later AV block may be mediated by increased concentrations of adenosine in the AV node released by the ischemic insult. Aminophylline (a competitive antagonist of adenosine) may be successful in treating atropine-resistant block, obviating the need for isoproterenol or temporary pacing.

Beta-Adrenergic Blocking Agents. Beta blockers are attractive agents for controlling supraventricular arrhythmias because they also have anti-ischemic effects (Table 8). Although its dosing schedule is somewhat complex, esmolol (Brevibloc) is especially useful in the intensive care setting because it has a half-life of only 10 minutes.

Calcium Channel Blockers. Verapamil (Calan, Isoptin) and diltiazem (Cardizem) can quickly control the ventricular rate in atrial fibrillation and are effective during periods of high adrenergic tone because they increase the AV node refractory period instead of working through indirect vagal effects as digitalis does. Verapamil is very effective in converting paroxysmal supraventricular tachycardia. Special caution is in order if beta blockers are also being used because both increase the risk for heart failure, hypotension, bradycardia, and heart block.

Digitalis. Digitalis can be used to control the ventricular rate during atrial fibrillation or to suppress atrial arrhythmias in patients with left ventricular dysfunction who may not tolerate beta-adrenergic blockers or calcium channel blockers. Disadvantages include a slow onset of action, an inability to control the rate during periods of enhanced sympathetic activity, a low threshold for toxicity, and a potential to increase myocardial oxygen demand, infarct size, or ventricular arrhythmias. Patients with renal insufficiency or concomitant therapy with quinidine, verapamil, or amiodarone require a downward adjustment of the maintenance dose because of decreased renal clearance.

Adenosine. Adenosine (Adenocard) has some advantages over beta blockers, verapamil, and digitalis for treating paroxysmal supraventricular tachycardia, but is relatively expensive. Its half-life is less than 20 seconds, so side effects are transient. Success rates of approximately 95% have been noted.

Lidocaine. Lidocaine is the agent of choice for complex ventricular ectopy, ventricular tachycardia, or ventricular fibrillation (see earlier).

Procainamide. Procainamide is the drug of second choice when lidocaine is unsuccessful in treating ventricular arrhythmias (Table 9). It also is effective

TABLE 8. **Pharmacologic Treatment for Supraventricular Arrhythmias**

Drug	Dose	Side Effects
Beta blockers		CHF, bronchospasm, hypotension, bradycardia, AV block
Esmolol (Brevibloc)	500 mcg/kg IV over 1 min repeated before each upward titration 50 mcg/kg min infusion increased by 50 mcg/kg every 5 min up to 250 mcg/kg/min	
Propranolol (Inderal)	1 mg/min IV up to 0.1 mg/kg	
Metoprolol (Lopressor)	5 mg IV over 2 min; repeated every 5 min × 2	
Atenolol (Tenormin)	5 mg IV over 2 min; repeated in 10 min	
Verapamil (Calan, Isoptin)	5 mg IV over 2 min, then 1–2 mg q 2 min up to 20 mg	CHF, hypotension, heart block, bradycardia
Diltiazem (Cardizem)	0.25 mg/kg IV over 2 min, then 5–15 mg/h	CHF, hypotension, heart block, bradycardia
Digoxin	0.5 mg IV over 5 min, then 0.25 mg IV q 4 h to 1 mg	Ventricular arrhythmia, heart block, increased infarct size
Procainamide (Pronestyl)	20 mg/min IV to 1 g, then 2–6 mg/min	Hypotension
Adenosine (Adenocard)	6 mg IV, then 12 mg IV if not effective	Flushing, chest pain, dyspnea, sinus pauses

Abbreviations: CHF = congestive heart failure; AV = atrioventricular.

TABLE 9. **Pharmacologic Treatment for Ventricular Arrhythmias**

Drug	Dose	Side Effects
Isoproterenol	2–20 mcg/min to HR higher than 90 bpm	Arrhythmia, increased infarct size, hypotension
Lidocaine	1 mg/kg IV, 1–4 mg/min infusion, 0.5 mg/kg IV q 10 min × 1–6	Nausea, numbness, confusion, slurred speech, respiratory depression, tremors, seizures, sinus arrest
Procainamide	20 mg/min IV to 1 g, then 2–6 mg/min	Hypotension
Bretylium	5–10 mg/kg IV every 15–30 min to 30 mg/kg, then 1–2 mg/min infusion	Tachycardia, hypertension, hypotension
Amiodarone (Cordarone)	600 mg orally × 4 daily × 10 days, then 200–400 mg PO daily	Hypotension, myocardial depression, bradycardia, conduction block
Magnesium	2 gm over 5 min, 8 gm over 24 h	Flushing, bradycardia

Abbreviations: HR = heart rate; bpm = beats per minute; IV = intravenous push.

in converting atrial fibrillation to sinus rhythm after rate control has been achieved with either beta blockers, calcium channel blockers, or digoxin. Downward titration of the drug is necessary when renal insufficiency is present.

Bretylium. Bretylium is used when ventricular tachycardia or fibrillation is refractory to lidocaine and procainamide therapy. Transient hypertension and sinus tachycardia may be followed by orthostatic hypotension. These effects are due to an initial release of norepinephrine from the sympathetic ganglia and later postganglionic blockade.

Amiodarone. Amiodarone (Cordarone) is the drug of last resort for refractory ventricular arrhythmias. It is approved only for oral use in the United States but has been effective when used intravenously.

Temporary Pacing

Prophylactic pacemaker insertion should be considered in patients with Mobitz II second-degree AV block, new-onset left bundle branch block, or new-onset bilateral bundle branch block (right bundle with left anterior or posterior hemiblock, or alternating bundle branch block) because of their frequent progression to third-degree block. Therapeutic indications include asystole, symptomatic sinus bradyarrhythmias unresponsive to atropine, symptomatic second- or third-degree AV block in inferior MI, and any second-or third-degree AV block in anterior MI. Additionally, overdrive pacing can occasionally convert ventricular tachycardia, inhibit torsades de pointes, or convert atrial flutter and paroxysmal supraventricular tachycardia to sinus rhythm.

CONCLUSION

The morbidity and mortality of MI are directly related to the duration of symptoms. Thus, the diagnosis of MI and the initiation of reperfusion therapy in appropriate candidates should be approached with the same sense of urgency directed toward major trauma victims. Administering thrombolytic therapy and aspirin saves 5 lives per 100 treated patients. Using accelerated tPA instead of streptokinase therapy saves 1 additional life, and 1 life is saved for every hour the time to treatment is reduced. Other interventions directed toward alleviating acute myocardial ischemia include oxygen, sublingual nitroglycerin, morphine, heparin, and intravenous nitroglycerin therapy. Appropriate patients may also benefit from beta-adrenergic blockers, intra-aortic balloon counterpulsation, and revascularization with either coronary angioplasty or coronary artery bypass graft surgery. Interventions directed toward assessing and treating acute left ventricular dysfunction include invasive hemodynamic monitoring and echocardiography; maximizing the preload; correcting blood gas, serum electrolyte, acid-base, or hemoglobin abnormalities; controlling the heart rate; and maintaining AV conduction. Pharmacologic agents to consider include diuretics, nitroglycerin, nitroprusside, dobutamine, dopamine, norepinephrine, and amrinone or milrinone. Support devices, coronary angioplasty, and cardiac surgery are also occasionally needed. Interventions directed toward preventing or treating arrhythmias and conduction disturbances include atropine, isoproterenol, beta blocker, calcium channel blocker, digitalis, adenosine, lidocaine, procainamide, bretylium, and amiodarone therapy; countershock; and cardiac pacing.

CARE AFTER MYOCARDIAL INFARCTION

method of
REGIS A. DESILVA, M.B., and
NATHANIEL C. EDWARDS, M.D.
Harvard Medical School
Boston, Massachusetts

In the United States, of the 1.5 million people who suffer acute myocardial infarction (MI) each year, 500,000, die within 1 year of the acute event; 412,000 have coronary angiography performed; 121,500 undergo coronary artery bypass grafting; and 97,500 undergo balloon angioplasty. Of the 1.3 million survivors of MI annually, only 150,000 enter a formal cardiac rehabilitation program. The majority of cardiac rehabilitation programs in current use employ a three-pronged approach that includes a graduated exercise program, education in dietary and lifestyle changes, and psychological and vocational counseling. Such programs are of proven benefit in improving exercise capacity and return to work and in reducing mortality. Risk-reduction programs involving exercise and modification of plasma lipoproteins through diet and drug therapy may also retard the progression of coronary atherosclerosis.

EXERCISE TRAINING

Supervised exercise training is the cornerstone of all cardiac rehabilitation programs. The beneficial effects of exercise training include an increase in arterial oxygen saturation and improved oxygen uptake by peripheral tissues. The improved efficiency of oxygen transport and utilization by peripheral tissues result in a decrease in the cardiac output required to perform a certain level of exercise. The ability to perform a greater level of activity at a given cardiac output is probably responsible for the decrease in anginal episodes after exercise training.

On the first hospital day in patients with uncomplicated MI, Phase I rehabilitation begins with range-of-motion exercises and progresses through assumption of an upright posture twice a day to slow walking. Heart rate, blood pressure, and the electrocardiogram (ECG) are monitored during exercise. Phase I rehabilitation is aimed primarily at preventing the physical deconditioning and decrease in plasma volume that occur with bed rest. Early mobilization also reduces the risk of development of thromboembolic complications and autonomic dysfunction. Furthermore, early Phase I rehabilitation provides an opportunity for the identification of early postinfarction patients with exercise-induced left ventricular dysfunction, angina, or arrhythmias, all of which may merit further evaluation. However, even patients with significant left ventricular dysfunction who are clinically stable and have no evidence of active ischemia on submaximal and symptom-limited exercise testing are candidates for exercise training.

Phase II cardiac rehabilitation commences after hospital discharge, following successful completion of a submaximal exercise stress test. The test is usually performed immediately before or within 1 week of hospital discharge. During Phase II cardiac rehabilitation, patients perform low-intensity aerobic exercise under monitoring. Patients usually perform exercise training in 1-hour sessions three times a week. Thirty minutes of the exercise period is devoted to warm-up and cool-down activities and 30 minutes to aerobic training.

The intensity of the training session is based, in large part, upon the results of the submaximal exercise test mentioned above. Because of baseline interindividual variability and frequent use of drugs that reduce heart rate in cardiac patients, the use of age-predicted maximal heart rate (220 minus age) to determine exercise intensity is not recommended. The Borg scale for rating perceived exertion, ranging from 6 (no exertion) to 20 (heavy exertion), is the other major tool used in determining the intensity of the training session. Although there is some interindividual variability, there is a nearly linear relationship between heart rate achieved and rating of perceived exertion, and ratings are consistent from test to test. Thus, the rating of perceived exertion is very useful in translating the degree of exertion during training sessions to those during daily activities at home. The initial intensity of training is 50 to 70% of maximal heart rate or a rating of perceived exertion of 12 or 13 on the Borg scale. The duration and intensity of exercise are gradually increased as tolerance improves.

The 1995 American Heart Association (AHA) exercise classification for activity and monitoring of post-MI patients depending on the risk profile is shown in Table 1. Medical supervision is recommended with ECG monitoring for the first 6 to 12 sessions in patients known to have cardiac disease who may be at risk for complications during exercise. Medical supervision is not necessary for Class A subjects (apparently healthy people); Class B patients require medical supervision only for the prescription session if there are no symptoms during that evaluation. A symptom-limited treadmill exercise test is performed approximately 6 weeks after hospital discharge and is used in risk stratification as well as in advancing the patient's exercise prescription. The target heart rate is gradually increased to 70 to 85% of maximal heart rate, or a score of 14 to 15 on the Borg scale. Training at heart rates above 85% of maximal heart

TABLE 1. **Medical Activity Classification for Exercise**

Class A Apparently Healthy

Activity guidelines:	No restrictions
ECG and BP monitoring:	None
Medical supervision:	None

Class B Known Stable Cardiac Disease

Activity guidelines:	Individualized with exercise prescription
ECG and BP monitoring:	Usually 6 to 12 sessions
Medical supervision:	During prescription session; self-monitoring during exercise

Class C Moderate to High Risk for Complications During Exercise or Unable to Self-Monitor or Understand Recommendations

Activity guidelines:	As for Class B
ECG and BP monitoring:	As for Class B
Medical supervision:	For all sessions or until safety is established

Class D Unstable Disease with Activity Restriction

Activity guidelines:	No activity recommended for conditioning until patient is treated

Abbreviations: ECG = electrocardiogram; BP = blood pressure.
From Fletcher GF, Balady G, Froelicher VF, et al: Exercise standards. A statement for healthcare professionals from the American Heart Association. Circulation 91:580–615, 1995. Reproduced with permission. Circulation. Copyright 1995 American Heart Association.

rate in post-MI patients has been associated with increased mortality and is therefore not recommended.

In many cardiac rehabilitation programs, moderate amounts of strength training are introduced 6 weeks after hospital discharge after successful completion of the symptom-limited exercise test. Training with light weights has been proved to be safe in the absence of uncontrolled blood pressure or arrhythmia in patients with an ejection fraction of greater than 35% who are able to exercise to a level of 6 to 8 metabolic equivalents on the symptom-limited exercise test. The American College of Sports Training recommends that 8 to 10 resistive exercises of the major muscle groups be included in the rehabilitation program 2 days per week. Strength training has been shown to reduce the degree of blood pressure elevation at a given submaximal workload and to raise anginal threshold during daily activities. Strength training is of particular importance to patients whose occupation involves physical labor.

Three months after discharge, or after Phase II is completed, patients enter Phase III of cardiac rehabilitation. The goal of this phase is to improve endurance, further modify risk factors, and develop a lifelong pattern of regular aerobic exercise. Phase III cardiac rehabilitation may be undertaken in community programs or at home. Periodic exercise testing is performed for purposes of risk stratification, to evaluate the effectiveness of the exercise program, to advance the exercise prescription, and to provide motivation for patients whose exercise tolerance has improved. Close follow-up by medical personnel by telephone contact and during office visits is important in aiding patients to continue regular exercise and thereby maintain the benefits accrued during the first two phases of cardiac rehabilitation.

DRUG THERAPY

Pharmacologic therapy with antiplatelet agents and beta-adrenergic blocking drugs, and with angiotensin-converting enzyme (ACE) inhibitors in patients with a left ventricular ejection fraction of less than 40%, reduces mortality after MI. Large clinical trials and meta-analyses of smaller trials show a consistent benefit of aspirin therapy after MI. Overall mortality is reduced 15 to 25%, and nonfatal stroke and reinfarction are reduced 30 to 50%, with little to no increase in major bleeding episodes. Oral anticoagulants of the warfarin class confer similar benefit. Overall mortality is reduced by approximately 25%, and nonfatal reinfarction and stroke are reduced 35 to 55%. However, oral anticoagulant therapy has shown a fourfold increase in major bleeding episodes compared with placebo. Despite what appears to be equal efficacy between aspirin and oral anticoagulant therapy, aspirin therapy is currently preferred because of a lower rate of bleeding complications.

Beta-adrenergic blocking agents have been shown to improve survival after MI. A review of the 15 largest long-term beta-blocker prevention trials shows a 22% overall reduction in total mortality, 20% in nonfatal reinfarction, and 33% in sudden death. Patients with left ventricular dysfunction or ventricular arrhythmias and those over 60 years of age appear to derive the greatest benefit from postinfarction beta-blocker therapy. The mechanisms by which beta blockers benefit the postinfarction patient probably include effects such as a reduction in myocardial oxygen demand, antiplatelet effects, antiarrhythmic effects, and a reduction in rates of rupture of atherosclerotic plaque. Selective and nonselective beta blockers as well as those with intrinsic sympathomimetic activity confer similar benefit. Based on current data, it is recommended that beta-blocker therapy be initiated before hospital discharge and continued for at least 2 years.

ACE inhibitors should be considered for all postinfarction patients with ejection fractions below 40%, whether or not there are symptoms or signs of congestive heart failure. In patients with MI and left ventricular ejection fraction of less than 40% but without clinical evidence of congestive heart failure, captopril (Capoten) produces a 17% reduction in overall mortality and a 19% reduction in hospitalizations for exacerbation of congestive heart failure. A similar reduction in mortality in patients with ejection fractions below 30% is seen in patients treated with enalapril (Vasotec). Questions remain to be answered regarding the optimal time to initiate therapy, the duration of therapy, and the possibility of differences in efficacy among the various agents in this class. For patients who cannot tolerate ACE inhibitors, the combination of the vasodilator hydralazine (Apresoline) and nitrate therapy appears to improve symptoms of congestive heart failure without increasing mortality.

RISK FACTOR MODIFICATION

Epidemiologic observations suggest that smoking doubles both total mortality and the risk of recurrent infarction and sudden death in post-MI patients. The risk of recurrent MI decreases immediately on smoking cessation and within 3 years reaches that of survivors of MI who have never smoked. The mechanisms by which smoking increases cardiac risk probably include increased platelet activation, decreased coronary and collateral flow reserve, and increased levels of plasma fibrinogen. Tobacco dependence has psychological and physiologic components, both of which must be addressed to optimize smoking cessation rates. Factors that have been found to be associated with low success rates postinfarction include the amount of tobacco consumption before infarction, increased age, higher rates of alcohol consumption, high anxiety levels, and a low sense of personal control over life events. Smoking cessation rates are highest among patients who receive strong and repeated advice to quit smoking from health care professionals. The nicotine withdrawal syndrome plays an important role in early failures and can be diminished in severity through the use of nicotine-containing gum or transdermal nicotine delivery systems.

Plasma lipid and lipoprotein profiles have a strong correlation with the development and progression of coronary atherosclerosis and with cardiac event rates. Secondary prevention is augmented by improvement in plasma lipid and lipoprotein profiles through diet, exercise, and drug therapy, as these measures lead to a reduction in cardiac event rates, slowing of progression of atherosclerotic lesions, and, in some cases, regression of coronary atherosclerotic lesions. Guidelines for diet and lipid-lowering therapy have been published by the National Cholesterol Education Program (NCEP) and the AHA. In general, postinfarction patients should follow an NCEP or AHA Step II diet in which daily cholesterol intake is less than 200 mg with less than 7% of total calories from saturated fat. For those patients with a low-density lipoprotein (LDL) cholesterol level greater than 130 mg per dL after maximal dietary therapy, drug therapy should be initiated to reduce the LDL-cholesterol level to less than 100 mg per dL. Weight reduction through diet and exercise also aid in blood pressure control in hypertensive patients and in glucose control in diabetics.

PSYCHOLOGICAL AND VOCATIONAL COUNSELING

Up to 30% of survivors of acute MI suffer from moderate to severe depression or anxiety. These disorders and overprotection by family members can inhibit the patient's return to normal domestic, vocational, and sexual function. In addition, depression, low morale and psychological distress are predictive of mortality following MI. Initial experience with patients receiving psychological interventions and support following MI appears to show improvement in return to work and sexual activity, greater domestic independence, and lower cardiac mortality.

Although invasive approaches to angina, which include angioplasty and coronary bypass surgery, have a valid place in management, their effect in reducing overall cardiac mortality is not large. Moreover, such approaches to the long-term management of the post-MI patient are associated with higher risks and costs. Despite information derived from pooled studies that indicate that patients in medically prescribed and supervised exercise programs show a 20 to 25% reduction in mortality, only about 15% of survivors of MI enter such programs. This low rate of enrollment may reflect factors such as low patient motivation, lack of physician referrals, financial and logistic considerations, and a lack of understanding of the benefits of such treatment. Secondary prevention of MI is extremely important since a comprehensive approach that includes an exercise prescription, dietary counseling, and vocational counseling coupled with appropriate beta blocker, aspirin, or ACE inhibitor therapy produces a large benefit in reducing all-cause and cardiovascular mortality. Thus, the principles of management for the post-MI patient outlined here have much to recommend them.

PERICARDITIS

method of
JOSEP GUINDO, M.D., and
ANTONIO BAYÉS DE LUNA, M.D., Ph.D.
Hospital de la Santa Creu i Sant Pau
Universitat Autònoma de Barcelona
Barcelona, Spain

Pericarditis is a relatively common disease and a frequent cause for consulting primary care physicians. Pericarditis should be kept in mind in the differential diagnosis of all chest pain syndromes. Although it is generally benign, hazardous complications may appear during the natural course of the disease. Of note, pericarditis may be the first manifestation of life-threatening disease (dissecting aneurysm). In this chapter we will focus on acute pericarditis, but sometimes (e.g., constrictive pericarditis, cardiac tamponade, congenital defects, etc.) pericardial disease may have an insidious presentation.

The pericardium is a fibrous structure that is attached to the heart in the mediastinum. It is composed of two layers, the parietal and the visceral pericardium, constituting a sac that normally contains up to 50 mL of clear fluid. The main functions of the pericardium are fixing the heart in position and controlling excessive cardiac motion with changes in body position; reducing the friction between the heart and surrounding organs; and acting as a barrier against extension of malignancy or infection from organs contiguous to the heart. Moreover, the pericardium may play a role in the distribution of hydrostatic forces on the heart, the prevention of acute cardiac dilatation (e.g., during acute mitral insufficiency), and the diastolic coupling of the two ventricles. Nevertheless, despite these functions the pericardium is not essential to life; congenital absence or surgical removal of the pericardium usually is not followed by adverse consequences.

ACUTE PERICARDITIS

Acute inflammation of the pericardium is characterized by chest pain, fever, pericardial friction rub, and electrocardiographic abnormalities. It is found in 2 to 6% of postmortem studies and in about 1 in 1000 hospital admissions, thus suggesting that many episodes are unrecognized clinically.

Etiology

Acute pericarditis may be caused by any one of a number of agents or circumstances listed in Table 1. The relative frequency of causes of pericarditis depends on the clinical setting. For primary care physicians and in the emergency rooms of community hospitals, idiopathic (presumably viral) pericarditis is responsible for most (more than 90%) cases. Pericarditis related to malignancy, acquired immune deficiency syndrome, uremia, connective tissue diseases, or other systemic diseases is more common in tertiary hospitals.

Diagnosis

The diagnosis of acute pericarditis is based mainly on the clinical history (chest pain, dyspnea, cough), physical

TABLE 1. Causes of Pericarditis

1. *Idiopathic* (nonspecific)
2. *Viral infections* (Coxsackie virus, adenovirus, echovirus, mumps virus, infectious mononucleosis, varicella, hepatitis, acquired immune deficiency syndrome)
3. *Tuberculosis*
4. *Acute bacterial infections* (pneumococcus, staphylococcus, Haemophilus influenzae, tularemia, meningococcemia, gonococcal septicemia, infective endocarditis or other septicemias)
5. *Fungal infections* (Candida, histoplasmosis, blastomycosis, coccidioidomycosis, sporotrichosis)
6. *Other unusual infections* (toxoplasmosis, amebiasis, mycoplasma infections, echinococcosis, Lyme disease)
7. *Malignancy* (lung cancer, breast cancer, melanoma, leukemia, lymphoma, Hodgkin's disease)
8. *Radiation injury*
9. *Uremia* (de novo, dialysis-associated)
10. *Inflammatory disease states* (systemic lupus erythematosus, rheumatoid arthritis, scleroderma, polyarteritis nodosa, mixed connective tissue disease, Wegener's granulomatosis, acute rheumatic fever, sarcoidosis, amyloidosis, inflammatory bowel disease, Whipple's disease, temporal arteritis, Behçet's disease)
11. *Drug reactions* (hydralazine, procainamide, phenytoin, isoniazid, phenylbutazone, dantrolene, doxorubicin, methysergide, cyclophosphamide, penicillin)
12. *Trauma* (chest trauma, thoracic surgery, insertion of pacemaker or other implantable devices, diagnostic cardiac catheterization)
13. *Dissecting aortic aneurysm*
14. *Acute myocardial infarction*
15. *Delayed postmyocardial or postpericardial injury syndromes* (postmyocardial infarction [Dressler] syndrome, postpericardiotomy syndrome and other postcardiac trauma syndromes)
16. *Miscellaneous* (myxedema, chylopericardium, esophageal–pericardial fistula, pancreatic–pericardial fistula)

examination (pericardial friction rub, fever) and electrocardiographic abnormalities (diffuse ST-segment elevation).

Chest pain is the most frequent symptom of acute pericarditis. Pain, generally described as dull or oppressive, is usually localized in the retrosternal and left precordial regions and frequently radiates to the scapular region and neck. In most cases the onset is insidious, persisting for hours or days, is aggravated by lying down, coughing, or deep inspiration, and is eased by sitting up or leaning forward. Differentiating chest pain secondary to pericarditis from chest pain secondary to myocardial ischemia is very important (Table 2).

Pleurisy frequently is present, which may explain the pleuritic nature of chest discomfort. It is not exertional in character.

Dyspnea may be related in part to the need to breathe shallowly to avoid chest pain. Nevertheless, the presence of severe pericardial effusion must be ruled out.

Other symptoms such as weight loss, cough, sputum production, or arthralgia may be related to the underlying systemic disease such as tuberculosis, malignancy, uremia, or inflammatory disease states.

The *physical examination* may reveal pericardial friction rub, fever, signs of right heart failure (if cardiac tamponade is present), and other signs related to the specific disorder associated with acute pericarditis (Table 1). In the auscultation, heart sounds may be muffled if significant pericardial effusion is present.

Pericardial friction rub is a scratching, grating, high-pitched sound found in most patients with acute pericarditis. Classically, it has three components related to (1) cardiac motion during atrial systole (heard before the first sound), (2) ventricular systole, and (3) rapid ventricular filling (early diastole). It is often transient and evanescent and may vary with breathing or changes in body position, so it is sometimes difficult to hear. It is important that the diaphragm of the stethoscope be firmly applied to the chest (avoiding the noise caused by the movement of skin or chest hair) and that the physician auscultate the patient in several body positions.

Fever, if present, is generally low-grade and transient. Occasionally, fever may be high-grade and persistent, but in these cases secondary forms of pericarditis should be investigated.

Pericardial effusion frequently is found in patients with acute pericarditis, but it is generally mild and rarely causes cardiac compression. In patients with acute pericarditis, the presence of sinus tachycardia, jugular distention, pulsus paradoxus (inspiratory decrease in the amplitude of the palpated pulse), and signs of low cardiac output, suggests cardiac tamponade. In the extreme cases, circulatory collapse may develop quickly.

Serial *electrocardiograms* are very useful, not only to confirm the diagnosis of acute pericarditis, but also to rule out other important causes of acute chest pain (e.g., myocardial infarction, pulmonary embolism). Electrocardiographic abnormalities are present in about 90% of patients with acute pericarditis. They may appear hours or days after the onset of pericardial pain. Diffuse, upwardly concave ST-segment elevation is highly suggestive of acute pericarditis. T waves are usually upright in the leads with ST-segment elevation. PR-segment depression is an early and characteristic sign of the disease that presents in up to 80% of cases. In typical cases, after several days the ST

TABLE 2. Differences Between Pericardial and Ischemic Chest Pain

Pain Characteristics	Pericarditis	Angina or Infarct
Location	Precordial	Precordial
Radiation	Scapular region	Shoulder, arms
Quality	Sharp, stabbing, dull ache	Pressure, burning oppression
Posture-related	Yes: aggravated by recumbency; relieved by leaning forward	No
Thoracic motion	Increased by breathing, rotating thorax	Not affected
Effort-related	No	Stable angina: usually Unstable angina or infarction: usually not
Time course	Hours or days	Minutes to hours
Pleurisy	Frequent	None
Fever	Common	Unusual
Related to concomitant disorders	May be	Rare

segment returns to baseline and T-wave inversion appears. Negative T waves may persist in the long-term follow-up or may return to normal after several months. Sinus tachycardia is relatively common. Premature beats or paroxysmal atrial tachyarrhythmias, particularly atrial fibrillation, are described. When voluminous pericardial effusion is present, low QRS voltage and electrical alternance are sometimes apparent.

The *chest x-ray film* is of little value in acute pericarditis but should be routinely obtained in all patients with acute chest pain. Cardiac enlargement or changes in the cardiac silhouette suggest large pericardial effusion. Chest x-ray examination may provide insight into the underlying cause of the pericarditis (e.g., tuberculosis, malignancy).

Echocardiography is the most sensitive and accurate method for detecting pericardial effusion. Whenever possible, it should be performed in all patients with pericarditis.

Blood tests demonstrate only nonspecific indicators of inflammation. Cardiac enzyme levels are generally normal.

When secondary forms of pericarditis are suspected, *specific diagnostic tests* may be indicated (e.g., blood cultures; a human immunodeficiency virus [HIV] test; serologic tests; measurements of immunofluorescent antibody titers, thyroid hormones levels, and blood urea nitrogen [BUN] and creatinine levels; a tuberculin skin test; a computed tomographic scan; and magnetic resonance imaging).

TREATMENT (Table 3)

Acute Pericarditis

Hospital admission for at least 48 to 72 hours is warranted for most patients with acute pericarditis. Initial management should include careful diagnostic evaluation, bed rest, relief of pain with nonsteroidal anti-inflammatory drugs (NSAIDs), and observation for possible complications. In most cases, pain responds well to oral *aspirin* (650 mg every 3 to 4 hours) or other NSAIDs such as *indomethacin* (Indocin) (25 to 50 mg orally every 6 hours) or *ibuprofen* (400 to 800 mg every 6 hours). In selected cases with severe pain, initial treatment with *meperidine* (50 to 100 mg intramuscularly) or *morphine* (8 to 15 mg intramuscularly) repeated every 4 hours may be justified. Empirical antibiotic therapy and oral anticoagulants should be avoided. *Antibiotics* are indicated only when purulent pericarditis is documented. Patients in whom *anticoagulants* are absolutely necessary (e.g., mechanical prosthetic heart valve) should receive continuous intravenous heparin. Most patients with uncomplicated idiopathic acute pericarditis can be discharged early (2 to 3 days after admission) (see Table 3).

In patients with severe, persistent chest pain and deterioration of general status who do not respond to a full dose of NSAIDs within 48 to 72 hours, *corticosteroids* may be required. However, there is substantial evidence that *corticosteroids increase the risk of recurrence* and steroid dependence. Thus, every effort should be made to avoid this therapy. When indicated, prednisone (20 to 40 mg every 8 hours) is recommended, with tapering-off of the dose until it is totally discontinued in about 3 weeks (see Table 3).

In the presence of mild to moderate *pericardial effusion,* physical examination and echocardiography

TABLE 3. Management of Acute Pericarditis

First Step
1. Hospital admission
2. Bed rest
3. Aspirin 650 mg PO q 3–4 h
   or
   Indomethacin 25 to 50 mg PO q 6 h
   or
   Ibuprofen 400 to 800 mg PO q 6 h
4. If severe chest pain:
   Meperidine 50 to 100 mg IM
   or
   Morphine 8 to 15 mg IM
5. Routine diagnostic assessment
6. Avoid corticosteroids, empirical antibiotic therapy, and oral anticoagulants
7. Uncomplicated idiopathic pericarditis:
   Early hospital discharge (48–72 h)
   Maintain nonsteroid treatment for 15 days

Second Step (Complications)
8. Prednisone if chest pain is severe and persistent:
   20–40 mg q 8 h for 5 days
   20 mg tid for 5 days
   10 mg daily for 5 days
   5 mg daily for 5 days
9. Significant pericardial effusion without cardiac compression:
   Frequent physical examination and echocardiography
   Pericardiocentesis *only* if purulent effusion is suspected
   Prednisone if persistent signs of inflammation are present
10. Cardiac tamponade:
    Intravenous fluid
    Inotropics: dobutamine, isoproterenol, norepinephrine
    Pericardiocentesis
    Pericardiotomy or pericardiectomy
11. Recurrent pericarditis:
    Nonsteroidal anti-inflammatory agents (similar to acute crisis)
    Colchicine (1 to 2 mg PO daily)
    Corticosteroids (similar to acute episode)
    Pericardiectomy, immunosuppressive agents
12. In all of these cases: careful and exhaustive diagnostic evaluation to rule out secondary forms of acute pericarditis

Third Step (Secondary Forms of Acute Pericarditis)
13. Specific evaluation and treatment according to cause

should be performed at short regular intervals. In the absence of cardiac tamponade, pericardiocentesis is not indicated unless bacterial pericarditis is suspected.

Cardiac tamponade is rarely seen in ambulatory patients with acute pericarditis, but it occurs in up to 15% of patients admitted to tertiary university hospitals. In these cases, patients should be referred to an intensive care unit for hemodynamic monitoring (thermodilution catheter). Hemodynamic support includes intravenous fluid administration and inotropic agents (dobutamine, isoproterenol, or norepinephrine). Pericardiocentesis should be scheduled and performed by trained personnel. Two-dimensional echocardiography may be very useful in guiding pericardiocentesis. An indwelling drainage catheter should be left in place for 24 to 48 hours. In case of recurrent tamponade, surgical resection (e.g., opening a pericardial window) is justified.

Recurrent Pericarditis

Recurrent pericarditis occurs in approximately 20% of patients. Most patients may be treated effectively by reintroducing NSAIDs in high doses. Occasionally, steroid administration is required. We have demonstrated that oral colchicine* (1 to 2 mg daily) may be very useful. Most of our patients received corticosteroids before colchicine therapy was initiated. In many patients, colchicine prevents new relapses. In the remaining patients, the interval between crises was lengthened and the dose of corticosteroids could be progressively reduced until withdrawal. In our series, no patient required surgical treatment or immunosuppressive agents. Our results have been confirmed by other authors. The drug is generally well tolerated and should be maintained for at least 6 to 12 months. In very selected cases, pericardiectomy has been attempted or immune suppressive agents have been administered. However, the results of such measures are controversial.

In all complicated cases, a careful diagnostic evaluation should be performed to identify specific causes of pericarditis (see Table 1). In this case, appropriate treatment depends on the cause (see Table 3). Discussion of these options exceeds the scope of this article.

PERIPHERAL ARTERIAL DISEASE

method of
JAMIE D. SANTILLI, M.D.,
STEVEN M. SANTILLI, M.D., Ph.D., and
JERRY GOLDSTONE, M.D.
University of California, San Francisco
San Francisco, California

Peripheral arterial disease is a common disorder affecting the lower extremities of many individuals in the Western world. It can be divided into subgroups consisting of occlusive disease, embolic disease, and aneurysmal disease. Although the vessels supplying the upper extremities can be affected, it is far more common for the infrarenal aorta and the vessels supplying the lower extremities to produce significant symptoms.

ATHEROSCLEROTIC OCCLUSIVE DISEASE OF THE LOWER EXTREMITIES

Atherosclerotic occlusive disease of the lower extremities is estimated to affect a large segment of the population. Approximately 10% of persons over the age of 70 years have symptoms of atherosclerotic occlusive disease of the lower extremities, and there are currently about 100,000 surgical procedures and another 100,000 interventional radiologic procedures performed in the United States each year for lower extremity ischemia. This disease process occurs primarily in elderly males who have other risk factors for atherosclerosis: hypertension, diabetes mellitus, cigarette smoking, or hypercholesterolemia. Patients may manifest symptoms of atherosclerosis in other vascular beds, most commonly the coronary or cerebral. There seems to be a genetic component to atherosclerotic occlusive disease of the lower extremities as well as a hydrodynamic component, in that this disease process is related to blood flow and its turbulence and is commonly found at branch points and bifurcations. This is a fortunate occurrence, because the disease tends to occur focally, which facilitates its treatment.

Symptoms of atherosclerotic occlusive disease of the lower extremities vary from intermittent claudication to pain at rest, nonhealing wounds, and gangrene. The most common symptom, claudication, is classically described as exercise-induced pain relieved by rest. The muscles most often affected are those in the calf. Patients with claudication typically describe a progression of their symptoms; they are able to walk shorter and shorter distances before experiencing pain, and longer periods of rest are required for complete recovery. In patients with more advanced disease, the symptom complex often includes ischemic pain at rest. This is described as a burning pain involving the toes and forefoot that awakens the patient at night and is relieved by dangling the feet over the side of the bed. It must be distinguished from night cramps that affect the foot and calves and are common in the same elderly patients. These patients may also have nonhealing wounds or areas of frank gangrene. Nonhealing wounds due to arterial occlusive disease are often painful, dry, clean wounds associated with little bleeding or granulation tissue. Gangrene commonly affects one or more toes and can be dry (mummified) or wet (infected).

Symptoms of atherosclerotic occlusive disease of the lower extremities depend on the segments of the arterial tree affected by disease. Patients with aorto-iliac occlusive disease present with symptoms first described by Dr. René Leriche in 1923. Intermittent claudication (usually involving the buttock and thigh), global atrophy of both lower limbs, some impairment in wound healing, and an inability to maintain a stable erection are consistent with a diagnosis of aortoiliac occlusive disease. Physical examination reveals absent or severely diminished pulses in both lower extremities beginning at the groin.

Patients with occlusive disease involving a femoral artery most commonly complain of calf claudication. These symptoms may worsen with time, but disease localized to the femoral artery does not commonly result in limb-threatening ischemia. Stenosis or occlusion of the superficial femoral artery is the most frequent pattern of arterial occlusive disease. Pulses distal to the femoral artery are diminished.

Diffuse tibial artery disease is most commonly found in patients with diabetes mellitus, but isolated short-segment tibial disease is rare. Most of these patients have more extensive disease extending distally to the pedal vessels and proximally to the aorta, femoral artery, or popliteal artery. Physical examination may reveal normal or diminished pulses in the groin and possibly the popliteal artery, with diminished or absent pedal pulses. The skin of the distal

---

*Not FDA-approved for this indication.

leg is shiny, thin, and hairless, and nail thickening may be present. Patients with severe limb-threatening ischemia—manifested by ischemic rest pain, non-healing wounds, or gangrene—almost always have occlusion or stenosis of multiple arterial segments. Single-level obstructions rarely produce symptoms of this severity.

The diagnosis of atherosclerotic occlusive disease is based on a careful history and physical examination, followed by appropriately indicated tests, varying from simple noninvasive evaluations to those of a more invasive nature. A reliable initial test to perform is Doppler segmental pressures, with calculation of the ankle-brachial index (ABI). This is a simple, quick, inexpensive, and noninvasive manner of assessing the location of occlusive lesions and their severity. Blood pressures are measured in the arm (brachial), proximal and distal thigh, proximal calf, and ankle. A blood pressure rise of less than 20 mmHg from the arm to the proximal thigh suggests significant aortoiliac occlusive disease. A pressure drop of more than 30 mmHg between any two pressures (cuffs) in the lower extremity is considered a sign of significant arterial occlusion. An ankle-brachial index of less than 0.85 is considered abnormal, between 0.5 and 0.75 is consistent with claudication, and a value less than 0.5 is indicative of severe ischemia. These measurements are unreliable in patients with calcified vessels (usually associated with diabetes mellitus), because blood pressures may be falsely elevated. In this setting, measurement of toe pressures can be valuable, because digital arteries are rarely calcified. A toe pressure less than 30 mmHg is consistent with severe ischemia. Arteriography may be indicated if the history and physical examination as well as the segmental pressures and indices suggest significant arterial occlusive disease that requires operative or interventional therapy. Arteriography has been the "gold standard" test with which all others have been compared. Angiography provides an accurate anatomic diagnosis and a road map to guide further therapy, but it is an invasive and expensive procedure and is associated with some risk. Therefore, a decision to treat the patient must be made prior to performing arteriography. In patients with renal failure, magnetic resonance angiography is now an alternative method for imaging the arteries of the lower extremity.

The decision to surgically treat a patient with arterial occlusive disease of the lower extremity is based on the nature and severity of presenting symptoms and knowledge of the natural history of claudication or limb-threatening ischemia. Intermittent claudication may not be a benign symptom, because a fair number of these patients go on to develop worsening ischemia. The risk of developing worsening symptoms must be weighed against the decreased long-term survival of patients with lower extremity occlusive disease. At the current time, the decision to treat patients with only claudication is made on an individual basis, taking into account overall patient well-being, severity of claudication, interference with lifestyle and activities of daily living, and estimated long-term survival. Usually the symptoms should be incapacitating or severely limiting before surgical intervention is recommended.

Amputation is often required in patients with limb-threatening ischemia unless some form of intervention is accomplished. Some patients with non-healing wounds and severe ischemia benefit from good wound-healing programs consisting of frequent dressing changes, antibiotics (if indicated), and wound protection with special shoes or braces. Surgical therapy, however, should not be dismissed and should be utilized in those patients with progressing gangrene, severe invasive infection, or failure to heal wounds with good medical therapy. All these recommendations need to be tempered with clinical judgment, taking into account operative morbidity and mortality.

Treatment for patients with atherosclerotic occlusive disease of the lower extremity varies from conservative medical management with an exercise program, drug therapy, and wound care to major aortic-based operative interventions. Patients with intermittent claudication who are well motivated may respond to a vigorous exercise program and risk factor modification, including cessation of cigarette smoking, control of diabetes and hypertension, and lowering of serum lipids. In some patients with mild to moderate claudication, pentoxifylline (Trental) has been shown to be effective therapy, allowing patients to increase walking distances. Patients with more advanced degrees of claudication (those not responding to conservative management of claudication, or those with limb-threatening ischemia) require intervention. Most patients with aortoiliac occlusive disease and some with femoropopliteal disease may be adequately treated with the minimally invasive techniques of angioplasty and/or stent placement. Patients with more extensive aortoiliac lesions requiring operation are best treated by an aorto-bifemoral bypass. Those patients with femoral, popliteal, and tibial disease can be treated with a bypass utilizing a reversed or in situ saphenous vein. Long-term clinical success with these procedures, as measured by graft patency and limb salvage rates, is quite good, but results may vary with distal bypasses, depending on vein quality and the extent of distal (outflow) disease. Operative intervention can usually be safely performed in these patients, with morbidity and mortality rates varying between 1 and 5%.

EMBOLIC OCCLUSIVE DISEASE OF THE LOWER EXTREMITIES

Acute embolic occlusion of the aorta or lower extremity vessels is a relatively rare cause of leg ischemia. The most frequent source of emboli is the heart, followed by the aorta and superficial femoral arteries. These emboli most commonly lodge in the femoral artery (40%), popliteal artery (20%), and aorta (10%). The symptom complex associated with acute embolic occlusion of a lower extremity artery is classically described as the five p's; pain, pallor, paresthesias, paralysis, and pulselessness. The pain is usually described as quite severe and is not relieved by large doses of narcotics. Patient mortality is 10 to 15%, usually due to underlying cardiac disease. If no therapy is instituted, further embolization commonly occurs, as well as limb loss from the acute occlusion.

The diagnosis can usually be made by history and physical examination. The clinical presentation of an acute embolic event is sometimes difficult to distinguish from acute thrombosis, but acute thrombosis usually occurs in a vessel with significant stenosis. These patients usually give a history of symptoms consistent with arterial occlusion.

After a diagnosis of acute arterial embolus is made, no further diagnostic tests are warranted if there appears to be critical ischemia of the limb (alterations in nerve function, including paresthesias and paralysis). With lesser degrees of ischemia and a question as to the location of the arterial occlusion, arteriography is the diagnostic procedure of choice.

Treatment most often includes use of a balloon catheter to remove emboli and all subsequently developed thrombus, with restoration of flow to the lower extremity. These procedures can usually be done under local anesthesia with an 80 to 90% success rate. Recent studies suggest that lytic therapy is as good as surgery in patients who do not have any decrease in neurologic function and that it should be considered as a treatment option. Immediately upon the diagnosis of an acute embolic arterial occlusion, the patient should be treated with systemic heparin, which should be maintained after the operative procedure. Postoperatively, the patient should be switched to long-term anticoagulation with warfarin (Coumadin) during the search for a source of the embolic material.

Some patients may present with a clinical syndrome of microemboli to smaller vessels in the calf and foot, which manifest clinically as critical ischemia of one or more toes. Arteriography is needed for source isolation as well as therapeutic decision-making. These patients often have occlusive disease of the distal tibial vessels (with reconstitution of the pedal vessels) and often require a distal saphenous vein bypass for limb salvage. The source of emboli in this setting is commonly a peripheral artery (i.e., popliteal aneurysm), which must be removed or excluded from the arterial tree.

ABDOMINAL AORTIC ANEURYSMS

Abdominal aortic aneurysms are a common clinical entity, and recent studies suggest that their incidence is increasing. An aneurysm is defined as a permanent focal dilation of the artery with an increase in diameter greater than 1.5 times the diameter of the normal adjacent arterial segment. Aneurysms of the abdominal aorta are most common in the arterial tree and are usually located below the renal arteries and above the iliac artery bifurcation. Men are affected more commonly than women in a ratio of 4:1, and abdominal aortic aneurysms are often associated with other aneurysms, including those in the common and internal iliac, femoral, and popliteal arteries. The pathogenesis and etiology of arterial aneurysms remain controversial. Atherosclerosis is usually present, but other factors—including genetic susceptibility, alterations in the quantities of elastin and collagen within the artery wall, and hemodynamic factors—play a role. Most patients with abdominal aortic aneurysms have risk factors for atherosclerosis, including cigarette smoking, hypertension, and hypercholesterolemia.

Abdominal aortic aneurysms are usually asymptomatic, being discovered as a pulsatile abdominal mass during a routine physical examination. Symptoms of expansion or rupture are those of severe unremitting abdominal, back, and/or flank pain associated with hypotension and shock when frank rupture occurs.

In the early 1950s, Estes described the natural history of patients with abdominal aortic aneurysms detected by physical examination. Mortality during the follow-up period was 100%, with most patients dying from aneurysm rupture. These findings suggest that most patients with abdominal aortic aneurysms should be considered for repair to prevent the highly lethal complication of rupture.

If widening of the normal aortic pulsation is suspected during a physical examination, the best screening test is abdominal ultrasonography. It is a relatively specific and sensitive test for detecting and determining the size of infrarenal abdominal aortic aneurysms. Additional diagnostic tests may be necessary, depending on the complexity of the aneurysm and the need for further information prior to operative therapy. Computed tomography scanning is also a sensitive and specific way to determine the size of abdominal aortic aneurysms and iliac arteries, as well as the proximal and distal extent of disease. The use of arteriography in the evaluation of abdominal aortic aneurysms has diminished in recent years. It is an expensive and invasive procedure with some risk, and it tends to underestimate the size of an aneurysm due to the dye column filling only the flow channel, whereas the abdominal aortic aneurysm frequently has thrombus lining its walls.

Currently, the decision to treat a patient with an abdominal aortic aneurysm is most dependent on its size, since risk of rupture is proportional to aneurysm diameter. The relative rupture risk of 5-cm aneurysms is 5 to 7.5% per year, and the risk of rupture increases exponentially with increasing aneurysm size. A ruptured abdominal aortic aneurysm carries a mortality of 78 to 90%, whereas elective surgical repair has an operative mortality between 1 and 3%. Aneurysms 5 cm or larger in diameter should be treated. Currently, aortic aneurysms less than 5 cm in diameter do not require therapy. This group of patients is being investigated in several prospective randomized clinical trials comparing operative and nonoperative therapy.

Surgical replacement of the abdominal aorta with a prosthetic graft has been the procedure of choice for nearly 40 years, but less invasive therapy is being investigated. Placement of an endovascular stented graft has been successful in small clinical trials and can be expected to achieve widespread clinical use within 2 to 3 years. The endovascular graft may result in lower operative morbidity and mortality and shorter hospital stays and reduce overall costs.

FEMORAL ARTERY ANEURYSMS

Femoral artery aneurysms are a relatively uncommon clinical entity, occurring in 3 to 7% of patients with abdominal aortic aneurysms. These aneurysms usually involve the common femoral arteries and are found in a male/female ratio of approximately 20:1. Patients with femoral aneurysms have the usual atherosclerosis risk factors, including hypertension, cigarette smoking, diabetes mellitus, and hypercholesterolemia.

The majority of patients with femoral aneurysms have symptoms of either local swelling or lower extremity ischemia. There may be a painful mass over the femoral artery or symptoms of distal ischemia secondary to recurrent embolization. Occasionally, patients with femoral artery aneurysms present with symptoms of venous occlusion due to the compression of nearby veins. Physical examination usually reveals a pulsatile groin mass in the femoral triangle. An ultrasound study confirms the presence of the aneurysm and documents its size. Since associated arterial aneurysms are found in up to 85% of these patients, they should also be screened for aneurysms in other areas of the arterial tree, most notably the aorta and popliteal arteries. The natural history of femoral artery aneurysms is unknown. Those that produce symptoms of either a mass effect or peripheral ischemia and those larger than 2.5 cm in diameter should be repaired unless the patient has prohibitive operative risks. If therapy is indicated, arteriography is recommended to allow determination of inflow and outflow arteries. The aneurysm is replaced by a prosthetic bypass graft. Most patients have an uncomplicated recovery and excellent long-term survival and limb salvage.

POPLITEAL ARTERY ANEURYSMS

Popliteal artery aneurysms are relatively common disorders of the vascular tree and are frequently found in patients with abdominal aortic aneurysms. A patient with an abdominal aortic aneurysm has a 25% chance of having a popliteal artery aneurysm. A patient with a popliteal artery aneurysm has a 50% chance of having a popliteal artery aneurysm on the contralateral side and a 30% chance of having an abdominal aortic aneurysm. Thus, finding any of these lesions warrants a search for the others. Men are affected in a ratio of approximately 15:1 over women. As with other arterial aneurysms discussed in this chapter, popliteal aneurysms are common in patients with risk factors for atherosclerosis.

The most frequent presentation is an asymptomatic, widened popliteal pulse. Despite current trends toward preventive medicine, far too many patients present with popliteal artery aneurysm thrombosis and a severely ischemic leg. Distal embolization can also occur. Rarely, a patient with a popliteal artery aneurysm presents with signs of venous compression due to a local mass effect.

The diagnostic work-up of a popliteal artery aneurysm is dependent on the presenting symptoms. Those patients diagnosed with an asymptomatic, widened popliteal artery should first undergo ultrasonography followed by arteriography if operative therapy is planned. Those patients with acute thrombosis and a threatened lower extremity often require urgent arteriography and occasionally thrombolytic therapy to determine inflow and outflow arteries for potential resection and bypass.

The decision to treat a popliteal artery aneurysm is based on the natural history of this disease process and the size of the aneurysm. Asymptomatic patients with small popliteal artery aneurysms not containing thrombus can be safely followed with ultrasonography. Asymptomatic patients with popliteal artery aneurysms greater than 2.5 cm in diameter should undergo operative therapy due to the high frequency of complications, including thrombosis, distal embolization, and limb loss. Those patients presenting with symptoms related to their popliteal artery aneurysms should undergo operative repair to prevent limb loss.

The only current established form of therapy for popliteal artery aneurysms is surgical repair by exclusion of the aneurysm (ligation of inflow and outflow arteries to the aneurysm) and bypass grafting. The preferred bypass conduit is reversed saphenous vein. Limb salvage rates of more than 95% can be anticipated with elective operative therapy. Emergency repair of a thrombosed popliteal artery aneurysm is associated with a high incidence of limb loss.

DEEP VENOUS THROMBOSIS OF THE LOWER EXTREMITIES

method of
R. JAMES VALENTINE, M.D., and
G. PATRICK CLAGETT, M.D.
*University of Texas Southwestern Medical
    Center*
Dallas, Texas

Venous thromboembolism is a major cause of death and long-term morbidity in the United States. It has been estimated that pulmonary embolus (PE) accounts for over 200,000 deaths each year in the United States; autopsy surveys suggest that the number of undiagnosed pulmonary emboli far exceeds that number. The direct and indirect costs associated with deep venous thrombosis (DVT) and nonfatal PE are substantial. In addition to increased hospital stays and the risks of long-term anticoagulation, more than 7 million Americans are estimated to be afflicted with chronic postphlebitic symptoms such as ankle ulcerations, pain, and edema.

Since venous thromboembolism is often clinically silent, it is incumbent on the clinician to institute preventive measures in patients who are at increased risk for DVT and PE. Fortunately, venous thromboembolic complications are largely preventable. A number of different agents have been shown to be efficacious in reducing the overall incidence of DVT and PE, and risk reduction can be tailored to each individual's clinical situation. In patients who develop venous thromboembolism, rapid and accurate diagnosis, coupled with institution of appropriate treatment, may prevent more serious sequelae.

CAUSE

The elements predisposing to the formation of DVT were first reported by Virchow in 1845 but are adaptable to modern clinical situations. Virchow's original triad of stasis of blood flow, endothelial damage, and hypercoagulability still represents the cornerstone for the known DVT clinical risk factors (Table 1).

Stasis of blood flow is common among hospitalized patients. Patients who are immobile or bedridden are known to be predisposed to DVT, especially those with congestive heart failure or spinal paralysis. Although pulmonary emboli may emanate from right heart chambers, leg veins are still the most common source of emboli in these patients. Direct and indirect endothelial damage accounts for much of the DVT risk associated with the postoperative state, but immobility during surgery and in the postoperative period is also a factor. The increased risk of DVT in patients with a history of venous thromboembolism and in those with varicose veins can be related to endothelial cell dysfunction as well as to stasis of blood flow in obstructed venous segments. Other risk factors are multifactorial, including obesity and advanced age. Oral contraceptive use is generally considered a risk for DVT, and the risk appears to be proportional to the dose of estrogen in the particular preparation.

Clinical risk factors are highly prevalent in hospital patients, and they are additive. For example, an elderly patient with a history of congestive heart failure has a higher risk of developing DVT after elective surgery than does a 30-year-old patient with varicose veins. Patients with hip fractures and those undergoing major orthopedic procedures have the highest risk of venous thromboembolism. This risk is attributable in part to additive risk factors

TABLE 1. Risk Factors for Development of Deep Venous Thrombosis

Clinical Conditions
Age > 40 yr
Immobility/paralysis
Congestive heart failure
Surgery and other trauma
Advanced age (>70 yr)
Prior venous thromboembolism
Malignancy
Operations on the pelvis or leg
Oral contraceptive use
Obesity
Varicose veins

TABLE 2. Hypercoagulable States

Hereditary Disorders	Acquired Disorders/ Secondary Hypercoagulable States
Antithrombin III deficiency	Myeloproliferative disorders
Protein C deficiency	Malignancy
Activated protein C resistance	Lupus anticoagulant
Protein S deficiency	Anticardiolipin antibodies
Congenital fibrinolytic disorders	Heparin-induced thrombocytopenia with thrombosis
Dysfibrinogenemia	Nephrotic syndrome
Homocystinuria	

of trauma, advanced age, and immobility. Extraskeletal trauma is also associated with high DVT risk. DVT has been shown to be a common complication following major trauma of all types, with up to 60% of patients having venographically proved leg DVT and 18% having proximal vein thrombosis. DVT risk is highest among trauma patients with injuries of the spinal cord, head, and lower extremities.

A number of congenital and acquired alterations in hemostatic mechanisms have been identified that also predispose patients to DVT. Collectively termed "hypercoagulable states," these disorders are disturbances in the normal balance between coagulation and fibrinolysis. Patients with so-called primary hypercoagulable states often have a familial history of venous thromboembolic disease. Many present with unusual clinical scenarios such as DVT at a young age, recurrent DVT, or venous thrombosis in unusual locations (e.g., mesenteric veins). Some remain asymptomatic for years. Others may never develop DVT. Nevertheless, identification of patients with primary hypercoagulable states is important because of the extremely high risk conferred in situations involving other known DVT risk factors, such as immobility.

The primary forms are listed in Table 2; most reflect flaws leading to an inability to inactivate the coagulation system or activate the fibrinolytic system. The secondary forms are much more common but less well understood. Secondary hypercoagulable states accompany clinical conditions such as malignancy, myeloproliferative disorders, pregnancy, and the nephrotic syndrome. These disorders are considered to have multiple causes related to hyperviscosity, elaboration of procoagulants, and inactivation of elements that lead to alterations in the balance between coagulation and fibrinolysis. In some cases, the development of DVT may precede the appearance of the associated medical condition: There is an important association between recurrent, idiopathic DVT and the subsequent development of clinically overt cancer.

Venous thrombi arise most often as small fibrin deposits in the soleal veins of the calf or behind valve cusps in the tibial veins. Although the risk of embolization in patients with isolated calf vein DVT is small, up to 25% of these patients experience propagation of thrombi into the popliteal or more proximal veins, where embolic potential becomes a significant risk. Not all DVT originates in calf veins. Thrombi may originate in the more proximal veins in up to 50% of patients with orthopedic trauma. The risk of venous thromboembolic complications has been reported with the use of meta-analysis in general surgery patients. The overall incidence of DVT in patients who do not receive antithrombotic prophylaxis is 25 to 30%, and 25% of these will extend proximal to the knee. This results in clinically significant PE in 2%, about 50% of which are fatal.

DIAGNOSIS

The clinical diagnosis of DVT is nonspecific, and objective vascular tests are required to confirm the diagnosis before therapy is instituted. Most DVT is clinically silent, and the first manifestation may be a fatal PE. The classic physical symptoms of pain, swelling, and erythema are unreliable. More than half of patients who are suspected of having DVT on clinical grounds do not have a confirmed diagnosis on objective testing. However, a careful history and physical examination are mandatory to exclude other causes for leg symptoms, such as infection, hematoma, or congestive heart failure.

The standard for diagnosis of DVT is the ascending phlebogram, which is highly accurate in detecting calf vein thrombi as well as thrombi involving the more proximal venous segments. Several technical considerations are crucial to the overall accuracy of this test. Phlebography is invasive, uncomfortable, and associated with contrast allergies in a small percentage of patients. In rare cases, it is known to cause DVT. Because phlebography cannot be used on a repeated basis, it is not appropriate for monitoring patients with serial studies.

Duplex scanning, with and without color-flow contrast, is highly accurate in the diagnosis of DVT and has replaced contrast venography in many medical centers. The duplex scan combines B-mode ultrasonography with a real-time, Doppler color-flow image to achieve a color-coded image of the tissue being examined. The overall sensitivity for detecting proximal DVT in *symptomatic* patients is greater than 95%, and the overall specificity is nearly 100%. It is much less sensitive in *asymptomatic* patients, probably because of partially occlusive thrombus, and is unreliable in screening patients after orthopedic surgery. Duplex scanning is also less accurate in detecting calf vein thrombi owing to technical factors. It is also problematic in imaging thrombi in iliac veins or the vena cava, since bowel gas interferes with direct visualization of these structures in many cases. However, Doppler flow patterns in the femoral veins may aid in the diagnosis of thrombi at more proximal levels. Most authorities consider duplex ultrasound to be sufficiently sensitive and specific to confirm or rule out proximal DVT in symptomatic patients. This test is an excellent choice for following patients with calf vein DVT to detect proximal extension of the thrombus.

Other objective tests for the diagnosis of DVT include fibrinogen scanning, impedance plethysmography, computer-assisted tomography (CT), and magnetic resonance imaging (MRI). Radiolabeled ^{125}I fibrinogen scanning has been widely used in the past, but it has been withdrawn from the market because of potential transmission of infectious agents from fibrinogen donor pools. Fibrinogen scanning is most sensitive in detecting distal thrombi; it is less sensitive in detecting DVT above the midthigh.

Impedance plethysmography has been recommended for detecting proximal DVT. However, it has been found to lack sensitivity when used as a screening test for patients at high risk for DVT because the test misses large thrombi that are not completely occlusive. Impedance plethysmography may still be useful for serial monitoring of patients with distal DVT in order to detect proximal propagation of thrombus. CT and MRI are not cost-effective for routine DVT screening or for serially monitoring patients with calf vein DVT. However, both may be useful in special cases. For example, CT is useful to detect thrombi in iliac veins and the vena cava. MRI has been found to have a nearly 100% sensitivity and specificity for proximal DVT, but it is unlikely to replace the less costly tests such as duplex ultrasonography and venography.

PREVENTION

Since DVT is a clinically silent disease, the concept of DVT prophylaxis is both rational and prudent. The efficacy of pharmacologic and physical measures to prevent DVT and PE has been reaffirmed on numerous occasions, and effective prophylaxis is available for nearly all patient groups. Despite the strong evidence supporting DVT prophylaxis, there are wide practice variations among clinicians. Recent hospital surveys suggest that approximately one-half of surgeons in the United States use specific prophylaxis in less than one-third of their patients. This is explained in part by the low frequency of fatal PE in an individual clinician's practice and by the misconception that antithrombotic therapy is associated with a high risk of bleeding complications. Since DVT risk factors are highly prevalent in hospitalized patients, it is incumbent on clinicians to increase the use of DVT prophylaxis to prevent PE and late sequelae of DVT.

Appropriate DVT prophylaxis is based on stratification of patients according to the presence of risk factors. Risk assessment has been evaluated in surgical patients and in patients with a number of medical conditions (Table 3). A combination of simple prophylactic techniques to avoid venous stasis may be successful in patients with low DVT risk. These include elevation of the extremities, early mobilization, and use of graduated compression stockings. Early mobilization or a combination of elevation and compression stockings will generally provide adequate prophylaxis in low-risk patients.

A number of antithrombotic regimens are effective among patients at moderate-to-high risk for DVT (Table 4). Although there is an associated increased risk of postoperative wound hematomas in surgical patients, major bleeding complications are rare. Small, fixed doses (minidose, 5000 U) of heparin administered subcutaneously either two or three times daily are effective in patients with moderate-to-high risk. It is not necessary to monitor activated partial thromboplastin time (aPTT) with this method. Minidose heparin has been shown to be beneficial in medical patients after acute myocardial infarction, congestive heart failure, and thrombotic stroke. It is also effective in patients undergoing general, thoracic, and urologic surgery. However, it is less effective in patients undergoing orthopedic procedures, particularly total hip and knee replacements. Wound hematomas occur in approximately 5% of patients receiving minidose heparin, but major bleeding complications are exceedingly rare. Another rare but important complication is the development of heparin-induced thrombocytopenia, which is sometimes associated with thromboembolism.

Heparin in adjusted doses appears to offer more

TABLE 3. **Classification of Level of Risk Based on Published Data**

Thromboembolic Event	Low Risk (%)	Moderate Risk (%)	High Risk (%)	Very High Risk (%)
	Uncomplicated surgery in patients <40 years old with no other risk factors	Major surgery in patients >40 years old with no other risk factors	Major surgery in patients >40 years old with additional risk factors or myocardial infarction	Major surgery in patients >40 years old plus previous thrombo/malignant disease or orthopedic surgery or hip fracture or stroke or spinal cord injury
Calf vein thrombosis	2	10–20	20–40	40–80
Proximal vein thrombosis	0.4	2–4	4–8	10–20
Clinical pulmonary embolus	0.2	1–2	2–4	4–10
Fatal pulmonary embolus	0.002	0.1–0.4	0.4–1.0	1–5

Modified from Gallus AS, Saltzman EW, Hirsh J: Prevention of venous thromboembolism. *In* Colman RW, Hirsh J, Marder VJ, Saltzman EW (eds): Hemostasis and Thrombosis: Basic Principles and Clinical Practice, 3rd ed. Philadelphia, JB Lippincott Co, 1994, p 1332.

protection against venous thromboembolism than minidose heparin in patients undergoing total hip replacements. In this regimen, the dosage of subcutaneous heparin is adjusted to keep the aPTT in the

TABLE 4. **Antithrombotic Regimens to Prevent Venous Thromboembolism**

Method	Description
Low-dose heparin	5000 U heparin given SC q 8–12 h, starting 1–2 h before operation
Adjusted-dose subcutaneous heparin	3500 U heparin given SC q 8 h with postoperative dose adjustments by ±500 U to maintain aPTT at high-normal values
Low-molecular-weight heparin and heparinoids	Various doses, depending on preparation, given SC once or twice daily
Moderate-dose perioperative warfarin	Start moderate daily dose (5 mg) the day of or the day after operation; adjust dose for prothrombin time ratio 1.3–1.5 (INR 2–3) by day 5
Pre- and postoperative two-step warfarin	Start 1–2.5 mg/day 5–14 days before operation, aiming for 2–3 s increase in prothrombin time at time of operation; give 2.5–5 mg/day, aiming for prothrombin of 1.3–1.5 (INR 2–3) in postoperative period
Minidose warfarin	Start 1 mg/day 10–14 days before operation, aiming for INR = 1.5 after operation
Dextran 40/70	500–1000 mL dextran 40 or 70 during operation, then 500 mL daily for 3 days, then every other day
Aspirin	325–3600 mg/day
Intermittent pneumatic compression/elastic stocking	Start immediately before operation, and continue until fully ambulatory

Abbreviations: aPTT = activated partial thromboplastin time; INR = international normalized ratio.

upper normal range (e.g., 31 to 36 seconds). The aPTT is measured 6 hours after the last heparin injection, and the adjusted heparin dosage is administered every 12 hours. Adjusted-dose heparin has been shown to reduce the rate of proximal and distal venous thrombi. However, the tedium of multiple laboratory determinations has probably limited the widespread acceptance of this regimen for DVT prophylaxis.

Low-molecular-weight heparin compounds (i.e., heparin species between 2 and 7 kD) and heparinoids have received increasing attention as prophylactic agents. Low-molecular-weight heparin has been shown to be superior to low-dose standard heparin in reducing the incidence of DVT in orthopedic patients. There is evidence from both animal and human studies that these agents have a lower incidence of hemorrhagic side effects compared with standard heparin. Low-molecular-weight heparin has a long biologic half-life, allowing it to be administered once or twice daily with predictable plasma concentrations. Laboratory tests are not needed. This form of prophylaxis appears to be best suited for patients undergoing hip or knee surgery, in whom other regimens are ineffective or labor-intensive. The high cost of available preparations has been an impediment to greater popularity.

Platelet antagonists may offer limited protection against DVT in selected patients. Aspirin has been shown to have a limited effectiveness in reducing DVT among orthopedic and general surgery patients, but other more efficacious agents are available. Low-molecular-weight dextran has also been shown to be an effective agent in prevention of PE by inhibition of platelet aggregation and decreasing blood viscosity. However, it is not as effective in preventing leg DVT as low-molecular-weight or minidose heparin. Since low-molecular-weight dextran must be given as a continuous intravenous infusion, it is relatively cumbersome. Use of this agent is further limited by the associated increase in plasma volume, which is an important issue in patients with cardiac disease.

Oral anticoagulants in adjusted doses represent another effective form of DVT prophylaxis. These agents are a highly satisfactory form of prophylaxis in orthopedic patients and currently represent the most cost-effective method in this group. Reported bleeding complication rates are acceptable when administration is carefully controlled and the prothrombin times are closely monitored. Warfarin (Coumadin) is generally given in one of two prophylactic regimens. In the two-step method, warfarin is administered preoperatively to maintain the prothrombin time between 1.5 and 3 seconds above normal at the time of operation, followed by an increased dosage to produce a prothrombin time ratio of 1.5 times the control value in the postoperative period. Alternatively, warfarin administration may be delayed until the postoperative period. This method can prevent late thromboembolic complications while reducing the risk of perioperative bleeding.

For patients in whom any bleeding is undesirable (e.g., neurosurgery or ophthalmology patients) and for those who have already experienced bleeding complications, anticoagulant prophylaxis may be contraindicated. Intermittent pneumatic compression (IPC) carries no risk of bleeding and is effective prophylaxis in moderate-risk patients. IPC may be used to augment other forms of prophylaxis in high- and very-high-risk patients who are also receiving anticoagulant prophylaxis. IPC represents an additive benefit without conferring a significant risk of complications in these patients. Occasionally, the presence of multiple injuries may contraindicate the use of anticoagulants and IPC. In patients considered to be at high or very high risk for DVT, the use of serial noninvasive tests is appropriate to detect the development of proximal DVT. Once venous thrombosis is detected, prophylactic placement of a vena cava filter device should be considered if contraindications to anticoagulation persist.

TREATMENT

The goals of treatment in patients with DVT are to prevent PE and to restore venous function. Maintenance of venous patency and valve competence are necessary to reduce postphlebitic sequelae. Therapeutic options depend on the clinical circumstances, including the presence of co-morbid conditions, the ability to use anticoagulants or fibrinolytic agents, and the extent of DVT. All patients with DVT should be placed at bed rest with the legs elevated until symptoms subside. Anticoagulation is the mainstay of treatment in proximal DVT. Isolated calf vein DVT that remains confined to the calf is associated with a low risk of clinically evident PE (less than 1%) or recurrent DVT (2%). However, most authorities feel that patients with symptomatic calf vein thrombosis should be treated with full anticoagulant therapy. Most patients with asymptomatic calf vein DVT can be managed with leg elevation alone if serial nonin-

vasive testing is used to detect proximal extension of the thrombus. Anticoagulation is instituted in patients who have proximal thrombus extension (approximately 20%). Anticoagulation should also be instituted in patients with isolated calf vein DVT in whom serial noninvasive testing cannot be performed.

All anticoagulant therapy is considered prophylactic, since the intention is to interrupt extension of the thrombus rather than to dissolve it. Anticoagulation should be initiated rapidly. Heparin is ideally suited for initial therapy because it has an immediate anticoagulant effect. Low-molecular-weight heparin administered subcutaneously at fixed intervals has recently been shown to be as effective as standard heparin in preventing the extension of existing thrombus and recurrent DVT. An appropriate intensity of anticoagulation should be reached as quickly as possible (within 24 hours) to avoid a high risk of recurrent DVT.

Conventional therapy begins with standard heparin, which can be administered either as a continuous intravenous infusion or as intermittent subcutaneous injections. A higher risk of bleeding has been reported with intermittent intravenous injections. When administered intravenously, a bolus of heparin at a dose of 100 U per kg of body weight gives immediate protection against PE and reduces the risk of recurrent DVT. This is followed by a continuous heparin infusion of 1000 U per hour. The aPTT is checked 4 to 6 hours after the initial bolus dose, and the hourly heparin dose is altered to maintain the aPTT at one and a half to two times the control value. Failure to obtain an adequate anticoagulant response is associated with a 20 to 25% risk of recurrent venous thromboembolism.

When heparin is given by the subcutaneous route, dosing should begin with 12,500 U every 12 hours. aPTT are drawn 6 hours after dosing, and the heparin dose is adjusted to maintain the aPTT in the therapeutic range (one and a half to two times control value). Heparin should be administered for at least 5 days; extending the course for longer periods has not been found beneficial. After that time, anticoagulation is continued with an oral agent such as warfarin. It should be noted that treatment of DVT with oral agents alone (i.e., without heparin) is inadequate, as it is associated with a higher risk of thrombus extension and recurrent DVT.

Warfarin is usually initiated as an oral dose of 10 mg per day for 2 days. There is a delay in the anticoagulant effect because time is required for clearance of normal coagulation factors already present in the plasma. To reduce the duration of hospitalization, warfarin can be started within 48 hours of admission and continued during the 5-day heparin infusion. The warfarin dose is adjusted according to the one-stage prothrombin time, which is now expressed according to an International Normalized Ratio (INR). Adjustments require intuitive planning based on the known delay in anticoagulant effect. The goal of warfarin therapy is to maintain the INR between 2.0 and 3.0. Oral anticoagulation should be maintained for at least 3 months to reduce the risk of recurrent DVT. Some patients require continued anticoagulation for up to 6 months or longer, depending on the degree of venous thrombosis and the presence of continued risk factors. A single DVT recurrence should probably warrant anticoagulation for 1 year. Patients with defined hypercoagulable states or multiple DVT recurrences may require life-long anticoagulation. The risk of bleeding is related more to the intensity of anticoagulation than to the duration of warfarin therapy.

Warfarin therapy is not appropriate in some patients. These include patients who are pregnant, those who experience multiple recurrences despite adequate warfarin dosage, and those who cannot take oral warfarin. These patients can be treated for 3 months with subcutaneous heparin administered every 12 hours in doses to maintain the aPTT one and a half to two times the control value. The aPTT should be measured 6 hours after the last dose of heparin. Once the optimal dose is found, the aPTT does not require further monitoring (except during pregnancy, when dosage requirements may change).

The indications for use of thrombolytic agents in the initial treatment of venous thromboembolism remain undefined. Thrombolytic agents have been associated with a more rapid restoration of vein patency compared with anticoagulants alone. However, a number of clinical trials have shown identical degrees of late postphlebitic sequelae in patients treated with thrombolytic agents and those treated with heparin alone. Following PE, initial lung scan improvement is more rapid with thrombolytic therapy, but subsequent scan improvement is no different than that seen in patients who receive heparin alone. Thrombolytic agents do not offer more protection than heparin against PE. The higher incidence of bleeding complications in patients receiving thrombolytic agents makes this option less attractive in most cases. A number of promising new agents under investigation have been associated with reduced systemic hemorrhagic effects and may be shown to be superior to anticoagulants in the future.

At the present time, thrombolytic therapy should be reserved for treating patients with massive PE who are hemodynamically unstable and do not appear to be at risk of bleeding. Thrombolytic agents should also be considered for use in patients with phlegmasia cerulea dolens who have not had symptomatic improvement after anticoagulation.

In patients who cannot receive anticoagulation or who experience recurrent DVT or PE while on adequate anticoagulant therapy, interruption or sieving of the inferior vena cava may offer protection against PE. A number of options are available, including surgical plication or interruption, placement of partially occluding external clip devices, transluminal balloon occlusion, and placement of intraluminal filter devices. Interruption of the inferior vena cava is associated with significant morbidity. Surgical plication and placement of partially occluding external

devices have a high risk of subsequent caval occlusion.

Since filter devices offer a high degree of protection against PE while maintaining caval patency, they have achieved an overwhelming popularity in PE prophylaxis. Current indications for insertion of a vena cava filter are listed in Table 5. Although there are a number of approved filter devices, the largest experience has been reported with the original stainless steel device developed by Greenfield. The Greenfield filter is associated with a long-term (12-year) caval patency of 98% and a recurrent PE incidence of 4%. The filter device is placed transvenously, either by venous cut-down or percutaneous introduction. The newer titanium Greenfield filter was developed for percutaneous insertion using a No. 12 French introducer through a No. 14 French sheath. A modification of the hook design has improved filter stabilization, reducing the incidence of filter migration and caval wall penetration.

The filter is usually deployed below the level of the renal veins, but it has also been placed without problems in the suprarenal vena cava and in the superior vena cava. Since the filter does nothing to treat leg vein DVT, it is desirable to maintain patients on long-term anticoagulation after filter placement to reduce the risk of developing the post-thrombotic syndrome.

Iliofemoral thrombectomy is largely of historical interest because it is generally associated with a high risk of recurrent DVT. There has been a resurrection of enthusiasm for this procedure in Europe, where creation of an arteriovenous fistula at the time of thrombectomy is reported to reduce DVT recurrence and increase vein patency. The renewed interest in iliofemoral venous thrombectomy has not been seen in the United States, however. This technique is cur-

TABLE 5. **Indications for Insertion of a Vena Cava Filter**

Absolute Indications
   DVT or documented thromboembolism in a patient who has a contraindication to anticoagulation
   Recurrent thromboembolism despite adequate anticoagulation
   Complications of anticoagulation requiring therapy to be discontinued
   Failure of another form of caval interruption
   Patient who has had a pulmonary embolectomy

Relative Indications
   High-risk patients with a free-floating iliofemoral and/or vena caval thrombus demonstrated on venography
   Patients with a propagating iliofemoral thrombus despite adequate anticoagulation
   Chronic pulmonary embolism in a patient with pulmonary hypertension and cor pulmonale
   Patient with occlusion of more than 50% of the pulmonary vascular bed and who would not tolerate any additional thrombus
   Presence of recurrent septic embolism

Abbreviation: DVT = deep venous thrombosis.
   Modified from Greenfield LJ, Whitehall TA: New developments in caval interruption: Current indications and new techniques for filter placement. *In* Veith FJ (ed): Current Critical Problems in Vascular Surgery, Vol 4. St. Louis, Quality Medical Publishing, 1992, pp 113–121.

rently reserved for the rare patient with phlegmasia cerulea dolens who fails to respond to standard anticoagulant or thrombolytic therapy.

LATE TREATMENT

During the late phases of DVT treatment, patient education and long-term avoidance of venous stasis are important to prevent recurrent DVT and minimize the risk of postphlebitic symptoms. Approximately 80% of patients will have some degree of edema, pigmentation, varicosities, and abnormal venous hemodynamics 5 to 10 years after a single episode of DVT. Five to 10% will develop ankle ulcerations. Avoidance of stasis is important to reduce venous hypertension and to control leg edema. Patients should be instructed to elevate the involved extremity whenever possible and to avoid extended periods of sitting with the legs dependent, such as on long car or airplane trips. The use of graduated compression stockings may be beneficial in controlling edema, which if untreated can lead to skin fibrosis and eventual ulceration. Since a history of venous thromboembolism is a lifelong risk factor for DVT, patients should be instructed to seek medical advice immediately should they develop recurrent symptoms.

The Blood and Spleen

APLASTIC ANEMIA

method of
STEPHEN D. NIMER, M.D., and
BARRETT H. CHILDS, M.D.
Memorial Sloan-Kettering Cancer Center
New York, New York

Aplastic anemia (AA) is characterized by pancytopenia and a hypocellular or acellular bone marrow. Congenital forms of AA occur, but AA is usually an acquired disorder. This discussion will focus on the management of patients with acquired AA.

The incidence of AA in the United States is approximately 2 to 10 cases per million population per year. Males and females are equally affected. Medications, chemicals, ionizing radiation, infectious agents, and autoimmune disorders have been associated with the development of aplastic anemia; however, most cases are idiopathic (Table 1). Drug-induced marrow suppression can be either dose-related (e.g., cancer chemotherapeutic agents) and usually reversible, or rare, idiosyncratic, and often irreversible. Pharmacologic agents that have been associated with the development of aplastic anemia are listed in Table 1.

The prognosis of patients with AA, which is directly related to the severity of the disease as estimated by the neutrophil count at presentation, has improved considerably over the past 2 decades, coincident with improvements in antibiotic and blood product support, as well as the establishment of effective treatment strategies.

A variety of pathophysiologic mechanisms, including immune suppression of hematopoiesis, intrinsic hematopoietic stem cell defects, marrow stromal cell (microenvironment) defects, and cytokine dysregulation, have been postulated to occur in patients with aplastic anemia. Most evidence favors immunologic suppression and/or stem cell defects as the most prevalent mechanisms. In many patients, T cells capable of suppressing hematopoiesis have been identified. This observation and the frequent response to immunosuppressive therapy suggest that immunologic suppression of hematopoiesis is a common event. Evidence for intrinsic stem cell defects in patients includes difficulties culturing AA hematopoietic progenitor cells in culture, the cure of AA with the infusion of syngeneic bone marrow, and the relatively frequent occurrence of myelodysplastic syndromes or acute leukemia after immunosuppressive therapy. It has been postulated that the development of an intrinsic stem cell defect induces a protective, immunologic suppression of hematopoiesis in some patients.

DIFFERENTIAL DIAGNOSIS

AA must be distinguished from other causes of pancytopenia, which are managed differently. These include myelodysplastic syndrome, paroxysmal nocturnal hemoglobinuria, Fanconi's anemia, aleukemic acute leukemia, hairy cell leukemia, other lymphoproliferative disorders (including T-gamma lymphocytosis), hypersplenism, and myelofibrosis. Tests that help to distinguish these conditions from AA are listed in Table 2. The presence of lymphadenopathy, splenomegaly, or an inaspirable ("dry") marrow argues against the diagnosis of AA and should prompt a search for an alternative explanation for the patient's pancytopenia.

TREATMENT

Bone marrow transplantation (BMT) and immunosuppressive therapy with equine antithymocyte glob-

TABLE 1. **Etiologic Agents in Acquired Aplastic Anemia**

Pharmacologic agents*
  Cancer chemotherapeutic agents
    Alkylating agents (e.g., busulfan), anthracyclines (e.g., daunorubicin), antimetabolites (e.g., methotrexate), antimitotic agents (e.g., colchicine), levamisole†
  Antibiotics
    Chloramphenicol, penicillins, cephalosporins, sulfonamides†
  Anti-inflammatory drugs
    Phenylbutazone, indomethacin, ibuprofen, sulindac, diclofenac, gold compounds, penicillamine
  Antiepileptic agents
    Phenytoin, carbamazepine, ethosuximide, and other minor anticonvulsants
  Antithyroid agents
    Methimazole, propylthiouracil
  Hypoglycemic agents
    Chlorpropamide, tolbutamide
  Antimalarial agents
    Quinacrine, chloroquine
  Neuroleptic agents
    Chlorpromazine,† clozapine†
  Cardiac medications
    Captopril,† procainamide†
Chemicals and toxins
  Pesticides, benzene, other aromatic hydrocarbons
Infections
  Viral hepatitis, Epstein-Barr virus (infectious mononucleosis), cytomegalovirus, brucellosis, miliary tuberculosis, parvovirus B19‡
Rheumatologic and autoimmune diseases
  Systemic lupus erythematosus (SLE), rheumatoid arthritis, cryoglobulinemia, graft-versus-host disease
Paroxysmal nocturnal hemoglobinuria
Ionizing radiation
Thymoma
Pregnancy
Idiopathic

*Listed are agents more commonly associated with aplastic anemia. The list is not intended to be exhaustive.

†More commonly associated with agranulocytosis than with aplastic anemia.

‡More commonly associated with aplastic crises in patients with underlying hemolytic disorders.

333

TABLE 2. **Differential Diagnosis of Pancytopenia**

Disorder	Distinguishing Feature(s)
Aplastic anemia	Hypocellular or acellular bone marrow
	Normal morphology or residual hematopoietic precursors
	Normal karyotype
Myelodysplastic syndrome	Dysplastic bone marrow morphology (especially RBC precursors)
	Karyotypic abnormality
Paroxysmal nocturnal hemoglobinuria	Abnormal acid ± sucrose hemolysis tests
Fanconi's anemia	Abnormal chromosomal fragility
Aleukemic acute leukemia	Increased percentage of bone marrow blasts
Hairy cell leukemia	Inaspirable bone marrow
	Splenomegaly
	TRAP stain of bone marrow and peripheral blood
T-gamma lymphocytosis	T cell–receptor genes rearranged
Myelofibrosis	Inaspirable bone marrow
	Increased reticulin ± trichrome staining of marrow biopsy
	Splenomegaly

Abbreviations: TRAP = tartrate-resistant acid phosphatase; RBC = red blood cell.

ulin (ATG) (Atgam) and/or cyclosporin A (CsA) (Sandimmune), are currently the major therapeutic options for patients with AA. All patients who are more than 45 years old should be treated with immunosuppression since the risks associated with BMT in this age group are quite high. In patients who are 45 years old or less, the existence of a histocompatible relative and the severity of the disease, as estimated by the absolute neutrophil count at the time of treatment, are the main criteria used to select a treatment strategy. Bone marrow transplantation should be recommended as the initial therapy for nearly all younger patients with severe or very severe AA and a human leukocyte antigen (HLA)–identical sibling.

Initial Evaluation and Management

The initial clinical and laboratory evaluation of the patient presenting with pancytopenia should proceed as rapidly as possible. Patients with symptomatic anemia, severe thrombocytopenia with bleeding, or febrile neutropenia must be treated immediately for these complications with red blood cell transfusions, platelet transfusions, or empirical broad-spectrum antibiotics, respectively. The essential laboratory studies (outlined in Table 3) should be completed within the first few days of presentation. Exposure to potential etiologic agents should be stopped immediately. In the case of mild drug-induced cytopenias, observation for a brief period of time (10 to 14 days) after withdrawal of potentially offending agents, with hematopoietic growth factor stimulation of residual progenitors, may be appropriate, with the

hope that hematologic recovery may spontaneously occur. Most patients with very severe neutropenia (fewer than 200 neutrophils per μL) do not spontaneously recover hematopoiesis despite withdrawal of potentially offending agents; thus therapeutic intervention in this setting should not be delayed once the diagnosis has been clearly established. In patients who are tolerant of their pancytopenia and who might be eligible for immediate BMT, blood and/or platelet transfusions should be avoided, if possible, until the existence of a histocompatible relative is determined, because untransfused or minimally transfused patients have better survival after BMT. In order to minimize the risk to minor transplantation antigens, family donors should not be used for transfusional support until it is determined whether the patient is a candidate for BMT. Once it is determined that no HLA-identical relative is available for BMT, this restriction no longer applies. In potential transplant recipients, only cytomegalovirus (CMV)-negative blood products should given (if possible) until the recipient's CMV serologic test results are available, to minimize problems with CMV infection after BMT. If the recipient is CMV-seropositive, this restriction is no longer necessary. For patients who have an HLA-identical sibling donor, irradiation of blood products or, alternatively, transfusions through leukocyte depletion filters may decrease sensitization to transplantation antigens. Prophylactic antibacterial agents should not be given routinely to afebrile patients with AA, and aspirin, rectal medications, or intramuscular injections should be avoided, as in all thrombocytopenic patients. Suppression of menses with conjugated estrogens is advisable to prevent menorrhagia in premenopausal female patients with severe thrombocytopenia.

Bone Marrow Transplantation

Transplantation of bone marrow from an identical twin or an HLA-identical sibling is curative in the majority of AA patients, with complete restoration of hematopoiesis. Immunosuppression of the recipient is required for allogeneic transplantation, and the complications of allogeneic BMT relate to the side effects of the immunosuppressive conditioning regimen (diminished pulmonary function, endocrine dysfunction, infertility, liver function abnormalities, and

TABLE 3. **Initial Laboratory Evaluation**

Complete blood count with differential and reticulocyte count
Bone marrow aspiration and 1-cm core biopsy
Bone marrow karyotype
HLA typing of patient and siblings (if patient < 45 years old)
CMV serologic examination (if potential BMT recipient)
Acid and sucrose hemolysis tests
Liver enzyme tests
Hepatitis serologic examination
EBV serologic test

Abbreviations: HLA = human leukocyte antigen; CMV = cytomegalovirus; BMT = bone marrow transplantation; EBV = Epstein-Barr virus.

secondary malignancies), to the duration of post-transplant neutropenia and thrombocytopenia that occur before engraftment, or to the development of graft-versus-host disease (GvHD). The risk of graft rejection relates to the degree of genetic disparity between the donor and the recipient, and to the intensity of the immunosuppression given to the recipient. The risk of graft failure may be increased if the recipient has already been sensitized to donor histocompatibility antigens by prior blood transfusions. Graft failure can usually be obviated by increasing the intensity of the immunosuppression (e.g., by adding total body or total lymphoid irradiation), but in general these manipulations have not improved overall survival. The main limitation to the success of bone marrow transplants in AA patients is complications related to GvHD, particularly in adult patients. The development of severe acute GvHD and/or chronic GvHD negatively affects survival.

Pretransplant immunosuppression with cyclophosphamide (Cytoxan), 200 mg per kg (usually delivered as four daily 50 mg per kg infusions), is sufficient for untransfused patients with AA. The incidence of graft rejection or GvHD in this cohort of patients is low, and current survival rates are 80 to 100% for all patients, with children having survival rates of 90 to 100%. Cyclophosphamide alone is not adequately immunosuppressive to ensure durable engraftment in multiply transfused patients. In these patients, the addition of ATG to the pretransplant cytoreductive conditioning appears to improve survival compared with cyclophosphamide alone, and survival rates in multiply transfused patients approach those of untransfused patients. Some combination of CsA (started at least 24 hours before marrow infusion) along with methotrexate and/or prednisone (administered post transplant) is used as GvHD prophylaxis in BMT recipients.

T cell depletion of the allograft has been attempted in older patients (over 40 years) with HLA-identical sibling donors to decrease or obviate manifestations related to GvHD. Although reductions in GvHD have been demonstrated with this approach, overall survival was not improved, because of graft rejection and increased infectious complications.

The survival of patients who have received allografts from partly HLA-matched relatives or from HLA-matched unrelated donors is low, so this approach should only be considered for patients in whom attempts to restore hematopoiesis using immunosuppressive therapy have failed.

Immunosuppressive Therapy

More than half of all patients with AA are ineligible for BMT either because of advanced age or the lack of availability of an HLA-compatible relative. ATG, with or without CsA, is the treatment of choice for these patients. Although such therapy is commonly referred to as "immunosuppressive therapy," it is not clear that the effectiveness of these agents relates solely to their immunosuppressive properties.

Corticosteroids and monoclonal antibodies directed against human T cells, though immunosuppressive, are ineffective treatments in AA. Numerous parameters have been reported to predict the response to ATG, but most have not been reproducibly predictive at different institutions. An exception is the severity of neutropenia, which has correlated with the response to ATG at many centers. In our series to date, approximately three-fourths of patients whose absolute neutrophil count (ANC) exceeded 200 per μL responded to ATG, whereas only one-third of patients whose ANC was 200 per μL or less responded. The severity of neutropenia at the time of treatment also correlates with long-term survival.

Treatment with ATG is associated with a 30 to 50% response rate, but only 10 to 25% of these responses result in complete restoration of hematopoiesis. Most responding patients have improvement in one or more cell lineages, resulting in transfusion independence and/or a normal risk of bleeding or infection. The side effects of ATG include the development of serum sickness, which can be largely prevented by the administration of corticosteroids for approximately 1 month from the start of ATG therapy. Because ATG can bind to all circulating blood cells, not only to T cells, patients commonly have increased transfusional needs during ATG treatment. A response to ATG typically takes 8 to 12 weeks, during which time significant morbidity or mortality may occur, primarily related to infectious complications. The use of granulocyte colony-stimulating factor (G-CSF) (filgrastim [Neupogen]) during this period to decrease the risk of serious infections is under investigation at several academic centers. Disease relapse and the development of clonal abnormalities can occur after ATG therapy, especially in partial responders. Approximately 20% of responders relapse between 4 and 12 months after ATG therapy, and 30 to 60% of patients develop hematologic and/or cytogenetic features of a myelodysplastic syndrome.

ATG is usually administered over 4 to 10 days, at a total dose of 160 mg per kg. Before the initiation of treatment, patients should be skin-tested with a dilute solution of ATG to determine whether they are allergic to the equine ATG antiserum. A wheal and flare reaction indicates the need for desensitization before ATG administration. More severe reactions may preclude the administration of ATG. Serum sickness, manifested by constitutional symptoms including a maculopapular exanthem, fever, arthralgias, myalgias, or gastrointestinal symptoms, occurs in virtually all patients beginning 7 to 10 days after ATG therapy is initiated, unless patients are given high-dose corticosteroid prophylaxis. For unexplained reasons, renal abnormalities are rarely seen with ATG-induced serum sickness.

The simultaneous use of ATG and CsA has been associated with an improved response rate at 3 and 6 months, when compared with ATG alone, but no survival benefit has been demonstrated. One limitation to the combined use of ATG and CsA is the potential for irreversible nephrotoxicity from CsA that could limit a subsequent attempt at BMT.

A randomized trial, conducted in France, compared CsA and ATG as initial therapy for AA and demonstrated equivalent response rates. Some patients who failed to respond to ATG responded to CsA, and vice versa, suggesting that at least in some patients these agents may restore hematopoiesis by different mechanisms.

Recombinant Human Hematopoietic Growth Factors

Recombinant hematopoietic growth factors have been used in AA in patients who have failed to respond to immunosuppressive therapy; as an adjunct to immunosuppressive therapy to hasten blood count recovery; for patients with frequent or severe recurrent bacterial infections; and in the management of patients with sepsis in addition to antibiotics and supportive measures. Although most patients have an increase in the number of circulating neutrophils while on G-CSF or granulocyte-macrophage colony-stimulating factor (GM-CSF) (sargramostim [Leukine]) therapy, neither of these cytokines, nor interleukin-3,* consistently increases platelet counts or hemoglobin levels. The effects of growth factor therapy are transient, and blood counts rapidly return to baseline once the cytokine therapy is stopped. The chronic administration of CSFs does not appear to be beneficial, although the selected use of CSFs may be beneficial in certain circumstances. The role of newer cytokines, such as recombinant human stem cell factor (SCF),* a growth factor with potential trilineage hematopoietic stimulatory capability, or the recently cloned thrombopoietin,* a glycoprotein that stimulates platelet production in mice and nonhuman primates, remains to be determined.

Treatment of Patients Refractory to Immunosuppressive Therapy

Patients who lack a related BMT donor and inadequately respond to immunosuppressive therapy can be supported by the judicious use of red blood cell and platelet transfusions. A formal search for an HLA-matched unrelated donor should be undertaken in patients 45 years old or less. Infectious complications of prolonged or severe neutropenia require immediate treatment with antibiotics and, in some patients, G-CSF. For the occasional patient in whom extended survival is expected and in whom extensive red cell transfusional support is anticipated, chelation therapy may prevent, delay, or reduce complications related to hemosiderosis.

---

*Investigational drug in the United States.

IRON–DEFICIENCY ANEMIA

method of
JAMES A. STOCKMAN III, M.D.
American Board of Pediatrics
Chapel Hill, North Carolina

Iron-deficiency anemia is defined as anemia that is caused by an inadequate availability of iron to sustain bone marrow erythropoiesis. Iron-deficiency anemia remains a worldwide problem, particularly in developing nations, because of the shortage of iron-rich food and the high incidence of gastrointestinal blood loss resulting from gastrointestinal parasites. Iron deficiency is also a significant problem in the United States and is particularly prevalent in certain populations and age groups. Infants who are born prematurely commonly develop iron deficiency unless they receive large supplemental doses of iron. This is because preterm delivery results in inadequate stores of iron at birth. Toddlers frequently develop iron deficiency because of a rapid increase in their red cell mass, which accompanies growth. Adolescents have unusual demands for iron because of the increase in red cell mass that accompanies sexual development. At this age, the diet is frequently marginal, and in adolescent girls the onset of menses further exacerbates the likelihood of iron deficiency. Highly trained athletes, particularly runners, sustain unusual degrees of iron loss, particularly in the gastrointestinal tract. Pregnant women are depleted of approximately 300 mg of iron as a consequence of a transfer of iron to their fetus. Women who breast feed lose approximately 1 mg of iron for every liter of breast milk produced.

IRON BALANCE

The average man has between 3500 and 4500 mg of total body iron. Two-thirds of this circulates in the form of porphyrin-bound iron within hemoglobin. Thus approximately 1000 to 2000 mg are stored in various reticuloendothelial sites. Women have approximately 80% of the total iron stores of men. Infants and children vary in the amount of storage iron they have. Newborns enter the world with a total iron endowment of approximately 75 mg per kg of body weight, with approximately two-thirds of the iron in circulating hemoglobin. Because of the rapid increase in red cell mass, which places demands on iron stores, most toddlers have marginal amounts of storage iron even though they show no clinical evidence of iron deficiency. In addition to the iron found in circulating hemoglobin and in iron stores, approximately 4 mg of iron is attached to the transport protein transferrin, 250 mg of iron is part of tissue myoglobin, and approximately 10 mg of iron is found in various respiratory enzymes. Although the amount of iron found in enzyme systems is quite small, in the presence of iron deficiency, inhibition of enzyme function may occur, resulting in a variety of nonhematologic manifestations of iron deficiency.

In men, slightly more than 1 mg of iron is lost from the body each day. This iron is lost in the form of iron contained within cells that are shed from the gastrointestinal tract, the skin, and the urinary tract. Women experience these same losses, but lose additional iron from monthly menstrual losses. On average, menstrual losses amount to the equivalent of 30 mL of packed red blood cells; 1 mL of packed red blood cells contains 1 mg of iron. Thus, menstrual losses represent an additional 1 mg of iron loss on average per day.

These losses of iron from the body are balanced by the absorption of corresponding amounts of iron from the diet. Each day the average adult American will ingest 10 to 20 mg of iron, approximately 10% of which is absorbed (1 to 2 mg of iron absorbed per day). Greater amounts of iron are absorbed in the presence of iron deficiency.

Term infants must take in 1 mg of iron per kg per day throughout the first year of life. Preterm infants require twice the amount. Thereafter, the average requirement per day from all food sources in the diet is approximately the same as for adults (10 to 20 mg per day).

The form of iron in the diet influences the percentage of iron that is assimilated. The average iron absorption from foods in general is approximately 10%. Although 50% of the iron in breast milk is absorbed, much less than 10% of the iron in cows' milk is absorbed. These are important considerations with regard to iron balance in the young. Vegetarians should be advised to eat ascorbic acid–containing vegetables or to supplement their meals with ascorbic acid, which markedly enhances iron absorption. On the other hand, the common beverage tea markedly inhibits iron absorption. Iron absorption from the gastrointestinal tract requires adequate stomach acid and a normal mucosal surface at the site of absorption, the upper small intestine. Chronic antacid ingestion diminishes iron absorption. Surgical operations that decrease gastric acidity result in both continued blood loss and decreased iron absorption.

CLINICAL SIGNS AND SYMPTOMS

Since iron is an essential element for normal cellular function, certain symptoms of iron deficiency are independent of the presence of an anemia. For example, iron deficiency without anemia can cause attention deficit, difficulty learning, lack of exercise tolerance, fissuring of the corners of the lips, abnormal growth of the fingernails, and the passage of red urine after the ingestion of beets. The tongue may become smooth. Pica may develop, particularly pica for dirt, clay, starch, and ice.

When anemia develops, other symptoms may be experienced. Some individuals develop extreme fatigue with activity when the hematocrit falls below approximately 25%. Very severe anemia produces shortness of breath, lassitude, confusion, and even congestive heart failure.

CAUSES OF IRON DEFICIENCY

In children, a common cause of iron deficiency anemia is inadequate iron in the diet. Even more common in the United States is the impact of acute and chronic infection. The latter conditions markedly impair the absorption of iron from the gut. Prolonged episodes of inflammation and/or infection can therefore result in iron deficiency.

In adults, iron deficiency anemia rarely occurs on a dietary basis alone. In the absence of unusual iron losses, even if no iron were absorbed from the diet, it would take many years for the onset of iron deficiency to be noticed. This leaves blood loss as the principal cause of iron deficiency in adults.

Iron-deficiency anemia can be caused by blood loss from a number of different sources, the most common being the gastrointestinal tract. Remarkable quantities of iron can be lost in the urine as hemosiderin. Intravascular hemolysis can cause deposition of hemosiderin into renal tubular cells, which are then shed into the urine, causing the hemosiderinuria. Paroxysmal nocturnal hemoglobinuria may also result in iron deficiency on the same basis. Internal bleeding within soft tissues may sequester iron, preventing its recycling for new blood formation. An example of this includes persons with hemophilia, who bleed into their joints and soft tissues. Individuals with idiopathic pulmonary hemosiderosis may additionally experience the onset of iron deficiency. In adolescent and adult women, menorrhagia commonly causes iron-deficiency anemia. Inadequate iron intakes can further hasten the onset of anemia in individuals who have such blood losses.

DIAGNOSIS

The diagnosis of iron-deficiency anemia should be made on the basis of a carefully performed history and physical examination, to determine whether or not diet or blood loss (or a combination of the two) is the cause of the iron deficiency, and the performance of certain diagnostic tests or a trial of iron therapy.

Iron deficiency leads to a progression of laboratory abnormalities. The first finding is a fall in serum ferritin levels, followed shortly thereafter by a decline in serum iron levels and a rise in serum iron-binding capacity. Concomitant with this is a rise in free erythrocyte protoporphyrin levels in the blood and a decline in red cell mean corpuscular volume (MCV). Finally, anemia develops. Laboratory tests for iron deficiency are based on these serially evolving abnormalities (Table 1). Unfortunately, each of these laboratory tests has certain aspects that affect either its sensitivity or its specificity. Serum ferritin values are unreliable in inflammatory states and in the presence of significant hepatocellular dysfunction, in which the values tend to be higher than expected. Determination of the percentage of transferrin saturation requires assessment of the serum iron concentration. The serum iron level has a diurnal variation. It tends to be lower than expected in the presence of inflammation. Thus it lacks sensitivity and specificity. Changes in the MCV occur late. The levels of free erythrocyte protoporphyrin may be affected by hemolytic anemia states, lead poisoning, and inherited metabolic disorders. In the presence of iron deficiency, a rise in the red cell distribution width (RDW) may be seen. An elevation in RDW may be noted in other disorders such as lead poisoning, and therefore it is a relatively insensitive and nonspecific indicator of iron deficiency unless correlated with other findings. The purest test of iron deficiency is the demonstration of the absence of bone marrow iron, but this procedure is rarely done for the purpose of determining whether an individual is iron deficient because of the discomfort associated with the procedure.

Given the many problems of sensitivity and specificity of the currently available studies for iron deficiency, a trial of iron is not only therapeutic, but diagnostic as well. There is much to be said for a clinical trial of therapy as a diagnostic test for iron-deficiency anemia.

IRON REPLACEMENT

The standard treatment for iron-deficiency anemia is the administration of oral iron salts. The available iron salts are ferrous sulfate, ferrous gluconate, and ferrous fumarate. The most commonly available iron preparations are in the form of ferrous sulfate. This iron salt is the cheapest and a very efficient way to replace iron. A 300-mg tablet of ferrous sulfate provides 60 mg of elemental iron. The standard management of iron-deficiency anemia using oral iron replacement therapy is a dose of oral iron equivalent

TABLE 1. **Readily Available Laboratory Tests Employed in the Evaluation of Disorders Producing Hypochromia and Microcytosis**

Disorder	Serum Iron Level	Iron-Binding Capacity	Ferritin Level	Free Erythrocyte Protoporphyrin	Hemoglobin Electrophoresis	Marrow Iron Stores
Iron deficiency	Decreased	Increased	Decreased	Increased	Normal	Decreased
Chronic disease anemia	Decreased	Decreased	Increased	Increased	Normal	Increased
Sideroblastic anemia	Increased	Normal	Increased	Decreased	Normal	Ring sideroblasts
Beta-thalassemia trait	Normal	Normal	Normal	Normal	Hemoglobin A_2 increased	Normal
Alpha-thalassemia trait	Normal	Normal	Normal	Normal	Normal	Normal

to 150 to 200 mg of elemental iron given daily in divided doses. As noted, ferrous sulfate tablets generally contain 60 mg of elemental iron, whereas ferrous gluconate tablets contain only about half this amount. Many pharmaceutical preparations of iron salts contain ascorbic acid. Ascorbic acid results in a higher amount of absorption of the ferrous salt. For practical purposes, however, the amount of iron available from tablets does not require assistance from ascorbic acid. Maximal iron absorption is obtained by taking the iron salts separately from meals. A standard recommendation would be to administer iron tablets 1 to 2 hours before meals. An additional dose may be given at bedtime. Such methods of administration may increase gastrointestinal side effects. Offering the tablets with meals may diminish such side effects, but results in a decrease in iron absorption.

In children, the dose of iron that seems to be capable of producing an adequate rise in hemoglobin concentration with the least side effects is 1.5 to 2 mg per kg of elemental iron administered three times daily between meals. The maximal dose of elemental iron necessary for most children is 180 mg per day. For infants and small children, a small calibrated dropper with a solution containing 15 mg of elemental iron per 0.6 mL can be used. Toddlers can take syrup or elixir containing 30 or 45 mg of elemental iron per 5 ml, and older children can be given tablets or capsules containing the usual adult dose of iron. Liquid iron preparations are tolerated no better or worse than tablet forms of iron. Liquid preparations stain clothing and teeth. Children should be advised to rinse or brush their teeth after each dose.

The major limitations to oral iron therapy are its gastrointestinal side effects, which include constipation, abdominal cramps, nausea, epigastric pain, and symptoms of heartburn. In some cases, vomiting and severe abdominal cramps may occur. Lower gastrointestinal symptoms appear unrelated to dose and, in placebo-controlled studies, occur at almost equal frequency in subjects receiving iron or placebo. The lower gastrointestinal side effects can be managed symptomatically and do not require alteration of the iron dosage. The upper gastrointestinal side effects are much more troublesome and do respond to a lowering of the dose or the administration of iron with meals. With all forms of medicinal iron, stools soon become black. Medicinal iron, however, does not cause guaiac positivity on stool examination.

There are preparations of iron on the market that allow a sustained release of the ferrous salt. These preparations limit some of the side effects of ferrous salt administration by delaying the release of iron until it passes the maximal site of iron absorption in the upper small intestine. Thus, although their use improves patients' symptoms, it should be recognized that a longer course of iron therapy may be needed because of the diminished iron absorption that is consequent to the use of such preparations.

RESPONSE TO ORAL IRON THERAPY

The response to oral iron therapy is usually prompt. Reticulocyte production begins approximately 3 days after the institution of therapy. A peak reticulocyte count response is seen at 7 to 10 days. At this time, one sees the maximal rate of rise in hemoglobin concentration. The peak rise may be as great as 0.4 gm per dL. The change in hemoglobin level actually observed in any particular patient depends on the initial level of hemoglobin and the duration of the observation period. The lower the hemoglobin concentration, the greater the rise per day. The shorter the observation period, the greater the calculated rise in hemoglobin concentration per day. If the initial hemoglobin concentration is very low, the daily rise in hemoglobin may be as much as 0.3 to 0.4 gm per dL or more for the first week of treatment and then fall off gradually to 0.1 gm per dL toward the end of treatment. Verification of an adequate response to treatment can be done by the notation of the increase in reticulocyte count at approximately 1 week from the start of treatment. Alternatively, the hemoglobin concentration may be checked in several weeks when the return to normal should have occurred.

Iron therapy should be continued until iron stores are totally replenished. This empirically means extending the course of iron therapy for several months beyond the point at which the hemoglobin deficit is fully corrected. If it is felt important to do so, one can verify the adequacy of iron stores by monitoring the serum ferritin concentration. A target serum ferritin level of 50 μg per L should be sought.

FAILURE TO RESPOND TO ORAL IRON TREATMENT

Oral iron therapy occasionally fails to correct iron deficiency anemia. In these instances, one should determine whether the diagnosis is correct. Other causes of failure to respond to oral iron therapy include the presence of mixed nutritional deficiencies, especially folic acid deficiency; failure of compliance; improper administration of iron; improper dosage; malabsorption of iron; and poor iron utilization. The latter generally results from concomitant chronic disease states. The iron deficiency associated with sideroblastic anemia and lead poisoning may fail to respond to treatment. Patients with a history of gastrectomy may absorb iron poorly if it is taken with food but respond when the iron is taken between meals. Patients who have had an upper small bowel resection, or who may have other disorders of the small intestine such as celiac, may fail to respond to oral iron therapy.

Failure to absorb iron may be assessed with a simple "oral iron absorption test." In children, this consists of the administration of 1 mg of elemental iron per kg of body weight in the fasting state. A rise in the serum iron level from an abnormally low value to greater than 100 to 200 μg per dL indicates an adequate absorption of iron. In adults, this same response is seen with the administration of 100 mg of elemental iron. These doses must be given in the fasting state and the rise in serum iron noted between 1 and 2 hours subsequent to the administration of the oral test dose of iron.

One last cause of failure to respond to oral iron is unsuspected, continuing blood losses in excess of what can be compensated for by the oral iron administered. Noncompliance, failure to absorb iron, or an iron requirement in excess of what can be absorbed orally may be indications for iron dextran administration.

PARENTERAL IRON THERAPY

Parenteral iron should not be administered routinely. Its usage should be restricted to those conditions in which oral iron therapy either has failed or would not be predicted to be effective. These conditions include, in part, noncompliance, failure of iron absorption, severe recurrent iron deficiency due to uncontrollable blood losses, and intractable severe gastrointestinal side effects of orally administered iron. The latter is a relative indication for parenteral iron since in most instances the gastrointestinal side effects of orally administered iron can be minimized or eliminated with a modification of the dosage regimen.

Various preparations have been used for the parenteral treatment of iron deficiency. With these preparations, iron is bound to a substance that stabilizes the iron in a complex form. Substances such as saccharose, dextrin, dextran, or modified dextran have been used as stabilizers. All these iron preparations are of high molecular weight. Recently, low-molecular-weight iron dextran complexes or iron–sorbitol–gluconic acid preparations have been investigated. Iron dextran (Imferon) is the most widely used parenterally administered iron preparation in the United States. Iron dextran contains 50 mg per mL of elemental iron.

The preferred route for administration of iron dextran is intravenous. Intramuscular administration is possible. With the intravenous route, a single infusion can be used to deliver the total quantity of iron required. The amount of iron needed is calculated from the deficit in circulating hemoglobin, assuming that 1 gm of hemoglobin per 100 mL of whole blood corresponds to 150 mg of iron in an average-sized male adult. An additional 500 mg is given to replenish stores. This can be calculated by the following formula:

$$\text{Total iron required (mg)} = 100 \, [\text{Hb deficit (gm/dL)} \times \text{estimated blood volume (mL)} \times 3.4] + 500$$

This amount of iron dextran is diluted in normal saline to a concentration not exceeding 5% and is administered slowly over 2 to 3 hours.

The dosage calculation for children is somewhat different. The calculation for the volume of iron dextran required, based on an average blood volume of 75 mL per kg, an additional iron replacement of 50% for replenishment of stores, and the fact that 1 g of hemoglobin contains 3.5 mg of iron, is as follows:

$$\text{Iron dextran (mL)} = \text{weight (kg)} \times \text{desired rise in Hb (gm/dL)} \times 0.076$$

Iron dextran therapy is not free of risks. Fatal anaphylactic reactions may occur. Parenteral administration of iron can also cause vomiting, chills, fevers, arthralgia, and urticaria. To safeguard against anaphylaxis, the rate of intravenous infusion should be kept at less than 10 drops per minute during the first 10 to 15 minutes of administration. If no reaction occurs, the rate of infusion can be increased. Patients who develop significant symptoms related to iron dextran administration may have worse reactions with subsequent therapy. Iron dextran administration may be contraindicated in patients with rheumatoid arthritis because it is known to exacerbate synovitis. Lastly, if iron is administered by the intramuscular route, it must be given by a deep zigzag intramuscular injection in order to avoid tattooing of the skin.

Parenteral iron therapy generally does not produce a more rapid response than does oral iron therapy except in conditions in which the orally administered iron has failed to be absorbed.

AUTOIMMUNE HEMOLYTIC ANEMIA

method of
RAJA MUDAD, M.D., and
MARILYN J. TELEN, M.D.
Duke University Medical Center
Durham, North Carolina

In normal adults, approximately 2×10^{11} new red blood cells, or erythrocytes, must be produced daily to maintain a constant circulating red cell mass. Red cells leave the bone marrow as reticulocytes and normally survive in the circulation for approximately 120 days. To achieve this degree of longevity, the erythrocyte must maintain the integrity of its membrane and cytoplasmic contents, protecting them from the various chemical and physical stresses that it encounters in the circulatory environment. Although much is known about why and how abnormal erythrocytes are destroyed, the signal that triggers the disappearance of normal senescent red cells from the circulating blood is still unresolved. It is thought that progressive decline in enzymatic activity within the red cell and selective binding of normal human immunoglobulin G (IgG) to senescent cells followed by their sequestration by the reticuloendothelial system (RES) both play a role. Hemolytic disorders are characterized by premature destruction of circulating red cells, either because the red cells are inherently defective or as a result of injury from extracellular events. Hemolysis can be extravascular, when the abnormal red cells are cleared from the circulation by the RES, or intravascular, when the red cells break down inside the blood vessels and release their hemoglobin into the circulation.

When the hematopoietic system is faced with accelerated red cell destruction, normal bone marrow responds by increasing the production of reticulocytes and by releasing them earlier into the circulation. The best estimate of this response is the absolute reticulocyte count. Normal bone marrow is capable of maximally increasing its red cell production approximately eightfold. However, in autoimmune hemolytic anemia, the compensatory response most often is incomplete and anemia ensues.

AUTOIMMUNE HEMOLYSIS

Definition

Autoimmune hemolytic anemia (AIHA) is a condition characterized by the accelerated destruction of red blood cells by autoantibodies. In a broader sense, it also includes conditions associated with cell-mediated red cell destruction. Autoantibodies against red cells may be found in persons without any signs of increased red cell destruction and in whom red cell survival may be normal; in patients with compensated increased red cell destruction; and in patients with overt hemolytic anemia. The mechanism of red cell destruction may be through complement activation and subsequent intravascular hemolysis or through clearing of IgG- and complement-coated red cells by the RES. AIHA is most often classified based on the type of immunoglobulin that initiates red cell destruction, as well as according to the conditions in which this antibody is maximally reactive.

Classification

Four forms of AIHA are recognized (Table 1): warm AIHA, cold AIHA (CAIHA), paroxysmal cold hemoglobinuria (PCH), and drug-induced hemolysis. Warm AIHA is characterized by the presence of an IgG antibody that reacts with red cells best at temperatures between 35° and 40° C. Once attached, this antibody promotes the accelerated clearance of red cells by the RES; phagocytosis and cytolysis may be induced by opsonization via the Fc receptors or complement receptors on cells of the monocyte-macrophage system. The IgG antibody may have blood group antigen specificity but most often recognizes nonpolymorphic determinants on the Rh, Band 3, or glycophorin A proteins. CAIHA is characterized by the production of an IgM antibody that reacts with red cells best at temperatures below 30° C. These antibodies more often activate the complement system directly and hence may lead to the destruction of red cells intravascularly. Their specificity is most commonly anti-I or anti-i, although other specificities have been described. PCH is characterized by the presence of an IgG biphasic hemolysin that binds to red cells at low temperatures but causes lysis at 37° C. The antibody specificity is typically against the P blood group antigen, and hemolysis is often intravascular. Finally, drug-induced hemolysis is characterized by the appearance, in the serum, of an antibody that mediates red cell destruction in the presence of a drug or that is induced by drug therapy.

CLINICAL RECOGNITION OF HEMOLYTIC DISORDERS

History

The patient's history usually contains several clues that aid in the recognition of a hemolytic process. Weakness, fatigue, lightheadedness, dizziness, palpitations, and angina, as well as symptoms of congestive heart failure or central nervous system ischemia, may be induced or aggravated by significant anemia of any cause. An acquired hemolytic process is suggested by the rapid appearance of symptoms and signs of anemia in a patient with no previous history of a similar condition and no evidence of blood loss. In contrast, anemias due to bone marrow failure are more often gradual in onset and better tolerated by the patient. The presence of other autoimmune diseases or lymphoproliferative disorders also increases the likelihood of an acquired hemolytic process. A history of drug exposure should raise the suspicion of drug-induced hemolysis, while a history of previous cardiac valve replacement should prompt the physician to investigate the possibility of mechanical he-

TABLE 1. **Classification of Autoimmune Hemolytic Anemias**

	Coombs-Reactive Component
Warm antibody	
Idiopathic	IgG ± C3
Secondary	
Hematologic malignancies (CLL, lymphoma)	IgG
Nonhematologic malignancies	IgG ± C3
Autoimmune disorders (SLE, RA)	IgG + C3
Cold antibody	
Idiopathic	C3
Secondary	
Lymphoproliferative disorders	C3
Infections (EBV, CMV, *Mycoplasma pneumoniae*)	C3
Drug-induced	
Drug-adsorption type (penicillin)	IgG
Immune complex type (quinidine)	IgG or IgM, ± C3
True autoantibody type (alpha-methyldopa)	IgG
Paroxysmal cold hemoglobinuria	C3 or negative

Abbreviations: CLL = chronic lymphocytic leukemia; SLE = systemic lupus erythematosus; RA = rheumatoid arthritis; EBV = Epstein-Barr virus; CMV = cytomegalovirus.

molysis. Specific symptoms pertaining to the particular type of hemolytic anemia will be discussed in the respective sections.

Physical Findings

Physical findings are usually related to the acuteness of the hemolytic process and may manifest as pallor, jaundice, dark urine, tachycardia, and signs of congestive heart failure. In addition, depending on the severity of the anemia, the patient may exhibit widened pulse pressure as well as postural hypotension. Organomegaly is common: splenomegaly is seen in 30 to 80% of patients, and hepatomegaly is seen in approximately 45%. Occasionally, findings related to an associated condition (such as lymphoma-related adenopathy or lupus-related rash) may suggest the cause of an autoimmune hemolytic anemia.

Laboratory Features

The hallmark of AIHA consists of anemia of varying severity. This is usually accompanied by reticulocytosis, unconjugated hyperbilirubinemia without bilirubinuria, decreased serum haptoglobin levels, and elevated lactate dehydrogenase (LD) levels. The single most helpful laboratory test is careful examination of the peripheral blood film. This usually reveals polychromasia, nucleated red cells, and microspherocytosis. In more than 95% of patients, the direct antiglobulin test (DAT) is positive (see Table 1). This test detects the presence of immunoglobulins and/or complement components bound in vivo to red cells. In general, the presence of IgG on the red cells suggests warm or drug-induced AIHA, whereas the presence of complement without IgG suggests CAIHA. In approximately 40% of warm AIHA cases, complement can be found on the red cells in addition to IgG. Occasionally, the standard DAT, performed by looking for agglutination in the presence of anti–human IgG or anti-C3, is negative. In such cases, more sensi-

tive tests for red cell–bound IgG can be performed. Various tests using either radiolabeled or enzyme-linked anti–human IgG may be used to detect the presence of low numbers of IgG molecules on the surface of the red cells and are more sensitive than the routine screening DAT. In 1% of cases, even an enhanced DAT is negative, and one has to embark on a Coombs-negative hemolytic anemia work-up. This may consist of performing diagnostic tests to rule out the presence of paroxysmal nocturnal hemoglobinuria (PNH), PCH, low-affinity IgG autoantibody, IgA-mediated AIHA, and other rare entities. Occasionally, one has to resort to measuring the patient's red cell survival and site of destruction using a ^{51}Cr-labeling technique. This technique documents the presence of rapid red cell destruction or sequestration and determines the site of sequestration (liver or spleen), which may be helpful in making a decision regarding splenectomy if nonsurgical therapies fail.

WARM AUTOIMMUNE HEMOLYTIC ANEMIA

The incidence of warm AIHA is estimated to be approximately 10 cases per million population per year. It is more common in women than in men and occurs at all ages, although the incidence peaks in midlife. About half the cases are idiopathic, and the rest are associated with other conditions, such as autoimmune disorders, B cell lymphomas, or chronic lymphocytic leukemia (CLL). The possible diagnosis of a lymphoproliferative disorder is of particular concern whenever autoimmune hemolytic anemia is diagnosed in an elderly person. In addition, the Coombs test is positive in 18 to 43% of patients with human immunodeficiency virus (HIV) infection and 15% of hospitalized patients receiving transfusions, although clinically significant hemolysis occurs in only a minority of these patients.

The cause of AIHA is not known. Although immune dysregulation is thought to be present, the events that lead to the production of antibody to autoantigens are for the most part unknown. In lymphoproliferative disorders, the antibodies produced are often polyclonal; in CLL in particular, they are usually not produced by the malignant clone.

Treatment

When the diagnosis of AIHA is first made, a careful history and physical examination should be performed to determine if an associated disorder such as tumor, lymphoma, or collagen vascular disease is likely to be present, since therapy for such a disorder may take precedence over treatment of the hemolytic process.

Blood Transfusion. Blood transfusion may be necessary as an emergency measure but is usually reserved for patients with severe and fulminant disease. Destruction of the transfused blood is usually as rapid as that of the patient's own blood. Transfusing blood lacking a particular antigen with which the patient's serum reacts strongly may be helpful but is not always possible. Crossmatching blood for a patient with AIHA can be very difficult, and the physician may have to accept blood that is incompatible in vitro. However, despite in vitro incompatibility, patients with warm AIHA are not at higher risk for alloimmunization than other patients, and their long-term outcome after a blood transfusion is not different from that of other multitransfused patients in at least one study. It is important to inquire about a history of previous blood transfusion or pregnancy in any patient requiring a transfusion, since antibody due to previous alloimmunization can be masked by the presence of an autoantibody. In this case, blood should be given slowly and under constant supervision.

Corticosteroids. The corticosteroid hormones constitute the initial therapy of choice for most patients with warm AIHA. Prednisone at a dose of 1 to 2 mg per kg per day suppresses hemolysis in 80% of patients, initially by inhibiting macrophage function and subsequently by decreasing autoantibody production. Responding patients usually show a benefit within 7 days, but full responses may require 4 to 6 weeks. Therapy is then usually tapered over several months, with careful observation for recurrent hemolysis. Only about 20% of patients are successfully weaned completely from steroid therapy; an equal number may maintain an adequate hematocrit on low or alternate-day doses. About 15 to 20% of all patients are completely unresponsive to steroid therapy; these individuals, as well as those requiring high maintenance doses of steroids, are candidates for other forms of therapy, such as cytotoxic drugs or splenectomy.

Splenectomy. Splenectomy is recommended for patients who are not responsive to steroids, those who require large doses of maintenance steroids, and those who have suffered serious complications from relatively low doses of steroids. It is less helpful in patients with cold antibodies and more helpful if splenomegaly is present. Splenectomy is felt to work by removing the site of clearance of IgG-coated red cells; however, it may also prompt a decrease in antibody production. Approximately 50 to 80% of splenectomized patients are able to reduce or stop prednisone therapy. The administration of pneumococcal vaccine is recommended before splenectomy, and empirical penicillin should be administered for febrile episodes thereafter until the source of fever is identified. Occasionally, an accessory spleen is present, and this can account for failure of splenectomy in some patients.

Cytotoxic Drugs. Many cytotoxic drugs are potently immunosuppressive, and this provides the basis for their use in patients with AIHA. However, their therapeutic effect does not depend on immunosuppression alone, since clinical success is not always accompanied by a reduction in the titer of anti–red cell antibodies. Cyclophosphamide (Cytoxan) 60 mg per m^2 per day and azathioprine (Imuran) 80 mg per m^2 per day are the most commonly used agents. Cyclophosphamide appears to be one of the most effective immunosuppressive agents available and may have a therapeutic index that is better than that of other drugs. About 40 to 60% of all patients who receive cytotoxic drug therapy show some measure of improvement. Steroids are usually administered concomitantly and tapered over a period of 3 months, while the cytotoxic drug is given for at least 6 months before gradual reduction of dosage is instituted. These agents are usually reserved for patients who are unresponsive to steroids or who require an unacceptably high maintenance dose. They can also be used in patients who are poor candidates for splenectomy or those in whom such treatment has failed. Immunosuppressive agents have multiple serious side effects; these should be discussed with the patient before initiation of therapy. Particular attention should be given to female patients of childbearing age, and adequate contraception should be discussed.

Danazol. Danazol (Danocrine), a modified androgen with reduced masculinizing effects, has also been used with varied success.

Intravenous Immune Globulin.* Intravenous immune globulin (IVIG) has been used with only modest success in different series. The dose required in AIHA is usually higher than that needed for idiopathic thrombocytopenic purpura (ITP). A dose of 5 grams per kg has been shown to be helpful in children with AIHA, but responses were limited to those with warm (IgG) antibody-mediated disease and were less frequent than responses in ITP. Maintenance therapy with 400 mg per kg every 3 weeks may be necessary to maintain the effect. In patients with AIHA secondary to lymphoproliferative disorders, IVIG has been shown to be helpful only in patients with hypogammaglobulinemia. The mechanism of action is thought to be blockade of the Fc receptors in the reticuloendothelial system.

---

*Not FDA-approved for this indication.

COLD AUTOIMMUNE HEMOLYTIC ANEMIA

AIHA caused by a cold-reacting antibody (CAIHA) can be classified into three main entities: postinfectious CAIHA, CAIHA associated with hematologic malignancies, and cold agglutinin disease (CAD). CAD represents a clonal disorder characterized by the production of a monoclonal antibody, usually of the IgM type, with I antigen specificity, occurring without a known antigenic stimulus. Postinfectious CAIHA typically follows infections with *Mycoplasma pneumoniae;* the antibody is usually polyclonal and has I antigen specificity but may be oligoclonal. Epstein-Barr virus is another agent described as causing CAIHA; the antibody in this case has i antigen specificity. Malignancies, mainly hematologic but occasionally nonhematologic, can be associated with the production of a cold-reacting antibody that is usually monoclonal and also of i specificity. The best example is CLL.

The degree of clinical relevance of a cold-reacting antibody is a function of its thermal amplitude, i.e., the temperature range through which the antibody binds to red cells, and its titer. Most naturally occurring cold agglutinins are present in low titer, do not react at physiologic temperatures, and thus are usually not clinically significant except in extremely cold conditions. When a cold agglutinin causes hemolysis, the direct Coombs test is positive for C3d and the cold agglutinin titer is usually greater than $\frac{1}{64}$ at 0° to 4° C.

Treatment

Treatment of CAD may consist primarily of maintenance of an ambient temperature sufficient to keep body temperature at all sites above the maximal temperature at which the antibody reacts. Many patients have a mild, chronic hemolytic process and do not require any specific therapy beyond control of the environmental temperature. Blood transfusions in patients with CAD may be associated with accelerated red cell destruction; crossmatching is often difficult, especially if the antibody has a high thermal amplitude, and a fraction of transfused cells may undergo rapid destruction until they become coated with complement degradation products. Splenectomy and corticosteroids are usually not effective as therapy for CAD, although some authors have reported success in some patients. When required, therapy for this syndrome relies on the suppression of antibody production, usually via cytotoxic chemotherapy. This can be accomplished using cyclophosphamide or chlorambucil (Leukeran), although the degree of success in reducing hemolysis is variable. Many drug schedules have been described. One often-used regimen is cyclophosphamide 250 mg per day orally together with prednisone 100 mg per day for 4 days, repeated every 2 to 3 weeks. Alternatively, intravenous cyclophosphamide 500 to 1000 mg given once and repeated every 2 to 3 weeks can be used. Chlorambucil 16 to 30 mg per m² orally once every 2 to 4 weeks can be used as well. Interferon-alpha has been used with some success in this disease.

PAROXYSMAL COLD HEMOGLOBINURIA

PCH is a rarely diagnosed entity characterized by the sudden passage of hemoglobin in the urine on exposure to cold. Historically, it was most commonly associated with syphilis, but now it is usually seen following other infectious processes, typically childhood viral exanthems. In PCH, hemolysis is caused by a cold-reacting IgG antibody with a high thermal amplitude. This antibody is usually directed against the P antigen on red cells. Physiologically, the antibody binds to red cells most avidly at low temperatures and then fixes complement, which goes on to cause hemolysis at higher temperatures. The Donath-Landsteiner (biphasic hemolysin) test reproduces this reaction in vitro and is used for diagnosing PCH. Acute PCH is usually self-limited, with rapid and complete recovery of the patient within days after treatment of the underlying infection. However, anemia can be severe, and blood transfusions may be necessary if the hemoglobin level drops precipitously. Some adults appear to develop PCH as a true autoimmune disease. In these patients, steroids may be helpful, although prednisone will not reduce immune adherence. With antibodies of high thermal amplitude, steroids have been reported to reduce the frequency of hemolysis.

DRUG-INDUCED IMMUNE HEMOLYSIS

An acquired hemolytic anemia can result after exposure to many different drugs. The mechanism of red cell destruction on exposure to the drug in question can be classified into three different types:

1. *Drug adsorption type* (example: penicillin). In this type, the offending drug binds to the surface of the red cells and induces the formation of an antibody that reacts with the drug only and not with any structures on the red cell membrane. Since the drug is bound to the red cells, its interaction with the antibody leads to clearance of the sensitized cells via antibody-mediated phagocytosis. The antibody in this case is usually a warm-reacting, non-complement-binding IgG that causes a positive direct Coombs test.

2. *Immune complex type* (example: quinidine). In this type, antibodies are generated against the offending, unbound drug, and the resulting immune complexes bind to red cells, leading to their destruction via complement fixation and cell lysis. The antibodies in this case may be IgG, IgM, or both. Although drug-related immune complexes have been thought to bind to red cells nonspecifically, recent evidence suggests that some of the antibodies generated may react with red cell surface structures. The Coombs test in this type is positive for complement.

3. *Autoimmune hemolytic anemia type* (example: alpha-methyldopa). In this type, the offending drug induces the formation of a warm antibody directed against the red cell. The target antigen is usually the proteins that bear Rh blood group antigens, and autoantibody may be detectable when the drug is no longer present in the serum. The picture is very similar to warm AIHA, and the Coombs test is positive. The exact mechanism by which antibody induction occurs is unknown. In the case of alpha-methyldopa, AIHA usually follows prolonged administration (more than 3 months) of the drug, and as many as 15% of patients taking this drug develop a positive Coombs test without overt hemolysis. Less than 5% of patients taking the drug develop hemolysis.

Treatment of drug-induced hemolysis consists of removing the offending drug and observation of the patient. In rare situations, blood transfusions may be necessary. In the type of AIHA caused by such drugs as alpha-methyldopa, the autoantibody may persist several months after cessation of drug therapy, although hemolysis ordinarily resolves much more quickly.

NONIMMUNE HEMOLYTIC ANEMIA

method of
PETER B. RINTELS, M.D., and
JAMES P. CROWLEY, M.D.
Brown University School of Medicine
Providence, Rhode Island

The term "nonimmune hemolytic anemia" implies a useful algorithm for evaluating a hemolytic process—that is, once it has been established that hemolysis may be taking place, a Coombs' test (direct antiglobulin test) should be performed. If antibody or complement is detected on the red blood cell (RBC) surface, the hemolysis is most likely due to an immune mechanism. If not, the constellation of Coombs'-negative nonimmune hemolytic anemias (NIHAs) needs to be considered. NIHAs can be divided into essentially five categories as outlined in Table 1: red cell enzyme disorders (G6PD being by far the most common), hemoglobin disorders, inherited or acquired red cell membrane disorders, microangiopathic processes such as thrombotic thrombocytopenic purpura (TTP), and toxin-mediated processes. True immune hemolysis with a negative Coombs' test is rare but has been reported with IgA antibodies; it may also be due to highly potent IgG hemolysins that may induce RBC destruction at densities on the RBC membrane that are too low to be detected by standard Coombs' agglutination testing. Some of the illnesses that cause Coombs'-negative hemolysis, such as sickle cell disease and TTP, are discussed in separate chapters.

The presence of hemolysis is established by the detection of elevations of lactate dehydrogenase (LD), most prominently isotype 2; elevation of the indirect (unconjugated) bilirubin, lowering of the serum haptoglobin, and elevation of the reticulocyte count. Hemolysis that takes place within the splenic sinusoids has historically been labeled extravascular, although anatomically this is somewhat arbitrary. Hemolysis that takes place in the intravascular space outside of the spleen, liver, and other reticuloendo-thelial organs is usually referred to as intravascular. In addition to the above findings, "intravascular" hemolysis is characterized by free serum hemoglobin, methemalbumin (which may impart a pink appearance to serum), and free urine hemoglobin or hemosiderin. Free hemoglobin appears in the urine when the amount of hemoglobin presented to the renal proximal tubule exceeds 150 mg per dL. Hemoglobin absorbed by the proximal tubule is metabolized to hemosiderin, a storage form of iron related to ferritin. Hemosiderin is subsequently shed by the proximal tubule and can be detected in the urine using the Prussian blue reaction, but it is present only in chronic and not acute intravascular hemolysis. In addition, hemosiderin breaks down rapidly, and false negatives may result if the testing is not done on a fresh specimen.

The "gold standard" test for hemolysis is the ^{51}Cr-labeled RBC survival study, although this is rarely necessary in clinical practice. Situations that can sometimes create confusion about the presence of hemolysis include illnesses associated with ineffective erythropoiesis, such as megaloblastic anemias, some cases of myelodysplasia, and reabsorption of a hematoma. Most markers of accelerated RBC breakdown are present in these situations. In addition, the reticulocyte count may be elevated in the setting of marrow recovery from a toxin (e.g., alcohol) or a deficiency state (e.g., folate or iron) and in subacute hemorrhage, but the reticulocyte count is usually higher in hemolytic states for any given level of hemoglobin than in these situations.

ENZYME DISORDERS

Glucose-6-Phosphate Dehydrogenase Deficiency

Glucose-6-phosphate dehydrogenase (G6PD) deficiency is by far the most common red cell enzyme abnormality in the world, affecting as much as 10% of the world's population. Like most of the common erythrocyte abnormalities, the incidence is highest in populations from the malaria belt, where it likely conferred a survival advantage. G6PD initiates the hexose monophosphate shunt, whose primary role is protecting the RBCs against oxidative insults. G6PD-mediated oxidation of glucose-6-phosphate simultaneously generates reduced NADP, which is required for the actions of glutathione peroxidase and catalase. These enzymes remove peroxide from the RBCs. In the absence of this "defense," oxidative destabilization of RBC proteins and phospholipids ensues. Key among the affected proteins is hemoglobin, which precipitates to form Heinz bodies. These remnants of oxidized hemoglobin attach to the membrane and are subsequently removed by the spleen, giving the characteristic "bite cell" appearance on the peripheral smear.

A recent review identified 299 G6PD variants, 60 of which have been defined at the molecular level. The gene is X-linked, hence males are more commonly affected. But because of X-chromosome inactivation, heterozygote women have a population of hemolysis-susceptible cells. A mild form is carried in approximately 10% of African-Americans, and the incidence runs as high as 70% in Kurdish Jews. Deficiency may be seen in populations throughout Africa, the Mediterranean basin, the Middle East,

TABLE 1. **Nonimmune (Coombs'-Negative) Hemolytic Anemias**

Cause	Diagnostic Evaluation

1. Microangiopathic hemolysis
    TTP–HUS
    DIC
    Pregnancy-related syndromes (eclampsia, HELLP
      syndrome, fatty liver of pregnancy)
    Mechanical heart valve/other intravascular "hardware"
    Vascular anomalies (e.g., cavernous hemangioma)
    Vasculitis
    Malignant hypertension
    Extrinsic injury: burns, March hemoglobinuria
	Peripheral blood smear review for presence of
	  schistocytes; other tests as indicated to establish
	  cause of microangiopathy

2. Enzyme disorders
    Glucose-6-phosphate dehydrogenase (G6PD)
 	
    Pyruvate kinase
 	
    Other enzymes of glycolytic/hexose monophosphate
      shunt pathways (extremely rare)
	Enzyme assay; Heinz body preparation will be
	  positive*
	Enzyme assay; Heinz body preparation will be
	  negative
	Enzyme assay (may require referral to reference
	  laboratory)

3. Hemoglobin disorders
    Hemoglobin SS/SC/S-beta-thalassemia
    Hereditary unstable hemoglobin disorders
 	
    Acquired methemoglobinemia
	Hemoglobin electrophoresis/clinical syndrome
	Heinz body preparation (screen), hemoglobin
	  electrophoresis (may be normal); may require
	  referral to reference laboratory
	Methemoglobin level; clinical picture of cyanosis
	  without hypoxemia

4. Membrane disorders
  Hereditary
    Hereditary spherocytosis
    Hereditary elliptocytosis (HE)/hereditary
      pyropoikilocytosis (HPP)
    Hereditary ovalocytosis
    Abetalipoproteinemia
 	
    Others (very rare)
  Acquired
    Paroxysmal nocturnal hemoglobinuria
 	
    Liver disease (spur cell anemia)
	
	Osmotic fragility test, peripheral blood smear†
	Peripheral blood smear (elliptocytes); osmotic fragility
	  is abnormal in HPP, often normal in HE†
	Osmotic fragility test, peripheral blood smear†
	Peripheral blood smear (acanthocytosis), lipoprotein
	  levels
	
	—
	
	Sucrose/acid hemolysis test, urine for hemosiderin;
	  leukocyte alkaline phosphatase score will be low;
	  flow cytometry for CD 59 on RBC, neutrophils
	Peripheral blood smear (acanthocytosis); biochemical
	  markers or hepatic failure

5. Infection/physical agents
    Clostridia
    Malaria
    Babesiosis
    Bartonellosis
    Haemophilus influenzae
    Arsine gas
    Copper
    Lead intoxication
    Severe hypophosphatemia
    Envenomations
      Cobra
      Brown recluse spider
	Cultures, smear evaluation
	
	Exposure history; levels as appropriate
	
	Exposure history

*Fluorescent spot test is a useful screen. In class 3 deficiency, it may be necessary to wait 8 to 12 weeks after the hemolytic episode.
†Rarely, molecular studies of membrane proteins will be helpful in confirming the diagnosis.
Abbreviations: DIC = disseminated intravascular coagulation; RBC = red blood cell; TTP–HUS = thrombotic thrombocytopenic purpura–hemolytic uremic syndrome; HELLP = *h*emolytic anemia, *e*levated *l*iver enzymes, and *l*ow *p*latelets.

southern Asia, the Pacific Islands, and Central America.

The World Health Organization has classified deficiency states according to degrees of severity: class 1, associated with baseline hemolysis (least common); class 2, severe and associated with potentially severe drug-induced hemolysis and favism; and class 3, mild deficiency associated with milder forms of drug-induced hemolysis. The common African A⁻ variant is class 3; many Mediterranean and Asian variants are class 2.

Hemolysis in G6PD deficiency is most commonly caused by infection, although the exact nature of the oxidative stressor in this situation is not completely understood. The early literature on G6PD includes many reports implicating drugs used to treat infection as inducers of G6PD hemolysis, but subsequent experience has found them to be innocent bystanders. Medications that have been reliably implicated in G6PD-related hemolysis are listed in Table 2. The degree of danger from drug-related hemolysis may not be predictable for individual patients and may

TABLE 2. **Medications That Should Be Used with Caution in Patients with G6PD Deficiency***

Dapsone
Methylene blue
Nalidixic acid
Isobutyl nitrite
Nitrofurantoin (Macrodantin)
Phenazopyridine (Pyridium)
Primaquine
Sulfacetamide
Sulfanilamide
Sulfapyridine
Sulfamethoxazole
Toluidine blue

*Medications should be used in class 3 (mild) deficiency with caution and avoided in class 1 and 2 deficiency.
Modified from Beutler E: Review: G6PD Deficiency. Blood *84*:3613–3636, 1994. With permission.

vary according to the severity of the deficiency and individual variations in metabolism of the drug. Drug-induced hemolysis typically starts 1 to 2 days after drug ingestion and may last for several days afterward. In class 3 (mild) variants, only older cells are affected; in more severe forms, all cells are affected and the hemolysis is more intense. Treatment during acute episodes is supportive. If a precipitating medication is essential and the hemolysis is not life-threatening, it may be reasonable to continue the medication and follow blood counts. Hemolysis may abate over 7 to 10 days in class 3 patients as G6PD-deficient older cells are replaced by hemolysis-resistant reticulocytes. Transfusion of blood *from* G6PD-deficient individuals may hemolyze in the recipient, and this possibility should be considered in appropriate settings. Splenectomy has little role in most common G6PD variants, but a benefit has been found in some cases of chronic hemolysis associated with class 1 deficiency.

Favism has historically been one of the more intriguing aspects of G6PD deficiency and represents severe hemolysis associated with the ingestion of fava beans by patients with class 2 (and on rare occasions class 3) G6PD abnormalities. Hemolysis does not necessarily occur with each ingestion and is presumably due to unique oxidants in these beans. The most dangerous hazard of G6PD deficiency is neonatal kernicterus, which appears to be due to a deficiency of G6PD in the livers of neonates with class 2 deficiency. Phototherapy, exchange transfusion, and phenobarbital may be helpful in preventing mental retardation.

The diagnosis of G6PD deficiency is not a problem in class 1 and 2 variants and is based on quantitative tests of G6PD activity. In class 3 patients, the diagnosis may be complicated by the disappearance of older G6PD-deficient cells during episodes of acute hemolysis. The remaining younger cells and reticulocytes may have normal levels. In this instance, it is reasonable to wait 8 to 12 weeks after the hemolytic event and repeat the testing. If this is not possible, more sophisticated techniques may be required. The fluorescent spot test is useful for screening. This test is based on the principle that NADP reduced in the presence of adequate G6PD levels will fluoresce under ultraviolet light. G6PD-deficient specimens will have either no or dull fluorescence.

Pyruvate Kinase

Deficiencies of enzymes in the glycolytic pathway may also cause hemolytic anemias, with deficiencies of pyruvate kinase accounting for 90% of this group. In contrast with G6PD, this abnormality is extremely rare, with described cases numbering in the hundreds (vs. hundreds of millions for G6PD). Inheritance is autosomal recessive, and the deficiency results in inadequate adenosine triphosphate (ATP) generation to maintain the Na^+/K^+ and other membrane pumps, leading to cellular dehydration, sometimes echinocyte formation, and hemolysis in the spleen. Splenectomy may be beneficial in severe cases.

Other enzyme deficiencies involving the hexose monophosphate shunt and the glycolytic pathway may cause hemolysis, but they are extremely rare.

MEMBRANE DISORDERS

Hereditary

The red cell membrane is composed of a phospholipid bilayer that is traversed by several transmembrane proteins, the most abundant and important for membrane stability being glycophorin and band 3. To this is attached a protein cytoskeleton made up of a highly organized latticework of intertwining strands of alpha and beta spectrin. Spectrin binding to the band 3 membrane protein is mediated by ankyrin and possibly protein 4.2; its binding to glycophorin is mediated by protein 4.1 and actin. These spectrin-membrane interactions serve to stabilize the RBC membrane while allowing sufficient membrane deformability to make it possible for the RBCs to traverse the microvasculature and especially the splenic sinusoids. The 1 to 3 μm slits in the splenic sinusoids represent by far the greatest obstacle to continued circulation of RBCs with either unstable or nondeformable membranes, hence the dramatic improvement seen in these disorders following splenectomy.

The most important of the inherited membrane disorders are those involving abnormalities of the protein cytoskeleton, resulting in hereditary spherocytosis (HS), hereditary elliptocytosis (HE), and hereditary pyropoikilocytosis (HPP). HS is a heterogeneous group of disorders at the molecular level that affect binding of the spectrin cytoskeleton to the phospholipid membrane. These have been referred to as "vertical" defects of the cytoskeleton. Abnormalities that can produce the HS phenotype have been identified in ankyrin, spectrin, band 3, and protein 4.2. The net effect of these abnormalities is to destabilize the RBC membrane, causing loss of phospholipids and hence membrane surface area. The membrane is thus forced to reconfigure to its lowest surface-to-volume ratio, that is, as a spherocyte. These spherocytes are nondeformable and are trapped by the splenic sinusoids, where interactions with the monocyte macrophage system and hypoxia (which results in failure of the ATP-requiring Na^+/K^+ pump) eventually cause premature RBC destruction. Splenectomy is therefore highly effective at improving RBC survival and is usually accompanied by cholecystectomy to prevent bilirubin gallstone formation. The inheritance pattern of HS depends on the specific molecular defect creating the phenotype. Most are autosomal dominant.

In patients with HE, the effect of the cytoskeleton protein defects is not membrane loss but abnormalities in the formation of the spectrin cytoskeleton latticework. These have been referred to as "horizontal" defects. Although the exact physiology of the formation of elliptocytes remains unclear, current speculation is that the abnormal spectrin lattice lacks plasticity and is less likely to return to its normal shape when subjected to shear stress or deformation on passage through the microvasculature. Abnormalities of spectrin self-association or of spectrin binding to ankyrin or protein 4.1, deficiencies of glycophorin C, and abnormalities of protein 4.2 have resulted in the HE phenotype. Hemolysis is usually mild and asymptomatic in HE patients, but, as in HS, splenectomy improves RBC survival, if indicated. Inheritance is autosomal dominant, and the incidence is highest in patients of African ancestry.

Patients with HPP are either homozygotes or double heterozygotes for an HE defect, resulting in more bizarre red cell morphology and more severe hemolysis. The RBCs are notable for their thermal instability (hence *pyro*poikilocytosis). Whereas in normal cells, fragmentation and spectrin denaturation occur at 49° to 50° C, in HPP, this takes place at 45° to 46° C. This phenomenon can occur in some cases of HE, however, and is occasionally absent in HPP.

Hereditary ovalocytosis (HO) may result from severe homozyous protein 4.1 deficiency. Heterozygotes have mild HE. Another form of HO is very common in some Asian populations (up to 30% in parts of Malaysia and New Guinea) and is due to a protein 3 abnormality that enhances the binding of the cytoskeleton to the membrane, increasing its rigidity.

Although none of these syndromes is common, several rarer hemolytic syndromes exist: hereditary stomatocytosis, hereditary xerocytosis, Rh deficiency syndrome, and the McLeod antigen syndrome. More detailed discussion of these and the molecular pathology of the RBC cytoskeleton is available in recent exhaustive reviews in standard hematology texts.

The diagnostic suspicion of HS, HE, HO, and HPP is based on characteristic morphology of the blood smear. The osmotic fragility is increased in HS, HO, and HPP, but not in milder forms of HE. The mean corpuscular hemoglobin concentration is characteristically increased in HS. The key therapeutic issues are the appropriateness of splenectomy and maintaining adequate marrow compensation for the hemolysis (see the discussion following).

Rarely, hereditary defects affect primarily the phospholipid membrane. Patients with abetalipoproteinemia lack B apolipoprotein, with consequent abnormalities in cholesterol and triglyceride transport. Circulating RBCs acquire an acanthocytic (knobby) appearance and become more fragile. This disorder is associated with a progressive neurologic syndrome that is clinically more serious.

Acquired

Liver Disease/Spur Cell Anemia

End-stage liver disease is often characterized by the appearance of numerous acanthocytes and significant hemolytic anemia. Its more severe form is referred to as "spur cell anemia," which affects a small percentage of severe liver disease patients, usually portending a poor prognosis. Physiologically, the RBCs have acquired increased amounts of cholesterol on the outer surface of the phospholipid membrane from circulating lipoproteins and possibly abnormal lipid metabolism. The imbalance of lipids between inner and outer membrane is accommodated by the acanthocytic change. Although the spleen plays a role in the hemolysis, splenectomy is rarely possible due to portal hypertension.

Zieve's syndrome is a mild spherocytic anemia associated with fatty metamorphosis of the liver and hyperglycemia and should be distinguished from spur cell anemia. Its physiologic basis is not well understood.

Paroxysmal Nocturnal Hemoglobinuria (PNH)

This rare but fascinating syndrome, of which it has been said (probably correctly) that "more people study it than have it," enters frequently into the differential diagnosis of unexplained nonimmune hemolysis, hypercoagulation syndromes (particularly hepatic vein and cerebrovenous thrombosis), unexplained iron deficiency, and pancytopenia. The primary abnormality in paroxysmal nocturnal hemoglobinuria (PNH) is an acquired mutation of the PIG-A gene, which codes an enzyme needed to synthesize the glycophosphatidylinositol (GPI) "anchor." This glycolipid attaches numerous proteins to hematopoietic cell membranes. All GPI-anchored proteins are absent from the membranes of affected cells. The defect is at the stem cell level; abnormalities of GPI-anchored proteins have been found in all hematopoietic cell lines in PNH patients. At least three RBC membrane proteins involved in preventing complement-mediated RBC lysis are affected: decay accelerating factor (DAF), membrane inhibitor of reactive lysis (MIRL), and homologous restriction factor (HRF). Together, these defects account for the marked increase in complement-mediated lysis seen in PNH RBCs.

Biochemical markers in PNH reflect intravascular hemolysis, most notably the urine hemosiderin. The sucrose hemolysis test and acid hemolysis (Ham) test demonstrate increased serum-mediated lysis of complement-sensitive PNH cells. More recently, flow cytometry using anti-CD59 (MIRL) antibody has been used diagnostically to identify GPI-deficient neutrophils and RBCs in PNH. The leukocyte alkaline phosphatase (LAP) score is also low, since LAP is a GPI-anchored protein.

Between 10 and 15% of patients presenting with aplastic anemia (AA) show evidence of PNH, and up to 50% of AA patients develop a PNH defect over the course of their illness. Conversely, patients with PNH may evolve an AA picture. Bone marrow transplant has been successfully performed in patients with PNH that has evolved to severe AA. Although bone marrow transplant is the only potential curative therapy available, its significant risks make its role in PNH without life-threatening aplasia a topic of controversy. Management of hemolysis in PNH requires judicious use of iron replacement. A too sudden rise in the number of PNH complement-sensitive erythrocytes may induce a hemolytic crisis and threaten renal function. Infection may also act as a stressor to induce a hemolytic crisis. In this situation, the most effective way to suppress the hemolysis is hypertransfusion. The role of steroids in PNH is debated. They are not a primary therapy. Patients with PNH are usually transfused with washed RBCs to decrease the amount of passenger complement, although the contribution of such plasma to in vivo hemolysis is probably minimal.

PNH may induce life-threatening thrombosis in the hepatic veins, for which thrombolytic therapy may be lifesaving. Although earlier reports suggested that heparin may increase complement-mediated hemolysis in PNH, in our experience and in that of others, it is safe.

HEMOGLOBIN DISORDERS

Hereditary

Several forms of mutations may result in unstable hemoglobins with subsequent hemolysis. The most common, hemoglobin S and thalassemia mutations, are discussed elsewhere. Mutations primarily causing oxidative instability of heme are uncommon but are important in the differential diagnosis of Coombs'-negative hemolysis. A common feature of the mutations causing unstable hemoglobins is that they affect heme-protein interactions in the heme pocket of the globin chains. Such mutations may directly involve heme-protein binding (e.g., hemoglobin Köln) or cause conformational changes in the folding of the hemoglobin that alter the stability of the heme pocket and its ability to exclude oxidants (e.g., hemoglobin Christchurch). When unstable hemoglobins are subject to oxidant stresses, hemoglobin is converted to methemoglobin (hemoglobin with iron oxidized to the Fe^{+++} state). Although normal hemoglobins can handle this challenge (methemoglobin reductase reduces the methemoglobin back to hemoglobin), in unstable hemoglobins, the methemo-

globin is more prone to denature and precipitate, resulting in the formation of characteristic Heinz bodies. Heinz bodies are aggregates of precipitated hemoglobin that attach to the RBC membrane at band 3 and are subsequently removed by splenic or hepatic macrophages, producing bite cells, as in G6PD deficiency (see the previous discussion). The precise mechanism of hemolysis is uncertain. Heinz bodies may impede passage of RBCs through the splenic sinusoids or, more likely, induce membrane changes that render the RBCs more susceptible to splenic destruction.

The degree of hemolysis in these syndromes varies significantly according to the specific mutation. It is often induced by the same oxidative stresses that induce G6PD deficiency—infection and medication. These syndromes can be screened for with a standard Heinz body preparation. (Heinz bodies cannot be seen on a standard Wright's stain smear.) Hemoglobin electrophoresis may identify an abnormal hemoglobin, but many unstable hemoglobins are electrophoretically silent, since the mutations do not necessarily affect the overall charge on the molecule. Diagnosis in this instance requires referral to a hemoglobin reference laboratory. A hemoglobin-oxygen dissociation curve is sometimes a helpful adjunct to diagnosis, since some of these hemoglobins are also high-affinity variants. Transfusion may be required during hemolytic episodes, but the hemolysis is usually well compensated. Splenectomy may be helpful if a clinically meaningful transfusion requirement develops.

Homozygous beta-globin variants may also induce mild hemolysis. Hemoglobin C ($\beta6$ glu $\rightarrow$ lys) forms intracellular crystals; in the homozygous state, a mild hemolytic anemia is present. Hemoglobin E ($\beta26$ glu $\rightarrow$ lys), which is common in Southeast Asians, is a beta-globin variant with decreased globin chain synthesis due to an unstable messenger RNA. The homozygous state resembles a beta-thalassemia minor. Hemoglobin E inherited with beta-thalassemia results in a beta-thalassemia major phenotype, with severe transfusion-dependent anemia.

Acquired

The pathologic significance of acquired methemoglobinemia is related more to its high oxygen affinity than to hemolysis, but it may induce Heinz body–related hemolysis and is reasonably considered to be an acquired hemoglobin disorder. Ferrous (Fe^{++}) iron is ordinarily oxidized to ferric (Fe^{+++}) iron at a low baseline rate, converting hemoglobin to methemoglobin. The reaction is reversed by methemoglobin reductase and other RBC antioxidants. Rarely, inherited hemoglobin (M hemoglobins) or enzyme disorders result in congenital methemoglobinemia, a clinically benign condition resulting in congenital cyanosis. More typically, methemoglobinemia is acquired in the setting of oxidant drug or toxin exposure. Important inducers include nitrates, nitrites (including nitroglycerin, nitroprusside, and some "recreationally" used drugs, such as amyl nitrite), sulfones such as dapsone, benzocaine (sometimes used to cut cocaine and possibly relevant in cocaine overdoses), phenazopyridine (Pyridium), and aniline dyes. Chronic hemolysis has been well described with methemoglobinemia due to chronic phenazopyridine use. However, the typical clinical picture of methemoglobinemia is cyanosis in the presence of normal oxygen saturation, since methemoglobin does not revert to a red color on binding oxygen. Clinical signs and symptoms are due to oxygen deprivation. Methemoglobin is a high-affinity hemoglobin that does not release oxygen to tissues. Treatment is methylene blue 1 to 2 mg per kg as a 1% solution in saline infused over 10 to 15 minutes, which acts as an electron donor to NADPH reductase, allowing conversion of methemoglobin back to hemoglobin. The dose can be repeated hourly up to 7 mg per kg. Since the action of NADPH reductase is dependent on G6PD, this treatment is not helpful in G6PD-deficient patients. Exchange transfusion may be indicated in this situation. Hypoxic symptoms typically start at methemoglobin levels of 30% and become life-threatening at 50%.

OTHER CAUSES OF NONIMMUNE HEMOLYSIS

Catastrophic intravascular hemolysis may be seen with infection due to *Clostridium welchii*, which releases a potent phospholipase. Mortality rates of greater than 50% have been reported, even with aggressive antibiotic treatment. Worldwide, the most common cause of infection-related hemolysis is malaria. Other infectious agents that may be associated with nonimmune hemolysis are *Bartonella baccilliformis* (bartonellosis), *Babesia* species (babesiosis, currently localized to the northeastern United States), and, rarely, *Haemophilus influenzae*. Venoms of the brown recluse spider and the cobra contain potent hemolysins. Other spider and snake envenomations rarely cause hemolysis except by precipitating disseminated intravascular coagulation (DIC). Arsine gas (AsH_3, a by-product of processing and manufacturing fertilizer) and copper exposures have also been associated with hemolysis; copper-mediated RBC damage is the likely cause of hemolysis associated with Wilson's disease. Mild hemolysis is also seen in lead intoxication, but the primary cause of the anemia is impaired heme production. Severe hypophosphatemia may also cause hemolysis due to the inability to make ATP and loss of Na^+/K^+ pump function.

Burns may be associated with microangiopathic hemolysis, as are some forms of vigorous exercise involving repetitive trauma to the soles of the feet (march hemoglobinuria). Other microangiopathic processes that can cause nonimmune hemolysis are outlined in Table 1 and should be considered when schistocytes are seen on the blood smear. The more serious causes—TTP, DIC, and pregnancy-related causes—are discussed in other chapters. Intravascular hardware such as mechanical heart valves and aortic balloon pumps also cause microangiopathy. Intravascular hemolysis associated with mechanical heart valves often precipitates iron deficiency due to urinary iron losses. A sudden rise in the degree of valve hemolysis should raise the suspicion for a perivalvular leak. Pharmacologic manipulation to decrease the number of RBCs crossing the valve (i.e., the cardiac output or regurgitant fraction) is the only nonsurgical management for this problem.

APLASTIC/HYPOPLASTIC CRISIS

In milder hemolytic syndromes, the increased destruction is well compensated by an increase in marrow production of RBCs, to a maximum of 10 times normal. Patients with shortened RBC survival are accordingly disproportionately affected by any condition that impairs marrow production of RBCs. Folate deficiency is a rare cause of this problem, but it is always a concern, because the increased RBC turnover increases folate requirements and stores are modest—2 to 4 months. However, patients eating an otherwise balanced diet rarely develop clinical folate deficiency, although supplementation is generally recommended as a precaution. Iron deficiency anemia should be considered in menstrual-age women and in patients with a source of chronic blood loss through the urine or gastrointestinal tract. Renal failure and consequent fall in erythropoietin levels should also be considered, especially in diabetic patients. If erythropoietin levels are low or normal, recombinant erythropoietin supplementation may obviate transfusion therapy.

Acute infection or any other cause of an inflammatory reaction also suppresses RBC production, which should return to normal once the inflammatory reaction has passed. The mechanism is identical to that of the so-called anemia of chronic disease, and this should not be confused with aplastic crisis.

True aplastic crisis is due to infection with parvovirus B19, an RNA virus that causes pure red cell aplasia for approximately 14 days in immunocompetent hosts. The reticulocyte count in parvovirus infection is typically 0 or very close to it—"mere" RBC hypoplasia is against parvovirus infection in our experience. The ability to weather 14 days of aplasia depends entirely on what the RBC survival is, but in clinically relevant chronic hemolytic syndromes, this usually results in life-threatening anemia. The clinical syndrome may consist of arthralgias and malaise and a "slapped face" rash on the cheeks, the so-called fifth viral exanthem of childhood (hence the name fifth disease). Many patients are asymptomatic, however, apart from the consequent anemia.

Diagnosis is established by detection of serum IgM antibodies against parvovirus. The illness is self-limited in otherwise immunocompetent patients and should require no therapy apart from transfusion support. In immunocompromised patients, such as those with HIV infection, parvovirus may cause a chronic pure red cell aplasia that responds dramatically to intravenous immune globulin infusions, 1 to 2 grams per kg every 3 weeks.

SPLENECTOMY

Potential clinical consequences of chronic hemolysis are transfusion requirement and the development of bilirubin (pigmented) gallstones. In syndromes characterized by destruction of RBCs in the spleen (HS, HPP, unstable hemoglobins), splenectomy may be beneficial. Gallstones often occur at a young age in patients with HS; this is generally considered an indication for splenectomy, since gallstones may recur despite cholecystectomy. A recent survey of 226 patients who had undergone splenectomy for HS found a rate of fatal sepsis of 0.73 per 1000 years. All cases were prior to the introduction of pneumococcal vaccine. All patients considered for splenectomy should be given pneumococcal, meningococcal, and *Haemophilus influenzae* vaccines. It is not our practice to give prophylactic antibiotics to adult patients, but we do advise them to keep penicillin or erythromycin available and to begin treatment immediately for fever. Postsplenectomy sepsis rates in children under age 6 years are higher, and splenectomy should be delayed if reasonable in this age group. Prophylactic penicillin (or equivalent) should be given to splenectomized children under age 6 years.

PERNICIOUS ANEMIA AND OTHER MEGALOBLASTIC ANEMIAS

method of
AŚOK C. ANTONY, M.D.
Indiana University School of Medicine
Indianapolis, Indiana

Both vitamin B_{12}, or cobalamin (Cbl), and folate are essential for DNA synthesis. Deficiency of either vitamin can lead to megaloblastosis, manifesting morphologically as a nuclear-cytoplasmic dissociation primarily affecting rapidly proliferating cells, and clinically as megaloblastic anemia. However Cbl deficiency can also lead to a neurologic syndrome involving cerebral, myelopathic, peripheral neuropathic, optic, and/or autonomic nerve dysfunction. In general, it is important to recognize megaloblastic anemia and/or neurologic disease, distinguish folate from Cbl deficiency and combined Cbl plus folate deficiency, and identify the mechanism leading to deficiency.

CLINICAL PRESENTATIONS WITH COBALAMIN AND FOLATE DEFICIENCY

Classic descriptions of Cbl (and folate) deficiency have stressed megaloblastosis presenting as pancytopenia with a megaloblastic bone marrow as early manifestations (other features can include glossitis, broad-spectrum malabsorption, cervical or uterine dysplasia, hyperpigmentation, and infertility). However, with Cbl deficiency it is now recognized that there is an inverse relationship between the degree of anemia and neurologic disease. Nearly one-

third of Cbl-deficient patients have neurologic disease without anemia, and almost one-half with neurologic manifestations have either mild or no anemia; thus only a *minority* have combined hematologic and neurologic disease.

DIAGNOSIS OF COBALAMIN AND FOLATE DEFICIENCY

Morphologic Evaluation

Macro-ovalocytes and hypersegmented polymorphonuclear leukocytes (PMNs) are the hallmark of megaloblastosis. Apart from drugs (phenytoin [Dilantin], azathioprine [Imuran], and occasionally zidovudine [Retrovir]) and alcohol, macrocytosis *without* megaloblastosis may be seen with reticulocytosis, liver disease, aplastic anemia, myelodysplastic syndromes, myeloma, and chronic obstructive pulmonary disease. The frequency of hypersegmented PMNs (5% with five lobes or 1% with six lobes) in patients with megaloblastic hematopoiesis is 98%. The sensitivity decreases to only 78% in alcoholics, although the specificity of this finding is approximately 95%. With combined hypersegmented PMNs and macro-ovalocytosis, the specificity is 96 to 98% and the positive predictive value of either folate or Cbl deficiency is approximately 94%. However, since these findings have been missed in approximately 33% by laboratory personnel, one must exert caution before eliminating Cbl and folate deficiency based on laboratory reports alone.

Megaloblastosis due to Cbl or folate deficiency may be reversed in 24 hours by the administration of folate (including a nutritious hospital meal); however, hypersegmented PMNs (when present) may be found in the circulation for up to 2 weeks after replacement with Cbl or folate.

When folate or Cbl deficiency coexists with anemias secondary to iron deficiency, chronic disease, or hemoglobinopathies, megaloblastic manifestations of red blood cells (RBCs) (but not white blood cells [WBCs]) may be masked. Appropriate replacement with Cbl or folate elicits maximal responses only when associated iron deficiency is corrected. Conversely, if combined iron and Cbl or folate deficiency is treated with iron alone, megaloblastosis is unmasked.

The need for a bone marrow test is often dictated by the urgency to diagnose megaloblastosis (results available in 1 hour). Thus, in outpatients, or with characteristic peripheral smears, or primary neuropsychiatric presentations, one can initiate diagnostic tests without a bone marrow test. Also, in pregnant patients with characteristic smears and a history of noncompliance with prenatal supplements, a bone marrow test is not necessary to initiate therapy for a strong presumptive diagnosis of pure folate deficiency.

Biochemical Evaluation

Serum and Red Blood Cell Folate Levels. When combined with a clinical picture of megaloblastic anemia and additional results of Cbl levels, the serum folate level is the cheapest and most useful initial biochemical test to diagnose folate deficiency (Table 1). However, false-positive reductions of the serum folate level occur in one-third of hospitalized patients with anorexia, after acute alcoholism, in pregnancy, and with anticonvulsant therapy. Conversely, in up to 50% of alcoholic patients with folate-deficient megaloblastosis, the serum folate levels may be low-normal or borderline (i.e., low-normal = 2 to 4 ng per mL) by radioassay. Thus, the serum folate level alone should never dictate therapy, and it is important to con-

TABLE 1. **Stepwise Approach to Diagnosis of Cobalamin and Folate Deficiency**

Megaloblastic anemia or neurologic and psychiatric manifestations consistent with Cbl deficiency

plus

Test results on serum Cbl and serum folate levels:

If Cbl is <200 pg/mL and serum folate level is normal, i.e., >2 ng/mL (and not low-normal, i.e., <4 ng/mL), diagnosis is consistent with Cbl deficiency.

If Cbl is 200–300 pg/mL and serum folate level is normal, i.e., >2 ng/mL (and not low-normal, i.e., <4 ng/mL), go to metabolite levels to rule out Cbl deficiency.

If Cbl is >300 pg/mL and serum folate level is <2 ng/mL, diagnosis is consistent with folate deficiency.

If Cbl is <200 pg/mL and serum folate level is <2 ng/mL, diagnosis is consistent with combined Cbl and folate deficiency, or isolated folate deficiency; go to metabolite levels.

If Cbl is >300 pg/mL and serum folate level is low-normal (i.e., 2–4 ng/mL), diagnosis could be either folate deficiency or anemia that is not related to vitamin deficiency; go to metabolite levels.

If serum Cbl is unavailable* and serum folate level is 2–4 ng/mL (borderline low), go to metabolites to rule out Cbl and/or folate deficiency.

If Cbl and folate test results suggest that additional testing with metabolites is warranted:

Test results on metabolites, MMA, and HCYS:

If MMA and HCYS levels are increased, Cbl deficiency is confirmed; folate deficiency still possible.

If MMA level is normal but HCYS level is increased, folate deficiency is likely; ~5% with Cbl deficiency have this combination.

If MMA and HCYS levels are normal, Cbl deficiency is excluded.

*Call laboratory for information they have on Cbl levels done at same time folate tests were generated.
Abbreviations: Cbl = cobalamin; MMA = methylmalonic acid; HCYS = homocysteine.

sider the clinical picture, peripheral smear, and bone marrow morphology, and to rule out underlying Cbl deficiency.

When tissue folate stores are exhausted, RBC folate levels fall to less than 150 ng per mL. However, RBC folate assays have generally been unreliable in alcoholic, pregnant, and Cbl-deficient patients. Current radioassays for RBC folate levels that have major problems with precision and accuracy have also not been clinically validated. This has led several experts to avoid the use of RBC folate levels until these issues are resolved. An approach that relies on serum Cbl and folate levels as initial tests is presented in Table 1.

Serum Cobalamin Levels. A low serum Cbl level (less than 200 pg per mL) plus clinical or morphologic evidence supporting Cbl deficiency confirms the diagnosis. However, there are well-recognized false-positive and false-negative results, and a low serum Cbl level is therefore not synonymous with Cbl deficiency.

The serum Cbl level is less than 300 pg per mL in 99% of patients *with* clinical hematologic or neurologic manifestations of Cbl deficiency. Conversely, a Cbl level greater than 300 pg per mL predicts folate deficiency, or another hematologic disease (see Table 1). Furthermore, despite Cbl deficiency, approximately 5% have normal Cbl levels, and approximately 10% of adults (approximately 15% of elderly persons) with true Cbl deficiency may have Cbl values in the low-normal (200 to 300 pg per mL) range.

These individuals should now be tested with more sensitive metabolite tests (methylmalonic acid [MMA] and serum homocysteine [HCYS] levels; discussed below), which can identify those with Cbl deficiency. The Cbl levels are also reduced in up to one-third of those with folate deficiency but normalize after therapy with folate. In the event they do not, the patient may have a combined Cbl deficiency.

Serum Homocysteine and Methylmalonic Acid Levels. Levels of the metabolites HCYS and MMA increase in the serum as a result of inhibition of Cbl- or folate-dependent enzymes. With Cbl deficiency, MMA levels are elevated in 98.4%, and HCYS in 95.9%, with levels of both metabolites elevated in 99.8% (a minority with Cbl deficiency have only increased HCYS levels). Thus, normal levels of both MMA and total HCYS rule out clinically significant Cbl deficiency with 100% certainty. With folate deficiency, HCYS levels alone are increased in 91%. Following appropriate Cbl replacement, the elevated HCYS and MMA levels drop and normalize after a week; they do not decrease with folate alone. Likewise, elevated HCYS levels from folate deficiency do not normalize until folic acid is correctly administered.

I recommend first using the cheaper serum folate and Cbl tests, which assist in diagnosis of the majority of obvious cases of Cbl and folate deficiency, and to restrict the use of serum MMA and HCYS tests for the following cases:

1. Those with borderline Cbl and folate levels (see Table 1).

2. Those in whom there are coexisting conditions known to falsely perturb folate or Cbl tests.

3. Those in whom both Cbl and folate levels are low; in such cases a high MMA level is useful in confirming Cbl deficiency (rather than attributing the condition to folate deficiency alone).

4. Those with low serum Cbl levels but in whom there is an alternative explanation for the syndrome that led to testing the serum Cbl level (i.e., in diabetic or alcoholic patients with a peripheral neuropathy, or in alcoholic patients with macrocytosis and low serum Cbl level without anemia).

ETIOPATHOGENESIS OF COBALAMIN AND FOLATE DEFICIENCY

Since humans are dependent on Cbl (and folate) from dietary sources, there are several potential mechanisms for the development of deficiency (Table 2). Cobalamin is extremely well conserved, and it takes several years to develop deficiency after insufficient intake or malabsorption. Consequently, clinical manifestations develop insidi-

TABLE 2. **Mechanisms Leading to Development of Cobalamin and Folate Deficiency**

Cobalamin	Folate*
Nutritional Cbl deficiency	*Decreased Supply*
Inadequate dissociation of Cbl from food protein	Intake
	Absorption
Absent IF secretion (pernicious anemia)	Transport
Usurpation of luminal Cbl	*Increased Requirement*
Inadequate ileal absorptive surface	Utilization or metabolic consumption
Inactivation of Cbl via N_2O exposure	Destruction
	Excretion

*Often in a given patient, there is a combination of mechanisms.
Abbreviations: Cbl = cobalamin; IF = intrinsic factor.

ously and additional tests are usually required to establish the cause. Pernicious anemia, the commonest cause for Cbl deficiency, is seen among all ethnic and age groups.

The Schilling test identifies the mechanism for malabsorption of Cbl and can suggest further diagnostic tests and specific therapy; this in turn dictates the duration of replacement therapy required. Normally, oral (crystalline) radiolabeled cyanocobalamin (CN[57Co]Cbl) first binds R protein, which on degradation by pancreatic proteases releases the radiolabeled Cbl for intrinsic factor (IF) binding and absorption via ileal IF-Cbl receptors. If the blood contains an excess of Cbl (from a "flushing" injection of Cbl), more than 8% of the CN[57Co]Cbl is normally excreted in the urine in 24 hours (*normal Stage I test*). With absent endogenous IF, as in pernicious anemia, less than 8% of the radiolabel is excreted; however, when IF is given with the CN[57Co]Cbl, this abnormality is corrected (*positive Stage II test*). With bacterial usurpation of Cbl, oral antibiotic therapy for 10 days corrects Cbl malabsorption (*positive Stage III test*); if not, then (with rare exceptions) Cbl malabsorption is localized to an ileal cause (*abnormal Stage I, II, and III Schilling tests*). If the Stage I test result is normal, as is observed in 10 to 20% of those with true Cbl deficiency, there may be an inability to release Cbl from food because of hypo- or achlorhydria. This is not identified by the standard Schilling test using *crystalline* CN[57Co]Cbl and is an indication for the food–CN[57Co]Cbl (food-Cbl) absorption test, in which the capacity to absorb protein-bound Cbl is tested (i.e., CN[57Co]Cbl bound to either egg yolk–ovalbumin or proteins in chicken serum). This test can be low in 25 to 50% of patients with low Cbl levels, normal Schilling tests, and adequate diet, especially in those over 70 years of age but is incompletely validated.

An intestinal cause for Cbl malabsorption may be (incorrectly) identified as the primary mechanism of Cbl malabsorption in pernicious anemia unless the Schilling test is delayed until after 2 months of Cbl replacement to ensure correction of any functional defects arising from intestinal megaloblastosis. Anti-intrinsic factor antibodies, which are highly specific for pernicious anemia, are present in the serum in only 60% of patients.

Since folate stores last approximately 4 months, the cause of folate deficiency can often be traced to the fairly recent past (see Table 2). However, multiple mechanisms may contribute to folate deficiency in the same patient, and causal assignment to one or more mechanisms is clinically based.

THERAPEUTIC ISSUES

Therapeutic Trials

The traditional therapeutic trial using physiologic doses of vitamins (100 μg of folate or 1 μg of Cbl given daily while monitoring the reticulocyte response) has given way to a modified therapeutic trial. Here, the intention is often not so much to make the diagnosis of a deficiency, but to confirm the clinical suspicion that the patient does not have a deficiency. This is demonstrated by a lack of response to full replacement daily doses of both vitamins (1 mg of folic acid orally for 10 days and 1 mg of Cbl intramuscularly for 10 days). Clinical scenarios in which such trials may be applicable (after drawing blood for serum Cbl and folate tests) are as follows:

1. When there is a clinical suspicion that the un-

derlying disease is *not* due to a vitamin deficiency, but this is not supported by clinical, morphologic, and biochemical evaluation. Such conditions include anemia with a megaloblastic bone marrow that may be secondary to chemotherapy, myelodysplastic syndromes, or acute myeloid leukemia; when either time is critical in making the diagnosis or the levels of Cbl are likely to be falsely abnormal because of these diseases; or when there is underlying dehydration or renal dysfunction that predictably gives falsely high levels of metabolites.

2. In other situations (i.e., pregnancy, acquired immune deficiency syndrome [AIDS], or alcoholism) with a multifactorial basis for anemia, in which the response (or lack thereof) to full doses can eliminate Cbl or folate deficiency from consideration and thereby narrow the (often extensive) differential diagnosis.

3. When severe anemia with megaloblastosis is clinically obvious but is also so serious that one cannot wait for the results of specific tests for deficiency. If there is a response to the *full doses,* manifested by brisk reticulocytosis by day 5 to 7, retrospective assignment of the deficiency is based on the results of blood samples drawn before beginning the trial.

In all therapeutic trials, if there is no evidence of response within 10 days, a bone marrow test is indicated to identify another primary hematologic disease.

Replacement Therapy

An appropriate replacement regimen is 1 mg of intramuscular cyanocobalamin (CN-Cbl) per day (week 1), 1 mg twice weekly (week 2), 1 mg per week for 4 weeks, and then 1 mg per month *for life.* Traditionally, patients have been managed by monthly self-administered Cbl injections. However, oral Cbl is a viable alternative to parenteral Cbl for maintenance therapy. Therefore, for those who refuse or cannot manage parenteral Cbl, or prefer daily oral therapy, 1-mg-per-day Cbl tablets are available for long-term administration. (Since approximately 1% of Cbl is passively absorbed across the gastrointestinal tract despite Cbl malabsorption, the use of *at least* 1 mg ensures adequate uptake daily.) A switch to oral Cbl should be considered only after replenishment of Cbl-deficient tissues and stores by parenteral Cbl therapy. The important issue is to ensure compliance by the demonstration of adequate serum Cbl levels and the resolution of hematologic and/or neurologic abnormalities on follow-up.

Oral folate (folic acid, 1 to 5 mg per day) results in adequate absorption (even when intestinal malabsorption of food folate is present). Therapy should be continued until complete hematologic recovery is documented, but if the underlying cause leading to folate deficiency cannot be corrected, folate therapy should be continued. Folinic acid (leucovorin), which is very expensive, should be reserved for rescue protocols involving antifolates (methotrexate, trimethoprim-sulfamethoxazole); for use as an adjunct to trimetrexate for *Pneumocystis carinii* pneumonia; for 5-fluorouracil modulation protocols; and for use after prolonged N_2O exposure.

Causes for nonresponsiveness to Cbl or folate (manifested by lack of reticulocytosis by day 10) include a wrong diagnosis, combined folate and Cbl deficiency treated with only one vitamin, or associated disease (iron deficiency, hemoglobinopathy, chronic disease, or hypothyroidism).

Transfusions and Adjunctive Therapy

In severely anemic patients with heart failure or imminent decompensation, transfusion of 1 U of packed RBCs *slowly,* with vigorous diuresis, can be lifesaving. Although transfusion does not alter serum folate or Cbl levels, the temptation to overtransfuse should be resisted. And in the absence of heart failure, the likelihood of a dramatic response in the sense of well being within hours and a hematopoietic response within days of appropriate vitamin replacement argues in favor of withholding transfusions.

Since the hematopoietic response to Cbl and folate therapy is invariably accompanied by early hypokalemia and hyperuricemia, any pre-existing potassium deficit or hyperuricemia must be corrected at the beginning of replacement therapy with Cbl or folate.

PROPHYLAXIS

Indications for routine supplementation with Cbl and folate are listed in Table 3. Apart from routine supplemental folic acid during pregnancy, it is now recognized that *periconceptional* folate supplementation (at least 400 μg per day) for *all normal women* reduces the incidence of neural tube defects (spina bifida, meningocele, anencephaly) in their babies. Also, women with a prior history of delivering a child with neural tube defects have a 10-fold increased

TABLE 3. **Indications for Prophylaxis with Cobalamin or Folate**

Prophylaxis with Cobalamin
Infants of mothers with pernicious anemia
Infants on specialized diets
Vegans
Those with total or partial gastrectomy with achlorhydria*

Prophylaxis with Folic Acid†
All women contemplating pregnancy (at least 400 μg/day)
Women during pregnancy and lactation, premature infants
Mothers at risk for delivery of infants with neural tube defects (4 mg/day)
Those with hemolytic anemias or hyperproliferative hematologic states‡
Patients with rheumatoid arthritis or psoriasis on therapy with methotrexate§

*Prophylaxis should include iron.
†One should ensure that the patient does not have cobalamin deficiency before initiating folate prophylaxis.
‡This is to prevent a reticulocytopenic crisis from superimposed megaloblastic changes.
§This is to reduce toxicity of the antifolate.

risk of delivering a subsequent child with the same disorder and should be given periconceptional folic acid in higher doses (4 mg per day), which protects approximately 75% of the fetuses of these women.

THALASSEMIA

method of
LAWRENCE WOLFE, M.D.
Boston Floating Hospital
Boston, Massachusetts

Thalassemia is a genetically determined illness affecting primarily (but not confined to) people of Mediterranean or Asian origin. An irreversible deficiency exists in the synthesis of either alpha- or nonalpha-globin chains of hemoglobin. Consequently, there is a decrease in the hemoglobin content of individual red cells, which leads to the formation of hypochromic microcytic red blood cells. At the same time, the excess normally produced chains precipitate in the absence of their corresponding globin chain, and these aggregates lead to premature red cell death, both in the marrow (ineffective erythropoiesis) and in the peripheral blood (hemolytic anemia). The severity of each component of the illness is directly proportional to the degree of chain imbalance.

Since there are two beta-globin genes, there are two major levels of gene output and hence severity of illness in beta-thalassemia. The heterozygote for beta-globin gene failure has a recognizable carrier state ("beta-thalassemia trait") characterized by mild anemia (hemoglobin ≥10 grams per dL), hypochromia, and microcytosis. Failure of both beta genes leads to a severely affected homozygote. Patients with no beta-globin production and no compensatory response of other nonalpha chains have the most severe illness ("thalassemia major"), requiring transfusion for day-to-day survival. If some beta globin is produced from the defective genes or if there is elevated production of gamma chain (hemoglobin F), the patient may maintain a hemoglobin level that permits life without transfusion ("beta-thalassemia intermedia").

There are four alpha-globin genes and, hence, greater heterogeneity in clinical alpha-thalassemia syndromes. Failure of a single alpha gene creates no recognizable clinical phenotype. When two alpha genes fail, the degree of globin-gene imbalance is analogous to the situation in which a single beta gene is defective, and thus the clinical picture is identical to that of beta-thalassemia trait. When three alpha genes fail, there is 25% of the normal gene output. This clinical syndrome is called "hemoglobin H disease," because the excess precipitated beta chains are called "hemoglobin H." Since there is decreased but *not* ablated alpha-chain production, this illness approximates mild beta-thalassemia intermedia. Complete failure of alpha-gene output is lethal and leads to spontaneous abortion or to the birth of a stillborn infant with hydrops fetalis and Bart's hemoglobin (precipitated gamma chains) in its red cells.

The degree of anemia that the untransfused patient manifests sets the pattern and tempo of an individual patient's disorder. In alpha- or beta-thalassemia trait there is virtually no anemia and hence no illness. When globin imbalance becomes more severe, the anemia induces the virtually malignant expansion of the ineffective bone marrow erythroid mass, which leads to the skeletal expansion and catabolism of the disease. Anemia-induced extramedullary hematopoiesis enlarges the liver and the spleen. This immense erythron is avid for iron, and gastrointestinal iron absorption increases 6- to 10-fold.

The chronically low hemoglobin level can also lead to life-threatening, high-output congestive heart failure. The reticuloendothelial blockage engendered by the peripheral hemolytic aspect of the anemia leads to susceptibility to infection. In fact, before the use of transfusion, congestive heart failure and infection were the cause of death in most patients.

By eliminating anemia, transfusion halts and reverses most of the signs and symptoms of thalassemia, leading to an improved quantity and quality of life. Unfortunately, treatment by transfusion is accompanied by the ongoing accumulation of iron and hence iron-induced organ failure. It is unfortunate that transfusion, the treatment that now prevents death in patients in their first decade, provides the major component of the iron poisoning that without treatment is so deadly in the third decade. In fact, transfusion-iron-induced organ failure (cardiac disease, liver disease, diabetes mellitus, and other endocrinopathies) constitutes almost all the aspects of disease in patients with thalassemia treated today. In the absence of current therapies directed at iron overload, chronically transfused patients with thalassemia major would die of a cardiac disorder, usually in the second or third decade.

DIAGNOSIS

Alpha-Thalassemia

There are four alpha genes; therefore four clinical pictures may develop. The loss of a single alpha gene has no effect. Deletion of two alpha genes, alpha-thalassemia trait, results in a hypochromic microcytic anemia. The specific diagnosis of the condition is made by (1) exclusion of other causes of hypochromic microcytic anemia (e.g., iron deficiency, beta-thalassemia trait, lead poisoning), (2) demonstration of a parent with hypochromic microcytic red cells satisfying condition 1, and (3) association with an ethnic group known to have a high incidence of alpha-thalassemia (blacks and people of Asian or Mediterranean descent). Occasionally, hemoglobin H (precipitated beta chains) can be found on staining of peripheral blood in patients with alpha-thalassemia trait. Hemoglobin H is far more apparent in the more severe hypochromic microcytic anemia (called "hemoglobin H disease"), which occurs with the loss of three alpha genes. Hydropic stillbirth is the usual outcome of complete loss of all four alpha genes.

Beta-Thalassemia

With two beta-globin genes functioning in the normal individual, the basic clinical syndromes observed relate to loss of one ("beta-thalassemia trait" or "minor") or two ("beta-thalassemia major") beta genes. The patient with beta-thalassemia trait has a mild anemia (hemoglobin ≥ 10 grams per dL) with hypochromic microcytic red cells and usually belongs to an ethnic group known to have an incidence of beta-gene deletion (blacks and people of Mediterranean or Asian descent). Confirmation of the diagnosis is made by hemoglobin electrophoresis. The hemoglobin A_2 level is moderately elevated (3.8 to 8% in most cases), and increased levels of fetal hemoglobin (1 to 10%) occur in approximately half the patients. Care must be taken not to perform hemoglobin electrophoresis on red cells from an individual with concomitant iron deficiency, as this may artificially lower the hemoglobin A_2 level. Beta-

thalassemia major is a life-threatening hypochromic microcytic anemia not present at birth but fully established before the first birthday. The peripheral smear usually contains strikingly hypochromic red cells, fragments, and some nucleated red cells. Hemoglobin electrophoresis shows primarily hemoglobin F. Both parents are found to have obvious thalassemia trait in most cases.

The Asian population has an important structural hemoglobin variant, hemoglobin E. Recent evidence has shown that the beta gene that produces hemoglobin E is also a thalassemia gene, producing less beta globin than normal. Although hemoglobin E trait and homozygous hemoglobin E disease are mild hypochromic microcytic anemias, the matching of a hemoglobin E gene and a beta-thalassemia trait gene leads to the clinical phenotype of a thalassemia major patient. Hemoglobin E can be detected on standard hemoglobin electrophoresis and is an important condition to detect, especially for issues of genetic counseling.

THERAPY

Thalassemia Major

The goals of therapy include (1) maintaining the hemoglobin at a level consistent with a high quality of life, (2) imparting as little transfusion-related iron as possible, and (3) inducing iron excretion to achieve negative iron balance (more iron excreted than ingested each day).

Transfusion

The evolution of transfusion for patients with thalassemia major began with its intermittent use to prevent death from anemia. As patients began to live longer, attempts to improve the quality of life led to so-called hypertransfusion programs aimed at maintaining hemoglobin levels between 10 and 11 grams per dL. Expected benefits of these programs include deceleration of bone marrow expansion and skeletal changes, as well as improvements in growth and development. The next step was "supertransfusion" (maintaining hemoglobin at ≥ 12 grams per dL), designed to suppress the iron-avid erythroid mass completely and theoretically to decrease gastrointestinal iron absorption. In a cohort of patients treated in this manner, blood volume decreased as well as plasma iron turnover. The decrease in blood volume in these patients permitted stabilization of the higher hemoglobin levels without an increase in the amount of blood (and therefore iron) transfused. We currently use supertransfusion for our patients, but centers that promote hypertransfusion have reported excellent results.

In the late 1970s, the use of red cell preparations enriched with young red cells ("neocytes") began to be explored. Most centers that have used these products have found them to decrease the amount of transfusion required to maintain a given hemoglobin level, but problems concerning a true cost/benefit analysis and increased donor exposure have prevented their widespread use.

The patient who depends on transfusion to sustain life is at risk for transfusion reactions of all sorts, red cell sensitization (as well as human leukocyte antigen [HLA] sensitization), and transmission of infection. Strict adherence to blood bank standards and regulations should dramatically reduce infectious risk and is critically important for these patients, who may face lifelong transfusion. Prevention of most transfusion reactions can be achieved by the use of an in-line white blood cell filter. Patients with febrile or allergic transfusion reactions to white cell–filtered erythrocytes may benefit from the use of frozen deglycerolized washed red cells.

Chelation

As humans tend to sequester iron so successfully, iron excretion must be promoted by the use of a chelator. Currently, deferoxamine (Desferal) is the drug of choice by virtue of its avidity for iron and its safety during chronic administration. Deferoxamine was initially given by daily or intermittent injection; however, the achievement of net negative iron balance was shown to require parenteral infusion.

Daily ambulatory 12-hour subcutaneous infusion is also effective and is now the most popular choice. A portable infusion pump delivers 5 mL of deferoxamine over 12 hours during the night. The drug is directed subcutaneously, using a 27-gauge needle on 12-inch tubing, and infusion is rotated daily among sites on the anterior thighs and abdomen. The appropriate dose is mixed with sterile water and administered as soon as possible after its preparation. Occasionally, even after mixing, the solution remains cloudy, and we choose not to infuse these vials. Local reactions to the infusion are common and usually take the form of redness, swelling, and sometimes a hard lump at the injection site. Often these are a result of improper subcutaneous positioning of the needle. If this is not the case, hydrocortisone (1 mg) is added to the deferoxamine solution, and warm soaks are applied to the injection site for 10 to 15 minutes at the end of the infusion. If this fails to improve local reactions, various antihistamine and anti-inflammatory creams can be applied or nonsteroidal anti-inflammatory agents can be taken for short periods of time in order to diminish reactions at all sites and allow more rapid healing. Portocaths can be implanted in patients whose reactions are so severe that adherence to the regimen is threatened. Because of the prolonged nature of deferoxamine infusion, concern about infection of implanted catheters should be heightened.

A dose of 25 to 50 mg of deferoxamine per kg per day is administered at least 5 days a week. Small children (approximately 5 years of age) generally receive a dose of about 500 to 750 mg per day, whereas larger children and adolescents approach our maximum dose, between 2.5 and 3 grams per day. Most side effects of deferoxamine have been seen with doses above 50 mg per kg per day. In addition, we give 500 mg of deferoxamine intravenously during transfusion to eliminate any free iron in the blood component.

To begin chelation, patients must meet the following criteria: (1) the serum ferritin level must be >1000 mg per dL, or the iron/iron-binding capacity ratio must be ≥80%, (2) a provocative deferoxamine challenge of 25 to 50 mg per kg must lead to a urinary iron excretion of at least 0.5 mg per kg per 24 hours, and (3) the parents of patients must be taught to give the subcutaneous infusions and must demonstrate the necessary proficiency.

The efficacy of a chelation program is judged by the ability to create negative iron balance. This, in turn, requires the calculation of iron intake and the measurement of iron excretion. Iron intake includes the transfusion iron load (165 mg of elemental iron per 220 mL of red cells) and an estimate of gastrointestinal iron absorption (at least 3 mg of iron per day in patients on such programs). An average teenager acquires 17 to 22 mg of iron per day. Once a year, urinary iron excretion is measured daily for 3 days at the patient's daily dose with 500 to 1000 mg more a day (up to a maximum of 3 grams per day) to determine whether a higher dose would be useful. (Urine alone is measured because the contribution of stool iron excretion has been thought to be quite small.) The mean iron excretion is then compared with iron intake to document whether negative iron balance has been achieved. Serum measurements that reflect iron stores (ferritin iron and total iron-binding capacity) may be followed every 3 to 6 months to establish a trend toward more or less iron loading and to help judge the adherence to an iron-chelation program. It has been shown that a negative iron balance in severely iron-overloaded patients can reduce hepatic iron and reverse hepatic fibrosis. It is now apparent that strict compliance with a chelation program (adequate doses for 5 days per week) can protect patients from iron-induced organ failure, especially cardiac disease.

In patients with established organ failure, aggressive chelation programs have shown real progress. Cardiac function can be improved significantly, to the point of reversal of clinical cardiac symptoms. As doses greater than 50 mg of deferoxamine per kg per day have been associated with ophthalmic disorders and ototoxicity, we have studied an approach using 25 to 50 mg per kg per day given as a 24-hour continuous intravenous or subcutaneous infusion. This program leads to iron excretion similar to that of high-dose programs and has improved severe cardiac disease in our patients.

Patients who continue to show problems with adherence (or excrete iron poorly) may be helped by a monthly intensification using high doses of deferoxamine. (We do this with an overnight stay at the time of transfusion.) These patients (often in their teen years) may receive up to 4 grams in 24 hours by continuous infusion without acute toxicity. Care must be taken to monitor for ophthalmic and otic toxicity during such a program.

Splenectomy

All patients with thalassemia major and thalassemia intermedia develop some degree of hypersplenism, usually after 5 years of age. Clinical hypersplenism is usually heralded by an increase in the transfusion requirement to 200 ml per kg of body weight per year, representing a serious increase in body iron loading (>25%). We recommend splenectomy when transfusion needs rise but try to avoid it if the child is less than 4 years old, as the risk of overwhelming postsplenectomy sepsis is so high.

To avoid postsplenectomy sepsis we give all patients pneumococcal (Pneumovax), *Haemophilus influenzae* (if not previously vaccinated) and meningococcal vaccine immunization before splenectomy. In addition, all patients are maintained on penicillin prophylaxis until the teenage years, when they are told to begin amoxicillin orally at the first sign of malaise or fever and to seek medical attention immediately. Fever greater than 38.5° C (101° F) without a source of infection is treated aggressively with intravenous antibiotics in the hospital until cultures are negative.

Additional Management

Infection. Clinical suspicion of septicemia in a febrile, splenectomized patient should be treated with intravenous ceftriaxone or other antibiotics with a suitable spectrum until cultures are negative at 72 hours or an organism is identified. We usually hospitalize such patients for at least 24 hours, holding those that remain febrile or appear toxic and considering ambulatory ceftriaxone therapy for those who are otherwise asymptomatic. In patients treated by a transfusion and chelation regimen, enhanced consideration should be given to the possibility of *Yersinia enterocolitica* infection in patients presenting with unexplained fever and toxicity, or fever and abdominal pain.

Pericarditis. Patients with thalassemia major are prone to develop a syndrome of benign pericarditis. No data currently reveal any specific cause, other than the usual infectious agents associated with the disease. Nonetheless, the frequency with which thalassemic patients acquire pericarditis has led some clinicians to suggest iron deposition as a causative factor. Treatment differs little from that of an otherwise normal patient with this illness. Bed rest with analgesics is the current management. The effect of nonsteroidal anti-inflammatory agents has yet to be ascertained, but steroids did not have a major impact in older studies. We currently use aspirin or a nonsteroidal anti-inflammatory agent, along with mild ambulatory narcotic therapy if necessary. If a pericardial effusion appears and is significant in the amount of effusion or rapidity of accumulation, the patient is hospitalized, observed, and treated aggressively.

Diabetes Mellitus. Patients should be treated with insulin when clinical signs appear or when fasting blood sugar levels are in a pathologic range. The oral glucose tolerance test may be abnormal for years before clinical symptoms appear. Deferoxamine therapy rarely reverses this complication.

Hypoparathyroidism. Patients with tetany from hypoparathyroid hypocalcemia have been reported.

We perform yearly clinical evaluations, examining serum calcium, phosphorus, ionized calcium, and vitamin D levels. In the presence of hypocalcemia, we give calcium or vitamin D (or vitamin D analogues) to maintain normal calcium levels.

Hypothyroidism. Although we monitor our patients yearly for evidence of thyroid dysfunction, none of our patients have ever required replacement therapy or demonstrated even mild thyroid failure.

Growth Failure and Delayed Puberty. Most patients with thalassemia major experience growth failure and late onset of puberty. Improvements in transfusion and chelation have not yet had a major impact on this problem. Studies have not revealed the mechanism involved, but current evidence favors hypothalamic dysfunction.

Our patients undergo a yearly endocrine evaluation, as serial analysis provides information on whether puberty should be expected. Prepubertal adolescent boys who desire secondary sexual characteristics and who are not expected to begin puberty within the near future (owing to bone age retardation and gonadal hormone levels prepubertally) are treated with testosterone or other gonadal hormone therapy. The same considerations apply for our female patients with amenorrhea. After careful endocrine evaluation, they may be treated with estrogen or gonadal hormones. To balance the desire for secondary sexual characteristics with that of attainment of maximal growth and preservation of fertility, the patients are followed jointly with an endocrinologist.

Coagulation Disorder. Older patients with thalassemia can have laboratory evidence of clotting factor deficiency, usually related to hepatic parenchymal disease. Although this rarely leads to clinical bleeding, it may be necessary to treat these patients with vitamin K or fresh-frozen plasma when they are exposed to a hemostatic challenge.

Cardiac Disease. The iron-induced cardiac disease seen in thalassemia major is usually complex and difficult to treat. The arrhythmias, which may occur in the presence or absence of congestive heart failure, consist of supraventricular or ventricular extrasystoles and tachycardia and are often difficult to control. Occasionally, serial noninvasive cardiac function tests can suggest the approach of cardiac disease. Usually, however, these patients manifest sudden, severe biventricular cardiac failure with the clinical picture of diffuse cardiomyopathy. Although digoxin, diuretics, afterload reducers, and antiarrhythmic drugs help, these patients require intensive state-of-the-art cardiac therapy. In addition, aggressive 24-hour-per-day chelation should be immediately begun.

Thalassemia Intermedia

Patients described as having thalassemia intermedia have the clinical syndrome of thalassemia major but with less anemia (hemoglobin level, 6.5 to 7 grams per dL); therefore, they do not require transfusion for survival. The severity of the anemia in thalassemia determines the tempo of the illness, and thus the "intermedias" have a thalassemia that might be described as occurring "in slow motion." At the start of their clinical course, these patients present at an older age (2 to 4 years). As time goes by, however, they may develop marked skeletal changes and hypersplenism. Still, they frequently enjoy better growth and more appropriate sexual maturation than patients with other forms of thalassemia. In addition, depending on severity, they have superior longevity (often surviving beyond their fourth decade) without chelation, since their iron accumulation results from gastrointestinal iron absorption only. We maintain these patients on folic acid, 1 mg per day, and monitor them yearly for hyperuricemia secondary to their massive bone marrow turnover.

Specific treatment of these patients involves intervention when the chronic anemia and ineffective erythropoiesis, along with the resulting skeletal disease and extramedullary hematopoiesis, lead to specific problems. Transfusion for aplastic or hypoplastic crises is occasionally required. When hypersplenism appears, the patient may acquire a new transfusion requirement, so splenectomy is performed (usually after the age of 4 years) to ameliorate the new need for transfusion. When skeletal disease leads to severe deformity, fractures, or growth failure, or in the face of severe chronic fatigue or cardiac disease, a temporary chronic transfusion program is begun. Since the effect of intermittent transfusion on the longevity of these patients is unknown, we place them on our usual chelation program during transfusion to attempt the maintenance of negative iron balance.

Hemoglobin H Disease

Hemoglobin H disease is a form of alpha-thalassemia and for most patients is clinically similar to mild beta-thalassemia intermedia (mean hemoglobin level, 7.8 grams per dL). Occasionally these patients have a syndrome similar to beta-thalassemia major. Except for the latter group, these patients rarely require regular transfusion. Most of them develop significant hypersplenism in the first decade of life, and after splenectomy their hemoglobin level improves by 2 to 3 grams per dL. They may develop mild thalassemic bone disease but rarely have the degree of deformity or growth failure seen in beta-thalassemia. Iron loading appears not to occur in these patients if they are not transfused, and their lifespan may be normal. The treatment is otherwise the same as that for mild beta-thalassemia intermedia.

Prenatal Diagnosis

The first prenatal diagnosis for thalassemia was by globin chain synthesis studies obtained from fetal blood by fetoscopy. This technique is accurate (error rate, 1.5%) but is limited by a 3% risk of abortion and an 8% chance of an inability to obtain an appropriate specimen. Fetoscopy is available in a limited number of centers across the United States. Newer DNA analysis techniques have made diagnosis by amniocentesis possible in over 75% of patients, provided the patterns of DNA restriction enzyme polymorphisms of the parents are known. Recently, other techniques using oligonucleotide libraries of known thalassemia mutations and fetal DNA mapping have become available and may permit the use of amniocentesis, with its lower morbidity (<0.5% abortion), to diagnose a larger percentage of cases. Amniocentesis can be done as early as 16 weeks, and if it is unsuccessful, fetoscopy can be performed at 18 to 20 weeks. Chorionic biopsy, which can supply large amounts of uncontaminated fetal DNA as early as 8 to 12 weeks, may simplify prenatal diagnosis even further, once maternal and fetal morbidity rates are determined to be acceptable.

NEWER THERAPIES

Bone Marrow Transplantation. Studies performed in Italy have demonstrated high rates of quality survival when HLA-matched siblings have given bone marrow to appropriately prepared children with thalassemia major. Consistently good results have been obtained in transplanted children who have no preoperative evidence of severe iron overload or hepatic involvement. In those patients without iron overload there is a 6% chance of mortality, compared with the excellent chance of survival into the third and fourth decades with conventional treatment. Nonetheless, transplantation must be considered as an option for patients with HLA-matched siblings, as "conventional" treatment for thalassemia major is arduous and has its own impact on the quality of life.

Increase in Activity of the Fetal Hemoglobin Gene. Scholarly clinical work has been performed in the attempt to increase hemoglobin F production and thus improve anemia and the sequelae of anemia in these and other patients. Drugs that affect DNA methylation (5-azacytidine) or cell cycle kinetics (hydroxyurea) have been shown to cause some (albeit variable) increase in hemoglobin F production. No treatment has yet ameliorated the transfusion requirement significantly enough to justify potential toxicity. Butyrate compounds have recently been tested with sometimes dramatic effects on hemoglobin F production when given intravenously. Clinicians who treat these patients anxiously await the formulation and testing of effective oral analogues of these drugs.

Genetic Manipulation. Changing the actual hemoglobin genes in the red cell precursors of thalassemia major patients has been a goal of many researchers. With so much work done on the beta-hemoglobin gene cluster and with emerging techniques for gene transfer into human cells, the day may come when patients can have normal hemoglobin genes implanted in their own bone marrow. This would cure or ameliorate the disease without the toxicity of transplantation or chronic medication.

Oral Chelation. In the absence of ameliorating the

disease itself, much investigation has sought oral alternatives to subcutaneous deferoxamine. A few oral chelators are in active clinical trials, but none have yet been able to meet the extraordinary efficacy/safety ratio that parenteral deferoxamine achieves.

SICKLE CELL DISEASE

method of
PAUL S. SWERDLOW, M.D.
Wayne State University School of Medicine
Detroit, Michigan

TYPES OF SICKLE CELL DISEASE

Sickle hemoglobin (HbS) is caused by a point mutation changing a single amino acid residue in the beta-globin chain of hemoglobin. Once deoxygenated, HbS polymerizes, wreaking havoc on first the red cells, then the body. Clinically, the disorders are inherited hemolytic anemias accompanied by pain and organ damage. In sickle cell anemia, both beta-globin genes have the mutation. Patients with one sickle gene and either an HbC or a thalassemic beta-globin mutation are also at risk for sickling (sickle–C disease or sickle–beta-thalassemia). Patients with one sickle beta-globin gene and one normal gene (sickle trait) are essentially normal, without hemolysis or anemia. They may have complications with extreme altitude (>2500 meters) or dehydration. They occasionally have hematuria. Hyphema requires ophthalmic intervention, since even trait cells in the anterior chamber sickle and can elevate optic pressures to dangerous levels.

DIAGNOSIS

The diagnosis can be made at birth by screening programs. Unscreened children who are at risk should be tested by age 4 months to allow timely institution of prophylactic penicillin. Definitive diagnosis requires hemoglobin electrophoresis or other direct techniques, not a sickle preparation or Sickledex test. Referral to a specialized center provides confirmation and facilitates consultation, should complications develop.

PEDIATRIC CARE

Follow-up every 2 months the first year and every 3 months the second year is needed, as mortality is high in untreated patients. A routine diet should be supplemented with folic acid. Iron supplements after the first year require evidence of low iron stores. Routine immunizations are encouraged. Pneumococcal vaccine, *Haemophilus influenzae* B conjugate, and hepatitis B are particularly important. A key intervention is prophylactic penicillin 125 mg orally twice daily to age 3 years, and 250 mg orally twice daily from ages 3 to 5 years. Children who are allergic to penicillin can be given erythromycin ethyl succinate, 20 mg/kg/day divided into two daily doses.

Parents and children must work to ensure adequate fluid intake and avoid extreme temperatures, especially swimming in cold water. Bed wetting may be due to hyposthenuria. Parents must learn to rec-ognize symptoms of anemia, take a temperature, and palpate the spleen so that they can determine when prompt medical attention is needed. In splenic sequestration, the spleen massively enlarges with sequestered blood, often leading to shock. Prompt transfusion is lifesaving. Routine ophthalmic examinations should begin at age 10 years.

ADOLESCENT CARE

Frank discussions are needed regarding limitations owing to disease, issues of retarded growth and delayed sexual development, avoidance of tobacco and street drugs, protection of ankles, contraception and protection from sexually transmitted disease, and any problems of low self-esteem and missed school. Discussion of role models may be helpful, as are support groups and academic and vocational counseling. Ideal jobs allow for intermittent absences and avoid severe physical effort. The difficult transition to adult medicine is eased by communication among pediatrician, internist, family, and patient.

ADULT CARE

Many adults benefit from discussing disease complications and preventive measures, such as drinking adequate fluids and avoiding prolonged cold. Vaccinations and routine health screens should be up to date, including visits with the dentist and ophthalmologist. Patients must know to present immediately when they have fever, cough, dyspnea, orthostasis, or neurologic symptoms. The physician should be supportive in the patient's dealings with prospective employers or with disability forms.

Many patients can control most pain at home. Some respond to nonsteroidal agents. Others require short-acting narcotics such as codeine or oxycodone. For many patients, small supplies last for months. Others who have daily pain need significant supplies of medication to avoid frequent visits to emergency rooms. To optimize care, it is important that one physician or group prescribe all pain medication. The patient must schedule an appointment for medication renewal before running out. Emergency requests for medication are discouraged. More severely affected patients have a poorer prognosis and a shortened survival. They need to be seen frequently and their pain taken seriously. Many qualify for hydroxyurea therapy.

Hydroxyurea, when used according to Table 1, reduces emergent pain by 44% and decreases acute chest syndrome and the necessity for transfusion. Patients whose dosage falls in between the 500-mg capsules can take the medication on alternating days. The physician and patient must carefully weigh the risks and benefits. Short-term toxicity is due to marrow suppression. It is strongly recommended that only 2-week supplies be prescribed and that toxicity criteria be strictly followed. Long-term safety remains unknown. An increased risk of leukemia is suggested by some but not all studies in cancer pa-

TABLE 1. **Hydroxyurea for Sickle Cell Anemia According to the Multicenter Study of Hydroxyurea (MSH) in Sickle Cell Anemia**

Eligibility
Age at least 18 years
More than three painful crises per year requiring hospital or emergency treatment
Reliable enough to take medication properly and follow up every 2 weeks
Not currently attempting to have children (male or female) or breast-feeding
Informed of long-term potential risks

Dosing
Start at 15 mg/kg/day as a single daily oral dose
Increase at 12-week intervals by 5 mg/kg/day to maximum of 35 mg/kg
If toxic:
Stop hydroxyurea until counts normal (generally by next visit)
Restart at a dose 2.5 mg/kg/day lower
If after 12 weeks no toxicity, increase by 2.5 mg/kg/day

Toxicity
Check for toxicity every 2 weeks until MTD,* then every 4 weeks
Any one of the following counts as toxicity:
ANC† less than 2,000/mm³
Platelets less than 80,000/mm³
Hb less than 4.5/mm³
Hb less than 5.0 with ARC‡ less than 320,000/mm³ if pretreatment Hb was more than 7.0
Hb less than 9.0 if ARC is less than 80,000/mm³

*MTD (maximal tolerated dose) is the highest dose that does not produce toxicity.
†ANC (absolute neutrophil count) is the number of neutrophils per mm³ of blood. It is reported directly by some laboratories. It is calculated as the total white count multiplied by (% polys + % bands)/100.
‡ARC (absolute reticulocyte count) is the number of reticulocytes per mm³ of blood. It is reported directly by some laboratories. It is calculated as the total red cell count per mm³ (not hemoglobin or hematocrit) multiplied by the % reticulocytes/100.
Abbreviation: Hb = hemoglobin in gm/dL.

tients. Hydroxyurea causes birth defects in animals, so neither men nor women attempting to have children should be on therapy. Use in children awaits controlled clinical trials, since pediatric toxicity is unknown.

EMERGENT PAIN EPISODES

Patients frequently present emergently with pain. A careful evaluation is imperative, since nearly a third of patients who die initially present with pain, acute chest syndrome, or stroke. A focused history and physical examination should ensure that there is no intercurrent infection and no other cause for pain and that the patient is not dehydrated, hypoxic, or having a stroke. Patients can often tell whether the pain is "sickle" pain or not. Hydration either orally or intravenously (5% dextrose at 3 to 5 mL per kg per hour) and oxygen are often begun routinely. Oxygen should be stopped if there is no hypoxia, since it can suppress erythropoiesis. Overhydration is of no benefit. Given the risks of infection, one should have a low threshold for ordering chest x-rays, urinalyses, and cultures. As early as feasible, the pain should be controlled.

Pain is poorly treated by most practitioners owing to a fear of narcotics and a lack of trust in the patient's perception of pain. There are no clinical or laboratory tests to indicate that a patient is having a pain episode. A patient's report of pain is the most accurate indicator. Initial doses for emergent treatment of severe sickle cell pain are presented in Table 2. Intravenous doses can be repeated every 10 minutes if needed. Subcutaneous and intramuscular doses can be repeated every 30 minutes or so. Avoiding intramuscular injections prevents sterile abscesses and preserves the patient's limited muscle mass. Patients who are narcotic-naive or elderly or who have liver disease or limited respiratory drive may need smaller doses. Tranquilizers should be avoided. Where available, patient-controlled analgesia (PCA) is useful both in an inpatient setting and emergently, as long as an adequate bolus is given.

Patients who regularly experience pain learn to use distraction (watching TV, talking on the phone) to avoid focusing on the pain. If interrupted, they again focus on the pain. This may be misinterpreted as "faking"—for example, an active patient who complains of pain when staff arrives. Few sickle patients are truly addicted to pain medication. Such a determination is best made on an outpatient basis by skilled personnel, not in an emergency room. The use of placebos is of no help, since they often work for known pain. The few patients who become addicted should be detoxified. Such patients may still receive narcotics in the hospital for pain, provided they are tapered off before discharge.

Nonaddicted patients who are tapered too rapidly may go through withdrawal and return with acute pain. The pain should be treated and the medication

TABLE 2. **Initial Doses of Narcotics Recommended for Acute Emergent Pain***

Medication	Adult Dose (Pediatric Dose in mg/kg)	Routes	Interval	PO Equivalent (mg/kg)	Comments
Morphine	10 mg (0.15)	IV, SC, IM	q 3–4 h	40 mg (0.6)	Drug of choice
Hydromorphone (Dilaudid)	1.5 mg (0.02)	IV, SC, IM	q 3–4 h	6 mg (0.04)	Expensive
Methadone	10 mg	IV, SC	q 6–8 h	20 mg	Mild withdrawal
Meperidine (Demerol)	75 mg (1.1)	IV, IM	q 2–3 h	300 mg	Seizure risk†

*If adequate relief is not obtained, doses can be repeated every 10 min for IV and every 30 min for IM or SC, with the patient being carefully monitored. Intervals shown maintain the pain relief achieved with the first dose. The elderly or those with liver disease or decreased respiratory drive may need lower doses.
†Normeperidine levels increase for many days with repeated use and can cause seizures. Normeperidine is contraindicated in those with a history of central nervous system disease or those on monoamine oxidase inhibitors.

tapered more slowly. Transferring such patients to oral medications, especially methadone, before discharge minimizes withdrawal symptoms. Although the government restricts the use of methadone for substance abuse treatment to approved programs, the use of methadone for pain control is not limited. Breaking cycles of withdrawal pain can dramatically improve a patient's well-being and decrease medication utilization.

TRANSFUSION

Transfusions are greatly overused in sickle cell disease, resulting in acute volume overload, chronic iron overload, and sensitization to blood group antigens. The need for each transfusion must be carefully considered, since sensitization may limit later transfusions. Careful matching of blood can delay sensitization but requires prior red cell typing. In life-threatening anemia, transfusion should always be performed with the most compatible blood available, even if it cannot be fully cleared by the blood bank.

Simple and exchange transfusions have different indications. Simple transfusion is indicated for *symptomatic* anemia. Patients with chronic anemia are not benefited by transfusions at arbitrary hemoglobin cutoffs. Patients who tolerate hemoglobin levels of 4 g per dL without ill effect should be allowed to do so. Angina, orthostasis, dyspnea, or neurologic symptoms attributable to anemia are good indications for transfusion. Despite popular wisdom, transfusions do not decrease pain or shorten established pain episodes. Generalized weakness, malaise, or a longer than usual hospital stay is *not* a sufficient indication for transfusion. Simple transfusion may be needed in patients with rapidly falling hemoglobins due to bleeding, splenic sequestration, or aplastic or hemolytic crises.

For stroke and uncontrollable hypoxia—and, less certainly, for persistent priapism and before certain surgeries—it is important to decrease the sicklable cells to less than 30% of the circulating pool while keeping the total hemoglobin around 10 grams per dL. Exchange transfusion via pheresis machine is an elegant way to achieve these goals. Instructions for manual exchange are found in an excellent monograph, "Management and Therapy of Sickle Cell Disease" NIH publication no. 91–2117.

CONTRACEPTION AND PREGNANCY

There are no contraindications to contraception in patients with sickle cell disease. Many patients find that medroxyprogesterone (Depo-Provera) or levonorgestrel (Norplant) helps minimize cyclical menstrual sickle pains. Pregnancy carries increased risk for mother and fetus, but the increase is modest, and positive outcomes are the rule. Nondirective genetic counseling should be offered, with hemoglobin typing of the partner. Prenatal diagnosis is feasible early in pregnancy. Ideally, folic acid, 1 mg per day, is begun before pregnancy. Frequent visits with an obstetri-

cian or clinic specializing in high-risk pregnancy are recommended. Patients should be screened for blood alloantibodies, and the pregnancy should be followed carefully for possible hemolytic disease in the fetus. Because of the frequency of iron overload, iron supplements should be withheld unless iron stores are low.

Pregnancy generally results in increased pain. Fortunately, there is no contraindication to narcotics. Unfortunately, transfusion is commonly performed for uncomplicated pain crises despite a randomized trial of transfusion in sickle cell disease, which found no difference in maternal or fetal outcome. Women with a repeated history of miscarriage may benefit from repeated exchange transfusions, but the risks must be weighed against the possible benefits.

INFECTION

Infection tends to occur in tissues damaged by sickling, such as lung, urinary tract, and bone. Infections must be treated rapidly to avert sickling complications and because patients are functionally asplenic. Temperatures above 101° F should be assumed to be due to infection and treated empirically. Urinary tract infections tend to recur. Repeating urine cultures 2 weeks and then several months after infection ensures complete eradication. Aplastic crises are often due to parvovirus B19, the causative agent of fifth disease. Owing to hemolysis, the hemoglobin falls dramatically when the reticulocyte count is suppressed. Transfusions are usually required. Folate deficiency is another cause of aplastic crisis.

LUNG PROBLEMS

Acute chest syndrome is a new segmental or larger pulmonary infiltrate accompanied by cough, wheezing, tachypnea, new chest pain, or a temperature above 38.5° C (101.3° F). This dangerous syndrome includes both pneumonia and pulmonary infarction, and elements of both may be present. Marrow fat embolism may contribute in many cases. Management includes antibiotics to cover common organisms (pneumococcus and mycoplasma) and careful attention to oxygenation. If there is doubt that the P_{O_2} can be maintained above 60 mmHg (70 mmHg in a child), exchange transfusion must be performed. Repeated episodes of acute chest syndrome can result in pulmonary hypertension with cor pulmonale. Chronic transfusions or night-time oxygen may help. A related syndrome of multiorgan failure involves some combination of the pulmonary, renal, central nervous, and hepatic systems. Patients who are exchange transfused often make a full recovery.

Splinting due to chest wall pain is a frequent cause of atelectasis, which may lead to acute chest syndrome. Patients with splinting need adequate pain relief to allow full and deep respiration, preferably with an incentive spirometer, to minimize atelectasis. Dyspnea due to chest wall pain is not a contraindication to narcotic use. Indeed, respiration increases as the pain is relieved.

STROKE

One in 15 sickle cell patients will suffer a stroke, the majority before age 18 years. Rapid exchange transfusion to less than 30% sicklable cells may prevent progression and should take precedence over imaging studies. For thrombotic strokes, the high risk of recurrence mandates transfusion for 3 to 5 years, at least in children. Exchange transfusion can minimize iron overload and may obviate the need for later chelation. Patients who have suffered two strokes are likely to need transfusions for life. Hemorrhagic stroke requires angiography, after exchange, to rule out surgically correctable lesions.

GALLBLADDER AND LIVER

Pigment gallstones affect most patients before age 30 years and many by age 10 years. Cholecystectomy should be performed in those with symptoms attributable to gallstones or with frequent abdominal pain. Some recommend that simple transfusion to a hemoglobin of 10 g per dL be performed before even laparoscopic cholecystectomy.

Acute sickle liver disease usually resolves within 2 weeks. It may be characterized by bilirubin values in the teens and elevated liver enzymes. Care must be exercised in evaluating lactate dehydrogenase (LDH), which may be due to red cell hemolysis, and alkaline phosphatase, which may be due to bony sickling. Rarely, liver disease is severe, with bilirubin values approaching 100 or evidence of hepatic failure. Exchange transfusions are then indicated. Chronic liver disease may be due to viral hepatitis, hemosiderosis, pulmonary hypertension, or repeated sickle infarcts. Liver biopsy may clarify the diagnosis.

LEG ULCERS

Leg ulcers commonly cause morbidity. Patients should be advised that wounds near the malleoli heal poorly, so they should keep these areas clean and well moisturized. Once an ulcer develops, local care is key. The wound must be kept clean and well débrided with regular dressing changes, such as wet-to-dry saline solution with fine mesh gauze, enzyme-based ointments (e.g., Elase), or whirlpool therapy. Moisturizing the surrounding skin with baby oil or Eucerin cream is helpful. Systemic antibiotics are indicated only for accompanying cellulitis. Edema is treated with elevation and compression stockings. Zinc supplements or hydroxyurea may help. As a last resort, hypertransfusion for 6 months with or without skin grafting may be tried.

BONY DISEASE

Many pain episodes focus on bones, but permanent damage does not usually result. Sickling of growth plates can cause uneven growth of bones. Osteomyelitis is not common, but when it occurs, it is often with salmonella or staphylococcus. Nuclear medicine scans do not easily differentiate osteomyelitis from bony infarcts, and plain films may prove more useful. It is important to obtain a biopsy of any affected bone to determine the appropriate antibiotics to use.

Both hips and shoulders are subject to avascular necrosis, which can lead to chronic arthritis and the need for joint replacement. Early diagnosis is often better with magnetic resonance imaging (MRI). Avoidance of weight bearing for several months may prevent collapse of the femoral head. Some advocate core decompression, but data on efficacy are lacking. Vertebrae are subject to central collapse, causing "fish mouth" or "Lincoln log" deformities, which can result in chronic arthritis.

Gout should be suspected if a joint is swollen, warm, red, and exquisitely tender. Aspiration is essential to document gout crystals and rule out septic arthritis. Acute therapy is with indomethacin (Indocin) 50 mg every 8 hours. Allopurinol (Zyloprim) 300 mg per day is used for prevention only after repeated episodes.

RENAL COMPLICATIONS

Hyposthenuria is nearly universal. To avoid dehydration, adults should drink at least 4 liters of fluid daily (150 mL per kg for children). Defects in secretion of acid and potassium may result in metabolic acidosis and hyperkalemia, but in severe cases, alternative causes should be sought.

Hematuria, usually painless, is common in sickle cell disease and trait. Evaluation should consider tumor, stones, glomerulonephritis, infection, and bleeding disorders, but papillary necrosis is most common. Most episodes clear spontaneously with good hydration. If hematuria persists, epsilon-aminocaproic acid 5 grams every 8 hours for four doses may be helpful, but the risk of clot formation in the renal pelvis and ureter requires careful monitoring in the hospital. DDAVP (1-deamino-8-D-arginine vasopressin) and cauterization of bleeding sites in the renal pelvis have also been reported to help. Transfusions may be needed, including exchange if hematuria remains refractory. Iron supplementation should be given only if stores are low. Nephrectomy should be avoided, as bleeding may occur in the remaining kidney.

Proteinuria greater than 2 grams per 24 hours may need biopsy for evaluation. Hypertension should be treated with nondiuretic medications. Neither dialysis nor transplantation is contraindicated in chronic renal failure, but those patients undergoing transplant should expect an increase in pain.

PRIAPISM

Priapism is a prolonged, painful erection that can be caused by sickling. There is no established effective therapy. Avoidance of prolonged sexual activity, alcohol, and dehydration may reduce the incidence. Home therapies include hot baths, exercise, or prostatic massage, which, although awkward, can be performed by most patients after brief instruction. Prolonged episodes require emergent evaluation. One must ensure adequate hydration, oxygenation, and pain control; the absence of infection; and the ability to urinate. A Foley catheter may be needed. Nifedipine (Procardia)* 10 mg or hydralazine (Apresoline)* 10 mg can be tried acutely. Irrigation of the corpora is a low-risk procedure that is easily performed by a urologist in the emergency room. After 12 to 24 hours, exchange transfusion is usually considered, but there are few data indicating that it helps. Shunt procedures are considered if this fails, but there remains an overall 25% risk of impotence. Those who develop impotence should be referred to a urologist. For patients with repeated episodes, nightly therapy with a nitroglycerine patch* (0.2 to 0.4 mg per hour) or hydralazine 10 mg before bedtime may help. Luteinizing hormone-releasing hormone (LHRH) agonists such as luprolide (Lupron)* may help by decreasing testosterone to castration levels.

SURGERY AND ANESTHESIA

A randomized multi-institutional study found that preoperative exchange transfusion was no better than simple transfusion to a hemoglobin of 10 g per dL in decreasing surgical complications. It is critical that good oxygenation be maintained throughout surgery and especially in the postoperative period. Aggressive pulmonary toilet with incentive spirometry helps minimize pulmonary complications. Surgery that is unlikely to cause respiratory splinting, such as hip replacement, may not require any transfusion pre-operatively. Dental procedures should be performed with nitrous oxide only if no good alternatives exist and the nitrous oxide is given with pure oxygen.

FUTURE THERAPY

Related bone marrow transplant can result in cure, but at the risk of substantial morbidity and mortality. Newer agents that increase fetal hemoglobin, block polymerization, alter oxygen affinity, or increase cellular water are being tested. Before any new drugs can be recommended, appropriate randomized trials must be performed. There is a great temptation to try anything in sickle cell disease because of the frustrations encountered in dealing with the disease or the patients. Outside of controlled clinical trials, such temptations must be resisted in the best interests of the patient.

---

*Not FDA-approved for this indication.

NEUTROPENIA

method of
GERALD ROTHSTEIN, M.D.
University of Utah School of Medicine
Salt Lake City, Utah

Neutrophils constitute an essential front line of defense against bacterial infection, and when the supply of neutrophils is deficient, host resistance and survival are critically challenged. One of the most important laboratory signs of a deficient neutrophil supply is neutropenia: a circulating neutrophil concentration below the levels found in normal persons.

PRODUCTION AND UTILIZATION OF NEUTROPHILS

The neutrophilic granulocytes are produced by the bone marrow and are stored there for 10 to 14 days before being released into the blood. Studies of the kinetics of neutrophil utilization have shown that the circulating half-life of neutrophils in normal humans is only 4 to 7 hours. Therefore, the entire population of circulating neutrophils must normally be replaced two to three times per day. During infection, the utilization of neutrophils is further increased by tenfold or more. Abrupt increases in the need for neutrophils demand that the marrow be capable of rapidly increasing the number of available neutrophils in response to physiologic challenges such as bacterial infection. It is believed that regulatory mechanisms, including the production of cytokines such as interleukin-3, granulocyte-macrophage colony-stimulating factor (GM-CSF), and granulocyte colony-stimulating factor (G-CSF) are instrumental in regulating neutrophil production by increasing cellular proliferation, and recombinant cytokines have been shown to be effective enhancers of neutrophil production in certain neutropenic states. In addition to cellular proliferation, the host's ability to supply large numbers of neutrophils immediately is bolstered by a reserve of cells within the marrow of 10 to 14 times the neutrophils in the circulation. These stored neutrophils can be released quickly from the marrow's reserve into the circulation during infectious challenge, in response to corticosteroids, or on activation of complement. Because many of the stored neutrophils are nonsegmented band forms, differential counts of blood neutrophils after acute release of marrow neutrophils usually reveal a "left shift."

DETECTION OF NEUTROPENIA

The concept of the *absolute neutrophil count* (ANC) is essential to recognizing neutropenia. The ANC is calculated by multiplying the nucleated cell count (from the complete blood count [CBC]) by the percentage of polymorphonuclear neutrophils (PMN and band forms) in the peripheral blood differential count.

ANC = "white cell count" × % neutrophils

If the differential count has been performed by microscopy, the sum of the percentage of PMN + percentage of bands should be used for the percentage of neutrophils. If an automated cell counter has been used to perform the differential count, the staining methods used for automation detect both PMN and band forms, and the percentage of neutrophils can be taken directly from the reported count. Once the ANC has been calculated, it should be recalled that the lower limits for ANC differ for infants. For example, the lower limit for ANC values is 3500 per mm³ immediately after birth for full-term infants and 5000 per mm³ at 12 hours of age. At 72 hours of age, the lower limit for ANC has fallen to 1800 per mm³ and remains at that level for the duration of childhood and adult life.

Once detected, even incidentally, a reduced ANC should be considered a signal of an increased risk of infection. Even so, reduced ANCs do not always reflect a reduced neutrophil supply. This is accounted by the distribution of total blood neutrophils into two "pools" of neutrophils: a freely *circulating pool* and another *marginal pool* of neutrophils located in the microvasculature. Only the circulating pool is detected by the CBC, and reduced ANCs can occur because the vast majority of neutrophils are located within the marginal pool, leaving a small circulating pool but a normal and functionally sufficient number of total neutrophils. When neutropenia has occurred because of margination, the reduced ANC is referred to as "pseudoneutropenia" and is not associated with reduced neutrophil supply or a risk of infection. Transient pseudoneutropenia can be induced by epinephrine or nicotinic acid, but it also may be chronic. However, most chronically reduced ANCs do reflect a reduced neutrophil supply.

EVALUATION

Neutropenia may be discovered as an incidental finding in a CBC, or it may be found because a subject displays the symptoms that occur because of neutropenia: painful stomatitis (agranulocytic angina), gingivitis, fever, pneumonia, sepsis, or perforation of the cecum (typhlitis). For neonates and elderly subjects, the febrile response to infection may be blunted or absent, and a high index of suspicion will be needed to detect unexpected infection in a timely fashion. A finding of a reduced ANC should prompt a consideration of the various causes of neutropenia (Table 1).

The clinical approach is initially to aggressively institute diagnostic measures and treatment if bacterial infection is suspected. In subjects with a reduced neutrophil supply, host resistance is impaired, thus interventions during infection should be prompt, broadly focused, and vigorous. The significance and cause of neutropenia must also be addressed. A careful history is obtained to determine the age at onset of the neutropenia, whether exposure to toxins or medicines has occurred, and whether the patient is known to have autoimmune disease, alcohol abuse, or a history of repeated infections. Physical examination focuses on the site and extent of any infection and the hemodynamic stability of the subject. The patient is examined

TABLE 1. **Causes of Neutropenia**

Congenital neutropenia
Neonatal sepsis
Overwhelming infection in debilitated patients
Infiltrative marrow disease (e.g., leukemia, myelofibrosis)
Chemotherapeutic agents, antimetabolites
Aplastic anemia
Autoimmune neutropenia
  Idiopathic
  Autoimmune diseases
Viral infection
Folic acid of B₁₂ deficiency
Alcoholism
Viral infection
Exposure to toxins (e.g., benzene)

for lymphadenopathy, arthritis, splenomegaly, bone tenderness, and stomatitis. If only one blood count has revealed neutropenia and the patient is not infected, a repeat count (or counts) is obtained before conducting further work-up. The CBC is reviewed for other cytopenias and the differential count examined for evidence of abnormal cells. In patients with chronic neutropenia, the marrow is examined by aspiration (and usually biopsy) for its content of mature neutrophils and their precursors, cellularity, and maturation of other cell lines. In some cases, chromosomal analysis of the marrow cells may be helpful. The work-up usually also includes assays of serum B₁₂ and folate concentrations.

TREATMENT OF INFECTION

The most immediate concern in neutropenic subjects is to determine whether infection is present. In general, the degree of neutropenia can be used as a guide for the potential risk for infection. Subjects with blood neutrophil concentrations of greater than 1000 per mm³ may resist infection relatively well; those with ANCs between 500 and 1000 per mm³ may display reduced host resistance; those with ANCs greater than 500 per mm³ usually experience a serious risk for infection, and those with counts over 250 per mm³ are the most likely to experience life-threatening infection and must be approached very aggressively. In subjects with ANC greater than 500 per mm³, a febrile state even in the absence of identified infection, hospitalization and empirical antibiotic treatment are provided as soon as examination is completed and appropriate blood and body fluid specimens for culture are obtained. A careful physical examination is carried out to identify the site of infection. In addition to evaluation of the lungs and urinary tract, attention is paid to the ears, sinuses, central nervous system, skin, and perianal and periodontal areas. In severely neutropenic subjects, it is advisable to avoid digital rectal examination because of the risk of inducing bacteremia by this maneuver. In the absence of sufficient numbers of neutrophils, signs of inflammation may be slight or absent, and PMN may be difficult to find even in infected body fluids. Consequently, treatment of infection may of necessity be empirical, and even multiple cultures may fail to identify the infectious agent.

General guidelines can be provided for the treatment of neutropenic subjects with presumed infection but no identified organism or source. The treatment is modified in the case of impaired renal function, and particular care must be taken to estimate creatinine function in elderly subjects in whom serum creatinine determinations alone are inaccurate predictors of renal function. When renal function is normal, an aminoglycoside is combined with an antibiotic with antipseudomonal activity, monitoring serum concentrations of aminoglycoside. If renal impairment is present, then a third-generation cephalosporin or ureidopenicillin may be more appropriate. Of course, the identification of a specific organism may focus therapy, and in subjects with indwelling intravenous catheters, the addition of vancomycin may be advisable to cover for staphylococci. In patients with identified infections, at least 2 weeks of therapy are generally recommended, or therapy for 7 days after the fever is resolved. The duration of therapy in patients without identified infection is less clear, but some recommend 14 days of treatment if the patient becomes afebrile after the first 5 days of therapy. In patients with persistent fever for 5 to 7 days in spite of antibiotic coverage, the possibility of fungal infection should be considered, and amphotericin may be initiated empirically. In subjects with recurrent infection, periodic prophylactic treatment with trimethoprim-sulfamethoxazole may be effective, and some patients may benefit from prolonged courses of oral antifungal treatment.

TREATMENT OF NEUTROPENIC STATES

In subjects with long-standing chronic neutropenia, cellular marrows, and an adequate number of mature and precursor neutrophils, treatment of the neutropenia itself is not indicated. In symptomatic neutropenias or when neutropenia is due to vitamin deficiency, a therapeutic intervention is initiated when possible. For example, specific therapy is employed to correct deficiency states of B_{12} or folic acid. In subjects whose neutropenia is associated with alcohol abuse, alcohol ingestion should be discontinued and folate supplementation begun. The deficiency of classic pernicious anemia dictates treatment for life with intramuscular B_{12}.

When neutropenia and infection are associated with specific medicines, the offending agent is discontinued. Successful treatment of autoimmune diseases may also be associated with resolution of the neutropenia. When neutropenia is associated with cytoreductive chemotherapy or antiviral agents such as zidovudine (AZT, Retrovir), return of the neutrophil counts to normal may be accelerated by the administration of the neutropoietic cytokines filgrastim (G-CSF, Neupogen) or sargramostim (GM-CSF, Leukine, Prokine). Cytokine treatment has also been effective in some subjects with cyclical neutropenia and Kostmann's syndrome (congenital neutropenia). However, the administration of these cytokines is not without adverse consequences. Treatment with G-CSF may induce bone pain and vasculitis, and GM-CSF therapy has been associated with pronounced eosinophilia, fluid retention, pleural effusion, respiratory distress, pericardial effusion, and a sometimes serious or fatal capillary leak syndrome. Since excessive elevations of total leukocyte or platelet counts are causes for discontinuing GM-CSF, treatment with it dictates frequent monitoring of blood counts.

HEMOLYTIC DISEASE OF THE FETUS AND NEWBORN
(Red Cell Alloimmunization)

method of
KENNETH J. MOISE, JR., M.D.
Baylor College of Medicine
Houston, Texas

Although the human maternal and fetal circulations are anatomically separate, small fetomaternal hemorrhages (FMHs) can be demonstrated in virtually all pregnancies. When fetal erythrocytes containing red cell antigens foreign to the mother gain access to the maternal circulation, antibody formation occurs, a condition known as "red cell alloimmunization." Since the placenta actively transports immunoglobulin G (IgG) antibodies into the fetal circulation, antibody-antigen interactions occur on the fetal red cells. Although most of these antibodies do not fix complement, cell-mediated destruction of antibody-opsonized erythrocytes is thought to take place in the fetal spleen, resulting in fetal anemia. Although the RhD antigen is the most common cause of red cell alloimmunization, a wide variety of red cell antigens have been implicated in hemolytic disease of the fetus and newborn. The antigens that produce severe fetal disease necessitating intrauterine transfusion are, however, limited in number. Often the D antibody is found in conjunction with other Rh antibodies (c, C, E, e) of weaker titer. Two other antibodies that cause severe in utero disease are c and Kell. Duffy (Fy^a) and Kidd (Jk^a, Jk^b) on rare occasions also cause severe fetal anemia.

PREVENTION

Before the use of Rh immune globulin (RhIG) (Rho-GAM, Gamulin Rh), approximately 1% of all Rh-negative pregnant women became alloimmunized after delivery. In 1968, RhIG was approved for clinical use in the United States. Thereafter, Rh-negative patients delivering Rh-positive infants were administered 300 μg of RhIG intramuscularly within 72 hours of delivery. A rapid fall in the incidence of Rh sensitization was noted as a result of this practice. Sensitization occurring before delivery became the primary cause of new cases of Rh disease. Further studies found that a single dose of RhIG administered at 28 weeks of gestation is effective in preventing almost all cases of antepartum alloimmunization. In 1984, the American College of Obstetricians and Gynecologists recommended routine antenatal prophylaxis in all Rh-negative women.

Current obstetric practice dictates that an indirect Coombs test should be obtained on all obstetric patients at the first prenatal visit. If no antibodies are detected in the Rh-negative patient, an indirect Coombs test is repeated at 28 weeks' gestation. This enables the detection of the rare patient who has become sensitized in the early phase of pregnancy. At the same clinical setting, before the completion of the laboratory testing, 300 μg of RhIG can be administered intramuscularly. If the indirect Coombs test returns negative, no further testing is necessary until delivery. With the onset of labor, a repeat indirect Coombs test is obtained. Since the half-life of RhIG is approximately 23 days, 15 to 20% of patients still have anti-D detected in their serum in a low titer (<4) at the time of delivery. Umbilical cord blood should be obtained at delivery for blood typing of the infant. In the case of an Rh-positive infant, a minimum of 300 μg of RhIG is administered within 72 hours of delivery. This dose is sufficient to neutralize an FMH of 30 mL. In a very small percentage of deliveries, an FMH in excess of 30 mL occurs. These cases are usually associated with a large placental mass or difficult removal of the placenta at the time of delivery. Examples include multiple gestations, placental abruption, placenta previa, and the need for manual removal of the placenta. Standards proposed by the American Association of Blood Banks call for routine screening of all patients at the time of delivery for excessive fetomaternal hemorrhage. Most centers use the rosette test for this purpose. The test is very sensitive for the presence of a bleed and is reported as positive or negative. An acid elution test, the Kleihauer-Betke stain, is then undertaken for quantitation of the FMH if the rosette test proves positive. If the volume of the hemorrhage is found to be in excess of 30 mL, the blood bank calculates the additional dose of RhIG necessary.

Several situations deserve special mention regarding the administration of RhIG. Amniocentesis for the assessment of fetal lung maturity is usually undertaken just before delivery. For this reason, it is suggested that RhIG be withheld unless more than 48 hours transpires between the procedure and delivery. If a patient has received a standard dose of RhIG less than 21 days before delivery and maternal testing does not reveal the presence of an FMH, a postpartum dose is not indicated. Alternatively, an indirect Coombs test can be performed 48 hours after delivery. If free anti-D is detected in the patient's serum, adequate protection is present and no further RhIG is necessary. On rare occasions, the patient may be inadvertently discharged from the hospital after delivery before the administration of RhIG. Consideration should be given to the administration of RhIG for as long as 28 days after delivery.

A variety of clinical situations can occur before 28 weeks' gestation that may lead to passage of fetal cells into the maternal circulation (Table 1). Chorionic villus biopsy or second-trimester amniocentesis is frequently used for genetic evaluation of the fetus. A standard dose of 300 μg of RhIG should be given after these procedures in Rh-negative patients. Patients receiving RhIG after prenatal diagnostic procedures should still receive a second dose of RhIG at 28 weeks' gestation and a third dose in the postpartum period. Spontaneous miscarriage, therapeutic abortion, and ectopic pregnancy are further indications for prophylaxis. The use of RhIG in cases of threatened first-trimester abortion or after the delivery of a hydatidiform mole should be strongly considered. Blunt trauma to the abdomen or motor vehicle accidents are associated with a significant incidence of FMH and warrant administration of RhIG in the Rh-

TABLE 1. **Indications for Rh Immune Globulin in the Unsensitized Rh-Negative Pregnant Patient**

1. Routine
   A. 28 weeks of gestation
   B. Within 72 h postpartum if neonate is Rh-positive
2. After invasive prenatal diagnostic procedures
   A. Chorionic villus biopsy
   B. Amniocentesis
3. Abnormal pregnancy
   A. Ectopic pregnancy
   B. Threatened abortion
   C. Spontaneous abortion
   D. Elective abortion
   E. Hydatidiform mole
4. Trauma
   A. Blunt trauma to the abdomen
   B. Motor vehicle accident
5. External cephalic version

negative patient. External cephalic version to turn a fetus from an abnormal position to vertex requires considerable manipulation of the maternal abdominal wall and may be associated with FMH. RhIG should be given post procedure in the Rh-negative woman.

The RhIG is ineffective once alloimmunization has occurred. Therefore, its use in the patient who already demonstrates anti-D antibody is unwarranted. A final area of confusion related to Rh prophylaxis involves the patient who is blood typed as D$_u$-positive. These individuals should be viewed as expressing a weak Rh-positive antigen on their red cell surfaces and therefore are not at substantial risk to become alloimmunized if exposed to fetal Rh-positive red cells. RhIG is therefore not indicated in these cases.

INCIDENCE

With the widespread use of immune globulin (IG), it was once thought that Rh alloimmunization in pregnancy could be eradicated in the United States. The rate of hemolytic disease of the newborn secondary to Rh antibody declined from 45.1 cases per 10,000 total births in 1970 to 15.6 cases per 10,000 total births in 1983. In 1986, the Centers for Disease Control and Prevention through their Birth Defects Monitoring Program reported that Rh hemolytic disease of the newborn affected approximately 1 in 1000 live births in the United States. Red cell alloimmunization involving irregular antibodies continues to be a problem since prophylactic IG is not available to prevent these cases. The majority of cases of Kell sensitization in the United States are secondary to incompatible red cell transfusions, since blood is not routinely crossmatched for the Kell antigen. Fetal or neonatal anemia secondary to maternal Kell alloimmunization occurs 10 times less frequently than Rh disease.

DIAGNOSIS

The approach used at our institution in the newly diagnosed alloimmunized pregnancy is depicted in

Figure 1. If an initial antibody screen returns positive, the antibody is identified and a titer performed. A detailed history regarding previous pregnancy outcome should then be obtained. As a general rule, a pregnancy-related event in a previous gestation is discovered as the cause of the sensitization. Only in the rarest of situations is intrauterine transfusion required in the first affected pregnancy. An early ultrasound examination to accurately establish gestational age should then be undertaken. Paternal blood type and genotype testing are obtained early in the course of evaluation. In cases of D alloimmunization, the blood bank is consulted for genotype testing. Based on paternal antigen testing at the remaining Rh antigen sites (C/c and E/e), a heterozygous or homozygous D status can be determined with a reasonable degree of certainty. If the paternal blood type is negative for the involved red cell antigen, the fetus will be unaffected and further testing is unnecessary. One should document in the medical record that thorough counseling regarding paternity has taken place. If there is any question regarding paternity, the diagnostic algorithm should be followed. If paternal blood typing reveals that the father of the fetus is positive for the involved red cell antigen, maternal antibody titers are repeated at monthly intervals until a critical titer of 16 is reached. This is the titer at which the fetus becomes at risk for anemia; further invasive fetal testing is then warranted.

If a heterozygous paternal genotype for the involved red cell antigen is noted, fetal blood for typing can be obtained through cordocentesis. In this procedure, a needle is directed into the umbilical vessels under continuous ultrasound guidance in order to obtain a sample of fetal blood. The procedure is associated with a 1 to 2% rate of loss and should only be performed by a perinatologist in a referral center. In 50% of cases of a heterozygous paternal genotype, the fetus is found to be antigen-negative and further evaluation of the pregnancy is unnecessary. More recently, several centers have developed DNA techniques using amniotic fluid obtained by amniocentesis to determine whether the fetus is Rh-positive. Although this technology is not yet widely available, it has the advantage of allowing blood typing of the fetus through a less risky procedure than cordocentesis.

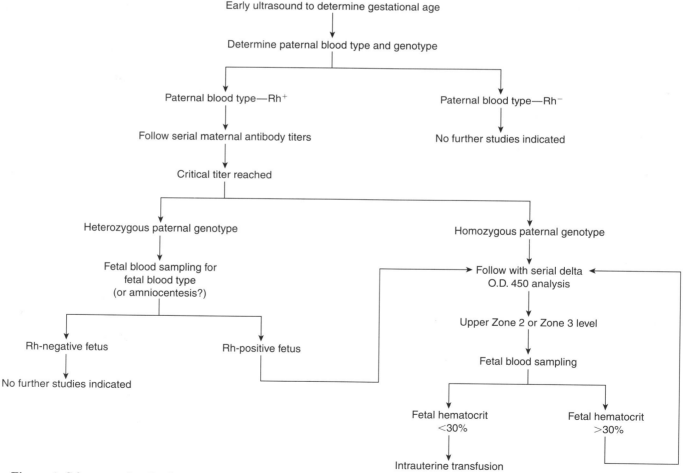

Figure 1. Scheme used at Baylor College of Medicine for management of newly diagnosed red cell alloimmunization in pregnancy. (Redrawn from Moise KJ: Changing trends in the management of red blood cell alloimmunization in pregnancy. Arch Pathol Lab Med *118*:421–428, 1994. Copyright 1994, American Medical Association.)

In cases of a homozygous paternal genotype or a fetus found to be positive for the red cell antigen at cordocentesis, serial amniocenteses to measure amniotic fluid bilirubin levels (delta O.D. 450) should be performed every 10 to 14 days. These values are plotted on a normative curve for gestational age called the "Liley graph." The graph consists of three zones: Zone 1 indicates no evidence of severe hemolytic disease in the fetus, Zone 2 is intermediate, and Zone 3 indicates significant ongoing fetal hemolysis and anemia. Although the original Liley graph was to be used in pregnancies after 26 weeks of gestation, "modified" Liley graphs have underestimated the severity of fetal disease in earlier gestational ages. When amniocentesis is undertaken at less than 26 weeks' gestation, recently published normative graphs should be used. A plateauing or rising trend into the upper portion of Zone 2 or into any portion of Zone 3 of the Liley graph warrants referral to a specialty center. There, cordocentesis with blood readied for intrauterine transfusion should be scheduled; intrauterine transfusion is undertaken when the fetal hematocrit is found to be less than 30%.

In the pregnant patient whose previous child required either intrauterine transfusions or exchange transfusions after birth, a more aggressive management scheme is used at our institution. Maternal antibody titers are less useful in predicting fetal disease after the first affected fetus or neonate. Approximately one-fourth of such pregnancies require invasive diagnostic techniques, with 50% of these subsequently requiring intrauterine transfusion. Serial ultrasound examinations are initiated at 16 weeks' gestation and repeated every 2 weeks. Ultrasound is a poor tool for the prediction of fetal anemia. Overt hydrops fetalis (scalp edema, pleural effusion, ascites) should be considered end-stage disease and is not evident on ultrasound until the fetal hematocrit is less than one-third of normal. At 20 to 22 weeks' gestation, serial amniocenteses are initiated to measure delta O.D. 450 values. The remainder of the diagnostic protocol is similar to that for the first affected gestation.

TREATMENT

Although a variety of treatments have been attempted to effect a decrease in maternal red cell antibody levels, only intrauterine transfusion has proved successful for fetal treatment. In the mid-1960s, the intraperitoneal transfusion of donor red blood cells under fluoroscopic guidance was the mainstay of therapy. Unfortunately, survival in cases of hydrops fetalis only approached 50%. Today, intrauterine transfusion at most perinatal centers consists of cordocentesis under ultrasound guidance with the intravascular transfusion of red blood cells. Other modifications in technique include the routine intraoperative use of short-term paralytic agents to prevent fetal movement and the use of maternal washed blood as the source of red cells for the transfusion. Intrauterine transfusions are continued every 2 to 4 weeks until 35 weeks' gestation. Vaginal delivery at term with a neonatal hospital course of only several days' duration is now the norm. Many of these infants do not require phototherapy for hyperbilirubinemia. Successful reversal of hydrops fetalis in utero with overall survival in 75 to 80% of cases can now be anticipated. Intravascular intrauterine transfusions produce profound suppression of fetal erythropoiesis in utero. Initial neonatal blood samples reveal an absence of reticulocytes and a blood type consistent with that of previous donor blood. When maternal blood has been used as the source of red blood cells, the neonatal blood type is equivalent to that of the mother. Neonates treated with intrauterine transfusions should undergo weekly hematocrit tests and reticulocyte counts in the first 6 to 8 weeks after birth. Approximately 50% require 1 to 2 "top up" transfusions in the neonatal period because of symptoms related to anemia. Once the maternal antibody levels that have been acquired transplacentally have decreased, the neonates begin to revert to their own blood type and replace donor red blood cells with their own.

The majority of cases of Rh alloimmunization can be prevented through the judicious use of RhIG. Inadvertent omission of prophylaxis or cases of hemolytic disease of the fetus and newborn secondary to red cell antigens for which no immune prophylaxis exists dictates that cases will continue to occur. The relative infrequency of this condition and the rapidly evolving technological breakthroughs call for consultation with a referral center that routinely treats this condition when the physician is confronted with a case of red cell alloimmunization in pregnancy.

HEMOPHILIA AND RELATED CONDITIONS

method of
W. KEITH HOOTS, M.D.
University of Texas M. D. Anderson Cancer Center
Houston, Texas

Hemophilia A (Factor VIII deficiency) and hemophilia B (Factor IX deficiency) are X-linked inherited hereditary bleeding disorders. By contrast, von Willebrand's disease (vWD) is autosomally inherited, so that males and females are affected equally. Hemophilias A and B present as clinically identical conditions; the primary morbid manifestations are joint bleeding (hemarthrosis) and joint destruction. The reason that the clinical findings are indistinguishable is that Factor VIIIc (hemophilia A) and Factor IX (hemophilia B) are essential cofactors for activating Factor Xa in the intrinsic clotting pathway. Each of these factors is primarily produced in the liver. Factor IX is a serine protease, and Factor VIIIc is a large glycoprotein essential for configuring the clotting enzymes on the platelet surface so that enzyme-substrate reactions occur at optimal maximal kinetics.

Both hemophilias A and B exhibit a range of clinical

severities that correlates fairly well with assayed factor levels. Specifically, severe disease is defined as less than 1% assayed clotting factor in plasma, whereas approximately 1 to 5% and greater than 5% of normal are defined as moderate and mild disease, respectively. Males within a family almost always have the same degree of impairment since they share the same defect in the DNA coding for the clotting protein.

Both hemophilia A and hemophilia B are coded for by DNA on the long arm (q) of the X chromosome. The Factor VIII gene, coding for a glycoprotein that is substantially larger than the Factor IX protein (approximately 340,000 vs. approximately 70,000 daltons), has been demonstrated to be highly susceptible to mutation events including deletions and missense and nonsense mutations. Though significantly smaller than the Factor VIII gene, the Factor IX gene has also been shown to be prone to new mutation events, particularly of the missense and nonsense type. In practical terms, this results in approximately 25 to 30% of newly diagnosed cases of either hemophilia A or hemophilia B representing a *new* mutation event within a family previously unaffected by hemophilia. This also accounts for the exceptional consistency of prevalence and incidence of both hemophilia A and hemophilia B across all racial and ethnic groups.

The incidence of hemophilias A and B together is between 1 in 5000 and 1 in 10,000 live male births. Approximately 80 to 85% of these affected neonates have heymophilia A. Approximately two-thirds of those with hemophilia A have severe or moderately severe ($\leq$1% Factor VIII) disease. By contrast almost half of hemophilia B patients have greater than 1% Factor IX levels. Hemophilias A and B of comparable severities bleed with similar frequency.

vWD results when there is a defect in the gene for Von Willebrand's factor (vWf), which is located on chromosome 12. The disease is among the most prevalent of genetic diseases. As high as 1% of certain cohort studies using molecular biologic analyses for gene mutation have shown abnormalities. The glycoprotein coded for by the vWf gene is a large subunit of approximately 226,000 daltons that multimerizes into large cell-adhesive molecules that are essential both for platelet aggregation via cross-linking of glycoprotein IB receptors between platelets and for platelet adhesion at the site of blood vessel endothelial cell injury. In addition, these vWf multimers that are secreted from both endothelial cells and platelets are essential for stabilizing Factor VIIIc from proteolysis in the circulating plasma. This explains the low level of Factor VIIIc seen in several types of vWD (see later) despite the fact that both the Factor VIIIc gene and its coded protein are entirely normal.

Unlike the pattern in hemophilias A and B, the clinical bleeding pattern of vWD is primarily localized to mucous membrane surface. Hence, epistaxis, menorrhagia, post–dental surgical, and gastrointestinal bleeding are common manifestations in individuals with vWD. Postsurgical bleeding or hemorrhage secondary to significant trauma occurs to differing degrees, depending on the qualitative or quantitative defect or deficiency in the circulating vWf molecule.

Despite the heterogeneity of the molecular defects of vWf, the categorization of clinical vWD is based on the amount and the functional capacity of the vWf protein in the plasma. Abnormalities have been divided into three major types based on the specific laboratory tests that assess both the quantity and the function of vWf in the plasma of an affected individual.

Type I (Type 1) vWD is a heterozygous state in which the genetic defect inherited from one parent (or representing a new mutation) is partially compensated for by normal vWf production directed by the normal gene from the other parent. This Type I, or classic, vWD is the clinical state most commonly diagnosed. *Quantitative* laboratory studies that measure vWf protein immunologically (Factor VIII–related antigen) are abnormal. The results of vWf (Factor VIII vWf: ristocetin cofactor activity [FVIII vWf:RCoF]) *functional* studies that measure qualitative function in the plasma are proportionally reduced. Further, as noted previously, the Factor VIIIc level in the plasma is frequently abnormal as well, since the diminished FVIII vWf:RCoF level results in a decreased plasma half-life of the Factor VIIIc molecules produced by the hepatocyte.

Type II (Type 2) vWD consists of multiple genetic defects sharing one common defining characteristic: there is normal production of vWf protein that is measured by protein antigen assays in the plasma; however, these vWf molecules are functionally defective to differing degrees. A comprehensive discussion of all the Type II variants of vWD is beyond the scope of this article. Nonetheless, several distinct categories that illustrate the heterogeneity can be listed: abnormalities in the multimerization of the vWf subunits, a defective Factor VIIIc binding site, and a defective secretion of vWf from platelets despite normal plasma vWf structure and function. Any and all may produce clinical bleeding syndromes. Further, as with vWD in general, there is often substantial clinical heterogeneity between individuals of the same Type II variant.

Persons with Type III (Type 3) vWD have a defect in the vWf genes of both chromosomes 12. In many cases, neither parent has a clinically significant bleeding history since subclinical disease among Type I heterozygotes is common. By contrast, the individual with Type III homozygous vWD has severe clinical bleeding since he or she has little if any vWf protein or circulating Factor VIIIc. The latter is deficient since a paucity of vWf in plasma results in rapid proteolysis of Factor VIIIc even though its production is normal. Hence, individuals with Type III vWD may experience both the mucous membrane hemorrhage pattern seen with vWD and bleeding into deep tissue or organs (e.g., hemarthroses) seen more commonly in hemophilic persons. Further, chronic morbidity is much more commonly observed in these individuals.

Inherited bleeding diatheses secondary to abnormalities of other plasma proteins, platelets, or blood vessels are much less common than either hemophilia or vWD. Genetic defects in Factors XI, prekallikrein, and high-molecular-weight kininogen result in prolongation of the activated partial thromboplastin time (aPTT) and may cause clinical bleeding syndromes, although usually less severe than in hemophilia A or B. By contrast, inherited Factor XII deficiency, although prolonging the aPTT, produces no clinical bleeding.

Autosomally inherited Factors V, VII, and X and prothrombin deficiencies are quite rare. When diagnosed they may produce a significant hemorrhagic state, the severity of which correlates inversely with the circulating plasma concentration of the deficient protease (Factors II [prothrombin], VII, and X) or glycoprotein (Factor V).

Factor VII deficiency is suggested when the prothrombin time (PT) is prolonged but the aPTT is normal. Homozygous autosomal afibrinogenemia, the clinical incidence of which is approximately 1 in 1 million live births, may present in the neonatal period with life-threatening hemorrhage necessitating emergent and aggressive replacement therapy with cryoprecipitate. Abnormalities in Factors II, V, and X and fibrinogen prolong both the PT and the aPTT.

Two inherited protein deficiencies are notable for their likelihood of producing hemorrhagic syndromes despite normal PT and aPTT screening tests. The first, Factor XIII deficiency, frequently presents with an indicative clinical history: delayed bleeding after initial adequate hemostasis. This occurs because Factor XIII is required for clot stabilization. The second, homozygous deficiency of the inhibitor alpha$_2$-antiplasmin, also produces a bleeding diathesis, since a dearth of this natural inhibitor of the fibrinolytic protein plasmin permits exaggerated clot lysis by plasmin, thus producing clinical bleeding after tissue injury. Inherited disorders of platelet and endothelial cell function do, in a number of circumstances, cause clinical bleeding.

TREATMENT

Hemostatic Abnormalities

Replacement Therapy

For the majority of inherited coagulation disorders, primary therapy consists of infusing a protein product that replenishes the deficient clotting component. Historically the source of these replacement clotting proteins has been human plasma. The majority of these clotting proteins have their hemostatic activity defined as units of clotting activity per milliliter of pooled normal human plasma. Hence, the blood bank and pharmaceutical strategy for improving the replacement capacity for the specific deficient factor has been to concentrate the specific protein. In some cases, similar proteins co-purify in the concentration process from the source plasma. The first successful strategy for concentrating such clotting proteins from source plasma was cryoprecipitate, which results from the slow thawing of freshly frozen plasma and results in a severalfold concentration of the following clotting proteins: Factor VIIIc, Factor VIII vWf, fibrinogen, Factor XIII, and fibronectin.

Commercial fractionation of cryoprecipitate yielded the first generation of lyophilized Factor VIII concentrates, which resulted in an approximate 100-fold increase in the concentration of Factor VIII per milliliter of infusate. This commercial scale-up resulted when source plasma from 5 to 25,000 donors was converted into lyophilized vials of Factor VIII. These vials ranged in potency from 200 to 1500 U (20 to 35 U per mg of protein) per vial. For the first time convenient home infusion for hemophilia-associated hemorrhage was feasible. Unfortunately, because of the number of donors contributing to the commercial plasma pool, transfusion-transmitted viral disease (particularly transfusion-associated hepatitis and human immunodeficiency virus [HIV] infection) became a common complication in the hemophilia A population. Purification strategies to alleviate or ultimately eliminate this viral risk awaited advances in technology.

Similar viral transmission risk existed for the fractionated therapeutic clotting factor produced for hemophilia B. Since cryoprecipitation does not enrich the product with Factor IX, the initial step in the fractionation of Factor IX clotting factor products has traditionally been barium or aluminum sulfate adsorption followed by further column fractionation. For therapies used in the 1970s and 1980s, this resulted in co-purification of all the molecularly similar vitamin K–dependent factors (II, VII, IX, and X), yielding a final product called prothrombin complex concentrates (PCCs). Like the production of Factor VIII products, the production of PCCs yielded a final vial concentration of 200 to 1500 U (20 to 40 U per mg of protein) per vial. Like the factor VIII products, these commercially produced factor concentrates were, in the years before more effective viral-attenuation techniques, almost invariably virally contaminated, notably with several species of hepatitis and with HIV (after 1979).

The co-purification of Factors II, VII, and X in the preparation of Factor IX concentrates sometimes resulted in the selective conversion of one or more of these protease zymogens to its active enzyme (e.g., Factor VII is converted in trace amounts to Factor VIIa). This trace contamination with active proteases means that PCCs have a thrombogenic potential. Indeed, PCCs given therapeutically in high and recurrent dosing schedules have produced significant and sometimes fatal clotting events in patients with hemophilia B—particularly in individuals receiving the PCCs to provide hemostasis in association with orthopedic surgery. Other clinical situations in which thrombogenesis may be associated with the infusion of PCCs include (1) sustained crush injuries, (2) large intramuscular bleeds (e.g., psoas or thigh), (3) the treatment of neonates with hemophilia B who have immature natural anticoagulation, and (4) hemostatic therapy given to individuals with severe chronic hepatitis (since this may adversely affect their ability to make antithrombin III and the Vitamin K–dependent inhibitors protein-C and protein-S in their hepatocytes). In its most severe manifestations, dosing with PCCs has produced acute myocardial infarction and disseminated intravascular coagulation. The latter risk may be mitigated by not infusing more than 75 U per kg per dose daily when recurrent dosing is required (e.g., after surgery or to treat life-threatening hemorrhage) and by adding small amounts of heparin to each infusion. Fortunately, more advanced purification technologies have resulted in the production of single-component Factor IX products that are free of any significant trace-activated proteases. These now provide the mainstay for therapy of hemophilia B patients when high-dose, recurrent infusion therapy is required.

Later-Generation Clotting Factor Concentrates

Therapeutic Options for Treatment of Hemophilias A and B in the mid-1990s

FACTOR VIII PRODUCTS

Because of the high frequency and profound impact of transfusion-associated transmission of hepatitis and HIV infection in the hemophilic population during the 1970s and 1980s, there were rapid and profound advances in the attenuation (and even elimination) of these and other viral contaminants. The first step in this evolution was heat treatment of Factor VIII products first licensed for use in 1983. Subsequent advances included pasteurization; solvent-detergent treatment to eliminate lipid-envelope viruses; advanced sepharose chromatography; affinity chromatography with monoclonal antibodies directed against the Factor VIIIc–Factor VIII vWf complex or against Factor IX; and most recently, the commercial production of a recombinant Factor VIIIc product in transfected mammalian cell systems. Each nonrecombinant clotting factor concentrate presently produced in the United States is made from a donor pool screened for HIV, hepatitis B virus, and hepatitis C virus. In addition, each of the currently marketed products undergoes either heating to high temperatures for a long time or solvent-detergent treatment. Both processes appear sufficient to remove the risk of HIV transmission but not necessarily the hepatitis risk particularly when concomitant donor screening is employed.

This degree of confidence that the product is safe in terms of HIV infection does not exist for cryoprecipitate and fresh-frozen plasma (FFP), which typically undergo no viral attenuation other than donor screening (an exception is the investigational pasteurized FFP product made by the New York Blood Center). Efficient donor screening has reduced the relative risk of infection from either of these single-donor products to between 1 in 40,000 and 1 in 100,000 per donor unit for HIV and to 1 in 3000 or less per donor unit for hepatitis C virus. Even though the risk of hepatitis B infection from single-donor cryoprecipitate or FFP is similarly low, anyone likely to be treated with *any* plasma-derived product (whether single-donor or pooled, attenuated product) *should* receive a full three-inoculation course of the hepatitis B vaccine.

Each one of the Factor VIII concentrates available at this time is considered safe in terms of transmission of HIV and similar retroviruses. However, they are not all free of hepatitis C transmission risk. Fortunately the relative risk that any single lot of any of the products will transmit hepatitis C appears low. Nonetheless, documentation of transmissions of hepatitis C virus, hepatitis A virus, and human parvovirus B19 from some existing Factor VIII products has been documented. Current products can be classified by relative product purity, although any comparisons may quickly become outdated as technology advances.

The intermediate-purity factor concentrates are so designated because even though they undergo aggressive viral inactivation with heat (even pasteurization) and/or solvent detergent, the final concentration of Factor VIII in the end product represents a small percentage of the total heterogeneous plasma proteins present (6 to 10 U of Factor VIIIc per mg of total protein excluding albumin).

High-purity products are factor concentrates that have at least 50 U (range: 50 to 150) of Factor VIIIc per mg of protein (excluding albumin for stabilization). In the majority of cases, specialized column chromatographic techniques (e.g., heparin sepharose) result in the significantly higher purity, although there still is trace contamination with immunoglobulins or other plasma proteins. The chromatographic technique provides some viral attenuation, but enhanced viral safety is dependent on postchromatographic pasteurization or solvent-detergent treatment. The end products are considered safe in terms of HIV and relatively but not absolutely safe in terms of hepatitis C virus.

Ultrahigh-purity products are the monoclonal antibody affinity–purified plasma-derived factor concentrates and the recombinant Factor VIII products. For the former the affinity chromatography step is not only efficient at removing all non–Factor VIIIc protein but is a very efficient viral attenuation process as well. Nonetheless, effective elimination of hepatitis C virus from the monoclonal products has required subsequent pasteurization or treatment with solvent detergent. The specific activity of the monoclonal preparations (before the addition of human serum albumin) is 3000 U of Factor VIIIc per mg of protein. This is essentially identical to the effective purity of the licensed recombinant products, which also require comparable dilution with albumin to maintain stability after lyophilization.

With regard to theoretical viral safety, a notable distinction must be made between the monoclonal and the recombinant products. Since the recombinant Factor VIII products are affinity-purified from the cell culture of transfected hamster-derived cell lines, there is no requirement for any further viral attenuation. The addition of human serum albumin constitutes the sole theoretical source of human viral contamination. A theoretical risk of contamination by other nonhuman mammalian viruses or other infective species remains.

Frequent infusions of ultrapure products (specifically the monoclonal products) have been shown to produce a stabilization of the CD4 count in HIV-infected hemophilic patients when compared with chronic infusion of similar amounts of intermediate-purity clotting factor concentrates. It is suspected that in these ultrapure products this results from the absence of other protein contamination rather than from greater purity in terms of viral contamination. Nonetheless, most physicians treating hemophilia have opted to use one of these ultrapure products to treat their HIV-infected patients. Many have also chosen to treat their previously untreated hemophilia A patients (particularly the young children) with these products because of a perceived theoretical viral safety. This safety margin is inferred from (1) studies showing an enhanced capacity to remove surrogate viruses during the monoclonal processing, and (2) the bypassing of a human plasma source (with the exception of the added human serum albumin) from the recombinant products.

It should be noted that there are ongoing clinical trials of a recombinant Factor VIIIc preparation from which the B domain of the gene has been removed before transfection of the hamster cell lines. The protein portion of Factor VIII coded for by the B domain of the gene is not required for efficient clotting function; further, its deletion confers greater stability on the resultant smaller Factor VIIIc molecule. Hence there is no requirement for human serum albumin to stabilize the final lyophilized product. This may provide a higher level of confidence that the product is safe from any future microbiologic contamination. It is not yet apparent when this product will be available for clinical use.

FACTOR IX PRODUCTS

The clotting factor products available for treating hemophilia B must be assessed for two potential factors: (1) theoretical viral safety and factor purity (activity per milligram of protein), and (2) thrombogenicity. The Factor IX products determined to be free of thrombogenic potential are those preparations that have effectively purified the Factor IX protein from the other prothrombin complex proteins (Factors II, VII, and X). Two technical strategies have been employed to purify Factor IX from the other vitamin K factors and thereby to remove the thrombogenic risk: (1) chromatographic partitioning followed by solvent-detergent treatment, *and* (2) monoclonal affinity purification of Factor IX. The product produced by the former process contains some residual nonclotting plasma proteins. By contrast the monoclonal product is free of other plasma proteins. Viral attenuation to remove HIV appears effective in both processes. The hepatitis virus risk is significantly reduced by both processes. However, studies using surrogate viruses imply greater safety from hepatitis C or similar viruses with the monoclonal Factor IX concentrate.

The other clotting factor concentrates available for treating hemophilia B patients are PCCs. They can produce thrombotic complications when given in high doses or after repeated or sequential dosing. Viral-attenuation strategies for PCCs are either solvent-detergent treatment or heating to 80° C for more than 10 hours. PCCs made by using the heat process may provide a greater viral attenuation for some viruses, although this has not been proved. Either of these PCCs may prove efficacious for treating moderate bleeding (e.g., hemarthrosis) in individuals with highly responsive Factor VIII inhibitors for whom Factor VIIIc concentrates are nonhemostatic because of the Factor VIII antibody.

ANTI-INHIBITOR CLOTTING PREPARATIONS

Since PCCs are thrombogenic because of their trace contamination with the active proteases (e.g., Factor VIIa or Factor Xa), they have been used for nearly 2 decades to treat bleeding in Factor VIII–deficient patients with high responsive (i.e., anamnestic) Factor VIII antibodies. Later manufacturers of PCCs increased the trace amounts of these active proteases to produce activated PCCs (aPCCs). There is no in vitro assay for either of the two licensed

aPCC products that correlates with in vivo hemostatic efficacy. Hence, it is often difficult to predict the hemostatic efficacy of aPCCs. Both the individual response and the therapeutic efficacy for specific hemorrhagic episodes vary widely. Stated another way, it is problematic, if not impossible, to predict a priori whether a given dose (units per kilogram of body weight) will provide the necessary hemostasis after a single infusion in a patient with no prior use of aPCC. This is true even though the aPCCs are supplied according to units of hemostatic activity (Factor VIIIc "bypassing" activity) per vial and are dosed accordingly (typical dosing for hemarthroses is 100 U per kg per dose.) To further complicate the issue, there are two aPCC preparations. One may be ineffective in a patient whereas the other may produce effective hemostasis for acute bleeding for that patient. Conversely, the alternative aPCC may prove superior in a second patient with a similar bleeding episode. Because of this capriciousness of aPCC therapy in patients with inhibitors, an individualized therapeutic plan must be established empirically. However, certain principles generally apply: (1) effective dosing of aPCCs is minimally 75 to 100 U per kg; (2) dosing frequency more often than every 6 hours predisposes to significant thrombogenicity, particularly after the third to fourth consecutive dose (hence monitoring for markers of disseminated intravascular coagulation is warranted when sequential dosing over several days is required), and (3) since the activated proteases that account for the procoagulant activity of aPCCs are short-lived, initial hemostasis may be followed by breakthrough bleeding between doses that may create difficulty for maintenance hemostatic therapy. Therapy with aPCCs is expensive, is less than reliable, and carries a risk of significant complications. Experience and expertise in their use help to mitigate these risks and to differentiate the appropriate use of aPCCs from the other alternatives for inhibitor therapy cited later.

One alternative therapy for treating patients with inhibitors is porcine Factor VIII. This product is produced from porcine plasma using a polyelectrolyte resin separation technology. The residual nonhuman protein is relatively low, although this does not completely eliminate the anaphylactoid potential of this product. Another characteristic of porcine Factor VIII often limits its efficacy in many individuals with inhibitors. In many cases the specific anamnestic antibody directed against the human Factor VIIIc glycoprotein cross-reacts with shared epitopes on the porcine molecule. Therefore, before the therapeutic efficacy of the product of porcine Factor VIII can be assessed in a patient, it is necessary to quantitate the neutralizing capacity of the antibody against both the porcine and the human Factor VIII product using the Bethesda assay. In those instances in which the anti–porcine product Bethesda unit titer is significantly lower (<10 Bethesda U) than the corresponding anti–human product Bethesda titer, therapy with porcine Factor VIII may be the therapy of choice.

Before infusing the first dose of porcine Factor VIII (at a starting dose of approximately 100 U per kg), there is need to infuse a test dose of approximately 100 U to ensure that there is no immediate hypersensitivity reaction. If none occurs, a slow infusion over 20 to 30 minutes with careful monitoring for allergic symptoms can proceed. Further, since the porcine Bethesda unit inhibitor assay provides an in vitro estimate of the neutralizing capacity of the anti–Factor VIII antibody against porcine Factor VIII, it is essential to monitor Factor VIII levels in these patients. As with most therapies for Hemophilia A patients with inhibitors, therapy with porcine Factor VIII is quite costly.

The indications for the use of other more esoteric and experimental therapies for Factor VIII inhibitors (e.g., Factor VIIa, immune tolerance induction, or antibody depletion using a staphylococcal protein A sepharose chromatographic column) are beyond the scope of this discussion. Comprehensive hemophilia treatment centers provide expertise for these specialized therapeutic procedures. Further, since optimal methodologies are still to be determined by collaborative research protocols, discussion with physician-scientists at these centers offers the best prospect for providing clinicians with up-to-date information about therapeutic options for treating complex inhibitor patients.

THERAPIES FOR VON WILLEBRAND'S DISEASE

Patients with Type I and most with Type II vWD may often be treated with desmopressin acetate (DDAVP), a synthetic analogue of the antidiuretic hormone 1-deamino-8-D-arginine vasopressin. Because of its efficacy in inducing the release of vWf multimers from endothelial cells, it results in a concomitant rise in Factor VIIIc levels (because vWf spares the latter molecule from rapid proteolysis in plasma). DDAVP at a dose of 0.3 μg per kg by slow intravenous infusion increases circulating vWf by approximately 250% in the average individual and increases Factor VIIIc approximately 300%. Therefore it becomes the treatment of choice for mild-to-moderate bleeding in most individuals with both mild hemophilia A (e.g., >5% Factor VIII activity) and Types I and II vWD. (Note: In Type IIb vWD, in which the largest vWf multimers are missing from plasma but are released in excess following DDAVP use, there is a theoretical risk of thrombocytopenia from excessive platelet aggregation. Hence its use in this subgroup must be evaluated on an individual case basis.) Since a two and one-half to threefold increase in both Factor VIIIc and Factor VII vWf is often sufficient to raise both to normal ranges in vWD patients, many such individuals may never require any other type of therapy for either acute hemorrhage or prophylaxis for surgical or dental procedures. Tachyphylaxis after repeated dosing with DDAVP can occur because of depletion of the vWf stores in the endothelial cells. Therefore, monitoring of in vivo clotting factor activity levels in those individuals requiring frequent dosing (i.e., daily or more often) is indicated.

Recently a highly concentrated (1500 μg per mL)

intranasal form of DDAVP (stimate) has been licensed in the United States. Two inhalations in a single nostril acutely in adults and one inhalation in children typically achieve approximately two-thirds of the therapeutic effect of the intravenous dosing. As with the intravenous preparation, facial flushing, mild to moderate blood pressure elevation, and antidiuresis are expected side effects.

For individuals with Type III vWD, for those with Types I and II who either fail to respond to DDAVP or do so to a degree inadequate to achieve complete and predictable hemostasis, and for those vWD patients who experience tachyphylaxis precluding required repeated therapy, other therapeutic options are needed. Traditionally, cryoprecipitate administered in a dose calculated to elevate either the Factor VIIIc, or the Factor VIII:vWf level or both to the normal range has been the most effective means for achieving hemostasis in such patients. However, as noted previously, single-donor cryoprecipitate has a very small but finite risk of causing hepatitis virus and even HIV infection.

Hence many hematologists have chosen to employ one of three intermediate- or high-purity Factor VIII concentrates that have been demonstrated to have most sizes of vWf multimers present after reconstitution. Unlike cryoprecipitate, these concentrates may not have the ideal ratio of vWf multimers when compared with the physiologic state. Nonetheless, the theoretical viral safety conferred by the attenuation they undergo in preparation more than compensates for this theoretical hemostatic deficit. Several studies have shown clinical efficacy to be good even when individuals with severe disease (Type III) have experienced potential or actual life-threatening hemorrhage.

ANTI-FIBRINOLYTIC AGENTS

Tranexamic Acid (Cyklokapron) and epsilon-aminocaproic acid (EACA) (Amicar) act by inhibiting plasminogen activation, thereby enhancing clot stability. These two agents are useful therapeutic adjuncts to stabilize clots that have formed after therapy in patients with underlying hemostatic defects. For patients with inherited clotting disorders, they have proved particularly efficacious for bleeding in the oral cavity (e.g., after dental or oral surgical procedures or trauma to the mouth) and for epistaxis. Dosing for oral tranexamic acid is 25 mg per kg per dose every 6 to 8 hours; for EACA it is 75 to 100 mg per kg per dose every 6 hours (maximal dose is 3 to 4 grams every 6 hours). For patients with hemophilia and vWD, treatment may be required for 7 to 14 days, depending on the amount of tissue injury. In hemophilia B, it is prudent to use a purified Factor IX preparation rather than PCC when concomitant antifibrinolytic therapy is contemplated because of the added thrombotic risks of the two latter agents together.

PREVENTIVE CARE

Male infants born to known or suspected hemophilic carrier mothers should not be circumcised until hemophilia in the infant has been excluded by laboratory testing. Blood for assay for aPTT and Factor VIII or Factor IX assay (or both if the family history is uncertain) should be obtained from cord blood. When a cord blood sample is not available, venipuncture should be performed in a superficial limb vein in order to lessen the likelihood of producing a hematoma that might then require the patient to have replacement therapy. Femoral and jugular sites must be avoided.

Routine immunizations requiring injection such as diphtheria-pertussis-tetanus (DPT) or measles-mumps-rubella (MMR) may be given in the deep subcutaneous tissue (rather than deep intramuscular as is the usual practice), using the smallest gauge needle that is feasible. Hepatitis B vaccine should be given as soon after birth as possible to all infants with confirmed diagnosis of hemophilia. The oral polio live attenuated viral vaccine should not be given to an infant whose hemophilic older brother (or grandfather in the household) is known to be HIV immune-suppressed; Salk vaccine may be substituted.

Early infant dental examination is recommended to teach proper teeth brushing and to ensure adequate household water fluoridation. In addition to education about hemophilia, both genetic and psychosocial counseling are important for the mother of a newborn with hemophilia. This is particularly true for the approximately 30% for whom the hemophilia represents a new mutation and for whom there is no previous family experience with the disease. Reluctance to clean the teeth routinely should be dispelled early, and anticipated problem areas for causing bleeding should be discussed.

Both parents should be encouraged to participate intensively in every part of the infant's care. Further, normal socialization opportunities must not be limited because of the hemophilia. Experienced personnel should discuss specifically what minimal limitations are reasonable versus what constitutes overprotection and therefore may jeopardize the child's normal development.

An appropriate exercise regimen that excludes "contact" sports (e.g., tackle football) should be encouraged as a daily routine. Further, the role of such a program for the child and adult following episodes of hemarthrosis is best discussed before the child has a joint bleed.

SPECIAL CONSIDERATION FOR HEMOPHILIC BLEEDING

It should be emphasized that early treatment improves the quality of life. It is not only necessary but in many cases diminishes the ultimate duration of therapy. For example, infusion for an acute hemarthrosis with an appropriate dose of factor concentrate (generally 15 to 25 U per kg of body weight) immediately on recognition of pain may obviate the need for a second infusion by forestalling the inflammatory response in the joint. This may curtail the predisposi-

tion for rebleeding in the same joint. Appropriate dosage is chosen to ensure some circulating factor level for at least 48 hours. The strategy for always maintaining such a minimal level is known as "prophylaxis" and has been demonstrated to be efficacious in preventing essentially all joint bleeding in patients with both hemophilia A and hemophilia B. A decision to undertake primary prophylaxis requires extensive prospective evaluation and is best done in close consultation between the parent of the hemophilic child and professionals in the comprehensive hemophilia treatment center.

For life-threatening bleeding in a hemophilic patient, the exigency for immediate infusion is superseded only by resuscitative requirements. Every effort should be made to keep the factor level in the normal range (i.e., >50%) until this bleeding emergency has passed. Further, an acutely hemorrhaging hemophilic patient should be transported, if at all possible, to an emergency center that stocks appropriate plasma products. All head injuries must be considered nontrivial unless proved otherwise by observation and computed tomography or magnetic resonance imaging scan. Late bleeding after head trauma can occur as long as 3 to 4 weeks after the injury. Hence, patients with head and neck injuries should be infused immediately unless one is totally convinced that the injury is insignificant. Additionally, if the patient is not hospitalized, the patient and his or her family should be instructed in the neurologic signs and symptoms of central nervous system bleeding so that the patient will return for reinfusion, clinical and radiologic reassessment, and hospitalization at the earliest manifestation of bleeding.

Bleeding from the floor of the mouth or the pharynx or epiglottic region frequently results in partial or complete airway obstruction. Therefore, such bleeding should be treated with an aggressive infusion program with extended clinical follow-up to ensure resolution. Such bleeding may be precipitated by coughing, tonsillitis, oral or otolaryngologic surgery (e.g., extraction of wisdom teeth, tonsillectomy, adenoidectomy), or regional block anesthesia. For surgery and anesthesia, prophylaxis with appropriate infusion therapy before the procedure usually obviates the need for further treatment.

Patients with hemophilia who have gastrointestinal lesions, such as ulcer, varices, or hemorrhoids, must be managed with an appropriate continuous infusion regimen that maintains nearly normal circulating levels of Factor VIIIc or IX until some healing has been achieved. Concomitant transfusions with packed red blood cells may also be required.

Selected types of hemarthroses may be particularly problematic. Hip joint or acetabular hemorrhages can be dangerous because increased intra-articular pressure from bleeding and the associated inflammation may lead to aseptic necrosis of the femoral head. Twice-daily infusion therapy designed to sustain a factor level above 10 U per dL for at least 3 days should be given, along with enforced bed rest that includes Buck's traction for immobilization.

A hemarthrosis of the hip may, at first appearance, be difficult to differentiate from a bleed in the iliopsoas muscle. The latter limits primary hip extension, whereas a bleed in the joint makes any motion of the hip excruciatingly painful. Further, an iliopsoas bleed may decrease sensation over the ipsilateral thigh because of compression of the sacral plexus root of the femoral nerve. Ultrasonography may demonstrate a hematoma in the iliopsoas region. Treatment of the two is similar, although rehabilitation from the hip bleed is more protracted. Both benefit from a physical therapy regimen that strengthens the supporting musculature while slowly mobilizing the affected area. Closed compartment muscle and soft tissue hemorrhages are dangerous because they frequently impinge on the neurovascular bundle. These can occur in the upper arm, forearm, wrist, and volar aspect of the hand as well as the anterior or posterior filial compartments. Swelling and pain precede tingling, numbness, and loss of distal arterial pulses. Infusion must maintain an adequate hemostatic level of Factor VIIIc or IX. Other possible therapeutic maneuvers include elevation to enhance venous return and, as a last resort, surgical decompression if medical therapy fails to forestall progression.

COMPREHENSIVE CARE

Special treatment centers have been established in the United States and many other countries to provide multidisciplinary care for patients with hemophilia and related disorders. Many patients infused with plasma-derived factor concentrates before 1984 to 1985 were infected with the HIV and/or one of the hepatitis viruses. The comprehensive hemophilia centers provide voluntary testing for these viruses, counseling of patients found seropositive for previous infection, and access to appropriate care and therapy. Risk reduction counseling and education are as essential elements of comprehensive treatment centers as is repeated testing for evidence of hepatitis infection.

Comprehensive hemophilia treatment centers are also the mainstay for ongoing education of patients and families about the management of their bleeding disorder. The centers coordinate home therapy and preventive services and work closely with hemophilia consumer organizations to advocate advances in therapy and care.

Further information about hemophiliac care, hemophilia centers, and HIV risk reduction and counseling is available through the National Hemophilia Foundation, The Soho Building, 110 Greene Street, Suite 303, New York, New York 10012 (telephone, 212–219–8180 or 800–424–2634) or from its local chapters.

PLATELET-MEDIATED BLEEDING DISORDERS

method of
ANNA JACQUELINE MITUS, M.D.
Brigham and Women's Hospital
Boston, Massachusetts

Normal hemostasis hinges on complex interactions among platelets, coagulation proteins, and the vessel wall. Formation of the initial platelet plug—primary hemostasis—is contingent on normal platelet number and function. Subsequently, the coagulation proteins stabilize this structure, producing a firm fibrin clot—secondary hemostasis. The clinical pattern of hemorrhage may suggest the underlying coagulation abnormality and direct further laboratory investigation (Table 1).

PRIMARY HEMOSTASIS

To fully understand platelet-mediated bleeding disorders, it is helpful to review briefly the steps involved in the formation of the platelet plug (Figure 1). On damage to the blood vessel wall, platelets *adhere* to exposed subendothelium, a process mediated by the "molecular glue" von Willebrand factor (vWf). Subsequently, in a complex series of events termed "activation," platelet receptors for fibrinogen are expressed, the contents of various granules are released, and the potent vasoconstrictor thromboxane A_2 is generated from arachidonic acid. Additional platelets are then recruited and *aggregated* through interlinking fibrinogen bridges. Defects anywhere in this pathway (adhesion, activation, or aggregation) can give rise to hemorrhage.

CLINICAL FINDINGS
(see Table 1)

When primary hemostasis is disturbed, bleeding occurs immediately after an inciting event and involves mucocutaneous surfaces (skin, nares, oral cavity, and genitourinary and gastrointestinal tracts). In contrast, defects in secondary hemostasis predispose to delayed hemorrhage into deep-seated spaces such as the joints or the retroperitoneum. Consequently, a patient complaining of menorrhagia, epistaxis, or petechiae most likely has a disturbance in platelet number or function. Physical findings vary according to the severity of the condition. Petechiae (reddish-purple, nonblanching skin lesions) usually indicate marked thrombocytopenia. They appear predominantly in the dependent regions of the body and reflect small hemorrhages into the skin. Blood-filled mucosal blisters in the mouth are particularly suggestive of an acute drop in platelet number.

TABLE 1. **Clinical Patterns of Hemorrhage**

	Primary Hemostasis (Platelet Plug Formation)	**Secondary Hemostasis (Fibrin Clot Formation)**
Onset	Immediate	Delayed
Site	Mucocutaneous (skin, mouth, gastrointestinal tract, genitourinary tract)	Deep-seated (joints, retroperitoneum)

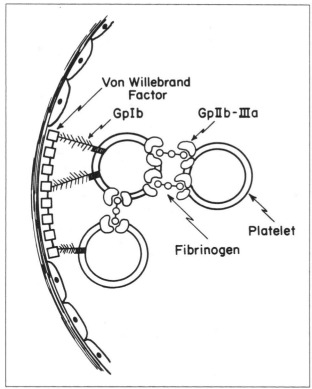

Figure 1. Diagrammatic representation of the platelet-vessel interaction. The "molecular glue" von Willebrand factor binds to subendothelial collagen and to platelet glycoprotein (GpIb), thereby ensuring adhesion of the platelet to the denuded vasculature despite high shear forces. Fibrinogen serves to interlock platelets via GpIIb-IIIa. (From Handin RI: Bleeding and thrombosis. *In* Braunwald E, Isselbacher KJ, Petersdorf RG, et al. [eds]: Harrison's Principles of Internal Medicine, 12th ed. Reproduced with permission of McGraw-Hill, Inc., New York, 1991, p 349.)

LABORATORY EVALUATION

The laboratory evaluation of the patient presenting with bleeding should include a general screen of the hemostatic mechanism, beginning with a complete blood count (CBC) with platelet count, prothrombin time (PT), and partial thromboplastin time (PTT). When a disorder in platelet function is suspected, additional studies can be ordered. The *bleeding time* (BT) is obtained by performing a small incision in the skin and absorbing blood with a filter paper disk at 30-second intervals. Platelet counts below 100,000 per µL or disruption of platelet function (thrombasthenia) prolong the BT beyond the normal range of about 8 minutes. In practice, the BT can be unreliable because it is highly operator dependent and affected by unrelated abnormalities of the skin (e.g., Ehlers-Danlos syndrome) or subcutaneous tissues (e.g., edema).

The integrity of aggregation mechanisms is assessed in the laboratory by *platelet function studies*. A series of pharmacologic agonists (epinephrine, thrombin, adenosine diphosphate [ADP], and so on) is added to platelet-rich plasma in an aggregometer, and the pattern of aggregation is observed. Defects in these tests pinpoint specific abnormalities in platelet surface receptors or in granular content or release. Quantitative or qualitative defects in vWf give rise to the most common inherited disorder of primary hemostasis, von Willebrand's disease. Diagnosis of this condition is confirmed by obtaining a *von Willebrand disease screen* (see later).

THROMBOCYTOPENIA

When the platelet count falls to about 100,000 per µL, a mild increased predisposition to hemorrhage develops, manifested by prolongation of the BT. Many patients remain asymptomatic or note only slight bruising. The frequency and severity of bleeding worsen as levels decline further, occurring spontaneously with severe thrombocytopenia (platelet count <20,000 per µL). The risk of hemorrhage for any given level of platelet count must be interpreted in the context of platelet function. With superimposed platelet dysfunction (e.g., aspirin consumption), bleeding may develop even when platelet counts exceed 50,000 per µL, whereas in consumptive thrombocytopenia, relatively young "superfunctioning" platelets are produced, and patients may have few or no symptoms even when markedly thrombocytopenic.

As with the approach to any cytopenia, thrombocytopenia can be considered as arising from decreased production or increased destruction (Table 2). The hematocrit and white blood cell count provide important clues about the nature of the process. Accompanying anemia and leukopenia are strongly suggestive of a primary marrow disturbance (aplasia, vitamin deficiency, infiltration by metastatic tumor, granuloma or fibrosis, replacement by leukemia or lymphoma) and must be assessed by obtaining a bone marrow aspirate and biopsy. Isolated thrombocytopenia arising from decreased production (amegakaryocytic thrombocytopenia) is extremely uncommon and is limited to rare congenital or acquired disorders. Uncommonly, alcohol and medications such as the thiazide diuretics and estrogens can directly suppress megakaryopoiesis.

Thrombocytopenia more frequently results from in-

TABLE 2. **Approach to Thrombocytopenia**

Decreased Production

Associated with Anemia, Leukopenia

Vitamin deficiency (folate, cobalamin)
Infiltration (fibrosis, metastatic cancer, granuloma)
Aplastic anemia
Primary hematologic disorder (acute leukemia, myelodysplasia)

Isolated Thrombocytopenia
Amegakaryocytic thrombocytopenia
Drug suppression (thiazide diuretics, estrogens)

Increased Destruction

Associated with Anemia, Leukopenia
Hypersplenism

Isolated Thrombocytopenia
Immune-mediated (ITP)
Drug-mediated
Consumptive (DIC, TTP)

Abbreviations: ITP = immune thrombocytopenic purpura; DIC = disseminated intravascular coagulation; TTP = thrombotic thrombocytopenic purpura.

creased destruction within the peripheral circulation or sequestration within the spleen. In these cases, the bone marrow shows normal or increased numbers of megakaryocytes.

Immune Thrombocytopenic Purpura

Immune (formerly idiopathic) thrombocytopenic purpura (ITP) is the disorder most likely to be encountered by the internist. It occurs two to three times more frequently in women than in men and sometimes is a manifestation of an underlying autoimmune disease (e.g., systemic lupus erythematosus) or lymphoproliferative disorder (e.g., chronic lymphocytic leukemia). Assays for antiplatelet antibodies are available but lack the sensitivity and specificity to render them clinically helpful. Instead, the diagnosis is one of exclusion, resting on elimination of other processes or medication associated with thrombocytopenia. Because ITP is a well-recognized complication of early human immunodeficiency virus (HIV) infection, viral serology should also be obtained at initial presentation.

Treatment with corticosteroids is the mainstay of therapy. Prednisone (1 to 2 mg per kg per day) is usually instituted when the platelet count falls below 50,000 per µL or if clinical bleeding develops, regardless of platelet number. Responses are seen within 7 to 10 days in most patients. High doses should be continued for at least 2 weeks before a slow taper (10 mg per week) is attempted. Corticosteroids alone are unlikely to cure ITP; many patients require splenectomy, which yields response rates of 60 to 80%. In steroid-refractory patients or in emergency situations, an infusion of intravenous gamma globulin (2 gm per kg intravenously [total] over 2 to 5 days) can rapidly improve thrombocytopenia. Its effects, however, are short-lived (about 2 to 3 weeks), and a single course of therapy is expensive. Other treatment modalities are generally reserved for the nonresponsive patient and include high-dose dexamethasone (40 mg orally daily for 4 days), danazol (Danocrine), vincristine, combination chemotherapy, and azathioprine (Imuran). In HIV infection, zidovudine somewhat paradoxically has been shown to improve the platelet number and should be considered among first-line interventions.

Drug-Mediated Thrombocytopenia

Numerous medications have been implicated in thrombocytopenia, and a detailed list of all drug ingestions (prescribed, over-the-counter, and illicit) must be obtained from the thrombocytopenic individual. Most drug-induced thrombocytopenia appears to be immune mediated. Heparin is a common offending agent, causing a fall in the platelet count in 1 to 5% of treated patients. Concomitant platelet activation can rarely lead to serious or life-threatening thrombosis. If thrombocytopenia is noted in a patient on heparin, even if the dose is small (subcutaneous administration or intravenous flushes), the drug should

be discontinued as soon as possible. Alternative therapeutic measures include a trial of porcine (rather than bovine) heparin, low-molecular-weight heparin, or experimental defibrinogenating agents such as ancrod (Arvin).*

Microangiopathic Thrombocytopenia

Disseminated intravascular coagulation (DIC) and thrombotic thrombocytopenic purpura (TTP) are characterized by abnormal consumption of platelets in the peripheral circulation. In the former condition, an inciting event, usually sepsis, promotes endothelial damage and subsequent activation of the coagulation cascade. Fibrin thrombi trap platelets, leading to thrombocytopenia and fragmentation of erythrocytes (microangiopathic hemolysis). In TTP, platelet-rich thrombi occlude the vasculature, leading to myriad clinical symptoms, including renal and neurologic dysfunction. These topics are covered in detail elsewhere in this volume.

Hypersplenism

In the normal steady state, approximately one-third of platelets are contained within the spleen, a percentage that can increase dramatically as the organ enlarges. Platelet counts lower than 50,000 per µL are unusual, and as a rule mild anemia and leukopenia are also noted. Most often, splenomegaly is a result of primary hepatic disease and secondary portal hypertension, but it can also develop as a consequence of lymphoma, storage diseases, and a multitude of systemic conditions. Therapy is directed at the underlying disorder, and only rarely is splenectomy indicated either for diagnosis or for amelioration of cytopenias.

QUALITATIVE DEFECTS OF PLATELETS

Inherited Disorders

Inherited causes of platelet-mediated bleeding can be classified as defects in platelet adhesion (e.g., von Willebrand's disease, Bernard-Soulier disease), activation and secretion (e.g., storage pool defects), and aggregation (e.g., Glanzmann's thrombasthenia).

Von Willebrand's disease is a common but heterogeneous disorder generally transmitted in an autosomal dominant pattern. Three major forms have been identified, based on whether there is mild or severe deficiency of the protein (Types I and III, respectively) or a qualitative abnormality (Type II). Typical of platelet-mediated bleeding disorders, epistaxis, menorrhagia, gingival hemorrhage, and easy bruising are common complaints and as expected, the BT is prolonged. Because symptoms can be mild, recognition of this disease may be delayed until adulthood. Diagnosis and subtyping are facilitated by

---

*Investigational drug in the United States.

measuring the antigenic level of the von Willebrand factor (vWf:Ag). In addition, because vWf circulates in the plasma as a complex with Factor VIII, a diminution in plasma vWf is usually accompanied by a parallel reduction in Factor VIII levels, leading to variable prolongation of the PTT. It is important to remember, however, that the finding of a normal PTT does not exclude the diagnosis.

The antibiotic ristocetin induces platelet aggregation and thrombocytopenia via an incompletely understood mechanism involving vWf. This observation led to the development of a third assay for this disease, the ristocetin cofactor activity (vWf:RCo). In this test, patient plasma is added to normal platelets in the presence of ristocetin, and the rate of agglutination is measured. Disproportionate lowering of the vWf:RCo correlates with qualitative abnormalities of the vWf protein and is characteristic of Type II disease.

Classification of von Willebrand's disease is important because therapy varies. In mild forms, treatment is indicated only for moderate-to-severe bleeding or for perioperative management. The synthetic vasopressin analogue desmopressin (1-deamino-[8-D-arginine]-vasopressin [DDAVP], 0.3 μg per kg) induces a rapid, transient rise in vWf and Factor VIII levels, presumably by stimulating secretion of vWf from storage organelles in the endothelial cell. Peak response is at 30 to 60 minutes and lasts about 6 hours. Flushing, tachycardia, hypertension, headache, nausea, and more rarely, hyponatremia and water intoxication are side effects. In addition, because tachyphylaxis develops after repetitive administration, DDAVP is usually employed when only a limited duration of therapy is needed. Recent availability of an intranasal preparation (Stimulate) will undoubtedly aid in the management of patients with mild disease. Cryoprecipitate and certain purified forms of Factor VIII concentrates (e.g., Humate-P) provide an exogenous source of vWf for patients with severe forms of this condition (Type III) or for those who are refractory to DDAVP.

Bernard-Soulier disease is a rare, autosomal recessive disorder usually presenting early in childhood. As in von Willebrand's disease, the primary hemostatic defect lies in the platelet–vessel wall interaction. In this condition, however, the vWf protein itself is quantitatively and qualitatively normal. Instead, the platelet receptor for vWf (GpIb) is absent. Clinically affected patients are homozygous for this defect and subject to serious hemorrhage. Laboratory data include a prolonged BT, mild thrombocytopenia, and large-appearing platelets on the peripheral smear. As in von Willebrand's disease, loss of response to ristocetin is the major aggregatory abnormality, whereas reactivity to ADP, epinephrine, and collagen remain normal. Platelet transfusion is the treatment of choice for severe hemorrhage, whereas DDAVP may be effective in nonacute settings.

Several rare inherited disorders of platelet activation and secretion have been described. Storage pool diseases are a well-defined subset of secretory abnormalities and represent a spectrum of platelet granule deficiency. In one such condition, isolated loss of alpha granules gives rise to mild thrombocytopenia and abnormal-appearing, agranular gray platelets, the gray platelet syndrome. Infusions of DDAVP and cryoprecipitate or platelet transfusion can be tried to control hemorrhagic symptoms in this disease and related disorders.

Loss of the platelet fibrinogen receptor (IIb/IIIa) causes abnormal platelet aggregation and a severe hemorrhagic disorder, Glanzmann's thrombasthenia. Like Bernard-Soulier disease, it is transmitted as autosomal recessive, and clinical symptoms are found predominantly in homozygote patients. In contrast, platelet morphology is normal in Glanzmann's thrombasthenia, and aggregation abnormalities reveal complete loss of response to ADP, epinephrine, collagen, and arachidonate, and preserved ristocetin activity (mirror opposite to Bernard-Soulier disease). The only effective therapy is platelet transfusion.

Acquired Defects

The most common cause of an acquired defect in platelet function is drug administration. Both aspirin and nonsteroidal anti-inflammatory agents interfere with the production of thromboxane A_2, a potent stimulant of platelet aggregation. Absent arachidonate, blunted collagen responses, and loss of second wave aggregation to epinephrine and ADP are characteristic findings. Cyclooxygenase, the enzyme responsible for converting arachidonic acid to thromboxane A_2, is irreversibly acetylated by aspirin, thus permanently inhibiting this synthetic pathway for the life span of the platelet (about 7 days). Consequently, patients on aspirin should discontinue therapy 5 to 7 days prior to elective procedures. In contrast, nonsteroidal anti-inflammatory medications have a reversible effect on cyclooxygenase, and their antiplatelet effect terminates with clearance of the drug from the circulation (about 6 hours). Antibiotics, particularly high-dose penicillins and cephalosporins, are among other commonly prescribed medications that cause abnormalities of platelets and prolongation of the BT.

The bleeding diathesis of renal failure remains poorly understood, manifested by an abnormal BT and variable aggregatory disturbances. Infusion of DDAVP or conjugated estrogens (0.6 mg per kg per day for 5 days) improves bleeding parameters and can be helpful in controlling hemorrhage or in perioperative management. It is postulated that the underlying pathogenesis is abnormal platelet–vessel wall interaction, but concomitant anemia may also play a role because normalization of the hematocrit can shorten the BT. Similarly, in hepatic failure, patients develop platelet dysfunction, which is not well defined but which may partially correct with DDAVP.

Hemorrhage and thrombosis are major complications of the myeloproliferative disorders. Despite the fact that platelet counts are often elevated, numerous structural and functional abnormalities have been described, none of which reliably predicts bleeding or thrombotic complications. Treatment is directed at the underlying condition and suppression of the malignant clone. In emergency situations, platelet transfusion can be given.

Rarely, patients with multiple myeloma or Waldenström's macroglobulinemia acquire qualitative platelet abnormalities. Usually nonspecific coating of the platelet by paraprotein is responsible, and lowering of the immunoglobulin level with chemotherapy improves bleeding parameters.

Approximately one-quarter of patients discovered to have a prolonged BT will have no identifiable defect in platelets. Depending on the clinical situation, an empirical trial of DDAVP or steroids (prednisone 20 to 60 mg daily) may be warranted.

DISSEMINATED INTRAVASCULAR COAGULATION

method of
JOHN J. BYRNES, M.D.
University of Miami School of Medicine
Miami, Florida

Disseminated intravascular coagulation (DIC) is a clinicopathologic syndrome that may occur secondary to a variety of disorders. The primary disorder causes either endothelial cell injury or the release of procoagulant material into the circulation. Thrombin is formed by activation of either the intrinsic or extrinsic coagulation pathway in excess of the capacity of normal counter-regulatory activities such as antithrombin III and protein-C. Excessive intravascular activation of thrombin leads to the formation of fibrin, which deposits as microthrombi in the smaller vessels of the circulation. In the process, fibrinogen and Factors II, V, VIII, and XIII are consumed. Platelets are trapped in the fibrin meshwork. In addition, exposure of platelets to thrombin causes their aggregation, which contributes to thrombocytopenia. Thrombin in lesser concentrations causes secretion of platelet granules, which leads to a functional defect of platelets remaining in the circulation. Fibrinolysis occurs as plasminogen is activated to plasmin in response to intravascular fibrin deposition. Plasmin also degrades fibrinogen and Factors V, VIII, and XIII, which causes even more severe depletion of coagulation factors. Degradation products of fibrinogen and fibrin inhibit fibrin polymerization and platelet-platelet interaction, further interfering with hemostasis. Consequently, a hypocoagulable state may result from the depletion of hemostatic elements, whereas inhibitors of hemostatic mechanisms, such as fibrin degradation products, exacerbate the hemorrhagic diathesis. Conversely, a hypercoagulable state may ensue because of activated procoagulant factors in the circulation and the depletion of counter-regulatory factors such as antithrombin III and protein-C and protein-S.

The clinical presentation of DIC may be either acute and fulminant or low grade and chronic, depending in large part on the initiating process. Thrombotic or hemorrhagic clinical manifestations may predominate in a given patient, or both manifestations may occur simultaneously. In general, hemorrhagic problems more often complicate acute DIC, whereas chronic DIC is more frequently associated with thrombotic disorders. In acute DIC, the precipitating disorder is generally readily evident and often catastrophic; common etiologies of intravascular coagulation are given in Table 1. Dysfunction of multiple organs due to thrombi in their microcirculation or generalized bleeding complicates an already difficult situation. Chronic DIC is more subtle and may be manifest long before or after the underlying disorder. Recurrent thromboses may be the clue that prompts the search for an occult cancer.

Hemorrhagic manifestations seen with DIC reflect associated trauma or breaches in skin or mucosal integrity that may be relatively minor. Organ systems that are often involved are the skin, gastrointestinal tract, lungs, and brain. Continued bleeding or rebleeding from sites of minor trauma such as venipunctures is typically seen. As previously mentioned, hemostatic failure is due to the depletion of coagulation factors and platelets, accompanied by the accumulation of inhibitors of hemostatic mechanisms and the activation of fibrinolytic mechanisms.

Thrombotic manifestations of DIC can result from widespread microthrombus formation, leading to impaired perfusion of multiple organs. Fulminant DIC can lead to occlusion of the terminal arterioles in the skin and thus to necrosis of digits, nose, and ears and occasionally diffuse skin infarction (purpura fulminans). Renal dysfunction may be extreme and may result in complete renal failure. Involvement of cerebral microvessels often produces nonfocal dysfunction or seizures. Occlusions in the pulmonary microcirculation may be manifest as the respiratory distress syndrome. The clinical syndrome in cancer patients of recurrent or migratory venous or arterial

TABLE 1. **Etiologies of Intravascular Coagulation**

Disseminated

Infections
  Gram-negative sepsis
  Meningococcemia
  Rocky Mountain spotted fever
  Postsplenectomy sepsis
Hypotension—shock
  Of any etiology
  Obstetric complications
  Abruptio placentae
  Amniotic fluid embolism
  Retained dead fetus
  Saline-induced abortions
Malignant disorders
  Mucin-producing adenocarcinomas, especially prostatic and gastric adenocarcinomas
  Promyelocytic leukemia
Injuries
  Extensive tissue damage
  Brain trauma
  Burns
  Snakebite
Metabolic disorders
  Hyperthermia
  Acidosis
Immunologic disorders
  Hemolytic transfusion reaction
  Anaphylaxis

Localized

Vascular malformations
  Giant hemangioma
  Aortic aneurysm

thromboses—Trousseau's syndrome—is due to the hypercoagulable state resulting from chronic low-grade DIC. Frequently, nonbacterial thrombotic endocarditis is associated, which leads to systemic emboli as well.

The laboratory picture of DIC may be unmistakable or subtle. In acute DIC, the platelet count is low; 50% of the time it is less than 50,000 per microliter. The prothrombin time (PT) and partial thromboplastin time (PTT) are prolonged, and the fibrinogen level is below normal. Fibrinogen levels may be normal if the patient initially had elevated levels because of pregnancy or a response to infection. Fibrin (and fibrinogen) degradation products are a hallmark of the disorder; cross-linked fibrin degradation products—D-dimer—indicate fibrin clot lysis. Impaired microvascular blood flow by fibrin strands leads to fragmentation of red blood cells, and microangiopathic hemolytic anemia may ensue, especially in severe acute DIC. Characteristic schistocytes or helmet cells may appear in the blood smear. In chronic DIC, fibrin degradation products are present, but the PT and PTT may or may not be prolonged; the PTT may actually be shorter than normal because of activated factors and depletion of antithrombin III. Liver failure may make it difficult to diagnose DIC, since clotting factor deficiency often occurs, together with thrombocytopenia and impaired clearance of fibrin degradation products, leading to elevated levels.

TREATMENT

In all instances, successful resolution of DIC depends ultimately on successful management of the initiating process. Thus, that is the first priority. It is also important to take supportive measures to maintain adequate blood pressure, hemoglobin concentration, oxygenation, and acid-base and electrolyte balances to minimize organ damage consequent to the impaired microvascular perfusion. Therapeutic intervention aimed at the coagulation disorder must be considered in the full clinical context, and the risks of therapy must, as usual, be weighed against the potential benefit. If there is only laboratory evidence of DIC but no significant hemorrhage or thrombosis, specific measures other than addressing the underlying process are not required. If bleeding is the predominant clinical problem, factor replacement with fresh-frozen plasma (FFP), cryoprecipitate, and platelet transfusion should be used to replenish diminished levels. FFP 2 to 4 U daily is generally adequate. A platelet count of at least 50,000 per microliter should be maintained if there is significant bleeding. Cryoprecipitate may be required in severe DIC to obtain a fibrinogen level higher than 100 mg per dL. If, despite these measures, the bleeding continues and the initiating process persists, disrupting the actions of thrombin with heparin should be considered. A continuous infusion of 600 to 1000 U per hour is generally recommended, with subsequent empiric adjustment. If this treatment is successful, the bleeding should diminish and the platelet count and fibrinogen level should stabilize or increase.

When thrombotic complications resulting in severe organ hypoperfusion occur, anticoagulation with heparin should also be considered. In adults, a loading dose of heparin 5000 U followed by the continuous intravenous infusion of 1000 U per hour is usually given to start. Adjustment of the dose of heparin is determined by the clinical and laboratory response. Improvement in organ perfusion and a rising fibrinogen level and platelet count with diminished signs of intravascular hemolysis point to a satisfactory response. If both thrombotic and bleeding manifestations occur simultaneously, FFP and platelets should be given concomitantly with heparin treatment. FFP also serves to replenish antithrombin III, protein-C, and protein-S. Often, less oozing from venipunctures is also seen as platelets regain hemostatic effectiveness. It must be realized that there are no properly controlled studies demonstrating the effectiveness of heparin in DIC or studies demonstrating the optimal dosing and modification. The evidence for effectiveness is limited to case reports. A specific contraindication to the use of heparin is DIC associated with head trauma or intracerebral hemorrhage.

Several circumstances require particular mention. Myeloid leukemia—especially acute promyelocytic leukemia—is associated with the release of lysosomal granule contents from the promyelocytes into the circulation, thus activating the coagulation cascade. Cytolysis caused by treatment of the leukemia releases even more granule contents into the circulation, which causes acceleration of DIC. In these patients, it has been common practice to treat DIC prophylactically with heparin before embarking on chemotherapy. However, an effect on the ultimate outcome has not been demonstrated. The thrombocytopenia is due partly to the leukemia, and platelet transfusions are usually required despite control of DIC. Remission induction in promyelocytic leukemia with all-*trans*-retinoic acid minimizes the occurrence and progression of DIC.

Acute DIC in pregnancy is caused most often by abruptio placentae. Mild DIC is common in patients in whom abortion is induced by intra-amniotic injection of hypertonic saline; severe DIC is relatively uncommon. In most obstetric patients, management of acute DIC consists of removing the products of conception and supportive care. Transfusions are used to replace clotting factor in patients with significant bleeding. The role of heparin remains controversial, and there are no control studies. However, several reports demonstrated the effectiveness of heparin in controlling bleeding manifestations when there was an unavoidable delay in the resolution of the underlying cause.

Certain disease states are associated with the consumption of platelet and clotting factors at localized anatomic sites. These states include aortic aneurysm, large hemangiomas (Kasabach-Merritt syndrome), and certain renal disorders, including hyperacute allograft rejection. The laboratory values are often compatible with disseminated consumption (DIC). The risk of not recognizing the limited nature of the disorder is that inappropriate therapy may be given for a presumed "disseminated" state. If surgery for an aortic aneurysm is to be done, stabilization of hemostasis is best obtained first. Most patients with chronic DIC of this nature respond to treatment with heparin and factor replacement. A new approach to the treatment of surgically unresectable hemangiomas is to purposely thrombose the vascular channels by using a fibrinolytic inhibitor.

Chronic low-grade DIC associated with venous thromboses, such as in Trousseau's syndrome, requires treatment with full-dose heparin, a loading dose of 5000 to 10,000 U followed by continuous intravenous infusion of 1000 to 2000 U per hour. After resolution of the venous thrombosis, 5000 U of heparin should be given subcutaneously every 8 or 12 hours to prevent recurrence; warfarin (Coumadin) is not as effective in this setting.

The protease inhibitors gabexate, nafamostat, and Trasylol, as well as concentrates of antithrombin III and protein-C, have been used to treat DIC. However, these are still in development and are not yet approved for this indication.

THROMBOTIC THROMBOCYTOPENIC PURPURA AND THE HEMOLYTIC–UREMIC SYNDROME

method of
JOHN J. BYRNES, M.D.
University of Miami School of Medicine
Miami, Florida

Thrombotic thrombocytopenic purpura (TTP) most often afflicts relatively young adults who are otherwise healthy. Platelets agglutinate and form microthrombi in arterioles and capillaries throughout the body. The cause of this agglutination is poorly understood; von Willebrand factor participates in the process and several other abnormalities of plasma factors have been described, but the pathogenetic significance of each is not clear. Endothelial injury, recanalization of the thrombi, endothelial cell proliferation, and microaneurysm formation occur. The consumption of platelets results in thrombocytopenia, and the thrombi disrupting the microcirculation cause fragmentation of red blood cells, which gives the characteristics of microangiopathic hemolytic anemia (MAHA).

Disturbance in the microcirculation of the brain is often manifested as symptoms and clinical findings. The unpredictable distribution of lesions leads to a diversity of neurologic manifestations. Impaired perfusion of the kidneys generally results in renal dysfunction, although it is often not severe. Other organs variably manifest clinical or laboratory abnormalities early in the disease. The triad of thrombocytopenia, fragmentation hemolysis, and bizarre neurologic abnormalities that wax and wane is highly indicative of TTP. In addition, the high incidence of renal impairment and fever at presentation has been noted. This pentad of findings has been popularized as constituting the syndrome. However, the patient with TTP may be virtually asymptomatic or may suffer from failure of virtually every organ system. Without effective treatment, the disorder is fatal because of progressive multiple organ failure or bleeding into the brain.

The outlook for patients with TTP was extremely poor until the beneficial effect of infusion of whole blood or plasma was recognized. A plasma factor, which is still poorly characterized, can neutralize abnormal platelet agglutination. A satisfactory clinical response to plasma therapy occurs in more than 70% of patients. Eventually, the syndrome passes and the plasma requirement abates. However, recurrent episodes occur in more than 30% of patients.

EVALUATION BEFORE INSTITUTING THERAPY

Alternative disorders with consumptive thrombocytopenia and MAHA may resemble TTP and should be excluded. Disseminated intravascular coagulation (DIC) often has to be considered. However, as the patient first presents, the clinical setting is generally not appropriate for DIC, and the fibrinogen level is typically normal in TTP. Furthermore, there is usually little or no evidence of coagulation factor consumption, fibrin deposition, or fibrinolysis. The prothrombin time and partial thromboplastin time are usually normal; the thrombin time, however, may be slightly prolonged. DIC may occur late in the course of inadequately treated TTP. The hemolytic-uremic syndrome (HUS) resembles TTP in many features but should be considered separately (see later section). The HELLP syndrome of pregnancy—hemolysis with schistocytes, elevated liver enzymes, and low platelets—is probably a variant of eclampsia. During the peripartum period, either HUS or the HELLP syndrome may be confused with TTP. Furthermore, there is an association of TTP with pregnancy. Severe vasculitis can resemble TTP; systemic lupus erythematosus, especially with cerebritis, can mimic TTP in many clinical features, but TTP also has an increased incidence in autoimmune disorders such as systemic lupus. Malignant hypertension can cause platelet consumption and fragmentation hemolysis, often with associated neurologic disturbance. Occasionally, these disorders and TTP cannot be distinguished, and empirical treatment for both must be considered.

The question of a tissue biopsy often arises to establish the diagnosis more firmly. TTP must be treated promptly. Biopsies in TTP, even in fulminant disease, have a substantial percentage of false-negative results. Thus, the biopsy result does not change the management; therapy should be instituted without delay.

It is important to assess the patient clinically and with laboratory measurements so that the response to therapy can be evaluated and adjustments made accordingly. The rapid reversibility of neurologic manifestations is often remarkable. Laboratory parameters that are especially important to follow are the platelet count, hematocrit, and serum lactate dehydrogenase (LDH) level. The serum LDH level reflects the combined hemolysis and other tissue injury, and as such, it is an excellent guide to the patency of the microcirculation and a good indicator of disease activity. These studies should be obtained daily during the acute phase of management.

TREATMENT

Diagnosing TTP is a medical emergency, whether or not the patient has critical manifestations. The cornerstone to the treatment of TTP is plasma therapy. Plasma infusion and plasmapheresis with plasma exchange are both highly effective; however, plasmapheresis has been shown to have an edge. Plasmapheresis is often more time consuming to initiate than plasma infusion. Consequently, once I suspect the patient has TTP, I immediately order plasma infusions at the rate of about 30 mL per kg daily, if the patient's condition does not otherwise preclude this, and initiate arrangements for plasmapheresis. The volume of plasmapheresis should be at least 1 plasma volume daily and preferably 1.5 plasma volumes; it should continue for at least 5 days. The replacement fluid should be platelet-depleted plasma.

Some patients have a reversal of the syndrome with the infusion of only a few units of plasma; most patients require much more. The daily dose of plasma and the duration of the requirement are separately variable. The amount of plasma or the number of plasmaphereses necessary to control the disorder and the duration must be empirically determined for each patient.

Plasmapheresis should be continued until the patient's clinical status has stabilized and the indicators of TTP have resolved—that is, the central nervous system and other organ dysfunction has reversed, the platelet count is normal, the serum LDH level is normal, and hemolysis is minimal. Plasmapheresis can be converted to plasma infusion at the rate of 1 U every 2 to 6 hours. As the patient improves, the rate of plasma therapy should be gradually tapered and discontinued. If the patient starts to relapse, the frequency of plasma infusions should be increased. If this does not control the relapse, then plasmapheresis should be resumed.

Antiplatelet agents have been used in the treatment of TTP. In general, I do not recommend their use, especially if the patient is severely thrombocytopenic. Their effectiveness in TTP is marginal, and they handicap the platelets' ability to prevent hemorrhage. Clinical experience suggests that patients with TTP are more likely to suffer bleeding complications if antiplatelet agents are used.

Corticosteroids are often used. They have an apparently beneficial effect, although this is not proved, especially when used in conjunction with other effective modalities. Because of this potentially ancillary benefit, I generally prescribe prednisone, 1 to 2 mg per kg daily, or equivalent. This agent is gradually stopped when the patient is in remission.

The requirement for plasma therapy generally lasts 1 week or more but may be extended for many months in some patients. If the patient is responding poorly to plasma therapy, I suggest the use of plasma from which the cryoprecipitate has been removed. This is depleted of the large forms of von Willebrand factor that agglutinate the platelets.

Various therapeutic modalities have been used in attempts to end plasma therapy. There are many reports of the disorder's abatement after the administration of agents such as vincristine (Oncovin),* cyclophosphamide (Cytoxan),* or azathioprine (Imuran).* There are also reports of TTP's resolution after splenectomy. If the course is becoming pro-

---

*Not FDA-approved for this indication.

tracted, I recommend the intravenous administration of vincristine (Oncovin) in standard dosage, 1.4 mg per m², not to exceed a 2-mg final dose. This treatment can be repeated weekly, with the usual precautions. Splenectomy is considered in a patient who responds poorly to continued plasma therapy and in whom several attempts to terminate the process with vincristine administration have failed.

Some physicians may be tempted to give platelet transfusions to a severely thrombocytopenic patient, especially if surgery is being contemplated. Several instances of severe neurologic deterioration and death immediately after platelet transfusion have been recorded. I believe that platelet transfusions in TTP are extremely hazardous and of unlikely benefit.

In all patients with TTP, a search for an exacerbating inflammatory process or associated illness should be undertaken, because addressing such problems may help alleviate the disorder. Some patients have a recurrence of TTP at the time of a subsequent illness. In fact, 30% or more of patients who recover from TTP have a subsequent episode. Therefore, any patient who recovers from TTP should be closely monitored, especially during illness.

The occurrence of TTP secondary to chemotherapy has been reported. Several of these patients have apparently benefited from plasma therapy, and the same therapeutic recommendations hold. However, because several reports were associated with chemotherapy regimens containing vinca alkaloids, use of these agents in TTP in this setting would not seem to be advisable.

THE HEMOLYTIC–UREMIC SYNDROME

HUS is characterized by MAHA, thrombocytopenia, and acute renal failure. As in TTP, microvascular thrombi are responsible, and von Willebrand factor appears to participate in the platelet agglutination. In contrast with TTP, the kidneys are virtually the only organs involved, but severely so. In children, the syndrome often is preceded by an episode of pneumonia or gastroenteritis. There is a seasonal prevalence, as well as small clusters of cases. Verotoxin produced by a strain of *Escherichia coli* has been implicated in HUS. The reservoir for this toxin-producing *E. coli* is the bovine large intestine. Epidemiologic studies should be undertaken; these often reveal poorly cooked, contaminated ground beef as the source. In adults, HUS occurs even more sporadically. Associations with pregnancy and chemotherapy (especially chemotherapy containing mitomycin) have been reported.

Treatment

Because of the resemblance of HUS to TTP, similar plasma therapy is often applied. Plasmapheresis rather than plasma infusions is generally the necessary mode of therapy because of oliguria or anuria. However, in childhood HUS, plasmapheresis has been shown not to be better than good supportive care. A number of adults with HUS have been reported to have responded to plasmapheresis. Because HUS is a more self-limited and less life-threatening disorder than TTP, it is difficult to draw firm conclusions about the effectiveness of therapy; most patients survive and improve as long as the complications of acute renal failure are adequately managed. I consequently recommend supportive care in childhood HUS and plasmapheresis in adult HUS if the disorder cannot be clearly differentiated from TTP, or if the thrombocytopenia, which is an indicator of active thrombi formation, persists for more than 3 days. The same guidelines for plasmapheresis are used as those described for TTP; plasma infusions generally cannot be given. Regeneration of renal function, which is usually the critical issue, is more likely to be adequate in children than in older adults.

HEMOCHROMATOSIS

method of
PAUL C. ADAMS, M.D.
University of Western Ontario,
London, Ontario, Canada

Hemochromatosis is a common genetic disease with a prevalence of approximately 1 in 300 in white populations. Despite the high prevalence compared with other genetic diseases (cystic fibrosis: 1 in 2500), awareness of this disease by physicians and the general public has been limited. Furthermore, although diagnostic tests are readily available, there have been problems in making a definitive diagnosis of hereditary hemochromatosis.

UNDERDIAGNOSIS IN PATIENTS WITH HEMOCHROMATOSIS

The prevalence of symptoms of hemochromatosis increases with age, and symptoms are more common in males than in females. The clinical symptoms of fatigue, arthritis, impotence, and diabetes are so common in the aging population that they do not immediately trigger an investigation for hemochromatosis. The presence of hepatomegaly or mild liver enzyme abnormalities should lead to further investigation with serum transferrin saturation (serum iron/total iron-binding capacity [TIBC]) and serum

TABLE 1. **Diagnosis of Hereditary Hemochromatosis**

> History and physical examination
> Transferrin saturation test
> Ferritin test
> Liver biopsy
> Hepatic iron concentration test
> Investigation of family members

ferritin tests. Patients with abnormalities in these tests and with a clinical suspicion of hemochromatosis should proceed to liver biopsy (Table 1). Imaging studies such as computed tomography (CT) or magnetic resonance imaging (MRI) do not replace the need for diagnostic liver biopsy. Disease in younger patients who are completely asymptomatic is unlikely to be detected unless these tests are ordered as part of an automated profile of screening tests. Of these tests, the transferrin saturation test is most likely to be abnormal in young adults with hemochromatosis, with the ferritin levels rising later as body iron stores increase. The serum iron level alone is an unreliable screening test for the disease. Although population screening has shown efficacy and cost benefits, it has not been widely implemented because of the initial cost of the screening programs. Once the diagnosis is confirmed, it is essential to test siblings who have a 1 in 4 chance of having hemochromatosis. Children are less likely than siblings to be homozygotes but should also be screened for hemochromatosis with serum transferrin saturation and ferritin tests.

OVERDIAGNOSIS IN PATIENTS WITHOUT HEMOCHROMATOSIS

The relationship between alcoholism and hemochromatosis has been overemphasized in the past because of an overlap between alcoholic siderosis of the liver and hereditary hemochromatosis (Table 2). The patient with heavy alcohol consumption and histologic features of alcoholic liver disease on liver biopsy (fat, polymorphonuclear infiltrate, Mallory's hyaline bodies, and patchy iron staining) usually does not have hereditary hemochromatosis. In this type of patient, the hepatic iron concentration is measured in a paraffin-embedded liver biopsy by atomic absorption spectrophotometry. The hepatic iron concentration (μmol per gram) divided by the patient's age is the hepatic iron index. If this index is greater than 2, it is very suggestive of hereditary hemochromatosis. In contrast, patients with alcoholic siderosis usually have an index less than 2. In other words, in two patients of similar age, the hemochromatosis patient will have acquired much more

TABLE 2. **Differentiation of Hemochromatosis from Alcoholic Siderosis**

Clinical Feature	Hemochromatosis	Alcoholic Siderosis
Distinguishing clinical symptoms	Arthritis Pigmentation	
Serum ferritin level (μg/L)	>1500*	<1500*
Transferrin saturation	>80%*	50–80%*
Liver pathologic examination	Hepatocyte iron	Fat, Mallory's hyaline, polymorphonuclear bodies, infiltration, pericentral fibrosis
Hepatic iron: μmol/gm	200–800	40–100
μg/gm	11,160–44,640	2232–5580
Hepatic iron index = [Liver Fe]/ age = (μmol/gm)/yr	>2	<2
HLA-identical sibling	Has hemochromatosis	Normal iron studies

*Serum ferritin level in hemochromatosis depends on age and sex of patient. Example shown would be typical for 50-year-old male patient.

hepatic iron than the patient with alcoholic siderosis. The iron index has not been fully validated in other types of secondary iron overload. The hepatic iron index may be less than 2 in young asymptomatic homozygotes. I do not consider the index to be the "gold standard" for the diagnosis and have seen young asymptomatic patients with a clear family history of disease in which the index is less than 2.

Another strategy for the discovery of hemochromatosis in siblings utilizes the close proximity of the hemochromatosis gene to the human leukocyte antigen (HLA) locus on chromosome 6. HLA typing (A and B) is performed on siblings of the initial patient in combination with serum ferritin and transferrin saturation tests. An HLA-identical nonalcoholic sibling with normal transferrin saturation and ferritin tests strongly suggests a diagnosis of alcoholic siderosis rather than hereditary hemochromatosis in the proband case. Patients with chronic hepatitis (B, C, autoimmune hepatitis) may present with abnormalities in transferrin saturation and serum ferritin levels. These patients usually do not have hemochromatosis. Heterozygotes have an abnormal transferrin saturation or ferritin level in only 15% of cases, but since the prevalence of heterozygotes has been estimated to be as has high as 1 in 10, this may explain results in patients with a mild elevation in serum ferritin levels (<1000 μg per liter) and mild iron deposition on liver biopsy. A true genetic test for hemochromatosis may eventually demonstrate that many of the patients with "secondary" iron overload, such as alcoholic siderosis, may be heterozygotes for hereditary hemochromatosis.

TREATMENT

The treatment of hemochromatosis relies on the medieval therapy of periodic venesections. Patients are initially treated with the removal of 500 mL weekly with a hemoglobin or hematocrit test done at each session. Mild anemia is common with therapy, and the treatment is continued if the hemoglobin level is above 10 grams per dL from the previous week. A serum ferritin test is done every 3 months, and venesections are continued until the serum ferritin level is less than 50 μg per liter. At that time, a maintenance program of one venesection every 3 to 4 months with an annual ferritin determination is started. The rate of iron reaccumulation is extremely variable between patients: some patients require a venesection every 2 months, and others have no venesections for years without a significant rise in the serum ferritin level. Deferoxamine (Desferal) therapy is reserved for patients with secondary iron overload from transfusions or anemia. New oral iron chelators have been successful in children with thalassemia and will likely become the treatment of choice for these anemic patients.

PROGNOSIS

The long-term outcome in patients with hemochromatosis depends on the stage at which the diagnosis is made. Patients with cirrhosis at the time of diagnosis are five and a half times more likely to die than noncirrhotic patients. A 20-year survival of 71% has been seen in our patients. Unfortunately, many symptoms such as arthritis, diabetes, and impotence do not improve with iron depletion therapy. It is unfortunate that many hemochromatosis patients are diagnosed for the first time at the time of liver transplantation, which is the only treatment for end-stage liver disease. Initial studies have suggested a slightly worse outcome for hemochromatosis after liver transplantation (1-year survival: 53%) with gradual reaccumulation of iron in the new liver. Hepatocellular carcinoma has been described in 18.5% of cirrhotic hemochromatosis patients. Although screening with periodic ultrasound examination and alpha-fetoprotein tests can detect early tumors, curative treatment options (transplantation, hepatectomy) are often limited.

HODGKIN'S DISEASE: CHEMOTHERAPY

method of
RALPH M. MEYER, M.D.
Hamilton Civic Hospitals
Hamilton, Ontario, Canada

The principles of curative cancer therapy are exemplified by strategies used in managing patients who have Hodgkin's disease. After appropriate investigations provide an accurate diagnosis and determine the extent of disease, optimum provision of radiation and/or chemotherapy can cure more than 80% of patients with limited-stage disease and 65% of those with advanced-stage disease. Strategies attempting to further improve outcomes must not only address the issue of disease eradication but must also reduce the long-term toxic effects of therapy.

To determine the best therapy, the clinician must first assess those factors that reflect the biology of the disease and measure the spread of the tumor. These factors include the histopathologic subtype of Hodgkin's disease and the disease stage assessed using the Ann Arbor classification. Prognostic factors such as patient age and gender, the presence of bulky mediastinal disease, the number of disease sites, and the erythrocyte sedimentation rate (ESR) can also be used to decide on the therapy, particularly when patients have limited-stage disease.

HISTOPATHOLOGY AND STAGING

The histologic diagnosis of Hodgkin's disease requires observation of the pathognomonic finding, the Reed-Sternberg cell, with background lymph node architecture showing proliferation of lymphocytes, plasma cells, eosinophils, granulocytes, or fibroblasts with associated fibrosis. The histopathologic assessment uses the Rye modification of the Lukes and Butler classification, which includes the lymphocyte predominance, nodular sclerosis, mixed cellularity, and lymphocyte depletion subtypes. Among these subtypes, nodular sclerosis and mixed cellularity are the most common and account for more than 80% of cases. The four subtypes can be associated with specific clinical features; for instance, lymphocyte predominance is associated with a limited disease burden and a favorable prognosis when treated with radiation therapy; nodular sclerosis is associated with mediastinal involvement; mixed cellularity commonly includes subdiaphragmatic spread of disease and, on histologic grounds, can be confused with peripheral T cell lymphoma; and lymphocyte depletion often presents with advanced-stage disease in an older patient and, on histologic grounds, can be confused with diffuse large cell or immunoblastic lymphoma.

The stage of Hodgkin's disease is described using the Ann Arbor classification, modified at the Cotswolds Meeting, as shown in Table 1. Determination of the stage requires a thorough history and physical examination with the appropriate use of laboratory and imaging tests. Important findings from the history include an unexplained fever of 38° C or more, drenching night sweats, or an unexplained loss of greater than 10% of body weight within the previous 6 months (the "B" symptoms of the Ann Arbor classification); unexplained pruritus; focal symptoms suggesting organ involvement (e.g., respiratory symptoms, back pain); changes in activities of daily living (often assessed as the "performance status," e.g., the Karnofsky performance status); and risk factors for exposure to the human immunodeficiency virus (HIV). The physical examination should include notation of the distribution and size of any palpable lymph nodes; measurement of the liver and spleen, if palpable; and any other findings associated with extensive disease (e.g., pleural effusion, spinal cord compression). Standard laboratory investigations include a complete blood count (CBC); ESR (particularly for patients with limited-stage disease); parameters of renal and liver function; serum calcium and lactate dehydrogenase levels; and, if appropriate, HIV serologic tests. All investigations may not directly influence the choice of therapy but may

lead to further investigations or suggest the need for additional supportive measures. Required imaging tests include a chest radiograph and computed tomographic (CT) scanning of the chest, abdomen, and pelvis. Additional studies may include bipedal lymphangiography (if CT scanning of the abdomen and pelvis is negative), gallium scanning (to determine pulmonary involvement in patients with bulky mediastinal disease), and other imaging tests required to assess findings gleaned from the history or physical examination. A bone marrow biopsy should be done if the CBC reveals a cytopenia, or if the patient has any features suggesting that the disease is not localized. Additional biopsies are not commonly needed but may be required if investigations result in diagnostic uncertainties that might influence therapy. A staging laparotomy should no longer be considered standard; a large randomized trial reported by the European Organization for Research and Treatment of Cancer has shown that staging laparotomy does not improve progression-free or overall survival.

TREATMENT

Chemotherapy Regimens

When choosing a management plan, the clinician must use information gained from the staging evaluation and consider factors specific to the individual patient. In addition to selecting the most appropriate chemotherapy regimen, consideration of whether treatment should be supplemented with radiation therapy is required. Commonly used chemotherapy regimens are shown in Table 2 and include mechlorethamine, vincristine (Oncovin), procarbazine, and prednisone (MOPP); doxorubicin (Adriamycin), bleomycin, vinblastine, and dacarbazine (ABVD); and a combination of both given in alternating cycles (MOPP-ABVD) or as a hybrid regimen (MOPP-ABV).

MOPP

The MOPP regimen was developed at the National Cancer Institute (U.S.A.) almost 3 decades ago. Although this was the first regimen shown to have curative potential for patients with advanced-stage disease, randomized trials have shown that remission rates and progression-free survivals are inferior to those achieved with ABVD or MOPP-ABV(D). In addition to toxicities commonly seen with most chemotherapeutic regimens, MOPP can lead to infertility (particularly in women older than 30 years and in males of any age) and may be leukemogenic. The use of MOPP is generally reserved for patients with underlying cardiac or pulmonary disease for whom doxorubicin and bleomycin would be contraindicated.

ABVD

Developed by investigators at the National Tumor Institute in Milan, ABVD was first described as second-line therapy for patients unsuccessfully treated with MOPP. In subsequent randomized studies assessing first-line therapy for patients with a variety of disease stages, progression-free survival was better with ABVD than with MOPP. The results of a randomized trial conducted by the Cancer and Leukemia Group B, which assessed patients with ad-

TABLE 1. **The Ann Arbor Staging Classification of Hodgkin's Disease (Modified at Cotswolds Meeting)**

Stage I: Involvement of single lymph node region, lymphoid structure (e.g., spleen, thymus), or extralymphatic site.

Stage II: Involvement of two or more lymph node regions on same side of diaphragm. Single extranodal site adjacent to, or extending from, regional lymph node can be included. Number of disease sites is indicated as subscript (e.g., II_2). Mediastinal nodes are one site; each hilar region is considered separate site.

Stage III: Involvement of lymph node regions on each side of diaphragm. Single extranodal site can be included as per Stage II. Stage III_1 refers to subdiaphragmatic disease including spleen, splenic hilar, celiac, or portal nodes; Stage III_2 refers to subdiaphragmatic disease including para-aortic, iliac, or mesenteric nodes.

Stage IV: Involvement of extranodal site(s) beyond that adjacent to, or extending from, regional lymph node (e.g., liver or bone marrow).

Specific Notations:

A: No symptoms

B: Fever, night sweats, or weight loss (see text)

X: Bulky disease defined as mediastinal mass measuring greater than one third of internal transverse diameter of thorax (measured at T5/6), or nodal mass of >10 cm

E: Limited involvement of extralymphatic tissue as only site of disease, or as site adjacent to, or contiguous with, involved regional lymph node

CS: Clinical stage

PS: Pathologic stage (requires staging laparotomy or biopsy confirming involvement of specific sites, e.g., positive liver or bone marrow biopsy)

Data from Lister TA, Crowther D, Sutcliffe SB, et al: Report of a committee convened to discuss the evaluation and staging of patients with Hodgkin's disease: Cotswolds meeting. J Clin Oncol 7:1630, 1989.

TABLE 2. **Chemotherapy Regimens for Hodgkin's Disease**

Regimen	Drug	Dose (per m²)	Schedule
MOPP	Mechlorethamine (Mustargen)	6 mg IV	Days 1 and 8
	Vincristine (Oncovin)	1.4 mg IV	Days 1 and 8
	Prednisone	40 mg PO	Days 1–14
	Procarbazine (Matulane)	100 mg PO	Days 1–14
ABVD	Doxorubicin (Adriamycin)	25 mg IV	Days 1 and 15
	Bleomycin (Blenoxane)	10 U IV	Days 1 and 15
	Vinblastine (Velban)	6 mg IV	Days 1 and 15
	Dacarbazine	375 mg IV	Days 1 and 15
MOPP–ABV	Mechlorethamine	6 mg IV	Day 1
	Vincristine	1.4 mg IV	Day 1
	Prednisone	40 mg PO	Days 1–14
	Procarbazine	100 mg PO	Days 1–7
	Doxorubicin	35 mg IV	Days 8
	Bleomycin	10 U IV	Days 8
	Vinblastine	6 mg IV	Days 8

All regimens are given as 28-day cycles. Doses and schedule are modified for toxic reactions (e.g., neutropenia, thrombocytopenia).

vanced-stage disease, suggested that ABVD and MOPP-ABVD produce similar outcomes. A large randomized trial involving multiple cooperative groups is currently comparing ABVD with MOPP–ABV. The special toxicities of ABVD include risks of congestive cardiomyopathy (from doxorubicin) and pulmonary fibrosis (from bleomycin [Blenoxane]). When chemotherapy is required, first-line therapy with ABVD is a reasonable option and is the treatment of choice for those patients in whom the maintenance of fertility is a high priority.

MOPP–ABV(D)

The Milan group was the first to compare alternating monthly cycles of MOPP–ABVD and MOPP in a randomized trial. They showed that outcomes were superior with MOPP–ABVD. Subsequent randomized trials have confirmed these findings; superior progression-free survival and a trend for superior survival are consistently observed. The MOPP–ABV hybrid regimen was developed at the British Columbia Cancer Agency in Vancouver and has been compared with alternating MOPP–ABVD in a randomized trial conducted by the National Cancer Institute of Canada; no differences in outcome were seen. As MOPP–ABV does not include dacarbazine, a potentially highly emetogenic drug, this regimen is often preferred to MOPP–ABVD. In comparison with ABVD, the number of patients treated and the duration of follow-up are greater with MOPP–ABV(D), thus providing more confidence in long-term results. Therefore, MOPP–ABV is considered standard first-line therapy for patients with advanced-stage disease, unless maintenance of fertility makes ABVD a preferred option.

Combined Modality Therapy

Combining chemotherapy and radiation may provide better disease control for patients with limited-stage disease associated with adverse prognostic factors, and when sites of bulky disease exist. Practice patterns may vary considerably, as randomized trials have not consistently demonstrated a survival advantage for this approach. For patients with advanced-stage disease, adding radiation therapy has not been shown to improve progression-free or overall survival and is usually reserved as supplemental treatment of sites of bulky disease.

Toxicities and Supportive Care

Potential toxicities common to all chemotherapy regimens include alopecia, nausea and vomiting, myelosuppression with risks of infection, and neuropathy (peripheral neuropathy with vincristine; autonomic neuropathy causing abdominal pain and constipation with vinblastine [Velban]). Prednisone can be associated with many side effects; common problems include mood changes, dyspepsia, and glucose intolerance. Osteonecrosis is an uncommon late complication of regimens that include prednisone. Procarbazine (Matulane) shares properties with monoamine oxidase inhibitors and when combined with alcohol or certain foods can lead to flushing, fever, and nausea with vomiting.

Attention to details of supportive care is an essential component of therapy. In addition to preventing or managing the above toxicities, health care professionals need to help patients in coping with the diagnosis of Hodgkin's disease and the psychosocial sequelae of therapy. Following successful treatment, issues of survivorship, including reintegration into school or employment, require ongoing assessment.

Current Treatment Recommendations

Clinical Stages I and IIA. This group is very heterogeneous, and management options are controversial. The practices described below can be expected to cure 80 to 90% of patients. Prognostic factors can be used to stratify patients into very favorable, favorable, and unfavorable categories.

Very favorable patients have all the following features: lymphocyte predominance or nodular sclerosis histologic type; small disease bulk (e.g., less than 3 cm); low ESR (e.g., less than 50 mm per hour); and disease confined to a unilateral high-neck or single epitrochlear region. These patients can be treated with involved-field or short mantle irradiation. Patients in the favorable category have all the following features: lymphocyte predominance or nodular sclerosis histologic type; age less than 40 years; ESR less than 50 mm per hour; and fewer than three sites of disease. These patients can be treated with radiation given to the mantle, splenic, and para-aortic regions. Patients in the unfavorable category have at least one factor making them ineligible for the favorable group and should receive combined modality therapy. Appropriate treatment includes an abbreviated course of chemotherapy (e.g., 2 to 3 cycles of ABVD) plus radiation as described for patients in the favorable category. In Canada, patients in the favorable and unfavorable groups are eligible for a randomized trial comparing the above therapies with ABVD (4 to 6 cycles) alone.

Clinical Stages IIB, III, and IV and Relapse After Radiation Therapy. These patients require a full course of chemotherapy consisting of eight cycles of MOPP–ABV or six cycles of ABVD; 65 to 80% of patients can be cured with this approach. As discussed earlier, MOPP–ABV is often considered standard therapy as there has been longer follow-up of patients treated with this regimen, particularly for those with Stages IIIB and IV disease. However, ABVD is a reasonable option and should be given when maintenance of fertility is a high priority.

Bulky Mediastinal Disease. Patients with a bulky mediastinal mass are at risk of disease progression at this site and within the lung parenchyma. These patients should receive a full course of chemotherapy, regardless of stage, and often need supplemental radiation to the site of the bulky mass. Selected patients may not require radiation if an excellent response has been achieved with chemotherapy, the response has been stable over repeated investigations performed during therapy, and gallium scanning is negative. As randomized trials have not thoroughly addressed this issue, optimum management remains controversial.

Relapse After Full-Course Chemotherapy. Treatment for relapse after chemotherapy depends on the specifics of the initial and recurrent patterns of disease. Many patients are candidates for high-dose chemotherapy with autologous bone marrow or peripheral blood stem cell reinfusion.

HODGKIN'S DISEASE: RADIATION THERAPY

method of
DAVID I. ROSENTHAL, M.D., and
ELI GLATSTEIN, M.D.
University of Texas Southwestern Medical Center at Dallas
Dallas, Texas

Hodgkin's disease (HD) is a malignant tumor of lymph nodes. Although as recently as the 1960s it was considered uniformly fatal, today most patients can be cured with radiation therapy (RT), chemotherapy (CT), or, in selected cases, combined modality therapy (CMT). HD spreads predictably through contiguous chains of lymph nodes, forming the basis for curative RT. Radiation is the oldest and single most effective therapeutic agent for HD and the treatment of choice for typical patients with Stages I and II disease. The median age at the diagnosis of HD is 26 years, and there is high expectation for long-term survival. Since outcomes have become so good, therapeutic decisions for patients with HD should now be driven equally by estimates of outcome, concerns about diagnostic and therapeutic morbidity, and the potential for salvage therapy.

PATHOLOGY

The malignant cells in HD are thought to be multinuclear Reed-Sternberg (RS) cells and/or their mononuclear predecessors. These cells are surrounded by a larger inflammatory milieu that is *not* thought to be neoplastic. RS cells are not pathognomonic of HD, so the diagnosis of HD requires the presence of both RS cells and a characteristic inflammatory infiltrate. The excisional biopsy of a lymph node with an intact capsule is the preferred diagnostic procedure because of the overall relative paucity of RS cells and the need to characterize both the inflammatory infiltrate and the nodal architecture. The high curability of HD is probably related to relatively small numbers of true tumor cells throughout an entire mass.

There are four histologic types of Hodgkin's disease as described in the modified Rye histologic classification: lymphocyte-predominant (LP), nodular sclerosing (NS), mixed cellularity (MC), and lymphocyte-depleted (LD). This division is based on relative compositions of RS cells and lymphocytes. Each histologic type has the tendency to present in certain age groups and at different stages, but the cure rates, stage for stage, are thought to be similar.

The LP histologic type occurs as early-stage disease in young adults, with infrequent systemic symptoms (about 10%). The NS variant is the most frequent (about 80%) and purest form of HD and has an intermediate frequency of systemic symptoms (about one in three). The NS form may respond slowly to treatment and leave a residual mass, perhaps reflecting the large collagen component of tumor volume. The nodal masses of the LP variant, in contrast, may resolve within days of the initiation of treatment, perhaps reflecting the lack of collagen matrix and the exquisite radioresponsiveness of normal lymphocytes. The MC variant tends to present in somewhat older patients, in a more advanced stage, and is the most frequent type among acquired immune deficiency syndrome (AIDS) patients. Finally, the lymphocyte-depleted variant is the least frequent, tending to present in advanced stages in the geriatric group. There is heterogeneity in clinical behavior within the groups of this classification schema, as recent studies suggest that patients with subtypes of LP and LD HD may have tumors that clinically and immunophenotypically resemble non-Hodgkin's lymphoma (NHL).

PROGNOSTIC FACTORS

Stage alone cannot always directly determine treatment, as not all prognostic factors are included in the staging system. The prognostic factors can be either patient-, disease-, or treatment-related.

Patient-related, pretreatment, prognostic factors include age, performance status, and gender. These factors also affect the suitability of specific treatment programs. The extremes of age have special treatment requirements. The natural history and outcome of HD in children and adults are similar, but the consequences of high-dose radiation on growing bone and soft tissues are so severe that radiation alone is virtually never used in children. At the other extreme, the typical aggressive staging and management programs may be inappropriate in the elderly with limited physiologic reserve and intercurrent diseases. In contrast to the prognosis in children, the prognosis in patients over the age of 65 is worse on a stage-for-stage basis. It is not clear whether this is due to intrinsic differences in HD in the elderly or simply a reflection of reduced tolerance for treatment.

Women have a slightly better prognosis than men; however, the differences are very small and generally do not influence the choice of treatment. The drug combinations that include alkylating agents such as MOPP (nitrogen mustard [Mustargen], vincristine [Oncovin], procarbazine [Matulane], and prednisone) virtually always lead to male sterility. Both pelvic irradiation and MOPP can cause infertility, especially in women older than 25 years.

Tumor-related prognostic factors include stage, tumor burden, and histologic type. It has also been suggested that low hemoglobin levels, high lactate dehydrogenase and serum copper levels and high erythrocyte sedimentation rates are less favorable. Staging is discussed in a later section. Tumor burden is reflected in the number of sites of involvement and their size. Bone marrow, lung, and liver involvement are unfavorable. A disease site is considered bulky if the nodal diameter is greater than 10 cm, or a mediastinal mass is greater than one-third the maximum transthoracic diameter on an upright posteroanterior chest teleradiograph. The histologic type was initially considered to be an important independent prognostic factor in HD, but when the histologic type is corrected for stage, it is not an independent prognosticator.

Treatment-related prognostic factors include response, but adequate RT doses and field limits, and the time–dose intensity of chemotherapy are critical.

PATTERNS OF INVOLVEMENT AND SPREAD: CONTRAST TO THE NON–HODGKIN'S LYMPHOMAS

Patients with HD tend to have axial nodal involvement. The majority of patients (80%) present with painless cervical lymphadenopathy, followed by involvement of mediastinal (50%), then periaortic, axillary, and groin lymph nodes. Other nodes may be involved, but it is uncommon for HD to involve epitrochlear and mesenteric nodes. Isolated extralymphatic involvement is extremely rare, but its presence does not adversely affect survival. HD can extend into contiguous tissues and can also spread through the bloodstream.

There is a rather orderly spread of HD to contiguous nodal groups, in distinction to the NHLs, in which initial nodal involvement is more random and spread does not often follow this contiguous pattern. Bone marrow and gastrointestinal (GI) involvement and direct involvement of the central nervous system (CNS), as opposed to extension from bony disease, are also very uncommon in HD, as is involvement of extranodal lymphatic sites such as Waldeyer's ring. This is in distinction to many of the NHL patients, who may more frequently have bone marrow, GI, CNS, or extranodal involvement. Extralymphatic involvement in Hodgkin's disease is, indeed, less common than in the other lymphomas, but it is important to note that if extralymphatic HD is localized, this is not a negative prognosticator, whether it is contiguous with an adjacent involved nodal site or completely separate. The probability of liver involvement is high when there is splenic involvement in HD, but with a negative splenectomy specimen the liver is unlikely to be involved.

STAGING AND FOLLOW–UP

The most important single prognostic factor in determining the choice of treatment for HD is the Ann Arbor anatomic stage (Table 1). The staging of HD is designed to guide radiation therapy and help select those who require systemic treatment. The diaphragm was an arbitrary point of division, but a convenient limit for sequential radiation fields, as high-dose radiation is not tolerated simultaneously on both sides of the diaphragm, since large volumes of bone marrow are encompassed. Details of our initial patient evaluation are outlined later (Table 2).

The use of surgical staging, particularly laparotomy, is controversial. We, however, find no better way to tailor treatment to an individual patient's needs than surgical staging (laparotomy or scalene node biopsy) in appropriate patients. Staging laparotomy should be used only when it would be the final determinate between RT alone versus systemic CT, and if the yield is expected to be at least 10 to 15%, there is no massive mediastinal disease, and the patient is not physiologically compromised. Children and

TABLE 1. **Ann Arbor Staging Classification**

Stage I	Involvement of single lymph node region (I), or single extralymphatic organ or site (IE)
Stage II	Involvement of ≥2 lymph node regions on same side of diaphragm (II), or localized involvement of extralymphatic organ or site and of one or more lymph node regions on same side of diaphragm (IIE)
Stage III	Involvement of lymph node regions on both sides of diaphragm (III), which may also be accompanied by involvement of spleen (IIIs), or by localized involvement of extralymphatic organ or site (IIIE), or both (IIIEs)
Stage IV	Diffuse or disseminated involvement of one or more extralymphatic ogans or tissues, with or without associated lymph node involvement

The absence or presence of fever, night sweats, and/or unexplained loss of ≥10% body weight in 6 months before diagnosis is denoted by suffix letters A or B, respectively.

Patients are assigned clinical stage (CS) based on initial biopsy and all subsequent nonsurgical staging studies. Pathologic stage (PS) is assigned based on all clinical studies as well as surgical staging procedures such as bone marrow biopsy, staging laparotomy with splenectomy, and scalene node biopsy.

TABLE 2. **Initial and Subsequent Evaluation for Hodgkin's Disease Patients**

	Initial	Subsequent‡‡
Pathology slide review	√	
History and physical examination	√	√
Chest x-ray	√	√
Chest CT scan	*	†
Abd & pelvic CT scan	√	†
LAG‡	√	
Alkaline phosphatase level	√	√
Hemogram	√	√
LD	√	††
ESR	√	††
Cu	√	††
BM Bx	§	
Surgical staging‖	√	
T4/TSH	¶	**

*If this is abnormal, obtain a chest x-ray film.
†Repeat post-treatment baseline at 2–4 months if initial study is abnormal.
‡Bipedal lymphangiography.
§Bone marrow aspirate and biopsy if there is infradiaphragmatic disease or "B" symptoms.
‖Scalene node biopsy or laporotomy for appropriate patients.
¶If neck is irradiated.
**Repeat q 6–12 months.
††Repeat only if initially positive.
‡‡Interval: Every 2–3 months × 2 years.
                Every 4–6 months × 2 years.
                Annually thereafter.
Abbreviations: CT = computed tomography; LD = lactate dehydrogenase level; ESR = erythrocyte sedimentation rate; BM Bx = bone marrow biopsies and aspirates; TSH = thyroid stimulating hormone; Cu = serum copper level; LAG = bipedal lymphangiography.

elderly, obese, and other medically compromised patients are not good candidates for an elective procedure such as this. Women desiring pregnancy should be evaluated for ovarian transposition at the time of the laparotomy.

Overall, 38% patients have staging changed by laparotomy: 25% are upstaged and 13% are downstaged, mostly because of the high rate of up to 40% false-positive lymphangiograms. Splenectomy is the most effective way to evaluate for splenic involvement and is the single most common site upstaging patients after positive laparotomy. If a patient has splenomegaly, the spleen is pathologically involved in half the cases, but if the laparotomy is positive, the spleen is involved in two-thirds of the cases. Independent of surgical complications, overwhelming sepsis with a roughly one-third mortality is the most feared long-term complication of splenectomy. This can be reduced with presplenectomy vaccination. There is no clear evidence linking splenectomy to an increased risk of secondary malignancy.

Most patients who relapse with HD will do so within 2 years, and the risk of relapse diminishes with time, but as many as 13% of those still in remission at 3 years go on to develop recurrent disease. Our post-treatment patient evaluation is tabulated (see Table 2). We recommend that the first relapse of HD be documented histologically, as reactive hyperplasia is common in unirradiated lymph nodes just beyond the limits of the irradiated fields.

RADIOTHERAPY

Radiation fields should be custom-shaped, requiring fluoroscopic simulation and verification of the port films by their relationship to simulator films.

Shielding of critical structures is accomplished by the use of diverging blocks cast from cerrubend, a lead alloy with a melting point of 56° C. When the shape of the block has been determined, the molten cerrubend can be poured into a polystyrofoam mold, allowed to cool, and then transferred to an acrylic tray and used to shape the field by careful placement under the head of the machine gantry. A linear accelerator using energies between 6 and 10 MV is now used for the treatment of HD. We prefer to use doses of 45 Gray for areas of known involvement, treating at the rate of 1.8 Gray per day 5 days per week, and 36 Gray to uninvolved contiguous sites for prophylaxis.

The mantle field is one of the largest fields used in conventional RT. It extends from the inferior surface of the mandible to just below the domes of the diaphragm, approximately T9, and encompasses all major nodal regions above the diaphragm. The shape of mantle fields is highly individualized and is dynamic, with planned additions of custom shielding to eliminate organs from the high-dose radiation field as the dose increases. The custom-shaped blocks are designed to protect the heart, lungs, occiput, spinal cord, larynx, and humeral heads. When radiation therapy alone is used, the mantle field can be modified or extensions added. It is typical to use a partial transmission block to deliver low-dose, 15 to 16.5-Gray, radiation to the entire lung(s) if there is hilar adenopathy, or if involvement of lung parenchyma is apparent. The entire cardiac silhouette is radiated to 15 Gray in the presence of any mediastinal involvement, and the subcarinal heart is blocked at 30 Gray. These reduced doses are well tolerated and appear adequate to control subclinical disease and reduce in-field failure. Preauricular fields are used to treat lymph nodes above the angle of the mandible therapeutically to 45 Gray if they are clinically involved, or prophylactically to 36 Gray if there is neck involvement above the thyroid notch. Today this is best accomplished by means of electron fields, in order to spare the contralateral parotid gland and avoid xerostomia.

Subdiaphragmatic radiation therapy fields include the "inverted 'Y,'" which extends from the diaphragm, matching the mantle field, down to the iliofemoral region, thus including the periaortic, splenic hilar, common and external iliac, and iliofemoral lymph nodes. Frequently it is not required to treat the pelvic nodes, and the anterior border of the subdiaphragmatic field can then be terminated at approximately the bottom of L4 (which represents the bifurcation of the periaortic nodes), or at the mid–sacroiliac joint level to also include the common iliac lymph nodes, termed a "spade" field. If the spleen has not been removed, it is included as an extension of these fields in addition to the splenic hilum. It is sometimes necessary to treat the whole liver, as is the case with splenic involvement when radiation is to be used alone. This is accomplished with a partial transmission block that delivers a full dose to the periaortic nodes, and one-half that to the liver. When the mantle and the full inverted Y and spleen are treated, this is considered to be "total lymphoid irradiation." When the pelvis is omitted, it is termed "subtotal lymphoid irradiation."

RADIATION THERAPY TOXICITY

Gonadal toxicity from treatment is an important issue with RT, and minimizing the risk requires careful shielding of the pelvis in all patients, the transposed ovaries in girls and women, and the testicles in boys and men. This results in a testicular dose of 3% or less and an ovarian dose of <10% of the nodal dose. Future parenting is documented in both men and women.

A variety of acute side effects are expected to occur during radiation treatment, including skin reactions, hair loss, odynophagia, nonproductive cough, and sometimes nausea and vomiting. These are typically mild, easily palliated medically, and resolve in the ensuing weeks.

Subacute and chronic or late complications also occur. Radiation pneumonitis can develop within the first 3 months after completion of the mantle radiotherapy in approximately 2 to 3% of patients. Radiation carditis occurs in about 1% of patients. Acute pericarditis can usually be managed by conservative means with nonsteroidal anti-inflammatory agents. The asymptomatic pericardial effusion typically clears slowly over a month to even a few years. Constrictive pericarditis may require surgical pericardiectomy. RT to the heart may also accelerate coronary atherosclerosis. Hypothyroidism occurs in approximately one-third of those treated with a mantle. Herpes zoster may affect 15 to 20% of patients.

Acute transient radiation myelopathy or Lhermitte's sign (paresthesias occurring down the dorsal portion of the extremities when the neck is flexed) occurs in about 10 to 15% of patients after mantle therapy. This particular complication typically occurs 6 weeks to 3 months after RT and is self-limited, resolving in weeks to months; it is *not* a harbinger of chronic myelopathy. Xerostomia can result from treatment, especially if care is not taken in setting up the upper edge of the mantle with respect to the teeth. Fluoride supplements are required to minimize the risks of radiation caries and other complications. We recommend oral surgery evaluation if the mandible is to be irradiated. If the spleen has been removed as part of a staging laparotomy, the risk of sepsis can be minimized by appropriate immunization.

The data on secondary solid tumors and leukemia are still emerging. Leukemia is very uncommon after RT, in contrast to CT. The solid tumors tend to occur in the second decade after treatment and thus far appear to represent a hazard of both RT and CT. The major risk appears to be lung cancer, mostly in smokers; breast and thyroid cancers are also a concern among women, especially when irradiated at a young age. Other cancers that have been associated with RT include salivary gland and skin cancers and sarcomas.

COMBINED MODALITY THERAPY

The most important indication for using CMT in the initial management of patients with HD is the presence of massive mediastinal or other massive nodal involvement. We prefer to use MOPP alone with radiation because of its diminished cardiopulmonary interactions, compared with ABVD (doxorubicin [Adriamycin], bleomycin, vinblastine, decarbazine). In general, for most other problems outside a study setting, we recommend the use of either RT or CT, but not both. For patients who achieve a complete remission with CT, there is no confirmation that the addition of RT is beneficial. We thus do not advocate the routine application of reduced-dose RT to all involved sites independent of initial bulk and response to CT. If the patient's tumor regression is less than complete, however, we prefer full-dose RT. We would prefer not to radiate at all in conjunction with CT, as long as the response appears to be complete. We do not advocate the use of combined attenuated CT and RT for HD except in a study setting, as this is investigational and not standard treatment.

THE TREATMENT OF HODGKIN'S DISEASE

We use the decision tree shown in Figure 1 as a general guideline for the treatment of HD. Once the diagnosis of HD is confirmed, the patient is staged clinically, possibly with the addition of a bone marrow biopsy. The first distinction is between Stages grouped I and II versus III and IV. We recommend CT, in general, for Stage III and IV patients and those Stage I and II patients who would not be suitable for RT, those at the age extremes or with medical contraindications. RT may be added later for less than a complete response to CT. This includes those with massive mediastinal presentations. Overall, approximately 80% of patients with Stage I and II HD are cured with RT, and more than 50% of those who later relapse are salvaged by CT, leading to an overall 10-year survival of approximately 90%.

All other Stage I and II patients are divided into supra- and infradiaphragmatic locations. Patients with Stage I disease below the inguinal ligament with a negative lymphangiogram are treated with extended-field RT without further staging. All other subdiaphragmatic Stage I and II patients with fewer than four sites of involvement undergo staging laparotomy. If this is negative, RT is appropriate; but if the laparotomy is positive, CT is recommended. If there are more than five sites of involvement, we consider these patients to have an unfavorable disease burden for RT and recommend CT.

Supradiaphragmatic Stage I patients with high neck only, or axilla only, or small mediastinal only involvement are considered to have favorable disease, and we recommend ipsilateral scalene node bi-

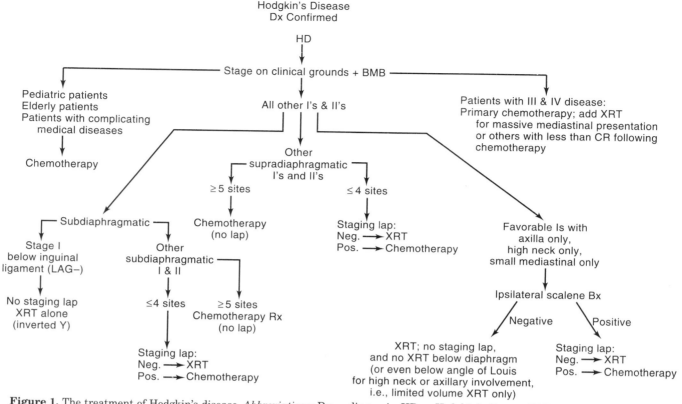

Figure 1. The treatment of Hodgkin's disease. *Abbreviations*: Dx = diagnosis; HD = Hodgkin's disease; BMB = bone marrow biopsy; XRT = external radiation therapy; CR = complete response; Lap = laparotomy; LAG = lymphangiogram; Rx = therapy; Bx = biopsy.

opsy. If this is negative, minimantle RT is appropriate, but if it is positive, a staging laparotomy should be performed.

All other patients with supradiaphragmatic Stage I and II disease are evaluated by the number of sites of involvement. Those with more than five sites are considered to have unfavorable disease, and we recommend CT directly. If there are fewer than four sites, then we recommend staging laparotomy.

SALVAGE TREATMENT

It is impossible to be dogmatic about second-line treatments. Induction failures or those with complete remissions (CRs) lasting less than 1 year have little chance for meaningful longevity. Patients in whom RT alone fails have a 50 to 80% initial salvage rate with multiagent CT. On the other hand, most patients in whom multiagent CT fails have a low salvage rate with RT, but those with lymph node disease on one side of the diaphragm who relapse after 1 year may have an RT salvage rate of more than 50%. The development of a platelet-stimulating factor may be able to ultimately improve results in this area, as it would allow high-dose radiation on both sides of the diaphragm. CT relapses may also be salvaged with further CT. Those with a MOPP-induced remission but who relapse more than 1 year later have a 90% chance of a second CR with the same drug regimen, and many CRs are durable. This has not

been improved by the use of non-cross-resistant regimens. We consider bone marrow transplantation to be investigational at this time.

ACUTE LEUKEMIA IN ADULTS*

method of
JUDITH E. KARP, M.D.
National Cancer Institute
Bethesda, Maryland

There are approximately 30,000 new cases of leukemia each year in the United States. About 90% of these arise in the adult; roughly 40% (or 11,000) are acute leukemias. The vast majority (80 to 85%) of acute leukemias in the adult population are acute myelogenous leukemias (AMLs), and the remainder are acute lymphocytic leukemias (ALLs) (the opposite distribution is seen in the childhood leukemias). Over the past 2 to 3 decades, the outlook for diverse types of acute leukemias has changed; diseases that were rapidly fatal are now potentially curable. This gratifying change is mainly applicable to childhood ALL, in which more than 70% are cured, but also holds true for some adult (in particular those under the age of 60 years) AMLs and ALLs. Still, even in the younger adult population, only about 30% are able to attain long-term disease-free survival (DFS). And unfortunately, even that degree

*This article is in the public domain.

of improvement has yet to be realized for older adults (aged over 65 years) and for those with therapy-induced leukemias or whose leukemias have evolved from a preleukemic myelodysplastic syndrome (MDS), in which cure rates are less than 10 to 15%. Thus, the leukemias continue to present a formidable challenge for which there is not yet a reliably curative "standard approach" for the majority of adults with this family of diseases.

The cornerstone of both present and future therapeutic advances is an understanding of leukemia biology on both the molecular and the clinical level, and continued progress will likely be linked to the exploitation of leukemia-associated molecular targets. As a case in point, the clinical application of polymerase chain reaction (PCR) based technologies is permitting the detection of small numbers of residual malignant cells persisting after therapy, a finding that is critical to overall therapeutic planning. Likewise, there are certain molecular and biologic features that may prognosticate overall clinical outcome with regard to potential curability with specific treatment modalities such as allogeneic bone marrow transplantation (BMT), autologous BMT with novel purging regimens, aggressive chemotherapies using non-cross-resistant agents with unique mechanisms of action, or new modalities (gene-directed approaches such as antisense or gene therapy, immunoconjugates, and agents aimed at abrogating drug resistance, for example).

MOLECULAR EPIDEMIOLOGY AND GENETICS OF ACUTE LEUKEMIAS

Lymphohematopoietic malignancies are frequently accompanied by nonrandom chromosomal abnormalities that represent a disruption in the normal structure and function of genes that control the balance of proliferation and differentiation. Duplications (e.g., trisomy 8) or losses of whole chromosomes (-5, -7) or chromosome segments ($5q-$, $7q-$, $20q-$) occur in many AML variants including those evolving from MDS, and gene point mutations (e.g., in tumor-suppressor genes RB, $p53$) are often associated with both lymphoid and myeloid malignancies. In addition, many leukemias are typified by specific gene rearrangements and reciprocal chromosome translocations. Such translocations can juxtapose two growth-promoting oncogenes, e.g., the Philadelphia (Ph) chromosome—t(9;22)(q34;q11), fusing the bcr and abl oncogenes—that typifies chronic myelogenous leukemia (CML) and also occurs in about 30% of adult ALL patients. In a similar vein, certain B cell ALLs, in particular the so-called L3 ALL that resembles Burkitt's lymphoma, are typified by translocations of the c-myc oncogene on chromosome 8q24 to immunoglobulin gene loci: the immunoglobulin heavy chain gene on 14q32, the kappa light chain gene on 2p11, or the lambda light chain gene on 22q11. Alternatively, an oncogene can recombine with a gene whose products encode factors influencing differentiation, as in acute progranulocytic leukemia (APL), in which the t(15;17) (q11;q11.2-12 or q21.1) fuses a rearranged PML (or "promyelocytic") oncogene encoding a transcription factor with a rearranged and truncated gene encoding the retinoic acid receptor–alpha. The resultant chimeric oncogenes in such translocations produce tumor-specific fusion mRNAs and proteins that, in turn, lead to dysregulated cellular proliferation and/or defective differentiation.

The cause of de novo acute leukemia is unknown, but both genetic and environmental factors are important. The etiologic linkages of ionizing radiation, benzene and other organic solvents, petroleum products, and pesticides with

AML have been established through epidemiologic studies of environmental and occupational exposures. The AMLs linked to such exposures constitute roughly 25 to 30% of all AMLs. They are often preceded by MDS and are characterized by one or more genetic abnormalities including trisomy 8, partial or complete deletions of chromosomes 5 and/or 7, point mutations and activation of ras oncogenes (N-ras and K-ras, in particular), and breaks and translocations of the EVI-1 (ecotropic virus integration site 1) gene located on chromosome 3q26.

The particular genetic lesion has major prognostic significance in terms of the initial response to therapy and the overall duration of that response. As a case in point, detection of the Ph chromosome in either AML or ALL portends a poor prognosis, whereas other translocations in AML, such as t(8;21), t(15;17), and inversions within the long arm of chromosome 16 (inv16), are associated with sensitivity to antileukemic therapy as manifested by achievement of complete remission (CR) in roughly 80% and prolonged DFS and cure in 40 to 60% with intensive therapies. On the other hand, trisomy 8 and partial or total deletions of chromosomes 5 or 7 reflect damage to a primitive stem cell and drug resistance. Likewise, the presence of 11q23 abnormalities in either de novo or therapy-induced ALL or AML with monocytic features connotes a very poor prognosis (see later). Unfortunately, current approaches in the MDS-related and induced AMLs yield CR rates of 40% or less, with CRs being brief (<6 to 12 months), and abysmally low cure rates, even with BMT.

THERAPY-RELATED ACUTE MYELOGENOUS LEUKEMIA: AN INCREASING CHALLENGE

The secondary, or therapy-related, AMLs currently account for roughly 15 to 20% of all AMLs. In many senses, the therapy-related AMLs can be viewed as a subset of environmental or occupational leukemias. Indeed, AMLs arising after DNA-damaging chemotherapeutic agents and the AMLs caused by diverse environmental factors are genotypically identical, the majority being characterized by deletions of all or part of chromosomes 5 and/or 7. In contrast, cytotoxic chemotherapeutic agents that target the intranuclear enzyme topoisomerase II—notably the epipodophyllins (e.g., etoposide [VP-16]) but also anthracyclines such as doxorubicin (Adriamycin) or epirubicin in concert with other DNA-damaging agents such as cis-platin and cyclophosphamide—induce single-strand breaks and produce characteristic lesions at other gene loci, in particular the MLL gene (mixed lineage leukemia, also known as ALL-1) on chromosome 11q23. This gene appears to have a pivotal role in controlling growth and differentiation in primitive hematopoietic stem cells. The disruption, translocation, and recombination of the MLL gene in stem cells, such as occurs in the t(4;11), t(6;11), t(9;11), and t(11;19), may impair orderly differentiation, thereby accounting for the occurrence of both ALL and AML (especially monocytic subtypes) among these 11q23-associated acute leukemias. In addition, the "partner genes" that recombine with MLL encode transcription factors, and resultant fusion proteins confer marked growth dysregulation as well as aberrant differentiation and leukemic transformation. The ability of these fusion proteins to drive cellular proliferation in an uncontrolled fashion on the molecular level is reflected in the clinical presentation of 11q23-linked leukemias, namely high peripheral blood blast counts with signs and symptoms of leukostasis (especially in monocytic variants) and the abrupt onset without the MDS prodrome that

TABLE 1. **Pathophysiology of Acute Leukemia**

Factor	Clinical Consequences	Time of Appearance During Therapy	Correction
Bone marrow failure	Anemia Bleeding Infection	Early and late	Restoration of normal hematopoiesis with functional differentiation
Leukemic clone	Leukostasis Disseminated intravascular coagulation Tumor lysis syndrome Hypermetabolic syndrome Extramedullary tissue infiltration	Early	Initial cytoreduction

commonly accompanies the induced AMLs associated with abnormalities of chromosomes 5 and/or 7.

PATHOPHYSIOLOGY AND CLINICAL PRESENTATIONS OF ACUTE LEUKEMIAS

In acute leukemia, unregulated accumulation of immature leukocytes compromises organ function most markedly in the bone marrow but also in other tissues that become infiltrated with the immature cells. The pathophysiology and clinical presentation of acute leukemia relate to two factors: bone marrow failure due to tumor-related suppression of normal hematopoiesis, and the clinical expression of the malignant hematopoietic clone (Table 1). The growth of blood cell precursors arrested at an immature stage of differentiation suppresses the production of normal bone marrow elements, resulting in anemia, infection, and bleeding. The increased growth of leukemic cells accompanied by the metabolic effects of increased cell turnover, and the infiltration of virtually all organ systems, complete the pathophysiologic complex. The signs and symptoms of bone marrow failure and infiltration of the central nervous system (CNS), liver, spleen, testes, ovaries, lymph nodes, skin, and gastrointestinal (GI) tract, with varied degrees of failure of each organ, may contribute to the constellation of symptoms and the protean clinical presentation.

Patients presenting with massive hyperleukocytosis (peripheral blast counts >100,000 per μL) are at high risk for life-threatening dysfunction of critical organs, namely, lung, heart, and CNS (Table 2). Those with monocytic phenotypes are especially vulnerable, with the risk beginning at peripheral blast counts as low as 50,000 per μL, since monocytes are large, "sticky" cells with great capacities for tissue invasion and adhesion. The majority of signs and symptoms of leukostasis relate directly to extramedullary leukemic cell aggregates with tissue infiltrates and small vessel leukothrombi that induce endothelial cell damage, tissue infarction and hemorrhage, organ barrier breakdown, and eventual multiorgan failure. Clinical stigmas include leukemic cell aggregation as manifested by skin chloromas, especially at sites of trauma (such as venipuncture), and gingival hypertrophy; hypermetabolism (fever, tachycardia); impaired oxygen transfer with hypoxemia (dyspnea, agitation, confusion, and eventual stupor); chest pain on the basis of myocardial ischemia and/or pericardial infiltration; and focal or diffuse neurologic deficits. These findings are often accompanied by metabolic derangements characteristic of the tumor lysis syndromes that attend massive tumor burdens with high cell turnover rates and bleeding diatheses, including a consumptive coagulopathy (see later for further discussion).

Patients with ALL have a striking incidence of CNS leukemia, and abnormal cells are often identified in the spinal fluid, even before the onset of symptoms. In contrast, the overall incidence of CNS involvement in AML is

TABLE 2. **Emergency Syndromes in Presentation of Leukemia**

Syndrome	Etiologic Factors	Manifestations

Tumor lysis	At presentation:
	  Massive tumor burden
	  Enzyme-rich cells
	  High cell turnover
	Rapid cytoreduction with initial cytotoxic therapy
		Hyperuricemia
		Hyperphosphatemia
		K^+ and Ca^{2+} imbalance
		Renal dysfunction
		Coagulopathy

Hyperleukocytosis with leukostasis	High blast count: Monoblast > myeloblast > lymphoblast Leukemic cell aggregates with tissue invasion Small vessel leukothrombi Endothelial damage	Whole blood hyperviscosity Pulmonary decompensation with hypoxemia (blockade of alveolar capillary oxygen transfer) CNS infiltration and hemorrhagic infarction Skin chloromata Gingival hypertrophy

Disseminated intravascular coagulation (APL, monocytic)	At presentation:
	  Proteolytic enzymes
	  Tissue thromboplastins
	  Profibrinolytic enzymes
	  Endothelial damage
	Rapid tumor lysis with initial cytotoxic therapy
		Consumptive coagulopathy with active bleeding diathesis
		Thromboembolic events

Abbreviations: APL = acute progranulocytic leukemia; CNS = central nervous system.

less than 10%, but AML occurs with significant frequency in the setting of hyperleukocytosis and in myelomonocytic and monocytic types, independent of peripheral blast counts. Both B and T cell ALLs are commonly attended by bulky extramedullary disease, with abdominal organ involvement especially prominent in B cell ALL and mediastinal masses typifying T cell ALL. Bone pain with infarction or marrow necrosis and attendant high fever (which may be impossible to distinguish from that of infection) are prominent in all variants of ALL but may occur also in certain AMLs, especially monocytic and megakaryocytic variants. Hyperuricemia and hyperphosphatemia are exceedingly common in all forms of ALL, with strikingly high levels the rule in B and T cell ALLs, and if not treated can result in obstructive uropathy. Hyperuricemia accompanies all types of full-blown AML as well, and hyperphosphatemia is often present in APL, monocytic subtypes, and those AMLs presenting with massive tumor burden. Additional renal problems may be present in AMLs with monocytic features. In these cases, the leukemic cell cohort produces excessive amounts of lysozyme, which, in turn, leads to hypokalemia without renal tubular acidosis, and with a defect in both glomerular filtration and proximal tubular function related to lysozyme-induced damage. These metabolic derangements are exacerbated transiently (but dramatically) with the initial cytoreduction of the leukemic cell mass. Additional treatment-related derangements such as hyperkalemia and hypercalcemia may ensue as a consequence of rapid cell death. This constellation of events, known as "tumor lysis syndrome," was first described in patients with ALL who experienced brisk increases in tumor cell lysis in response to steroids, but it occurs to differing degrees in all types of acute leukemia, particularly in concert with intensive cytotoxic antileukemic therapy.

Acute leukemias are often accompanied by bleeding diatheses of diverse causes. Thrombocytopenia on the basis of marrow failure is common in all forms of acute leukemia. In addition, virtually all patients with APL, the majority with monocytic subtypes, and some with certain ALL subtypes (L3, Ph+) are at major risk to develop a consumptive coagulopathy that has the clinical and laboratory hallmarks of disseminated intravascular coagulation (DIC). The cause of this DIC relates to numerous proteolytic and profibrinolytic enzymes and tissue-active factors (e.g., tissue thromboplastins and acid mucopolysaccharides) secreted by the leukemic cell cohort, with ensuing activation of the clotting cascade. In turn, the resultant formation of thromboemboli, and widespread thrombosis with surrounding hemorrhage, cause consumption of platelets and coagulation factors and stimulate fibrinolytic mechanisms—in short, a fulminant DIC picture that further augments the underlying thrombocytopenia and can be exacerbated by concomitant infection (see Table 2). The laboratory manifestations of this coagulopathy include prolongation of the prothrombin time (PT), partial thromboplastin time (PTT), and thrombin time; decreases in circulating levels of several clotting factors including X, V, VII, VIII, II (thrombin), and especially I (fibrinogen); and activation of fibrinolytic pathways with concomitant elevated levels of fibrinogen-fibrin degradation products (FDPs). Importantly, the institution of cytoreductive chemotherapy and the consequent rapid tumor lysis acutely exacerbate the coagulopathy. Even in those who do not evince DIC initially, initial cytoreduction may precipitate active DIC that persists until the period of initial drug-induced tumor lysis is over.

Thus, the combination of marrow failure and organ barrier breakdown from tumor invasion determines the clinical presenting features of acute leukemia. Certain elements of disease expression—tumor mass, cellular biochemistry, and the rate of cell turnover—determine both the need for prompt intervention and the initial therapy-related complications. Paradoxically, a rapid cell kill with intensive drug treatment results in the appearance or exacerbation of severe metabolic imbalances and coagulopathies that are self-limited but may be fatal if not prevented or rapidly reversed. The recognition of both disease- and treatment-related complications and the rational use of supportive measures are key to treatment survival and disease eradication. We discuss the management of metabolic, hemostatic, and infectious complications later.

DIAGNOSIS AND INITIAL EVALUATION

The diagnosis of acute leukemia is usually easily established by the demonstration of marrow replacement by immature cells. This finding effectively eliminates a leukemoid reaction, but problems may arise occasionally in distinguishing a leukemic marrow from that of megaloblastic anemia or a marrow recovering from aplasia caused by a drug, hepatitis, or infection, particularly viral. Classification of the specific cell of origin and lineage of the leukemic process is accomplished by Wright-Giemsa staining of the bone marrow aspirate and biopsy. The bone marrow biopsy is especially useful for detecting myelofibrosis, but the aspirate is essential for specific morphologic diagnosis and molecular characterizations. In addition, histochemical stains such as specific and nonspecific esterases, periodic acid–Schiff (PAS), acid phosphatases, and Sudan black are helpful in determining specific diagnosis. The combination of morphologic characteristics and histochemical staining patterns is the basis for the French-American-British (FAB) classification. This system, introduced almost 20 years ago, was the first attempt to categorize the acute leukemias for the purpose of improving scientific communication about and understanding of the biology, prognosis, and therapy of specific leukemia subtypes. As new insights have emerged regarding both unique determinants and common threads among the many leukemia variants, the FAB classification has been expanded and modified accordingly, including the development of morphologic criteria to categorize MDS. To date, eight AML categories (M0 to M7) and three ALL categories (L1 to L3) are defined on the basis of cell lineage, differentiation status, and degree of maturational impairment. Moreover, it is now possible to place the FAB system into a proper perspective as one of several complex determinants of leukemia prognosis and therapy by linking morphology with molecular immunology and genetics.

The ability to determine the immunophenotype of individual leukemic populations through identification of specific surface antigenic markers provides crucial diagnostic and prognostic information. These markers, detected by monoclonal antibodies (MoAbs) directed against cell surface proteins, can define both the lineage and the level of differentiation of the leukemic population. Asynchronous surface antigen expression reflecting aberrant differentiation states, mixed lineage clones, or primitive stem cell involvement can be associated with disease that is refractory to antileukemic therapy. For instance, in AML, aberrant expression of lymphoid markers (especially those of T lineage), the monocytic marker CD11b, or the stem cell marker CD34 may be associated with a decrease in remission achievement and duration, and a shortened survival. In ALL, a B cell phenotype (defined by the presence of surface immunoglobulin) confers a similar poor prognosis, especially in conjunction with certain genetic lesions such as the Ph chromosome, 6q−, and 14q+.

As discussed before, detailed chromosomal analysis provides pivotal information on diagnosis and prognosis. Further, the initial genetic lesion serves as the fundamental marker by which to measure persistent minimal residual disease, relapsing leukemia, and clonal evolution with the acquisition of new lesions, for instance multidrug resistance. Thus the genetic complexion of the leukemia has potential major impact on present-day therapeutic decision making, an impact that will grow as we become more sophisticated in exploiting leukemia-specific molecular aberrations for therapeutic advantage.

A comprehensive evaluation of specific metabolic parameters, including uric acid and phosphate; and all coagulation parameters, including clotting factors, fibrinolysis, and evidence for fibrinogen-fibrin degradation, is an essential part of the initial assessment. In addition, renal and hepatic dysfunctions have important bearing on the metabolism of antileukemic agents, and the detection of intrinsic abnormalities may dictate adjustments in drug dosing to avoid multiple organ toxicities. However, part or all of such abnormalities on admission may be caused by leukemic cell infiltration and/or tumor-related metabolic derangements that will resolve after the initial cytoreduction. Of special importance is the evaluation of myocardial function, as the anthracyclines (daunorubicin in particular) possess myocardial toxicity and can lead to potentially fatal cardiac insufficiency in patients with intrinsically compromised cardiac status. Histocompatibility (HLA) typing should be performed in every new patient to identify potential bone marrow donors among the patient's siblings (or even from unrelated donor data banks) and to provide HLA-matched platelet transfusions if and when the patient becomes refractory to unmatched platelet transfusions because of alloimmunization. Lastly, full microbiologic assessment is a crucial part of the initial evaluation of these highly compromised hosts. To this end, baseline surveillance cultures of blood, urine, stool, and various mucosal surfaces should be obtained even in the absence of fever or overt infection. The management of infectious complications is surveyed later.

ANTILEUKEMIA THERAPEUTIC STRATEGIES

Most adult patients with newly diagnosed acute leukemia are able to achieve a CR in response to induction chemotherapy. The long-term clinical results of BMT and dose-intensive chemotherapy in the first CR continue to improve in several leukemia patient subgroups. The advances achieved in DFS are in large part attributable to the intensive cytoreductive therapies that have been made possible only by aggressive support measures. There is no question that intensive cytotoxic therapy is accompanied by a heightened risk of widespread mucosal and nonhematopoietic multiorgan toxicities as well as profound marrow aplasia. With an increasing ability to manage and in some instances circumvent diverse cytotoxic complications, the full antileukemic potential of aggressive cytoreductive therapy can be evaluated.

The most appropriate forms of remission induction therapies and potentially curative postremission therapies continue to be controversial with respect to treatment modalities, drug doses, and schedules. As a case in point, the overall treatment strategies pioneered in adult AML differ considerably from the approaches commonly used in adult ALL (see Table 3 for overview). In AML, induction chemotherapy is followed by short-term, intensive therapy (either chemotherapy or BMT) in early first CR, at the time of minimal residual disease. In counterpoint, the approach to adult ALL has been modeled after the successes in childhood ALL, in which post-CR therapy is given over a prolonged time period. Yet the relatively low cure rate in adult ALL has prompted the investigation of approaches that parallel those of adult AML, namely the application of dose-intensive modalities in early CR. Thus the disease-specific treatments of adult acute leukemias remain investigative and should be undertaken in the setting of active clinical-laboratory correlative research.

Initial Management: Preparation for Cytoreductive Therapy

In general, the institution of antileukemic therapy should begin promptly (but not emergently) once the diagnosis is established, the specific cell lineage defined, and the pretreatment evaluations completed. Measures aimed at averting tumor lysis syndrome should be implemented in preparation for cytoreductive therapy. Specifically, hydration and allopurinol (Zyloprim) 300 mg per day orally should be instituted at least 24 hours before chemotherapy in order to prevent the hyperuricemia and urate nephropathy that accompany massive cell death. Allopurinol should be continued until the period of cell lysis ends (generally 8 to 10 days). The amelioration of hyperphosphatemia is equally important, but there is no intervention of comparable efficacy. Still, in the presence of pretreatment hyperphosphatemia or with a diagnosis in which hyperphosphatemia is likely to ensue with tumor lysis, the use of a phosphate-binding compound such as an aluminum hydroxide gel (Amphojel) may attenuate the risk. Should massive hyperphosphatemia or other tumor lysis–related metabolic derangements precipitate acute renal failure, early institution of hemodialysis is indicated. Additionally, the correction of severe anemia and thrombocytopenia with packed red blood cell (RBC) and platelet transfusions, respectively, is essential to optimize intravascular volume and prevent life-threatening hemorrhage. The use of a white blood cell (WBC) filter with the administration of blood products and the avoidance of transfusions from potential allogeneic BMT donors are important steps that should be taken to reduce the risk of alloimmunization.

Management of Emergency Syndromes

A number of clinical constellations (see Table 2) constitute medical emergencies demanding rapid recognition and intervention. Of special importance is hyperleukocytosis, in which the immediate institu-

TABLE 3. **Selected Commonly Used Induction and Postremission Therapeutic Regimens for Adult Acute Leukemias**

	Acute Myelogenous Leukemias	Acute Lymphocytic Leukemias
Induction therapy	Cytarabine (ARA-C) 100–200 mg/m²/day for 7 days IV by continuous infusion *plus* daunorubicin (Cerubidine) 45 mg/m²/day or idarubicin (Idamycin) 12 mg/m²/day IV on days 1–3 ("7 + 3" regimen)	Prednisone 40–60 mg/m²/day PO for 21 days Vincristine (Oncovin) 1.4 mg/m² IV days 1, 8, 15, and 22 Daunorubicin 45 mg/m²/day IV on days 1–3 or days 16–18
Additional options	Etoposide (VP-16) (VePesid) 150–300 mg/m²/day for 3 days IV over 4–6 h/dose or by continuous infusion Hematopoietic growth factors (e.g., GM-CSF [Leukine], IL-3) used as "priming agents" (before and concomitant with cytotoxic chemotherapy) For acute progranulocytic leukemia, *all trans*-retinoic acid (ATRA) 45 mg/m²/day PO until normal hematopoiesis is achieved For high-risk AML, high-dose ara-C 2–3 gm/m² IV over 4–6 h and every 12 h for 4–8 doses *plus* daunorubicin (or idarubicin) as above, with optional inclusion of VP-16 or other non-cross-resistant agents	Cyclophosphamide (Cytoxan) 1 gm/m² IV on Day 1 L-Asparaginase (Oncaspar) 5000 IU/m²/day IM for 10–14 days or 10,000 IU/m² sc weekly for 3 weeks High-dose ara-C 1–3 gm/m² IV over 4–6 h and given every 12 h for 4–8 doses
CNS prophylaxis		Intrathecal methotrexate 12 mg/m² (maximum 15 mg) *or* ara-C 30–45 mg/m² weekly for 6 weeks *plus* cranial irradiation 18–24 Gy in 10 fractions over 2 weeks
Postremission therapy	Intensive chemotherapy: high-dose ara-C plus daunorubicin (as above) *or* Myeloablative therapy (cyclophosphamide plus busulfan or total body irradiation) followed by allogeneic or autologous bone marrow transplantation	Cyclical consolidation and maintenance chemotherapies consisting of multiple agents, administered over 1.5–3 years: Consolidation: 2–4 alternating cycles of noncross-resistant therapies: e.g., prednisone, vincristine, daunorubicin plus L-asparaginase; ara-C plus teniposide (VM-26) (Vumon); methotrexate, 6-mercaptopurine, cyclophosphamide (Cytoxan), and dactinomycin (Cosmegen) *followed by* Maintenance therapy: e.g., 6-mercaptopurine 40–60 mg/m²/day PO, methotrexate 10 mg/m² twice weekly PO ± vincristine and prednisone *or* Myeloablative therapy (cyclophosphamide plus total body irradiation) followed by allogeneic or autologous bone marrow transplantation

Abbreviations: GM-CSF = granulocyte-macrophage colony-stimulating factor; AML = acute myelogenous leukemia; IL-3 = interleukin-3; CNS = central nervous system.

tion of cytoreductive therapy is essential in order to lower the WBC count acutely and thereby avoid death from pulmonary or CNS leukostasis. An overall strategy for the management of this potentially highly fatal situation is suggested in Table 4. In AML, especially with monocytic features, the rapid institution of definitive cytotoxic therapy (e.g., within 2 hours of presentation) is imperative and crucial to the killing of both circulating and tissue-sequestered leukemic cells. However, extensive CNS infiltration with cranial nerve involvement may require CNS irradiation and intrathecal administration of cytarabine (ara-C) and/or methotrexate, in addition to systemic therapy. The resultant rapid cell death will be complicated by massive tumor lysis with exaggerated metabolic derangements and coagulopathy. To this end, aggressive hydration and measures to abrogate hyperuricemia and hyperphosphatemia are mandatory. In addition, vigorous support of hemostasis to maintain a platelet count of roughly 50,000 per μL

will attenuate the tumor lysis–aggravated coagulopathy and decrease the propensity for hemorrhagic necrosis at sites of small vessel leukothrombi (especially in the CNS). However, the transfusion of RBCs should be avoided until the WBC falls below the range in which leukostasis occurs, since elevation of the total cytocrit by RBC transfusion will aggravate the already-existing hyperviscosity and enhance small vessel sludging.

Mechanical removal of circulating blasts by leukapheresis can be performed at the bedside. This procedure lowers the peripheral WBC count acutely and, by virtue of decreasing the tumor load, may potentially reduce the magnitude of tumor lysis syndrome once chemotherapy is instituted. However, without the addition of cytotoxic therapy, the effects are transient and have no impact on tissue infiltrates. In addition, leukapheresis may be attended by volume shifts in an already hemodynamically compromised patient and by alterations in drug

TABLE 4. **Key Strategies in Management of Leukostasis**

Rapid referral to treatment center
Immediate cytoreductive measures
  Chemical: cytotoxic antileukemic therapy
  Mechanical: leukapheresis
Vigorous hydration plus measures to enhance renal blood flow to
  maintain brisk urine output
Antitumor lysis syndrome measures (e.g., allopurinol, Amphojel)
Close monitoring of metabolic and hemostatic parameters
  P_{O_2}
  Serum urate, phosphate, potassium levels
  Renal function
  Clotting and fibrinolytic factors
Vigorous support of hemostasis to maintain platelet count
  >50,000/μL
Resisting temptation to transfuse RBCs until WBC level falls
  below range of whole blood hyperviscosity

pharmacokinetics. Thus the procedure should be performed in a manner that does not delay the institution of, or have adverse impact on the net efficacy of, definitive cytotoxic therapy. Leukapheresis may be most useful in hyperleukocytotic ALL, in which there is less urgency to initiate chemotherapy because the somewhat smaller size of the leukemic lymphoblast (with less tissue infiltrative capabilities) poses a relatively lesser risk for leukostasis and hyperviscosity.

Another situation that demands quick recognition and urgent intervention is DIC. As noted earlier, this potentially fatal consumptive coagulopathy commonly accompanies APL (and monocytic subtypes as well) at presentation and is exacerbated during chemotherapy-induced tumor lysis. Two major approaches to interdicting the bleeding diathesis are vigorous platelet support and heparinization. Heparinization is aimed at abrogating the constitutive activation of the clotting cascade and the consequent consumption of clotting factors, including platelets. Heparinization should begin 6 to 12 hours before the institution of chemotherapy with a bolus of 5000 U intravenously followed by a continuous infusion of 8 to 10 U per kg per hour. The infusion is maintained until the period of maximal tumor lysis ends and active DIC dissipates, as evidenced by disappearance of FDPs and the normalization of levels of fibrinogen and other soluble clotting factors (in general, 5 to 8 days after chemotherapy onset). Frequent monitoring of coagulation parameters (every 8 hours) is essential in order to titrate heparin dosage in the setting of fluctuating DIC activity and thereby avoid excessive anticoagulation or insufficient blockade of clotting cascade activity.

Acute Myelogenous Leukemia

Recent clinical trials in adults with AML indicate that CRs can be achieved in roughly 70% of those receiving intensive induction chemotherapy with cytarabine (cytosine arabinoside; ara-C) (Cytosar-U) plus daunorubicin (Cerubidine) or plus the newer anthracyclines mitoxantrone (Novantrone) or idarubicin (Idamycin). The most common regimen employs ara-C 100 to 200 mg per m² per day given by continuous infusion for 7 days plus daunorubicin 45 mg per m² or idarubicin 12 mg per m² per day for 3 days, the so-called "7 + 3" regimen, with CR achieved after 2 to 3 cycles. The anthracycline dose should be attenuated by about 30% or an alternative anthracycline such as mitoxantrone should be used in patients aged 70 years or older and in patients with known underlying cardiac compromise, in order to avoid dose-limiting, irreversible cardiac toxicity. More intensive induction regimens combining ara-C and daunorubicin with non-cross-resistant agents with different mechanisms of action (e.g., VP-16) and, in some cases, growth factor stimulation (see later) yield equivalent CR rates of roughly 70% after a single course of therapy.

Further intensive therapy administered early in first CR, at the time of minimal residual disease, has resulted in prolonged (>5 years) DFS and cure in 35 to 50% of patients treated in this manner. Less aggressive therapies that use prolonged maintenance approaches consisting of low-dose or moderate-dose chemotherapy have not yielded such prolongations of CR and survival. These curative approaches can employ three distinct modalities: (1) intensive chemotherapy, e.g., one to three short courses of intensive chemotherapy with high-dose ara-C (2 to 3 grams per m² administered over 4 to 6 hours and given every 12 hours for 4 to 8 doses) plus daunorubicin; (2) myeloablative therapy with cyclophosphamide (Cytoxan) plus busulfan (Myleran) or with cyclophosphamide with total body irradiation, followed by allogeneic BMT; or (3) myeloablation followed by autologous BMT, using bone marrow (or in some instances peripheral blood stem cells) harvested during CR and commonly purged ex vivo with one or more cytotoxic agents. At present, each of these approaches yields comparable results in the younger adult population with de novo AML. Hypothetically, allogeneic BMT may have a particular role in the treatment of the highly refractory "stem cell leukemias," as exemplified by those AMLs evolving from an antecedent MDS or induced by prior cytotoxic therapies. Novel approaches to the purging of residual AML cells from marrow harvested in CR for future autologous BMT include the use of monoclonal antibodies (MoAbs) targeting myeloid surface antigens that are highly expressed on AML populations (e.g., CD33, CD14, CD15), and the use of gene-directed constructs (e.g., antisense molecules) designed to target and neutralize the expression of certain genes (e.g., the *myb* oncogene or the abnormal fusion *bcr-abl* gene). These molecular therapies and certain types of gene therapy technologies aimed at replacing or correcting defective genes are entering the clinical testing arena. Nevertheless, aggressive cytoreductive therapy with or without BMT is not now curative for the majority of adults with AML. Further, these aggressive approaches, especially BMT modalities, are difficult to deliver in patients over the age of 60 years; however, low-dose regimens or attempts to induce differentiation with biomodulatory approaches have not yet met with success.

One of the consistent characteristics of leukemic cells is their inability to undergo normal differentiation and maturation. A significant step in the treatment of leukemias during the last decade is the development of differentiation therapy, in which dividing tumor cells are moved into a pathway of growth inhibition and maturation in response to differentiating agents. The first successful application of differentiation therapy is the treatment of APL with *all-trans*-retinoic acid (ATRA), a biologically active metabolite of vitamin A that promotes morphologic and functional differentiation of APL in vitro and in vivo and produces dramatic clinical responses without causing overt cytotoxicity in some patients. The unique sensitivity of APL to ATRA is integrally related to the underlying genetic basis of the disease, namely the pathognomonic t(15;17), discussed earlier, which produces an abnormal retinoic acid receptor–alpha with unusual affinity for ATRA. Initial therapy with ATRA 45 mg per m^2 per day induces remissions with re-emergence of normal hematopoiesis in roughly 80% of APL patients, similar to the CR rate achieved with cytotoxic therapy. The median time to CR is roughly 40 days, although remissions have ensued as early as 18 days and as late as 80 days of daily ATRA therapy. ATRA-induced remissions, however, are short-lived and must be followed with chemotherapy incorporating ara-C plus daunorubicin in order to achieve prolonged DFS and cure. In addition, ATRA induction therapy can be associated with the so-called retinoic acid syndrome consisting of fever and diffuse capillary leak with adult respiratory distress syndrome (ARDS) and multiorgan failure. This constellation of findings is precipitated by ATRA when the presenting WBC count is 20,000 per μL or more, which occurs in 40 to 50% of all APL patients, or when ATRA induces a rapid outpouring of cells (which occurs in 15 to 20%). Thus, roughly half of all APL patients are at risk for developing this syndrome, which ultimately occurs in 25 to 30% and is fatal in 10 to 15% of the ATRA-treated APL population. Early intervention with a brief course of high-dose steroids (e.g., dexamethasone 10 mg intravenously every 12 hours for 3 days) or cytotoxic therapy in the face of a rapidly rising WBC count (e.g., hydroxyurea; ara-C plus daunorubicin) reverses the clinical syndrome and prevents a fatal outcome.

The clinical availability of recombinantly produced hematopoietic growth factors—granulocyte (G-CSF; filgrastim) (Neupogen) and granulocyte-macrophage colony-stimulating factors (GM-CSF; sargramostim) (Leukine, Prokine) and interleukins (ILs)—opens several new therapeutic avenues. One such avenue is the potential to "prime" tumor cells in order to enhance their sensitivity to cytotoxic agents. Cytotoxic agents preferentially destroy actively dividing tumor cells but do not kill tumor cells that are in the quiescent phase of the cell cycle. As a case in point, ara-C is a cell cycle–dependent, phase-specific drug,

highly cytotoxic to proliferating cells undergoing DNA synthesis (S phase) but not to nonproliferative cells. The fraction of nondividing cells in many cancers, including leukemias, can, in fact, be very high. Hematopoietic growth factors can bring leukemic cells into the cell division cycle and thereby increase the fraction of dividing leukemic cells. The administration of a growth factor for several days before treatment with such chemotherapeutic agents is being explored with the expectation that this sequencing of growth factor followed by chemotherapy may enhance the effectiveness of the chemotherapeutic drugs. Clinical trials are now in progress to define the optimal roles for G- and GM-CSF, interleukin-3 (IL-3), or the fusion IL-3–GM-CSF protein (PIXY 321) in augmenting the antileukemic effects of ara-C plus daunorubicin in the treatment of AML in both de novo and poor-prognosis types such as the therapy-related variants and the AMLs evolving from MDS. In addition, the ability of the CSFs and IL-3 to promote morphologic and functional differentiation of the aberrant clone in MDS is under study.

Treatment for AML that is primarily refractory to induction or that relapses after initial CR is generally not curative. Reinduction with high-dose ara-C plus anthracycline and/or non–cross-resistant agents (e.g., VP-16, amsacrine,* cyclophosphamide) may yield CR in 40 to 50%, with BMT resulting in prolonged DFS in 20 to 35% of those achieving second CR. Given the generally poor outcome, this population should be considered strongly for testing of new (Phase I) agents and new modalities (growth factors, gene therapies, and inhibitors of drug-resistance pathways).

Acute Lymphocytic Leukemia

Initial chemotherapy with vincristine, prednisone, and daunorubicin induces CR in roughly 70 to 80% of adults with ALL. As in childhood ALL, vincristine 1.4 mg per m^2 is administered weekly for three doses with concomitant prednisone 40 to 60 mg per m^2 per day for 21 days. This combination yields CR in 80 to 90% of all children with ALL, but in only 40 to 50% of adults (although roughly 75% evince objective response with re-emergence of normal hematopoiesis). Nonetheless, the addition of daunorubicin 45 mg per m^2 per day for 3 days results in a marked increase in the adult CR rate to 70 to 80%. Some induction regimens also incorporate L-asparaginase (Elspar), the latter based on its efficacy in childhood ALL, although its precise contribution to the CR rate and duration in adults is not clear. The incorporation of additional cytotoxic agents—cyclophosphamide 1 gram per m^2, high-dose ara-C 1 to 3 grams per m^2 given every 12 hours for 4 to 8 doses, and the epipodophyllin VM-26 (teniposide) (Vumon)—may improve both the achievement and the duration of CR in particularly aggressive ALL variants, namely those presenting with peripheral blast counts greater than

---

*Investigational drug in the United States.

25,000 per μL, L3 morphology, pure B or T cell markers, and unfavorable chromosomal translocations, e.g., Ph chromosome or t(4:11). Importantly, the customarily held notion that T cell ALL connotes a poor clinical outcome has been overcome to a large degree by employing intensive cytotoxic chemotherapy with the above agents early in the course of the disease.

ALL in both the adult and the child is accompanied by a significant incidence of CNS leukemia. In this regard, it is customary to administer "CNS prophylaxis" after initial CR induction, even in the absence of documented involvement or high-risk features on disease presentation. After induction therapy, prophylactic treatment of the CNS with intrathecal methotrexate and/or ara-C, sometimes in combination with cranial irradiation, should be undertaken. Systemic therapies that cross the blood-brain barrier—for example, high-dose methotrexate given in combination with leucovorin to "rescue" the bone marrow from myelotoxicity—can be employed. After CNS prophylaxis, cyclical courses of moderately intensive consolidation and maintenance therapies consisting of multiple, non-cross-resistant agents are administered during first CR for a period of 1.5 to 3 years. Drugs commonly used in this cyclical approach include cyclophosphamide, methotrexate, 6-mercaptopurine, vincristine and prednisone, daunorubicin, and, perhaps of special importance in aggressive disease, ara-C and the epipodophyllin VM-26 (teniposide).

However, although CR is attained in the majority of adults with ALL, the durations of those CRs are relatively brief (median 15 to 18 months), and the subsequent achievement of CRs of meaningful duration is low (30% or less). In contrast to adult AML, where more than 5-year DFS and cure are realized in 35 to 50% of those achieving CR, the overall cure rate in adult ALL remains substantially lower: 15 to 25% of those achieving CR, especially with prolonged (1.5 to 3 years) multiagent maintenance chemotherapy approaches alone. Thus, at present, a major thrust of clinical investigation is the exploration of the roles of intensive chemotherapy with non-cross-resistant drugs and BMT (allogeneic and autologous) in prolonging the DFS in adult ALL. In this regard, allogeneic BMT performed in first CR achieves prolonged DFS in 30 to 40% of adults under 50 years of age. In contrast, the clinical outcomes of autologous BMT (with purged or unpurged marrow) and cyclical consolidation and maintenance chemotherapies are less salutary, with both modalities yielding DFS of more than 2 years in only 25 to 30%, late (>3 years) relapses (mainly in the chemotherapy-treated patients), and overall cure rates less than 20%. The ability to monitor minimal residual disease on the molecular level by using PCR to measure the persistence of small numbers of cells containing immunoglobulin gene or T cell receptor gene rearrangements or other leukemia-specific translocations will define the efficacy of aggressive therapies delivered with curative intent and will identify those adults who might benefit from further intensive therapeutic interventions, including the testing of new agents with unique mechanisms of action.

MANAGEMENT OF INFECTIOUS COMPLICATIONS OF LEUKEMIA AND ANTILEUKEMIC THERAPY

The patient with acute leukemia is at exceedingly high risk for the development of life-threatening infection on the bases of both the underlying marrow failure and the hematopoietic and mucosal toxicities of cytoreductive therapies. Fever acts as the "surrogate marker" for infection. Because the patient is highly compromised due to both disease- and treatment-related bone marrow failure and attendant profound neutropenia, any unexplained fever demands the immediate institution of antibiotic coverage. This emergent response is necessary because many of the signs and symptoms of infection in acute leukemia are typically muted by a lack of the expected inflammatory response. The rapid recognition and treatment of infection is essential to a successful outcome of intensive antileukemic chemotherapy. Prophylaxis against GI-based infection with oral antibiotics that act against aerobic bacteria, such as norfloxacin (Noroxin),* prevents infection with endogenous host gram-negative organisms emanating from the GI tract (in particular, *Pseudomonas aeruginosa, Escherichia coli* and *Klebsiella* spp). Periodic surveillance cultures of blood, urine, stool, and mucosal surfaces may give advanced warning of colonization by new or resistant organisms that may subsequently cause local or systemic infection. The febrile neutropenic patient should be treated with an antibiotic regimen that provides broad coverage against gram-negative bacteria—either a combination of a beta-lactam (e.g., ticarcillin [Ticar] or piperacillin [Pipracil] plus an aminoglycoside or one of the newer extended-spectrum agents (ceftazidime [Fortaz] or imipenem-cilastatin [Primaxin])—and the antibiotic therapy should be continued until the recovery of normal hematopoiesis. Further, beta-lactam-resistant gram-positive organisms including staphylococci, streptococci (including enterococci) and corynebacteria from both cutaneous and mucosal sources continue to emerge as important pathogens and prompt the addition of vancomycin. Therapy with the antiviral agent acyclovir (Zovirax) abrogates any recrudescence of latent herpes simplex during marrow aplasia. For patients with defective lymphocyte function (e.g., ALL patients receiving high-dose steroid therapy for prolonged periods or allogeneic BMT patients receiving immunosuppressive therapies for graft-versus-host disease), *Pneumocystis carinii* is an important pathogen; infection with *P. carinii* can be successfully treated with trimethoprim-sulfamethoxazole (TMP–SMX) (Bactrim) and, more importantly, can be prevented with the prophylactic use of TMP–SMX in high-risk immunocompromised individuals.

Continuing or recrudescing fever despite full anti-

---

*Not FDA-approved for this indication.

bacterial coverage should prompt consideration for systemic antifungal coverage with amphotericin B. Systemic prophylaxis with the newer azoles, fluconazole and itraconazole, can suppress colonization and infection by *Candida albicans* and *Candida tropicalis* but not by filamentous fungi such as *Aspergillus* and *Fusarium*. The new azoles may also be attended by the emergence of resistant yeasts such as *Candida krusei* and *Torulopsis glabrata*. A clinical and radiographic picture consistent with invasive fungal infection of the lung or paranasal sinuses, commonly caused by *Aspergillus* spp, or the appearance of fungal skin emboli or other evidence of disseminated fungal infection caused by relatively resistant fungal pathogens (*C. krusei, C. parapsilosis, Trichosporon,* or *Fusarium*) may dictate the need for high doses of amphotericin B (at least 1 mg per kg daily) and addition of another antifungal agent such as 5-flucytosine (5FC). An approach to the management of presumed and documented infections in the profoundly compromised leukemia patient is delineated in Table 5.

The colony-stimulating factors and ILs, discussed before, are also adjuncts in infection management, enhancing cellular and humoral host defense mechanisms. To this end, the administration of G-CSF and GM-CSF during cytotoxic chemotherapy with or without BMT accelerates bone marrow recovery in terms of decreasing the duration (but not depth) of the low granulocyte counts (but not platelet counts); decreases the incidence and severity of antibiotic-requiring fevers and documented infections; and in some cases decreases the duration of hospitalization. There is no evidence that G-CSF or GM-CSF given in this manner has a negative impact on the underlying leukemia. Further, early data suggest that some colony-stimulating factors might protect against the mouth sores and diarrhea that arise from therapy-induced mucosal toxicities. Indeed, a randomized, placebo-controlled clinical trial of GM-CSF in older adults (aged 55 to 70 years) with de novo AML undergoing 7 + 3 induction therapy demonstrates that GM-CSF administration results in an improved overall survival in this high-risk population, because of a more rapid recovery of normal granulocytes and a concomitant attenuation of mucosal and infectious complications of cytotoxic therapy. IL-3 stimulates the growth and differentiation of multipotential hematopoietic precursors, leading to an increase in multiple lineages including granulocytes, monocytes, eosinophils, lymphocytes, and platelets. On the basis of its ability to recruit monocytes, eosinophils, and lymphocytes as well as granulocytes, IL-3 might have a special role in the management of fungal and perhaps viral infections. Similarly, monocyte-macrophage colony-stimulating factor (M-CSF) specifically stimulates the proliferation, survival, and functional activation of monocytes and macrophages. Recent trials in allogeneic BMT patients demonstrate that M-CSF in conjunction with amphotericin B yields up to

TABLE 5. **Suggested Schema for Prevention and Management of Infections in Neutropenic Hosts**

Prophylaxis Started at Day 0 or at Day of granulocytes <500 × 10⁹/L Maintain throughout granulocytopenia	Norfloxacin (Noroxin) 400 mg PO every 12 h for prevention of GN sepsis Acyclovir (Zovirax) 250 mg/m² IV every 8 h for prevention of HSV reactivation
Additional Options	1. Addition of GP coverage, e.g., vancomycin 500 mg IV every 12 h if GP infection rate is high 2. Addition of antifungal prophylaxis, e.g., low-dose amphotericin B, azoles 3. Addition of cytokines, e.g., G-CSF (Neupogen), GM-CSF (Leukine), IL-3, M-CSF (especially for fungal infections)
First Infectious Fever	*Antipseudomonal penicillin,* e.g., ticarcillin (Ticar) 270 mg/kg/24 h (continuous infusion) provides GN, anaerobic, and some GP coverage; *and aminoglycoside,* e.g., gentamicin 2 mg/kg IV every 6 h provides broad-spectrum coverage and synergistic effect with penicillins; *or* single-agent, new beta-lactam antibiotics, e.g., ceftazidime (Fortaz) 2 g every 8 h or imipenem-cilastatin (Primaxin) 500 mg every 6 h for broad GN coverage.
Progressive Disease No response within 48–72 h of starting first fever coverage	1. With clinical suspicion of smoldering bacterial infection: substitute TMP–SMX for gentamicin. Add vancomycin if not already started. 2. With clinical evidence of more rapidly deteriorating condition: substitute amikacin 8 mg/kg IV every 6 h and piperacillin 270 mg/kg/24 h (continuous infusion). 3. With clinical suspicion of fungal infection (~5–10% of first fever), add amphotericin B 0.5 mg/kg/day IV.
Recrudescent Fever >72 h after starting first fever coverage without microbial documentation	1. Add amphotericin B (0.5 mg/kg/day) IV if not started already. 2. Switch to amikacin plus piperacillin if bacterial sepsis suspected.
Specific Treatment of Microbiologically Documented Infection	1. Bacterial-specific antibiotic or combinations of antibiotics 2. Fungal species-dependent: Amphotericin B 0.5 mg/kg/day Amphotericin B 1.0–1.25 mg/kg/day + 5-flucytosine 25 mg/kg PO every 6 h* for more refractory yeast species and all filamentous mycoses

*To achieve serum level of 30–60 μg/mL to avoid 5-flucytosine-related toxicity.
Abbreviations: CSF = colony stimulating factor (G = granulocyte; GM = granulocyte-macrophage; M = monocyte-macrophage); GN = gram-negative; GP = gram-positive; HSV = herpes simplex virus; IL = interleukin; TMP–SMX = trimethoprim-sulfamethoxazole (Bactrim).

fivefold improvements in survival because of long-lasting suppression of fungal infection and an associated 50% survival rate for M-CSF-treated patients with *Candida*, but unfortunately not *Aspergillus*, infections.

FUTURE DIRECTIONS: ADDRESSING CONTINUING CHALLENGES

We began this chapter by noting the significant progress that has been made in the face of acute leukemia in the adult, changing it from a family of diseases that were uniformly fatal to one in which there are realistic possibilities for cure in a substantial number of adults with certain distinctive subtypes of disease. Although this degree of progress is encouraging, it is clearly not enough, and we need to continue our research efforts on all levels—molecular, cellular, and clinical—with active cross-talk among all these diverse investigative components. The coupling of basic and clinical investigation in a fashion that fosters a bidirectional exchange of information and the translation of basic discoveries into clinical advances can be performed only in a research setting that is committed to the support of such multidisciplinary approaches. The critical portions of the "translational research equation" are twofold: a clinical milieu that fosters the development and implementation of innovative clinical investigative protocols and is equipped with specialized nursing units to provide the complex supportive therapies that must accompany aggressive interventions in critically ill patients; and an intellectual and infrastructural commitment to basic laboratory investigation devoted to the study of human leukemia biology. It is only through the vigorous pursuit of both facets in an integrated fashion that we will continue to make real progress with real increases in DFS and cure in these devastating diseases. Until cures can be realized in the majority of adults with acute leukemia, there is no such entity as "standard therapy" and we must continue to approach these diseases with an investigative mentality.

ACKNOWLEDGMENT

I am indebted to Dr. Robert B. Geller, Director, Leukemia Program, Emory University School of Medicine, for his critical review and insightful suggestions.

ACUTE LEUKEMIA IN CHILDHOOD

method of
GRETCHEN M. EAMES, M.D., and
MARK E. NESBIT, JR., M.D.
University of Minnesota
Minneapolis, Minnesota

Leukemias are the most common childhood malignancies, accounting for 30% of all cancer diagnoses among persons zero to 14 years of age. There are approximately 2500 new cases diagnosed annually in the United States. Leukemia is a malignancy of the hematopoietic system and is characterized by the diffuse replacement of the bone marrow by neoplastic hematopoietic cells. Acute leukemias are classified into two main types based on morphology, cytochemistry, and immunophenotyping, with approximately 85% of childhood cases classified as acute lymphoblastic leukemia (ALL) and 13% as acute myeloid leukemia (AML).

Before the early 1960s, a child with ALL lived only 6 to 8 weeks, but as of 1990, approximately 75% of children treated for ALL are without evidence of disease at 5 years, with the vast majority of these cases representing cures. The dramatic improvement in survival of children with ALL has occurred as a result of progressive intensification of treatment with multiagent chemotherapeutic regimens, improvements in supportive care, improved therapy for infectious complications, better infection prophylaxis, and therapy directed at the biologically classified subgroups of leukemia.

The incidence of childhood ALL peaks between the ages of 3 and 5 years. As of 1990 in the United States, the overall annual age-adjusted incidence rate of ALL in children aged zero to 14 years was 35 per million. During the period 1973 to 1990, the overall incidence has escalated by 27%. This increase may be an artifact due to other factors, or it may be a genuine increase in the incidence, reflecting possibly new or changing exposures to environmental or infectious carcinogens.

AML, a malignancy much more commonly seen in adults, has an annual age-adjusted incidence rate in children aged zero to 14 years of 5.8 and 4.8 per million for whites and blacks, respectively. With the exception of a modest peak in adolescents, the incidence of childhood AML remains relatively constant until the age of 20 years. Also, unlike the increased incidence of ALL, the incidence of childhood AML has not increased in the United States over the last 2 decades. Unfortunately, the 5-year survival rates for children diagnosed with AML have not improved as dramatically as for ALL. In 1990, the overall probability of survival for children with AML was only 28% at 5 years. Recent data with shorter follow-up has shown an improvement, with 40 to 50% surviving at 3 years.

Although a number of studies have addressed the cause of childhood leukemia, there has been a lack of strong, consistent association with environmental and genetic risk factors. It is the hope that future studies will place higher priority on clinical information to allow studies of epidemiologic factors within the different biologically identified subgroups.

CLINICAL PRESENTATION

Symptoms and signs of acute leukemia, which often develop over several weeks, are related to the proliferation of malignant cells in the bone marrow at the expense of normal hematopoiesis as well as to the extent of extramedullary disease spread. In clinically overt ALL there are approximately 10^{12} leukemic cells in the marrow. The two most common clinical manifestations of acute leukemia are fever and hepatosplenomegaly. Bone pain may also be an early symptom in 27 to 33% of children with leukemia and is more common in ALL than in AML. Arthritic symptoms may be a prominent feature of acute leukemia and can be mistaken for various rheumatic diseases. Anemia resulting in pallor and fatigue, and increased bruising, bleeding, or petechiae due to thrombocytopenia are also quite common.

In the newly diagnosed patient, bleeding can also be related to platelet dysfunction if the patient has been receiving aspirin or nonsteroidal anti-inflammatory drugs for fever or bone pain. Although lymphadenopathy is a common presentation in ALL, it is more common in benign conditions. Lymphadenopathy in the posterior auricular, epitrochlear, or supraclavicular area or other nodes more than 10 mm or inguinal nodes greater than 15 mm should raise concern. Also, patients with acute leukemia usually present with generalized rather than localized adenopathy. Those patients with mediastinal lymphadenopathy may present with symptoms related to compression or erosion of adjacent organs, such as the respiratory tract producing cough, stridor, or hemoptysis. Unusual presentations of ALL include aplastic anemia, cyclic neutropenia, eosinophilia, bone marrow necrosis, pulmonary nodules, pericardial effusion, hemophagocytosis syndrome, and skin nodules. Unusual presentations of AML can include an ovarian or testicular mass or bone and soft tissue masses (chloromas). Signs or symptoms of central nervous system (CNS) involvement are rarely a presenting feature for either type of leukemia.

Pancytopenia consisting of anemia, leukopenia, and thrombocytopenia can occur in both lymphoblastic and myeloid leukemia. Less common is leukocytosis. An initial white blood cell (WBC) count of less than 10,000 per mm^3 is seen in 53% of children with ALL; 30% have a count between 10,000 and 50,000 per mm^3, and 17% present with a WBC count of greater than 50,000 per mm^3. Exaggerated leukocytosis is most often seen in newly diagnosed cases of childhood AML, with 21% having an initial WBC count greater than 100,000 per mm^3. Other laboratory features may include elevations of liver enzyme levels, hyperuricemia, hypocalcemia, hyperphosphatemia, and hyperkalemia.

DIAGNOSIS

The diagnosis of cancer in a child begins with a thorough history and physical examination; the chief complaint is the most important initial clue. The family medical history is also a key element, as certain familial and genetic diseases are associated with an increased risk of leukemia and should be documented. These include Down's syndrome, which has a 15- to 30-fold risk of leukemia above that of the general population, as well as genetic disorders associated with chromosomal fragility (ataxia-telangiectasia, Bloom's syndrome, and Fanconi's anemia). Other diseases associated with a higher risk of acute leukemia include neurofibromatosis and some immunodeficiency disorders. Also, siblings of a child with leukemia have a higher risk of leukemia (two- to fourfold) than children in the general population.

In a child presenting with abnormal peripheral blood counts, a bone marrow examination is indicated to rule out leukemia or another malignancy when (1) atypical or blast cells are present on the peripheral smear, (2) significant depression of more than one blood cell element is seen, (3) unexplained lymphadenopathy or hepatosplenomegaly is present, and/or (4) an infectious cause of the blood abnormality is not found. Abnormal clotting studies can be associated with acute leukemia, especially T cell ALL and some types of AML. Initial evaluation of all patients, especially those who present with bleeding, should include a prothrombin time (PT), activated partial thromboplastin time (aPTT), thrombin time (TT), fibrinogen level, and serum fibrin-fibrinogen degradation products (FDPs). The diagnostic work-up for a child suspected to have acute leukemia

TABLE 1. **Diagnostic Work-Up**

History and physical examination
Complete blood count with differential
Peripheral smear
Test for levels of electrolytes, including phosphorus, calcium, and magnesium
Test for ALT, total bilirubin, LDH, alkaline phosphatase, serum creatinine, and uric acid levels
Urinalysis
Test for PT, PTT, TT, and levels of fibrinogen and FDPs
Test for immunoglobulin levels (G and subclasses A, M, and E)
Chest x-ray examination
Lumbar puncture for cell count, cytospin and glucose and protein levels
Bone marrow biopsy and aspirate: morphology with cytochemistry, cytogenetics, immunophenotyping, and heparinized marrow to be saved for further studies

Abbreviations: ALT = alanine aminotransferase; LDH = lactate dehydrogenase; PT = prothrombin time; PTT = partial thromboplastintime; TT = thrombin time; FDPs = fibrin-fibrinogen degradation products.

is listed in Table 1. The need for special studies done on the bone marrow at diagnosis as well as many other tests that are prognostically important warrants prompt referral to a center that specializes in pediatric oncology. Although the incidence of malignancy in children is low, the impact of cancer makes it imperative that all health care professionals taking care of children have a high index of suspicion of cancer.

COMPLICATIONS AND INITIAL MANAGEMENT

The initial hours of management of patients with suspected or newly diagnosed acute leukemia involve recognition and prevention or treatment of life-threatening complications. Potential problems include bleeding, infection, hyperleukocytosis, severe anemia, and tumor lysis syndrome.

Bleeding

Bleeding is usually the result of thrombocytopenia or coagulopathy. Spontaneous bleeding rarely occurs until the platelet count is below 20,000 per mm^3, but infection or disseminated intravascular coagulopathy (DIC) may predispose to hemorrhage at higher platelet counts. Platelet transfusions should be given to maintain the platelet count above 15,000 to 20,000 per mm^3 or a higher target count if the patient is actively bleeding. If DIC is present, aggressive replacement of clotting factors with cryoprecipitate and fresh-frozen plasma is recommended. All blood products should be irradiated and cytomegalovirus-negative, if available.

Fever and Infection

Fever is seen at diagnosis in 60% of children with ALL and in 30 to 40% of children with AML. Although infection is usually present, it is documented in less than 50% of cases and should be considered as the cause of fever until proved otherwise. Infection rates are much higher in those who are severely neutropenic (less than 500 neutrophils per mm^3); thus febrile, neutropenic patients should receive empirical broad-spectrum antibiotics after appropriate cultures are obtained. Gram-positive bacteria and enteric gram-negative bacilli are responsible for the majority of infections at diagnosis.

Hyperleukocytosis

"Leukostasis" is the term used to describe intravascular clumping of blasts, with the resultant risk of hypoxia, hemorrhage, and infarction of the affected tissues. This rarely occurs unless the WBC count is greater than 150,000 per mm³. The brain and lungs are the most commonly affected organs. Tachypnea and oxygen need may herald lung involvement, and CNS symptoms may include somnolence, headache, vision changes, stroke, or coma. Leukaphoresis or exchange transfusion is the therapy of choice to rapidly lower the WBC count, but these methods are only transiently effective until cytotoxic therapy is initiated.

Anemia

Hemoglobin values of less than 7.0 gm per dL are seen in approximately 40% of newly diagnosed cases of childhood ALL. If clinical symptoms of cardiac failure or respiratory compromise exist because of the degree and duration of anemia, then packed red blood cell transfusions should be given over 3 to 4 hours. The anemia associated with acute leukemia is usually chronic unless significant bleeding is present, and thus most patients have adapted well to their degree of anemia.

Tumor Lysis Syndrome

"Tumor lysis syndrome" is the metabolic consequence of the release of the cellular contents of dying leukemia cells, which can occur before or during cytotoxic chemotherapy. This results in hyperuricemia with potential risk of renal failure, hyperkalemia, hyperphosphatemia, and secondary hypocalcemia. Patients with large tumor burdens such as massive lymphadenopathy, mediastinal masses, and/or high WBC counts are at the greatest risk. It is imperative that all children receive aggressive hydration, alkalinization of the urine with intravenous bicarbonate, and allopurinol (Zyloprim) therapy. Careful monitoring of serum electrolyte levels, urine output, and renal function is important during the initial few days of evaluation and therapy.

ACUTE LYMPHOBLASTIC LEUKEMIA

ALL is a clinically and biologically heterogeneous disease. Immunologic classification of ALL has become more and more sophisticated over recent years and involves the use of a wide range of monoclonal antibodies that identify cell surface antigens. Based on these results, lymphoblastic leukemia is subdivided into two broad categories dependent on whether the cells are of T or B cell lineage. Approximately 90% of childhood ALL originate from the monoclonal proliferation of B cell–committed progenitors, and 10% have T cell ALL as determined by

positivity with the monoclonal antibodies CD2 and CD7. Mature B cell leukemias have surface immunoglobulin detectable, account for only 1 to 2% of ALL cases in children, and are associated with a poor prognosis. In pre-B cells that are arrested at earlier stages of differentiation, cytoplasmic immunoglobulin is detectable, and these patients also have a poor prognosis, especially when there is an associated t(1;19) chromosomal translocation. The most favorable prognosis is for patients with cells arrested at the earliest stage of differentiation (pre-pre-B cell ALL). Now that monoclonal antibodies are widely available, there are increasing reports of patients with ALL in whom the blast cells express one or more myeloid antigens, and these cases have been termed "mixed lineage" leukemia. It is estimated that up to 10 to 20% of childhood ALL may express one or more myeloid antigens. Although co-expression of myeloid antigens in adult ALL has been shown to be associated with a poor prognosis, there is no firm evidence that this is the case in childhood ALL.

Morphologic characteristics are used to classify lymphoblasts according to the French-American-British (FAB) cooperative group criteria. Approximately 85% of ALL cases have L1 lymphoblasts, which are small with regularly shaped nuclei, indistinct nucleoli, and scanty cytoplasm and are associated with the best prognosis. L2 morphology is found in 14% of childhood cases. These cells are more heterogeneous, have a low nuclear/cytoplasmic ratio and prominent nucleoli and are associated with a poorer prognosis. The L3 lymphoblasts are large, homogeneous cells resembling those in Burkitt's lymphoma; they account for only 1% of cases and have the worst prognosis.

Cytogenetic analysis places patients in prognostic categories and has allowed investigators to focus on areas of the genome that may be important in leukemogenesis. The chromosome number has been shown to be important in that children with hyperdiploid ALL or a high DNA index have a good prognosis, whereas those with pseudodiploid ALL have a poorer prognosis. Chromosomal translocations that are consistently associated with a poorer prognosis include t(9;22) or Philadelphia-positive (Ph⁺), t(4;11), t(8;14), and t(1;19).

Patients are assigned to risk groups on the assumption that children at highest relative risk of relapse benefit from more intensive therapy than those at lower risk. The definition of risk groups in ALL varies between institutions and cooperative groups. The Children's Cancer Group (CCG) now defines *lower risk* patients as those between the ages of 1 and 9 years, with non–T cell disease, and with a presenting WBC count of less than 50,000 per mm³, representing approximately 60% of all children diagnosed with ALL. Patients who do not fit this criteria as well as those who have greater than 25% of blasts with L3 morphology, CNS involvement at diagnosis, or with t(9;22) or t(4;11) chromosomal translocations are considered *higher risk* patients (Table 2). The age

TABLE 2. **Children's Cancer Group Risk Group Definitions**

Lower risk	Age 1–9 years Initial WBC count <50,000 Non–T cell disease
Higher risk	Age <1 or ≥9 years Initial WBC count ≥50,000 T lineage disease >25% L3 blasts CNS disease at diagnosis Specific chromosomal abnormalities 　　Hypodiploid 　　t(9;22), t(4;11)

Abbreviations: WBC = white blood cell; CNS = central nervous system.

TABLE 3. **Prognostic Factors for Acute Lymphoblastic Leukemia**

Age	Cell surface markers
Initial white blood cell count	B or T lineage
Leukemic cytogenetics	Myeloid
Chromosomal translocations	Response to initial therapy
DNA content	

and extent of disease at presentation, specifically the WBC count, are factors that nearly all investigators agree are prognostically important. Children aged 2 to 10 years do better than adolescents. Infants of less than 1 year, who account for approximately 3% of children with ALL, consistently do poorly. Boys also relapse more frequently than girls. Treatment is the most important factor influencing survival, and thus the prognostic factors listed in Table 3 may lose their significance with treatment.

Treatment

Recent years have seen a great success story in the treatment of ALL, but nearly one-third of children with ALL still relapse and only a small percentage of these can be cured. These cures in relapsed patients are often at the expense of long-term physical and psychological sequelae that can adversely affect the patient's quality of life. Thus there is a strong need to continue to develop more effective forms of therapy that can be more specific and lead to less long-term toxicity. Recent methods to detect minimal residual disease may make it possible to identify both children who have received insufficient therapy and may need additional therapy and children who may have received adequate therapy and can possibly have their treatment reduced.

The standard approach to treatment of ALL (Table 4) involves four components: induction, consolidation,

some form of delayed intensification, and maintenance therapy. Table 5 lists the adverse effects of antineoplastic agents commonly used to treat acute leukemia.

Induction

The well-established induction therapy for childhood ALL consists of the combination of vincristine (Oncovin), prednisone, and L-asparaginase (Elspar), which induces a remission in over 95% of children by Day 28 of therapy. CCG studies have shown that children not in marrow remission by Day 14 have a worse disease-free survival rate. Adding a fourth drug such as daunorubicin, an anthracycline, improves the remission induction rate in high-risk groups and may improve their survival. During this phase of therapy it is also conventional to start CNS therapy with intrathecal methotrexate.

Consolidation

Once complete remission has been achieved, continuation of therapy is required. The consolidation phase is important in the eradication of lymphoblasts that remain undetected. This phase minimizes the development of drug cross-resistance by the use of several agents and concentrates on sanctuary sites such as the CNS. Long-term neuropsychological sequelae as a result of CNS-directed therapy are of great concern, but the fact remains that up to 50% of children with ALL develop overt CNS involvement if this sanctuary goes untreated. The type of CNS therapy varies with the age and risk group of the patient and includes periodic intrathecal chemotherapy with methotrexate with or without other drugs, intravenous methotrexate, and cranial irradiation. For nearly 2 decades cranial or cranial-spinal irradiation was felt to be the most effective form of pre-

TABLE 4. **Sample Approach to Treatment of Acute Lymphocytic Leukemia**

Induction (1 month)	Consolidation (3 Months)	Delayed Intensification (2 Months)	Maintenance (Males, 32 Months) (Females, 20 Months)
PRED VCR L'ASP IT MTX	PRED VCR 6 MP IT MTX PO MTX	DEX VCR L'ASP DOX CPM 6 TG ARA-C IT MTX	PRED VCR 6 MP IT MTX PO MTX

Abbreviations: PRED = prednisone; VCR = vincristine; L'ASP = L'Asparaginase; IT MTX = intrathecal methotrexate; 6 MP = 6-mercaptopurine; PO MTX = oral methotrexate; DEX = dexamethasone; DOX = doxorubicin; CPM = cyclophosphamide; 6 TG = 6-thioguanine; ARA-C = cytarabine.
Adapted from Children's Cancer Group Protocol No. 1922. Randomized comparison of intravenous vs. oral mercaptopurine and dexamethasone vs. prednisone for favorable and intermediate acute lymphocytic leukemia. Arcadia, CA, Children's Cancer Group (unpublished).

TABLE 5. **Adverse Effects of Drugs Commonly Used to Treat Acute Leukemia**

Drug	Toxicity
Vincristine (Oncovin)	Jaw pain, alopecia, peripheral neuropathy, constipation, SIADH, cellulitis with extravasation
Prednisone	Hyperglycemia, hypertension, increased appetite and weight gain, fluid retention, mood changes, myopathy, cushingoid features
L-Asparaginase (Elspar)	Anaphylaxis, hyperglycemia, coagulation defects, pancreatitis
Methotrexate	Nausea, rash, stomatitis, hepatic toxicity, myelosuppression
6-Mercaptopurine (Purinethol)	Myelosuppression, hepatic toxicity, cholestasis
Doxorubicin (daunorubicin)	Nausea, myelosuppression, cardiomyopathy, alopecia, stomatitis, cellulitis with extravasation
Cyclophosphamide (Cytoxan)	Nausea, myelosuppression, alopecia, stomatitis, hemorrhagic cystitis, pulmonary fibrosis, SIADH
Cytarabine (Cytosar-U)	Nausea, myelosuppression, diarrhea, hepatic toxicity, stomatitis
Thioguanine	Nausea, myelosuppression, hepatic toxicity
VP-16 (etoposide) (VePesid)	Nausea, myelosuppression, hypotension, allergic reactions, alopecia, peripheral neuropathy, stomatitis, hepatic toxicity

Abbreviations: SIADH = syndrome of inappropriate secretion of antidiuretic hormone.

symptomatic CNS therapy. However, a CCG randomized study recently found that cranial irradiation is not essential for CNS treatment in children in lower-risk categories, and these patients could be successfully treated with intrathecal methotrexate alone. Children in higher-risk categories need additional CNS protection with aggressive combinations of intrathecal chemotherapy, intravenous methotrexate, and/or cranial irradiation.

Delayed Intensification

A German Berlin-Frankfurt-Münster (BFM) study as well as a CCG randomized trial have shown that some form of intensification during the first 6 months of therapy is of benefit to both high- and low-risk groups and is associated with a 15% improvement in the 5-year event-free survival in those less than 10 years of age at diagnosis. Many intensification schedules of differing complexity and composition have been designed and include such drugs as those listed in Table 4. This phase is usually given after an approximately 2-month period of maintenance-type therapy.

Maintenance

Initial therapy protocols for ALL, which consisted of combination chemotherapy for only 12 to 15 months, were associated with a high relapse rate after completion of therapy. Strong evidence now exists that continuing treatment with mercaptopurine and methotrexate for a period of at least 2 years from diagnosis is beneficial. ALL appears to be unique in

this requirement for long-term therapy, and it is felt that maintenance therapy not only suppresses leukemic growth, but also provides continuing leukemic cytoreduction of ALL cells that cycle slowly without permitting emergence of drug-resistant clones. Additional pulses of vincristine and prednisone during this phase may also decrease the relapse rate. Therapy is continued for at least 20 months in females and 32 months in males, and CCG has found that 3 years of therapy is equivalent to 5 years of therapy.

Infants and Adolescents

Children of less than 1 year of age as well as those over 10 years have a poorer outcome. Infants often present with very high WBC counts, significant thrombocytopenia, hepatosplenomegaly, and CNS involvement. Blast cells often express myeloid antigens. There is also a high incidence of associated chromosomal abnormalities; the most common are t(4;11) or other translocations involving 11q23. Treatment for infants involves very intensive regimens using multiple drug combinations as well as bone marrow transplantation (BMT) in some cases.

About 20% of children with ALL are over 10 years of age. Adolescents with ALL are more likely to be male, have a higher WBC count, have L2 morphology, and less frequently show hyperdiploidy on chromosomal analysis, all associated with a higher risk of relapse. In addition, adolescents are less compliant with therapy, which may contribute to their poor response. The use of intensive multiagent therapy is also indicated in this subgroup of patients.

Relapse

Therapy for children who relapse continues to be unsatisfactory in a high percentage of cases, and not only are the chances of cure dramatically reduced, but retreatment is often associated with significant morbidity. The most common site of relapse is the bone marrow. Although it may be easy to achieve a second remission in most cases, the chances of a durable remission in patients relapsing during or soon after the completion of therapy are small. Despite therapy attempts with a variety of complex and intensive regimens, very few of these children can be cured with conventional chemotherapy. For these children, BMT is the most effective treatment if they have a histocompatible sibling donor. However, 30% of children who have an isolated bone marrow relapse more than 6 months after the completion of therapy can achieve a prolonged remission with intensive chemotherapy and a second course of CNS therapy.

Even with presymptomatic CNS treatment, between 5 and 10% of children with ALL develop CNS leukemia. In general, a patient who experiences a CNS relapse has a poor prognosis; approximately 65% die within 3 years after a CNS relapse.

Testicular relapse in boys with ALL occurs most often in the first year after completion of therapy in approximately 5 to 15% of patients. These children often respond to further chemotherapy and local irradiation, whereas overt testicular relapse during treatment has a poorer prognosis.

Bone Marrow Transplantation

The selection of appropriate patients for BMT is not yet clear. Cases in which there is a clear indication for allogeneic BMT in first remission include those with Ph⁺ ALL, those with t(4;11) ALL, and the 1 to 2% who have none of these features and yet fail to respond to induction therapy. However, alternative preparative regimens that do not include total body irradiation in order to spare the deleterious late effects of radiotherapy in the very young child need to be developed. As stated previously, patients who relapse while on therapy or within 6 months of stopping primary therapy should also be considered for BMT. A 35 to 40% long-term disease-free survival can be achieved in patients in second remission and a 20 to 35% survival for those in third remission. Autologous BMT may be considered for relapse patients who do not have a sibling donor. After successful reinduction, the marrow can be harvested and immunochemical methods can be used to purge the marrow *in vitro* before reinfusion after ablative chemoradiotherapy. This can result in a 3-year disease-free survival of 20 to 25%.

ACUTE MYELOID LEUKEMIA

AML classification into subtypes is determined by the type of leukemic "stem cell" that clonally expands and is based on morphologic considerations, histochemical staining, specific cell surface markers, and occasionally, electron microscopy. The FAB cooperative group classifies AML into seven subgroups: acute myelogenous leukemia (M1 and M2), which accounts for 50 to 70% of children with AML; acute promyelocytic leukemia (M3); acute myelomonocytic leukemia (M4), accounting for 20 to 40% of childhood cases; acute monocytic leukemia (M5); acute erythroleukemia (M6); and acute megakaryocytic leukemia (M7). Approximately 25% of cases with AML can possess lymphoid-associated surface antigens.

Since the advent of chromosome banding studies, it has become evident that up to 50 to 60% of children with AML have chromosome abnormalities. The most frequent abnormalities seen include trisomy 8, t(8;21), t(15;17), the loss of a sex chromosome, and 11q abnormalities. A large study reported by CCG correlating cytogenetic findings and prognosis found that trisomy 8 and t(8;21) were associated with a high complete remission (CR) rate (>90%), whereas abnormalities of chromosome 7 were associated with a low CR rate (28%). Further studies of cytogenetic analyses may more precisely classify patients into distinct clinical and hematologic subgroups with differing prognoses and responses to therapy.

The cause of AML in humans is unknown, and the vast majority of children with AML have no obvious predisposing factors. However, as with ALL, certain inherited disorders and congenital conditions associated with chromosome instability predispose patients to AML. These include Down's syndrome, Fanconi's anemia, Bloom's syndrome, Kostmann's syndrome, and Diamond-Blackfan anemia. Exposure to certain drugs (benzene, alkylating agents) and ionizing radiation are also predisposing factors. Children with preleukemic syndromes such as myelodysplasia, chronic myelomonocytic leukemia, and monosomy 7 are also at risk for the development of AML. The clinical course of these syndromes is variable, but nearly 90% ultimately develop AML, most within a few months to a few years of diagnosis.

Contrary to what has been found in ALL, many pediatric and adult studies have failed to identify consistent prognostic factors for childhood AML.

Treatment

The treatment of AML has slowly improved over the past 15 years, and modern intensive chemotherapy, BMT, and advances in supportive care have all contributed to the improved outlook for children with AML. Transplantation remains the treatment of choice for children with AML in first remission, and 45 to 60% of those with a matched sibling or parent donor achieve long-term remissions. For the remaining children without matches, intensive chemotherapy after induction can lead to long-term remissions in 25 to 50% of individuals. The benefits of maintenance therapy after intensive consolidation are still widely debated.

Induction

Two important principles have been established regarding induction therapy for childhood AML: combination chemotherapy is more effective than single agents, and drug dosages must be high enough to achieve bone marrow aplasia for best results. The two most effective drugs for remission induction appear to be daunorubicin (Cerubidine), an anthracycline, and cytarabine (ara-C), an antimetabolite. Recent regimens have added other drugs, such as 6-thioguanine, steroids, and epipodophyllotoxins such as etoposide (VePesid), in hopes to improve induction success rates. During induction, two cycles of therapy including these drugs are given 6 days apart regardless of the degree of myelosuppression already present. This "intensive timing" has improved remission rates to 80 to 85% and leads to an improved event-free survival rate at 3 years. The 15 to 20% of children in whom induction fails either have drug-resistant leukemia or die of hemorrhage, infection, or leukostasis.

Intensification

Without further therapy after induction more than 90% of children relapse within 1 year. Trials in CCG are assessing the efficacy of three different approaches during intensification: allogeneic BMT versus autologous BMT versus non-marrow-ablative aggressive chemotherapy. If a matched sibling donor is available, allogeneic transplantation is used for (1) patients in first complete remission, (2) patients in whom initial induction therapy fails, and (3) patients who have relapsed and are in either untreated first relapse or second remission. Because only one-third of children are likely to have a matched sibling donor, the use of autologous transplant with *in vitro* purged marrow in first remission is being evaluated, and preliminary results suggest a similar disease-free survival. The intensive chemotherapy arm revolves around the use of higher doses of ara-C.

Presymptomatic Central Nervous System Therapy

Previous studies have shown that without specific presymptomatic CNS therapy, isolated CNS relapse can occur in up to 20% of children with AML. The majority of patients with CNS relapse develop a subsequent bone marrow relapse. Current protocols consist of intrathecal ara-C given periodically.

Relapse

Limited success had been seen in children who relapse or fail initial induction therapy. Several intense regimens have been used in these patients; however, second remissions maintained with chemotherapy are relatively brief. Autologous or allogeneic BMT offers somewhat better long-term survival in relapsed patients.

LATE EFFECTS OF THERAPY

With the aggressive use of multimodal therapy, more children than ever are being cured of leukemia. Current estimates suggest that by the year 2000, one in every 5500 persons less than 35 years of age in the United States will be a survivor of childhood leukemia. Unfortunately, these cures are often at the expense of long-term physical and psychosocial sequelae that can affect the patient's quality of life. Potential late sequelae can involve almost any organ system but can be predicted, in part, by the chemotherapy or radiation that individuals may have received as well as their age at the time of treatment. Table 6 lists the potential long-term deleterious effects of therapy for acute leukemia. All health care professionals involved in caring for leukemia survivors need to be alert to the possible toxicities likely to be encountered and should provide anticipatory guidance and surveillance depending on the specific therapy and history of each patient.

Cranial irradiation therapy in childhood ALL has been associated with adverse neuropsychological effects. The risk of long-term cognitive defects increases with the increasing dose of cranial irradiation and with the decreasing age of the patient at the time of therapy. The incidence of neuropsychological sequelae has varied from 30 to 78%; however, most studies have found that nonverbal skills are the most frequently and severely affected, in particular memory tasks. Cranial irradiation has also been associated with growth failure during and after treatment and with thyroid disease, including thyroid malignancies.

TABLE 6. **Potential Late Effects of Therapy**

Altered growth and/or development	Impaired cognitive development
Cardiac abnormalities	Osteoporosis and/or other bony abnormalities
Cataracts	
Delayed sexual maturation	Psychosocial difficulties
	Renal abnormalities
Hepatitis and/or cirrhosis	Second tumors
	Thyroid abnormalities
Infertility	

Second malignancies can occur after therapy for acute leukemia in 5 to 10% of long-term survivors. Brain tumors, leukemias, and lymphomas are the most common second malignancies in leukemia survivors. Radiation therapy and leukemogenic antineoplastic drugs such as alkylating agents (cyclophosphamide) and epipodophyllotoxins (etoposide) are felt to be the most important contributing factors.

Delayed sexual maturation as well as sterility in males can be seen after testicular irradiation and can be seen in both genders after therapy with alkylating agents.

Anthracycline-associated congestive heart failure and/or cardiomyopathy has been recognized for a number of years. Most data show that the likelihood of dysfunction is directly associated with the cumulative dose (>500 mg per m^2), the age at the time of treatment, and the length of follow-up. The occurrence of acute toxicity does not necessarily predict long-term effects, and, conversely, late abnormalities can develop in those who show no signs of acute toxicity.

It is becoming readily apparent that the long-term care of the childhood cancer survivors is quickly becoming as complex as the acute treatment. Equally important to the late effects mentioned above are the psychosocial sequelae that may occur, including problems in employment, insurability, and marriage. It is imperative that institutions treating children with childhood malignancies develop long-term follow-up clinics in order to educate clinicians to the needs of cancer survivors, foster an awareness of the needs of the patients, and develop a broad-based evaluation of patients involving multiple subspecialists, social workers, and pediatric oncologists.

CHRONIC LEUKEMIAS

method of
SERGIO A. GIRALT, M.D., and
HAGOP M. KANTARJIAN, M.D.

The University of Texas
M. D. Anderson Cancer Center
Houston, Texas

CHRONIC MYELOGENOUS LEUKEMIA

Clinical Features, Diagnosis, and Natural History

Chronic myelogenous leukemia (CML) is characterized by leukocytosis and the presence of immature white blood cells (WBCs) in the peripheral blood with all maturation stages present. Bone marrow examination reveals a hypercellular marrow with myeloid hyperplasia. With conventional cytogenetic analysis and sensitive molecular techniques, the Philadelphia chromosome is found in more than 95% of the patients in either peripheral blood or bone marrow.

The presenting features of CML have changed over time. In the past most patients presented with fatigue, fever, or other features related to leukostasis and splenomegaly (i.e., right upper quadrant pain and focal neurologic abnormalities). In recent studies many patients are diagnosed in an asymptomatic phase as a result of an increased WBC count discovered during a routine physical examination.

The natural history of CML is to inexorably progress from the chronic indolent phase, which is easily controllable with oral chemotherapy, to the transformed accelerated and blastic phases. The definitions of the CML phases are shown in Table 1. The median duration of these phases has traditionally been reported to be 3 years, 6 to 18 months, and 2 to 6 months, respectively. Earlier diagnosis, better supportive care, and newer treatment strategies have had an impact mainly on the duration of the chronic phase. Clinical features at diagnosis help segregate patients into different prognostic categories. These prognostic groups have been useful in patients treated with conventional chemotherapy, interferon-alfa (IFN-α), and bone marrow transplantation (BMT). The prognostic classification used at the M. D. Anderson Cancer Center is summarized in Table 2.

Initial Evaluation and Management of the Newly Diagnosed Patient with Chronic Myelogenous Leukemia

The initial goals of treatment in patients with newly diagnosed CML are to prevent organ damage from leukostasis by rapid reduction of the WBC count with chemotherapy or, if needed, with leukopheresis, and to prevent tumor lysis syndrome by adequate hydration and allopurinol (Zyloprim) therapy. An approach to the work-up and management of patients with newly diagnosed CML is summarized in Table 3.

Long-Term Treatment of Chronic Myelogenous Leukemia

The mainstay of therapy for CML had been conventional chemotherapy with hydroxyurea (Hydrea) or busulfan (Myleran) to control the WBC count and the symptoms generated by the myeloid hyperplasia and splenomegaly. These therapies are successful for a variable period of time, but the disease always progresses to the blastic phase, which ultimately kills the patient.

High-dose chemoradiotherapy followed by syngeneic or allogeneic BMT is able to cure 40 to 70% of the patients with CML. IFN-α can delay the progression to the blastic phase in the majority of patients and may induce long-term durable major cytogenetic remissions in 20 to 25%. The new goals of therapy for

TABLE 1. **Diagnostic Criteria for Chronic Myelogenous Leukemia Phases**

Chronic phase
  None of the criteria for accelerated phase or blastic phase
Accelerated phase
  Established criteria
    Peripheral blasts ≥15%
    Peripheral blasts plus progranulocytes ≥30%
    Basophilia ≥20%
    Platelets <100 × 10⁹/L unrelated to therapy
    Cytogenetic clonal evolution
  Other common criteria
    Increased drug requirement
    Increasing splenomegaly
    Marrow fibrosis
    Marrow or peripheral blasts ≥10%
    Basophils plus eosinophils >10% in blood or bone marrow
    Unexplained fever or bone pain
Blastic phase
  ≥30% blasts in blood or bone marrow
  Extramedullary disease with localized immature blasts

TABLE 2. **Prognostic Staging of Chronic Myelogenous Leukemia**

Stage	No. of Poor Prognostic Features	Median Survival with Interferon Therapy (Months)
1	0 or 1	102
2	2	95
3	≥3	62
4	Any accelerated-phase characteristic	41

Poor Prognosis Characteristics
Age ≥60 years
Spleen ≥10 cm
Blasts ≥3% in blood or bone marrow
Basophils ≥7% in blood or ≥3% in bone marrow
Platelets ≥700 × 10⁹/L

Accelerated-Phase Characteristics
Cytogenetic clonal evolution
Blasts ≥15% in blood
Blasts plus progranulocytes ≥30% in blood
Basophils ≥20% in blood
Platelets <100 × 10⁹/L

TABLE 3. **Evaluation and Management of the Patient Newly Diagnosed with Chronic Myelogenous Leukemia**

Initial Evaluation

History:	Visual disturbances, neurologic symptoms, abdominal pain, weight loss, or fever
Physical examination:	Degree of splenomegaly, signs of leukostasis (visual abnormalities, priapism, focal neurologic deficits), chloromas
Laboratory:	CBC with differential, blood chemistry analysis, coagulation profile, and HLA typing of patient and family
Bone marrow:	Morphology, cytogenetics, molecular studies (BCR/ABL)

Initial Management

1. If there are signs or symptoms of leukostasis: give hydration and allopurinol therapy and emergency leukapheresis, and initiate hydroxyurea (Hydrea) therapy, 3–6 PO gm daily.
2. If WBC count > 20 × 10⁹/L, give hydration and allopurinol therapy and begin hydroxyurea therapy 3–6 gm PO daily and dose-adjust.
3. Treat patients with WBC count >20 × 10⁹/L as outpatients with careful monitoring of WBC count on a weekly or biweekly basis until WBC count < 20 × 10⁹/L, when IFN-α therapy is begun.
4. With patients with WBC <20 × 10⁹/L immediately begin IFN-α-based therapy.

Subsequent Management

1. Allogeneic BMT is offered as initial therapeutic option if appropriate. Other patients are offered IFN-α-based regimens.
2. Periodic follow-up and quarterly bone marrow examination with cytogenetic analysis are done to assess response to IFN-α-based therapy. If there is progression or no cytogenetic response within 12 months, patients are offered allogeneic BMT, or other strategies.

Abbreviations: BCR/ABL = breakpoint cluster region/Abelson oncogene; WBC = white blood cell; IFN-α = interferon-alfa; HLA = human leukocyte antigen; CBC = complete blood count; BMT = bone marrow transplantation.

CML should therefore focus on long-term cytogenetic remissions achieved either through allogeneic BMT or IFN-α therapy, or possibly through new investigational approaches.

Treatment of Chronic Myelogenous Leukemia

Conventional Chemotherapy

Conventional chemotherapy with hydroxyurea or busulfan can control the signs and symptoms of CML in over 80% of patients treated at diagnosis. The most commonly used dose regimens, toxicities, and guidelines for treatment monitoring are outlined in Table 4.

Hydroxyurea therapy is associated with better survival than is busulfan therapy. Busulfan therapy should be limited to patients in whom close monitoring will be difficult or in the elderly patient.

Interferon-Alfa Therapy

Therapy aimed at changing the natural history of CML requires a significant reduction in the leukemic burden as determined by the presence of Ph-positive cells by conventional cytogenetic techniques. The cytogenetic response has been defined according to the percentage of residual Ph-positive cells (Table 5). IFN-α therapy can improve survival in patients with CML by inducing durable major cytogenetic responses and delaying progression of the disease to the blastic phase.

Treatment with IFN-α regimens in CML at the M. D. Anderson Cancer Center consists of a combination of daily IFN-α (5 × 10⁶ U per m² subcutaneously) and low-dose cytarabine (ara-C) (10 mg daily subcutaneously). This combination has been well tolerated and may be more effective than IFN-α alone in inducing hematologic and cytogenetic remissions. Other combinations may include IFN-α plus hydroxyurea. Combining IFN-α and busulfan should be avoided because of unpredictable profound myelosuppression that may occur.

Early side effects of IFN-α therapy such as fever, chills, postnasal drip, and anorexia are usually not dose-limiting. Serious toxicities usually occur late, the most common being fatigue, depression, insomnia, and weight loss. Autoimmune disorders are noted in 5% of patients. Practical guidelines to IFN-α therapy are outlined in Table 6.

TABLE 4. **Guidelines for Treatment of Chronic Myelogenous Leukemia with Hydroxyurea or Busulfan**

	Indications	Usual Dose Schedule	Dose Modifications	Side Effects
Hydroxyurea (Hydrea)	Initial cytoreduction Combination therapy with interferon Sole treatment for patients intolerant to interferon	1.0–5.0 gm PO daily in 2–3 divided doses	50% dose reduction with each 50% reduction of the WBC count; hold when WBC count <2.0 × 10⁹/L	Leukopenia Stomatitis Nausea Diarrhea
Busulfan (Myleran)	Cytoreductive therapy for elderly patients, or patients in whom close monitoring is needed	2.0–6.0 mg PO daily	Discontinue when WBC count <20.0 × 10⁹/L	Prolonged myelosuppression Pulmonary fibrosis Veno-occlusive disease

TABLE 5. **Response Assessment in Chronic Myelogenous Leukemia**

Response	Definition
Complete hematologic response	Normal platelet count, leukocyte count, and differential without splenomegaly
Partial hematologic response	50% decrease in leukocyte count from pretreatment levels to $\leq 20 \times 10^9$/L
	Persistent splenomegaly despite normalization of peripheral blood
Complete cytogenetic response	0% Ph$^+$ cells on cytogenetic analysis
Partial cytogenetic response	1–34% residual Ph$^+$ cells on cytogenetic analysis
Minor cytogenetic response	35–95% residual Ph$^+$ cells on cytogenetic analysis

Allogeneic Bone Marrow Transplantation

Allogeneic BMT is an established curative strategy for patients with CML. Almost 4000 transplants for CML were reported to the International Bone Marrow Transplant Registry (IBMTR) between 1988 and 1990. The numbers will increase with the availability of alternative donors. The best results are reported for young patients (≤ 20 years) transplanted early in chronic phase with a disease-free survival (DFS) of approximately 70%. The overall DFS is 40 to 60% with a 10 to 20% leukemic relapse rate. Allogeneic BMT cures leukemia through two mechanisms: (1) marrow-ablative chemoradiotherapy and (2) immune-mediated graft-versus-leukemia effect.

Allogeneic BMT is associated with serious morbidity and an early mortality rate of 20 to 30%. Major complications include graft-versus-host disease (GVHD), interstitial pneumonitis, serious viral and fungal infections, severe organ damage from the conditioning regimen, and bleeding. Improvements in supportive care have decreased the treatment-related mortality but have not affected relapse rates. Mortality is higher with older age, and many transplant centers limit allogeneic BMT to patients younger than 55 years of age.

Allogeneic BMT is only available to 15 to 25% of patients because of age limitations and human leukocyte antigen (HLA) compatible donor availability. Transplants using alternative donors (i.e., unrelated donor transplantation, mismatched donor transplantation) will make the procedure more available. Referral to specialized centers and careful discussions with patients eligible for transplantation regarding the risks versus benefits of BMT in different CML phases are warranted.

Treatment of Accelerated-Phase Chronic Myelogenous Leukemia

Allogeneic BMT should be considered the first treatment approach for patients if an HLA-identical donor is available. This approach can produce long-term disease control in up to 30% of patients treated. Patients ineligible for allogeneic BMT should be considered candidates for investigational protocols. Patients treated with IFN-α-based regimens have had transient benefit.

Treatment of Blastic-Phase Chronic Myelogenous Leukemia

Allogeneic BMT is the only therapeutic strategy that can achieve long-term disease control in patients

TABLE 6. **Practical Guidelines to Interferon Therapy**

Therapy Initiation
Give hydroxyurea to obtain initial cytoreduction (WBC: 10–20 $\times$ 10^9/L).
Slow dose escalation: 3 $\times$ 10^6 U daily for a week; then 5 $\times$ 10^6 U daily for a week; then 5 $\times$ 10^6 U/m^2 daily or maximally tolerated individual dose.
Educate patients and family members.

Improve Tolerance
Premedicate with acetaminophen.
Give tricyclic antidepressants for neurologic side effects (insomnia, depression, fatigue).

Therapeutic Monitoring
Do CBCs weekly until counts are stable, then biweekly. Do blood chemistry tests monthly. Keep WBC count between 2 and 4 $\times$ 10^9/L and platelets >50 $\times$ 10^9/L.
Do cytogenetic evaluation on bone marrow aspirate every 3 months in first year then every 4–6 months.

Dose Modifications
Interrupt IFN-α therapy for Grades 3–4 toxicities; then resume at 50%.
Reduce dose schedule by 25% for Grade 2 persistent chronic toxicities.
Do not reduce IFN-α dose schedule for "low counts" unless WBC count is <2 $\times$ 10^9/L or platelets <50 $\times$ 10^9/L. A 25% dose reduction is then appropriate.
Hold IFNα therapy for moderate acute intercurrent diseases.

Efficacy Assessment
Hematologic remission at 3–8 months
Cytogenetic response by 12 months
Major cytogenetic response by 18 months

Abbreviatons: WBC = white blood cell; IFN-α = interferon-alfa; CBC = complete blood count.

whose disease has progressed to the blastic phase. Even with this therapy only 10% of the patients are long-term survivors. Leukemic relapse is the most important cause of treatment failure.

Patients unable to undergo allogeneic BMT should be considered for investigational protocols. In patients with myeloid or undifferentiated blastic-phase CML, intensive combination chemotherapy with anthracycline and ara-C produces response rates of 0 to 40%, but the median survival is about 2 to 6 months.

Patients with lymphoid blastic-phase CML have a better prognosis and can be treated with anti–acute lymphocytic leukemia therapy. The combination of vincristine, doxorubicin (Adriamycin), and dexamethasone can induce a second chronic phase in 40 to 50% of patients. The median survival of patients with lymphoid blastic-phase CML is about 9 to 12 months.

Summary

Physicians caring for patients with Ph-positive CML have to choose among various strategies as best treatment options for their patients. Allogeneic BMT offers the greatest potential for cure but is only available to patients younger than 55 years of age with an HLA-compatible donor and is associated with significant morbidity and mortality among older patients.

The majority of patients with CML are ineligible for allogeneic BMT because of either age or lack of a histocompatible donor. IFN-α therapy, either alone or in combination with other agents, should be the treatment of choice. Patients who fail to achieve a meaningful cytogenetic response may continue on this therapy as their best potential approach or may be offered investigational therapies with potential benefit (new agents, autologous stem cell transplantation, mismatched or unrelated donor transplantation).

For patients with an HLA-compatible donor, the timing of BMT remains controversial. Younger patients have a low transplant-related mortality (5 to 10%) and should undergo allogeneic BMT as their initial therapeutic option. Older patients may have up to a 30% transplant-related mortality rate and may be offered a trial of IFN-α-based therapy. Patients who achieve a significant cytogenetic response continue on IFN-α therapy until the response is lost. Patients with late-chronic-phase CML or advanced phases of CML, or those failing IFN-α therapy, should be offered an allogeneic BMT as soon as a donor is available; otherwise investigational options may be considered.

CHRONIC LYMPHOCYTIC LEUKEMIA

Clinical Features, Diagnosis, and Natural History

Chronic lymphocytic leukemia (CLL) is the most common leukemia in the Western world. It is more

frequent in males and has a median age of onset of 55 years. CLL is characterized by the progressive accumulation of mature lymphocytes, and 95% of the cases are of B cell origin (B cell CLL). The malignant cell in CLL has a characteristic immunophenotypic pattern that is useful in differentiating it from other chronic lymphoproliferative disorders. Our current approach to the management of B cell CLL is the focus of this article.

The diagnosis of CLL is made serendipitously in more than 40% of the patients, as a result of an abnormal routine complete blood count (CBC) in an otherwise asymptomatic patient. Fever, weight loss, diffuse adenopathy, history of multiple infections, and splenomegaly are hallmarks of a more advanced stage of the disease. A minority of patients present with symptoms due to autoimmune-induced phenomena (anemia and/or thrombocytopenia) that occur with this disease.

The National Cancer Institute Working Group on CLL has formulated the following diagnostic criteria for CLL:

1. Absolute lymphocytosis of $\geq 5 \times 10^9$ per liter of morphologically mature lymphocytes sustained over a period of at least 4 weeks
2. $\geq 30\%$ lymphocytes in a normocellular or hypercellular bone marrow
3. A monoclonal B cell phenotype with coexpression of CD5 and low levels of surface immunoglobulins

Two staging systems for CLL are routinely used throughout the world. These staging systems segregate patients into different prognostic groups and are useful in making therapeutic decisions. These staging systems are summarized in Table 7. Other prognostic factors useful in CLL include the lymphocyte doubling time, the beta$_2$-microglobulin level, the pattern of bone marrow infiltration (diffuse vs. nodu-

TABLE 7. **Staging Systems for B Cell Chronic Lymphocytic Leukemia**

Stage	Description	Median Survival (Years)
Rai Staging System		
0	Lymphocytosis	>10
1	Lymphocytosis and lymphadenopathy	>8
2	Lymphocytosis and splenomegaly ± lymphadenopathy	6
3	Lymphocytosis and anemia (hemoglobin <11 gm/dL), ± lymphadenopathy or hepatosplenomegaly	2
4	Lymphocytosis and thrombocytopenia (platelets <100 × 10⁹/L) ± anemia, lymphadenopathy, or hepatosplenomegaly	2
Binet Staging System		
A	≤2 lymphoid-bearing areas	>10
B	>2 lymphoid-bearing areas	6
C	Anemia (hemoglobin <10 gm/dL) and/or thrombocytopenia (platelets <100 × 10⁹/L)	2

lar), cytogenetics, and the lactate dehydrogenase level.

The natural history of CLL with conventional therapy is to become increasingly more refractory to therapy. Patients progressively deteriorate from cytopenias and infections. Many patients succumb to infectious complications as a result of the underlying immunodeficiency and hypogammaglobulinemia. Transformation to large cell lymphoma (Richter's transformation) occurs in approximately 10% of the patients and is almost uniformly fatal. New therapeutic modalities are now becoming available that may change the natural history of the disease.

Initial Evaluation and Management of the Patient Newly Diagnosed with Chronic Lymphocytic Leukemia

In contrast to patients with CML, patients with CLL rarely require emergency cytoreductive therapy. Leukostasis occurs rarely, and most patients do not require hospitalization for initial management unless infected. The initial evaluation of patients with CLL is aimed at defining the extent of the disease and determining the need for cytotoxic therapy or other therapeutic maneuvers. A possible approach is summarized in Table 8.

Long-Term Treatment of Chronic Lymphocytic Leukemia

When to Treat

Treatment of CLL with conventional chemotherapy during the early phases of the disease has not improved survival. Therefore the decision to treat needs to be balanced against the potential side effects of therapy. Outside a clinical trial setting the standard indications for treatment of CLL are (1) disease-related symptoms (fever, night sweats, weight loss), (2) progressive cytopenias (immune- and nonimmune-mediated) with progression to advanced stages, (3) bulky lymphadenopathy, (4) massive splenomegaly, (5) short lymphocyte doubling time (≤ 12 months), (6) absolute lymphocyte count $>150 \times 10^9$ per liter, or (7) recurrent infections.

Conventional Chemotherapy

Physicians caring for patients with CLL should encourage their patients to participate in ongoing clinical trials. For patients unwilling to participate in these trials, standard initial therapy consists of oral alkylating agent therapy with or without steroids. Chlorambucil (Leukeran) and cyclophosphamide (Cytoxan) are the most widely used agents. Chlorambucil has a better side effect profile than cyclophosphamide and is considered the therapeutic agent of choice for patients with CLL treated outside a clinical trial. The most common conventional chemotherapeutic regimens used for the treatment of CLL are summarized in Table 9. The response to treatment should be assessed regularly using standard criteria such as those stated in Table 10.

Nucleoside Analogues

Fludarabine monophosphate (Fludara) has recently been approved by the Food and Drug Administration for the treatment of CLL refractory or relapsing after therapy with oral alkylators. It is administered intravenously at a dose of 25 to 30 mg per m^2 daily for 5 days every 3 to 4 weeks. Most common toxicities are myelosuppression and infections, with nausea, vomiting, stomatitis, diarrhea, and peripheral neuropathy occurring in less than 5% of patients. The addition of steroids to fludarabine does not enhance the therapeutic effect but increases the incidence of opportunistic infections.

Frontline therapy of CLL with fludarabine as a

TABLE 8. **Management of the Patient Newly Diagnosed with Chronic Lymphocytic Leukemia**

Initial Evaluation

History:	Abdominal pain, weight loss, fever, bleeding, fatigue, history of recurrent infections, rate of growth of adenopathy, prior blood work
Physical examination:	Extent of lymphadenopathy; degree of splenomegaly; signs of infection, bleeding, or anemia
Laboratory:	CBC with differential; blood chemistry analysis; tests for LDH and beta$_2$ microglobulin levels; coagulation profile; immunophenotyping; and HLA typing.
Bone marrow:	Morphology and immunophenotyping

Initial Management
1. Determine need for therapy (symptoms, stage, lymphocyte doubling time).
2. If WBC count $>200 \times 10^9$/L, consider admission, hydration, allopurinol therapy, and emergent leukopheresis followed by chemotherapy.
3. Treat patients with autoimmune disorders with corticosteroids.

Subsequent Management
1. Patients are encouraged to participate in clinical trials.
2. Patients requiring therapy and ineligible for investigational therapy can receive oral chlorambucil (Leukeran) or other conventional chemotherapeutic regimen.
3. Patients relapsing or refractory to alkylating agents should be considered for allogeneic BMT if eligible or for fludarabine (Fludara) based salvage therapy.
4. There should be a high incidence of suspicion for recurrent infections, hypogammaglobulinemia, immune cytopenias, and transformation

Abbreviations: CBC = complete blood count; LDH = lactate dehydrogenase; HLA = human leukocyte antigen; WBC = white blood cell; BMT = bone marrow transplantation.

TABLE 9. **Chemotherapy Regimens for Chronic Lymphocytic Leukemia**

Chlorambucil + prednisone
  Chlorambucil: 0.3 mg/kg PO daily on Days 1 through 5
  Prednisone: 40 mg/m² PO daily on Days 1 through 5
  Repeat monthly

Cyclophosphamide, vincristine (Oncovin), prednisone (COP)
  Cyclophosphamide: 300 mg/m² PO on Days 1 through 5
  Vincristine: 1 mg/m² IV on Day 1
  Prednisone: 40 mg/m² PO daily on Days 1 through 5
  Repeat monthly

Cyclophosphamide, doxorubicin, vincristine, prednisone (CHOP)
  Cyclophosphamide: 300 mg/m² PO on Days 1 through 5
  Doxorubicin: 25 mg/m² IV on Day 1
  Vincristine: 1 mg/m² IV on Day 1
  Prednisone: 40 mg/m² PO daily on Days 1 through 5
  Repeat monthly

Fludarabine
  Fludarabine: 30 mg/m² IV daily on Days 1 through 5

single agent or in combination should be limited to clinical trials until its superiority over more conventional therapies is demonstrated in this setting.

Other purine analogues such as 2-CDA and deoxycoformicin have also shown activity in CLL, but their use should still be considered investigational.

Bone Marrow Transplantation

Allogeneic BMT can induce complete remissions and long-term disease control in selected patients with relapsing or refractory CLL. This treatment option should be considered for all patients under 55 years of age with advanced refractory CLL.

Special Problems in Chronic Lymphocytic Leukemia

Immune-Mediated Cytopenias

Autoantibodies can be detected in up to 75% of patients with CLL. The incidence increases with the

TABLE 10. **NCI Criteria for Response Assessment in Chronic Lymphocytic Leukemia**

Site	CR	PR
Physical examination		
Nodes	None	≥50% decrease
Liver or spleen	Not palpable	≥50% decrease
Symptoms	None	Not applicable
Peripheral blood		
Granulocytes	≥1.5 × 10⁹/L	≥1.5 × 10⁹/L or >50% improvement above baseline
Platelets	≥100 × 10⁹/L	≥100 × 10⁹/L or >50% improvement above baseline
Hemoglobin	>11 gm/dL	>11 gm/dL or >50% improvement above baseline
Lymphocytes	≤4.0 × 10⁹/L	≥50% decrease from baseline
Bone marrow		
Lymphocytes	<30%	Not applicable

Abbreviations: R = complete remission; NCI = National Cancer Institute; PR = partial remission.

disease stage. The diagnosis of autoimmune hemolytic anemias and immune thrombocytopenia in patients with CLL is similar to that in non-CLL patients. Treatment with steroids (i.e., prednisone 60 to 100 mg daily) should be instituted once the diagnosis is suspected with slow tapering after a clinical response is obtained. Steroid-refractory patients have occasionally responded to splenectomy or intravenous immunoglobulin therapy.

Pure red cell aplasia occurs in less than 1% of patients with CLL and is characterized by severe anemia, reticulocytopenia, and less than 0.5% mature erythroblasts in the bone marrow. Cyclosporine has been of benefit in this setting. Other autoimmune diseases associated with CLL include systemic lupus erythematosus, rheumatoid arthritis, and Sjögren's syndrome.

Recurrent Infections

Infections are an important cause of morbidity and mortality in patients with CLL. The susceptibility of these patients is in part due to markedly decreased levels of serum immunoglobulins G, A, and M (IgG, IgA, IgM). Replacement therapy with intravenous immunoglobulin (500 mg per kg every 3 to 4 weeks for 12 months) has been shown to decrease subsequent infections in patients with a prior history of a major bacterial infection or with very low baseline IgG levels. Lower dosages (200 to 250 mg per kg monthly) have also been used with equal therapeutic benefit and lower cost.

Disease Transformation

Transformation to large cell lymphoma (Richter's transformation) occurs in 10% of patients with CLL and is usually accompanied by fever, increasing adenopathy, and hepatosplenomegaly. Response to combination chemotherapy is poor, and the median survival ranges from 2 to 4 months after transformation. Rarely (2 to 5%) does CLL transform to prolymphocytic leukemia characterized by the presence of 30% prolymphocytes, to acute leukemia, or to multiple myeloma.

Summary

Therapy for CLL is evolving; the discovery of new active agents capable of inducing complete remissions and the increasing use of allogeneic BMT for this disease may change the natural history of the disease. Patients should be encouraged to participate in clinical trials to further define the role of these new therapies. Patients who require therapy and are unwilling or ineligible to participate in investigational protocols should receive conventional therapy with chlorambucil; fludarabine should be reserved for the time of relapse. Patients younger than 55 years with refractory or relapsing disease should be considered for allogeneic BMT if a histocompatible donor is available.

NON–HODGKIN'S LYMPHOMAS

method of
BRUCE D. CHESON, M.D.
National Cancer Institute
Bethesda, Maryland

The non-Hodgkin's lymphomas (NHLs) are a heterogeneous group of lymphoid malignancies that differ with respect to their histologic, immunologic, molecular biologic, and clinical characteristics, and to their outcome with therapy.

DIAGNOSIS

An accurate diagnosis requires excision of a lymph node and its evaluation by an experienced pathologist. If a definitive diagnosis cannot be made, a repeat biopsy may be needed. A needle biopsy is generally not adequate since it may not provide sufficient information on the malignant cell type or architecture of the node. In 10 to 25% of patients with NHL there may be different histologic findings in different nodes (discordant), different histologic findings in the same node (composite), or a transformation of a low-grade to a high-grade NHL. For example, of patients with large cell lymphoma in the lymph nodes and bone marrow involvement, 40 to 50% may have a small cleaved cell lymphoma in the bone marrow. Although response rates may be unaffected by the discordance, late relapses are more common with involvement of the bone marrow of the low-grade histologic type.

CLASSIFICATION

The most commonly used classification of the NHL is the Working Formulation (WF), which was introduced more than a decade ago as a means of improving communication among the various classification schemes in use at that time. The WF organized NHL into three histologic grades on the basis of nodal architecture, cell type, and clinical behavior (Table 1). Although still useful, the WF has serious deficiencies. There are histologic types within grades that differ in their clinical course and treatment. A more practical approach is to separate the NHLs into those types that are indolent, that is, they are associated with a relatively long survival, but with no plateau of the survival curve, and those that are aggressive, i.e., a short natural history if untreated but a significant cure rate with current therapy.

The WF also does not incorporate the immunophenotypic or biologic features of the lymphomas. Moreover, new clinical and pathologic entities have been identified that are not included in the WF and account for a significant proportion of cases. Mantle cell lymphomas (MCLs), previously called "intermediately differentiated lymphomas," are derived from lymphocytes in the mantle zone of the lymphoid follicles. They have been misdiagnosed in the past as chronic lymphocytic leukemia or small cleaved cell NHL since their histologic appearance is intermediate between that of a small lymphocyte and that of a small cleaved cell. Distinguishing features of MCLs are the expression of CD5$^+$ and the expression of the *bcl*-1 oncogene.

Mucosa-associated lymphoid tissue lymphomas (MALTomas) and monocytoid B cell lymphomas are derived from cells in the marginal zone of lymph nodes and probably represent variants of the same disease. MALTomas generally involve the lung or the gastrointestinal tract, and more than 90% of gastric MALTomas have been associated with infection with *Helicobacter pylori*; in several reported cases they have been responsive to antibiotic therapy. Monocytoid B cell lymphomas commonly involve the salivary glands. Both disorders have a high incidence of Sjögren's syndrome. The natural history of the marginal zone lymphomas is more consistent with indolent NHL.

Sclerosing B cell lymphoma of the mediastinum is a large cell lymphoma characteristically seen in young women. Significant peripheral lymphadenopathy is often absent, but unusual extranodal sites may be involved, including the kidneys and adrenal glands. The *c-myc* rearrangement is present in a substantial number of patients. A significant proportion of these patients are curable with intensive multiagent chemotherapy regimens.

The peripheral T cell lymphomas are a heterogeneous group of diseases that are usually of large cell or mixed small lymphocytic and large cell histologic type. Cutaneous T cell lymphomas (i.e., mycosis fungoides) and T cell lymphoblastic lymphomas (LBLs) are not included in this category.

Angiocentric lymphoproliferative lesion (AIL) is characterized by vascular invasion and necrosis. It may involve the lungs (lymphomatoid granulomatosis) or nasopharynx and sinuses (lethal midline granuloma) and is graded, by the number of large lymphoid cells, from "suspicious," which may not initially require aggressive treatment, to an overtly malignant lymphoma that requires systemic chemotherapy or interferon-alpha therapy.

Anaplastic large cell lymphoma (Ki-1) is an immunoblastic lymphoma characterized by large, pleomorphic cells that express CD30 (Ki-1). Almost all patients have lym-

TABLE 1. **Classification of Non-Hodgkin's Lymphomas According to the Working Formulation**

Grade	Subtype	Frequency (%)
Low	Small lymphocytic, diffuse	6
	Follicular small cleaved cell	16
	Follicular mixed small cleaved and large cell	6
Intermediate	Follicular large cell	3
	Diffuse small cleaved cell	6
	Diffuse mixed small cleaved and large cell	5
	Diffuse large cell	26
High	Immunoblastic	9
	Lymphoblastic	1
	Small noncleaved cell	
	Burkitt's	1
	Non-Burkitt's type	1

phadenopathy, with extranodal disease in half of the patients, often limited to the skin. Although the bone marrow is generally not involved, most patients are Stage III or IV at diagnosis. The diagnosis may be confused with Hodgkin's disease since typical Reed-Sternberg cells may be seen; malignant histiocytosis; or even anaplastic carcinoma. One-half to two-thirds of the patients express a T cell phenotype, almost one-third express a B cell phenotype, and the remainder are unclassifiable. Although Ki-1 NHL may be quiescent and spontaneous regression may occur, the disease more often behaves as an aggressive lymphoma. Almost half the patients achieve a complete remission with intensive chemotherapy. The 2-year survival rate is 75%, but only 20 to 40% are free of disease.

Adult T cell leukemia-lymphoma (ATLL) is an uncommon form of lymphoma initially described in Japan and the Caribbean, although cases have also been identified in the United States. It is associated with infection with the human T cell lymphotropic virus Type I (HTLV-I) retrovirus. ATLL exhibits a wide clinical spectrum from an indolent disease to a highly aggressive lymphoma characterized by hypercalcemia, bone disease, and central nervous system, skin, and blood involvement. Responses are transient even with aggressive multiagent chemotherapy.

STAGING

Careful clinical staging determines the extent of involvement of the lymphoma, provides prognostic information, and helps the physician select the most appropriate form of therapy. The NHLs are generally staged according to the Ann Arbor classification, similar to that for Hodgkin's disease. The Ann Arbor classification has been modified to include bulk greater than 10 cm in the single widest diameter, or a mediastinal mass greater than one-third the maximum thoracic diameter. A staging laparotomy is generally not performed in NHL because these tend to be disseminated diseases at the time of presentation, often with malignant cells circulating in the peripheral blood (particularly the NHLs with indolent histologic findings), and most require chemotherapy as part of their treatment. It is more useful to categorize patients with NHL as having limited (nonbulky Stage I or IIA) or advanced (IIB, bulky Stage II, III or IV) disease.

The appropriate evaluation of a patient with NHL should include a careful history to elicit the presence of symptoms referable to lymphoma, which are associated with a poor prognosis: fevers without apparent infection, chills, or unexplained weight loss greater than 10% of body weight (Table 2). During the physical examination, the size and distribution of enlarged lymph nodes should be precisely recorded, as well as liver and spleen size. Laboratory evaluation should include a complete blood count with careful examination of the peripheral blood smear for the presence of circulating lymphoma cells; serum chemistry studies, including tests for calcium levels; kidney and liver function studies, particularly measurements of lactate dehydrogenase (LDH) levels, which also correlate with tumor burden. A test for serum beta₂-microglobulin levels may also have prognostic value. Bilateral bone marrow biopsies are needed to evaluate the possibility of bone marrow involvement. A chest radiograph and computed tomography (CT) scan as well as an abdominal CT scan should be performed. Neither a gallium scan nor a lymphangiogram, although useful in Hodgkin's disease, is part of the routine management of NHL. In the absence of physical signs or symptoms, a lumbar puncture is not necessary in the low- or intermediate-grade NHL; however, it is an important

TABLE 2. **Staging of Patients with Non-Hodgkin's Lymphoma**

History (with particular attention to constitutional symptoms)
Physical examination
Chest x-ray examination
CT scans of chest, abdomen, and pelvis
CBC with platelet count
Examination of peripheral blood smear for lymphoma cells
Bilateral bone marrow biopsies
Serum creatinine, BUN, transaminase, lactate dehydrogenase, and calcium level tests
Beta₂-microglobulin assay
Serum protein electrophoresis, beta₂-microglobulin
HIV testing (for patients with intermediate- or high-grade NHL)

Abbrevations: CT = computed tomography; CBC = complete blood cell count; BUN = blood urea nitrogen; HIV = human immunodeficiency virus; NHL = non-Hodgkin's lymphoma.

part of the evaluation of patients with lymphoblastic lymphoma and small noncleaved cell NHL.

Specific clinical situations may require additional staging studies. For example, the cerebrospinal fluid (CSF) should be examined in patients with involvement of the peripheral blood, bone marrow, or sinuses by intermediate- or high-grade NHL because of a greater than 50% likelihood of central nervous system (CNS) involvement.

INDOLENT NHL

The indolent NHLs include those with low-grade histologic findings and diffuse small cleaved cell NHL (Table 3). These B cell disorders have a relatively prolonged median survival in the range of 5 to 10 years. Waldenström's macroglobulinemia and MCLs are included with the indolent lymphomas; however, their survival tends to be shorter: 4 to 5 and 2 to 3 years, respectively.

In most patients, indolent NHL eventually transforms to an aggressive, high-grade NHL, generally presenting with rapidly enlarging lymphadenopathy, hepatosplenomegaly, a rising LDH level, and disease-related symptoms. In that clinical setting a repeat lymph node biopsy should be performed.

Biology

In more than 80% of follicular lymphomas, overexpression of the *bcl*-2 oncogene can be demonstrated. The *bcl*-2 oncogene is responsible for normal B and T cell development as well as homeostasis of normal

TABLE 3. **"Indolent" Non-Hodgkin's Lymphomas**

Low-Grade (per Working Formulation)
Diffuse small lymphocytic
Follicular, small cleaved cell
Follicular, mixed small cleaved and large cell
Intermediate-Grade
Diffuse small cleaved cell
Others
Marginal zone (MALT, monocytoid B cell)
Mantle cell
Waldenström's macroglobulinemia

Abbreviation: MALT = mucosa-associated lymphoid tissue.

tissues such as the gastrointestinal epithelium and skin. It confers longevity on tissues by interfering with apoptosis, or programmed cell death. The *bcl*-2 oncogene may also be a mechanism of acquired drug resistance in malignant lymphocytes. Overexpression of the *bcl*-2 gene may occur in patients with large cell NHLs, some of which have most likely transformed from a low-grade NHL. Mutations of p53 appear to correlate with aggressive transformation.

Prognostic Factors

Clinical and laboratory features that separate patients into risk groups include age, clinical stage, histologic findings, performance status, LDH levels, bone marrow involvement, and molecular biologic findings. For a classification to be clinically meaningful, however, therapies should be differentially effective for each of the risk groups, which is often not the case.

Therapy

Only 10 to 15% of indolent NHLs are considered localized after careful staging. Appropriate therapy for patients with Stages I or IIA disease includes subtotal nodal irradiation, total lymphoid irradiation, or a combination of radiation therapy and chemotherapy (Figure 1). At 10 years, approximately 60% of these patients remain in remission, and more than 80% are still alive.

Between 30 and 70% of patients with advanced-stage disease achieve a remission with conventional forms of therapy, depending on how carefully staging is carried out. Remissions generally take a year or longer to occur and last 1 to 3 years. Complete clinical remissions are uncommon, and molecular remissions are rare.

Conventional treatments have included single alkylating agents (e.g., chlorambucil or cyclophosphamide), combinations of alkylating agents with vincristine and prednisone (e.g., CVP [cyclophosphamide, vincristine, prednisone]), or radiation therapy. Combination regimens may be useful in patients who require a more rapid response; however, there is no apparent survival advantage from any of these approaches. The incurability of patients with advanced-stage indolent NHL has led to the opinion that it is appropriate to defer treatment of these patients,

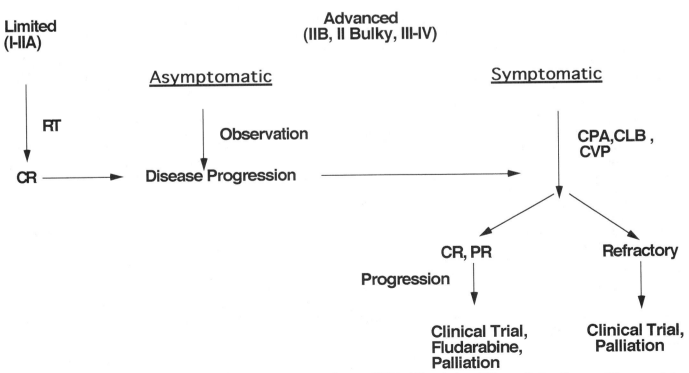

Figure 1. Therapeutic approach to indolent non-Hodgkin's lymphomas (NHL). *Abbreviations*: RT = radiation therapy; CR = complete remission; CPA = cyclophosphamide; CLB = chlorambucil; CVP = cyclophosphamide, vincristine, prednisone; PR = partial remission.

particularly if they are elderly or ill, until there are clear indications for treatment: fevers, chills, weight loss, cosmetic or mechanical problems with enlarged nodes, or hepatosplenomegaly. Treatment should be discontinued when the maximum response has been achieved to minimize the potential risks of cumulative toxicity.

More intensive regimens such as CHOP (cyclophosphamide, hydroxydaunomycin [doxorubicin], Oncovin [vincristine], prednisone) as used in a large trial conducted by the Southwest Oncology Group failed to demonstrate an advantage over historical controls treated with less intensive chemotherapy. A National Cancer Institute study that randomized patients either to no initial therapy at presentation ("watch and wait") or to the intensive ProMACE–MOPP (prednisone, methotrexate, Adriamycin [doxorubicin], cyclophosphamide, etoposide–mechlorethamine, Oncovin [vincristine], procarbazine, prednisone) regimen with total nodal irradiation in those who achieved a complete response failed to identify a difference in survival.

Relapsed Disease

Once a patient with an indolent NHL relapses, the median survival is 5.2 years if the first complete remission was at least a year, 4.6 years in those with a partial remission longer than a year, but only 2.6 years in those with a complete or partial remission lasting less than a year. Although subsequent remissions may be achieved, they are less durable. Therefore, those with brief initial responses should be considered candidates for clinical trials evaluating new approaches to therapy.

Therapeutic options for patients with an indolent NHL who are refractory to initial therapy or who have relapsed after an initial response are unsatisfactory. In general, patients without signs or symptoms referable to their disease are not treated because the potential for benefit may be less than the side effects of the treatment. If treatment is indicated, patients should be considered for a clinical trial. If that is not an option, palliative treatment with an alkylating agent or other single active agent is acceptable. One of the most active agents in the treatment of indolent NHL is fludarabine (Fludara), a purine analogue that achieves responses in 50 to 60% of relapsed patients, with responses often lasting a year or longer.

A related drug, 2-chlorodeoxyadenosine, or cladribine (CdA) (Leustatin), achieves similar response rates, but these do not appear to be as durable. Both fludarabine and CdA are very active in previously untreated patients. Side effects of both drugs include myelosuppression and immunosuppression with an increased susceptibility to infections, notably with opportunistic organisms. Neurotoxicity with the recommended doses is sporadic, mild to moderate in severity, and generally reversible. Combinations of these drugs with other active agents are in development.

Radiation therapy is generally only considered for patients with limited disease or in the palliative setting (e.g., relief of symptoms, ureteral obstruction).

INTERMEDIATE–GRADE NHL

An analysis of data from 2031 patients with large cell NHL treated with an anthracycline-containing regimen was the basis for the International Index. Patients can be classified into four risk groups based on their number of adverse features: age, stage, LDH level, performance status, and number of extranodal sites. Overall 5-year survival rates were 73, 51, 43, and 26%. The 5-year survival rates in patients 60 years of age or younger were 83, 69, 46, and 32%. The increased risk in the poorer-outcome group resulted from both lower response rates and higher rates of relapse.

Whether patients with T cell lymphomas have a worse prognosis than those with B cell lymphomas is a subject of controversy. When patients with a similar age, performance status, and histologic picture are compared, the outcome of the two types appears to be similar.

More biologically relevant factors are also being examined, such as the Ki-67 proliferation index, adhesion molecules, regulators of immune surveillance, acquired drug resistance, and others. In about 30% of patients with diffuse large cell NHL, *bcl*-6 gene rearrangements occur and may be associated with a favorable outcome.

Therapy

Only 20 to 30% of patients with intermediate- or high-grade NHL present with early-stage disease. Patients with Stage I disease after careful staging have more than an 80% likelihood of cure with either radiation therapy or chemotherapy (Figure 2). Between one-third and one-half of patients with Stage II disease relapse. Generally, three to four courses of multiagent chemotherapy are given, followed by involved field radiation. However, various combinations of chemotherapy and radiation therapy are currently being evaluated to determine the optimal strategy. This approach may be modified in certain situations, such as in patients with salivary gland tumors, who may be treated with chemotherapy alone to preserve gland function.

The optimal strategy for patients with primary gastric lymphoma is controversial. The standard approach is a gastrectomy followed by either radiation therapy or chemotherapy. Although those with bulky disease, bleeding, or signs or symptoms of perforation may first require surgery to reduce the risk of tumor necrosis and perforation, recent data suggest that many other patients can be managed without surgery, using combination chemotherapy. The association of marginal zone lymphomas of the stomach with *H. pylori* infection (see previous discussion) has led to an evaluation of antibiotic therapy in these patients.

Therapeutic Approach to NHL

Aggressive

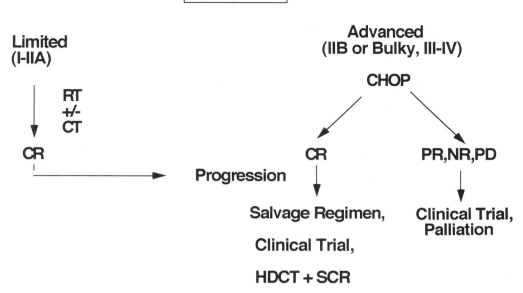

Figure 2. Therapeutic approach to aggressive NHL (intermediate-grade and immunoblastic). *Abbreviations*: RT = radiation therapy; CT = chemotherapy; CR = complete remission; CHOP = cyclophosphamide, doxorubicin, vincristine, prednisone; PR = partial remission; NR = no response; PD = progressive disease; HDCT + SCR = high-dose chemotherapy with stem cell rescue.

The first major advance in the therapy of advanced-stage intermediate-grade NHL was the introduction of doxorubicin into combination with other agents to form CHOP (see previous definition). A series of more intensive regimens appeared to achieve a higher response rate and longer disease-free survival than CHOP. However, a large randomized study conducted by the Southwest Oncology Group with collaboration from the Eastern Cooperative Oncology Group was unable to identify any benefit for m-BACOD (methotrexate, bleomycin, Adriamycin [doxorubicin], cyclophosphamide, Oncovin [vincristine], dexamethasone), Pro-MACE–CYTABOM (cytarabine, bleomycin, Oncovin, mechlorethamine), or MACOP-B (methotrexate, Adriamycin, cyclophosphamide, Oncovin, prednisone, bleomycin) compared with CHOP, which was also the least toxic and, therefore, remains the standard (see Fig. 2). Six to eight courses are generally administered, with no evidence for benefit from continuing therapy. Complete remissions can be achieved in 50 to 70% of patients with any of these regimens, and 30 to 40% of patients are cured.

Therapy for Relapsed Disease

Patients whose disease fails to be cured with initial therapy remain a difficult challenge. Options include a clinical trial of a new agent, a salvage chemotherapy regimen, bone marrow transplantation in appropriate cases (see below), or palliative care. Participation in a clinical trial should be encouraged. Commonly used salvage regimens include MIME (mitoguazone, ifosfamide, methotrexate, etoposide), IMVP-16 (ifosfamide, methotrexate, etoposide),

DHAP (dexamethasone, high-dose cytarabine, Platinol [cisplatin]), ESHAP (etoposide, Solu-Medrol, high-dose cytarabine, cisplatin), and EPOCH (continuous infusion of etoposide, Oncovin [vincristine], and doxorubicin with bolus cyclophosphamide and oral prednisone) (Table 4). Each of these programs achieves responses in 40 to 60% of relapsed patients, less often in refractory cases, with a median duration of response of 12 to 15 months, and no plateau on the survival curve. Radiation therapy may be needed for control of pain or to relieve an obstruction.

Bone Marrow Transplantation and High-Dose Chemotherapy

Autologous bone marrow or peripheral blood stem cell transplantation has been used for NHL more often than allogeneic transplantation, and generally in patients with relapsed rather than refractory dis-

TABLE 4. **Salvage Chemotherapy Regimens for Relapsed and Refractory Aggressive Non-Hodgkin's Lymphoma**

DHAP: dexamethasone, high-dose cytarabine, Platinol (cisplatin)
ESHAP: etoposide, Solu-Medrol, high-dose cytarabine, cisplatin
IMVP-16: ifosfamide, methotrexate, etoposide
MIME: mitoguazone, ifosfamide, methotrexate, etoposide; or methotrexate, ifosfamide, Novantrone (mitoxantrone), etoposide (also called MINE)
FND: fludarabine, mitoxantrone, dexamethasone
EPOCH: infusional etoposide, doxorubicin, and Oncovin (vincristine), with bolus cyclophosphamide and oral prednisone

ease. Of patients with an intermediate-grade NHL who are still sensitive to standard-dose chemotherapy, 40% may achieve long-term disease-free survival with high-dose chemotherapy and autologous stem cell support; 15 to 20% of those with a resistant NHL relapse, and virtually no patient with primary refractory disease benefits from this therapy. However, whether high-dose therapy is better than other salvage approaches in similar patients is an unanswered question. Preliminary data from a randomized trial (the Parma study) suggest superiority for autologous transplantation. There is no apparent benefit from high-dose therapy to consolidate an initial complete remission or in those patients who respond slowly to induction chemotherapy.

Initial results suggesting long-term benefit from high-dose therapy in patients with indolent NHL have deteriorated with longer follow-up. Whether there is meaningful clinical benefit from this approach is still unclear. Data for patients treated in first complete remission also do not support long-term benefit in the majority of cases. This form of therapy should be restricted to clinical trials.

A newly recognized complication of high-dose chemotherapy for lymphomas is secondary myelodysplasia and acute myeloid leukemia, which may occur with a frequency of 6 to 18%.

Biologic Therapies

The largest experience with biologic therapies has been in patients with low-grade NHL treated with interferon-alpha (IFN-α).* Responses occur in 20 to 30% of patients, but less than 10% of these are complete and they are not durable. IFN-α used in combination with other chemotherapy drugs, or as a form of maintenance, does not improve the response rate, but there is an apparent prolongation of disease-free survival. Unfortunately, the data do not support a prolongation of overall survival.

Monoclonal antibodies directed at B cell antigens have had limited effectiveness. Monoclonal antibodies used to deliver drugs or toxins to the tumor have demonstrated promise in pilot studies. Immunoconjugates under investigation include interleukin-2 (IL-2)–diphtheria toxin,† anti-CD19 (B4) conjugated to ricin,† and a number of anti–B cell antibodies conjugated to ^{131}I or ^{90}Y.†

Preliminary studies suggest a possible future role for active specific immunotherapy. Patients with minimal residual disease after chemotherapy may generate a humoral or cell-mediated response to subcutaneous injections of immunoglobulin–idiotype protein resulting in regression of measurable disease.

HIGH-GRADE LYMPHOMAS

The high-grade lymphomas include immunoblastic lymphoma (IL), lymphoblastic lymphoma (LBL), and

---

*Not FDA-approved for this indication.
†Investigational drug in the United States.

diffuse small noncleaved cell lymphoma (DSNCL). IL behaves clinically like diffuse large cell lymphoma (DLCL) and is treated in a similar fashion. LBL can be distinguished from other NHLs by its T cell phenotype and the presence of terminal deoxynucleotidyltransferase (TdT), although 10 to 20% of patients exhibit a pre–B cell phenotype and 20% of patients are biphenotypic. Presenting symptoms of LBL generally relate to the presence of a mediastinal mass in 75 to 80% of cases. CNS involvement is uncommon in newly diagnosed LBL, although it is frequently present at relapse. The malignant cells in LBL and T cell acute lymphoblastic leukemia (T–ALL) have similar histologic, immunophenotypic, and cytogenetic characteristics. LBL and T–ALL can be distinguished by the characteristic mediastinal mass in the former, and more frequent extensive bone marrow infiltration in the latter.

Factors that predict outcome in LBL include the serum LDH level, age, and the presence of extranodal disease. Intensive, multiagent chemotherapy is required for LBL. Approximately 90% of patients in the low-risk category (Stage I-III, or IV with an LDH level <1.5 times normal) respond, and 80% of these remain free of disease at 5 years using an aggressive regimen including induction and consolidation with cyclophosphamide, doxorubicin, vincristine, prednisone, and L-asparaginase with CNS prophylaxis using intrathecal methotrexate, followed by prolonged maintenance with methotrexate and 6-mercaptopurine. In contrast, those with high-risk disease (Stage IV with bone marrow or CNS involvement, or with other extranodal sites and an LDH level >1.5 times normal) have a complete remission rate of 50 to 60%, but with only 20% free of disease at 5 years. This high-risk group should receive an aggressive ALL-like regimen and be considered for bone marrow transplantation.

Small noncleaved cell lymphomas (SNCLs) are uncommon B cell NHLs in adults that are characterized by rapid growth and extensive disease at diagnosis. They are subclassified into Burkitt's and non-Burkitt's types. The characteristic cytogenetic abnormality, t(8;14)(q24;q32), involves the c-myc oncogene. Half the patients present with Stage IV disease, with bone marrow involvement in 20%, although CNS involvement is uncommon. The most important determinant of survival is tumor burden, indirectly measured by the serum LDH level. No large-scale clinical trials have been conducted in SNCL, and the optimal therapy is unknown. Treatment of patients with Stage I-III disease with an intensive chemotherapy regimen incorporating such agents as high-dose methotrexate, cyclophosphamide or ifosfamide, vincristine, and prednisone, along with CNS prophylaxis, produces complete remission rates of 80 to 100% and a 5-year relapse-free survival of 80 to 90%. Complete remissions may be achieved in half of patients with Stage IV disease, but with only a 25% freedom from progression at 5 years. Patients with advanced disease are candidates for bone marrow transplantation or experimental therapies.

Patients with high-grade NHL, particularly Burkitt's and LBL, are susceptible to rapid tumor lysis on initiation of chemotherapy. Prophylaxis against tumor lysis syndrome should include alkalinization of the urine, hydration with forced diuresis, and allopurinol therapy. Serum electrolyte levels and renal function should be monitored closely. Hemodialysis may be indicated in cases of severe deterioration.

PRIMARY CENTRAL NERVOUS SYSTEM LYMPHOMA

Primary CNS lymphoma is rare, accounting for only 1% of newly diagnosed lymphomas, and only 2% of primary brain tumors. Predisposing factors include congenital immune deficiency syndromes, human immunodeficiency (HIV) infection, and immune suppressive therapy, particularly in the setting of organ transplantation. Symptoms include headache and meningismus, and otherwise generally reflect the area of CNS involvement. The role of surgery is primarily for diagnosis, with radiation therapy the standard treatment. If untreated, the median survival is 2 months. Corticosteroids are effective in reducing symptoms, but with little influence on survival. Radiotherapy achieves complete responses in the majority of patients, with a prolongation of the median survival to about a year. High-dose systemic methotrexate or cytarabine may induce responses in radiation failures. A number of combination chemotherapy regimens (e.g., CHOP, DHAP) appear to prolong survival in uncontrolled series, although all patients eventually die from their disease. The best sequence of chemotherapy and radiation as well as the optimal chemotherapy program remains unknown.

ACQUIRED IMMUNE DEFICIENCY SYNDROME–RELATED NON–HODGKIN'S LYMPHOMA

The incidence of AIDS-related NHL is showing a dramatic increase, which is likely due to prolonged survival of AIDS patients related to the availability of antiretroviral agents. More than 30% may develop NHL after 3 years, and patients with CD4 counts less than 50 per μL appear to be at the greatest risk. From 80 to 90% of AIDS-related lymphomas are high-grade B cell tumors, which account for only 10 to 15% of the NHLs in HIV-negative patients. The AIDS-related lymphomas are similar to NHLs observed in other patients with chronic immune suppression. There are case reports of AIDS-associated low-grade NHLs, plasmacytomas, and multiple myelomas, although their relationship to the HIV infection is unclear. Patients with NHL tend to exhibit constitutional symptoms, and up to 98% have widespread extranodal involvement, particularly in the CNS, gastrointestinal tract, bone marrow, and liver. The prognosis of primary CNS NHL is poor, with a median survival of less than 6 months. Treatment of systemic NHL has also been disappointing, with low complete remission rates (40 to 50%), frequent opportunistic infections, and a median survival of less than 6 months; fewer than 40% survive beyond a year. Small series suggest that low-dose chemotherapy may be effective. Whether the addition of myeloid growth factors (e.g., granulocyte colony-stimulating factor [G-CSF]) will improve on these results by permitting more intensive therapy is under evaluation. CNS prophylaxis is an essential component of a treatment program.

MULTIPLE MYELOMA

method of
MALCOLM R. MACKENZIE, M.D.
University of California, Davis
Davis, California

Multiple myeloma is a neoplastic disease of B cells, primarily manifested by an expansion of the plasma cell in the bone marrow compartment. Symptoms are caused by both local expansion of the plasma cells and remote effects of the biologic material secreted by the plasma cell. The disease has an incidence of 5 per 100,000 individuals and reaches a peak in the sixth decade of life. The disease is uncommon before the age of 40 years. It is characterized by the secretion of a single (i.e., monoclonal) immune globulin species in serum or urine, or both. In only extremely rare instances do the plasma cells fail to secrete immune globulin molecule.

The local effects of plasma cell expansion include the development of multiple osteolytic lesions, best appreciated by routine radiographs or computed tomography, but rarely by bone scan, and localized pressure, from an expanding mass of plasma cells, those of most concern involving the spinal cord or the roots of peripheral nerves. The erosion of bone, which is mediated by a set of materials known as "osteoclast-activating factors," including some of the tumor necrosis factor family, results in unopposed activity of osteoclasts and the frequent production of hypercalcemia. Unrestrained hypercalcemia for a prolonged period of time will produce renal lesions. The secretion of the immune globulin molecule, particularly the light chain component—that is, Bence Jones proteins, which are then secreted by the kidney—produces a varied amount of renal (glomerular and tubular) damage, providing further insults to the kidneys. Secretion of products, either by the plasma cell or by lymphocytes and macrophages in response to plasma cell proliferation, results in a suppression of normal primary immune responses and leaves the patient particularly vulnerable to recurrent infections.

Finally, the suppression of normal hematopoiesis by the plasma cells residing within the bone marrow compartment leads to anemia, thrombocytopenia, and granulocytopenia.

The mere presence of a monoclonal peak in serum or urine is insufficient information on which to base the diagnosis of multiple myeloma. A wide spectrum of disorders must be differentiated by the physician. Myeloma itself also has a wide spectrum of stages in which symptoms develop, and there is a variable rate of progression in an individual patient. It is important, then, that the clinician adhere to diagnostic criteria for the various conditions described later, and once one has decided the patient has myeloma, to stage them.

Major diagnostic criteria for multiple myeloma are the identification of a plasmacytoma on tissue biopsy, a bone marrow plasmacytosis with greater than 30% plasma cells, and the presence of a monoclonal immune globulin peak on serum or urine electrophoresis that exceeds 3.5 grams per dL for IgG or 2.0 grams for IgA and greater than 1 gram per 24 hours of light chain excretion in the urine. At times, a patient will not fulfill these criteria.

Minor criteria are considered to be a bone marrow plasmacytosis with 10 to 30% plasma cells, documented to be monoclonal preferably by immunoperoxidase studies; a monoclonal globulin peak of less than the values given earlier; the presence of multiple lytic bone lesions; and finally, the depression of normal immune globulin values—that is, of those immune globulins not represented in the monoclonal peak, with IgM less than 50 mg, IgA less than 100 mg, or IgG less than 600 mg per dL.

The diagnosis of myeloma requires a minimum of one major criterion and one minor criterion, or all the minor criteria present in obviously symptomatic patients. Once the diagnosis of myeloma is established by the criteria listed earlier, the patient's disease should be staged.

In Stage I, thought to represent a low tumor cell mass group, patients should have all the following three criteria: hemoglobin greater than 10 grams per dL, serum calcium less than 12 mg per dL, and a normal skeleton roentgenogram or a solitary lytic lesion. If there is an IgG peak, the component should be less than 5 grams per dL; if an IgA peak is less than 3 grams per dL, the urine light chain M component should be greater than 4 grams per 24 hours.

The patient with a high tumor mass, in essence being in a poor-risk group (Stage III), should have one or more of the following characteristics: hemoglobin less than 8.5 grams per dL, serum calcium above 12 mg per dL, and advanced and multiple lytic bone lesions. IgG protein should be greater than 7 grams per dL, an IgA protein should be greater than 5 grams per dL, and a urine light chain immune globulin peak should be greater than 12 grams per 24 hours.

Note that Stage I requires all the criteria to be present; Stage III requires only one. Patients who do not fulfill either low-stage or high-stage group criteria are considered to be in Stage II.

A further important modification of the staging is division into A or B, with individuals who clearly have normal renal function as A, and those with abnormal function who have a blood urea nitrogen of greater than 30 mg per dL or a serum creatinine greater than 2 mg per dL as B. Once it has been determined that a patient has Stage I myeloma, one must be sure that one is not dealing with two entities that have been described in recent years: indolent myeloma and smoldering myeloma. Indolent myeloma criteria are the same as those of myeloma, with the following modifications: There are either no or only limited bone lesions (i.e., less than three lytic lesions), there are no compression fractures, there are no symptoms, the hemoglobin is greater than 10 grams per dL, and renal function is normal. Smoldering myeloma has similar criteria, except there should be no demonstrable bone lesions and the bone marrow plasma cells should be between 10 and 30%. These individuals can be followed closely, with determination of their hemoglobin, renal function, and serum M component performed at bimonthly intervals during the first 6 to 12 months, and perhaps every 3 months thereafter as long as the situation remains stable.

Individuals with Stage I myeloma have a median sur-

vival of at least 5 years, and frequently no therapeutic intervention is required. These patients must be differentiated from those with monoclonal gammopathy of undetermined significance (MGUS). The latter are asymptomatic and have an M component level with an IgG of less than 3 grams per dL, IgA less than 2 grams per dL, and Bence Jones protein level of less than 1 gram per 24 hours. The bone marrow plasma cells are less than 10%, and there are no bone lesions. These individuals' M components are usually an incidental finding. Only about 20% of patients initially felt to have MGUS will progress to overt myeloma. MGUS requires evaluation and follow-up but no therapy.

Prognosis in myeloma is related to stage and to two other simple measurements: (1) the serum albumin level at presentation and (2) the serum beta$_2$ microglobulin levels. Those with serum beta$_2$-microglobulin levels of less than 4 µg per mL and a concomitant serum albumin level of greater than 3 grams per dL have an excellent prognosis. Patients with beta$_2$-microglobulin levels of greater than 4 µg per mL and with a serum albumin of less than 3 grams per dL have an exceedingly poor prognosis without intervention. Serial determinations of beta$_2$-microglobulin levels appear not to add any information to this classification.

TREATMENT

Once the decision is made to treat a myeloma patient, the following principles should be kept in mind: (1) Although it is a readily treatable malignant disease, it is not (with our current methodologies) a curable malignant disease. (2) It is almost always a disseminated malignant disease, so that local measures should be used only to alleviate local and severe problems, such as (a) bones that are in immediate danger of fractures, like the femur or humerus; (b) significant impingement on the spinal cord; or (c) painful lesions that appear to be relatively refractory to systemic chemotherapy. Younger individuals with this disease—under the age of 50 years—should be considered for more radical therapies such as allogeneic bone marrow transplant, if a suitable donor is available, or autologous bone marrow or peripheral stem cell transplant with high-dose radiation and combination chemotherapy, as is being explored in various centers.

Chemotherapy

Chemotherapy can be divided basically into two major categories: induction and maintenance. The choice of agents for induction, despite 2 decades of systemic studies, remains moderately controversial. The standard care during the 1970s was the administration of oral melphalan (Alkeran) in combination with oral prednisone. Although a variety of schedules have been published, I prefer an intermittent schedule: melphalan at 0.25 mg per kg per day for 4 days, in association with prednisone, 1 mg per kg per day for the same 4 days, with the cycle repeated every 4 to 6 weeks, depending on the patient's hematologic toxicity. It is important when administering oral melphalan to recognize that it is inconsistently absorbed. In the early cycles, it is important to document that there has been a drop in the white blood cell count to 2000 to 3000 per mm^3 at approximately 2 weeks after the initiation of therapy. If the count fails to demonstrate drug action, the drug should be increased. Conversely, if there is an excessive induction of leukopenia, i.e., white cell counts below 1000 to 1400 per mm^3 or the granulocyte count dropping below 500 to 750 per mm^3, the dose should be lowered.

A response is defined by the diminishment of the serum protein electrophoretic and monoclonal spike to 50% of the pretreatment value, as defined by the Myeloma Task Force in 1973. A more stringent criterion has been suggested by the Southwest Oncology Group of 75% in the serum and/or urine abnormality, but it is not clear that this standard has yielded substantial therapeutic benefit. Both criteria are clearly partial responses, with a complete response being defined as the diminishment of all protein abnormalities to a normal baseline and the correction of anemia to normal values. In patients who have achieved a response, investigative studies with anti-idiotype reagents indicate that there still is residual disease; thus, it is doubtful that a complete response has ever been achieved with our current agents.

In a series of studies during the late 1970s, the Southwest Oncology Group presented evidence that the more complicated regimens that included alternating cycles of multiple-agent chemotherapy were more effective. These include vincristine (Oncovin), 1.0 mg intravenously on day 1; melphalan, 6 mg per m^2 orally on days 1 through 4; cyclophosphamide (Cytoxan), 125 mg per m^2 orally on days 1 through 4; and prednisone, 50 mg per m^2 orally on days 1 through 4; alternating with vincristine, 1 mg intravenously on day 1; bis-chloroethyl-nitrosurea (BCNU; carmustine), 30 mg per m^2 intravenously on day 1; doxorubicin (Adriamycin), 30 mg m^2 orally on day 1; and prednisone, 60 mg per m^2 orally on days 1 to 4. Each cycle is repeated at 3- to 4-week intervals for 6 to 12 cycles. The maximal lifetime dose of doxorubicin is 480 mg per m^2.

A second intensive regimen that has been suggested is the use of melphalan, 0.25 mg per kg per day, days 1 through 4; prednisone, 1 mg per kg per day, days 1 through 7; vincristine, 0.03 mg per kg, day 1; BCNU, 1.0 mg per kg per day, day 1; and cyclophosphamide, 10 mg per kg per day on day 1; the last three all being given intravenously. This cycle is repeated every 5 weeks. American studies of these combination agents in head-to-head trials with melphalan and prednisone have indicated substantial increase is response rate and survival statistics. This has not been true in European trials with similar or identical regimens, thus raising the question, "Is the substantial increase in expense and morbidity that the multiple-agent regimens inevitably require justified over standard melphalan and prednisone?" Now that these studies have had a chance to "mature"—that is, have long-term follow-up—it is clear that with the more intensive regimen, in those individuals who do respond, a substantial number (20 to 25%) demonstrate a prolonged survival, al-though the median survival rate may not be substantially different worldwide. Survival rates of 8 to 10 years are now being seen in this treated group. The VAD regimen of an intravenous infusion of vincristine (Oncovin), 0.1 mg per day, and doxorubicin (Adriamycin), 4 mg per m^2 per day, with dexamethasone given orally, 40 mg a day, for 4 days, repeated on days 9 and 17 of a 28-day cycle, originally described as salvage therapy, gives a rapid response (within three cycles) in 55% of newly diagnosed patients. It is particularly useful in patients with severe hypocalcemia and/or renal failure. Recent data suggest that the addition of higher doses of a glucocorticosteroid, such as prednisone, 50 mg every other day, between courses of chemotherapy has survival value.

Current clinical research has explored the use of high-dose chemotherapy with autologous stem cells derived from peripheral blood as rescue from bone marrow toxicity. In newly diagnosed patients, there appears to be a survival value, but all patients eventually relapse. The proper role of this modality remains to be defined.

My approach to therapy is as follows: Individuals under the age of 50 years and with Stage III disease receive VAD therapy, and if they respond are considered candidates for inclusion in the clinical studies on high-dose therapy. Individuals between 50 and 70 years of age and in Stage III disease receive any of the described therapies with which the treating physician is familiar. Individuals over 70 years of age receive standard melphalan and prednisone. It is important to note that individuals who have renal disease, with blood urea nitrogen (BUN) concentrations of 30 to 49 mg per dL and creatinine levels of 2.0 to 2.9 mg per dL, should receive only 50% of their theoretical calculated alkylating agent dose. For patients with more severe impairment of renal function (i.e., BUN concentrations of greater than 50 mg per dL or creatinine levels greater than 3 mg per dL), only 25% of the calculated dose will be given initially. As the individual's tolerance for this chemotherapy is assessed, the doses can be adjusted upward toward the full dose. It is clearly important to get adequate doses of these therapeutic agents to the patient to get maximal results.

Several studies have now shown that once maximal tumor reduction has been achieved, continuing with the induction regimen provides little survival value. Such patients, however, should be monitored closely, and if their monoclonal abnormalities should increase to greater than 25 to 30% of the nadir value, reinstitution of therapy should be considered. Expanded studies of interferon alfa-2 (Roferon-A) or interferon alfa-2b (Intron A) have not confirmed its activity in routine maintenance therapy.

Relapse

The problem of patients with refractory disease and those who experience relapse is severe, with only limited options. If the patient has received only melphalan and/or prednisone, responses have been achieved by the use of the vincristine, carmustine, doxorubicin, and prednisone regimen outlined earlier. If the patient is refractory to initial therapy or has received other combination drugs, one can use a regimen of infusional (i.e., a continuous infusion over 4 days) vincristine (Oncovin), 0.4 mg per day, and doxorubicin, 9 mg per m² per day, with dexamethasone given orally, 40 mg a day, for 4 days, and then again on day 9 and day 17 of a 28-day cycle. About 25% of patients previously refractory to other regimens will respond to this therapy, and 50 to 60% of patients with relapse have been noted to respond.

Because these agents (vincristine and doxorubicin) are highly toxic if given outside the venous system, such therapy requires a central indwelling catheter. I prefer to use a single-lumen Hickman catheter because of the potential danger of a needle being dislodged from a subcutaneously placed catheter system during the period of the 4-day infusion. Infusion may be given as an outpatient procedure, using infusion pumps, and is exceedingly well tolerated by most patients.

With patients with very refractory disease, particularly those with severe bone pain, one may consider giving sequential hemibody or even total body irradiation. These maneuvers have been successful in relieving pain in carefully selected patients. As indicated earlier, local irradiation can be utilized to relieve areas of obvious plasmacytoma involvement, particularly those threatening neurologic catastrophes, but it is important to limit radiation exposure, at least early in the course of patients with myeloma, owing to the substantial damage to bone marrow with subsequent inability to receive adequate doses of systemic chemotherapy. Relapsed and refractory patients are not candidates for high-dose therapy.

Supportive Therapy for Complications

Hypercalcemia. Hypercalcemia should be treated with initial isotonic saline diuresis, furosemide (Lasix) in doses of 40 to 80 mg or higher, as required, and prednisone, 40 mg per m² per day. Obviously, if this is an initial presentation, specific chemotherapy should be started as soon as possible. Unresponsive patients may require pamidronate (Aredia), 60 to 90 mg intravenously over 24 hours, or etidronate (Didronel), 7.5 mg per kg in 250 mL of saline intravenously for 3 to 5 days. Calcitonin has given only transient benefit and is not regularly employed.

Hyperuricemia. Hyperuricemia, owing to either tumor proliferation or induction chemotherapy, can be reduced or prevented by use of allopurinol (Zyloprim), 300 to 500 mg per day, and if hyperuricemia is severe, urine should be alkalinized with sodium bicarbonate, 1 to 2 grams orally every 6 hours.

Neurologic Defects. As indicated earlier, patients with spinal cord involvement should be evaluated promptly. Extradural compression of the spinal cord is common from vertebral collapse. Prompt evaluation with either computed tomography or magnetic resonance imaging should be undertaken to ascertain whether there is bone involvement secondary to vertebral collapse, or plasmacytoma. Plasmacytomas should then be treated with radiation therapy; on some occasions, neurosurgical intervention to relieve bone compression may be required.

Hyperviscosity. Hyperviscosity is relatively uncommon in multiple myeloma, although it does occur more frequently in patients with increased levels of IgA or in those with very high concentrations of IgG, such as 12 to 14 grams per dL. It should be suspected in patients with visual difficulty, severe bleeding diathesis, or altered mental status when the physical finding is of "box-car" or sausage-shaped abnormalities of the retinal veins. Plasmapheresis is highly effective in temporary relief of these symptoms and should be combined with systemic chemotherapy.

Amyloidosis. Amyloidosis may occur in 10 to 20% of patients with myeloma and should be considered in individuals with carpal tunnel syndrome, peripheral neuropathy, or unexplained nephrotic syndrome. Unfortunately, this complication does not respond well to therapy, so it is important that patients be so informed.

Acute Renal Failure. Acute renal failure can be managed aggressively with interim dialysis while one awaits a response to systemic chemotherapy.

Infections. As indicated earlier, life-threatening infections with pneumonia, septicemia, and so on are markedly increased in patients with myeloma. They are due to gram-positive encapsulated organisms, but with a substantial contribution of gram-negative bacteria. Appropriate cultures should be obtained and patients treated with broad-spectrum antibiotics. Prophylactic gamma globulin is administered only to those patients who have responded to therapy in the plateau phase and who demonstrate recurrent bacterial infections.

Anemia. Severe anemia may respond to erythropoietin (Epogen or Procrit), 4000 units subcutaneously three times a week, especially in those patients with some element of renal failure.

POLYCYTHEMIA VERA

method of
DILIP PATEL, M.D., and
KANTI R. RAI, M.D.
Long Island Jewish Medical Center
New Hyde Park, New York

DIAGNOSIS

We use the diagnostic guidelines recommended by the Polycythemia Vera Study Group (PVSG) detailed in Table 1, with a few minor modifications. Recognizing that measurement of serum erythropoietin levels was not a readily available test 2 decades ago when these guidelines were developed, we use this assay to determine whether absolute erythrocytosis is from secondary causes. Thus, in the presence of an abnormally high red cell mass and splenomegaly, if the serum erythropoietin level is low, we

TABLE 1. **Polycythemia Vera Study Group Diagnostic Criteria for Polycythemia Vera***

A1. Increased red cell mass Males ≥36 mL/kg Females ≥32 mL/kg	B1. Thrombocytosis (Platelets >400,000/μL)
A2. Normal arterial oxygen saturation	B2. Leukocytosis (>12,000/μL, no infection or fever)
A3. Splenomegaly	B3. Increased leukocyte alkaline phosphatase (>100, no fever or infection) Increased serum B_{12} (>900 pg/mL) or Increased unbound B_{12} binding capacity (>2200 pg/mL)

*Either A1 + A2 + A3 or A1 + A2 + any two from category B; but see the text for modification of these criteria.

do not insist on obtaining arterial oxygen saturation. Leukocyte alkaline phosphatase (LAP) is a crucial test to differentiate chronic myelocytic leukemia (CML), another chronic myeloproliferative disorder that may have features very similar to those of polycythemia vera at the time of initial presentation. In CML, the LAP score is very low or even zero, whereas it is markedly elevated in polycythemia. Although serum B_{12} and unbound B_{12} binding capacity is elevated in polycythemia, their measurements are no longer considered of critical importance.

CLINICAL FEATURES

In polycythemia vera, the presenting symptoms and physical findings are a direct consequence of a hypercellular marrow with an abnormal increase in all the cellular elements of the blood, but especially of erythrocytes. Although some patients may be asymptomatic and a diagnosis of polycythemia is made because a blood count was obtained for another reason, a large majority of patients present with any number of complaints, such as headache, generalized itching, weakness, dizziness, bone and joint pains, epigastric pain, and visual disturbances. Upon physical examination, the most frequently observed abnormalities include ruddy facial coloration, bright red conjunctiva, hypertension, and enlarged spleen. Patients with polycythemia vera are at an increased risk for spontaneous hemorrhage as well as for thromboembolic events. Bone marrow examination reveals hypercellularity with evidence of pan-myelosis and decreased or absent iron stores. Evidence of increased reticulin fibers may or may not be present initially. There are no characteristic cytogenetic abnormalities associated with polycythemia vera, but +1, +8, +9, and 20q- have been found in some cases.

TREATMENT

Although the therapeutic trials conducted by the PVSG have resulted in significant improvement in the overall duration of survival as compared with historical controls, treatment of polycythemia vera should be chosen according to the individual patient's clinical findings and risk status.

Initial Phlebotomies

We initiate a program of phlebotomies in all patients once a diagnosis of polycythemia vera has been established. The objective is to reduce the hematocrit to a range of 42 to 45% with as rapid a series of phlebotomies as the patient can tolerate. Usually a phlebotomy of 450 mL every 5 to 7 days is recommended until the hematocrit is stabilized within the desired range. Depending on how elevated the hematocrit is at baseline, it is usually necessary to perform four to eight phlebotomies during this initial phase.

All patients return to the clinic at monthly intervals for follow-up, and the rate of increase in hematocrit levels is observed. Additional phlebotomies are performed as needed to maintain the hematocrit between 42 and 45%. If more than three or four additional phlebotomies are required during a 12-month period, we recommend myelosuppressive therapy.

Myelosuppressive Therapies

Hydroxyurea (Hydrea)*

Hydroxyurea is our first choice among myelosuppressive agents. This drug is an S phase–specific ribonucleotide reductase inhibitor and is believed to have much less leukemogenic and oncogenic potential than alkylating agents and portosystemic radioactive phosphorus (^{32}P). The initial dose is 1.0 to 1.5 gram orally per day, with adjustment upward or downward, depending on reductions in hematocrit, platelet, and leukocyte levels. Some patients may need larger doses to 3 or 3.5 grams, whereas others may show a satisfactory response at a much lower dosage. We discontinue hydroxyurea after stabilizing the patient's clinical status and again try to maintain the hematocrit within the desired range with occasional phlebotomies, thereby using hydroxyurea on only an intermittent basis. Allopurinol (Zyloprim) 300 mg per day orally is used concomitantly with hydroxyurea or other myelosuppressive agents to prevent excess uric acid–related complications.

Radioactive Phosphorus

Elderly patients whose natural life expectancy is not very long may be treated with ^{32}P. Although use of ^{32}P and alkylating agents carries up to a 10% risk of developing acute leukemia or other secondary malignancies upon a long-term follow-up, these agents offer a significant protection from the thromboembolic complications that are expected in the natural course of polycythemia vera. In addition, usually only one or two doses of ^{32}P are needed to achieve an adequate level of myelosuppression, in contrast with the requirement of daily doses of hydroxyurea and frequent blood testing. The usual dose of ^{32}P is 2.3 mCi/m^2 intravenously; this dose may be repeated after 12 weeks if blood counts are not approaching satisfactory levels.

Busulfan (Myleran)*

We have not used busulfan for the treatment of polycythemia vera during the past decade, but this

*Not FDA-approved for this indication.

alkylating agent can be beneficial for patients who require myelosuppressive therapy but do not tolerate hydroxyurea. The busulfan dose is 2 to 6 mg daily, orally, for 4 to 8 weeks.

Interferon-Alfa*

Although the Food and Drug Administration has not approved the use of interferon-alfa for polycythemia vera, there have been a few reports of its efficacy in reducing hematocrits and platelets in some patients.

ADDITIONAL CONSIDERATIONS
Thrombocytosis

Most patients with polycythemia vera start with elevated platelet counts that may increase to levels approaching or exceeding 1 million per μL following institution of initial phlebotomy therapy. Such thrombocythemia puts the patient at increased risk of thrombotic complications. Therefore, hydroxyurea therapy should be initiated early during the phlebotomy process. Although controlled clinical trials failed to demonstrate a benefit from anti-platelet-aggregating agents such as aspirin and dipyridamole (Persantine), we use these drugs in all polycythemia vera patients with marked degrees of thrombocytosis.

Pruritus

Many patients with polycythemia vera suffer from intense generalized pruritus. We use histamine (H_1 or H_2) antagonists (cyproheptadine [Periactin] 4 to 8 mg per day orally) to control pruritus. If such therapy fails to control severe itching, myelosuppressive therapy is added to phlebotomy.

Surgery

Patients with uncontrolled polycythemia vera are at high risk of excessive bleeding and thrombosis following major surgery. Therefore, all elective surgical procedures should be put off until blood counts have been normalized with phlebotomy and myelosuppressive therapy.

Pregnancy

Female patients of childbearing age with polycythemia vera should be advised to refrain from having children while receiving myelosuppressive therapy. Phlebotomy alone is the recommended therapy for those patients who do plan to have children. Hematocrit values tend to normalize in some women during the course of pregnancy, but it is advisable to be alert to early signs of excessive hemorrhage or venous thrombosis as complications after delivery.

*Not FDA-approved for this indication.

LATE COMPLICATIONS OF POLYCYTHEMIA VERA
Postpolycythemic Myeloid Metaplasia

As part of the natural history of polycythemia vera, some patients develop the "spent phase" of the disease, characterized by marked degree of anemia (usually transfusion dependent) with progressive and massive splenomegaly. These patients have profound degrees of weakness and tend to have increased susceptibility to bleeding and infections. Myeloid metaplasia (with bone marrow fibrosis) is the cause of liver and spleen enlargement. There is no satisfactory treatment available for this complication, but some responses have been noted with one or more of the following: transfusions, androgens, glucocorticoids, busulfan, hydroxyurea, interferon-alfa, splenic irradiation, splenectomy, and erythropoietin.

Acute Leukemia

Acute leukemia occurs in a small proportion of patients as part of the natural history of polycythemia vera, but its incidence increases significantly among long-term survivors who previously received chlorambucil (Leukeran) or ^{32}P therapy. A majority of patients have myeloid leukemic transformation, but lymphoid leukemia has also been reported. These patients do not respond to acute leukemia chemotherapy protocols and have a very short life expectancy.

ACKNOWLEDGMENT

This work was made possible with grant support from Helena Rubinstein Foundation, Leon Lowenstein Foundation, Inc., Joel Finkelstein Foundation, United Leukemia Fund, Inc., and Wayne Goldsmith Leukemia Fund.

THE PORPHYRIAS
method of
YVES NORDMANN, M.D.
Hôspital Louis Mourier
Paris, France

The porphyrias are a group of inherited metabolic disorders of heme biosynthesis in which specific patterns of overproduction of heme precursors are associated with characteristic clinical features. Each type of porphyria is the result of a specific decrease in the activity of one of the enzymes of heme biosynthesis (Figure 1).

Porphyrias are presently classified as *erythropoietic* or *hepatic*, depending on the primary organ in which the excess production of porphyrins or precursors takes place.

The porphyrias are inherited as dominant autosomal characters, except congenital erythropoietic porphyria and Doss porphyria (both extremely rare), which are inherited as recessive autosomal characters.

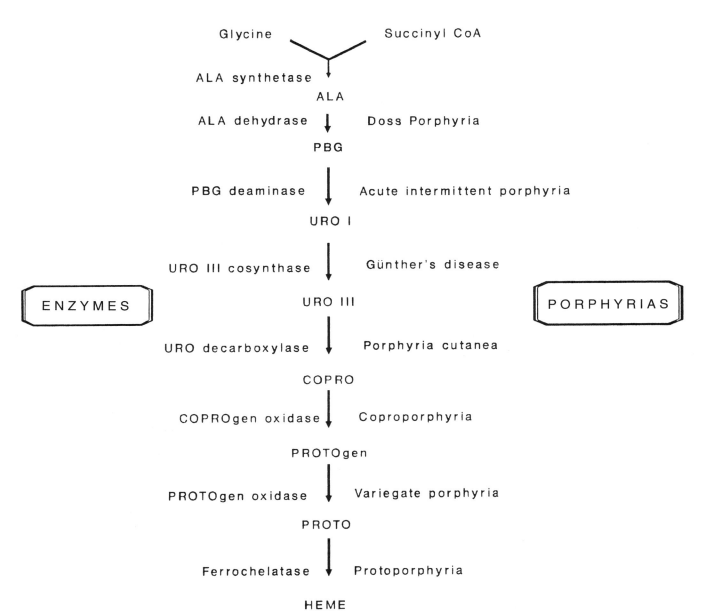

Figure 1. Inherited enzyme deficiencies in the porphyrias. *Abbreviations*: CoA = coenzyme A; ALA = alpha-aminolevulinic acid; PBG = porphobilinogen; URO = uroporphyrinogen; COPRO = coproporphyrinogen; PROTO = protoporphyrinogen.

THE ACUTE PORPHYRIAS

Typical, identical attacks of acute abdominal pain with vomiting and constipation occur in the four acute hepatic porphyrias: acute intermittent porphyria (AIP), hereditary coproporphyria (HC), variegate porphyria (VP), and Doss porphyria (DP); the attacks are sometimes associated with psychiatric manifestations such as anxiety, depression, disorientation, confusion, and delirium. Neurologic manifestations such as peripheral neuropathy with occasional cranial nerve involvement, respiratory distress, and grand mal seizures are most often caused by treatment errors. Despite the autosomal character of the traits of acute porphyrias, more than 80% of the patients showing acute attacks are women

(18 to 45 years old), and in fact, sex steroids are among the most important factors that result in clinical expression of acute porphyrias.

Darkening of urine (which may look like port wine) is attributed to nonenzymatic conversion of porphobilinogen (PBG) to a porphyrin-like compound and is common to all acute porphyrias. Cutaneous abnormalities (which are described later), though sometimes concurring with abdominal pain in HC and/or VP, may be absent in these acute porphyrias; they are never observed in AIP.

Precise identification of the type of acute porphyria by clinical examination alone is very difficult. Diagnosis is therefore primarily based on analysis of heme precursors in urine. In all acute attacks, large amounts of alpha-aminolevulinic acid (ALA) and

PBG—except in Doss porphyria—are excreted in the urine (20- to 200-fold elevated above normal levels). Stool porphyrins show usually a typical profile for each porphyria. However, as specific enzyme assays these investigations should be done after treatment has been started.

As soon as an attack has been diagnosed, a careful search should be made for any precipitating factor, especially drugs (including oral contraceptives), underlying infection, and a hypocaloric diet. Agitation and other psychiatric manifestations are usually controlled with chlorpromazine. Treatment of severe pain requires morphine-like drugs such as meperidine, but the danger of addiction (in patients experiencing frequent attacks) has always to be kept in mind. We usually combine chlorpromazine with meperidine and give the patient a quiet room.

Drug treatment is now superseded by glucose and hematin therapy. Adequate administration of glucose (300 to 400 grams per day), usually by slow intravenous perfusion, frequently leads to a reduction in the urinary excretion of heme precursors by still-undefined mechanism(s).

Treatment of a porphyric attack has been greatly improved with the introduction of hematin, which is superior to glucose because all patients respond favorably to hematin, whereas several do not respond favorably to glucose. Two preparations are available: lyophilized hematin (Panhematin)* and heme arginate (Normosang).* The latter is more stable and may produce fewer side effects, but it is not licensed for use in the United States. Hematin is given intravenously over a period of about 30 to 45 minutes, from a vial protected from light; doses up to 3 to 4 mg per kg of body weight per 24 hours are needed, usually during 4 days. Hematin probably replenishes the depleted hepatic pool of heme; the fact that urinary ALA (and PBG) levels decrease dramatically within 2 to 3 days shows that it exerts feedback on ALA synthase; most patients given heme arginate feel healthy within 3 to 4 days. It is important that all treatments be used early in the attack, before any nervous or respiratory complication arises; otherwise a biochemical response without concomitant clinical amelioration may be the only result.

Although the side effects of hematin such as coagulopathy or phlebitis have never been associated with real hemorrhage, hematin should not be used in conjunction with anticoagulant therapy (and a different vein must be used for infusion each day).

Recently, women with cyclical perimenstrual acute attacks have benefited from the administration of agonists of luteinizing hormone–releasing hormone (LHRH). These factors allow one to inhibit ovulation and are extremely well tolerated by the patients.

Tachycardia and hypertension are usually controlled with propranolol. Hyponatremia must be treated by fluid restriction. Of course balance has to be kept between the intravenous fluid therapy required to treat denutrition and/or dehydration and the fluid restriction needed by hyponatremia. Seizures are best treated with sodium valproate.

Prevention of acute attacks is one of the most important aspect of the treatment of acute porphyrias: affected individuals should keep in mind the known precipitants, mainly drugs and alcohol (a list of safe and unsafe drugs should be given to each patient and to each healthy genetic carrier).

Clinically latent individuals among relatives of patients must be detected (mainly by specific enzyme assays and/or by molecular biologic techniques).

PORPHYRIA CUTANEA TARDA

Porphyria cutanea tarda (PCT) is the most common form of porphyria. Cutaneous photosensitivity is the predominate clinical feature. Acute attacks with abdominal pain, psychiatric, and/or neurologic manifestations are never observed. *Skin fragility* is perhaps the most specific feature. Bullae, hypertrichosis, and pigmentation are very common. Among the precipitating factors, alcohol, estrogens, and other types of liver disease such as hepatitis C are most frequently incriminated. One must remember that most of the drugs classified as porphyrinogenic may have been used for several years before PCT develops.

Abnormal iron metabolism appears to be another precipitating factor: the serum iron level is frequently elevated, and a mild hepatic siderosis has been described in at least 80% of the patients.

Patients should first be advised to avoid all precipitating factors (alcohol, pills, drugs, etc.) and also exposure to sunlight until clinical and biologic remissions have been obtained by treatment.

Presently, phlebotomy is the treatment of choice in PCT, even when serum iron or ferritin levels are not increased. Venesections of 300 mL spaced at 10- to 12-day intervals are performed during 2 months until the serum iron level falls to 60 to 70% of its original value. The urinary uroporphyrin level should be measured every 2 months; clinical remission and normalization of urinary porphyrin levels are usually obtained within 4 to 6 months, but in the feces, copro- and isocoproporphyrin levels may remain elevated for a long time.

When phlebotomy is contraindicated (anemia, cardiac or pulmonary disorders, age), low-dose chloroquine (Aralen)* therapy (125 mg twice weekly for adults) is the favored alternative therapy. The duration of treatment and relapse rate are only marginally higher than with venesection. High-dose therapy has to be avoided because it causes a hepatitis-like syndrome in PCT patients. During remission, patients can be monitored by measuring urinary uroporphyrin excretion, and treatment can be restarted if concentrations reach around 200 nmol per mmol of creatinine.

---

*Investigational drug in the United States.

*Not FDA-approved for this indication.

ERYTHROPOIETIC PORPHYRIAS

Protoporphyria

Photosensitivity is the major clinical manifestation in erythropoietic protoporphyria (EPP): short exposure to sunlight induces painful burning sensations in the sun-exposed areas of the skin. The symptoms occur without any immediately observable change in the appearance of the skin, but several hours later they are usually followed by edema and erythema. Quite typically, facial skin appears normal. However, it bears a few shallow, circular scars often scattered over the bridge of the nose, forehead, and cheeks. The onset of cutaneous symptoms is usually in early childhood (3 to 5 years of age). Elevated protoporphyrin levels in erythrocytes and plasma are characteristic.

EPP is generally a benign disease, although a number of cases associated with abnormalities of the biliary tract and/or the liver have been reported: cholelithiasis often requires cholecystectomy. Chemical analysis of the gallstones reveals high levels of protoporphyrin. In rare cases (2 out of 150 patients in our study) fatal liver disease with cirrhosis may develop.

Oral administration of beta carotene (100 to 150 mg per day in adults) may afford photoprotection, resulting in improved tolerance to the sun. (The beta carotene would prevent the photosensitivity reaction by quenching the singlet oxygen or the triplet states of protoporphyrin [porphyrin concentrations remain unchanged].) However, results are variable. Whereas several patients report increased tolerance to light, a few patients (around 20%) seem to show no improvement.

The therapy of liver disease in EPP has included several trials such as the ingestion of cholestyramine resin to try to interrupt the enterohepatic recirculation of protoporphyrin to the liver, and the administration of bile salts to mobilize protoporphyrin directly from the liver. Liver transplantation is the therapy of last resort in irreversible liver damage.

Congenital Erythropoietic Porphyria

Congenital erythropoietic porphyria (CEP), or Günther's disease, is one of the rarer inherited porphyrias; the occurrence of severe photosensitivity may progress to mutilations of ears, nose cartilage, and digits. Hypertrichosis, erythrodontia, and splenomegaly with hemolytic anemia of varying severity are common.

General treatment includes minimal exposure to the sun, avoidance of trauma to the skin, and careful treatment of any skin infection. Packed erythrocyte transfusions markedly reduce excessive hemolysis and its stimulation of increased erythropoiesis. It also decreases porphyrin excretion. However, it is well known that multiple transfusions can be harmful.

Splenectomy is not necessarily recommended. Bone marrow transplantation might represent an effective treatment for these patients.

THERAPEUTIC USE OF BLOOD COMPONENTS

method of
IRMA O. SZYMANSKI, M.D.
University of Massachusetts Medical Center
Worcester, Massachusetts

With the advent of plastics technology, blood component preparation and transfusion was introduced in the 1950s. Although clinicians initially resisted giving up whole blood transfusions, availability of blood components has improved several aspects of medical care. It allows each component to be stored under the specific, optimal conditions that best maintain the viability and function of blood cells and plasma. Further, it allows a therapeutic dose of the required component to be given in a relatively pure form and in small volume, facilitating precise transfusion therapy and decreasing the rate of transfusion-associated complications.

In addition to the advances in blood component therapy, great strides have been made during the last decade toward improvement of transfusion safety because new methods have been developed to identify evidence of retroviral infections and hepatitis in donated blood. The chance of contracting acquired immune deficiency syndrome (AIDS) from a blood transfusion is now as low as 1 in 400,000 per unit of blood. Introduction of new tests for detection of hepatitis C virus (HCV) antibodies in donor blood has reduced the risk of post-transfusion HCV infection to about 1 in 6000 per unit of blood component given.

PREPARATION OF BLOOD COMPONENTS

The following blood components are prepared from anticoagulated whole blood by centrifugation techniques: packed red blood cells (RBCs), platelets, and plasma. Depending on the method of component preparation, the amount of other, contaminating blood elements will vary. In the United States, components are usually prepared by the differential centrifugation method, a process involving two centrifugation steps. First, the unit of whole blood is subjected to a low centrifugal force to separate platelet-rich plasma (PRP) from RBCs. After being expressed into a satellite bag, next the PRP is exposed to a relatively high centrifugal force to concentrate the platelets. The platelet-poor plasma is then expressed into another bag, yielding a unit of plasma and a platelet concentrate.

Although this is an efficient method, a large fraction of the leukocytes present in the original unit of whole blood remains in the cellular blood components. A different method of component preparation has gained a foothold in Europe. It involves the separation of whole blood into RBCs, plasma, and buffy coat following a high-speed centrifugation. The platelets are isolated from the buffy coat after a light-force centrifugation, and the buffy coat is discarded. The cellular components prepared by the buffy coat method contain significantly fewer leukocytes than those prepared by the "standard" method just described. The benefits of the buffy coat method include a low leukocyte-containing blood component supply, benefiting all transfusion recipients. The components prepared by centrifugation techniques can be further purified.

Red Cell Concentrates

Packed RBCs can be stored at 4° C for up to 42 days. Several approaches are available to purify the RBC concentrates further. The specific uses of these products are listed in Table 1.

Washed RBCs are prepared by washing the packed RBC concentrate with 0.9% sodium chloride. Since the RBCs are washed in an "open system," the product is good only for 24 hours after preparation. A bag of washed RBCs contains only a minimal amount of plasma and platelets and about 20% of the original white blood cells (WBCs).

Previously frozen RBCs are prepared from RBCs that have been stored in glycerol at −80° C for up to 10 years. Following thawing, the RBCs are deglycerolized, after which they may be stored at 4° C for up to 24 hours. The final product contains only negligible amounts of plasma and platelets and about 5% of the original WBCs. The concentration of 2,3-diphosphoglycerate (2,3-DPG) and adenosine triphosphate (ATP) in the deglycerolized RBCs is similar to what it was at the time of freezing. Thus, if a unit of RBCs is frozen within a week of collection or if stored RBCs have been *rejuvenated* by incubating them in a special "rejuvenation solution," they will have a high level of RBC 2,3-DPG, which confers to the RBCs a normal or higher than normal ability to release oxygen. Transfusion of RBCs with a high level of 2,3-DPG might be beneficial for surgical patients with decreased cardiac and pulmonary functions. Further, RBC freezing is a useful method to inventory autologous and rare cells.

Leukodepleted RBCs may be prepared by high-efficiency filtration of packed RBCs. The filtration can be done in the laboratory prior to storage or at the bedside by transfusing blood through a special filter. In the laboratory, using the latest-generation filtration technology, it is possible to remove over 99.9% of WBCs from the unit of RBC concentrate so that less than 1×10^6 WBCs per unit remain. This can be done in a "closed system" so that the expiration date of the product does not change. The poststorage filtration of the RBC product at the bedside at slow flow produces an acceptable product less consistently than the filtration in the laboratory at fast flow. The filtered RBC concentrates, however, still contain plasma.

Platelet Concentrates

In addition to *random platelet concentrates* prepared from units of whole blood by the centrifugation methods just described, platelets can be collected from donors directly by an apheresis procedure *(apheresis platelets)* without removing significant amounts of other blood elements. Both products are stored at 22° C for up to 5 days. One unit of random platelet concentrate contains at least 5.5 $\times 10^{10}$ platelets in a volume of about 50 mL, whereas an apheresis unit contains at least 3×10^{11} platelets in an approximate volume of 300 mL. A unit of random platelets contains about 2 to 4×10^7 contaminating WBCs, whereas the total amount of WBCs in a unit of apheresis platelets may be as low as 1×10^6. A therapeutic dose of platelets for adults may be delivered in 1 unit of apheresis platelets or in a pool of 6 to 8 units of random donor platelets. Transfusion of a unit of apheresis platelets, derived from a single donor, is associated with a lower risk of infectious disease transmission than is transfusion of a pool of random platelet concentrates. A therapeutic dose of human leukocyte antigen (HLA)–matched platelets can be obtained only by the apheresis procedure.

Both random and apheresis platelet concentrates can be filtered to reduce the WBC contamination. However, it should be noted that a unit of unfiltered apheresis platelets collected by the Cobe Spectra technology usually contains less than 1×10^6 WBCs. On the average, the platelet loss due to filtration is about 20 to 24%.

Washed platelets are prepared by subjecting a pool of random platelet concentrates or an apheresis platelet concentrate to wash cycles with 0.9% sodium chloride and 0.2% dextrose. About 35% of platelets are lost mechanically during washing.

White Cell Concentrates

Granulocytes, collected by an apheresis method, have been given in the past to neutropenic patients with gram-negative infections. However, such therapy is not very effective because the product contains too few granulocytes, and the transfusions are frequently associated with adverse effects. Besides, because of the effectiveness of newer antimicrobial therapies, granulocyte transfusions are now rarely even considered. However, granulocyte transfusions are still an adjunctive therapeutic modality in neonatal sepsis.

Peripheral Blood Stem Cells

Currently there is an increasing interest in peripheral blood stem cell (PBSC) therapy in the setting of both autologous and allogeneic bone marrow transplantation. Transplantation of autologous stem cells permits the use of intensive chemotherapy for certain tumors, such as breast cancer. The recovery of a patient's platelets and WBCs is more rapid after bone marrow repopulation with PBSC than it is after standard bone marrow transplantation. Many bone marrow transplantation centers are becoming interested in performing even the allogeneic bone marrow transplantation with PBSC.

Mobilized PBSC are harvested by an apheresis method from either a small (10 to 12 liters) or a large (20 to 28 liters) volume of the patient's/donor's blood. Progenitor cells are mobilized into peripheral blood during the early

TABLE 1. **Specific Uses and Advantages of "Purified" Red Blood Cell Concentrates**

Product	Specific Uses and Advantages
Washed RBCs	Prevention of allergic and febrile reactions
Previously frozen RBCs	Prevention of allergic and febrile reactions
	Prevention of CMV infection
	Salvage of outdated RBCs following rejuvenation
	Storage of autologous RBCs
	Storage of rare RBCs
	Preparation of RBCs with high 2,3-DPG content
	Prevention of TA-GvHD
Prestorage filtered RBCs	Prevention of immunization to HLA
	Prevention of CMV infection
	Prevention of febrile reactions

Abbreviations: RBCs = red blood cells; 2,3-DPG = 2,3,-diphosphoglycerate; TA-GvHD = transfusion-associated graft-versus-host disease; HLA = human leukocyte antigen; CMV = cytomegalovirus.

phase of bone marrow recovery from chemotherapy or, alternatively, after administration of growth factors (filgrastim [G-CSF, Neupogen] or sargramostim [GM-CSF, Leukine, Prokine]) or following the use of both chemotherapy and growth factors. A total of about 6×10^8 mononuclear cells or between 3 to 5×10^6 CD34-positive WBCs per kilogram of the patient's body weight should be collected to achieve engraftment.

Plasma Products

Cryoprecipitated antihemophilic factor (AHF) is prepared from fresh-frozen plasma (FFP) thawed at 4° C. The cryoprecipitable plasma proteins remain insoluble at that temperature, and after isolation by centrifugation, the precipitate is suspended in 10 to 20 mL of plasma to be stored frozen at −20° C for up to 1 year. One bag of cryoprecipitated AHF contains about 80 IU of Factor VIII and von Willebrand's factor (vWF), between 100 and 350 mg of fibrinogen, and about 50% of the Factor XIII and fibronectin originally present in the unit of FFP.

Plasma derivatives (albumin, immunoglobulin, coagulation factor concentrates, and antithrombin III) are prepared commercially from pooled plasma derived from thousands of blood donors. The plasma is initially fractionated by the Cohn-Oncley cold ethanol method, following which the fractions are further processed into specific derivatives. Since microorganisms present in any unit of plasma become uniformly distributed in a pool, products prepared from pooled plasma can be highly infectious. To prevent this, the current practice is to expose the plasma derivatives to one or more viral inactivation processes. Albumin production has always included a pasteurization step at 60° C for 10 hours. Heat or solvent/detergent treatments, the latter of which inactivates lipid-envelope viruses, are also used. Therefore, the currently prepared derivatives are safe products, although transmission of hepatitis A (which is not a lipid envelope virus) has occurred following transfusion of solvent/detergent–treated products.

Coagulation factor concentrates may be isolated from plasma fractions by immunoadsorption, but AHF may also be synthesized by recombinant methods. Although most brands of Factor VIII concentrate contain only the AHF, preparations enriched in vWF are also available (Humate-P). The recombinant Factor VIII is safe and effective, but also expensive.

The prothrombin complex (Profilnine), for treatment of Factor IX deficiency, actually contains the vitamin K–dependent Factors II, VII, IX, and X. Its use has been associated with disseminated intravascular coagulation (DIC) and thrombotic episodes owing to the presence of activated coagulation factors. Purified Factor IX concentrates (Alphanine and Mononine) contain less thrombogenic material than the prothrombin complex.

INDICATIONS FOR TRANSFUSIONS
Red Blood Cell Transfusions

To avoid transfusion-related complications, RBC transfusions should be given only when absolutely necessary. The National Institutes of Health (NIH) has published guidelines that state in general terms when and when not to transfuse RBCs. Although the need to transfuse depends on many clinical factors, hematocrit or hemoglobin values are commonly used as transfusion triggers. According to NIH guidelines,

RBC transfusions are necessary only if the hematocrit falls below 21%. However, in certain clinical situations, the hematocrit can be within normal range while the patient has a decreased RBC mass (following traumatic injuries or orthopedic surgery), or the hematocrit may be falsely low because of plasma volume expansion. Therefore, the decision to transfuse must be based on clinical evaluation of the patient. The indications of RBC transfusions following acute blood loss and for chronic anemia are discussed separately.

Acute Blood Loss

Patients who experience acute blood loss require surgical care and transfusion therapy. When the blood volume loss exceeds 15%, symptoms of hypovolemia occur. If more than 30% of blood volume is lost, cardiac output decreases by about 50% and the state of consciousness is affected. Hypovolemia must be corrected promptly, usually with crystalloid infusions. The patient may be considered normovolemic when vital signs, tissue perfusion, and urine output have become normal. Recent interesting reports suggest that when adult patients with penetrating injuries to the torso were not given intravenous fluids until the time of surgery, they tolerated the hypovolemic insult better and had a higher survival rate than patients who received the traditional fluid resuscitation prior to surgery. However, when the blood loss is extensive, fluid resuscitation and RBC transfusions are required.

It may not be advisable to be overly restrictive in RBC transfusions during surgery, as studies involving Jehovah's Witnesses showed an increased perioperative mortality rate when the preoperative hematocrit was less than 24% and operative blood loss exceeded 500 mL. Furthermore, it should be pointed out that although RBC transfusions primarily increase the RBC volume, they secondarily also increase plasma volume.

Chronic Anemia

When anemia is caused by chronic blood loss, its cause should be determined and appropriate treatment instituted. Some patients tolerate chronic anemia well because of development of compensatory mechanisms, such as an increase in the RBC 2,3-DPG level and an increase in cardiac output. Therefore, unless the hematocrit is below 18%, the decision to transfuse should be based on the symptoms present rather than on the level of hematocrit alone.

Patients with cardiovascular, cerebrovascular, or pulmonary diseases may not tolerate even mild anemia. RBC transfusions should not be given if anemia can be corrected with either hematinics (iron, vitamin B_{12}, or folic acid) or erythropoietin (EPO). EPO is approved by the U.S. Food and Drug Administration for treatment of anemia in chronic renal failure and in AIDS following zidovidine (AZT, Retrovir) treatment. Studies have shown improvement in the functional status of patients following EPO treatment because of the increase in the RBC mass. However, it is not known whether these conclusions apply to a transfusion situation. Nevertheless, it could be argued that patients who require chronic transfusion therapy should be maintained at a hematocrit level of about 30%, particularly since the total number of RBC units transfused to these patients is similar regardless of the level of hematocrit maintained.

When the decision to transfuse RBCs is made, one must consider what kind of RBC product is needed and how many units should be given. Although packed RBCs are most commonly used, some patients require WBC-depleted products or RBCs with a high level of 2,3-DPG. The number of units required for each transfusion may be estimated on the basis of the initial and desired hematocrit. One unit of packed RBCs is expected to increase the hematocrit by 2 to 3% in an average adult, although this might not be the case owing to an increase in plasma volume induced by the RBC transfusion. Previously it was thought that 1-unit RBC transfusions were unnecessary. According to current concepts, however, 1-unit transfusions are acceptable, even preferable to giving more blood. The usual infusion rate is 2 to 4 mL per kg per hour. In patients at risk for circulatory overload, the rate should not exceed 1 mL per kg per hour. In actively bleeding patients, the unit can be administered as rapidly as physically possible. The effectiveness of RBC therapy should be evaluated on the basis of clinical improvement and increase in hematocrit.

Platelet Transfusions

Platelets are given either prophylactically to prevent bleeding or therapeutically to stop bleeding caused by thrombocytopenia or, rarely, thrombocytopathy. In the United States, prophylactic platelet transfusions have been administered when the platelet count was less than 20,000 per μL. However, this transfusion trigger has been challenged, since data show that a striking increase in stool blood loss occurs only when the platelet count decreases below 5000 per μL. Table 2 provides currently accepted guidelines for prophylactic platelet transfusions on the basis of platelet counts and associated conditions. Platelet transfusions are contraindicated in autoim-

mune thrombocytopenic purpura, thrombotic thrombocytopenic purpura, and post-transfusion purpura except when life-threatening bleeding is present. Under these conditions, the transfused platelets are destroyed rapidly and may aggravate the disease process.

The major problem in platelet therapy is the development of nonresponsiveness to transfusions. This can have an immune or a nonimmune basis. The immune response is usually directed to HLAs as a result either of pregnancy or of previous transfusions containing white cells. About 10% of HLA-alloimmunized patients also have antibodies to a human platelet antigen (HPA), further interfering with response to platelet therapy. Fever, sepsis, and DIC cause refractoriness on a nonimmune basis.

The usual therapeutic dose of platelets for an adult is either a pool of 6 to 8 units of random donor platelets or 1 unit of apheresis platelets. It is necessary to evaluate the response to platelet transfusions by measuring the platelet count within 60 minutes of transfusion or 24 hours later, or both. In a stable, adult leukemic patient, 1 unit of apheresis platelets will increase the platelet count by 20,000 to 30,000 per μL. In nonresponsive patients who have developed alloantibodies, transfusion of HLA-matched or HLA- and HPA-matched platelets may be effective. Because of the heterogeneity of the HLA system, it is often difficult to provide apheresis platelets that have the same HLA type as the patient. However, immunized patients may also respond to transfusions of platelets with cross-reactive HLA antigens. Of course, transfusion of HLA-matched platelets is not necessary in responsive patients. To prevent alloimmunization, patients who are candidates for long-term platelet support should receive only leukodepleted blood products.

Transfusion of Plasma and Derivatives

Fresh-Frozen Plasma

FFP contains all normal plasma constituents, such as immunoglobulins, stable and labile coagulation factors, albumin, complement components, and so on. FFP is indicated for the treatment of acquired or congenital coagulation factor deficiencies, except Factor VIII or IX, when bleeding is present or surgery is scheduled. FFP is not recommended for blood volume expansion. The current guidelines recommend FFP infusions only when the prothrombin time or partial thromboplastin time is at least one and a half times over the control value. This usually translates to 16 seconds for the former and 60 seconds for the latter test. The usual dose of FFP is 10 to 20 mL per kg. In the future, solvent/detergent–treated pooled plasma, free from lipid-envelope viruses, may be available.

Cryoprecipitated Antihemophilic Factor

Cryoprecipitated AHF is used to treat congenital or acquired afibrinogenemia, vWF deficiency, and Factor XIII deficiency. DIC is an acquired fibrinogen

TABLE 2. **Recommended Triggers for Prophylactic Platelet Transfusions***

Patient's Platelet Count/μL	Associated Conditions
<5000	None
5000–10,000	Fever or minor hemorrhage
10,000–20,000	Heparin therapy, coagulation disorder
<60,000	Surgery contemplated
>100,000	Bleeding time >15 min and surgery contemplated

*Based on platelet count and associated conditions.

deficiency for which cryoprecipitate infusions are helpful. Usually, multiple doses of 10-unit pools of cryoprecipitated AHF are required for therapy. Fibrin glue, produced by mixing cryoprecipitated AHF with bovine thrombin and calcium, is intended for topical use in some surgical procedures.

Albumin

Albumin, available as 5 and 25% solutions, is an effective plasma volume expander and is used to treat hypovolemia following hemorrhagic shock and albumin loss following burn injuries. To reduce the costs of medical care, interest has focused on the use of crystalloids or synthetic colloids in place of albumin. Controlled clinical trials in settings of extensive vascular surgery or trauma have shown that patient outcomes were similar regardless of whether albumin or crystalloids were used. In patients with thermal injuries, albumin infusions are considered beneficial when given 24 hours after the injury. It is generally accepted that albumin should not be used to treat malnutrition.

Intravenous Immunoglobulin

Intravenous immunoglobulin (IVIG) is used to treat agammaglobulinemia and certain immune disorders, such as autoimmune thrombocytopenic purpura, Kawasaki's disease, and some neurologic diseases (acute Guillain-Barré syndrome). The beneficial effects are thought to result from the blockade of the reticuloendothelial system by the infused immunoglobulin, immunomodulation through anti-idiotype antibodies, or prevention of binding of the activated complement component C3 to target cells. The usual dose is 0.4 gram per kg per day for 5 days, although smaller doses have also been effective.

PREVENTION OF TRANSFUSION COMPLICATIONS

Autologous Blood

Many risks of transfusion can be eliminated by using autologous rather than homologous blood. All patients scheduled for an elective surgery for which blood use is anticipated should donate their own blood prior to surgery. Contraindications include a hematocrit of less than 33%, unstable angina, severe aortic stenosis, and the possibility of existing bacteremia (e.g., osteomyelitis). Intra- and postoperative salvage of autologous blood and preoperative hemodilution are other strategies to reduce homologous blood transfusions.

Some patients want to provide their own donors, a procedure known as "directed donation." This practice does not increase the safety of donated blood.

Blood Substitutes

Perfluorocarbons and modified hemoglobin solutions have been studied intensely as possible blood substitutes. Although these products have a potential to reduce the complications associated with the use of homologous blood, their efficacy and safety have not yet been demonstrated.

Special Blood Products

The use of special blood products may help prevent transfusion complications in patients who need allogeneic blood and who have a history of certain transfusion-related complications. For instance, allergic reactions can be prevented by giving plasma-free blood products (washed cellular components) or selecting plasma from donors that the patient has previously tolerated. Febrile reactions may be preventable by administration of leukodepleted cellular blood products. Reactions to platelet concentrates caused by the presence of bioreactive substances (interleukin-1-beta and interleukin-6), generated by mononuclear cells during storage, are avoided by transfusing packed or washed platelets.

Patients who are IgA-negative and have a history of anaphylactic transfusion reactions due to anti-IgA should receive blood products from IgA-deficient donors. These patients may experience an adverse reaction even when they receive an RBC product from which most of the plasma has been removed (e.g., previously frozen RBCs). This could be due to the presence of IgA on the surface of RBCs. Some donors have very small amounts of IgA on the RBC membrane, consequently, such RBCs, following a thorough washing, may be a safe product for immunized IgA-deficient patients.

Special categories of patients, regardless of previous history of transfusion complications, are nevertheless at risk for transfusion-associated graft-versus-host disease (TA-GvHD), cytomegalovirus (CMV) infection, and spread of AIDS. The use of special blood products to prevent these complications is discussed next.

Transfusion-Associated Graft-Versus-Host Disease

Immunoincompetent patients, who lack the ability to eliminate donor lymphocytes, are at risk of developing TA-GvHD when they receive immunocompetent donor lymphocytes in blood products (Table 3). It is of interest that patients with AIDS are not susceptible to TA-GvHD, nor has this complication been reported in patients with most solid tumors or aplastic anemia. But in a suitable setting, the donor lymphocytes may proliferate after transfusion and mount an attack against the patient's tissues. Typically, within 10 days after transfusion, such patients will develop persistent fever and a rash that eventually becomes generalized. Liver function tests become abnormal, and diarrhea may develop. Because of the ensuing bone marrow aplasia, the patient is susceptible to secondary infections. Eventually, multiorgan failure sets in, and the outcome is fatal in most cases. The diagnosis may be difficult and is often confused

TABLE 3. Risk Diseases and Conditions for Transfusion-Associated Graft-Versus-Host Disease

Developmental immunoincompetency (fetus, premature infant)
Hereditary immunodeficiency
    Wiskott-Aldrich syndrome
    Severe combined immunodeficiency
    Thymic dysplasia
Bone marrow transplantation
Hematologic malignancies
    Acute lymphocytic leukemia
    Acute nonlymphocytic leukemia
    Hodgkin's disease
    Non-Hodgkin's lymphoma
Other malignancies
    Neuroblastoma
    Glioblastoma
Patients receiving transfusions from relatives

with drug-induced aplastic anemia or various infectious diseases.

TA-GvHD has also been reported in recent years in immunocompetent patients if the lymphocytes present in the donor blood are homozygous for one of the patient's HLA haplotypes. The donor lymphocytes in this setting are not recognized as foreign by the patient's immune system and consequently are not eliminated. However, the donor lymphocytes recognize as foreign the patient's HLA haplotype that is different from theirs. TA-GvHD in immunocompetent patients is more common in populations that are genetically homogeneous, such as in Japanese, or in blood relatives of the patient.

TA-GvHD is preventable by irradiation of all cellular blood components given to patients in the risk groups (Table 3). The method of irradiation must provide a minimal dose of 15 Gy to all parts of the blood bag. It should be noted that there is no need to irradiate FFP. Previously frozen RBCs have not been shown to cause TA-GvHD.

Transfusion-Associated Cytomegalovirus Infection

Transfusion of CMV-seropositive cellular blood products may cause a serious infection in low-birthweight infants of CMV-seronegative mothers and in CMV-seronegative patients undergoing bone marrow transplantation. This complication can be prevented by transfusing CMV-seronegative blood products. Sufficient numbers of CMV-seronegative blood products may not always be available, since a large proportion of blood donors have had CMV infection. Alternatively, it was found that low-birthweight infants born to CMV-seronegative mothers who received previously frozen RBCs did not develop CMV infection. Recent clinical trials in both the autologous and the allogeneic bone marrow transplantation setting have demonstrated that cellular blood products that have been depleted from WBCs by high-efficiency filtration are as effective in preventing CMV infection as CMV-seronegative blood products.

Blood Transfusion for AIDS Patients

Co-culture of peripheral blood mononuclear cells from AIDS patients with normal WBCs induces a dose-related activation of human immunodeficiency virus type 1 (HIV-1) expression in in vivo infected cells and dissemination of the infection into previously uninfected patient cells. Thus it seems prudent to transfuse AIDS patients with leukocyte-depleted blood products. Multicenter clinical trials are now in progress to provide definitive explanations of these provocative data.

ADVERSE REACTIONS TO BLOOD TRANSFUSION

method of
JEFFERY S. DZIECZKOWSKI, M.D.
Wayne State University School of Medicine
Detroit, Michigan,

and

KENNETH C. ANDERSON, M.D.
Dana Farber Cancer Institute
Boston, Massachusetts

Adverse reactions to the transfusion of blood components are common despite multiple tests, inspections, and checks. The incidence of some reactions can be reduced or prevented with the use of modified (washed, filtered, or irradiated) blood components. Fortunately, the most frequently encountered complications are not life-threatening; however, serious reactions may present with similar, seemingly benign, signs and symptoms. Discontinuing the transfusion is critical to limiting and preventing additional adverse sequelae. The prudent clinician reports all suspected reactions to the transfusion service so that the reactions may be thoroughly investigated and documented.

Transfusion-transmitted infections are often considered the major risk of transfusion by the patient and clinician. These infections, which are often serious and possibly fatal, are fortunately becoming less frequent. Improved donor screening and testing have dramatically reduced the incidence of transfusion-related infections. These infections, like any adverse transfusion reaction, must also be brought to the attention of the blood bank for appropriate "lookback" studies.

Transfusion reactions are classically grouped into those mediated by immune and nonimmunologic mechanisms. Immune-mediated reactions are most often the result of antibody interaction, of either recipient or donor origin. However, cellular components of the donor or recipient's immune system may also cause transfusion complications. The chemical and physical properties of stored blood and its additives can also lead to unwanted reactions, which are often mild but may be life-threatening.

IMMUNE-MEDIATED REACTIONS

Acute Hemolytic Transfusion Reactions

Acute immune-mediated hemolytic reactions occur when the recipient has preformed antibodies that bind and lyse the donor red blood cells (RBCs). The ABO isoagglutinins, which are present in all individuals except those of blood type AB, are responsible for the majority of these reactions. Immediate hemolytic reactions may also be caused by preformed alloantibodies directed against other antigens found on RBCs, e.g., Rh, Kell, and Duffy.

The signs and symptoms of an acute hemolytic reaction include hypotension, tachypnea, tachycardia, fever, chills, hemoglobinemia, hemoglobinuria, chest and/or flank pain and discomfort at the catheter or infusion site. Monitoring the patient's vital signs at the beginning of the transfusion, particularly in the comatose patient, is important to identify these reactions promptly. When an acute hemolytic reaction is suspected, the transfusion must be immediately stopped and intravenous access maintained. The reaction must be immediately reported, and any untransfused blood component, along with a correctly labeled post-transfusion blood sample, sent to the blood transfusion service for investigation. Laboratory tests to determine whether hemolysis has occurred include haptoglobin, lactate dehydrogenase (LDH), and indirect bilirubin, and these should be monitored.

Late complications of hemolytic reactions may occur and can be fatal. The immune-mediated destruction of RBCs can result in renal compromise and subsequent failure. These complications are prevented or minimized by inducing diuresis with furosemide or mannitol and intravenous fluids. Disseminated intravascular coagulation (DIC) may also develop from the immune-mediated lysis of RBCs. Baseline coagulation studies, including prothrombin time (PT), activated partial thromboplastin time (aPTT), fibrinogen, and platelet count, and subsequent monitoring are warranted in patients transfused with incompatible blood.

Each hospital has policies and procedures for investigating suspected transfusion reactions. The task is to determine whether incompatible RBCs have been transfused, once the patient is stable. If an error has occurred, it is important to identify its source, so that errors do not recur (Mr. Jones received Mr. Smith's intended blood and, it is hoped, not vice versa). Examining the pre- and post-transfusion samples for evidence of hemolysis, retyping the patient, and performing a direct antiglobulin test (DAT) on the post-transfusion sample; re-crossmatching the blood component; and checking all clerical records for errors will determine whether a hemolytic reaction has occurred and often point to the source of the error. The majority of these reactions are the result of clerical error at the patient's bedside, such as mislabeled samples or an incorrectly identified patient.

Delayed Hemolytic and Serologic Transfusion Reactions

Delayed hemolytic transfusion reactions (DHTR) or delayed serologic transfusion reactions (DSTR) oc-

cur in patients previously sensitized to an RBC antigen who have no detectable alloantibody at the time of the alloantibody screen and crossmatch. The patient is transfused with antigen-positive blood to which she or he has been sensitized. An anamnestic response results in the early production of the alloantibody with possible hemolysis of the transfused RBCs. Soon after the transfusion the alloantibody screen becomes positive, and a positive DAT may be found in a post-transfusion sample.

Since DHTR develop slowly, 1 to 2 weeks after the transfusion, the patient has often been discharged. Thus these reactions often go undiagnosed. The diagnosis is made most frequently in the blood bank where a subsequent blood sample, often a sample for additional crossmatch, reveals a positive alloantibody screen or a new alloantibody. Aliquots from the transfused unit or records of the donor RBC phenotype may be available to confirm the source of antigenic rechallenge and thus confirm the diagnosis.

These reactions are mediated by alloantibodies that coat the antigen-positive transfused RBCs. The antibody-coated RBCs are removed by the reticuloendothelial system, and the hemolysis is extravascular. No specific therapy is usually required, although additional RBC transfusions may be necessary to replace those that have been removed. DSTR are similar to DHTR; however, there is no evidence of RBC destruction or removal.

Febrile Nonhemolytic Transfusion Reactions

Febrile nonhemolytic transfusion reactions (FNHTR) are the most frequent reaction associated with the transfusion of cellular blood components. The recipient experiences a rise in temperature of at least 1° C, often accompanied by chills and at times rigors. These reactions can be mediated by recipient antibodies directed against donor leukocyte antigens. Patients previously exposed and sensitized to multiple leukocyte antigens, such as the multiparous or multiply transfused, are at increased risk. The incidence and severity of these reactions may be decreased by premedicating the patient with acetaminophen or other antipyretic agents. Alternatively, transfusing leukocyte-reduced blood products reduces the frequency of FNHTR by preventing sensitization and exposure to those already sensitized. Recent studies suggest that cytokines that accumulate within stored cellular blood components may play a role in FNHTR.

The laboratory identification of recipient leukoagglutinins is possible, although it is not often readily available or necessary. FNHTR are primarily diagnoses of exclusion, once serologic tests and clerical checks have ruled out the possibility of a hemolytic reaction and other sources of fever have been considered.

Allergic Reactions

Hypersensitivity reactions to plasma proteins found in transfused components are common. These reactions present as urticaria or rash with itching, edema, headache, and dizziness, which are often mild. The mild reactions may be treated symptomatically by slowing or temporarily stopping the transfusion and administering antihistamines (diphenhydramine, 50 mg orally or intramuscularly). Once the medication has reversed the signs and/or symptoms, the transfusion may be completed. If a patient has a history of allergic transfusion reactions, prophylactic antihistamine administration is practical. Washing cellular components, which removes the offending plasma component, may be required to prevent this reaction in the extremely sensitive patient requiring packed RBC (PRBC) or platelet transfusion.

Anaphylactic Reactions

Anaphylaxis in any setting is a medical emergency. This severe reaction presents after a few milliliters of the blood component have been transfused. The patient may complain of difficulty in breathing, coughing, nausea and vomiting with hypotension, bronchospasm, respiratory arrest, shock, and loss of consciousness. Treatment begins by stopping the transfusion, maintaining vascular access with normal saline, and administering epinephrine (0.5 to 1.0 mL of 1:1000 dilution subcutaneously). In severe cases, corticosteroids may be required.

Anaphylactic reactions caused by transfusion are classically seen in the sensitized IgA-deficient patient who is transfused with IgA-containing plasma. Patients who have repeated allergic reactions to blood components should be tested for IgA deficiency. Individuals with severe IgA deficiency are at risk and should receive IgA-deficient plasma products. Cellular components may be washed, and fresh-frozen plasma or cryoprecipitate from IgA-deficient donors is available.

Graft-Versus-Host Disease

Graft-versus-host disease (GVHD) is a frequent complication of allogeneic bone marrow transplantation (ABMT), in which setting viable lymphocytes derived from donor bone marrow cannot be eliminated by an immunodeficient host. GVHD is mediated by donor T lymphocytes that recognize host human leukocyte antigens (HLA) as foreign and mount an immune response, which is manifested clinically by the development of fever, a characteristic cutaneous eruption, diarrhea, and liver function abnormalities. GVHD can also occur when blood components that contain donor T lymphocytes are transfused to immunodeficient recipients or to immunocompetent recipients who share HLA with the donor. In addition to the aforementioned clinical features, transfusion-associated (TA)–GVHD is further characterized by marrow aplasia and pancytopenia. In contrast to GVHD that develops in the setting of ABMT, TA–GVHD is notoriously resistant to treatment with immunosuppressive therapies, including corticosteroids, cyclosporine, antithymocyte globulin, and abla-

tive therapy followed by ABMT. Clinical manifestations and death occur at 8 to 10 days and 3 to 4 weeks post-transfusion, respectively. The resistance to treatment and fatal outcome highlight the need for identification of patient groups at risk for TA–GVHD and use of methods for its prevention.

TA–GVHD can be prevented by irradiation of cellular components (minimum of 2500 cGy) before transfusion to patients at risk. At present, patients at risk for TA–GVHD include fetuses receiving intrauterine transfusions, selected immunocompetent or immunocompromised recipients, recipients of donor units known to be from a blood relative, and recipients who have undergone bone marrow transplantation.

Transfusion-Related Acute Lung Injury

This rare reaction results from the transfusion of plasma containing high titers of anti-HLA antibodies reactive with the corresponding antigen(s) on recipient leukocytes. Unexpected pulmonary symptoms and signs of noncardiogenic pulmonary edema, including "white out" on chest radiograph, may occur in the recipient, and the alert clinician will consider this reaction. Treatment is supportive, and the patients usually recover without sequelae.

Reporting this reaction to the transfusion service is important, since testing of the transfused plasma may identify and document the source of the recipient's pulmonary reaction. In addition, plasma from donors with high titer anti-HLA antibodies, frequently multiparous women, may be withheld from future transfusion.

Post-Transfusion Purpura

This rare complication, manifesting as thrombocytopenia 7 to 10 days after platelet transfusion, occurs predominantly in women. This reaction is due to the production of platelet-specific antibodies by the recipient. The antibodies raised in response to the donor's platelets are thought to cross-react with the recipient's platelets, resulting in the increased destruction of platelets. Treatment, when necessary, is directed at neutralizing the recipient's antibodies. Intravenous immune globulin (IVIG) is thought to reduce the effects of these autoantibodies. Plasmapheresis to remove the offending antibodies may also be considered. Further platelet transfusions should be avoided.

Alloimmunization

Recipient alloimmunization may occur in response to antigens found on transfused RBCs, leukocytes, and platelets.

Approximately 1% of all patients transfused with allogeneic RBCs will develop alloantibodies. Patients with alloantibodies present problems to the blood bank in trying to identify compatible blood for future transfusion, and delays in providing crossmatch-compatible products may be encountered. In addition, women of childbearing age who become sensitized to RBC antigens (e.g., D, c, E, Kell, or Duffy) are at risk for bearing a fetus with hemolytic disease of the newborn.

Patients who are sensitized to antigens found on donor leukocytes or platelets may become refractory to further platelet transfusions. Identifying and supplying compatible platelets is difficult, requires recruitment of donors who share antigens with the recipient, and is often futile. Therapy is therefore directed at preventing sensitization through the use of leukocyte-reduced cellular components and limiting the number of donor exposures by using single-donor apheresis platelets plus the judicious use of transfusions.

NONIMMUNOLOGIC REACTIONS

Fluid Overload

Blood components are excellent volume expanders, and their transfusion may quickly lead to fluid overload. This complication can be easily prevented or treated with the use of diuretics and monitoring the rate and volume of the transfusion.

Hypothermia

Most blood components, with the exception of platelets, are stored refrigerated (4° C) or frozen (− 18° C or below). Hypothermia may develop with the rapid infusion of these cold components. Caution is required when transfusing via a central line since cardiac dysrhythmias can result from exposing the sinoatrial node to cold fluid. Warming the components with the use of an in-line warmer prevents this complication.

Electrolyte Toxicity

Prolonged storage of RBCs leads to an increase in the plasma concentration of potassium in the unit. Neonates and patients in renal failure are at risk for becoming hyperkalemic. The diagnosis is readily made by measuring the serum potassium or recognizing the characteristic electrocardiographic changes found with hyperkalemia. This complication can be fatal in neonates; thus preventive measures are used, such as transfusing fresh or washed RBCs.

Citrate, the most commonly used anticoagulant in blood components, acts by chelating calcium and thereby inhibiting the coagulation cascade. The transfusion of multiple units may lead to hypocalcemia, which is manifested by circumoral numbness and/or tingling sensations of the fingers and toes. Since citrate is quickly metabolized to bicarbonate, calcium supplementation is seldom required in this setting. Should calcium be required, it must be infused through a separate intravenous line. No medication should ever be added to the blood component bag or administered through the transfusion set.

Iron Overload

Chronic transfusion with PRBCs will result in iron overload. The body's affinity for iron and the lack of an effective clearance mechanism causes the total body stores of iron (1 to 3 grams) to steadily increase approximately 200 to 250 mg with each unit. The number of units transfused until signs and symptoms of iron overload present varies; however, it is not uncommon after 100 units have been transfused. Chelating agents, such as deferoxamine (Desferal), are available to reduce the body's burden of iron; however, their efficacy is suboptimal. Preventing this complication through alternative therapies (e.g., erythropoietin) and the judicious use of transfusion is preferable and cost effective.

Infectious Complications

Specific therapies related to infectious diseases should be consulted. However, it behooves the clinician who prescribes transfusion therapy to be aware of the infectious risks and to discuss these with the recipient.

Viral Infections

Hepatitis C Virus. The major etiologic agent of what was designated "non-A, non-B hepatitis" remains the most common viral infection of clinical significance. The testing of donated blood for the presence of antibodies to hepatitis C virus (HCV) has reduced the incidence to 3 in 10,000 transfusion episodes. Infection with HCV may be asymptomatic or may lead to chronic active hepatitis, cirrhosis, and liver failure.

Hepatitis B Virus. Increased and improved donor selection and screening, along with increased hepatitis B virus (HBV) vaccinations, has made transfusion-associated HBV infections rare. The current calculated risk of acquiring HBV through transfusion is 1 in 200,000 transfusions. Individuals who require long-term transfusion therapy should be vaccinated for HBV to prevent this complication.

Human Immunodeficiency Virus Type 1. Intensive donor screening and testing have dramatically reduced the risk of human immunodeficiency virus Type 1 (HIV-1) infection via blood transfusion. The risk of HIV-1 infection is approximately 1 in 250,000, although this estimate is based on data from the late 1980s. Current risk may in fact be lower.

Since 1992, all donated blood has been tested for HIV-2. There have been no reported cases in the United States of this infection related to transfusion.

Cytomegalovirus. This ubiquitous virus may be transmitted by the infected passenger white blood cells found in transfused PRBC components. Not all donor blood is tested for serologic evidence of donor exposure; however, seronegative, or cytomegalovirus (CMV)–safe, products are provided to those at risk for CMV complications. Cellular products that are depleted of leukocytes are considered to have decreased infectious risk. Patients at risk include immunosuppressed patients, CMV-seronegative transplant recipients, and neonates.

Human T Lymphotropic Virus–Type I. Human lymphotropic virus Type I (HTLV-I) is associated with adult T cell leukemia/lymphoma and tropical spastic paraparesis in a small percentage of those infected. HTLV-II may also be transmitted by blood products; however, no disease state has been associated with this virus. The reported risk of infection via transfusion is 1 in 50,000.

Parvovirus B-19. Blood components and products derived from pooled plasma can transmit this virus. The virus is the etiologic agent of erythema infectiosum, fifth disease, in children. Parvovirus B-19 shows tropism for erythroid precursors and inhibits RBC production and maturation. Pure red cell aplasia, presenting as either acute aplastic crisis or chronic anemia with shortened RBC survival, may occur in individuals with an underlying hematologic disease, in pregnant women, in patients with disorders involving increased red cell production, and those with congenital or acquired immunodeficiency.

Bacterial Contamination

Bacterial contamination of blood components may occur as a result of inadequate skin cleansing for venipuncture preparation, during postcollection component processing, or from the bacteremic donor. Since most bacteria do not grow well in a refrigerated or frozen environment, PRBCs and frozen plasma are not a common source of bacterial contamination. However, some gram-negative bacteria can grow at 1 to 6° C, including species of *Yersinia* and *Pseudomonas*. Platelet concentrates, which are stored at room temperature, are more likely to be contaminated with gram-positive skin contaminants and coagulase-negative *Staphylococcus*.

Recipients who are transfused with bacteria-contaminated units develop fever and chills, which may progress to septic shock and DIC. The reactions may occur suddenly, within minutes of initiating the transfusion, or after several hours. Characteristically, the onset of symptoms and signs is sudden and fulminant, which will aid in clinically differentiating bacterial contamination from FNHTR. The reactions, particularly those related to gram-negative contaminants, are the result of endotoxins infused within the contaminated stored component.

When contaminated transfusions are suspected (e.g., the sudden development of shock), the transfusion must be stopped immediately. Therapy is directed at supporting the recipient's blood pressure, pulse, oxygenation, and renal function. The laboratory investigation should include the usual checks and serologic tests. Cultures of any untransfused blood component and the recipient's blood may prove diagnostic. Broad-spectrum antibiotics should be started immediately and may be adjusted after the culture and sensitivity reports are available.

PARASITES

A number of parasites have been reported or are theoretically capable of being transmitted by blood transfusion. Among these parasites are *Babesia microti* (babesiosis), *Trypanosoma cruzi* (Chagas' disease), *Plasmodium* species (malaria), *Borrelia burgdorferi* (Lyme disease), and *Treponema pallidum* (syphilis).

The Digestive System

GALLSTONES AND GALLSTONE SYNDROMES

method of
WILLIAM C. MEYERS, M.D.
Duke University Medical Center
Durham, North Carolina

Stone formation within the gallbladder continues to be an extremely common condition that can cause a number of clinical problems of importance to primary care physicians and surgeons. Once gallstones have formed, the condition rarely resolves spontaneously, which leads directly to the question of treatment. Since 1990, no medical procedure has impacted surgery as much as laparoscopic cholecystectomy. The new technique greatly enlarged the entire field of minimally invasive surgery and has also stimulated a new look at cost-effectiveness and outcomes research in medicine. This subsection re-evaluates the traditional conditions in the light of new therapy.

GALLSTONES

The incidence of cholelithiasis in the United States remains about 10%, with some 800,000 new cases seen annually. In the United States, 80% of stones are thought to be of the cholesterol type, but the incidence of bilirubinate stones may be unexplainedly increasing. Cholesterol and pigment stones have individual risk factors, although some overlap exists (Table 1). The most prevalent risk factors for cholesterol stones are increasing age and female sex. In nearly all populations studied, the rate of increase with age decreases pronouncedly after 50 or 60 years of age, and the sex difference also fades with age. The newest recognized risk factors are total parenteral nutrition (TPN) and solid organ transplantation (best recognized in heart transplant recipients). Liver transplant recipients are also at risk for primary ductal stones. Much current research in cholesterol and bilirubinate gallstone formation continues to focus on possible nucleating factors.

Diagnosis

Although the oral cholecystogram (OCG), first introduced by the St. Louis surgeons Ewarts Graham and Warren Cole in 1924, was formerly the diagnostic "gold standard," the accuracy and practicality of ultrasonography became apparent in the late 1970s and has emerged as the preferred test. Ultrasonography has the advantages of being quick, cheap, and capable of evaluating the liver, common duct, pancreas, and other areas of the abdomen. Hepatobiliary scintigraphy has generally fallen into disfavor because of the associated time and cost, although occasionally this test definitively rules out the diagnosis of acute cholecystitis. A nuclear study showing a gallbladder ejection fraction of less than 50% is occasionally used as a warrant to operate on patients with classic biliary colic but no documentable cholelithiasis. Other diagnostic or complementary tests include the traditional OCG, plain abdominal radiography, examination of duodenal drainage for crystals, intraoperative palpation, abnormal liver function tests, upper gastrointestinal series, barium enema, upper endoscopy, colonoscopy, esophageal pH measurements, pancreatic function tests, intravenous pyelography, or spinal films. Endoscopic retrograde cholangiopancreatography (ERCP) and percutaneous transhepatic cholangiography (PTC) are generally more helpful in the diagnosis of choledocholithiasis or other biliary lesions than in the diagnosis of cholelithiasis per se.

Management

The most important consideration in the management of patients with gallstones is the natural his-

TABLE 1. **Risk Factors for Gallstones**

Cholesterol Stones
Known Risk Factors
Age
Sex (female)
Ethnic predisposition
Obesity
Clofibrate
Impaired ileal absorption
Heart transplantation
Possible Risk Factors
Diet
Oral contraceptives
Pregnancy
Vagotomy
Diabetes
Total parenteral nutrition
Dyskinesia
Pigment Stones
Age
Hemolysis
Geographic (Far East)
Cirrhosis
Total parenteral nutrition
Duodenal diverticula

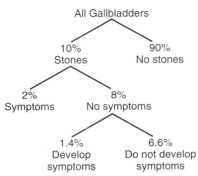

Figure 1. Natural history of gallstones. Data based on lifetime risk, compilation of studies from the literature. (From Meyers WC, Jones RS: Textbook of Liver and Biliary Surgery. Philadelphia, JB Lippincott, 1990, p 237.)

tory of the condition (Figure 1). Once gallstones are present, the predisposition for the gallbladder to develop more stones does not go away naturally unless the gallbladder is removed. However, autopsy studies indicate that most gallstones do not cause clinical problems and in fact never come to the attention of physicians. The number of diagnoses seems to be increasing, probably due to more comprehensive technology such as ultrasonography. In a Duke University study of 100 patients with gallstones detected coincidentally on ultrasonography performed for unrelated reasons, 19 clearly had episodes of right upper quadrant epigastric pain at the time of gallstone discovery, and an additional four patients developed symptoms over a 2-year follow-up. Also, the 20-year study of Gracie and Ransohoff on a predominantly male population with asymptomatic stones found an 18% incidence of symptom development. However, the vast majority of patients discovered clinically to have gallstones have some degree of upper abdominal pain, although not necessarily classic biliary colic.

The natural history of symptomatic gallstone disease is as follows. About two-thirds of patients have chronic pain only. The remaining one-third develop some acute problem such as acute cholecystitis, gallstone pancreatitis, or cholangitis. Most asymptomatic gallstones remain asymptomatic. Patients with asymptomatic gallstones develop symptoms at a rate of about 2% per year up to about 10 years, when the rate probably declines considerably. Fortunately, present data indicate that death from gallstones is exceedingly uncommon, particularly in the absence of acute complications. Once gallstone symptoms develop, however, there appears to be about a 50% chance that a significant clinical problem will develop in the next year.

Treatment Options

Cholecystectomy, specifically laparoscopic cholecystectomy, is presently the treatment of choice for the vast majority of patients with symptomatic cholelithiasis. Cholecystectomy usually relieves the preop-

erative symptoms and removes the source of stones, making a stone recurrence unlikely. An adjunctive procedure such as intraoperative cholangiography or common duct exploration may be necessary to eliminate concurrent stones in the common duct. The mortality from cholecystectomy and the risk of bile duct injury are both generally less than 0.1%, provided the procedure is performed by an experienced, fully trained surgeon. The risk increases in elderly patients, but it is still less than 1%. Cardiopulmonary complications are the principal cause of significant morbidity, but these have decreased considerably with the laparoscopic technique.

Laparoscopic cholescystectomy offers the advantages of reduced postoperative pain, decreased hospitalization, early return to full activity or employment, a lower incidence of cardiovascular complications, and a better cosmetic result. Most of the initial contraindications to laparoscopic cholecystectomy have disappeared. The operation is now regularly performed in patients with a prior history of abdominal surgery, obesity, acute cholecystitis, or suspected common duct stone or cirrhosis. The overall conversion rate (to the traditional approach) remains about 5%, although it may be higher in some groups. Other methods of gallstone treatment such as oral chemical dissolution, intracholecystic infusion agents, or shock wave lithotripsy have had some degree of success but are generally not recommended.

With otherwise uncomplicated cholelithiasis, pain is the first indication for cholecystectomy, if there is a high likelihood that stones are causing the pain. Pathologic evidence of chronic inflammation is so common with cholelithiasis, even in the absence of symptoms, that it should not be listed as the primary indication. Once present, pain is likely to recur, and patients are at high risk for the development of acute complications. Ample data support the safety of temporary, expectant therapy when there is little suspicion of acute inflammation and the clinical situation warrants it. It also seems logical to presume that the younger and healthier the patient, the longer he or she may live, and therefore the more likely that acute complications will develop.

The second indication for cholecystectomy is the development of acute complications such as acute cholecystitis, gallstone pancreatitis, or acute cholangitis. These complications carry a definite mortality, and the patient is at risk as long as the gallbladder remains in place.

The third indication is the development of a chronic complication (exclusive of chronic cholecystitis), such as fistula or cancer. This indication is uncommon, and gallbladder cancer is rarely resectable. The frequency of gallbladder cancer is so small (0.1%) that prophylactic cholecystectomy for this reason alone is not justified. However, some evidence suggests that patients with gallbladder wall calcification and certain other population groups may be at particularly high risk for the development of gallbladder cancer. In one study, Native Americans had 12 times the risk of control populations for the development of gallbladder cancer.

The fourth indication for cholecystectomy may be the presence of stones. Cholelithiasis alone is a sufficient indication when (1) stones are encountered coincidentally at laparotomy performed for another reason and the clinical situation is appropriate, (2) a patient is extraordinarily fearful of developing complications of the condition, or (3) special conditions are present that predispose to the development of acute complications. An example of situation (3) is the presence of gallstones in an organ transplant recipient or stones in a diabetic with minimal symptoms. Patients with sickle cell anemia and a history of abdominal crises should generally undergo elective cholecystectomy in centers familiar with the perioperative considerations in these patients. Uncomplicated cholelithiasis as an indication for cholecystectomy clearly requires the most judgment of the four indications listed. In addition, cholelithiasis is sufficiently common that screening the population for this condition is not justified. Other treatment options such as dissolutional agents or lithotripsy are best administered in a controlled setting as part of an investigational effort, so that results can be carefully evaluated. A reasonable approach to a patient with asymptomatic cholelithiasis, when there are no other indications for cholecystectomy, is a period of expectant management by the primary care physician.

GALLSTONE SYNDROMES

Acute Cholecystitis

Acute cholecystitis occurs in 15% of symptomatic patients. The primary pathophysiologic mechanism is cystic duct obstruction by a stone, which causes, to varying degrees, objective signs of acute infection such as right upper quadrant tenderness, fever, or an elevated white blood cell count. Acute acalculus cholecystitis accounts for up to 9% of all cases of acute cholecystitis. Nearly half of these cases are recognized as disorders occurring in patients who are critically ill from other conditions such as multiple trauma, major surgery, sepsis, drug overdosage, or multisystem failure. In general, this condition is treated like calculus cholecystitis, except that there would be a lower threshold for performing radiologically directed tube cholecystostomy.

For the demonstration of acute cholecystitis, ultrasonography is highly accurate in demonstrating gallstones or gallbladder wall thickening but provides little information about the patency of the cystic duct. However, in combination with clinical assessment, ultrasonography is highly accurate in the diagnosis of cholecystitis, and most physicians prefer this method over OCG or biliary scintigraphy. Most studies of the management of cholecystitis have focused on the timing of cholecystectomy; although most episodes of acute cholecystitis can be treated nonoperatively, the gallbladder will have to be removed at some point as definitive therapy.

The most important issue in management is weighing the risks of acute cholecystitis and of early versus delayed cholecystectomy. A predominance of evidence suggests that early cholecystectomy is just as safe or safer and more cost effective in the treatment of acute cholecystitis. Delayed therapy remains a reasonable clinical alternative, provided the patient gets over the episode. We usually delay several days after the initial presentation before performing laparoscopic cholecystectomy, because resolution of much of the initial edema makes the procedure technically easier. Relatively absolute indications for immediate cholecystectomy are emphysematous cholecystitis and the suspicion of gallbladder perforation. The former suggests the presence of a particularly toxic anaerobic infection. The latter occurs in 2% of patients with symptomatic cholelithiasis. Risk factors for the development of gallbladder perforation include advancing age, male sex, diabetes mellitus, and gallbladder cancer. Duration of cystic duct obstruction is also a contributing factor.

For patients with acute cholecystitis and severe illness, we now prefer radiologically placed tube cholecystostomy as the initial treatment. The procedure can be done by an experienced radiologist with a high degree of safety. The tube is usually placed through the liver side of the gallbladder to avoid peritoneal spillage. Elective laparoscopic or open cholecystectomy can be performed at a later date with relative safety.

Mirizzi's Syndrome

Mirizzi's syndrome is a rare cause of common duct obstruction occurring in 0.5% of patients who are symptomatic from gallstones or in 0.2% of all patients with gallstones. This syndrome is defined by common hepatic duct obstruction resulting from a stone impacted in the cystic duct or neck of the gallbladder. The associated fibrosis is severe and usually requires open cholecystectomy for diagnosis as well as treatment.

Gallbladder Hydrops

Hydrops of the gallbladder is defined as unusual gallbladder enlargement in the absence of acute or chronic inflammation. This condition is unusual in patients with only gallstones, occurring in 0.7% of symptomatic patients. The presence of hydrops should raise the suspicion of neoplasm.

Gallstone Pancreatitis

The clinical features of gallstone pancreatitis resemble those of other acute abdominal processes, such as perforated ulcer or mesenteric ischemia. The most important feature of gallstone pancreatitis is the radiologic demonstration of biliary stones. Historic factors, such as the absence of alcohol ingestion, are also important to rule out other causes. However, the diagnosis of gallstone pancreatitis is a highly judgmental one based on available historic data and the demonstration of biliary stones. ERCP is now considered safe in patients with gallstone pancreatitis if careful attention is given to the use of clean instruments, the avoidance of pressure injection of contrast material, and sphincterotomy. In addition to aiding in the diagnosis of common duct calculi, biliary dilation, or cystic duct obstruction, ERCP may also provide evidence of recent passage of stones through endoscopic visualization of an edematous papilla. ERCP may also help differentiate other causes of recurrent pancreatitis such as cancer, papillary stones, choledochal cyst, cystic fibrosis, or trauma.

Clinically, we divide these patients into those having "mild" and those having "severe" pancreatitis. In the vast majority of patients with gallstone pancreatitis, the acute illness resolves quickly, within several days. In fact, the pancreas in these patients frequently appears normal or only mildly enlarged at early surgery, despite recent, marked hyperamylasemia. A minority of patients fail to recover and develop a more severe form. The latter patients also have a more diffuse abdominal tenderness at initial presentation. If the pancreatitis does resolve quickly, one-half to two-thirds of nonoperatively managed patients develop recurrent pancreatitis within months.

On the basis of these observations of pancreatitis, the following recommendations are made: A short, 1- to 3-day period of observation is appropriate if the pancreatitis is clinically mild. Early operation is generally recommended to minimize the total duration of the illness and to avoid repeat attacks. Rapid resolution of marked hyperamylasemia can be used as a clinical guide in some cases. If the pancreatitis is severe, three options are available: early surgery, early ERCP, or delay. Early surgery in these cases is usually reserved for patients with Ranson's criteria of severe pancreatitis or other indications for exploration, such as hemorrhage.

Biliary Fistulas

Most biliary fistulas are caused by cystic duct obstruction and penetration of a stone through the gallbladder into an adjacent organ. The classic situation is a large stone fistulizing through the duodenum and becoming lodged in the distal ileum (gallstone ileus). In this syndrome, the recommended treatment is first to fix the small bowel obstruction, that is, remove the stone. The inflammation in the right quadrant is usually severe, and it is hazardous to correct the biliary tract abnormality initially. The treatment of other types of biliary fistulas should be individualized.

Common Duct Stones

Diagnosis of common duct stones is initially based on a history and physical examination consistent with chronic gallstone disease or biliary obstruction and laboratory tests suggestive of biliary obstruction or pancreatitis. In the presence of obstructive jaundice,

the best clinical predictor of choledocholithiasis, as opposed to malignant biliary obstruction, is a history of pain. A number of blood tests may suggest a diagnosis of choledocholithiasis. However, stones can be present in the common duct without biliary obstruction or any abnormality in the liver function tests. Incidental choledocholithiasis is found in about 10% of clinical gallstone patients, although studies of laparoscopic cholecystectomy underestimate this incidence.

With laparoscopic cholecystectomy and the increasing experience with laparoscopic common duct exploration, we have changed our approach to the majority of patients with symptomatic gallstones and enzyme abnormalities suggesting choledocholithiasis. Formerly, preoperative ERCP was the rule. Now we can avoid ERCP in over 90% of these patients. In the absence of a demonstrable stone in the common duct by ultrasonography or persistent, marked elevation in liver function test results, ERCP is of low yield. Intraoperative cholangiography is important, however. Occasionally, a stone is encountered that cannot be removed at surgery. We are confident that postoperative ERCP in skilled hands is successful and safe. Conversion to open common duct exploration is another alternative (Figure 2). Preoperative ERCP is clearly indicated if a diagnosis other than choledocholithiasis is suspected.

A patient with clear evidence of cholangitis should routinely undergo preoperative decompression of the biliary system by either ERCP or percutaneous cholangiography. Presently, open or laparoscopic cholecystectomy is rarely indicated for acute cholangitis. There are three parts to the treatment of cholangitis: general supportive measures, antibiotics, and biliary decompression. Many cases of mild cholangitis resolve with antibiotics and simple supportive measures.

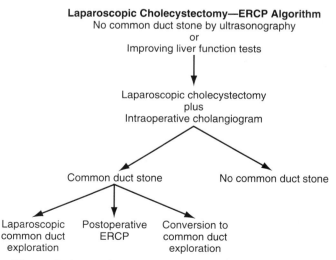

Laparoscopic Cholecystectomy—ERCP Algorithm

No common duct stone by ultrasonography
or
Improving liver function tests

↓

Laparoscopic cholecystectomy
plus
Intraoperative cholangiogram

Common duct stone   No common duct stone

Laparoscopic common duct exploration   Postoperative ERCP   Conversion to common duct exploration

Figure 2. Approach to patients with symptomatic gallstones and enzyme abnormalities suggesting choledocholithiasis. *Abbreviation*: ERCP = endoscopic retrograde cholangiopancreatography.

Primary Recurrent Cholangitis

With the increased immigration of people from Asia, primary hepatic duct stones, or cholangiohepatitis, is being seen with increasing frequency. The primary pathophysiology is probably related to parasitic infestation. The patients usually present in the emergency room with cholangitis. Unfortunately, in most cases, the hepatic biliary radicals are diffusely involved, making definitive treatment difficult. Efforts are focused on biliary decompression. Rarely, the disease is confined to one segmental duct, in which case the patient can be cured with hepatic resection.

CIRRHOSIS

method of
CARLOS GUARNER, M.D.
Hospital de Sant Pau
Barcelona, Spain

and

BRUCE A. RUNYON, M.D.
University of Louisville
Louisville, Kentucky

Cirrhosis is defined as irreversible fibrosis of the liver with nodular regeneration. Although the modifier "liver" is frequently used in conjunction with "cirrhosis," this is unnecessary and redundant. The liver is the only organ to develop cirrhosis. Other causes of cirrhosis, such as cardiac cirrhosis, are now rare enough to be anachronisms. Cirrhosis was the ninth leading cause of death in the United States in 1993. Cirrhosis is the final common pathway of many different chronic insults to the liver. Acute liver injury does not lead to cirrhosis. Regardless of the cause of the insult, the liver's response to various injurious agents is similar. Liver necrosis is followed by collapse of hepatic lobules, formation of fibrous septa, and nodular regrowth of liver cells, with disturbance of the architecture of the hepatic acini. Sinusoids persist at the periphery of the nodules at the site of the central-portal fibrous bridges, creating portal-systemic shunts and vascular insufficiency at the center of the nodules. "Capillarization" of the sinusoids impedes normal metabolic exchanges with liver cells.

Cirrhosis has been classified anatomically into three categories: micronodular, macronodular, and mixed. Although active alcohol abuse usually leads to a micronodular liver and cessation of drinking frequently permits conversion to a macronodular appearance, this is not always the case. Classification by etiology rather than nodule size seems to be more appropriate. The most common causes of cirrhosis are related to alcohol abuse and chronic viral hepatitis, in particular hepatitis C (Table 1). Prior to the availability of hepatitis C testing, alcohol was thought to be the most common cause of liver disease in the United States. Now it appears that hepatitis C, with or without the additional insult of excessive alcohol, is the most common cause of cirrhosis.

The prognosis of patients with cirrhosis depends on the severity of the liver disease. Forty percent of patients with cirrhosis may be diagnosed at the time of autopsy, with no signs or symptoms of liver disease during life. The Pugh modification of Child's original classification of the severity of liver disease has proved to be useful in predicting short-term prognosis (Table 2). Long-term prognosis varies, depending on the patient's state of "compensation." Patients with any major complication of liver disease (ascites, gastrointestinal hemorrhage related to portal hypertension, hepatic encephalopathy) are considered to be "decompensated." Five-year survival probability in compensated and decompensated patients with cirrhosis is 60 and 20%, respectively. The rate of decompensation of compensated patients is 5 to 10% per year. In addition, cirrhotic patients have a high risk of developing hepatocellular carcinoma. This complication has a profound negative impact on survival.

MANAGEMENT OF PATIENTS WITH CIRRHOSIS

In the management of patients with liver disease, one should consider general support measures, specific treatments according to the etiology of the liver disease, and prevention and treatment of complications of cirrhosis.

General Supportive Measures (Table 3)

Compensated patients should receive a well-balanced diet with 1 gram of protein per kg of body weight. Indiscriminate protein restriction may worsen malnutrition. Patients need not be put on sodium-

TABLE 1. **Causes of Cirrhosis in Adults**

Cause	Percentage
Chronic hepatitis C virus infection	45
Chronic hepatitis C virus infection plus alcohol	20
Alcohol abuse alone	10
Chronic hepatitis B virus infection	7
Chronic hepatitis B virus infection plus alcohol	3
Several virus infections (C and B with or without D)	3
Other causes	7
Primary biliary cirrhosis	—
Secondary biliary cirrhosis	—
Sclerosing cholangitis	—
Autoimmune hepatitis	—
Hereditary hemochromatosis	—
Wilson's disease	—
Alpha$_1$-antitrypsin deficiency	—
Drug-induced cirrhosis	—
Cryptogenic cirrhosis	5

TABLE 2. **Child-Pugh Score**

Parameter	Points		
	1	*2*	*3*
Encephalopathy (grade)	None	1–2	3–4
Ascites	Absent	Slight	Moderate
Bilirubin (mg/dL)	<2.0	2.0–3.0	>3.0
Albumin (gm/dL)	>3.5	2.8–3.5	<2.8
Prothrombin time (s prolonged)	1.0–4.0	4.0–6.0	>6.0

Class A: 5–6 points; Class B: 7–9 points; Class C: 10–15 points.

TABLE 3. **General Supportive Measures**

Abstinence from alcohol
Well-balanced diet with 1 gm protein per kg body weight and no
  restrictions of sodium or water in compensated patients
Additional calorie supplements in malnourished patients
Total enteral nutrition in hospitalized, severely malnourished
  patients.
Vitamin replacement in alcoholic patients and in patients with
  chronic cholestatic liver disease
Hepatitis B vaccination in seronegative patients

TABLE 4. **Drugs to Avoid in Patients with Cirrhosis**

Drug	Potential Problem
Sedatives	Coma or precoma
Narcotics	Coma or precoma
Nonsteroidal anti-inflammatory drugs	Fluid retention and gut bleeding
Nephrotoxic agents, particularly aminoglycosides	Renal failure

restricted diets until they develop ascites or edema. Calorie supplements added to a standard diet can be useful in malnourished cirrhotic patients, but supplemental branched chain amino acids are seldom, if ever, indicated because of their expense and unproven efficacy. Total enteral nutrition should be considered in hospitalized, severely malnourished cirrhotic patients, since it improves short-term outcome. Total parenteral nutrition is seldom, if ever, needed. Vitamin deficiencies are common in alcoholic patients and in patients with chronic cholestatic liver disease; when suspected or documented, these deficiencies should be appropriately corrected.

Abstinence from alcohol is the most effective therapy for patients with liver disease caused by alcohol. Alcoholic liver disease may have the most reversible component of all chronic liver diseases. Although it is impossible to prove in controlled trials, it appears that abstinence decreases morbidity and improves survival. Patients with cirrhosis in the setting of hepatitis C *and* alcohol abuse should also be advised to cease alcohol consumption. It is probably prudent for patients with nonalcoholic cirrhosis to abstain as well. Some authors recommend hepatitis B vaccination for seronegative patients with cirrhosis in order to prevent fatalities from superimposed acute viral hepatitis. However, patients with cirrhosis may not develop an antibody response to the vaccine.

Philosophy of Drug Use in the Setting of Cirrhosis

The cirrhotic liver's ability to metabolize drugs is limited. This frequently leads to a prolonged half-life of these drugs and the possibility of increased drug toxicity. Also, peculiarities of hepatic blood flow and renal function limit the drugs that can be safely given to patients with cirrhosis. Decompensated patients have more advanced disease and exhibit even more drug intolerance. In fact, drugs frequently precipitate decompensation. In the consultative practice of hepatology, one of the first steps in the evaluation and treatment of a patient with decompensated cirrhosis is to accurately determine the current drug list and discontinue all unnecessary or problematic drugs (Table 4). For example, the sleep-wake disturbance (insomnia at night with drowsiness during the day) of early hepatic encephalopathy may be misinterpreted by a physician as an indication for sedation. Sedative use precipitates near coma or frank

coma in these patients. Similarly, narcotics may precipitate or aggravate hepatic encephalopathy. These patients are exquisitely sensitive to the sedating effect of these agents. Sedatives and narcotics should be avoided in the treatment of patients with cirrhosis. Natriuresis is maintained in the setting of cirrhosis by increased renal prostaglandin secretion. Use of prostaglandin inhibitors (e.g., aspirin, ibuprofen) precipitates or aggravates fluid retention and may cause azotemia. Also, these drugs may precipitate gut mucosal injury and bleeding. Cirrhotic patients also appear to be exquisitely sensitive to nephrotoxic drugs. Because of the frequency with which these patients develop bacterial infections, antibiotics are regularly needed. However, the nephrotoxic potential of aminoglycosides precludes their use in this population.

Specific Treatment (Table 5)

With a better understanding of the causes and pathogenesis of cirrhosis, we can attempt to delay or perhaps even reverse fibrosis and its complications.

TABLE 5. **Specific Treatments**

Condition	Treatment
Alcoholic cirrhosis	Colchicine
	? Propylthiouracil*
	? S-adenosylmethionine
	? Polyunsaturated lecithin*
Acute alcoholic hepatitis	Corticosteroids (some indications)
Chronic viral hepatitis	Interferon alfa-2b (Intron A) (some indications)
Primary biliary cirrhosis	Ursodeoxycholic acid (Actigall)*
	? Colchicine
	? Methotrexate (Rheumatrex)*
	? Drug combinations
Primary sclerosing cholangitis	Ursodeoxycholic acid (Actigall)*
Autoimmune hepatitis	Corticosteroids
	Azathioprine (Imuran)*
	Cyclosporine (Sandimmune)* (few indications)
Hereditary hemochromatosis	Phlebotomy
	Deferoxamine (Desferal) (patients with anemia)
Wilson's disease	Penicillamine (Cuprimine, Depen)
	Trientine (Syprine)
	Zinc acetate† or sulfate (Eldercaps, Eldertonic)

*Not FDA-approved for this indication.
†Investigational drug in the United States.

Colchicine* inhibits collagen synthesis and procollagen secretion and enhances collagenase activity. One study demonstrated that colchicine decreased the incidence of major complications of liver disease and increased survival in alcoholic patients with cirrhosis compared with placebo-treated patients. Histologic improvement was reported in some patients treated with colchicine. Although this study has been subjected to considerable criticism, it has opened a new era of controlled trials of antifibrotic agents. The results of ongoing colchicine studies are required before the place of this agent in our treatment armamentarium becomes clear.

Propylthiouracil* is an antithyroid drug that has been evaluated in patients with alcoholic liver disease. The goal has been to reduce the alcohol-induced hepatic hypermetabolic state. One study reported a 60% reduction in the 2-year mortality in patients treated with propylthiouracil. Subsequent controlled trials have not been confirmatory. Neither colchicine nor propylthiouracil has enjoyed widespread enthusiasm or use.

Special nutrients such as S-adenosylmethionine and polyunsaturated lecithin support certain metabolic cellular functions and may be useful in protecting the liver from alcohol-induced damage and in preventing fibrosis. Results from experimental models are encouraging, and clinical trials are under way.

Because of the high short-term mortality associated with severe alcoholic hepatitis, controlled trials of many treatments have been performed. Even at the time of first decompensation, many of these patients have underlying cirrhosis. Mortality correlates with depth of jaundice, presence of encephalopathy, presence of ascites, and coagulopathy. These patients are frequently vitamin deficient and should receive oral or parenteral multivitamins (B complex, A, C, D, and folate). One subcutaneous injection of vitamin K is sufficient. There is no evidence that three doses are superior to one, and the injections frequently lead to a discolored plaque that may last for months at the injection site. Patients with severe alcoholic hepatitis usually do not take in sufficient calories spontaneously. Enteral caloric supplementation through a small bowel feeding tube to achieve a positive nitrogen balance should be considered. Enteral supplementation has been shown to reduce morbidity and improve short-term survival in the most seriously ill patients.

Anabolic steroids have been assessed in patients with alcoholic hepatitis. Oxandrolone (Oxandrin)* 80 mg per day orally in combination with an enteral food supplement (1200 kcal per day and 45 grams of protein per day) decreased mortality at 1 and 6 months in a subset of moderately malnourished patients in one study. Oxandrolone has not been widely used for this indication and is currently not available. In contrast, treatment with testosterone was not demonstrated to be effective and should not be used.

The role of corticosteroids in the therapy of alcoholic hepatitis continues to be controversial. Controlled trials of prednisolone (Prelone, Hydeltrasol) 40 mg per day or methylprednisolone (Medrol) 40 mg per day for 1 month have shown reduced short-term mortality in a subgroup of seriously ill patients characterized by deep jaundice and severe coagulopathy (i.e., if the sum of [4.6 multiplied by the prothrombin time in seconds] + [bilirubin in mg per dL] is >91) or by the presence of spontaneous hepatic encephalopathy and the absence of gastrointestinal hemorrhage. However, other controlled trials have been negative. Meta-analyses have demonstrated statistically significant increased short-term survival with steroids, but long-term survival is not affected, and the true clinical utility of steroids in this setting is probably small. These patients are immunocompromised, and use of corticosteroids may worsen host defenses against infection as well as precipitate pancreatitis and other complications of steroids.

Alternative therapies for alcoholic hepatitis, such as colchicine or insulin-glucagon infusions, have not been demonstrated to be of benefit. The severe hypoglycemia reported in some patients treated with insulin-glucagon precludes its use.

Chronic viral hepatitis is the most common cause of cirrhosis in the United States. A number of antiviral agents, including acyclovir (Zovirax),* adenine arabinoside monophosphate (Vira-A),* and interferon alfa-2b (Intron A), have been studied in an attempt to decrease viral replication and halt progression of liver disease caused by chronic hepatitis B or C. At present, interferon alfa-2b is the only drug approved by the Food and Drug Administration for the treatment of chronic viral hepatitis. Interferon alfa-2b treatment should be considered in the subset of patients with compensated chronic hepatitis B who have significant aminotransferase activity, active hepatitis on liver biopsy, and serologic evidence of viral replication (i.e., positive hepatitis B e antigen and/or hepatitis B virus [HBV]–DNA positivity). Treatment with 4.5 to 5 million U daily or 9 to 10 million U three times a week given either subcutaneously or intramuscularly for 4 to 6 months has been shown to be effective in inducing a remission in 30 to 40% of patients with chronic hepatitis B. Optimally, remission involves disappearance of serum hepatitis B e antigen and clearance of HBV–DNA from the serum, normalization of serum transaminases, and cessation of liver histologic activity. Unfortunately, clearance of hepatitis B surface antigen from the serum is very unusual, and even treated patients who clear all antigens from serum may still harbor viral genome in the liver when sophisticated testing is performed. Patients who have already developed cirrhosis usually do not tolerate standard doses of interferon, and the efficacy of treatment is lower in patients with cirrhosis compared with patients with hepatitis in the absence of cirrhosis. Compensated patients with cirrhosis can be treated if the degree

---

*Not FDA-approved for this indication.

*Not FDA-approved for this indication.

of activity warrants treatment. In this setting, dosing should be started at approximately 1 to 2 million U interferon-alfa-2b (Intron A) three times a week. Side effects of this drug are very common (Table 6). Frequent (initially weekly) monitoring of laboratory parameters is required. Mood disturbance and suicide have been reported in patients receiving the drug, even in the absence of a prior psychiatric history. Patients with known depression should probably not be treated with interferon alfa-2b. The side effects of treatment as well as the costs of the drug plus the costs of physician visits and laboratory testing must all be considered before a decision is made to begin therapy. Decompensated patients may develop frank liver failure and fatal bacterial infection if treated with interferon. In addition, these patients usually cannot tolerate a high enough dose of the drug to have an impact on the virus. Treatment of these patients with interferon should be reserved for research protocols.

Chronic hepatitis C virus (HCV) infection tends to be a silent but slowly progressive disease leading to cirrhosis and its complications in only a minority of patients after decades of infection. Survival after 20 years of infection is identical to that of normal control patients. Patients who drink alcohol in excess in the presence of hepatitis C develop cirrhosis more rapidly than they would with either single insult to the liver. The treatment of these patients should focus on abstinence from alcohol, not interferon. The prolonged asymptomatic natural history of hepatitis C, the low response rate to antiviral therapy, the side effects, and the cost of treatment all make it difficult to select patients for treatment. It is hoped that reducing the degree of abnormality of the aminotransferases and reducing the level of viral replication will lead to a delay in the development of cirrhosis and ultimately to improved survival. There are no convincing data to support these hopes to date. Interferon treatment should probably be reserved for precirrhotic patients with significant aminotransferase abnormalities, biopsy evidence of activity, and active viral replication as evidenced by a positive quantitative HCV-RNA test. The initial multicenter trial demonstrated that interferon alfa-2b given in doses of 2 to 5 million U three times a week for 6 months could induce an initial response (normalization of aminotransferases) in 38% of patients with chronic hepatitis C. Unfortunately, the relapse rate once therapy is stopped is higher than 50% in these patients. Transient normalization of aminotransferases in response to interferon may not have much clinical relevance. In addition, many investigators and practitioners have been unable to duplicate the results of the original studies. A realistic figure for durable normalization of aminotransferases is probably 10 to 15%. Patients with established cirrhosis have an even lower response rate and should probably not be treated with interferon alfa-2b. Treatment of decompensated cirrhotics with interferon should be reserved for research protocols.

Other antiviral and immunomodulatory agents that are currently being evaluated in the treatment of patients with chronic hepatitis B or C include levamisole (Ergamisol),* interleukin-2,† interferon-gamma-1b (Actimmune),* and nucleoside analogues. Some investigators have proposed using granulocyte-macrophage colony-stimulating factor to help prevent the cytopenias associated with interferon alfa-2b. Cost-effectiveness analysis will be required before this incredibly expensive combination could be advocated.

Primary biliary cirrhosis is an autoimmune disease that typically affects middle-aged women. These patients have chronic cholestasis, almost always associated with the presence of antimitochondrial antibodies in serum. As in other chronic cholestatic conditions, patients with primary biliary cirrhosis should be treated with fat-soluble vitamins (A, D, E, and K). A monthly dose of 100,000 IU of vitamin A (Aquasol A), 100,000 IU of vitamin D_2 (Calciferol), and 10 mg of vitamin K_1 (AquaMEPHYTON, Konakion) given parenterally seems to be appropriate. Vitamin E is not absorbed, and DL-tocopherol acetate (ANTIOX, Centrum Singles Vitamin E) is given orally at a dose of 200 mg daily. Calcium gluconate (Calcet) 6 grams per day or effervescent calcium tablets 30 grams per day help prevent hepatic osteodystrophy in these patients. Several drugs have been used to relieve the severe pruritus that is characteristic of this disease, including cholestyramine, histamine antagonists, phenobarbital, ursodeoxycholic acid,* and, most recently, rifampin.* Cholestyramine (Questran) 12 grams per day and ursodeoxycholic acid (Actigall) 10 to 15 mg per kg per day are the drugs most commonly used. Rifampin (Rimactane) 10 mg per kg per day relieves pruritus in 80% of patients, but these patients should be carefully monitored, because rifampin can be hepatotoxic. This drug should be considered a second-line alternative for patients who do not respond to cholestyramine and/or ursodeoxycholic acid. The drugs that have been tested in randomized trials of patients with primary biliary cirrhosis in-

TABLE 6. **Side Effects of Interferon alfa-2b (Intron A)**

Flulike symptoms
Myalgia
Headache
Nausea
Fatigue
Irritability
Anorexia
Weight loss
Alopecia
Bone marrow depression
Mood disturbance
Anxiety disturbance
Anxiety and depression
Suicide
Autoimmune disease
Hypothyroidism
Bacterial infection

*Not FDA-approved for this indication.
†Investigational drug in the United States.

clude corticosteroids, colchicine,* d-penicillamine,* chlorambucil,* cyclosporine,* malotilate,† and methotrexate.* No survival advantage has been demonstrated. Some of these drugs cause significant side effects. Steroids should not be used in these patients because of the worsening of bone thinning. Less toxic drugs should be used in this disease, since life expectancy of symptomatic patients with primary biliary cirrhosis is about 7 years, and that of asymptomatic patients is more than 10 years. Ursodeoxycholic acid replaces hydrophobic "hepatotoxic" bile acids with nonhepatotoxic bile acids and has been shown to be safe and to improve pruritus and liver tests in patients with primary biliary cirrhosis, when given at a dose of 10 to 15 mg per kg per day. There is some evidence of a survival advantage. Theoretically, ursodeoxycholic acid may prevent cirrhosis in early-stage, asymptomatic patients, but the drug would probably have to be taken for decades. This will be more practical after it becomes available in generic form. Combining a water-soluble bile acid, such as ursodeoxycholic acid, with an immunomodulatory or antifibrotic agent, such as methotrexate or colchicine, is a promising treatment and may be more effective than either agent alone. Randomized trials are ongoing. Patients with pruritus refractory to medical therapy, decompensated patients, and those with persistent serum bilirubin levels greater than 6 mg per dL should be considered for liver transplantation. Survival after transplantation is much higher than the natural history of patients with such evidence of advanced disease.

Primary sclerosing cholangitis is a chronic idiopathic inflammatory disease involving the intra- and/or extrahepatic bile ducts and resulting in fibrosis, strictures, and cirrhosis. This disease is usually associated with chronic inflammatory bowel disease, especially ulcerative colitis. These patients frequently develop pruritus, recurrent cholangitis, and cirrhosis with its complications. As in patients with primary biliary cirrhosis, replacement of fat-soluble vitamins is important. Pruritus can usually be controlled with cholestyramine and/or ursodeoxycholic acid. Recurrent cholangitis is usually caused by bile duct strictures with or without stones and requires antibiotic treatment and endoscopic management. Use of endoscopic sphincterotomy, dilation of biliary strictures, and placement of endoprosthesis should be considered. Surgical treatment of biliary strictures should be avoided, since right upper quadrant surgery can make future liver transplantation more difficult because of adhesions. The incidence of cholangiocarcinoma in patients with primary sclerosing cholangitis is increased, but early detection can be very difficult. Endoscopic cytology of strictures can be useful.

The drugs that have been used to try to delay the development of cirrhosis and its complications in patients with primary sclerosing cholangitis include prednisone,* prednisone plus colchicine,* azathioprine,* penicillamine,* colchicine,* and methotrexate.* A convincing benefit has not been demonstrated. Treatment with ursodeoxycholic acid* 10 to 15 mg per kg per day has been shown to improve pruritus and liver tests. More studies are needed to determine whether this drug prevents cirrhosis and prolongs survival. Ursodeoxycholic acid has also been used to treat other chronic cholestatic diseases, such as cystic fibrosis and graft-versus-host disease.

Autoimmune "lupoid" hepatitis is an uncommon inflammatory liver disease, usually occurring in young woman with hyperglobulinemia and autoantibodies. Corticosteroid treatment prolongs life in these patients, especially if they are diagnosed in the precirrhotic phase. The initial doses of prednisone (Deltasone, Sterapred) or prednisolone vary from 20 to 40 mg per day, depending on the severity of presenting symptoms and laboratory abnormalities. The dose is rapidly reduced to whatever will maintain remission, as defined by aminotransferases less than 100 IU per liter and normal bilirubin. Even a few milligrams per day may be enough. A dramatic improvement in symptoms and laboratory abnormalities is usually observed within a few days of initiating treatment. Azathioprine (Imuran) 50 mg per day can be added for its "steroid sparing" effect. Relapse of hepatitis is common after corticosteroid withdrawal. Patients whose disease activity flares on steroid withdrawal should be retreated and should probably remain on maintenance doses of steroids for life. Cyclosporine* should be considered for treatment of the small percentage of steroid-resistant patients. An even smaller subset of patients fails medical therapy and requires liver transplantation.

Hereditary hemochromatosis is an autosomal recessive disease characterized by elevated serum iron, ferritin, and transferrin saturation. Iron is deposited in the liver, joints, myocardium, and pancreas and can seriously injure each of these tissues. Early diagnosis is crucial, since treatment in the precirrhotic stage leads to normal life expectancy. Treatment consists of phlebotomy of 500 mL of blood once or twice a week until iron deficiency is documented. This may take 1 or even 2 years. Once iron deficiency is achieved, maintenance phlebotomy (about every 3 months) continues for life. Administration of parenteral deferoxamine (Desferal) is less effective than phlebotomy and quite expensive. Oral iron chelating drugs are under investigation. The risk of developing hepatocellular carcinoma in patients with hereditary hemochromatosis is 200 times that of the normal population; it usually develops in patients who are diagnosed after cirrhosis has occurred. Screening for this tumor with serial ultrasonography and alpha-fetoprotein levels may lead to earlier detection. First-degree relatives of hemochromatosis probands should be screened for iron overload with serum ferritin and iron levels. Those with abnormal values should undergo liver biopsy.

---

*Not FDA-approved for this indication.
†Not available in the United States.

*Not FDA-approved for this indication.

Wilson's disease is a congenital disease of copper metabolism characterized by low serum levels of ceruloplasmin and high levels of copper in urine, liver, and brain. The disease can be manifested as fulminant hepatic failure, chronic active hepatitis, or cirrhosis. Again, early diagnosis is crucial, since neurologic disorders and liver damage can be prevented by use of an appropriate copper chelating agent. Penicillamine (Cuprimine, Depen) is the drug with which we have the most experience and is the drug of choice. It chelates copper and increases urinary copper excretion. The initial dose is 1 to 2 grams per day divided in four doses and taken before meals. The maintenance dose is 0.5 to 1 gram per day. Oral pyridoxine hydrochloride 25 mg daily should be added to counteract the antipyridoxine effect of penicillamine. Thirty to 40% of treated patients develop severe side effects from penicillamine, including hypersensitivity reactions and autoimmune syndromes. Despite its lower cupriuretic effect, trientine (Syprine) is a good alternative therapy for these patients. An adequate dose is 750 mg to 2 grams per day in three doses. Zinc acetate* or sulfate (Eldercaps, Eldertonic) induces intestinal metallothionein, which blocks intestinal copper absorption and promotes fecal copper excretion. Oral doses of 25 to 50 mg per day in two divided doses can safely substitute for patients who are intolerant to penicillamine or trientine. Zinc has been advocated as first-line therapy, but more data are required before it can be recommended. Emergent liver transplantation should be considered in patients with Wilsonian fulminant hepatic failure that is unresponsive to intensive medical therapy and in patients with decompensated cirrhosis who are unlikely to respond fully to medical therapy alone. Liver transplantation cures the defect in copper metabolism, but severe neurologic deficits will probably not reverse with transplantation.

Prevention and Treatment of Complications of Cirrhosis (Table 7)

Unfortunately, despite general supportive measures and specific treatment, cirrhosis may develop, along with complications that shorten life expectancy. Many patients do not come to medical attention until they develop a complication of their previously silent liver disease. Major complications develop during follow-up of compensated patients at

---

*Not FDA-approved for this indication.

TABLE 7. **Management of Complications of Cirrhosis**

Treatment and prevention of gastrointestinal hemorrhage secondary to portal hypertension
Treatment of ascites
Treatment and prevention of spontaneous bacterial peritonitis
Treatment of umbilical hernia
Treatment of hepatorenal syndrome
Treatment of acute and chronic hepatic encephalopathy
Treatment of coagulation abnormalities

TABLE 8. **Ten-year Cumulative Probability of Developing Complications of Cirrhosis**

Complication	Probability of Developing (%)
Ascites	55
Hepatic encephalopathy	50
Jaundice	45
Gastrointestinal hemorrhage	40

a rate of 5 to 10% per year. Major complications include ascites, portal hypertension with gastrointestinal hemorrhage, hepatic encephalopathy, bacterial infections (in particular, spontaneous bacterial peritonitis), and hepatorenal syndrome (Table 8). These complications are landmarks in the natural history of cirrhosis and predict short life expectancy or directly lead to the patient's death. These complications, together with hepatocellular carcinoma, are the causes of death in more than 90% of patients with cirrhosis (Table 9). Over the past few years, significant advances have been made in our knowledge regarding the pathogenesis of the complications of cirrhosis. This knowledge has permitted a more rational approach to the prevention and treatment of these complications.

Portal Hypertension

Portal hypertension is a common complication of cirrhosis. It leads to the development of esophageal and gastric varices and portal hypertensive gastropathy. Gastrointestinal hemorrhage and death frequently follow. This subject is discussed in another section.

Ascites

Ascites formation is the most common complication of cirrhosis (see Table 8), and development of ascites is a marker of a poor prognosis. The probability of survival after the onset of ascites has been estimated to be 50% at 1 year and 20% at 5 years of follow-up. However, it is important to recognize that ascites is not synonymous with cirrhosis. Other causes of ascites include peritoneal carcinomatosis, heart failure, tuberculosis, and pancreatitis. Approximately 5% of patients have two or more causes of ascites.

Analysis of ascitic fluid obtained by abdominal paracentesis is the first step in the differential diagnosis of ascites. Cell count and differential, bacterial

---

TABLE 9. **Causes of Death in Patients with Cirrhosis**

Cause	Percentage
Liver failure*	49
Hepatocellular carcinoma	22
Gastrointestinal hemorrhage	13
Hepatorenal syndrome	8
Bacterial infection	3
Other causes	5

*Many patients have multiple possible causes of death and are simply diagnosed as dying of liver failure.

TABLE 10. **Ascitic Fluid Testing**

Routine Tests	Optional Tests	Unusual Tests
Cell count	Glucose	Tuberculosis smear and culture
Albumin (1st specimen)	Lactate dehydrogenase	Cytology
Culture (in blood culture bottles)	Amylase	
Total protein	Gram's stain	

From Runyon BA: Paracentesis and ascitic fluid analysis. *In* Yamada T, Alpers D, Owyang C, et al. (eds): Textbook of Gastroenterology. Philadelphia, JB Lippincott, 1991, pp 2455–2465.

culture, Gram's stain, albumin, and total protein concentration of the fluid should be routinely performed in patients with new-onset ascites and at the time of admission to the hospital in cirrhotic patients with ascites. These tests should be repeated in cirrhotic patients whose clinical condition deteriorates during hospitalization, especially when they develop signs or symptoms of bacterial infection (Table 10). Additional tests should be ordered in specific circumstances when there is high suspicion of other causes of ascites (see Table 10). It is not cost effective to order every test on every specimen. Cytology and culture for tuberculosis may cost $400 each. The cell count is probably the single most helpful test performed on ascitic fluid and provides relatively immediate information regarding the likelihood of bacterial infection, the most acutely life-threatening complication of ascites. Bacterial culture and Gram's stain provide confirmatory evidence for bacterial peritonitis. However, cultures do not grow bacteria for 12 to 48 hours, and infected patients may die before there is evident growth of bacteria. Gram's stain is less than 10% sensitive in detecting bacteria in patients with spontaneous bacterial peritonitis. Therefore, empirical antibiotic treatment for suspected bacterial peritonitis should be started when the absolute neutrophil count is 250 per mm³ or greater (Table 11).

The exudate-transudate system of classifying ascites was based on total protein concentration or ascitic fluid/serum ratios of protein and lactate dehydrogenase. This concept was extrapolated from pleural fluid analysis and has proved to be more confusing than helpful in the setting of ascites. The serum-ascites albumin gradient is a more useful parameter for classifying ascites, because it indicates whether portal hypertension is present. Serum and ascitic fluid specimens obtained should be tested for albu-

min concentration in the same laboratory with accuracy at low range. The ascitic fluid value is simply *subtracted* from the serum value to calculate the gradient. If specimens are collected several days apart or sent to laboratories with different normal ranges or inaccuracy at low range, results are uninterpretable. Patients with gradients of 1.1 gram per dL or greater have portal hypertension, and patients with gradients less than 1.1 gram per dL do not (Table 12). A high gradient only rules in portal hypertension; it does not rule out a second cause for ascites formation. For example, some patients with cirrhosis and ascites develop tuberculous peritonitis. These patients with portal hypertension and another cause for ascites formation have a high gradient, reflecting their high portal pressure. More than 80% of patients who develop ascites have cirrhosis and portal hypertension. Total protein concentration of ascitic fluid is inversely related to the risk of developing spontaneous bacterial peritonitis and is useful for differentiating spontaneous from secondary bacterial peritonitis.

Recently, a new theory of ascites formation in the setting of cirrhosis has been proposed. It postulates that the initial events in ascites formation are splanchnic and peripheral arteriolar vasodilation. The expansion of these vascular beds leads to an underfilling of the arterial compartment, with secondary activation of vasoconstrictor systems such as the sympathetic nervous system, renin-angiotensin-aldosterone system, and antidiuretic hormone. In turn, this neurohumoral excitation leads to renal retention of sodium and water and overfilling of the vascular system. Consequently, the sodium and water retained by the kidneys accumulate in the abdominal cavity.

Ascites warrants treatment for the following reasons: to relieve abdominal discomfort, respiratory compromise, and early satiety; to avoid formation of abdominal wall hernias; and to prevent rupture of the right hemidiaphragm due to elevated intra-abdominal pressure. Spontaneous bacterial peritonitis

TABLE 11. **Indications for Empirical Antibiotic Treatment of Suspected Bacterial Infection**

High clinical suspicion of bacterial infection (after culturing ascitic fluid, blood, urine, and sputum)
Ascitic fluid polymorphonuclear count ≥250 cells/mm³ in the absence of another explanation for neutrocytic ascites
Symptomatic bacterascites

TABLE 12. **Classification of Ascites According to the Level of Serum-Ascites Albumin Gradient**

High Gradient (≥1.1 gm/dL)	Low Gradient (<1.1 gm/dL)
Cirrhosis	Peritoneal carcinomatosis
Alcoholic hepatitis	Peritoneal tuberculosis
Cardiac failure	Pancreatic ascites
Massive liver metastases	Biliary ascites
Fulminant hepatic failure	Nephrotic syndrome
Budd-Chiari syndrome	Serositis
Portal vein thrombosis	Bowel obstruction or infarction
Veno-occlusive disease	
Fatty liver of pregnancy	
Myxedema	
"Mixed" ascites*	

*Found in patients with portal hypertension and another cause of ascites formation (e.g., cirrhosis plus peritoneal tuberculosis).
From Runyon BA: Paracentesis and ascitic fluid analysis. *In* Yamada T, Alpers D, Owyang C, et al. (eds): Textbook of Gastroenterology. Philadelphia, JB Lippincott, 1991, pp 2455–2465.

develops only in pre-existing ascitic fluid; eliminating ascitic fluid prevents this infection.

Based on the pathogenesis of ascites formation in the setting of cirrhosis, the aim of medical treatment is to mobilize the ascitic fluid by creating a negative sodium balance. Water follows passively. A negative sodium balance is accomplished by reducing sodium intake in the diet and increasing urinary sodium excretion. In afebrile patients without diarrhea, urinary excretion is the only significant route of sodium removal.

Cirrhotic patients with ascites should be treated initially by dietary sodium restriction (50 to 88 mEq per day) and diuretics (Table 13). A more severe restriction of sodium intake can be imposed, but this may worsen the anorexia and malnutrition that are usually present in these patients. Outpatient treatment can be attempted, but it usually fails. A short hospitalization to obtain an accurate diagnosis, monitor electrolytes, and determine appropriate diuretic doses is usually required. Diet education for the patient is crucial to successful treatment. In 15 to 20% of patients, a negative sodium balance can be achieved with dietary sodium restriction alone. Water restriction is not necessary unless the serum sodium concentration drops below 120 mEq per liter. Indiscriminate fluid restriction is unnecessary and poorly tolerated by patients, and it may lead to hypernatremia. Since 80 to 85% of patients require diuretics to achieve an adequate natriuresis, it is reasonable to start diuretics in all patients. To initially withhold diuretics from all patients in order to find the few patients who do not need diuretics only delays a successful response. Spironolactone (Aldactone) and furosemide (Lasix) are the diuretics most frequently used in cirrhotic patients. Spironolactone, an antagonist of aldosterone, inhibits sodium reabsorption in the collecting tubule, and furosemide impairs sodium reabsorption in the ascending limb of the loop of Henle. Although furosemide is a more potent diuretic than spironolactone in patients without cirrhosis, randomized trials have demonstrated that spironolactone is more useful than furosemide as a single agent in the setting of cirrhosis. However, because of its very long half-life in patients with cirrhosis, single-agent spironolactone is slow to begin natriuresis. Spironolactone is potassium sparing; furosemide is potassium wasting. Using both agents speeds the onset of natriuresis and helps maintain normokalemia. Some alcoholics with new-onset ascites have spontaneous hypokalemia; these patients should receive single-agent spironolactone until nor-mokalemia is achieved. Then furosemide is added. Spironolactone or another distal potassium-sparing diuretic such as amiloride should be routinely used in the initial regimen. The starting doses of diuretics should be 100 mg of spironolactone and 40 mg of furosemide; all pills are given orally in the morning. Dividing doses decreases compliance and is not helpful. If the patient's body weight does not decrease or the 24-hour urinary sodium excretion does not exceed the dietary intake after 2 or 3 days of treatment, the dose of both diuretics should be progressively increased, usually in simultaneous 100 mg and 40 mg per day increments, respectively, until urinary excretion of sodium is greater than dietary intake. Most patients achieve negative sodium balance on 200 mg and 80 mg per day. The highest doses of spironolactone and furosemide used are 400 mg and 160 mg per day, respectively. Serial monitoring of urinary sodium excretion and daily weighing of the patient are the best ways to determine the optimal dose of diuretics. Random measurements of urinary sodium concentration are of some value, but 24-hour collections are optimal. Once ascites has been mobilized, the diuretic dosage should be individually adjusted to keep the patient free of ascites. After a steady state has been reached with spironolactone (2 to 4 weeks), the diuretic doses can frequently be reduced. A few days in the hospital with careful outpatient follow-up yields optimal results. Weight, serum and urine electrolytes, and renal function are monitored.

Unfortunately, many patients treated with diuretics develop side effects and complications of treatment, including painful gynecomastia, muscle cramps, potassium imbalance, encephalopathy, and azotemia. Most patients find the spironolactone-induced gynecomastia tolerable; if not, amiloride (Midamor) 10 to 40 mg orally every morning can be substituted. Muscle cramps almost always respond to oral quinine sulfate (Quinamm) 200 mg as needed. Normokalemia can almost always be achieved by adjusting the ratio of potassium-sparing versus potassium-wasting diuretics. Patients with intrinsic renal disease, e.g., diabetic or IgA nephropathy, have a tendency toward hyperkalemia and usually tolerate only small doses of potassium-sparing diuretic. The development of mental status change or azotemia warrants careful analysis of the situation. A creatinine greater than 2 mg per dL should prompt discontinuation of diuretics. The most sodium-avid patients may achieve no natriuresis and only azotemia on diuretics. These patients, as well as those with an inadequate response to salt restriction and high-dose diuretic treatment, should be labeled diuretic resistant or refractory and should be evaluated for alternative therapies (Table 14). However, before proceeding to second-line therapies, excessive sodium intake, bacterial infection, occult gastrointestinal hemorrhage, and intake of prostaglandin inhibitors (e.g., aspirin) should be excluded. Less than 10% of cirrhotic patients with ascites are refractory to standard medical therapy. Patients with refractory ascites have "pre-

TABLE 13. **Treatment of Ascites in the Setting of Cirrhosis**

Dietary sodium restriction (50–88 mEq/day)
Fluid restriction if serum sodium concentration <120 mEq/L
Spironolactone (Aldactone) 100 mg/day and furosemide (Lasix) 40 mg/day orally
Increase diuretic doses to achieve weight loss and negative sodium balance

TABLE 14. **Treatment Options for Patients with Cirrhosis and Diuretic-Resistant Ascites**

Evaluation for liver transplantation
Chronic outpatient paracenteses
Peritoneovenous shunt
? Transjugular intrahepatic portosystemic stent-shunt (TIPS)

hepatorenal syndrome" and a poor prognosis; 1-year survival is less than 20%.

Large-volume paracentesis is an ancient (circa 20 B.C.) procedure that mobilizes ascitic fluid in cirrhotic patients. There has been renewed interest in this procedure in the last decade, as well as proof of its safety and efficacy. Therapeutic paracentesis has additional beneficial effects on the hemodynamic status of patients with tense ascites by means of decreasing intra-abdominal pressure and increasing venous return from the lower extremities. However, repeated large-volume paracenteses deplete proteins, including antibacterial proteins such as complement. Protein depletion aggravates malnutrition and, theoretically, could predispose to bacterial infection. Therefore, therapeutic paracentesis should not be used as a first-line treatment of cirrhotic patients with ascites; it should be reserved for patients with tense and/or refractory ascites.

Plasma volume expansion after large-volume paracentesis remains controversial. Albumin infusion (6 to 8 grams per liter of fluid removed) has been advocated to correct protein losses and avoid theoretic hemodynamic disturbances that could develop after therapeutic paracentesis of 5 or more liters of ascitic fluid. However, albumin infusion enhances albumin degradation and excretion. In addition, increasing albumin concentration in hepatocyte cell culture media results in decreased albumin synthesis. Although postparacentesis albumin infusion has been demonstrated to decrease the frequency of (asymptomatic) laboratory abnormalities compared with paracentesis without albumin infusion, no impact of albumin infusion on clinical morbidity or survival has been demonstrated. The cost of albumin is extremely high—$5 to $25 per gram; in comparison, the cost of gold is about $13 per gram. Therefore, albumin or less expensive volume expanders, such as dextran, should be viewed as optional until it is demonstrated that volume expansion after therapeutic paracentesis is cost effective.

Peritoneovenous shunt was introduced for the treatment of cirrhotics with refractory ascites in 1974 by LeVeen and associates. Peritoneovenous shunt increases plasma volume and inhibits vasoconstrictor systems, leading to a marked diuresis and natriuresis. However, it is associated with a large number of complications, especially in those patients with severe hepatocellular insufficiency. Early complications such as bacterial infection, fluid overload, and disseminated intravascular coagulation can be prevented by preoperative prophylactic antibiotics (cloxacillin 1 gram every 6 hours) and intraoperative evacuation of ascitic fluid. Shunt occlusion is the most frequent late complication of peritoneovenous shunt and usually requires reoperation and replacement of the occluded portion of the shunt. Addition of a titanium tip to the venous end of the prosthesis does not prevent shunt obstruction. Shunting does not improve long-term survival in cirrhotic patients. Therefore, peritoneovenous shunt should probably be reserved for the small subset of cirrhotic patients (<1%) with refractory ascites who are not liver transplant candidates and in whom large-volume paracentesis is difficult to perform.

Transjugular intrahepatic portosystemic stent-shunt (TIPS) is an interventional radiologic technique that consists of creating a fistula between the hepatic venous system and the portal venous system and then placing an expandable metal stent in the balloon-dilated fistula to maintain patency. This technique was introduced to treat patients with recurrent variceal hemorrhage by decreasing portal pressure. Initial results have demonstrated that TIPS can be useful in the treatment of cirrhotics with refractory ascites. However, the cumulative risk of shunt occlusion and hepatic encephalopathy due to this side-to-side portacaval shunt is greater than 50%. Controlled trials are required to establish the place of this new technique in the treatment of cirrhotics with refractory ascites.

Patients with cirrhosis who develop ascites should be considered for liver transplantation, especially when they develop refractory ascites, since 1-year survival after liver transplantation is higher than natural outcome (>75% vs. <20%, respectively).

Spontaneous Bacterial Peritonitis

Spontaneous bacterial peritonitis (SBP) is a frequent and severe complication of ascites in patients with cirrhosis. Recent studies have shown that the 1-year cumulative probability of the first episode of SBP developing in cirrhotics with ascites is approximately 10%, and in those patients with an ascitic fluid total protein less than 1 gram per dL, it is 50%. Moreover, patients with cirrhosis who recover from SBP have a cumulative probability of SBP recurrence of 69%. The short-term survival of patients with SBP during the last 15 years has dramatically improved as a consequence of a higher index of suspicion of infection, earlier diagnosis, and the use of non-nephrotoxic antibiotics. However, the long-term survival continues to be extremely poor: only 30 to 40% of patients are alive 1 year after the first episode of SBP.

The diagnosis of SBP is based on the results of ascitic fluid analysis. Based on ascitic fluid culture and polymorphonuclear (PMN) cell count of ascitic fluid, three different variants of ascitic fluid infection have been described in cirrhotic patients during the last decade (Table 15). SBP is defined as an ascitic fluid PMN count of 250 or more cells per mm^3 with a positive ascitic fluid culture (usually for a single organism). Culture-negative neutrocytic ascites is defined as an ascitic fluid PMN count of 250 or more

TABLE 15. **Variants of Ascitic Fluid Infection**

Spontaneous bacterial peritonitis: ascitic fluid PMN $\geq$250 cells/mm^3 and positive culture

Culture-negative neutrocytic ascites: ascitic fluid PMN $\geq$250 cells/mm^3 and negative culture

Bacterascites: ascitic fluid PMN <250 cells/mm^3 and positive culture

Abbreviation: PMN = polymorphonuclear.

cells per mm^3 with a negative ascitic fluid culture. Bacterascites is defined as an ascitic fluid PMN count of less than 250 cells per mm^3 with a positive ascitic fluid culture for a single organism.

Although more than 90% of ascitic fluid infections in cirrhotic patients are spontaneous (without a surgically treatable source), it is important to differentiate spontaneous from secondary peritonitis, because SBP is always treated medically and secondary peritonitis usually requires surgical intervention. Analysis of ascitic fluid is helpful in differentiating these entities. Secondary bacterial peritonitis should be suspected when ascitic fluid analysis shows two or three of the following criteria: total protein greater than 1 gram per dL, glucose less than 50 mg per dL, and lactate dehydrogenase (LDH) greater than 225 mU per mL (or higher than the upper limit of normal for serum). Most ascitic fluid cultures in secondary peritonitis are polymicrobial, whereas in SBP the infection is usually monomicrobial. Patients with suspected secondary peritonitis must be evaluated by emergency radiologic techniques to confirm and localize possible visceral perforation. In patients with nonperforation secondary peritonitis, these criteria are not as helpful as in those with free perforation, and paracentesis should be repeated after 48 hours of antibiotic treatment to assess the effect of treatment on ascitic fluid PMN count and culture. In patients with nonperforation secondary peritonitis, the ascitic fluid PMN count increases beyond the pretreatment value, and the ascitic fluid culture remains positive. Conversely, ascitic fluid PMN cell count decreases rapidly and ascitic fluid culture becomes sterile in appropriately treated patients with SBP.

Empirical antibiotic treatment must be started as soon as possible to improve survival (see Table 11). Therefore, it is important to perform routine bacterial cultures of ascitic fluid, blood, urine, and sputum and an ascitic fluid PMN count when any hospitalized patient with ascites develops clinical signs of possible infection (fever, abdominal pain, encephalopathy) or shows a deterioration in laboratory parameters (azotemia, acidosis, leukocytosis). Also, analysis of ascitic fluid and urine should be performed when any cirrhotic patient with ascites is admitted to the hospital, as about 20% of such patients are infected at this time. Immediately after cultures and cell counts are obtained, empirical antibiotics should be started whenever bacterial infection is suspected. An ascitic fluid PMN count of 250 or more cells per mm^3 is also an indication for empirical treatment.

Patients with symptomatic bacterascites or culture-negative neutrocytic ascites must be treated with antibiotics, because approximately 40% of the former and 70% of the latter progress to SBP. In contrast, asymptomatic bacterascites may resolve spontaneously and may not require treatment with antibiotics. However, before a decision can be made to withhold treatment, paracentesis must be repeated to recheck ascitic fluid neutrophil count and culture.

In the remote past, the antibiotic combination of an aminoglycoside plus ampicillin was used to treat cirrhotic patients with suspected SBP. However, because of the high risk of nephrotoxicity in this population, aminoglycosides are avoided. Third-generation cephalosporins are effective against most of the flora (70% gram negative) responsible for SBP and are not nephrotoxic. Recently, it has been demonstrated that 2 grams of cefotaxime (Claforan) given intravenously every 8 to 12 hours is as effective as every-6-hour dosing. Also, the length of antibiotic therapy has recently been clarified; a short course of therapy (5 days) has been shown to be as effective as a long course (10 days). Other third-generation cephalosporins such as ceftriaxone (Rocephin) (2 grams per day) or cefonicid (Monocid) (2 grams every 12 hours) are good alternatives. Oral quinolones such as pefloxacin* or ofloxacin (Floxin) are currently under investigation and may be effective for treating patients with noncomplicated SBP.

Prophylaxis of bacterial infection should be considered in patients with liver disease who are at high risk of infections, including SBP. Selective intestinal decontamination consists of the inhibition of the gram-negative flora of the gut with preservation of gram-positive cocci and anaerobic bacteria. Preservation of the anaerobes is important in preventing intestinal colonization, overgrowth, and subsequent extraintestinal dissemination of pathogenic bacteria. Several trials have shown that selective intestinal decontamination with oral norfloxacin (Noroxin) is very effective in preventing bacterial infections, including SBP, in cirrhotic inpatients with gastrointestinal hemorrhage (400 mg twice daily) or with low ascitic fluid protein concentration (400 mg per day) and in patients with fulminant hepatic failure (400 mg per day) (Table 16). Although short-term prophylactic treatment (400 mg of oral norfloxacin per day)

*Not available in the United States.

TABLE 16. **Indications for Selective Intestinal Decontamination Using Oral Norfloxacin (Noroxin)**

Cirrhotics with gastrointestinal hemorrhage: 400 mg bid for 7 days

Cirrhotics with ascitic fluid protein concentration <1 gm/dL: 400 mg/day during hospitalization

Patients with fulminant hepatic failure: 400 mg/day during hospitalization

Cirrhotics who have survived an episode of spontaneous bacterial peritonitis: 400 mg/day indefinitely or until liver transplantation has been shown to be effective in preventing SBP recurrence, some authors do not consider long-term therapy to be appropriate because of the selection of resistant flora. More trials are needed. However, patients with cirrhosis recovering from an SBP episode should be considered for liver transplantation, and treatment with norfloxacin should be considered while patients await liver transplantation.

Umbilical Hernia

Umbilical hernia is a common problem in cirrhotic patients with tense ascites. The prevalence is almost 20%, and more than 50% of patients with umbilical hernia develop complications during follow-up, including incarceration, skin ulceration, and rupture. Control of ascites with paracentesis and diuretics is important to prevent rupture of the hernia. Rupture is fatal in more than one-third of patients. Prevention of hernia formation is more effective than treatment of the hernia once it has developed. Hernias repaired in the presence of ascites almost always recur. Incarceration should be treated medically if possible. Emergency surgery should be performed in patients with rupture or medically resistant incarceration of the hernia.

Hepatorenal Syndrome

Hepatorenal syndrome may be defined as renal failure that occurs in patients with liver disease in the absence of known clinical causes of renal failure and without anatomic or urinalysis evidence of renal damage. Pathogenesis remains uncertain, but it involves mechanisms that lead to renal vasoconstriction and cortical hypoperfusion, resulting in the development of progressive renal failure. The onset may be insidious and slowly progressive over a few months, or it may be rapidly progressive over days or weeks with a fatal outcome. Ninety-five percent of cirrhotic patients with hepatorenal syndrome die within 1 month of the onset of renal failure. Hepatorenal syndrome is characterized by asymptomatic inexorable increase in serum urea and creatinine, low urinary sodium concentration (usually <10 mEq per liter), urinary osmolality greater than serum osmolality, normal urinalysis, and no response to volume expansion. Most patients diagnosed erroneously with hepatorenal syndrome actually have prerenal azotemia or iatrogenic tubular necrosis from nephrotoxins.

Therapeutic approaches to hepatorenal syndrome have included hemodialysis, peritoneal dialysis, infusion of intrarenal or systemic vasodilators (acetylcholine, prostaglandins), vasoconstrictor blockade (phentolamine,* saralasin,† captopril*), volume expansion with peritoneovenous shunt, and TIPS (Table 17). None of these maneuvers has demonstrated a consistent benefit in these patients. The problem is the liver, not the kidney. Kidneys removed from patients with hepatorenal syndrome function well when transplanted into a recipient without liver failure.

---

*Not FDA-approved for this indication.
†Not available in the United States.

TABLE 17. Treatment of Hepatorenal Syndrome

Unproven Approaches
Hemodialysis
Peritoneal dialysis
Infusion of intrarenal or systemic vasodilators
Vasoconstrictor blockade
Peritoneovenous shunt
Transjugular intraheptic stent-shunt
Effective Approach
Liver transplantation

Attention should be focused on the liver. Liver transplantation is currently the only effective therapy in cirrhotic patients with hepatorenal syndrome.

Hepatic Encephalopathy

Hepatic encephalopathy is characterized by a broad spectrum of neuropsychiatric disturbances that occur in patients with advanced liver disease. Recently, the prevalence of latent or "subclinical" hepatic encephalopathy in cirrhotic patients has been estimated to be 71% by sensitive psychomotor testing. The degree of hepatocellular insufficiency and the presence of portocollateral shunts are the determining factors in the development of hepatic encephalopathy. Several theories have been proposed in the pathogenesis of hepatic encephalopathy: Neurotoxins of intestinal origin (ammonia) are not detoxified by the damaged liver, or false neurotransmitters (including gamma-aminobutyric acid [GABA]) are synthesized as a consequence of an increase in aromatic amino acids and a decrease in branched chain amino acids.

Hepatic encephalopathy in cirrhotic patients can be acute, and usually reversible with appropriate treatment, or chronic. Acute hepatic encephalopathy can be precipitated by sedatives, gastrointestinal hemorrhage, bacterial infection, electrolyte imbalance, azotemia, and constipation. Management of acute encephalopathy is based on correction of any precipitating factor, restriction of protein intake, gut cleansing, and the administration of nonabsorbable disaccharides or neomycin (Table 18).

Patients who are frankly comatose should receive tap-water enemas until mental status improves, usu-

TABLE 18. Treatment of Hepatic Encephalopathy

Acute Encephalopathy
Correction of any precipitating factor
Restriction of protein intake
Gut cleansing
Oral nonabsorbable disaccharides (lactulose) or oral nonabsorbable antibiotics (neomycin)
Chronic Encephalopathy
Restriction of animal protein intake
Vegetarian or lactovegetarian protein diet
? Oral branched chain amino acid supplements
Oral nonabsorbable disaccharides (lactulose)
Evaluation for liver transplantation

ally in 24 to 48 hours. Lactulose enemas are very expensive and should be reserved for patients refractory to water enemas. Nothing should be given by mouth until mental status improves. Aspiration pneumonia is the most common cause of death in patients with hepatic encephalopathy. Dietary protein should be restricted to 0.5 gram per kg body weight per day for only a few days. After improvement in mental status, protein should be reintroduced to the level of a non-protein-restricted diet, i.e., 1 gram per kg body weight per day. Very few patients require chronic restriction of dietary protein. Unnecessary restriction aggravates malnutrition.

Lactulose (Cephulac) given orally at a dose of 30 mL every 6 to 12 hours, adjusted to achieve two soft bowel movements per day, is the drug treatment of choice after enemas have improved mental status. Beneficial effects of oral disaccharides are related to inducing osmotic diarrhea and increasing fecal nitrogen excretion by acidification of the colon, decreasing intestinal bacteria's generation of ammonia, and stimulating the incorporation of ammonia into bacterial proteins.

Oral absorbable or nonabsorbable antibiotics are also useful in the treatment of patients with hepatic encephalopathy, since they reduce colonic bacterial flora that produce ammonia. Neomycin (Neobiotic) is the most commonly used antibiotic at a dosage of 2 to 6 grams per day. This is as effective as lactulose but may induce bacterial or fungal overgrowth and cause ototoxicity.

Recently, the efficacy of sodium benzoate has been assessed. Sodium benzoate decreases serum ammonia levels by increasing waste nitrogen excretion by alternative pathways, such as binding to the nitrogenous compounds glycine and glutamine to form hippurates, which are excreted in the urine. Sodium benzoate given orally at a dose of 5 grams twice daily seems to be as effective as lactulose in cirrhotics with acute encephalopathy, but the cost is 30 times lower. However, many patients have gastrointestinal intolerance that requires acid suppression therapy.

Intravenous administration of branched chain amino acids or flumazenil (Romazicon),* a benzodiazepine antagonist, is generally unnecessary and can be reserved for special cases.

Patients with chronic hepatic encephalopathy that is resistant to lactulose alone should also receive chronic dietary protein restriction. This situation is unusual and is most commonly encountered after surgical portacaval shunt. In these patients, vegetarian or lactovegetarian proteins and possibly oral branched chain amino acids may permit more protein intake and prevent protein malnutrition. Lactulose is given in the same dosage as in acute hepatic encephalopathy. Other therapies such as bromocriptine (Parlodel),* l-dopa, and zinc supplementation have not been clearly effective. Finally, patients with

chronic or recurrent hepatic encephalopathy should be considered for liver transplantation.

Coagulation Abnormalities

Cirrhotic patients frequently have coagulation abnormalities. In fact, a platelet count less than 100,000 per mm³ in a patient with liver disease should raise the suspicion of cirrhosis and associated hypersplenism. The liver is the site of synthesis of almost all coagulation proteins. In addition, some patients with cirrhosis malabsorb fat-soluble vitamins. Fat-soluble vitamin K is indispensable for hepatic synthesis of several clotting factors. Therefore, cirrhotic patients with prolonged prothrombin time should receive 10 mg of vitamin K_1 subcutaneously. Intramuscular injections can lead to soft tissue hemorrhage. There is no evidence that two or three injections are better than one. Vitamin K will correct only hypoprothrombinemia that is related to its deficiency. It is especially important in patients with chronic cholestatic liver disease. In most patients with cirrhosis, vitamin K does not improve the coagulopathy, because the coagulopathy is due to the damaged liver, not the vitamin deficiency.

Cirrhotic patients with active bleeding (usually gastrointestinal hemorrhage) and coagulopathy should receive fresh-frozen plasma in a dose of 2 U every 3 to 6 hours until hemorrhage ceases. Prothrombin time seldom normalizes with plasma infusion because the cirrhotic liver cannot clear fibrin monomer. Cryoprecipitate is seldom, if ever, needed.

Platelet concentrates should be administered to cirrhotic patients with severe thrombocytopenia (<50,000 cells per mm³) when an invasive procedure is performed. Desmopressin (DDAVP) is a vasopressin analogue that can transiently improve platelet function in the setting of renal failure. It can be administered in a slow intravenous infusion of 0.3 μg per kg body weight diluted in 50 mL of sterile saline to cirrhotic patients with renal failure prior to invasive procedures. Diagnostic or therapeutic paracentesis does not require these measures.

Hepatocellular Carcinoma

Hepatocellular carcinoma is a frequent complication of cirrhosis. More than 90% of these tumors are associated with cirrhosis. Prognosis in the United States is very poor, probably because the diagnosis is usually made very late, when therapeutic options are unable to modify the outcome. However, serial monitoring of alpha-fetoprotein and sequential ultrasonography studies during follow-up of cirrhotic patients at risk of developing hepatocellular carcinoma permit an earlier diagnosis and improved therapeutic options.

The approach to patients with hepatocellular carcinoma can be surgical or medical. Surgical treatment should be the first option considered, because it provides the only chance for cure. Unfortunately, most patients with hepatocellular carcinoma have underlying cirrhosis and develop fatal liver failure if a large resection is performed. Liver transplantation

---

*Not FDA-approved for this indication.

may be the only surgical option for cirrhotic patients with hepatocellular carcinoma. However, since the tumor recurrence rate is very high, only patients with tumors less than 4 cm and without vascular invasion by the tumor should be considered for liver transplantation. In these patients, the recurrence rate of the tumor is less than 30% after 3 years of follow-up. Chemoemobilization as adjuvant therapy prior to liver transplantation can be performed to avoid tumor growth while awaiting surgery.

Medical treatment of hepatocellular carcinoma should be considered in patients who are not surgical candidates. However, decompensated patients with hepatocellular carcinoma have a very poor prognosis and should probably receive no treatment for the tumor. Currently, several therapies are under investigation, including intralesional alcohol injection, arterial embolization, hormonal manipulation, chemotherapy, immunotherapy, and radiotherapy. Intralesional injection of absolute alcohol causes tumor necrosis and is a good therapeutic option for patients with tumors less than 4 cm. Prognosis is similar to that of surgical resection. This option is probably the most practical worldwide, because it requires only ultrasound guidance, syringes, and needles. Arterial embolization with Lipiodol and gelatin with or without chemotherapeutic agents may be helpful in reducing the size of large tumors. However, controlled trials are needed. Antiestrogen drugs such as tamoxifen (Nolvadex)* 10 mg every 8 hours may improve survival in patients with large tumors who are not candidates for other therapies. Combined medical treatments are currently under investigation.

LIVER TRANSPLANTATION

Orthotopic liver transplantation is the only treatment that has been convincingly demonstrated to improve survival in cirrhotic patients. During the last decade, survival of liver transplant patients has improved dramatically; more than 70% are alive 5 years later. These improved results can be attributed to more careful patient selection, better surgical techniques and postoperative care, and better immune suppression.

Liver transplantation should be considered in any patient with end-stage liver disease of any etiology for which there is no acceptable alternative therapy. The optimal timing for transplantation is difficult to define. In general, cirrhotic patients who have suffered a major complication of liver disease should be evaluated for liver transplantation (Table 19). Contraindications to liver transplantation include psychological, physical, or social inability to tolerate transplantation; active sepsis; acquired immune deficiency syndrome; and advanced cardiopulmonary disease. Advanced age (more than 60 years), portacaval shunt, portal vein thrombosis, and prior complex hepatobiliary surgery are relative contraindications. Alcoholism is currently considered a temporary contraindication. Alcoholic patients are usually evaluated after a period of 6 to 12 months of alcohol abstinence. If a psychosocial evaluation predicts a significant risk of recidivism, transplantation is denied. Liver transplantation in patients with chronic liver disease related to hepatitis B virus with active replication (serum HBV-DNA positive) should be considered investigational, since the incidence of aggressive recurrent disease is very high. Results of antiviral therapy prior to and after liver transplantation and/or immunotherapy have been disappointing. The incidence of recurrence of hepatitis C virus infection is also very high, but rapid progression to cirrhosis seems to be less frequent than in patients with hepatitis B virus–related cirrhosis. The number of cirrhotic patients with hepatocellular carcinoma submitted to liver transplantation is decreasing due to the recognized high rate of tumor recurrence. In general, the number of candidates for liver transplantation is increasing continuously, but not the number of human donors. Therefore, other sources of liver donors are currently being explored.

TABLE 19. **Indications for Liver Transplantation in Patients with Cirrhosis**

Ascites, especially when diuretic resistant
Variceal hemorrhage, especially when resistant to medical treatment
Hepatic encephalopathy, especially when resistant to medical treatment
Incapacitating fatigue
Incapacitating pruritus in the setting of primary biliary cirrhosis

BLEEDING ESOPHAGEAL VARICES

method of
ALBERT J. CZAJA, M.D.
Mayo Clinic
Rochester, Minnesota

Bleeding from esophageal varices accounts for only 10% of all cases of gastrointestinal hemorrhage, but it has the highest immediate mortality. From 30 to 80% of patients with cirrhosis who experience their first variceal hemorrhage die, and of those who survive, bleeding recurs in 33 to 70%, typically within 6 weeks of the first occurrence. The mortality of each recurrent hemorrhage averages 50%. Prompt diagnosis and expeditious effective intervention undoubtedly improve these outcomes.

The immediate objective of treatment is to restore and maintain hemodynamic stability. Mortality increases markedly after 48 hours of continuous bleeding, and treatment efforts must be vigorous to control the hemorrhage quickly. Fortunately, 90% of patients stop bleeding spontaneously or with conventional nonoperative measures within this interval. Once acute bleeding has been controlled, the next objective is to prevent rebleeding long term. The severity of the underlying liver disease is the most important determinant of longevity, and this realization influences the long-term treatment strategy. Individuals with advanced decompensated liver disease are candi-

---

*Not FDA-approved for this indication.

dates for expeditious liver transplantation, whereas patients with early-stage cirrhosis or nonhepatic causes of portal hypertension are candidates for pharmacologic, endoscopic, or surgical interventions.

Varices bleed because increased intravascular pressure stretches and thins the vessel wall until rupture occurs. Variceal hemorrhage is not due to acid-peptic injury of the mucosa or direct mechanical injury. Indeed, patients who bleed typically have large varices and portal pressures that exceed 12 mmHg. Logically, therefore, management strategies should be directed at eliminating the varices or reducing their size and/or lowering portal pressure below 12 mmHg. Ideally, in patients with advanced liver disease, implantation of a new liver treats the primary disease (cirrhosis) and its immediate life-threatening manifestation (variceal hemorrhage).

IMMEDIATE MANAGEMENT

Resuscitation

Clinical Assessment

A systolic blood pressure of less than 100 mmHg and a pulse rate of greater than 100 beats per minute connote a reduction in blood volume of at least 20%. An orthostatic blood pressure drop of more than 10 mmHg reflects a blood loss of at least 1 liter, and it correlates more closely with volume changes than the pulse rate. Under such circumstances, intravenous replacement is essential to preserve renal perfusion and minimize liver cell anoxia. Too vigorous resuscitation, however, can be hazardous, especially in the elderly patient with precarious cardiac function. Additionally, overexpansion may prolong bleeding or precipitate rebleeding by increasing portal pressure. Large volumes of crystalloid solution can aggravate ascites, peripheral edema, and pleural effusions as well as promote hyponatremia in patients with cirrhosis.

Volume Replacement

Intravenous access must be established immediately, and a large-bore catheter is preferred (Table 1). At least two access lines are ideal in the vigorous unstable bleeder. The mean number of blood transfusions during the first 24 hours is 3.8 U, and the mean total during hospitalization is 11 U. Consequently, large volumes of blood must be ready for delivery, and at least 3 U of stored packed red blood cells should be available at all times (see Table 1). Access to fresh-frozen plasma and platelets should also be ensured. Crystalloid solutions (isotonic saline or Ringer's lactate) are appropriate until blood typing and crossmatching are completed (see Table 1). Initial blood studies should include the hemoglobin level, a platelet count, the creatinine level, the prothrombin time, the activated partial thromboplastin time, electrolyte levels, and the glucose concentration.

Monitoring Mechanisms

All patients with active variceal bleeding should be managed in an intensive care setting (see Table 1).

TABLE 1. Supportive Measures for Acute Variceal Hemorrhage

Supportive Measures	Individual Aspects
Intensive care monitoring	Arterial blood pressure Urinary catheter Central venous pressure or Swan-Ganz catheter
Intravenous lines	Large-bore venous catheter (preferably two)
Intravenous fluids and blood products	Crystalloid (Ringer's lactate, isotonic saline) Packed red blood cells (at least 3 U available) Fresh-frozen plasma (2 U q 2–3 h until bleeding stops or prothrombin time improves; 1 U after every 5 U of packed red blood cells) Platelets (2 U every 5 U of packed red blood cells or if platelet count low or function impaired)
Vitamin K₁	10 mg daily IM
Endotracheal tube	Obtundation and/or vomiting
Lactulose	Oral regimen (30 mL q 6–8 h) Retention enema regimen (300 mL in 700 mL tap water q 8 h)
Nutrition	PO and/or IV (25 kcal/kg/day and 80–120 gm amino acids/day)

Blood replacement should be guided by hemodynamic assessments rather than hematocrit determinations. Arterial blood pressure and urine output must be monitored closely and a central venous pressure line placed if bleeding is active. If hemodynamic instability is evident, renal function is impaired, cardiac failure is imminent, or pulmonary congestion is apparent, a Swan-Ganz catheter should be positioned to assess the pulmonary artery and wedge pressures, the cardiac index, and the peripheral vascular resistance (see Table 1). When the blood pressure is restored to low-normal and urine output is increased to 50 mL per hour, the volume of intravenous infusions can be reduced to match losses. A hematocrit between 30 and 35 is adequate for oxygen transport.

Hemostasis

Stored bank blood provides factors VII, IX, and X and prothrombin, but transfusions of fresh-frozen plasma and platelets are necessary to restore the more labile factors. Fresh-frozen plasma supplements factors V, VII, VIII, X, and XI and prothrombin. Two units of platelets and 1 U of fresh-frozen plasma should be administered after every transfusion of 5 U or more of stored packed red blood cells as a minimum replacement (see Table 1). For severe hypoprothrombinemia and active bleeding, 2 U of fresh-frozen plasma should be given every 2 to 3 hours until bleeding stops or the prothrombin time is within 3 seconds of normal. Platelet transfusions can also be administered to ensure adequate platelet function even in patients with normal platelet counts. Vitamin K_1 (AquaMEPHYTON, Konakion), 10 mg daily, should be administered intramuscularly (see Table 1).

Supportive Measures

An endotracheal tube should be inserted in patients with active bleeding who are obtunded and at risk for aspiration (see Table 1). This is an especially important precaution before gastric lavage, endoscopic examination, or balloon tamponade. After the acute bleeding has stopped, efforts should be directed to the treatment or prevention of hepatic encephalopathy. Purgation of the gastrointestinal tract with cleansing saline enemas reduces the protein catabolism and ammonia production associated with residual blood in the gastrointestinal tract. Lactulose (Cephulac), 15 to 30 mL every hour until loose stools and then 30 mL every 6 to 8 hours thereafter to maintain at least three bowel movements daily, can be given by mouth or nasogastric tube (see Table 1). Neomycin, even as a retention enema, should be avoided if possible because of the risks of nephrotoxicity, ototoxicity, and intestinal malabsorption. In patients in whom oral therapy is difficult or hazardous, lactulose (300 mL in 700 mL of tap water) can be administered every 8 hours as a retention enema (see Table 1). Solutions containing high concentrations of branched chain amino acids and low levels of aromatic amino acids (HepatAmine) are useful in maintaining positive nitrogen balance in individuals who can tolerate the fluid volume, and they should be used mainly for this purpose rather than as a principal treatment for hepatic encephalopathy. Nutritional support is essential, and at least 25 kcal per kg of body weight should be provided daily, mainly as an intravenous glucose infusion. From 80 to 120 grams of amino acids (HepatAmine) can be given daily, but regimens must be modified according to tolerance for intravenous fluids (see Table 1).

Control of Bleeding

Gastric Lavage

A nasogastric tube should be placed to assess the activity of bleeding, decompress the stomach, and prepare the upper gastrointestinal tract for endoscopic examination. Vigorous bleeding justifies passage of an orogastric tube (No. 36 French Ewald tube) to evacuate large clots (Table 2). Tube placement has not been shown to aggravate the varices or perpetuate the bleeding. Lavage should be performed with saline or tap water that is at room temperature. Iced water can lower the patient's core body temperature, and it may impair the clotting mechanisms. The contribution of lavage to hemostasis is uncertain, but over 30% of patients stop bleeding during this procedure.

Endoscopic Examination

Emergency fiberoptic examination of the upper gastrointestinal tract is essential to establish the site

TABLE 2. **Initial Strategies for Active Variceal Bleeding**

Treatment Measures	Individual Aspects
Nasogastric or orogastric tube	No. 36 French Ewald tube for large clots
Gastric lavage	Saline or tap water at room temperature
Intravenous drug therapy	Terlipressin (Glypressin) (2-mg bolus, then 1 mg q 4 h for 24 h) *or* Somatostatin (Zecnil)* (250 μg bolus, then infusion of 250 μg/h for 24 h) *or* Octreotide (Sandostatin)† (25–50 μg/h infusion) *or* Vasopressin (Pitressin) (20 U in 100 mL of 5% dextrose, then 0.2–0.4 U/min infusion adjusted to maximum dose of 1 U/min) *plus* Nitroglycerin† (40 μg/min infusion with maximum dose of 400 μg/min or 0.4 mg sublingual q 30 min)
Endoscopic sclerosis or banding	Preferably during bleeding-free interval on drug therapy

*Investigational drug in the United States.
†Not FDA-approved for this indication.

of bleeding and define the proper therapeutic action (see Table 2). In many instances, prompt and effective therapy can be rendered directly through the endoscope at the time of the examination. Portal hypertension predisposes to congestive gastropathy and gastric varices as well as esophageal varices. Other nonliver and nonportal hypertensive causes of bleeding must also be excluded. As many as 50% of patients with cirrhosis and esophageal varices are bleeding from nonvariceal sites.

The overall diagnostic accuracy of endoscopic assessment during active bleeding is 67%. Identification of the bleeding site is most likely if the examination is performed within 3 hours after the onset of bleeding. Vigorous hemorrhage and patient instability can preclude immediate passage of the scope. Gastroesophageal balloon tamponade should *never* be attempted as an interim measure before endoscopic confirmation of variceal bleeding. If a diagnosis cannot be established because of brisk hemorrhage, emergency visceral angiography should be performed.

Drug Therapy

Vasopressin (Pitressin) should be administered during active bleeding and after restoration of hemodynamic stability. It must never be given to individuals in shock or near shock. An intravenous bolus of 20 U in 100 mL of 5% dextrose should be followed by a continuous intravenous infusion at a rate of 0.2 to 0.4 U per minute. The rate can be adjusted each hour by increments of 0.1 to 0.2 U per minute until bleeding stops, side effects develop, or a maximum dose of 1 U per minute is achieved. Adjunctive use of nitroglycerin,* preferably as an intravenous infusion (40 µg per minute, starting dose; 400 µg per minute, maximum dose), improves the hemodynamic response and reduces the frequency of ischemic complications. Alternatively, sublingual nitroglycerin can be given (Nitrostat, 0.4 mg) every 30 minutes for up to 6 hours (see Table 2).

Vasopressin reduces portal pressure by vasoconstricting the splanchnic arteries and decreasing splanchnic blood flow. It may also diminish flow through the varices by contracting the esophageal musculature. A continuous infusion reduces the wedged hepatic vein pressure by 29%, and it terminates bleeding in 50 to 86% of patients. Peripheral intravenous infusion is as effective as selective intraarterial infusion and more effective than intermittent intravenous bolus therapy.

Bleeding is usually controlled soon after institution of the vasopressin infusion, and this therapy should not be continued indefinitely in the absence of a clinical response. The infusion should be maintained for at least 6 hours after cessation of bleeding, and ideally it should be continued for at least 24 hours after successful endoscopic sclerotherapy or banding. The infusion can then be discontinued in a gradual tapered dose fashion over a 6-hour period.

Complications of vasopressin infusion reflect mainly the drug's systemic circulatory effects. Reductions in hepatic blood flow and cardiac output may result in hepatic ischemia, abdominal cramps, bowel ischemia, cardiac arrhythmia, or myocardial infarction. Enhancement of peripheral vascular resistance may increase arterial blood pressure and reduce heart rate. Tissue extravasation of the drug may produce a gangrenous extremity, and excessive antidiuretic activity may contribute to hyponatremia.

Side effects can be minimized if vasopressin is administered in a low dose under close supervision to adequately resuscitated patients. Continuous electrocardiographic monitoring is advisable during the infusion, and the drug should not be given to individuals with myocardial ischemia or disturbances in cardiac rhythm.

Terlipressin (Glypressin)† is a synthetic vasopressin analogue that has a biologic activity of 3 to 4 hours. This duration of action contrasts with the few minutes of efficacy associated with vasopressin administration, and it allows intravenous bolus injections of the drug. Studies have indicated that it is superior to placebo and vasopressin in the management of variceal hemorrhage and that it is comparable to treatment with somatostatin. Since it does not activate plasminogen or have serious cardiac consequences, terlipressin has fewer side effects than vasopressin. The drug is administered as an initial 2-mg intravenous bolus. Thereafter, a 1-mg bolus is injected intravenously every 4 hours for 24 hours (see Table 2). Terlipressin should be used in preference to vasopressin if a choice is possible.

Somatostatin (Zecnil)* reduces splanchnic blood flow and portal pressure in a highly selective fashion. It also inhibits gastric acid secretion, and it may enhance platelet aggregation. These advantages have been exploited in the treatment of variceal hemorrhage, and somatostatin infusions have been shown to be as effective as balloon tamponade and terlipressin and superior to vasopressin in randomized controlled clinical trials. Somatostatin has a plasma half-life of 2 to 6 minutes depending on its molecular form, and it must be administered as a continuous intravenous infusion. Efficacy has been demonstrated with a 250-µg intravenous bolus followed by a continuous infusion of 250 µg per hour for 24 hours (see Table 2). Treatments with somatostatin and terlipressin are comparable in efficacy, and preferences reflect differences in availability, expense, and personal experience.

The synthetic analogue, octreotide (Sandostatin),† has a plasma half-life of 113 minutes after a single subcutaneous injection, and hepatic excretion is 30 to 40% in healthy volunteers. In patients with cirrhosis, arterial blood levels of the drug can be achieved with only half the dose required in normal individuals. Portal pressure is decreased mainly by splanchnic vasoconstriction, and intravenous infusions of octreotide as low as 25 to 50 µg per hour have had favorable hemodynamic effects in patients with cirrhosis (see Table 2). Many medical centers now use octreotide as the preferred pharmacologic agent for bleeding esophageal varices.

Metoclopramide (Reglan)† reduces transmural variceal pressure in cirrhosis without affecting portal hemodynamics. A 10-mg intravenous bolus decreases variceal pressure by 16% when compared with saline infusions. Presumably, the tightening of the lower esophageal sphincter has a local effect on variceal filling and pressure. Future studies will need to determine if this action has a therapeutic advantage.

Endoscopic Sclerotherapy or Variceal Banding

Variceal sclerosis or banding is regarded as the definitive primary treatment for acute variceal hemorrhage, whereas supportive and pharmacologic measures are considered to be expedient but temporary actions (see Table 2). Variceal sclerosis using sodium tetradecyl sulfate (Sotradecol), ethanolamine oleate (Ethamolin), polidocanol, or ethanol, or banding (using small elastic O rings), should be done at the time of the initial endoscopic examination and preferably after the institution of pharmacologic therapy and the induction of a bleeding-free interval. The efficacy of emergency sclerotherapy ranges from 65 to 95% depending on hemorrhagic activity. Rebleeding after treatment is also less frequent if the initial procedure is performed in the absence of active hemorrhage (30 vs. 50%). Follow-up sclerotherapy or banding sessions sustain control and reduce the immediate re-

---

*Not FDA-approved for this indication.
†Investigational drug in the United States.

*Investigational drug in the United States.
†Not FDA-approved for this indication.

bleeding frequency to 10% or less. These follow-up sessions should aim at obliteration of the remaining visible vessels. Pharmacologic treatment complements endoscopic treatment by limiting hemorrhagic activity during the procedure and maintaining a lowered portal pressure after it. Ideally, drug therapy should be continued for at least 24 hours after the initial sclerosis or banding.

Endoscopic ligation or banding of varices was introduced in 1986, and it has supplanted variceal sclerosis in many centers (see Table 2). As a mechanical method of variceal obliteration, it has few systemic sequelae such as pneumonia or infection, and since the quantity of tissue ligated is restricted by the design of the device, local complications such as esophageal stricture are also reduced. In a randomized trial comparing endoscopic ligation with sclerotherapy, active bleeding at the first treatment was controlled more commonly (86 vs. 77%), bleeding recurred less often (36 vs. 48%), treatment sessions for variceal obliteration were less numerous (four ± two vs. five ± two sessions), mortality was lower (28 vs. 45%, p = .04), and the frequency of complications (2 vs. 22%, p < .001) was less with ligation than with sclerotherapy. The major survival advantage for ligation is in patients with Child-Pugh Classes A and B, in whom there is a lower frequency of death by exsanguination than with sclerotherapy. The few complications associated with ligation include pneumonia and bacterial peritonitis, and these are unrelated to the Child-Pugh class.

Endoscopic variceal sclerosis may worsen portal hypertensive gastropathy during a 6- to 9-month period after eradication of the esophageal varices, and gastric varices may appear or enlarge during this period in 12 to 20% of patients. It is uncertain that these endoscopic changes contribute to morbidity or mortality. Typically they improve spontaneously after 9 months, presumably because collateral channels develop to decompress the gastric mucosa. The long-term use of propranolol (160 to 320 mg per day as a slow-release preparation of Inderal) after endoscopic sclerotherapy and variceal obliteration can reduce variceal recurrence from 73 to 15% during the first year after treatment. It may also have an advantage in reducing bleeding from esophageal varices and congested gastric mucosal vessels.

Transjugular Intrahepatic Portal Systemic Shunts

Refractory variceal bleeding or hemorrhage from inaccessible gastric or intestinal varices occurs in 10 to 15% of patients. Placement of a transjugular intrahepatic portal systemic shunt (TIPS) should be considered in such patients if they are poor risks for shunt surgery and they are candidates for liver transplantation (Table 3). The right internal jugular vein is punctured and an angiographic catheter and guidewire are manipulated into the middle or right hepatic vein before the catheter is exchanged for an angiographic sheath with a hemostasis valve. A transjugular needle is then passed through the

TABLE 3. **Salvage Therapies for Acute Variceal Bleeding**

Salvage Measures	Individual Aspects
Repeat endoscopic sclerosis or banding	Reasonable but temporary option High mortality after second failure
Balloon tamponade	Modified Sengstaken-Blakemore or Minnesota tube (4 lumens) Gastric balloon first (150 mL) Esophageal balloon last (pressure, 25–40 mmHg) Periodic deflation (every 6–12 h) of esophageal balloon Discontinue within 36 h
Transjugular intrahepatic portal systemic shunt (TIPS)	Interim measure in liver transplantation candidates
Emergency portosystemic shunts	End-to-side portocaval, interposition mesocaval, or distal splenorenal shunts Best in Child-Pugh Class A or B with good hepatic functional reserve in whom immediate liver transplant is unlikely
Esophageal transection and devascularization	Emergency control measure for elective shunt or liver transplant candidates
Selective injection to induce sclerosis or embolization	Child-Pugh Class C patients who are not candidates for liver transplantation but whose status can be upgraded for elective shunt
Liver transplantation	Possible but not advisable during active hemorrhage Can usually be temporarily deferred by endoscopic treatment or TIPS

sheath and directed out of the hepatic vein anteriorly through the liver tissue into the right portal vein under ultrasonographic guidance. The tract is dilated with a balloon catheter, and a self-expanding metallic stent is then positioned to stent the hepatic and portal veins. The mean duration of the procedure is 121 ± 29 minutes, and hemorrhaging patients must be stabilized before and during TIPS placement. Fortunately, the stent can usually be placed under local anesthesia or sedation.

Successful placement of the stent is manifested by an immediate drop in portal pressure from an initial average of 34 ± 9 cmH$_2$O to a post-treatment average of 22 ± 5 cmH$_2$O and rapid control of hemorrhage. In experienced medical centers, the technical success rate for stent placement is 92 to 96%, and the mortality within 30 days is 0 to 14%. Importantly, the procedure-related mortality is less than 3%, and the stent remains patent in 90% of instances. Stent closure can be diagnosed by Doppler ultrasonography and treated successfully with low-dose urokinase, dilation of the stent, or replacement. Stent migration is infrequent, and endothelialization of the shunt occurs within 7 to 10 days. Ascites resolves in 80 to 90% of patients, treatable encephalopathy develops in 9%, and rebleeding occurs in 14%. TIPS is not yet endorsed as a permanent treatment measure for bleeding varices, and therefore its use should be coupled with a long-term treatment strategy that includes liver transplantation (Table 4).

Balloon Tamponade

Balloon tamponade is a standard treatment for refractory bleeding from esophageal varices (see Table 3). Placement of a four-lumen balloon tube (modified Sengstaken-Blakemore or Minnesota tube) is justified if bleeding persists despite pharmacologic and endoscopic measures or if stabilization is required before the TIPS procedure, shunt surgery, or liver transplantation.

Tolerance for the tube is best when it is introduced through the nasal passage, but it can be inserted through the mouth. The stomach should be emptied before insertion, and the airway should be protected by endotracheal intubation if the sensorium is impaired. Placement in the stomach must be verified by auscultation over the area during air insufflation. The gastric balloon can then be partially inflated with 50 mL of air. The balloon position is confirmed by roentgenography before inflation to its full capacity of 150 mL. The distended gastric balloon is then drawn up tightly against the gastroesophageal junction, where it is secured under 1 pound of tension by tape to the nose or face mask of a football helmet. If bleeding continues, the esophageal balloon is inflated to the minimal pressure that exceeds variceal pressure (25 to 40 mmHg), and its position is confirmed by chest roentgenography. The pressure in the esophageal balloon must be monitored continuously by an attached pressure gauge during the entire period of inflation. Strong traction on the tube is not necessary, and it may be harmful. Suction on the tube above the esophageal balloon is essential to reduce secretions and reduce the risk of pulmonary aspiration. A pair of scissors should be taped to the bedpost for rapid transection of the tube and defla-

tion of the balloons in the event of respiratory distress (see Table 3).

Balloon tamponade stops bleeding in 70 to 88% of patients, especially if instituted within 6 hours after onset. Control is obtained more frequently after the first bleed than after recurrences. Complications develop in 9 to 39% of patients, and these include aspiration, esophageal rupture, pressure necrosis, esophageal stenosis, and respiratory obstruction. Risks increase with the duration of balloon inflation, and the tamponade should not be sustained for more than 36 hours. Indeed, the esophageal balloon should be deflated for short periods every 6 to 12 hours (see Table 3).

Rebleeding occurs after deflation in 24 to 64% of patients, and when this occurs, the mortality is 60%. Because balloon tamponade achieves only temporary control of bleeding, it must be coupled with a long-term management strategy that includes endoscopic sclerosis or banding, TIPS placement, shunt surgery, or liver transplantation.

Removal of the tube should be in staged fashion. The esophageal balloon should be deflated first after bleeding has been controlled for at least 24 hours. The gastric balloon should then be deflated if stability has been maintained over the next 6 hours. The entire tube can be withdrawn after another 24 hours of quiescence.

Emergency Shunts

Surgical decompression or elimination of esophageal varices is a consideration if the other treatment maneuvers fail (see Table 3). Emergency portocaval anastomosis is the most effective method of lowering portal pressure acutely, but operative mortality is fivefold greater than that of an elective procedure. The risk of surgery must be balanced against the probable life expectancy after the operation. In patients with adequate hepatic functional reserve (Child-Pugh Classes A and B), the operative mortality of 20% may be an acceptable risk for the years of life gained. In patients with poor hepatic reserve (Child-Pugh Class C), the surgical procedure with its mortality of 87% may not offer an advantage over nonoperative measures. Indeed, if surgery is undertaken in such patients, expeditious liver transplantation rather than shunt surgery is a better choice.

The surgical options are an end-to-side portocaval shunt, an interposition mesocaval shunt, or a distal splenorenal shunt, and shunt selection is determined by the surgical experience, vascular anatomy, hepatic functional reserve, direction of portal vein blood flow, and likelihood of subsequent liver transplantation (see Table 3). In patients with Child-Pugh Class A and B cirrhosis, interposition mesocaval and distal splenorenal shunts are less likely to complicate future efforts at liver transplantation. In patients with Child-Pugh Class C, a mesocaval or interposition shunt is associated with less ascites postoperatively, and it can be ligated if severe encephalopathy develops. In patients with minimal hepatopedal flow and/or unstable clinical condition, an end-to-side portoca-

TABLE 4. **Long-Term Management of Acute Variceal Hemorrhage**

Long-Term Measures	Individual Aspects
Repeated endoscopic therapy and indefinite drug treatment	Repeat sclerosis or banding (sessions every 1–4 weeks until obliteration, then every 3–6 months for 1 year, then every year thereafter) *plus* Propranolol* (20–180 mg orally twice daily titrated to pulse rate and tolerance, then long-acting drug to maximum dose of 320 mg daily)
Distal splenorenal shunt	Child-Pugh Class A or B patients with good hepatic reserve who rebled after endoscopic and drug therapy Patients in whom liver transplantation is not possible
Liver transplantation	Patients with progressive liver disease who rebled after endoscopic and drug therapy

*Not FDA-approved for this indication.

val shunt is preferable, whereas in patients with frank hepatopedal flow, a distal splenorenal shunt preserves portal perfusion of the liver and hepatic function.

Emergency portocaval shunts stop bleeding in 95% of instances, but the complications in survivors include encephalopathy (up to 40%) and shunt thrombosis (10 to 24%).

Emergency Nonshunting Procedures

Transabdominal esophageal transection and devascularization involves the use of a stapling device that simultaneously resects a ring of esophageal wall and reanastomoses the esophagus (mucosa-to-mucosa) by means of 12 to 14 tantalum staples. When the procedure is combined with ligation of the left gastric vein and periesophageal collaterals, the 1-year rebleeding frequency can be reduced to 20% and the 1-year survival can be increased. Operative mortality under emergency circumstances, however, exceeds 30%. In patients with reversible hepatic decompensation who are candidates for an elective shunt procedure or liver transplantation, esophageal transection and stapling with lower esophageal devascularization is a mechanism to control life-threatening hemorrhage without disruption of hepatic blood flow and subsequent hepatic encephalopathy (see Table 3). Prospective randomized trials comparing sclerotherapy, esophageal transection, and distal splenorenal shunt for bleeding varices in patients with Child-Pugh Class A and B cirrhosis have shown that the three procedures are comparable in cumulative rebleeding rates (0 vs. 6 vs. 13%) and survival (88 vs. 84 vs. 74%) during 6 to 72 months of follow-up. These findings endorse sclerotherapy as the initial treatment strategy, but they do not apply to patients who have been selected for surgical intervention by virtue of the failure of previous therapies.

Selective injection of embolic or sclerosing substances into the variceal tributaries is another method to achieve hemostasis in the recalcitrant bleeder. The left gastric or coronary vein and the short gastric veins that communicate with the gastroesophageal varices can be catheterized using the percutaneous transhepatic route, and the vessels can be occluded with gelatin foam, autogenous blood clots, sodium tetradecyl sulfate, thrombin, steel coils, metal clips, or synthetic polymer (isobutylcyanoacrylate). The procedure lasts 2 to 5 hours, but varices are obliterated in 80% of cases. Rebleeding occurs in 65% of patients within 5 months, and the procedure cannot be repeated long term. Collateralization eventuates in 76% of patients, and this may enhance hepatofugal blood flow and further compromise liver function. Most importantly, portal vein thrombosis, which may preclude liver transplantation and reduce shunt options, develops in 36%, and gastrointestinal ischemia and necrosis are other possible consequences. The complications and impermanence of transhepatic variceal obliteration warrant the restriction of its use to patients with poor hepatic functional reserve (Child-Pugh Class C) who are not candidates for liver transplantation but whose Child-Pugh classification can be improved sufficiently to justify a shunt procedure later (see Table 3).

Transesophageal ligation of varices through a left thoracotomy has a high operative mortality (30%), disappointing rebleeding rate (33%), and dismal 1-year survival expectation (5%). It is a procedure that has now been supplanted by other better options.

LONG–TERM MANAGEMENT

Prevention of rebleeding is the main objective of long-term management. The follow-up strategy depends on the type of therapy required to control the initial hemorrhage. In most instances, it entails repeated endoscopic examinations to obliterate residual or recurrent varices by injection or banding.

Repeated Endoscopic Sclerosis or Banding

Endoscopic variceal sclerosis or banding can eliminate varices after a median of four sessions in 90% of patients (see Table 4). These sessions are scheduled at 1- to 4-week intervals to decrease the incidence of rebleeding. Short intervals are preferred because rebleeding may occur in 48 to 58% of individuals awaiting variceal obliteration (see Table 4). New varices develop in 67% of patients, and rebleeding occurs in 19%, usually within 12 months after initial obliteration. Follow-up endoscopic examinations are necessary to treat recurrent varices every 3 to 6 months for 1 year after initial eradication and then once each year thereafter (see Table 4). The morbidity of sclerosis (fever, chest pain, pleural effusion, injection ulcers, bacteremia, esophageal stricture, pneumonia, and bacterial peritonitis) is 9% per procedure and 19% per patient (mortality, 0.7 to 2%). Gastric varices cannot be obliterated by this procedure, and successful eradication of esophageal varices may actually increase the propensity for fundic varices or congestive gastropathy to bleed. Banding has fewer complications than sclerosis, and it is as effective. Two studies have indicated a survival benefit from sclerotherapy, but other studies have been contradictory. Ultimately, survival reflects the severity of the underlying liver disease.

Propranolol (Inderal)* and Nadolol (Corgard)*

Propranolol and nadolol are nonselective beta blockers that decrease portal pressure by reducing cardiac output, inducing splanchnic vasoconstriction, and impairing vasodilation. These hemodynamic effects produce a reduction in azygos blood flow and intravariceal pressure. Multiple controlled trials and meta-analyses have indicated that propranolol and nadolol are effective in reducing the frequency of rebleeding from esophageal varices (66 to 45%), but no studies have demonstrated an improvement in survival. Treatment with propranolol or nadolol can also prevent rebleeding from portal hypertensive con-

---

*Not FDA-approved for this indication.

gestive gastropathy, and these drugs may be of value in the management of gastric varices.

Propranolol is administered in a divided dose that is sufficient to reduce the resting pulse rate by 25% (dose range, 20 to 180 mg twice daily) (see Table 4). A long-acting, once-a-day preparation (Inderal LA) can be introduced later when drug tolerance and efficacy have been established (maximum dose, 320 mg per day) (see Table 4). Unfortunately, propranolol has a highly variable effect on portal pressure. The average decrease is only 15%, and 30 to 50% of patients have no response. Additionally, there may be a progressive decrease in hepatic perfusion with chronic administration, and this may facilitate the late development of hepatic encephalopathy.

The portal vein has only alpha adrenoreceptors and beta blockade in patients with decompensated cirrhosis may intensify the alpha effect on portal vasoconstriction and not lower portal pressure. Perhaps this explains reports of treatment efficacy mainly in patients with good hepatic functional reserve (Child-Pugh Class A). Cardioselective beta blockers (atenolol [Tenormin],* betaxolol [Kerlone]*) can also reduce azygos vein blood flow, but they do not have an advantage over propranolol in decreasing portal pressure.

Propranolol is probably less effective than sclerotherapy in preventing rebleeding, although only one of six controlled studies has demonstrated a statistically significant difference between these two strategies (rebleeding frequency, 54% after propranolol vs. 45% after sclerotherapy, p < .05). The combination of propranolol and sclerotherapy, however, is more effective than propranolol (45 vs. 65%) or sclerotherapy (20 vs. 75%, p < .05) alone, and one study has demonstrated a survival advantage for combination treatment (mortality, 55 vs. 81%, p < .05). Consequently, repeated endoscopic sclerosis or banding in conjunction with long-term propranolol therapy is a preferred regimen (see Table 4).

Distal Splenorenal Shunt

Portosystemic shunts are associated with lower frequencies of rebleeding than endoscopic sclerosis or banding and beta blockade, but they have a higher mortality (10%) and frequency of hepatic encephalopathy (20%). Since they do not treat the underlying liver disease, their ability to improve long-term survival remains uncertain and their use has declined as liver transplantation has evolved. Patients with good hepatic functional reserve (Child-Pugh Class A or B) who have recurrent variceal bleeding despite sclerotherapy or banding and beta blockade are the principal candidates for shunt surgery. In these patients, liver transplantation may be too early, not available, or contraindicated (see Table 4).

The distal splenorenal shunt is the preferred procedure, although studies comparing it with total shunts have been contradictory. Three studies in the United States have indicated a lower incidence of hepatic

encephalopathy after distal splenorenal shunt than after total shunt, but three other studies have not found this advantage. Prevention of rebleeding was similar to total shunt in five studies but not in a sixth study, in which rebleeding occurred in 30% of those undergoing selective shunt. Properly chosen patients for such surgery have a 1-year survival of 90% and a 3-year survival of 77%, liver function is maintained, and liver transplantation is required in only 2% over a median follow-up of 2.5 years.

The distal splenorenal shunt separates the splanchnic circulation into portomesenteric and gastrosplenic components, which in selected patients has the advantage of preserving portal perfusion of the liver and decompressing the esophageal varices. The operative mortality is low; rebleeding occurs in 10%; hepatic encephalopathy develops in less than 15%; and shunt occlusion occurs in less than 10%. Ideal circumstances for performance of the procedure include an intact spleen, favorable renal and splenic veins, hepatopedal portal blood flow, and the absence of ascites. Additionally, patients with nonalcoholic liver disease fare better. Unfortunately, progressive systemic collateralization occurs in time, converting the selective shunt to a total shunt. Hepatic portal perfusion can be maintained in only 42% of patients, and the complications of liver failure and hepatic encephalopathy may develop later.

Liver Transplantation

Long-term survival of patients who have bled from esophageal varices is related to hepatic functional reserve, and in many instances liver transplantation is the only means of improving that reserve and "curing the disease." Every patient who presents with variceal hemorrhage should be considered as a potential transplant candidate, and the strategies to control bleeding in the acute and convalescent period should be chosen to protect and facilitate the transplantation option. The stage and the expected course of the underlying liver disease are major determinants of the management algorithm, and patients who rebleed after other measures, force the transplantation issue (see Table 4). Patients with Child-Pugh Class C cirrhosis are candidates for expeditious liver transplantation, and these patients may require TIPS if other measures fail to bridge the period until elective transplantation. Patients with less advanced disease can be managed with repeated endoscopic variceal obliteration or surgical shunt until liver transplantation is indicated. The failure of a second endoscopic sclerosis or banding to prevent rebleeding is associated with a mortality of 66%, and this occurrence compels a surgical decision.

The operative risk for shunt surgery and liver transplantation are comparable in emergency (30 to 50%) and elective (10 to 15% or less) situations. Rebleeding (10 to 20%), shunt thrombosis (2 to 30%), and hepatic encephalopathy (10 to 40%) can complicate shunt surgery, whereas recurrence of the original disease, consequences of immunosuppressive therapy (including hypertension, nephrotoxicity, in-

---

*Not FDA-approved for this indication.

fection, and malignancy), and chronic rejection can complicate liver transplantation. The cost of liver transplantation is greater than that of shunt surgery, but shunt surgery may be associated with repeated hospitalizations and eventual liver transplantation. The 1-year (80 to 90% vs. 70 to 90%) and 5-year (60 to 70% vs. 40 to 60%) survivals are better after liver transplantation than after shunt surgery, but the differences are not dramatic, and they probably reflect patient selection rather than treatment efficacy. Importantly, shunts require no specialized facilities and no waiting time, whereas liver transplantation must be done in a committed center and it depends on donor organ availability. The approach to each patient must be individualized and reflect the available facilities and expertise. Shunt and transplantation surgery can each have an important role in different patients or at different times in the same patient, and they should be regarded as complementary procedures. Previous shunt surgery does not preclude liver transplantation.

DYSPHAGIA AND ESOPHAGEAL OBSTRUCTION

method of
MARIA A. GEORGSSON, M.D., and
DOUGLAS L. BRAND, M.D.
State University of New York at Stony Brook
Stony Brook, New York

Dysphagia, or difficulty with passage of food from the mouth to the stomach, is quite specific for esophageal disorders. It refers specifically to the complaint of food or fluid "sticking" or "hanging up" after a swallow. It is distinct from globus hystericus, which is a constant sensation of a "lump" in the throat. It is also separate from odynophagia, or pain on swallowing, usually a symptom of esophageal mucosal disease, such as carcinoma or moniliasis.

Dysphagia denotes one of two situations: obstruction of the esophageal lumen or abnormal function of the esophageal neuromuscular apparatus (esophageal motility disorder). The medical history can separate these possibilities 80% of the time (Figure 1). Dysphagia only for solid food suggests a mechanical obstruction, a peptic stricture, an esophageal ring or web, or a carcinoma. Progressive dysphagia with a history of long-standing heartburn and without weight loss is characteristic of a benign peptic stricture, whereas rapidly progressive dysphagia with a history of anorexia and weight loss is more consistent with an esophageal ring or web.

The first test to order in the work-up of dysphagia is the barium esophagogram, which is superior to endoscopy in evaluating esophageal strictures or rings and in the preliminary assessment of peristaltic abnormalities. A double-contrast study improves the sensitivity of detecting mucosal lesions. If an obstruction or mucosal abnormality is seen, a flexible endoscopy with possible biopsy should be done. Manometry is useful in detecting motility disorders of the esophageal body and lower esophageal sphincter.

OROPHARYNGEAL DYSPHAGIA

Difficulty initiating swallows defines oropharyngeal or transfer dysphagia, a symptom of a neuromuscular disorder affecting the hypopharynx and upper esophagus. Sometimes a liquid or food bolus may enter the trachea or the nose, producing coughing or choking. The possible causes of oropharyngeal dysphagia include

1. In the central nervous system: a cerebrovascular accident, Parkinson's disease, a brain stem tumor, or amyotrophic lateral sclerosis, and
2. In the skeletal and muscular systems: dermatomyositis or polymyositis.

The initial test to order is a barium swallow with videofluoroscopy, which will characterize the mechanical difficulty.

ESOPHAGEAL DYSPHAGIA

Mechanical Obstruction

Peptic Stricture. Chronic gastroesophageal reflux not infrequently produces narrowing of the distal esophagus to a degree sufficient to cause dysphagia. Progressive stricturing implies active esophagitis from ongoing reflux, whether or not the symptoms of heartburn and regurgitation are prominent. Management of peptic strictures consists of strict adherence to an antireflux regimen, pharmacologic intervention, and esophageal dilatation. An antireflux regimen includes dietary adjustment to avoid foods that decrease esophageal sphincter pressure, such as fatty foods, chocolates, and alcohol. The patient is also advised to avoid cigarettes, wear loose-fitting clothing, eat small meals, and observe the usual postural precautions, which are avoidance of the supine position for 3 hours after eating and elevation of the head of the bed on 4- to 6-inch blocks.

Medications used to treat reflux include antacids, which buffer acid; sucralfate (Carafate), 1 gram orally four times daily, which protects against mucosal damage; histamine$_2$ receptor antagonists such as ranitidine (Zantac), 150 mg orally twice daily, or cimetidine (Tagamet), 400 mg orally twice daily, and omeprazole (Prilosec), 20 mg orally daily, which suppress acid release; and prokinetic agents such as metoclopramide (Reglan), 10 mg orally four times daily, and cisapride (Propulsid), 10 mg orally four times daily, which increase lower esophageal sphincter pressure, enhance gastric emptying, and improve esophageal peristaltic function. Rarely, a surgical antireflux procedure will be required to prevent restricturing.

Nearly all peptic strictures can be successfully dilated to full size and kept there with infrequent or no maintenance dilatations. The technique of dilatation depends on the tightness of the stricture. For strictures of 30-caliber French or larger, rubber mercury-filled dilators with a tapered (Maloney) or blunt (Hurst) tip are suitable. For tighter (less than No. 30 French), long and segmental (over 2 cm), or tortuous

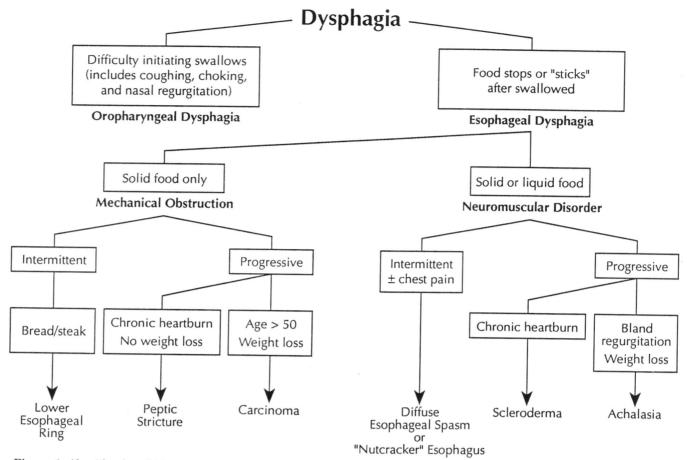

Figure 1. Algorithm by which patient's symptoms can be used to predict the underlying disorder and choose the initial diagnostic test. (Modified from Castell DO, Donner MW: Evaluation of dysphagia: A careful history is crucial. Dysphagia 2:65, 1987.)

strictures, hard plastic dilators (Savary) are often necessary; however, it is reasonable to try the rubber dilators first, since they are less uncomfortable.

All strictures should be dilated under fluoroscopy at first, to ensure safe passage of the dilator into the gastric lumen. It is advisable to dilate strictures to full size (No. 50 French or greater). Dilating sessions are carried out weekly, then every 2 weeks, then every month, and so on. If full size cannot be maintained at a given dilatation interval, the interval must be shortened.

In the special instance of Barrett's epithelium (columnar epithelium replacing squamous epithelium in the esophagus) associated with an esophageal stricture, periodic (every 1 to 3 years) endoscopy with biopsy and cytology, in addition to dilatation, is advisable because of the risk (1 to 10%) of the development of adenocarcinoma within the columnar epithelium.

Neoplasms. When dysphagia occurs as a result of malignant obstruction, the disease is usually advanced with little chance of cure. In general, esophageal cancer is a late diagnosis. When there is evidence of metastatic spread, aggressive surgical intervention should be discouraged and palliation en-

couraged. Computed tomography scanning and endoscopic ultrasound are frequently used to determine the extent of local spread of disease and assess operability.

Treatment of dysphagia associated with malignancy involves peroral dilatation. The safety of dilating malignant strictures is comparable to that of benign ones, providing an important method of palliation. Dilatation is successful in over 90% of cases, enabling the patient to swallow food, fluids, and saliva and preventing the aspiration of secretions. Dilatation can be safely carried out during and after radiation therapy. Patients whose esophageal lumens cannot be kept open by dilatation or who have a fistula from the esophagus to the trachea or a bronchus may be helped by the endoscopic peroral placement of a polyvinyl prosthesis, which remains in place for the rest of the patient's life to maintain a patent lumen and/or seal off a fistula. Transendoscopic laser ablation of obstructing lesions is another method of relieving dysphagia, usually requiring two to six treatments, with retreatment required every 3 months, on average. The combination of a peroral prosthesis and laser treatment successfully treats dysphagia in over 95% of cases.

Rings and Webs. An esophageal ring is a thin layer of mucosa, submucosa, and muscle that should be considered as an unlikely cause of dysphagia; other causes must be ruled out. Once this is done, dilatation is easily performed and is usually effective. Rarely, the symptom will return; if this happens, pneumatic dilatation (see "Achalasia," next) should be done. Webs are thin structures composed of mucosa and submucosa that can occur anywhere in the esophagus but are most common in the cervical portion, where an association with carcinoma necessitates endoscopic inspection and possible biopsy. Treatment is by dilatation, often by using a single large dilator.

Neuromuscular Disorders

Dysphagia for both liquids and solids suggests a neuromuscular disorder.

Achalasia. Characterized in its complete form by a hypertensive lower esophageal sphincter that fails to relax completely with swallowing and absent peristalsis in the esophageal body, achalasia is treated with pharmacotherapy, pneumatic dilatation, and myotomy. Medications that relax the smooth muscle of the lower esophageal sphincter, such as isosorbide dinitrate (Isordil), 5 to 10 mg sublingually before meals, or the calcium channel blockers diltiazem (Cardizem), 30 mg orally three times daily, or nifedipine (Procardia), 10 mg orally three times daily, are initially used to alleviate symptoms; however, dilatation is generally required.

Pneumatic dilatation is the initial method of choice to treat achalasia. This treatment gives results comparable to those of surgical myotomy in approximately 75% of patients and is much simpler. Pneumatic dilatation differs from standard dilatation in that the goal of therapy is to partially disrupt the esophageal circular muscle, which is necessary to produce a lasting effect. Using fluoroscopy, an inflatable bag is endoscopically placed at the level of the gastroesophageal junction, where it is inflated to a designated pressure. Because of the necessity of disrupting muscle fibers, perforation is more common (3 to 5% of cases) than in the dilatation of peptic strictures (1%). However, most of these cases (about 80%) can be treated conservatively.

Failure to respond to two or three dilatations is an indication for surgical myotomy. Other relative contraindications for pneumatic dilatation are a tortuous "sigmoid" esophagus or a patient too young or too apprehensive to cooperate with the procedure.

Diffuse Esophageal Spasm. This uncommon entity, diagnosed by radiography or manometry, can produce dysphagia and chest pain. If searched for, gastroesophageal reflux frequently is present; if it is, an antireflux regimen is appropriate as first-line treatment. Other approaches are isosorbide dinitrate, helpful in one-third to one-half of cases, calcium channel blockers (see earlier), and dicyclomine (Bentyl), 20 mg orally three times daily. If medications fail, periodic passage of a large dilator may

help. Many of these patients need no treatment beyond knowledge of the correct diagnosis; the reassurance of knowing that their chest pain is not angina pectoris makes the symptoms tolerable.

Scleroderma. The smooth muscle region of the esophagus is frequently affected in this connective tissue disorder, with resultant disordered motility and lower esophageal sphincter incompetence. There is often significant gastroesophageal reflux because of inefficient esophageal clearance. Dysphagia occurs as a result of the motility disorder and/or peptic strictures from reflux disease. Management is directed at treating the gastroesophageal reflux because of the potential complications. Antireflux precautions and medications are utilized. Antireflux surgery is generally not recommended because of the potential for worsening the dysphagia.

DIVERTICULA OF THE ALIMENTARY TRACT

method of
HARRIS R. CLEARFIELD, M.D.
Hahnemann University—Medical College of
Pennsylvania
Philadelphia, Pennsylvania

Diverticula are often asymptomatic but may produce symptoms if they distend with food or liquid and compress the lumen (Zenker's and epiphrenic diverticula), harbor sufficient organisms to produce a bacterial overgrowth syndrome (jejunal diverticula), or become inflamed or bleed (Meckel's and colonic diverticula).

ESOPHAGEAL DIVERTICULA

Hypopharyngeal Diverticula

The hypopharyngeal diverticulum (Zenker's diverticulum) is found in approximately 2% of patients presenting with dysphagia, and the majority of cases occur in patients beyond the seventh decade of life. The diverticulum generally protrudes between the cricopharyngeus muscle (superior esophageal sphincter) and the inferior constrictor muscle. Small diverticula are asymptomatic, but progressive enlargement can occur as a result of food-induced stretching. The opening to the diverticulum may become larger than the lumen of the esophagus, so that food and liquid preferentially enter the diverticulum and subsequently spill over into the lumen, and the progressively enlarging diverticulum may exert sufficient pressure on the esophagus to produce dysphagia. Inadequate or uncoordinated relaxation of the superior sphincter is thought to result in sufficient pharyngeal pressure to force mucosa between the muscle bundles to form the diverticulum. Symptoms include cervical dysphagia, coughing while eating, bad breath from the fermenting food, a swelling in the neck caused by the enlarging diverticulum, and nocturnal wheezing resulting from aspiration. Medications may also accumulate in the diverticulum causing erratic absorption. These symptoms may be suggestive, but barium upper gastrointestinal tract x-ray films usually establish the diagnosis. If Zenker's diverticulum is suspected, upper endoscopy, if necessary, should be accomplished by inserting the instrument under direct vision to reduce the likelihood of perforation.

Treatment

No treatment is needed for asymptomatic diverticula, but those producing symptoms often require surgery. A myotomy of the superior esophageal sphincter is advocated for small diverticula; larger lesions are generally resected.

Midesophageal Diverticula

Midesophageal diverticula were once thought to represent a fibrotic "pull" or "traction" from an adjacent mediastinal inflammatory reaction, but this theory has been largely replaced by the observation that many diverticula are associated with motility abnormalities, such as achalasia or esophageal spasm. The diverticula are usually small and wide-mouthed, so that food trapping rarely occurs and symptoms are unusual. If chest pain is associated with these diverticula, esophageal motility studies should be performed. No treatment is usually required for the diverticula.

Epiphrenic Diverticula

Epiphrenic diverticula occur in the distal esophagus and are thought to result from high pressure generated by a motility disorder of the lower esophageal sphincter or distal esophagus, such as achalasia or esophageal spasm. Most diverticula are symptomatic, but an occasional diverticulum may progressively distend and begin to trap food and secretions, leading to dysphagia, substernal discomfort, or vomiting (often nocturnal). The diagnosis is usually established by barium upper gastrointestinal studies but upper endoscopy will also reveal the lesion.

Treatment

No treatment is required for small asymptomatic outpouchings, but detailed motility studies should be performed for larger diverticula. Symptomatic diverticula associated with esophageal spasm or achalasia have been treated pharmacologically with calcium channel blockers but medical therapy is usually ineffective. If surgery is required, diverticulectomy is often combined with a lower esophageal myotomy that extends to the cardia of the stomach (Heller's procedure). Some surgeons advocate the addition of an antireflux procedure to prevent the complications associated with a relaxed lower esophageal sphincter.

SMALL INTESTINAL DIVERTICULA

Duodenal Diverticula

Duodenal diverticula are noted in approximately 5% of patients studied with barium upper gastrointestinal x-rays. These diverticula are exceeded in frequency only by colonic diverticula. They usually occur within the "C loop," often adjacent to the ampulla of Vater, and are rarely found on the lateral wall of the duodenum. The diverticula increase in frequency with advancing age. They are usually composed of mucosa without muscle fibers, which suggests that they are the result of duodenal pressure, but congenital diverticula may also occur. There appears to be no increased incidence of colonic diverticula in patients with duodenal lesions, thus negating the concept of a general gastrointestinal predisposition to diverticular formation.

Duodenal diverticula are described more frequently by barium x-ray films than by endoscopy because the narrow or slitlike ostia may be missed during the endoscopic examination. Because the upper gastrointestinal x-rays are usually obtained as a result of upper abdominal symptoms, it is tempting to ascribe such symptoms to the presence of the diverticula. However, it is difficult to establish a correlation between these occasionally encountered diverticula and a variety of dyspeptic or aerophagic complaints. There does appear to be an increased frequency of bacterial isolates from the bile of patients with juxtapapillary duodenal diverticula, raising the possibility that the diverticula may affect the flow in the bile duct by extrinsic pressure. Extrinsic pressure could also lead to the increased incidence of common duct stones in these patients. Dysfunction of the spincter of Oddi has been ascribed to the presence of adjacent diverticula and could lead to reflux of duodenal content and bacteria into the biliary tree. The presence of juxta-ampullary diverticula may complicate diagnostic and therapeutic endoscopic retrograde cholangiopancreatography (ERCP) procedures.

Treatment

Duodenal diverticula rarely produce symptoms and therefore usually require no therapy. Upper gastrointestinal tract bleeding, brisk rather than occult, may arise from these lesions but efforts should be made to define some other, more likely cause. A causal relationship between diverticula and bleeding should be established only with convincing endoscopic or angiographic findings. The management of the bleeding is similar to that of other causes of upper gastrointestinal tract hemorrhage but emergency excision of the diverticulum could be required if supportive measures are unsuccessful. Diverticular perforation and abscess are even more uncommon and would prompt computed tomography (CT) scan, ultrasonography, or surgical exploration to establish the diagnosis. Diverticulectomy would be required for such patients.

Jejunal and Ileal Diverticula

Jejunal and ileal diverticula are uncommon and are thought to be primarily of the acquired type. They tend to occur on the mesenteric border of the small bowel, where blood vessels penetrate from the serosal surface, thus creating a potential weakness in the musculature. Multiple large diverticula, usually jejunal, may permit sufficient bacterial overgrowth to result in a malabsorption syndrome. This complication may be associated with a more generalized bowel motility disorder, such as scleroderma. The symptoms are those of other malabsorption syndromes and include megaloblastic anemia secondary to vitamin B_{12} or folate deficiency, steatorrhea, diarrhea, weight loss, and fat-soluble vitamin deficiency. Jejunal diverticula have also been associated with intestinal pseudo-obstruction, although the retrospective nature of the published reports does not permit an estimate of the frequency of this relationship. The diverticula appear to be a manifestation of the pseudo-obstruction rather than the cause. The generalized nature of the small bowel motility disorder in these patients is illustrated by such associated findings as esophageal dysmotility, the CREST syndrome (calcinosis cutis, Raynaud's phenomenon, esophageal dysfunction, sclerodactyly, and telangiectasia), and degenerated smooth muscle cells consistent with a visceral myopathy. True mechanical obstruction has also been reported as a result of diverticulitis (sometimes with perforation), volvulus, or adhesions.

Treatment

The bacterial overgrowth of small bowel diverticulosis often responds to antibiotic therapy. Tetracycline, 250 mg four times daily, or other broad-spectrum antibiotics for 7 to 10 days may be effective. Unfortunately, relapse is common and some patients benefit from 1 week of antibiotic therapy each month. A promotility agent, such as cisapride (Propulsid), 10 to 20 mg three times daily may be helpful. Vitamin B_{12}, folic acid, and fat-soluble vitamins should be provided, and dietary fat and milk products should be reduced. Resection of the small bowel containing the diverticula has been suggested for patients with chronic symptoms, but this may prove to be ineffective if the diverticula are the result of a generalized neuropathic or myopathic process. Surgery should be reserved for acute complications, such as bleeding, diverticulitis, or volvulus. It is therefore important to consider an associated motility disturbance in patients with symptomatic small bowel diverticula.

Meckel's Diverticulum

Meckel's diverticulum, which is present in 1 to 3% of the population, represents the failure of the intestinal end of the primitive yolk duct (vitelline duct) to close completely. The diverticula usually occur on the antimesenteric surface of the ileum, approximately 60 to 80 cm from the ileocecal valve, but they may occur as far as 200 cm proximal to the valve. The diverticulum is usually several centimeters in size, but diverticula measuring up to 10 cm have been described. The majority of the diverticula are asymptomatic.

The major complications of bleeding, inflammation, and obstruction are seen most commonly in infants and young children, with a male predominance. Bleeding generally results from the presence of ectopic gastric mucosa within the sac, a finding in approximately 60 to 70% of symptomatic patients. The acid production leads to ulceration and bleeding from within or adjacent to the diverticulum. The bleeding is more frequently maroon or red than tarry and is more likely to be brisk than occult. Obstruction, with or without a fibrous attachment to the umbilicus, can result from volvulus or intussusception and may be of the closed-loop type. Inflammation of the diverticulum (diverticulitis) is less common than appendicitis because of the diverticular wide neck that permits the fecal stream to exit easily. The motility of the ileum decreases the likelihood that the inflammation will be sealed off, increasing the possibility of perforation should diverticulitis occur. The presence of painless, massive lower gastrointestinal tract bleeding in an infant or child should suggest the possibility of Meckel's diverticulum. Bowel obstruction or peritonitis in this age group should also raise this suspicion. Although less common, the preceding complications can also occur in adults.

The diagnosis of Meckel's diverticulum is rarely made by barium small bowel examination, although this study (or small bowel enema) may be useful in selected patients to exclude other disorders. The ^{99m}Tc pertechnetate isotope is taken up by Meckel's diverticula containing gastric mucosa and may be helpful for establishing the diagnosis, but a negative examination does not exclude the possibility. Mesenteric angiography may be useful during active bleeding; intestinal obstruction is diagnosed on the basis of clinical and radiographic criteria; and peritonitis in an infant or child should suggest appendicitis or diverticulitis.

Treatment

The treatment of bleeding from Meckel's diverticula requires blood replacement, localization of the bleeding point if possible by isotope scan or angiography, and diverticulectomy if the lesion can be identified. Occasionally patients, both young and old, may bleed intermittently, posing diagnostic problems if the preceding localizing efforts prove to be fruitless. Bowel obstruction requires immediate surgery, and inflammation or a diverticulum usually requires exploration. An incidental Meckel diverticulum discovered during abdominal surgery for some other disorder should be removed if there is no contraindication.

DIVERTICULAR DISEASE OF THE COLON

Diverticula occur in two rows on either side of the colon, with a distinct clustering in the sigmoid colon.

Although diverticula may also be observed in the proximal colon, it is most unusual for patients to have right-sided or transverse colon diverticula in the absence of sigmoid involvement. The frequency of diverticula formation is almost directly related to age, so that the condition is uncommon before age 40 years and is found in approximately 50% of individuals in their ninth decade of life.

The diminished frequency of diverticula among individuals from Africa, Asia, and certain areas of South America has been attributed to a high-fiber diet, which tends to decrease transit time in the gut, to increase stool frequency, and to result in softer, larger stools. This is an attractive hypothesis, but recent studies indicate difficulty in distinguishing normal persons from those with diverticulosis on the basis of stool weight and frequency. Another theory regarding the cause of colonic diverticula relates to the high sigmoid pressure observed in patients with the irritable bowel syndrome. This is the basis of the supposition that increased intraluminal pressure forces the mucosa to protrude through the relatively weak areas of the colonic musculature adjacent to the blood vessels that penetrate from the serosal surface. This explanation seems reasonable, but diverticula have been found in patients with no history of irritable bowel symptoms. A convincing and unifying explanation for the development of colonic diverticula is not yet available.

Diverticulosis

Uncomplicated diverticula do not produce symptoms, but in patients with the irritable bowel syndrome, colonic diverticula may be revealed by barium enema examination or colonoscopy. Treatment, therefore, is not directed to the diverticula but focuses on the predominant symptoms, such as pain, diarrhea, or constipation. Consider therapy with a high-fiber diet, psyllium preparations (Metamucil, Konsyl) or methyl cellulose (Citrucel) for constipation, antispasmodic medications such as dicyclomine (Bentyl) for crampy pain, or antidiarrheal agents such as loperamide (Imodium) or diphenoxylate (Lomotil). Patients with diverticula and the irritable bowel syndrome should not be informed that they have diverticular disease or diverticulitis because these labels may induce added anxiety and create confusion for physicians who may subsequently evaluate the patients.

Diverticular Bleeding

Diverticula are one of the major causes of massive colonic hemorrhage. The bleeding is usually painless and rarely accompanies clinical diverticulitis. It is thought to result from the presence of an inspissated diverticular fecalith that erodes or ulcerates into an adjacent penetrating artery. The close relationship of the diverticula to these arteries explains why bleeding may be more severe than that encountered from an arteriovenous malformation (AVM). Although it has been stated that right-sided diverticula are more prone to bleed than sigmoid diverticula, colonoscopic examinations suggest that the AVM is a more common cause of bleeding from the right colon. The bleeding site (but not the cause) may be established by a technetium isotope bleeding study (usually an initial study) or by angiography, but these studies must obviously be performed during the bleeding episode if localization is to be made with confidence. Cleansing of the colon with a lavage solution (Go-LYTELY, Colyte) can be accomplished in selected patients during the bleeding episode if hemodynamic stability can be achieved, permitting a colonoscopic examination that can often determine the site of bleeding and the cause (diverticula, AVM, or neoplasm).

Treatment

It is more important to determine which segment of the colon is the site of brisk bleeding (sigmoid, left, transverse, or right colon) than to identify the specific diverticulum or other cause at fault. Hemodynamic stability should be achieved before time-consuming diagnostic studies are initiated. The most common cause for death resulting from gastrointestinal hemorrhage is inadequate transfusions. An isotope bleeding study may demonstrate the area of colonic bleeding but will be helpful only if the patient is bleeding actively during the study. Angiography permits the most precise localization of bleeding points but many patients bleed intermittently, which may negate the value of the study.

If a bleeding diverticulum is identified, vasopressin infusion may cause sufficient local vasoconstriction to permit cessation of bleeding. Colonoscopy during a colonic hemorrhage can be achieved if the patient is stable and capable of tolerating the cleansing preparation. The examination may show evidence of vascular lesions, "oozing," from a presumably culpable diverticulum, or neoplasms (benign polyps rarely bleed massively). If major bleeding continues and the diagnostic strategies outlined earlier are unrewarding, a subtotal colectomy with ileorectal anastomosis should be considered. A "blind" left-sided colectomy in patients with known diverticular disease may be disastrous if the bleeding originates from the right colon. If diverticular bleeding stops with conservative measures, elective surgery need not be immediately considered because there is a reasonable possibility that bleeding will not recur. Recurrent bleeding should be approached surgically if the site is identified.

DIVERTICULITIS

Diverticulitis results from a microperforation of a single diverticulum, usually into pericolic tissues. The inflammatory reaction is generally walled off by surrounding omentum or adjacent bowel loops but may progress to an abscess or phlegmon (marked cellulitis without pus). If the inflammatory process is not sealed, a free perforation may rarely occur. Diverticulitis usually involves the sigmoid colon, but instances of right-sided diverticulitis have been encountered.

The patient usually complains of left lower quadrant or suprapubic pain, which may be accompanied by back pain, nausea, vomiting, dysuria, or fever. Gross rectal bleeding is unusual. Physical examination generally reveals tenderness over the left lower area or the suprapubic area, or both. Muscle guarding or rebound tenderness may be elicited.

An elevated white blood cell count has little localizing value but can be useful in distinguishing between the irritable colon (normal count) and diverticulitis (leukocytosis is common). A urinalysis may reflect the presence of cystitis secondary to an adjacent inflammatory reaction or a true colovesical fistula (ask the patient about the passage of gas during urination). An obstruction series may provide little information, but a sigmoid obstruction secondary to edema and inflammation may occur, or a partial small bowel obstruction may result from a segment of distal jejunum or proximal ileum that becomes surrounded by the pericolonic inflammatory reaction. If the clinical picture of left lower abdominal pain and tenderness, fever, and leukocytosis is convincing, additional imaging studies may not be urgently required. Ultrasound may demonstrate an abscess but overlying bowel gas frequently negates the value of the procedure. If necessary, a CT scan is more likely to show an abscess or a pericolonic inflammatory reaction, but the study may be normal if the process is in the early stages. Blood cultures should be obtained in febrile patients.

Sigmoidoscopy and colonoscopy should be avoided during the acute process so that free perforation secondary to air insufflation can be avoided. Contrast x-ray films of the colon are ordinarily deferred for the same reason, but early imaging may be required if the clinical picture is atypical, perhaps raising the possibility of ischemia, acute colitis, or perforated neoplasm. In such circumstances, diatrizoate (Gastrografin) administration given without air insufflation is usually sufficient to outline the pathology. A barium enema should be obtained after 7 to 10 days of therapy. This may show a fistula, partial obstruction, or evidence of an extrinsic mass effect. Colonoscopy is less useful for the diagnosis of recent diverticulitis but can be helpful in the differential diagnosis.

The differential diagnosis may include the irritable bowel syndrome, but the presence of fever, leukocytosis, and/or peritoneal signs should suggest an inflammatory reaction. Ovarian pathology, appendicitis (the appendix may extend down into the pelvis), inflammatory bowel disease, and ischemic colitis should be considered. A confined perforation of a colonic carcinoma is more difficult to exclude during the acute process. Even the surgeon may have problems making the diagnosis during emergency exploration because the surrounding inflammatory reaction may be intense.

Complications include fistulas to the bladder (less common in women since the uterus "protects" the bladder), small bowel, or vagina. Free perforation, which is rare but significantly increases the morbidity and mortality rate, abdominal abscess, partial or complete obstruction of the small or large bowel, and septicemia may occur. Another serious complication of diverticulitis is spread of the bacteria through the portal vein to the liver, leading to pylephlebitis (pus in the portal vein) and suppurative liver abscess.

Treatment

Mild cases of diverticulitis with low-grade fever, tenderness without peritonitis, and modest leukocytosis may be treated on an ambulatory basis with clear liquids and oral antibiotics such as amoxicillin-clavulanate (Augmentin). More severe cases require hospitalization. The bowel should be kept at rest and intravenous fluids given. Nasogastric suction should be used if peritonitis or obstruction is present. Parenteral broad-spectrum coverage against both aerobic and anaerobic bacteria should be provided. Although combinations of aminoglycosides (gentamicin) and antianaerobic agents (clindamycin [Cleocin], metronidazole [Flagyl]) have been popular, the trend is toward using single agents such as cefotetan that provide both aerobic and anaerobic coverage.

If the patient fails to improve, as judged by the white blood cell count, fever status, and abdominal findings, surgical intervention may be required. A one-stage procedure with resection of the inflamed bowel and reanastomosis is more often performed now, but a staged procedure with a diverting colostomy is preferable if significant peritonitis or infection is present in the area of the planned anastomosis or if the anastomosis cannot be accomplished without tension. Preoperative percutaneous aspiration of a diverticular abscess may sufficiently reduce the surrounding inflammatory process to permit a one-stage resection and reanastomosis rather than require a staged procedure.

If the patient responds to medical therapy, diet is gradually advanced, but the patient is instructed to avoid small, hard particles such as seeds, nuts, corn, and fish bones to prevent their entrapment in diverticula. It is also prudent to avoid constipation by increasing the fiber content of the diet, using either bran cereals, psyllium products such as Metamucil, or Konsyl or methyl cellulose (Citrucel). Elective resection of the sigmoid colon after the diverticulitis has resolved with medical therapy was once advocated but current experience indicates that approximately 50% of patients have no further symptoms. A recurrence of diverticulitis, however, should suggest consideration of surgery in view of the potential complications. Elective resection should be considered after a first attack in patients younger than 50 years of age (their recurrence rates are higher) and in those patients who have experienced a particularly severe first attack.

ULCERATIVE COLITIS*

method of
DOUGLAS S. LEVINE, M.D.
University of Washington
Seattle, Washington

ETIOLOGY

Ulcerative colitis and Crohn's disease are the most common forms of idiopathic inflammatory diseases affecting the human alimentary tract. These two diseases share many clinical, pathologic, and epidemiologic features, but there are usually sufficient differences to allow their separation as distinct clinical entities. However, in some patients with idiopathic colitis, differentiation between these two categories is not possible. The causes of these idiopathic inflammatory bowel diseases are unknown.

Ongoing research suggests that several sequential and/or interactive pathogenetic mechanisms are responsible and involve genetically based regulatory disturbances of the intestinal mucosal or systemic immune response, including (1) stimulation by luminal antigens, (2) dysfunction of the mucosal barrier, (3) disordered regulation of mucosal and systemic immune systems, (4) generation of proinflammatory mediators within intestinal mucosa, and (5) other local intestinal physiologic and anatomic factors. These hypothesized mechanisms of idiopathic inflammatory bowel diseases form the basis for several empirical therapies for affected patients (Figure 1).

What we diagnose as "ulcerative colitis" may in fact be several different diseases that ultimately may become defined molecularly with both genetic and subclinical markers. Ongoing immunogenetic and clinical investigations of ulcerative colitis may confirm observations suggesting that patients conform to a wide variety of subsets with different clinical presentations, pathologic manifestations, medical or surgical treatment responses, and tendencies toward disease recurrence.

DIAGNOSIS

Ulcerative colitis is generally limited to the superficial portion, or mucosa, of the large intestine. This disease may vary in both the inflammatory intensity and the total surface area of involvement of the large intestine. In its most limited form, only a small portion of the rectum may be involved, and in its most severe form, a large portion or the entirety of the colon is affected. Therefore, the spectrum of clinical symptoms and diagnostic abnormalities, which reflect these differing pathologic manifestations, is diverse. In some patients, inflammation may be so minimal it may only be detectable by endoscopic visualization and biopsy. In other patients severe ulceration and hemorrhage are obvious, and in others inflammation may involve the entire large bowel wall thickness, leading to the formation of strictures or progression to perforation with the potential for septicemia.

The symptoms of ulcerative colitis result from disturbances of normal colorectal function and the typical intestinal mucosal erosions involving the rectum and a variable extent of the large intestine proximal to the rectum. The most common symptoms include tenesmus, hematochezia, crampy abdominal pain, and diarrhea. In health, the distal colonic property of receptive relaxation permits subconscious accumulation of feces until sufficient mass is present to produce conscious awareness, leading to voluntary defecation or a decision to postpone this activity. Distal colonic inflammation, which is typical of ulcerative colitis, disrupts storage function and produces tenesmus, or urgency to defecate, as well as fecal incontinence on occasion. The fluid and electrolyte reabsorption function of the more proximal colon is perturbed by more extensive colonic inflammation, leading to diarrhea.

Symptoms of ulcerative colitis are mild or moderate in the majority of patients, with some increase in the number of bowel movements per day, clinically insignificant intestinal blood loss, and tolerable levels of crampy abdominal pain. For others, symptoms are severe with disabling diarrhea, anemia due to intestinal blood loss, abdominal pain, fevers, and/or significant extraintestinal manifestations. Fulminant disease occurs in the minority of patients who must be hospitalized for a variety of complications, including severe intestinal hemorrhage, vomiting, abdominal pain, fevers, malnutrition, dehydration, electrolyte imbalances, and infection. A subset of this group may develop toxic colitis, sometimes accompanied by gross colonic dilatation (megacolon) or intestinal perforation, and require emergent surgical intervention to prevent peritonitis and sepsis.

Ulcerative colitis generally is most easily and safely diagnosed using rigid or flexible sigmoidoscopy with superficial mucosal biopsies to differentiate this disease from other forms of. colitis. Other diagnostic tests that provide imaging of the entire large intestine, such as air contrast barium enema examination or colonoscopy, are potentially hazardous and more uncomfortable for patients with active disease. However, such examinations may become necessary in some patients to allow differentiation between ulcerative colitis and Crohn's disease, or to assess the proximal extent of large intestinal involvement and the intensity of mucosal inflammation as part of therapeutic planning and monitoring. These examinations also identify complications of colitis such as strictures, pseudopolyposis, or adenocarcinoma. Diffuse, contiguous colonic mucosal involvement is characteristic of ulcerative colitis. Patients with active disease have loss of normal mucosal vascular detail, mucosal friability, erosions, and/or ulcers, and the presence of an inflammatory exudate composed of pus, mucus, and blood.

The loss of mucosal integrity, as demonstrated endoscopically and histologically, is perhaps the most obvious feature of the inflamed intestinal mucosa in patients with idiopathic inflammatory bowel diseases. The differentiation between Crohn's disease and ulcerative colitis is difficult if Crohn's disease involvement is limited to the large intestine. However, radiologic and endoscopic observations and certain histologic features of mucosal biopsies may help differentiate these two disorders. Barium enema examination and total colonoscopy establish the presence of a diffuse, contiguous mucosal inflammatory process consistent with ulcerative colitis. Histologic evaluation of colonic mucosal biopsies from patients with ulcerative colitis reveals diffuse inflammatory involvement with increased mucosal neutrophils, plasma cells, lymphocytes, and eosinophils. Crypt architecture is distorted, the epithelial surface loses its integrity and develops erosions, and crypt abscesses appear.

NATURAL HISTORY AND PROGNOSIS

The clinical courses among patients with ulcerative colitis are highly variable and usually relate in part to the

*Supported in part by Food and Drug Administration Office of Orphan Products Development grant FD-R-000827.

Idiopathic Inflammatory Bowel Disease

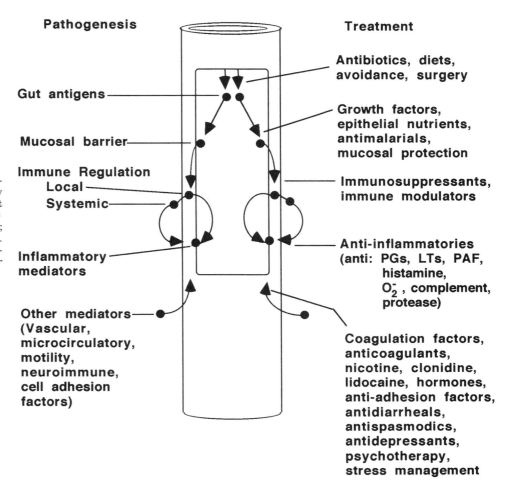

Pathogenesis

Gut antigens

Mucosal barrier

Immune Regulation
Local
Systemic

Inflammatory
mediators

Other mediators
(Vascular,
microcirculatory,
motility,
neuroimmune,
cell adhesion
factors)

Treatment

Antibiotics, diets,
avoidance, surgery

Growth factors,
epithelial nutrients,
antimalarials,
mucosal protection

Immunosuppressants,
immune modulators

Anti-inflammatories
(anti: PGs, LTs, PAF,
histamine,
O_2^-, complement,
protease)

Coagulation factors,
anticoagulants,
nicotine, clonidine,
lidocaine, hormones,
anti-adhesion factors,
antidiarrheals,
antispasmodics,
antidepressants,
psychotherapy,
stress management

Figure 1. Hypothetical mechanisms of idiopathic inflammatory bowel diseases paired with treatment strategies. *Abbreviations:* PGs = prostaglandins; LTs = leukotrienes; PAF = platelet activating factor. (From Levine DS: Medical and surgical options for ulcerative colitis. *Curr Opin Gastroenterol 11*:29–35, 1995.)

proximal extent of colonic involvement and the intensity of inflammation. Most patients have disease limited to the left colon and give a history of periodic exacerbations of disease interspersed with complete remissions or near-normal health during time intervals that vary from months to several years. In other patients, their disease is chronic and unremitting with severe tenesmus, bloody diarrhea, anemia, abdominal discomfort, and generalized or constitutional symptoms. If medical therapy fails to significantly reduce or eliminate these symptoms, colectomy will be required. Rarely, patients present with severe, acute pancolitis that may require prompt surgical intervention. Some patients develop large intestinal epithelial dysplasia and adenocarcinoma independent of the inflammatory intensity and their disease course.

The prognosis for individual patients with ulcerative colitis is most easily assessed after the patterns of disease exacerbations and responsiveness to medical treatment have been observed for at least 2 years after the onset of symptoms and diagnosis. These patterns of disease activity and treatment response tend to be consistent for the majority of patients. However, the development of more proximal colonic inflammation of significant intensity in patients with mild or moderate distal disease is generally a poor prognostic sign, signaling the need for more aggressive medical therapy or surgical intervention.

MEDICAL TREATMENT

A variety of empirical therapies have been used for treating patients with ulcerative colitis (see Figure 1), but the most well established interventions include anti-inflammatory drugs, immune-modulating agents, and surgical resection. The choices of therapies in individual patients vary depending on disease severity (e.g., symptoms reflecting distal versus more proximal colonic disease involvement, and differing intensity of inflammation), patient status (e.g., ambulatory versus hospitalized for ulcerative colitis), and disease activity (e.g., treatment of active disease versus therapy for maintenance of remission). Initial patient management should include counseling about the natural history of the disease, explanations of the anatomic and physiologic basis of symptoms, and discussion of the spectrum of available therapies, including their potential benefits and side effects.

Usually, the safest, least toxic drugs are used to initiate medical treatment for ulcerative colitis. It is not unusual for patients to require concurrent therapy with multiple drugs of different classes administered by different routes (oral, rectal, or parenteral) to achieve remission of disease activity. Most patients can be prescribed simpler, single-drug treatment to maintain remission, and others may enjoy long periods of disease remission without medications.

Anti-Inflammatory Drugs

Aminosalicylates function as topical anti-inflammatory agents and are used in oral formulations for the treatment of acute ulcerative colitis and the maintenance of disease remission. These drugs may be used successfully in patients with differing proximal limits of colitis, but their onset of action is not as prompt as that of corticosteroids. Sulfasalazine (Azulfidine) is the oldest product and is a prodrug consisting of sulfapyridine chemically linked to mesalamine (5-aminosalicylic acid). The majority of orally administered sulfasalazine survives transit to the colon, where bacteria hydrolyze the prodrug to release pharmacologically active mesalamine. Doses range from 1 to 4 grams per day administered in divided doses twice daily, and supplemental folic acid is recommended. Side effects are common and probably dose-related; they include nausea, headache, rash, dyspepsia, fever, arthralgias, and folate deficiency. Less common adverse effects that require discontinuation of the drug include hepatitis, pancreatitis, pericarditis, pneumonitis, bone marrow suppression, lupus-like syndrome, male infertility, and exacerbation of colitis.

The side effects of sulfasalazine, which are most often attributable to the sulfapyridine moiety, limit dosing or preclude its use in many patients. Fortunately, several other aminosalicylate products that omit sulfapyridine are available for use, including olsalazine (Dipentum), a chemically linked pair of mesalamine molecules, and controlled-release formulations of mesalamine (Asacol, Pentasa), designed to release pharmacologically active drug at different small intestinal sites for flux into the colon. These drugs may be administered in doses as high as almost 5 grams per day for the treatment of acute disease. Unfortunately, these products, particularly olsalazine, may produce diarrhea. In addition, some patients may develop side effects similar to those found with the use of sulfasalazine. Moreover, high-dose treatment with the controlled-release products may be associated with nephrotoxicity because of systemic absorption. Balsalazide (Colazide),* which is undergoing clinical testing in the United States, is a prodrug consisting of an inert carrier molecule linked to mesalamine and has more colon-specific drug delivery than the controlled-release formulations of mesalamine. Para-aminosalicylic acid (PASA), or 4-aminosalicylic acid, an antitubercular drug, is sometimes used but has not been extensively tested as a therapy for ulcerative colitis.

Rectal formulations of mesalamine (Rowasa) are available as 500-mg suppositories (for twice-daily ad-

ministration) and 4-gram retention enemas and are usually used for the treatment of acute proctitis, proctosigmoiditis, or disease confined to the left colon, and in alternate-day or every-third-day schedules for the maintenance of disease remission. PAS enema formulations have also been shown to be effective for distal colitis. These products may be used in conjunction with other oral therapies for the treatment of more extensive colitis. Enemas are difficult to retain unless the patient remains recumbent and are thus usually recommended for use once daily, usually at bedtime. Patients benefit from instructions to change body position after their administration to enhance more proximal flow of the fluid vehicle and to reduce rectal urgency.

Corticosteroids are used in retention enema formulations for the treatment of acute disease in a manner analogous to that of mesalamine products. Although such steroids have topical anti-inflammatory activity, the products that are currently available by prescription in the United States are absorbed systemically, potentially producing adverse side effects. Therefore, these should not be used chronically for the maintenance of disease remission. Hydrocortisone formulated in a 100-mg liquid retention enema (Cortenema) or as an 80-mg foam preparation (Cortifoam) are recommended for use once daily at bedtime for no more than a few weeks, but if more prolonged therapy is necessary patients should discontinue use gradually by alternate-night use. A variety of other corticosteroids, such as prednisolone in a 20- to 40-mg dose, may be formulated for once-nightly enema administration.

More potent, topically active corticosteroids with less potential for systemic toxicity should become available by general prescription in the near future as preferred retention enema products for ulcerative colitis. Budesonide (Entocort) retention enema has been shown to be at least as effective as standard corticosteroid enema formulations but lacking in systemic steroid side effects in European and North American clinical trials. As of mid-1995, budesonide is not yet commercially available in the United States. Other steroids with similar properties, such as beclomethasone dipropionate, fluticasone, and other conjugated steroids have been investigated less extensively and are not commercially available in the United States.

Oral prednisone is indicated as acute treatment in patients with more severe forms of ulcerative colitis, or in patients with more moderate disease symptoms that do not abate with oral aminosalicylate, rectal mesalamine, and rectal steroid therapy. Interestingly, oral prednisone is often ineffective in patients with distal proctitis that is unresponsive to rectally administered anti-inflammatory agents. When prednisone is used for relatively severe left-sided colitis or more proximal disease, initial dosing of approximately 1 mg per kg (40 to 80 mg) per day is recommended for 3 to 5 days. Many patients enjoy a very prompt recovery during this short treatment period

---

*Investigational drug in the United States.

and remain stable as the prednisone is rapidly tapered and discontinued, such as by decreasing the daily dose by 5 to 10 mg on consecutive days. If there is a lack of response to such short-term, high-dose prednisone therapy, or if symptoms rapidly recur during the tapering course, more prolonged treatment, a slower tapering regimen, or alternate-day dosing regimens may be necessary. The chronic use of oral prednisone, even at low doses, is not recommended for the maintenance of disease remission because of the potential for side effects.

The risk of adverse side effects associated with prednisone use is generally associated with both the duration of drug use and the dose. However, there is considerable interindividual variation in susceptibility to these adverse effects. Short-term, high-dose prednisone therapy may produce intolerable side effects, including psychological disorders such as anxiety, mania, mood swings, depression, and suicidal ideation, a variety of sleep disturbances, and cosmetic changes resulting from hyperphagia with weight gain, fluid retention, acne, capillary fragility, and hirsuitism. Other serious side effects may result from longer-term use of prednisone, including profound suppression of the hypothalamic-pituitary-adrenal axis; immunosuppression, electrolyte imbalances; hypertension; glucose intolerance and diabetes; osteoporosis with pathologic fractures and aseptic necrosis; cataracts; glaucoma; and myopathy.

One of the most dangerous adverse effects of oral prednisone use is adrenal insufficiency resulting from premature discontinuation of steroid therapy. This complication can be life-threatening because of hypotension and electrolyte disturbances. Therefore, patients who are on high doses of prednisone for more than 2 weeks should be informed of the importance of complying with a dose-tapering regimen. If patients are on high doses of prednisone for several months, they should be informed that relative adrenal insufficiency may persist for as long as 1 year after therapy is discontinued and that they may require treatment with steroid supplements during that time period for severe illnesses, trauma, or surgical procedures.

High-dose intravenous methylprednisolone or corticotropin therapy is used for up to approximately 2 weeks for patients hospitalized for severe ulcerative colitis or toxic colitis. Patients who respond may be switched to oral prednisone and other anti-inflammatory agents. Patients who fail to improve significantly with parenteral steroid treatment become candidates for surgical therapy or acute immunosuppressive treatment.

Immune-Modulating Agents

Antimetabolites, such as azathioprine (Imuran)* and 6-mercaptopurine (Purinethol),* are effective in inducing or maintaining remission of ulcerative colitis and limiting or eliminating concomitant systemic corticosteroid use. The onset of action of these drugs may be very slow in some patients, taking up to 6 months, and thus they cannot be used as reliable acute monotherapy. Doses should be lowered if patients are using allopurinol coincidentally. The initiation of therapy and dosage increments require blood parameter monitoring because bone marrow suppression can result in a dose-related manner. Other side effects of these agents include pancreatitis; hepatitis; infectious complications due to immunosuppression; drug fever; and arthralgias. The risk of neoplastic complications resulting from iatrogenic immunosuppression with these drugs remains theoretical based on the most recent investigations. Only a limited number of investigations suggest that these immune-suppressive agents may be safe for use during pregnancy.

Other immune-modulating agents are under active investigation. Parenteral administration of the *cyclic polypeptide* cyclosporine (Sandimmune)* can produce improvement during several days in severely ill patients hospitalized with ulcerative colitis. Parenteral and oral treatment with the *folic acid antagonist* methotrexate* can produce clinical improvement during several weeks in ambulatory patients. Cyclosporine and methotrexate may produce nephrotoxicity and hepatotoxicity, respectively, as well as predispose patients to infection. The roles of these drugs in the long-term management of ulcerative colitis remain to be defined.

Other Medical Therapies

Several other medical treatment approaches have been investigated in a limited number of studies and should be considered only for individual patients with caution because of the comparative lack of more general experience with them (see Figure 1). The following therapies are attracting the attention of clinicians who care for patients who fail to respond to standard treatment. The rectal administration of short-chain fatty acids, such as acetate, propionate, and butyrate, may ameliorate distal colitis by the provision of essential nutrients for colonocytes. The rectal administration of the local anesthetic lidocaine is reported to improve distal colitis in open-label trials. Recent reports of the effectiveness of nicotine patches and subcutaneous administration of heparin require further study. Broad-spectrum antibiotics are anecdotally reported to be effective in ulcerative colitis, but randomized controlled trials have failed to confirm the open-label observations.

Symptomatic and Supportive Measures

Several adjunctive measures can be used together with the more specific anti-inflammatory and immune-modulating therapies in patients with ulcera-

---

*Not FDA-approved for this indication.

*Not FDA-approved for this indication.

tive colitis to diminish associated functional symptoms and to enhance coping skills for living with this chronic disease.

Bowel rest and hyperalimentation, as an accompaniment to intravenous steroid treatment, have not been shown to improve severe colitis. However, chronically ill, nutritionally depleted patients should receive enteral or parenteral nutritional supplementation as judged necessary. In ambulatory patients, specific dietary recommendations are limited. Avoidance of foods, spices, and beverages that produce symptoms should be the general rule. Patients who have constipated bowel function in association with exacerbations of ulcerative colitis may benefit by increased fiber intake. Other patients with tenesmus and diarrhea often feel better with less fiber intake because of a decrease in the gas and water production that results from fermentation of these complex carbohydrates by the colonic bacterial flora.

Judicious use of *antispasmodics, analgesics,* or *antidiarrheal drugs* may be helpful to some patients experiencing symptoms of abdominal pain or diarrhea as part of acute exacerbations of ulcerative colitis. In the outpatient setting, anticholinergics and narcotics should be limited to patients who have been demonstrated to have left-sided colitis because the use of such intestinal motility–modifying agents in more extensive colitis or pancolitis may precipitate complications such as toxic colitis or megacolon. Such comfort measures can be made available to hospitalized patients with extensive colitis, provided they are monitored carefully. Tenesmus accompanying distal colitis can improve with the use of low-volume retention enemas containing tincture of opium.

Every effort should be made to identify and manage psychosocial, emotional, and dysfunctional problems in conjunction with the symptoms and complications of ulcerative colitis. It is important to develop an appropriate approach to the patient with regard to eliciting information about health and life circumstances, providing a therapeutic relationship, involving family members as appropriate, and counseling about problems and expectations. Health care workers should be prepared to assess the degree of disability associated with exacerbations of ulcerative colitis so that they may communicate effectively with third parties, such as employers and insurers, on their patients' behalf. Some patients may benefit from participating in self-help and support group activities organized through local hospitals and the Crohn's and Colitis Foundation of America (CCFA), or from learning about ulcerative colitis from brochures, newsletters, and books prepared specifically for patients.

SURGICAL TREATMENT

Surgical resection of the large intestine is performed on patients with ulcerative colitis for the following indications: (1) urgent management of complications of ulcerative colitis, such as toxic colitis, megacolon, perforation, or hemorrhage, (2) elective

management of benign inflammatory disease that is unresponsive to medical treatment or associated with drug-induced adverse effects, or (3) treatment or prevention of colorectal adenocarcinoma.

Patients should be counseled about the availability of surgical treatment for ulcerative colitis for several reasons. Surgical removal of the large intestine is essentially curative for this disease, whereas no medical therapy can provide a definitive cure. Therefore, patients who are not responsive to medical treatment and who are unaware of the surgical options may suffer needless frustration and depression over their failure to improve clinically. Patients may not realize that the large intestine is unessential for survival, and they may not be aware of the most modern practices of medical centers that emphasize safe anesthetic practice, humane and effective management of postoperative pain, and a variety of surgical techniques, all of which may influence a decision about undergoing colectomy.

The standard and most common surgery offered to patients with ulcerative colitis is *total proctocolectomy with ileostomy.* The advantages of this procedure, when it is performed electively, are that it is completed in one stage and ensures continence with the use of an ileostomy appliance. Although the ileostomy does not produce any functional disability, it may appear unsightly and perhaps frightening to some patients, leading to their refusal to undergo surgery. The frequency of this latter circumstance has led to the development of alternative surgical procedures. One is the *continent ileostomy,* after total proctocolectomy, which involves the creation of an ileal pouch that requires intermittent catheterization for emptying rather than the use of an external fecal collection appliance. A more aesthetically pleasing, flesh-toned button is placed at the abdominal skin site of the channel opening to the ileal pouch between catheterizations.

Another surgical alternative is the *ileal pouch anal anastomosis* (IPAA) after subtotal colectomy and rectal mucosectomy. This procedure allows perianal defecation by preservation of the otherwise normal anus and rectal and perianal musculature. Patients who require surgery for ulcerative colitis may elect this procedure largely to avoid having a permanent ileostomy and should be alerted to some potential disadvantages. IPAA should be performed by surgeons who are experienced in this technique. The ultimate completion of the procedure may require two stages, or three stages in severely ill patients, during which the patient is required to have a temporary diverting ileostomy. With the takedown of the ileostomy and the initiation of use of the pouch, patients often experience large numbers of stools per day, nocturnal stools, and fecal soilage or overt incontinence. Fortunately, considerable improvement in function evolves during a period of several months after the initiation of pouch use. Satisfaction ratings for this procedure performed at specialty centers is very high. The increasing ability to perform colon resection and IPAA in one stage, coupled with laparoscopy-assisted surgical approaches may further patient acceptance of surgery as a therapeutic intervention for ulcerative colitis.

Approximately 25% of patients with ileal pouch procedures (IPAA or continent ileostomy) develop pouchitis, an inflammatory process of the distal ileal pouch, leading to diarrhea and bleeding. The basis for this postoperative complication is not well understood. Fortunately, the majority of cases of pouchitis are promptly responsive to treatment with antibiotics, such as metronidazole.

OTHER ISSUES IN ULCERATIVE COLITIS

Pregnancy

Pregnancy may be associated with exacerbations of, improvement in, or no effect on ulcerative colitis disease activity in an unpredictable and inconsistent manner in individual patients. Very mild distal disease may go untreated but should be carefully monitored clinically. Moderate disease that could potentially threaten the fetus should be treated, preferably with standard oral aminosalicylates, with folate supplementation, and/or with corticosteroids as necessary because of their lack of teratogenic effects. The use of rectally administered agents, as well as sigmoidoscopy, should be avoided because of their potential for inducing premature labor. Severe disease that threatens the mother should be treated as necessary with hospitalization, supportive care, corticosteroid therapy, antimetabolite immunosuppressive therapy, or surgery, all of which may be able to preserve the pregnancy and result in the delivery of a healthy baby.

Risk of Colorectal Cancer

The risk of colorectal adenocarcinoma in ulcerative colitis increases with the proximal extent and duration of the disease but is probably not associated with the inflammatory intensity. In this disease, the progression to colorectal adenocarcinoma occurs as a morphologically recognizable multistep process via a dysplasia intermediate, but without necessarily involving a polypoid intermediate, as is usually the case in the common variety of colorectal cancer. Patients with ulcerative colitis documented to extend proximal to the splenic flexure, and with a history of this disease for at least 10 years' duration, are often referred for colonoscopic biopsy surveillance at 1- to 2-year intervals to detect precancerous dysplasia or early, treatable cancer. The benefits of colonoscopic biopsy surveillance as a method of cancer control is debated. The explanations for the variance in opinion on this issue probably include a lack of certainty about the magnitude of risk of colorectal cancer in different subsets of patients with ulcerative colitis, as well as differences in patient selection and surveillance practices among several research studies.

Extraintestinal Manifestations

Perhaps as many as 40% of patients with ulcerative colitis have associated nonintestinal complications that may arise, worsen, or improve in conjunction with colitis disease activity. Alternatively, extraintestinal manifestations of ulcerative colitis may have independent courses that are unrelated to the course of colitis and require separate therapeutic interventions. Patients should be evaluated routinely for these complications because a delay in detection and treatment can lead to significant morbidity. The following extraintestinal manifestations are associated with ulcerative colitis: erythema nodosum; pyoderma gangrenosum; uveitis; iritis; episcleritis; peripheral arthritis; sacroiliitis; ankylosing spondylitis; pericholangitis; sclerosing cholangitis; bile duct carcinoma; hepatitis; fatty liver; thrombocytosis; venous thrombosis; embolic disease; amyloidosis; hemolytic anemia; psychiatric disorder associated with chronic disease; narcotic abuse; and suicidal ideation.

CROHN'S DISEASE

method of
STEPHEN B. HANAUER, M.D.
University of Chicago Medical Center
Chicago, Illinois

Crohn's disease, in distinction from ulcerative colitis, is a chronic, panenteric inflammatory bowel disease manifested by focal, asymmetric, transmural, and, occasionally, granulomatous inflammation involving any portion of the gastrointestinal tract from the mouth to the anus. The pattern of gastrointestinal involvement, including the location within the digestive tract (e.g., ileitis, ileocolitis, colitis) and subtype of inflammation (e.g., inflammatory, fibrostenotic, fistulizing), persists within an individual and recurs in the same pattern after intestinal resection. The management of patients presenting with Crohn's disease depends on the location, severity, complicating features, and response to prior intervention. There has been an evolution of medical therapies for Crohn's disease, with a recent emphasis on the avoidance of corticosteroids or the withdrawal of steroids in corticosteroid-dependent patients. In addition, recent advances in maintenance therapy (the prevention of relapse) afford long-term symptom-free intervals. Because of the poor correlation between symptoms and endoscopic or pathologic findings, the primary focus of Crohn's disease therapy is to minimize symptoms and complications.

THERAPEUTIC OPTIONS

Nutritional Therapies

Although no dietary factor has been proved to initiate or exacerbate Crohn's disease, diet can be used in two ways for treatment: to minimize symptoms or to treat inflammatory features. Dietary considerations include an assessment for lactose intolerance and the avoidance of nonabsorbed carbohydrates to minimize diarrhea and gaseousness. Generally, a low-residue diet is advisable for patients with intestinal narrowing; conversely, bulking agents may be useful for patients with constipation. Extensive ileal disease often leads to bile salt or fat malabsorption, which benefits from a low-fat diet. Postoperative diarrhea after short ileal resections often responds to cholestyramine in divided doses to minimize bile salt–related diarrhea.

More extensive dietary therapies, including elemental diets or liquid polymeric diets, have been equivalent to steroids in inducing clinical remission and lowering inflammatory mediators. When employed, these treatments are quite successful but are compromised by lack of compliance, high cost, and recurrence after the return to a more generalized diet. Similarly, total parenteral nutrition and bowel rest are effective for nutritional restoration and minimizing or eliminating symptoms and inflammatory sequelae; however, maintenance therapy is necessary to prevent recurrence after cessation of the nutritional intervention.

Aminosalicylates

Sulfasalazine (Azulfidine) has long been recognized as an initial approach for mild to moderately active ileocolonic or colonic Crohn's disease. It is now recognized that patients who respond to sulfasalazine therapy benefit from long-term maintenance treatment continued after symptom resolution. Generally, doses between 3 and 6 grams daily are required but may be complicated by by sulfa-induced intolerance. More recently, the mesalamine (5-ASA) derivative (Asacol, Pentasa)* has been effective in high doses for the treatment of ileal and ileocolonic or colonic Crohn's disease. Preferably, the mesalamine preparation should be targeted to the site of disease activity (e.g., Asacol for ileal disease, and Pentasa for more extensive ileal, ileocolonic, or colonic disease). Doses between 4 and 5 grams daily are effective in inducing clinical remission and in preventing relapse when the drug is continued after symptomatic improvement or when initiated after surgical resection.

Corticosteroids

Corticosteroids administered orally (prednisone), parenterally (hydrocortisone or methylprednisolone), or via adrenocorticotropic hormone (ACTH) stimulation have been effective for the short-term treatment of Crohn's disease. However, the facile short-term treatment is usually compromised by long-term steroid dependency. Between one-third and one-half of patients started on prednisone therapy become dependent on continued steroid administration or their disease becomes refractory to treatment. Therefore, the introduction of steroid therapy requires consideration of the length of treatment and potential mechanisms for steroid withdrawal. Steroids have not been effective for the maintenance of Crohn's disease, and there is often confusion between recurrent inflammatory symptoms and symptoms of steroid withdrawal (e.g., malaise, fatigue, depression, diarrhea, and arthralgias). Patients receiving long-term steroid therapy should be monitored for systemic sequelae, primarily accelerated osteoporosis. All attempts should be made to minimize steroid exposure, and patients who fail to taper completely should be considered candidates for surgical resection or long-term immune suppression therapy.

Immune Suppressants

The value of azathioprine (Imuran)* and 6-mercaptopurine (Purinethol)* has been recognized in Crohn's disease for over 2 decades. However, concern regarding the potential risks based on the experience in organ transplant patients has inhibited more extensive use of these agents. Recently, accumulating clinical and safety experience has broadened the use of these drugs for steroid-refractory or steroid-dependent Crohn's disease and for long-term maintenance of clinical remission. The benefits of azathioprine and 6-mercaptopurine may require up to 6 or even 12 months to become evident. Generally, patients respond to low doses (50 to 100 mg daily), and controversy remains whether leukopenia is necessary to provide optimal benefits. In general, we advance to leukopenic doses only in patients who fail to respond over 6 months to initial intervention at 1 to 2 mg per kg per day. The benefits of these agents are long term, and relapses occur when therapy is withdrawn, even after several years. Although there is some controversy regarding the safety of these agents in pregnancy, most clinicians continue treatment in patients who would otherwise relapse after withdrawal.

Intravenous cyclosporine and parenteral methotrexate have recently been evaluated in Crohn's disease. Intravenous cyclosporine provides initial therapeutic benefit and heals fistulas but requires long-term therapy to provide maintenance benefits. Studies are under way to determine whether substituting a more traditional immune suppressant can prolong the short-term benefits of cyclosporin. Intramuscular or subcutaneous methotrexate, at a dose of 25 mg per week, has been shown to be effective in withdrawing steroids from dependent patients. The long-term benefits of methotrexate therapy are currently being evaluated.

Antibiotics

Clinical trials have demonstrated that metronidazole (Flagyl)* is of therapeutic benefit (comparable to sulfasalazine) in the treatment of mild to moderate Crohn's disease. Many clinicians use alternative antibiotics (e.g., trimethoprim-sulfamethoxazole [Bactrim, Septra],* cephalosporins,* or ciprofloxacin [Cipro]*) that have not been adequately studied in controlled trials. Long-term therapy is usually necessary to control perianal drainage and may be complicated by peripheral neuropathy secondary to metro-

*Not FDA-approved for this indication.

*Not FDA-approved for this indication.

nidazole. Metronidazole should be avoided in the first trimester of pregnancy due to teratogenic effects in animals. Patients respond to 10 to 20 mg per kg, and the dose should be tapered to the lowest effective level that maintains symptomatic improvement. Metronidazole may also be beneficial in preventing the short-term relapse of Crohn's disease after surgical resection, although further long-term studies are necessary to define the postoperative maintenance benefits.

TREATMENT OPTIONS

Gastrointestinal Crohn's Disease

Gastrointestinal Crohn's disease is uncommon, presenting with either peptic-like symptoms or gastric outlet obstruction. The former respond to acid-reduction therapy with high-dose H_2 receptor antagonists or a proton pump inhibitor. Often, gastrointestinal lesions are asymptomatic. Gastric outlet obstruction requires a short course of corticosteroids in conjunction with acid-suppressive therapy, but it ultimately requires immune suppression treatment with azathioprine or 6-mercaptopurine to prevent recurrent obstructions. Failure of maintenance therapy necessitates a gastrojejunostomy bypass procedure.

Jejunoileitis

Jejunoileitis presents with extensive small intestinal Crohn's disease and is often complicated by fibrostenotic strictures. It tends to be a corticosteroid-resistant variant of Crohn's disease. Patients present with diarrhea, weight loss, and hypoalbuminemia. The course is often complicated by small bowel bacterial overgrowth. Initial therapeutic approaches include nutritional support via an elemental diet to minimize symptoms and improve inflammatory features (erythrocyte sedimentation rate, C-reactive protein) and broad-spectrum antibiotics to minimize bacterial overgrowth. A continuous-release mesalamine preparation (e.g., Pentasa 4 grams daily) is a safe initial intervention. The nutritional complications are often resistant to corticosteroids, and many patients require long-term immune suppression therapy with azathioprine or 6-mercaptopurine. Obstructing strictures should be treated by surgical stricturoplasty rather than extensive resections.

Ileitis

Terminal ileitis is a more common presentation of Crohn's disease that may be inflammatory, stenosing, or fistulizing. The length of ileal disease remains constant and recurs at approximately the same length after resection. Hence, in patients with short-segment disease, the ileitis tends to persist or recur with short segments, and vice versa with long-segment disease. Patients presenting with mild to moderate nonobstructing ileitis can be managed with an aminosalicylate (sulfasalazine 4 grams daily, mesala-

mine 4 grams daily), antibiotics (e.g., metronidazole, trimethoprim-sulfamethoxazole, or ciprofloxacin), or an elemental diet. Moderate to severe illness requires a short course of steroids (prednisone 40 mg daily), tapered according to the time required to induce improvement. Approximately one-third to one-half of patients managed with corticosteroids become either steroid resistant or steroid dependent. In patients with short-segment ileitis, a surgical resection is warranted. Patients with more extensive disease benefit from long-term immune suppression therapy with azathioprine or 6-mercaptopurine. There is increasing evidence that maintenance therapy with high-dose mesalamine (3 to 4 grams daily) prevents a significant proportion of relapses after medical induction of remission or surgical resection.

Ileocolitis

Involvement of the ileum and right colon is the most common subtype of Crohn's disease and can be complicated by either stricture formation or fistulization. Uncomplicated ileocolitis responds to elemental diets, aminosalicylates, or antibiotics, but moderate to severe disease necessitates a course of steroids to induce clinical remission. Maintenance therapy is beneficial with either the inductive agent (continuation of antibiotics or aminosalicylates) or with the substitution of an immune suppressant for steroid withdrawal. Prevention of postoperative recurrence can be achieved with high-dose mesalamine, or possibly an immune suppressant initiated at the time of surgery.

Colonic and Perianal Crohn's Disease

Crohn's colitis occurs in approximately 20% of patients and must be distinguished from ulcerative colitis based on relative rectal sparing, focality, cobblestone ulcerations, and the presence of perianal skin tags, abscesses, or fistulas. Mild to moderate disease responds to sulfasalazine or an alternative aminosalicylate and equally well to metronidazole or an alternative antibiotic). Patients with colonic Crohn's disease also respond to nutritional interventions with an elemental diet. Again, after initial improvement, the patient should be continued on treatment to prevent clinical relapse. Moderate to severe disease necessitates steroid-inductive therapy with the substitution of a high-dose aminosalicylate or immune suppressant for maintenance benefit. The co-occurrence of perianal disease requires surgical drainage of suppuration, antibiotics such as metronidazole to control fistula output, or long-term immune suppression to minimize recurrence and provide long-term relief of symptoms.

Pregnancy

The principles of treating pregnant patients with Crohn's disease are not dissimilar from those for treating nonpregnant patients, except for the avoidance of metronidazole in the first trimester. Active disease should be controlled with aminosalicylates or with steroids for more severe symptoms. Careful attention is paid to maintaining adequate nutrition and weight gain, and either enteral or parenteral supplements may be utilized to ensure nutritional intake. Immune suppressants should be continued if required to maintain stability of the inflammatory sequelae.

IRRITABLE BOWEL SYNDROME

method of
ARISTOTLE J. DAMIANOS, M.D., and
KENNETH L. KOCH, M.D.
The Pennsylvania State University
Hershey, Pennsylvania

The irritable bowel syndrome (IBS) is a chronic gastrointestinal disorder consisting of abdominal pain and altered bowel habits. Despite the frequency with which it is seen by both primary care physicians and subspecialists, the pathophysiology of IBS is poorly understood. Earlier theories invoking intestinal dysmotility are being discarded in favor of newer hypotheses focusing on visceral hypersensitivity. Specific diagnostic criteria for IBS were not agreed on until 1990, making review of the literature especially difficult. Prior to this, many studies involved small groups of patients with heterogeneous disorders that would not satisfy today's more stringent definition of IBS. Adequate trials of treatment regimens have not been conducted. Since the cause of IBS is unknown, and treatment regimens are nonspecific, the cornerstone of successful therapy is a strong physician-patient relationship.

EPIDEMIOLOGY

IBS is extremely common. The disorder accounts for roughly 12% of primary care visits, and 20 to 50% of referrals to gastroenterologists. In the United States, up to 20% of the population has symptoms of IBS, with twice as many women reporting the disorder as men. Similar prevalences have been identified in non-Western countries as well, although in some cultures the gender ratio is reversed. In the United States, 75 to 80% of patients seeing a physician for IBS are female. IBS can be found in all age groups, but is most common between the ages of 15 and 45 years.

Only a minority of subjects with symptoms of IBS ever seek medical attention for their symptoms. The high prevalence of IBS, however, makes this a significant public health issue, especially in light of the large number of diagnostic tests that are often ordered to exclude other diagnoses. After the common cold, IBS is the leading cause of health-related absenteeism from work or school. IBS patients have more physician visits for both gastrointestinal and nongastrointestinal complaints than patients without abdominal symptoms.

PATHOPHYSIOLOGY

Intestinal and Colonic Dysmotility

The term "spastic colon" is often used by physicians to refer to IBS, reflecting the long-held belief of many clinicians that the abdominal pain, diarrhea, and constipation of IBS are the result of altered motility of the large intestine. In fact, abnormal motility patterns have been found in IBS patients not only in the colon but also in the small intestine and in the esophagus. Abnormalities in colonic myoelectric activity, contractile activity, and colonic transit times have been described in patients with IBS, mostly in response to a meal or to a stressor such as balloon inflation in the rectosigmoid. Many of the studies have been marred, however, by imprecise subject selection, lack of appropriate controls, and our poor understanding of normal colonic motility. A consistently described dysmotility pattern has not been discovered in IBS, and many subjects with symptoms of IBS have no demonstrable intestinal motor abnormality.

Psychosocial Factors

Abnormalities in psychoneurotic profile have been described in some, but not all, patients with IBS. As a group, patients with IBS score in the abnormal range on tests such as the Minnesota Multiphasic Personality Inventory. Psychiatric diagnoses including major depression, personality disturbance, hysteria, anxiety, and somatization disorder have been found in up to three-quarters of patients with IBS. In the majority of these patients, the psychiatric illness has been found to predate the onset of irritable bowel.

It must be remembered that studies that have found such a high incidence of psychiatric disease in IBS were based on *patients* with IBS, most of whom were seen in referral centers. This referral bias overestimates the degree to which psychosocial factors are involved in all persons with IBS, since 80% of persons with IBS do not seek medical attention for their symptoms. People with IBS who do not consult a physician for their bowel complaints have psychoneurotic profiles that are similar to those of healthy controls, and do not have a higher rate of physician visits or absenteeism. Therefore, there appears to be a difference in psychosocial factors between those who consult physicians for IBS symptoms and those who do not. A recent study of women at a university clinic found that nearly 45% of females with IBS had a history of abuse. This again is a select population, but it suggests that some type of psychological trauma may influence the decision to seek medical care for IBS.

Visceral Hypersensitivity

Pain is the predominant symptom in patients with IBS, many of whom do not exhibit colonic dysmotility or abnormalities in psychoneurotic profile. Subjects with IBS are more sensitive to visceral stimuli, as evidenced by a lower pain threshold to balloon distention of the rectum. This, however, is not a generalized decrease in pain threshold, as IBS subjects appear to have a higher pain threshold to nonvisceral stimuli. These findings have led to the concept of visceral hypersensitivity, or hyperalgesia. Attention currently is focused on visceral afferent pathways. The afferent input from the gut travels via spinal pathways to the brain, where central processing of the input takes place. Pain, therefore, may result either from an abnormal afferent input that is perceived normally or from a normal afferent input that is abnormally processed (Figure 1).

Unifying Hypothesis

It is not known why patients with IBS have pain. One hypothesis is that subjects with IBS have visceral hyper-

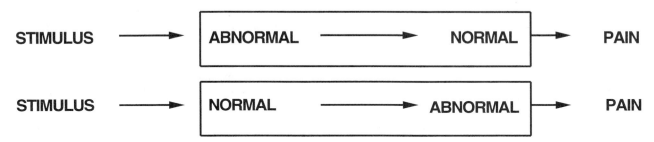

Figure 1. Proposed mechanism of pain in irritable bowel syndrome. The visceral afferent input from a stimulus may be abnormal, with this abnormal input perceived appropriately. Conversely, the afferent input may be normal but may be processed abnormally, leading to pain.

sensitivity based on either abnormal afferent input from gut stimuli or abnormal central processing. In some subjects, this hypersensitivity may trigger various forms of intestinal dysmotility. The majority do not seek medical attention. A variety of psychosocial stressors may influence the decision to consult a physician. This hypothesis is currently an area of considerable investigation.

NATURAL HISTORY

Most patients with IBS remain symptomatic for many years, although symptoms may wax and wane. Quiescent periods during which bowel function is normal may alternate with periods of abdominal pain and irregular bowel habits. One-third of patients will become symptom free over time. A small minority progress to daily symptoms.

There is no increase in mortality associated with IBS. Of patients diagnosed with IBS and followed over time, few are found to have actually had organic disease. Thus, once the diagnosis is established, there is no role for continued diagnostic testing unless symptoms change. Patients must be reassured that IBS does not progress to cancer, inflammatory bowel disease, or any other organic illness. It should be remembered that patients are not protected from these other conditions either, and a change in the symptom complex should prompt further appropriate investigation.

DIAGNOSIS

Symptoms

Functional gastrointestinal disorders encompass a wide spectrum of symptoms in which no pathologic lesion can be found despite the suggestion of altered function of the digestive tract (Table 1). IBS is a functional bowel disorder defined by a specific symptom complex. The diagnosis of IBS is made by the presence of an appropriate history and the absence of findings to suggest organic disease. In 1990, an international working team meeting in Rome developed specific criteria for the diagnosis of functional gastrointestinal disorders, including IBS. IBS is defined as a chronic

or recurrent symptom complex consisting of abdominal pain and disturbed defecation (Table 2). The pain must be either relieved with defecation or associated with a change in the frequency or consistency of stool. Patients may have

TABLE 1. **Functional Gastrointestinal Disorders**

A. Esophageal disorders
   A1. Globus
   A2. Rumination syndrome
   A3. Functional chest pain of presumed esophageal origin
   A4. Functional heartburn
   A5. Functional dysphagia
   A6. Unspecified functional esophageal disorder
B. Gastroduodenal disorders
   B1. Functional dyspepsia
      B1a. Ulcer-like dyspepsia
      B1b. Dysmotility-like dyspepsia
      B1c. Unspecified dyspepsia
   B2. Aerophagia
C. Bowel disorders
   C1. Irritable bowel syndrome
   C2. Functional abdominal bloating
   C3. Functional constipation
   C4. Functional diarrhea
   C5. Unspecified functional bowel disorder
D. Functional abdominal pain
   D1. Functional abdominal pain syndrome
   D2. Unspecified functional abdominal pain
E. Biliary disorders
   E1. Gallbladder dysfunction
   E2. Sphincter of Oddi dysfunction
F. Anorectal disorders
   F1. Functional incontinence
   F2. Functional anorectal pain
      F2a. Levator ani syndrome
      F2b. Proctalgia fugax
   F3. Dyschezia
      F3a. Pelvic floor dyssynergia
      F3b. Internal anal sphincter dysfunction
   F4. Unspecified functional anorectal disorder

From Thompson, WG: Functional bowel disorders and functional abdominal pain. *In* The Functional Gastrointestinal Disorders, edited by Douglas Drossman. New York, Little, Brown, 1994. Published by Little, Brown and Company.

TABLE 2. **Rome Criteria for Diagnosis of Irritable Bowel Syndrome**

Continuous or recurrent symptoms for at least 3 months of:
A. Abdominal pain, relieved with defecation, or associated with a change in frequency of consistency of stool; and
B. An irregular (varying) pattern of defecation at least 25% of the time (2 or more of):
   Altered stool frequency
   Altered stool form (hard or loose/watery stool)
   Altered stool passage (straining or urgency, feeling of incomplete evacuation)
   Passage of mucus
   Bloating or feeling of abdominal distention

Adapted from Drossman DA, et al: Identification of subgroups of functional gastrointestinal disorders. Gastroenterol Int 4:159–172, 1990.

alternating diarrhea and constipation, or they may have diarrhea or constipation as predominant symptoms. Painless diarrhea, painless constipation, and chronic abdominal pain in the absence of altered bowel habits are classified as separate functional disorders, and are not considered IBS.

In a prospective study of patients referred for abdominal pain and altered bowel habits, Manning and colleagues evaluated 15 symptoms to differentiate IBS from organic disease. Four of these were found to be highly discriminatory in favor of IBS. These 4 historical markers were looser stools at the onset of pain, more frequent stools at the onset of pain, pain eased by bowel movements, and the presence of abdominal distention (Table 3). The findings of mucus per rectum or the sense of incomplete evacuation were less predictive. The validity of the Manning criteria in men has been questioned. Weight loss, rectal bleeding, and nocturnal symptoms are generally not seen in IBS and should suggest organic disease, with the caveat that weight loss is often a prominent symptom of psychiatric illness such as major depression.

Physical Examination

Three-quarters of IBS patients complain of tenderness to palpation on physical examination, particularly in the left lower quadrant. Especially in patients with abdominal scars, an attempt should be made to identify abdominal wall pain using Carnett's test. In this maneuver, the abdomen is palpated to discern the minimal amount of pressure required to elicit pain. The patient is then asked to flex the neck, raising the head off the bed, or to flex at the hips, raising the legs off the bed, thereby tightening the abdominal musculature. The abdomen is then palpated again using the same amount of pressure. Abdominal wall pain will be more severe with the muscles of the abdomen taut, requiring less pressure to provoke it.

Laboratory Studies

Biochemical markers, radiographic studies, and histopathology are all normal in IBS. Laboratory evaluation should be aimed at excluding other causes of abdominal pain or altered bowel habits. Complete blood count with differential and erythrocyte sedimentation rate both screen for anemia and inflammation. Stool should be tested for occult blood. Flexible sigmoidoscopy should be performed on all patients during the initial evaluation. This limited initial work-up, when combined with the appropriate clinical history, has been shown to have a diagnostic accuracy of 95%.

Further diagnostic testing may be pursued in a minority of patients, as indicated by history or by clinical suspicion for organic disease. A lactose tolerance breath test should be performed in patients with complaints of bloating and diarrhea. It is important to make the diagnosis of lactase deficiency not only because the treatment differs from that of IBS but also to exclude the diagnosis in women who may unnecessarily be avoiding calcium-rich dairy products. A small bowel series may be necessary in some patients to exclude inflammatory bowel disease. Patients with watery diarrhea should also undergo endoscopic biopsies of the colon to rule out collagenous or lymphocytic colitis. Stool examination to exclude giardiasis may also be warranted. Full colonoscopy should be reserved for patients over age 40 years, patients at risk because of family history, or patients with occult blood in the stool. Again, most patients can be successfully evaluated with a limited work-up. Further testing may raise doubts in patients' minds as to the clinicians' confidence in the diagnosis. IBS is a chronic disease. The continued presence of symptoms after long-term follow-up does not justify further or repeated testing.

TREATMENT

A solid physician-patient relationship is the cornerstone to successful treatment of IBS. Many patients will have seen a number of physicians, with disappointing results. A review of the frequency of IBS and a brief explanation of proposed pathophysiology will help assure the patient that the symptoms are not "in her head." It is important to discover the patient's agenda: many fear they have cancer or other organic illnesses. Simple reassurance may be all that is needed. Others may be seeking secondary gain.

A plethora of therapeutic modalities have been used to treat IBS, all with varying success. These include fiber supplements, anticholinergics, barbiturates, antidepressants, dopamine antagonists, benzodiazepines, and opioids. A critical review of the literature has demonstrated that no single pharmacologic therapy has proved more effective than placebo in treating IBS. Most investigations have been marred by flawed study designs, including small subject groups, and the inclusion of subjects with functional bowel disorders that do not meet current diagnostic criteria for IBS. The overall response rate to placebo is 40 to 70%, perhaps in part reflecting the waxing and waning nature of the symptoms. This high rate

TABLE 3. **Manning Criteria for the Diagnosis of Irritable Bowel Syndrome**

Symptom	Organic Disease*	IBS	Significance
Looser stools at onset of pain	8/30	25/31	p <.001
More frequent stools at onset	9/30	25/31	p <.01
Pain eased after defecation	9/30	22/31	p <.01
Visible distention	7/33	19/32	p <.01

*Number of patients with symptoms/total number of patients.
Abbreviation: IBS = irritable bowel syndrome.
Adapted from Manning AP, Thompson WG, Heaton KW, Morris AF: Towards positive diagnosis of the irritable bowel. Br Med J 2:653–654, 1978.

TABLE 4. **Fiber Supplements Commonly Available**

Trade Name	Type of Fiber	Form	Fiber Content
Metamucil	Psyllium	Powder, sugar-free flavors, orange and citrus flavors, effervescent powders, wafer	3.4 gm/tsp 3.4 gm/tbsp 3.4 gm/packet 3.4 gm/2 wafers
Mylanta Natural Fiber	Psyllium	Powder	3.4 gm/tbsp
		Sugar-free powder	3.4 gm/tsp
Perdiem Fiber	Psyllium	Granules	4.03 gm/tsp
Citrucel	Methylcellulose	Powder	2 gm/tbsp
Fiberall	Polycarbophil	Tablet	1 gm tablet
	Psyllium	Wafer, powder	3.4 gm/wafer, tsp
FiberCon	Polycarbophil	Tablet	0.5 gm/tablet

of placebo response also makes it difficult to statistically demonstrate true superiority of regimens if they do exist. Although no treatment is of proven benefit for the global syndrome of IBS, certain therapies may help alleviate specific symptoms.

Fiber supplementation often improves symptoms of constipation by drawing water into the colon, lubricating, and increasing stool volume. It can also aid as a bulking agent in diarrhea. The average American diet contains only 19 grams of fiber per day. Thirty to 40 grams of indigestible fiber is recommended per day; therefore most patients will need to ingest an additional 10 to 20 grams of fiber daily. Although some patients will be willing to alter their dietary habits and consume a diet higher in fiber, most will not, and these will require commercially prepared supplements (Table 4). Patients taking psyllium-based preparations should be warned that an increase in bloating, gas, and cramping may initially occur secondary to bacterial degradation of fiber, but that this improves over time. Side effects may also be reduced by initiating therapy with a single daily dose, increasing every few days as tolerated. To ensure an adequate trial, fiber supplementation should be continued for at least 1 month, titrating the amount until stools are bulky, soft, and easily passed. Too little fiber for too little time is a frequent cause of treatment failure.

Most patients seen in a primary care setting have mild symptoms and little psychopathology. Reassurance and instructions to avoid obvious stressors often suffice. A trial of fiber supplementation to achieve a soft, bulky bowel movement is generally safe and inexpensive. In persistent diarrhea, loperamide (Imodium), an opioid antagonist that does not cross the blood-brain barrier, may also be helpful. The initial dosage is 4 mg. Additional doses of 2 mg may be taken as needed up to a maximum of 16 mg per day. This may be especially helpful in situations when it will be difficult for the patient to reach a bathroom. Diphenoxylate (Lomotil) does cross the blood-brain barrier, and may be habit-forming.

Abdominal pain is more difficult to treat. Some patients may respond to anticholinergic agents such as dicyclomine (Bentyl), or hyoscyamine (Levsin). Studies that have reported pain relief using anticholinergics also included fiber supplementation rather than anticholinergics alone. High doses of anticholinergics (e.g., dicyclomine 10 to 40 mg four times a day) may be used to reduce symptoms. Compliance may, however, be limited by side effects. Blurred vision and dry mouth are common; urinary retention and tachycardia may occur. Care must be taken with these agents in elderly patients. Just as fiber supplementation is instituted gradually, so too should the dose of anticholinergics be slowly increased over time. Patients may be advised that the development of dry mouth signals the onset of therapeutic drug levels. The pain pattern should dictate the timing of medication. Those patients with postprandial pain should take their medication ½ hour before meals. Patients with an unpredictable pain pattern may benefit from taking a faster-acting sublingual preparation (Levsin/SL) at the first onset of pain.

Patients with severe symptoms have a higher degree of psychopathology. They are often referred to subspecialists, or even tertiary care centers. Their course is frustrating to both patient and physician, and outcomes tend to be poor. Proper expectations must be set. The clinician must strive to orient the patient away from "cure" and toward "coping" with symptoms. Tricyclic antidepressants and serotonin reuptake inhibitors are useful. In patients who continue to have disabling symptoms, referral for biofeedback training should be pursued.

Most patients with IBS can be successfully managed by their primary care physician. Improvement in our understanding of the pathophysiology of IBS, and refinements in the definition of the syndrome, may lead to more definitive treatments in the future.

HEMORRHOIDS, ANAL FISSURE, AND ANORECTAL ABSCESS AND FISTULA

method of
YANEK S. Y. CHIU, M.D.
California Pacific Medical Center
San Francisco, California

The general public tends to attribute any anorectal symptom to "hemorrhoids." This is certainly not correct.

After a careful history and physical examination are done, it is found that half the patients who claim to have hemorrhoidal symptoms simply do not have any hemorrhoids at all. Their symptoms are due to other anorectal diseases. Hemorrhoids will be found to be the cause of the complaints in the remaining half, but only one-tenth of these patients will require surgical treatment. Symptoms from anal fissure and anorectal abscess and fistula may overlap those from hemorrhoids at first glance, but a good history-taking will separate them out, and a gentle anorectal examination will confirm the diagnosis without any ambiguity.

In taking the history, symptoms of pain, bleeding, swelling, prolapsing tissue, drainage, or leakage must be touched on (Table 1). Questions should be asked whether these symptoms are related to the act of defecation or afterward, whether the symptoms start abruptly or insidiously, and are continuous or intermittent, and whether the symptoms may be the result of recent medical or surgical treatment of any anorectal disease. The proctologic examination should be preceded by words of reassurance (vocal anesthesia) and should be conducted in a comfortable setting with good nursing assistance. Good lighting is mandatory, and the left or right lateral decubitus position is preferred by most patients. Simple inspection of the perianal skin and gentle spreading of the buttocks will reveal vital information, and this step is far too often neglected. Gentle and slow insertion of a well-lubricated gloved index finger will elicit important data without patient apprehension. If the diagnosis, such as an acute anal fissure or an obvious abscess, can be made at this point, anoscopy or sigmoidoscopy will not be necessary and can be deferred to a later time after resolution of the painful process. Additional investigations such as barium enema or colonoscopy should be ordered as appropriate.

HEMORRHOIDS

External Hemorrhoids

Hemorrhoids are simply dilated veins of the anorectum. The external ones are those below the dentate line, covered by the stratified squamous epithelium of the skin. The skin is rich in somatic nerve fibers and therefore is very sensitive to noxious stimuli. At the same time, the stratified squamous epithelium provides strong tensile strength, thus protecting the external hemorrhoids. External hemorrhoids usually are asymptomatic, as long as the overlying skin is in good condition. However, bad hygiene may cause perianal itching and burning, which are symptoms related to the skin rather than to the external hemorrhoids themselves. The only clinically significant entity involving external hemorrhoids is acute thrombosis.

Acute Thrombosed External Hemorrhoid

This term is a misnomer, because it is really a perianal hematoma. There is no thrombosis of the external hemorrhoidal vein. There is no need for any anticoagulation (as in deep vein thrombosis of the lower extremities). In fact, heparin therapy is contraindicated. What actually happens is that the veins rupture under excessive straining, such as heavy lifting or with constipation, and blood extravasates into the perianal tissue, forming a hematoma and causing an isolated painful perianal swelling that is usually of sudden onset. (Occasionally the hematomas can be multiple, as in pregnancy or the immediate postpartum period.) The pain is excruciating, reaching a peak between 24 and 48 hours. The hematoma has stretched the perianal skin, firing off the numerous somatic nerve fibers. The characteristic single tender perianal swelling with a bluish-purple hue under the skin is seen. The size of the hematoma varies, but it is usually not much bigger than 1.5 cm.

If the acute episode of thrombosed hemorrhoid is diagnosed within the first 24 or 48 hours, if the skin is quite stretched and shiny, and if the patient is experiencing a great deal of pain, immediate excision under local anesthesia will give prompt relief. Lidocaine 1% with epinephrine in a 5-mL syringe with a 27- or 30-gauge needle is injected into the base of the swelling and into the overlying skin. The skin is excised together with the clots, leaving a small denuded area for drainage. A sitz bath followed by a perianal topical local anesthetic such as Prax or a cleansing lotion such as Balneol on a daily basis will lead to complete healing of the wound within a week. Constipation should be corrected by proper diet and water intake, and stool softener can be added as indicated. The patient is advised against strenuous exercise during the recovery period. Only in severe cases of multiple thrombosis will a formal hemorrhoidectomy under regional anesthesia be necessary.

However, most of the time the patient will seek medical advice 4 to 5 days after the acute episode. By then, the skin is usually not so stretched. The pain is starting to subside, and it will not be necessary to perform any minor surgical procedure. The best approach then is the use of sitz baths and a soothing perianal cleansing lotion, correction of constipation, and avoidance of strenuous exercise. The

TABLE 1. **Anorectal Symptoms and Diagnosis**

Diagnosis	Symptoms				
	Bleeding	Prolapse	Pain	Swelling	Drainage
Internal hemorrhoids	+ + + +	+ + + +			+ +
Thrombosed external hemorrhoid			+ + + +	+ + + +	
Anal fissure	+ +		+ + + +		
Acute abscess			+ + + +	+ + + +	+ +
Anal fistula	+		+	+	+ +

acute episode will then subside within 2 weeks. Repeated thrombosis in the same location will result in the formation of a chronic skin tag that may at times be inflamed and tender, and it may also occasionally be the cause of difficulty with good anal hygiene. If the skin condition cannot be improved on with the usual lotion, then excision of the chronic skin tag under local anesthesia in the office or the clinic can be very cost-effective.

Internal Hemorrhoids

The most common symptoms of internal hemorrhoids are bleeding and prolapse with bowel function. The blood is usually bright red, even though it is coming from the venous system, because of a certain amount of arteriovenous shunting. The bleeding can be profuse, as seen in the water, and characteristically spraying around the sides of the toilet bowel. It may be on the toilet paper on wiping only, or it may even stain the patient's underwear afterward, which indicates large, prolapsing tissues trapped outside the rectum after defecation. A careful history will define clearly that bleeding is hemorrhoidal in origin. As a precaution, in individuals over the age of 50 years, especially with a family history of colorectal cancer or polyps or if the bleeding symptom is atypical of hemorrhoids, additional work-up such as flexible sigmoidoscopy or even colonoscopy or barium enema must be carried out.

Physical examination should always start with inspection, which can reveal the chronically prolapsed internal hemorrhoid with the exposed rectal mucosa. However, this is not often seen; usually internal hemorrhoids are hidden from direct inspection of the perianal skin and they are not usually palpable on digital rectal examination. A slotted anoscope is useful in diagnosis and treatment. Internal hemorrhoids are usually located over the right anterior, right posterior, and left lateral quadrants. By gently rotating the anoscope, the three groups of tissue can be inspected for size, the degree of erosion of the overlying rectal mucosa, the tendency to protrude with slight straining, and even bleeding under direct vision.

Based on the extent of prolapse, internal hemorrhoids are categorized into first, second, third, and fourth degrees. There is no classification on the amount of bleeding. Small internal hemorrhoids, such as the first-degree type, can bleed, whereas a chronic prolapsing fourth-degree hemorrhoid may not. Treatment should be individualized (Table 2).

Treatment modalities for internal hemorrhoids include cryosurgery, sclerotherapy, rubber band ligation, laser and infrared coagulation, and surgical hemorrhoidectomy. Cryosurgery has fallen out of favor. Laser is hospital based and expensive and no more effective than hemorrhoidectomy. Infrared coagulation with a hand-held machine is imprecise and expensive, although it is easily used in the office or clinic setting. Sclerotherapy, using 5% phenol in cottonseed oil in a 5-mL syringe, is a safe, effective, and inexpensive method of submucosal injection,

TABLE 2. **Degree of Internal Hemorrhoids and Recommended Treatment**

Degree	Definition	Treatment
First	No prolapse; dilated veins seen on anoscopy	None
Second	Prolapse with spontaneous reduction	Sclerotherapy or band ligation
Third	Prolapse requiring manual reduction	Sclerotherapy or band ligation
Fourth	Chronic prolapse	Hemorrhoidectomy

with prompt shrinkage of the internal hemorrhoidal vascular cushions. Five milliliters is sufficient for a three-quadrant injection treatment, and the injection can be repeated once every 4 weeks with minimal side effects. It is particularly useful in stopping hemorrhoidal bleeding and is quite effective against prolapse as well.

Rubber band ligation has gained widespread acceptance and popularity over the last 20 years. It is the most often used office procedure for the treatment of internal hemorrhoids in the United States. A tight rubber band is placed at the base of the internal hemorrhoid to be treated. The pinched-off tissue will slough through tissue necrosis. The scarring at the base will result in fixation of the adjacent rectal mucosa. It is most often used for prolapsing symptoms. Although popular, rubber band ligation carries the small risk of severe infection, rectal pressure, or pain; urinary retention; delayed hemorrhage; or perianal thrombosis. Banding should never be done in the presence of acute anorectal infection. The tissue banded should be clearly above the dentate line to minimize the chance of discomfort or pain sensation from the somatic nerve fibers that are so great a part of the perianal skin. If a patient experiences excruciating pain with the banding, the band must be removed immediately.

Evidence of urinary retention postbanding is an ominous sign of severe retroperitoneal infection. The band should be removed immediately and high-dose triple antibiotics instituted intravenously without delay to avoid the dire consequence of synergistic gangrene in the anorectum.

When the bleeding is profuse and unrelenting despite repeated sclerotherapy, or if the prolapse is large and chronic even with several attempts at banding, then surgical hemorrhoidectomy is the treatment of choice. Surgery for hemorrhoidal disease is now performed primarily as an outpatient procedure. The improved anesthesia, as well as better pain medications and more conservative surgical excision, has made the transition to outpatient surgery possible.

The goal of treatment for hemorrhoidal disease is to eliminate the symptoms, not necessarily to eliminate all the hemorrhoids. The end point is when the patient is asymptomatic, even if on examination large external or internal hemorrhoids are still seen. By using this approach and individualizing the various treatment modalities, patients with this common ailment will be well served, and they are usually very grateful and satisfied.

ANAL FISSURE

Anal fissure, or anal ulcer, is a tear on the anoderm just below the dentate line or mucocutaneous junction. It is most commonly located at the posterior midline, although it can occur at the anterior midline, particularly in women. In the majority of cases, the cause is repeated trauma to the anal canal, usually due to chronic constipation and, occasionally, severe diarrhea. The symptom is the characteristic sharp, knifing pain with defecation, with or without bleeding, which is usually minor. It is the severe pain that makes the patient afraid to have a bowel movement. In the acute case, the ulcer is sharply defined, but in the chronic type, there is the associated skin tag and hypertrophied anal papilla.

The diagnosis of acute anal fissure should be entertained by simply taking a careful history. The physical examination will confirm the diagnosis if performed appropriately and with minimal trauma or discomfort to the patient. Gentle spreading of the buttocks will reveal the sentinel tag over the posterior midline in most cases, or the everting of the anal canal will demonstrate the anal ulcer associated with involuntary sphincter spasm. Once the diagnosis is made, there is no need to proceed with any further investigation at the initial visit. The history should alert the clinician to the possibility of acute anal fissure being the diagnosis. Anoscopy and sigmoidoscopy, however, add little. The instruments will actually miss the fissure, and they cause considerable discomfort to the patient.

Initial treatment of an anal fissure consists of the proper diet of high fiber with plenty of water intake. Stool softener such as docusate sodium (Colace) may be added. Sitz baths provide sphincter relaxation and good anal hygiene, and topical hydrocortisone cream reduces the inflammatory reaction at the ulcer site. A follow-up visit in 3 weeks is essential. If the fissure has healed, a careful digital rectal examination should be carried out, as well as anoscopy (and if appropriate, flexible sigmoidoscopy) to rule out other anorectal and colonic pathology. The anal sphincter tone should be assessed; if it is normal, anal fissure should not recur given the proper diet.

However, if the anal ulcer persists despite adequate medical management, then the cause is internal sphincter hypertrophy or spasm, or both. This will happen in about 10% of all anal fissure patients. The spasm quite often lasts for hours after defecation, which explains the biphasic pain pattern seen in these individuals. The high-toned involuntary internal sphincter spasm is best appreciated with a gentle digital rectal examination, with the patient totally relaxed in the lateral decubitus position. Surgical treatment should be recommended, consisting of partial lateral internal sphincterotomy and mini-mal fissurectomy (primarily to remove any scar tissue, sentinel tag, and hypertrophied anal papilla).

With the patient under local or regional anesthesia, a small radial incision is made below the dentate line, and the whitish-yellow internal sphincter band is divided partially under direct vision, thus releasing the spasm. Bleeding is controlled by electrocautery, and the skin incision is left open. The subcutaneous approach to cutting of the internal sphincter, popularized by British surgeons, appears to be imprecise and may predispose to hematoma or abscess formation. If at the time of surgery no hypertrophied or tight internal sphincter is encountered, no sphincterotomy should be carried out because of the potential postoperative complication of anal incontinence. In such a case, a minimal fissurectomy should be performed to remove any scar tissue, and the anal sphincter gently dilated with anal retractors.

Surgical treatment for anal fissure is almost always performed as an outpatient procedure. Complications are infrequent, consisting of wound hematoma or abscess formation, or temporary incontinence of gas. If properly performed, the benefit is immediate, with the next bowel movement causing little or no pain. These patients are invariably very grateful. Recurrence is rare. However, it is important to differentiate anal fissure from Crohn's disease, tuberculosis, and syphilis, which present with lateral or multiple anal ulcers; squamous cell carcinoma in immunosuppressed or elderly patients; or benign fissure from anal stenosis from previous extensive hemorrhoidectomy.

With the stress of modern society, anal fissure secondary to internal sphincter hypertrophy or spasm appears to be on the rise. The patients often have high-strung personalities. A careful scrutiny of the social and personal history in these patients is very illuminating.

ANORECTAL ABSCESS

Over 90% of anorectal infection is of the cryptoglandular variety. The infection arises from the anal glands at the crypts at the dentate line. Once these crypts are plugged by stool laden with bacteria, mucus provides a ready medium for bacterial growth and the abscess will fester for a short time before it breaks into the perianal, perirectal, or ischiorectal space. Involvement of the skin will produce the usual redness, induration, pain, swelling, heat, and at the later stage, fluctuance. An acute abscess usually takes a few days to come to a point. The patient will notice the insidious onset of some nonspecific discomfort in the anorectum, but when the skin is involved and pain is increasing to an intolerable level, the patient will seek urgent medical care, often in the emergency room setting after hours.

Once the diagnosis is made, prompt surgical drainage is mandatory. This can be accomplished with the patient under local anesthesia using 1% lidocaine with epinephrine and a 30-gauge needle, infiltrating the skin over the most fluctuant part of the abscess.

A small incision made with a No. 11 knife blade will bring forth the pus. The skin opening should be enlarged slightly to allow adequate drainage. It is not always necessary to probe or break up all the loculations, because most abscesses have one large cavity. The patient is advised to have frequent sitz baths and to return for follow-up within 48 to 72 hours to make sure there is marked clinical improvement. Occasionally further drainage in the office under local anesthesia is necessary.

If the abscess is extensive, involving a large surface area, and if the patient appears toxic, suggestive of systemic sepsis, the abscess is best drained in the operating room under proper regional anesthesia. Antibiotic treatment has no role in the initial management of anorectal abscess, except in cases of obvious systemic toxicity. Prompt and adequate surgical drainage remains the treatment of choice. Occasionally a deep-seated ischiorectal abscess may not have any skin manifestation, but if the abscess is suspected, examination under anesthesia and surgical drainage will often yield dividends.

ANAL FISTULA

Once the abscess has been drained, a fistula may form. This is the case in about 50% of the time. The incision made on the skin for the abscess drainage becomes the secondary opening, and the primary opening where the infection originates is somewhere among the crypts at the dentate line. The fistula will drain intermittently, usually a small amount of purulent fluid or blood, and the patient will notice a slight lump adjacent to the anal opening, often staining the underwear. The symptoms are usually mild, and the patient will seek medical attention in a much more leisurely manner. Conceptually, abscess is the acute phase, and fistula is the chronic phase.

If the fistula is symptomatic enough, surgical treatment should be recommended. It consists of either anal fistulotomy or fistulectomy. In the former, the overlying skin and subcutaneous tissue are unroofed. The skin edges are trimmed back for adequate drainage, and the bottom of the fistulous tract is simply curetted clean of any granulation tissue and left intact. Fistulectomy is the complete excision of the fistulous tract down to soft pliable muscle. Fistulectomy is preferred when the tract is superficial, with only partial involvement of the deep external sphincter. This leads to good healing without any residual scar tissue from the fibrous fistulous tract. However, in deep fistula, when there is concern for sphincter damage, fistulotomy is preferred to spare as much of the remaining deep external sphincter as possible to maintain continence. These procedures can be carried out with the patient under local or regional anesthesia, and most patients go home the same day postoperatively with minimal discomfort.

In surgery for anal fistula, the primary opening must be sought, identified, and destroyed. In the unusual case of a deep or supralevator fistula in which the entire thickness of the deep external sphincter is involved, a seton can be placed to identify the track and allow for adequate drainage. Using the seton to cut through the muscle in stages is still a popular practice, but most experienced specialists prefer the rectal wall advancement flap to cover and repair the primary opening, leaving the external tunnel as a sinus tract to heal spontaneously. Over the past 2 years, fibrin glue repair of such deep anal fistulas has yielded satisfactory results and may be the future procedure of choice in these difficult cases.

The complications from surgical treatment of anal fistula consist of recurrence (owing to the inability to identify and eradicate the primary opening) and anal sphincter incontinence (from extensive cutting of the deep external sphincter). However, with experience and the selection of the appropriate surgical technique in each case, the incidence of complications should be below 3 to 5%.

Hidradenitis suppurativa is a chronic indolent infection of the apocrine sweat glands of the perianal skin. It can produce a small, firm, subcutaneous nodule at first, with occasional discharge of a small amount of yellowish, thick, creamy pus. With time, the infection can affect a large area of the perianal skin, with the nodules fusing together to form a cord-like structure, with severe undermining of the skin. Superficial fistulas are present, and in neglected cases a deep fistula can extend into the anal canal, simulating an anal fistula. Wide excision of the affected skin with the patient under local or regional anesthesia will bring about a complete cure.

GASTRITIS

method of
CHARLES BRADY, M.D.
University of Texas Health Science Center at San Antonio
San Antonio, Texas

The very word "gastritis" conjures up images of a variety of upper gastrointestinal symptoms, as well as a host of radiologic, endoscopic, and histologic abnormalities. Although acute gastritis may produce vague and nonspecific symptoms that are almost always self-limited, chronic gastritis without ulcer formation rarely causes symptoms. Because of the poor correlation among the clinical picture, radiologic, endoscopic, and histologic features, it has become popular to denote the clinical symptom complex as "nonulcer dyspepsia." However, a universally agreed definition of dyspepsia is lacking, but it is probably best defined as persistent or recurrent abdominal discomfort centered in the upper abdomen or epigastrium. Other clinical manifestations, such as distention, feeling of fullness or bloating, early satiety, and nausea, may be present.

Although symptom clusters can be clinically identified in dyspepsia, the pathophysiologic mechanisms generating these symptoms are imperfectly understood. Thus, the mere presence of gastritis should not be construed to be the cause of a particular set of symptoms in such patients. Gastritis is best defined from a histologic standpoint, and numerous classification systems have been proposed but lack universal agreement. Two important discoveries have changed many of our concepts concerning gastritis. First is the recognition of *Helicobacter pylori* as the cause of most cases of nonerosive chronic active gastritis. The second discovery has been the recognition that in some types of mucosal injury, epithelial or vascular changes dominate with trivial inflammatory cell infiltrates. The term "gastropathy" is used to describe these features.

From a clinical standpoint, gastritis can be classified into three major groups based on pathogenesis and/or associated clinical conditions: (1) erosive and hemorrhagic gastritis, (2) nonerosive nonspecific gastritis, (3) specific (distinctive) gastritis. Erosive or hemorrhagic lesions are typically seen in patients undergoing endoscopy for gastrointestinal bleeding. Stress lesions, nonsteroidal anti-inflammatory drug (NSAID) gastropathy, and portal hypertensive gastropathy account for the majority of lesions in this group and are discussed in the sections dealing with peptic ulcer disease and bleeding esophageal varices, respectively. The term "alcoholic gastritis" is commonly used in a clinical or endoscopic context to explain abdominal pain or gastric lesions in alcoholic patients. However, alcohol is more typically associated with subepithelial hemorrhage, and any inflammatory cell infiltrate is likely to be from some other cause, such as *H. pylori*.

H. pylori is the most common cause of nonerosive nonspecific gastritis. Although linked closely to chronic active (infiltration by neutrophils) gastritis, especially of the antrum, the importance of *H. pylori* at present is in regard to peptic ulcer pathogenesis and the potential for therapy and is covered in the article "Peptic Ulcer Disease." The source of *H. pylori* is unknown and it is found only in gastric-type mucosa. Person-to-person spread is important, as exemplified by data on intrafamilial clustering and a high prevalence by serologic testing in institutionalized persons. *H. pylori* has worldwide distribution and is found in 20 to 90% of various populations, depending on age, and social and hygienic status. Most people with *H. pylori* gastritis are asymptomatic and have normal-appearing gastric mucosa at endoscopy. Symptoms attributed to *H. pylori* gastritis are vague and similar to symptoms produced by other gastric conditions, including peptic ulcer and gastric malignancy. Evidence is accumulating that *H. pylori* may be linked to gastric adenocarcinoma and the low-grade B cell active lymphoma of mucosa-associated lymphoid tissue (MALT) type or gastric MALToma, previously known as pseudolymphoma. Preliminary data suggest that eradication of *H. pylori* in gastric MALToma may lead to regression of the lymphoma.

Direct and indirect methods exist to detect *H. pylori*. The direct methods are clinically the most commonly employed and require endoscopy with biopsy. The organism can be detected in a majority of cases on routine hematoxylin and eosin (H&E) stain, but occasionally special stains are required (Giemsa, Warthin-Starry). Culture of biopsy tissue is highly specific, but has a low yield in many clinical laboratories and is not widely done. Indirect methods make use of the urease enzyme produced by *H. pylori*, which splits urea into CO_2 and ammonia with a resultant increase in pH. The rapid urease tests require tissue to be placed on plates with urea and pH color indicator that changes from yellow to red as the pH rises. Urea carbon breath tests (^{13}C, ^{14}C) utilize the same chemical reaction to detect labeled CO_2 in the breath. Although highly specific and sensitive, they are not yet readily available for routine clinical use. Serologic tests can be obtained and are highly specific and sensitive for *H. pylori*. They are better suited for epidemiologic purposes than for assessing response to treatment, as titers may take months to decline.

Other disorders associated with nonerosive nonspecific gastritis include autoimmune gastritis and the reactive gastropathy seen in the postoperative stomach attributed to alkaline reflux. Autoimmune gastritis primarily affects the body and fundus, sparing the antrum with resultant achlorhydria. Some patients have pernicious anemia owing to inability to secrete intrinsic factor and may have other autoimmune disorders. More common is a state, usually in the elderly, with severe atrophic gastritis without pernicious anemia. In both entities, serology suggests that infection with *H. pylori* may play a role in pathogenesis, even though the organism is no longer present. The postoperative stomach has some degree of chronic inflammation, although this is not usually marked. The epithelial changes are the most striking with elongated foveolae, cuboidal epithelial cells with loss of mucin, and reactive changes.

"Specific or distinctive gastritis" refers to distinctive histologic and sometimes endoscopic features that are either diagnostic of a condition or markedly narrow the differential. Such abnormalities may be both erosive and nonerosive. Infectious agents in this group include bacteria (tuberculosis, syphilis), viruses (cytomegalovirus, herpes simplex virus), fungi (candidiasis, histoplasmosis), and parasites (cryptosporidium). Specific gastritis may occur as a part of generalized gastrointestinal disease (Crohn's disease, eosinophilic gastroenteritis) or as part of systemic disease (sarcoid, graft-versus-host disease). Miscellaneous types of gastritis—usually of unknown cause, but having distinctive features—are among this group. Menetrier's disease is one such example. Focal gastric lymphoid hyperplasia used to be of unknown cause, but is now known to be a result of *H. pylori* infection.

TREATMENT

Since symptoms of the entities included in this section are so vague and nonspecific, treatment starts with a thorough history and physical examination followed by appropriate laboratory, radiographic, and endoscopic procedures as indicated. Most of the lesions in the erosive and hemorrhagic group are readily apparent based on their clinical features and endoscopic findings. The treatment of stress-related lesions, NSAID gastropathy, and portal hypertensive gastropathy is covered in the articles "Peptic Ulcer Disease" and "Bleeding Esophageal Varices."

Most of the entities in the nonerosive nonspecific group are asymptomatic and require no treatment. Thus, when symptoms are present, it is difficult to attribute them to the inflammatory infiltrates and other histologic features of gastritis. It is important to exclude other causes for the patient's symptoms, such as biliary, pancreatic, or dysmotility disorders. Once this is done, treatment is usually empirical. If symptoms sound acid-peptic in nature, then a trial of antacids or an H_2 blocker is indicated. If symptoms or findings are suggestive of delayed gastric emptying or other dysmotility, a prokinetic agent such as cisapride (Propulsid)* 10 to 20 mg orally before meals and at bedtime may be beneficial. Metoclopramide

---

*Not FDA-approved for this indication.

(Reglan)* is less frequently used owing to its significant side effect profile.

The mere presence of *H. pylori* in the absence of ulcer disease does not constitute an indication for eradication therapy. The majority of people with *H. pylori* gastritis are asymptomatic, and eradication of *H. pylori* in those with symptoms (nonulcer dyspepsia) has not been shown to significantly improve symptoms. Should empirical therapy and reassurance fail and other causes for the patient's continued symptoms are excluded, an attempt to eradicate *H. pylori* may be justified. The most effective treatment to date still remains the 2-week triple therapy regimen of tetracycline* 500 mg four times daily, metronidazole (Flagyl)* 250 mg three times daily, and a bismuth compound, bismuth subsalicylate (Pepto-Bismol),* in a dose of 2 tablets four times daily. With good compliance, this regimen should have an eradication rate over 90%. Omeprazole (Prilosec),* 20 mg twice daily for 2 weeks, may enhance this eradication rate somewhat, but all four medications need to be started simultaneously. Amoxicillin,* 500 mg four times daily, plus omeprazole* 20 mg twice daily, both for 2 weeks, is a popular alternative regimen, but eradication rates are somewhat lower. The role of clarithromycin (Biaxin)* is being clarified, but it may be substituted for metronidazole and given as 500 mg three times daily for 2 weeks along with the other agents of a particular regimen. Treatment of the specific or distinctive forms of gastritis is that of the underlying infection or disease with surgery as an option for Crohn's disease, eosinophilic gastroenteritis, and Menetrier's disease, should medical therapy fail.

---

*Not FDA-approved for this indication.

ACUTE AND CHRONIC VIRAL HEPATITIS

method of
TONY LEMBO, M.D., and
PAUL MARTIN, M.D.
UCLA School of Medicine
Los Angeles, California

There are five major hepatotropic viruses, A through E. Although all these hepatitis viruses can cause acute viral hepatitis, only hepatitis viruses B, C, and D cause chronic liver disease. Cytomegalovirus (CMV) and Epstein-Barr virus (EBV) are less common causes of acute viral hepatitis and are not discussed here.

HEPATITIS A VIRUS

The hepatitis A virus (HAV) is a small RNA virus that causes acute hepatitis only. A serum antibody (anti-HAV) appears before symptoms begin and is present at the time of presentation. Immunoglobulin M (IgM) anti-HAV indicates a recent infection, whereas IgG anti-HAV, appearing 2 to 6 months later, provides immunity (Table 1).

Epidemiology

HAV is spread almost exclusively by the fecal-oral route. Since the hepatitis virus has a viremic phase of only several hours, parenteral transmission is extremely rare and accounts for less than 1% of cases. HAV has been detected in saliva, urine, and semen, but these bodily fluids probably do not transmit the virus. Vertical transmission has not been reported. Children are the principal group affected; in underdeveloped countries that are densely populated and have poor sanitation, up to 95% of young adults are IgG anti-HAV positive. In the United States, the age-adjusted prevalence of anti-HAV is 42% and is inversely associated with personal income. Waterborne and food-borne epidemics also occur. The modes of transmission in these outbreaks include raw food such as shellfish harvested from sewage-contaminated areas, and food contaminated by infected food handlers.

Clinical Course

The incubation period after HAV infection is 2 to 6 weeks. The virus appears in the stool in high concentrations toward the end of the incubation period but before the onset of symptoms. Viral shedding in the stools continues until the peak of symptoms, which is usually 1 to 2 weeks after presentation. The IgM anti-HAV is usually detectable in serum at the onset of symptoms (Table 2). Typically, the IgM anti-HAV antibody persists for 3 to 6 months after the acute illness and rarely up to 12 months. The IgG anti-HAV antibody appears within the first 2 months of the convalescent stage. The IgG anti-HAV provides lifelong immunity to the hepatitis A virus. False-positive IgM anti-HAV tests are very rare but occasionally are found in the presence of a positive rheumatoid factor antibody or hypergammaglobulinemia.

HAV infection is often clinically silent in children. Symptoms when they do occur in children are often mistaken for a viral gastroenteritis. Adults, who often are more symptomatic, can rarely develop fulminant hepatic failure. Hepatitis A symptoms resemble those of other viral hepatitis infections and typically include nausea, vomiting, low-grade temperature, anorexia, and fatigue. Right upper quadrant discomfort is often present because of stretching of the hepatic capsule. Darkening of the urine and lightening of stool color precede the onset of jaundice.

Elevation of the serum aminotransferase levels always precedes symptoms. The alanine aminotransferase (ALT) level is usually greater than the aspartate aminotransferase (AST), though the alkaline phosphatase level is near normal. Most patients recover within 1 to 2 months; biochemical abnormali-

TABLE 1. **Comparison of Hepatitis Viruses A, B, C, D, and E**

	HAV	HBV	HCV	HDV	HEV
Genome	RNA	DNA	RNA	RNA	RNA
Incubation (days)	15–45	30–180	15–150	30–180	15–60
Transmission	Fecal-oral	Blood and sexual	Blood	Blood (in the presence of HBV only)	Fecal-oral
Severity	Mild (worse with age)	Often severe	Mild (often insidious)	Moderate to severe	Mild (20% mortality rate in pregnant women)
Progression to chronicity	None	5–10%	>50%	Seen in HBV carriers	None

Abbreviations: HAV = hepatitis A virus; HBV = hepatitis B virus; HCV = hepatitis C virus; HDV = hepatitis D virus; HEV = hepatitis E virus.

ties, however, may persist for several months. In a small percentage of cases, patients may develop a prolonged cholestatic phase or relapse 1 to 3 months after an apparent recovery. The relapse resembles the original attack, and HAV is again found in the stool. In less than 1% of cases, fulminant hepatic failure occurs and orthotopic liver transplantation needs to be considered. Signs of impending fulminant hepatic failure include a markedly prolonged prothrombin time, hypoglycemia, disorientation, and a serum bilirubin level greater than 10 mg per dL.

Treatment

Since hepatitis A is not a chronic infection, alleviation of symptoms and not a cure of the disease is the goal of treatment. A low-fat, high-carbohydrate diet should be followed. Alcohol should be avoided. Sedatives and analgesics should not be taken unless essential. Hospitalization may be required for intravenous hydration, changes in mental status, or hypoglycemia.

Prevention

HAV is excreted in the stools of afflicted patients for as long as 1 to 2 weeks before the onset of symp-

TABLE 2. **Viral Hepatitis Serologic Findings**

	Acute Hepatitis	Chronic Hepatitis	Immunity
HAV	IgM anti-HAV		IgG anti-HAV
HBV	IgM anti-HBc	*Low-Level Replication*	anti-HBs
	HBsAg	HBsAg	
		IgG anti-HBc	
		anti-HBe	
		High-Level Replication	
		HBsAg	
		IgG anti-HBc	
		HBeAg or anti-HBe	
		HBV, DNA	
HDV	IgM anti-HDV	IgM anti-HDV *or*	
	IgM anti-HBc	IgG anti-HDV	
HCV	anti-HCV	anti-HCV	

Abbreviations: HAV = hepatitis A virus; HBV = hepatitis B virus; HCV = hepatitis C virus; HDV = hepatitis D virus; anti-HAV = antibody to HAV; anti-HBc = antibody to HBV core antigen; HBsAg = hepatitis B surface antigen; anti-HBs = antibody to HBsAg; HBeAg = hepatitis B e antigen; anti-HBe = antibody to HBeAg; anti-HCV = antibody to HCV; anti-HDV = antibody to HDV.

toms. Thus, spread of the virus usually occurs before knowledge of the disease. A single dose of immune serum globulin (ISG) administered within 2 weeks of exposure at a dose of 0.02 mL per kg prevents infection in 80 to 90% of patients. ISG is recommended for all household and intimate contacts of the patient with hepatitis A; age and pregnancy are not contraindications. Prophylaxis for school or work contacts is not recommended unless several cases have been identified. ISG should be administered before exposure for travelers to endemic areas. ISG provides protection from HAV for 4 to 6 months; repeat administration should be given for longer stays. Testing for anti-HAV in travelers, however, can reduce the need for ISG, particularly in those who are likely to have the antibody and thus have immunity (Table 3).

An HAV vaccine has been developed and is highly efficacious in preventing infection before exposure. Its efficacy in the postexposure setting is not known. The vaccine will be commercially available in the United States in the latter half of 1995, and guidelines for its use should be established by then.

HEPATITIS B VIRUS

The hepatitis B virus (HBV), a DNA virus, is a major cause of acute and chronic hepatitis, cirrhosis, and hepatocellular carcinoma in over 300 million infected people throughout the world. In the United States the chronic carrier rate of HBV is 0.1 to 0.5% of the population, whereas in Asia the rate may exceed 10%. In some isolated communities, such as Australian aborigine communities, the carrier rate is as high as 85%. The risk of developing chronic HBV infection after acute infection is greatest in infants infected at birth and declines with age.

Epidemiology

Transmission of HBV is primarily parenterally or by intimate contact (see Table 1). Vertical transmission from mother to newborn occurs in 70 to 90% of mothers who are positive for hepatitis B e antigen (HBeAg). HBeAg-negative mothers have a 10 to 40% risk of infecting their neonate. HBV is sexually transmitted; risk factors include multiple sexual partners,

TABLE 3. **Immunoprophylaxis and Vaccination Against Hepatitis A and B**

	Pre-Exposure	Post-Exposure
HAV	ISG (0.02 mL/kg). Repeat every 6 months if anti-HAV test is negative. Vaccine available in U.S. (1995)	ISG (0.02 mL/kg) within 2 weeks.
HBV	Recombinant HBV vaccine (10 μg or 1 mL) at 0 and 1 month and booster at 6 months. If anti-HBs test is negative and patient is high-risk, repeat booster.	HBIG (0.05 mL/kg) as soon as possible (preferable within 24 h) combined with the first of three HBV vaccine doses. Previously vaccinated patient should receive complete course unless anti-HBs test is positive.

Abbreviations: HAV = hepatitis A virus; HBV = hepatitis B virus; anti-HBs = antibody to hepatitis B surface antigen; anti-HBc = antibody to hepatitis B core antigen; HBIG = hepatitis B immune globulin; ISG = immune serum globulin.

a history of sexually transmitted diseases, and homosexuality (especially with receptive anal intercourse). Percutaneous exposures such as sharing of hypodermic needles and inadvertent needle sticks also result in HBV transmission. Blood transfusion has become an extremely rare cause of HBV infection since screening of all donors with hepatitis B surface antigen (HBsAg) began over 20 years ago. The presence of the HBeAg in serum correlates with greater infectivity. In the United States, 30 to 40% of patients with HBV infection do not acknowledge any risk factors for such infection, and at least some presumably acquire the disease from inapparent parenteral contact (Table 4).

Clinical Course

Less than 5% of adult patients with acute HBV infection develop a chronic infection; the remainder resolve their infection. The clinical course of acute hepatitis B is similar to that of other types of viral hepatitis. Subclinical infections are common. The nonicteric patient is more likely to develop chronic infection than the icteric one as the inflammatory activity and associated liver injury correlate with an enhanced immunologic host response. On rare occasions, patients with chronic hepatitis B can develop immune complex diseases such as polymyalgia rheumatica, polyarteritis, essential mixed cryoglobulinemia, glomerulonephritis, and myocarditis.

Three different HBV-associated viral antigens or their corresponding antibodies are available for routine serologic testing: HBsAg and its corresponding antibody (anti-HBs), HBeAg and its corresponding an-

TABLE 4. **People at Risk for Hepatitis B**

IVDA or people with other percutaneous exposures such as tattoos
Homosexuals (especially with receptive anal intercourse), or heterosexuals with multiple sexual partners
Neonates born to mothers with hepatitis B: 20–40% transmission rate if mother is HBsAg-positive only; 70–90% if mother is HBeAg-positive
Health care workers exposed to blood products
Institutionalized patients
Patients on hemodialysis
Natives of endemic areas such as Australia, Asia, Africa

Abbreviations: HBsAg = hepatitis B surface antigen; HBeAg = hepatitis B e antigen; IVDA = intravenous drug abusers.

tibody (anti-HBe), and antibody to hepatitis B core antigen (anti-HBc) (see Table 2). Hepatitis B core antigen is found only in infected liver cells and is not detectable in serum. The presence of IgM anti-HBc in serum implies acute HBV infection. Since HBsAg is found in both acute infection and chronic HBV infection, its presence does not necessarily indicate an acute infection, whereas the presence of IgM anti-HBc does indicate an acute infection. HBeAg correlates with ongoing viral synthesis and with infectivity. HBsAg usually is detectable during the clinical illness and disappears during convalescence. Recently, assays to detect HBV DNA by molecular hybridization and the polymerase chain reaction (PCR) have become available. Molecular hybridization techniques can detect DNA concentrations of 10^6 genomes per mL, and such detection signifies ongoing replication of HBV in hepatocytes. The PCR technique is more sensitive and can detect HBV DNA in quantities as low as 10 to 50 genomes per mL. Detection of HBV DNA by the PCR technique, but not by the molecular hybridization technique, signifies ongoing HBV infection with little active replication. The persistence of HBsAg for more than 12 weeks after the onset of HBV-related symptoms is a predictor of chronic infection, whereas the presence of HBsAg for 6 months or longer indicates chronicity. The presence of anti-HBs indicates resolution of infection and provides immunity to HBV.

When HBsAg persists without abnormal ALT levels or other signs of liver disease, the term "healthy carrier" can be used. Healthy carriers without markers of replication such as HBeAg or HBV DNA appear to have few significant sequelae of chronic liver disease. Although HBsAg usually persists in chronically infected individuals, approximately 1% of HBsAg-positive patients lose their HBsAg each year. The HBeAg tends to disappear in about 50% of chronically infected patients with active replication over time; loss of HBeAg is often accompanied by a transient rise in ALT levels and worsening of symptoms. Anti-HBe production can be transient, and it is often not detected in serum. Reactivation of hepatitis B can occur spontaneously or after treatment with immunosuppressive agents such as steroids or chemotherapy.

Prognosis

Patients who acquired chronic HBV infection during childhood have a 300-fold increase in the risk of developing hepatocellular carcinoma. This risk appears to be increased in men, with the presence of cirrhosis, and with increasing duration of disease. An annual surveillance program including serial serum alpha-fetoprotein levels and right upper quadrant ultrasound examinations should be undertaken in patients who are felt to have acquired HBV infection in childhood.

Treatment and Prevention

As with HAV infection, treatment of acute HBV infection consists mainly of alleviation of symptoms. Persons who have been exposed to HBV, either through blood products (e.g., needle stick) or through sexual contact should be offered hepatitis B immune globulin (HBIG) at a dose of 0.05 mL per kg, preferably within 24 hours of exposure. This should be followed by a course of recombinant HBV vaccine (Table 3).

Recently, recombinant interferon-alfa-2b (Intron A) has been approved for the treatment of chronic hepatitis B. The usual dose is 5 million U subcutaneously daily for 16 weeks. Approximately 40% of patients lose HBeAg, and 10% of patients subsequently lose HBsAg after clearance of HBeAg. Side effects include hair loss, leukopenia, flulike symptoms, diarrhea, fatigue, thrombocytopenia, and mood changes. Predictors of response are a relatively short duration of HBV infection, raised pretreatment ALT levels, and low HBV DNA levels. Patients with decompensated cirrhosis should not receive interferon, as the immune-mediated flare in disease activity may cause worsening of hepatic function.

The HBV vaccine is effective in preventing HBV infection. Pre-exposure immunization with recombinant HBV vaccine should be considered in high-risk groups such as homosexuals or promiscuous heterosexuals, intravenous drug abusers, hemodialysis patients, institutionalized patients, close family and sexual contacts of chronic hepatitis B patients, and health care workers. Furthermore, the Centers for Disease Control and Prevention (CDC) now recommends that all children be vaccinated against HBV regardless of their exposure risk. The vaccine is given at a dose of 10 μg intramuscularly at 0, 1, and 6 months. If serum HBsAb is not detected after 5 to 7 years, a further booster dose of the vaccine should be considered.

HEPATITIS D VIRUS (DELTA VIRUS)

The hepatitis D virus (HDV), or delta virus, is a defective RNA virus that requires the HBV genome to replicate, and thus HDV infection can occur only in patients who are also infected with HBV. HDV infection can be acquired simultaneously as co-infection with HBV or by superinfection of a patient already HBV-infected. Co-infection by HBV and HDV leads to more severe acute disease and a higher risk of fulminant hepatic failure (2 to 20%). Chronic HBV carriers who acquire superinfection with HDV have a higher incidence of chronic liver disease with cirrhosis (70 to 80%) compared with HBV infection alone (15 to 30%) (see Table 1).

The modes of transmission of HDV are similar to those of HBV. Parenteral transmission from shared needles by intravenous drug abusers is the most common route, whereas sexual transmission of HDV appears to be significantly less efficient. Serologic tests for IgM and total anti-HDV are commercially available. Since HDV antigen (HDAg) is found infrequently in serum, anti-HDV is often the only indicator of an HDV infection. IgM anti-HDV appears 10 to 15 days after the onset of jaundice, and therefore repeat testing for IgM anti-HDV is recommended if initial testing is negative.

Interferon therapy is less successful with HDV-HBV co-infection than in HBV infection alone. Relapses are frequent after cessation of therapy, and treatment for longer periods of time may be necessary than with HBV alone. Vaccination against HBV prevents HDV infection in the individual who has not yet acquired HBV. HBV carriers should reduce potential risk factors of acquiring HDV, especially continued drug abuse.

HEPATITIS C VIRUS

The hepatitis C virus (HCV) is a single-stranded RNA virus that was first discovered in 1989. It is responsible for most cases of what was previously known as non-A, non-B hepatitis. Approximately 1 to 2% of the world population is chronically infected with HCV. Unlike hepatitis B, in which only 5 to 10% of patients develop chronic hepatitis, the majority of patients with acute HCV infections develop chronic hepatitis (see Table 1). HCV is also a major cause of hepatocellular carcinoma.

Epidemiology

HCV is transmitted by infected blood, such as transfused blood, infected donor organs, or blood from needles shared by intravenous drug abusers (Table 5). Approximately 10% of health care workers who are exposed to HCV through needle sticks develop the disease. Although studies have not been conclusive, sexual transmission of HCV probably does occur, albeit at a very low rate. Perinatal transmission of HCV is also uncommon. In general, HCV is much less infectious than HBV.

Clinical Course

The clinical picture of acute hepatitis C is usually mild. The virus has an incubation period of 2 to 21 weeks, after which only 25% of patients become jaundiced. Indeed, many patients with acute hepatitis C are minimally symptomatic. Serum aminotransferase levels increase after 7 to 8 weeks but are only mildly elevated (10 to 15 times normal). Most patients with acute hepatitis C develop chronic disease. Typically the course of chronic hepatitis C is

TABLE 5. **Prevalence of Hepatitis C**

Risk Factor	Anti-HCV-Positive (%)
IVDA	60–90
Hemophilia	50–90
Hemodialysis	20
High-risk sexual behaviors	1–10
Health-care work	1
Volunteer blood donation (in the U.S.)	0.5

Abbreviations: Anti-HCV = hepatitis C virus antibody; IVDA = intravenous drug abuse.

characterized by slightly abnormal aminotransferase levels (2 to 3 times normal), which fluctuate over time. Cirrhosis develops in 10 to 25% of patients with chronic infection followed over several years. Cirrhotic patients are at increased risk of developing hepatocellular carcinoma.

In 1990 a serologic first-generation enzyme-linked immunosorbent assay (ELISA) became available commercially; it detected antibodies against C100-3, a recombinant polypeptide derived from a nonstructural region of the HCV genome. In 1992, the second-generation serologic ELISA, which is more sensitive and specific, became available. It detects antibodies to structural and nonstructural HCV antigens 5-1-1, C-22, C-33, and C100-3. With the second-generation test, antibodies to HCV can be detected as early as 6 weeks after infection and are almost always detected within 20 weeks of an infection. The recombinant immunoblot assay (RIBA) uses similar HCV antigens (C100-3, 5-1-1, C33c from the nonstructural region, C22-3 from the HCV core-associated region, as well as superoxide dismutase). The major use of RIBA testing is to confirm a positive ELISA result. Detection of small amounts of HCV RNA by the PCR technique is also possible and is used at present mainly as a research tool.

Since anti-HCV seroconversion can occur weeks after the onset of symptoms, it often cannot be used to make the initial diagnosis of acute HCV. The anti-HCV antibody is non-neutralizing. Multiple strains of the virus exist, and there is a high mutation rate. The anti-HCV antibody can persist in patients who apparently do not have chronic infection, often for many years. False-positive antibody tests occasionally occur in autoimmune hepatitis and hypergammaglobulinemia. A small percentage of the normal population also have false-positive assays. In these patients, the HCV antibody titer is usually low.

Prevention

Routine screening of blood donors for anti-HCV as well as the previously introduced screen of ALT and anti-HBc by blood banks has reduced the incidence of post-transfusion hepatitis. A vaccine is not yet available.

Treatment

Currently, recombinant interferon-alfa-2b is the only approved treatment for HCV. After a 6-month course of 3 million U given three times per week, approximately 50% of patients have a biochemical and histologic response. Unfortunately, 50% of the responders relapse after the completion of therapy. Currently, trials of longer-term therapy and different dosing regimens of interferon are under way. Contraindications to treatment include thrombocytopenia, decompensated liver disease, autoimmune diseases, and psychiatric conditions. Patients most likely to respond to therapy include those with a low viral load and, probably, those with certain strains of HCV.

HEPATITIS E VIRUS

Hepatitis E virus (HEV) is an RNA virus that is spread through the fecal-oral route. It is most commonly found in developing countries including India and Mexico, and in Central and South America, and North Africa. The clinical features of hepatitis E are similar to those of hepatitis A, although it is associated with a high mortality (20%) in pregnant women in their third trimester. HEV is not indigenous to the United States, but cases have been reported in travelers from third-world countries. The incubation period is 2 to 8 weeks, and chronic infection does not occur. Anti-HEV antibodies are now available in research laboratories.

MALABSORPTION SYNDROMES

method of
CHRISTOPHER F. SCHULTZ, M.D., and
GARY R. LICHTENSTEIN, M.D.
University of Pennsylvania
Philadelphia, Pennsylvania

NORMAL DIGESTION AND ABSORPTION

Normal digestion begins in the mouth with mastication and secretion of salivary amylase and acid-resistant lipase. As the food bolus enters the stomach, it causes gastric distention and stimulates the release of hydrochloric acid, pepsinogen, gastric lipase, and intrinsic factor. The stomach functions as a reservoir capable of segregating chyme along a pH gradient that allows for digestion by pH-sensitive peptides. The slow release of small food particles into the duodenum and the selective retention of larger pieces of food are accomplished by the concerted action of both phasic and tonic contractions of the stomach, the ability of the pylorus to control flow, and the receptive capacity of the small bowel. In the proximal small intestine, digestion continues through the action of pancreatic enzymes (amylase, lipase, trypsin, chymotrypsin, and carboxypeptidase), bile salts, and brush border enzymes.

Absorption of nutrients occurs throughout the length of the small intestine with certain substrates having preferred regions of absorption. Monoglycerides, fatty acids, iron, calcium, and water-soluble vitamins are primarily absorbed in the proximal small bowel. Absorption of vitamin B_{12}–intrinsic factor complexes and intraluminal bile salts, however, requires specific receptors located in the terminal ileum.

Impairment of either the normal intraluminal digestion of food or the intestinal absorption of nutrients is commonly referred to as "malabsorption."

PATHOGENESIS

Syndromes of malabsorption can be classified on the basis of the predominant pathophysiologic mechanism: (1) impaired intraluminal digestion (maldigestion), (2) impaired nutrient absorption, and (3) impaired delivery to tissues. Maldigestion (of proteins, lipids, and carbohydrates) may result from either low intraluminal concentrations of pancreatic enzymes or inactivation of normally secreted digestive enzymes. Chronic pancreatitis subsequent to alcoholism, hereditary pancreatitis, traumatic pancreatic duct disruption, idiopathic pancreatitis, cystic fibrosis, tropical pancreatitis, protein-calorie malnutrition, isolated pancreatic enzyme deficiency (e.g., lipase, colipase), trypsinogen-enterokinase enzyme deficiency, pancreatic and duodenal neoplasms, pancreatic resection, hemochromatosis, Shwachman-Bodian syndrome (pancreatic insufficiency and bone marrow dysfunction), and Johanson-Blizzard syndrome (multiple developmental abnormalities and pancreatic insufficiency) can result in reduced secretion of pancreatic enzymes with subsequent maldigestion. Alternatively, acid-hypersecretory states, such as Zollinger-Ellison syndrome, are associated with malabsorption by luminal inactivation of normally secreted acid-labile pancreatic enzymes (such as lipase and colipase).

Once digestion has occurred and fats are broken down into their constituent components (fatty acids and monoglycerides), conjugated bile salts are necessary for the formation of mixed micelles and the solubilization of these components. A reduction in the intraluminal concentration of bile salts can result in fat maldigestion and/or malabsorption. Inadequate intestinal bile salt concentrations may be seen secondary to (1) decreased synthesis in acute and chronic hepatocellular disease, (2) impaired excretion in the setting of intrahepatic or extrahepatic cholestasis, (3) bile salt depletion with biliary drainage, terminal ileal disease, or resection (typically in excess of 90 cm) resulting in interruption of the enterohepatic circulation, and (4) deconjugation of bile salts by a reduction in luminal pH (Zollinger-Ellison syndrome) or metabolism by bacteria in disease states predisposing to bacterial overgrowth (such as the blind loop syndrome, scleroderma, intestinal pseudo-obstruction).

Mucosal dysfunction is a common mechanism for a large, diverse group of disease processes and predisposing conditions resulting in nutrient malabsorption. Deficiencies in brush border enzymes (e.g., lactase) cause malabsorption of specific nutrients. Diffuse small bowel mucosal injury caused by inflammatory or infiltrative disorders such as Crohn's disease, infectious enteritis, tropical sprue, radiation enteritis, eosinophilic enteritis, amyloidosis, scleroderma, and lymphoma can result in poor translocation of intestinal contents. Gluten-sensitive enteropathy (celiac sprue) with severe effacement of intestinal microvilli and short bowel syndrome secondary to surgical resection decrease the absorptive surface area available to luminal contents and frequently cause malabsorption. A reduction in intestinal transit time is seen with intestinal bypass surgery for morbid obesity, enteroenteric fistulous disease secondary to regional enteritis, and postgastrectomy syndromes.

After uptake of nutrients by intestinal enterocytes, malabsorption of fat and/or protein-losing enteropathy may still occur with lymphatic obstruction secondary to intestinal lymphangiectasia, Whipple's disease, and lymphoma. Abetalipoproteinemia, a disease that typically presents in young children, is associated with steatorrhea secondary to impaired chylomicron synthesis.

CLINICAL PRESENTATION

Whereas the pathologic processes leading to malabsorption are so disparate, and the associated symptom complexes so variable, it is reassuring to note that initial complaints of many patients are often related to common functional abnormalities of the bowel. Diarrhea is most common and may be secondary to one or several mechanisms including the impaired absorption of water and electrolytes, hypersecretion of gastric acid, diffuse small intestinal exudative inflammation, the osmotic effect of unabsorbed carbohydrates, or fat maldigestion/malabsorption and resultant steatorrhea. Patients with steatorrhea may describe loose or watery, voluminous stools that are often foul-smelling and may be oily in appearance. Excessive flatus owing to bacterial fermentation of undigested carbohydrate reaching the colon is also common.

Other, less-specific symptoms are frequently reported with a more indolent presentation. Cachexia and malnutrition can result from anorexia and fecal loss of calories. Edema secondary to hypoalbuminemia may be seen in patients with protein malabsorption and protein-losing enteropathy. Fatigue and malaise are commonly observed in association with anemia (impaired assimilation of iron, vitamin B_{12}, and folic acid). Deficiencies in fat-soluble vitamins may result in purpura and ecchymoses (vitamin K deficiency); xerophthalmia, follicular hyperkeratosis, night blindness (vitamin A deficiency); osteomalacia/osteoporosis and tetany/paresthesias (vitamin D deficiency); or neurologic symptoms mimicking spinocerebellar degeneration (vitamin E deficiency). Peripheral neuropathy may be a manifestation of vitamin B_{12} or thiamine malabsorption. Dermatologic abnormalities including dermatitis, glossitis, cheilosis, and stomatitis complicate a variety of vitamin deficiencies.

Alternatively, specific signs and symptoms can suggest certain pathologic processes and allow for a more directed diagnostic evaluation. Constant, midepigastric, abdominal pain radiating through to the back and a history of alcohol abuse suggest chronic pancreatitis. Severe peptic ulcer disease and/or gastroesophageal reflux disease unresponsive to acid suppression may be seen with the Zollinger-Ellison syndrome. Jaundice and other signs of chronic liver disease are prominent findings in patients with hepatocellular dysfunction and a reduction in bile salt synthesis. Arthritis, cardiac abnormalities, and neurologic deficits in persons with malabsorption should suggest Whipple's disease.

DIAGNOSIS

Evaluation for suspected malabsorption must begin with a detailed history. A previous diagnosis of inflammatory bowel disease, pancreatitis, alcoholism, chronic liver disease, connective tissue diseases, or human immunodeficiency virus (HIV) infection should be sought. Previous surgery for peptic ulcer disease, large resections of small bowel, surgery for obesity, and previous radiotherapy are important predisposing conditions that must be elicited. If diarrhea is a prominent complaint, an attempt to characterize the frequency, appearance, and amount of stool and the duration of increased stool output is essential. The response to fasting, the relationship to meals, the presence or absence of mucus or blood in the stool, and an association with certain foods (dairy products, sorbitol-containing food products) or medicines (lactulose, cathartics) are important historical considerations. Finally, a detailed history of HIV risk factors and recent or past travel may also yield useful information suggesting potential causes (e.g., giardiasis, tropical sprue).

Initial screening tests in a patient with suspected malabsorption may include (1) complete blood count (CBC) with differential and mean corpuscular volume (MCV), (2) serum iron, ferritin, transferrin, or total iron-binding capacity (TIBC), (3) vitamin B_{12} and folate levels, (4) liver-associated enzymes, albumin, cholesterol, (5) calcium, prothrombin time, serum carotene, and (6) abdominal radiographs (which may demonstrate pancreatic calcifications in patients with chronic pancreatitis).

Because the majority of disorders causing malabsorption result in the fecal loss of fat, if initial screening tests are suggestive of malabsorption, a Sudan stain for fecal fat should be performed (Figure 1). The specimen is ideally collected while the patient is eating a regular diet over a course of several days prior to testing. A small amount of feces is treated with two drops of 36% acetic acid and stained with Sudan III stain. The sample is then heated to boiling and immediately examined for the presence of orange-red fat globules. A strongly positive Sudan stain is recorded if 100 or more fat globules measuring 6 to 75 μm in diameter are present per high-power field (HPF). A positive test demonstrates more than 100 fat globules measuring 4 to 8 μm in diameter per HPF. A negative Sudan stain should contain no more than a very few, very small fat droplets. Properly performed, the Sudan stain is highly sensitive and specific (~90%) for the detection of fat malabsorption. Occasionally, a patient with malabsorption will have a negative Sudan stain because the dietary fat intake has been inadequate (false-negative) or because the subject has a specific malabsorptive disorder of protein (protein-losing enteropathy) or carbohydrate (lactase or sucrase-isomaltase deficiency) resulting in a true-negative test for fat malabsorption.

The quantitative stool fat measurement is the most sensitive test for lipid malabsorption. It is indicated in the evaluation of individuals in whom the suspicion for steatorrhea is high and who have an equivocal or negative Sudan III stain assessment. The test requires that the patient consume a 100-gram fat diet for 5 days with complete stool collection occurring over a 72-hour period on days 3, 4, and 5. Stool fat in excess of 7 grams over 24 hours indicates an abnormality in fat absorption (coefficient of fat absorption <93% is abnormal).

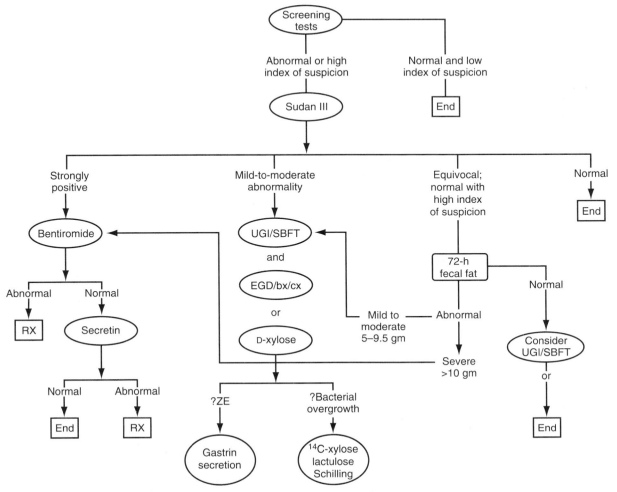

Figure 1. Algorithm for the diagnosis of malabsorption. *Abbreviations*: UGI/SBFT = upper gastrointestinal series with small bowel follow-through; EGD/bx/cx = esophagogastroduodenoscopy, biopsy, and culture; RX = treatment; ZE = Zollinger-Ellison syndrome.

Once the presence of steatorrhea has been confirmed, it is necessary to determine whether the abnormality involves a defect in the luminal digestion of nutrients or an insult to the integrity of the absorptive surface of the small intestine. An appropriate first study in mild-to-moderate fat malabsorption is the upper gastrointestinal series with a small bowel follow-through (UGI/SBFT) that will delineate the anatomy and may guide further diagnostic studies (i.e., esophagogastroduodenoscopy and small bowel biopsy). Aphthous ulcerations, thickening of folds, a cobblestone appearance, fissures, strictures, or fistulas suggest small bowel Crohn's disease. An abnormal separation of jejunal folds (three folds or valvulae conniventes per inch of jejunum instead of the normal five) may be seen in celiac disease. Anatomic abnormalities predisposing to stasis and possible bacterial overgrowth such as surgical blind loops, duodenal-jejunal diverticular disease, obstruction, and pseudo-obstruction should be easily demonstrated. Other nonspecific findings (fold thickening, nodular mucosa, mild dilatation) may also be found in the presence of mucosal disease.

In patients with mild-to-moderate steatorrhea (>7 grams of stool fat but <9.5 grams over 24 hours on a 100-gram fat diet), with or without findings on UGI/SBFT, upper endoscopy with small bowel biopsy (plus, in experienced institutions, quantitative anaerobic proximal small intestinal cultures) is probably the next most appropriate diagnostic study. Characteristic endoscopic mucosal changes may be observed and histopathology can be diagnostic or strongly suggestive of certain disease states. Microscopic study of mucosal biopsies is diagnostic in Whipple's disease, *Mycobacterium avium-intracellulare* (MAI) infection (pseudo-Whipple's), abetalipoproteinemia, and agammaglobulinemia. Although sometimes limited by the patchy nature of the mucosal involvement, histopathology may be diagnostic in intestinal lymphangiectasia, lymphoma, eosinophilic enteritis, amyloidosis, Crohn's disease, and giardiasis. Strongly suggestive mucosal changes are seen in celiac sprue, tropical sprue, collagenous sprue, radiation enteritis, bacterial overgrowth, and infectious enteritis.

The D-xylose absorption test is performed in the evaluation of possible small intestinal mucosal disease when (1) upper endoscopy with biopsy is not available or contraindicated, (2) small bowel biopsy is normal but UGI/SBFT demonstrates distal disease, or (3) clinical suspicion for mucosal disease is high but other tests are negative. A five-carbon nondietary sugar, D-xylose, is primarily absorbed by passive diffusion and its uptake reflects the absorptive surface area of the small intestine and epithelial cell membrane permeability. The test is performed after an overnight fast. The patient first voids to empty the bladder and 25 grams of D-xylose is given orally with water. The patient is encouraged to drink fluids to ensure good urine output. All urine is collected for the next 5 hours and blood is drawn for serum D-xylose concentration at 1 and 2 hours after the oral dose. A normal urine D-xylose output is 5 grams over 5 hours and the peak serum concentration is greater than 25 mg/dl. A low urine or serum D-xylose level is consistent with the diagnosis of a mucosal abnormality. False-positive test results can occur with inadequate urine collection or renal insufficiency. Abnormally low levels are also seen in patients with ascites or massive edema secondary to third-spacing of D-xylose. Nonsteroidal anti-inflammatory drugs may also result in poor uptake or reduced urinary excretion of D-xylose.

If historical information strongly suggests pancreatic exocrine insufficiency, if steatorrhea is severe (>10 grams of stool fat over 24 hours), or if small bowel disease has been satisfactorily ruled out by the aforementioned tests, it is appropriate to consider evaluation for pancreatic exocrine dysfunction. The bentiromide (Chymex) test is a noninvasive, simply performed assessment of pancreatic chymotrypsin release. Bentiromide, or N-benzoyl-L-tyrosyl-p-aminobenzoic acid, is a synthetic peptide that is cleaved by chymotrypsin to release para-aminobenzoic acid (PABA). Following the oral administration of 500 mg of bentiromide, free PABA is absorbed in the proximal small intestine, partially conjugated in the liver, and excreted in the urine. An excretion of less than 50% in 6 hours is diagnostic of pancreatic insufficiency. Unfortunately, the test is not very sensitive for mild-to-moderate degrees of pancreatic insufficiency and may give false-positive results with severe mucosal disease, severe hepatocellular disease, renal disease, and diabetes mellitus. The most sensitive test currently available to assess exocrine function of the pancreas is the secretin stimulation test. Secretin is a very potent stimulator of pancreatic bicarbonate secretion and when administered intravenously in a dose of 2 U per kg should result in pancreatic secretions with a bicarbonate concentration of greater than 90 mEq/L. The test does require duodenal intubation and is not available at all centers.

If the UGI/SBFT demonstrates abnormalities predisposing to stasis or if there is a history of scleroderma, a disorder of intestinal motility, resection of the ileocecal valve, or achlorhydria, the diagnosis of bacterial overgrowth syndrome should be entertained. The 1-gram ^{14}C-xylose breath test demonstrates excellent sensitivity and specificity for the presence of bacterial overgrowth. This compound is not normally metabolized by humans but is metabolized by gram-negative aerobes, which are always part of the overgrowth flora. Radiolabeled CO_2 is then absorbed and the expired $^{14}CO_2$ is measured. The exhaled $^{14}CO_2$ will reach a diagnostic level in 85% of patients with bacterial overgrowth within 60 minutes. Because the ^{14}C-xylose breath test requires exposure to small amounts of radiation, it is not recommended for children or pregnant women. In this clinical setting, the hydrogen breath test (with a sensitivity of 90% and a specificity of 78%) is the most appropriate means of evaluation. The test involves the ingestion of a nonabsorbable carbohydrate (e.g., lactulose), which is metabolized by bacteria to H_2 (not a by-product of human metabolic processes) and can be measured in the expelled air within the first 2 hours. Abnormalities of the rate of intestinal transit can confuse the interpretation of tests for bacterial overgrowth. Delayed gastric emptying can result in the late release of $^{14}CO_2$ or H_2. Rapid intestinal transit may cause early delivery of substrates to normal colonic bacteria, producing an earlier than expected rise in expired $^{14}CO_2$ or H_2. Finally, the Schilling test, performed before and repeated after the administration of oral antibiotics, is available at all centers for the diagnosis of bacterial overgrowth.

SPECIFIC DISORDERS AND THEIR MANAGEMENT

Impaired Luminal Digestion

Pancreatic Insufficiency

Pancreatic exocrine insufficiency is usually secondary to chronic pancreatitis, which in Western society, is due to alcoholism in 70% of cases. Recurrent episodes of severe abdominal pain or reports of constant epigastric pain will predate steatorrhea, which is not observed until pancreatic lipase output is less than 10% of normal. In this setting salivary amylase and lipase have clinically significant activity but are ultimately insufficient in preventing malabsorption. Cachexia and malnutrition ensue. The 24-hour fecal fat content is abnormal and can reach 30 to 40 grams. The bentiromide test should be abnormal and the Schilling test may demonstrate mild vitamin B_{12} malabsorption.

Treatment consists of oral enzyme replacement (and, in the setting of chronic pancreatitis, pain control). Malabsorption does not occur if more than 5% of normal maximal postprandial enzyme activity is delivered to the duodenum. This level is achieved if oral enzyme supplements can provide approximately 30,000 IU of lipase per meal to the small intestine. A number of commercially available preparations are now in general use. Clinicians should choose preparations with higher lipase activity to enable patients to reduce the number of pills they must take with each meal (improving compliance) and maximize duodenal delivery. Because pancreatic enzymes are inactivated by the action of gastric acid and pepsin, several approaches have been designed to protect capsules or tablets with acid-resistant and alkali-sensitive coatings. To date, no single preparation design has been clearly demonstrated to be superior. If several different preparations have failed to alleviate steatorrhea and the patient has documented acidic duodenal pH, a trial of acid suppression with H_2 receptor antagonists is indicated.

Zollinger-Ellison Syndrome

Diarrhea occurs in approximately 33 to 50% of patients with gastrinoma and it may be the presenting symptom in up to 35% of these individuals. The diarrhea may be the product of one or several mechanisms: (1) the secretion of large volumes of gastric acid, (2) the osmotic effect of steatorhhea secondary to deconjugation of bile salts and the denaturation of pancreatic enzymes, and (3) the exudative inflammatory changes seen with severe peptic ulceration. The diagnosis is generally established by the demonstration of fasting hypergastrinemia (>1000 pg/ml) and gastric acid hypersecretion or a gastric pH of less than 3. Provocative testing is indicated and necessary in patients with a nondiagnostic fasting level of hypergastrinemia or if the cause of hypergastrinemia is in question. The intravenous injection of secretin (2 U/kg) should produce an increase of at least 200 pg/ml over baseline serum gastrin levels. This increase usually occurs within the first 10 minutes following the intravenous administration of secretin.

The medical management of gastric acid hypersecretion in the Zollinger-Ellison syndrome has been revolutionized by the substituted benzimidazoles such as omeprazole (Prilosec), which covalently bind to the H^+K^+/ATPase proton pump and dramatically inhibit acid secretion. A median daily dose of 40 mg orally in one or two divided doses is effective in the majority of Zollinger-Ellison syndrome patients. Tachyphylaxis, historically a problem with H_2 receptor antagonists, seems to be observed less frequently with omeprazole. The potency, efficacy, long duration of action, and desirable safety profile of these agents make proton pump inhibition with omeprazole the treatment of choice for peptic ulcer disease and diarrhea associated with the Zollinger-Ellison syndrome. Total gastrectomy should be considered only in patients who are noncompliant with medical therapy or who do not have access to routine medical follow-up.

An increasing appreciation for the presence of extrapancreatic primary neoplasms (perhaps as high as 66%) and improved diagnostic modalities in specialized centers now allow potentially curative resection in up to 30% of patients. The precise role of chemotherapy, hepatic artery embolization, debulking of tumor, and use of somatostatin analogues in the treatment of metastatic gastrinoma has not been defined.

Bacterial Overgrowth Syndrome

Some of clinical conditions most often associated with bacterial overgrowth have been mentioned previously and a more comprehensive list can be found in Table 1. Bacterial overgrowth is defined as the demonstration of greater than 100,000 organisms per ml of small intestinal luminal aspirate. The flora is polymicrobial and often a predominance of facultative anaerobes and/or strict anaerobes is seen. Common clinical features of bacterial overgrowth include (1) vitamin B_{12} deficiency and a macrocytic anemia, the result of cobalamin uptake by gram-negative anaerobes, (2) fat malabsorption and diarrhea secondary to the deconjugation of bile salts, (3) bloating and

TABLE 1. **Conditions Predisposing to Bacterial Overgrowth**

Anatomic Abnormalities Producing Stasis
Strictures
   Crohn's disease
   Radiation enteritis
   Vasculitis
Duodenal-jejunal diverticular disease
Afferent loop of Bilroth II and other surgical blind loops
Anatomic Abnormalities Allowing Proximal Migration of Distal Bowel Flora
Fistulas
   Gastrocolic
   Jejunocolic
   Gastroileal
   Jejunoileal
Resection of ileocecal valve
Motor Abnormalities
Scleroderma
Diabetic visceral neuropathy
Idiopathic intestinal pseudo-obstruction
Reduced Host Defenses
Hypochlorhydria or achlorhydria
   Pernicious anemia
   Medical therapy to suppress acid
Immunodeficiency syndromes
Cirrhosis
Miscellaneous
Pancreatic insufficiency

abdominal pain, and (4) hypoproteinemia, guaiac-positive stools, and a hypochromic microcytic anemia with small intestinal mucosal damage in the blind loop syndrome. The diagnosis, as described previously, can be made by culture, ^{14}C-xylose breath test, H$_2$ breath test, or the Schilling test.

Treatment is directed at reducing the degree of bacterial overgrowth, with either antimicrobial agents or reversal of the condition predisposing to intestinal stasis. Traditionally, tetracycline 250 mg orally four times daily, trimethoprim-sulfamethoxazole (TMP–SMX) (Bactrim DS) one tablet by mouth twice daily, or metronidazole (Flagyl) 250 mg orally three times a day have been used. Problems with resistance (particularly to tetracycline) have resulted in the use of newer agents such as amoxicillin-clavulanate (Augmentin) 250 to 500 mg three times daily. Initial therapy should continue for 7 to 10 days. If symptoms do not resolve, patients may require continuous treatment for 1 to 2 months. With symptoms that recur frequently, cyclical therapy (antibiotics for 1 week of every 4) may provide long-term symptomatic relief. Nutritional support should be aggressive. Deficiencies of specific vitamins require correction. Promotility agents and somatostatin analogues have not been demonstrated to be reliable therapeutic options; however, they may be considered in refractory cases.

Impaired Nutrient Absorption

Celiac Disease (Gluten-Sensitive Enteropathy)

Celiac sprue is characterized by the development of villous atrophy in response to ingestion of dietary proteins contained in cereal grains such as wheat, rye, barley, and oats. The offending agent has been shown to be gliadin, the alcohol-soluble component of the water-insoluble protein gluten found in these grains. The actual mechanism of disease is unknown but several theories have been postulated. Enzyme deficiency leading to accumulation of "toxic peptides," genetic predisposition, autoimmune processes, and environmental factors have all been implicated. Patients classically present with diarrhea, flatulence, weight loss, and fatigue, but symptoms can vary tremendously and some individuals will present with only iron deficiency, folate malabsorption, or hypocalcemia. Steatorrhea is usually present but the diagnosis requires (1) demonstration of characteristic histologic changes (villous atrophy, damage to enterocytes, crypt hyperplasia, and increased mitoses) on small bowel biopsy, (2) unequivocal clinical response to gluten withdrawal, and (3) reversal of the mucosal lesion with avoidance of gluten. The diagnosis should be confirmed by rechallenge with gluten and repeat biopsy in all children and any adult in whom the diagnosis is in question. Antigliadin and antiendomysial antibodies may be positive.

Treatment consists of a gluten-free diet (avoidance of all foods containing wheat, rye, barley, and oats).

Corn, rice, buckwheat, soybean, and potato products are reasonable substitutes. Celiac sprue usually responds rapidly to gluten withdrawal. Failure to improve may suggest (1) an incorrect diagnosis, (2) noncompliance with diet, (3) concomitant lactase deficiency, (4) nongranulomatous ulcerative jejunoileitis, (5) collagenous sprue, or (6) celiac sprue–associated intestinal T cell lymphoma. Other conditions associated with celiac disease include dermatitis herpetiformis, insulin-dependent diabetes mellitus, and selective IgA deficiency.

Collagenous Sprue

This entity is characterized by the progressive deposition of large amounts of collagen within the small intestinal lamina propria of celiac sprue patients. These individuals can become refractory to dietary therapy and may respond only to corticosteroids or other immune suppressive agents (or, rarely, nothing at all). Subepithelial collagen deposits, however, do not preclude response to dietary therapy. Consequently, all patients with a new diagnosis of collagenous sprue should initially be treated with gluten withdrawal.

Idiopathic Ulcerative Jejunoileitis

This chronic nongranulomatous ulcerative process is believed to be a complication of gluten-sensitive enteropathy. These patients no longer respond to a gluten-free diet and may not improve with corticosteroids. The ulcers can bleed or perforate and this decompensation of previously controlled celiac disease may herald the development of an intestinal lymphoma.

Giardiasis

Giardia lamblia is a protozoan, with worldwide prevalence, that is transmitted by oral ingestion of fecally contaminated water (people living in or visiting developing countries, backpackers in wilderness areas) or person-to-person fecal-oral contact (children in daycare centers, homosexual men, institutionalized patients). After dormant cysts are ingested, gastric acid promotes excystation and release of trophozoites, which colonize the proximal small bowel. Adherence to the brush border of intestinal epithelial cells results in a syndrome of diarrhea, malabsorption, and weight loss through poorly understood mechanisms. An incubation period of 1 to 2 weeks follows ingestion of *G. lamblia* cysts. Symptoms may then begin acutely and can persist for weeks to months before the process resolves spontaneously or definitive therapy is instituted. Diagnosis can be made by demonstrating the organism in stool, a duodenal aspirate, or small bowel biopsy. Treatment with quinacrine (Atabrine) 100 mg orally four times daily or metronidazole 250 mg orally three times a day for 7 to 10 days is effective in 90% of cases. Individuals with IgA or IgA and IgM deficiency may have recurrent episodes of *G. lamblia* infestation.

Tropical Sprue

Primarily a disease of adults, tropical sprue occurs only in persons with exposure to certain regions of the tropics (Cuba, Puerto Rico, Haiti, Dominican Republic, Southeast Asia, and Indonesia). The disease can begin abruptly or it may take several weeks or months to develop symptoms following arrival in an endemic area. Rarely, individuals who have since returned to more temperate climates may not manifest evidence of disease until several years after their last possible exposure. Contamination of the small bowel with toxigenic strains of coliform bacteria is believed to be the mechanism of disease. Patients present with watery diarrhea and abdominal cramps. Weight loss and steatorrhea are often present. The D-xylose test is abnormal and vitamin B_{12} and folate are poorly absorbed. The diagnosis is made by eliciting a history of travel to an endemic tropical area and demonstrating characteristic changes on jejunal biopsy.

Initial therapy includes the replacement of folate (5 mg orally daily) or vitamin B_{12} (1000 µg subcutaneously or intramuscularly each week). In early disease, this treatment alone may be curative. With more chronic symptoms, antimicrobial therapy is necessary to eradicate the coliforms. Tetracycline 250 mg four times daily or TMP–SMX (Bactrim DS) one tablet twice a day is equally efficacious. Treatment for up to 6 months is often needed for chronic disease.

Mycobacterium avium-intracellulare

MAI infection can involve the small intestine in persons with acquired immune deficiency syndrome (AIDS), producing a syndrome of watery diarrhea and malabsorption. Small intestinal biopsies demonstrating periodic acid–Schiff (PAS)–positive macrophages in the lamina propria resulted in this disorder being confused with Whipple's disease (hence, the term "pseudo-Whipple's disease"). Although there are subtle differences on PAS staining that allow an accurate diagnosis to be made, differentiation of these two disease states is made easier with acid-fast staining of MAI. Treatment with multiple antituberculous medications including amikacin (Amikin) 7.5 mg/kg intravenously daily for 4 weeks, ciprofloxacin (Cipro) 750 mg orally twice daily for 12 weeks, ethambutol (Myambutol) 1000 mg by mouth daily for 12 weeks, and rifampin (Rifadin) 600 mg a day orally for 12 weeks has shown some benefit.

Radiation Enteritis

Abdominopelvic radiotherapy may cause acute radiation injury to the small bowel that can present with a watery, self-limited diarrhea. Symptoms usually begin during treatments or shortly after the completion of therapy and resolve spontaneously within a few weeks. Alternatively, a chronic form of radiation injury can occur months to years later. This later form is the result of an ischemic vasculitis that can lead to stricture formation, fistulas, or obstruction. Bacterial overgrowth can develop in this setting of distorted anatomy/intestinal stasis and produce malabsorption. Bacterial overgrowth is treated as described under the "Bacterial Overgrowth Syndrome," earlier in this article.

Eosinophilic Enteritis

This syndrome is characterized by recurrent attacks of abdominal pain, diarrhea, steatorrhea, and protein-losing enteropathy. Patients may demonstrate peripheral eosinophilia in 20 to 90% of cases. At endoscopy, the mucosa appears friable, granular, and edematous with a patchy pattern of involvement. The mucosal layer, muscularis propria, or subserosal layer may be involved with dense eosinophilic infiltrates, which can be so massive as to create large pale plaques seen at endoscopy. The clinical presentation varies with the layer of the intestinal tract involved (e.g., eosinophilic ascites may be seen with subserosal involvement). Diagnosis is dependent on the presence of symptoms, the characteristic findings on mucosal biopsy, and the absence of parasitic or other systemic illnesses. Treatment consists of corticosteroids, usually administered orally, to abort acute attacks.

Impaired Delivery to Tissues

Whipple's Disease

Whipple's disease is a systemic bacterial infection, predominantly of middle-aged white men and is now known to be caused by the bacterium *Tropheryma whippelii*. Whipple's disease is characterized by arthralgias, diarrhea, malabsorption, abdominal pain, weight loss, lymphadenopathy, fever, cardiac abnormalities, and central nervous system dysfunction. The diagnosis is confirmed by small bowel biopsy showing clubbed villi and PAS-positive macrophages in the lamina propria. Therapy should consist of 1.2 million U of procaine penicillin G given intramuscularly plus 1 gram of intramuscular streptomycin daily for 2 weeks followed by oral TMP–SMX (Bactrim DS) one tablet twice daily for 1 year. For patients allergic to sulfonamides, penicillin VK 250 mg orally four times daily for 1 year may be substituted for TMP–SMX.

Miscellaneous

Malabsorption in AIDS

Weight loss, diarrhea, and malabsorption can frequently be encountered in patients with AIDS, especially when the disease is advanced. Many opportunistic infections and the direct effect of HIV on the intestinal mucosa may account for this. Diarrhea may result from protozoal disorders (cryptosporidiosis, coccidiosis, microsporidiasis, giardiasis, amebiasis, leishmaniasis, *Blastocystis hominis* infection), viral disorders (cytomegalovirus [CMV], herpes simplex, adenovirus, and HIV itself), intestinal neoplasms (lymphoma, Kaposi's sarcoma), pancreatic insufficiency (infectious pancreatitis [CMV, MAI infection], drug-related pancreatitis [pentamidine], tumor infiltration [Kaposi's sarcoma, lymphoma]), bacterial infections (salmonellosis, shigellosis, campylobacteriosis, MAI infection, tuberculosis, small bowel bacterial overgrowth), fungal (histoplasmosis, coccidiomycosis), or idiopathic ("AIDS enteropathy"). Those agents that are small bowel pathogens or affect the pancreas may cause malabsorption or maldigestion. After initial evaluation of stool specimens for enteric pathogens, ova, parasites, and acid-fast bacilli, consideration should be given to perform flexible sigmoidoscopy with biopsy and/or culture of tissue (for viruses, protozoa, and bacteria), especially if the individual has rectal bleeding and/or tenesmus. If no insight is gained, then consideration should be given to the performance of esophagogastroduodenoscopy with aspiration of small bowel secretions for ova and parasites, bacterial culture, and biopsy of the small bowel mucosa for routine histologic evaluation and for performance of electron microscopy.

ACUTE PANCREATITIS

method of
CHARLES J. YEO, M.D.
Johns Hopkins University School of Medicine
Baltimore, Maryland

Acute pancreatitis includes a broad spectrum of pancreatic abnormalities ranging from mild interstitial edema to severe hemorrhagic gangrene and necrosis. The clinical presentation can vary from mild, self-limited abdominal discomfort to severe illness with hypotension, metabolic derangements, and sepsis.

ETIOLOGY

Many stimuli have been implicated as causes of acute pancreatitis (Table 1). In industrialized countries, more than 90% of the cases are related to biliary tract disease or to excessive alcohol intake. Gallstone-associated pancreatitis is initiated by the migration of a gallstone down the distal common bile duct with either passage through or impaction at the ampulla of Vater. Alcohol is implicated as the etiologic agent in many patients with acute pancreatitis. Although the exact mechanism of alcohol-related pan-

TABLE 1. **Causes of Acute Pancreatitis**

Biliary tract disease	Pancreatic duct obstruction
Alcohol	Tumor
Hyperlipidemia	Pancreas divisum
Hypercalcemia	Ampullary stenosis
Familial cause	*Ascaris* infestation
Trauma	Duodenal obstruction
External	Viral infection
Operative	Scorpion venom
Retrograde pancreatography	Idiopathic cause
Ischemia	Drugs
Hypotension	
Cardiopulmonary bypass	
Atheroembolism	
Vasculitis	

TABLE 2. **Drugs Implicated in the Initiation of Acute Pancreatitis**

Definite Association	Probable Association
Azathioprine (Imuran)	Thiazide diuretics
Estrogens	Furosemide (Lasix)
	Ethacrynic acid (Edecrin)
	Sulfonamides
	Tetracycline
	L-Asparaginase (Oncaspar)
	Corticosteroids
	Phenformin
	Procainamide
	Valproic acid (Depakote)
	Clonidine (Catapres)
	Pentamidine (Pentam)
	Dideoxyinosine (Videx)

creatitis is unknown, several theories have been proposed: alcohol-related pancreatic hypersecretion in the presence of partial ampullary obstruction, alcohol-induced protein plugging of the pancreatic duct, and alcohol-induced hypertriglyceridemia.

A number of drugs (Table 2) have been linked to the initiation of acute pancreatitis, with the most substantive evidence implicating azathioprine (Imuran) and estrogens.

Despite the large number of inciting events known to cause acute pancreatitis, the cellular and molecular mechanisms involved in the actual process of pancreatic parenchymal injury have not been clearly defined.

CLINICAL PRESENTATION

In most patients with acute pancreatitis, the predominant clinical feature is abdominal pain, characteristically centered in the midepigastrium, and reaching its maximal intensity several hours after the start of the illness. Paroxysms of pain are uncommon. In up to 50% of patients the pain may have a boring or penetrating quality, with radiation to the back. Nausea and vomiting generally accompany the abdominal pain. Common physical findings include fever, tachycardia, epigastric tenderness, and abdominal distention. In less than 3% of patients, severe hemorrhagic pancreatitis may result in a bluish discoloration in the left flank (Grey Turner's sign) or in the periumbilical region (Cullen's sign). Jaundice is an unusual finding at initial presentation, although it may be present with gallstone-associated pancreatitis. In patients with severe pancreatitis, abnormalities such as hypotension, hypoperfusion, and obtundation may be present. Extra-abdominal manifestations may include pleural effusion (usually left-sided), tachypnea, dyspnea, cyanosis, cerebral abnormalities, and findings of disseminated intravascular coagulation.

DIAGNOSIS

Diagnosis is made on the basis of the clinical presentation combined with appropriate laboratory and radiographic findings (Table 3). The most widely used laboratory test is the determination of serum amylase levels. Hyperamylasemia is observed generally within 24 hours of the onset of symptoms, with a gradual return to normal levels over the ensuing days. Persistent elevations in amylase levels may indicate the development of pancreatic necrosis, pseudocyst, or abscess. The degree of initial hyperamylasemia does not reliably predict the severity of the pancreatic

TABLE 3. Diagnosis of Acute Pancreatitis

Laboratory Tests	Radiographic Procedures
Serum amylase levels	Plain chest x-ray
Serum amylase isoenzyme levels	Plain abdominal x-ray
Urinary amylase levels	Ultrasound examination
Amylase/creatinine clearance ratio	Computed tomography
Serum lipase levels	Magnetic resonance imaging

injury. Amylase is not an ideal marker for the diagnosis of pancreatitis, as many other causes of hyperamylasemia exist (Table 4). Improved accuracy in the diagnosis of acute pancreatitis can be achieved by the measurement of levels of amylase isoenzyme components, urinary amylase, or serum lipase, or by measurement of the amylase creatinine clearance ratio. Unfortunately, none of these tests are totally specific for acute pancreatitis.

Multiple radiographic procedures can support the clinical and laboratory suspicion of acute pancreatitis. Findings on chest x-ray examination such as left pleural effusion or left basilar atelectasis are suggestive. Abdominal x-ray films may reveal nonspecific abnormalities including the "sentinel loop sign" or the "colon cutoff sign," as well as evidence of cholelithiasis, a nonspecific ileus pattern, or the presence of pancreatic calcifications. Abdominal computed tomography (CT) is currently the most sensitive noninvasive method available to confirm the diagnosis. The findings in acute pancreatitis can be divided into pancreatic and peripancreatic changes (Table 5). A correlation exists between the degree of CT abnormality and the clinical course and severity of the acute pancreatitis. Magnetic resonance imaging (MRI) appears to give information similar to that of CT. Endoscopic retrograde cholangiopancreatography (ERCP) is not recommended for the routine diagnosis of acute pancreatitis; however, it may be useful in patients who have recurrent attacks without an obvious cause.

CLINICAL COURSE

Ninety percent of patients with the diagnosis of acute pancreatitis have a mild, self-limited illness and require

TABLE 4. Disorders Associated with Hyperamylasemia

Intra-Abdominal	Extra-Abdominal
Pancreatic disorders	Salivary gland disorders
Acute pancreatitis	Mumps
Chronic pancreatitis	Parotitis
Trauma	Trauma
Neoplasm	Calculi
Pseudocyst	Irradiation sialoadenitis
Pancreatic ascites	
Abscess	Impaired amylase excretion
	Renal failure
Nonpancreatic disorders	Macroamylasemia
Biliary tract disease	
Intestinal obstruction	Miscellaneous
Mesenteric infarction	Pancreatic pleural effusion
Perforated peptic ulcer	Pneumonia
Peritonitis	Mediastinal pseudocyst
Afferent loop syndrome	Cerebral trauma
Acute appendicitis	Severe burns
Ruptured ectopic pregnancy	Diabetic ketoacidosis
Salpingitis	Pregnancy
Ruptured aortic aneurysm	Drugs
	Bisalbuminemia

TABLE 5. Computed Tomographic Findings in Acute Pancreatitis

Pancreatic changes	Peripancreatic changes
Parenchymal enlargement	Blurring of fat planes
Diffuse	Thickening of fascial planes
Focal	Presence of fluid collections
Parenchymal edema	
Necrosis	Nonspecific findings
	Bowel distention
	Pleural effusion
	Mesenteric edema

only simple supportive care. The remaining patients may develop a severe form of the disease with the potential for complications, lengthy hospital stay, and significant mortality. One of the most widely used prognostic classification schemes is the one proposed in 1974 by Ranson (Table 6), which allows prediction of the severity and prognosis of an attack of pancreatitis by using routinely available clinical and laboratory determinations. Patients who present with from zero to two Ranson prognostic signs have a near zero mortality rate and typically require only simple supportive care. Patients with three or four signs may have a mortality rate of 15%, and 40% of these patients require intensive care support. Patients with five or more prognostic signs can have mortality rates up to 50% and almost universally require intensive care support. Universal application of this prognostic scoring system to all patients with acute pancreatitis permits the early identification of patients with severe disease (three or more prognostic signs). Although the Ranson criteria have gained widespread use, other predictive systems exist, such as the second version of the Acute Physiology and Chronic Health Enquiry (APACHE II), the Simplified Acute Physiology (SAP) score, and the Medical Research Counsel Score (MRCS).

NONOPERATIVE MANAGEMENT

After clinical assessment, diagnosis, and prediction of prognosis using the Ranson criteria, the initial management of each patient with acute pancreatitis is nonoperative (Table 7). All patients are initially treated with intravenous fluids, electrolyte replacement, and analgesics. Patients with a severe attack of pancreatitis (three or more Ranson criteria) may require nutritional support by parenteral alimenta-

TABLE 6. Ranson's Early Prognostic Signs of Acute Pancreatitis

At Admission	During Initial 48 h
Age over 55 years	Hematocrit fall >10 percentage points
WBC >16,000 cells/mm^3	
Blood glucose level >200 mg/dL	BUN level elevation >5 mg/dL
Serum lactate dehydrogenase level >350 IU/L	Serum calcium level fall to <8 mg/dL
AST level >250 U/dL	Arterial P$_{O_2}$ <60 mmHg
	Base deficit >4 mEq/L
	Estimated fluid sequestration >6 L

Abbreviations: WBC = white blood count; BUN = blood urea nitrogen; AST = aspartate aminotransferase (formerly SGOT).

TABLE 7. **Proposed Nonoperative Therapies for Acute Pancreatitis**

Supportive measures
    Intravenous fluid therapy
    Electrolyte replacement
    Analgesia
    Nutritional support*
    Antibiotics*
    Respiratory support*
Pancreatic exocrine secretion suppression (unproven)
    Nasogastric suction
    Histamine H$_2$-receptor antagonists
    Antacids
    Anticholinergics
    Glucagon
    Calcitonin (salmon) (Calcimat)
    Somatostatin analogue (Octreotide)
    Peptide YY
    Cholecystokinin-receptor antagonists
Pancreatic enzyme inhibition (unproven)
    Protease inhibitors
        Aprotinin (Trasylol)
        Gabexate
        Camostat
        Fresh-frozen plasma
    Antifibrinolytics
    Chloroquine (Aralen)
    Phospholipase A inhibitors
Pancreatic protection from oxygen-derived free radicals (unproven)
    Free radical scavengers
    Xanthine oxidase inhibitors
    Isovolemic hemodilution
Elimination of toxic intraperitoneal compounds (unproven)
    Peritoneal dialysis

*Needed or recommended for patients with severe pancreatitis, defined as three or more Ranson prognostic signs.

tion; antibiotic administration for the prevention or treatment of septic complications; or respiratory support in the face of pancreatitis-associated pulmonary dysfunction.

Fluid sequestration caused by acute pancreatitis can be massive. Generous fluid resuscitation with correction of hypovolemia and restoration of circulating blood volume is an essential step in therapy. The volume of intravenous fluid necessary for adequate fluid repletion varies. The adequacy of volume replacement must be assessed by evaluation of the heart rate, blood pressure, and urinary output. The use of crystalloid solutions such as intravenous Ringer's lactate or saline-containing solutions is usually adequate replacement therapy for acute pancreatitis. Patients with severe hemorrhagic pancreatitis may require the transfusion of blood or blood products to replace losses. Patients with severe pancreatitis or patients with pre-existing cardiopulmonary or renal disease may require invasive monitoring to include urethral catheterization, central venous pressure measurement, or measurement of cardiac output and cardiac filling pressures with a Swan-Ganz catheter. Persistent shock despite adequate fluid resuscitation may require the use of potent vasopressors such as phenylephrine (Neo-Synephrine) or norepinephrine (Levophed).

A variety of electrolyte abnormalities may be encountered with acute pancreatitis. Hypernatremia may be observed, usually resulting from intravascular volume contraction, and it should be treated with isotonic volume replacement and free water if necessary. Persistent emesis, with loss of the hydrogen cation (H$^+$) and the chloride anion (Cl$^-$), may lead to a severe hypochloremic contraction alkalosis. Treatment consists of volume replacement with normal saline, supplemented with exogenous potassium chloride (KCl) to accelerate the correction of the alkalosis. Abnormalities of the divalent cations calcium and magnesium may also occur. Patients with subnormal ionized calcium or magnesium levels require exogenous calcium or magnesium administration. Blood glucose levels are often elevated in acute pancreatitis, as a manifestation of the catecholamine-mediated stress response combined with the increased secretion of glucagon from pancreatic islet alpha cells and relative insufficiency of insulin from pancreatic islet beta cells. Treatment of marked hyperglycemia or glycosuria requires cautious exogenous insulin administration combined with volume repletion.

Narcotic analgesics should be administered in cautious doses to relieve the abdominal pain that is the clinical hallmark of acute pancreatitis. Morphine is generally avoided because of its potential for causing sphincter of Oddi spasm, which could theoretically potentiate ongoing pancreatic injury. Meperidine (Demerol) is the preferred drug, with parenteral administration preferred. We favor intravenous administration using approved patient-controlled analgesia devices. Oral intake of all liquids and solids is typically prohibited in patients with acute pancreatitis. Both reactivation of pancreatic inflammation and the formation of pancreatic abscess have been associated with premature return to oral intake. In most patients, the symptoms of acute pancreatitis persist for only a short period, and oral intake can be resumed when pain, tenderness, and ileus have resolved. In a few patients, oral refeeding must be delayed as a result of persistent pain, tenderness, or ileus. Parenteral nutritional support is indicated for these patients.

Antibiotics are not indicated in the routine treatment of mild to moderate pancreatitis. However, in patients with severe pancreatitis (Ranson scores of 3 or greater and CT scans demonstrating necrotizing pancreatitis), a recent prospective, randomized multicenter trial comparing no antibiotics to imipenem-cilastatin (Primaxin), 500 mg intravenously every 8 hours for 2 weeks demonstrated that the incidence of culture-proven pancreatic and nonpancreatic sepsis was significantly lower in the imipenem-cilastatin group. Based on these data and past clinical practice, we advise the use of prophylactic broad-spectrum antibiotic therapy in patients with severe pancreatitis (defined as three or more Ranson prognostic signs).

Pulmonary complications may occur in up to 50% of patients with acute pancreatitis. Treatment is generally supportive and includes supplemental oxygen administration, physical therapy, treatment of infection, and avoidance of volume overload. Endotracheal intubation and positive end-expiratory pressure ventilation are indicated in the face of progressive pulmonary insufficiency that does not respond to other treatment modalities.

At the current time, specific therapies to treat pancreatitis based on its presumed pathogenesis remain unproved. Such therapies include pancreatic exocrine secretion suppression, pancreatic enzyme inhibition, pancreatic protection from oxygen-derived free radicals, and elimination of toxic intraperitoneal compounds (Table 7). Although much experimental and clinical work has been performed in testing these therapies, there are no substantive data applicable in all settings to support the use of any of these specific therapies in the treatment of patients with acute pancreatitis.

OPERATIVE MANAGEMENT

Accumulated experience now supports operative intervention for acute pancreatitis for four specific indications (Table 8):

1. Uncertainty of clinical diagnosis. It may be difficult to rule out other diagnoses that mimic acute pancreatitis, such as perforated viscus or mesenteric ischemia. If the diagnosis remains cryptic, exploratory laparotomy may be indicated to rule out a surgically correctable disease with a potentially fatal outcome in the absence of operative intervention.

2. Treatment of secondary pancreatic infections. Secondary pancreatic infections are a serious and life-threatening complication of acute pancreatitis, occurring in 2 to 5% of patients. These secondary pancreatic infections include infected pancreatic pseudocyst, pancreatic abscess, and infected pancreatic necrosis. These infections are believed to occur by secondary infection of necrotic pancreatic and peripancreatic tissues. The development of such an infection should be suspected in all patients with severe pancreatitis (three or more Ranson signs), in patients with clinical deterioration after the first week of illness, and in patients with documented bacteremia. At present, dynamic contrast-enhanced CT is the radiographic investigation of choice to evaluate for potential secondary pancreatic infection. The combination of abdominal CT and CT-guided percutaneous needle aspiration appears to reliably differentiate infected from sterile peripancreatic necrosis. In selected cases, percutaneous catheter drainage of a solitary spherical pancreatic abscess may be successful. In patients with infected pancreatic necrosis, surgical drainage and débridement are required.

TABLE 8. **Indications for Operation in the Management of Acute Pancreatitis**

Uncertainty of clinical diagnosis
Treatment of secondary pancreatic infections
Correction of associated biliary tract disease
Progressive clinical deterioration despite optimal supportive care

3. Correction of associated biliary tract disease. Gallstone-associated pancreatitis is a clear indication for a definitive biliary tract procedure intended to reduce the risk of recurrent attacks of pancreatitis. Biliary tract surgery within 3 to 5 days of admission, performed as a laparoscopic cholecystectomy, has proved to be safe and cost-effective for the treatment of these patients. Visualization of the biliary tree by preoperative ERCP or intraoperative cholangiography has been used to evaluate the biliary tree in patients with gallstone-associated pancreatitis.

4. Progressive clinical deterioration despite optimal supportive care. The most controversial indication for surgery involves patients with deteriorating clinical status who fail to respond to nonoperative supportive care. Specific recommendations for the extent of pancreatic resection in these cases range from total pancreatectomy to only limited débridement of obvious necrotic tissue (necrosectomy).

CHRONIC PANCREATITIS

method of
L. WILLIAM TRAVERSO, M.D., and
RICHARD A. KOZAREK, M.D.
Virginia Mason Medical Center
Seattle, Washington

Progressive destruction of the pancreas characterizes the natural history of chronic pancreatitis. The chronic variety differs from acute pancreatitis because the inflammatory lesion persists even when the cause is removed. Historically, acinar atrophy first appears in isolated focal areas. The spotty fibrosis ultimately coalesces to result in exocrine and then endocrine atrophy. The most common cause is long-standing alcohol abuse. With continued follow-up, it is not difficult to make the diagnosis of chronic pancreatitis just on clinical grounds.

Malabsorption results when 90% of a patient's exocrine tissue has been replaced by scar. Chemical diabetes occurs when more than 80% of the islet tissue has been destroyed by the encroaching fibrosis. Insulin-dependent diabetes ensues after approximately 90% of a patient's functional islet cell mass has been destroyed by the encroaching fibrosis. Some individuals have occult chronic pancreatitis, because major portions of pancreatic tissue must be destroyed before clinical symptoms are observed. Some patients may have just malabsorption and/or diabetes. An unfortunate number of patients, however, develop the severe complications of chronic pancreatitis, which are usually associated with either intermittent or continuous midabdominal pain, often radiating to the back. A patient with chronic pancreatitis may require no treatment, treatment for malabsorption alone, diabetes alone, or both clinical sequelae of chronic pancreatitis. Any of the above possibilities may be associated with chronic abdominal pain. This pain requires treatment that is a coordinated team effort between physician, psychiatrist, interventional radiologist, therapeutic endoscopist, and pancreatic surgeon.

MEDICAL TREATMENT (Table 1)
Malabsorption

Even though a patient may not describe steatorrhea or severe weight loss, malabsorption is usually

TABLE 1. **Medical Treatment of Chronic Pancreatitis**

Alcohol interdiction	
Therapy for exocrine insufficiency	Pancreatic enzymes
Therapy for endocrine insufficiency	Diet
	Oral hypoglycemics
	Insulin
Analgesia	Alcohol interdiction
	Narcotics
	± celiac plexus block
	Inhibitors of neurotransmission (e.g., tricyclics)

present when a patient with chronic pancreatitis seeks medical care. The diagnosis can be confirmed by doing a qualitative or 72-hour stool fat study. Also a study of para-aminobenzoic acid (PABA) excretion in the urine after the oral administration of PABA linked to a synthetic peptide can be performed. Restricting dietary fat is the initial treatment, but if weight loss and/or diarrhea are still significant after such restriction, then oral enzymes therapy should be provided. Oral pancreatic extract tablets should not be used. Enteric-coated microspheres of animal-derived pancreatic enzymes (Pancrease, Creon) have been found to be more effective than conventional enzyme tablets (even if enteric coating is present) for weight gain, decreasing stool frequency, and decreasing fecal fat. The microsphere (not necessarily the enteric coating) is the key to the improved exocrine enzyme replacement. Particles greater than 3 mm in diameter remain in the stomach, while masticated foods with microspheres easily enter the duodenum through the pylorus. Microspheres allow even dispersal of the enzymes within gastric chyme and simultaneous delivery of enzyme and chyme into the duodenum.

Treatment with these modern enzyme supplements consists of two or occasionally three capsules with each meal and one capsule with each snack. One capsule should be taken at the beginning and the end of a meal, and, if necessary, at the middle of each meal.

Diabetes

When a patient has sustained approximately a decade of alcohol abuse and develops chronic pancreatitis, the first metabolic complication is diabetes, followed in several years by exocrine insufficiency. Although a fourth of these patients present with diabetes (as determined by an increased fasting glucose level), far more are found to have an abnormal glucose tolerance test. As scattered areas of acinar atrophy coalesce to replace pancreatic parenchyma with areas of sclerotic fibrosis, diabetes ultimately develops. Diabetes of chronic pancreatitis is not more difficult to control than adult-onset diabetes provided the physician has a cooperative patient willing to control both malabsorption and diabetes. The patient

must understand the need for and follow a regimen of a constant diet, daily self-performed glucose determinations, and reliable insulin administration.

Pain

The nonoperative treatment of pain involves abstinence from all alcohol or alcohol-containing products (e.g., cough syrup) plus the judicious use of oral analgesics. However, many patients with chronic pain have stopped alcohol use voluntarily. Alcohol initially relieves the abdominal pain but ultimately exacerbates the discomfort. This is the time when the patient seeks medical advice. Analgesics are progressively ineffective, leading to narcotic addiction. Therefore, it is not surprising that the patient's last drink will have been between 1 to 3 years before an operation to treat a pancreatitis complication and that patients have usually substituted narcotics for alcohol.

Almost every patient with the severe complications of chronic pancreatitis has the concomitant symptoms of abdominal pain. The pain is the result of chronic fibrosis with nerve entrapment or, more commonly, the sequelae of ductal obstruction or pancreatic ductal disruption. Therefore, to understand the mechanism of disease in each patient, the physician requires information derived from radiologic and endoscopic diagnostic techniques.

The patient who ultimately requires some form of interventional therapy does not just have abdominal pain but also has concomitant severe complications as a result of disrupted pancreatic anatomy (obstructed biliary or pancreatic ducts with or without pancreatic duct disruption). These potentially fatal complications can be divided into four groups: (1) pancreatic ductal obstruction alone (usually in the head), (2) pancreatic duct plus common bile duct obstruction with or without duodenal stenosis, (3) single or multiple pseudocyst formation from pancreatic duct disruptions in one or more of the following areas: over the portal vein, midbody, or tail, and (4) the potentially immediately fatal complication of pseudoaneurysm or arteriovenous connections in the inflammatory tissue—usually in the head—associated with splenic vein and/or portal venous occlusion.

Identifying the anatomic situation is paramount to making decisions about therapy. The anatomy is best understood by drawing a "composite" picture using information from computed tomography (CT) scans, endoscopic retrograde cholangiopancreatography (ERCP), and operative findings. Therefore the anatomic picture can best be obtained by using the team approach, with the cooperation of the departments of radiology, endoscopy, and surgery.

The CT scan remains the primary method of determining the presence and location of the following indicators of severity: pseudocysts, ductal dilatation, calcifications, splenic vein occlusion with prominent gastric varices, the extent of inflammation associated with ductal disruption, and biliary dilatation. Patients with severe complications of chronic pancreati-

TABLE 2. **Endoscopic Treatment Modalities in Chronic Pancreatitis**

Stricture	Endoprosthesis ± dilatation
Bile duct	
Pancreatic duct	
Ductal disruption	Endoprosthesis
Ascites	
Pleural effusion	
Fistula	
Pseudocyst (persistent	Cystogastrostomy
ductal disruption)	Cystduodenostomy
	Transpapillary stent
Stone	Pancreatic sphincterotomy ±
	ESWL, stone retrieval

Abbreviaton: ESWL = extracorporeal shock wave lithotripsy.

tis in the head of the gland benefit by mesenteric arteriography to determine the presence of arteriovenous malformation or arteriovenous fistulas. In addition, the added information from the portal venous phase illustrates the frequent presence of splenic vein occlusion leading to left-sided portal hypertension or even to the more uncommon but most severe association of portal vein occlusion.

ENDOSCOPIC DIAGNOSIS AND TREATMENT (Table 2)

ERCP has been used primarily as a diagnostic tool. It may be used simply to confirm a diagnosis suspected on ultrasound or CT examination, to define a complication (e.g., duodenal or biliary obstruction or pancreatic ductal disruption with pseudocyst, pancreatic ascites, pleural effusion, or fistula) or as a preoperative "road map." Classic findings in chronic pancreatitis include ductal ectasias with beading and irregularity, inflammatory strictures, and pancreatic calculi. Concomitant and not uncommon findings include gastric varices (splenic vein occlusion), mucosal changes in the gastric antrum (antral pad) and duodenal C loop, and variable degrees of bile duct stenosis or displacement.

More recently, ERCP has been utilized therapeutically in selected patients with chronic pancreatitis. Treatment has primarily been directed toward stenoses or ductal disruption. For instance, patients who develop jaundice or cholangitis as a consequence of bile duct cicatrization as the duct traverses the pancreatic head can be temporarily decompressed by the placement of an endoprosthesis. The same rationale has led to the use of pancreatic stents to bypass a tight and obstructing pancreatic ductal stenosis. Because stents occlude and may themselves induce lesions within the pancreatic duct, their use presupposes a degree of reversibility of the inflammatory process, or they may be used to convert an urgent surgical condition into an elective one. Ductal disruptions can also be treated endoscopically. For instance, patients with pancreatic ascites, fistulas, or pleural effusions may have an anatomy that allows stent placement across an area of ductal disruption. Endoprostheses divert pancreatic secretions and allow

healing of the disruption in a significant subset. Pseudocysts, also a consequence of ductal disruption, can occasionally be treated by transpapillary prostheses. Alternatively, pseudocysts contiguous with the stomach or duodenum can be drained by fistulizing through gut wall using a needle-knife sphincterotome. Chronic drainage is ensured by the placement of a stent between the stomach or duodenum and the fluid collection. Such stents are usually retrieved 4 to 6 weeks later. This therapy must be placed into the perspective of alternative methods of pseudocyst drainage to include percutaneous (radiologic) and surgical cyst decompression.

Finally, pancreatic calculi, usually the consequence of chronic pancreatitis, can at times obstruct the duct and cause chronic pain or relapsing attacks of pancreatitis. Stones within the major ductal system, particularly those within the head, can be removed after pancreatic duct sphincterotomy using balloon or basket technology. Because these stones frequently are adherent to the duct wall or tightly impacted, calculus fragmentation with extracorporeal shock wave lithotripsy (ESWL) is not infrequently used as an adjunct to removal. Long-term follow-up is required to determine the role of these newer approaches, but they have proved useful in our experience.

SURGERY (Table 3)

Once all prior treatments have been discarded or have failed, surgical options are considered. If the ductal system is shown to be dilatated, treatment is designed to relieve obstruction of the entire major ductal system. If the duct is obstructed throughout the head of the gland, an intestinal drainage procedure to decompress the ductal system in the body or tail will not be sufficient to prevent continued problems. The head of the pancreas can be thought of as the "pacemaker of pancreatitis" as persistent inflammation, calcification, and duct obstruction in the head totally block the upstream flow of pancreatic juice from the body and tail. Besides the main pancreatic duct, the ductal systems in the uncinate pro-

TABLE 3. **Surgical Modalities in Chronic Pancreatitis**

Ductal obstruction	
Chain of lakes type but open into duodenum	Longitudinal pancreaticojejunostomy (Puestow procedure)
In head	Resection of head (Whipple)
Ductal disruption	
With or without pseudocyst	Segmental resection
	Cystenterostomy
Pseudocyst only	Cystenterostomy
	Segmental resection
	External drainage
Contiguous organ obstruction	Choledochojejunostomy
	Gastrojejunostomy
	Whipple procedure
	Splenectomy (splenic vein occlusion)

cess as well as those areas drained by the superior head through the duct of Santorini must also be decompressed. If these ducts are obstructed, they cannot be successfully decompressed by a drainage procedure and the surgical options in this area are narrowed to resection.

In our experience, the Puestow procedure or lateral pancreaticojejunostomy (the side of the entire pancreatic duct in the body and tail is decompressed by anastomosis to the side of a jejunal limb) has proved very effective in continued pain relief when the pancreatic duct in the head is open and there are no other severe complications of pancreatitis, e.g., pseudocyst, duodenal and/or bile duct stenosis, or pseudoaneurysm. Not only can pain be alleviated but also the progression of pancreatic exocrine and endocrine insufficiency appear to be interrupted by the drainage procedure in selected patients undergoing long-term follow-up. Once destruction of endocrine and exocrine function has occurred, the drainage procedure cannot be expected to improve function.

When a patient has any of the severe complications of chronic pancreatitis listed earlier, they usually reside in the head of the gland, and removal of the head solves the vexing and serious medical problem. With appropriately selected patients, despite the severity of their illness, we have found almost all are relieved of the potentially fatal complications of chronic pancreatitis and almost all have a total relief of pain by a pylorus-preserving pancreaticoduodenectomy (Whipple procedure). In up to 10 years of follow-up, this relief of pain has persisted even though the inexorable fibrosis continues within the pancreatic remnant (pancreatic tail and body). Evidence for progressive fibrosis in the remaining pancreas is seen because diabetes (if not present before resection) develops in approximately one-half of these patients beginning 1 to 2 years after surgical therapy.

Splenectomy is performed as an additional procedure when significant gastric varices are associated with splenic vein occlusion. The spleen is removed at the time of a Puestow or a Whipple procedure to eliminate the "left-sided" portal hypertension and potential gastric variceal complications.

Surgery is necessary only for the severe complications of chronic pancreatitis. Almost without exception, pain is associated with these anatomic complications. Therefore, surgery is not for the pain but rather for one of the severe complications listed earlier. The use of the Puestow procedure alone or resection of the head of the gland (pancreaticoduodenectomy) in our experience results in interruption of the complications of severe chronic pancreatitis and ameliorates the associated chronic abdominal pain in almost all patients. Since alcohol is the cause in the majority of patients, the main reason for recurrence of symptoms is a return to alcohol abuse. No treatment can overcome continued pancreatic insult in the patient who continues to abuse alcohol.

GASTROESOPHAGEAL REFLUX DISEASE

method of
REZA SHAKER, M.D.
Medical College of Wisconsin
Milwaukee, Wisconsin

The entry of gastric contents into the esophagus (i.e., gastroesophageal reflux) occurs in differing degrees in symptomatic as well as asymptomatic individuals. Depending on a variety of factors including, but not limited to, the frequency of reflux episodes and the composition of the refluxed material; the effectiveness of the esophageal clearance mechanism; and esophageal mucosal resistance and regeneration capability, gastroesophageal reflux events may lead to inflammation, mucosal disruption, ulceration, stricture, bleeding, and the premalignant condition of gastric metaplasia of the esophageal mucosa, namely, Barrett's esophagus.

The term "gastroesophageal reflux disease" (GERD) is commonly used to describe any symptomatic clinical condition or histologic changes that result from a backward flow of the gastric contents into the esophagus. Thus, GERD presents as a spectrum of conditions. Individuals with symptoms of reflux, but without macroscopically detectable lesions, occupy one end, and patients with severe reflux esophagitis and its consequent complications occupy the other end of the spectrum. Symptomatic GERD is the most common disease of the esophagus. Heartburn (pyrosis), the cardinal symptom of GERD, is reported to occur in 10 to 20% of the general population. From 4 to 7% of the population are reported to experience daily heartburn. Other symptoms of GERD include regurgitation, hypersalivation (water brash), sour taste (sour brash), frequent belching, and epigastric pain.

Currently, the pathogenesis of GERD is believed to be multifactorial. These factors include (1) those affecting the antireflux mechanism (such as lower esophageal sphincter [LES] tone, the frequency of inappropriate LES relaxation, the angle of the esophagogastric junction, and the presence or absence of hiatal hernia), (2) the volume of the gastric contents (balance between intake and gastric secretion against gastric emptying), (3) the composition and potency of the refluxed material (the presence of acid, pepsin, bile salts, pancreatic enzyme, by-products of digestion, etc.), (4) the efficiency of the esophageal clearance mechanisms (primary and secondary esophageal peristalsis, saliva and its bicarbonate content), and (5) esophageal mucosal resistance to injury and its reparative abilities. Each of these factors or a combination of them may play the predominant role in inducing reflux injury in a given patient. For example, during pregnancy the commonly reversible reflux disease is believed to be due to the low LES tone induced by the large amount of circulatory progesterone as well as the presence of increased intra-abdominal pressure. Other conditions that may predispose to reflux by either reducing the LES tone, provoking LES relaxation, or impairing the esophageal clearance mechanism include unconsciousness, head injury, mental retardation, and nasogastric intubation. Systemic sclerosis especially predisposes the patient to reflux injury and its complication of stricture. This is due to the negligible LES tone and impaired esophageal peristalsis and possibly the presence of delayed gastric emptying and decreased salivary production.

Recent clinical observations indicate that the extent of

reflux injury is not limited to the esophagus and that supraesophageal complications of reflux disease are more prevalent than previously thought. In this regard, GERD is becoming a disease attended by physicians of various disciplines including otolaryngologists, pulmonologists, and pediatricians, in addition to gastroenterologists and internists. A multitude of airway and aerodigestive disorders have been attributed to GERD (Table 1). The most common clinical symptom of GERD is heartburn, or pyrosis, which is described as a retrosternal burning sensation or discomfort; however, heartburn may be absent in a substantial percentage of GERD patients with esophageal injury as well as those with supraesophageal complications of GERD. Similarly, severe heartburn sensation may not be accompanied by any detectable macroscopic changes.

Other symptoms of GERD include retrosternal chest pain, regurgitation, sour brash, water brash, dysphagia, and, rarely, painful swallowing, or odynophagia. However, GERD-induced odynophagia is uncommon, and the presence of this symptom should prompt investigation for infectious esophagitis such as those symptoms induced by *Candida*, herpes simplex virus, or cytomegalovirus infection of the esophageal muscosa. Similarly, pill-induced esophageal lesion must be considered. Reflux-induced chest pain may be caused by the acid stimulation of the pain receptors and possibly by acid-induced spastic esophageal contraction. However, extreme caution must be exercised in attributing chest pain to reflux disease even when conventional cardiac work-up such as angiography is reported normal, since abnormalities of microvascular cardiac circulation that escape detection by conventional methods may exist. Difficulty swallowing reported by reflux patients generally indicates the presence of an esophageal stricture. However, dysphagia may also be caused by abnormal esophageal motor function induced by GERD. Gastrointestinal (GI) blood loss due to esophagitis generally presents itself as occult GI blood loss, but occasionally it may induce frank upper GI bleeding. The severity of various symptoms of reflux disease varies widely among patients but does not correlate closely with the degree of severity of esophageal injury.

There is wide variation in the clinical course of reflux symptoms; in some patients they undergo spontaneous remission, and in others they become intractable and are accompanied by complications. A large majority of patients, however, have mild disease with differing degrees and frequency of symptoms. These patients respond to medical therapy. In some patients, reflux symptoms respond favorably to aggressive therapy, but symptoms recur soon after the therapy is stopped. In a minority of patients, reflux symptoms are refractory and may require surgical therapy.

ESOPHAGEAL COMPLICATIONS OF GASTROESOPHAGEAL REFLUX DISEASE

Stricture. About 10% of patients with severe reflux esophagitis develop peptic stricture during the course of their disease. About 40% of all peptic strictures are accompanied by Barrett's esophagus. Although peptic esophageal strictures are nearly always located in the distal esophagus where the acid exposure is maximal, they may occur in the proximal esophagus and present with symptoms of cervical dysphagia. Distal esophageal stricture presents with gradually developing solid food dysphagia. With stricture formation, reflux symptoms may abate. In severe cases, liquid dysphagia may be present. In reflux patients without heartburn, solid food dysphagia due to stricture formation may be the presenting symptom. The benign nature of these strictures needs to be verified by endoscopy and biopsy.

Barrett's Esophagus. Barrett's esophagus is defined as replacement of the esophageal squamous cell epithelium by metaplastic columnar-type epithelium occurring as a result of reflux injury. Because of malignant potential, the development of Barrett's esophagus is clinically significant and needs to be followed closely. About 10 to 20% of patients with reflux esophagitis develop Barrett's epithelium. It is found in about 40% of patients with peptic strictures. The actual incidence of adenocarcinoma arising from Barrett's esophagus is not known. However, the risk has been reported to be between a few percent and 10%. Barrett's esophagus is commonly seen in patients older than 40 years, but it is also seen in young adults and children.

In the early fetal stage, the esophageal lumen is lined by columnar epithelium, but during the later fetal stage, this epithelium is replaced by squamous epithelium. However, this transformation may not be complete, and in about 4% of adult patients who undergo upper GI endoscopy, an islet of columnar epithelium may be found in the proximal esophagus. In a minority of instances this aberrant mucosa may be found in the distal esophagus. These epithelia are different from reflux-induced metaplastic columnar epithelium in their lack of inflammation and other evidences of reflux disease.

Although symptoms of patients with Barrett's esophagus are no different from those of "garden variety" severe peptic esophagitis, in some patients the symptoms may be more severe initially. However, the heartburn may reduce in severity as the columnar epithelium extends more proximally. Odynophagia and chronic substernal chest pain in Barrett's patients may indicate the development of ulceration. Barrett's ulcer develops most often on the posterior or posterolateral esophageal wall and may result in significant bleeding or perforation. Stricture may also develop in Barrett's esophagus. Barrett's esophagus is considered a premalignant condition. The transformation of the columnar epithelium of Barrett's esophagus into the stages of mild dysplasia, then severe dysplasia, and eventually frank adenocarcinoma is a time-dependent process. An estimated 5 to 10% of all esophageal malignancies are

TABLE 1. **Extraesophageal Complications of Gastroesophageal Reflux Disease**

Buccal burning	Contact granulomas of TVCs
Dry or sore throat (discomfort)	Cricopharyngeal dysfunction
	Torticollis (Sandifer's syndrome)
Hoarseness	Loss of dental or gingival structure
Globus sensation	Posterior laryngitis
Regurgitation	Recurrent respiratory disease
Vomiting	Apneic episodes
Aspiration	Otitis media
Lung abscess	Subglottic stenosis
Pulmonary fibrosis	Noncardiac chest pain
Chronic cough	Asthma
"Hyperphlegmia"	
Lateral cervical pain	
Laryngospasm	
Otalgia	
Bad breath	
Pharyngeal tightness	
Choking sensation	
"Losing voice"	

Abbreviation: TVC = true vocal cord.

thought to be due to adenocarcinoma developed in Barrett's esophagus. Adenocarcinoma in Barrett's epithelium may be multifocal and is often well advanced at the time of diagnosis.

DIAGNOSTIC EVALUATION

Most patients with simple heartburn, especially of a mild nature and transient or short duration, do not require any diagnostic test and are easily managed medically. However, patients with severe and/or long-standing heartburn, dysphagia, atypical symptoms such as chest pain, GI bleeding, and supraesophageal complaints require one or more diagnostic tests to determine the extent and severity of the disease and to tailor their therapy. Endoscopy with and without biopsy is the diagnostic modality of choice. It helps determine the presence or absence of Barrett's mucosa, significant stricture, and the extent and severity of the mucosal injury.

A barium esophagram is helpful in patients with dysphagia, when the possibility of the presence of a distal esophageal ring exists, as well as for preoperative evaluation. Atypical symptoms of GERD, such as chest pain and pressure, and wheezing, can be elicited by the Bernstein test. Manometry can help evaluate reflux-associated dysphagia. It is also useful in preoperative evaluation of esophageal peristaltic function.

Concurrent ambulatory pH monitoring of the esophagus and pharynx helps detect pharyngeal acid reflux. It also helps evaluate the correlation between reflux episodes and the patient's atypical symptoms. It has also been used to assess the efficacy of the acid-suppressive or surgical therapy. Ambulatory manometry can potentially detect abnormal esophageal motor function that has escaped short-term stationary studies.

MANAGEMENT OF GASTROESOPHAGEAL REFLUX DISEASE

The management of GERD needs to be tailored to the disease of each individual patient. General precautionary measures include (1) elevation of the head of the bed (6 to 8 inches), (2) dietary measures such as avoiding fats, chocolate, alcohol, cigarettes, peppermint, and caffeine, which are known to decrease the LES resting pressure. Other measures include weight loss. Since reflux episodes occur most frequently 1 to 3 hours after a meal, refraining from eating for 2 to 3 hours before retiring is helpful. However, these measures are not usually sufficient to remedy moderate to severe reflux symptoms. Although dietary discretion may reduce the frequency of symptoms, it is ineffective in treating esophagitis. Antacids work primarily by their acid-neutralizing capacity, but this effect is temporary. Antacid in large doses (30 minutes and 3 hours after each meal and at bedtime) has been used to treat GERD. However, its superiority over placebo in treating esophagitis has not been clearly established. Alginic acid, present in some aluminum hydroxide antacids, acts as a mechanical barrier by forming a highly viscous solution that floats over the gastric contents and may reduce the number of reflux episodes. Acid-suppressive agents, either H_2-receptor antagonists such as rani-

tidine (Zantac), cimetidine (Tagamet), nizatidine (Axid), famotidine (Pepcid), or a proton pump inhibitor such as omeprazole (Prilosec), are the mainstay of the medical management of gastroesophageal disease. The healing rate varies among these two classes of agents. Omeprazole has been shown consistently to be superior to ranitidine (150 mg orally twice daily) and cimetidine (800 mg orally twice daily) in healing reflux esophagitis and relieving its symptoms.

Mild to moderate esophagitis responds favorably to H_2-receptor antagonists in 75 to 90% of patients. However, with severe reflux esophagitis, frequently a proton pump inhibitor, such as omeprazole (20 to 40 mg orally twice daily for 8 to 12 weeks), is needed to achieve healing.

One of the characteristics of moderate to severe reflux disease is its tendency to recur. Over 80% of the esophageal mucosal lesions recur within 6 months of the termination of pharmacologic antireflux therapy. For this reason, maintenance therapy is needed to sustain healing. Maintenance therapy for these patients requires the use of therapeutic agents in full dose. Prokinetic agents such as cisapride (Propulsid), 10 mg orally twice a day in combination with acid-suppressive therapy, may improve results by enhancing esophageal motility, LES tone, and gastric emptying.

Surgical therapy (conventional or laparoscopic fundoplication) is reserved for patients in whom medical management fails, such as young patients in whom lifetime therapy is undesirable, and reflux patients with supraesophageal manifestation of reflux disease such as asthma and laryngitis that do not respond adequately to acid-suppressive therapy.

PEPTIC ULCER DISEASE

method of
COLIN W. HOWDEN, M.D.
University of South Carolina School of Medicine
Columbia, South Carolina

Conventional thinking about peptic ulcer disease has changed dramatically in the last few years. Few areas of internal medicine, let alone gastroenterology, have witnessed such a profound change in thinking. Once regarded as a chronic, relapsing, and possibly lifelong condition of unknown cause, peptic ulcer is now recognized as being most often due to chronic infection with the bacterium *Helicobacter pylori*. This has completely altered our perspective on the cause of peptic ulcer disease and is having a tremendous influence on approaches to treatment. There is now the real possibility of curing peptic ulcer disease with medication, in at least some patients.

A number of drugs introduced over the years are effective in healing peptic ulcers. These include antacids, the histamine H_2-receptor antagonists, sucralfate, and the H^+/K^+-ATPase inhibitors, or acid pump inhibitors. Physicians have grown accustomed to prescribing antiulcer medication for patients with a variety of dyspeptic complaints, including those associated with peptic ulcer. Indeed, the safety and efficacy of these drugs when used appropriately are so impressive that many patients receive empirical therapy without prior recourse to endoscopic diagnosis. This has long been considered a safe and efficient way to treat young, otherwise healthy patients with a brief history of dyspepsia. However, opinion on the appropriateness of this approach is changing since it has become increasingly important to document accurately the presence of an ulcer and of *H. pylori* infection before definitive treatment. The successful treatment of infection can have a dramatic effect on the long-term prognosis of patients with ulcer disease. Empirical therapy may continue to have a role in the management of some dyspeptic patients presenting to a primary care physician. However, endoscopic confirmation of a clinical suspicion of peptic ulcer is now strongly recommended. This is essential if treatment aimed at eradicating *H. pylori* infection is planned. As is seen later, such therapy is strongly recommended for all ulcer patients who have this infection.

Older patients (such as those over 50 years) and patients with additional symptoms such as weight loss, persistent vomiting, or dysphagia should also be promptly investigated. This is because there is a greater probability of finding more serious organic disease in such patients.

PATHOGENESIS

The traditional explanation for the cause of peptic ulcers was that they represented the result of an imbalance between aggressive and defensive factors in the upper gastrointestinal tract. The aggressive factors are principally acid and pepsin, which are normal secretory products of the stomach. As a group, patients with duodenal ulcer have higher mean levels of gastric acid secretion compared with matched controls. However, there is also a large degree of overlap with control subjects. This means that patients with duodenal ulcer can have "normal" levels of gastric acid secretion. In the rare condition Zollinger-Ellison syndrome (ZES), excess secretion of gastric acid may be sufficient to cause ulceration of the gastric or duodenal mucosa (or elsewhere in the gastrointestinal tract) with apparently normal mucosal defense. However, in the vast majority of patients with peptic ulceration, it is impairment of mucosal defense mechanisms that allows gastric acid and pepsin to damage the mucosa and lead to ulceration. The two principal factors that impair mucosal defense mechanisms in humans are *H. pylori* infection and the use of aspirin or nonsteroidal anti-inflammatory drugs (NSAIDs). Cigarette smoking is an additional factor in many patients.

Helicobacter pylori *Infection*

Since the gram-negative bacterium *H. pylori* was identified in the early 1980s, a great deal has been discovered about its role in the etiology of gastritis and peptic ulcer. The organism may also be involved in the etiology of adenocarcinoma and lymphoma of the stomach, but discussion of these topics is beyond the scope of this article. Over 90% of patients with duodenal ulcer, as well as up to 80% of patients with gastric ulcer, are infected with *H. pylori*. However, the infection is also very common in asymptomatic individuals.

Helicobacter pylori is the commonest chronic bacterial infection to afflict humans. Millions of patients are infected worldwide, with the prevalence generally higher in underdeveloped nations. In the United States, the prevalence of the infection increases with advancing age and is higher in individuals from lower socioeconomic backgrounds. The exact route of infection is unknown, but it is likely to be fecal-oral. In developing nations, where there is associated poverty, poor sanitation, and overcrowding, many individuals become infected in childhood. Once infection is established, it usually becomes chronic unless specific eradication treatment is administered. The bacterium colonizes only gastric-type mucosa. It induces a local inflammatory reaction in the stomach (gastritis), and a systemic immune response. Circulating antibodies to *H. pylori* can be used to diagnose the presence of the infection.

Although many millions of patients worldwide have this chronic bacterial infection of the stomach with associated gastritis, only a minority become symptomatic or develop an ulcer. The explanation for this observation has not been completely determined. There may be strain differences so that certain types of the bacterium are more closely linked to ulcer development, or there may be certain factors in the host response to the infection that are associated with ulceration. Nonetheless, it remains true that the majority of infected patients are asymptomatic despite having chronic inflammation of the gastric mucosa. Therefore, the somewhat loose use of the term "gastritis" as a clinical diagnosis for a patient presenting with dyspepsia should be abandoned; most patients with true gastritis have no symptoms.

When it initially infects the stomach, *H. pylori* has a predilection for the gastric antrum. Here it lies in close apposition with the gastric epithelium beneath the mucus layer. It may form adhesion pedicles to the gastric epithelium and may also be found in the antral gastric glands, but it only rarely invades the gastric mucosa. Since it lies beneath the mucus layer, into which the gastric epithelium secretes bicarbonate ions, it is protected from the bactericidal effects of gastric acid. The pH microclimate at the site of the bacteria is around 6, while the pH in the gastric lumen is around 2.

Once infection is established, the bacterium induces an acute and chronic inflammatory response. It secretes a number of putative virulence factors that may cause superficial damage to the gastric mucosa and weakening of the tight junctions between adjacent epithelial cells. *Helicobacter pylori* produces urease, enabling it to break down urea, which is normally present in gastric juice, to produce ammonia and carbon dioxide. Although other bacteria, such as *Proteus*, also produce urease, *H. pylori* appears to be the most potent urease producer of all known bacteria. This may be a factor in its pathogenicity, since ammonia and ammonium ions are potentially toxic to the gastric mucosa.

It has been difficult to explain how a chronic bacterial infection of the gastric mucosa is related to ulceration of the duodenal mucosa, particularly since the bacterium colonizes only gastric-type epithelium. *Helicobacter pylori* cannot survive on normal duodenal epithelium. However, there are usually foci of gastric metaplasia in the duodenum in patients who have duodenal ulceration. Many years of excessive exposure of the duodenal mucosa to excess gastric acid may induce this type of metaplasia. Once there is gastric-type epithelium in the duodenum, *H. pylori* can migrate from the gastric antrum to colonize these areas. There, it induces an inflammatory reaction just as it does in the stomach. The resulting duodenitis disrupts the integrity of the mucosa and may allow the back-diffusion of acid that leads to the formation of a duodenal ulcer.

Thus, most cases of duodenal ulcer result from a complex inter-relationship between gastric acid secretion and the effects of *H. pylori* infection. It should be stressed that it is rare to find a duodenal ulcer without *H. pylori* infection.

If this situation is encountered in clinical practice, other rarer causes of duodenal ulceration should be considered. These include ZES, Crohn's disease, cytomegalovirus infection in immune-suppressed patients, and the possibility of surreptitious aspirin or NSAID use. However, it is clear that *H. pylori* infection is an essential cofactor in the vast majority of cases of duodenal ulcer. The situation is slightly different in gastric ulcer, in which *H. pylori* infection is only present in around 80% of patients at most. In gastric ulcer, the other important etiologic agent is aspirin or NSAID use.

Aspirin and Nonsteroidal Anti-Inflammatory Drugs

Aspirin and NSAIDs are directly toxic to the gastric mucosa. They are inhibitors of prostaglandin synthesis within the upper gastrointestinal tract and elsewhere. Prostaglandins may play some physiologic role in the upper gastrointestinal tract in regulating cell turnover and the maintenance of mucosal defense through modulation of gastric mucosal blood flow and stimulation of mucus and bicarbonate secretion.

Acute ingestion of aspirin or an NSAID usually causes subepithelial hemorrhages and superficial gastric erosions. Usually, these phenomena are asymptomatic, although erosions may be associated with overt gastrointestinal bleeding. With continuous use, there is usually some degree of adaptation to the effects of aspirin or NSAIDs in most patients. However, if this adaptation is ineffective, chronic ingestion can be associated with the development of ulceration, which is most often found in the gastric antrum.

Current thinking about gastric ulceration is that it is due either to the effects of *H. pylori* infection or to aspirin or NSAID use. If both these factors exist together, there does not appear to be any additive risk of gastric ulcer. Aspirin or NSAID use may not be reported by the patient or may be completely surreptitious. This should be considered in any patient with an unexplained benign gastric ulcer, particularly without *H. pylori* infection, or if a gastric ulcer persistently fails to heal on medical therapy.

Cigarette Smoking

It has been known for some time that smoking is adversely associated with peptic ulceration. Although it is not regarded as causal, smoking is associated with a more rapid recurrence of peptic ulcer after healing. In addition, it has been postulated that the therapeutic efficacy of some of the agents used for peptic ulcer, such as the H_2-receptor antagonists (see later), is impaired. This latter point remains controversial.

The reason for the adverse influence of smoking is not entirely clear. Smoking has no consistent effects on gastric acid secretion. It may impair bicarbonate secretion by the pancreas and the duodenal mucosa which normally neutralizes some of the acid delivered from the stomach. Smoking may also accelerate gastric emptying, thereby promoting the delivery of acid to the duodenum.

Psychological Stress

Although many patients perceive an association between stress and ulcers, there is no hard evidence for this. Some patients may report a temporal relationship between ulcer symptoms and episodes of stress. It is difficult to offer any firm or useful advice about this.

DIAGNOSIS OF PEPTIC ULCER

Some patients with dyspeptic symptoms receive empirical therapy without any diagnostic work-up. This approach is only suitable for some young, otherwise healthy individuals with minor or moderate symptoms of short duration. If dyspepsia is associated with more alarming symptoms such as dysphagia, weight loss, persistent vomiting, or gastrointestinal bleeding, then prompt referral is indicated. Older patients, such as those aged 50 years or above, should also be referred for further evaluation.

If peptic ulcer is suspected as the cause of dyspepsia, and if empirical therapy is not being considered, the physician has the choice of upper gastrointestinal endoscopy or barium radiologic examination as a method of investigation. Endoscopy is more sensitive and more specific than barium radiologic examination and allows biopsies to be taken. There is no indication to use barium radiologic examination for the investigation of dyspepsia. Some patients who have barium radiologic examinations still require endoscopy. These include patients with an apparently normal barium study, and also those found to have gastric ulceration. All patients with gastric ulcer should have endoscopy with biopsies and brushings taken from around the ulcer crater and from the ulcer base to exclude the possibility of malignancy.

Another excellent reason for recommending endoscopy to confirm the clinical diagnosis of peptic ulcer is that it allows prompt and easy identification of *H. pylori* infection. Both the infection and its associated gastritis can be detected on routine histologic evaluation of gastric mucosal biopsies taken at endoscopy. *Helicobacter pylori* may also be cultured from gastric mucosal biopsies and its antibiotic sensitivities determined. However, these steps are not performed routinely, since they are both expensive and largely unnecessary.

Some diagnostic tests for *H. pylori* rely on its urease activity. A simple urease test on a gastric mucosal biopsy, such as the commercially available "Clo-test," gives prompt and reliable confirmation of infection. Since the human gastric mucosa does not normally contain urease, any urease activity detected in the biopsy is derived from *H. pylori*. In the Clo-test, a gastric mucosal biopsy is placed in a gel on a plastic slide. The gel contains urea and a pH indicator. If *H. pylori* is present in the biopsy material, its urease breaks down the urea to release ammonia. This causes a rise in the pH and a change in the color of the pH indicator from yellow to red or pink. A biopsy urease test, such as the Clo-test, is cheap and adds very little to the cost of endoscopy. It is the method of choice for detecting *H. pylori* infection at endoscopy. False-negative results may be found if the patient has been taking antibiotics, bismuth-containing medications, or acid-suppressing drugs.

Since those peptic ulcer patients who have *H. pylori* infection are likely to benefit from its successful eradication (see later), it is important that both the ulcer and the infection be correctly diagnosed and documented before attempted treatment. A biopsy urease test should be performed if a patient is found at endoscopy to have a gastric or duodenal ulcer. The probability of a positive test is high in routine clinical practice (about 80% for gastric ulcer and 95% for duodenal ulcer). However, it is important to document the infection before treatment, and it is also important to correctly identify those rare patients with duodenal ulceration unrelated to *H. pylori* infection. This should lead to a consideration of other potential diagnoses such as those already described. In patients with gastric ulcer unrelated to *H. pylori* infection, one should strongly suspect aspirin or NSAID use. Although some patients are aware of using one of these medications, others may not know that their analgesic preparation contains aspirin, or they may not choose to inform their physician that they are taking aspirin. Although not recommended for routine clinical use, a simple in vitro test of platelet adhesiveness reliably indicates whether or not a patient has been taking aspirin.

Once treatment to eradicate *H. pylori* infection is completed, it is reasonable to want to perform some sort of test to see if the treatment has been effective. Repeated endoscopy would be a very expensive option and might not be acceptable to the patient. Serologic analysis for antibodies to *H. pylori* is unreliable in this situation, since antibody titers fall very slowly after successful eradication. To check for successful eradication of *H. pylori*, a radiolabeled urea breath test is probably the method of choice but is not yet routinely available. In these tests, the patient is given a small oral dose of urea labeled with ^{13}C or ^{14}C. If *H. pylori* infection is still present in the stomach, its urease breaks down the urea to produce ammonia and carbon dioxide. The carbon dioxide carrying the radiolabeled carbon atom diffuses into the circulation and is excreted by the lungs, where it can be detected in the breath. A negative urea breath test 4 weeks after stopping therapy for *H. pylori* infection indicates successful eradication.

TREATMENT

It is relevant first to explore the general advice that should be offered to patients with peptic ulceration before specific therapeutic agents are considered. All ulcer patients should be strongly advised to stop smoking, both for their ulcer disease and for their general health.

However, patients with peptic ulcer do not require any specific advice on diet. There is no rationale for recommending the bland diets used in the past. Patients may eat what they want, with the physician stressing the importance of a nutritious and well-balanced diet. Obviously, the patients will avoid specific foodstuffs that they associate with ulcer pain.

Similarly, no specific advice on alcohol use is necessary unless a patient is drinking excessively. In that case, advice on reducing or discontinuing alcohol consumption is necessary for general health concerns rather than for peptic ulcer per se. There is no hard evidence that alcohol plays any role in the etiology of peptic ulcer. Some clinical trials have even suggested that a moderate intake of alcohol may be beneficial in promoting ulcer healing, although this is not established. Of the different types of alcoholic beverages, there may be differences with respect to their effects on gastric secretion. Wine and beer have the greatest stimulant effects on gastric acid secretion, whereas more concentrated forms of alcohol, such as distilled liquor, may not produce any measurable effect. It is only necessary to recommend avoidance of a specific form of alcoholic beverage if the patient has noticed a temporal relationship between its ingestion and symptoms.

It is important to know if the patient is taking aspirin or NSAIDs. Generally, patients should be advised to avoid these agents. Small doses of aspirin, such as those used as prophylaxis against cardiovascular problems, are probably unimportant. If the patient is taking an NSAID, a decision must be made on whether this needs to be continued. This is discussed in more detail later.

Traditionally, the goals of treatment for peptic ulcer have been defined as

Alleviation of symptoms
Healing of the ulcer
Prevention of complications
Prevention of recurrence

The first two of these goals are relatively easy to achieve, with many effective drugs currently available. There is little evidence to suggest that peptic ulcer treatment is effective in the primary prevention of ulcer complications. Medical treatment is effective in the secondary prevention of bleeding. Continuous use of the H_2-receptor antagonist ranitidine (Zantac) after ulcer healing has been shown to reduce the rate of recurrent ulcer hemorrhage.

The continuous use of H_2-receptor antagonists, sucralfate (Carafate), or acid pump inhibitors after ulcer healing is effective in reducing the rate of ulcer recurrence. However, once such maintenance treatment is stopped, ulcers recur with the same frequency as before. Eradication of *H. pylori* infection is the only medical treatment to have had a major impact on the natural history of peptic ulceration. This is now regarded as an effective long-term treatment for peptic ulcer and offers the possibility of a cure in at least some patients.

Treatment of peptic ulcer used to consist of short-term management designed to relieve symptoms and heal the ulcer, followed by long-term management in an attempt to prevent ulcer complications or recurrence. However, this approach is likely to change with the introduction of treatment regimens that heal the ulcer and eradicate *H. pylori*, thereby also providing effective long-term management (see pp. 510–511 for specific treatment).

With short-term treatment, there are no important differences between duodenal and gastric ulcers, although endoscopic biopsy is essential for the latter, as already discussed. The same drugs and the same dosage regimens are used for both duodenal and gastric ulcer. A brief discussion of the available drugs follows.

Antacids

Antacids are frequently used by patients with dyspepsia. Most of these patients either have self-limiting symptoms or gastroesophageal reflux disease rather than peptic ulcer. However, antacids are effective symptomatic treatment for the pain of peptic ulceration. Indeed a clinical history of epigastric pain that awakens a patient and is relieved by an antacid is circumstantial evidence of peptic ulceration.

Antacids are weak bases that neutralize gastric acid. In addition, they may have some other properties such as stimulating the production of endogenous prostaglandins and growth factors around ulcer craters. Such properties have been defined in experimental studies but have not been confirmed to be important in routine clinical use.

Most of the antacids in use are nonsystemic and contain either aluminum or magnesium or a combination of the two. Since these agents are not absorbed from the gastrointestinal tract to any appreciable extent, their adverse effects are concentrated on the gut. Antacids containing aluminum may cause constipation, whereas those that contain magnesium may cause diarrhea. Some antacids are freely absorbable and may influence systemic acid-base balance if taken in excessive quantities. An example is sodium bicarbonate, which is a highly effective antacid but which may produce systemic alkalosis and sodium overload if taken in sufficient quantities. It should not be taken over prolonged periods and should be avoided by patients with cardiac or hepatic insufficiency.

As well as being effective for the control of ulcer symptoms, it is clear that antacids can also heal peptic ulcers. In controlled studies performed in the United States, high doses of magnesium-containing liquid antacids have been shown to be more efficacious than placebo in this regard. However, diarrhea was a frequent and troublesome side effect. Since large doses of antacids are cumbersome to take and are associated with the side effect of altered bowel habit, they are not recommended for the routine treatment of peptic ulcer.

Histamine H₂-Receptor Antagonists

Since the introduction in the late 1970s of cimetidine (Tagamet), the first commercially available H₂-receptor antagonist, these drugs have been extensively used for the treatment of peptic ulcer. They are effective for the relief of ulcer pain as well as for healing the ulcer. In addition, their continued use after ulcer healing reduces the rate of ulcer recurrence. As a group, the H₂-receptor antagonists are remarkably safe and well tolerated. Four H₂-receptor antagonists are available in the United States: cimetidine, ranitidine, famotidine (Pepcid), and nizatidine (Axid).

In pharmacologic terms, these agents are competitive antagonists for histamine at the H₂-receptor site. Although this type of receptor is widely disseminated in the body, its only defined physiologic role is in the stimulation of gastric acid secretion by parietal cells in the oxyntic mucosa of the stomach. Therefore, the H₂-receptor antagonists inhibit gastric acid secretion. In this regard, they are more effective in inhibiting acid secretion in the basal state, such as occurs with fasting or overnight, than in response to food ingestion. In patients with duodenal ulcer, there is often a relative and inappropriate hypersecretion of gastric acid during the overnight period. The use of an H₂-receptor antagonist at night before retiring is effective in controlling this hypersecretion and is sufficient to heal most duodenal ulcers. Typically, a standard single daily dose of an H₂-receptor antagonist taken at bedtime (e.g., cimetidine 800 mg, ranitidine 300 mg, famotidine 40 mg, or nizatidine 300 mg) should heal about 80% of duodenal ulcers after 4 weeks, increasing to 95% after a total of 8 weeks. Healing of gastric ulcers takes longer, but typical expected healing rates are 65 to 70% at 4 weeks increasing to 85 to 90% after 8 weeks. Although most duodenal and gastric ulcers heal satisfactorily on an H₂-receptor antagonist, patient compliance is an important factor. Patients usually notice improvement in their symptoms within a few days of starting treatment. However, they should be advised not to discontinue treatment at that point but to complete the prescribed course.

In the case of duodenal ulcer treated with a single evening or bedtime dose of an H₂-receptor antagonist, it is important that patients are advised not to have anything by mouth once they have taken their dose. Ingestion of food after taking an H₂-receptor antagonist is associated with stimulation of gastric acid secretion by gastrin and vagal pathways such that the pharmacologic effect of the H₂-receptor antagonist is largely overcome.

Although there have been some reports of pharmacologic tolerance to H₂-receptor antagonists developing with their continuous use, this has not been a problem in the treatment of patients with peptic ulcer. Indeed, continuous use of an H₂-receptor antagonist after initial ulcer healing is effective in preventing ulcer recurrence. However, despite the strenuous marketing efforts of the pharmaceutical industry, not all patients with duodenal ulcer require this form of maintenance treatment. Although most patients with duodenal ulcer eventually experience a recurrence, most have a maximum of two episodes of recurrence in the year after initial ulcer healing, and many have none or one. These patients can be managed with intermittent courses of medication when they develop a recurrence. Continuous maintenance treatment probably does have a role in sick, elderly patients with other concomitant illnesses and in patients with a previous episode of hemorrhage or perforation. In addition, some patients with aggressive ulcer disease associated with frequent episodes of recurrence and possible complications might be managed better with an H₂-receptor antagonist in its full dose rather than the traditional half doses recommended for maintenance. The same may be true for ulcer patients who are unwise enough to continue smoking cigarettes. Traditional half-dose maintenance treatment with an H₂-receptor antagonist is often ineffective in smokers, although full doses may produce better results.

Despite the efficacy of maintenance treatment with the H₂-receptor antagonists in preventing ulcer recurrence, success is not guaranteed. Typically, 20% of patients on maintenance H₂-receptor antagonists experience an ulcer recurrence within the next 12 months compared with up to 80% on no treatment. Attention has now switched from the concept of maintenance treatment to that of perhaps curing the ulcer diathesis with effective eradication of *H. pylori* infection. However, for those patients who had sustained a complication of peptic ulceration, continuous maintenance treatment with an acid-suppressing drug is still considered appropriate even after attempted eradication of *H. pylori* infection.

The H_2-receptor antagonists are extremely safe in routine clinical practice. Few side effects have been described, and these are usually mild and self-limiting. There are few important differences between the agents of this class with respect to their safety and tolerability. Cimetidine may be associated with antiandrogenic side effects such as impotence, gynecomastia, and loss of libido. However, these are all extremely rare. Cimetidine and ranitidine have been associated with reversible mental confusion, particularly in sick, elderly patients in the intensive care unit who were receiving high doses of these drugs. Ranitidine has been associated with headache and with mild, transient elevations in the levels of some liver enzymes. Again, these side effects are generally mild and not serious. Apparent differences between agents may simply reflect reporting bias rather than true pharmacologic differences.

Many drug interactions have been reported with various H_2-receptor antagonists, with the majority attributed to cimetidine. However, most of the interactions are of no clinical relevance and concern alteration in pharmacokinetics only. Cimetidine is a nonspecific inhibitor of the hepatic cytochrome P-450 system. It therefore reduces the metabolism of a number of drugs that are cleared from the body via this route. The only important interactions involving cimetidine are with phenytoin (Dilantin), theophylline, and warfarin (Coumadin). These three drugs are extensively metabolized in the liver and have narrow therapeutic indices. If their metabolism is reduced through concomitant use of cimetidine, their steady-state plasma concentrations increase and may reach the toxic range. Other H_2-receptor antagonists, such as ranitidine, also bind to hepatic cytochrome P-450 but with much less propensity to cause interactions. There are no important drug interactions reported with ranitidine or the other H_2-receptor antagonists in current use.

Sucralfate

Sucralfate (Carafate) is a complex salt of aluminum and sucrose octasulfate. Its exact mode of action is unknown. It does not suppress gastric acid secretion but heals peptic ulcers at rates that are very similar to those of the H_2-receptor antagonists. In experimental studies, sucralfate can be shown to bind to ulcer bases. The insoluble coating it produces is thought to be capable of preventing further damage from gastric acid and pepsin. In addition, it may stimulate the local production of prostaglandins and endogenous growth factors around ulcers.

The standard clinical dose of sucralfate is 4 grams daily—either 1 gram four times daily or 2 grams twice daily. After ulcer healing, sucralfate may be continued in half its initial healing dose as maintenance therapy. At the time of writing, sucralfate was not approved for the treatment of gastric ulcer. The most frequent side effect associated with sucralfate is constipation, by virtue of its aluminum content. A number of drug interactions have been reported with sucralfate, since it is capable of binding a number of other agents within the gastrointestinal tract before their absorption. However, these are rarely of clinical importance and can be avoided by administering sucralfate at times separate from those of other drugs that patients may be receiving.

Acid Pump Inhibitors

Acid pump inhibitors, including omeprazole (Prilosec) and lansoprazole (Prevacid), are irreversible inhibitors of the enzyme H^+/K^-–ATPase that is found in the secretory canaliculi of parietal cells. That enzyme, the acid pump, is responsible for the final step in the process of acid secretion by the parietal cell, namely the active transport of hydrogen ions into the gastric lumen. Irreversible blockade of this enzyme leads to marked suppression of acid secretion by the cell, irrespective of any stimulus. However, inhibition of acid secretion is never complete, since new molecules of H^+/K^-–ATPase are constantly being synthesized. Acid pump inhibitors do not, therefore, induce achlorhydria.

Since these drugs produce a greater degree of inhibition of gastric acid secretion than conventional doses of the H_2-receptor antagonists do, they are associated with higher rates of ulcer healing. Looked at in a slightly different way, they heal peptic ulcers faster than the H_2-receptor antagonists. Typically, an acid pump inhibitor heals as many duodenal ulcers in 2 weeks as an H_2-receptor antagonist does in 4 weeks. Proportions of healed ulcers increase with the duration of therapy, so healing rates on an acid pump inhibitor after 4 weeks approximate those seen on an H_2-receptor antagonist after 8 weeks. Although ulcers heal faster on acid pump inhibitors, there is no associated increase in the rate of ulcer recurrence after healing. Similarly, there is no rebound hypersecretion of acid after discontinuing an acid pump inhibitor.

The acid pump inhibitors are safe in routine use. Few adverse events have been recorded, and as with the H_2-receptor antagonists, these drugs are generally very well tolerated. Diarrhea, which is usually mild and self-limiting, is probably the most frequently observed adverse event in routine clinical practice. At the time of writing, the acid pump inhibitors had not received FDA approval for continuous long-term use except in ZES.

When given to rats in very high doses over prolonged periods, these drugs have been associated with the formation of nonmetastasizing gastric carcinoid tumors derived from enterochromaffin-like (ECL) cells. The mechanism for the formation of these tumors, which have not been observed in any other species studied, is through extreme hypergastrinemia. When gastric acid secretion is inhibited, the natural brake on endogenous gastrin release is removed, allowing gastrin levels to increase. The gastrin response in rats is extremely sensitive to reduced acidity, and the rat mounts an excessive gastrin response to this. In turn, the ECL cell in the rat appears to be very sensitive to the trophic effects of gastrin.

ECL cell carcinoid tumors have not been encountered in humans during the routine clinical use of acid pump inhibitors. Such tumors do occur sporadically in humans, especially in association with hypergastrinemia as in pernicious anemia or ZES. In ZES, patients may be successfully managed with high doses of acid pump inhibitors over many years. Even in that situation, there has been no increased rate of ECL cell gastric carcinoid tumors.

In controlled clinical trials, omeprazole, 20 mg daily, or lansoprazole, 15 mg daily, heals over 90% of duodenal ulcers and around 90% of gastric ulcers in 4 weeks. Acid pump inhibitors are also extremely effective in relieving the pain of peptic ulceration. Indeed, they may be more effective in this than the H_2-receptor antagonists. There is also a limited amount of data to suggest that the acid pump inhibitors are superior to the H_2-receptor antagonists in healing unusually large peptic ulcers, in healing ulcers in patients who continue to smoke cigarettes (although all patients must be advised to stop smoking), and in healing ulcers in patients who continue to use NSAIDs.

A SYSTEMATIC APPROACH TO THE TREATMENT OF PEPTIC ULCER

Let us assume that the diagnosis of duodenal or gastric ulcer has been confirmed endoscopically, that malignancy has been appropriately excluded in the case of gastric ulcer, and that a biopsy urease test has been performed to check for *H. pylori* infection. The patient should receive the appropriate advice about smoking and should be advised to avoid taking aspirin and NSAIDs.

If the patient has *H. pylori* infection, this should be addressed. The National Institutes of Health (NIH) Consensus Development Conference of February 1994 recommended that all infected ulcer patients receive antimicrobial treatment aimed at eradicating *H. pylori*. This should be done whether on the first or a subsequent presentation with ulcer. Specific eradication regimens are discussed later.

If the patient does not have *H. pylori* infection, consideration should be given to other causes of ulceration. In the case of gastric ulcer, this is most likely to be the use of aspirin or NSAIDs. If a patient with a gastric ulcer is taking one of these agents, a careful review of the indication and justification for it must be made. The aspirin or NSAID therapy should be stopped if it is not for a valid reason. Many patients, especially the elderly, take these drugs for inappropriate reasons and might obtain equal benefit from a simple analgesic such as acetaminophen.

However, if the patient has a truly inflammatory arthropathy such as rheumatoid arthritis, it is likely that there will be continued need for an NSAID. It is important, however, to ensure that the patient is receiving the lowest effective dose of the NSAID consistent with an acceptable quality of life. Whether the NSAID therapy can be discontinued or not, almost all these ulcers heal satisfactorily with any of a number of available agents including H_2-receptor antagonists, sucralfate, or acid pump inhibitors. Limited data suggest that the acid pump inhibitors are the most effective in this situation, although this requires confirmation. Ulcer healing is more rapid if the NSAID therapy can first be stopped.

HELICOBACTER PYLORI ERADICATION MEASURES

The majority of patients with peptic ulcers are infected with *H. pylori*, which plays a major role in the etiology of the ulcer. There is now incontrovertible evidence that successful eradication of this infection is associated with a major reduction in the rate of ulcer recurrence, possibly even constituting a cure of the ulcer diathesis in some patients. However, a number of problems are encountered in attempting to eradicate this infection.

To date, no single agent has proved effective in eradicating *H. pylori* infection. Even the combination of two antibiotics given together is unlikely to prove efficacious. For that reason, three drugs are often combined in what has become known as triple therapy. This combination usually consists of a bismuth salt (such as Pepto-Bismol), metronidazole (Flagyl, Protostat), and an additional antibiotic such as amoxicillin (Amoxil, Moxilin, Wymox) or tetracycline (Achromycin). Appropriate doses would be Pepto-Bismol two tablets four times daily, metronidazole 250 mg three or four times daily, and tetracycline or amoxicillin 500 mg four times daily. If taken together for 2 weeks, this therapy can be successful in eradicating *H. pylori* in 80 to 90% of infected patients. Compliance with the medication is important for treatment to be successful. If the patient takes less than 60% of the prescribed medication, the chances of successful eradication drop dramatically.

Triple therapy is difficult and cumbersome for patients to take. It involves a large number of tablets taken at frequent intervals during the day, which may further limit compliance. Adverse effects have been reported in between 30 and 50% of patients. These may include taste disturbance and diarrhea but are only rarely serious. If a regimen containing metronidazole is used, patients should be advised to abstain from alcohol because of the unpleasant interaction. *Helicobacter pylori* may rapidly acquire resistance to metronidazole.

In view of the problems associated with triple therapy, alternative regimens have been developed and studied. The combination of amoxicillin and metronidazole with the H_2-receptor antagonist ranitidine was found to be highly effective in one trial. The combination of an acid pump inhibitor and one or two antibiotics may also be particularly effective. These approaches have the added advantage that they will effectively heal an active ulcer as well as address the underlying *H. pylori* infection. Triple therapy is unlikely to produce ulcer healing unless combined with an acid-suppressing medication such as an H_2-receptor antagonist or acid pump inhibitor. In that event, triple therapy effectively becomes quadruple therapy.

Omeprazole or lansoprazole may suitably be combined with an antibiotic such as amoxicillin or clarithromycin (Biaxin), although acquired resistance may be a problem with the latter. Many different regimens have been studied, and the optimum dosages have yet to be defined. However, it appears that the acid pump inhibitor should be prescribed twice daily and should be started at the same time as the antibiotic. Since these regimens do not contain metronidazole, they should be effective even if the bacterium is resistant to metronidazole. In addition, if eradication is unsuccessful, patients can receive treatment with a more traditional triple therapy approach.

No firm recommendations can be given about checking for successful eradication. The radiolabeled urea breath test should become more widely available. If the costs of such tests are not too high, they would be appropriate in this context, with patients being tested about 4 to 6 weeks after stopping their eradication regimen.

Currently available data suggest that true reinfection with *H. pylori* is rare after successful eradication. There are no firm guidelines as to how patients should be treated if they become reinfected. However, in some studies documented reinfection with the bacterium was not necessarily associated with recurrence of peptic ulcer.

SUMMARY

The importance of *H. pylori* cannot be overemphasized; it has had enormous influence on how peptic ulcer is perceived and managed. Research is extremely active in this area, and the optimum treatment for the infection remains to be discovered. The conclusions of the 1994 NIH Consensus Development Conference provide valuable recommendations about management of peptic ulcer patients in this new and exciting era.

TUMORS OF THE STOMACH

method of
H. RICHARD ALEXANDER, JR., M.D.
National Cancer Institute
Bethesda, Maryland

At the beginning of the twentieth century, adenocarcinoma of the stomach was the leading cause of cancer death in the United States, and until 1988 it was the leading cause of cancer death worldwide. The annual incidence of gastric adenocarcinoma decreased significantly in the United States from 33 per 100,000 persons in 1935 to 9 per 100,000 persons in the early 1980s. However, the National Cancer Institute (NCI) SEER (surveillance, epidemiology, and end results) program has shown that the incidence of gastroesophageal adenocarcinomas and gastric adenocarcinomas arising in the cardia has increased dramatically over the past 15 years. Between 1976 and 1987 the annual rate of increase of adenocarcinoma of the gastric cardia was 5.6% for black women, 4.3% for white men, 4.1% for white women, and 3.6% for black men. This rate of increase during the late 1970s and through the mid-1980s was greater than that of any other cancer. In Japan, Eastern Europe, and portions of South America, particularly Chile and Costa Rica, gastric cancer is epidemic.

Stomach cancers occur approximately twice as often in men as in women, and the incidence of stomach cancer increases with advancing age. In 1965, Lauren described two distinct histologic types of stomach adenocarcinoma. The glandular form is also known as "intestinal" or "differentiated cancer" and is typically diploid. This is the most frequent type of gastric cancer seen in populations in which the disease is epidemic; it has a slightly greater incidence in males and is typically antral. The second form is called "diffuse" or "undifferentiated cancer" and is typically aneuploid. This type of gastric adenocarcinoma is most frequently seen in populations in which the disease is endemic; it has an equal distribution between males and females, is most frequently seen in patients who have familial predisposition to gastric cancer, and is more commonly proximal.

It has been clearly shown that certain environmental and nutritional factors are associated with increased risk of developing stomach adenocarcinoma. Populations that have diets low in animal protein and fat and high in complex carbohydrates and that use salted meats or fish have a higher incidence of gastric adenocarcinoma. Diets that are typically rich in vitamins A and C are associated with a low risk of gastric adenocarcinoma. Environmental factors that are predisposed to the development of gastric cancer include poor food preparation, including the use of smoked food; a lack of refrigeration; and poor-quality drinking water (which may have high levels of nitrates). To a lesser degree smoking has been associated with the increased risk of stomach cancer. Recently it has been appreciated that chronic *Helicobacter pylori* infection is associated with a higher incidence of gastric adenocarcinoma. In addition, a history of prior gastric resection for benign disease is also associated with an increased risk of developing gastric stump adenocarcinoma. Currently available information suggests that normal gastric mucosa may undergo atrophic changes secondary to chronic exposure to diet as described above, high salt intake, or a prior vagotomy. Gastric atrophy with an increase in intragastric pH leads to chronic bacterial overgrowth within the stomach, resulting in chronic atrophic gastritis. Subsequently, the gastric epithelium may undergo metaplasia with subsequent dysplastic changes ultimately leading to frank carcinoma.

Unfortunately, most patients in the United States with gastric cancer are diagnosed with advanced-stage disease because many of the symptoms associated with gastric adenocarcinoma are nonspecific. Patients may have a combination of signs and symptoms including weight loss, anorexia, fatigue, and vague abdominal discomfort. Early satiety is an infrequent symptom of gastric cancer but usually indicates a diffusely infiltrating tumor and loss of distensibility of the gastric wall. Persistent vomiting may be a reflection of gastric outlet obstruction secondary to a large antral tumor. On physical examination, signs of advanced gastric cancer include the presence of ascites, a palpable abdominal mass, or the presence of metastatic lymph nodes around the umbilicus, the left supraclavicular fossa, or the left axilla. In addition, metastatic deposits in the ovary or a pelvic mass on rectal examination may be present.

If a diagnosis of gastric carcinoma is suspected, an upper endoscopy with biopsy should be performed. After the diagnosis is established, staging procedures include careful physical examination, routine blood screening tests, and abdominal and chest computed tomography (CT) scanning. CT is useful for assessing the lateral extension of the primary tumor and for identifying systemic metastases. However, up to 50% of patients who have localized disease based on preoperative CT scanning have more extensive disease found at laparotomy. There has been recent interest in the use of endoscopic ultrasonography (EUS) for the staging of gastric adenocarcinoma. EUS uses a high-frequency transducer that is attached to the end of an upper endoscope; it allows the accurate staging of the depth of penetration of the primary tumor and is more accurate than CT scan for the staging of lymph node disease. However, the vast majority of metastatic nodes in gastric cancer are less than 3 to 4 mm in diameter and therefore are difficult to distinguish by EUS. In the future, laparoscopic staging in patients with apparently localized gastric cancer may become more commonly used.

The staging of gastric adenocarcinoma follows the tumor, node, metastases (TNM) classification (American Joint Cancer Commission, 1988). The 5-year survival for patients with Stage IA or IB disease is approximately 85%; only between 1 and 5% of all patients are diagnosed with this stage disease. Another 10 to 15% of patients are diagnosed with Stage II disease, defined as a primary tumor that penetrates the gastric wall to the serosa with or without the presence of regional metastatic lymph nodes. The 5-year overall survival for patients with Stage II disease is only about 50%. The remainder of patients, approximately 70 to 85%, are diagnosed with Stage III or Stage IV disease, for which the 5-year survival is at best 10%.

TREATMENT

Localized Gastric Adenocarcinoma

The only potentially curative modality for localized gastric adenocarcinoma is surgery. The current areas of debate include the potential therapeutic benefit of an extended lymphadenectomy, the use of a total versus subtotal gastrectomy for tumors of the body and antrum of the stomach, and the use of prophylactic splenectomy for tumors not adjacent to the splenic hilum. When the type of gastric resection for gastric adenocarcinoma is considered, the location of the primary tumor is critical. A proximal margin less than 7 cm from the gross edge of the tumor results in an increased incidence of an anastomotic recurrence secondary to the very rich submucosal lymphatics of the stomach wall. In contrast, the pylorus is a remarkably effective barrier against the prograde extension of gastric cancer, and duodenal stump recurrences of stomach cancer are extremely rare. The

French Association for Surgical Research published a prospective controlled trial of total versus subtotal gastrectomy for adenocarcinoma of the gastric antrum and showed that there was no difference between the two techniques with respect to 5-year survival. The Norwegian Stomach Cancer Trial showed that complications and mortality in patients undergoing total gastrectomy for stomach cancer were significantly higher than those undergoing less-than-total gastrectomy. However, a proximal gastric resection for tumors of the body or cardia was associated with the highest rate of postoperative complications. Others have shown that the functional results of a proximal gastric resection are considerably poorer than those of a total gastrectomy. Therefore, for lesions of the body and antrum a subtotal gastric resection confers the same survival advantage as a total gastrectomy with fewer attendant complications. For tumors of the body or cardia a total gastrectomy is preferable to a proximal gastric resection.

Prophylactic splenectomy has been advocated in the past as a technique to facilitate the lymphadenectomy of the perigastric nodes that are residing adjacent to the splenic hilum. The weight of current data indicates that splenectomy has no effect on the length of survival in patients undergoing potentially curative gastric resection and may be associated with increased perioperative complications, primarily of the infectious type.

Prospective randomized trials designed to evaluate the potential therapeutic effect of an extended lymphadenectomy in patients with potentially curable gastric cancer are under way in Europe. A large number of retrospective series, primarily from Japan, have reported that more extensive lymphadenectomy is associated with improved survival in patients with N_0 or N_1 disease. In a single small prospective random-assignment trial comparing limited lymphadenectomy with an extended lymphadenectomy, there was no difference in the probability of 3-year survival between the more limited and the extended lymphadenectomy. The extended lymphadenectomy was associated with a longer operating time, a higher transfusion requirement, and a longer postoperative stay. However, a more recent interim report from the Multicenter Nationwide Random Assignment Trial comparing limited versus extended lymphadenectomy in Dutch patients with gastric cancer has reported no significant differences in the length of hospital stay or types of complications with the two procedures.

Finally, various innovative treatment strategies are being evaluated because of the extremely poor prognosis for patients with gastric cancer even after potentially curative surgery. These approaches include the use of neoadjuvant chemotherapy and intraperitoneal treatment strategies. More than 12 prospective random-assignment trials show no consistent benefit with postoperative adjuvant combination chemotherapy, most commonly using a 5-fluorouracil regimen for patients with resected gastric cancer.

Primary Gastric Lymphoma

Approximately 60% of all primary gastrointestinal lymphomas involve the stomach. There is recent epidemiologic evidence from the NCI SEER program that the age-adjusted incidence of gastric lymphoma has increased twofold from 1973 to 1986. Numerous studies have demonstrated superior survival for patients undergoing resection of a primary lesion followed by systemic chemotherapy. However, inherent in these studies may be a selection bias related to selecting patients with a more favorable prognosis for surgery. Although surgical resection should be considered for patients with localized primary gastric lymphoma and for some patients with poor prognosis factors such as bulky disease, B symptoms, poor performance status, or high serum lactate dehydrogenase levels, the treatment of choice may be systemic chemotherapy and radiation therapy.

TUMORS OF THE COLON AND RECTUM

method of
NANCY KEMENY, M.D.
Memorial Sloan-Kettering Cancer Center
New York, New York

and

OMAR T. ATIQ, M.D.
University of Arkansas for Medical Sciences
Little Rock, Arkansas

Colorectal cancer is the second leading cause of cancer death in the United States. It is estimated that 55,000 people will have died of colorectal cancer in 1995, accounting for 10% of cancer-related mortality. Approximately 138,000 new cases will be diagnosed, with no sex predilection. The incidence and survival rates following surgical resection, the only known curative treatment, have not improved significantly in the last 40 years; however, there has been a slight trend toward decline in the incidence and mortality from colorectal cancer more recently. Future improvements will include earlier recognition of the disease and more aggressive therapy. Early recognition involves careful screening of the general population over 50 years of age and especially of high-risk groups.

ETIOLOGY

Numerous factors contribute to the development of colorectal cancer. The most important of these are genetic, environmental, and dietary factors.

Genetic Factors

Patients with hereditary gastrointestinal polyposis syndromes have a very high incidence of colorectal malignancies. Adenomatous polyposis coli is a rare disease characterized by the presence of over 100 adenomatous polyps scattered throughout the large bowel. If untreated, the disease leads to the development of carcinoma in nearly 100% of affected individuals. When polyposis is the only manifestation of disease, the patient has the autosomal dominant familial polyposis coli syndrome. In Gardner's syndrome, polyposis is associated with osteomas, epidermoid cysts, and soft tissue tumors and is also characterized by autosomal dominant inheritance. Turcot's syndrome is an autosomal recessive disease in which polyposis is associated with central nervous system malignancies.

The age of onset of polyposis syndromes ranges from 7 to 60 years, demonstrating the need for early and frequent screening of all family members of affected patients. Colectomy is the treatment of choice for affected individuals; however, the appropriate time for this intervention is controversial.

The hereditary nonpolyposis colon cancer syndrome is characterized by an excess of proximal colonic involvement, an early age of cancer onset, an excess of multiple primary tumors, and a frequent association with other tumors, especially those of the endometrium and ovary. This syndrome is seen more frequently in relatives of patients with transverse and sigmoid primary tumors than in those with cecal or descending colon tumors.

Peutz-Jeghers syndrome and juvenile polyposis manifest polyps that are not considered premalignant, but recent evidence suggests a greater risk for malignancy in patients with these syndromes and therefore screening and close follow-up are advised.

There is also a three- to fivefold increase in the risk of colon cancer among first-degree relatives of colon cancer patients. However, no similar relationship has been seen in spouses, who presumably share a similar environment but differ genetically.

Patients with ulcerative colitis have an increased risk of developing colon cancer. The most important factors appear to be the extent of involvement and the age of onset, with extensive colitis and earlier onset resulting in a higher risk. Estimates of risk vary from 4.7 to 50% at 30 years. Crohn's disease also increases the risk of colon cancer by 4 to 20%. Colon cancer in these patients occurs at an earlier age and with a higher prevalence of mucinous carcinoma when compared with colon cancer in the general population (Table 1).

Environmental and Dietary Factors

There is evidence indicating that environmental and dietary factors play a role in the etiology of colon cancer. Industrialized nations show markedly elevated incidence rates of colorectal cancer compared with those of developing countries. It is interesting that migrants moving from low-risk to high-risk countries acquire the level of risk that exists among people born in the adopted country. Dietary differences in these countries are believed to be the predominant environmental risk factors. High-fat and low-fiber intake are major features of the Western diet, whereas high-fiber, low-fat diets prevail in Africa, Asia, and other areas where the risk of colon cancer is low. An inverse relationship between colon cancer incidence and

TABLE 1. **Risk Factors for Colorectal Carcinoma**

Familial polyposis syndromes	Inflammatory bowel disease
Gardner's syndrome	Ulcerative colitis
Turcot's syndrome	Crohn's disease
Juvenile polyposis	Family history
Inherited adenomatosis	Past history of colorectal, breast, or endometrial cancer

fiber intake has been more consistent for fruits and vegetables than for cereals.

Other dietary agents that may be implicated in the prevention of colorectal carcinoma are selenium, vitamin C, vitamin A, and flavones and indoles. These substances are present in such vegetables as Brussels sprouts, cabbage, and broccoli. Calcium may be another protective agent.

In addition to diet, other epidemiologic and environmental factors have been suggested as contributors in the development of colon cancer; these include decreased physical activity, increased parity, and occupational exposure to various materials, including asbestos and organic solvents. There are studies suggesting that aspirin and other nonsteroidal anti-inflammatory drugs provide a protective effect by inhibition of prostaglandin synthesis, which decreases the development of colonic polyps.

SCREENING

The rationale for screening is based on the hypothesis that most colorectal cancers are the end result of an orderly progression from normal colonic mucosa to adenomatous polyp, early and surgically curable cancer, and finally advanced and incurable cancer. Screening is intended to detect and remove precancerous polyps as well as early cancers.

To be effective, screening should distinguish people with a high probability of disease from those with low probability through the use of rapid, simple tests. The benefits of screening should include a cost reduction based on diagnosis of the disease at an early stage when treatment is more effective and likely to offer a cure.

The three screening tests commonly used to detect colon cancer are the fecal occult blood test, the digital rectal examination, and sigmoidoscopy. The fecal occult blood test has most frequently involved the use of the Hemoccult card in which the peroxidase-like activity of hemoglobin catalyzes the phenolic oxidation of guaiac-impregnated paper to an easily recognizable blue compound. False-negative results can occur in the presence of dietary vitamin C, which inhibits the chemical reaction. However, the most important reason for the occurrence of false-negative results is that not all colon cancers bleed sufficiently to generate positive test results. Blood losses of more than 20 mL per day are necessary to produce a reliably positive result. Smaller lesions, particularly adenomas, are less likely to bleed. Because hemoglobin is degraded within the bowel lumen, bleeding from right-sided lesions is less likely to be detected than the same amount of bleeding from left-sided lesions. Even in lesions that do bleed, the blood loss may be intermittent, requiring repeated tests.

False-positive results can be caused by ingestion of various fruits and vegetables whose peroxidase activity can mimic that of hemoglobin. Rare beef and iron supplementation can cause a positive result. Positive results can also be obtained by physiologic blood loss, benign bleeding from hemorrhoids, diverticulosis, and peptic ulcers. The number of false-positive results may be reduced by combining a sensitive guaiac test with a specific new quantitative test that detects human hemoglobin through an immunologic assay. A recent randomized trial demonstrated a 33% reduction in 13-year cumulative mortality from colorectal cancer with annual fecal occult blood testing with rehydration of the samples.

Digital rectal examination is a simple method of screening for colorectal cancer, but it is of limited efficacy. Approximately 10% of colorectal cancers are detectable by this method.

Sigmoidoscopy is a screening test that requires more time, costs more, and causes more patient discomfort, compared with the two tests just described. Currently, the National Cancer Institute and the American Cancer Society advocate screening asymptomatic patients over the age of 50 years with digital rectal examination and a fecal occult blood test annually and sigmoidoscopy every 3 to 5 years. However, there is evidence to suggest that screening sigmoidoscopy once every 10 years may be nearly as effective as more frequent screening. Flexible sigmoidoscopy has been shown to detect 2.5 times the number of adenomas and carcinomas detected with the older 25-cm rigid sigmoidoscope and to cause less patient discomfort as well.

Cancer screening should be distinguished from early case finding in patients with risk factors other than age. In patients who may have hereditary colorectal cancer, screening should begin several years earlier, before the earliest age of onset of colorectal cancer in affected family members. In such patients, colonoscopy every 1 to 3 years may be appropriate. Individuals with symptoms or signs suggestive of colorectal cancer should have appropriate evaluation based on their individual circumstances. Such patients are not candidates for screening programs.

Adenomatous polyps of the colon and rectum are regarded as precursors of cancer, and their removal with colonoscopic polypectomy has been shown to decrease the incidence of colorectal cancer in such patients. Recent data suggest that colonoscopy performed 3 years after complete removal of such polyps is as effective as a repeat colonoscopy done after a year.

SYMPTOMS IN COLORECTAL CANCER

The manner in which colorectal cancer presents depends to a large degree on the location of the primary tumor. Right-sided lesions are often insidious in onset. Vague abdominal discomfort, unexplained iron-deficiency anemia, and a positive occult blood test result on screening may be the earliest indication of a tumor.

Lesions of the left colon are more likely to cause colicky abdominal pain, alterations in bowel movements, or other evidence of partial or even complete obstruction leading to a surgical emergency. Rectal lesions may present with tenesmus, frank hematochezia, or pelvic pain.

A very short duration of symptoms (less than 1 week), particularly in those presenting with surgical emergencies, is usually more ominous than a longer duration of symptoms. However, a delay in diagnosis resulting from external factors other than the patient's symptoms does result in a poor prognosis.

PATHOLOGY

The overwhelming majority of malignant colorectal tumors are adenocarcinomas. In addition to the common type, which most closely resembles normal colonic mucosa, four other subcategories are recognized. Signet ring adenocarcinoma, frequently seen in younger patients, is associated with extremely poor prognosis. Mucinous or colloid, scirrhous, and carcinoma simplex are other subtypes. Rare histologic types include squamous carcinoma, undifferentiated carcinoma, leiomyosarcoma, lymphoma, and carcinoid tumors.

STAGING

Staging systems are devised to separate patients with a high probability of relapse from those with a low probability in order to guide further therapy (Table 2). In addition, accurate staging systems are required to permit comparability of treatment results obtained by different authors. Many staging systems are available; Dukes' and TNM (tumor, nodes, and metastases) classifications are the most commonly used.

PROGNOSTIC FACTORS

In addition to the stage and histologic grade of the tumor, the preoperative laboratory test results shown to predict a poor prognosis are a low serum protein level and a high carcinoembryonic antigen (CEA) level. Once colon cancer has recurred, several factors are predictive of response to therapy and survival. Serum lactate dehydrogenase level, performance status, weight loss, and tumor burden are important in determining the prognosis in such patients.

MANAGEMENT

Surgery. Surgical resection generally provides the only opportunity for cure. It may be undertaken for palliation in order to prevent or treat obstruction, perforation, or hemorrhage. A curative operation involves en bloc removal of the primary tumor, along with the regional lymph nodes. Surgery may also be curative for selected patients with Stage IV disease. Candidates for such resection usually have one to four liver metastases that can be completely resected with a good surgical margin. Similar operation can occasionally be undertaken for limited pulmonary metastases, with the best results seen in patients with solitary lesions. The 5-year survival in such patients is approximately 30%.

Adjuvant Therapy

Adjuvant therapy is given to patients who have undergone complete resection of colorectal cancer with curative intent but have a high risk of relapse. The most useful predictors of relapse are stage and site of the primary tumor within the large bowel. Stage I tumors of the colon and rectum have a low risk of relapse and are managed with surgery alone. Adjuvant therapy is recommended for patients with higher-stage colorectal adenocarcinomas.

Colon Cancer. In 1990, a National Cancer Institute Consensus Development Conference recommended that patients with Stage III colon adenocarcinoma be considered for 1 year of adjuvant therapy with 5-fluorouracil (5-FU) and levamisole (Ergamisol) following tumor resection. This recommendation

is still valid in 1995. A statistically significant survival advantage has not yet been documented in patients with Stage II disease. 5-FU plus leucovorin (Wellcovorin) may be considered as an alternative regimen for patients who cannot tolerate levamisole. Adjuvant radiation therapy is not recommended in colon cancer.

Rectal Cancer. Stage II and Stage III rectal adenocarcinomas tend to recur locally in the pelvis, as well as spread to distant sites despite potentially curative resection. Adjuvant therapy for rectal adenocarcinoma involves combined modality therapy with 5-FU and pelvic irradiation. Besides 5-FU being administered concomitantly with radiation, it is also given prior to and following concomitant therapy.

Treatment of Metastatic Disease

5-FU is the mainstay of systemic chemotherapy for patients with metastatic colorectal cancer. The overall response rate with the single agent 5-FU is 15 to 20%. Biochemical modulation of 5-FU with leucovorin increases the response rate significantly (30 to 40%); however, there is no improvement in survival. Other 5-FU modulating agents such as alpha-interferon, methotrexate, and phosphonacetyl-L-aspartic acid (PALA) are also used, as are other combination chemotherapy regimens employing 5-FU. There is a suggestion of improved response to prolonged continuous infusion rather than bolus 5-FU. Because of the modest response rates of currently available agents, efforts are under way to identify more active compounds.

Treatment of Isolated Unresectable Liver Disease. Isolated recurrences in the liver are common in colorectal cancer, many being unresectable. Because of its high hepatic extraction ratio and rapid total body clearance, fluorodeoxyuridine (FUDR) given directly into the hepatic arterial circulation has shown significant improvement in the tumor regression rate compared with systemic chemotherapy (40 to 60% versus 10 to 20%). Patients with hepatic metastases who have failed systemic chemotherapy may also respond to the intra-arterial therapy.

Palliative radiation therapy is generally reserved for painful pelvic or bone disease or brain metastases. Since there is no effective treatment for advanced colorectal cancer, patients should be encouraged to participate in well-designed clinical trials.

INTESTINAL PARASITES

method of
MURRAY WITTNER, M.D., PH.D.
Albert Einstein College of Medicine of Yeshiva University
Bronx, New York

Parasitic diseases, which are caused by helminths, protozoans, and arthropods, often cause chronic debilitating dis-

TABLE 2. **Staging and Survival in Colorectal Cancer**

AJCCS Stage	Dukes' Stage	5-Year Survival (%)
I	A, B1	85–95
II	B2, B3	60–80
III	C	30–60
IV	D	<5

Abbreviation: AJCCS = American Joint Committee on Cancer Staging.

ease and death. They are encountered more frequently in tropical and subtropical areas, where they constitute the leading cause of serious infectious diseases. A warm, moist climate, poor sanitation, low socioeconomic status, and inadequate diet contribute to the prevalence of parasitic diseases in these areas. Many diseases that were previously regarded as tropical are in reality cosmopolitan. The rise in immigration from tropical and subtropical areas and the advent of worldwide tourism have contributed to the increasing incidence of parasitism in temperate climates. Every patient's history, therefore, must include the question, "Where have you been and when?" The answer will often suggest the solution of a patient's clinical problem.

ENTAMOEBA HISTOLYTICA

Entamoeba histolytica is a ubiquitous organism that has been estimated to infect at least 10% of the world's population. The diagnosis of amebiasis requires confirmation by identifying the parasite in stool or sigmoidoscopy samples or by serologic evidence of infection. *E. histolytica* must be differentiated from *E. hartmanni*, which is nonpathogenic, and other nonpathogenic intestinal amebas such as *Entamoeba coli, Endolimax nana,* and *Iodoamoeba buetschlii* must be correctly diagnosed. *E. dispar* cannot be differentiated from *E. histolytica* morphologically.

Serologic methods are useful, particularly in extraintestinal disease. Treatment of benign cyst passers is with iodoquinol (Yodoxin), 650 mg three times daily for 20 days. Because of the rare possibility of optic neuritis, the recommended dosage should not be exceeded. Paromomycin (Humatin), 10 mg per kg three times daily for 7 days, or diloxanide furoate (Furamide),* 500 mg three times daily for 10 days, is an alternative. For the treatment of invasive intestinal amebiasis, metronidazole (Flagyl) should be used in addition to iodoquinol. Three weeks after therapy is completed, follow-up stool examination should be done to ascertain cure. Most hepatic abscesses will respond dramatically to metronidazole therapy with a decrease in the size of the abscess. In a small percentage of cases, relapse may occur. In cases that fail to respond to therapy within 48 hours, surgical intervention or percutaneous drainage, using computed tomography scan or ultrasound guidance, may be warranted. Resolution of the hepatic lesion may be assessed with ultrasound or technetium liver scan, but the defect often persists for months. To be certain that no intestinal infection remains, a luminicidal drug such as iodoquinol or diloxanide furoate should be given as well. Ameboma or extraintestinal disease usually will respond to metronidazole.

Prophylaxis of "traveller's diarrhea" with a variety of amebacides, usually iodochlorhydroxyquinoline (Entero-Vioform), is to be condemned. This drug has been implicated in reports of subacute myelo-optic neuropathy.

---

*Investigational drug in the United States.

GIARDIA LAMBLIA

Giardia lamblia is a flagellated protozoan that is one of the major causes of parasitic diarrhea in the United States. Approximately 4% of the population is said to harbor this parasite. Diagnosis of a *Giardia* infection is usually made by stool examination. Trophozoites can be found in diarrheic stools, whereas cysts are encountered in formed or semiformed stools. A concentration technique should be employed to enhance the chances of finding the cysts. Trophozoites must be found on direct examination, however, as they do not survive concentration techniques. Cyst excretion can be sporadic, and in low excreters only 40% of stools will be positive. It seems reasonable to conclude that if the parasite cannot be found after four or five stool examinations, alternative diagnostic techniques may be needed. The use of a weighted duodenal gelatin capsule containing 140 cm of 3-ply nylon string (Entero-Test) or duodenal aspiration may also be effective in recovering the organism. Purgatives have not proved useful in increasing the number of positive stools. Indirect fluorescent antibody or enzyme-linked immunosorbent assay (ELISA) antigen systems are currently being used to enhance the detection of *Giardia* in the stool. These tests may be used as valuable adjuncts in the diagnosis of giardiasis.

Therapy for giardiasis should be provided for all individuals, including asymptomatic cyst passers. Quinacrine is curative but is no longer available. Metronidazole, 250 mg three times daily for 7 days, is now the drug of choice, although the cure rate is somewhat lower. Furazolidone (Furoxone), 100 mg four times daily for 10 days, is less effective than metronidazole, but it is available as a suspension for young children.

COCCIDIOSIS

Recent recognition of the severe enteritis produced by *Cryptosporidium* spp in patients with human immunodeficiency virus (HIV) infection has awakened interest in the gastrointestinal manifestations of the coccidian parasites. The subclass includes several genera pathogenic for humans: *Sarcocystis, Cryptosporidium, Cyclospora, Toxoplasma, Plasmodium,* and *Isospora.*

In immunocompetent hosts the organism causes a self-limited illness characterized by colicky abdominal pain, flatulence, and diarrhea lasting 2 to 3 weeks. Rarely a chronic malabsorption syndrome has resulted. In the immunocompromised host, the disease presents as a chronic diarrhea with severe weight loss and malabsorption, and the illness can be fatal if untreated.

Oocysts of *I. belli* appear in the stool at a variable interval after the onset of infection and may be excreted for up to 3 months in the normal host. Diagnosis is made by examination of stool concentrated by flotation techniques. Like the oocysts of *Cryptosporidium*, these are also acid-fast. In rare patients the diagnosis may be made by duodenal aspiration or Entero-Test when the stool examination is negative. Small bowel biopsy may reveal organisms present in mucosal epithelium.

Recommended therapy for this infection is trimethoprim-sulfamethoxazole (Bactrim, Septra), 160 mg of the former and 800 mg of the latter four times daily for 10 weeks, then twice daily for 3 weeks, or pyrimethamine-sulfadoxine (Fansidar). These drugs produce a rapid response, usually within 48 hours. There have been reports of cure with metronidazole and furazolidone. In the author's experience in patients allergic to sulfa drugs, high-dose pyrimethamine (Daraprim) alone (50 to 75 mg per day) has produced a rapid response whereas metronidazole and furazolidone have not. In the immunocompetent host, the disease does not recur after treatment, but in acquired immune deficiency syndrome (AIDS) patients a 50% recurrence rate 8 weeks after stopping therapy is reported. In these patients, maintenance therapy to prevent recurrence and to allow the small bowel to repair itself is indicated.

CRYPTOSPORIDIUM

Cryptosporidium, like the other coccidia, is a parasite of importance in veterinary medicine. The advent of the AIDS epidemic has called attention to its widespread distribution and the capacity of *Cryptosporidium* to produce human disease. Cryptosporidiosis in the setting of AIDS has led to the emergence of new and simple diagnostic techniques that have aided diagnosis. Presently, diagnosis of cryptosporidiosis rests on the demonstration of oocysts in stool specimens or the presence of the organism in biopsy specimens. The modified Ziehl-Neelsen hot acid-fast stain is considered to be the best for overall sensitivity and morphology in conjunction with an initial potassium hydroxide digestion. Utilizing this stain, the oocyst appears bright-pink and red with a green background. Yeast forms stain green. The most sensitive diagnostic method employs a murine monoclonal antibody to the oocyst wall, but this method will miss cases of isosporiasis that are also positive by the acid-fast technique. *Cyclospora* can be differentiated from *Cryptosporidium* by measurement of the oocyst (4 to 6 μm vs 8 to 10 μm).

No effective therapy has been found for cryptosporidiosis despite the screening of a large number of medical and veterinary drugs. Spiramycin* has shown some antiparasitic activity, but the clinical response to this drug has been disappointing. High-dose azithromycin (Zithromax), about 2 grams daily, has been effective in some AIDS patients. Symptomatic therapy of immunocompetent hosts with fluid replacement and antimotility drugs is presently recommended. In the immunocompromised host, parenteral nutrition may be required.

---

*Not available in the United States.

BLASTOCYSTIS HOMINIS

The precise classification and clinical importance of this organism have been controversial since its initial description in the early 1900s. Although originally believed to resemble a yeast, some workers have concluded that *Blastocystis hominis* should be classified a protozoan. The great majority of patients are asymptomatic; others may have mild-to-moderate nonspecific gastrointestinal signs and symptoms that may include cramping, abdominal pain, and diarrhea. An occasional patient may present with recurrent diarrhea, which is usually not associated with fever or bloody stools. In vitro and limited clinical experience suggest that iodoquinol therapy, 650 mg three times daily for 20 days, may result in a 60 to 70% cure rate. Metronidazole, 750 mg three times daily for 7 to 10 days, has also been reported to give similar results. Cases unresponsive to iodoquinol may respond to metronidazole.

BALANTIDIUM COLI

Balantidium coli is a large, ciliated protozoan parasite, the largest protozoan parasite of humans. The diagnosis of *B. coli* infection rests on finding organisms in the patient's feces. Trophozoites are short-lived and will disintegrate unless stool specimens are examined promptly. Cysts are sometimes found in formed stools.

The usual treatment is with tetracycline, 500 mg four times daily for 14 days, or iodoquinol, 650 mg three times daily for 20 days.

DIENTAMOEBA FRAGILIS

Dientamoeba fragilis was first described in 1911. Although considered to be an ameba by many protozoologists, most recently it has been classified as a flagellate with close affinities to such parasitic flagellates as *Trichomonas*.

It is not clear how *D. fragilis* is transmitted, but a number of investigators have suggested that it is transmitted with the egg of the pinworm *Enterobius vermicularis*. Patients with *D. fragilis* may have frank diarrhea, with soft or normally formed stool. They complain most frequently of mild-to-severe diarrhea, abdominal pain, pruritus, abdominal distention, and flatulence. The diagnosis of *D. fragilis* infection depends on finding the parasite in a stool sample that has been collected and promptly examined. Patients with *D. fragilis* infection should be examined for pinworm infection.

Treatment is recommended for all patients with a positive diagnosis. The treatment of choice is iodoquinol, 650 mg three times daily for 20 days. Alternatively, tetracycline, 500 mg four times daily for 10 days, or paromomycin, 10 mg per kg three times daily for 10 days, may be used.

MICROSPORIDIA

The microsporidia are very primitive, eukaryotic, obligate, intracellular protozoan parasites, infecting every major animal group, especially insects, fish, and mammals. The majority infect the digestive tract and/or related organs, but reproductive, excretory, and nervous system infections are well documented, as well as those in connective and muscle tissues.

Since 1985 many cases of microsporidiosis in AIDS patients have been recognized; the great majority were intestinal infections. In the United States, most cases of intestinal microsporidiosis have been caused by *Enterocytozoon bieneusi*. Recently, another new microsporidian, *Septata intestinalis*, has been found in an AIDS-wasting syndrome of a patient with chronic diarrhea. The latter organisms were also found in enterocytes, but they were more invasive and developed differently.

Currently, definitive diagnosis of microsporidiosis requires biopsy and electron microscopic visualization of spore ultrastructure. The small intestine has provided the highest diagnostic yield, and organisms tend to be most numerous in the jejunum. Because of multiple developmental stages, intracellular location, the small size of the organisms, and variable staining characteristics, the diagnosis of intestinal microsporidiosis can be difficult. In paraffin-embedded sections, spores of *E. bieneusi* are sometimes discernible with hematoxylin-eosin stain, and sometimes they can be seen with Brown-Brunn or Brown-Hoops tissue Gram's stains. Giemsa-stained touch preparations and stained semithin plastic sections may also be helpful, but specific identification of microsporidian species still depends on ultrastructural characteristics, although skilled personnel are able to recognize the organisms in stool or urine.

Treatment with albendazole,* 400 mg twice daily for 3 or more weeks, although experimental, has been shown to be effective for *S. intestinalis* and *Encephalitozoon* infections. Treatment of *E. bieneusi* infections with this compound has not been as successful.

HELMINTIC INFECTIONS

Ascariasis

Ascaris lumbricoides is the largest intestinal roundworm infecting humans. In very light cases, it is possible to have an infection with a single-sex organism, and thus ova may be absent. Fertilized ova may survive in the soil for years.

Diagnosis is established by finding ova in the feces or by the identification of a spontaneously passed adult worm. Occasionally, worms will be discovered during a small bowel radiographic series. Several drugs are available for the treatment of this infection. Mebendazole (Vermox), 100 mg twice daily for 3 days, is the standard treatment for adults and children. Pyrantel pamoate (Antiminth), 11 mg per kg once (maximum, 1 gram), or albendazole,* 400 mg once, is alternative therapy for all age groups. Therapy may be accompanied by migration of the *Ascaris* through the mouth and nose.

Trichuriasis

Trichuriasis is caused by the whipworm *Trichuris trichiura*, a roundworm that inhabits the large intestine, producing mild-to-severe abdominal symptoms. The golden-brown eggs are typically barrel-shaped.

The diagnosis is made by stool examination. Treatment is usually successful. Mebendazole, 100 mg twice daily for 3 days, or albendazole,* 400 mg once, is highly effective in curing *Trichuris* infection in both adults and children. Rectal prolapse usually does not require surgery.

Strongyloidiasis

Strongyloides stercoralis is a small nematode that can exist as both a free-living organism and a tissue parasite localized to the mucosa of the duodenum or upper jejunum.

Strongyloidiasis can be diagnosed by finding rhabditiform larvae in stool. In 10 to 30% of cases, sampling of duodenal contents by a string test or duodenal aspiration by endoscopy may be needed to demonstrate the organism. In the hyperinfection syndrome, adult worms and eggs as well as larvae may be seen in sputum or bronchial washing. Centrifuged cerebrospinal fluid (CSF) specimens may also demonstrate filariform larvae on staining of the cell pellet. Serology is available and may be helpful in diagnosis and serologic testing for the presence of *Strongyloides*-specific IgG.

Strongyloidiasis responds to treatment with thiabendazole (Mintezol), 50 mg per kg per day in two divided doses (maximum of 3 grams per day for 2 days) for both adults and children. In patients with uncomplicated strongyloidiasis, 2 days is sufficient for a 95% cure rate. In the management of patients with disseminated disease, steroids should be discontinued and antiparasitic treatment should be continued for at least 5 days or until the stool examination demonstrates the absence of larvae. Thiabendazole causes nausea and vomiting, and occasionally it is associated with rash and fever. Albendazole,* 400 mg per day for 3 days, is effective. Recently, ivermectin has been shown effective in normal hosts with a dose of 200 μg per kg per day for 1 to 2 days. It is particularly useful in hyperinfection syndrome. In one case, ivermectin cleared the cerebrospinal fluid of filariform larvae.

Hookworm Disease

Hookworm disease is the result of small bowel infection with the nematodes *Necator americanus* and *Ancylostoma duodenale*. Finding of ova in a direct or unconcentrated stool examination suggests a clinically important hookworm infection. In mild infections, it may be necessary to obtain multiple stool examinations and employ concentration techniques.

---

*Not available in the United States.

*Not available in the United States.

Mebendazole, 100 mg twice daily for 3 days, or pyrantel pamoate (Antiminth), 11 mg per kg daily for 3 days (1 gram per day maximum), is recommended for adults and children. Albendazole,* 400 mg once, is alternative therapy for adults or children. In clinically significant infection, correction of nutritional deficiency is always indicated.

Enterobiasis

Enterobiasis is caused by the pinworm *Enterobius vermicularis*. Enterobiasis is a ubiquitous infection that is often more prevalent in temperate and colder climates where individuals, especially children, may live, play, and sleep closer to one another, thus facilitating the ready transfer of eggs from one child to the next. In the United States, infection rates in young school children may vary from 10 to 45%, and family infections are common, especially in young women. Nocturnal perianal pruritus, especially in children, strongly suggests pinworm infection. Small, creamy-white worms will often be found on examination of the perianal and perineal region when the child is awakened by itching. Inasmuch as ova are seen infrequently in the stools, the Scotch tape swab technique is the diagnostic method of choice.

Treatment of pinworm infection has become relatively simple and effective since a number of highly efficacious drugs have become available. It is important to remember that infection is often present in several members of a household, if not the entire family. Therefore, if each family member cannot be examined, it is important to treat the entire family simultaneously. When therapy is instituted, it is important to instruct the patient and/or parents on the nature of pinworm infection and on the usual widespread dissemination of the ova throughout the household. Initially, bed sheets, underwear, and night clothes should be washed and the household vacuum cleaned and/or damp mopped to reduce the number of ova.

Mebendazole, 100 mg once, and pyrantel pamoate (Antiminth), 11 mg per kg (maximum of 1 gram) once, are equally effective. An alternative is albendazole,* 400 mg once. In each instance, therapy for the entire household should be repeated after 2 weeks to assure almost 100% cure.

Anisakiasis and Other Parasitic Nematodes of Fish

Infection of the human gastrointestinal tract with the intermediate larval stages of several parasitic marine nematodes is termed "anisakiasis."

In humans, infection is usually caused by larvae belonging to the genera *Anisakis, Phocanema*, or *Contracaecum*. Infection results from the ingestion of raw, salted, pickled, smoked, marinated, or poorly cooked fish. Clinical disease is caused by the penetration of the larvae into the gastrointestinal mucosa,

*Not available in the United States.

resulting in either gastric or intestinal anisakiasis. Diagnosis of infection can be difficult. The clinical history of ingestion of raw fish associated with the onset of symptoms allows a presumptive diagnosis. Eosinophilia is sometimes seen, and in 40% of cases occult blood is present in the stool or gastric juices. An upper gastrointestinal series may demonstrate the outline of a worm associated with mucosal edema or tumor. Serodiagnosis has been reported to be useful in some cases. Identification and removal of the worm by endoscopy is both diagnostic and therapeutic. No specific treatment exists for these parasites other than endoscopic removal.

In addition to the saltwater fish–associated nematodes, infection of humans with freshwater nematodes of the genus *Eustrongylides* has been reported after eating raw minnows or "home-made" sushi. These patients have had intestinal perforation due to migration of the larval nematode out of the gastrointestinal tract. No specific treatment exists other than surgical removal of the worm and repair of the perforated bowel.

CESTODE INFECTIONS

Infection with tapeworms is one of the oldest recognized afflictions of humanity. The tapeworms' huge size and, at times, untimely egress from the body, could hardly go unnoticed.

Diphyllobothriasis

The fish or broad tapeworm *Diphyllobothrium latus* is a frequent human intestinal parasite in many areas where uncooked freshwater fish are consumed. The infection can be diagnosed readily by finding characteristic ova in the feces. Concentration methods are usually unnecessary since the numbers of eggs present are often so great that direct examination of a small amount of patient's feces in a drop of saline is usually sufficient. In addition, a strobila may be expelled in the feces, and on rare occasions portions of worm may be vomited. The treatment of choice for adults is praziquantel. Praziquantel (Biltricide) is given as a single dose of 10 to 20 mg per kg for both adults and children.

Taeniasis

The pork tapeworm *Taenia solium* and the beef tapeworm *Taenia saginata* are the common tapeworm parasites of humans. These infections have been known since ancient times and occur whenever infected, insufficiently cooked beef or pork is consumed. Human infection caused by larvae of *T. solium*, known as "cysticercosis," is a common clinical problem.

T. saginata infection occurs among those who prefer to eat raw or insufficiently cooked beef. In the United States, it is common to find raw beef included on menus as "steak tartare" at "chic" metropolitan restaurants, indicating the extent of the popularity of this food.

Since the finding of *Taenia* eggs in the stool is not sufficient to make a specific diagnosis, a gravid proglottid must be obtained for this purpose. This is not difficult, since proglottids are passed in the stool or emerge on the perianal or perineal region frequently and spontaneously but at irregular intervals.

Identification of a proglottid is done by pressing the segment between two glass microscope slides and counting the main lateral branches of the uterus. *T. solium* has fewer primary branches, usually 7 to 13 on each side; *T. saginata* usually has 15 to 20 lateral primary branches per side. Fecal examination, especially in the case of *T. saginata*, is often an unrewarding test inasmuch as gravid proglottids tend to be eliminated or "crawl" out on the perianal area prior to ovipositing. Thus, anal swabs such as the Scotch tape method, as usually done for the diagnosis of pinworm, are recommended in order to discover the ova. Serologic tests are useful in making the diagnosis of cysticercosis.

The treatment of both tapeworm infections is similar. Since the advent of praziquantel, paromomycin and dichlorophen are very rarely prescribed. In the treatment of *T. solium* infections, precautions should be taken to prevent autoinfection or dissemination to others. Drugs that induce vomiting should be avoided, since retrograde peristalsis might bring gravid proglottids into the gastroduodenal area, resulting in their subsequent digestion followed by egg hatching, penetration, and cysticercosis. In addition, since praziquantel kills the worm but not the eggs released from the disintegrating gravid segments, cysticercosis is theoretically possible following treatment. It is also unknown whether larvae released from eggs in the colon are capable of penetrating the intestinal wall. However, no cases of cysticercosis have been reported by this mechanism. As a precaution, however, some clinicians advise that for the treatment of *T. solium* infections, a purge be given 2 hours after treatment to eliminate all mature segments before eggs can be released. The patient should be followed to ensure prompt evacuation. Post-treatment follow-up stool examination should be performed after approximately 5 weeks and again at 3 months.

Hymenolepiasis

Two species of small tapeworms of the genus *Hymenolepis* infect humans. The dwarf tapeworm, *H. nana*, is a common infection, especially of children, throughout the world and can be passed from human to human. In moderate-to-heavy infections, it may cause a variety of abdominal and neurologic symptoms. *H. diminuta* is primarily a parasite of rodents and infrequently also of humans. The diagnosis is made by identifying the characteristic ova in a fecal specimen. Proglottids are usually not found because they degenerate before passage.

Successful therapy depends on understanding the life history of the carriers of this infection, and there-fore one should recall that the larval stage, or cysticercoid, is buried in the intestinal mucosa and presumably not killed by the drugs ordinarily employed. The treatment of choice is praziquantel, as it is lethal to both the cystcercoid stage within the tissue and the worm in the lumen. The recommended dose for adults and children is 25 mg per kg in a single dose.

Dipylidiasis

Dipylidium caninum is a cestode of dogs, cats, and wild carnivores that occasionally infects humans. Adult tapeworms inhabit the small intestine. Treatment is the same as that discussed for *D. latum* infections.

TREMATODE INFECTIONS

Clonorchiasis

The Chinese liver fluke *Clonorchis sinensis* is found throughout most of eastern Asia, especially Hong Kong, southern China, Taiwan, Japan, and Korea. Clonorchiasis can be treated successfully with praziquantel,* 25 mg per kg three times in 1 day. Because praziquantel has not been approved for this use informed patient consent should be obtained.

Fascioliasis

Fasciola hepatica, the sheep liver fluke, is found wherever sheep are raised. The diagnosis can be made when the characteristic ova are found on stool examination or duodenal aspiration; a concentration method should always be used. Serologic methods are not generally available, although the complement-fixation test is said to be helpful.

The author has encountered people who have eaten infected liver and have passed eggs of *Fasciola* as well as other liver flukes such as *Dicrocoelium* in their feces. This can be mistaken for actual infection unless care is taken to ensure that the infection is spurious. The patients are placed on a liver-free diet for 4 to 5 days, and their stools are re-examined; the eggs are not found again. The eggs of the giant intestinal fluke *Fasciolopsis buski* are very similar to those of *Fasciola*, and this infection must be ruled out by the clinical features and the likely region where the infection was acquired. Bithionol (Lorothidol, Bitin),† 30 to 50 mg per kg on alternate days for 10 to 15 doses, is recommended for therapy. Other anthelmintics are being tried. A veterinary fasciolicide, triclabendazole,* has been used in humans with excellent results.

Fasciolopsiasis

In Asia and the southwest Pacific, *Fasciolopsis buski* is one of the more frequently encountered intestinal flukes of humans and swine. Eggs are continuously passed in the feces and cannot be distin-

---

*Not FDA-approved for this indication.
†Investigational drug in the United States.

guished from those of *Fasciola hepatica*. Recent limited information suggests that praziquantel, 25 mg per kg three times daily for 2 days, effectively eliminates this infection without significant toxicity.

Schistosomiasis

Large intestinal infections caused by *Schistosoma mansoni* are the most frequently encountered form of schistosomiasis in the United States. On occasion, *S. japonicum* and *S. mekongi* are seen. In about 15% of *S. haematobium* cases, the large intestine is also involved. Treatment with praziquantel, 40 mg per kg in two divided doses on one day, is recommended for *S. mansoni* and *S. haematobium*. However, *S. japonicum* and *S. mekongi* cases require higher doses of 60 mg/kg/day in three divided doses in 1 day.

Section 7

Metabolic Disorders

DIABETES MELLITUS IN ADULTS

method of
ROBERT R. HENRY, M.D., and
STEVEN V. EDELMAN, M.D.
Veterans Affairs Medical Center
San Diego, California

There are currently an estimated 12 to 15 million Americans with diabetes, greater than 90% of whom have the adult-onset form termed "Type 2" or "non–insulin-dependent diabetes mellitus" (NIDDM). Of this number, approximately one-half are undiagnosed. Seventy to 80% of NIDDM patients are obese. Infrequently, insulin-dependent diabetes mellitus (IDDM) does develop in adults but this situation is not addressed further in this article. In patients with NIDDM, both micro- and macrovascular complications may be present at the time of diagnosis, implying that the diabetic state often develops many years earlier than when it is recognized. At the current time, the incidence of NIDDM in the United States is stable at 650,000 new cases per year. NIDDM aggregates within families and has a strong genetic component as well as contributing environmental determinants. Factors that are known to influence the development of NIDDM include obesity, sedentary lifestyle, high-fat low-fiber diets, previous gestational diabetes, impaired glucose tolerance, lipid abnormalities, hypertension, and aging. The risk of developing diabetes is greatly increased in minority populations such as African Americans, Hispanic Americans, Native Americans, Asian Americans, and Pacific Island Americans. In these groups, diabetes is approaching or has reached epidemic proportions, and its occurrence is strongly related to cultural changes in lifestyle and economy.

In the United States, diabetes is the seventh leading cause of death and a major contributor to an additional 300,000 deaths. Diabetes is associated with specific long-term microvascular complications that include retinopathy, neuropathy, nephropathy, and a markedly increased risk of premature atherosclerotic vascular disease. In adults, diabetes is the most common cause of end-stage renal disease, new-onset blindness, and lower extremity amputations. Compared with their nondiabetic counterparts, men with NIDDM have a two- to threefold increased risk and women a four- to fivefold increased risk of cardiovascular disease. The economic burden imposed by diabetes is immense, accounting for one-seventh of the total annual health care expenditure in the United States.

PATHOPHYSIOLOGY

Hyperglycemia develops in NIDDM from three basic abnormalities: excessive hepatic glucose production, impaired pancreatic insulin secretion, and resistance to insulin action occurring principally in liver and muscle tissue. This contrasts with IDDM in which the sole cause of hyperglycemia is insulinopenia due to autoimmune destruction of the pancreatic beta cells of the islets of Langerhan. A number of secondary causes of diabetes, such as hemochromatosis, hypercortisolism, and chronic pancreatitis, can be biochemically similar to NIDDM and need to be considered when the diagnosis of diabetes is made. In NIDDM, the degree of hyperglycemia varies considerably between individuals owing to differences in the severity of these three contributing abnormalities. Such differences are best exemplified by the lean and obese varieties of NIDDM, which exhibit the same underlying pathophysiologic basis but differ in the extent to which each abnormality contributes to the development of the hyperglycemic state. In lean patients with NIDDM, impaired insulin secretion is the predominant defect, whereas insulin resistance tends to be less severe than in the obese form. On the other hand, insulin resistance and hyperinsulinemia are the classical abnormalities of obese individuals with NIDDM. When obesity and diabetes coexist, insulin secretion is often excessive compared with the nondiabetic situation, but it is still insufficient to overcome the peripheral insulin resistance that is present. It is important to understand and appreciate these fundamental differences when considering the therapeutic options available and the likelihood of their success—for example, when insulin is used, it can often be predicted with considerable certainty that lean Type II diabetic subjects, in whom insulin resistance is mild or moderate in severity, will require considerably less insulin to control their hyperglycemia than obese subjects. In contrast, large doses of exogenous insulin are the rule in obese patients with this disorder to achieve near normal glucose levels.

Individuals with insulin resistance, including those with NIDDM, are also at increased risk of developing a constellation of abnormalities that make up the insulin resistance syndrome or syndrome X. It is generally believed that insulin resistance and/or hyperinsulinemia are the underlying basis of this disease complex and exert a major role in the development of the associated disorders that include hypertension, dyslipidemia, and premature cardiovascular disease.

DIAGNOSIS

The diagnosis of diabetes in adults can be suspected based on obvious signs and symptoms of hyperglycemia such as blurred vision, polyuria, polydipsia, or weight loss but measurement of plasma glucose is required for confirmation. In nonpregnant adults, the diagnosis of diabetes can be made if one or more of the following criteria are met: a fasting plasma glucose value of 140 mg per dL or greater on at least two separate occasions, a random plasma glucose level of 200 mg per dL or greater with signs and symptoms of diabetes, or a fasting plasma glucose level less than 140 mg per dL but a 2-hour glucose concentration of 200 mg per dL or greater during a 75-gram oral glucose tolerance test. Although the oral glucose tolerance test is usually not necessary for the diagnosis of diabetes, it can be used for those individuals at particularly high risk of developing diabetes so that preventive measures such as diet modification, weight loss, and an exercise program can be instituted at an early stage. Individuals at increased risk of developing NIDDM include those with a strong family history, previous gestational diabetes, obesity, or impaired glucose tolerance. In addition, a number of factors including certain medications, stress, carbohydrate restriction, and physical inactivity can adversely influence carbohydrate metabolism and need to be considered when interpreting plasma glucose levels.

TREATMENT OVERVIEW

The primary objectives of management of NIDDM are to achieve and maintain normal metabolic and biochemical status in order to reduce hyperglycemic symptoms and prevent or delay the development of micro- and macrovascular complications. Despite a clear understanding of the pathophysiologic mechanisms contributing to the development of hyperglycemia in NIDDM and the availability of therapeutic agents to control this disorder, most patients remain under less than ideal metabolic control. The failure to achieve optimal glycemic regulation is multifactorial in origin, but is rooted to some extent in the long-held misconception that NIDDM is a mild disease that is easily treated. In addition, the metabolic nature and ramifications of NIDDM have only recently been fully recognized and appreciated. The hyperglycemia of NIDDM is often associated with numerous other metabolic abnormalities that also favor the development of diabetic complications and premature cardiovascular disease. Furthermore, hyperglycemia itself contributes to perpetuating hyperglycemia through the effects of so-called glucose toxicity. This refers to the ability of glucose to be toxic to multiple organ systems and to further impair the pathophysiologic abnormalities causing NIDDM. Any approach that is used to optimally manage NIDDM must consider all of these aspects and be multifaceted in nature.

In the past, definitive data confirming the benefits of near-normal glucose levels on microvascular complications of diabetes has been lacking. The Stockholm Diabetes Intervention Study and the Diabetes Control and Complications Trial (DCCT) are recently completed long-term studies that provided compelling evidence that glycemic control does matter and that near-normalization of blood glucose levels can delay the development and progression of retinopathy, nephropathy, and neuropathy in IDDM patients. A major issue derived from these studies is whether the conclusions about the benefits of aggressive glycemic management are equally applicable to those individuals with NIDDM. At the present time, unequivocal data on this issue are not available. However, there is substantial evidence indicating that the severity and duration of hyperglycemia are critical factors in the pathogenesis of microvascular complications in both forms of diabetes. This has led to the

TABLE 1. **Target Levels of Glucose Control**

Biochemical Measurement	Normal	Acceptable
Preprandial glucose (mg/dl)	<115	80–120
Bedtime glucose (mg/dl)	<120	100–140
Glycated hemoglobin (%)*	<6	<7

*Normal reference range: 4–6%.

current recommendation by the American Diabetes Association (ADA) that even in the absence of confirmatory data, it is warranted to expect that NIDDM patients will also benefit from improved glycemic control. Therefore, the ADA advises that management should be directed at safely achieving the best possible glycemic control in this group as well.

GLYCEMIC OBJECTIVES

Based on evidence that good glycemic control reduces the risks of complications in diabetes, the goals of therapy have been recently redefined and are shown in Table 1. Although treatment goals should be individualized, the glycemic targets for diabetes reflect the belief that efforts to achieve near-normal glucose levels should be attempted whenever possible. The current glycemic goals to strive for are a fasting and preprandial glucose level of 80 to 120 mg per dL, a bedtime or evening glucose of 100 to 140 mg per dL, and a glycosylated hemoglobin of less than 7%. Normalizing glycemia and glycosylated hemoglobin is not only difficult to attain but also must be done while minimizing weight gain and hypoglycemia and maintaining a reasonable quality of life. Reducing cardiovascular risk factors is important in NIDDM owing to the high incidence of macrovascular disease, and this can be achieved by optimizing diet, body weight, blood pressure, and lipoproteins to levels shown in Table 2. Patients should also be encouraged and assisted with discontinuing cigarette smoking.

Both glycemic control and cardiovascular risk factors should be managed initially by dietary modification and exercise therapy. Even though these modalities do not usually result in complete normalization of metabolic abnormalities by themselves, they are

TABLE 2. **Cardiovascular Risk Factor Reduction**

1. Systolic/diastolic blood pressure less than 130/85 mmHg
2. Ideal body weight approached or maintained
3. Low-cholesterol low-saturated-fat diet
4. Regular exercise routine
5. Lipoprotein levels optimized:
   A. Triglycerides less than 200 mg/dL
   B. HDL cholesterol greater than 35 mg/dL
   C. LDL cholesterol less than 130 mg/dL (less than 100 mg/dL if coronary heart disease already present)
   D. Total cholesterol less than 200 mg/dL
6. Cigarette smoking cessation

Abbreviations: HDL = high-density lipoprotein; LDL = low-density lipoprotein.

beneficial and adherence should be constantly encouraged and reinforced since the response to the subsequent institution of pharmacologic therapy will be enhanced. Not only must every effort be made to optimally control glycemia in NIDDM but major macrovascular risk factors such as hypertension and dyslipidemia must be also promptly identified and aggressively treated.

METHODS TO IMPROVE DIABETES TREATMENT EFFICACY

The most effective management of diabetes is achieved when a coordinated team approach that involves active participation and encouragement by the physician, diabetes nurse educator, and dietician with the diabetic patient and family members is utilized. The achievement of normal or near-normal glucose levels requires comprehensive training in self-management and monitoring of blood glucose levels. Continuing education and reinforcement is necessary to ensure that treatment goals are understood and that appropriate attention is given to meal planning, exercise, and therapeutic regimens including the prevention and treatment of hyperglycemia and other acute and chronic complications. Self- or home glucose monitoring (HGM) of capillary blood glucose is one of the most significant recent developments available to improve glycemic control. This technique enables the patient to be involved in self-management and to understand the influence of therapy on blood glucose levels. Since HGM facilitates glycemic control and reinforces adherence to therapy, virtually all diabetic patients should perform HGM at least once daily. In patients achieving acceptable control on diet, exercise, and oral hypoglycemic agents, a daily overnight fasting or bedtime measurement may be sufficient. When less than optimal control is achieved or intensive management with oral antidiabetic and/or insulin is instituted, four to six daily measurements should be made and recorded. In this situation, the recommended times for self-monitoring are before each meal and at bedtime. To assess the glucose response to food intake, intermittent measurements can be made 1 to 2 hours after meals. Measurements should also be made anytime the patient suspects hypoglycemia including if he or she awakes during the night.

DIABETES MANAGEMENT

Nonpharmacologic Methods

Nutrition Therapy

Nutrition therapy should be tailored to the individual needs and requirements of the patient. An appropriate diet should account for factors such as age, sex, activity level, degree of obesity, presence of complications, medications, and current nutritional status of the patient. Cultural, ethnic, and socioeconomic status must also be considered when formulating a diet. Following the diagnosis of diabetes, a dietician or nutritionist should be involved in the management to record a diet history including lifestyle and eating habits, review basic principles of diet therapy, and develop a meal plan. If the fasting glucose level is less than 200 mg per dL, diet manipulation alone may be sufficient. When the blood glucose is above this level, patients tend to be symptomatic and diet must usually be combined with pharmacologic therapy. In obese adults with diabetes, caloric restriction and increased physical activity to achieve weight loss, as well as optimal dietary composition, are necessary. Even small amounts of weight loss can have dramatic benefits on metabolic control.

To improve glycemic control, meals should be spaced throughout the day to allow sufficient time for insulin to be effective. Large caloric loads at any one time tend to produce large glycemic excursions. Considerable controversy continues about the optimal diet composition for adults with diabetes. In the most recent recommendations of the ADA, emphasis has been placed on diets that achieve and maintain a reasonable body weight and reduce both blood glucose and cholesterol levels. The basic recommendation is to limit dietary cholesterol to less than 300 mg per day and to restrict saturated fat intake to less than 10% of calories and protein to 10 to 20% of total daily calories. Dietary fat intake is discussed in greater detail under "Dyslipidemia," later in this article. In contrast to previous recommendations, the absolute intake of carbohydrate and fat in the diet should be based on an individual nutritional assessment and metabolic response to diet. In general, reduction of carbohydrate intake is probably best offset by increasing the monounsaturated fat intake.

Exercise

Unless contraindications exist, exercise should be an integral component of the treatment program for adults with diabetes. Exercise increases energy expenditure and enhances the response to dietary and pharmacologic therapy. An exercise program must be individually planned and tailored to meet physical limitations. Many adults with diabetes are sedentary and deconditioned. Therefore, exercise should be started at a low level and gradually increased to limit adverse effects such as physical injury, cardiac problems, or hypoglycemia. Before initiating an exercise program in most adults with diabetes, an exercise stress test should be performed to rule out significant cardiovascular disease or silent ischemia. To avoid hypoglycemia in patients treated with oral antidiabetic agents or insulin, blood glucose should be self-monitored both pre- and postexercise with consumption of appropriate snacks, as necessary. A regular exercise routine also minimizes the likelihood of exercise-induced hypoglycemia. Walking, stationary cycling, aerobic water exercises, or lap swimming three to four times per week for 20 to 30 minutes expends 100 to 200 kcal per session and are safe and effective activities. Any increase in exercise intensity needs to be closely monitored to allow for adjustment of medication. A more intensive program should be managed by a physical therapist knowledgeable in exercise therapy for diabetes.

Pharmacologic Methods

Oral Antidiabetic Agents

When diet and exercise are unable to maintain plasma glucose levels within the glycemic objectives shown in Table 1, oral antidiabetic agents are usually instituted. Oral medication should be used not as a substitute for diet and exercise but rather as adjunctive therapy. Currently available therapy includes the first- and second-generation sulfonylureas and the recently approved biguanide metformin (Glucophage). Both of these two classes of drugs are effective in management of glycemia but differ in their mechanism of action. Sulfonylureas work primarily by stimulating pancreatic insulin secretion, whereas the main effect of metformin is to suppress excessive production of glucose by the liver. The sulfonylureas and metformin also improve lipid parameters. Whereas sulfonylureas tend to cause some weight gain, metformin use in obese adults with diabetes is reported to result in significant weight loss. Sulfonylureas are capable of producing severe hypoglycemia but this side effect is rare with metformin, since this agent does not stimulate endogenous insulin secretion. Unlike the previous biguanide phenformin, which was associated with a substantial incidence of lactic acidosis that led to its withdrawal from clinical use, this complication is uncommon with metformin. Both of these agents should be used with caution when evidence of significant hepatic or renal dysfunction is present.

Some of the more commonly used oral antidiabetic agents currently available in the United States are shown in Table 3. There is little difference in the efficacy between first- and second-generation sulfonylureas but the first-generation agents are less expensive. The second-generation sulfonylureas are more potent on a per-milligram basis and tend to have fewer side effects. These medications should be started at the lowest possible dose and given before breakfast, with progressive increments every 1 to 2 weeks until the desired therapeutic response is achieved. When the daily dose approaches 50% or more of the maximal recommended dose, these agents are usually given twice daily, before breakfast and supper.

Both the sulfonylureas and metformin can be used alone, but the likelihood of therapeutic success with these agents declines when the fasting plasma glucose level is above 200 mg per dL. They are unlikely to be effective when given alone for fasting glucose levels above 300 mg per dL. Below a fasting glucose of 300 mg per dL, oral medication is usually still tried, with a strong likelihood that supplemental insulin may also be required. When primary or secondary sulfonylurea failure occurs, it is usually not advantageous to switch to another oral agent. Weight gain often occurs with sulfonylureas but not with metformin use. Metformin has beneficial effects when combined with sulfonylureas and can be effective at improving glycemic control when given in combination to patients failing maximal doses of sulfonylureas.

Insulin

Insulin therapy should be reserved for patients who have failed an adequate trial of diet, exercise, and oral antidiabetic agents according to the stepwise approach advocated by the ADA. A number of insulin treatment regimens, shown in Table 4, are commonly used in the treatment of adults with diabetes. The primary objective of insulin treatment is to achieve the best possible glycemic control with the least risk of hypoglycemia using the simplest regimen.

The starting dose of insulin is highly variable in adult diabetes and is usually lowest in lean elderly patients and greatest when obesity is present. The usual initial dose ranges from as little as 0.1 to 0.3 U per kg body weight with dosage increments of 0.05 to 0.1 U every 3 to 5 days until the fasting glucose measured by self-monitoring is less than 140 mg per dL. Insulin is given 15 to 30 minutes before meals and the dose is usually split if more than 30 U per day is required. Fine-tuning of insulin administration requires frequent HGM. Measurements are usually made before meals, at bedtime, 1 to 2 hours after meals, and during the night between 2 and 4 A.M. Measurements should be recorded in a log book and brought to each physician visit so that appropriate insulin dosage adjustments can be made. Between office visits, the physician may wish to make dosage adjustments by phone on the basis of HGM results.

SINGLE-INJECTION THERAPY

The use of one injection of intermediate insulin (NPH [neutral protamine Hagedorn] or Lente) or an intermediate-regular combination before breakfast or supper is easy to administer but it is unlikely to

TABLE 3. **Oral Antidiabetic Agents Commonly Used in Adult Diabetes**

Agent	Recommended Starting Dose (mg)*	Recommended Maximal Dose (mg)
Sulfonylureas		
FIRST-GENERATION		
Tolazamide (Tolinase)	100	1000
Acetohexamide (Dymelor)	250	1500
SECOND-GENERATION		
Glyburide (DiaBeta, Micronase)	2.5	20
Glipizide (Glucotrol)	5	40
Biguanide		
Metformin (Glucophage)	500	2550

*Starting dose for elderly and lean adults with diabetes may need to be reduced by up to 50%.

TABLE 4. **Common Insulin Regimens Used in Adult Diabetes**

Regimen	Administration	Comment
Single insulin injections	NPH or Lente alone or with regular insulin at breakfast, supper, or bedtime	Increase dose every 3–5 days; glucose control usually inadequate
Insulin and oral agents	NPH or Lente at bedtime or before supper added to maximal dose oral antidiabetic agents	Total oral dose given before breakfast
Multiple insulin injections	NPH or Lente with regular insulin prebreakfast and supper; regular insulin before meals and NPH, Lente, or Ultralente at bedtime or late afternoon	Premixed 70/30 useful Four daily injections

Abbreviation: NPH = neutral protamine Hagedorn.

achieve optimal glycemic control. One scenario in which one daily injection may be effective is in the patient who eats the largest meal of the day in the evening and has a light breakfast and lunch. In this situation, a single predinner injection of intermediate-regular combination can be effective in controlling both the postdinner glycemic rise and overnight glucose levels. Administration of intermediate insulin alone prior to bedtime (9 to 11 P.M.) can also be used in circumstances in which the primary abnormality is an elevated prebreakfast glucose level. When intermediate insulin is given in this fashion, its effects tend to peak just prior to breakfast when it is needed most. However, as with the other single-injection regimens, day-long glycemia is not usually well controlled.

INSULIN AND ORAL AGENTS

Most adult diabetics requiring insulin have failed to achieve optimal glycemic control on maximal doses of oral agents. In this situation, the addition of intermediate-acting evening or bedtime insulin to the oral agents is an easy and often highly effective method to regain glucose control. When evening insulin is added, the total dose of the oral agent can be given in the morning before breakfast. In this manner, the evening insulin can be used to control the early morning hyperglycemia, whereas the oral agents exert their effects on daytime glycemia. In some patients, it is occasionally better to move the bedtime evening insulin injection to before supper for optimal benefits. In this situation, the intermediate insulin can be given alone or with regular insulin to control postprandial glycemia following the evening meal. The addition of bedtime insulin can often prevent or delay the need for multiple daily insulin injections. This technique also allows the patient to gradually become accustomed to the use of insulin should a multiple-injection regimen become necessary. When the addition of bedtime insulin to maximal doses of oral agents is not effective, the transition to a twice or more daily insulin regimen is reasonably smooth and does not necessarily require that evening insulin be stopped.

MULTIPLE INSULIN INJECTIONS

When insulin is required more than once daily to achieve glycemic control, it is most commonly admin-

istered either as an intermediate-regular combination given before breakfast and supper or with regular insulin before breakfast, lunch, and supper with intermediate or long-acting insulin given in the evening. Both of these regimens can be highly effective but require frequent monitoring. These regimens are also associated with a higher incidence of side effects such as hypoglycemia and weight gain. When an intermediate-regular combination is used, premixed 70% intermediate and 30% regular insulin can simplify matters. The insulin dose is adjusted keeping in mind that long-acting insulin peaks in about 4 hours and has a duration of 30 hours, intermediate insulins peak at 5 to 10 hours with a duration of approximately 18 hours, and regular insulin action peaks at 2 to 4 hours and its effect is complete by 6 to 8 hours.

There are many acceptable methods to initiate insulin therapy in adults with diabetes but none is uniformly effective in all patients. With twice-a-day insulin before breakfast and supper, about one-half to two-thirds of the total daily insulin dose is given before breakfast.

CARDIOVASCULAR RISK MANAGEMENT

Hypertension

Any evidence of hypertension in NIDDM should lead to prompt and effective management since its presence accelerates cardiovascular and renal complications. The systolic and diastolic blood pressure should be maintained below 130 and 85 mmHg, respectively, in NIDDM. If isolated systolic hypertension is present, the pressure should be reduced to 160 mmHg or less. Further reductions below 140 mmHg may be indicated if well tolerated. Except when hypertension is severe, management should be initiated using a low-salt diet with weight loss if the patient is obese and combined with exercise when possible. Often, one or more antihypertensive medications are also required to achieve acceptable blood pressure control.

Hypertension in NIDDM should be vigorously treated using initial therapy with calcium channel blockers, angiotensin-converting-enzyme (ACE) inhibitors, or alpha-adrenergic blockers, either alone or in combination. ACE inhibitors are frequently the first medication used to treat hypertension in NIDDM because of their efficacy and low incidence of side effects. The ACE inhibitors do not exhibit deleterious effects on carbohydrate or lipid metabolism and have been shown to slow the rate of progression of proteinuria in diabetic nephropathy. Serum potassium should be closely monitored if ACE inhibitors are used in NIDDM patients suspected to have hyporeninemic hypoaldosteronism (Type IV renal tubular acidosis) owing to the possibility of developing severe hyperkalemia. Although controversial, low-dose thiazides and beta blockers can sometimes be carefully used with minimal adverse effects. These agents reduce the complications of hypertension but can worsen glucose intolerance and lead to a more atherogenic lipid profile.

Dyslipidemia

Lipid abnormalities are more common in NIDDM patients than in the nondiabetic population and contribute to accelerated atherosclerosis. The characteristic profile includes hypertriglyceridemia that is due primarily to increased triglyceride-rich very-low-density lipoprotein (VLDL) levels and decreased high-density lipoprotein (HDL) levels. Low-density lipoprotein (LDL) levels are highly variable and can be low, normal, or elevated. In NIDDM, the composition of lipoprotein particles may also be abnormal with increased concentrations of small, dense LDL and IDL particles. The presence of excessive amounts of small, dense LDL and IDL has been termed the "phenotype B pattern" and appears to be associated with an increased risk of cardiovascular disease. A fasting lipid profile including serum triglyceride, total cholesterol, HDL cholesterol, and LDL cholesterol should be performed during the initial evaluation of every NIDDM patient. LDL cholesterol is not routinely measured in most laboratories but can be accurately estimated when the serum triglyceride is less than 400 mg per dL using the following equation:

$$\text{LDL cholesterol} = \text{total cholesterol} - [(0.2 \times \text{triglycerides}) + \text{HDL cholesterol}]$$

Since NIDDM patients are at high risk of premature cardiovascular disease, any abnormality of lipid levels should be initially treated with prompt institution of diet and exercise and intensification of glycemic control. If these modalities are ineffective, pharmacologic therapy should be administered.

The most effective dietary regimen for dyslipidemia in NIDDM primarily involves limitation of calories, fat, and cholesterol intake and a diet high in soluble fiber. Diets high in soluble fiber from oat and bean products can have beneficial effects primarily on LDL cholesterol levels. Diets should be stepped in their degree of fat and cholesterol restriction, along the lines suggested by the National Cholesterol Education Program (NCEP) Step 1 and Step 2 diets, modified as necessary for overall optimal diabetes nutrition. The Step 1 diet recommends that saturated fat intake be 8 to 10% of total daily calories with 30% or less of calories from total fat and less than 300 mg of cholesterol per day. If a diet of this nature proves inadequate to achieve the desired goals, a Step 2 diet should be instituted. This diet recommends a further reduction in saturated fat intake to less than 7% of total daily calories and cholesterol intake less than 200 mg per day. The Step 1 and Step 2 diets advised by the NCEP for adults with high blood cholesterol are very similar to those currently recommended by the ADA and are shown in Table 5. When serum triglyceride levels are greater than 1000 mg per dL, all forms of dietary fats should be reduced to lower circulating chylomicrons. Diets of these types are best instituted with the involvement or assistance of a registered dietician or other qualified nutrition professional.

When lipid-lowering drugs are required, they should be instituted in combination with diet and exercise and efforts to improve glycemic control. Although the exact level of serum triglyceride required to reduce atherogenic risk is unknown, persistent elevation above 1000 mg per dL, which is primarily due to excessive chylomicron particles, increases the risk of pancreatitis and warrants treatment with a low-fat diet and medication, usually with the fibric acid derivative gemfibrozil (Lopid) 600 mg twice daily given before breakfast and supper. In susceptible individuals, alcohol ingestion and other agents such as estrogen therapy can precipitate hyperchylomicronemia and should be considered in the cause. When triglyceride levels are the primary lipid abnormality and are consistently above 400 mg per dL, with or without low HDL levels, therapy with gemfibrozil at the same dose as indicated previously is also probably justified. This agent is particularly effective at decreasing hepatic VLDL production and enhancing VLDL-triglyceride clearance. Nicotinic acid, although highly effective and often beneficial at improving all lipoprotein parameters, is frequently not used in NIDDM, or is done so cautiously, primarily owing to adverse effects on glycemia.

When the primary lipoprotein abnormality is an elevated LDL cholesterol level, bile-acid sequestrants

TABLE 5. **Recommended Dietary Fat and Cholesterol Intake in Patients with Diabetes Mellitus**

Fat Intake

Saturated fat: <10% of daily calories; <7% when LDL elevated

Polyunsaturated fat: ≤10% of daily calories

Total fat intake varies with lipid treatment goals
~30% when lipids and weight normal
<30% when obese and/or LDL elevated
<40% when triglycerides elevated and unresponsive to fat restriction and weight loss efforts; liberalize monounsaturated fat intake

Cholesterol Intake

<300 mg/day

Abbreviation: LDL = low-density lipoprotein.

and/or 3-hydroxy-3-methylglutaryl-coenzyme A (HMG-CoA) reductase inhibitors that reduce cholesterol synthesis are recommended. Bile acid binders should be instituted gradually, as colestipol (Colestid) 5 grams or cholestyramine (Questran) 4 grams mixed with water or juice given before supper. If well tolerated, the dose can be doubled in 1 to 2 months and also be given before breakfast or lunch to enhance bile excretion. Gastrointestinal complaints are frequent with these agents and compliance tends to be poor. To prevent interference with drug absorption, bile acid binders should not be administered when oral medications such as anticoagulants and those for cardiac or blood pressure management are taken. Use of bile acid binders may also lead to elevation of triglyceride levels.

If HMG-CoA reductase inhibitors are necessary, they are most effective when given at bedtime or with the evening meal. The usual starting doses are lovastatin (Mevacor) 20 mg, simvastatin (Zocor) 5 to 10 mg, or pravastatin (Pravachol) 10 to 20 mg once daily. The maximal recommended daily doses are lovastatin 80 mg, simvastatin 40 mg, and pravastatin 40 mg. The main adverse effects of these compounds are abnormal liver function tests, particularly increased transaminase levels, and myopathy. Serum transaminase levels and creatine phosphokinase (CPK) levels should be monitored periodically and more frequently in the 3 to 6 months following initiation of therapy. The risk of myopathy is increased when the other hypolipidemic agents gemfibrozil and nicotinic acid as well as erythromycin and cyclosporine are administered concomitantly with HMG-CoA reductase inhibitors. The combination of these medications should be used with caution. If HMG-CoA reductase inhibitors are combined with any of these other agents, patients must be carefully monitored for evidence of myopathy.

MANAGEMENT OF MICROVASCULAR AND NEUROPATHIC COMPLICATIONS

Diabetic Retinopathy

More than 80% of patients with diabetes for 15 years or longer have evidence of retinopathy, and diabetes is a leading source of new-onset blindness in the United States. Loss of vision and blindness from proliferative retinopathy and macular edema can be drastically reduced or delayed when laser photocoagulation is utilized in a timely manner. Therefore, all patients with diabetes should be seen annually by an ophthalmologist with expertise in the eye diseases of diabetes. Between the annual visits to the ophthalmologist or whenever symptoms indicate, diabetics should have a complete ocular evaluation that includes assessment of visual acuity and examination with the pupil dilated. If there is any question about the possible progression of retinopathy, referral to an ophthalmologist is indicated. Since the development and progression of retinopathy is adversely influenced by hyperglycemia, a concerted effort should be directed at achieving the best possible glycemic control in all persons with diabetes. Adequate control of hypertension may also be beneficial in reducing the development of diabetic retinopathy. In addition to proliferative retinopathy and macular edema, patients with NIDDM develop cataracts more frequently and at an earlier age than those without diabetes. Patients should be informed and reassured that changes in visual acuity most commonly result from fluctuating glucose levels but should still be encouraged to report any new visual symptoms promptly.

Diabetic retinopathy is classified into nonproliferative or background, preproliferative, and proliferative types. Background changes are the earliest and are characterized by microaneurysms and intraretinal "dot" and "blot" hemorrhages. Often, these findings do not progress and visual acuity is unaffected. Hard exudates may be present and reflect leakage of serous fluid from abnormal vessels. Macular edema cannot be seen by direct ophthalmoscopy. Therefore, when hard exudates are located in close proximity to the macula, they are suggestive of possible edema and warrant prompt referral to an ophthalmologist to preserve vision. The preproliferative stage is an advanced form of background retinopathy and is distinguished by "beading" of retinal veins as well as abnormalities that include soft exudates or "cotton-wool" spots from ischemic infarcts and irregular, dilated, and tortuous capillaries with occasional early intraretinal new vessel formation. Any of these findings requires referral to an ophthalmologist for further evaluation. The proliferative phase demonstrates neovascularization on the surface of the retina that may extend into the posterior vitreous. These new vessels are fragile and are prone to bleed, posing a threat to vision. Active bleeding may manifest as "floaters," "cobwebs," or sudden, painless loss of vision. Retinal detachment can result from contraction of fibrous tissue from preretinal or vitreous bleeds.

There is no standard therapy for background retinopathy other than optimizing metabolic control. If macular edema occurs, photocoagulation may slow progression of visual loss. Photocoagulation can reduce visual loss by more than 50% when it is used to prevent neovascularization and recurrent vitreal hemorrhages that can lead to irreversible damage. Retinal detachment and large vitreous hemorrhages may require vitrectomy to relieve retinal traction and partially restore sight.

Diabetic Nephropathy

More than 20% of adults with diabetes for 20 years or more will display evidence of overt nephropathy that may progress to end-stage renal failure. Approximately 30% of end-stage renal disease requiring dialysis is due to diabetes. The development of nephropathy in diabetes patients is insidious in onset and requires laboratory evaluation for detection. Microalbuminuria is the first sign of nephropathy and may progress to the "overt" or "clinical" stage, which is defined by persistent proteinuria of greater than 500 mg per day of total protein or greater than 300 mg per day of albumin. Hypertension is invariably present when proteinuria occurs and may play a role in the development and acceleration of renal insufficiency. Other factors that may influence the course of renal function deterioration in diabetes include concomitant urinary tract infection and obstruction and the use of nephrotoxic drugs and radiocontrast dyes. Persons with diabetes should be carefully evaluated for the presence of neurogenic bladder, occult urinary tract infection, and use of agents that accelerate the progression of renal failure such as nonsteroidal anti-inflammatory drugs and chronic analgesic abuse. Dye-contrast studies should be performed only when adequate hydration and diuresis can be ensured and if there is no suitable alternative diagnostic procedure.

An evaluation of renal function should be carried out initially and then at yearly intervals in all new adult diabetic patients. This should include a serum creatinine and urea, a urinalysis with microscopic analysis and a 24-hour urine collection for microalbuminuria, proteinuria, and creatinine clearance. Urinary tract infection, if present, should be promptly treated before the degree of proteinuria can be accurately evaluated. To retard or prevent further development of nephropathy, glycemic control should be optimized and hypertension aggressively treated as indicated earlier. A diet low in protein of 0.8 grams per kilogram body weight per day or approximately 10% of daily calories may also be of value in reducing the rate of progression of nephropathy. Consultation with a nephrologist is indicated when proteinuria is persistent or progressive, hypertension is unresponsive to treatment, or serum creatinine continues to rise.

Diabetic Neuropathy

Neuropathy is commonly encountered in diabetes, is highly variable in its presentation, and is often difficult to treat. Diabetic neuropathy is generally categorized into the sensorimotor peripheral neuropathies and autonomic neuropathies. Sensorimotor neuropathies include those of the symmetrical, distal, and bilateral type of the upper and lower extremities, various specific mononeuropathies, and diabetic amyotrophy. Autonomic neuropathies include gastroparesis diabeticorum, diabetic diarrhea, neurogenic bladder, impaired cardiovascular reflex responses, and impotence.

Symmetrical distal sensorimotor neuropathy is more common in the lower than the upper extremities and usually causes numbness, tingling, or a "pins and needles" sensation. Occasionally, these dysesthesias may be painful with burning or stabbing discomfort that can significantly affect quality of life and be associated with the so-called diabetic or neuropathic cachexia syndrome that includes anorexia, depression, and weight loss. Numerous medications have been tried for these neuropathies, particularly the painful variety, with variable efficacy. These include the tricyclic antidepressants, carbamazepine, phenytoin, and counterirritants such as topical capsaicin. At the present time, no form of therapy has been uniformly beneficial but the painful component of these neuropathies may subside within 6 to 12 months. In severe cases, narcotic analgesics can be used to control pain but the risk of addiction with chronic use is substantial.

Several mononeuropathies are classic in diabetes and include the cranial nerves, particularly the third and sixth, that result in extraocular muscle motor paralysis and peripheral palsies involving the peroneal, median, and ulnar nerves. Although certain nerves are more prone to involvement, mononeuropathy can occur in virtually any cranial or peripheral nerve. In the majority of cases, spontaneous recovery is usual over 3 to 6 months. Diabetic amyotrophy is often asymmetrical, more common in men, and associated with lower extremity weakness and wasting of the proximal muscles of the lower extremity with minimal or modest sensory involvement. The pelvic girdle and quadriceps muscles tend to be most severely affected with atrophy and absent patellar tendon reflexes. Despite the severity of the features, there is usually complete recovery in 6 to 12 months. Treatment involves maintenance of metabolic control as well as symptomatic and physical therapy.

Gastroparesis should be suspected in diabetic patients who experience nausea, vomiting, early satiety, abdominal distention, and bloating following food ingestion. It often occurs in concert with other forms of autonomic neuropathy and results from delayed emptying and retention of gastric contents. Metoclopramide can be beneficial but use of this medication has recently been discouraged owing to the irreversible side effect of tardive dyskinesia. Cisapride (Propulsid) 10 to 20 mg before meals and at bedtime is often helpful.

Diabetic diarrhea can be extremely difficult to treat and may be intermittent or alternate between constipation and diarrhea. High fiber intake can be of value as can diphenoxylate (Lomotil) 2.5 to 5 mg four times daily or loperamide (Imodium) 2 to 8 mg daily. Not uncommonly, patients will respond transiently for several weeks to therapy with ampicillin, tetracycline, or other broad-spectrum antibiotics. In otherwise refractory cases of diabetic diarrhea, intermittent therapy with varying antibiotic regimens can be effective. The somatostatin analogue octreotide (Sandostatin) 100 to 200 μg in two to four divided doses has also been used with benefit but requires subcutaneous or intravenous injection.

The most troublesome and potentially disabling autonomic symptom involving the cardiovascular system in diabetes is orthostatic or postural hypotension. This abnormality may cause light-headedness, syncope, and in rare instances, sudden death. A fixed tachycardia may also be present, and it is not uncommon for such patients to be hypertensive when sitting or lying. Treatment usually involves elevating the head of the bed on blocks, lower limb and torso compression stockings, supplementary salt intake and in some cases use of fludrocortisone (Florinef Acetate) beginning at 0.05 mg with gradual increments as necessary up to 0.5 to 1.0 mg. Therapy with fludrocortisone should be used cautiously since supine hypertension can be exacerbated with this medication and fluid retention may occur with precipitation of congestive heart failure.

The diagnosis of neurogenic bladder should be considered in any diabetic patient with neuropathy or when complaints of increased urinary frequency of small amounts or incontinence are elicited. Confirmation of neurogenic bladder requires the demonstration of cystometric abnormalities and large residual urine volume. Not uncommonly, bladder dysfunction escapes detection until urinary retention or a urinary tract infection develops. Treatment is generally unsatisfactory but some benefit can be derived by scheduling frequent voids (every 3 to 4 hours) combined with the administration of bethanechol 10 to 50 mg three to four times a day supplemented with small doses of phenoxybenzamine (Dibenzyline) to enhance bladder contractility and emptying. In men, concomitant prostatic hypertrophy or other causes of outflow obstruction should be treated. Prophylactic antibiotic therapy with trimethoprim-sulfamethoxazole may prevent recurrent urinary tract infection.

Impotence occurs frequently in men with diabetes and may be of neurogenic or vascular origin. Usually, libido is intact but there is inability to sustain a firm erection and retrograde ejaculation may occur. Impotence unrelated to diabetes, especially of psychological or endocrinologic cause, must also be considered in the differential diagnosis. Another common cause of impotence in males with diabetes is antihypertensive medications. Various external and implantable penile devices are now available to assist with resumption of sexual intercourse in some cases.

Diabetic Foot Disorders

Diabetes accounts for more than one-half of all nontraumatic amputations in the United States, and the majority of these are preventable with proper care. The most important aspect of diabetic foot care is prophylaxis to prevent development of problems. Both the physician and the patient must be diligent about regularly examining the feet to detect redness or other signs of trauma. Foot lesions usually begin because of lack of pain, position, and vibratory sensation from neuropathy, associated deformities, and vascular ischemia. Abnormal distribution of foot pressure from proprioceptive defects predisposes to pressure ischemia and skin breakdown. Autonomic neuropathy contributes to decreased sweating and dry skin that can become cracked and thickened with increased potential for infection and ulceration.

Patients must be educated to inspect their feet daily, to recognize early skin lesions, and to avoid situations that might increase their likelihood of developing a sore. Education about the risks and prevention of foot problems needs to reinforced on a regular basis. Proper footwear and foot care can minimize the appearance of problems. Assistance from specialized health care professionals with expertise in diabetic foot care, such as podiatrists, should be sought. High-risk patients need regular care of their nails and calluses and may require special shoes and inserts. Once an ulcer develops, pressure must be alleviated, the site débrided, and if an infection is present, antibiotic therapy should be instituted after appropriate cultures have been obtained. X-rays are helpful to detect foreign bodies, soft tissue gas, or bony abnormalities. To assist healing, patients should be off their feet or alternately can be placed in a well-fitting orthopedic walking cast to relieve pressure but permit mobility. A combination of distal arterial revascularization and local foot-sparing surgery is often necessary to prevent amputations.

DIABETES MELLITUS IN CHILDREN AND ADOLESCENTS

method of
JOSEPH I. WOLFSDORF, M.B., B.CH., and
CHRISTINA LUEDKE, M.D., PH.D.
Children's Hospital
Boston, Massachusetts

Type I diabetes mellitus or insulin-dependent diabetes mellitus (IDDM) results from insulin deficiency caused by chronic progressive autoimmune destruction of the insulin-producing beta cells of the islets of Langerhans. In the United States, the prevalence of IDDM in people younger than 20 years is about 1.7 cases per 1000; it is estimated that there are about 125,000 children and teenagers with IDDM.

Hyperglycemia occurs when at least 90% of the beta-cell mass has been destroyed. The most common symptoms are polyuria, polydipsia, and weight loss. Dehydration results from the osmotic diuresis induced by hyperglycemia. More severe insulin deficiency causes unrestrained lipolysis and ketoacid production that leads to an anion gap acidosis characterized by nausea, vomiting, abdominal pain, and hyperpnea (Kussmaul's respiration).

At diagnosis, most children have residual beta cells whose function is impaired by hyperglycemia. Reversal of the metabolic derangements restores function of the remaining beta cells for months to years until they are destroyed by progression of the autoimmune process. Similarly, correction of hyperglycemia restores tissue sensitivity to insulin. These two factors account for the period of partial remission, often called the "honeymoon," during which normal or nearly normal glycemic control is easily maintained with a relatively low dose of insulin, on the order of less than 0.3 to 0.5 U per kg per day. After destruction of the remaining beta cells, the insulin dose gradually increases until the full replacement dose is reached.

At our center, most children are briefly hospitalized to initiate therapy. Even when the child is not gravely ill, the emotional impact of the diagnosis on the child and family often causes great distress. Therefore, we prefer to begin the program of diabetes education and self-care training in a safe and supportive environment. This enables grieving and overwhelmed parents to acquire survival skills while they are coping with the emotional upheaval caused by the crisis resulting from the discovery of this incurable disease in their child.

The initial goals of therapy are to stabilize the metabolic state with insulin, fluid, and electrolyte replacement and to provide basic diabetes education and self-care training to the patient, in an age-appropriate fashion, and to parents and other important caregivers.

DIABETIC KETOACIDOSIS

Approximately one-third of newly diagnosed children referred to Children's Hospital, Boston, arrive in diabetic ketoacidosis (DKA). The principles of the treatment protocol used at this center are presented here.

Initial Evaluation

1. Perform a clinical evaluation to establish the diagnosis and determine its cause (especially any evidence of infection) and to assess the patient's degree of dehydration. Weigh the patient and measure height or length.
2. With a glucose meter, determine the blood glucose concentration at the bedside.
3. Obtain a blood sample for measurement of plasma glucose, electrolytes, total CO_2, BUN, serum osmolality, arterial or venous pH, PCO_2, PO_2, hemoglobin, hematocrit, white blood cell count and differential, calcium, magnesium, and phosphorus. Calculate the anion gap.
4. Perform a urinalysis and obtain appropriate specimens for culture (blood, urine, throat) even if the patient is afebrile.
5. Perform an electrocardiogram for baseline evaluation of potassium status.
6. Determine baseline neurologic status.

Supportive Measures

1. In semiconscious or unconscious patients, secure the airway and empty the stomach by nasogastric suction to prevent aspiration.
2. Give supplementary oxygen to patients who are cyanosed or in shock or when the PaO_2 is less than 80 mm Hg.
3. Measure urine output accurately; use bladder or condom catheterization if necessary.
4. Record in a flow chart the patient's clinical and laboratory data, details of fluid and electrolyte therapy, administered insulin, and urine output. Successful management of diabetic ketoacidosis requires meticulous monitoring of the patient's clinical and biochemical response to treatment so that timely adjustments in the treatment regimen can be made when necessary.

5. Measure plasma glucose, serum electrolytes (and corrected sodium), pH, PCO_2, TCO_2, anion gap, calcium, and phosphorus every 2 hours for the first 8 hours and then every 4 hours until they are normal.
6. Admit to an intensive care unit infants, toddlers, and severely ill older children with DKA, especially those with central nervous system obtundation or cardiovascular instability.
7. Administer broad-spectrum antibiotics to febrile patients after appropriate cultures of body fluids have been obtained.

Fluid and Electrolyte Treatment

All patients with DKA are dehydrated and suffer total body depletion of sodium, potassium, chloride, phosphate, and magnesium. Patients with mild-to-moderate DKA are usually about 5% (50 mL per kg) dehydrated, and those with severe DKA are up to 10% (100 mL per kg) dehydrated.

1. Start an intravenous infusion using a large-bore cannula and infuse 10 mL per kg of isotonic saline solution (0.9%) within 60 minutes. In the severely dehydrated patient or the patient in shock, initially give 20 mL per kg followed by an additional 10 mL per kg over 60 minutes if hypotension or shock persists.
2. Once the circulation has been stabilized, change to half-normal saline solution and aim to replace the calculated fluid deficit at an even rate over 24 to 36 hours. Aim to achieve slow correction of the serum hyperosmolality and to avoid a rapid shift of water from the extracellular to the intracellular compartment. The sodium concentration of the solution should be increased to 100 to 130 mEq per liter if the corrected serum sodium concentration fails to rise as the plasma glucose concentration decreases. The corrected sodium is calculated:

$$Na^+ + (1.6 \times [\text{plasma glucose mg per dL} - 100]/100)$$

3. Maintenance fluid is given as half isotonic saline solution at a rate of 1500 mL per m^2 per day.
4. Add 5% dextrose to the infusion fluid when the plasma glucose concentration reaches 300 mg per dL and attempt to maintain the plasma glucose concentration at approximately 200 mg per dL for the first 36 to 48 hours. To avert hypoglycemia, 10% dextrose may be needed.
5. Continue intravenous fluid administration until acidosis is corrected and the patient can eat and drink without vomiting.

Insulin

After an intravenous priming dose of 0.1 U per kg, insulin is diluted in saline solution (50 U regular insulin in 50 mL saline solution) and is given intravenously at a rate of 0.1 U per kg per hour, controlled by an infusion pump. Insulin has a serum half-life of approximately 5 to 7 minutes; therefore, insulin deficiency develops rapidly if the insulin infusion is interrupted. Intravenous insulin therapy should not be used unless it can be closely supervised.

When DKA has resolved (venous pH greater than 7.32, total CO_2 greater than 18 mEq per liter) and the change to subcutaneous insulin is planned, the first injection should be given 60 to 120 minutes before stopping the infusion, to allow sufficient time for the injected insulin to be absorbed.

Potassium Replacement

All patients with DKA are potassium depleted (4 to 6 mEq per kg) despite an initial serum potassium concentration that may be normal or increased. With the administration of fluid and insulin, serum potassium may decrease abruptly, predisposing the patient to cardiac arrhythmias. Patients whose serum potassium level is initially low are the most severely depleted. They should receive potassium after urinating, and the serum potassium concentration should be measured hourly. The serum potassium level should be maintained in the normal range. Half the potassium is given as potassium acetate and the other half as potassium phosphate; this reduces the total amount of chloride administered and partially replaces the phosphate deficit.

Acidosis

Routine administration of bicarbonate neither hastens resolution of acidosis nor improves survival and may impair tissue oxygenation and cause hypokalemia. Its routine use is not recommended; however, when acidosis is severe (arterial pH less than 7.0) or there is hypotension, shock, or an arrhythmia, sodium bicarbonate, 1 to 2 mEq per kg or 40 to 80 mEq per m², is infused over 2 hours.

Cerebral Edema

This is an uncommon complication of DKA that can cause acute brain herniation and death. It typically develops abruptly within 2 to 12 hours of starting treatment and manifests as headache, vomiting, altered level of consciousness, delirium or restlessness, incontinence, bradycardia, increased blood pressure, unequal pupils, papilledema, respiratory arrest, and sudden onset of polyuria from acute diabetes insipidus. Computed tomography scan of the brain confirms brain swelling. When cerebral edema is suspected, the following steps should be taken immediately: administer mannitol, 1 gram per kg intravenously, and repeat as necessary; reduce the rate of fluid administration; insert an endotracheal tube; and hyperventilate the patient.

INSULIN THERAPY

The three major categories of insulin preparations differ in their absorption kinetics (Table 1). Several insulin regimens can be used: each has the same goal, namely, to provide basal insulin throughout the day and more with meals (Table 2). The most commonly used regimen consists of a combination of short- and intermediate-acting (NPH or lente) insulin given twice daily, before breakfast and before the evening meal. A modification of this regimen that

involves three doses per day, with intermediate-acting insulin given at bedtime instead of before supper, is especially recommended for adolescents. The child's age, weight, and pubertal status guide the initial choice of dose.

Subcutaneous insulin is started in a newly diagnosed child who is not significantly dehydrated, is not vomiting, and either does not have ketoacidosis or has mild ketoacidosis (arterial pH greater than 7.25, venous pH greater than 7.20). In a child diagnosed early with moderate hyperglycemia and no ketonuria, the recommended starting dose of insulin is 0.3 to 0.5 U per kg per day. When metabolic decompensation is more severe (ketonuria but without acidosis or dehydration), the initial dose is 0.5 to 0.75 U per kg, supplemented, if necessary, with 0.1 U per kg of regular insulin subcutaneously at 4- to 6-hour intervals. The upper end of each suggested range is used for pubertal patients and for those who are physically inactive and overweight. The total daily dose (TDD) is divided so that two-thirds is given before breakfast and one-third in the evening. The ratio of short- to intermediate-acting insulin at both times is 1 : 2. Target blood glucose levels for different ages are shown in Table 3. The insulin dose is adjusted until satisfactory blood glucose control is achieved.

For toddlers and young children, we use U10 (U100 insulin diluted 1:10) regular insulin; children of this age typically require a smaller fraction of regular

TABLE 1. **Insulin Preparations***

Type	Action	Onset of Action (h)	Peak Action (h)	Duration of Action (h)
Regular	Short-acting	0.5	2–4	6–8
NPH (isophane)	Intermediate-acting	1–2	6–12	18–24
Lente	Intermediate-acting	1–3	6–12	18–24
Ultralente	Long-acting	4–6	8–20	24–28

*These figures are for human insulins and are approximations from laboratory studies in test subjects. The times of onset, peak, and duration of action vary greatly within and between patients and are affected by many factors, including size of dose, site of injection, exercise of the injected area, temperature, and insulin antibodies.

TABLE 2. **Insulin Regimens**

Doses	Breakfast	Lunch	Dinner	Bedtime
Two	R + NPH/L		R + NPH/L	
	R + NPH/L		R + UL	
	R + UL		R + UL	
Three	R + NPH/L		R	NPH/L
	R + UL	R	R + UL	
Four	R	R	R	NPH/L
	R + NPH/L	R	R	NPH/L

Abbreviations: R = regular insulin; L = lente insulin; UL = ultralente insulin. NPH/L = either intermediate-acting insulin may be selected for use with this regimen.

TABLE 3. **Target Blood Glucose Levels for Children and Adolescents***

	Fasting (mg/dL)	Premeal (mg/dL)	2–4 A.M. (mg/dL)
Infant/toddler	80–180	100–200	80–180
School-age	80–150	80–180	80–150
Adolescent	70–120	70–180	70–150

*Target blood glucose levels for patients with normal counterregulatory mechanisms who practice intensive insulin therapy are 70–120 mg/dL fasting and before meals, <180 mg/dL 90–120 minutes after meals, and 70–100 mg/dL at 2–4 A.M.

insulin (10 to 20%) with proportionately more intermediate-acting insulin.

The optimal ratio of rapid- to intermediate-acting insulin for each patient is determined empirically, guided by the results of frequent blood glucose measurements. Five measurements daily: before each meal, before the bedtime snack, and at 2 to 4 A.M., are initially required to determine the effects of each prescribed dose. Adjustments are made to each dose at 3- to 5-day intervals, usually in 10% increments or decrements, in response to patterns of consistently elevated or low blood glucose levels, respectively. The daily insulin requirements of patients with complete insulin deficiency ("total" diabetes) is 0.5 to 1.0 U per kg before puberty and 0.8 to 1.5 U per kg during puberty.

Good glycemic control is impossible to achieve without strict attention to the other important factors that influence blood glucose levels: namely, diet and physical activity.

NUTRITION

Attention must be paid to the timing and content of meals in order to match food intake with the availability of injected insulin. The registered dietitian is an important member of the diabetes treatment team. Starting with the initial hospitalization and continuing with intermittent visits in the outpatient setting, the dietitian is responsible for instructing patients on the principles of nutritional management of diabetes and formulating an individualized meal plan that attempts to minimize postprandial hyperglycemia and avoid hypoglycemia between meals.

General Principles

The nutritional needs of children with diabetes do not differ from those of healthy children. Newly diagnosed children, however, typically have lost weight, and the initial diet prescription aims to restore a desirable weight for height. Once this has been achieved, the total intake of calories and nutrients must be sufficient to balance the daily expenditure of energy and satisfy the requirements for normal growth and development. A method commonly used to estimate energy requirements is based on age and is useful as a crude approximation for children up to 12 years of age: to 1000 kcal, add 100 × the patient's age in years.

The American Diabetes Association currently recommends that carbohydrate provide 50 to 60% of the total calories, with protein and fat making up 15 and 30%, respectively. The diet prescription has to be periodically adjusted to achieve an ideal or desirable body weight and to maintain a normal rate of physical growth and maturation. The main objective of dietary therapy in obese patients is to lose weight.

People with diabetes are predisposed to atherosclerosis and should follow a prudent fat diet; the amount of fat should not exceed 30% of the total daily calories. Dietary cholesterol is reduced to 300 mg per day or less and saturated fat to less than 10% of calories by consumption of less beef and pork and leaner cuts of meat, chicken, turkey, fish, low-fat milk, and vegetable proteins.

Dietary fiber may benefit the diabetic patient by blunting the rise in blood glucose after meals. Unrefined or minimally processed foods, such as grains, legumes, and vegetables, should replace highly refined carbohydrates. To avoid abrupt increases in blood glucose, children should eat fruit whole and avoid fruit juices, which should be reserved for treating episodes of hypoglycemia.

Because insulin is released continuously from the injection site, hypoglycemia, exacerbated by exercise, may occur if snacks are not eaten between the main meals. Hence, most children who receive twice-daily injections of insulin (split-mixed insulin regimen) have a snack between each meal and at bedtime; adolescents usually prefer to omit the midmorning snack. Meals and snacks should be eaten at approximately the same time each day, and the total consumption of calories and the proportions of carbohydrate, protein, and fat in each meal and snack should be consistent from day to day.

Exchange System

The meal plan is formulated using the system of food exchanges and is individualized to meet the ethnic, religious, and economic circumstances of each family and the food preferences of the individual child. The diet prescription must take into account the child's school schedule, gym classes, and after-school physical activity. The exchange system is based on six food groups—milk, fruit, vegetable, bread/starch, meat/protein, and fat—and the meal plan contains the number of exchanges from each food group to be included in each meal and snack. Parents should learn to calculate exchanges from the information on food labels.

EXERCISE

Exercise acutely lowers the blood glucose concentration by increasing utilization of glucose to a variable degree, depending on the intensity and duration of physical activity and the concurrent level of insulinemia. Children and teenagers with diabetes are encouraged to participate in sports and to exercise throughout the year. In addition to normalizing the child's life and promoting a positive self-image, exercise promotes good health practices, facilitates weight control, and may improve glycemic control.

Young children's activities tend to be spontaneous; bursts of activity are covered with a snack before and, if the exercise is prolonged, during the activity. A useful guide is to provide 15 grams of carbohydrate (one bread or fruit exchange) per 30 to 60 minutes of vigorous physical activity. Strenuous exercise in the afternoon or evening should be followed by a 10 to 20% reduction in the presupper or bedtime dose of intermediate-acting insulin and a larger bedtime snack, to reduce the risk of nocturnal or early-morning hypoglycemia from the lag effect of exercise.

Acute vigorous exercise in the face of poorly controlled diabetes can aggravate hyperglycemia and ketoacid production. Therefore, a child with ketonuria should not exercise. Exercising the limb into which insulin has been injected accelerates the rate of insulin absorption. If exercise is planned, it is recommended that the preceding insulin injection be given in a site that is least likely to be affected by exercise. Youngsters who participate in organized sports are advised to reduce the dose of insulin predominantly active during the period of sustained physical activity. The size of such reductions is determined by measuring blood glucose levels before and after exercise and are generally in the range of 10 to 30% of the usual insulin dose.

DIABETES CARE IN THE OUTPATIENT SETTING

The child is discharged from the hospital as soon as she or he is medically stable and the parents (or other care providers) have learned the essentials of diabetes management: insulin administration, self-monitoring of blood glucose (SMBG), urine ketone measurement, basic meal planning, and recognition and treatment of hypoglycemia. Frequent telephone contact, often daily, is initially needed to help parents interpret SMBG data and adjust insulin dose(s) necessitated by the home schedule of activity and meals. Within the first few weeks of diagnosis, two-thirds of children enter partial remission, and the dose of insulin usually has to be reduced considerably.

The patient is seen frequently in the first month, primarily by the nurse specialist/educator and dietitian, to review and consolidate the skills and principles taught in the hospital. Thereafter, follow-up visits with members of the diabetes team occur every 3 months. The purpose of regular clinic visits is to ensure that the child's diabetes is being appropriately managed at home and that the goals of therapy are met. A focused history should obtain information about self-care behaviors, the child's daily routines, the frequency, severity, and circumstances surrounding hypoglycemic events, and evidence of hyperglycemia (polyuria, polydipsia, nocturia, weight loss, blurry vision, perineal candidiasis).

At every visit, height and weight are measured and plotted on a growth chart. The weight curve is especially helpful in assessing adequacy of therapy, since a significant weight loss usually indicates that the prescribed dose is insufficient or the patient is omitting injections. A physical examination should be performed at least twice per year and includes measurement of blood pressure, pubertal staging, signs of thyroid disease, skin examination, and an evaluation of the organs most affected by long-standing diabetes. The injection sites are inspected for evidence of lipohypertrophy from overuse of the site.

Insulin therapy must be viewed as a dynamic process that takes into account growth and development, changes in lifestyle and activity, intercurrent illness, and other factors that influence insulin requirements. Doses are adjusted with the goal of maintaining blood glucose levels within the target range as much as possible. The target range varies with the age of the patient (see Table 3). For infants and toddlers, who cannot understand or easily express symptoms of hypoglycemia, the target range is higher to minimize the risk of severe hypoglycemia.

Regular clinic visits are opportunities to reinforce and expand on the diabetes self-care training that began in the hospital. Optimal care of diabetes depends on the patient's intimate understanding of the interplay of medication and lifestyle. At each visit, the goal is to increase the patient's and family's understanding of diabetes management, so that as the child becomes more independent, he or she can assume increasing responsibility for daily self-care. Mature and motivated teenagers are encouraged to use intensified insulin management techniques that involve multiple daily insulin injections, use of algorithms for insulin dose selection, and target blood glucose levels in or near the normal range (see Table 3).

Self-Monitoring of Blood Glucose

This is routinely taught to all patients with IDDM, and the ability of patients to obtain accurate results is confirmed at clinic visits, when patients are asked to compare results obtained with their meters with simultaneous blood glucose determinations in the clinical chemistry laboratory. SMBG is the cornerstone of any intensive diabetes management program, and frequent SMBG in conjunction with urine tests for ketones is essential to manage intercurrent illnesses and prevent ketoacidosis. A variety of meters with a digital display are available that enable the user to obtain measurements of blood glucose concentration within 10% of the value obtained in a clinical chemistry laboratory.

Patients ideally should test before each meal and at bedtime. If this is impractical or intolerable, patients should be encouraged to test before each dose of insulin and perform additional tests before lunch and at bedtime at least twice each week. Alternatively, for patients who cannot tolerate such frequent monitoring or who cannot afford the cost of the reagent strips, a period of intensive monitoring before each meal, at bedtime, and between 2 and 4 A.M. for several consecutive days before an office visit often provides sufficient information to confirm satisfactory control or serve as a basis for modifying the insulin regimen.

Urine should be tested for the presence of *ketones* whenever the child is sick, when the blood glucose level exceeds 250 mg per dL, and when blood glucose levels are high before breakfast and the possibility of unrecognized nocturnal hypoglycemia is suspected.

Glycosylated Hemoglobin (Hemoglobin A_1 or A_{1c}). The level of glycosylated hemoglobin, formed when glucose is bound nonenzymatically to the hemoglobin molecule, is directly proportional to the time-integrated mean blood glucose concentration over the preceding 2 to 3 months. Quarterly determinations of glycosylated hemoglobin should be used to provide an objective measure of average glycemia in the intervals between office visits.

PSYCHOSOCIAL ISSUES

A social worker performs a psychosocial assessment on all newly diagnosed patients and their families. Thereafter, patients are referred to the mental health specialist on the diabetes team when emotional, social, or financial concerns are identified that may be obstacles to achieving and maintaining acceptable glycemic control. Common problems encountered in a diabetes clinic are financial hardship affecting the ability to purchase costly supplies, parental guilt, the child's rebellion against treatment, noncompliance with medication, family adjustment problems, and frequently missed appointments. Recurrent ketoacidosis is the most extreme indicator of psychosocial stress.

HYPOGLYCEMIA

Occasional episodes of hypoglycemia are an unavoidable consequence of insulin therapy aimed at maintaining blood glucose levels near normal. The goal is to minimize the frequency and severity of hypoglycemia while maintaining the best possible glycemic control.

Patients and family members must be taught to recognize the early symptoms of hypoglycemia and to treat it promptly with a suitable form of concentrated carbohydrate. Because infants and toddlers may be unable to recognize the symptoms of hypoglycemia and cannot verbalize their symptoms, parents are advised to measure the blood glucose concentration whenever the child's behavior is unusual. Most episodes of hypoglycemia are satisfactorily treated with 10 to 20 grams of glucose; 5 grams is sufficient for an infant or toddler. Suitable forms of rapidly absorbed carbohydrate for treatment of hypoglycemia are glucose tablets (each contains 5 grams of glucose), Lifesavers candy (3 grams each), granulated table sugar (4 grams per teaspoon), orange or apple juice (10 to 12 grams per 120 mL). Family members are taught

to use glucagon (which should be available at home) to treat an episode of severe hypoglycemia in which the child is unconscious or unable to swallow or retain ingested carbohydrate. Glucagon (0.02 to 0.03 mg per kg, maximal dose 1.0 mg) is injected intramuscularly or subcutaneously and raises the blood glucose level within 5 to 15 minutes. Nausea and vomiting may follow the administration of glucagon. After consciousness has been regained, oral carbohydrate should be given to prevent further hypoglycemia. If the patient cannot take it orally or retain sugar-containing fluids, glucose, 0.5 gram per kg, is injected intravenously followed by a continuous infusion at a rate that maintains a normal blood glucose concentration.

A Medic Alert bracelet or necklace should always be worn to identify the patient as having diabetes mellitus.

SCREENING FOR COMPLICATIONS

The organs most affected by diabetes are the eyes, kidneys, circulatory system, and peripheral nervous system. Diabetic complications develop insidiously but can be detected years before they become symptomatic. Systematic screening is performed to detect abnormalities early, when intervention to arrest, reverse, or retard complications is most beneficial. Both diabetic retinopathy and nephropathy are rare before puberty and in patients who have had IDDM for less than 5 years. Therefore, beginning 5 years after diagnosis, patients annually should have a dilated retinal examination and measurement of albumin and creatinine concentrations in a timed overnight or first-morning urine specimen to detect microalbuminuria. Circulatory and neurologic complications of diabetes are seldom clinically significant in the pediatric and adolescent population.

CONCLUSION

Advances in the treatment of diabetes in children in the past 2 decades now make it possible to ensure normal growth and development and safely achieve a level of blood glucose control that previously was unattainable. It is reasonable to expect that the benefits of sustained improvement in glycemic control will prevent, or at least delay, the appearance of the chronic complications of diabetes. It is important, however, to remember that the arduous task of controlling blood glucose in a child is difficult and frustrating. The members of the diabetes team must set realistic and attainable goals for each patient and constantly provide encouragement and support. The resources of a multidisciplinary health care team— physician, nurse educator, dietitian, mental health specialist, and ophthalmologist—are essential for the successful management of IDDM by the child or adolescent and family.

DIABETIC KETOACIDOSIS

method of
MICHAEL E. MAY, Ph.D., M.D., and
CONNIE YOUNG, R.N., M.S.N.
Vanderbilt University Medical Center
Nashville, Tennessee

Diabetic ketoacidosis is a severe metabolic disturbance resulting from absolute deficiency of insulin or severe resistance to insulin action. It is fatal if untreated. Mortality from diabetic ketoacidosis has decreased over past decades but remains at 3 to 5% of cases. Many patients respond rapidly to treatment. The length of hospital stay for ketoacidosis is about 5 to 6 days in adults. Diagnosis Related Group guidelines for length of stay for ketoacidosis state 4.4 days for those under 35 years of age and 5.9 days for those aged 35 years or over.

Treatment of ketoacidosis is simplified by separation of the hospital course into three phases (Table 1): recognition, treatment of acidemia, and discharge planning. Goals, diagnostic actions, and physician orders are different for each phase. Each phase includes direct patient care, laboratory tests, fluid administration, insulin administration, and other actions.

Phase A demands clinical suspicion of diabetic ketoacidosis. Ketoacidosis should be considered for

Every patient with diabetes mellitus and uncontrolled emesis
Every patient with diabetes mellitus with acute illness
Every patient with unexplained coma or acute mental status changes
Every patient with severe malaise or severe dehydration

Symptoms of diabetic ketoacidosis reflect basic physiology. Hyperglycemia leads to polyuria, nocturia, and blurred

TABLE 1. Phases of Diabetic Ketoacidosis

Phase A: Recognition

Goals:
1. Stabilize circulation and airway
2. Diagnose diabetic ketoacidosis
3. Assess patient for major co-diagnoses
4. Initiate fluid and insulin therapy

Exit: Diagnosis of ketoacidosis has been made, fluid therapy started, first dose of insulin given, and care transferred to an inpatient care team

Phase B: Acidemia

Goals
1. Restore blood buffering to total $CO_2 \geq 20$ mEq/L (20 mM)
2. Keep serum glucose in range of 90–200 mg/dL (5–11 mM)
3. Maintain serum potassium of 3.5–5.5 mEq/L (3.5–5.5 mM)
4. Partial replacement of fluid deficit
5. Appropriately treat co-diagnosis

Exit: $TCO_2 \geq 20$ mEq/L (20 mM) and glucose < 300 mg/dL (16.7 mM)

Phase C: Discharge Planning

Goals
1. Make diet transition to oral food
2. Start routine insulin therapy
3. Treat co-diagnosis
4. Arrange follow-up care for diabetes and for co-diagnosis
5. Teach outpatient survival skills

Exit: Hospital discharge

TABLE 2. Diagnosis of Diabetic Ketoacidosis*

1. Serum or blood glucose $\geq$ 200 mg/dL (11.0 mM) for nonpregnant subjects
   or Blood glucose $\geq$ 150 mg/dL (8.3 mM) for pregnant subjects
2. Urine ketones positive at small, moderate, or large
   or Serum acetone titer $\geq$ 1:2
3. Venous total CO_2 < 20 mEq/L (20 mM)
   or calculated bicarbonate from arterial blood gas < 20 mEq/L (20 mM)
   or Arterial base excess $\leq$ −2.0 mEq/L (−2.0 mM)
   or Blood pH < 7.30
   or Anion gap $\geq$ 20 mEq/L (20 mM)

*Diabetic ketoacidosis is present when one criterion is met for each of the three components listed.

vision. Volume depletion leads to thirst, weakness, dizziness, and syncope. Electrolyte depletion causes weakness, muscle cramps, and palpitations. Ketosis causes nausea and emesis. Metabolic acidemia increases respiratory drive and hence may cause chest muscle pain.

Symptoms from an accompanying condition may dominate patient complaints. Common co-diagnoses include infections (bacterial, viral, fungal), inflammations (burns, postoperative state, acute asthma, esophagitis), and toxic states (cocaine overdose). Infarctions (cardiac, peripheral vascular, cerebral) may precipitate ketoacidosis but are less common than acute infections. Omission of insulin shots leads to ketoacidosis in Type I diabetes. Medical noncompliance and substance abuse are usually denied. New diabetes may present with ketoacidosis in both children and adults.

Physical examination routinely discloses lethargy and tachycardia. Signs of dehydration (hypotension, orthostasis, tenting skin) or acidemia (Kussmaul's breathing) are supportive but not sensitive markers of ketoacidosis. Most subjects with ketoacidosis are not hypotensive on presentation. Kussmaul's breathing is deep and regular. It may be missed by inexperienced clinicians because the respiratory rate may not be striking. Abdominal ileus, tenderness, and rigidity are caused by ketoacidosis. Surgical causes of an acute abdomen are not excluded until the abdominal examination improves with metabolic treatment.

Table 2 lists criteria for diagnosis of diabetic ketoacidosis. Multiple measures of acidemia are not needed. Each physician must use the most convenient and rapid tests available. A urine dipstick plus the Chemistry 6 stat panel is adequate. We have noted Kussmaul's breathing only when the serum TCO_2 is less than 13 mM. Thus, treatment is started immediately if the history is appropriate, tachycardia and Kussmaul's breathing are present, and the urine dipstick is positive for glucose and ketones. The differential diagnosis of diabetic ketoacidosis includes pregnancy, renal failure, and toxins such as ethanol, methanol, ethylene glycol, and organic solvents. Routine tests should cover pregnancy, cocaine use, renal failure, and hypoxemia. Other tests are added as indicated by the clinical situation.

PHASE A: RECOGNITION

Table 3 shows essential actions in Phase A diabetic ketoacidosis. Diabetic ketoacidosis includes whole-body depletion of water, sodium, and potassium. Intravenous fluids are started before laboratory test results are known. The absolute fluid infusion rate is 300 to 500 mL per hour for most adults. We recom-

TABLE 3. **Actions in Phase A Ketoacidosis: Recognition**

Patient Care

1. Assess breathing and secure airway
2. History: Ask about nausea, emesis, abdominal pain, respiratory difficulty, polyuria, dysuria, sinus pain, headache, fever, ulcer, cough, chest pain, ethanol use, cocaine ingestion, diabetes care practices
3. Assess vital signs, respiratory pattern, peripheral perfusion, mental status, peripheral edema, pulmonary auscultation, oral examination, focal signs of infection, estimated body weight
4. Place intravenous infusion line(s)
5. Place bladder catheter only if patient unable to void

Important: Unresponsive patients need immediate dextrose, 25 gm; thiamine, 100 mg; and naloxone, 0.4 mg IV, without waiting for tests

Laboratory Tests

1. Urine dipstick
2. Serum Chemistry 6 panel (sodium, potassium, chloride, total carbon dioxide, urea nitrogen, glucose)
3. Blood cell count
4. Serum creatinine, serum phosphorus, serum acetone titer
5. Urine pregnancy test in postpubertal females
6. Urine microscopic analysis
7. Pulse oximetry or arterial blood gas for oxygen saturation
8. Urine toxicology screen
9. Cultures, if appropriate
10. Electrocardiogram and radiographs, if appropriate

Fluid

Lactated Ringer's solution, 7 mL/kg/h if no edema or rales

Insulin

Insulin, regular, 0.1 U/kg IM, plus 0.3 U/kg SC

Diet

Ice chips by mouth as tolerated

---

mend a 1-liter bag for initial fluid in adults and a 500-mL bag for initial fluid in adolescents. Normal saline solution is an acceptable alternative to lactated Ringer's solution for the first infusate. Higher rates of fluid infusion are not advantageous. About one-fifth of adults with diabetic ketoacidosis have partial or total renal insufficiency. Thus, minimal intravenous fluid is given in the face of rales or peripheral edema. An intravenous bolus of regular insulin disappears very rapidly. We begin insulin intramuscularly plus subcutaneously and decide on use of an insulin drip later.

Most patients with diabetic ketoacidosis are admitted to the hospital. The median time for metabolic recovery is 22 to 24 hours. The time required to treat the precipitating cause is longer. Only a few patients may be treated fully in an emergency department or office. The extent of hyperglycemia and acidemia do not predict mortality nor length of hospital stay. Hence, metabolic status does not dictate where to admit the patient. Children are admitted to an intensive care unit. Patients with chest pain, cardiac arrhythmia, severe hypotension, probable septic shock, full coma, and respiratory failure are put in the intensive care unit. Patients on renal dialysis are admitted directly to a hemodialysis unit. Pregnant women with ketoacidosis are admitted to a delivery unit for continuous fetal monitoring. All other adults are admitted to a general care floor, provided infusion therapy and bedside glucose monitoring are available and reliable.

PHASE B: TREATMENT OF ACIDEMIA

Treatment of Phase B ketoacidosis is outlined in Table 4. Water, salt, potassium, and insulin are needed to resolve hyperglycemia and acidemia. Routine use of infusates with a sodium-to-chloride ratio greater than 1.0 reduces postrecovery hyperchloremic acidosis. After the first bag of fluid (usually 1 liter) has infused, we halve the infusion rate. If serum potassium is less than 6.0 mEq per liter (6 mM) and urine output is present, we increase infused potassium in the second bag of intravenous fluids. Dextrose is also added to the second bag. Postponing addition of dextrose until the blood glucose level is less than 250 mg per dL (14 mM) leads to hypoglycemia if there are any communication delays. There are champions of routine magnesium therapy, routine thiamine therapy, and routine sodium bicarbonate therapy in selected cases. No studies prove benefit for these actions. Specifically, we do not use sodium bicarbonate except during cardiopulmonary resuscitation.

Insulin doses include two components: the fasting insulin requirement and the extra insulin needed to reverse ketoacidosis. The latter may be given by continuous infusion or by intramuscular plus subcutaneous injections. Typical doses are shown in Table 4. Infused insulin should be pumped separately and piggybacked into the main intravenous infusate. The infusion method is simple to remember. It depends on close control of low-volume fluid delivery and reliable preparation of the infusate. Mixing of all medications by a central pharmacy may cause delay in starting insulin infusions. The injection method requires simpler infusion apparatus. The injection method described in Table 4 is easy to switch to routine insulin therapy on resolution of acidemia. Rapid resolution of acidemia is anticipated by giving intermediate-acting insulin (NPH or human Ultralente), dosed for the fasting state, at the next usual dose time (morning or bedtime).

Bladder or nasogastric catheterization is not routinely needed. Usually the patient requests more oral intake as acidemia resolves. The diet order during this phase is liquids as tolerated. Acidemia resolves, on average, about 24 hours after initial presentation.

Asymptomatic cerebral edema occurs in many cases of ketoacidosis. Symptomatic brain edema occurs several hours after therapy for ketoacidosis. Mild changes in mental status or irritability may be the first symptoms. Progressive brain swelling leads to emesis, seizures, or autonomic instability. Brain stem herniation causes coma, fixed pupils, cranial nerve palsy, and cardiorespiratory arrest. Therapy of cerebral edema includes mannitol, 0.5 to 1.0 gram per kg (up to 50 grams) intravenously, intubation for mechanical hyperventilation, and high-dose glucocor-

TABLE 4. **Treatment of Phase B Ketoacidosis:
Acidemia**

Patient Care

1. Assess vital signs and urine output every 4 h
2. Assess mental status every hour in children

Laboratory Tests

1. Bedside blood glucose every 2 h (with IV regular insulin) or every 4 h (with IM and SC regular insulin injection)
2. Serum Chemistry 6 panel; phosphorus every 8 h
3. Serum acetone and blood count every day
4. Bacterial cultures, if clinically appropriate

Fluid

Dextrose 5%—lactated Ringer's solution with 40 mEq/L of potassium acetate at 3.5 mL/kg/h

Insulin

1. Maintenance: 0.1–0.15 U/kg morning and bedtime; NPH insulin or human Ultralente insulin, SC
2. Extra insulin:
   a. IV infusion method
      Begin insulin regular, 0.1 U/kg/IV, THEN ADJUST rate of insulin drip every 2 h based on bedside glucose as follows:

Glucose Level	Change in Insulin Dose
<60	Stop drip 30 min, give 25 gm of glucose (1 amp D50) IV, resume insulin at a rate 2.5 U/h less than prior rate
60–79	Stop drip 30 min, resume insulin at a rate of 2 U/h less than prior rate
80–109	Reduce rate by 1.3 U/h
110–140	Reduce rate by 0.5 U/h
141–170	No change in drip rate
171–200	Increase rate by 0.3 U/h
201–250	Increase rate by 0.7 U/h
251–349	Give insulin regular, 4 units IV push, and then increase drip rate by 1.1 U/h
>350	Give insulin regular, 10 units IV push, and then increase drip rate by 1.1 U/h

   b. Injection method
      ADJUST insulin dose every 4 h based on bedside glucose as follows:

Glucose Level	Insulin Dose
< 50	Give 25 gm of glucose (1 amp 50% dextrose) IV, page physician
50–89	Give 25 gm of glucose (1 amp 50% dextrose) IV, plus 2 units insulin regular SC
90–119	Insulin regular, 0.05 U/kg SC
120–149	Insulin regular, 0.10 U/kg SC
150–179	Insulin regular, 0.20 U/kg SC
180–209	Insulin regular, 0.30 U/kg SC
210–239	Insulin regular, 0.40 U/kg SC
240–299	Insulin regular, 0.10 U/kg IM plus 0.3 U/kg SC
> 300	Page physician

Diet

Liquids as tolerated

Co-Diagnosis

Treat appropriately

---

ticoids. Prediction of cerebral edema is poor. There are anecdotal impressions that rapid correction of hyperosmolality is causative. Retrospective reviews have not proved that rate or type of fluid replacement predicts cerebral edema. Nevertheless, infusion rates in Tables 3 and 4 are deliberately conservative in an attempt to forestall cerebral edema. Unexpected cerebral edema during ketoacidosis rarely has been reported in adults. Thus, recommended monitoring is more stringent in children.

Aggressive therapy with insulin and dextrose promotes intracellular movement of potassium. Waiting until the plasma potassium level has fallen low before replacement carries the risk of cardiac arrhythmia and pulmonary arrest. Intravenous potassium at concentrations greater than 40 mEq per liter causes infusion site pain and thrombosis. The method described in Table 4 leads to a cumulative dose of 2.8 to 3.3 mmol of potassium per kg per day. We have not found any severe hypokalemia (serum potassium less than 3.0 mEq per liter [3.0 mM]) when potassium supplementation is at least 2.0 mmol per kg per day. Serum potassium must be monitored to avoid hyperkalemia with renal insufficiency and to diagnose unusual potassium needs.

The serum phosphorus level also falls with treatment of ketoacidemia. Two prospective trials found no benefit in routine phosphate replacement during ketoacidosis. Neither trial included any subject with severe hypophosphatemia (serum level less than 1.0 mg per dL [0.32 mM]). Hypophosphatemia may be treated orally or intravenously. Each 15 mmol of potassium phosphate contains 22 mEq of potassium. Potassium phosphate should not be added to lactated Ringer's solution, which contains calcium. The serum calcium level may fall with intravenous phosphorus therapy and hence must be monitored. Oral potassium sodium phosphate solution (Neutra-Phos), 75 mL in 4 oz of orange juice by mouth three times a day, provides 750 mg of phosphorus and 39 mEq of potassium.

Since only a minority of cases have bacterial infection, we do not use antibiotics in every case. The failure of blood glucose to fall or the failure of serum TCO_2 to rise is most often due to untreated infection or ongoing infarction. The failure of a response demands reconsideration for an underlying co-diagnosis.

PHASE C: DISCHARGE PLANNING

The longest period of a hospital admission for ketoacidosis is the discharge planning phase. Treatment is summarized in Table 5. The frequency of patient monitoring is reduced. Intravenous fluids are reduced to 1.5 mL per kg per hour and then stopped. Additional potassium can be given orally. Intermediate-acting insulin is needed twice a day. Regular insulin is needed to cover meals and to cover extra requirements during infection. A patient who has been on insulin before is restarted on prior doses. The dose estimate for other patients is 0.1 to 0.15 units per kg twice a day for maintenance (NPH or human Ultralente), plus 0.1 unit per kg per meal to cover food intake (regular insulin). The dose for the lunch meal can be added to the morning NPH for a twice-a-day insulin regimen. Patients who have never taken insulin (new diagnosis of diabetes or

TABLE 5. **Treatment of Phase C Ketoacidosis: Discharge Planning**

Patient Care

1. Monitor vital signs every 4–8 h
2. Teach or review self-monitoring of diabetes
3. Review outpatient sick day self-care
4. Teach insulin administration technique

Laboratory Tests

1. Capillary glucose before meals and at bedtime
2. Serum potassium and acetone every day

Fluid

Dextrose 5%—lactated Ringer's solution with 40 mEq/L potassium acetate at 1.5 mL/kg per h with taper to zero

Insulin

1. Maintenance: NPH or human Ultralente insulin twice a day (0.1 U/kg SC A.M. + HS or resume prior doses)
2. Meal coverage: Insulin regular SC premeals (0.1 U/kg/meal or resume prior doses)
3. Sliding scale: Insulin regular SC premeals and bedtime, 1 U per change of glucose of 50 mg/dL beginning at 150 mg/dL, in addition to meal coverage

Diet

Solid food, 30 cal/kg

---

patients formerly on pills) need instruction in insulin administration before discharge.

All patients need a review of sick day management of diabetes. It is impractical to provide a comprehensive inpatient diabetes education program to every patient admitted with ketoacidosis. Every patient needs clear delineation of follow-up care for diabetes. Ideally, educational issues raised during hospitalization are communicated to the outpatient diabetes educator.

The co-diagnosis or precipatating cause of diabetic ketoacidosis is treated so that it no longer interferes with outpatient functioning. Occasionally, localizing symptoms and signs of infection are not evident until after recovery from ketoacidemia. Patients with positive bacterial cultures stay about twice as long as those with other cases of ketoacidosis. Inadequate insulin or inadequate treatment of an infection during this phase leads to recurrent ketoacidemia. Such patients stay an extra 1 to 3 days in the hospital.

Hypoglycemia is not limited to Phase B. During an entire hospital stay, hypoglycemia occurs at least once in about 30% of cases of ketoacidosis. Delay in giving intravenous dextrose risks early hypoglycemia. Older age, hepatic and renal insufficiency, and inappropriate continuation of aggressive insulin are risk factors for late hypoglycemia.

Arterial thrombosis and venous thrombosis are recognized complications of ketoacidosis. Clinical recognition may be delayed until the discharge planning phase. Delay in recognition and treatment of cerebral edema in children leads to severe permanent neurologic impairment in survivors. Proper long-term care must be arranged for treatment of all complications and co-diagnoses.

PREVENTION

Many subjects with Type I diabetes mellitus never have ketoacidosis, whereas some subjects have multiple episodes of it. Recurrent ketoacidosis reflects either a flawed management plan, an underlying infection (abscess), an undiagnosed co-morbidity (such as cocaine use), or a psychosocial disturbance leading to lack of patient self-care. Ketoacidosis secondary to infection is potentially preventable by vigorous outpatient management of sick days. Patients must be taught never to omit insulin, to replace solid food with liquids during nausea, to maintain noncaffeinated fluid intake during illness, and to call for telephone assistance before becoming moribund. However, an incidence of 2.0 cases of ketoacidosis per 100 patient-years was reported in the Diabetes Control and Complications Trial. Subjects in that trial had extensive cost-free care by diabetes specialty care teams. Thus, ketoacidosis may not be a totally preventable disorder.

HYPERURICEMIA AND GOUT

method of
KAM SHOJANIA, M.D., and
JOHN P. WADE, M.D.
University of British Columbia
Vancouver, Canada

Gout is a disease in which monosodium urate crystals precipitate into tissue because of supersaturation of extracellular fluid. The peak incidence of gout occurs in the fifth decade of life. It predominantly occurs in men and is unusual in adolescents or in premenopausal women. The range of clinical manifestations of gout includes acute inflammatory arthritis (acute gout), chronic articular and periarticular inflammation, accumulation of crystalline aggregates in tissue (chronic tophaceous gout), uric acid urolithiasis, and rarely, renal impairment (gouty nephropathy). Although hyperuricemia is the common denominator for the various manifestations of gout, it is asymptomatic in most cases. Hyperuricemia is therefore not a disease state unless accompanied by clinical symptoms and signs of gout.

The lack of the enzyme uricase in humans makes uric acid the end product of the breakdown of purines. Uric acid is sparingly soluble in body fluids, and more than 90% of the uric acid is resorbed by the kidneys. Uric acid secretion usually is able to balance production and keep the uric acid concentration below the limit of solubility of monosodium urate in plasma. Genetic and environmental factors increasing the production or decreasing the excretion of uric acid may cause hyperuricemia. Problems associated with gout include alcohol use, obesity, diabetes mellitus, hypertension, and atherosclerosis. It is important to consider drugs like thiazide diuretics or low-dose salicylates as a contributory factor in the gouty attack.

Hyperuricemia can be conveniently classified into (1) uric acid overproduction and (2) uric acid undersecretion. About 10% of patients with hyperuricemia are overproducers of uric acid, such as with inherited enzyme deficiencies or myeloproliferative disorders. Underexcretion of uric acid is sometimes due to renal insufficiency or drugs but is often idiopathic.

Asymptomatic Hyperuricemia

The prevalence of asymptomatic hyperuricemia among adult men is 5 to 8%. Fewer than one in five people with hyperuricemia will ever present with clinical gout. There is no evidence to suggest that asymptomatic hyperuricemia should be treated unless the levels are above 12.8 mg per dL (760 μmol/liter) for men or 10.0 mg per dL (600 μmol/liter) for women. At these high levels, there is increased risk of renal complication such as nephrolithiasis.

CLINICAL MANIFESTATIONS

The classic three phases of clinical gout are acute gouty arthritis, intercritical gout, and chronic tophaceous gout.

Acute Gout

Acute gouty arthritis is an acute monoarticular or oligoarticular arthritis involving the joints of the lower limbs, with the first metatarsophalangeal (MTP) joint involved at some point in 75% of patients. Attacks frequently begin at night. Affected joints are usually red, swollen, and exquisitely tender. Early attacks usually subside spontaneously after 3 to 10 days, with some desquamation of the skin overlying the joint. Typically, untreated patients will have more frequent attacks that last longer. Acute gout is often precipitated by events such as surgery, myocardial infarction, trauma, alcohol use, or drugs such as diuretics. The differential diagnosis always includes septic arthritis or pseudogout; therefore, the diagnosis should always be confirmed by joint aspiration and examination of synovial fluid.

In acute gout, polarizing microscopy of the synovial fluid will demonstrate monosodium urate crystals (needle-shaped, intracellular, negatively birefringent crystals). The value of a serum uric acid level is limited because it can be normal at the time of an acute attack in up to 25% of patients. The serum uric acid level is useful in following response to long-term treatment. A 24-hour urine measurement of uric acid will help in determining whether the patient is a uric acid overproducer or an undersecretor.

Intercritical Gout

Intercritical gout describes the asymptomatic period between acute gouty attacks of arthritis. During this time, monosodium urate crystals can be aspirated from most previously involved joints and even some joints that have never been involved. Over 50% of patients who have had an episode of acute gout will have a recurrence within the year. The attacks will become more frequent, longer-lasting, and often polyarticular. Eventually, the patient will not have pain-free intercritical periods, and bony erosions may occur.

Chronic Tophaceous Gout

This is now less frequently seen with the use of hypouricemic agents. It is characterized by gouty tophi, which are the deposition of clinically evident subcutaneous monosodium urate crystals. The tophi occur an average of 10 years after the initial clinical symptoms of untreated gout. Typically, they are seen over the olecranon bursa, in subcutaneous tissues over the extensor surfaces of the forearms and the Achilles tendons, and on the helix of the ear. Monosodium urate crystals also deposit in periarticular and articular structures with the development of a destructive arthropathy and eventually degenerative changes in the joint. Tophi may be confused with rheumatoid nodules unless they are aspirated for diagnosis.

Renal Disease

Uric acid stones comprise about 5 to 10% of renal stones in North America. The risk of urolithiasis is three times more common in people with asymptomatic hyperuricemia and nine times more common in people with clinical gout. Calcium stones are also more common in people with gout, with uric acid forming a nidus for the calcium crystals. Urate nephropathy describes the deposition of uric acid in the renal tubules. This occurs with very high serum levels of uric acid, often associated with the treatment of hematologic malignancies, and is prevented by the administration of allopurinol.

TREATMENT OF GOUT

The goal of treatment of gout is to provide relief of acute attacks safely, to prevent further attack, to prevent the destructive arthropathy, and to prevent the formation of tophi and renal stones.

Treatment of the Acute Attack

Treatment of acute gout includes nonsteroidal anti-inflammatory drugs (NSAIDs), corticosteroids, and colchicine. Remember that the acute attack of gout is painful, but it is a self-limiting and not life-threatening disease. If left untreated, the acute attack usually resolves in 7 to 10 days. Treatment such as rest, ice, and analgesics is acceptable for an acute attack of gout, particularly if significant contraindications to other therapies exist.

NSAIDs

Usually, NSAIDs are started at the first sign of a gouty attack and are given at high dose initially and continued at a lower dose until the attack has resolved. There is no good comparison of the effectiveness or toxicity of the various NSAIDs, but many physicians use indomethacin (Indocin), for acute gouty arthritis at a dose of 50 mg three to four times daily for several days until there has been improvement, then continued at a lower dose for 10 to 14 days. Significant side effects of NSAIDs include gastritis and peptic ulcer disease, renal dysfunction, sodium retention, headache, and confusion. Caution should be used in particular with elderly people or in patients who have acute gout precipitated by events such as surgery or myocardial infarction. A few commonly used NSAIDs and the doses used for gout are in Table 1. It is also important to remember that low-dose salicylates suppress tubular secretion of uric acid and can increase hyperuricemia whereas high-dose salicylates also suppress reabsorption and can result in hyperuricosuria.

TABLE 1. **Nonsteroidal Anti-Inflammatory Drugs (NSAIDs) Useful in Acute Gout**

Drug	Dose
Indomethacin (Indocin)	50 mg tid–qid
Naproxen (Naprosyn)	500 mg bid–tid
Ketoprofen (Orudis)	50–75 mg tid
Diclofenac (Voltaren)	50–75 mg tid
Tolmetin (Tolectin)	400–600 mg tid

Colchicine

Colchicine is effective in the treatment of acute gout, but it may cause gastrointestinal toxicity, including nausea, vomiting, and diarrhea in up to 80% of patients at higher doses. The intravenous route avoids the gastrointestinal toxicity, but the higher blood levels increase the possibility of bone marrow toxicity, and we do not recommend its use if other options are available. The dose of colchicine is 0.6 mg four times daily for 2 to 3 days, then continue at a twice-daily schedule for 1 to 2 weeks. Some investigators recommend oral colchicine at doses of 0.6 mg every 1 to 2 hours until symptoms improve or gastrointestinal symptoms occur. The maximal dose of 6 mg (10 tablets) over 24 hours should not be exceeded, and no further colchicine should be given over the next 7 days. If used, intravenous colchicine may be given at an initial dose of 1 to 2 mg intravenously followed by 1 mg at 6 and 12 hours intravenously. The maximal dose should be 4 mg over 24 hours, and no further colchicine should be given over the next 7 days. If there is any renal or hepatic dysfunction, a maximum of 2 mg intravenously should be given over 24 hours. Colchicine can cause local phlebitis and skin sloughing if given intravenously. By any route, colchicine can cause bone marrow suppression, renal failure, disseminated intravascular coagulation, hypocalcemia, seizures, and death. Chronic use of colchicine can cause a neuromuscular syndrome resembling polymyositis.

Corticosteroids

Corticosteroids are effective in the treatment of gout and can be given orally, intra-articularly or parenterally. A typical oral dose is 20 to 40 mg of prednisone over the first 2 to 4 days, tapered over 2 weeks. Individual response to steroids is highly variable. Intra-articular steroids are useful when only one or two joints are involved. Intravenous steroids such as methylprednisolone can be used in equivalent doses or one dose of intramuscular adrenocorticotropic hormone (ACTH, corticotropin [Acthar]) at a dose of 40 to 80 IU. There is no advantage in using ACTH over corticosteroids over the short term.

Special Considerations in the Critically Ill Patient

Acute gout may be precipitated by major illness. Unfortunately, these patients often are unable to take oral medications, have compromised renal and hepatic function, and are on multiple medications. NSAIDs and colchicine are often contraindicated in these patients. Probably the best alternative is to use intra-articular corticosteroids. If multiple joints are involved, one may use a single dose of intramuscular methylprednisolone, 40 mg, or oral prednisone at 20 to 40 mg daily for 2 days tapered over 2 weeks. If there are significant contraindications to the use of any of these medications, it is reasonable to treat with analgesics and to wait for the natural resolution of the acute gouty attack in 7 to 10 days. There is no place for uric acid–lowering therapy in the critically ill patient. This treatment should be delayed until the patient is stable.

Prophylactic Treatment of Intercritical and Chronic Tophaceous Gout

General Considerations

After the acute attack has resolved, the decision to treat the intercritical periods prophylactically must be made. It is agreed that patients with recurrent attacks of gout, chronic tophaceous gout, or renal disease should be treated prophylactically, but there is debate whether one should treat someone prophylactically who has had only one or two acute attacks.

Prophylactic treatment should always include weight and blood pressure control, a low-purine diet, and education about the disease, its complications, and avoidance of precipitating factors. Patients also should be instructed to avoid thiazide diuretics and low-dose salicylates. The choice of a hypouricemic agent is either a uricosuric drug or a xanthine oxidase inhibitor. A 24-hour urine uric acid should be obtained to help guide the selection of the most appropriate urate-lowering treatment. The 10% of patients who are uric acid overproducers and thus have increased urinary uric acid should not be on a uricosuric agent. Other patients who should not be given a uricosuric agent include those with a history of nephrolithiasis or poor renal function and those over 60 years of age. Before starting any uric acid–lowering treatment, the criteria listed in Table 2 should be met.

When using either agent, it is useful to follow the serum uric acid level at about 3 to 6 months after starting the medication and after dose changes to determine the optimal dose of the hypouricemic

TABLE 2. **Criteria Before Starting Hypouricemic Therapy**

1. Signs of acute inflammation should be absent
2. The patient should be aware of precipitating factors
3. Prophylactic colchicine may be started at 0.6 mg one to two times daily and continued for 3–6 months or until tophi are gone (may use low-dose NSAIDs instead)
4. If one elects not to use prophylactic treatment, the patient should be warned that an acute attack may be precipitated by initiation of hypouricemic therapy
5. The patient should be provided with an anti-inflammatory drug and instructions regarding what to do in the event of an acute attack

agent and to verify compliance. The goal should be to decrease the serum uric acid to well into the normal range.

Uricosuric Agents

The uricosuric most often used is probenicid (Benemid), which is started at a dose of 0.5 mg daily and increased to a maximum of 1 gram two to three times daily or until the target serum uric acid is reached. Sulfinpyrazone (Anturane) is the alternative and can be started at 50 mg twice daily and increased to a maximum of 200 mg two or three times daily. Common side effects of each are rash or gastrointestinal toxicity. An important side effect of uricosuric agents is urate nephrolithiasis that may occur despite encouraging the patient to drink fluids. It is important to remember that these agents also interfere with the excretion of other medications.

Allopurinol

Allopurinol (Zyloprim), a xanthine oxidase inhibitor, is clinically indicated for uric acid overproducers and patients with nephrolithiasis or other contraindications to uricosuric therapy. It is also used frequently in preference to uricosuric agents because of the ease of administration. It should be used if there is renal insufficiency, but at a reduced dose. Typically, the initial dose is 300 mg per day and can be increased up to 800 mg per day, but in elderly people or in patients with decreased renal function, one should use a starting dose of 100 mg per day. Common side effects are headache, dyspepsia, and diarrhea. A pruritic rash may develop in about 5% of patients, and in a small percentage of these patients, a syndrome of allopurinol hypersensitivity may occur with fever, acute renal failure, and toxic epidermal necrolysis. There are significant drug interactions, in particular with purine analogues such as azathioprine (Imuran) and oral anticoagulants, and there is increased toxicity from cytotoxic drugs.

The optimal duration of uric acid–lowering therapy is not clear. It is possible that after years of treatment and normouricemia, the total body urate stores are low, and it would be reasonable to discontinue therapy for periods of time.

Other Considerations

The Patient with Renal Insufficiency

Serum uric acid is often elevated in these patients, but clinical gout is unusual and occurs in less than 1% of uremic patients. If there is no evidence of clinical gout, the hyperuricemia should not be treated. Caution should be used in the treatment of acute gout in these patients because all NSAIDs can decrease renal function. Colchicine and allopurinol doses should be reduced, and the uricosuric agents should not be used. Often, corticosteroids or low-dose colchicine for the acute attack, followed by a reduced dose of allopurinol, is the best treatment.

The Patient with Malignancy

The very high serum uric acid of some patients with malignancy puts them at risk of developing acute gouty nephropathy. This is a particular risk when the patient is treated with chemotherapy or radiotherapy. Prophylactic allopurinol should be started before chemotherapy if possible. Remember that allopurinol may potentiate the toxic effects of cyclophosphamide.

The Transplant Patient

These patients are often on multiple medications, including azathioprine (Imuran). They also may have impaired renal function that may prohibit the use of uricosuric agents, and dose adjustments of colchicine and allopurinol should be made. Allopurinol increases the half-life of azathioprine and potentiates the therapeutic and toxic effects. Remember that these patients are immunocompromised and are particularly susceptible to septic arthritis.

Coexisting Infection and Gout

Patients with underlying joint disease such as gout are at greater risk of septic arthritis, which should be considered in any patient with an acute arthritis. The synovial fluid of all patients with an acute arthritis should be evaluated with Gram's stain, cultures, and polarized microscopy. This includes patients with known gout who are having an acute attack. It is possible that septic arthritis may mimic an acute gouty arthritis in a joint that has pre-existing gout.

HYPERLIPOPROTEINEMIA

method of
NEIL J. STONE, M.D.
Northwestern University School of Medicine
Chicago, Illinois

Convincing evidence now exists to show that aggressive lipid and lipoprotein treatment can retard progression of atherosclerotic plaques on serial angiograms and result in improved survival and fewer cardiovascular events. Extrapolation of clinical trial data suggests that the decrease in myocardial infarction, angioplasty, and coronary bypass surgery realized with such therapy makes it cost effective.

The interaction of risk factors with vessel wall or endothelium plays a key role in the atherosclerotic process. Many investigators feel that the key event in atherosclerotic progression to coronary accidents is the rupture of the cholesterol-rich fibrous plaque. Stabilization of the plaque through lipid lowering is the putative answer to explain the remarkable decrease in subsequent coronary events in several clinical trials despite the finding of only minor changes on angiography. This improvement does not appear to be the result of a specific intervention but has been seen with diet; drugs such as cholestyramine and colestipol, niacin, lovastatin, pravastatin, and simvastatin; and partial ileal bypass surgery.

A high cholesterol level can cause vasoconstriction—a

reversal in the usual vasodilatation that occurs with acetylcholine infusion. Moreover, cholesterol-lowering therapies can reverse such early changes in vessel wall reactivity.

Cholesterol and triglycerides are blood lipids. Cholesterol is vital for animal life because of its key role in cell membranes, adrenal hormone and sex hormones, and the various forms of vitamin D. It is not found in vegetable products. Triglycerides are sources of storage fat. Fatty acid chains are attached to the glycerol backbone of triglycerides. Saturated fatty acids have no double bonds in these chains and generally raise blood cholesterol (stearic acid is an exception). Cholesterol levels are generally lowered when saturated fatty acids are replaced in the diet with monounsaturated fats (e.g., olive oil and canola oil) or polyunsaturated fats (e.g., corn oil, safflower oil, sunflower oil). Consumers are cautioned to avoid excessive amounts of polyunsaturated oils, as they increase the risk of cholelithiasis, lower high-density lipoprotein cholesterol (HDL-c), and appear to make low-density lipoprotein cholesterol (LDL-c) more oxidizable. There are unnatural forms of monounsaturated fats called "trans" fatty acids, which appear to raise LDL-c and lower HDL-c when ingested in large amounts. This is usually not a problem for those on a fat-controlled diet.

Cholesterol and triglycerides, however, are insoluble and exist in the inner core of large macromolecular complexes called "lipoproteins." Successful treatment is often based on hyperlipidemia being envisioned as lipoprotein excess or deficiency. There are four major lipoprotein classes. Chylomicrons and very-low-density lipoproteins (VLDL) are triglyceride-rich lipoproteins. The former carry dietary lipid and the latter are produced in the liver. Insulin deficiency can impair chylomicron removal and cause triglyceride levels that exceed 1000 mg per dL. Obese patients with insulin resistance often have accompanying hypertension and hypertriglyceridemia. Here elevated triglyceride levels are most often due to an excess of VLDL production. Triglyceride-rich remnant lipoproteins can accumulate and aggravate atherosclerotic risk.

Low-density lipoproteins (LDLs) and high-density lipoproteins (HDLs) carry most of the plasma cholesterol. LDLs either are produced from the intravascular conversion of VLDL or are secreted from the liver. HDLs are secreted as cholesterol-poor precursors from the liver and intestines. Protein subunits or apolipoproteins (apo) are present on all the lipoproteins and play an essential role in guiding the lipoproteins to their metabolic fates or serving as cofactors for important metabolic steps. Lp(a) has some sequences similar to those seen in plasminogen but is devoid of fibrinolytic activity. Its localization in atherosclerotic plaques suggests an important role that is still not clearly defined.

The LDLs are small, cholesterol-rich particles that depend on cell surface receptors called "LDL receptors" for clearance. The function of these receptors is to maintain an adequate supply of cholesterol for the cell. A molecule of apo B is present on each LDL (and VLDL). The liver, which is the major site for LDL removal, has LDL receptors that recognize at least two kinds of these surface components of LDLs, called "apo B 100" and "apo E." Raised levels of LDL cholesterol (LDL-c) are caused either by too few receptors (genetic or diet-induced) or by abnormal apo B (genetic). When functioning LDL receptors are reduced, there is a rise in LDL-c and a proportionate increase in risk of coronary artery disease (CAD). Efforts at reducing LDL-c focus on inhibiting the enzyme controlling the rate-limiting step of cholesterol synthesis (3-hydroxy-

3-methylglutaryl-coenzyme A [HMG-CoA] reductase) or depleting the cell of cholesterol by interrupting bile acid reabsorption in the intestine.

Dietary cholesterol packaged in remnants of chylomicron metabolism interacts with the LDL receptor and affects blood cholesterol levels. Humans show great variability to dietary cholesterol loads. LDL that has been modified by oxidation appears to be particularly atherogenic. Individuals with inherited high levels of small, dense LDLs (determined by a research technique) are at high risk for premature CAD. This can be suspected clinically by those with a family history of premature CAD and features of insulin resistance (abdominal obesity, high triglycerides, glucose intolerance, and low HDL-c).

HDL is an even smaller lipoprotein than LDL. The function of this protein-rich class of lipoproteins is to remove cholesterol from tissues and transport it to the liver. It also provides cholesterol to lipoproteins and acts as a reservoir for apoproteins needed in metabolism of triglyceride-rich lipoproteins. Commonly, when triglyceride levels are high owing to impaired catabolism, HDL-c levels are low. Reduced levels of HDL-c contribute greatly to the development of CAD. Families with inherited raised levels of HDL-c appear to have low rates for CAD. Looking at HDL-c levels in isolation, however, can be confusing, since a high-fat, atherogenic diet raises HDL-c levels, and a low-fat, vegetarian diet lowers HDL-c levels. In the former case, however, LDL-c levels are high, whereas in the latter example, they are invariably low (along with levels of blood pressure and usually low cardiac risk).

For men and women, ratios of total cholesterol/HDL-c levels above 6 : 4 and 5 : 6, respectively, identify groups at increased risk for CAD. Ratios can mislead if you do not consider the entire risk factor profile (including age, other risk factors, and CAD status) in your evaluation of the patient.

DETECTION AND ASSESSMENT OF HYPERCHOLESTEROLEMIA

The National Cholesterol Education Program (NCEP) has provided guidelines for screening that follow these basic principles:

1. The intensity of evaluation and treatment depends on the patient's risk status.
2. Those shown to be at high risk for developing coronary heart disease (CHD) events in the near term are evaluated for more intensive intervention than those patients at lower risk for near-term events of CHD.

Table 1 shows the three general categories of risk for CHD. For the highest risk group, the Simvastatin Scandinavian Survival Study demonstrated that cholesterol low-

TABLE 1. **Risk Categories for Coronary Heart Disease Events**

Very high risk	Those with CHD or other atherosclerotic vascular disease
High risk	No overt CHD, but with two or more risk factors (diabetes counts as two risk factors)
Low risk	Those with less than two risk factors

From Second Report of the Expert Panel on Detection, Evaluation, and Treatment of High Blood Cholesterol in Adults (Adult Treatment Panel II). Washington, DC, National Institutes of Health, National Heart, Lung, and Blood Institute, NIH Publication 93-3095, September 1993.

TABLE 2. **Risk Factors for Coronary Heart Disease (Other Than LDL-Cholesterol)**

Positive Risk Factors

Age:
  Male: ≥45 years
  Female: ≥55 years or premature menopause without estrogen replacement therapy

Family history of premature CHD:
  Definitive myocardial infarction or sudden death before age 55 years in father or other male first-degree relative;
  OR
  before 65 years of age in mother or other female first-degree relative

Current cigarette smoking

Hypertension (≥140/90 or on antihypertensive medications)

Low HDL-c levels (<35 mg/dL)

Diabetes mellitus

Negative Risk Factor

High HDL-c level (>60 mg/dL)

ering in those with CHD will significantly reduce total mortality as well as new events of CHD. This approach is known as "secondary prevention." Clinical judgment is required for those with multiple risk factors (Table 2) who do not have established CHD and yet may be at high risk for cardiac events. Since we do not know whether aggressive cholesterol lowering with drug therapy will reduce total mortality in those without CHD and multiple risk factors, a more conservative approach is favored, with the major emphasis on diet and physical activity.

Primary Prevention

In the Multiple Risk Factor Intervention Study, observation of 350,000 persons showed that with increasing cholesterol levels, the risk of CHD rose in exponential fashion, with strikingly higher rates at levels above 240 mg per dL. There was no clear threshold above which risk commenced. A total cholesterol level, however, is not a good discriminator between those patients who are likely to have CAD and those who are not. Studies of hospitalized patients with angiographic CAD show that roughly one-third have a cholesterol level of under 200. In these patients, almost three-fourths will have an HDL-c level of less than 35 mg per dL. A low HDL-c level and a family history of premature CHD are important clues that CAD may be found despite a total cholesterol level of less than 200 mg per dL.

For primary prevention, the best screening tests are a total cholesterol level and an accurate measurement of HDL-c. The patient does not need to be fasting. Patients with a total cholesterol level of under 200 mg per dL and an HDL-c level of above 35 mg per dL should have repeat total cholesterol and HDL-c studies within 5 years or with a physical examination. These low-risk individuals need only information on healthy eating patterns, advice on pursuing an active lifestyle, and correction of any abnormal risk factors.

Those with a borderline cholesterol level of between 200 and 240 mg per dL and an HDL level of 35 or more mg per dL, as well as fewer than two risk factors, should be given the preceding advice and be retested in 1 to 2 years. This leaves for more careful scrutiny those patients with a total cholesterol level of above 240 mg per dL, two or more risk factors, or an HDL-c level of less than 35 mg per dL

(Table 3). For further evaluation, a 12- to 14-hour fasting lipoprotein analysis is required. Total cholesterol, triglyceride, and HDL-c studies are ordered. The following formula is used to calculate LDL-c:

$$LDL\text{-}c = Total\ cholesterol - (HDL\text{-}c) - (triglyceride/5)$$

(This assumes a fasting specimen with a triglyceride level of less than 400 mg per dL and absence of the rare Type 3 or familial dysbetalipoproteinemia disorder.)

The LDL-c level, if elevated, should be repeated within 1 to 6 weeks to provide a more reliable baseline measurement. If values differ by more than 30 mg per dL, then a third determination is ordered.

LDL-c levels are classified as desirable (below 130 mg per dL), borderline high-risk (130 to 159 mg per dL), and high-risk (160 mg per dL or greater). If the LDL-c level is under 130 mg per dL and the HDL level is over 35 mg per dL, patients can be given the aforementioned general advice (including treatment of risk factors) and can be retested within 5 years. For those with borderline LDL-c and with fewer than two risk factors, the same advice and repeat lipoprotein analysis in 1 year are appropriate. For example, normal LDL-c and low HDL-c levels are seen in those who have adopted a vegetarian lifestyle and are otherwise at low risk for CHD. Other factors associated with a low HDL-c level that should be corrected, if possible, include cigarette smoking, sedentary lifestyle, weight excess, or hypertriglyceridemia.

A borderline LDL-c level with two or more risk factors or a high-risk LDL-c level warrants a complete evaluation that considers secondary causes (Table 4), familial disorders (Table 5), and the influence of age, sex, and other CHD risk factors. Once this is done, a goal LDL-c level can be set and nonpharmacologic therapy begun, with emphasis on reducing excess weight, adopting an active lifestyle, and eating a low-saturated-fat, low-cholesterol diet (Table 6). Note that the total cholesterol level can serve as a surrogate for LDL-c in monitoring. Drug therapy is deferred for at least 6 months until the results of this can be adequately assessed. In those with severe familial elevations of LDL-c resistant to diet (LDL-c > 220 mg per dL), a shorter interval before drug therapy is utilized is reasonable.

Secondary Prevention

For those with established atherosclerotic disease, an LDL-c goal of 100 mg per dL or less is optimum. Many patients with CHD also will have a low HDL-c level and multiple risk factors (see Table 2). A consideration of secondary causes should be carried out as discussed earlier. For patients suffering an acute myocardial infarction, lipids checked within the first 24 hours can indicate pre-event dyslipidemia, but after 24 hours the decline in cholesterol

TABLE 3. **Evaluation of Hypercholesterolemia: Primary Prevention**

	Total Cholesterol	HDL-c	Risk Factors	What to Do Next
If	<240	≥35	<2 risk factors	Diet, exercise, repeat within 5 yr
If	>240			Lipoprotein analysis
If		<35		Lipoprotein analysis
If			≥2 risk factors	Lipoprotein analysis

TABLE 4. **Secondary Causes of Abnormal Lipid Profiles**

Most Common Causes	
High cholesterol	*Diet*
	Rich in total fat, saturated fat, and cholesterol
	Diseases/Conditions
	Nephrotic syndrome
	Hypothyroidism (particularly subclinical hypothyroidism in which T_4 is low-normal and TSH is elevated)
	Obstructive liver disease, e.g., primary biliary cirrhosis
	Drugs
	Anabolic steroids, diuretics, progestins, cyclosporine, amiodarone
High triglycerides	*Diet*
	Rich in extra calories, sugar, and alcohol
	Diseases/Conditions
	Obesity
	Type II diabetes
	Chronic renal failure
	Pregnancy (3rd trimester)
	Drugs
	Estrogen, cholestyramine (both also elevate HDL-c levels)
	Beta blockers, diuretics, retinoic acid
Low HDL-c	*Diet*
	Low-fat diet
	Diseases/Conditions
	Obesity
	Sedentary lifestyle
	Cigarette smoking
	Hypertriglyceridemia
	Drugs
	Beta blockers (beware of ophthalmic beta blockers)

levels and the rise in triglyceride levels obscure the patient's prior lipid status. Often it is easiest to initiate family screening for dyslipidemia while the patient is recovering from the acute myocardial infarction. Parents, siblings, and children need a fasting lipoprotein analysis to see whether an inherited lipid disorder is present and who might be possible candidates for intervention.

Some lipid experts advocate measurement of apolipoproteins such as apo B, apo A1, and Lp(a), when they can

TABLE 5. **Familial Disorders**

Familial Disorder	Clinical Features
Familial hypercholesterolemia	Tendon xanthomas; cholesterol values 325–500 mg/dL untreated
Familial combined hyperlipidemia	No xanthomas; often with associated high triglycerides; elevated apo B; increased diabetes, BP
Primary moderate hypercholesterolemia	No xanthomas; cholesterol 240–300 mg/dL
Familial dysbetalipoproteinemia	High triglycerides and high cholesterol the rule; tuboeruptive xanthomas; associated hypothyroidism seen
Familial hypertriglyceridemia	No xanthomas; no increase in diabetes seen; no increase in CHD risk

TABLE 6. **Level Goals for Primary Prevention**

Status	Initiation Level for Dietary Treatment (LDL-c) (mg/dL)	Goal of Therapy (LDL-c) (mg/dL)	Monitoring Goal (Total Cholesterol) (mg/dL)
Without CHD and < two risk factors	≥160	<160	<240
Without CHD and ≥ two risk factors	≥130	<130	<200

be done accurately. They may be useful in those with a personal or family history of premature coronary disease who would not normally be candidates for drug therapy under the current NCEP guidelines. Available evidence is insufficient to recommend these tests routinely.

HYPERTRIGLYCERIDEMIA

Elevated triglyceride levels may be important for several reasons. They may indicate increased levels of atherogenic "remnant" lipoproteins; they may signal an inherited atherogenic trait in which small, dense LDL levels with less cholesterol are found; they may be associated with coagulation abnormalities; or they may indicate such a substantial circulating lipid load, e.g., over 1000 mg per dL, that the patient is at risk for acute pancreatitis. Single values are not reliable, as triglycerides vary greatly depending on factors such as stress, dietary carbohydrate or alcohol ingestion, and activity. Thus, repeat values under stable conditions are preferred, unless the levels are above 1000 mg per dL, which should prompt immediate attention. Values of 200 to 400 mg per dL are considered borderline, and values of 400 to 1000 mg per dL are considered high.

Secondary causes of high triglyceride levels are numerous and must be considered carefully (see Table 4). Changes in lifestyle have an appreciable impact on triglycerides—adoption of regular exercise and weight control can result in dramatic improvement. Alcohol excess, estrogen use, and cholestyramine or colestipol therapy also elevate triglycerides but raise HDL-c levels, whereas weight gain, a sedentary lifestyle, and many medications lower HDL-c levels. Restriction of alcohol intake, at least on a trial basis, is often useful if excess use is suspected. Triglyceride values of over 1000 mg per dL, precipitating acute pancreatitis, have been seen in patients with an underlying lipid disorder who have had as triggers an alcoholic and dietary fat binge, the third trimester of pregnancy, or estrogen or steroid therapy.

NONPHARMACOLOGIC TREATMENT

Effect of Diet on CHD

The link between diet and CHD is inferred from a wealth of experimental, epidemiologic, and clinical investigations. In primary prevention, the Oslo Diet and Smoking study was a large, randomized trial of smoking cessation and a low total (27.9%) and saturated fat (8.9%) diet in men with hypercholesterolemia. Although not a "pure" diet trial, total mortality was improved in long-term follow-up of the intervention group. A secondary prevention trial of hypercholesterolemic British men showed that a low total fat (27%) and saturated fat (8 to 10%) diet was associated with a 16% reduction in LDL levels and insignificant changes in HDL-c levels. There was no change in the mean absolute width of the coronary arteries, but there was improvement in clinical event rates. There was a strong in-study relationship with small, dense LDL levels.

This improvement in clinical event rates was also seen in two trials of exercise and very-low-fat diets that restricted fat to either 20% or less than 10% of energy. The loss of angina early in such trials suggested a mechanism other than atherosclerosis regression. The demonstration in men that the lowering of cholesterol levels by diet or drug therapy, or both, can reverse endothelial dysfunction suggests a plausible answer to why lipid lowering improves symptoms so early and underscores the importance of the lipid-lowering diet.

Diet and Management of Hyperlipidemia

Cholesterol-lowering diets are primary therapeutic interventions for those at risk of CHD. Clinical studies in high-risk subjects have shown reductions of 4 to 17% in total cholesterol levels. No loss of effectiveness was seen in those trials in which dietary counseling was maintained. An associated loss of weight suggests that the patient actually had a lower fat intake, which is associated with increased efficacy. Since the HDL-c level often falls upon a switch to a low-fat diet, the addition of regular aerobic exercise to a prudent weight-reducing diet often lowers the triglyceride level and increases HDL-c levels in men and prevents a reduction in HDL-c levels in women.

The Step One diet is the primary prevention diet. It is recommended for the entire population. It is reduced in total fat, saturated fat, and dietary cholesterol. The Step Two diet requires individual counseling and frequent feedback for optimal effectiveness. It is particularly restricted in saturated fat and dietary cholesterol (Table 7). For those with hypertriglyceridemia, low HDL-c, or both, weight reduction and regular aerobic exercise are crucial for effective therapy.

Meat fat, dairy fat, commercial baked goods, egg fat, and fat used in the preparation and processing of foods represent the major suppliers of saturated fat and dietary cholesterol in the diet. To change

dietary habits, patients need more than a positive attitude; they require knowledge and skill to succeed. It is useful to ask whether they can read food labels, can order a low-fat meal when dining out, or know how to alter favorite recipes when cooking at home. Table 8 can be photocopied and patients can fill in the answers in the waiting room. Those who require an upgrade in knowledge or skill levels should be referred to a dietitian.

If triglycerides are high, alcohol may need to be restricted. Epidemiologic data suggest that low amounts (one to two drinks in men, less in women) are associated with a reduction in CHD, compared with teetotalers. At least part of the benefit is related to an increase in HDL-c levels, with an effect on fibrinolytic activity as well. The negative aspects of alcohol, however, increase dramatically with consumption. Three or more drinks per day exacerbate hypertension and increase the risk of stroke, cerebrovascular accidents, liver disease, and for those who start drinking habitually, alcoholism. The public health message is clear: we have no basis for recommending that patients start to drink or increase their current intake of alcohol to raise their HDL level or lower their CHD risk.

How long should a trial of diet and exercise last? Generally an effect is seen in 6 to 8 weeks in the well-motivated patient. Although there are no definite rules, 6 months is a minimal time to allow for dietary adherence for primary prevention. As a general rule, those who respond with lower triglycerides and undergo some weight loss are usually adhering well to the diet. Those at highest risk, e.g., those with LDL-c levels of over 220 mg per dL or with existing atherosclerotic vascular disease, may need concomitant drug therapy started sooner.

DRUG THERAPY

As a general rule, consider drug therapy by weighing the severity of the LDL-c level abnormality and the patient's risk of CHD. The major drugs used are the resins (cholestyramine [Questran] and colestipol [Colestid], niacin (nicotinic acid), and the statins (fluvastatin [Lescol], lovastatin [Mevacor], pravastatin [Pravachol], simvastatin [Zocor]). Each has particular advantages, depending on the age of the patient and the severity and nature of the lipid abnormality.

Resins. The bile acid–sequestering resins are cholestyramine and colestipol. They bind bile acids in the gut, prevent their enterohepatic circulation, and promote their fecal excretion. The depletion of the bile acid pool redirects cholesterol to bile acid production, stimulating an increase in LDL receptors with resultant LDL-c level lowering. The usual starting dose is 4 grams of cholestyramine or 5 grams of colestipol powder, which is gradually increased. Because of their safety, they are often the drugs of first choice for premenopausal women and young adult men who require therapy owing to an adverse risk factor profile.

TABLE 7. **Main Features of the Step One and Step Two Diets**

Constituents of Diet	Step One Diet	Step Two Diet (As % of Calories)
Total fat	30% or less	
Saturated fatty acids	8–10%	Less than 7%
Polyunsaturated fat	Up to 10%	
Monounsaturated fats	Up to 15%	
Dietary cholesterol	<300 mg/day	<200 mg/day
Total calories	To achieve and maintain desirable weight	

TABLE 8. **Diet Modifications to Achieve a Low-Fat Diet (Medics)**

Category	Ask Regarding	Skills to Learn
Meal frequency	How many meals per day?	Eat regular, balanced meals
Meat ingestion	Beef, pork, lamb, or veal? Portion size? Liver or organ meats? Fowl or fish meals? Hot dogs or sausages?	Learn to order leaner cuts of meats Restrict portions to 4 oz or less Avoid organ meats Use skinless poultry; avoid frying fish Use more sparingly
Egg yolks	How many per week? (Four for Step 1, two for Step 2)	Use egg whites for omelettes and recipes Consider egg substitutes
Dairy products	Whole milk products? Cheeses? Ice cream? Cream cheese?	Use skim milk or 1% milk Use low-fat cheeses like mozzarella Use no- or low-fat yogurt Use no-fat cream cheese
Invisible fats in baked goods	Doughnuts, coffee cakes, pies, muffins, cakes, cookies?	Read labels and use no-fat items; watch muffins, which can be high fat. Learn to bake with low-fat recipes
Snacks	Ice cream, cake, candy bars, cookies, snack chips?	Consider pretzels if salt is not an issue. Use more fruits and vegetables as snacks
Spirits	How many drinks of alcohol per week? (A drink is 1 oz of liquor, one glass of wine, one can of beer)	Limit alcohol to 1–2 drinks per day Restrict if triglycerides are high

EFFICACY. In those with diet-resistant familial hypercholesterolemia (FH), 4 scoops of resin lower the total cholesterol level 20% and the LDL-c level 27%. The HDL-c level is also raised slightly. For those with milder forms of hypercholesterolemia, lower doses (2 scoops per day) can lower LDL-c levels about 10 to 20%. With time, there can be a waning of lipid-lowering effects. Efficacy against CHD was shown in the Lipid Research Centers Primary Prevention trial, where for every 1% of cholesterol lowering there was a 2% decline in CHD events.

TOXICITY. These are safe drugs because they are not absorbed. Gastrointestinal side effects such as constipation, aggravation of hemorrhoids, bloating, distention, and cramping are frequently seen and are more likely with higher dose levels. Before starting resins, it is helpful to increase fiber in the diet or add a psyllium powder (which by itself can lower cholesterol modestly). For those who do not tolerate full dosages, 1 to 2 scoops of resin daily may still give reasonable cholesterol lowering. Do not give these drugs to patients with triglyceride levels above 250 mg per dL, as these agents increase triglyceride levels.

TOLERABILITY. The resins are gritty powders supplied in cans (cheapest form), packets, and most recently in tablets. They need to be mixed with liquids, like fruit juice, skim milk, or water, or with applesauce or yogurt. Resins interfere with the absorption of other medications such as digoxin, antibiotics, thiazides, warfarin, and thyroxine. They should be taken 1 hour after other medications or at least 3 to 4 hours before other medications. Taking resins 1 hour after breakfast when other medications are taken can be inconvenient, so some physicians prescribe digoxin and other drugs at noon and give resins alone in the morning and 1 hour after supper (if other medications are taken with supper).

Niacin. This is vitamin B_3, or nicotinic acid. Avoid niacinamide (nicotinamide); it is another form of the vitamin that is not effective in lowering lipids. Niacin inhibits fatty acid release from adipose tissue and decreases secretion of VLDLs from the liver. It causes a decrease in the fractional catabolic rate of HDLs, leading to higher serum levels of HDL-c. It is available in both immediate-release and sustained-release forms. The latter form causes more hepatotoxicity and should not be used routinely. The initial dosage is 100 or 250 mg with a gradual increase to 1.5 grams or 3.0 grams per day. It should be taken in divided dosage with meals. Rarely, patients require higher dosages for greater LDL-c lowering, which are associated with a greater incidence of side effects.

EFFICACY. Niacin lowers total cholesterol, LDL-c, and triglyceride levels in a dose-dependent fashion. It is the most useful drug for raising the HDL-c level, which may increase by as much as 30%. In the Coronary Drug Project, men who had had infarctions were given 3 grams daily of niacin and had significantly reduced nonfatal rates of myocardial infarction at 5 years and 11% lower total mortality at 14 years, compared with the placebo group.

TOXICITY. Niacin can cause abnormal liver tests, aggravate peptic acid disease, increase glucose values and markedly worsen control in diabetics, and precipitate gout in hyperuricemic patients. Dry skin or acanthosis nigricans is occasionally seen. These effects are usually reversible with cessation of the drug. Hepatotoxicity has been reported when patients were switched from immediate-release to timed-release niacin and the dosage was not reduced. Patients should not change brands of niacin, as some appear to be better tolerated than others.

TOLERABILITY. About one-third of patients cannot tolerate niacin, most often because of the dramatic vasodilatory effect of facial and truncal flushing and itching. Tachyphylaxis eventually develops in response to this in most patients. Since the vasodilatation is prostaglandin mediated, a useful trick is to take a 5-grain aspirin tablet about 1 hour before the day's first dose of niacin. Patients should take niacin with food, but they should avoid very hot foods or alcohol, as these accentuate flushing.

Statins. These are competitive inhibitors of HMG-CoA reductase, the enzyme catalyzing the rate-limiting step in cholesterol synthesis. Lovastatin was the first agent on the market and has been followed by pravastatin, simvastatin, and fluvastatin. These drugs cause marked reductions in LDL-c; they also raise HDL-c and mildly lower triglyceride levels.

EFFICACY. All these drugs show a log dose-response curve. This means that the biggest drop in the LDL-c level comes from the first 10 to 20 mg. Higher dosages give progressively smaller increments of LDL-c level lowering. Simvastatin is roughly twice as potent as lovastatin and pravastatin for LDL-c level lowering. Fluvastatin does not seem quite as potent as lovastatin and pravastatin. Available data from long-term clinical trials show that 40 mg of lovastatin or pravastatin or 20 mg of simvastatin lowers the LDL-c level about 30%, and 80 mg of lovastatin or 40 mg of simvastatin lowers the LDL-c level about 35%. (LDL-c level lowering is less dramatic than in the shorter trials that are often quoted, but these figures probably more closely represent clinical practice.) HDL-c levels are raised about 8 to 10%. Fluvastatin data from long-term double-blind clinical trials are not yet available. A 20-mg dose of this water-soluble synthetic drug lowers LDL-c levels about 22% on average.

Several double-blind randomized angiographic trials have shown that statin monotherapy causes a reduction in angiographic progression and, most importantly, a striking reduction in clinical event rates. The Simvastatin Scandinavian Survival Study showed that 40 mg of simvastatin monotherapy lowered the LDL-c level 35% on average and was associated with a 30% reduction in total mortality as well as improvements in cardiovascular end points, including stroke. The improvement in cardiovascular end points pertained to women as well as men.

TOXICITY. The incidence of hepatic side effects is dose dependent. In one large study of lovastatin, the incidence was 0.1% for 20 mg; 0.9% for 40 mg; and 1.5% for 80 mg. An increased likelihood of hepatotoxicity can occur when statins are combined with other drugs like niacin or there is excess alcohol usage. Myositis is a rare occurrence with monotherapy. It is more likely to occur if gemfibrozil, cyclosporine, or niacin is added to the statin regimen. Patients who require such combinations (they should be given only to those at high cardiovascular risk, with no other good therapeutic options, who agree to close follow-up) should be warned about prolonged muscle soreness or tenderness with marked fatigue. If this occurs, the drug should be stopped and the creatine phosphokinase (CPK) checked. Values above 10 times the upper limits of normal indicate myositis. If

not detected promptly, this can lead to rhabdomyolysis and attendant renal failure. If cyclosporine is given, limit dosages of the statin to no more than 20 mg of lovastatin or its equivalent. No increase in lens opacities with statin therapy has been found, and routine eye examinations are not required.

TOLERABILITY. The statins are all remarkably well tolerated. Although twice-a-day dosage may give slightly greater improvements in LDL-c level for the statins, single drug dosage is possible for many patients who do not have very high LDL-c levels and need LDL-c level lowering for secondary prevention. At this writing, there are cost differences between the statins that should be considered as well.

Gemfibrozil (Lopid). This is a second-generation fibric acid derivative. It is the drug of first choice for those who present with triglyceride values of above 800 mg per dL (signifying a problem with removal of triglyceride-rich chylomicrons and VLDLs). It appears to increase the enzyme needed for triglyceride removal—lipoprotein lipase. The initial dosage and the maintenance dosage are 600 mg twice a day.

EFFICACY. The Helsinki Heart Trial showed that gemfibrozil therapy, compared with placebo, resulted in significantly fewer fatal and nonfatal coronary events. There was no effect on total mortality, but the trial was not powered to show such an effect. It lowered cholesterol and triglyceride levels by approximately 10% and 35%, respectively, and raised HDL-c levels by approximately 10%. The gemfibrozil-associated reduction in the incidence of definite coronary events varied according to lipid values at baseline and their changes during treatment. The greatest reductions were seen in subjects with low initial HDL-c levels and hypertriglyceridemia. In those with pure hypercholesterolemia, gemfibrozil lowers LDL-c levels on the order of 5 to 15%. When used to treat those with hypertriglyceridemia and borderline LDL-c, levels of LDL-c actually can rise. Because of its modest effects on LDL-c levels, it is not listed as a major drug in secondary prevention.

TOXICITY. Gemfibrozil increases biliary saturation in healthy persons, and there may be a small increase in cholesterol gallstones. It is much safer than clofibrate in this regard. Myopathy can be seen in rare patients. Avoid gemfibrozil in those with renal impairment. Be careful about combining with a statin because of the increased likelihood of myositis (see preceding section on "statins").

TOLERABILITY. It is well tolerated with only mild gastrointestinal distress noted.

Probucol (Lorelco). Probucol lowers both LDL-c and HDL-c levels by stimulating LDL receptor activity. This nonreceptor-mediated mechanism may account for its success in mobilizing tissue cholesterol from xanthomas. It is a powerful antioxidant. It comes in 250-mg tablets. The dosage is 500 mg twice daily.

EFFICACY. Probucol appears to lower LDL-c levels by 10 to 15%. It has no effect on triglycerides. The decline in HDL-c levels seen with this drug is a concern, since clinical trial data do not support its

TABLE 9. **Guide for Selecting Lipid Lowering Therapy**

Category	Choices (Listed in Order of Potency—Largest Effects First)
Lower LDL-c	Statins (simvastatin [Zocor], lovastatin [Mevacor], pravastatin [Pravachol], fluvastatin [Lesco]), resins,* niacin, estrogens in postmenopausal women
Raise HDL-c	Niacin, gemfibrozil (Lopid), estrogen, statins, resins*
Lower triglycerides	Gemfibrozil, niacin, statins (do not use statins if triglyceride level is over 800 mg/dL)
Raise triglycerides	Resins,* estrogens
Safest	Resins* (not absorbed, although gastrointestinal side effects limit use)
Cheapest	Unmodified niacin, fluvastatin
Ease of use	Statins, gemfibrozil
Require patient counseling	Niacin, resins*
Combinations to try in familial hypercholesterolemia	Resin* and statin, resin* and niacin; stubborn cases require triple therapy with resin,* statin, and niacin
Combinations to avoid	Lovastatin and gemfibrozil (increases risk myositis)
Not recommended	Clofibrate (Atromid-S) (adverse effects in WHO trial); lorelco (Probucol) (not shown to be efficacious against atherosclerotic vascular disease in clinical trials)

*Resins are cholestyramine (Questran) and colestipol (Colestid).

efficacy in patients with atherosclerotic vascular disease.

TOXICITY. Probucol prolongs the QT interval, which could be a problem in patients prone to arrhythmia. Probucol is stored in adipose tissue and slowly excreted in the bile.

TOLERABILITY. Mild diarrhea is seen in some patients. Until clinical trials are available to document its efficacy and long-term safety, it is not a drug to be recommended for either primary or secondary prevention.

Estrogen Replacement Therapy. Hormone replacement therapy reverses the loss of estrogen-stimulated LDL receptor synthesis after menopause. Clinical trial data show that estrogen, as well as estrogen plus progesterone (for those with an intact uterus), improves cardiovascular risk factors. Moreover, prospective cohort trials suggest that a significant reduction in CHD is attainable with estrogen use. Emerging evidence suggests that estrogen therapy reverses endothelial dysfunction associated with cholesterol-induced atherosclerosis. Estrogen therapy should be considered before drug therapy in most cases. In those with LDL-c levels under 200 mg per dL, it may obviate the need for additional lipid-lowering drugs.

EFFICACY. Estrogen causes a fall in total cholesterol and LDL-c levels, whereas HDL-c and triglyceride levels rise. Fibrinogen levels fall. Progestins cause changes in LDL-c, HDL-c, and triglyceride levels that are opposite to those seen with estrogens. The osteoporosis risk is decreased if estrogens are started soon after the menopause.

TOXICITY. If unopposed estrogens are given to women with a uterus, about one-third develop an adenomatous or atypical endometrial hyperplasia. No excess of thrombophlebitis, gallbladder disease, or cancer was seen in one large clinical trial. The link between estrogen and breast and uterine cancer should be discussed individually with each woman. In women with genetic hypertriglyceridemia (often obese, diabetic, or both), unopposed estrogen can cause a marked rise in triglyceride levels (over 1000 mg per dL) and increase the risk of pancreatitis.

TOLERABILITY. Estrogen usually is well tolerated. Some women prefer estrogen patches, but these do not affect blood lipids as do oral preparations.

Summary of Drug Therapy

Although individualized clinical judgment is important for each patient, certain generalizations may prove useful for clinicians (Table 9). As noted earlier, patients at highest near-term risk of CHD events should receive the most aggressive care. The converse also makes sense—those who are younger and have fewer than two risk factors should receive more conservative care, with more emphasis on diet and exercise. *Resins* are a good choice for younger patients owing to their overall safety. *Statins* are a good choice for those with higher LDL-c levels, as are statins plus resins for those with the most severe elevations of LDL-c levels. After cigarette cessation, correction of obesity, and regular exercise, *niacin* is a good choice for those with low HDL-c levels associated with high triglyceride or elevated LDL-c levels. Drug therapy for "isolated" low HDL-c levels is of unproven value. A high triglyceride level is a concern if it is associated with atherogenic lipoproteins or a low HDL-c level. Weight reduction and regular exercise are initial steps, with *gemfibrozil* or *niacin* being good choices for additional efficacy. When triglyceride levels exceed 400 mg per dL, *gemfibrozil* becomes the first choice. Above 1500 mg per dL, severe fat and alcohol restriction as well as gemfibrozil is needed to prevent acute pancreatitis.

OBESITY

method of
DONALD F. KIRBY, M.D.
Medical College of Virginia Hospitals
Richmond, Virginia

Obesity is a chronic medical disorder with multiple etiologies and is of national concern. Approximately one-third of men and two-thirds of women are 20% or more over

TABLE 1. MetLife Height and Weight Tables

Men*					Women*				
Height		*Small Frame*	*Medium Frame*	*Large Frame*	*Height*		*Small Frame*	*Medium Frame*	*Large Frame*
FEET	INCHES				FEET	INCHES			
5	2	128–134	131–141	138–150	4	10	102–111	109–121	118–131
5	3	130–136	133–143	140–153	4	11	103–113	111–123	120–134
5	4	132–138	135–145	142–156	5	0	104–115	113–126	122–137
5	5	134–140	137–148	144–160	5	1	106–118	115–129	125–140
5	6	136–142	139–151	146–164	5	2	108–121	118–132	128–143
5	7	138–145	142–154	149–168	5	3	111–124	121–135	131–147
5	8	140–148	145–157	152–172	5	4	114–127	124–138	134–151
5	9	142–151	148–160	155–176	5	5	117–130	127–141	137–155
5	10	144–154	151–163	158–180	5	6	120–133	130–144	140–159
5	11	146–157	154–166	161–184	5	7	123–136	133–147	143–163
6	0	149–160	157–170	164–188	5	8	126–139	136–150	146–167
6	1	152–164	160–174	168–192	5	9	129–142	139–153	149–170
6	2	155–168	164–178	172–197	5	10	132–145	142–156	152–173
6	3	158–172	167–182	176–202	5	11	135–148	145–159	155–176
6	4	162–176	171–187	181–207	6	0	138–151	148–162	158–179

*Weight at ages 25–59 years based on lowest mortality. Weight in pounds according to frame (in indoor clothing weighing 5 lb for men and 3 lb for women; shoes with 1″ heels).

To Approximate Your Frame Size

Bend forearm upward at a 90° angle. Keep fingers straight and turn the inside of your wrist toward your body. Place thumb and index finger of other hand on the two prominent bones on either side of the elbow. Measure space between your fingers on a ruler. (A physician would use a caliper.) Compare with tables below listing elbow measurements for *medium-framed* men and women. Measurements lower than those listed indicate small frame. Higher measurements indicate large frame.

Elbow Measurements for Medium Frame

Men		Women	
HEIGHT†	ELBOW BREADTH (INCHES)	HEIGHT†	ELBOW BREADTH (INCHES)
5′2″–5′3″	2½–2⅞	4′10″–4′11″	2¼–2½
5′4″–5′7″	2⅝–2⅞	5′0″–5′3″	2¼–2½
5′8″–5′11″	2¾–3	5′4″–5′7″	2⅜–2⅝
6′0″–6′3″	2¾–3⅛	5′8″–5′11″	2⅜–2⅝
6′4″	2⅞–3¼	6′0″	2½–2¾

†In shoes with 1″ heels.
Reprinted Courtesy of Metropolitan Life Insurance Company.

their ideal body weight (IBW) and are considered obese, with minority women most severely affected. Six of the 10 leading causes of death in the United States are diet-related. Medical science is now able to achieve 5-year cures for many cancers, but most people who lose weight fail to keep it off for 5 years. The failure of present treatment methods is due, in part, to the American people's desire for a quick and easy solution to a long-standing, chronic problem. Billions of dollars are spent each year on suspect methods of weight loss, and each week the tabloids feature another new diet used by celebrities to attain weight loss.

One obstacle in obesity treatment is the physician. Most physicians receive minimal or no training in nutrition, leaving them ill equipped to deal with certain nutrition-related problems. Many physicians themselves have been shown to practice poor nutritional habits, making them inadequate role models for patients. The first hurdle to clear is that of convincing both physician and patient that obesity is a chronic disorder, similar to hypertension, that requires long-term planning and treatment for weight loss to be successful.

How is obesity defined and why is it a health problem?

Obesity is an excess of body weight, mostly fat tissue, that develops from excess energy intake compared with energy expenditure. Interestingly, a new weight plateau may be attained when intake balances output. To lose weight, a caloric deficit must be produced from either decreased intake or increased output (exercise), or a combination of both. Our modern mobile society is often very concerned about body image and a clear understanding of the concepts of weight control should be given to interested patients. The most frequently quoted weight-for-height tables are those of the 1983 Metropolitan Life Insurance Company (Table 1). This information should be available in every practitioner's office. Deviations of less than 20% above or below the IBW are generally considered acceptable; however, above 20% IBW correlates with increasing patient morbidity and mortality.

Another weight comparison method is the body mass index (BMI). BMI is the weight in kilograms divided by the height in meters square (kg/m^2). Some believe that this is a superior method of identifying excess weight, and there are nomograms available to make the calculation less intimidating. Distribution of the excess fat is also an important factor. Truncal obesity (central and upper body fat = beer belly = apple shape) is riskier than lower body obesity (peripheral fat = thighs and buttocks = pear shape). Truncal obesity is more highly associated with hypertension, hyperlipidemia, diabetes mellitus, and heart disease.

Obesity is a major health problem that precipitates or aggravates many other diseases including coronary heart disease, diabetes mellitus, gallbladder disease, gout, hyperlipidemia, hypertension, infertility, osteoarthritis, restrictive lung disease, sleep apnea, and thromboembolic disease. Weight loss may benefit those patients already suffering from those conditions. In addition, several cancers (e.g., breast, ovarian, uterine, biliary tree, and gallbladder cancer in women and colorectal and prostate cancer in men) have a higher incidence in the obese population. The psychosocial trauma to the obese person also cannot be ignored. Job issues are important because many obese persons suffer job discrimination. They are perceived as slow, lazy, or lacking willpower, and in certain jobs, appearance rather than performance may dictate hiring practices.

TREATMENT

Setting Reasonable Goals

Setting a goal near IBW is generally unreasonable. Patients between 30 and 95% over IBW should strive for 20% above IBW. Patients who are more than 100% above IBW should aim to lose 50% or more of their excess body weight, but rarely do they attain IBW. A new trend has suggested that the obese person focus on just enough weight loss to ameliorate medical problems such as hypertension or hyperlipidemia. It may be easier for some people to lose 10 to 30 pounds, which might be medically beneficial, and to keep this amount off. This trend has not been validated by enough data to offer it as standard practice.

Unfortunately, there are data to warn against habitual weight loss followed by repeated weight gain—the "yo-yo effect." This may actually be worse because the body becomes more efficient in using a given set of calories, requiring the person to eat less and exercise more to get the excess weight off and keep it off on the next attempt at weight loss. This often leads to more patient frustration, but it helps validate the concept of the need for prolonged treatment regimens. However, this concept of the yo-yo effect has recently been challenged and is believed not to be a major problem.

For each pound that is to be lost, approximately 3500 kilocalories must be used. Spread over a week, this translates to a deficit of 500 kcal per day to lose 1 pound per week. To accomplish this, the obese person must either ingest fewer calories than required or increase exercise, or both. Although this concept sounds simplistic, it is also very difficult to put into practice on a long-term basis. Thus, to achieve lasting weight loss, people must understand that they need to change their basic attitudes and behavior toward eating, not for just a few weeks, but for a lifetime.

Diet

Diet is generally considered the cornerstone of any weight-loss program. Unfortunately, most people equate the word "diet" with weight loss; however, a "diet" means a manner of living with regard to food. A weight-loss diet, perceived as the enemy, is only one of many dietary options. The role of a registered dietitian (R.D.) in an overall weight-loss program cannot be underestimated. Performing a food-habits inventory—including examining a food diary, 24-hour recall, food frequency checklist, and general diet-related issues—begins a proper assessment that helps the clinician plan a meaningful treatment plan for an individual patient. Ethnic and socioeconomic factors must also be considered so that individualized treatment plans can be fashioned rather than depending on preprinted diet sheets that are routinely never followed. For the clinician not presently utilizing the services of an R.D., this should become a management priority. If the clinician is unfamiliar with services locally available, then a toll-free call to the American Dietetic Association Hotline might be valuable (1-800-366-1655).

One of the first goals is to categorize the degree of obesity (for this discussion we shall use IBW, not BMI). Mild obesity is considered weight less than 30% above IBW; moderate obesity is weight between 30 and 100% above IBW; and severe obesity is weight greater than 100% above IBW. Mild-to-moderate levels of obesity are more likely to respond to nonsurgical intervention whereas more severe levels of obesity may require seemingly more drastic treatment approaches.

The next goal is to determine the patient's baseline caloric needs. In a relatively healthy, ambulatory patient, equations such as the Harris-Benedict method will approximate a reasonable caloric level, but in this population this method should be used in conjunction with diet recall/food frequency information. If available, indirect calorimetry by a metabolic cart is more accurate, but more expensive. By establishing the person's daily caloric needs, a proper caloric level can be set for a weight-reduction diet. These diets may be as simple as making some lifestyle changes, to have a person eat a low-fat, high-carbohydrate diet while watching for empty calorie choices such as alcohol and sweets, or more severe restrictions that may include special low-calorie diets utilizing liquid supplements exclusively. Metabolically, it is easier to take fat calories and store excess calories as fat as opposed to carbohydrate calories, which require considerable energy expenditure to be converted into fat to be stored. Also, fat calories contain 9 kcal per gram compared with 4 kcal per gram for carbohydrate and protein sources. Thus, the composition of a meal *does* matter when planning a diet. To offset feelings of hunger, eating a low-fat, high-complex carbohydrate diet is an excellent strategy.

The clinician must understand that a diet routinely less than 1600 kcal per day will tend to be deficient in the recommended dietary allowances

(RDA) for many of the macronutrients (sodium, potassium, magnesium, and calcium) and micronutrients (vitamins and minerals). These will need to be carefully supplemented, and the lower the caloric intake, the more intense should be the patient monitoring. Very-low-energy diets (VLED) range from 300 to 800 kcal per day. This type of diet should be medically supervised. If done improperly, protein depletion can occur, which can lead to cardiac problems, and electrolyte depletion may also result, which has been associated with fatal arrhythmias. The ultimate goal is to lose excess fat and not lean body tissue so that proper protein intake on any planned weight-loss diet must be a priority. This is another reason why having a skilled R.D. assist in a weight-loss plan is essential.

Almost all weight-loss diets (and surgery) are associated with decreased gallbladder emptying, which can lead to cholelithiasis and possibly cholecystitis. Ursodiol (Actigall) 300 mg twice daily can significantly reduce cholelithiasis compared with placebo. VLED programs such as HMR (Health Management Resources, Boston, Massachusetts) and Optifast (Sandoz Nutrition, Minneapolis, Minnesota) are liquid diets that have the advantage of achieving rapid initial weight loss. However, a liquid diet does not reflect the real world, so the patient must be taught dietary principles and practices to reassimilate to real world food choices and caloric levels; otherwise, the patient is doomed to regain the lost weight as soon as he stops the liquid diet. Commercial programs, such as Nutri/System, rely on selling the client foods that are considered better choices for individuals. Other organizations like Weight Watchers, TOPS (Take Off Pounds Sensibly), and Overeaters Anonymous offer group self-help and dietary advice. These groups can offer continued motivation and support when patients feel themselves slipping into old habits and are particularly beneficial to those with mild to moderate obesity.

Behavior Modification Therapy

The premise of behavior modification is that most obese persons have learned certain behaviors related to both eating and activity that have either caused or perpetuated that person to be obese. By examining a patient's behavior of when, why, how much, and under what circumstances he or she eats, patterns may emerge that will help a skilled behavior therapist assist in planning specific areas for patients to explore. Approaches to overcome low activity levels or aversions to exercise are also important. Behavioral approaches are good in that they put the patient in charge of his destiny, and group sessions also help patients feel that there are other people with similar problems and that they are not isolated.

Used by itself, behavior modification can obtain good initial weight loss over a prolonged period of therapy, usually 18 weeks or more. However, most weight is regained in 1 to 5 years. Better results have been seen when behavior modification therapy

is part of a more structured program that involves diet and exercise interventions. More attention should be paid to the first phase where there is reintroduction of foods after a liquid diet program. Behavioral approaches that encompass a long maintenance phase might be more beneficial in reacclimating patients to make sensible choices for long-term success. It cannot be overstressed that obesity is a chronic problem that requires prolonged treatment.

Exercise

Exercise should be considered another major cornerstone to any weight-loss program. This is a natural conclusion since exercise increases caloric consumption. Many obese persons are chronically inactive and avoid opportunities to exercise. For moderately and severely obese persons, this may be due to orthopedic-related problems from their chronic obesity. As a weight-loss plan is formulated, hip, knee, and foot problems should be identified. Treatment and exercise plans can often be created around them. The easiest exercise to *prescribe* is walking. Initially, distances should be modest while focusing on working up to 45 to 60 minutes 5 to 7 days a week. As exercise tolerance increases, so can the walking pace or time interval. Some patients may feel pressured to begin jogging; however, more orthopedic problems occur in this population, and the concept of physical activity should be stressed more than the actual activity. For those patients with more severe orthopedic problems, swimming and aqua aerobics are good ways to increase caloric utilization and minimize the stress to the joints. Other printed materials list the calorie-burning potential of an individual exercise activity, and these should be made available to patients.

Exercise also has medical benefits besides expending calories. Increases in lean body tissue and high-density lipoproteins are associated with exercise programs. Patients who incorporate and continue an exercise program as a lifestyle change are much more likely to maintain their weight loss over a prolonged period of time. It is also a false perception that modest exercise increases appetite, so patients should not fear this. The value of a continuous exercise plan outweighs any potential minor increase in caloric intake.

The Role of Medications

Medications presently play a minor role in the treatment of obesity. One major reason for this is the strict prescribing policies involved with many of the drugs. Treatment is often limited to a few weeks, and longer use may be cause for review by state medical review boards. Much of the concern regarding drug therapy for obesity grew from use, abuse, and the addictive potential of the amphetamine family of drugs (Schedule II drugs), which are no longer suggested for obesity. Medications should never be the

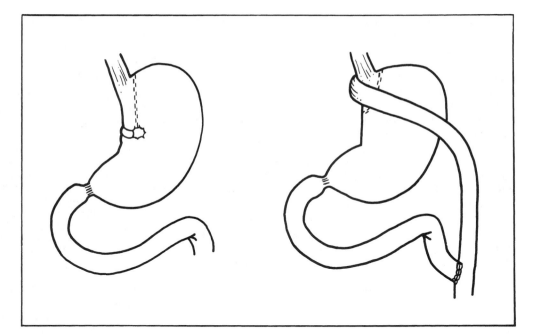

Figure 1. Currently practiced operations for obesity include vertical-banded gastroplasty *(left)*, and Roux-en-Y gastric bypass *(right)*. (From Apovian CM, Jensen GL: Overnutrition and obesity management. *In* Kirby DF, Dudrick SJ [eds]: Practical Handbook of Nutrition in Clinical Practice. 1994, p 43. Reprinted by permission of CRC Press, Boca Raton, Florida.)

sole therapy, but rather part of a program of diet and exercise.

Available obesity medications are broken into two broad categories—adrenergic and serotonergic compounds. Phenylpropanolamine is an adrenergic compound that binds to alpha₁ receptors. It has minimal side effects and is the active ingredient in many over-the-counter medications (e.g., Dexatrim). Other centrally acting adrenergic agents bind to beta receptors, reduce hunger and food intake, and have low abuse potential. The major side effects are tremor and nervousness. Examples of these drugs are diethylpropion mazindol (Sanorex, Mazanor—Schedule IV drugs); and phentermine (Fastin, Adipex-P—Schedule IV drugs).

Fenfluramine (Pondimin—Schedule IV drug) is a serotonergic agent that reduces hunger and enhances satiety. It is unclear whether it also has a role in increasing energy expenditure. Fluoxetine (Prozac)* and sertraline (Zoloft)* are other serotonergic agents used for depression and are not controlled substances. These drugs are being evaluated in the treatment of obesity.

The National Institutes of Health (NIH) Workshop on Pharmacologic Treatment of Obesity concluded that drugs should presently be only one component of a weight-control program. Further research and more flexibility in prescribing available drugs are needed. Studies on long-term use, combination therapy, and biochemical mechanisms are essential. In Virginia, the limitation on prescribing medications for a long-term problem has been lifted, and I now use pharmacologic agents with dietary counseling, exercise prescriptions, and a firm patient contract.

---

*Not FDA-approved for this indication.

Surgery

The thought of surgical intervention for obesity might seem drastic to some. However, for patients who are morbidly obese (>100% above IBW) or are moderately overweight and have significant co-morbid medical conditions, this may be their last chance, especially if they have failed multiple nonsurgical approaches at weight loss. Surgery has undergone many different forms over the past 40 years. Regrettably, it developed a bad reputation from the jejunoileal bypass procedure, which was associated with many complications and even death. This procedure is no longer practiced. The NIH Consensus Conference on Obesity has recommended only two procedures, the vertical-banded gastroplasty and the Roux-en-Y gastric bypass operation (Figure 1).

Data from our institution show that a careful preoperative dietary evaluation helps to select the most appropriate procedure. The vertical-banded gastroplasty creates a small gastric pouch, making it difficult for the patient to ingest large quantities of food. The procedure has no effect on digestion or absorption. However, it can be defeated by a person with a sweet-eater's dietary history. Such an individual can consume several thousand calories in liquids such as sodas, sweetened fruit punches, or even milk shakes. The liquids flow easily through the created pouch and then are digested and absorbed normally.

The Roux-en-Y gastric bypass not only makes a small gastric pouch but also bypasses the stomach, duodenum, and part of the jejunum. This leads to superior weight loss compared with that attained with the vertical-banded gastroplasty, but it is technically more difficult to perform. Deficiencies in calcium, iron, and vitamin B₁₂ absorption resulting from the changes in anatomy must be anticipated and supplemented. The sweet-eater who has a bypass procedure and ingests sugar-sweetened beverages is likely to suffer symptoms of dumping syndrome with malaise, dizziness, abdominal cramping, or diarrhea. These symptoms act as a method of surgical behavior modification; to avoid these symptoms, the patient must change his dietary intake.

Significant improvements in surgical technique and especially postoperative management have lowered the mortality risk to between 1 and 2%. Surgical morbidity rates vary, but most problems are handled readily. Surgery can usually be expected to ameliorate many of the co-morbidities associated with obesity such as diabetes mellitus, hyperlipidemia, hypertension, and respiratory problems. The success of this type of intervention can be seen in a higher number of patients who have maintained their weight loss at 5 years and generally lost 50% of the excess body weight. Refinements of the techniques and operative care are being studied.

VITAMIN DEFICIENCY

method of
DEMETRE LABADARIOS, M.B., Ch.B., Ph.D.
*University of Stellenbosch and Tygerberg Hospital
Tygerberg, South Africa*

and

JOHN M. PETTIFOR, M.B., B.Ch., Ph.D.
*University of the Witwatersrand
Johannesburg, South Africa*

Vitamins are organic catalysts necessary for growth maintenance and health; they cannot be endogenously synthesized at all or in sufficient amounts to meet daily needs; as such, they must be supplied, by definition in small amounts, by food. Vitamin status and its role in the prevention of disease, especially of chronic degenerative diseases, is currently the subject of intense debate. The focus of debate is not so much on the treatment of clinical vitamin deficiencies per se but rather on the daily requirements of these nutrients for optimal health. In this regard, the concept of "marginal vitamin status or subclinical deficiency" has gained added momentum, but the term itself, and its possible implications for health, is in urgent need of a more objective definition. However, whereas the totality of scientific evidence must be awaited before making recommendations on the role of antioxidant micronutrients (especially vitamins E, C, selenium, and the carotenoids) in the prevention of a number of degenerative diseases (cardiovascular disease, certain types of cancer, cataracts, and age-related macular degeneration), there exists little doubt at present about the major benefits accrued, in terms of survival and health, from targeted high-dose vitamin A supplementation in children under 6 years of age with low blood vitamin A levels but without signs of clinical deficiency; similarly, folic acid supplementation in high-risk pregnancies has been shown to be beneficial in the prevention of neural tube defects.

In general, clinical vitamin deficiencies do certainly occur among poor people in developing countries. However, although such deficiencies are not common in normal populations of Western societies, they do occur especially, for instance, among individuals who abuse alcohol, food faddists, malnourished patients, patients with gastrointestinal pathology, and patients with inborn errors of metabolism or those receiving incomplete or inadequate total parenteral nutrition (TPN) or pharmacotherapy. The safe and effective practice of clinical vitaminology, therefore, entails knowledge of physiology and nutrition, a high index of suspicion because of the insidious onset of deficiency symptoms, as well as awareness of the coexistence of multiple rather than single vitamin deficiencies. Moreover, vitamins in large doses should be considered as pharmacologic agents rather than as essential nutrients, and the potential toxicity or interactions that may arise from the administration of large supplemental doses should be borne in mind. Further, nutrition education regarding the principles of eating a varied and balanced diet should accompany the treatment of deficiency states, as appropriate, and the need for prophylactic vitamin supplements should be established.

In considering the pathophysiology of vitamin deficiencies, five main etiologic factors should be remembered: decreased dietary intake, impaired absorption, increased excretion, impaired utilization, and increased requirements consequent to acute or chronic disease or to physiologic states such as growth, pregnancy, and lactation. Additionally, one should be aware that deficiency can and does occur in the short term (2 to 4 weeks), especially in the case of some water-soluble vitamins, whereas inadequate dietary intake for 3 or more years is necessary before clinical vitamin B_{12} deficiency manifests. Nevertheless and as a general rule, when deficiency is suspected, it should be treated immediately; confirmation of the diagnosis can be based on the therapeutic response following supplementation or on biochemical assessment when possible.

THIAMINE DEFICIENCY

Yeast, wheat germ, rice husk, offal (liver and kidney), and some fruits and vegetables are good dietary sources of thiamine. Absorption takes place in the duodenum and jejunum by passive diffusion (high concentrations) or by active transport (low concentrations). The total body content of thiamine has been calculated to be approximately 30 mg for an average adult. The Recommended Daily Allowance (RDA) for thiamine is related to energy intake (0.5 mg per 1000 kcal) and is 0.3 to 0.4 mg for infants, 0.7 to 1.3 mg for children 1 to 14 years of age, 1.3 to 1.5 for male adolescents and adults, and 1.1 mg for women; a higher intake is recommended for pregnancy (1.5 mg) and lactation (1.6 mg).

The active coenzyme form of the vitamin, thiamine pyrophosphate, catalyzes the oxidative decarboxylation of alpha-ketoacids (pyruvate, alpha-ketoglutarate) and ketoanalogues (leucine, isoleucine and valine) and the utilization of pentose in the hexose monophosphate shunt (the transketolase reaction). Additionally, thiamine is present in axonal membranes, and nerve stimulation is associated with the release of thiamine diphosphate and triphosphate.

Thiamine deficiency can commonly occur in populations consuming milled rice as a staple or consuming foods (shellfish, raw fish) containing thiaminase, an enzyme that inactivates the vitamin; tannins, as found in tea and coffee, are also known to oxidize the vitamin. Deficiency is also commonly encountered among individuals who abuse alcohol, which primarily impairs thiamine absorption and makes an excessive contribution to the total daily energy intake. In the clinical setting, patients on diuretic therapy, peritoneal dialysis, or hemodialysis, with thyrotoxicosis, diabetes, trauma, and fever, may become deficient because of increased thiamine requirements. Iatrogenically, thiamine deficiency may be induced in patients on TPN, during refeeding after starvation, or in asymptomatic patients who are thiamine-depleted and in whom glucose is administered without thiamine supplements.

Resting tachycardia, weakness, muscle tenderness, decreased deep tendon reflexes, and even sensory neuropathy have been demonstrated within 1 week of consuming a thiamine-free diet. The cardiovascular system (wet beriberi) and the nervous system (dry beriberi; neuropathy, Wernicke's encephalopathy, and Korsakoff's syndrome) are profoundly affected by clinical deficiency, with a lesser involvement of the gastrointestinal system (anorexia and constipation). Beriberi heart disease is characterized by a high-output state due to peripheral vasodilatation, biventricular heart failure, and edema secondary to sodium and water retention. The neuropathy is characterized by impaired sensory, motor, and reflex function and is predominantly distal and symmetrical and may be painful. Wernicke's encephalopathy usually presents with ophthalmoplegia (unilateral or bilateral), horizontal (most common) nystagmus, fever, ataxia, vomiting, and mental deterioration that may progress to global confusion, coma, and death; thiamine administration may change the clinical picture to Korsakoff's syndrome (retrograde amnesia, impaired learning ability, and confabulation).

In the absence of laboratory facilities, response to treatment is the only criterion that can be used for confirming the clinical diagnosis. Treatment-induced clinical improvement in cardiovascular beriberi can usually be seen within 8 to 16 hours and a reduction in heart size within 2 to 3 days. Biochemically, although blood concentrations of thiamine, pyruvate, lactate, and glyoxylate, and urinary excretion of thiamine and its metabolites have been used for diagnostic purposes, the most accepted method of assessment is the measurement of transketolase activity in whole blood or washed erythrocytes. The in vitro addition of thiamine pyrophosphate (TPP) increases the activity of the enzyme, the so-called TPP effect; an increase in the enzyme activity that exceeds 25% (some authorities use 15%) is, together with the clinical response to treatment, usually confirmatory of the diagnosis.

Treatment. Treatment, apart from the necessary support for heart failure, consists of the prompt administering of 50 to 100 mg of thiamine intravenously or intramuscularly for 5 days, followed by 5 to 10 mg orally for 10 days. Multivitamin supplements (containing two to five times the RDA) should also be administered, orally or intravenously as appropriate, and alcoholic cardiomyopathy should be excluded.

Toxicity. Although cases of an anaphylactic type of reaction (the ill-defined and so-called thiamine shock) have been reported, thiamine toxicity per se has not been described in humans with doses up to 200 times the RDA.

NIACIN (NICOTINIC ACID, NIACINAMIDE) DEFICIENCY

Niacin is widely distributed, in most cases in small amounts, in foods of plant and animal origin. Meat products, especially offal (liver, kidney), are the richest sources of the vitamin. In some foods, especially in maize, bound forms of niacin are not nutritionally available. Niacin is absorbed from the whole gastrointestinal tract by passive diffusion and active transport. The RDA for niacin is influenced by energy intake (6.6 mg per 1000 kcal) and by the quantity and quality of dietary protein, because of the endogenous synthesis of niacin from tryptophan (on average, 1 mg of niacin is formed from 60 mg of tryptophan). Infants require 5 to 6 mg of Niacin Equivalents (NE); children 1 to 14 years of age, 9 to 17; male adults and adolescents, 15 to 20; and women, 15; 17 and 20 mg of NE is recommended for pregnant women and lactating mothers, respectively.

The active coenzyme forms of the vitamin, niacin adenine dinucleotide (NAD) and niacin adenine dinucleotide phosphate (NADP), participate in oxidation-reduction reactions involved in aerobic oxidation, fatty acid oxidation, and glycolysis, and steroid, pyrimidine, amino acid, and glucuronide biosynthesis. Additionally, large doses of nicotinic acid (3 to 6 grams per day), but not niacinamide, lower serum cholesterol levels, but amounts greater than ten times the RDA can cause flushing and peripheral vasodilatation.

Pellagra is usually, but not invariably, found in populations whose major source of protein is food grains (maize or millet). They have a low NE content, and niacin may be unavailable depending on the method used in their preparation; an imbalance in essential amino acids (tryptophan and leucine), as found in maize and millet, may also exacerbate the deficiency. Pellagra is also seen in chronic alcoholics, food faddists, and patients with malabsorption. A deficiency state is occasionally encountered in patients with malignancy and prolonged febrile illness and less frequently in patients with the carcinoid syndrome (in which tryptophan is converted to serotonin rather than niacin), Hartnup's disease (in which tryptophan absorption and other amino acid absorption is impaired), and secondary to vitamin B_6 deficiency (in which the conversion of tryptophan to nicotinic acid is impaired). Iatrogenically, the deficiency has been induced in asymptomatic but malnourished patients by the intravenous administration of glucose without niacin supplements.

The 3D symptoms and signs involving the skin (*d*ermatitis), the gastrointestinal tract (*d*iarrhea) and the central nervous system (*dementia*) are the main characteristics of pellagra (4Ds if *death* is added). The dermatitis is symmetrical and bilateral, has clearly defined borders, and is seen in the sun-exposed areas of the body; hyperkeratosis, hyperpigmentation, and desquamation are characteristic of the skin lesions. The diarrhea, which results from inflammatory changes of the gastrointestinal mucosa, is recurrent with watery and occasionally bloody stools; other mucosal signs include stomatitis, glossitis, and vaginitis. Anorexia, vomiting, and indigestion may be present. The dementia usually includes fatigue and insomnia as well as apathy and may progress to encephalopathy; the latter is characterized by memory loss, confusion, disorientation, hallucination, and eventually psychosis.

The most reliable method of diagnosis is the response to treatment. The available biochemical tests are laborious and, at best, questionable. Nevertheless, plasma tryptophan and erythrocyte NAD and NADP concentrations as well as urinary niacin and tryptophan metabolites have been shown to be low in the presence of established deficiency.

Treatment. Oral daily supplements (50 to 150 mg) lead to clinical improvement within a week, but the resolution of the dementia may follow a more protracted course. Larger doses (200 mg) may be necessary for patients with Hartnup's disease or the carcinoid syndrome.

Toxicity. Niacin toxicity is associated only with large doses of nicotinic acid and presents as flushing (it can occur with as low as 50 to 100 mg), nausea, dizziness, diarrhea, abdominal pain, exacerbation of asthma and pre-existing gastrointestinal ulceration, hyperuricemia, hyperglycemia, cardiac arrhythmias, cholestatic jaundice, and abnormal liver function; all symptoms and signs resolve on discontinuation of the vitamin.

RIBOFLAVIN DEFICIENCY

Milk, eggs, liver and kidney, and green leafy vegetables are rich dietary sources of riboflavin. The vitamin is absorbed from the upper small intestine by an energy-dependent process. The body content of riboflavin, mainly in the form of flavin adenine dinucleotide (FAD) and flavin mononucleotide (FMN) has been calculated to be in the region of 15 mg. The RDA for infants is 0.4 to 0.5 mg; for children 1 to 14 years of age, 0.8 to 1.5 mg; for male adolescents and adults, 1.5 to 1.7 mg; and for females, 1.3 mg; the RDA for pregnant and lactating women is 1.6 and 1.7 to 1.8, respectively.

FMN and FAD, the active coenzyme forms of the vitamin, catalyze oxidation-reduction reactions involving electron transport systems, including succinic dehydrogenase, amino acid oxidases, xanthine oxidase, glutathione reductase, and fatty acid synthesis and oxidation.

Deficiency of riboflavin alone is rather uncommon and usually occurs in combination with that of other vitamins, especially among individuals who do not consume adequate amounts of dairy products. Alcohol is known to impair the digestion and absorption of the vitamin, and cancer chemotherapeutic agents, phenothiazines, and tricyclic antidepressants inhibit the biosynthesis of its active coenzymes. Phototherapy as used in the treatment of neonatal jaundice is thought to induce deficiency, as is hemodialysis, peritoneal dialysis, thermal injury, trauma, malignancy, and chronic debilitating illness.

Deficiency presents with cheilosis, angular stomatitis, glossitis (magenta tongue), seborrheic dermatitis (around the nose, ears, mouth, eyes, and/or scrotum), corneal neovascularization, and a normochromic, normocytic anemia.

Clinical response to treatment is a useful diagnostic tool, and generally clinical improvement can be seen within a week of the initiation of treatment. Biochemically, the riboflavin coefficient is currently used for diagnostic purposes; the coefficient is based on the increase in the activity of erythrocyte glutathione reductase by the in vitro addition of FAD; a coefficient greater than 1.2 is suggestive of deficiency.

Treatment. Oral (6 to 15 mg) or intramuscular (25 mg; where available) daily riboflavin supplements are generally adequate in treating the deficiency.

Toxicity. Riboflavin toxicity has not been described in humans.

PYRIDOXINE (VITAMIN B$_6$) DEFICIENCY

Pyridoxine is widespread in nature but yeast, wheat, corn, egg yolk, legumes, nuts, offal, and meat products are some of the more concentrated dietary sources. The vitamin is absorbed from the upper gastrointestinal tract by passive diffusion and possibly an active transport mechanism. The RDA for infants is 0.3 to 0.6 mg; for children 1 to 14 years of age, 1.0 to 1.7 mg; and 1.6 to 2.0 mg for adult women and men, respectively; the RDA is increased in pregnancy (2.2 mg) and lactation (2.1 mg). Requirements depend on the protein content of the diet (0.016 mg per gram of protein).

Vitamin B$_6$ vitamers (pyridoxine, pyridoxal, pyridoxamine, and their phosphate esters) are converted to pyridoxal-5'-phosphate (PLP), the active coenzyme form of the vitamin. PLP participates in a number of metabolic transformations of amino acids (for example, serine, glycine, glutamate, tryptophan, methionine, cysteine), in heme synthesis, in neuronal excitability, and in stabilizing phosphorylase in muscle; more recently, a regulatory role in steroid hormone action has been postulated.

Primary pyridoxine deficiency is rare in humans. It does, however, occur with severe dietary deprivation, in patients with celiac sprue, malabsorption, renal or hepatic disease, and pharmacotherapy (isoniazid, cycloserine, hydralazine, penicillamine). A number of pyridoxine-responsive genetic disorders with aberrant enzyme structure-synthesis (glutamic acid decarboxylase, kynureninase, cystathionine synthetase) have been described.

Pyridoxine deficiency is associated with symptoms and signs in the skin and central nervous system and with erythropoiesis. Skin lesions include seborrheic dermatitis, glossitis, cheilosis, and angular stomatitis, which are often indistinguishable from lesions of niacin and riboflavin deficiency. Somnolence, depression, irritation, and convulsions, the latter especially in infants, make up the central nervous system symptoms of the deficiency. Several cases of pyridoxine-responsive microcytic hypochromic anemia have been reported.

Apart from a favorable therapeutic response to supplemental therapy, several biochemical procedures have been used for the assessment of pyridoxine status in humans; these include the tryptophan- or methionine-loading test, the increase in the activity of glutamic-pyruvic transaminase by the in vitro addition of PLP, and plasma PLP alone or in conjunction with plasma pyridoxal and albumin concentrations. At present there is considerable disagreement as to which of these parameters is the best criterion of pyridoxine status.

Treatment. Treatment consists of the oral administration of pyridoxine (25 mg); higher doses (100 to 500 mg) have been used for the treatment of anemia and in patients on penicillamine therapy. Pyridoxine supplements may impair the efficacy of L-dopa, phenytoin, and phenobarbital.

Toxicity. A reversible peripheral neuropathy (ataxia, poor coordination of the hands and feet, loss of position and vibration sense, perioral numbness with intact reflex and sensory function) has been reported in individuals ingesting high doses (2 grams) of pyridoxine over a prolonged period; paresthesia and muscle weakness have also been reported with lower (greater than 120 mg) doses.

FOLIC ACID DEFICIENCY

Good sources of folic acid include green leafy vegetables, legumes, whole grain cereals, nuts, liver and kidney, and yeast. Folic acid is primarily absorbed in the upper third of the small intestine, although absorptive capacity has been demonstrated over its entire length. Total body stores in an average individual range from 5 to 20 mg, of which approximately half is found in the liver. The RDA for infants is 25 to 35 μg; for children 1 to 14 years of age, 50 to 150 μg; and 200 and 180 μg for men and women, respectively. In pregnancy and lactation, 400 and 260 to 280 μg are recommended, respectively.

Folic acid, in its active coenzyme form [tetrahydrofolic acid (THFA)], participates in the transfer of 1-carbon units in thymidylate synthesis (the rate-limiting step in DNA synthesis), in the catabolism of tryptophan, serine, glycine, and histidine, as well as in purine and protein synthesis. In the presence of insufficient vitamin B_{12}, "trapping" of folic acid in the methyl THFA form limits the regeneration of THFA, thus compromising DNA synthesis and cell proliferation.

Folic acid deficiency is probably the most common deficiency in humans. Etiologically, inadequate dietary intake is a major contributing factor, especially among alcoholics and elderly people. A number of diseases (malignancy, thermal injury, surgical trauma, sepsis, chronic hemolytic anemias and exfoliative skin disorders, hepatic disease or failure, renal failure requiring hemodialysis) and physiologic states (pregnancy, lactation, growth) precipitate deficiency by increasing folic acid requirements. Further, deficiency is also common in patients with malabsorption (inflammatory bowel disease, diverticulosis, small bowel resection, sprue, gluten enteropathy, anticonvulsant medication) or in those in whom folic acid metabolism is impaired (alcoholism; pharmacotherapy with methotrexate, pyrimethamine, triamterene, oral contraceptives, and anticonvulsants).

Macrocytic anemia and megaloblastosis of the bone marrow are the most common findings in folic acid deficiency. Thrombocytopenia, leukopenia, diarrhea, glossitis, anorexia, and weight loss are also frequently present.

Megaloblastic anemia is suggested by an increased mean corpuscular volume (MCV of greater than 100 to 110 fL); marked anisocytosis, poikilocytosis, and macro-ovalocytes are typically seen in the blood smear. Reticulocyte count is low. A bone marrow examination is very helpful in the diagnosis. Moreover, low serum (less than 4 ng per mL; indicative of recent inadequate intake) and erythrocyte (less than 150 ng per mL; indicative of longer-term inadequate dietary intake) folate concentration is invariably present.

Treatment. Oral folic acid supplements (1 mg daily) are efficacious in correcting the deficiency. A marked reticulocytosis is usually seen by the end of the first week of supplementation, and the anemia is corrected over the ensuing 1 to 2 months. Larger doses (5 mg daily) may be necessary in the presence of markedly increased requirements. An adequate dietary intake or a daily oral supplement of 0.4 mg of folic acid preconceptually and throughout pregnancy is recommended for the prevention of neural tube defects.

Toxicity. Some cases of hypersensitivity have been reported, especially with intravenous folic acid supplements. However, no adverse effects have been reported with oral doses of 15 mg for a month. It should be borne in mind that high supplemental doses of folic acid can partially overcome its "trapping" in the presence of vitamin B_{12} deficiency and thus, in the absence of vitamin B_{12} supplements, contribute to the deterioration of the neurologic symptoms of vitamin B_{12} deficiency.

VITAMIN B_{12} (COBALAMIN, CYANOCOBALAMIN) DEFICIENCY

Vitamin B_{12} is found only in foods of animal origin (meat and dairy products). Its absorption in the distal ileum requires the intrinsic factor (IF), which is secreted by the parietal cells of the gastric mucosa; approximately 1% of free vitamin B_{12} can be absorbed by passive diffusion over the entire length of the small bowel. Vitamin B_{12} body stores range from 1 to 10 mg of which 50 to 70% are found in the liver. Requirements for infants vary from 0.3 to 0.5 µg and for children 1 to 14 years of age from 0.7 to 2.0 µg; adults require 2.0; pregnant women, 2.2; and lactating mothers, 2.6 µg.

Adenosylcobalamine and methylcobalamine are the active forms of the vitamin. Methylcobalamine is involved in the conversion of homocysteine to methionine; this reaction is of crucial importance in (1) the regeneration of tetrahydrofolate, which is required for DNA synthesis and cell maturation, and (2) the synthesis of choline and choline-containing phospholipids. Adenosylcobalamine is involved in the conversion of methylmalonyl coenzyme A to succinyl coenzyme A. The impairment of both these conversions is thought to contribute to the neurologic damage seen in vitamin B_{12} deficiency. Vitamin B_{12} is also important in the functioning of many sulfhydryl (SH)–activated enzyme systems.

Deficiency is occasionally seen in strict vegetarians; the slow onset of the deficiency in the presence of no dietary intake in these individuals is attributed to the enterohepatic circulation and efficient conservation of cobalamin. Malabsorption is the main etiologic factor of the deficiency; it can be due to inadequate production of IF (pernicious anemia, gastrectomy, congenital IF defects), disorders of the terminal ileum (resection, regional enteritis, sprue, malignancy), competition for cobalamin (fish tapeworm, blind loop syndrome), or pharmacotherapy (colchicine, para-aminosalicylic acid, neomycin).

The most important manifestations of the deficiency involve hematopoiesis, the gastrointestinal tract, and the nervous system. The hematologic manifestations are those of macrocytic anemia, which may be accompanied by thrombocytopenia, and megaloblastosis of the bone marrow; gastrointestinal symptoms and signs include anorexia, nausea, vomiting, weight loss, glossitis (beefy red), and diarrhea. Demyelination and axonal degeneration involving peripheral nerves, the lateral and posterior columns of the spinal cord, as well as the cerebrum, characterize the neurologic abnormalities; additionally, position sense and vibration sense are usually diminished, sphincter disturbances may be present, and reflexes may be absent or increased. Mental changes include irritability, memory loss, depression, and psychosis.

In addition to the hematologic investigations (see section on folic acid), serum cobalamin concentration is low (less than 80 pg per mL). The Schilling test is helpful in elucidating the pathogenesis of the deficiency.

Treatment. The hematologic response to intramuscular cyanocobalamin administration (100 µg daily for a week, total of 2 mg for the first 6 weeks) is similar to that of folic acid deficiency (see section on folic acid); neurologic symptoms may persist even with long-term adequate supplementation. Oral supplements (1 mg daily) can be given but are not generally recommended, especially for severe deficiency. Lifelong intramuscular supplements (100 µg monthly or 1 mg every 6 months) are necessary to prevent relapse.

Toxicity. Vitamin B_{12} toxicity has not been reported in humans.

VITAMIN C DEFICIENCY

Citrus fruit, broccoli, green peppers, tomatoes, and cabbage are some of the richer sources of the vitamin; their vitamin C content is greatly diminished with prolonged storage and prolonged cooking. Vitamin C is absorbed from the upper third of the small bowel. Body stores are in the region of 1.4 to 3 grams in an average individual. The RDA for infants ranges from 30 to 35 mg; for children 1 to 14 years of age, from 40 to 50 mg; and is 60 mg for adults. Requirements are increased in pregnancy (70 mg) and lactation (90 to 95 mg). There is, however, considerable controversy on the issue of requirements, and some suggest that 100 and 180 mg for adults who do not and do smoke, respectively, is a truer reflection of daily needs.

Vitamin C is a powerful water-soluble antioxidant and does not function as a conventional coenzyme. The best-defined function of the vitamin is in collagen synthesis, specifically in the hydroxylation of proline and lysine. Other functions include the regulation of body iron storage and distribution, promotion of nonheme iron absorption, and maintenance of folic acid in the reduced tetrahydrofolate form. Currently, the antioxidant functions of the vitamin are intensely debated, especially in relation to the prevention of cardiovascular disease and certain types of cancer.

An increased incidence of deficiency occurs among infants, individuals on very restricted diets, and elderly people—especially among elderly men living alone. It is also occasionally seen among alcoholics and in diarrheal disease. It is interesting that a decrease in plasma vitamin C levels occurs in the presence of the acute phase response, but whether deficiency occurs under these circumstances remains to be elucidated. Nevertheless, thermal injury, surgical trauma, thyrotoxicosis, malignancy, infectious diseases, and hemodialysis increase vitamin C requirements.

Early symptoms and signs in infancy and childhood include decreased appetite, poor weight gain, and irritability; at a more advanced stage of deficiency, tenderness of the legs, pseudoparalysis of the lower extremities, hemorrhage into the periostium of long bones, epiphyseal separation, and elevation of the rib margins (scorbutic rosary) are seen. Purpura, ecchymoses, and bleeding gums (if teeth are present) occur. Intracerebral, subarachnoid, and retrobulbar hemorrhages may occur and be fatal. In adults, weakness, irritability, lassitude, muscle tenderness, painful joints, and weight loss are followed by a tendency to hemorrhage; perifollicular hemorrhage, purpura, bleeding gums (if teeth are present), and hemorrhage into muscles, joints, and nail bed (splinter hemorrhage) are usually seen. Anemia (normocytic, normochromic) as a result of blood loss is often present; macrocytic and/or megaloblastic anemia may also be present secondary to folic acid deficiency. Wound healing is impaired, and wound dehiscence may occur. Edema, fever, jaundice, convulsions, and hypotension may develop at an advanced stage of the deficiency.

Apart from the clinical presentation and a favorable response to treatment, leukocyte vitamin C concentration (less than 25 μg per 10^8 WBC) can be diagnostically helpful; plasma vitamin C concentration (less than 0.25 mg per dL) is less specific. In infants, radiologically detected skeletal changes may be diagnostic.

Treatment. Prompt therapeutic response is seen with supplemental vitamin C (250 mg twice daily in adults; 10 to 25 mg three times daily in infants and children). Lesions usually disappear within 2 weeks, although cutaneous pigmentary changes may persist longer.

Toxicity. Although serious toxicity from high doses of vitamin C is uncommon, acidification of the urine may promote the precipitation of cystine or oxalate stones in the urinary tracts of susceptible individuals.

VITAMIN A DEFICIENCY

Dietary vitamin A is obtained mainly from animal foods (dairy products, offal [liver, kidney, and so on], fish, fish oils, egg yolk) but is also endogenously synthesized from plant carotenes, mainly beta-carotene (yellow-pigmented and green leafy vegetables and fruit). The absorption of vitamin A and beta-carotene depends on the presence of bile and lipase and takes place in the upper half of the small bowel. The body stores of an average individual have been calculated to be in the region of 0.3 to 1.0 gram, and hepatic stores (storage capacity, 300 mg per gram) can supply the body's needs for approximately 1 year. Retinol-binding protein (RBP) is the vitamin's specific carrier protein, and its release from the liver is inhibited in vitamin A deficiency. The RDA for infants is 375 μg Retinol Equivalents (RE); for children 1 to 14 years of age, 400 to 1000 μg RE; and for male and female adults, 1000 and 800 μg RE, respectively. Requirements in pregnancy are 800 μg RE, whereas in lactating mothers the recommended intake ranges from 1200 to 1300 μg RE. One microgram RE equals 1 μg of retinol, 6 μg of beta-carotene, 12 μg of other provitamin carotenoids, or 3.3 International Units (IU). The efficiency of conversion of beta-carotene to vitamin A is, however, variable.

Vitamin A is an important component of the visual pigment in the visual cycle; it also plays an important role in growth, tissue differentiation, lysosomal membrane stabilization, and the maintenance of the integrity of epithelial tissues. The vitamin has been shown to have an immunostimulatory effect,

and very high doses (100,000 to 200,000 IU) have consistently been reported to decrease mortality by 25 to 40%, and to a lesser extent morbidity, from respiratory and diarrheal disease in children younger than 6 years of age. In children with measles, such high doses have also been reported to decrease mortality, complications and their severity, and the duration of hospitalization.

Primarily in developing countries, half a million children become blind annually because of vitamin A deficiency, which is mainly due to inadequate dietary intake of the vitamin or the provitamin beta-carotene. In other countries, vitamin A deficiency occurs in premature infants, or in patients with malabsorption (sprue, intestinal bypass surgery, chronic pancreatitis, cystic fibrosis) or liver disease, or in association with pharmacotherapy (mineral oil and laxative abuse, cholestyramine, neomycin). Decreased plasma vitamin A levels are also seen in association with the acute-phase response and include patients with thermal injuries, surgical trauma, and sepsis. In chronic alcohol abuse, "pseudo"–vitamin A deficiency is due to zinc deficiency, which interferes with the release of vitamin A from hepatic stores.

The symptoms of the deficiency are multisystemic in nature, with vision impairment being its chief characteristic. The earliest manifestation of deficiency is night blindness, followed by conjuctival xerosis and Bitot's spots, which are reversible with prompt intervention. Ulceration and necrosis of the cornea (keratomalacia), with perforation and endophthalmitis, occur in severe deficiency and lead to blindness. Follicular hyperkeratosis and dryness of the skin are usually present. A reduced number of goblet cells have been demonstrated in the gastrointestinal mucosa, and this has been proposed to be of importance in necrotizing enterocolitis, stress ulceration, surgical trauma, and thermal injury. Further, keratinization of epithelial tissues is thought to be associated with bronchitis and urinary tract stone formation and infection.

Dark adaptation measurements, rod scotometry, or electroretinography may be employed, when available, to confirm the clinical diagnosis. The most practical and generally accepted biochemical method used for diagnosis, however, is the determination of serum retinol; a serum concentration of less than 10 μg per dL, in conjunction with the clinical picture and history, is strongly indicative of vitamin A deficiency; serum levels of less than 20 μg per dL are considered indicative of marginal vitamin A status. It should nevertheless be borne in mind that serum levels of retinol decrease in the presence of the acute-phase response, a limitation that also applies to such newer proposed methods of assessment of vitamin A status as the modified relative dose response (MRDR) test.

Treatment and Toxicity. For practical reasons, current treatment for children older than 1 year of age and adults, except for women of childbearing age, consists of the oral administration of 200,000 IU on 2 consecutive days, followed by a similar dose every

6 months. Half this dose is administered to children under 1 year of age. These doses are well tolerated, with a reported prevalence of toxicity of less than 2%. Dietary diversification and promotion of breast-feeding should form part of the longer-term treatment; targeted supplementation and food fortification have been implemented as preventive strategies with varying success. However, vitamin A supplements may and do induce acute and/or chronic toxicity in well-nourished individuals. In fact, toxicity has been reported with as low a supplemental vitamin A dose as 5000 IU taken over a prolonged period.

Special attention should be paid to supplements during pregnancy because of the congenital malformations that have been reported with daily doses of 25,000 to 50,000 IU. For women of childbearing age, the currently recommended safe supplementary dose ranges from 5000 to 10,000 IU daily. Patients with chronic renal failure and women on oral contraceptives as a rule do not need supplements because of their elevated plasma levels of retinol-binding protein.

Toxicity presents with anorexia, nausea, vomiting, headache, weight loss, pseudotumor cerebri, muscle and bone pains, muscle fasciculation, pruritus, paresthesia, dry skin, desquamative dermatitis, alopecia, hypercalcemia, and hepatotoxicity; in neonates, irritability, drowsiness, vomiting, and bulging of fontanelles are seen. Most of the symptoms subside within a few weeks following discontinuation of the supplements. Caution is recommended against the use of high-dose beta-carotene supplements until the long-term safety has been fully established. In this regard, a significantly higher (18%) prevalence of lung cancer and cancer mortality has recently been reported in the alpha-tocopherol and beta-carotene cancer prevention trial in Finland among smokers receiving beta-carotene supplements (20 mg).

VITAMIN D DEFICIENCY

Vitamin D exists in nature in one of two major forms: vitamin D_2 (ergocalciferol), which is formed by the ultraviolet (UV) irradiation of the plant sterol, ergosterol; or vitamin D_3 (cholecalciferol), which is formed by the UV irradiation of 7-dehydrocholesterol in the skin of animals. Although classified as a vitamin, vitamin D should be regarded instead as a pro-hormone, as the normal diet contains only small amounts, which are usually insufficient to meet nutritional requirements. Further, vitamin D is biologically inactive until hydroxylated in the liver and the kidney, after which the metabolite has actions on a number of tissues.

The first step in the activation pathway of vitamin D takes place in the liver, where it is hydroxylated to 25-hydroxyvitamin D (25-OHD). This latter compound is the major circulating form of the vitamin, and its serum concentration is a good indicator of the vitamin D status of an individual. The final hydroxylation step occurs in the proximal tubule of the kidney, where 25-OHD is converted to 1,25-dihydroxyvitamin D (1,25-$(OH)_2D$) or 24,25-dihydroxyvitamin D (24,25-$(OH)_2D$) under the influence of parathyroid hormone and serum phosphate concentrations.

At physiologic concentrations, 1,25-$(OH)_2D$ is thought to be the only active metabolite of vitamin D. It plays a major role in serum calcium homeostasis, through increasing intestinal absorption of calcium and the mobilization of mineral from bone. In situations of increased calcium demands associated with a fall in ionized calcium concentrations, increased parathyroid hormone secretion stimulates the formation of 1,25-$(OH)_2D$, with the resultant increase in calcium absorption from the intestinal tract and an increase in bone resorption thus correcting the hypocalcemia.

A deficiency of vitamin D manifests biochemically with features of disturbed calcium homeostasis (low serum calcium and phosphorus concentrations, and elevated serum alkaline phosphatase and parathyroid hormone levels), whereas clinically vitamin D deficiency presents typically as rickets or osteomalacia, although features of hypocalcemia and myopathy may also be present.

Vitamin D deficiency classically results either from inadequate formation of vitamin D in the skin or from a dietary lack of vitamin D. Unless foods are vitamin D–fortified, meeting the nutritional requirements for vitamin D by dietary means is difficult; thus most individuals are dependent on the formation of vitamin D in the skin to meet the metabolic requirements.

Consequently, vitamin D deficiency is most prevalent in persons at the two extremes of life: in the first year of life prior to the infant being able to walk outdoors, and in the geriatric age group, in whom illness and infirmity confine individuals indoors. Other factors that predispose to the development of vitamin D deficiency include decreased intestinal absorption from intestinal malabsorption syndromes (e.g., celiac disease) and gastric surgery, low dietary calcium intake or impaired calcium absorption as might occur in vegetarianism or high-phytate-containing diets, increased vitamin D catabolism (due to drugs such as anticonvulsant medication), and decreased cutaneous vitamin D synthesis due to a decrease in the substrate 7-dehydrocholesterol that occurs with aging.

Clinical and biochemical features similar to those of vitamin D deficiency are also typical of a number of conditions in which there is a failure to form the active metabolite 1,25-$(OH)_2D$, despite an adequate intake of vitamin D and normal levels of 25-OHD. This occurs in renal failure or in vitamin D–dependency rickets type 1. Recently, a similar picture has also been described from genetic abnormalities of the intracellular vitamin D receptor (hereditary hypocalcemic vitamin D–resistant rickets).

The RDA for vitamin D is 400 IU (10 μg) for children and 200 IU for adults. A higher intake of vitamin D (800 to 1000 IU) has been recommended for premature infants during their hospitalization, as they are prone to develop rickets due to a number of factors, including vitamin D deficiency and lack of dietary calcium and/or phosphorus.

Characteristically, vitamin D deficiency is a disease of populations living in countries of high latitude, where during the winter months very little UV radiation reaches the earth, or of communities whose social customs, such as purdah, preclude UV exposure of the skin. Considerable strides have been made in reducing the prevalence of vitamin D deficiency in at-risk communities or groups either by fortifying foods such as milk with vitamin D (400 IU per quart as in the United States) or by providing vitamin D supplements. In a number of countries, mothers are encouraged to provide vitamin D supplements (400 IU per day) to breast-fed infants. In some Eastern European countries, regular oral doses of vitamin D (200,000 to 600,000 IU every 4 to 6 months) (Stoss Therapy) are recommended to prevent vitamin D deficiency in infants, although some studies have documented transient hypercalcemia following the use of high doses of vitamin D.

In healthy individuals, vitamin D supplements are probably unnecessary, as vitamin D synthesis in the skin in response to UV irradiation is very efficient. Only the face and hands need to be exposed to summer sunshine for a short period each day to maintain an adequate vitamin D status. Like other fat-soluble vitamins, vitamin D is stored in the body, thus stores can be built up during summer to last over the winter months.

Treatment. Treatment of vitamin D deficiency has two major objectives: first, to correct the underlying deficiency of vitamin D, and second, to correct the acute symptoms of hypocalcemia if they should be present.

In situations of privational vitamin D deficiency (due to a lack of sunlight or dietary intake) vitamin D, 1000 to 5000 IU (25 to 125 μg) per day for 6 to 8 weeks, rapidly corrects the abnormality. Biochemically, early signs of response to therapy include a rise in serum phosphorus and calcium values, which should occur within 1 to 2 weeks. Serum alkaline phosphatase concentrations, which are already elevated, may rise further on initiation of therapy and take many months to return to normal; thus, they are not a useful measure of the early response to therapy. Radiologic evidence of response to therapy may be seen within 2 to 4 weeks in children with rickets, but it may take much longer in adults with osteomalacia.

An adequate calcium intake should be ensured during the treatment of vitamin D deficiency. In infants and children, a calcium intake of between 800 and 1000 mg per day is recommended; adults should ingest between 1000 and 1500 mg. Hypocalcemia, if it manifests clinically (as in convulsions or tetany), should be managed as a medical emergency.

In the treatment of privational vitamin D deficiency, there is no advantage in using the newer vitamin D analogues or metabolites over the parent compound, as the oral administration of vitamin D leads to a rapid and sustained rise in serum levels of 1,25-$(OH)_2$D. However, if intestinal malabsorption is a factor, then parenteral vitamin D could be considered in the place of large doses of vitamin D (10,000 to 25,000 IU daily) orally. Water-soluble forms of vitamin D are available in some countries and may be of value in managing vitamin D deficiency in patients with fat malabsorption. In malabsorption disorders, care should be taken to address possible associated calcium and/or magnesium deficiencies, which might delay the response to vitamin D therapy.

A clinical and biochemical picture similar to that of vitamin D deficiency may be seen in a number of conditions associated with abnormalities of vitamin D metabolism or action.

VITAMIN E DEFICIENCY

Vitamin E is widely distributed in plant and animal foods; some of the richer dietary sources include vegetable oils, margarine, beans, nuts, cereals, and whole grain products. There are eight naturally occurring tocopherols, of which alpha-tocopherol is biologically the most active. The percentage of the vitamin absorbed is inversely related to the dose administered; absorption is maximal in the middle portion of the small bowel and depends on the presence of fat bile salts. Once in the bloodstream, the vitamin is associated with chylomicrons and beta-lipoproteins. Body stores are considered to be large, and plasma levels do not decline until months after a deficient diet is instituted. The RDA, in milligrams of alpha-tocopherol equivalents (1 mg α-TE = 1 mg d-α-tocopherol), for infants is 3 to 4; for children 1 to 10 years of age, 6 to 7; and 10 and 8 for male and female adults, respectively. Pregnancy increases requirements to 10 and lactation to 11 to 12 mg α-TE. Selenium is known to have a sparing effect on vitamin E requirements.

The lipid-soluble antioxidant properties of the vitamin relate to its function in preventing lipid peroxidation of unsaturated fatty acids in cell membranes. In this regard, increased erythrocyte fragility has been demonstrated in subjects consuming a vitamin E–deficient diet and also in newborn infants, especially those born prematurely and/or with low (less than 1500 grams) birthweight. Vitamin E is also thought to be important in the development and maintenance of nerve function as well as in prostaglandin synthesis.

In the absence of disease, vitamin E status can be generally assumed to be adequate. However, increased susceptibility to deficiency has been documented in patients with gastrointestinal disorders (gastrectomy, biliary atresia, liver disease, cystic fibrosis, chronic pancreatitis, pancreatic malignancy, gluten enteropathy, regional enteritis), in abetalipoproteinemia, and in premature infants. The totality of evidence in the future will better define the role of vitamin E status, together with other antioxidant vitamins, in the prevention of chronic degenerative diseases. However, a daily oral intake of 100 IU has been shown to be beneficial, but the long-term safety of such a dose is not known.

Clinical vitamin E deficiency has not been demonstrated in normal people but has been described in pathologic conditions. Apart from oxidant-induced increased erythrocyte fragility, other manifestations include muscle weakness, ataxia, decreased reflexes, ophthalmoplegia, decreased proprioceptive and vibratory sense, degeneration of the posterior columns of the spinal cord, and loss of large-caliber myelinated axons in peripheral nerves. In premature infants, the reported association between vitamin E deficiency and such conditions as retrolental fibroplasia, bronchopulmonary dysplasia, necrotizing enterocolitis, and hemorrhagic tendency is in need of better definition.

Plasma vitamin E concentration is currently the most widely used method of assessing status (less than 6.0 μg per mL is suggestive of deficiency and more than 11 μg per mL, optimal status). The additional use of the ratio of serum vitamin E to total lipids (normal range, 0.6 to 0.8 mg per gram) affords greater specificity in identifying vitamin E deficiency.

Treatment. The treatment of deficiency is usually in the form of oral supplements. Although a variety of therapeutic doses have been used, daily supplements of 25 IU in infants, 50 to 100 IU in 1- to 10-year-old children, 100 IU in 11- to 18-year-olds, and 200 IU in adults have proved adequate. High doses of vitamin E are better tolerated than those of other fat-soluble vitamins. However, good data on the long-term safety of pharmacologic doses of the vitamin are needed; fatigue, muscular weakness, creatinuria, and elevated serum creatinine, thyroid hormone, and fasting serum triglyceride levels have been reported. Moreover, high doses may act antagonistically to coumarin anticoagulants and can exacerbate coagulation defects in vitamin K–deficient individuals.

VITAMIN K DEFICIENCY

method of
MAMMO AMARE, M.D., and
JOHN V. COX, D.O.
Texas Oncology, P.A.
Dallas, Texas

Vitamin K exists in two natural forms differing from one another in the structure of their side chains. Phylloquinone (vitamin K_1) is mainly found in green plants, and the menaquinones (vitamin K_2), which include a spectrum of molecular forms, are produced by intestinal flora. Menadione (vitamin K_3) is a synthetic vitamin that is converted in the liver to vitamin K_2.

Vitamin K is a cofactor in the gamma carboxylation of a diverse group of proteins present in various tissues. The most widely known vitamin K–dependent proteins are the four clotting factors—Factors II, IX, X, and VII—and the natural inhibitors of coagulation proteins C and S. After being assembled in the liver as inert precursor molecules, these coagulation factors undergo post-translational modi-

fications in hepatocytes including a unique vitamin K–dependent gamma carboxylation of specific glutamic acid residues. Gamma-carboxyglutamic acid confers metal-binding properties to the proteins, which, in the presence of calcium, attach to cell membranes, especially platelet surfaces, where they form complexes with other clotting factors to carry out their biologic activity.

The carboxylase that catalyzes the gamma carboxylation of vitamin K–dependent proteins requires a steady supply of reduced vitamin K, derived from two sources. First, vitamin K obtained from the diet and intestinal bacteria is reduced in the liver by hydroquinone reductase to functionally active vitamin K hydroquinone. Second, during the process of carboxylation, reduced vitamin K is oxidized to vitamin K epoxide. A liver microsomal epoxide reductase then converts vitamin K epoxide to vitamin K quinone, which is reduced and recycled in the carboxylation process. Oral anticoagulants produce their effect by inhibiting vitamin K reductases, particularly epoxide reductase. Inhibition of the reductases depletes reduced vitamin K and curtails gamma carboxylation of the vitamin K–dependent clotting factors, which accumulate as nonfunctional uncarboxylated forms, collectively known as "protein induced by vitamin k antagonists" (PIVKAs).

Vitamin K is also necessary for the functional integrity of noncollagenous proteins, particularly osteocalcin, important for bone formation. Hence the distinct chondrodysplasia seen in infants born to women exposed to warfarin during early pregnancy is believed to be due to the drug-induced vitamin K deficiency leading to the formation of defective hypocarboxylated osteocalcin. A similar embryopathy has been described in an infant with a congenital absence of vitamin K epoxide reductase, the enzyme selectively inhibited by warfarin, in the liver.

The daily requirement of vitamin K is unknown, but it is generally recommended that adults consume 70 to 200 μg per day. Green leafy vegetables such as spinach, broccoli, brussels sprouts, and lettuce are important sources of phylloquinone, which accounts for the major portion of the vitamin normally found in the liver. Menaquinones (vitamin K_2) synthesized by intestinal bacteria may be additional sources of the vitamin.

The precise mechanisms of absorption of vitamin K are not fully understood. Dietary vitamin K_1, phylloquinone, is mainly absorbed from the proximal small bowel in the presence of bile salts. Animal studies have shown that menaquinones may be absorbed by simple diffusion in the distal ileum and the colon. Recent observations, however, suggest that a bile-mediated absorption from the terminal ileum may be more important. Once absorbed, vitamin K is mostly transported by chylomicrons via lymphatics to its primary storage site in the liver. The storage pool is small and may be depleted within days to weeks.

CAUSES OF VITAMIN K DEFICIENCY

The major categories of vitamin K deficiency are listed in Table 1. Sensitive assays indicate that poor dietary intake leads to a progressive depletion of vitamin K, despite the lack of clinically overt vitamin deficiency. When poor intake coexists with a reduced endogenous bacterial source, clinical deficiency occurs more rapidly. The contribution of menaquinones to the overall body store of vitamin K remains controversial, and it is uncertain if selective depletion of menaquinones results in clinically significant vitamin K deficiency. The hypoprothrombinemic coagulopathy seen with certain antibiotics that contain the methyltetrazole thiol (e.g., aztreonam, cefoperazone) results

TABLE 1. **Causes of Vitamin K Deficiency**

Decreased ingestion
   Poor dietary intake
Decreased endogenous (intestinal) production
Impaired absorption
   Obstructive biliary disease
   Intrinsic intestinal disease; short bowel syndrome
Impaired utilization
   Oral anticoagulant
   Anticonvulsant

from direct inhibition of vitamin K rather than from alteration in the intestinal flora.

Diseases associated with disruption of bile flow to the intestinal lumen (e.g., obstructive biliary disease) and malabsorptive disorders due to intrinsic small intestinal disease or short-bowel syndrome lead to vitamin K deficiency of variable severity within days or weeks.

Vitamin K antagonists block the conversion of vitamin K to its biologically active reduced form (see earlier), in effect producing a vitamin K–deficiency state.

HEMORRHAGIC DISEASE OF NEWBORN

Hemmorrhagic disease of the newborn (HDN) is a self-limited but at times fatal bleeding disorder caused by deficiency of vitamin K–dependent factors. Three clinical forms are known: early, classic, and late. Early HDN occurs within the first 24 hours of birth and is frequently associated with exposure of the mother to vitamin K antagonists such as warfarin or anticonvulsants. Classic HDN has its onset in the first 7 to 14 days after birth. Bleeding commonly occurs from the skin, gastrointestinal tract, and circumcision site. Inadequate intake, poor transplacental transfer of vitamin K, a lack of intestinal bacteria, and immaturity of the liver may contribute to the negative vitamin K balance. Late HDN becomes manifest between 2 and 12 weeks after birth and is associated with a higher incidence of intracranial bleeding.

LABORATORY TESTS

The prothrombin time (PT) and activated partial thromboplastin time (aPTT) are standard screening tests for coagulopathy of vitamin K deficiency. Prolongation of the PT occurs early, and abnormality of the aPTT indicates a more severe deficiency. Correction of the PT and aPTT when the patient's plasma is mixed with an equal volume of normal plasma confirms the deficiency of factor(s) and excludes the presence of inhibitor. Direct measurement of individual vitamin K–dependent clotting factors shows a variable decrease in the functional activities of Factors II, VII, IX, and X, and proteins C and S.

Routine laboratory tests do not discriminate between early hepatocellular disease and vitamin K deficiency. The distinction can be made by measuring both factor activity and antigen level. Vitamin K deficiency shows a decreased factor activity and a normal antigen level, whereas liver disease is manifested by a proportional decrease in the antigen and functional activity level. "Ecarin test" provides similar information. Ecarin, a snake venom, converts normal and uncarboxylated prothrombin molecules to thrombin. The test is normal in vitamin K deficiency and prolonged in liver disease. Diagnosis of the coagulopathy induced by the accidental ingestion or surreptitious use of warfarin may require measurement of the plasma drug level.

PREVENTION

The routine administration of vitamin K_1, 0.5 to 1 mg parenterally or 2 to 5 mg orally, to newborn babies has significantly reduced the incidence of HDN. Repeated doses may be necessary with oral prophylaxis.

Patients with poor oral intake or on long-term parenteral nutrition benefit from vitamin K supplementation, especially if they are concurrently receiving a broad-spectrum antibiotic. In patients with malabsorption syndrome the periodic (every 1 to 4 weeks) administration of vitamin K_1, 5 to 10 mg intramuscularly or subcutaneously, is appropriate. When clinically applicable, oral vitamin K, 5 to 10 mg daily, may be used.

TREATMENT

The treatment of the coagulopathy caused by vitamin K deficiency is dependent on the site and severity of the bleeding. For a patient who has active bleeding or needs an immediate correction of the coagulopathy, the therapeutic options include fresh-frozen plasma (FFP) and/or vitamin K replacement. FFP is usually reserved for life-threatening bleeding and is infrequently used for surgical emergencies when prompt control of the coagulopathy is critical. It is administered at a dose of 15 to 20 mL per kg of body weight together with parenteral vitamin K. If the PT remains prolonged at 6 to 8 hours, a second dose may be necessary. FFP carries the risk of viral transmission and should be used with caution.

Vitamin K_1 (AquaMEPHYTON), 5 to 10 mg intramuscularly, is sufficient to correct the PT within 6 to 24 hours. An identical dose of intravenous vitamin K_1 is used if there is a contraindication to intramuscular injection or if a more rapid correction of the coagulopathy is desired. Intravenous vitamin K has been associated with anaphylactic reaction and should be given with care after the necessary precautions are taken. Oral vitamin K (Mephyton), 10 to 20 mg, may be used for less severe bleeding.

In a patient on oral anticoagulant therapy, withholding the drug corrects the prolonged PT and PTT within hours to days. In contrast, treatment of the coagulopathy caused by ingestion of long-acting "superwarfarins" (e.g., brodifacoum) may require the administration of high daily doses of vitamin K_1 over weeks to months for normalization of the PT.

OSTEOPOROSIS

method of
MARCELA FISHER-TABUENCA, M.D., and
DAVID J. BAYLINK, M.D.
Loma Linda University
Loma Linda, California

Osteoporosis is a metabolic bone disease characterized by a generalized decrease in bone density, which results in increased susceptibility to fragility fractures. This disease afflicts more than 20 million people, mostly women, in the United States, at a total cost of approximately $10 billion a year.

Osteoporosis can be classified as either primary or secondary. Primary osteoporosis includes postmenopausal osteoporosis (type 1) and senile osteoporosis (type 2). Although the causes of primary osteoporosis are not completely understood, it is by far the most common type. Secondary osteoporosis is marked by a low bone density due to acquired or inherited disorders.

The principles of prevention and treatment of primary osteoporosis in women apply as well to men and to both sexes with secondary osteoporosis. The goal of the therapeutic program is to prevent future fractures.

THERAPEUTIC PRINCIPLES

1. Patients with calcium malabsorption must be treated with either large amounts of calcium or with 1,25-vitamin D (calcitriol).

2. Patients with high urine calcium or a history of kidney stones should be given calcium supplements with caution.

3. All patients should be placed on an exercise program that should include walking as well as upper body exercise, within the limits of the patient's disability.

4. Patients with a high bone resorption rate, as determined by biochemical markers, should be placed on antiresorptive therapy, such as estrogen replacement, etidronate (Didronel),* or calcitonin.

5. A patient who has a bone density below the fracture threshold should be referred to a treatment center where fluoride therapy will be available.

6. If the patient has bone pain, injectable calcitonin should be considered.

THERAPEUTIC STRATEGIES

The first step in selecting the most appropriate therapy is to measure the spinal bone density (Figure 1) to determine whether the patient has osteopenia or osteoporosis.

Spinal bone density can be measured by either dual-energy roentgenographic absorptiometry (DXA) or quantitative computed tomography (QCT). The fracture threshold has been defined for both these approaches: 100 mg per mL for QCT; 0.80 mg per cm² for Hologic DXA; and 0.74 gram per cm² for Lunar DXA†. DXA can also be applied to measure hip bone density, which is a useful alternative site if the patient has severe spinal degenerative joint disease that can spuriously increase the spinal bone density.

Measurements of the spine can give the following densities of bone:

---

*Etidronate (Didronel) has been approved by the FDA for the treatment of Paget's disease, but not for the treatment of osteoporosis. Thus, our use of etidronate is acknowledged as an off-label use.

†Fracture threshold for QCT varies in different laboratories from about 70 to 100 mg per mL.

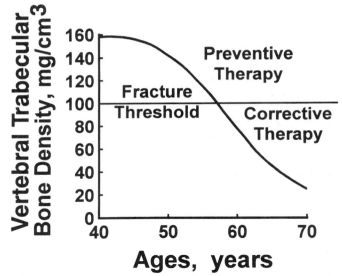

Figure 1. Schema of quantitative computed tomography (QCT) for spinal bone density as a function of age. This schematic model illustrates our strategy for treating patients on the basis of their bone density. Those subjects with bone densities above the fracture threshold are treated with preventive therapy, and those subjects with densities below the fracture threshold are treated with both preventive and corrective therapies.

1. Bone density that is above the fracture threshold and within 1.5 standard deviations of peak bone density (normal).

2. Bone density that is above the fracture threshold but is 1.5 standard deviations or more below the peak bone density (osteopenia).

3. Bone density that is below the fracture threshold (osteoporosis).

Preventive Therapy

If the patient has normal bone density, we recommend preventive therapy using estrogen, adequate calcium intake, and exercise (Figure 2). Preventive therapy is also recommended for patients with osteopenia or osteoporosis. Patients with osteoporosis require corrective as well as preventive therapy. To ensure prevention of further bone loss in these patients, we recommend screening for calcium malabsorption, hypercalciuria, and increased bone resorption, with corrective action(s) as appropriate.

Exercise. Based on recent studies, the exercise protocol we recommend includes walking 2 miles daily and engaging in some type of upper body exercise, such as weight-lifting. For example, in a standing position with the back extended, the patient holds a 1- to 2-pound weight in each hand and lifts them over the head. Eventually, the patient should use 5-pound weights in each hand for this type of exercise. It is emphasized that all exercise should be designed to avoid injury.

Evaluation of Calcium Absorption. The prevalence of calcium malabsorption is unknown but is expected to be relatively high in patients over 70 years of age, since the efficiency of calcium absorp-

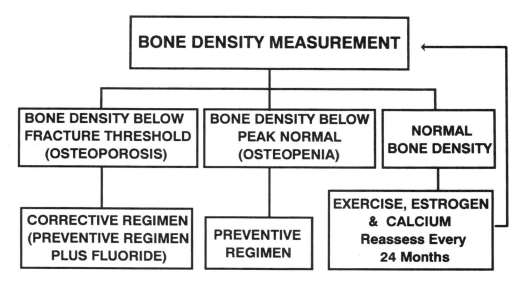

Figure 2. Algorithm for the treatment of osteopenia and osteoporosis (see text).

tion declines with age, and the serum parathyroid hormone (PTH) increases with age. To assess calcium absorption, a 24-hour urine specimen for calcium determination is collected while the patient is on a total (diet plus supplements) calcium intake of 1500 mg a day for at least 1 week. (In patients with either known primary hyperparathyroidism or a past history of kidney stones, the 24-hour urine specimen should be collected while the patient is on a low-calcium diet of 400 mg per day.)

The rationale for this test is as follows: When the patient is on a high-calcium intake (1500 mg per day), a 24-hour urine calcium level of less than 100 mg suggests calcium malabsorption.* This level of 100 mg per day is an arbitrary value based on the facts that (1) urinary excretion of 50 mg or less of calcium per day on a regular diet containing calcium is low, reflecting calcium deficiency or vitamin D deficiency; and (2) a urinary calcium level of 100 mg per day is substantially below the upper normal limit of 250 mg per day and thus would not be associated with increased risk of renal stones. Therefore, we have defined 100 mg per day as a safe value to achieve with the calcium intake described.

Serum PTH levels may or may not be elevated above the normal range in patients with impaired calcium absorption. However, we have observed hyperparathyroidism in a surprisingly large number of osteoporotic patients, and this can be attributed to calcium deficiency in approximately 10% of our clinic population.

Patients with a low urine calcium level, even when the PTH is normal, are treated as if they had calcium malabsorption, with the exception of patients with familial hypocalciuric hypercalcemia (FHH). FHH is a rare autosomal disorder that is usually asymptomatic and that presents with a normal or slightly elevated PTH level, a low or normal urine calcium level, and a mild-to-moderate *hypercalcemia*. This disorder needs to be ruled out before calcium therapy is initiated.

The first step to correct calcium malabsorption is a measurement of serum 25-OH-vitamin D, to determine whether the malabsorption is due to classic vitamin D deficiency. In such cases, the level of 25-OH-D is below normal, and the patient should be treated with vitamin D, 50,000 U daily for 1 month. At this time, the serum 25-OH-D should be normal, and the calcium absorption test (i.e., the urine calcium in response to 1500 mg of total dietary calcium) should be repeated.

If the 25-OH-D level was normal to begin with, or if after vitamin D supplementation the urine calcium level remains below 100 mg per 24 hours, the next step is to increase the calcium intake to 2000 to 2500 mg per day. In addition, rather than using the most common forms of calcium supplements (calcium carbonate or calcium phosphate), a more soluble form of calcium (calcium citrate) may be prescribed. If increasing the dose of calcium and/or changing to a different calcium salt fails to increase the urine calcium and to decrease the serum PTH (if high) after 3 months of supplementation, calcitriol (Rocaltrol), 0.25 µg per day, along with a total (diet plus supplements) calcium intake of 800 mg per day, is prescribed. If, after 1 week on this therapy, the 24-hour urine calcium level remains below 100 mg per day, the dose of calcitriol is increased to 0.50 µg per day. Larger doses of calcitriol and/or calcium are not recommended because of the risk of hypercalcemia. To avoid hypercalcemia, patients on calcitriol therapy are monitored by measuring the serum calcium level 1 week after starting therapy (or changing the dose). Subsequently, serum and urine calcium levels are monitored every 3 to 6 months.

Evaluation of Bone Resorption. Bone resorption is assessed by 24-hour urine measurements of the hydroxyproline/creatinine. This can be measured in the same urine sample that is used for the

---

*Note that there is no clinically available test to measure calcium absorption; what we describe is a rational approach that has not been validated.

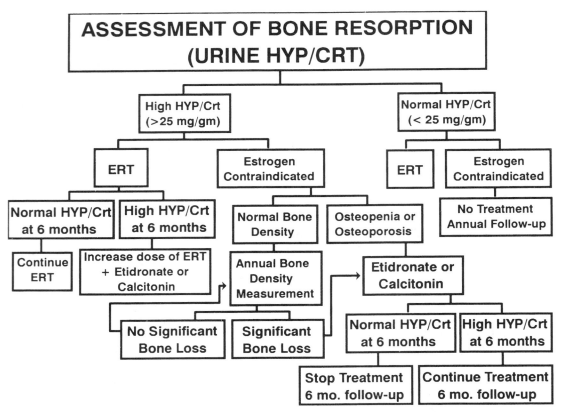

Figure 3. Algorithm for the prevention of osteoporosis by antiresorptive therapy. See text for details of how the urine hydroxyproline/ creatinine (HYP/Crt) ratio can be used to monitor the response to antiresorptive therapy. Low bone density (i.e., osteopenia) is defined as a value at least one standard deviation below the peak bone density in young, normal subjects but above the fracture threshold. *Abbreviation*: ERT = estrogen and progesterone therapy.

24-hour calcium assessment (Figure 3). Because the diet normally contains hydroxyproline, the patient is placed on a hydroxyproline-free diet for the meal prior to the day of the urine collection and the day itself.

The normal range for the urine hydroxyproline/ creatinine ratio is quite broad, and there is no general agreement about what value indicates high bone resorption. Since bone loss is not significant in premenopausal women, we have arbitrarily selected the mean of the normal premenopausal range, plus two standard deviations, as the acceptable upper limit in developing therapeutic strategies to prevent bone loss. This value is equal to 25 mg of hydroxyproline per gram of creatinine. Thus, any patient with a value greater than 25 mg per gram is considered to have increased bone resorption and to require antiresorptive therapy. In patients with severe osteoporosis, we have even greater concern for preventing further bone loss, and we attempt to achieve a hydroxyproline/creatinine value of 12.5 mg per gram, which is the premenopausal mean level.

Tests other than hydroxyproline can be used to assess bone resorption. These include measurements of the pyridinoline/creatinine (PYD/Crt) and deoxypyridinoline/creatinine (DPD/Crt) levels in urine. These tests are more accurate and more specific as indices of bone resorption than is hydroxyproline,

and, of the two, the DPD is most specific. The premenopausal mean, plus or minus two standard deviations, for PYD/Crt is 44 plus or minus 34 nanomoles per millimole, and for DPD/Crt is 10 plus or minus 9 nanomoles per millimole.

Our approach to the detection and correction of high bone resorption is summarized in Figure 3. It is important to detect elevated bone resorption, because it can be effectively treated with either estrogen replacement therapy, etidronate, injectable calcitonin, or a combination of these therapies. (It is anticipated that *nasal* calcitonin will be available in 1995.) If it is not contraindicated, estrogen is always prescribed (even to postmenopausal patients with a normal bone resorption rate), because of its positive cardiovascular actions.

Because the most rapid phase of menopausal bone loss occurs in the early stages of menopause, the earlier estrogen replacement therapy is initiated, the more effective it will be to prevent the development of osteoporosis. This also holds for the other antiresorptive agents. Although estrogen has its greatest effect in preserving bone density when given at the time of the menopause, even patients who are 70 years of age or older will benefit. However, such patients are seldom inclined to tolerate the attending menses that occur in many patients on estrogen therapy. Therefore, we frequently give etidronate or injectable calcitonin therapy to elderly osteoporotic patients with an intact uterus.

Our protocol for estrogen replacement therapy is as follows:

1. Baseline mammograms are obtained before estrogen therapy is initiated and annually thereafter.

2. The starting dose of estrogen is equivalent to 0.625 of conjugated estrogens (Premarin, Ogen). Several types of estrogens are available, including the oral (Estrace) and transdermal estradiol (Estraderm), all of which are effective in reducing bone resorption.

3. To prevent endometrial cancer, progesterone is prescribed for patients with an intact uterus. The equivalent of 2.5 mg per day of medroxyprogesterone acetate (Provera) is used. Both estrogen and progesterone are given daily in an attempt to avoid menstrual bleeding. However, bleeding still occurs in 25% of patients, which may be possible to reduce by treating for 3 weeks per month, instead of 4 weeks, with the combination therapy. (If these approaches are ineffective, a gynecologist should be consulted.)

4. Patients who have undergone hysterectomy are not given progesterone.

5. Patients who have a history of either breast or uterine cancer are not treated with estrogen unless so advised following consultation with their gynecologist.

Although we employ a dose of 0.625 mg per day of conjugated estrogens at the beginning of therapy, we have found that this dose is not adequate in all patients to reduce the bone resorption rate to the premenopausal value. With estrogen therapy, the nadir for the change in urine hydroxyproline/creatinine is at about 6 months. At this time, if we do not find a normal (premenopausal) bone resorption level, we either increase the dose of estrogen or, if this is not tolerated, add another antiresorptive agent at a low dose and re-evaluate after another 6 months of therapy. It is emphasized that, because the time-dependent variation in the urine hydroxyproline/creatinine assay is large, the physician should make therapeutic decisions based on two or more similar results.

When estrogen is contraindicated or ineffective at the highest tolerated dose—for example, some patients complain of breast tenderness at high doses of estrogen—we use either etidronate or injectable calcitonin. The recommended dose of etidronate (Didronel) is 400 mg daily for 2 weeks out of 12 weeks. It has not as yet been established that this dose is effective for all patients. It is not known when the nadir for hydroxyproline/creatinine is reached on this therapeutic regimen, so we suggest sampling at 6-month intervals after commencing therapy. Although it may be necessary to use higher doses (i.e., more continuous treatment) of etidronate to achieve a premenopausal urine hydroxyproline/creatinine level, this should be done with some caution, since larger doses of etidronate may cause osteomalacia. If higher doses are used, etidronate should still be given intermittently to allow for healing of any osteomalacia

that could be caused by etidronate. It is also recommended that etidronate be taken on an empty stomach, no food for 2 hours before or for 2 hours after the dose, since it is poorly absorbed and any calcium in the gastrointestinal tract will precipitate the etidronate. Side effects of this therapy are minor; we have observed only an occasional complaint of lower gastrointestinal discomfort.

The other alternative agent for antiresorptive therapy is injectable salmon calcitonin (Miacalcin, Calcimar). The dose we use is 50 U subcutaneously daily for 3 of every 4 months. The recommended dose is 100 U daily. We are concerned that high daily injections may cause resistance. Thus, we give lower, cyclical doses. Some experts prescribe even less drug (e.g., 50 U three times weekly instead of daily). However, the theoretical advantage of these therapeutic regimens using less than 100 U per day of calcitonin has not been experimentally validated. The nadir for the urine hydroxyproline/creatinine level following calcitonin therapy is at approximately 3 months, at which time the dose can be adjusted as necessary.

Corrective Therapy

In those patients with established osteoporosis (i.e., bone density below the fracture threshold and/or fragility fractures), prevention of bone loss by antiresorptive therapy as just described is insufficient to eliminate the fracture risk. Ideally, these patients should be treated with both preventive therapy and an agent that stimulates bone formation. Unfortunately, there are no FDA-approved agents that stimulate bone formation. The agent we use for this purpose is fluoride, in the form of monofluorophosphate, at a dose of 20 mg of elemental fluoride per day. Although the use of fluoride as a treatment for osteoporosis has been approved in Europe and South America, it has not received general acceptance in the United States because of the conflicting results obtained with fluoride therapy. Some clinical studies have found that fluoride therapy has significant side effects and thus poor antifracture efficacy, whereas other studies have shown very few side effects, together with significant antifracture efficacy. We believe that whether side effects occur and whether antifracture efficacy is seen very much depend on the dose of fluoride employed and whether the patient has adequate calcium absorption (e.g., a fluoride-induced increase in bone formation can cause significant calcium deficiency in a patient with poor calcium absorption). In practical terms, the information on fluoride emphasizes that the management of fluoride therapy is somewhat complicated, and therefore, we recommend that patients who require a stimulator of bone formation be referred for evaluation to a center that is authorized to use fluoride.

Treatment of Vertebral Compression Fractures

Patients who sustain an atraumatic spinal compression fracture that is attended by substantial pain should be at bed rest with bathroom privileges for a minimum of 3 to 4 days. Analgesics should be used as needed. In addition, injectable calcitonin at a dose of 100 U per day may substantially reduce the pain. If the calcitonin skin test is positive, the patient should not receive calcitonin therapy. The potential side effects of the injectable calcitonin are flushing and nausea. If this occurs, the dose should be reduced to 50 U per day. If the lower dose is tolerated, then the dose can be gradually increased to 100 U per day.

PAGET'S DISEASE OF BONE

method of
LORRAINE A. FITZPATRICK, M.D.
Mayo Clinic and Mayo Foundation
Rochester, Minnesota

Paget's disease is a localized focal disorder of bone remodeling. Paget's disease is common, and it has been estimated that 3% of people in the United States over age 55 years have Paget's disease. There are interesting geographic, ethnic, and genetic data that lend insight into the possible etiology of Paget's disease. Genetic analysis suggests an autosomal dominant pattern of inheritance, and 15 to 30% of patients with Paget's disease have positive family histories of the disorder. Paget's disease is seven times more likely to develop in a person with a family history of the disorder. Other data have suggested an increased frequency of specific HLA antigens in patients with Paget's disease.

Ethnic and geographic data provide further understanding of the nature of the disorder. The disease is most common in Europe, North America, Australia, and New Zealand. Prevalence rates in England in patients over 55 years of age have been estimated at 4.6%. Prevalence rates decrease when moving from north to south in Europe, and Paget's disease is distinctly rare in Asia. Prevalence rates are very low in areas of sub-Saharan Africa and select areas of the Middle East. In general, most Americans with Paget's disease are white and Anglo-Saxon or European descent. Paget's disease has been described in African Americans, but the actual prevalence of the disease is unknown.

The hallmark of the disease is an increase in bone remodeling, resulting in a mosaic of woven and lamellar bone and increased vascularity. The osteoclast is enlarged and may contain over 100 nuclei. The initial abnormality involves a marked increase in the rate of bone resorption at localized sites. In the early osteolytic stages, resorption progresses and may result in decreased trabecular volume. In response to the rapid resorption, recruitment of osteoblasts occurs, and new bone formation is initiated. The haphazard arrangement of the collagen fibrils results in woven bone, and numerous osteoblasts line formation surfaces. This phase is often termed the osteoblastic or "mixed" phase of the disorder. In the final stages, dense bone is present and cellular activity is reduced. This osteosclerotic phase is termed the "burned out" phase of the disorder. In an individual, lytic and blastic lesions often occur at adjacent sites.

ETIOLOGY

Sir James Paget named the disorder "osteitis deformans" and suggested that the disease was due to inflammatory and infectious processes. The etiology of Paget's disease remains unclear, and there are several interesting observations that have provided intriguing theories about its pathogenesis. Some data support a viral etiology. Inclusions that resemble viral nucleocapsids have been described in the nuclei and cytoplasm of osteoclasts at sites of pagetic involvement. The particles resemble members of the paramyxovirus family, which includes respiratory syncytial (RS), measles, and canine distemper viruses. It was proposed that Paget's disease was due to a slow viral infection of bone, and this hypothesis is consistent with the long clinically latent period. Other data in support of a viral etiology include increased measles antibodies in subjects with Paget's disease, but this finding was not confirmed in some studies. Cultures of bone biopsy specimens revealed immunologic evidence of measles and RS virus antigens in pagetic bone. Studies utilizing in situ hybridization have lent support to the concept that paramyxoviruses may be present in the bone cells of affected patients. These studies are not entirely specific, and further confirmation is necessary to prove the hypothesis. Utilizing reverse-transcriptase polymerase chain reaction, transcripts encoding for canine distemper virus were detected in bone cells obtained from a group of patients from northwest England. Other investigators have not confirmed this finding. Further evidence for a viral etiology was suggested in a study that evaluated long-term human marrow cell cultures from affected and unaffected patients. Measles viral transcripts were detected in precursor cells, and these cells form osteoclasts at a more rapid rate than normal osteoclast precursors. Increased levels of interleukin-6 and interleukin-6 receptor mRNA have been detected in pagetic bone, and IL-6 may represent an autocrine or paracrine factor associated with the aberrant remodeling seen in Paget's disease. Other investigators have described abnormalities in matrix production by osteoblasts obtained from patients with Paget's disease.

DIAGNOSIS

Paget's disease may be asymptomatic and detected by an increase in serum alkaline phosphastase (bone origin) on a chemistry panel. This parameter reflects the increased bone formation in patients with the disorder and is the most commonly used test for patient monitoring. Urinary hydroxyproline—or the newer biochemical markers of bone resorption, urinary deoxypyridinoline and pyridinoline—is also elevated, reflecting the rapid rate of bone resorption. These indices rise in proportion to each other, and the severity of the disease is usually reflected in the degree of abnormality. These tests are useful to monitor the progress of the disease and the response to therapy, although the serum alkaline phosphatase is usually the most convenient measurement of disease activity. Serum osteocalcin measurements are usually less sensitive than those of serum bone-specific alkaline phosphatase. Serum calcium is usually normal but may become elevated in a patient with Paget's disease who becomes immobilized or has coexisting hyperparathyroidism. There is a 15 to 20% incidence of secondary hyperparathyroidism with normal serum calcium levels and increased parathyroid hormone levels. This phenomenon is due to the increased calcium need during rapid bone formation.

Paget's disease affects both men and women, with a slight male predominance. Paget's disease is most common in subjects over the age of 55 years and rarely occurs before age 25. The disorder may be monostotic or polyostotic; sites are usually asymmetrical. The most commonly involved sites are the pelvis, femur, spine, skull, and tibia (Table 1). Bones of the upper extremity are less often involved, and bones of the hand and feet are rarely affected. Presentation may be variable, and frequently an asymptomatic patient comes to the attention of a physician because of the typical appearance on a radiograph taken for some other indication or the elevated serum alkaline phosphatase noted on a routine chemistry panel.

Bone pain is the most common symptom and occurs at rest or with motion. The pain is nonspecific and is often described as a "dull ache" that may occur at night. The pain may be due to the increased vascularity, microfractures, small lucencies associated with expanded cortices of weight-bearing bones, or the lytic, blade-of-grass lesion. Deformity of the femur or tibia can produce pain, and it may be difficult to distinguish whether the pain is due to the pagetic process or to osteoarthritis of the joints adjacent to the pagetic bone. Involvement of the spine can cause severe kyphosis, vertebral compression fractures, nonspecific aches, and spinal cord compression with sensory and motor changes. A vascular steal syndrome has also been noted in cases of neurologic deficit. Changes in the skull include an increase in head size or frontal bossing. Some patients complain of a headache that feels like a band tightened around the head. Hearing loss may be due to isolated or combined conductive or neurosensory abnormalities. Rarely, platybasia with basilar invagination can lead to more serious complications with obstructive hydrocephalus or brain stem compression. Other complications of skull involvement include tinnitus, vertigo, and a "rushing" sound in the head. Visual loss may be due to angioid streaks or optic nerve compression. Oral pathology may result in loss of teeth and facial deformity. Gait disturbance may represent bone involvement, with deformity due to Paget's disease, osteoarthritis of the involved or uninvolved side, or altered weight bearing due to pain.

Metabolically active pagetic bone is highly vascular and can lead to a high cardiac output and congestive heart failure. The increased blood flow can produce palpable warmth in the involved area. Patients with Paget's disease have a higher incidence of calcific aortic stenosis. Gout, pseudogout, and nephrolithiasis are increased in incidence, and osteoarthritis is common.

Atraumatic or pathologic fracture of pagetic bone may occur and is a serious complication of the disease. The most common site of fracture is the femoral shaft or subtrochanteric area. The increased vascularity of the site may lead to substantial blood loss, and nonunion has been estimated at 10 to 40%. Fractures may herald the development of malignant degeneration.

Neoplastic degeneration is a rare complication and occurs in less than 1% of cases. Clinical presentation is frequently that of pain at a new site, and the prognosis is grave. The tumor may be classified as osteogenic sarcoma, fibrosarcoma, or chondrosarcoma. Pulmonary metastasis or disease extension limits life expectancy to 1 to 3 years, even with aggressive treatment.

Diagnosis is usually confirmed by the typical radiographic appearance and elevated biochemical markers. Bone scans are a sensitive method of identifying sites of involvement but are nonspecific and can reflect degenerative changes unrelated to Paget's disease or metastatic disease. Radiographs of the involved areas confirm the sites of involvement by their pathognomonic appearance. Enlargement or expansion of the bone, coarsening of trabecular markings, and lytic or sclerotic changes may be noted. Skull involvement may be reflected by a "cotton-wool" appearance or osteoporosis circumscripta. Once the diagnosis is confirmed, repeat scans or radiographs are indicated when new symptoms occur or with exacerbation of current symptoms. Bone biopsy is indicated if malignant transformation or metastatic tumor to bone is suspected.

TREATMENT

Treatment is indicated for relief of symptoms and to prevent future complications. Symptoms include bone pain, headache due to skull involvement, radiculopathy due to nerve involvement, and excessive warmth over bone. Pain due to arthritis may or may not respond to treatment. Treatment is also indicated in patients who develop hypercalcemia in response to immobilization. Marked deformity may not respond to treatment, although in some instances, bone remodeling can produce dramatic changes. Involvement of Paget's disease in a weight-bearing area or where fracture could occur is another indication for therapy, although there is not complete consensus on when therapy should be initiated in asymptomatic patients. There are no uniformly accepted guidelines for patients who are asymptomatic and do not have involvement of weight-bearing areas. In addition, there are no studies that prove the efficacy of therapy prior to elective surgery on pagetic bone, although the reduced vascularity that occurs with treatment may be helpful in preventing blood loss. The most reliable and convenient biochemical marker is serum alkaline phosphatase, which correlates directly with urinary markers.

Therapy is directed toward suppression of osteoclastic activity, which reduces the bone remodeling rate. This results in the production of lamellar bone instead of the less structurally stable woven bone. Inhibitors of bone resorption include the calcitonins, bisphosphonates, and plicamycin.

Calcitonin

Calcitonin inhibits osteoclast function and reduces blood flow. At present, the only forms of calcitonin that are commercially available in the United States must be administrated subcutaneously or intramus-

TABLE 1. **Sites of Involvement of Paget's Disease***

Site	% of Patients
Pelvis	76
Lumbar spine	33
Sacrum	28
Femora	25
Skull	28
Scapula	26
Dorsal spine	20
Cervical spine	14
Ribs	3

*Sites of bone involvement with Paget's disease at the time of diagnosis in 1864 patients.
Adapted from Guyer PB, Chamberlain AT, Ackery DM, Rolfe EB: The anatomic distribution of osteitis deformans. Clin Orthop Rel Res 156:141–144, 1981.

cularly. Nasal spray preparations of calcitonin are widely available in Europe and are anticipated to be available in the United States soon (Miacalcin nasal spray).* Calcitonin is available as synthetic salmon calcitonin from Sandoz Pharmaceuticals (Miacalcin) or Rhone-Poulenc-Rorer Pharmaceuticals (Calcimar). Salmon calcitonin is administered at a dose of 100 U daily initially, and symptomatic relief occurs in the first few weeks; reduction of biochemical indices may take longer. Following adequate reduction of symptoms and suppression of serum alkaline phosphatase to approximately 50% of the initial value, the dose may be reduced to 50 to 100 U two to three times per week. Patients with monostotic disease may continue to experience relief from symptoms after calcitonin is discontinued; patients with severe disease may need continuous treatment. The most common adverse reaction is nausea, which can usually be prevented by initiating treatment with 25 U daily and increasing the dose over 7 to 10 days. Other side effects include abdominal pain, cramps, flushing, metallic taste, and numbness or tingling of the hands or feet, but most patients develop tolerance to these reactions rapidly. Escape from the beneficial effects or resistance to calcitonin may occur after a variable time period. The decreased efficacy may be due to the development of anticalcitonin antibodies or to receptor down-regulation.

Bisphosphonates

Bisphosphonates are pyrophosphate analogues that inhibit calcification and bone resorption. Treatment of Paget's disease with these agents results in reduced osteoclastic resorption and replacement of woven bone by lamellar bone. Etidronate disodium, or EHDP, is a commonly used bisphosphonate for the treatment of Paget's disease. EHDP is commercially available as Didronel. The amount of drug and timing of administration are limited by the fact that this agent inhibits both bone resorption and bone formation. Prolonged administration can result in impaired new bone formation; therefore, careful cyclical management (6 months on, 6 months off) is recommended. Prolonged clinical and biochemical remission occurs even during the "off" period. Many studies have demonstrated the efficacy of this compound in the treatment of Paget's disease. Side effects include abdominal cramps, diarrhea, increasing bone pain (especially with prolonged, noncyclical administration), and hyperphosphatemia. Another bisphosphonate, pamidronate (Aredia), has recently been approved for use and provides substantial reduction in alkaline phosphatase levels after intravenous or oral administration. Pamidronate has the advantage over EHDP of inhibiting bone resorption without impairing mineralization. The optimal regimen for pamidronate remains controversial, and numerous approaches have been studied. One recommendation is to provide an intravenous dose of 30

mg per day infused over 4 hours for 3 days (total dose 90 mg) for patients with moderate to severe disease. For mild disease, a single infusion of 60 mg over 3 to 4 hours has been useful. Treatment can be repeated if the patient does not respond by a lowering of the biochemical parameters. Suppression of urinary markers is noted immediately, but serum alkaline phosphatase levels may take longer to respond. In one study, 10 months after the infusion, 50% of patients remained in remission. Oral administration of pamidronate is limited by gastrointestinal absorption. Oral doses of 300 to 600 mg daily in divided doses, 30 minutes before meals, have produced favorable results. Pamidronate has been noted to be efficacious in patients whose disease is refractory to treatment with calcitonin or EHDP. Bisphosphonates have been combined with calcitonin in patients with severe disease; the combination of calcitonin and EHDP resulted in improved reduction in biochemical parameters compared with either agent alone. Several new bisphosphonates are under clinical review and may become available in the near future.

Plicamycin

Plicamycin (Mithracin; formerly mithramycin) is not approved for use in the treatment of Paget's disease, but it has been used for particularly refractory patients or those with acute neural compression. Plicamycin suppresses osteoclast activity and may also alter osteoblast action. This drug is a potent but toxic medication; at the doses used for Paget's disease (15 to 25 μg per kg infused over 6 to 8 hours), marrow toxicity and thrombocytopenia are uncommon. Hypocalcemia is a frequent side effect, but it responds to supplemental calcium and vitamin D. It is anticipated that the newer bisphosphonates may supersede the use of plicamycin, although it has been used successfully in a patient whose disease was refractory to both calcitonin and pamidronate.

Other Treatment Options

Analgesics and nonsteroidal anti-inflammatory agents may be useful to relieve pain, especially that associated with osteoarthritis. Other options include the use of orthotics or canes and walkers to aid in gait stability. Because immobilization is associated with the development of hypercalcemia in patients with Paget's disease, continued mobility is important.

Orthopedic surgery may be indicated for correction of a severely impaired gait. Osteotomy or hip or knee replacement may be indicated. Although well-defined studies have not been performed, most clinicians recommend medical therapy to reduce bone vascularity prior to orthopedic surgery. Controversy exists regarding postoperative management due to the possible inhibition of mineralization by the bisphosphonates. Some advocate the use of calcitonin in this situation due to its ability to rapidly reduce vascu-

---

*Investigational drug in the United States.

larity and because it does not impair bone mineralization.

In summary, Paget's disease of bone is a common disorder of bone remodeling. Genetic predisposition exists, and studies suggest a viral etiology. Diagnosis is confirmed by elevated serum alkaline phosphatase and pathognomonic radiographic appearance. Bone scans are useful in assessing the extent of disease. Indications for treatment are variable, but most agree that treatment should be initiated to relieve symptoms or when the disease extends into weight-bearing areas to prevent future complications. The bisphosphonates are the most promising class of compounds for treatment of the disorder, and pamidronate has been approved for use by the Food and Drug Administration. The newer bisphosphonates have fewer side effects and do not impair bone mineralization. Calcitonin is efficacious and reduces vascularity and pain. For acute intervention or prior to orthopedic surgery, calcitonin is recommended. Combination therapy of bisphosphonates and calcitonin may be necessary if the patient's disease becomes refractory to a single agent. Due to its high toxicity, plicamycin should be reserved for emergency situations. A multidisciplinary approach by physical therapists, orthopedic surgeons, and internists usually helps symptomatic patients, and pharmacologic intervention prevents long-term complications of the disorder.*

---

*The Paget's Foundation (200 Varich Street, Suite 1004, New York, NY 10014) is a nonprofit organization that provides patient-oriented literature and supports research on Paget's disease.

PARENTERAL NUTRITION IN ADULTS

method of
THOMAS R. ZIEGLER, M.D.
Emory University School of Medicine
Atlanta, Georgia

GENERAL GUIDELINES

The primary focus of nutritional support in patients with pre-existing malnutrition or with illness-related catabolic stress is to supply adequate micronutrients (vitamins, minerals, electrolytes) and to maintain or increase the body's lean tissue via provision of adequate energy and protein. Protein is critical for tissue structure and function; thus, erosion of lean tissue is clearly associated with worsened clinical outcomes, including diminished immune function, increased infection rates, increased postoperative morbidity, decreased tissue repair and wound healing, skeletal muscle dysfunction, and delayed convalescence. Direct cause-and-effect relationships between nutritional status and patient outcomes are difficult to prove because malnutrition may reflect, in part, the severity or nature of the underlying illness. Nonetheless, it is reasonable to assume that maintenance of nutritional status in both adult and pediatric patients is generally beneficial.

The overall goal of nutritional support is to maintain organ structure and function and to support metabolism and protein synthesis. The major objectives of nutritional and metabolic support in malnourished or catabolic patients are to detect and correct pre-existing malnutrition, prevent progressive protein-calorie malnutrition, optimize the patient's metabolic state (including fluid and electrolyte status), and reduce morbidity related to malnutrition. Parenteral and enteral nutritional support is adjunctive to such primary therapies as fluid resuscitation, oxygen delivery, abscess drainage, and provision of antibiotics. However, parenteral nutrition (PN) and tube feedings have become the standard of care in most intensive care units (ICUs) throughout the world, and few objective data from properly designed, randomized, controlled studies are available to determine the true efficacy of and the indications for nutritional support in critical illness. Nonetheless, a number of clear indications exist for the use of PN in adults (Table 1). A limited number of well-designed studies in surgical and medical patient subsets indicate that PN administration reduces overall morbidity, but only in individuals with pre-existing moderate-to-severe malnutrition.

NUTRITIONAL ASSESSMENT

Detailed nutritional assessment in the general hospital ward and ICU setting involves (1) physical examination; (2) evaluation of weight loss and dietary history; (3) evaluation of the type and severity of underlying illness, including organ function and fluid status; (4) determination of selected serum biochemical values; (5) estimation of energy, protein, and micronutrient needs; and (6) determination of the type of access available for nutrient delivery (Table 2). The basic premise in considering PN therapy is that the patient is unable to achieve adequate energy, protein, and micronutrient intake via the enteral route (oral food, liquid supplements, or tube feedings). Compared with PN, enteral feeding is much less expensive, maintains intestinal mucosal structure and function, is safer in terms of mechanical and metabolic complications, and is associated with reduced rates of nosocomial infections. Thus, the enteral route of feeding should be utilized whenever possible, with the energy and protein intake derived from PN correspondingly reduced.

Circulating protein concentrations (e.g., albumin, transferrin, retinol-binding protein) are generally not useful as indices of underlying nutritional status, especially in ICU patients, because protein levels are markedly affected by non-nutritional factors such as fluid status, altered hepatic synthesis due to inflammation or infection, and body losses via the kidney or the gut. Albumin levels in particular may remain low during adequate feeding because of the long circulating half-life of this protein (≈ 21 days).

TABLE 1. **Indications for Parenteral Nutrition in Adults**

Enteral feeding not possible for >5–7 days due to underlying illnesses or disorders:
  Severe catabolic stress (e.g., burns, trauma, sepsis)
  Gastrointestinal operations
  Bone marrow transplantation
  Inflammatory bowel disease
  Acute or chronic pancreatitis
  High-output enterocutaneous fistula
  Severe nausea or vomiting, diarrhea, ileus, bowel obstruction
Short bowel syndrome, with inability to maintain adequate nutrition enterally
Pre-existing moderate-to-severe protein-energy malnutrition and adequate enteral feeding to promote anabolism not possible

---

TABLE 2. **Nutritional Assessment in Hospitalized Patients**

1. **Perform Detailed Physical Examination**

   Skeletal muscle wasting
   Loss of fat stores
   Skin lesions suggestive of micronutrient deficiency

2. **Obtain Information on Preadmission Body Weight Pattern**

   Current body weight
   Usual body weight
   % weight loss past 2 weeks and past 3–6 months
   Ideal body weight

3. **Establish Preadmission Dietary Intake Pattern**

   General food intake pattern
   Previous intravenous or enteral nutritional support
   Use of nutritional supplements

4. **Estimate Overall Preadmission Functional Status**

   Ability to perform daily activities
   Muscle weakness and fatigue

5. **Determine If Intestinal Tract Is Totally or Partially Functional**

   Gastrointestinal symptoms (nausea, emesis, diarrhea, steatorrhea)
   Delayed gastric emptying, gastroparesis
   Ileus
   Obstruction
   Intra-abdominal infection, perforation, etc.
   Acute gastrointestinal bleeding

6. **Assess Intravenous Access**

   Central or peripheral venous catheter
   Peripherally inserted central venous catheter (PICC line)
   Dedicated port for parenteral nutrition available?

7. **Determine Fluid Status**

   Euvolemic
   Dehydrated
   Fluid overloaded
   Capillary leak syndrome

8. **Evaluate Selected Serum or Plasma Biochemistries**

   Standard organ function indices
   Electrolytes, including calcium, magnesium, and phosphorus
   Triglycerides
   Vitamins and minerals, if suggested by physical examination, diet history, or underlying illness (serum zinc and iron status most useful)
   Serum proteins often not helpful, especially in the ICU setting

ACCESS FOR PARENTERAL NUTRITION ADMINISTRATION

Hypertonic nutrient solutions ($\geq$10% dextrose or $\geq$4% amino acids) must be given via a high-flow, large-diameter vein such as the subclavian or internal jugular vein. The femoral vein is narrower and thus more susceptible to mechanical catheter injury and subsequent thrombosis. Available data suggest that the internal jugular and especially the femoral vein catheter sites for PN administration are riskier in terms of catheter sepsis compared with the subclavian site. Although the data are empirical, most specialists in nutrition support mandate that PN, especially solutions containing hypertonic dextrose, be infused via an inviolate, dedicated infusion port to minimize the risk of catheter-related infection. Thus,

a maximum of 10% dextrose should be used when a dedicated PN infusion port is not available. Hospital nutrition support teams, whose members include nurses with responsibilities for PN catheter care and continuing education of hospital staff, have dramatically reduced PN catheter–related infection rates in hospital settings.

PROTEIN AND ENERGY ADMINISTRATION

Studies on nutrient utilization efficiency in catabolic patients suggest that lower amounts of total energy (calories) and protein should be administered than were routine in the past. Excessive dietary calories and protein loads (hyperalimentation) may induce metabolic complications, including carbon dioxide overproduction, azotemia, hyperglycemia, electrolyte alterations, and hepatic dysfunction. Energy intake should be advanced slowly over several days after the initiation of specialized feeding, to provide maintenance energy intake. Energy requirements may be estimated using standard equations, such as the Harris-Benedict equation, which incorporate the patient's age, sex, weight, and height to determine basal energy expenditure (BEE):

Males (kcal per 24 hours)
$$= 66.5 + (13.8 \times \text{kg body weight}) + (5.0 \times \text{height in cm}) - (6.8 \times \text{age in years})$$

Females (kcal per 24 hours)
$$= 655.1 + (9.6 \times \text{kg body weight}) + (1.8 \times \text{height in cm}) - (4.7 \times \text{age in years})$$

The BEE is then multiplied by factors to account for activity (1.2 to 1.3 times BEE, unless the patient is sedated) and illness severity (usually an additional 25% to a maximum of 50%) to arrive at the energy prescription. The estimated maintenance energy requirement is usually between 1.3 and 1.7 times BEE. In obese subjects (>20% above ideal body weight), "adjusted" body weight should be used in the calculation of energy and protein needs (see the later discussion). Adjusted body weight = (current weight − ideal body weight [from standard tables or equations] $\times$ 0.25) + ideal body weight.

It is important to consider that energy expenditure varies considerably from day to day, especially in ICU patients. In light of complications related to overfeeding, energy provision in the range of 25 to 30 kcal per kg per day is generally safe for most ICU patients and for stable patients without severe malnutrition. In clinically stable individuals with severe malnutrition who require nutritional repletion, it is possible to provide 35 to 40 kcal per kg per day, with careful monitoring of serum chemistries, as outlined later. Carbon dioxide overproduction (evidenced by respiratory quotients $\geq$ 1.0) was not uncommon in earlier decades, when ICU patients routinely received much higher energy doses (e.g., >40 kcal per kg per day); however, this complication is now unusual, as lower nutrient loads are being administered.

Dextrose in PN should be given at a dose not to exceed 4 to 6 mg per kg per minute (400 to 600 grams per day in a 70-kg person). Studies demonstrate that catabolic patients are unable to efficiently oxidize larger carbohydrate loads, which may induce hyperglycemia, hepatic steatosis, and/or excessive carbon dioxide production. Dextrose should provide about 70 to 80% of nonprotein energy, unless the patient is hyperglycemic. The dextrose load should be reduced and/or regular insulin should be provided in parenteral feeding or as a separate insulin drip to maintain blood glucose between 100 and 200 mg per dL.

Intravenous lipid emulsions are used to provide essential fatty acids (e.g., 250 mL of a 20% lipid emulsion twice a week) or as an energy source (with lipid provided as about 20 to 30% of nonprotein energy), generally infused over a 24-hour period in patients requiring PN. Although more expensive, the use of total nutrient admixtures (or "3 in 1") may be helpful in fluid-restricted patients, but lipid emulsions are often given over 12 to 24 hours as separate infusions in many centers. The maximal recommended rate of fat emulsion infusion is 1.0 to 1.5 grams per kg per day (700 to 1000 fat kcal per day or 350 to 500 mL of the 20% emulsion, which provides 2 kcal per mL). Excessive doses of fat emulsion are associated with impaired reticuloendothelial function and possibly immune suppression. It is important to monitor serum triglyceride serially to assess clearance of the intravenous fat emulsion, and triglyceride levels should be maintained below 400 to 500 mg per dL. ICU patients generally clear intravenous fat emulsions well from plasma. However, administration of fat emulsion as an energy source in ICU patients with severely diminished pulmonary diffusion capacity may be contraindicated to avoid possible worsening of hypoxia.

Guidelines for protein administration are given in Table 3. Studies in ICU patients indicate that protein loads of more than 2.0 grams per kg per day are not efficiently utilized for protein synthesis but may be oxidized for energy and contribute to azotemia. Thus, protein should be provided at doses of about 1.5 grams per kg per day in most catabolic patients with normal renal function. The protein dose should be lowered or raised to the target range as a direct function of the degree of azotemia and hyperbilirubinemia. This strategy takes into account the inability of some patients to efficiently utilize exogenous nutrients during severe catabolic illness, as well as the knowledge that most protein and lean tissue repletion occurs over a period of several weeks during convalescence. Adequate nonprotein energy is essential to allow amino acids to be effectively utilized for protein synthesis. The nonprotein calorie/nitrogen ratio used in most centers ranges from 100:1 to 150:1 (nitrogen = protein/6.25). Highly catabolic patients are given protein loads at the lower end of this range, assuming near-normal renal and hepatic function. Branched chain amino acid (BCAA)–enriched PN solutions ($\approx$50% of protein as BCAA) improved short-term nitrogen balance in some studies. BCAA may also be useful in some patients with hepatic encephalopathy who demonstrate low plasma levels of BCAA and elevations in plasma aromatic amino acids. However, BCAA has not improved clinical outcomes in either encephalopathic or critically ill patients. Therefore, standard amino acid formulations should generally be used pending the results of ongoing research on newer amino acid formulations (see later section).

Because fluid restriction and/or the need for intravenous pressor, blood product, or drug administration often precludes the use of large fluid volumes for intravenous or enteral feedings, peripheral vein PN solutions (which provide low concentrations of dextrose [generally 5%] and amino acids [generally 3%] and a large proportion of energy as fat [50 to 65% of PN calories]) are generally not indicated in ICU patients. Rather, central venous administration of PN usually allows maintenance energy and protein intake in 1- to 1.25-liter volumes.

MICRONUTRIENT ADMINISTRATION

It is important to maintain blood glucose and serum electrolytes within the normal range during administration of specialized feeding. Malnourished patients frequently exhibit whole-body depletion of intracellular electrolytes (potassium, phosphorus, and magnesium), and levels of these may rapidly fall to dangerously low levels during nutritional repletion (refeeding syndrome). The dosage of electrolytes required to maintain normal plasma levels, particularly phosphorus and magnesium, appears to be directly related to the dose of administered dextrose in patients with normal renal function. In addition, studies indicate that maintenance of intracellular potassium, phosphorus, and magnesium concentrations in muscle is essential for normal protein synthesis and the ability to achieve neutral or positive nitrogen balance. Typical ranges for daily PN electrolyte administration in central venous PN solutions (which contain concentrated dextrose) or peripheral vein PN solutions (with 5% dextrose) are shown in Table 4.

Specific requirements for intravenous trace elements and vitamins in various catabolic states have

TABLE 3. **Guidelines for Protein Administration**

Condition	Protein Intake Goal* (gm/kg/day)
Encephalopathy	0.6
Hepatic failure	0.6–1.0
Renal failure, not dialyzed	0.6–0.8
Renal failure, dialyzed	1.2
Malnourished, clinically stable	1.5–2.0
Mild-to-moderate catabolic stress	1.5
Critically ill	1.5

*Protein load is adjusted based on hepatic and renal function studies.

TABLE 4. **Guidelines for Electrolyte* and Micronutrient Administration in Parenteral Nutrient Solutions**

Element	Peripheral PN	Central Venous PN
Sodium (mEq/L)	30–40	50–60
Potassium (mEq/L)	30–40	50–60
Chloride (mEq/L)	45	60
Acetate (mEq/L)	45	60
Phosphorus (mEq/L)	5–8	12–18
Calcium (mEq/L)	5	5
Magnesium (mEq/L)	5–8	10–15
Multivitamins	Standard products available to admix	
Trace elements	Standard products available to admix†	
Vitamin K (mg/day)	1	1

*Electrolytes are adjusted as indicated to maintain serum levels within the normal range; the percentage of salts as chloride is increased with metabolic alkalosis, and the percentage of salts as acetate is increased with metabolic acidosis.

†A standard trace element formulation (M.T.E.-6, Lyphomed) is composed of zinc 5 mg, copper 1 mg, manganese 0.5 mg, chromium 10 µg, selenium 60 µg, iodide 75 µg/mL.

Abbreviation: PN = parenteral nutrition.

not been defined, and therapy is directed at meeting the recommended dietary allowances (RDA) for micronutrients, with adjustments for PN, as published by the American Medical Association. Supplemental zinc (and possibly other trace elements such as selenium) should be provided in patients with burns, large wounds, severe pancreatitis, and/or significant gastrointestinal fluid losses. Approximately 12 mg of zinc are lost per liter of small bowel fluid, and urinary excretion of zinc increases dramatically as a function of the degree of catabolic stress. Zinc is an important nutrient for immune function, wound healing, protein synthesis, and gastrointestinal mucosal regeneration. Thus, using serum zinc levels and/or urinary excretion as a guide to therapy, administration of 5 to 10 mg per day of additional zinc intravenously (or 200 to 400 mg of zinc sulfate per day enterally) during severe catabolic illness reduces the risk of continued total body zinc depletion.

BIOCHEMICAL MONITORING

It is imperative to closely monitor plasma glucose, electrolytes (including magnesium), and triglycerides and to assess renal, hepatic, and pulmonary function on a daily basis in ICU patients and 2 to 3 times a week in non-ICU patients on PN to determine the metabolic response, especially during periods of clinical instability. The nutrient mix is adjusted to maintain normal blood concentrations of standard chemistries and minimize metabolic complications. When the patient is extremely unstable, it may be necessary to provide a lowered amount of parenteral diet or to simply give intravenous low-dose dextrose with vitamins and minerals until organ function stabilizes.

TIMING OF ADMINISTRATION

Few objective, clinical data are available to guide the timing of PN administration. The current stan-

TABLE 5. **General Guidelines for Parenteral Nutrition Use in Clinical Care**

Perform detailed nutritional assessment
Use enteral feeding whenever possible
Use a dedicated port for central venous parenteral nutrition
Avoid excessive energy and protein intake
Decrease protein load proportional to degree of renal or hepatic dysfunction
Provide dextrose at a dose not to exceed 4–5 mg/kg/min
Maintain blood glucose >100 and <200 mg/dL by providing adequate insulin and/or altering dextrose load
Normal serum electrolytes, including magnesium
Be aware of "refeeding syndrome" in severely malnourished patients, especially when given concentrated dextrose (follow electrolytes closely)
Administer adequate zinc

dard of care in most units is to provide specialized PN (if enteral feeding is not indicated) at least within 5 to 7 days after admission, although, in clinical practice, nutritional support is often provided several days sooner. Many specialists suggest that feeding be instituted within 48 to 72 hours after ICU admission of critically ill patients, after standard resuscitation therapy to achieve hemodynamic stability. Recently, some clinicians have advocated provision of only electrolytes, vitamins, minerals, and other trace elements during the initial 1 to 3 days after ICU admission. Full PN, providing about 50% of energy and protein needs, is then given for several days and advanced to achieve "maintenance" energy and protein intake by day 5 to 7 after admission. This more conservative approach reflects the known metabolic complications of aggressive feeding and the lack of demonstrated improved outcomes with early PN support, but no randomized trials have been performed on this practice. General guidelines for the administration of specialized PN are summarized in Table 5.

NEW DIRECTIONS IN NUTRITIONAL AND METABOLIC SUPPORT

Nutritional and metabolic support modalities are rapidly evolving. Current practices emphasize feeding via the intestinal tract and provision of lower amounts of energy and protein than were routinely provided in the past. These changes reflect, in part, the recognition that "more is not better" and an appreciation of the potential complications of specialized PN. However, several promising new strategies designed to improve the clinical and metabolic efficacy of PN are being actively investigated in the clinical setting. These approaches include the use of recombinant growth factors; administration of specific nutrients, including dietary fiber, short chain fatty acids, glutamine, arginine, and dipeptides; use of modified lipid products and nutrient antioxidants; and, finally, combinations of these therapies (Table 6). At present, many clinicians provide supplemental antioxidant nutrients during severe catabolic stress (e.g., vitamins C and E, glutamine by the intravenous

TABLE 6. **New Approaches in Nutritional and Metabolic Support**

Administration of growth factors (e.g., growth hormone, insulin-like growth factor-I)
Administration of conditionally essential amino acids (e.g., glutamine, arginine)
Use of specialized lipid products (e.g., medium chain triglycerides, short chain fatty acids)
Provision of nutrient antioxidants (e.g., vitamin E, vitamin C, glutamine)
Emphasis on enteral feedings designed to maintain intestinal absorptive, immune, and barrier functions
Combination therapies

or enteral route). Doses of oral or intravenous vitamin C in the range of 500 mg to 2 grams per day and vitamin E in the range of 400 to 800 IU per day have been used without evident untoward effects in selected subgroups of patients.

Administration of specific nutrients and recombinant hormones may reduce or alter protein-catabolic responses, influence metabolism, and facilitate uptake of conditionally essential substrates into cells and tissues. However, these approaches are currently being evaluated in randomized, controlled clinical trials and cannot be recommended routinely. Further clinical investigation is required to define the safety, clinical and metabolic efficacy, and cost effectiveness of these new approaches in specialized nutrition.

PARENTERAL FLUID THERAPY FOR INFANTS AND CHILDREN

method of
JONATHAN D. HEILICZER, M.D.
University of Illinois College of Medicine
Chicago, Illinois

When considering intravenous fluid therapy in any patient, we can divide the body into two parts: solids and body water. The water component is further divided by membranes into a series of compartments. Intravenous (IV) fluids allow access to the plasma compartment only. Therefore substances in relatively high concentration in plasma can change and be changed rapidly (minutes to hours). Intracellular substances must be manipulated more slowly (hours to days).

Na^+, the major plasma cation, can change and be changed rapidly. Conversely, the extracellular concentration of K^+ (the major intracellular cation) can only be changed slowly, as K^+ must pass through several membranes before reaching its area of highest concentration.

Keeping everything in place, maintaining compartment concentrations, are osmotic gradients. These are regulated by osmolality, the first line of cellular defense. Osmolality, defined as the number of particles dissolved per unit of fluid, can be measured in the laboratory by freezing point depression. Simply, a substance freezes at a higher temperature if it has more particles dissolved in its fluid state. One can calculate osmolality in clinical medicine by the following formula:

$$Osm = 2 \times Na + \frac{glucose}{20} + \frac{BUN}{3}$$

$$= (2 \times 140) + \frac{100}{20} + \frac{9}{3}$$

$$= 280 \ mOsm/L$$

Two times Na equaling 280 mOsm per liter can estimate osmolality when blood urea nitrogen (BUN) and glucose contribute very little to the overall osmolality. Therefore, under normal conditions, Na is the body's "osmometer," or put another way, the body's "hydrometer." The major etiology of hyponatremia is *dilutional,* caused by an excess of free water, whereas hypernatremia is due to *contraction,* losses of free water. However, in three situations hyponatremia occurs without an excess of free water. The first situation occurs during hyperlipidemia. The laboratory directly measures the Na^+ found in plasma water and then indirectly determines the Na^+ in the solid (cells) phase of blood, to arrive at a total serum Na. In hyperlipidemia, there are three phases of blood (solids, water, and lipid), and only the Na^+ in the water can be measured directly. The Na^+ "trapped" in the lipid phase cannot be measured, yet the laboratory still uses the smaller measurement over the entire volume. This is "factitious" hyponatremia and does not signify actual loss of Na^+. The other two conditions causing hyponatremia are chronic hyperglycemia and uremia; they occur because of Na^+ shifts to maintain osmolar integrity. Again, this may not signify actual loss of Na^+.

Beyond the cellular level, a number of organ groups account for control of normal fluid and electrolyte homeostasis (Table 1).

With this very basic understanding of normal homeostasis, we can now contemplate IV maintenance fluids. The goal in maintenance is to maintain euvolemia. Recognizing that all the formula calculations for maintenance are estimates of the fluid needs of the average-sized patient, it is very important that the following three statements be documented as correct for each individual patient:

Child is neither wet nor dry, but in *zero* water balance.

TABLE 1. **Normal Homeostasis**

Kidney	Renin
Liver	Angiotensin I
Lung	Angiotensin II
Adrenal	Aldosterone
Hypothalamus/pituitary	Antidiuretic hormone
Heart	Atrial natriuretic peptide

TABLE 2. **Methods of Calculating Maintenance Fluids**

Milliliters per Kilogram of Body Weight	
100 mL/kg for each of the first 10 kg	
50 mL/kg for each kg from 10.1–20 kg	
20 mL/kg for each kg over 20 kg	
Milliliters per Square Meter	
Metabolic loss	1000 mL/m²/day
Insensible loss	400 mL/m²/day
Fecal loss	100 mL/m²/day
Minimal urine loss	400 mL/m²/day
TOTAL	1900 mL/m²/day (~2000)

Child has a normal *cardiovascular system*, able to pump and retain within the system the fluid you are going to deliver.

Child has a normal *renal-endocrine system*, able to "fine-tune" the fluid you deliver.

If these statements describe your patient, then whichever method is used will get the patient "into the ball park" and the patient's organ-hormonal system will balance things appropriately. Two methods are in popular use: milliliters per kilogram of body weight and milliliters per square meter of body area. Either is correct (as long as the preceding three statements are also correct).

Pediatrics is a growth and development specialty, and fluid-electrolyte balance in children is therefore similar. Both methods of fluid calculation take the fluid changes during growth into account, varying with age (growth) and development.

We first review maintenance fluid (i.e., water) requirements and then add electrolytes to the fluid.

MAINTENANCE FLUID CALCULATIONS

The milliliters per kilogram of body weight method and the milliliters per square meter method are outlined in Table 2. Surface area can be calculated by a nomogram found in many pediatric reference texts, or it can be estimated using the following formula:

$$m^2 = \frac{4 \times (\text{wt in kg}) + 7}{90 + (\text{wt in kg})}$$

If our three statements are true, then either is correct. The difference in a 7-kg child who is 0.36 m² is less than 1 mL per hour (Table 3) and can easily be retained in the cardiovascular system and fine-tuned by the kidney and endocrine system.

If the three statements cannot be affirmed, then an alternative method for maintenance fluids must be used. One can examine the patient and determine

TABLE 3. **Fluid Maintenance Calculations**

7-kg child = 0.36 m²	
mL/kg	mL/m²
7 × 100 = 700 mL/day	0.36 × 1900 = 684 mL/day

TABLE 4. **The Safest Maintenance for Fluids**

Insensible H₂O loss = 400 mL/m²/day
plus
All output—urine, nasogastric, diarrhea, etc.
Insensible loss contains no electrolytes; therefore use D5W solution and then
Replace output with "appropriate" fluid

that the child is neither wet nor dry. Then maintaining that zero balance state can be accomplished by estimating any ongoing losses and replacing those losses (Table 4). The appropriate output replacement fluid can be scientifically determined by sending an aliquot to the laboratory for electrolyte determinations. A reasonable starting estimate for urine and gastrointestinal fluid is 0.45 normal saline (NS), which contains 77 mEq of NaCl (see next section). Replacement of cerebrospinal fluid (e.g., lost through ventricular drains) is best accomplished with NS.

ELECTROLYTE REQUIREMENTS

To this point we have dealt mainly with water. Now something needs to be mixed into the maintenance water, namely Na and K as cations, in addition to Cl as the major anion. Following are the maintenance requirements for Na and K (each usually balanced with Cl):

Na: 3 to 4 mEq/kg/day
K: 1 to 2 mEq/kg/day

However, a maximum of only 40 mEq per liter of K is used clinically, K being an intracellular ion, and therefore its extracellular concentration can be changed only slowly (over hours to days). Additionally, K is very caustic to peripheral veins in concentrations greater than 40 mEq per liter.

Therefore, a 7-kg child would require the following to be mixed into the daily maintenance water of 700 mL per day (using mL per kg for water):

7 kg × 3 mEq Na/day = 21 mEq NaCl
7 kg × 2 mEq K/day = 14 mEq KCl

Although one could ask the pharmacist to place the sodium chloride concentration into a liter bag of a D5W solution, economic necessity requires that we use some commercial solutions. The most common shelf solutions are

0.9% NaCl = 154 mEq Na per liter
0.45% NaCl = 77 mEq Na per liter
0.3% NaCl = 51 mEq Na per liter
0.2% NaCl = 34 mEq Na per liter

In our example, the closest fluid would be D5.2NS. As long as the *three statements are true*, then the small amount of extra Na per day is not a problem. Bear in mind that D5.2NS is the most commonly used pediatric solution because it fits the majority of children requiring intravenous fluids. However, in older (larger) children, the correct fluid might be 0.45

TABLE 5. **Calculations for Electrolytes**

$$\frac{21 \text{ mEq/NaCl}}{700 \text{ mL H}_2\text{O}} = \frac{X \text{ mEq/NaCl}}{1000 \text{ mL H}_2\text{O}} = X = 30 \text{ mEq NaCl/L}$$

$$\frac{14 \text{ mEq/KCl}}{700 \text{ mL H}_2\text{O}} = \frac{X \text{ mEq/KCl}}{1000 \text{ mL H}_2\text{O}} = X = 20 \text{ mEq KCl/L}$$

Abbreviation: X = total amount of Na per liter.

NS (containing 77 mEq per liter). In the example, our final order would be D5.2NS adding 20 mEq KCl per liter (after the child voids) to run at 29 mL per hour (Table 5).

Adding the potassium chloride after the child voids assures us that there is continued good renal function. Again, with the three statements being true and K being an intracellular ion (changing over hours to days), adding maintenance K later poses no risks.

Remember, maintenance fluid calculations are estimates, all based on the average-sized child under "ideal" conditions. Therefore, one cannot just "set it and forget it" but must reassess the patient to see that the fluid estimates remain reasonable in what might be a changing situation. The following conditions might alter fluid requirements and should be considered at the initial assessment and the frequent reassessments:

Fever will increase fluid requirements (12% for each 1° over 37.8° C, or 8% for each 1° over 100° F); hypothermia will similarly decrease needs.

Seizures due to constant and repetitive muscle activity will increase fluid requirements.

Changes in insensible losses will increase with tachypnea, low humidity, or burns and will decrease with mechanical ventilation, high humidity, or extensive casting.

Unusual sweating, such as with cystic fibrosis patients, will need increased water (10 to 25 mL per kg per day) and Na (1 to 2 mEq per kg per day). However, alterations in urine volume (increased in glycosuria, diabetes insipidus, and sickle cell disease and decreased in the syndrome of inappropriate antidiuretic hormone [SIADH]) require previously noted "safest maintenance."

Again, anyone without a normal renal-endocrine axis should not be placed on maintenance fluids.

DEFICITS

Fluid deficits are the most common reason that children require hospitalization. Gastrointestinal disorders (mostly viral) can cause rapid fluid losses. These losses are magnified in the pediatric patient, who is proportionately "wetter" and has larger fluid requirements relative to adults. Being able to determine deficit fluid requirements added to maintenance fluids is an important pediatric skill.

To determine a fluid deficit accurately, subtract the patient's dry weight from the preloss weight. Thus a child who weighed 10 kg yesterday and is 9.5 kg today has a fluid deficit of 500 mL (i.e., 0.5 kg

TABLE 6. **Evaluation of Fluid Deficits**

Deficit History

Fluid loss from vomiting, diarrhea
Frequency
Amount
Most recent weight
Replacement fluids/diet

Physical Examination

Tears and saliva	Skin color
Skin turgor	Peripheral perfusion
Mucous membranes	Anterior fontanelle
Blood pressure	Heart rate
Respiratory rate	Urine

Laboratory Evaluation

Hgb, Hct	HCO₃
K	BUN/creatinine
Serum osmolality	VBG
Na (plus Cl)	

Abbreviations: Hgb = hemoglobin; Hct = hematocrit; HCO_3 = bicarbonate; BUN = blood urea nitrogen; VBG = venous blood gas.

equals 0.5 liter). However, this ideal situation is rarely encountered clinically. In most cases, the fluid (and electrolyte) deficit will need to be estimated.

Any clinical problem requires a good history and physical examination. The child's hydration status is emphasized, as outlined in Table 6. In laboratory evaluation of children with fluid and electrolyte deficits, the laboratory value of water or the effect of water loss is the major issue. In evaluating hemoglobin (Hgb) and hematocrit (Hct), we look at the ratio of solids (Hgb) to fluid (Hct). The normal ratio is 1:3 (i.e., 12 grams to 36%). In dehydration, the Hct will theoretically rise because of concentration (less fluid). The reverse would be true in fluid overload situations. Serum osmolality and Na (and Cl) are the body's hydrometers. BUN will vary more with water content than will creatinine. Creatinine should in theory rise only when the glomerular filtration rate (GFR) falls. In simple dehydration, the GFR should remain relatively constant until fluid loss is severe enough to drop blood pressure (and thus renal blood flow). BUN, however, is a function not only of production (liver) and excretion (kidney) but also of volume concentration (hydration).

During fluid depletion, peripheral perfusion decreases in an effort to preserve the central circulation. Peripherally, O_2 delivery decreases and an increase in anaerobic metabolism occurs. The by-product of anaerobic metabolism is lactic acid. Thus, the possibility of a metabolic acidosis during dehydration requires evaluation of acid-base status. Checking a blood pH by venous blood gas (VBG) and either a bicarbonate (HCO_3) (from the VBG) or a TCO_2 (from a sequential multiple analyzer) allows us to further assess the severity of dehydration. Clinically, there is no need to use an arterial blood gas determination unless the child is suspected to have a concurrent pulmonary or cardiac problem.

Usually no accurate weight change is available to calculate deficits, so a *subjective* estimate must be

TABLE 7. **Estimating Isotonic Deficits**

	5%	10%	15%
Urine specific gravity	>1.030	>1.035	anuric
Membranes	moist	dry	parched
Skin color	pale	mottled	cyanotic
Heart rate	+ +	+ + +	+ + + +, thready
Peripheral perfusion	±	−	almost none
Fontanelle	within normal limits	±	sunken
Blood pressure	within normal limits	Low	*SHOCK*

TABLE 8. **Shock (Deficit 15% or Over)**

Rx: *Immediately treat with isotonic solution*
        and

Blood
Lactated Ringer's solution
Albumin
Normal saline

At a rate of at least 20 mL/kg/h until blood pressure is adequate

made. Table 7 is a general guideline for this estimate, which will vary from observer to observer. The goal is to estimate a deficit so as to calculate a replacement plus maintenance fluid requirement. We assume (from the history) that prior to the acute illness the child had normal water balance, a normal cardiovascular system, and a normal renal-endocrine axis. We want to get the child back to the starting point. Again, this estimate must be re-evaluated periodically to ensure that the child is responding appropriately.

The majority of deficits are isotonic (e.g., normal serum sodium). However, this can be determined only by laboratory evaluation.

For our purpose, the estimate of "% dry" can be used to obtain the milliliters of fluid deficit by multiplying the percent by the child's weight in kilograms. Example: a child weighing 7 kg and estimated at 10% dry has a fluid deficit of 700 mL (i.e., 7 kg × 10% = 0.7 kg; or, since a kilogram equals a liter, then 0.7 liter, or 700 mL). This is a subjective estimate, but if the assessment is 15% or more, the patient is in shock! A patient in hypovolemic shock has a deficit of at least 15%. Hypovolemic shock must be treated (as in Table 8) immediately via a large-bore IV line *(not a 25-gauge butterfly)*.

Isotonic Dehydration

When calculating fluid requirements in any deficit condition, the patient requires a deficit replacement plus usual maintenance and may also require concurrent replacement of ongoing losses. In the previous example, 7 kg × 10% dry, the child will need a maintenance of 700 mL per day (mL/kg method) and

need to make up a deficit of 700 mL (10% of 7 kg) (Table 9). The total fluid for 24 hours is 1400 mL. The child will also require maintenance Na (21 mEq per liter) and deficit Na.

Deficit losses (most commonly gastrointestinal) can be estimated as requiring 0.45 NS (77 mEq per liter). In our example, 700 mL of 0.45 NS contains 54 mEq of sodium chloride. This, added to maintenance Na, totals 75 mEq of sodium chloride added to 1400 mL for the day. The initial order would be D5.3NS per liter and add 10 mEq of potassium chloride per liter after the child voids twice. Start at 88 mL per hour for 8 hours, then 44 mL per hour for the balance of the 24 hours. Once again, this is an estimate, and you should reassess the patient's response.

Hypertonic Dehydration

The problem in hypertonic (hypernatremic) dehydration is essentially a greater amount of solvent (water) loss than solute (Na) loss. The major issue is, what fluid replacement would be best to utilize? Historically, this clinical entity accounted for approximately one-third of dehydrated children. However, with better oral replacement regimens that avoid the use of hypertonic solutions such as boiled milk, hypertonic dehydration has become less common. Physical examination in these children discovers extreme irritability and a lesser degree of circulatory collapse than one might expect because of the hypertonicity. The clinical problem is as follows:

$$\text{Osmolality} = (2 \times \text{Na}) + \frac{\text{Glucose}}{20} + \frac{\text{BUN}}{3}$$

TABLE 9. **Isotonic Deficit Calculations for a 7-kg Child Estimated 10% Dry**

	Water	Na	K
Maintenance	7 × 100 = 700	7 × 3 = 21	2 × 7 = 14
Deficit	7000 × 10% = 700	$\frac{77}{1000} = \frac{X}{700} = \sim 54$	*None*
Total	700 + 700 = 1400 *mL*	54 + 21 = 75	$\frac{14}{1400} = \frac{X}{1000} = 10$
		$\frac{75}{1400} = \frac{X}{1000} = 54/L$	*Add 10 mEq of KCl after 2 voids*
		or D5.3NS	

Replace half in the first 8 h
Replace the second half in the next 16 h

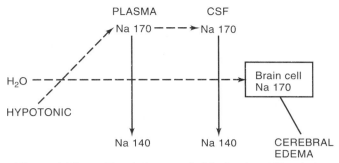

Figure 1. The problem in hypertonic dehydration. *Abbreviation*: CSF = cerebrospinal fluid.

that is, $= (2 \times 170) + \dfrac{100}{20} + \dfrac{30}{3} = 355 \text{ mOsm}$

As noted in Figure 1, the serum Na concentration can easily be decreased using a hypotonic solution (D5W or D5.2NS). However, the resulting rapid fluid shifts to other compartments will potentially cause cerebral edema, seizures, and death! Therefore, one must decrease the Na slowly at a rate no faster than 10 mEq per liter per day, using a solution allowing for a much more gradual gradient. Of the most common commercially available fluids, NS (154 mEq per liter) and 0.45 NS (77 mEq per liter) have the least steep gradients. Figure 2 illustrates this gradient differential.

D5.2NS, the most commonly used "pediatric" fluid, has an extremely steep and dangerous gradient if used in hypertonic dehydration. Thus a good rule to follow is: if you do not yet have the electrolyte results from the laboratory, use *normal saline* as the initial fluid. No one will ever be harmed by NS—the rate the fluid is given might be harmful (too fast or too slow), but not the content. The same cannot be said for any other fluid.

The goal is to lower serum Na slowly to less than 150 mEq per liter at a rate of approximately 10 mEq per liter per day. In a child with a serum Na of 170 mEq per liter, fluid calculation is based on the percent deficit plus two times the maintenance (water, sodium chloride, and maintenance K) to be replaced over 48 hours (half given in the first 16 hours, the rest over the following 32 hours). The initial fluid should be either NS (if the Na is greater than 170) or 0.45 NS (if the Na is less than 170). When the Na has decreased to less than 150, then the Na content should be adjusted for the amount that would be given in an isotonic patient. It is important to follow

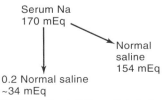

Figure 2. Fluid gradient differentials in hypernatremia.

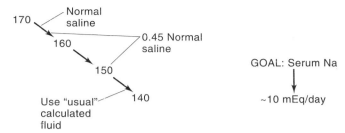

Figure 3. Treatment plan in hypernatremia.

electrolytes and make frequent clinical reassessments so as not to allow the Na to drop too fast (Figure 3).

Hypotonic Dehydration

The problem in these patients is the theoretical loss of more solute (Na) than solvent (water). In actuality this rarely causes hypotonic dehydration in pediatric patients. Rather, children develop fluid loss, and the fluid is abnormally replaced. This is the mother who takes the advice to place her child on a "clear fluid" diet to the extreme, using water exclusively (or forms of water such as tea or Kool-aid). Clinically, such a child may be profoundly hypotensive due to the low serum osmolality.

Treatment depends on symptoms and the serum Na level. Without central nervous system (CNS) symptoms and a serum Na level of more than 120 mEq per liter, replacement with NS over a period of 24 hours will suffice. However, if the child manifests CNS symptoms (particularly seizures) or the serum Na is less than 120 mEq per liter, then hypertonic 3% sodium chloride should be infused rapidly to raise the serum Na to approximately 125 mEq per liter. This is accomplished as in Table 10. Since fluid is not as significant an issue as osmolar content, rapid repletion of the initial Na deficit is possible. Full correction for fluid is then made over 48 hours.

ACID–BASE THERAPY

Our emphasis here is to address *acute* acid-base disturbances. Chronic pH, H^+ ion, or P_{CO_2} changes and their work-up are involved subjects beyond the scope of the present review. This includes chronic

TABLE 10. **Hypotonic Dehydration**

Amount of Na required: weight in kilograms × Na space (0.6) × deficit = mEq Na

10-kg child with Na level of 115 mEq/L: deficit here is 10 mEq/dL (the Δ of 125 − 115)

$$10 \times 0.6 \times 10 = 60 \text{ mEq Na}$$
or

$$\frac{X}{60} = \frac{1}{0.518} = \text{approximately 116 mL of 3\% NaCl}$$

Given over 60–90 minutes

metabolic acidosis (e.g., inborn errors of metabolism, renal tubular acidosis, renal failure).

The first step in evaluating any acid-base problem is differentiating respiratory etiology from metabolic causes. We essentially evaluate lung function (Pco_2) and kidney function (HCO_3).

$$(7.4) \; \text{Serum pH} = \frac{HCO_3}{Pco_2} = \frac{\text{Kidney}}{\text{Lung}}$$

$$7.3 - 7.49 = \frac{18 - 24}{35 - 45}$$

Clinical acid-base concerns differ from academic theory. Not every pH abnormality needs to be immediately corrected. For example, the most common type of metabolic acidosis encountered in pediatrics occurs during routine fluid-losing illnesses such as gastroenteritis. As previously discussed, in "clamping down" on the peripheral circulation to maintain central perfusion, lactic acid is produced. In most cases, just stopping the fluid loss by stopping any oral intake and beginning to replenish the deficit will be sufficient to shut off the lactic acid production and resolve the acidosis. Therefore, in most clinical pediatric situations, treatment with alkali is not undertaken unless the serum pH is less than 7.20.

Clinical Acid-Base Determinations

Respiratory Acidosis

$$\text{pH} < 7.30 = \frac{HCO_3}{Pco_2} = \frac{\text{nl or} > 24}{> 45}$$

Respiratory Alkalosis

$$\text{pH} > 7.45 = \frac{HCO_3}{Pco_2} = \frac{\text{nl or} < 24}{< 35}$$

Metabolic Acidosis

$$\text{pH} < 7.30 = \frac{HCO_3}{Pco_2} = \frac{< 18}{\text{nl or} < 45}$$

Metabolic Alkalosis

$$\text{pH} > 7.45 = \frac{HCO_3}{Pco_2} = \frac{> 24}{\text{nl or} > 35}$$

In respiratory acidosis, a ventilator may be needed but *not* HCO_3. Unless one suspects a pulmonary or cardiac problem (when an accurate Po_2 is necessary),

VBGs are sufficient for our purpose, namely serum pH. Alkalosis is just as harmful to body homeostasis as is acidosis; therefore a pH of over 7.49 should be addressed with the same degree of urgency as a pH of less than 7.20 (more on alkalosis later).

TREATMENT OF UNCOMPENSATED METABOLIC ACIDOSIS

pH < 7.2   Kg × 0.6 × deficit

deficit to >18 mEq/dL

Give only partial correction

When you have decided to help the patient compensate for an acute metabolic acidosis, the deficit is the difference between the child's present HCO_3 and the lower normal for HCO_3 of 18 mEq per dL. Only a third or a fourth of the calculated deficit is given over the first hour. Sodium bicarbonate ($NaHCO_3$) should not be given very rapidly as it is very hyperosmolar. In any event, with the most common form of metabolic acidosis—that due to poor peripheral perfusion—reversing the perfusion problem with rehydration will resolve the acidosis.

Metabolic alkalosis is most commonly seen in the following pediatric conditions: chronic vomiting (e.g., pyloric stenosis, anorexia or bulimia), nasogastric suction, and chronic diuretic therapy. Each of these conditions has as major components loss of Cl^- and K^+, in addition to H^+. Thus the usual treatment is Cl^- and K^+. These children will need higher concentrations of Cl^- as supplied by NS and probably a higher amount of KCl.

The preceding pages have been meant as an overview of parenteral fluid therapy in children. The clinician is cautioned to use this as a guideline. Specific clinical problems may require more complex solutions.

The Endocrine System

ACROMEGALY

method of
ANNE E. DE PAPP, M.D., and
PETER J. SNYDER, M.D.
University of Pennsylvania School of Medicine
Philadelphia, Pennsylvania

DIAGNOSIS

Acromegaly is the clinical syndrome caused by excessive growth hormone (GH) secretion; it can be recognized clinically and confirmed biochemically. A somatotroph adenoma of the pituitary is almost always the cause of the excessive GH secretion, but rarely a pancreatic islet or carcinoid tumor secreting growth hormone–releasing hormone may be the cause. Approximately 250 new cases of acromegaly are diagnosed in the United States each year, with equal frequency in men and women. The disease is insidious in onset and is often present for many years before diagnosis. Common clinical features include coarse facial features, wide hands and feet, headaches, arthralgias, paresthesias, hyperhidrosis, and skin tags. The best biochemical test for acromegaly is the serum concentration of insulin-like growth factor-1 (IGF-1; somatomedin C), the target gland hormone that is stimulated by GH and mediates many of GH's effects. IGF-1 is elevated in virtually all cases of active acromegaly and reflects integrated GH secretion over the previous several days. The diagnosis can be confirmed by showing a failure of serum GH concentrations to suppress to less than 2 ng per mL within 2 hours of an oral glucose load of 75 to 100 grams after an overnight fast. Random, isolated GH concentrations are usually not helpful in the diagnosis of acromegaly, because they fluctuate spontaneously in response to many physiologic stimuli. Somatotroph adenomas can usually be demonstrated by gadolinium-enhanced magnetic resonance imaging.

TREATMENT

Rationale

Although acromegaly does not pose an immediate threat to life, it is associated with increased morbidity and mortality. Acromegaly is associated with a two- to threefold increase in mortality compared with age-matched controls. Long-term medical sequelae include sleep apnea due to upper airway obstruction, hypertension, cardiomyopathy, glucose intolerance, degenerative arthropathies, compressive neuropathies (e.g., carpal tunnel syndrome), and a threefold increase in the risk of certain malignancies. Reducing GH secretion, in one study, was associated with lower mortality and, in another study, with improvement in cardiomyopathy.

Surgical Treatment

Trans-sphenoidal resection of as much of the adenoma as possible is the best initial treatment for most patients with acromegaly, because it results in a rapid reduction of the serum concentrations of GH and IGF-1 (Table 1). This treatment is usually best for the majority of patients who are not elderly, do not have contraindications to surgery, or have clear evidence of morbidity of the disease. The frequency with which surgery reduces GH and IGF-1 to normal levels depends on the size of the adenoma: this occurs in more than 80% of cases when the adenoma is less than 1 cm, and in less than 30% when the adenoma is greater than 1 cm. Even when the serum GH and IGF-1 are normal shortly after surgery, however, they may rise again within the next few years. Surgery also usually reduces the neurologic consequences of large adenomas, such as visual impairment and headache. Potential complications of surgery include cerebrospinal fluid leak and subsequent meningitis, impaired vision, diabetes insipidus, and hypopituitarism, but these occur infrequently when the procedure is performed by an experienced trans-sphenoidal surgeon. Hormonal function should be reevaluated 4 to 6 weeks after surgery by measurement of thyroid and adrenal function and by serum IGF-1 or postglucose GH concentrations. If the IGF-1 or GH values are still higher than normal, further treatment should be considered.

TABLE 1. **Summary of Therapeutic Options in Acromegaly**

Treatment	Advantages	Disadvantages
Surgery	Rapid reduction of GH levels; rapid resolution of neurologic compromise	Invasive procedure; curative in <30% of macroadenomas
Radiation	Normalizes IGF-1 in 60–70%	>10 years for maximum benefit; hypopituitarism in 50%
Dopamine agonists	Oral administration	Effective in only 20–30%; require high doses; cause nausea, postural hypotension
Octreotide (Sandostatin)	Effective in 70–80%	Frequent injections; high cost; gastrointestinal side effects

Radiation Therapy

Conventional supervoltage external radiation may be used as an adjunct to surgery or as a primary treatment in patients who are poor operative candidates (see Table 1). Conventional protocols deliver 45 Gy over a 4- to 6-week period. Radiation reduces serum GH and IGF-1 concentrations to normal in 60 to 70% of patients, but usually not for 10 to 20 years. Short-term side effects of radiation treatment include fatigue, nausea, loss of taste and smell, and loss of hair at the radiation portals; these effects almost always remit spontaneously in 1 to 3 months. The most common long-term side effect of radiation is the development of hypopituitarism, which occurs in approximately 50% of patients within 10 years of the treatment. Patients should therefore be screened annually and indefinitely for hypothyroidism, hypoadrenalism, and hypogonadism, as well as for IGF-1, or GH, or both. Because the GH and IGF-1 concentrations fall so slowly after radiation, other treatments can be considered in the interim.

Medical Therapy

The dopamine agonists bromocriptine (Parlodel) and pergolide (Permax)* reduce serum IGF-1 and GH concentrations in 20 to 30% of acromegalic patients and may therefore be tried as adjuvant therapy to surgery or radiation. Relatively high doses (20 to 30 mg daily of bromocriptine or 0.25 to 0.75 mg daily of pergolide) are necessary to achieve significant GH suppression. The most common side effects are nausea, postural hypotension, nasal stuffiness, and fatigue. The chance of these side effects occurring can be reduced by beginning with very low doses (1.25 mg of bromocriptine twice a day or 0.025 mg of pergolide once a day) and increasing the dose gradually over the course of several months. Pergolide's advantages over bromocriptine are a much lower cost and once-a-day dosing, but experience with pergolide is more limited, and it is not approved by the Food and Drug Administration (FDA) for use in acromegaly.

Octreotide acetate (Sandostatin, Sandoz) is a long-acting somatostatin analogue that is more effective than dopamine agonists in inhibiting GH secretion and was recently approved by the FDA for treatment of acromegaly. It is administered by subcutaneous injection in doses of 100 to 500 mcg every 8 hours, although it is not clear if the higher doses are more effective than 100 mcg. Octreotide can be used as primary treatment or as an adjunct to surgery or radiation. The major disadvantages of this treatment are the need for frequent injections and the cost—about $9000 a year for the 100-mcg dose. Short- and long-term gastrointestinal side effects also occur. The short-term side effects include abdominal cramps, nausea, diarrhea, steatorrhea, and flatulence, which occur in 30 to 50% of patients following initiation of

---

*Not FDA-approved for this indication.

therapy and usually remit within 10 days. The long-term side effect is gallstone formation, which occurs in 20 to 30% of patients within 2 years of treatment. Abdominal ultrasonography should therefore be performed prior to initiating therapy and periodically during therapy.

Observation

Because the deleterious effects of acromegaly usually take many years to develop, observation alone can be considered in patients who are elderly, whose life expectancy is relatively short, or who have relatively little morbidity from the disease.

ADRENOCORTICAL INSUFFICIENCY

method of
RITVA KAUPPINEN-MÄKELIN, M.D., PH.D.
Peijas Hospital
Vantaa, Finland

and

MATTI VÄLIMÄKI, M.D., PH.D.
Helsinki University Central Hospital
Helsinki, Finland

CAUSES OF ADRENOCORTICAL INSUFFICIENCY

Inadequate function of the adrenal cortex may be primary (Addison's disease) or central (deficient secretion of pituitary adrenocorticotropic hormone [ACTH] or hypothalamic corticotropin-releasing hormone [CRH]). In developed countries, the most important cause of Addison's disease is autoimmune damage of the adrenal cortex. Two-thirds of patients have antibodies to the adrenal cortex. Many patients have concomitant autoimmune phenomena, most commonly thyroid antibodies. Recently, the autoantigen has been discovered to be the 21-hydroxylase enzyme, prominent in the glomerular zone of the adrenal cortex. Tuberculous destruction of the adrenal glands accounts for only about 20% of cases today. However, in underdeveloped countries, most cases of Addison's disease are still caused by tuberculosis. The infection is usually hematogenic, and the patients have concomitant genitourinary or bone tuberculosis. Other causes are metastatic destruction of the glands and a variety of rare diseases (Table 1). Many pituitary and hypothalamic disorders can cause inadequate secretion of ACTH or CRH (Table 2). The most common cause of central adrenal hypofunction is hypothalamic-pituitary-adrenal axis suppression due to the use of exogenous glucocorticoids.

SYMPTOMS AND SIGNS OF ADRENOCORTICAL INSUFFICIENCY

Typical symptoms are fatigue, loss of appetite, and nausea. Diffuse myalgias and arthralgias are common. Salt craving should arouse suspicion for Addison's disease. Almost all patients with primary adrenal insufficiency lose weight and are hypotensive. Because of an elevated ACTH level, they have hyperpigmentation, especially in palmar creases, elbows, and knees. Typically, patients have hypo-

TABLE 1. **Causes of Addison's Disease**

Autoimmune Addison's disease
Tuberculosis
Malignancies with metastases to adrenal glands
Rare causes
    Histoplasmosis
    Blastomycosis
    Coccidioidomycosis
    Hydatid cyst
    Moniliasis
    Torulosis
    Cytomegalic inclusion disease
    Syphilis
    Acquired immune deficiency syndrome
    Hemorrhage
    Amyloidosis
Drugs
    Metyrapone
    Mitotane
    Ketoconazole
    Aminoglutethimide
Rare inherited disorders

natremia and hyperkalemia, but electrolyte disturbances are not always present. Because of impaired gluconeogenesis, many patients, especially insulin-treated diabetics, are prone to hypoglycemia. Patients are usually also anemic.

Patients with secondary hypocortisolism are less symptomatic and often have lethargy as their only major complaint. They may also have hypoglycemia as the primary manifestation. Patients with secondary hypocortisolism do not have hyperpigmentation, since the plasma ACTH concentration is not elevated. Because renin-angiotensin-aldosterone physiology is maintained, they usually do not have electrolyte disturbances or show only mild hyponatremia.

DIAGNOSIS OF ADRENOCORTICAL INSUFFICIENCY

If morning plasma cortisol concentration is more than 19 µg per dL (500 nmol per liter), adrenal cortex function is normal and no further tests are required. However, if the concentration is in the normal range but less than 19 µg per dL (500 nmol per liter), adrenocortical insufficiency is not excluded, and an ACTH test may be needed. Patients with morning plasma cortisol concentration of less than the lower normal limit (9 µg per dL or 200 nmol per liter) usually have adrenal hypofunction, and an ACTH test should be done. Morning plasma cortisol concentration of 3 µg per dL (100 nmol per liter) or less is always diagnostic of impaired cortisol production. The ACTH test is an excellent diagnostic test except in patients with recent pituitary

TABLE 2. **Major Causes of Central Adrenocortical Insufficiency**

Tumors
Infiltrative diseases
Pituitary or hypothalamic trauma
Pituitary apoplexy
Pituitary surgery or radiation therapy
Autoimmune hypophysitis
Congenital deficiency of pituitary hormones
Pituitary hypoplasia
Hypothalamic-pituitary-adrenal axis suppression owing to use of exogenous glucocorticoids

or hypothalamic damage, in which case results can be normal even though ACTH or CRH secretion is impaired. In the ACTH test, serum cortisol is measured before the injection of 250 µg synthetic ACTH intravenously and then 30 and 60 minutes after. A peak cortisol concentration of 18 µg per dL (500 nmol per liter) is an adequate response. It should be noted that hydrocortisone, prednisone, and methylprednisolone—but not dexamethasone—cross-react with cortisol measurement. Therefore, it is not possible to assess endogenous cortisol production in patients taking prednisone or methylprednisolone or in those taking suppressive doses of dexamethasone.

Once the diagnosis of adrenal insufficiency has been confirmed, the site of the defect must be determined. Plasma ACTH level is a good test to distinguish between primary and central adrenal insufficiency. Thereafter, the exact cause of the disease, whether localizing in the adrenal glands (morning plasma ACTH concentration high) or in the pituitary gland or hypothalamus (ACTH level normal or low), must be sought.

TREATMENT OF ACUTE ADRENAL CRISIS

Most patients who develop adrenal crisis have primary adrenal insufficiency. Patients with secondary hypocortisolism are less prone to developing crisis. In acute adrenal crisis, the patient is severely ill, and prompt treatment is mandatory. Blood samples are taken for future determinations of cortisol and ACTH. Thereafter, the patient is immediately given hydrocortisone 100 mg intravenously. The dose is repeated every 6 hours for the first day. During the following days, the dose is tapered off, as shown in Table 3. In addition to cortisol replacement, the patient in adrenal crisis must be given physiologic sodium chloride and glucose infusions to correct hypovolemia and hypoglycemia. The triggering factor for the crisis must be sought. It may be an infection, acute myocardial infarction, or surgery, among other causes.

TREATMENT OF CHRONIC ADRENOCORTICAL INSUFFICIENCY

In primary adrenal insufficiency, both cortisol and almost always mineralocorticoids must be replaced. In central adrenocortical insufficiency, only cortisol replacement is required, since aldosterone secretion

TABLE 3. **Treatment of Addison's Crisis**

Hydrocortisone 100 mg IV immediately after taking blood samples for cortisol and ACTH determination

First day: hydrocortisone 100 mg IV/IM × 4

Second day: hydrocortisone 50 mg IV/IM × 4

Third day: hydrocortisone 25–50 mg orally × 3

Thereafter, the dose can be reduced to an oral maintenance dose, unless there is a major complicating disease

In cases of primary adrenal insufficiency, a mineralocorticoid should be started when the hydrocortisone dose is less than 50 mg/day

TABLE 4. **Glucocorticoid Replacement Therapy**

Hydrocortisone 20–30 mg/day
  15–20 mg in the morning and 5–10 mg at 4–6 P.M.
  or
  15–20 mg in the morning, 5 mg at 2–4 P.M., and 10 mg at
    6 P.M.
Prednisone 5–7.5 mg/day
  5–7.5 mg late in the evening
  5–10 mg hydrocortisone at 2–4 P.M. if needed
Dexamethasone 0.5–0.75 mg/day
  0.5–0.75 mg late in the evening
  5–10 mg hydrocortisone at 2–4 P.M. if needed

continues under the control of renin. Lack of adrenal androgens need not be treated.

Cortisol can be replaced with hydrocortisone or with longer-acting glucocorticoids such as prednisone or dexamethasone (Table 4). The usual dosage of hydrocortisone is 20 to 30 mg per day, divided into two or three doses. Two-thirds is given early in the morning, and one-third is given in the afternoon, no later than 6 P.M. After the morning dose, the cortisol concentration rises rapidly to supraphysiologic levels and then declines, with a half-time of 1½ hours. Thus, the cortisol concentration is often subnormal in the afternoon as well as during the early morning hours. Many patients complain of fatigue and nausea on awakening. Therefore, it may be better to give longer-acting glucocorticoids as a single dose late in the evening. However, some patients develop insomnia when taking glucocorticoids at bedtime. For these patients, prednisone or dexamethasone can be given in the morning. The usual doses are prednisone 5 to 7.5 mg per day and dexamethasone 0.5 to 0.75 mg per day. Some patients may need a small dose of hydrocortisone (5 to 10 mg) in midafternoon, especially when using prednisone.

Prednisone or dexamethasone is a particularly good choice for diabetics or patients with congenital adrenocortical hyperplasia. Hypocortisolism impairs gluconeogenesis and makes insulin-treated diabetics prone to hypoglycemia. Patients with congenital adrenocortical hyperplasia need to get their plasma ACTH concentrations normalized. This is more easily achieved with prednisone or dexamethasone than with hydrocortisone.

As a mineralocorticoid replacement, fludrocortisone acetate is given for patients with primary adrenocortical hypofunction. The half-life of fludrocortisone is long (18 to 36 hours); therefore, one daily dose (usually 0.05 to 0.2 mg) is enough.

MONITORING THE DOSE

The dose of glucocorticoid is assessed mostly by clinical criteria. Increasing weight and rounding and reddening of the face indicate too high a dose. If the dose is too small, patients complain of fatigue and nausea. It is not worth measuring serum cortisol concentration. When prednisone or dexamethasone is used, it is possible to measure morning plasma ACTH concentration when treating patients with pri-

mary adrenal hypofunction. ACTH levels should be kept in the normal range.

Too high a dose of mineralocorticoid increases blood pressure, causes edema, and reduces serum potassium concentration. Salt craving, orthostatic hypotension, and an elevated serum potassium concentration indicate too small a dose. Stable weight, normal blood pressure, and normal serum electrolytes signify a proper dose. If plasma renin activity is measured, it should be in the upper normal range. However, renin determination is not usually needed.

INCREASING THE REPLACEMENT DOSE

The glucocorticoid dose must be increased during stressful events and illnesses. Drugs that stimulate hepatic microsomal enzymes, such as rifampicin, phenytoin, carbamazepine, phenazone, and mitotane, increase cortisol metabolism, necessitating an increase in the replacement dose. Alcohol also stimulates hepatic microsomal enzymes and may therefore increase the need for cortisol. When the patient takes hydrocortisone in two daily doses, an extra 5 to 10 mg may be needed in the evening if the patient is going to stay up late. During febrile illnesses, the glucocorticoid dose should be doubled. During severe acute diseases and surgery, the need for cortisol increases markedly. The generally accepted protocol for major surgery is shown in Table 5. Replacement needs are overestimated because too low a replacement dose increases mortality, but there are no reported hazards from high doses. During minor procedures under local anesthesia, no extra glucocorticoid is needed, but the oral glucocorticoid dose can be doubled before the procedure. Before endoscopic examinations and radiologic studies with contrast media, 100 mg of hydrocortisone is given intravenously. During pregnancy, cortisol needs usually remain stable, but for many patients, the hydrocortisone dose must be increased by 5 to 10 mg per day during late pregnancy.

The need for mineralocorticoid is increased when salt is lost. Because hydrocortisone has some miner-

TABLE 5. **Glucocorticoid Replacement Therapy During Major Surgery**

Day of operation
Hydrocortisone 100 mg IV/IM 1–2 h before; thereafter,
  hydrocortisone 100 mg IV/IM × 4

First postoperative day
Hydrocortisone 100 mg IV/IM × 4

Second to third postoperative days
Hydrocortisone 50 mg IV/IM × 4

Fourth to fifth postoperative days
Hydrocortisone 25 mg orally × 3

Sixth postoperative day
Hydrocortisone 20 mg + 10 mg

alocorticoid activity, no separate mineralocorticoid is needed when the hydrocortisone dose is more than 50 mg per day. The mineralocorticoid effect is very small for prednisone and is lacking for dexamethasone.

PATIENT EDUCATION AND MEDIC ALERT BRACELET

Patients with adrenocortical insufficiency need a Medic Alert bracelet describing their disorder and the appropriate medical treatment. They need to be taught when to increase the dose and how to handle different situations. They should also be given injectable hydrocortisone and taught how to use it.

CUSHING'S SYNDROME

method of
WILLIAM F. YOUNG, JR., M.D.
Mayo Clinic and Mayo Foundation
Rochester, Minnesota

Cushing's syndrome is a symptom complex that results from prolonged exposure to supraphysiologic concentrations of glucocorticoids. It is associated with an unmistakable phenotypic picture and, when correctly diagnosed and properly treated, is curable. When undiagnosed or improperly treated, it can be fatal. The source of excess glucocorticoids may be exogenous (iatrogenic) or endogenous. Endogenous Cushing's syndrome is caused by hypersecretion of corticotropin, or adrenocorticotropic hormone (ACTH) (ACTH-dependent Cushing's syndrome), or by primary adrenal hypersecretion of glucocorticoids (ACTH-independent Cushing's syndrome) (Table 1). The overall treatment program for patients with the Cushing syndrome includes the resolution of hypercortisolism, the concomitant treatment of the complications of Cushing's syndrome (i.e., hyperten-

---

Copyright 1996, Mayo Foundation.

TABLE 1. Causes of the Cushing Syndrome

Exogenous Glucocorticoid Administration (Most Common Cause)

Endogenous
ACTH-dependent
  Pituitary
    Corticotrope adenoma (80%)
    Corticotrope multinodular hyperplasia (rare)
  Ectopic
    Ectopic ACTH-secreting tumor (20%)
    Ectopic CRH-secreting tumor (rare)
    Ectopic ACTH- and CRH-secreting tumor (rare)
ACTH-independent
  Unilateral adrenal disease
    Adenoma (40–50%)
    Carcinoma (40–50%)
  Bilateral adrenal disease
    Massive macronodular hyperplasia (rare)
    Primary pigmented nodular adrenal disease (rare)

Abbreviations: ACTH = adrenocorticotropic hormone; CRH = corticotropin-releasing hormone.

TABLE 2. Diagnostic Evaluation of Cushing's Syndrome

1. Confirmation of hypercortisolism
  a. Clinical assessment
  b. Baseline glucocorticoids (serum cortisol levels, urinary free cortisol excretion) and low-dose dexamethasone suppression test
2. Subtype diagnosis
  a. Plasma ACTH
  b. High-dose dexamethasone suppression test
3. Localization studies
  a. Directed computed imaging
  b. Inferior petrosal sinus sampling for ACTH with oCRH stimulation

Abbreviations: ACTH = adrenocorticotropic hormone; oCRH = ovine corticotropin-releasing hormone.

sion, osteoporosis, and diabetes mellitus), and following definitive treatment, the management of glucocorticoid withdrawal and hypothalamic-pituitary-adrenal (HPA) axis recovery.

PRESENTATION

Typical signs and symptoms of the Cushing syndrome include weight gain with central obesity, facial rounding and plethora, dorsocervical fat pad, easy bruising, fine "cigarette paper" skin, poor wound healing, purple striae, proximal muscle weakness, emotional and cognitive changes (e.g., irritability, crying, depression, restlessness), hypertension, osteoporosis, opportunistic and fungal infections (e.g., mucocutaneous candidiasis, tinea versicolor, pityriasis), altered reproductive function, and hirsutism. These clinical features may develop slowly over time, making comparison of the patient's current appearance with old photographs invaluable. Standard laboratory studies may reveal fasting hyperglycemia, hyperlipidemia, and leukocytosis with relative lymphopenia.

Iatrogenic Cushing's syndrome, more common than the endogenous forms, is usually due to the known administration of glucocorticoids. Excess ACTH secretion by a pituitary tumor or by another neoplastic source is the cause of endogenous Cushing's syndrome in 85% of patients. ACTH-independent forms of Cushing's syndrome (adrenal adenoma, adrenal carcinoma, and adrenal nodular hyperplasia) are responsible for 15% of the endogenous cases (see Table 1).

DIAGNOSIS

Accurate diagnosis of the Cushing syndrome and subtype is essential to direct the appropriate treatment program. The diagnostic evaluation of Cushing's syndrome typically proceeds as outlined in Table 2. Because of the known manifestations of the disorder, hypercortisolism must be suspected and then confirmed with measurements of serum and 24-hour urine cortisol concentrations. Autonomous hypercortisolism (Cushing's syndrome) is confirmed with the low-dose dexamethasone suppression test (dexamethasone 0.5 mg orally every 6 hours for 48 hours); a 24-hour urinary cortisol excretion of 20 µg or more confirms the diagnosis. The plasma ACTH concentration classifies the subtype of hypercortisolism as ACTH-dependent (normal to high levels of ACTH) or ACTH-independent (undetectable ACTH).

Unfortunately, diagnosis of the Cushing syndrome is not always straightforward. The baseline 24-hour urinary cortisol measurements may be elevated by alcoholism, depression, and severe illness. In addition, all forms of endogenous Cushing's syndrome can produce cortisol in a cyclical fashion that confounds the biochemical documentation and interpretation of suppression testing.

In patients with ACTH-dependent hypercortisolism, the high-dose dexamethasone suppression test (dexamethasone 2 mg orally every 6 hours for 48 hours) helps differentiate pituitary from ectopic ACTH hypersecretion; a 24-hour urinary cortisol excretion that decreases 50% or more from baseline values is consistent with pituitary-dependent disease (Figure 1). However, because some types of ectopic ACTH-secreting tumors (e.g., bronchial carcinoid) may also suppress with high-dose dexamethasone administration, computed imaging of the chest is frequently indicated. When a pituitary tumor is not found on computed pituitary imaging, further evaluation is indicated, including computed lung imaging and inferior petrosal sinus sampling (IPSS) for ACTH with ovine corticotropin-releasing hormone (oCRH) stimulation (see Figure 1).

In patients with ACTH-independent hypercortisolism, the high-dose dexamethasone suppression test shows no suppression in urinary cortisol excretion (see Figure 1). In these patients, computed imaging of the adrenal glands usually indicates the type of adrenal disease (see Table 1).

PRINCIPLES OF TREATMENT

Selective pituitary adenectomy by transsphenoidal surgery (TSS) is the treatment of choice for patients with pituitary-dependent disease. The long-term surgical cure rate for ACTH-secreting microadenomas is approximately 90%. If pituitary surgery is not curative, bilateral adrenalectomy and pituitary irradiation are adjunctive treatment options. Surgical extir-

pation of an adrenal adenoma or carcinoma or the source of ectopic ACTH production is the treatment of choice for patients with primary adrenocortical disease or ectopic ACTH production. Bilateral adrenalectomy is the preferred treatment for patients with ACTH-independent bilateral macronodular or micronodular hyperplasia. Pharmacologic therapy is reserved for patients who are not cured with these surgical approaches.

Iatrogenic Cushing's Syndrome

Usually, iatrogenic Cushing's syndrome is the unfortunate accompaniment of the appropriate treatment of a life-threatening or debilitating inflammatory disorder (e.g., vasculitis, severe asthma) with supraphysiologic doses of glucocorticoids. The most frequently used preparation is prednisone (Deltasone). It has been suggested, but not proved, that alternate-day steroid therapy results in fewer side effects and less suppression of the HPA axis. HPA suppression can occur with high-dose (>100 mg hydrocortisone or equivalent per day) glucocorticoid therapy for more than 1 week or lower doses (>50 mg hydrocortisone or equivalent per day) for more than 4 weeks. If glucocorticoid therapy must be continued, the lowest possible dose that effectively treats the underlying disorder should be sought.

Pituitary-Dependent Cushing's Syndrome

The treatment of choice for pituitary-dependent Cushing's syndrome is transsphenoidal selective ad-

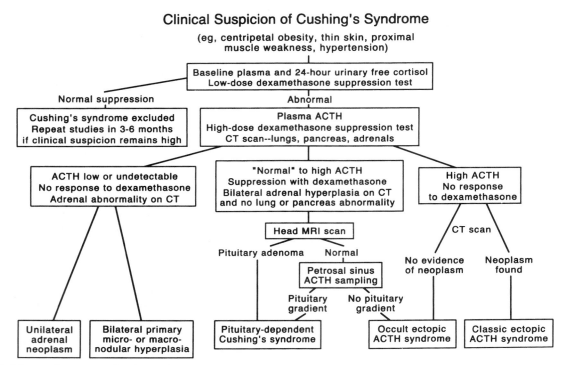

Figure 1. Diagnostic strategy for the evaluation of Cushing's syndrome. The details are discussed in the text. *Abbreviations*: ACTH = adrenocorticotropic hormone; CT = computed tomography; MRI = magnetic resonance imaging.

enectomy performed by an experienced neurosurgeon. IPSS for ACTH should be considered in patients with no obvious pituitary tumor on sellar magnetic resonance imaging (MRI). In cases in which an obvious tumor is not found at surgery, lateralization of ACTH secretion from the preoperative IPSS study guides the surgeon for a hemihypophysectomy. The goal of surgery is to remove the adenoma selectively and preserve normal pituitary tissue. At pituitary surgery centers, the mortality of TSS is 1% or less. The incidence of perioperative morbidity is approximately 10%; postoperative problems include transient diabetes insipidus, cerebrospinal fluid leak, and meningitis. Potential permanent complications are infrequent (<5%) and include diabetes insipidus, partial or complete anterior pituitary failure, and injury to the carotid arteries, optic nerve, or cavernous sinus cranial nerves.

Postoperative Management

Patients who are cured with TSS develop sudden secondary adrenal insufficiency. For this reason, all our patients receive a standard glucocorticoid preparation preoperatively of 40 mg methylprednisolone sodium succinate (Solu-Medrol) administered intramuscularly the morning of the operation and again the evening of the operation; the dose is tapered to 20 mg every 12 hours on the first postoperative day and to 10 mg on the morning of the second postoperative day. Plasma cortisol concentrations are measured at 8 A.M. and 4 P.M. on the third postoperative day. Most patients who are cured will develop symptoms of adrenal insufficiency 24 to 36 hours after the last dose of methylprednisolone. Patients are cautioned about these symptoms and advised to report them promptly—at which time a blood sample is obtained for cortisol measurement and 10 mg of methylprednisolone is administered intramuscularly. If the plasma cortisol concentrations are less than 3 μg per dL, a short-term cure is assured. We have observed some patients with long-term cures who had postoperative plasma cortisol concentrations between 3 and 20 μg per dL. Observation and reevaluation several weeks later with baseline 24-hour urinary cortisol and low-dose dexamethasone suppression are indicated in this setting.

Most patients have had endogenous hypercortisolism for many years, and abrupt postoperative institution of replacement doses of glucocorticoids is accompanied by significant withdrawal symptoms. Typically, patients are dismissed from the hospital on prednisone (Deltasone) 5 mg orally in the morning and 5 mg orally before the evening meal; 1 to 2 weeks later, the dosage is decreased to 5 mg in the morning and 2.5 mg in the afternoon. Even with this cautious tapering program, all patients have withdrawal (recovery) symptoms of myalgia, depression, and fatigue. This anticipated recovery phase is discussed with the patient preoperatively.

Full HPA axis recovery may require 6 to 24 months. The recovery of hypothalamic CRH secretion is the primary and limiting determinant for recovery.

Some degree of adrenal insufficiency must occur during recovery from HPA axis suppression. Two to 3 months after surgery, it is important to change the dosing to a single morning dose of a short-acting glucocorticoid (e.g., 20 mg hydrocortisone). This lower dose of hydrocortisone facilitates HPA recovery by causing relative cortisol deficiency in the afternoon and evening. If the symptoms of adrenal insufficiency cannot be tolerated, then 5 to 10 mg of hydrocortisone may be added at 4 P.M. daily for 2 to 3 weeks. Morning plasma cortisol concentrations are measured every 1 to 2 months to assess HPA axis recovery. When the daily dose of hydrocortisone is at 20 mg, it is rarely necessary to taper this dose further. When the basal level of plasma cortisol is 10 μg per dL or more, therapy may be discontinued. Depending on the degree of HPA suppression, it may take up to 2 years before the plasma cortisol concentration normalizes. Cosyntropin stimulation testing is superfluous in this setting. Also, alternate-day glucocorticoid administration is usually not necessary or helpful in the withdrawal process. Patients should receive stress glucocorticoid coverage and wear Medic Alert identification for 1 year after the use of exogenous glucocorticoids has been discontinued.

Finally, it is important to assess the status of the pituitary-thyroid and pituitary-gonadal axes 6 to 12 weeks postoperatively.

Failed Transsphenoidal Surgery

During the past decade, selective transsphenoidal adenectomy was curative in 202 patients with pituitary-dependent Cushing's syndrome operated on at the Mayo Clinic. However, another 24 patients (10%) were not cured with this operation owing to incomplete resection of a microadenoma (46%), an inability to locate a small microadenoma (33%), or incomplete resection of an invasive macroadenoma (21%). One-third of these patients subsequently developed the Nelson-Salassa syndrome, with hyperpigmentation and pituitary macroadenoma.

If TSS fails to cure the Cushing syndrome, a second operation should be considered. The role of total hypophysectomy in this situation is controversial, and many factors, such as hypopituitarism and desire for future reproductive function, should be considered.

In patients with severe Cushing's syndrome in whom TSS has failed (and in certain patients with mild to moderate persistent disease), I favor a quick and definitive cure of the hypercortisolism with bilateral adrenalectomy. Although this surgery may seem aggressive and directed at the "wrong gland," it can be a lifesaving maneuver.

In patients with mild Cushing's syndrome who have persistent disease following TSS, combined sellar irradiation and pharmacotherapy may be considered. Radiation therapy consists of 4500 to 5000 cGy over three fields in 25 fractions over 33 days. The disadvantages of conventional radiation therapy include a slow onset of action (1 to 2 years), temporal hair loss, and hypopituitarism.

Until radiation therapy is effective, some form of

pharmacotherapy must be continued. Drugs targeted at decreasing pituitary tumor ACTH secretion (e.g., cyproheptadine, bromocriptine, valproic acid, octreotide) are rarely effective. The two most commonly used agents that inhibit steroidogenesis are ketoconazole (Nizoral) and mitotane (1,1-dichloro-2[o-chlorophenyl]-2-[P-chlorophenyl]-ethane, o,p′DDD; Lysodren). Ketoconazole inhibits 17,20-desmolase, 11-beta-hydroxylase, and other enzymes in the adrenal cortex. Dosages range from 300 to 600 mg administered twice daily on an empty stomach. Since drug absorption requires an acidic environment, antacids and agents that decrease stomach acidity should be avoided. Side effects include hepatic dysfunction, renal dysfunction, gynecomastia, and gastrointestinal upset. Liver function, serum creatinine, and urinary cortisol excretion should be followed every 6 to 8 weeks. The use of mitotane is discussed in the later section on adrenocortical malignancy.

Ectopic ACTH Syndrome

The optimal treatment in patients with ectopic ACTH syndrome is to completely resect the ACTH- or CRH-secreting tumor. However, this may not be possible for two reasons: (1) in 20% of the cases, the source of ectopic ACTH production cannot be localized at the time Cushing's syndrome is diagnosed; and (2) the ectopic ACTH-secreting tumor may be metastatic or incompletely resectable.

Occult Ectopic ACTH

In a patient with an occult ectopic source of ACTH and moderate-to-severe Cushing's syndrome, I favor a quick, definitive cure with bilateral adrenalectomy. Pharmacotherapy in these patients rarely completely controls the hypercortisolism, and the associated morbidity and risk of mortality persist.

In a patient with an occult ectopic source of ACTH and mild disease, a reasonable approach is to treat the hypercortisolism with ketoconazole or mitotane and evaluate the patient every 6 months (for up to 2 years) with computed imaging (e.g., MRI of the chest and upper abdomen) and octreotide scintigraphy. If the ectopic source of ACTH is found, surgery is usually curative. The dosage of ketoconazole or mitotane is adjusted to maintain the 24-hour urinary cortisol at the low end of the normal range. To prevent symptomatic adrenal insufficiency, I treat these patients with low doses of dexamethasone (e.g., 0.25 to 0.5 mg daily). Owing to hepatic and renal toxicity associated with ketoconazole, liver function tests and serum creatinine should be checked every 6 to 8 weeks. This drug should be discontinued if evidence of hepatic or renal toxicity is found.

Metastatic or Unresectable ACTH-Secreting Tumor

In a patient with an unresectable or metastatic ACTH-secreting tumor, a quick, definitive cure with bilateral adrenalectomy is the treatment of choice. Although pharmacotherapy appears to be an attractive option in these cases, drug therapy rarely controls the hypercortisolism, owing to the markedly elevated levels of plasma ACTH. In some cases, such as small cell lung carcinoma, tumor-directed chemotherapy may result in a hormonal cure.

The perioperative glucocorticoid therapy for patients undergoing bilateral adrenalectomy is the same as that discussed previously for patients treated with TSS. However, since these patients no longer have adrenal glands that will recover, prednisone, or an equivalent of hydrocortisone, at a dose of 5 to 7.5 mg daily is continued for life. In many cases, the full replacement dosage is not needed because of a small amount of residual functioning adrenocortical tissue. We instruct patients about stress steroid coverage and the need to wear medical identification. In addition, orally administered mineralocorticoid replacement in the form of fludrocortisone (Florinef) at a dosage of 0.05 to 0.1 mg per day is started before discharge from the hospital. The proper dosage is determined by serum electrolytes and supine and standing blood pressures.

Adrenocortical Carcinoma

The treatment of choice for adrenocortical carcinoma is complete surgical resection through the anterior abdominal approach. This malignant tumor should be suspected in patients with marked hypercortisolism (24-hour urinary cortisol >1000 μg) and adrenal tumors greater than 6 cm in largest lesional diameter on computed imaging. Even when the resection is apparently complete, the recurrence rate is high, and the 5-year survival rate is approximately 20%. Treatment with mitotane should be used in patients with incomplete tumor resection. This drug is an adrenal cytolytic agent that inhibits adrenal steroid synthesis and destroys normal and neoplastic adrenocortical cells. The initial dosage is one 500-mg tablet with food twice daily. The total dosage is increased by 500 mg weekly until the maximal tolerated dosage or a maximal dose of 10 grams daily is attained. In most patients, the dosage is limited by nausea, anorexia, diarrhea, somnolence, skin rash, and pruritus. Mitotane is lipophilic and has a long half-life (2 weeks to 6 months). Therefore, mitotane is contraindicated in women desiring fertility within 2 to 5 years of treatment. This drug also destroys the normal contralateral adrenal gland, and concomitant therapy with dexamethasone 0.5 mg daily should be administered. In addition, low-dose mineralocorticoid replacement may be needed, which is determined by periodic measurement of serum potassium concentration. If hyperkalemia develops, treatment with fludrocortisone 0.05 mg daily is started and the dosage adjusted to maintain the serum potassium level in the normal range.

Because of the high recurrence rate of adrenocortical carcinoma, I favor adjuvant treatment with mitotane in patients who have apparently been cured surgically. Reevaluation with computed abdominal imaging is done at 3, 6, and 12 months after surgery.

If recurrent disease is not evident at 12 months postoperatively, the mitotane treatment is discontinued. This adjuvant treatment is controversial, and benefit has not been proved.

Adrenal Adenoma

Patients with Cushing's syndrome caused by an adrenal adenoma are cured with unilateral adrenalectomy. This surgery is usually performed using the traditional posterior approach or the more recently developed laparoscopic approach. The patient should be cautioned that it may take 4 to 18 months before the HPA axis recovers. The rate-limiting step in axis recovery is in the hypothalamic CRH neuron or higher regulatory inputs. At approximately 6 weeks following surgery, patients are switched to a single 20-mg morning dose of the shorter-acting glucocorticoid hydrocortisone. The single morning dosage allows for relative nocturnal glucocorticoid insufficiency and stimulation of the hypothalamic neurons. The concentration of plasma cortisol at 8 A.M. (prior to hydrocortisone administration) is measured every 6 to 8 weeks. Hydrocortisone treatment may be discontinued when the plasma cortisol concentration is 10 μg per dL or more. Patients are cautioned on the need for stress steroid coverage for approximately 1 year after exogenous treatment is discontinued. Mineralocorticoid replacement is usually not required in patients following unilateral adrenalectomy.

Complications of Cushing's Syndrome

Hypertension

Hypertension is present in approximately 75 to 80% of patients with Cushing's syndrome. The mechanisms of hypertension include increased production of deoxycorticosterone, increased vascular reactivity to catecholamines, and overload of cortisol inactivation with stimulation of the mineralocorticoid receptor. Deficient cortisol ring A reduction due to overload of metabolizing enzymes results in a Type II variant of "apparent mineralocorticoid excess" in patients with severe hypercortisolism. The hypertension associated with Cushing's syndrome should be treated until a surgical cure is obtained. Spironolactone (Aldactone), at dosages used to treat primary aldosteronism, is effective in reversing the hypokalemia (see "Primary Aldosteronism"). Second-step agents include thiazide diuretics, beta-adrenergic receptor blockers, angiotensin-converting enzyme inhibitors, and calcium channel antagonists. The hypertension associated with hypercortisolism usually resolves over several weeks after the surgical cure, and antihypertensive agents can be tapered and withdrawn. Approximately 26% of patients have persistent hypertension despite cure of the hypercortisolism.

Osteoporosis

In patients with iatrogenic Cushing's syndrome, it is important to quantitate and follow bone mineral density. If long-term glucocorticoid treatment is planned, it is important to optimize several factors in an attempt to preserve bone density: (1) increase daily elemental calcium ingestion to 1500 to 2000 mg daily; (2) follow 24-hour urinary calcium excretion and, if it exceeds 300 mg, consider thiazide diuretic therapy to prevent renal lithiasis; (3) ensure adequate daily vitamin D intake with one or two multiple vitamin tablets daily; (4) initiate estrogen replacement therapy in postmenopausal women; and (5) decrease the glucocorticoid dosage to the lowest effective single daily dose. Although bone-directed pharmacologic therapy has not been proved to be beneficial in these patients, several agents are under investigation. Until these become available, it is reasonable to consider treatment with antiresorptive agents such as calcitonin or a bisphosphonate.

A quick, complete cure of hypercortisolism is the best therapy for osteoporosis in patients with endogenous Cushing's syndrome.

Hyperglycemia

Diabetes mellitus secondary to hypercortisolism is common in Cushing's syndrome. Insulin therapy is frequently indicated and may need to be continued indefinitely in patients who have iatrogenic Cushing's syndrome because of planned long-term glucocorticoid administration. A quick, complete cure of hypercortisolism is the best therapy for diabetes mellitus in patients with endogenous Cushing's syndrome, and insulin treatment can frequently be tapered over several weeks following surgery and discontinued.

DIABETES INSIPIDUS

method of
PAUL M. PALEVSKY, M.D.
*University of Pittsburgh School of Medicine and
    Veterans Affairs Medical Center*
Pittsburgh, Pennsylvania

and

MALCOLM COX, M.D.
University of Pennsylvania School of Medicine
Philadelphia, Pennsylvania

Diabetes insipidus results either from failure of the hypothalamic-pituitary axis to synthesize or release adequate amounts of vasopressin (hypothalamic diabetes insipidus) or from failure of the kidney to produce a concentrated urine despite appropriate circulating vasopressin levels (nephrogenic diabetes insipidus). In both forms of diabetes insipidus, the inability of the kidney to concentrate the urine leads to polyuria, and osmotic stimulation of the hypothalamic thirst center results in secondary polydipsia. If water intake is inadequate to replace urinary electrolyte-free water losses, hypertonicity and hypernatremia ensue.

Diabetes insipidus may occur in either complete or partial form. In complete hypothalamic diabetes insipidus, vasopressin secretion is absent, resulting in the excretion of large volumes of dilute urine (urine osmolality <150 mOsm per kg water). In partial hypothalamic diabetes insipidus, vasopressin secretion is detectable but subnormal, and a less severe defect in renal water conservation is present. Similarly, in complete nephrogenic diabetes insipidus, renal responsiveness to the hydro-osmotic effect of vasopressin is absent, whereas an impaired response occurs in partial nephrogenic diabetes insipidus.

Any pathologic process involving the hypothalamic-pituitary axis may produce hypothalamic diabetes insipidus. Common causes include pituitary surgery, head trauma, tumors, hemorrhage, thrombosis, infarction, and granulomatous disease. Idiopathic hypothalamic diabetes insipidus also occurs, probably on an autoimmune basis. A rare hereditary form results from mutations in the vasopressin gene, leading to abnormal structure or processing of the vasopressin prohormone.

Nephrogenic diabetes insipidus may be congenital or acquired in origin. Severe nephrogenic diabetes insipidus is usually congenital, resulting from mutations in the vasopressin V_2-receptor gene or, in rare patients, from mutations in the aquaporin-2 water channel gene. Obstructive uropathy or therapy with lithium or demeclocycline may cause an acquired form severe enough to require specific therapy. Less severe nephrogenic diabetes insipidus may result from hypokalemia or hypercalcemia and usually responds to correction of the underlying disorder.

Diabetes insipidus needs to be differentiated from other causes of polyuria, including primary polydipsia, solute diuresis secondary to glucosuria, mannitol or diuretic therapy, or resolving acute renal failure. Solute diuresis can be excluded by demonstrating that the urine osmolality is less than 150 mOsm per kg of water. Formal dehydration testing to confirm diabetes insipidus is usually unnecessary and may cause severe hypernatremia. However, such testing may be required to diagnose partial diabetes insipidus. The urinary response to exogenous vasopressin usually differentiates between the hypothalamic and the nephrogenic forms of diabetes insipidus. Plasma vasopressin levels, although confirmatory and important in equivocal cases, are not available on a routine basis.

TREATMENT

Since polyuria is the primary manifestation of diabetes insipidus, water intake in sufficient quantity to maintain water balance and prevent hypernatremia is the mainstay of therapy. Specific therapeutic interventions are dependent on the particular clinical situation. In ambulatory patients with normal thirst, significant water deficits are uncommon, and therapy is directed at reducing the polyuria and polydipsia. In contrast, comatose patients with acute post-traumatic diabetes insipidus are unable to drink in response to thirst and may develop progressive, life-threatening hypernatremia. Therapy for these patients must first be directed at correcting the existing water deficit and replacing ongoing urinary water losses.

Correction of Water Deficits

In patients with diabetes insipidus, hypernatremia results when renal water losses are not matched by water intake. Assuming that total body solute has not changed and that total body water is usually 60% of body weight, the water deficit may be estimated as:

$$\text{Water Deficit} = 0.6 \times \text{Usual Weight} \times (1 - 140/[\text{Na}^+])$$

where the water deficit is measured in liters, the usual weight is expressed in kg, and $[\text{Na}^+]$ is the serum sodium concentration in milliequivalents per liter. Despite inherent inaccuracies in this formula (resulting from the fact that the usual weight is rarely known and that total body water is not always 60% of body weight), it provides an approximation of the water deficit, which can be used in planning therapy.

In hypertonic states, to protect against excessive shrinkage, the solute content of brain cells increases—both through uptake of extracellular sodium chloride and by the production of a variety of organic osmolytes. Because this solute cannot be immediately dissipated, the rapid replacement of large water deficits carries the risk of acute cerebral edema and may precipitate seizures, coma, permanent neurologic sequelae, or death. For this reason, although prompt therapy should be instituted to reduce the risk of central nervous system damage from protracted hypernatremia, no more than one-half of the estimated water deficit should be replaced during the first 6 to 12 hours. The patient's neurologic status should be monitored carefully and water repletion halted if neurologic deterioration occurs. The remainder of the deficit can be replaced over the ensuing 24 to 48 hours.

In addition to repairing the existing water deficit, ongoing water losses must be replaced. Enteral water administration, either orally or via feeding tube, is always preferable, provided that the risk of pulmonary aspiration is minimal. If enteral repletion is not possible, 5% dextrose in water can be administered intravenously. Urine volume and serum and urine electrolyte concentrations should be used to guide the prescription for water replacement.

Pharmacologic Agents

Pharmacologic therapy of diabetes insipidus has the goal of decreasing the polyuria, thereby permitting maintenance of water balance with a more tolerable level of water intake. Hormone replacement is used for patients with hypothalamic diabetes insipidus. In patients with nephrogenic diabetes insipidus, who are by definition resistant to vasopressin, pharmacologic management attempts to mitigate the polyuria by decreasing solute excretion and increasing vasopressin-independent water reabsorption. The agents and dosages currently recommended are listed in Table 1.

Vasopressin and Vasopressin Analogues

Arginine Vasopressin (Pitressin). Arginine vasopressin is a synthetic form of the naturally occuring human hormone. The aqueous solution, containing 20 IU per mL, is usually administered subcutaneously. Intravenous administration should be avoided because of undesired pressor and vaso-

TABLE 1. **Pharmacologic Treatment of Diabetes Insipidus**

Drug	Dose	Onset of Action (h)	Duration of Action (h)	Comments
Vasopressin Analogues				
Arginine vasopressin (Pitressin)	5–10 IU subcutaneously	0.5–1	2–8	Avoid IV use because of risk of acute hypertension and coronary vasospasm
Desmopressin (DDAVP)	5–20 μg (50–200 μL) intranasally	0.5–1	6–24	Drug of choice for chronic treatment of hypothalamic diabetes insipidus; larger doses may be beneficial in some patients with nephrogenic diabetes insipidus
	1–2 μg intravenously or subcutaneously	0.5–1	6–24	
Thiazide Diuretics				
Chlorthalidone (Hygroton)*	50–100 mg/day	2–4	24–48	Thiazide diuretics, when combined with dietary sodium restriction, ameliorate polyuria; useful in nephrogenic diabetes insipidus; comparable doses of other thiazides are equally effective; must be used with caution in patients taking lithium
Hydrochlorothiazide (Esidrix, HydroDIURIL)*	50–100 mg/day	2–4	6–12	
Nonsteroidal Anti-Inflammatory Drugs				
Indomethacin (Indocin)*	100–150 mg/day	2–4	6–8	Increases vasopressin-independent water reabsorption; useful adjunctive therapy in nephrogenic diabetes insipidus; other inhibitors of prostaglandin synthesis may also be effective
Tolmetin (Tolectin)*	1200–1800 mg/day	2–4	6–8	
Amiloride				
Amiloride (Midamor)*	10–20 mg/day	Delayed	Prolonged	Inhibits lithium entry into renal tubular cells; useful in lithium-induced nephrogenic diabetes insipidus

*Not FDA-approved for this use.

spastic effects. This agent is generally used in acute situations, such as postoperative diabetes insipidus, because of its relatively short duration of action. Repeated dosing is required, and the dose must be titrated to achieve the desired reduction in urine output.

Desmopressin Acetate. DDAVP (1-deamino-8-D-arginine vasopressin) is a synthetic analogue of arginine vasopressin. Because it is devoid of pressor activity and has a longer half-life than the native hormone, it is the drug of choice for the chronic management of hypothalamic diabetes insipidus.

Desmopressin is usually administered intranasally, either as an aqueous solution containing 100 μg per mL or as a metered-dose nasal spray delivering 10 μg in 0.1 mL per actuation. The solution is administered using a calibrated rhinal tube, which is filled to the appropriate graduated line and bent in a U shape. One end is placed in the mouth and the other end into the anterior nares; the drug is then puffed into the nasal cavity deeply enough to avoid runoff out of the nose but not so far back as to pass down into the throat. Patients require training in how to use the catheter to reliably deliver the prescribed dose. The metered-dose spray greatly simplifies administration but has the disadvantage of providing a fixed dose.

A parenteral formulation of desmopressin, containing 4 μg per mL, is available for intravenous or subcutaneous administration. Bioavailability is 5 to 10 times greater with parenteral administration as compared with nasal insufflation. This formulation is useful for hospitalized patients in whom intranasal administration is difficult (e.g., during the perioperative period) and in patients in whom intranasal pathology causes erratic or unreliable drug absorption. Oral administration of desmopressin has been demonstrated to be effective, but the doses required for antidiuresis are approximately 10 times higher than those required with intranasal administration, and the duration of action is only about 6 hours.

Lypressin (Diapid). Lypressin (8-L-lysine vasopressin) is structurally identical to bovine and porcine vasopressin and is available as a nasal solution containing 185 μg per mL. Each spray delivers approximately 7 μg of lypressin, with a biologic activity equivalent to approximately 2 IU of arginine vasopressin. Its use in the treatment of chronic hypothalamic diabetes insipidus has been largely supplanted by desmopressin, which lacks lypressin's pressor effects and has a substantially longer duration of action.

Thiazide Diuretics

Thiazide diuretics are the mainstay of therapy for nephrogenic diabetes insipidus. Thiazides inhibit sodium transport in the cortical diluting segment of the nephron and reduce urinary diluting capacity.

When combined with dietary sodium restriction, thiazide diuretics also produce mild hypovolemia, thereby enhancing proximal tubular fluid reabsorption, diminishing delivery to the distal nephron, and moderating the polyuria. Monitoring for hypokalemia is necessary. and potassium supplementation is often required. In patients with lithium-induced nephrogenic diabetes insipidus, thiazide diuretics must be used with caution, because volume contraction decreases lithium excretion and may result in lithium toxicity.

Amiloride (Midamor)

Amiloride is useful in the treatment of lithium-induced nephrogenic diabetes insipidus. Amiloride inhibits sodium reabsorption in the collecting duct by blocking the apical membrane conductive sodium channel. Since lithium is also transported by the sodium channel, amiloride inhibits the uptake of lithium, decreasing its intracellular concentration and restoring vasopressin responsiveness.

Nonsteroidal Anti-Inflammatory Drugs

Nonsteroidal anti-inflammatory agents, including indomethacin (Indocin), tolmetin (Tolectin), and ibuprofen (Motrin), have utility as adjunctive therapy in the treatment of nephrogenic diabetes insipidus. By increasing renal medullary blood flow, prostaglandins reduce the corticopapillary osmotic gradient for water reabsorption. Prostaglandins also inhibit vasopressin-stimulated adenylate cyclase activity, thereby directly antagonizing the hydro-osmotic effect of the hormone. By blocking renal prostaglandin synthesis, nonsteroidal anti-inflammatory drugs both enhance vasopressin-independent water reabsorption and improve the responsiveness of the collecting duct to vasopressin.

Other Agents

Chlorpropamide (Diabinese) enhances the hydro-osmotic effect of vasopressin and may also stimulate the release of residual vasopressin from the pituitary gland. For these reasons, it has been used as adjunctive therapy in patients with partial hypothalamic diabetes insipidus. However, because of the risk of hypoglycemia and the availability of effective hormone replacement therapy, its use is not advocated. Clofibrate (Atromid) and carbamazepine (Tegretol) also augment the release of vasopressin from the pituitary gland, but significant side effects preclude recommending their routine use.

Clinical Situations

Acute Hypothalamic Diabetes Insipidus

Acute hypothalamic diabetes insipidus is a frequent complication of pituitary surgery or severe head trauma. Because these patients are unable to increase water intake in response to thirst, hypernatremia may develop rapidly. Specific therapy to replace pre-existing water deficits and ongoing urinary water losses should be promptly initiated. Hormone replacement with arginine vasopressin (5 IU subcutaneously) or desmopressin (1 to 2 μg intravenously or subcutaneously) should be started to reduce polyuria and simplify fluid management. Frequent monitoring of urine output and serum electrolytes is required.

After the initial acute phase, partial or complete resolution of diabetes insipidus often occurs. In some patients, a triphasic course may occur, consisting of an initial phase of diabetes insipidus, followed by axonal necrosis of vasopressin-secreting neurons, with uncontrolled vasopressin release, and finally axonal death, with cessation of vasopressin secretion. To ensure detection of recovery from diabetes insipidus, the dosage interval for hormone replacement should be empirically tailored to allow intermittent recurrence of polyuria. Patients who do not recover require long-term management with desmopressin.

Chronic Hypothalamic Diabetes Insipidus

Unless there is concomitant involvement of the hypothalamic thirst center, severe hypertonicity rarely occurs in alert, ambulatory patients with hypothalamic diabetes insipidus who have free access to water. Although polyuria and polydipsia are inconvenient and disruptive, they are not life-threatening. Hormone replacement with intranasal or subcutaneous desmopressin has the goal of decreasing the polyuria and polydipsia, but it must be carefully titrated to prevent inappropriate antidiuresis and water intoxication. It is therefore best to permit brief periods of hormone withdrawal (ideally on a daily basis, but at least weekly) to prevent hormone over-replacement and iatrogenic hyponatremia.

Treatment must be individualized, usually with an in-hospital trial to determine the optimal dosage and dosing interval. This also permits careful education of patients about how to administer the drug intranasally and how to prevent water intoxication. The usual initial dose is 5 μg administered in the evening. The dose should be titrated upward to achieve satisfactory control of nocturia to permit sleep. If daily urine volume remains greater than 2 to 3 liters, a morning dose should be added and the dose titrated to achieve a urine volume of 1.5 to 2 liters per day. An afternoon dose may occasionally be necessary. Because increasing the administered dose generally prolongs the duration of antidiuresis rather than increasing its magnitude, titrating the dose may obviate the need for increasing the frequency of administration.

Nephrogenic Diabetes Insipidus

As with hypothalamic diabetes insipidus, the mainstay of therapy for nephrogenic diabetes insipidus is adequate water intake. As would be expected, patients with nephrogenic diabetes insipidus generally do not respond to hormone replacement therapy. Reversible etiologies (e.g., hypokalemia, hypercalcemia, urinary tract obstruction) should be treated, and offending drugs (e.g., lithium, demeclocycline) should be discontinued, if possible. Useful treatment measures include dietary protein restriction to decrease obligate urinary solute excretion, sodium restriction and thiazide diuretics to reduce steady-state solute excretion and electrolyte-free water clearance, and nonsteroidal anti-inflammatory drugs to increase vasopressin-independent water reabsorption. Although thiazides and nonsteroidal anti-inflammatory agents will not elevate urine osmolality above that of plasma, the increase in urine osmolality toward isosthenuria will nonetheless significantly ameliorate the polyuria. Amiloride may be beneficial in restoring vasopressin responsiveness in patients with lithium-induced polyuria. Although desmopressin is usually not effective in nephrogenic diabetes insipidus, occasional patients have partial responses with supraphysiologic doses of this agent.

GOITER

method of
AMY L. O'DONNELL, M.D., and
STEPHEN W. SPAULDING, M.D.
State University of New York at Buffalo
Buffalo, New York

Although any enlargement of the thyroid gland can be considered a goiter, this article focuses on simple nontoxic goiter and excludes goiters due to autoimmune thyroid disease, subacute thyroiditis, or cancer. The most common cause of goiter worldwide is iodine deficiency, the effects of which are often exacerbated by dietary goitrogens (particularly thiocyanate from cassava or millet). However, when dietary iodine is sufficient, excess iodine (from foods rich in iodine such as kelp, or from iodide-containing drugs such as amiodarone) may occasionally induce goiter. Lithium is another common goitrogenic drug. Familial defects in thyroid hormonogenesis are rare causes of goiter, but subtle defects may be uncovered with prolonged physiologic stimulation (such as pregnancy) and result in goiter formation. In iodine-sufficient areas, the etiology of most cases of nontoxic goiter remains unknown.

EVALUATION OF PATIENTS WITH NONENDEMIC GOITER

Asymptomatic thyroid enlargement (diffuse or nodular) is a common finding on routine physical examination. A patient with a large or substernal goiter, however, may first present with obstructive symptoms such as difficulty swallowing, shortness of breath, or a change in voice or hoarseness owing to compression of the recurrent laryngeal nerve. These symptoms may be exacerbated by the patient's raising his or her arms over the head. Once a goiter has been identified, the history and physical examination should be directed toward identifying signs or symptoms of hyperthyroidism, hypothyroidism, or malignancy. The patient should be questioned specifically about family history of thyroid problems or a history of exposure to radiation during childhood, to iodine deficiency or excess, or to drug or food goitrogens. The size, consistency, and nodularity of the thyroid gland as well as evidence concerning adenopathy should be documented.

Laboratory studies should include measurement of thyroid-stimulating hormone (TSH, thyrotropin) with a sensitive (third-generation) assay as well as either the free thyroxine level or the thyroxine level and thyroid hormone–binding capacity. Antithyroglobulin or antithyroid peroxidase (antimicrosomal) antibody assays can provide useful information concerning the possibility of autoimmune thyroid disease as a cause of the goiter, even if the patient is euthyroid. Ultrasonography of the thyroid may be helpful in assessing the size and extent of the goiter, as well as its nodularity. For a substernal goiter, a computed tomography (CT) scan may be necessary to evaluate the full extent of the gland. Pulmonary function testing, including flow-volume loops, can be helpful in determining the degree of functional tracheal compression by a large or substernal goiter.

TREATMENT OF NONTOXIC, NONENDEMIC GOITER

Five therapeutic options for treating a nontoxic goiter are: withdrawing any goitrogens, following the patient at regular intervals without any initial treatment, treatment with thyroid hormone to suppress TSH levels, surgery, and radioactive iodine therapy.

A careful patient history may reveal that the patient has been exposed to goitrogens. In some cases, it will not be possible to discontinue the use of a goitrogenic drug, such as amiodarone or lithium, without exacerbating the patient's other medical problems. Furthermore, these drugs may cause changes within the thyroid gland that are irreversible even after withdrawal of therapy.

If no identifiable goitrogen is found and the laboratory tests are normal, the physician must first decide whether treatment of the goiter is desirable or necessary and establish the goal of such therapy. If a long-standing multinodular goiter is an incidental finding on routine physical examination, particularly in an elderly patient with no complaints due to mass and no worrisome physical findings, it may be preferable to avoid thyroid hormone suppression therapy with its attendant cardiovascular effects. Follow-up visits are crucial to watch for the development of signs of hypothyroidism or hyperthyroidism or of new growth. If a patient presents with complaints of enlargement or pain in the region of a palpable nodule in a goiter, the suspicion of malignancy is raised, although hemorrhage into a nodule may result in similar symptoms. Patients with multinodular goiters may not have an increased risk of malignancy, but having a goiter does not confer "protection" from thyroid cancer.

Suppression of TSH by treatment with thyroid hormone is more likely to be effective in patients with diffuse goiters (uniform radioiodine uptake) than in patients with multinodular goiters. Reducing the TSH level will cause a reduction in volume only in tissue that is TSH sensitive. A multinodular goiter may well have some regions that are TSH sensitive, but it will also contain fibrous tissue and inactive follicles that are unlikely to respond to thyroid hormone therapy. Furthermore, nodules within a multinodular goiter may function autonomously and can grow independent of TSH stimulation. Although TSH is a potent growth factor for the thyroid gland, many other factors (cytokines, growth factors, autocrine or paracrine factors, growth-stimulating immunoglobulins, or other unrecognized goitrogens) also appear to play important roles in the development of a goiter. In some instances, however, thyroxine (Synthroid) treatment may be useful even in nodular goiters, depending on the therapeutic goal. Some multinodular goiters may decrease in size by as much as 30%, which may be an adequate response when one is trying to prevent worsening of compressive symptoms without resorting to more aggressive therapy. TSH suppression may also prevent the formation of new nodules or further growth of a multinodular goiter, although the efficacy of this treatment remains a focus of debate. Up to half of patients with multinodular goiter may show some response to suppressive therapy, but it is not possible to predict which patients will respond.

There are risks associated with thyroid hormone treatment of multinodular goiters, especially in elderly patients. Since some of the nodules in the goiter may be functioning autonomously, the addition of exogenous thyroid hormone may result in higher thyroid hormone levels and thus could precipitate angina, cardiac arrhythmias, or even frank hyperthyroidism. In general, the dose of thyroxine should be regulated to keep the TSH level in the low normal range, avoiding complete suppression of TSH into the hyperthyroid range, since even mild, asymptomatic (subclinical) hyperthyroidism may have long-term detrimental effects on the cardiovascular system and bones. The dose of thyroxine necessary to achieve this goal must be tailored to the individual patient but usually ranges from 100 to 150 μg per day. Another drawback to thyroxine therapy is that it is usually necessary to treat goiter patients for the rest of their lives; goiters usually resume their growth after treatment is stopped. For this latter reason, young patients with nodular goiters are more often treated with surgery.

Fine-needle aspiration of the thyroid may be indicated for a single dominant or growing nodule within a multinodular goiter. If the aspirate is clearly benign, the nodule may be observed for further growth, or the patient may be given a trial of thyroxine therapy to suppress TSH. If the nodule continues to grow on suppressive therapy, it should be surgically removed.

The other major indication for surgery is a large goiter with obstructive or compressive symptoms, such as dyspnea from tracheal compression, progressive dysphagia, or vocal cord paralysis. Substernal goiters causing outflow tract compression also may require surgical treatment. Near-total thyroidectomy is usually performed, since the goiter may recur from the thyroid remnant, but a subtotal thyroidectomy may be adequate if all palpable abnormal tissue is resected at the time of surgery. Following surgery for goiter, thyroid hormone treatment should be insti-tuted at least at replacement dosages—keeping the TSH at the low end of the normal range may help prevent goiter recurrence.

Radioactive iodine therapy has traditionally been used for hyperthyroidism or cancer. But if a patient presents with a large multinodular goiter, particularly one associated with obstructive symptoms, and is a poor surgical candidate, administration of iodine 131 may destroy enough functioning tissue to relieve the obstructive symptoms. Large doses of radioactive iodine may be required for a satisfactory response, which may necessitate the patient's admission to the hospital for treatment. The risk of transient worsening of obstructive symptoms following radioiodine therapy due to swelling of the thyroid tissue appears to be relatively small compared with the risk of no treatment.

HYPERPARATHYROIDISM AND HYPOPARATHYROIDISM

method of
LAWRENCE E. MALLETTE, M.D., PH.D.
Baylor College of Medicine
Houston, Texas

DIAGNOSIS

Primary Hyperparathyroidism

Primary hyperparathyroidism arises from the intrinsic hyperfunction of one or more of the parathyroid glands. Its hallmark is hypercalcemia. In mild cases or early in the course of more severe cases, the elevation in the total serum calcium level may be borderline or intermittent. Total serum calcium values that lie near the upper limit of normal should be checked by direct estimation of the free calcium ion concentration with an ion-selective electrode. In primary hyperparathyroidism, the ionized calcium value is often elevated when the total serum calcium value is in the upper part of the normal range.

To confirm that the cause of hypercalcemia is parathyroid hyperfunction, serum parathyroid hormone (PTH) levels can be measured. The availability of biterminal, or sandwich, assays that measure only the intact PTH molecule (but not the circulating catabolic fragments of PTH that are devoid of calcemic activity) has simplified diagnosis. Renal dysfunction has only a mild effect on the intact PTH value, and false-positive elevations are rare. The normal range for intact PTH is from 10 pg per mL to approximately 55 to 65 pg per mL. In approximately 80% of patients with primary hyperparathyroidism, the intact PTH value lies above 65 pg per mL. The remaining patients have values between 25 and 65 pg per mL. In patients with nonparathyroid hypercalcemia, the intact PTH value is usually suppressed below 20 pg per mL, unless renal dysfunction is present, in which case the intact PTH value may be as high as 25 pg per mL.

When the intact PTH value of a hypercalcemic patient lies between 25 and 65 pg per mL, presumably signaling a lack of suppressibility of PTH secretion, it may be helpful to measure the midregion PTH value by radioimmunoassay (RIA), as long as renal function is normal. Parathyroid adenomas may secrete both intact PTH and noncalcemic fragments of the hormone (both of which contain the midregion epitopes read by the RIA). Thus, midregion PTH values may be elevated when the intact PTH value is normal. Two factors must be borne in mind when interpretting midregion PTH RIA values, however. First, nonparathyroid hypercalcemia does not suppress serum midregion PTH values as fully as it does the intact PTH value, since the parathyroids continue to release fragments when intact hormone secretion has been fairly completely inhibited. Second, the midregion fragments are cleared largely by the kidneys, so renal dysfunction can increase the midregion PTH value even in patients with nonparathyroid hypercalcemia.

Secondary Hyperparathyroidism

Secondary hyperparathyroidism represents the expected physiologic response of the parathyroid glands to hypocalcemia or a decrease in vitamin D metabolites, or both. Both play a role in inhibiting PTH synthesis and secretion, and deficiency of either can increase PTH secretion and produce parathyroid hyperplasia. The most common settings for clinically evident secondary hyperparathyroidism are renal failure and intestinal malabsorption of fat-soluble vitamins. An increasingly common cause of subtle or subclinical secondary hyperparathyroidism is a failure of adequate vitamin D nutrition in the confined geriatric population, where the risk factors can include poor sun exposure, an inefficient cutaneous formation of vitamin D, an age-related inefficiency of intestinal absorption of vitamin D and its metabolites, and defective renal 1-alpha hydroxylation of 25-hydroxyvitamin D, related to the decline in renal function with age. In these patients secondary hyperparathyroidism increases fracture risk by accelerating bone loss and producing muscle weakness.

As vitamin D deficiency develops, the serum calcium level tends to be well maintained by the secondary rise in the PTH level. Serum phosphate levels fall in response to the increase in the PTH level. At this stage the patient may show only an increase in the serum PTH value, with normal total calcium values, low-normal ionized calcium values, and a drop in serum phosphate values within the normal range. Serum 25-hydroxyvitamin D values are usually below 15 ng per mL but often are above the formal lower limit of normal. Serum 1,25-dihydroxyvitamin D values are often normal or even slightly increased, since renal formation of this metabolite, although limited by a low substrate (25-hydroxyvitamin D) concentration, is stimulated by the increase in the PTH level and the fall in the calcium and phosphate levels. Bone remodeling is accelerated by the increase in the PTH level, whereas both bone synthesis and mineralization may be relatively inhibited by the drop in vitamin D metabolite levels and in serum calcium-phosphate product. Patients may be largely asymptomatic at this stage but show accelerated bone loss. This is the ideal time for diagnosis and intervention, but this stage of the disease can be detected only by measurement of PTH values (with confirmation by ionized calcium and 25-hydroxyvitamin D measurements). More severe vitamin D deficiency eventually decreases serum phosphate levels below normal and finally causes overt hypocalcemia. By this stage of the deficiency, histologic evidence of osteomalacia is present, and the patient has bone pain, muscle weakness, an increase in serum alkaline phosphatase levels, and hyperchloremic acidosis due to the proximal renal tubular effects of the hypocalcemia and increased PTH

level. Intervention is also rewarding at this stage, but the goal should be earlier diagnosis.

Secondary hyperparathyroidism occurs in renal failure as a function of the drop in serum 1,25-dihydroxyvitamin D levels engendered by the rise in serum phosphate levels, the decline in functional renal mass, and perhaps the acidosis. Hypocalcemia produced by the decline in intestinal calcium absorption and increase in the serum phosphate level also contributes. By the time the renal patient has developed symptomatic hyperparathyroid bone disease, intact PTH values are usually above 300 pg per dL, and midregion PTH values are more than 40-fold elevated.

Tertiary Hyperparathyroidism

Tertiary hyperparathyroidism is defined as hypercalcemia produced by parathyroid autonomy that has developed on a background of long-standing secondary hyperparathyroidism. Tertiary hyperparathyroidism usually develops in the setting of chronic dialysis therapy but may also occur in patients with a malabsorption syndrome. It is often manifested clinically as severe hyperparathyroid bone disease but in renal patients may be associated with widespread focal cutaneous calcification and infarction (calciphylaxis). Hypercalcemia can also be superimposed on secondary parathyroid hyperplasia by excessive treatment with a vitamin D congener, excessive oral calcium supplements, the sudden institution of effective restriction of total intestinal phosphate absorption, or a concomitant disease such as sarcoidosis. The parathyroid-independent hypercalcemias should not be confused with tertiary hyperparathyroidism. In these cases, the serum PTH level is less elevated than it was just before the hypercalcemia developed and usually lies in the lower part of the expected range for all secondary hyperparathyroid patients. In tertiary hyperparathyroidism the PTH values should be even more elevated than in secondary hyperparathyroidism.

Hypoparathyroidism

Hypoparathyroidism is characterized by hypocalcemia and hyperphosphatemia with inappropriately low or undetectable serum PTH levels. In total hypoparathyroidism, serum PTH levels remain undetectable in the face of hypocalcemia. In partial hypoparathyroidism, serum PTH levels are inappropriately normal or only mildly elevated despite hypocalcemia. Parathyroid loss can be due to autoimmunity, surgery or other trauma, infiltrative diseases, or congenital deficiency. Functional hypoparathyroidism also occurs in magnesium depletion, which is known to inhibit PTH secretion and action. Measurement of serum PTH levels with an adequately sensitive RIA or biterminal assay should establish the diagnosis.

Pseudohypoparathyroidism

Hypocalcemia and hyperphosphatemia also accompany pseudohypoparathyroidism, but PTH secretion and serum PTH levels are increased by the hypocalcemia and low 1,25-dihydroxyvitamin D levels. When renal function is normal, the finding of increased PTH values in the presence of hyperphosphatemic hypocalcemia suggests pseudohypoparathyroidism. False-positive elevations of PTH RIA values can occur (in less than 2% of patients), probably arising from antibodies in the patient's serum that interfere with the binding of tracer to the assay (anti-PTH) antibody. Thus, the increased PTH value should be confirmed in a second assay system, such as a biterminal intact PTH assay. In general the 70% of pseudohypoparathyroid patients who manifest brachydactyly and/or subcutaneous ossifications have Type 1 pseudohypoparathyroidism, but PTH infusion with measurement of urinary phosphate and cyclic adenosine monophosphate (AMP) responses is needed for the formal differentiation of Type 1 from Type 2 pseudohypoparathyroidism. Patients with pseudohypoparathyroidism should usually be referred to an academic center with interest in the disease and its genetics, so that the individual family's pathophysiology can be fully characterized, together with genetic screening and counseling.

TREATMENT

Primary Hyperparathyroidism

Selection of Therapy

Selection of optimal therapy for primary hyperparathyroidism remains an art as well as a subject of scientific inquiry. Surgical intervention is safe and highly effective, curing the disease permanently in over 95% of patients. On the other hand, mild primary hyperparathyroidism may cause minimal morbidity that for some patients may not outweigh the cost and risk of surgery. Surgical treatment is usually recommended when the patient's serum calcium values lie more than 1.0 mg per dL above the upper normal limit, since the risk of complications is increased. Patients with mild hypercalcemia present a more difficult decision, as many seem to be asymptomatic and there is little evidence for significant long-term morbidity. Factors favoring surgical intervention include a younger age (greater time over which morbidity might accumulate), a low bone mass, especially at the hip, and the presence of symptoms (even nonspecific ones) that might be ameliorated by surgery.

Before electing medical follow-up, it must first be established that the hyperparathyroidism is of the stable variety, i.e., the time course of the disease must be characterized. The vast majority of patients have stable hypercalcemia, caused by an adenoma that arose from a set point error in calcium detection in the clone of cells that now constitutes the tumor. When this clone has expanded to the point that it is able to produce enough PTH to increase serum calcium values to the new inhibitory set point, the stimulus to growth of the tumor is removed and the serum calcium level will remain stable indefinitely. A small number of parathyroid tumors arise on a different basis and produce a slow but steady increase in the serum calcium and PTH levels that becomes evident over weeks or months. These tumors are analogous to other endocrine neoplasms and grow steadily regardless of the ambient calcium level. Serial measurements of serum calcium and PTH levels identify these patients (both calcium and PTH levels should increase steadily). At the extreme end of this spectrum of tumors is the rare (<0.5% of all cases) parathyroid carcinoma, which usually has increased serum calcium levels to more than 13.5 mg per dL by the time it is discovered.

Patients who otherwise seem to be candidates for medical management should be screened for cortical bone loss (measurement of bone mass at the forearm or femoral neck). Mild primary hyperparathyroidism does not decrease spinal bone mass significantly but does compromise cortical bone mass. Patients with a critically low bone mass may benefit from parathyroidectomy, since a moderate increase in bone mass (10 to 15%) occurs during the first 6 months after parathyroidectomy. The added bone mass may protect against fracture in patients whose skeleton is nearing their own "fracture threshold." A radiographic or sonographic examination of the renal beds should also be done before medical management is elected as the long-term strategy. Nephrocalcinosis, nephrolithiasis, or even a staghorn calculus can develop without symptoms and must be excluded before electing to delay surgery.

Medical Management

In the past it was traditional to restrict dietary calcium intake in primary hyperparathyroidism. This is a rational step to minimize hypercalcemia in preparation for surgery or lessen hypercalciuria in a patient with nephrolithiasis. There is, however, the risk that the restriction of calcium intake on a chronic basis will accelerate bone loss. The resulting higher serum PTH values would accelerate bone resorption, especially from the endosteal envelope, where the osteoclasts may be more sensitive to PTH, and contribute to cortical osteopenia. The secondary decrease in serum phosphate levels would also tend to slow bone formation. Until long-term studies of the relationship of dietary calcium levels to skeletal health in hyperparathyroidism are available, it would seem prudent for patients to avoid excessive levels of dietary calcium but to maintain the same calcium intake that would normally be recommended for their age.

A feared complication of hyperparathyroidism is the hypercalcemic crisis. This constitutes a risk regardless of the severity of current symptoms. It is most likely to occur when an intercurrent illness decreases renal perfusion (decreased renal calcium clearance) or immobilizes the patient in bed (increased bone resorption). Examples of such intercurrent illnesses include myocardial infarction, gastroenteritis, cholecystitis, and an automobile accident with multiple fractures. Dehydration can also occur in elderly patients because of their impaired thirst mechanism, combined with the decreased renal concentrating ability produced by the hypercalcemia. Patients with primary hyperparathyroidism must develop a system for ensuring adequate fluid intake on a daily basis. Another potential cause of severe hypercalcemia is the abuse of calcium carbonate antacids by patients with dyspepsia to the extent of producing the equivalent of the milk-alkali syndrome. Patients with primary hyperparathyroidism may be predisposed to this complication because of their increased intestinal calcium absorption. Patients who are to be followed medically must be educated to avoid over-the-counter antacids that contain calcium and to report to an emergency facility if a severe bout of gastroenteritis or other illness predisposing to dehydration should ever occur, or if the patient develops severe lethargy or somnolence.

Medical ablation of the parathyroid adenoma is not yet possible, and no medication has been established as effective for most patients with primary hyperparathyroidism. Certain medications can be directed at protecting the skeleton or minimizing the rise in either serum calcium or PTH levels. A basic problem is that hypercalcemia and the increase in PTH levels (which usually vary inversely in each patient) probably contribute independently to symptoms and morbidity. Hypercalcemia predisposes to ectopic calcification, renal stones, pancreatitis, and gastric hypersecretion and may accelerate the development of atherosclerosis. The rise in PTH levels is probably responsible for the neurologic complications of hyperparathyroidism, including decreased memory, depression, and muscle weakness. Lowering serum calcium levels increases the patient's PTH levels, which would tend to exacerbate the neuromuscular symptoms.

Estrogen replacement therapy is indicated for the postmenopausal woman with primary hyperparathyroidism, to protect the skeleton and lessen the skeletal contribution to hypercalcemia. As for any postmenopausal woman, estrogen is of course most effective if instituted during the early postmenopausal period of rapid bone loss, but even later effects on cortical bone mass should not be considered unimportant. Estrogen may also tend to lessen the degree of hypercalcemia engendered by a given excess of PTH, by blunting the skeletal contribution to hypercalcemia. Addition of a progestagen to protect the endometrium does not seem to blunt the effectiveness of estrogen.

Other antiresorptive agents have also been advocated, such as calcitonin or a bisphosphonate. I use these agents only for patients with severe hyperparathyroidism who are not surgical candidates because of a concomitant serious illness that prevents surgical intervention. For example, a recent patient with terminal rheumatic heart disease and severe obstructive pulmonary disease whose serum calcium values tended to range above 13 mg per dL was successfully managed for more than 18 months with intermittent outpatient pamidronate infusions given whenever the serum calcium value exceeded 12.7 mg per dL.

Neutral phosphate taken orally has been proposed as a treatment to minimize the risk of nephrolithiasis. Few primary hyperparathyroid patients are candidates for this therapy, since nephrolithiasis is a strong indication for parathyroid surgery. The use of neutral phosphate in an attempt to prevent the formation of a first kidney stone is probably unnecessary, since most hyperparathyroid patients who are destined to be stone formers have already formed a stone by the time their hypercalcemia is discovered. Preventive therapy is important, however, for patients with known stone disease who are not surgical

candidates. Neutral potassium phosphate in divided doses (at a level of 1.0 to 1.5 grams per day) can be used to decrease serum 1,25-dihydroxyvitamin D values, intestinal calcium absorption, and urinary calcium excretion. I prefer the potassium salt to the mixed sodium and potassium salt, since sodium has a calciuric effect. Oral phosphate therapy should be undertaken only with great caution when the serum calcium value exceeds approximately 11.5 mg per dL, since the calcium phosphate product can be increased enough to cause ectopic calcification in the kidney and elsewhere, and injury to the kidney could result. Renal insufficiency is also a contraindication to neutral phosphate therapy, since no additional risk of renal injury can be tolerated and since the poor renal clearance of phosphate can predispose to hyperphosphatemia.

Surgical Treatment

Surgical treatment of hyperparathyroidism is elected for many patients with primary (and tertiary) hyperparathyroidism. The risk of parathyroid surgery is essentially the risk of a general anesthetic, plus the small risk of recurrent laryngeal nerve injury or hypoparathyroidism. For those who are not good candidates for inhalation anesthesia but are cooperative and relaxed about the idea of surgery, parathyroidectomy can be carried out under regional (cervical block) anesthesia.

When the operation is performed by a surgeon experienced in parathyroid surgery, the cure rate is approximately 95%, and in the absence of prior neck surgery, damage to the recurrent nerve is rare indeed. The preoperative assessment and preparation are no different from those of any other general anesthesia, except that patients with serum calcium values above 12 mg per dL should be given intravenous hydration overnight, rather than simply being kept "nothing by mouth." Mobilization after the procedure and recovery from the procedure itself are usually rapid, since the patient is not handicapped in the postoperative period by a painful thoracic or abdominal incision.

Although relatively safe and easy for the patient, parathyroid surgery can be quite involved and complicated for the surgeon, since parathyroid glands lie ectopically in a fairly high percentage of cases. Knowledge of the common "hiding places" and experience in approaching and exploring them is essential. Assessment of the size and consistency of the parathyroid glands at the time of surgery is essential to the differentiation of adenoma from hyperplasia, and this requires experience. The parathyroid carcinoma must be recognized at the time of surgery and treated properly, by en bloc resection of the parathyroid tumor and surrounding tissues, if the patient is to have any chance of cure. Thus, parathyroid surgery should be undertaken only by those experienced in the procedure. The surgeon should have "scrubbed" with a more experienced parathyroid surgeon many times before attempting to carry out the procedure on his or her own.

The use of preoperative localization studies is an evolving area of practice. For patients without prior neck surgery, preoperative localization studies in general are not necessary, since the success rate is already 95% without such studies. Thus, I reserve the use of nuclear thyroid scans, computed tomography (CT) scans, magnetic resonance imaging (MRI) scans, arteriography, or venous sampling procedures for patients with prior cervical surgery or with persistent or recurrent hyperparathyroidism. The exception to this general rule is ultrasonography of the thyroid bed, which should either be performed preoperatively or be available intraoperatively in all cases. The procedure is painless, relatively inexpensive, and risk-free. If the preoperative sonogram fails to show a candidate lesion, the surgeon may elect to set aside more time for the procedure, since a prolonged exploration is more likely to be required, or to perform additional localization studies preoperatively. Also, it is wise to know the internal details of thyroid anatomy while performing a parathyroid exploration, for several reasons. First, a parathyroid adenoma or one or more hyperplastic glands can be located within the thyroid gland. When exploration of the neck fails to uncover an adenoma or at least four hyperplastic glands, any hypoechoic lesion found on a thyroid sonogram is a likely candidate for resection. Since 15% of persons have five or more parathyroid glands, a fifth hyperplastic gland located intrathyroidally can be missed if ultrasonography is not performed. Actually, an argument can be made for resection of any isolated thyroid nodule larger than approximately 1 cm, even if it is not palpable and even if all parathyroid tissue has apparently been identified surgically. This would avoid repeat operation in the few cases in which the lesion proves to be a thyroid neoplasm.

A thorough family history concerning parathyroid disease and other endocrine disorders can be important to the surgical management of the patient, since surgical treatment of the hyperparathyroidism is often modified for familial parathyroid disease. Total parathyroidectomy with autogenous parathyroid grafting is favored by many specialists for the patient with multiple endocrine neoplasia Type 1 or Type 2. The other familial form of parathyroid disease that is well characterized is the hereditary cystic parathyroid adenoma–fibro-osseous jaw tumor syndrome, a dominant trait that is carried on chromosome 1. For this syndrome, bilateral inferior parathyroidectomy may be favored, since metachronous second adenomas are common and the adenomas tend to occur most often in the inferior parathyroid glands. Parathyroid tissue from familial cases should be preserved for possible use in future autotransplantation or for genetic studies of the mechanisms of tumorigenesis.

Postoperative Course

After resection of a parathyroid tumor, the serum calcium level usually falls slowly and steadily, either back to normal or below, usually reaching a nadir the evening of surgery or a day or two later. An occasional patient with more severe preoperative hypercalcemia may develop a positive Chvostek sign or circumoral paresthesia before the serum calcium level has fallen to normal, perhaps as a function of the rapidity of the drop. These symptoms need not be treated with intravenous calcium and usually resolve spontaneously, without risk that frank tetany will develop. Serum magnesium values may be low in some of these cases, in which case magnesium should then be administered parenterally. Serum calcium levels fall below normal in less than half the patients. Hypocalcemia indicates either transient or permanent hypoparathyroidism or the "hungry bones" syndrome: the skeleton goes into strong positive balance as bone turnover is returning to normal, since increased bone formation persists longer than the increased resorption. The osteoblasts continue to synthesize bone for several weeks, while the osteoclast count goes rapidly to normal. The serum phosphate level remains low in the hungry bones syndrome but increases in hypoparathyroidism. Measurement of PTH itself gives a more accurate differentiation, however. The hungry bones phenomenon is often accompanied by a transient rise in serum alkaline phosphatase values, and sometimes by an increase in bone pain. A transient rise in the serum creatinine level is also not unusual in the few days after surgery for moderate or severe primary hyperparathyroidism, its basis unknown.

The hungry bones syndrome may persist for several weeks. It can usually be treated satisfactorily with calcitriol (Rocaitrol) in doses of approximately 1 μg per day, plus oral calcium supplements. When the skeletal mineralization process nears completion, however, the need for the supplements may abate rather suddenly. Thus, close monitoring of serum calcium values is needed to avoid iatrogenic hypercalcemia.

Patients cured by resection of an adenoma should have normal serum calcium and PTH values by 6 months. Calcium metabolism requires only infrequent monitoring after this, since the risk of later recurrence is only approximately 0.5%.

Parathyroid Crisis

Primary hyperparathyroidism occasionally presents as life-threatening hypercalcemia, with serum calcium values above 14.0 mg per dL and major alterations in mentation, or nausea and vomiting. The emergent treatment of parathyroid crisis is similar to that of any form of severe hypercalcemia, except that oral neutral phosphate can be very effective. To eliminate the element of increased renal calcium retention due to volume contraction, the patient should be volume-repleted with normal saline, followed by volume expansion to increase proximal tubular rejection of calcium. This may require several liters of fluid. If renal function is adequate, these measures usually stop the upward spiral of calcium values and may lower serum calcium levels significantly. Oral administration of neutral phosphate is also effective. Doses of 1000 to 1500 mg per day safely lower serum calcium values in most patients. The dosage must be moderated if renal function is compromised, and phosphate therapy is contraindicated if the serum phosphate level is above the middle of the normal range. Oral phosphate of course cannot be used if the patient is vomiting or has depressed mentation. Hypokalemia can complicate oral phosphate therapy, so close monitoring of the serum potassium level is important.

When oral phosphate therapy cannot be used, I usually begin antiresorptive therapy early during treatment, in order to eliminate any skeletal contribution to the hypercalcemia, which may have been further increased by immobilization. As soon as I am confident, from the blood chemistry values and adequate urinary flow, that renal function is not severely compromised, an intravenous infusion of pamidronate (Aredia) is begun (usually 60 mg over 4 to 6 hours). If the serum creatinine value is above 5 mg per dL, I usually start antiresorptive therapy with subcutaneous salmon calcitonin (200 U every 12 hours).

Now that highly effective antiresorptive agents are available, emergency parathyroid exploration is seldom needed. The intact PTH assay can be performed in a very short time, requiring no longer than overnight, to provide rapid confirmation of the diagnosis in those rare cases in which emergency neck exploration is contemplated. To remove the risk of another crisis, elective parathyroid exploration should be carried out in most cases soon after the hypercalcemia has been controlled and the diagnosis confirmed.

Secondary Hyperparathyroidism

Secondary hyperparathyroidism is treated by provision of the missing vitamin D metabolite(s). For those with intestinal malabsorption, ergocalciferol (Drisdol) can be given orally in doses that usually range from 50,000 U weekly to daily. Alternately, ergocalciferol can be given intramuscularly (1 million U in 1 mL given monthly) to circumvent problems from variable intestinal absorption and decrease the number of oral medications the patient must contend with. There is no rationale for the use of the more expensive vitamin D congeners, such as calcifidiol, calcitriol, or dihydrotachysterol, in malabsorption or vitamin D–deficient patients. The skeletal lesions of patients who have symptomatic hypocalcemia and osteomalacia probably heal faster when oral calcium and phosphate supplements are given during the early few weeks of treatment, when skeletal remineralization is consuming large amounts of substrate.

Renal hyperparathyroidism can be such a devastating complication that treatment should begin with preventive measures at an early stage in the evolution of renal insufficiency. Dietary phosphate restriction, phosphate binders, and assurance of adequate calcium and vitamin D nutrition are important in slowing the development of secondary parathyroid hyperplasia, but now are known to be inadequate

alone. As the renal insufficiency advances and 1,25-dihydroxyvitamin D values decline, an active form of vitamin D must be provided to prevent parathyroid hyperplasia by keeping the parathyroid glands supplied with an active vitamin D metabolite. Oral calcitriol has recently seen heavy usage in renal insufficiency and is very effective in stimulating intestinal calcium absorption. It is not well absorbed, however, and may not reach the parathyroid glands in sufficient amounts. One of four strategies can be used to circumvent this problem. Calcitriol itself can be delivered to the parathyroid glands in increased amount either by giving it intravenously at the time of each hemodialysis or by giving it intermittently in large oral doses (3 to 5 μg given every 3 to 4 days). The third strategy is the use of dihydrotachysterol. This congener must be absorbed and 25-hydroxylated in the liver to acquire biologic activity but thereafter has "equal" effects on the parathyroid glands and intestinal tract. Historically, this was the first vitamin D congener found clinically to have biologic potency in uremia, but for unclear reasons it seems to have been largely forgotten in recent years. A compound with a similar pathway of activation and spectrum of action, but somewhat less fat-soluble, is 1-alpha-hydroxycholecalciferol. Hepatic 25-hydroxylation of this compound forms 1,25-dihydroxycholecalciferol (calcitriol), which then enters the circulation to have "equal" intestinal and parathyroid effects. This precursor is used in Europe but is not yet available in the United States. All these approaches must be monitored carefully to avoid inducing untoward rises in serum calcium and phosphate levels, with the risk of ectopic calcifications. In some patients these measure are insufficient to prevent or reverse severe parathyroid hyperplasia, and subtotal parathyroidectomy may become necessary.

Tertiary Hyperparathyroidism

In tertiary hyperparathyroidism, attempts at controlling the degree of hyperparathyroidism by medical means usually meet with little success, and while awaiting control of the hyperfunction, the patient often develops severe skeletal disease. This state of true parathyroid autonomy is therefore best managed by parathyroid surgery, assuming that the diagnosis has been confirmed by demonstrating the expected markedly elevated serum PTH value.

Hypoparathyroidism

Acute Hypocalcemia

Hypocalcemia requires emergency treatment when it produces overt tetany, laryngospasm, or seizures. I use intravenous calcium gluconate as a bolus of 5 mg of elemental calcium per kg of body weight over 3 to 5 minutes, followed by infusion of 5 mg per kg per hour for 3 or 4 hours. This usually raises the serum calcium level by 2 to 3 mg per dL. The infusion without the bolus can be used for severe symptoms without overt tetany. The change in the serum calcium level is confirmed at 2 hours and intermittently thereafter. I avoid the use of intravenous calcium chloride, which some have advocated as a better treatment because more free calcium ion is immediately available. The subcutaneous infiltration of calcium chloride may cause skin necrosis, which is not seen with the gluconate salt, which itself produces a rapid clinical response. If hypocalcemia is associated with magnesium depletion, parenteral magnesium therapy is mandatory and produces a much better and more complete response than intravenous calcium therapy alone.

Surgical Management

Parathyroid tissue implanted with proper technique into a muscle bed will survive and function well enough to maintain calcium homeostasis. Successful transplantation of parathyroid tissue between identical twins has been reported once, and parathyroid homografts have been carried out successfully in a small number of immunosuppressed renal transplant recipients. Prevention of hypoparathyroidism during thyroid surgery is important. Muscle implantation of questionably viable parathyroid glands or of glands recovered from the resected thyroid specimen (by dissection in a sterile field under a dissecting microscope) markedly reduces the incidence of hypoparathyroidism. I believe too few surgeons employ these stratagems.

Medical Therapy

The most important long-term goal of treatment is the prevention of tetany and seizures. This can be accomplished by keeping serum calcium levels above approximately 7.0 to 7.5 mg per dL unless the patient has an independent seizure disorder that is exacerbated by hypocalcemia. Additional goals are the prevention of premature cataract formation and calcifications of the central nervous system, especially the basal ganglia. These goals can be accomplished by keeping serum calcium values near or just below the lower limit of normal. Maintenance of *normal* serum calcium values is not necessary and is in fact detrimental.

For any given degree of hypocalcemia, the patient with hypoparathyroidism has a greater urinary calcium excretion than the patient with intact parathyroids, in whom the renal tubular reabsorption of calcium is stimulated by the increased PTH level. Returning the filtered calcium load entirely to normal in a hypoparathyroid patient often renders the patient hypercalciuric. The therapeutic goal is to keep the serum calcium level as close to normal as possible without producing hypercalciuria. Before the physiology of this situation was understood, patients were often overtreated and many developed the severe complications related to nephrocalcinosis and the concomitant hypertension.

The rare patient with partial hypoparathyroidism may be maintained on an oral calcium supplement alone (1000 to 2000 mg daily in divided doses). Most

hypoparathyroid patients, however, require additional therapy. Until a long-acting and easily administered congener of PTH is available, treatment of hypoparathyroidism will rely on the use of vitamin D congeners. Ergocalciferol, vitamin D_2 itself, increases intestinal calcium absorption enough to maintain a satisfactory serum calcium level. The usual dosage range is 50,000 to 100,000 U per day, although a few patients with partial hypoparathyroidism require less. Patients taking these doses of ergocalciferol usually have serum 25-hydroxyvitamin D values several-fold elevated, and normal 1,25-dihydroxyvitamin D values. Doses above 100,000 U per day often produce hypercalcemia within a few weeks. Ergocalciferol has a long half-life, so equilibrium is not reached for several weeks after a prescribed change in dosage, making management a bit clumsy. An advantage of the long half-life is that if the patient runs out of medicine, there is a several-week grace period before tetany becomes a risk. Ergocalciferol is several-fold more economical than other vitamin D congeners.

Dihydrotachysterol is a by-product of the photoactivation step that forms ergocalciferol, being formed when the B ring opens differently to rotate the steroid A ring 180 degrees, placing the original 3-beta hydroxy group in the 1-alpha steric position. Dihydrotachysterol must undergo only 25-hydroxylation in the liver to be biologically active, so its activity is independent of renal function. The compound is of similar polarity and fat solubility to ergocalciferol, so the above comments about frequency of dosage changes and duration of action pertain to dihydrotachysterol as well.

Calcitriol, or 1,25-dihydroxycholecalciferol, is also effective. It is not well absorbed orally, but produces a great enough increase in intestinal calcium absorption to maintain the serum calcium level. The compound has the advantage of a rapid onset of action and the potential disadvantage of a rapid dissipation of its action. I use it in two ways. It can be used as the chronic maintenance agent, usually in doses of 0.5 to 1.5 μg per day. It can also be used as a bridge in a newly diagnosed patient for whom the long-term agent is ergocalciferol: the patient is begun initially on ergocalciferol 50,000 U daily, plus calcitriol 1 μg daily, with an oral calcium supplement. The calcitriol increases the blood calcium level within just 2 or 3 days, allowing more rapid discharge from the hospital. Close monitoring of the serum calcium level is mandatory for the first 2 or 3 weeks to avoid hypercalcemia. Starting at about 3 weeks, the calcitriol dosage is tapered, the goal being to discontinue the agent by about 6 to 18 weeks. Meanwhile, the ergocalciferol dosage is increased slowly as needed to eventually stabilize the serum calcium level near the lower limit of normal. The time to equilibrium can be shortened by giving a large dose of ergocalciferol, 300,000 U daily, for the first 3 days, to "fill up the fat stores of the vitamin" more rapidly. The same "bridge" and "loading" strategies can also be used while initiating therapy with dihydrotachysterol.

I often prescribe a calcium supplement in the

range of 1000 to 2000 mg per day in hopes of lowering the requirement for the vitamin D congener. I generally use calcium carbonate and recommend that it be taken with meals to ensure a more predictable calcium absorption and maximize the desired phosphate-binding activity of the calcium (see later). The calcium supplement is not essential; a few of my patients did not wish to contemplate a lifetime of taking tablets several times a day and have maintained themselves in stable fashion for many years on the vitamin D congener alone, with a normal dietary intake of calcium.

Women with hypoparathyroidism may show a symptomatic drop in serum calcium values with the onset of menses. The addition of an oral calcium supplement during the menses is a useful means of minimizing this change without varying the dosage of the vitamin D congener.

Once treatment has established the desired serum calcium value, I check urinary calcium excretion. The goal is to show that the fasting morning urinary calcium/creatinine ratio lies below 0.15, or the 24-hour urine calcium value is less than 4 mg per kg of body weight per day. If there is hypercalciuria despite the desired simultaneous serum calcium value, I first prescribe a low-sodium diet. Then, especially if the patient has been thyroidectomized, I decrease the amount of calcium supplement, increasing the dosage of vitamin D congener to maintain the same fasting serum calcium value. It has been shown that thyroidectomized patients (lacking calcitonin) show a greater rise in serum calcium values after an oral calcium dose than do thyroid-intact subjects (thus having a higher 24-hour filtered load of calcium for any given fasting serum calcium value). Sometimes the calcium supplement must be discontinued altogether to avoid hypercalciuria. Even then, an occasional patient is able to avoid hypercalciuria only by maintaining a total serum calcium value closer to 8.0 mg per dL than to the usual target of 8.8 mg per dL.

The use of a thiazide diuretic has been advocated in an effort to reduce urinary calcium excretion, but thiazides are less effective in lowering urinary calcium levels in hypoparathyroid patients. The thiazide can also complicate matters by worsening the metabolic alkalosis that these patients usually show (due to loss of the PTH stimulation of renal bicarbonate excretion).

The dosages of vitamin D and calcium that are needed to maintain the desired serum calcium value may vary over a period of months. Episodic ethanol binges can lead to hypocalcemia in an otherwise stable patient, either by producing magnesium deficiency or perhaps by interfering with the activation of ergocalciferol. Other reasons for changing dosage requirements have not been identified. Thus, to minimize the risk of complications, serum calcium levels should be monitored at least every 3 or 4 months in most patients. Even a single bout of hypercalcemia produces nephrocalcinosis and permanent renal scarring. Experiments in laboratory animals have shown that systemic alkalosis predisposes to the development of nephrocalcinosis at any given level of hypercalcemia. Since the damage done by nephrocalcinosis is only partly reversible, hypercalcemia must be avoided.

Serum phosphate values should also be monitored in hypoparathyroid patients. The calcium ion itself stimulates renal phosphate clearance, so serum phosphate levels decline as the serum calcium level comes back toward normal with the initiation of treatment. I prefer to maintain the phosphate values below approximately 5.5 mg per dL. Whereas the cataracts that can complicate hypoparathyroidism are caused by the hypocalcemia, central nervous system and other ectopic calcifications probably arise more from unchecked hyperphosphatemia. In a rare patient it is necessary to prescribe a lower protein diet or to add a phosphate-binding agent (first calcium carbonate, then aluminum hydroxide) to ensure the desired normophosphatemia.

Pseudohypoparathyroidism

The treatment of pseudohypoparathyroidism is similar to that of hypoparathyroidism. The doses of vitamin D that are required are usually less, since the resistance to PTH does not seem to be complete. In Type 1 pseudohypoparathyroidism the renal tubule is usually not resistant to the effects of PTH on renal tubular calcium reabsorption, so normal serum calcium values can be maintained without a risk of hypercalciuria. This should, of course, be verified in each individual patient before undertaking a lifetime of treatment.

PRIMARY ALDOSTERONISM

method of
ANDREW J. NORTON, M.D., and
THEODORE A. KOTCHEN, M.D.
Medical College of Wisconsin
Milwaukee, Wisconsin

Primary aldosteronism is a hormonally mediated clinical syndrome characterized by increased aldosterone secretion despite suppressed plasma renin activity (PRA), hypokalemia, and hypertension. The prevalence of this disorder in hypertensive patients is less than 5%, with most estimates between 0.5 and 2.0%. Since primary aldosteronism is potentially a surgically curable cause of hypertension, it is important to identify and evaluate patients in whom this diagnosis is suspected. However, several apparently different adrenal pathologies may account for this syndrome, and the appropriate therapy depends on the identification of the specific adrenal disorder. The diagnosis of primary aldosteronism can be established in most patients with relatively simple outpatient testing. Subsequent definition of the specific form of hyperaldosteronism may be more difficult and requires additional testing.

CLINICAL SYNDROME

The age at the time of diagnosis is generally in the third through fifth decades, and equal numbers of men and women are affected. Most patients are asymptomatic, although infrequently polyuria, polydipsia, paresthesias, and rarely weakness progressing to tetany or paralysis may occur as a consequence of hypokalemic alkalosis and hypomagnesemia. The hypertension is usually mild to moderate, although isolated patients with malignant hypertension have been described. Unprovoked hypokalemia, profound hypokalemia with diuretic use, or hypokalemia resistant to replacement are important clues to the diagnosis. Additional abnormalities may include metabolic alkalosis, mild hypernatremia, hypomagnesemia, and glucose intolerance. Primary aldosteronism is diagnosed in up to 50% of hypertensive patients with this constellation of abnormalities.

Primary aldosteronism is caused by increased aldosterone production, independent of the renin-angiotensin system. Several distinct adrenal pathologies may culminate in this clinical syndrome (Table 1). Sixty to 70% of patients have an adrenal aldosterone-producing adenoma (APA). The tumor is almost always unilateral and most are small, measuring less than 3 cm in diameter. Twenty to 30% have bilateral adrenocortical hyperplasia (idiopathic hyperaldosteronism [IHA]). Several rare causes of primary aldosteronism are also listed in Table 1. As discussed subsequently, it is important to exclude or confirm these diagnoses before initiating therapy.

DIAGNOSIS

Approximately 25 to 30% of patients with essential hypertension also have suppressed PRA; consequently, low PRA by itself is not sufficiently specific or sensitive to be useful as a screening test.

In practical terms, the finding of unprovoked hypokalemia (serum K^+ <3.5 mEq per liter) or profound hypokalemia with diuretic use (serum K^+ <3.1 mEq per liter) in patients with hypertension should trigger an evaluation for primary aldosteronism. However, up to 20% of patients with primary aldosteronism, particularly patients with glucocorticoid-suppressible primary aldosteronism, may be either intermittently or persistently normokalemic unless exposed to the stress of diuretics. Inappropriate kalliuresis (urine K^+ >30 mEq per 24 hours) in the presence of hypokalemia also suggests mineralocorticoid-induced hypertension.

TABLE 1. **Causes of Primary Aldosteronism**

Type	% of Cases	Primary Therapy
Common		
Aldosterone-producing adenoma	60–70	Surgical
Bilateral adrenocortical hyperplasia (idiopathic hyperaldosteronism)	20–30	Medical
Uncommon		
Unilateral adrenal hyperplasia (primary adrenocortical hyperplasia)	<1	Surgical
Aldosterone-producing–renin-responsive adenoma	<1	Surgical/medical
Glucocorticoid-suppressible hyperaldosteronism	<1	Medical
Aldosterone-producing adrenocortical carcinoma	<1	Surgical/medical
Ectopic: ovarian arrhenoblastoma	<1	Surgical

TABLE 2. **Differential Diagnosis of Hypertension Associated with Hypokalemia**

Primary aldosteronism
Secondary aldosteronism
　Malignant hypertension
　Renovascular hypertension
　Renin-secreting tumor
Enzyme deficiencies
　11-beta-hydroxylase
　17-alpha-hydroxylase
　11-hydroxysteroid-dehydrogenase
　　Congenital (Ulicks' syndrome)
　　Acquired (glycyrrhizic acid–containing substances, e.g., licorice, chewing tobacco, some antacids)
Cushing's syndrome
Deoxycorticosterone-secreting adrenal tumors
Liddle's syndrome

As listed in Table 2, several other hypertensive diseases are also associated with hypokalemia, and these disorders must be considered in the differential diagnosis of patients suspected of having primary aldosteronism. Secondary aldosteronism should be considered in patients with accelerated or malignant hypertension, patients suspected of having renovascular hypertension, and young patients with severe hypertension (renin-secreting tumor). In contrast to low PRA in patients with primary aldosteronism, PRA is elevated in patients with secondary aldosteronism. Cushing's syndrome is usually suspected on the basis of a characteristic clinical presentation and may be screened with either an overnight dexamethasone suppression test or measurement of 24-hour urine free cortisol excretion. Deficiencies of several enzymes involved in the biosynthesis and metabolism of adrenal steroids also cause mineralocorticoid hypertension and hypokalemia. The 11-beta-hydroxylase deficiency is associated with inappropriate virilization, and the 17-alpha-hydroxylase deficiency is associated with failure of sexual maturation. Both PRA and plasma aldosterone (PA) are suppressed in patients with these enzyme deficiencies, as well as in patients with congenital and acquired 11-hydroxysteroid-dehydrogenase deficiency, deoxycorticosterone (DOC)-secreting adrenal tumors, and Liddle's syndrome. Consequently, these disorders should be considered in hypokalemic, hypertensive patients with low PRA and low plasma and/or urine aldosterone.

The evaluation of a patient with suspected primary aldosteronism can be accomplished in an outpatient setting. In patients on medications, spironolactone should be withheld at least 4 weeks before study, and angiotensin-converting enzyme inhibitors, other diuretics, beta blockers, and calcium antagonists should be withheld for at least 2 weeks. Peripherally acting alpha blockers can be used to control significant hypertension. Patients should consume a regular salt diet, and hypokalemia should have been corrected with potassium supplementation. In testing carried out under these conditions, 24-hour urine aldosterone excretion rates are abnormally elevated over 90% of the time and, in the presence of low PRA, are highly suggestive of the diagnosis.

After the patient has spent 2 hours in the upright position, PRA and PA may be diagnostic. Since aldosterone concentrations in patients with APA tend to fall during the day in concert with adrenocorticotropic hormone (ACTH), the blood sample should be obtained early in the morning, if possible. The findings of a PA:PRA ratio greater than 30:1, with an absolute PA concentration greater than 20 ng per dL, have the following test characteristics: sensitivity, 90%; specificity, 91%; positive predictive value, 69%; negative predictive value, 98%. In patients with an elevated PA:PRA ratio, false-positive results may be minimized by repeating measurements 60 minutes after a 25-mg dose of captopril. In patients with primary aldosteronism, the elevated ratio remains unaltered by captopril, whereas the ratio declines in patients with essential hypertension. However, this additional testing with captopril is generally not required.

Confirmation of primary aldosteronism is accomplished by demonstrating the failure to suppress urine aldosterone excretion to less than 14.0 μg per 24 hours after 5 to 7 days of a high-salt diet (addition of 10 to 12 grams of sodium chloride to the usual diet) or, more practically, after failure to suppress PA concentrations to less than 10 ng per dL after infusion of 2 liters of isotonic saline over 4 hours. In the presence of low PRA, this is diagnostic of primary aldosteronism. However, some patients with IHA may suppress to a level between 5 and 10 ng per dL after saline infusion.

IDENTIFICATION OF SPECIFIC ETIOLOGY

After confirming a diagnosis of primary aldosteronism, the next step in the evaluation is to identify the cause. In most cases, this means differentiating APA from IHA. Although the hormonal and metabolic abnormalities of APA are more marked than those of IHA, the considerable overlap does not permit reliable discrimination between these two syndromes. Further, the better detail provided by newer imaging procedures may lead to confusion, because hyperplasia may accompany an adenoma, and macronodularity may be seen with hyperplasia. Consequently, anatomic evidence must be correlated with functional data to ensure the correct diagnosis (Table 3 and Figure 1).

Steroid hormone synthesis differs in patients with APA and IHA, and this may assist in the differential diagnosis. The steroid 18-hydroxycorticosterone (18-OHB) is a by-product of aldosterone biosynthesis, and patients with APA generally have plasma 18-OHB concentrations above 65 ng per dL, whereas those with IHA do not. However, this test is not completely reliable. Recent evidence suggests that patients with APA excrete metabolites of C-18 oxygenated cortisols (18-hydroxycortisol and 18-oxocortisol) in their urine, whereas patients with IHA do not. The potential of these latter steroid measurements to distinguish between APA and IHA requires confirmation.

Aldosterone biosynthesis tends to be more responsive to ACTH in patients with APA and more responsive to renin-angiotensin in patients with IHA. Consequently, patients with IHA tend to have a postural increase in PA, whereas PA tends to decrease during the day (reflecting the circadian rhythm of ACTH) in patients with APA. However,

several patients with "aldosterone-producing, renin-responsive adenomas" have recently been described. In these patients, the aldosterone response to upright posture is similar to that in patients with IHA. In addition, the plasma 18-OHB concentrations in these patients are in the lower range generally observed in IHA.

Two other causes of primary aldosteronism merit brief mention—adrenal carcinoma and glucocorticoid-suppressible hyperaldosteronism. In contrast to patients with APA and IHA, most, but not all, patients with carcinoma overproduce other steroids in addition to aldosterone. Consequently, plasma dehydroepiandrosterone sulfate (DHEA-S) and 24-hour urinary excretion of cortisol and 17-keto steroids should be measured.

Glucocorticoid-suppressible aldosteronism is an inherited, autosomal dominant disease. Hypertension appears at young ages and is linked to a gene duplication arising from unequal crossing over, fusing the 5′ regulatory region of 11-beta-hydroxylase to the 3′ coding sequences of aldosterone synthetase. The chimeric 11-beta-hydroxylase/aldosterone synthetase gene produces an enzyme that catalyzes the formation of 18-hydroxylated steroids in the zona fasciculata. Consequently, in addition to aldosterone, serum 18-oxocortisol and 18-hydroxycortisol concentrations may be increased, and this diagnosis can be confirmed by correction of hypokalemia and hypertension in response to dexamethasone therapy (0.5 mg every 6 hours) within 7 to 10 days. It is likely that genetic screening will become available to evaluate family members.

To assist in defining the adrenal pathology, an abdominal computed tomography (CT) or magnetic resonance imaging (MRI) scan should be carried out in all patients diagnosed as having primary aldosteronism. These procedures will detect most adenomas greater than 1.0 cm in diameter, although smaller tumors may be missed. When a unilateral adenoma is the cause of primary aldosteronism, the CT scan will be positive 90% of the time; if an adenoma is present, it should be considered diagnostic. If the CT or MRI scan is not diagnostic, an adenoma may be detected by adrenal scintiscanning with the isotope 6-beta-[131I]-iodomethyl-19-nor-cholesterol (NP-59), after dexamethasone suppression (0.5 mg every 6 hours for approximately 7 days). When these scans are inconclusive, bilateral adrenal venous sampling for aldosterone and cortisol levels, in response to ACTH stimulation, should be carried out. When technically successful, this results in lateralization in 95% of patients with APA. Ipsilateral-to-contralateral aldosterone ratios greater than 10 (with symmetrical ACTH-stimulated cortisol levels) are considered diagnostic.

TREATMENT

Despite some overlap of hormonal responsiveness between adenomas and hyperplasia, the prudent ap-

TABLE 3. **Techniques to Differentiate Aldosterone-Producing Adenoma (APA) from Bilateral Idiopathic Hyperaldosteronism (IHA)**

	APA	IHA	Discriminating Value*
Plasma 18-OHB	>65 ng/dL	<65 ng/dL	82%
Postural increase of plasma aldosterone	<30%	>30%	85%
Adrenal CT or MRI	Unilateral mass	Bilaterally enlarged	90%
Adrenal scintiscan with dexamethasone suppression	Unilateral uptake	Uptake suppressed	90%
Bilateral adrenal venous sampling with ACTH stimulation	Unilateral increase in aldosterone	Aldosterone equal bilaterally	95%

*Data from Young WF, Hogan MJ, Klee GG, et al: Primary aldosteronism: Diagnosis and treatment. Mayo Clin Proc 65:96–110, 1990.

Diagnose Primary Aldosteronism
Upright PRA and PA
or
24-hr urine aldosterone level with PRA

Confirm Primary Aldosteronism
PRA and PA after 2 L saline infusion
or
24-hr urine aldosterone after salt loading

Differentiate Cause

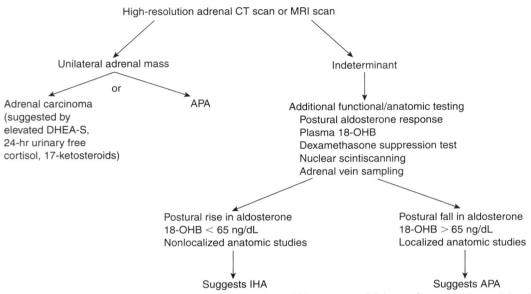

Figure 1. Diagnosis and differentiation of primary aldosteronism. *Abbreviations*: PRA = plasma renin activity; PA = plasma aldosterone; CT = computed tomography; MRI = magnetic resonance imaging; APA = aldosterone-producing adenoma; DHEA-S = dehydroxyepiandrosterone sulfate; 18-OHB = 18-hydroxycorticosterone; IHA = idiopathic hyperaldosteronism.

proach is to remove adenomas (whether renin-responsive or not) and to treat hyperplasia medically.

For patients with a unilateral APA, unilateral adrenalectomy (either via a flank incision or using a laparoscopic approach) is the recommended therapy and is curative in 40 to 70% of patients. However, even among "cured" patients, hypertension may persist for several months following surgery. The cure rate in response to unilateral adrenalectomy is higher in younger patients and lower in patients who have coexistent macronodules or micronodular hyperplasia in addition to an adenoma in the same gland.

Preoperative management should include correction of hypertension and potassium repletion with the aldosterone antagonist spironolactone (Aldactone), 200 to 400 mg per day, and cautious potassium supplementation, if necessary, for 1 to 2 months. Other metabolic abnormalities, including hypomagnesemia and diabetes, should be treated appropriately. Postoperative hypoaldosteronism, owing to suppression of the contralateral zona glomerulosa, may occur and persist for up to several months. This complication is recognized by hyperkalemia and orthostatic hypotension. Hyperkalemia may be treated with furosemide or thiazide diuretics; occasionally, short-term mineralocorticoid treatment with low doses of fludrocortisone may be required.

Medical therapy is the only accepted treatment for IHA, since hypertension is cured by surgery, including bilateral adrenalectomy, in only 20% of patients. Medical therapy is also indicated for patients with APA who are poor surgical candidates and for patients with bilateral APAs (approximately 6% of patients with APA). Potassium-retaining diuretics, either spironolactone or the renal sodium transport inhibitors amiloride (Midamor) and triamterene (Dyrenium), are the cornerstone of drug therapy. Treatment with spironolactone may be initiated with relatively high doses (200 to 400 mg per day), and the dose may subsequently be reduced after blood pressure is controlled and hypokalemia is corrected. Twice-daily dosing is probably adequate. Similar doses are used in chronic treatment of APA and IHA, and in these disorders, hyperkalemia rarely if ever occurs. In addition to competitive binding of mineralocorticoid receptors, spironolactone exhibits potent antiandrogenic activity at the dihydrotestosterone receptor. This explains the side effects of gynecomastia, decreased libido, and impotence. The combination of spironolactone and a thiazide diuretic may provide better blood pressure control and allow lower doses of spironolactone and hence fewer side effects. Aspirin should be avoided, since it antagonizes the effect of spironolactone.

Amiloride and triamterene inhibit sodium transport in the distal renal tubule, where sodium reabsorption is accompanied by potassium excretion. Both agents cause only modest increases of sodium excretion, but they significantly decrease high rates of potassium excretion. This effect is independent of aldosterone, and these agents are not aldosterone antagonists. Amiloride may be administered in a once-daily dose of 5 to 30 mg and is about 10 times more potent than triamterene. Consequently, higher doses of triamterene are required. These agents may be less effective than spironolactone in controlling hypertension, but they also have fewer side effects and are appropriate alternatives if side effects limit the use of spironolactone.

In the event that blood pressure cannot be adequately controlled with one of the potassium-retaining diuretics alone, a second drug should be added. A calcium entry blocker such as nifedipine (Procardia, 30 to 90 mg per day) or amlodipine (Norvasc, 5 to 10 mg per day) should be considered. Agonist-induced stimulation of aldosterone biosynthesis is dependent on increases in intracellular calcium, and limited evidence suggests that nifedipine inhibits aldosterone production. Alternatively, in patients with IHA, an angiotensin-converting enzyme inhibitor might be added to the potassium-retaining diuretic. In contrast to patients with APA, IHA patients have an enhanced aldosterone response to angiotensin II and a greater hypotensive response to captopril.

Surgery is indicated for treatment of aldosterone-producing adrenocortical carcinomas. Preoperative management is similar to that of patients with APA. Postoperatively, patients may be treated with the adrenolytic agent o,p'-DDD. Mean survival for combined surgical resection and o,p'-DDD treatment is approximately 6 years, compared with 2 years for patients treated with o,p'-DDD alone and less than 1 year for those treated with surgery only. Survival of patients with untreated disease averages less than 3 months.

Patients with glucocorticoid-suppressible primary aldosteronism may be treated with 0.5 to 1.0 mg per day of dexamethasone, although higher doses are occasionally required. To avoid the side effects of higher steroid doses, potassium-retaining diuretics may be useful adjuncts or alternatives.

HYPOPITUITARISM

method of
BLANCA N. OCAMPO-LIM, M.D., and
ARIEL L. BARKAN, M.D.
*Veterans Affairs and University of Michigan
Medical Centers
Ann Arbor, Michigan*

The pituitary gland is regulated by a variety of hypothalamic releasing factors, and it, in turn, releases a number of trophic hormones that increase the function of several target endocrine glands. There are complex feedback loops involving the hypothalamus and the target endocrine glands, which in turn modulate pituitary function. Hypopituitarism implies loss of function of the pituitary gland, either partial or complete. A variety of pathologic processes may affect the pituitary gland either directly or indirectly by influencing hypothalamic function. Clinical manifestations vary, depending on the rapidity of onset (acute vs. slowly progressing), the pituitary hormone lacking, and the severity of the hormonal deficiency. Patients may present with subtle, vague complaints of fatigue or malaise or with profound adrenal insufficiency or circulatory collapse. The more common picture is one of insidious onset with gradual loss of hormonal function, leading to multiple endocrine abnormalities such as growth failure, sexual dysfunction, hypothyroidism, hypoadrenalism, and diabetes insipidus. A thorough history and physical examination are crucial in the diagnosis of hypopituitarism. The integrity of the hypothalamic-pituitary system may be assessed by basal hormone studies and further stimulation or suppression tests for each of the pituitary hormones, if warranted. Radiologic or neuro-ophthalmologic testing may be required. Treatment options include surgical intervention and hormonal replacement therapy, which is usually lifelong.

ETIOLOGY

There are many etiologic factors in the pathogenesis of hypopituitarism (Table 1). The most common cause is the presence of a pituitary tumor, which is usually benign. Whether hormonally silent or not, such a tumor is capable of disrupting normal hypothalamic-pituitary function and producing clinical signs and symptoms of hypopituitarism. A sudden bleeding into a large pituitary tumor with subsequent loss of normal pituitary tissue is termed pituitary apoplexy. Sheehan's syndrome is the development of hypopituitarism after postpartum hemorrhage or infarction and shock. Radiation therapy given for pituitary or extrasellar brain tumors or for head and neck cancer almost invariably disrupts the hypothalamic function, with ensuing hypopituitarism. These conditions—pituitary or parapituitary tumor with or without preceding surgery, cranial radiation, and pituitary apoplexy—constitute the absolute bulk of all cases of true hypopituitarism seen in clinical practice. Less frequent causes are infiltrative, inflammatory, or metastatic diseases of the hypothalamic-pituitary area, traumatic hypopituitarism (most often stalk section), empty-sella syndrome, and drug-induced pituitary hormone deficiency. In addition, some systemic conditions can either

TABLE 1. **Causes of Hypopituitarism**

Tumors	Infiltrative diseases
Pituitary adenoma— functioning or nonfunctioning	Granulomatous diseases
	Sarcoidosis
	Eosinophilic granuloma
Craniopharyngioma	Hemochromatosis
Parasellar lesion	Wegener's granulomatosis
Hypothalamic tumor	Autoimmune
Pituitary radiation	Lymphocytic hypophysitis
Pituitary surgery	Infection
Vascular/infarction	Tuberculosis
Sheehan's syndrome	Fungal
Carotid aneurysm	Syphilis
Pituitary apoplexy	Metastatic tumor
	Other
	Trauma
	Empty sella

mimic hypopituitarism or cause functional and, as a rule, transient pituitary hormonal abnormalities. The possibility of nutritional abnormalities (obesity or malnutrition, including anorexia nervosa), psychosocial problems, or systemic disease should always be kept in mind. Elderly individuals generally have functional growth hormone, and old men often have gonadotropin deficiency.

CLINICAL APPROACH

When dealing with any patient with suspected hypopituitarism, several questions should be answered. The value of a careful history and clinical examination cannot be overemphasized.

1. Is hypopituitarism truly present? Short stature in a grossly neglected child or amenorrhea in an anorectic or overexercising young woman is, as a rule, due to functional causes and abates after correction of the underlying cause.

2. What is the likely cause of hypopituitarism? Isolated hypogonadism of prepubertal onset with anosmia is virtually always due to congenital gonadotropin-releasing hormone (GnRH) deficiency. A history of severe postpartum bleeding and shock strongly suggests Sheehan's syndrome. Amenorrhea and galactorrhea in a woman taking tricyclic antidepressants suggest a drug effect.

3. Are there any mass effects? Signs of intracranial hypertension (headache and vomiting) and/or papilledema indicate the presence of a large intracranial mass. Visual field defects (most often, superotemporal cuts) suggest compression of the optic chiasm, and ophthalmoplegia may be due to cavernous sinus invasion.

4. Is there any evidence of hormone hypersecretion? Clinical symptoms and signs of Cushing's syndrome, acromegaly, and hyperprolactinemia should be actively sought. If present, they indicate the diagnosis of a hormonally active pituitary tumor.

5. Is there any evidence of hormone deficiency? This is determined clinically and confirmed by baseline measurements or dynamic tests.

Once a clinical diagnosis of true hypopituitarism is made, a radiologic visualization of the hypothalamic-pituitary area should be accomplished. Brain magnetic resonance imaging (MRI) with and without a gadolinium contrast is the preferred method. It allows accurate definition of the pituitary margins, including potential extrasellar expansion (cavernous sinus, compression of the optic chiasm), and differentiation between solid and cystic lesions, and it demonstrates the presence of old pituitary hemorrhages or pituitary stalk integrity. Most important, this study can identify a carotid artery aneurysm that would otherwise require angiography and may obviate the need for neuro-ophthalmologic study. Whether only basal hormone levels are measured or dynamic tests performed as well is a clinical decision based on the patient's status and plans for subsequent therapy.

HORMONAL DEFICIENCY

The pituitary gland is very resilient to damage, and about 95% of it may be destroyed before clinical hormone deficiency occurs. Usually, there is a reasonably predictable order in which pituitary hormones disappear: growth hormone (GH), followed by luteinizing hormone (LH), follicle-stimulating hormone (FSH), thyroid-stimulating hormone (TSH), adrenocorticotropic hormone (ACTH), and prolactin. However, in practice, any combination and permutation of hormone deficit can occur.

Each pituitary hormone deficiency is discussed separately, with emphasis on clinical features, diagnostic work-up, and treatment.

Growth Hormone Deficiency

GH is usually the first hormone that disappears in hypopituitarism. In children, this manifests as growth failure and short stature. Growth deficiency among adults may be missed clinically, although patients may complain of decreased muscle strength, decreased exercise capacity, increased abdominal fat deposition, and altered psychosocial performance. Since GH is secreted in a pulsatile fashion with low or undetectable levels during most of the day and nocturnal augmentation usually during Stages 3 and 4 of sleep, measurement of basal GH levels is usually not informative. Measurement of the GH-dependent insulin-like growth factor-1 (IGF-1) may aid in the diagnosis of GH deficiency, but low levels of IGF-1 can also be caused by poor nutritional status or occur in the elderly. The IGF-1 level may even be "normal" in patients with GH deficiency. Certain stimulatory tests are used to evaluate GH secretory reserve. These include insulin-induced hypoglycemia and the administration of levodopa, arginine, clonidine, or growth hormone–releasing hormone (GHRH). Blunted GH responses to at least two agents are usually required to establish the diagnosis of GH deficiency. Insulin hypoglycemia (0.05 to 0.15 U per kg intravenously) is a "gold standard" of GH testing. Although there is no universal agreement on what constitutes the normal response, an increase of plasma GH above 7 μg per liter is likely to indicate an intact somatotropic axis. Achievement of adequate hypoglycemia (<40 mg per dL) is a necessary prerequisite. The same value (7 μg per liter) is also used for all other tests. The response may be artificially blunted in patients taking high doses of glucocorticoids, in hypo- and hyperthyroid subjects, and, most importantly, in obese patients.

GH treatment is usually indicated in GH-deficient children. This should be carried out only by an experienced pediatric endocrinologist. The use of GH therapy in GH-deficient adults* has always been questionable, but recent data suggest that the use of GH in this population may be beneficial, with resultant improvement in exercise capacity, normalization of body composition, and increased muscle strength, bone mineral mass, and cardiac performance. Presently, GH is too expensive to be routinely given to GH-deficient adults.

Gonadotropin Deficiency

The presence of normal menstrual cycles in females and normal spermatogenesis in males almost always indicates adequate gonadotropin reserve. In

---

*Not FDA-approved for this indication.

such cases, basal gonadotropin measurements are not taken. However, if clinical manifestations of gonadotropin deficiency are evident, then basal testing is recommended. Women present with menstrual dysfunction, decreased libido, or signs of genital atrophy. With concomitant ACTH deficiency, pubic and axillary hair may be lost. Men have loss of potency and libido. Clinically, hypogonadal subjects have decreased muscle mass, atrophic skin, decreased bone density, and lack of pubic hair. In men, fine radial wrinkling around the mouth is almost always present. Most hypogonadal subjects have soft and occasionally small testes. Small penis and testes indicate that the onset of gonadotropin deficiency dates back to before puberty. To establish the diagnosis of gonadotropin deficiency, serum FSH and LH, together with the gonadal steroid (testosterone in males and estradiol in females), are taken. In primary gonadal failure, one would expect the presence of high gonadotropins and low testosterone or estradiol because of the absence of negative feedback of the gonadal steroid. Secondary hypogonadism, whether from pituitary or hypothalamic cause, is present when both gonadotropins and gonadal steroid are low. Both FSH and LH secretion are modulated by hypothalamic GnRH. Since FSH and LH are secreted in a pulsatile fashion, isolated measurement of either hormone may show low levels in the face of normal GnRH secretion; therefore, assessment of the gonadotropin reserve may require the administration of exogenous GnRH. A blunted or absent LH or FSH response to a single bolus of GnRH, however, cannot definitely distinguish between primary pituitary disease and hypothalamic disease.

Premenopausal hypogonadal women are treated with estrogen-progesterone combinations. Usually, conjugated estrogens such as Premarin 0.625 to 1.25 mg per day or 17-B-estradiol such as Estrace 1 to 2 mg per day is given for the first 25 days of the month or even continually. In women who have already had hysterectomy, the addition of progesterone is not needed. Otherwise, medroxyprogesterone (Provera) 5 to 10 mg per day is given on days 16 through 25 of each cycle. Transdermal estrogens (Estraderm) can be used instead of oral preparations and seem to have fewer side effects in terms of coagulation profile and lipid metabolism. Affected men are given testosterone to restore libido, well-being, and potency. Long-acting preparations are commonly used, usually in the form of testosterone esters administered at a dose of 200 to 300 mg every 2 to 3 weeks. Side effects may include benign prostatic hypertrophy, polycythemia, or altered lipid profile. Restoration of fertility in both sexes is possible but often difficult. If the pituitary itself is damaged, sequential administration of human chorionic gonadotropin (hCG) and human menopausal gonadotropin (hMG) is needed. The availability of GnRH has made fertility induction easier by successfully restoring ovulation in females and sperm production in males, but it is effective only in patients with a hypothalamic origin of the disease. These treatments should be prescribed only by physicians specializing in reproductive endocrinology.

Thyroid-Stimulating Hormone Deficiency

As metabolism slows down with TSH deficiency, patients experience weakness, tiredness, sleepiness, and slowing of mentation and speech. Marked cold intolerance, constipation, weight gain, hoarseness, and paresthesias may occur. Physical findings include thickened, puffy features; hypothermia; bradycardia; yellowish, dry skin; and slow return of deep tendon reflexes. Low or normal TSH in the presence of low thyroid hormone levels indicates either pituitary or hypothalamic disease. The thyrotropin-releasing hormone (TRH) stimulation test may be used to assess the functional integrity of pituitary thyrotroph. A low or absent TSH response to TRH in the face of low plasma thyroxine (T_4) suggests pituitary disease. Patients with hypothalamic hypothyroidism may have a normal TSH response to TRH but with a delayed peak, about 60 minutes or more following TRH injection, presumably reflecting a deficiency of TRH secretion. The overlap between the pituitary and hypothalamic types of response makes the TRH test unreliable as a diagnostic tool. A simple documentation of low T_4 and TSH values in a patient with clinical hypothyroidism is sufficient to make the diagnosis of secondary hypothyroidism. However, one has to bear in mind that certain medical illnesses, such as Cushing's syndrome or malnutrition of any origin, and certain drugs, such as propranolol, corticosteroids, or dopamine, may interfere with the TSH response to TRH stimulation. The possibility of the so-called euthyroid sick syndrome should always be kept in mind.

Rapid correction of hypothyroidism is not advocated in the elderly or in those with a history of ischemic heart disease. Thyroid hormone replacement in these groups is initiated at a lower dose (25 μg of L-thyroxine [Synthroid] per day), which is gradually increased every week until a full maintenance dose is achieved with normalization of serum-free T_4. Younger and healthier patients may be started at a higher dose (50 μg of L-thyroxine per day) and advanced by 25-μg increments every week until the desired free T_4 level is attained, or they may be given the full replacement dose right away. Usually, 1.6 μg of L-thyroxine per kg of body weight is required as a replacement dose. Importantly, in patients with panhypopituitarism, T_4 replacement should always be started after cortisol replacement is initiated. Otherwise, increased metabolism of cortisol may precipitate adrenal crisis.

Corticotropin Deficiency

ACTH deficiency leads to adrenal insufficiency, with symptoms of fatigue, decreased appetite, nausea, vomiting, abdominal pain, changes in mental status, and intolerance to stress. Hyperpigmentation of the skin and mucous membranes does not occur in secondary adrenal insufficiency, since ACTH levels are low, but this is a usual manifestation in patients with primary adrenal insufficiency. Electrolyte imbalance in the form of hyponatremia and hyperkalemia is also not characteristic of secondary adrenal insufficiency, since aldosterone production depends mainly on renin and angiotensin, which are not disrupted in this condition. Long-standing ACTH deficiency combined with gonadotropin deficiency results in loss of axillary and pubic hair.

Assessment of the adequacy of ACTH secretion is usually difficult and indirect. The most commonly employed test to assess ACTH secretion is the cosyntropin stimulation test, which involves measurement of serum cortisol before and then 30 and 60 minutes after the intravenous administration of 250 µg of corticotropin. The normal response is a rise in serum cortisol to 20 µg per liter or higher. A blunted cortisol response indicates chronic ACTH deficiency, with resultant adrenal atrophy. However, partial ACTH deficiency may still maintain the normally trophic adrenal cortex, and the response to a large bolus of ACTH will be normal. In stressful situations, these patients will still be unable to mount a sufficient ACTH-cortisol response. Thus, although an unquestionably abnormal cosyntropin test (peak cortisol <10 to 15 µg per dL) is helpful in identifying patients with the most severe and long-standing forms of ACTH deficiency, a borderline or even normal response may be misleading. One dynamic test that is employed to test the entire hypothalamic-pituitary-adrenal axis is the insulin hypoglycemia test. Insulin, at a dose of 0.15 U per kg, is given intravenously, with the aim of producing adequate hypoglycemia when the serum glucose falls below 40 mg per dL. The normal response is a rise of plasma cortisol to greater than 20 µg per dL, indicating adequate ACTH reserve. The metyrapone test may also be used to assess the integrity of the pituitary-adrenal axis. Metyrapone (Metopirone), which blocks the final step in cortisol synthesis, is given 30 mg per kg orally at bedtime, with measurement of 11-deoxycortisol and ACTH at 8 A.M. the next day. A normal response is a rise in the 11-deoxycortisol level to 8 µg per dL or greater and a doubling of the ACTH value.

Cortisol replacement is most important and should be initiated promptly. In order to simulate the normal diurnal rhythm of cortisol secretion, physiologic doses of various glucocorticoid preparations may be used twice a day, with two-thirds of the dose in the morning (to account for the cortisol peak in the early morning) and the remaining one-third in the evening. Prednisone 5 mg in the morning and 2.5 mg in the evening or hydrocortisone 20 mg in the morning and 5 to 10 mg in the evening are used for this purpose. Supraphysiologic doses are required during times of stress. Doses are typically doubled or tripled during minor stress, such as the common cold or dental extraction; three- to fivefold increases are needed during severe stress, such as major surgery or serious infection or injury. Patients with ACTH deficiency are advised to wear a Medic Alert necklace or bracelet that states the need for steroids in emergencies.

Prolactin Deficiency

Deficiency of serum prolactin is rare and is usually of no clinical consequence. It may be responsible for the failure of lactation in Sheehan's syndrome in the postpartum period. A single low level does not confirm prolactin deficiency because of the episodic nature of its secretion. Measurement of prolactin response to TRH stimulation may be used; however, a blunted or absent response is seen not only in pituitary lactotroph failure but also in other conditions such as anorexia nervosa, malnutrition, chronic disease, and thyrotoxicosis.

PRACTICAL APPROACH TO THE MOST FREQUENT CAUSES OF HYPOPITUITARISM

Isolated Gonadotropin Deficiency

Isolated gonadotropin deficiency (with or without anosmia) is usually diagnosed as an absence of pubertal development. Biochemically, there are low plasma gonadotropin and gonadal steroid levels. Thyroid function (free T_4 level) and random prolactin are normal. Administration of GnRH as a single bolus may be helpful in establishing the ability of the pituitary to secrete gonadotropins in response to a "missing hormone" (GnRH), but the response is often very small or altogether absent. Priming with pulsatile GnRH may be needed before LH and FSH responses become normal. This test is useful if pulsatile GnRH therapy is contemplated. A computed tomography (CT) or MRI scan must be done to exclude a morphologic abnormality such as craniopharyngioma. If no anatomic abnormality is found, dynamic testing of ACTH, TSH, and GH secretion is not indicated. Initially, treatment consists of the administration of gonadal steroids. hCG-hMG or pulsatile GnRH therapy is reserved for specific periods to induce fertility.

Isolated Growth Hormone Deficiency

Slow statural growth with progressive deviation downward from the predicted growth percentile prompts medical attention. Careful history and physical examination are mandatory to uncover the possibility of physical and emotional neglect and to exclude chronic illnesses (diarrheal disease, diabetes, heart or respiratory failure, immunologic abnormality, chronic infection, and so on). Every girl with short stature should have a chromosomal study to exclude Turner's syndrome. Particular attention should be given to the child's neurologic status to exclude an intracranial tumor. Thyroid function should be tested. A single GH measurement is of limited value, and frequent blood sampling over 24 hours or at least overnight may be performed in the appropriate hospital setting. Since such a study can be done only as part of a defined research protocol, assessment of GH responses to various dynamic stimuli should be conducted. Insulin hypoglycemia (0.1 U per kg intravenously), oral clonidine (Catapres 0.25 mg) or levodopa (500 mg), and intravenous arginine infusion (30 grams over 30 minutes) are all used, and plasma GH should normally rise above 7 μg per liter in response to each stimulus. Absent GH responses to at least two stimuli are needed to make the diagnosis. A single low plasma IGF-1 concentration is helpful, but values often overlap with the normal range. A pituitary CT scan should be done in every patient to exclude a structural intracranial lesion. Only when the diagnosis is firmly established should therapy be prescribed. Reassessment of GH status should be done a year or two later, since as many as 30% of children with unequivocally abnormal results at diagnosis prove to have normal GH secretion later. A child with suspected GH deficiency should always be referred for final diagnosis and therapy to a qualified pediatric endocrinologist.

Pituitary Tumor

Pituitary tumors can cause hypopituitarism by one of a number of mechanisms or a combination thereof. Macroadenomas or craniopharyngiomas may actually destroy healthy pituitary tissue, and the ensuing hypopituitarism is irreversible. Alternatively, large or even relatively small tumors may impair the hypothalamic-pituitary circulation, with the resultant "stalk section" effect. This may cause functional deficiency of one or several pituitary hormones and, often, moderate hyperprolactinemia (<200 ng per mL). Prolactinomas almost invariably cause isolated gonadotropin deficiency by inhibiting GnRH secretion. Large pituitary tumors may cause neurologic deficits by compression of the optic chiasm or, when extended laterally, palsies of the third, fourth, and sixth cranial nerves. Careful neurologic examination, including visual field testing, is required. MRI with and without contrast is the optimal neuroimaging study.

The extent of the endocrine testing depends on the planned therapy. If no intervention is contemplated, a combined pituitary function test (insulin hypoglycemia, TRH, and GnRH) should be done at diagnosis, and appropriate replacement therapy should be started. If pituitary surgery is planned, sophisticated testing is not required, since tumor removal will either relieve the deficit or introduce a new one. Baseline assessment of thyroid function (free T_4 and TSH), gonadal function (gonadal steroid, LH, and FSH), and a single prolactin measurement will suffice. Adrenal function need not be tested, since steroid coverage will be started anyway prior to surgery and continued at least temporarily after the operation. About 2 months after surgery, hydrocortisone is stopped overnight and a combined test is performed. The pituitary status at that point represents the final result of surgery and determines the subsequent permanent replacement therapy.

Radiation Therapy

Radiation damage leading to hypopituitarism may occur after radiotherapy for pituitary lesions, head and neck cancer, supratentorial malignant tumors, posterior fossa tumors (often in children), and prophylactic radiation in children with lymphoblastic leukemia. The pituitary itself is quite resistant to radiation injury and remains functional unless it absorbs 15,000 to 20,000 cGy. In contrast, the hypothalamus may be damaged by as little as 400 to 500 cGy. Thus, even when the radiation beam is carefully aimed, scatter radiation of the hypothalamus may occur. Radiation-induced hypopituitarism is, by definition, almost always hypothalamic in origin. Although GH deficiency almost always occurs within the first year after radiation therapy, damage to other neuroendocrine systems is usually delayed and may become manifest up to 5 years later. Radiation therapy for pituitary tumors, for example, leads to gonadotropin deficiency in about 50 to 60% of cases and to ACTH and TSH deficiencies in about 30 to 50% of cases 5 years later. Continual follow-up of patients, with repeat assessment of pituitary function, is thus necessary. In cases in which supratentorial tumors are removed, an epileptogenic focus is created, and the patient is put on phenytoin (Dilantin) or carbamazepine (Tegretol). In this case, assessment of the ACTH reserve becomes difficult. An insulin hypoglycemia test may provoke a seizure. Metyrapone testing may be unreliable because the previously mentioned antiepileptic drugs induce hepatic cytochrome P-450 enzymes that accelerate the degradation of metyrapone. Often, a physician must rely on less than precise information to initiate steroid replacement. If there is biochemical evidence of hypogonadism and especially hypothyroidism (low T_4 and TSH) and the prolactin is even mildly elevated, the diagnosis of hypothalamic damage is made and an ACTH deficiency is presumed to exist.

Pituitary Apoplexy

Pituitary apoplexy may occur in women as a result of obstetric catastrophe (Sheehan's syndrome) or in patients of both sexes after a profound circulatory shock, especially if small blood vessels are already damaged (vasculitis, diabetic micro- or macroangiopathy). The ensuing hypopituitarism is immediate and irreversible. Pituitary function testing is done and replacement therapy is started and continued for life.

HYPERPROLACTINEMIA

method of
CHRISTOPHER M. CORSI, M.D., and
ALAN DALKIN, M.D.
University of Virginia Health Sciences Center
Charlottesville, Virginia

Hyperprolactinemia, defined as a persistently elevated serum prolactin (>25 ng per mL in most laboratories) in a man or in a nonpregnant, nonlactating woman, is a common endocrine abnormality. Prolactin is normally secreted by the pituitary lactotroph in both men and women. Dopamine, synthesized and secreted from the hypothalamus, is the primary regulator of prolactin release and maintains an inhibitory tone. Compounds that increase prolactin release have also been identified, such as thyrotropin-releasing hormone (TRH). Excess secretion of TRH, as in primary hypothyroidism, is one mechanism whereby hyperprolactinemia is manifest. Alternatively, prolactin levels display physiologic variation throughout each day and are generally maximal (often between 25 and 40 ng per mL) between 6 and 8 A.M. Therefore, when morning samples are minimally increased, we routinely repeat prolactin measurements in the late afternoon.

Although there is considerable overlap, gender plays a significant role in the clinical presentation of hyperprolactinemia. The most common signs and symptoms in women are oligo- and amenorrhea, galactorrhea, and infertility. Prolactin alters reproductive function predominantly via a central nervous system action whereby it inhibits the release of gonadotropin-releasing hormone (GnRH), resulting in hypogonadotropic hypogonadism. Because the production of breast milk requires the presence of both prolactin and estrogen, it is not surprising that the incidence of galactorrhea in women with hyperprolactinemia is quite variable. Women with mild or moderate degrees of hyperprolactinemia, irregular menses, and some endogenous estrogen secretion may have marked galactorrhea, whereas women with serum prolactin levels in excess of 1000 ng per mL but with minimal estrogen production and amenorrhea may have no demonstrable breast discharge. Prolactin does not act directly at the ovary; hence, infertility in the presence of *normal* menses is rarely the result of hyperprolactinemia. Men more commonly present with symptoms of mass effect (if the etiology of their hyperprolactinemia is a pituitary adenoma), although a history of diminished libido and impotence can often be elicited. Because the dynamic patterns of hormone release seen in the menstrual cycle do not occur in men, the duration of hyperprolactinemia preceding diagnosis is likely prolonged, thereby explaining their larger pituitary adenomas. Finally, *hyper*prolactinemia does not exclude *hypo*pituitarism. We therefore evaluate all patients with macroadenomas for secondary hypothyroidism and hypoadrenalism.

The possible causes of hyperprolactinemia are extensive (Table 1), and our approach in evaluating patients (Figure 1) accounts for this degree of complexity. The principal consideration in diagnosis is to differentiate intrinsic hypothalamic-pituitary disease from other causes. The degree of hyperprolactinemia is often helpful in this regard, since levels greater than 200 ng per mL virtually always represent a prolactin-secreting pituitary adenoma. Furthermore, the size of the tumor generally correlates with the degree of hyperprolactinemia. Macroadenomas (>1 cm in diameter) often present with severe hyperprolactinemia (values in excess of 1000 ng per mL are not uncommon), whereas microadenomas (<1 cm) are associated with lesser degrees of hyperprolactinemia and must be distinguished from other pathologic causes. Both primary hypothalamic disease and large pituitary tumors (of any cell type) that impinge on the vascular supply from the hypothalamus to the pituitary can prevent delivery of dopamine and are associated with serum prolactin levels between 50 and 200 ng per mL. Numerous medications increase prolactin secretion as a result of their antidopaminergic properties. In our experience, prolactin levels in medication-induced hyperprolactinemia rarely exceed 100 ng per mL. As noted

TABLE 1. Etiology of Hyperprolactinemia

Pituitary Disease

Tumors
1. Prolactin-secreting
   <10 mm—microadenoma
   >10 mm—macroadenoma
2. Multiple hormone-secreting adenomas
   (e.g., adrenocorticotropic hormone, growth hormone)
3. Other—nonfunctioning pituitary tumors, craniopharyngiomas, metastatic (breast, lung) tumors (causing stalk compression)
Empty sella syndrome
Pituitary stalk section

Hypothalamic Disease

Infiltrative disorders—tuberculosis, histiocytosis X, sarcoidosis
Tumors—craniopharyngiomas, germinomas, hamartomas, gliomas
Postcranial irradiation

Medications

Tricyclic antidepressants—amitriptyline, imipramine
Phenothiazines—perphenazine, chlorpromazine
Butyrophenones—haloperidol
Dopamine receptor blockers—metoclopramide, domperidone, cisapride
Antihypertensive agents—methyldopa, reserpine
Estrogen

Endocrine

Primary hypothyroidism
Polycystic ovary disease

Neurogenic

Chest wall trauma
Herpes zoster
Nipple stimulation

Other

Renal failure
Cirrhosis

Physiologic

Pregnancy
Lactation
Stress

Idiopathic

earlier, hypothyroidism is a reversible cause of hyperprolactinemia. Therefore, we routinely check levels of thyroid-stimulating hormone (TSH), as the clinical signs of hypothyroidism may be subtle. Chronic renal failure and hepatic disease reduce prolactin clearance and are associated with mild hyperprolactinemia. Hyperprolactinemia is occasionally seen in polycystic ovary disease, although the mechanism whereby this occurs is uncertain. In summary, the possible causes of an elevated serum prolactin are numerous. Medications and prolactin-secreting tumors are the most common causes; hence, if a careful history fails to implicate a pharmacologic cause, the most likely cause is a prolactinoma.

In cases of suspected pituitary adenomas, magnetic resonance imaging (MRI) of the pituitary with gadolinium enhancement is the procedure of choice. MRI has a greater sensitivity in detecting small lesions, but a high-resolution contrast computed tomography (CT) scan with thin sections through the pituitary can also be used. Intrasellar pathology seen on imaging procedures in the work-up of hyperprolactinemia does not always represent a prolactinoma. In particular, the finding of a serum prolactin value between 50 and 100 ng per mL with a macroadenoma

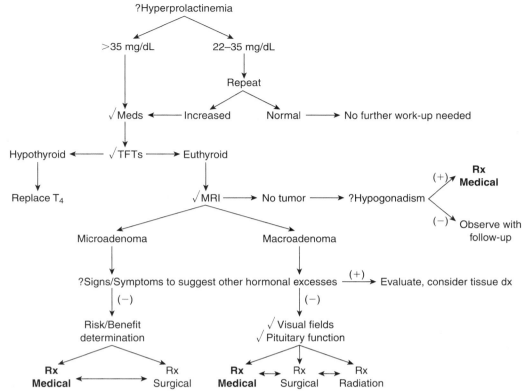

Figure 1. Approach to patient evaluation in hyperprolactinemia. *Abbreviations*: TFTs = thyroid function tests; MRI = magnetic resonance imaging; Rx = treatment; Dx = diagnosis.

should be cause for caution. Other types of pituitary adenomas, such as nonfunctioning adenomas or those producing growth hormone (acromegaly) or adrenocorticotropic hormone (Cushing's disease), are considered and ruled out with appropriate testing, if indicated. Similarly, we recognize that imaging alone cannot always distinguish primary pituitary adenomas from other causes of intrasellar pathology such as granulomatous disease, craniopharyngioma, meningioma, or metastatic disease (e.g., breast cancer). Clearly, in certain clinical settings, further extensive evaluations (not covered here) or even a pituitary biopsy may be needed to establish a firm diagnosis. However, when our clinical suspicion is toward the diagnosis of prolactinoma, the evaluation described previously is generally sufficient, and there are a number of specific therapeutic alternatives that may be employed for treatment.

TREATMENT

There is little evidence that hyperprolactinemia itself is deleterious. Galactorrhea is problematic but does not confer a greater risk of breast cancer. In contrast, hypogonadism can be a serious health risk with consequences (in both men and women), including osteoporosis. Therefore, the clinician should carefully review the indications of treatment for each patient. Our general goals include:

1. Restoration of gonadal function and fertility
2. Reduction or cessation of galactorrhea
3. Shrinkage of tumor mass (prolactinomas)

Occasionally, hyperprolactinemia as a result of mi-

croadenoma, medication, or an idiopathic etiology may be asymptomatic. Simple observation is a reasonable approach in these patients. In microadenomas, tumor enlargement is rare and is nearly always associated with increasing prolactin. If no intervention is indicated, we recommend semiannual serum prolactin levels with annual MRI for 2 to 3 years and then annual serum prolactin levels. Visual field examinations are not needed in idiopathic hyperprolactinemia or when microadenomas are stable and distant from the optic chiasm.

Microadenomas

In patients with microprolactinomas and symptoms as a result of the hyperprolactinemia, medical therapy with dopamine agonists is our first choice. These agents, bromocriptine (Parlodel) and pergolide (Permax), reduce both synthesis and secretion of prolactin. As of this writing, pergolide is not approved by the U.S. Food and Drug Administration for use in hyperprolactinemia. Prolactin declines rapidly (hours), with a duration of action for bromocriptine of approximately 6 to 8 hours. Tumor shrinkage occurs over days to weeks. Normalization of prolactin, restoration of the eugonadal state, cessation of galactorrhea, and some degree of reduction in tumor size can be anticipated in at least 70% of patients. Adverse effects include headache, nausea, dizziness, nasal congestion, orthostatic hypotension, and rarely hallucinations, confusion, and seizures. Most side effects are minimized by starting therapy at low doses and taking the medication with meals or at bedtime. With bromocriptine, we typically begin with one-fourth of a 2.5-mg tablet at bedtime and then increase to half a tablet within 3 to 5 days. This is then increased to twice daily, then every-8-hour dosing every 3 to 5 days; thereafter, the milligram per dose is increased until 2.5 mg every 8 hours is tolerated. Higher doses are only rarely more effective and are more likely to be associated with adverse effects. Bromocriptine can be taken for many years, and its long-term safety in the treatment of hyperprolactinemia is well known. Pergolide is a newer drug with less long-term experience, but its efficacy and incidence of side effects appear similar to those of bromocriptine. Also, pergolide is significantly less expensive than bromocriptine.

For patients on medical therapy, serum prolactin levels are repeated once the patient is on bromocriptine 1.25 mg every 8 hours. If the prolactin value has normalized, therapy is continued at that dose, with repeat measurements at 6 and 12 months. For patient convenience, we tried 2.5 mg twice daily as an alternative, with slightly less efficacy. For those patients who progress to higher doses of bromocriptine, levels are repeated 3 to 4 weeks after dosage adjustments. As there have been reports of spontaneous "cures" on bromocriptine, we discontinue these agents for 2 weeks annually (for the first 2 years) and obtain a prolactin level and repeat the imaging study.

Surgical resection through the trans-sphenoidal approach can also be considered for patients with microprolactinomas. This procedure is associated with very low risk in the hands of an experienced surgeon. Indeed, our "cure" rate for microprolactinomas at the University of Virginia (as defined by normal prolactin level 5 years after surgery) is nearly 80%. However, since potential complications include hypopituitarism, iatrogenic damage to the optic nerves, meningitis, and even death, surgery is reserved for patients who have either failed or not tolerated medical treatment. Informed patients occasionally prefer surgical intervention as the initial approach, citing their concerns about long-term use of medication. Postoperative follow-up includes serum prolactin levels 3, 6, and 12 months after surgery. Of interest, surgical responses in some patients may not be observed immediately after resection. Imaging studies are performed annually until any residual abnormalities are stable for 2 years.

Macroadenomas

Our approach to large pituitary tumors almost universally entails therapy with a dopamine agonist. Surgery, although effective in reducing tumor burden, is rarely if ever curative and should be considered as primary therapy only in special circumstances (discussed later). At least two-thirds of patients with macroprolactinomas will have a diminution on serum prolactin and tumor size in response to bromocriptine. Moreover, visual field defects, which are commonly found in patients with larger tumors, improve in over 80% of patients; responses are commonly noted within a few days. Although tumor reduction continues in some patients for months or even years, "cure" from bromocriptine is quite rare, and we advise patients that therapy is likely to be lifelong. We utilize a similar dosing regimen for bromocriptine as outlined earlier for microadenomas and generally attempt to attain a similar total daily dose (7.5 mg per day).

We limit the use of surgery for these large tumors to three general clinical categories:

1. Patients with tumors obstructing the flow of cerebrospinal fluid, resulting in hydrocephalus
2. Patients who fail to respond to dopamine agonist therapy within 8 to 12 weeks on maximal doses
3. Patients whose tumors progress while on dopamine agonist therapy

Although we do not generally recommend it, an occasional patient who is given a short course of bromocriptine will have remarkable tumor shrinkage and be a candidate for a curative surgical resection. In our clinics, this is not often observed, however. Conversely, there are data to suggest that bromocriptine given for long periods of time (months to years) may induce fibrotic changes within the tumor, thereby making surgical resection difficult. Thus, we do not prolong therapy more than 2 to 3 months if the patient fails to respond appropriately.

An additional therapeutic alternative for macroadenomas is radiation therapy. Although effective for long-term suppression of tumor growth and prolactin secretion, it often takes years for a benefit to be observed. Radiation therapy is also complicated by a high rate (>50%) of side effects, including hypopituitarism, optic nerve damage, and memory loss. Moreover, these adverse consequences may present as late as 10 years after therapy. Therefore, radiation therapy is generally reserved for patients whose tumors do not respond to medical therapy and are not amenable to surgery. At the University of Virginia, a technique of delivering focused radiation through multiple ports, known as the gamma knife, is often used. This method appears to minimize radiation exposure to normal tissues and is therefore expected to be better tolerated. Additionally, the treatment is administered in a single session, thereby avoiding multiple visits over an extended time. The long-term outcome of this procedure is currently being evaluated and compared with that of conventional radiation.

Follow-up for these patients is lifelong, with annual serum prolactin levels. We routinely follow annual imaging studies for 2 to 3 years. We continue these studies until tumor shrinkage is maximal, and they are not repeated thereafter unless symptoms of mass effect return or serum prolactin increases.

Special Considerations

Since many patients found to have hyperprolactinemia are diagnosed during an evaluation for infertility, it should be mentioned that subsequent pregnancy influences our management. Bromocriptine, although posing no demonstrable risk to the fetus, is discontinued when pregnancy is documented in women with microadenomas. Although the normal pituitary (and microadenomas) increases in size by nearly 50% during pregnancy, these smaller tumors only infrequently become problematic in terms of mass effect. We follow these women with visual field studies and serum prolactin levels each trimester. In women with macroadenomas, the risk of tumor growth is increased, and we generally continue the medication through pregnancy.

HYPOTHYROIDISM

method of
KELLY D. DAVIS, M.D., and
MITCHELL A. LAZAR, M.D., PH.D.
University of Pennsylvania School of Medicine
Philadelphia, Pennsylvania

Hypothyroidism, the clinical syndrome that results from deficiency of thyroid hormone (TH), is a highly variable disease, depending on the age of onset, duration, and severity of TH deficiency. Hypothyroidism in infants and children results in growth retardation and abnormal brain development, leading to short stature and mental retardation (cretinism) if undiagnosed. Fortunately, neonatal screening is standard in the United States, allowing early diagnosis. Children treated before symptoms develop have IQs that are indistinguishable from those of matched controls. In adults, overt hypothyroidism affects almost 2% of women and 0.2% of men. Deficiency of TH leads to a generalized slowing down of metabolic processes. Myxedema, the life-threatening syndrome caused by severe prolonged hypothyroidism, is now a very rare presentation of hypothyroidism, largely because of widespread availability of sensitive assays for thyroid-stimulating hormone (TSH), which has facilitated earlier diagnosis (discussed later). More often, patients have few or very mild manifestations of hypothyroidism that are recognized only retrospectively after appropriate hormone replacement.

ETIOLOGY

Hypothyroidism may result from defects in the hypothalamic-pituitary-thyroid axis, but in the vast majority of cases the thyroid itself is at fault (primary hypothyroidism). The causes of hypothyroidism are outlined in Table 1.

The most common cause of hypothyroidism in iodine-sufficient areas of the world is *chronic autoimmune (Hashimoto's) thyroiditis*, which results from cell- and antibody-mediated thyroid destruction. The cause of the autoimmune reaction is unknown. Approximately 3 to 4.5% of the population has some compromise in thyroid function from autoimmune thyroiditis. The disease is most common between the ages of 40 and 60 years, and women are affected at least five times more often than men. Hypothyroidism due to chronic autoimmune thyroiditis is irreversible and usually progressive. Chronic autoimmune thyroiditis has a hereditary component and patients with the disease may have a personal or family history of other autoimmune diseases. However, most cases of autoimmune

TABLE 1. Causes of Hypothyroidism

Primary (Thyroidal)
Chronic autoimmune thyroiditis*
Thyroidectomy
S/P radioiodine therapy or external irradiation
Congenital (thyroid dysgenesis or defects in hormone biosynthesis*)
Infiltrative diseases*
Drugs (thionamides, amiodarone, lithium)*
Iodine (deficiency or excess)*
Recovery from thyroiditis
Hypothalamic or Pituitary Disease
Generalized Thyroid Hormone Resistance*

*Associated with goiter.

thyroiditis are sporadic. Occasionally, autoimmune thyroiditis occurs as part of an autoimmune polyglandular syndrome in association with primary adrenal insufficiency, insulin-dependent diabetes mellitus, hypoparathyroidism, and other disorders. More than 90% of patients with autoimmune thyroiditis have elevated titers of autoantibodies to thyroglobulin or thyroid peroxidase (also called the "microsomal antigen"), but their role in the pathogenesis of the hypothyroidism is unclear. The majority of patients have a goiter, but other clinical findings vary depending on the severity of hormone deficiency at the time of diagnosis.

Iatrogenic hypothyroidism after *thyroidectomy* usually occurs within several months but can occasionally occur much later owing to superimposed autoimmune thyroiditis in the remaining thyroid tissue. *Radioactive iodine* (^{131}I) therapy for Graves' hyperthyroidism results in hypothyroidism within a year in the majority of patients; subsequently it occurs at a rate of 0.5 to 2.0% per year. Discontinuation of thyroid replacement, by either the patient or a physician unfamiliar with the patient's history, may lead to gradual development of hypothyroidism years after thyroidectomy or radioablation. *External irradiation* of the neck or upper chest (dosages of greater than 25 cGy) also causes hypothyroidism that develops slowly over several years. This occurs most commonly in young patients who receive mantle irradiation for Hodgkin's lymphoma.

Iodine deficiency is the most prevalent cause of hypothyroidism worldwide, but it is very uncommon in North America because of adequate dietary intake. *Excessive iodine* also can cause hypothyroidism by inhibiting triiodothyronine (T_3) and thyroxine (T_4) biosynthesis. Normal patients generally escape from this effect (known as the "Wolff-Chaikoff effect"), but this is often not the case for patients with decreased thyroid reserve (secondary to chronic autoimmune thyroiditis or a history of thyroidectomy or ^{131}I treatment for Graves' disease), who are therefore more susceptible to iodine-induced hypothyroidism. Excessive iodine is usually ingested in the form of contrast dyes used for radiographic studies, health tonics and dietary supplements available at health food stores, or drugs such as amiodarone.

A careful medication history should be taken in all patients with hypothyroidism, because many *drugs* interfere with TH synthesis and secretion by the thyroid gland. Propylthiouracil (PTU) and methimazole (Tapazole) are both used to treat thyrotoxicosis and are the most potent antithyroid agents. Lithium, which interferes with TH synthesis and release, induces development of goiter with or without hypothyroidism in patients with bipolar affective disorder. In one study, 15% of patients who took lithium for an average of 5 years developed overt hypothyroidism. Many patients who develop hormone deficiency on lithium are middle-aged women who have high titers of antithyroid antibodies, suggesting that chronic autoimmune thyroiditis predisposes them to the development of lithium-induced hypothyroidism. Patients who take lithium chronically should be monitored routinely every 6 to 12 months for development of hypothyroidism.

Infiltrative diseases, such as hemochromatosis, sarcoidosis, and amyloidosis, cause injury and hypofunction of the thyroid. *Subacute thyroiditis* causes mild thyrotoxicosis accompanied by pain and tenderness of the thyroid gland. About 20 to 30% of patients go on to develop transient hypothyroidism that lasts for about 1 to 3 months. Subacute thyroiditis rarely causes permanent hypothyroidism. *Silent thyroiditis* follows a similar course, except that the thyroid gland is nontender and the transient hypothyroidism may persist for up to 1 year. *Developmental defects*, usually agenesis of the thyroid gland, are the most frequent cause of hypothyroidism in the newborn. *Inherited defects in hormone biosynthesis* occur rarely. Most of these are transmitted via an autosomal recessive pattern of inheritance and, if left untreated, are associated with development of a goiter owing to increased TSH secretion.

Hypothalamic and Pituitary Disease

Insufficient secretion of thyrotropin-releasing hormone (TRH) and TSH by the hypothalamus and pituitary can cause secondary hypothyroidism, but this is relatively unusual compared with primary hypothyroidism. Any disorder of the pituitary (adenoma, infarction, previous surgery, or radiation) or hypothalamus (craniopharyngioma or granulomatous diseases) potentially can cause secondary (pituitary) or tertiary (hypothalamic) hypothyroidism, either alone or in combination with other hormonal deficiencies (see "Hypopituitarism" article for additional discussion). It is especially important to consider the possibility of associated adrenal insufficiency prior to initiating T_4 replacement in patients with secondary hypothyroidism, as discussed in the later section dealing with treatment.

Generalized Resistance to Thyroid Hormone

Generalized resistance to TH (GRTH) is a rare disorder characterized by reduced tissue responsiveness to circulating levels of THs that would ordinarily be excessive. It is usually inherited as an autosomal dominant disorder. Most patients with GRTH have mutations in one of the two alleles encoding a T_3 receptor, TRβ. The abnormal T_3 receptors bind T_3 poorly or not at all and cause the resistance by inhibiting the function of the remaining normal T_3 receptors. This dominant inhibition explains the inheritance of the disorder.

Clinical hallmarks of GRTH are elevated serum levels of free T_3 and T_4, nonsuppressed TSH (the resistant pituitary fails to respond to high levels of THs by shutting off TSH secretion), the absence of typical manifestations of hyperthyroidism, and thyroid gland enlargement. Abnormalities in patients with GRTH are mostly cognitive, especially attention deficit disorder and learning disabilities. Symptoms of hypothyroidism are usually minor or even absent, because normal receptors are present and competing with the mutant inhibitor. Treatment is indicated only when the TSH is elevated or if symptoms of hypothyroidism develop. Indeed, in some patients certain peripheral tissues display evidence of response to the high circulating TH levels. For example, a subset of patients with GRTH are tachycardic, not bradycardic as would be expected if the heart were resistant to the effects of TH.

DIAGNOSIS

Clinical evaluation, including history, physical examination, and laboratory tests, should be directed toward identifying the cause of hormone deficiency. The medical history may uncover past treatment of thyrotoxicosis with thyroidectomy or ^{131}I, or use of drugs that affect synthesis of THs. An old thyroidectomy scar or thyroid enlargement (goiter) may be detected on physical examination, which is often helpful in distinguishing the various causes of hormone deficiency. Measurement of the TSH concentration is helpful in distinguishing primary hypothyroidism (elevated TSH) from that due to underlying hypothalamic or pituitary disease (inappropriately normal or low TSH).

In adults, many of the common symptoms of hypothyroidism, such as fatigue, cold intolerance, weight gain, constipation, muscle cramps, depression, and menstrual irregularities, are nonspecific. Delay in the relaxation phase of the deep tendon reflexes is the most specific physical finding in hypothyroidism—others, such as puffiness of the hands and face, bradycardia, and dry skin, occur in association with many other diseases. Therefore, accurate tests to definitively determine serum concentrations of T_4 and TSH are crucial for making a diagnosis of hypothyroidism. As sensitive assays for T_4 and TSH have become widely available, patients diagnosed with hypothyroidism frequently have mild symptoms or only a single symptom because of recognition earlier in the course of the disease. Initiation of therapy when relatively mild thyroid function abnormalities are identified prevents morbidity associated with development of severe hypothyroidism.

The serum TSH is the most sensitive test for detecting hypothyroidism. Even though the normal range for T_4 is wide (about 4 to 11.5 μg per dL), each person has an endogenous set point dictating her or his optimal serum concentration. When the serum T_4 is decreased below that level, the TSH rises—for example, if a patient's serum T_4 concentration falls from 10 μg per dL (that person's normal set point) to 8 μg per dL (low for this patient, but still within the normal range), the TSH would be expected to rise well above normal, because a small reduction in T_4 concentration results in a large increase in TSH. Therefore, since primary hypothyroidism is the most common form of the disease, the serum TSH is an excellent screening test for thyroid dysfunction in patients evaluated in an ambulatory care setting who complain of nonspecific symptoms such as fatigue, depression, or menstrual irregularity. If pituitary or hypothalamic disease is known or suspected, TSH should not be used as a screening test (see "Treatment of Secondary Hypothyroidism" later). Also, TSH should not be used to screen for thyroid disease in hospitalized patients, since many other factors in acutely or chronically ill euthyroid patients influence TSH. In addition to changes in serum TSH associated with nonthyroidal illness itself, its secretion is suppressed by drugs such as dopamine, glucocorticoids, and somatostatin and may be increased after acute administration of dopamine antagonist drugs such as metoclopramide or domperidone (see "Thyroid Function in Nonthyroidal Illness" later and Figure 1).

When an elevated TSH is discovered during routine screening, it should be repeated with a total T_4 concentration and T_3 resin uptake. Occasionally the second TSH will be entirely normal, indicating that the initial *abnormal* value was due to laboratory error or a transient case of

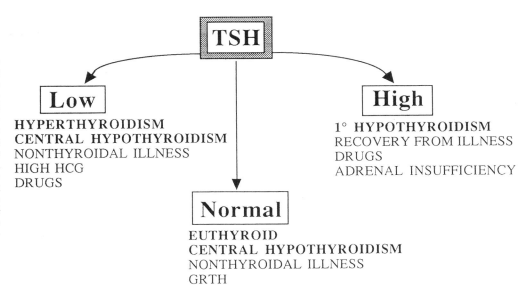

hypothyroidism. If the T_4 is frankly low, with low resin uptake and high TSH, the diagnosis is primary hypothyroidism, and appropriate replacement therapy should be initiated. If repeat TSH is high but the T_4 is within the normal range, this indicates subclinical hypothyroidism, and the decision about whether to prescribe thyroid hormone must be made on a case-by-case basis (see later section on "Subclinical Hypothyroidism"). Since the development of sensitive TSH assays, TRH testing is now unnecessary for diagnosing primary hypothyroidism.

In patients with hypothalamic or pituitary disease, the TSH does not increase appropriately as the T_4 falls, and clinical symptoms and the serum T_4 concentration must be used to make the diagnosis. The TSH may be either frankly low, inappropriately normal (for the low T_4), or slightly high (owing to secretion of biologically inactive TSH). Occasionally, pituitary enlargement will be discovered in a patient with severe primary hypothyroidism and very high TSH and be mistaken for a pituitary adenoma. This results from physiologic hyperplasia and hypertrophy of thyrotroph cells and is reversible with appropriate T_4 replacement. It is important to distinguish between this entity and a pituitary adenoma so that unnecessary surgery can be avoided.

TREATMENT

Unless hypothyroidism is transient (as after subacute thyroiditis) or reversible (owing to a drug that can be discontinued), treatment almost always requires use of synthetic TH to restore the euthyroid state. In virtually all cases, the drug of choice for treatment of hypothyroidism is levothyroxine (T_4 [Synthroid]), which because of its long serum half-life (7 days) can be administered once a day with maintenance of very constant serum levels. Thyroxine is actually a prohormone that is converted by the patient's 5'-deiodinase to T_3, which is the active form due to its higher affinity for the T_3 receptor. Many experts prefer the use of brand name preparations because of documented variation in generic formulations.

Other TH preparations, including liothyronine (T_3 [Cytomel]), desiccated thyroid, thyroglobulin (Pro-

loid), and mixtures of T_3 and T_4 (liotrix [Euthroid, Thyrolar]) should be avoided for routine treatment of hypothyroidism. Great variability from lot to lot has been reported with biologic preparations of T_3 and T_4. Patients treated with T_3-containing preparations have wide fluctuations in serum T_3 concentrations throughout the day because of rapid gastrointestinal absorption and its relatively short half-life in serum. Furthermore, it is difficult to interpret routine thyroid function tests, other than the TSH, to monitor the adequacy of therapy. In one clinical situation, however, T_3 (Cytomel) is routinely used as the primary TH replacement. In patients about to receive radioiodine ablation for thyroid carcinoma, T_4 is discontinued and T_3, which has a much shorter half-life, is given while the serum T_4 concentration is falling. Such temporary treatment with T_3 reduces the length of time that patients must remain hypothyroid prior to the ^{131}I treatment dose.

Replacement dosage of T_4 can be estimated at 0.075 mg per 100 pounds of body weight. Patients who are treated with T_4 usually begin to notice improvement in their symptoms within 2 weeks, but if hypothyroidism was severe, complete recovery can take several months. After beginning a new dose of T_4, the serum levels of T_4 and TSH should be measured in approximately 8 weeks and the dose adjusted accordingly. Increases in the amount prescribed should not be made before the T_4 levels have achieved steady state (approximately 5 weeks). In patients with more severe hypothyroidism accompanied by a very high serum TSH concentration, even 8 weeks may not be a sufficient interval to gauge the eventual effects of a particular T_4 dose. (For additional information on the treatment of life-threatening hypothyroidism, see the end section on "Myxedema Coma".)

The goal of treatment is to maintain the patient's sense of well-being and to keep the serum TSH concentration within the normal range. An additional goal of therapy in the patient with thyroid enlarge-

TABLE 2. **Drug Effects on Thyroid Function**

Drugs Causing Hypothyroidism	
Reduces Absorption	*Iodine-Containing*
Cholestyramine (Questran)	Amiodarone
Aluminum hydroxide	IV contrast dye
Sucralfate (Carafate)	Expectorants
Iron sulfate	
Blocks T_3/T_4 Synthesis and Release	
Lithium	

Drugs Causing Abnormal Thyroid Function Tests Without Hypothyroidism	
Reduces TBG	*Increases TBG*
Androgens	Estrogen
Glucocorticoids	Tamoxifen (Nolvadex)
	Clofibrate (Atromid-S)
Increases T_4 Clearance	Heroin/methadone
Phenytoin (Dilantin)	5-Fluorouracil
Carbamazepine (Tegretol)	
Rifampin (rifabutin)	*Suppresses TSH*
Phenobarbital	Glucocorticoids
	Dopamine
Blocks $T_4 \rightarrow T_3$ Conversion	Phenytoin
Amiodarone (Cordarone)	Octreotide
Glucocorticoids	
Oral cholecystogram dye	*Increases TSH*
	Domperidone* (Motilium)
Decreases T_4 Binding to TBG	Metoclopramide (Reglan)
Phenytoin	Oral cholecystogram dye
Salicylates	
NSAIDs	
Furosemide (Lasix)	

*Investigational drug in the United States.

ment due to autoimmune (Hashimoto's) thyroiditis is reduction in the size of the gland. Treatment with T_4 is effective in 50 to 75% of cases, although the decrease in the size of the goiter lags behind normalization of the TSH. After identification of the proper maintenance dose, the serum TSH may be monitored once a year; it usually does not require adjustment except in the case of pregnancy or institution of drugs that affect TH absorption, binding, or metabolism (Table 2).

Because many symptoms of hypothyroidism are nonspecific, patients often think that their T_4 replacement dose is inadequate when they feel tired or gain weight. In one study in which patients did not know the exact amount of T_4 they were taking, they preferred a dose that was on average 0.05 mg higher than the one that normalized their serum TH concentrations, TSH response to TRH, and basal TSH. In other words, most patients preferred a T_4 dose that rendered them mildly thyrotoxic. It is important, therefore, to educate patients about the possible adverse consequences of mild overtreatment, which include increased incidence of atrial fibrillation and potential acceleration of osteoporosis. The insufficiency of the current T_4 dose should be verified by measuring TSH before making adjustments because of subtle symptoms of hypothyroidism. Conversely, when the patient is clinically euthyroid on a stable T_4 replacement dose and the TSH is only slightly above the normal range, the dose need not be altered.

Borderline TSH elevations may be due to laboratory error or normal fluctuations in the serum concentration and should be repeated prior to changing a patient's T_4 dose.

Elderly Patients or Those with Coronary Artery Disease

Selected patients require more gradual restoration of the euthyroid state. Thyroid hormone increases myocardial oxygen demand and can precipitate cardiac arrhythmias, angina pectoris, or myocardial infarction in the predisposed patient. Therefore, elderly individuals or those with coronary artery disease, cardiac arrhythmias, or even those with multiple cardiac risk factors should be treated initially with 0.025 mg of T_4, and this dose is increased by 0.025 mg every 6 weeks until full replacement and normal serum TSH are attained.

Treatment During Pregnancy

Women have a higher requirement for TH during pregnancy, and those with hypothyroidism are unable to compensate for this by increasing TH production. The greater need for TH is only partially explained by the estrogen-mediated rise in serum TBG (thyroxine-binding globulin) levels; it is due also to enhanced clearance, metabolism, and passage of T_4 to the fetus. This is an important clinical issue for hypothyroid women who have been maintained on a stable amount of T_4 and become pregnant; the majority will have a rise in their TSH while taking their original maintenance dose. Thus, the average woman with primary hypothyroidism needs a 25 to 50% increase in her T_4 dose during pregnancy to maintain the TSH within the normal range. To avoid hypothyroidism during pregnancy, thyroid function should be checked every 2 months and the dose of T_4 increased if necessary.

Surgical Patients

Several studies have investigated the safety of general anesthesia and surgery in patients with hypothyroidism. Surprisingly few adverse effects were reported, although hypothyroid patients had a higher incidence of ileus, perioperative hypotension, hyponatremia, and central nervous system dysfunction than euthyroid controls, as well as failure to mount a febrile response in the presence of serious infection and enhanced sensitivity to anesthesia and narcotic pain medications. In general, surgery probably should not be postponed in hypothyroid patients who have an urgent indication for it, but they should be managed expectantly for the aforementioned complications. When hypothyroidism is discovered in a patient being evaluated for elective surgery, it is wisest to postpone the operation until the euthyroid state is restored.

Perioperative patients receiving chronic T_4 replacement may have their oral T_4 discontinued for several days without significant adverse effects. If it is necessary for the patient to have nothing by mouth for a more lengthy period, T_4 can be administered intravenously. The dosage should be adjusted to approximately 75% of the oral dose, however, to compensate for differences in absorption of the parenteral and oral preparations.

Subclinical Hypothyroidism

Patients who have normal serum concentrations of T_3 and T_4 but an elevated TSH have subclinical hypothyroidism. The normal range for the total T_4 concentration is wide, but each person's serum concentration is tightly regulated. The sensitivity of the TSH response allows the diagnosis of hypothyroidism to be made while the serum level of T_4 is still within the normal range, because even a small reduction in the serum T_4 is accompanied by a comparatively large increase in the serum TSH. Mild abnormalities of thyroid function can be caused by any of the processes listed in Table 1, the most prevalent being chronic autoimmune thyroiditis. As the name indicates, most patients with subclinical hypothyroidism are asymptomatic, and some have nonspecific symptoms such as fatigue, cold intolerance, constipation, or depression.

Randomized, double-blind, placebo-controlled trials of subclinically hypothyroid patients treated with T_4 indicate that about half noticed improvement in nonspecific indicators such as dry skin, poor energy level, and general sense of well-being. Other studies have shown improvement in cognitive function, cardiac indices (such as left ventricular ejection fraction and systolic time interval), and serum cholesterol and triglyceride concentrations in patients with subclinical hypothyroidism treated with T_4.

Lifelong T_4 treatment of subclinically hypothyroid patients probably should be reserved for those who have a significant chance of progressing to overt hypothyroidism. Those with positive antithyroid antibodies are one such group; prospective studies have shown that 5 to 20% annually will develop clinically significant hypothyroidism. Other groups of patients likely to develop more severe hypothyroidism in the future are those with serum TSH concentrations of between 10 and 20 μIU per mL and those with goiter at the time hypothyroidism is detected. Subclinically hypothyroid patients with borderline elevations of the TSH and negative antithyroid antibodies are unlikely to develop overt hypothyroidism during long-term follow-up, and in the majority the TSH abnormality resolves entirely.

We recommend T_4 replacement in patients with subclinical hypothyroidism who have positive antithyroid antibody titers or a persistently elevated serum concentration of TSH greater than 10 μIU per mL. Reduction of the serum TSH concentration is at least partially effective in reducing the size of a goiter in the majority of patients with autoimmune thyroiditis, and we recommend this for those who have compressive symptoms or are bothered by the appearance of the goiter. A trial of T_4 treatment in subclinically hypothyroid patients with nonspecific symptoms is also reasonable. The trial can be continued for several months to assess the clinical response. If there is no clinical improvement, the therapy can be discontinued and the thyroid function retested. Asymptomatic patients with negative antibodies and very slight elevations of TSH should simply have their thyroid function tested once a year. In summary, the decision to treat or not to treat subclinical hypothyroidism must be considered with each individual case, taking into account the patient's symptoms and predictors of progression to more severe hypothyroidism (Figure 2).

Treatment of Secondary Hypothyroidism

Patients who have hypothyroidism because of defective hypothalamic or pituitary function are at risk of having other hormonal deficiencies. Thyroxine replacement in patients with unsuspected secondary adrenal insufficiency can precipitate an acute addisonian crisis. Prior to initiating T_4 replacement in a patient with secondary hypothyroidism, a test of ACTH/adrenal reserve should be performed. If adrenal insufficiency is present, glucocorticoid replacement should be given prior to T_4. In patients with secondary hypothyroidism, one does not have the benefit of the serum TSH concentration to assist in titration of the T_4 dose. The dose should be adjusted according to the patient's symptoms, aiming to maintain the serum T_4 concentration in the upper part of the normal range.

Patients Taking T₄ for Unclear Indication

Occasionally patients will be identified who are taking TH replacement for uncertain or questionable indications. One can initially measure serum TSH concentration while the patient is taking T_4. If it is high, it indicates that the patient probably does have hypothyroidism, and the dosage can be adjusted accordingly. If, however, the TSH is normal or low, the T_4 supplement can be discontinued and the TSH measured in 4 to 6 weeks to verify the diagnosis of hypothyroidism. Most patients with hypothyroidism will begin to develop clinical symptoms and elevation in TSH during the first month after discontinuation of T_4. Many patients will be reluctant to discontinue their T_4 replacement for definitive testing, especially after years of taking it. In this case, the principal

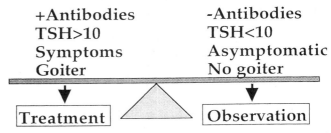

Figure 2. Approach to the Treatment of Patients with Subclinical Hypothyroidism. Patients more likely to progress to overt hypothyroidism should be given thyroxine (T_4) replacement. This includes those with positive antithyroglobulin or antimicrosomal antibody titers and higher TSH. A trial of T_4 replacement is also justified in patients with goiter or symptoms possibly caused by hypothyroidism.

goal should be to provide an appropriate T_4 dose, avoiding overtreatment and the potential adverse effects of thyrotoxicosis on the cardiovascular system and bone mass.

Thyroid Carcinoma

Patients taking thyroid hormone after thyroidectomy for thyroid carcinoma, with or without ^{131}I, deserve special mention because they take T_4 not only as TH replacement but also to prevent recurrence of thyroid cancer. Thyroxine replacement should be lifelong in these patients and should not be discontinued even if sufficient residual normal thyroid tissue remains to provide adequate hormone secretion. The goal of treatment is suppression of the TSH. It is not clear whether the end point should be complete suppression or suppression to levels below the normal range, which can now be distinguished by supersensitive TSH assays. At the present time, we recommend suppression to undetectable levels in those patients with the greatest risk of recurrence of thyroid cancer. Extensive discussion of these prognostic factors is beyond the scope of this article, but they generally include follicular carcinoma, large tumors, or tumors that extend through or outside the thyroid capsule. Patients with the best prognosis (young individuals with a small papillary carcinoma, for example) probably can be maintained on a T_4 dose that reduces the serum TSH to the low but detectable range. Less complete suppression also may be a compromise in elderly patients with a contraindication to induction of subclinical hyperthyroidism.

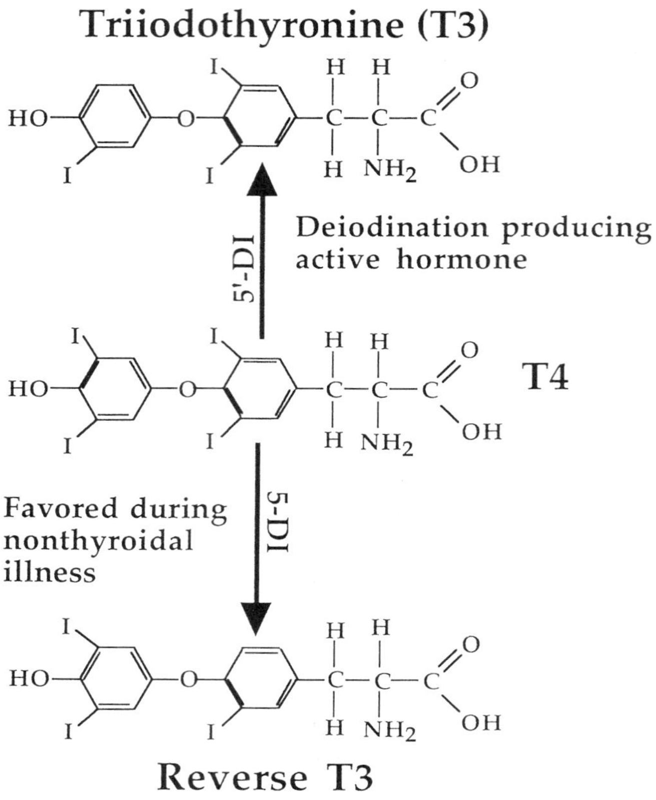

THYROID FUNCTION IN NONTHYROIDAL ILLNESS

A wide variety of abnormalities in thyroid function occur during severe illness, including changes in hormone binding to serum transport proteins, alterations in concentrations of the hormones and binding proteins themselves, and rerouting of T_4 deiodination to alternative pathways. In general, thyroid function and economy during illness tend to decrease the concentrations of biologically active THs, and the reduction in hormone concentrations is generally proportional to the severity of the illness. These changes have collectively been referred to as the "euthyroid sick syndrome" or the "low T_3 state of nonthyroidal illness." Despite extensive description and documentation of this phenomenon, the physiologic significance of the changes and their cause is unknown. They are believed to be adaptive in the setting of physiologic stress due to virtually any type of illness or starvation.

The earliest and most universal abnormality in sick patients is a low serum T_3 concentration resulting from decreased peripheral T_4 to T_3 conversion (5'-monodeiodination). Both the total hormone and the free hormone are diminished. Under normal conditions, T_4 is deiodinated primarily to T_3 (Figure 3), an active TH, whereas in nonthyroidal illness it is

Figure 3. Thyroxine Metabolism. Under normal physiologic conditions, T_4 is deiodinated by 5'-deiodinase (5'-DI) to biologically active triiodothyronine (T_3) and by 5-deiodinase (5-DI) to inactive reverse T_3 (rT_3). The activity of the type I 5'-DI, which provides T_3 to the plasma, is reduced during starvation or illness, thereby favoring deiodination to rT_3.

preferentially deiodinated to biologically inactive reverse T_3 (rT_3). In patients who are even more critically ill, usually those in intensive care units, the serum total T_4 is often low (less than 1 to 2 µg per dL). Individuals with low serum T_4 concentrations are generally more severely ill than those who have only decreased serum T_3 levels, and the degree of reduction in serum T_4 concentration parallels the severity of the nonthyroidal illness. This is due in part to decreased T_4 binding by TBG and other TH-binding proteins, and in part to decreased T_4 production because the hypothalamic pituitary axis fails to respond by increasing TRH and TSH. The high normal or increased T_3 resin uptake usually observed in critically ill patients can be explained by their low serum TBG concentrations and possibly a circulating inhibitor of binding to T_4/TBG. The TSH is typically normal or even subnormal, indicating that the pituitary is not responding appropriately to the low T_3–low T_4 state, much as would be observed in hypothyroidism due to hypothalamic or pituitary dysfunction. This is compounded by administration of drugs known to suppress its secretion, such as glucocorticoids and dopamine.

Several studies have shown that euthyroid hypothyroxinemia in the setting of severe illness has a dismal prognosis. It is often a great challenge to exclude or confirm concurrent hypothyroidism in severely ill patients. Most important is to limit evaluation of thyroid function to patients in whom there is reasonable suspicion on clinical grounds. Probably the best test is the free T_4 measured by an accurate method such as equilibrium dialysis, which should be low in hypothyroidism but normal or even slightly increased in nonthyroidal illness. Attempts have been made to treat critically ill patients with TH, but this is ineffective in improving the outcome and can potentially be harmful.

MYXEDEMA COMA

Myxedema coma, although very rare, is a medical emergency that usually results in death if left untreated. It generally occurs in elderly patients and may be the spontaneous end stage of long-standing untreated hypothyroidism or precipitated by another acute event, such as infection, myocardial infarction, cold exposure, or administration of narcotics. When a history can be obtained from family members, often noted were antecedent symptoms of hypothyroidism with progressive lethargy, stupor, and coma. Observation of a thyroidectomy scar on the neck or discovery of a history of ^{131}I therapy or hypothyroidism can be a clue to the diagnosis.

Patients with myxedema coma have hypothermia due to extreme metabolic slowing, which may be quite severe. Hyponatremia is also frequently present and is caused by excessive secretion of adrenocorticotropic hormone (ADH). Hypoventilation with respiratory acidosis is multifactorial, owing to central depression of ventilatory drive, mechanical obstruction by a large tongue, and/or respiratory muscle weakness. Hypoglycemia may be caused by hypothyroidism alone or coexistent adrenal insufficiency, and seizures and hypotension also frequently occur.

Aggressive treatment is required in patients suspected of having myxedema coma, because the mortality rate is high. Serum should be drawn for measurement of T_4, TSH, and cortisol prior to treatment. The T_4 is usually extremely low, and an elevated TSH confirms the diagnosis of primary hypothyroidism. However, the hypothyroidism may be secondary to hypothalamic or pituitary dysfunction, in which case the TSH will not be elevated. The exact mode of replacement is controversial, with some experts favoring administration of T_3 and others advocating treatment with T_4, allowing the patient's own deiodinase to produce T_3. Immediate restoration of serum TH levels is essential, but this carries a risk of precipitating cardiac arrhythmias or myocardial infarction. We recommend intravenous T_4, because of its wider availability in parenteral forms and smoother onset of action, in an initial dose of 0.3 to 0.6 mg intravenously. Daily doses of 0.05 to 0.1 mg should be given thereafter. Supportive measures are extremely important, including mechanical ventilation, appropriate fluid replacement, and correction of hyponatremia and hypothermia. Until coexisting adrenal insufficiency can be excluded, patients with life-threatening hypothyroidism should be treated with glucocorticoids in stress doses (hydrocortisone, 100 mg every 8 hours). After the patient has clinically improved and is alert, the daily replacement can be converted to an equivalent oral dose and given by mouth. The serum T_4 and TSH should be monitored to avoid overtreatment, comparing with the pretreatment results.

THYROTOXICOSIS

method of
JOHN C. MORRIS, M.D.
Mayo Medical School
Rochester, Minnesota

Thyrotoxicosis is a clinical and biochemical syndrome that results from exposure of tissues to excessive levels of thyroid hormones. The condition usually occurs because of excessive secretions of thyroid hormones directly from the thyroid gland *(hyperthyroidism)*, but it may sometimes be caused by ingestion of excessive amounts of exogenous thyroid hormones (iatrogenic or factitious) or, rarely, by hormone secretion from ectopic thyroid tissue (struma ovarii or metastatic thyroid cancer). Hyperthyroidism can be caused by several pathologic processes involving the thyroid, including (1) activation of the thyroid-stimulating hormone (TSH) receptor by stimulating substances (TSH receptor antibodies of Graves' disease, pituitary hypersecretion of TSH, or the excessive human chorionic gonadotropin (hCG) levels seen with trophoblastic tumors); (2) autonomous hypersecretion of thyroid hormones by thyroid cells in the absence of a known stimulator (toxic uni- or multinodular goiter, iodine-induced thyrotoxicosis, functional thyroid malignancy); or (3) discharge of preformed thyroid hormones into the circulation due to the inflammation and follicular disruption of subacute thyroiditis (discussed in a separate article). Effective management of the condition intimately depends on correct diagnosis of the underlying cause.

DIAGNOSIS

Whatever the cause, the clinical manifestations of thyrotoxicosis are similar. Symptoms include weight loss (despite increased appetite), heat intolerance, excessive sweating, tachycardia, palpitations, tremor, insomnia, anxiety, muscle weakness, increased defecation, and oligoamenorrhea. Findings related to the infiltrative disorders, ophthalmopathy, and pretibial myxedema are confined to those patients with Graves' disease. A history of current or recent neck or throat pain suggests subacute (granulomatous) thyroiditis.

Elevated concentrations of circulating thyroid hormones (total and free thyroxine [T_4] and triiodothyronine [T_3]) and suppressed TSH levels highlight the biochemical findings. Increased thyroidal uptake of a tracer dose of radioactive iodine (^{131}I) indicates that thyrotoxicosis is the result of excessive manufacture and secretion of thyroid hormones by the thyroid gland itself (i.e., hyperthyroidism). In this setting, the presence of a diffuse goiter implies Graves' disease, the most common form of thyrotoxicosis. Toxic nodular goiter is characterized by the presence of a palpably irregular gland in the setting of a normal or elevated radioactive iodine uptake (RAIU) and clinical thyrotoxicosis. Together, these two disorders account for more than 90% of cases of hyperthyroidism. A reduced RAIU (in the absence of recent iodine exposure such as administration of x-ray contrast media) indicates either an exogenous or an ectopic source of thyroid hormone or subacute thyroiditis, with suppression of the iodine-trapping mechanism because of reduced pituitary secretion of TSH.

TREATMENT

Graves' Disease

The cause of the hyperthyroidism of Graves' disease is stimulation of the TSH receptor on thyroid follicular cells by antibodies of the IgG class that are referred to as "thyroid-stimulating immunoglobulins" (TSI or TSAb). By way of activation of the TSH-sensitive adenylate cyclase system, the TSI–TSH receptor interaction leads to increased thyroid cellular iodine uptake, thyroglobulin and thyroid hormone synthesis and release, and cellular hypertrophy and hyperplasia. Unfortunately, specific immune therapy directed at the antigen-antibody interaction or at the production of TSI is not available. Current forms of treatment, therefore, are centered on the disruption of the thyroid response to the abnormal stimulator by the following means: (1) surgical ablation of the thyroid gland, (2) radioiodine ablation of the thyroid gland, or (3) antithyroid (thionamide) medication. Because none of these forms is completely satisfactory for all circumstances, each has a definite role in the management of selected patients.

Radioiodine Therapy

Radioiodine therapy using ^{131}I has been used successfully for over 50 years in the treatment of thyroid disorders and is the most common form of treatment for Graves' disease. Orally administered ^{131}I is rapidly trapped by the thyroid, and the resultant thyroid inflammatory response leads to progressive disruption of thyroid cellular activity and, ultimately, glandular atrophy. In some centers, a "lower-dose" regimen is followed, designed to deliver 50 to 80 μCi per gram of thyroid tissue (3 to 5 mCi total) and aimed at restoring euthyroidism, while avoiding hypothyroidism. With this regimen, the incidence of persistence or recurrence of thyrotoxicosis with the first dose is greater than with regimens using larger doses, and thus, multiple doses may be needed to achieve disease control. Although the incidence of early hypothyroidism is lower than with higher dose regimens (approximately 10% at 1 year), thyroid function may continue to decline, and late hypothyroidism occurs in about 2 to 5% of patients each year thereafter.

In recent years, "higher-dose" [131]I therapy, delivering approximately 200 μCi per gram of thyroid tissue (10 to 15 mCi total), has been given more often. This regimen usually results in early and predictable hypothyroidism, and the patient is then managed with appropriate thyroid hormone replacement. This procedure obviously exchanges one disease, thyrotoxicosis, for another, hypothyroidism. However, the latter is very easily managed and, in following such a regimen, hypothyroidism occurs within an expected time period (usually 2 to 6 months following treatment), thus avoiding the prolonged periods of symptomatic hormone deficiency that may occur with late-onset hypothyroidism.

Beta-adrenergic blocking drugs can be administered (discussed later) for relief of thyrotoxic symptoms while one is waiting for the therapeutic effects of [131]I. In extremely symptomatic patients, or those with thyroid storm, more rapid restoration of the euthyroid state may be desirable. Thionamides or stable iodine (both discussed later) can be added 3 to 5 days after [131]I (in this case, stable iodine must be withdrawn for at least 1 month and thionamides should be withheld for 3 to 5 days before administration of the radionuclide). Within 3 months of treatment, most patients are biochemically and clinically hypothyroid, at which time thyroid hormone replacement is begun. In patients still thyrotoxic after 3 to 6 months (less than 5% with higher-dose ^{131}I), a second dose can be administered. Some patients will become euthyroid after this treatment regimen and will not develop early hypothyroidism. These patients should be monitored at intervals of 3 to 4 months for the first year and at least yearly thereafter to observe for late hypothyroidism.

Adverse effects of ^{131}I therapy include both immediate reactions and the theoretical risks associated with radiation exposure. The most common adverse effect is the development of hypothyroidism, as just discussed. However, many view hypothyroidism after this form of treatment as a goal, rather than a complication. Rarely, exacerbation of thyrotoxicosis occurs following treatment; it is likely due to release of preformed hormone from the inflamed gland. Beta-adrenergic blocking agents or thionamide therapy, or both, can be used successfully for this problem. Pain and erythema in the region of the thyroid gland may rarely develop within the first few days after ^{131}I therapy as a manifestation of radiation thyroiditis. This complication is self-limited and can be managed with anti-inflammatory medications given symptomatically.

Theoretical complications of ^{131}I therapy include the concern about both radiation-induced malignancy and possible genetic alterations related to gonadal exposure. Several large studies involving tens of thousands of patients have addressed the issue of radiation-induced malignant disease, both thyroid cancer and leukemia. No increase in the rate of either has, to date, been detected in patients who received ^{131}I therapy when compared with patients with Graves' disease treated with surgery. It has been determined that the radiation dose delivered to the ovary with ablative ^{131}I therapy is essentially equivalent to that delivered by a diagnostic barium enema and is considered to pose acceptable risk to a woman of childbearing age. Because of the theoretically increased risk of gonadal damage in children, most centers prefer to avoid ^{131}I treatment in this age group. However, in recent years, some have pursued this method of management in children without reported adverse effects.

Antithyroid Medication (Thionamides) Therapy

Propylthiouracil (PTU) and methimazole (Tapazole) are the only thionamide compounds possessing antithyroid activity that are clinically available in the United States. Both exert blocking activity on the synthesis of thyroid hormones by inhibiting iodine organification and the coupling of iodothyronines. In addition, PTU inhibits the conversion of T_4 to T_3 by the deiodinase enzyme of extrathyroidal tissues, an action not shared with methimazole. Although these blocking actions have long been believed to be the only mechanism of action of these compounds, recent evidence suggests that these drugs may also modulate the function of the immune system, reducing the levels of thyroid-stimulating immunoglobulins and thereby reducing the stimulus to the development of hyperthyroidism.

The usual strategy of therapy is to begin with a larger dose of drug until euthyroidism is achieved and then reduce the dose to a lower, maintenance level. A guideline for daily doses is listed in Table 1. In general, the lowest possible dose that achieves and maintains euthyroidism should be used. Both drugs are avidly concentrated in thyroid tissue, and their durations of action are considerably longer than their respective half-lives. Methimazole can be effectively given as a single daily dose. PTU, with its shorter half-life, is usually given in three equally divided doses, but it has also been used successfully as a single daily dose. Reduction in goiter size, relief of thyrotoxic symptoms, and normalization of T_4 levels are typically achieved within 4 to 8 weeks, at which time the drug dose can usually be reduced by 50%. Persistence of hyperthyroidism necessitates the continuance of higher doses. Enlargement of the thyroid, after hyperthyroid symptoms have been controlled, suggests overtreatment and glandular growth resulting from elevated TSH levels. Recently, it has been suggested that the addition of T_4 replacement and continuance of higher doses of thionamides in this setting may increase the chances of long-lasting remission of Graves' disease, but results with this approach have been variable and its practice is not widely recommended at present.

Antithyroid drug therapy is generally maintained for at least 1 year in patients with established Graves' disease, after which the decision is usually made to discontinue the medication. Approximately 50 to 60% of patients so treated will experience relapse of hyperthyroidism within the first year, the majority occurring in the first 3 to 6 months. The remaining 40 to 50% of patients experience remission of their disease for a longer duration. However, it is not clear just how many will relapse given longer follow-up and how many may enjoy a "permanent" remission. Radioreceptor assays (TBII) or bioassays (TSI) for TSH receptor autoantibodies have been said to be of use in predicting the likelihood of relapse after 1 year of antithyroid drug therapy. However, results have varied widely among laboratories. It thus appears that no test currently available can consistently and reliably predict recurrence of hyperthyroidism or the likely duration of remission.

Adverse reactions to thionamide drugs may occur in up to 5% of patients treated. The most common side effects are those related to hypersensitivity: skin rash, pruritus, fever, and less commonly, arthralgias and serum sickness. These are self-limited on discontinuation of the drug and, although some cross-sensitivity may be seen, generally do not recur when treatment is switched to the other compound. The most serious adverse reaction is granulocytopenia, occurring in 0.2 to 0.3% of patients. Since the white blood cell counts fall precipitously, regular monitoring of patients receiving antithyroid medications is not likely to be of predictive value. Rather, patients should be warned to report promptly the onset of symptoms such as fever, pharyngitis, or stomatitis. Should granulocytopenia occur, the thionamide should be promptly discontinued and antibiotic therapy initiated for any evidence of infection. Fortu-

TABLE 1. **Thionamide (Antithyroid) Drugs**

| Drug | Half-Life | Dose (mg/day) | | Adverse Effects | |
		Initial	Maintenance	Effect	Incidence
Propylthiouracil (PTU)	2 h	300–600	50–200	MAJOR	
				Agranulocytosis	0.2–0.3%
				Hepatitis	Rare
				Cholestasis	Rare
				Lupus-like syndrome	Rare
Methimazole (Tapazole)	6–13 h	5–20	5–20	MINOR	
				Skin rash	3–5%
				Fever	Rare
				"Serum sickness"	Rare
				Arthralgias	Rare
				Arthritis	Rare

nately, white blood cell counts generally rise within 7 to 14 days. Other rare adverse reactions have been reported, including rhinitis, conjunctivitis, lymphadenopathy, hypoprothrombinemia, diarrhea, hepatitis, cholestasis, vasculitis, lupus-like syndrome, alopecia, and ageusia. If one of the more serious reactions occurs, another mode of therapy should be pursued because of the high risk of cross-sensitivity with other similar compounds.

Surgical Therapy

Of the three methods of management of hyperthyroidism, surgical ablation of the gland results in the swiftest resumption of the euthyroid state. The most common procedure is subtotal thyroidectomy, leaving behind only the posterior capsule and small portions of the inferior poles of the gland. It is of extreme importance that the procedure be performed by a surgeon experienced in thyroidectomy, as the incidence of surgical complications is quite low in seasoned hands. The incidence of recurrence of hyperthyroidism depends on the thoroughness of the thyroidectomy, as expected, and is around 10% in most centers. Recurrence is most common within 5 years of initial surgery and rarely occurs later. Because of the increased risk of complications during a thyroid reoperation, ^{131}I therapy is the treatment of choice for recurrence after thyroidectomy.

Adequate preparation of the thyrotoxic patient for surgery is of the utmost importance, because surgical morbidity and mortality are greatly increased without it, owing especially to the occurrence of thyroid storm or crisis. Seven to 10 days of preoperative stable iodine (such as Lugol's solution, 3 to 5 drops three times daily) serves to reduce thyroid vascularity, as well as to reduce thyroid hormone levels (see later). Propranolol (Inderal), 40 to 80 mg orally four times daily, inhibits the effects of excess thyroid hormones at the tissue level, thus abating the peripheral, especially cardiac, manifestations of hyperthyroidism. As noted earlier, when given for adequate periods of time, thionamides can be used to return the patient to the euthyroid state. Combinations of these regimens can be used as needed, with the choices depending on the severity of hyperthyroidism and the stability of the patient's clinical status. Many feel it necessary to achieve euthyroidism with several weeks of thionamide therapy before surgery, but most centers have found that 7 days of stable iodine plus adequate doses of propranolol (Inderal) serves adequately in all but the most extreme cases. Whatever regimen is used, the preoperative goal should be a comfortable patient without significant tachycardia, dehydration, or other significant signs of thyrotoxicosis. Postoperative fever and tachycardia in the absence of infection suggest impending thyroid storm and should be promptly treated with beta blockers and other measures as indicated (see later).

In the hands of an experienced thyroid surgeon, the incidence of operative complications from subtotal thyroidectomy for Graves' disease should be less than 1%, and mortality should approach zero. Aside from the usual risk of general anesthetic effects and bleeding, hypoparathyroidism and vocal cord paralysis are the major complications specific to the procedure. The incidence of both these complications rises with reoperation in the neck but should remain less than 2 to 5%. Postoperative hypothyroidism occurs with variable frequency and is related to the aggressiveness of the thyroidectomy. Generally, its incidence is inversely related to the incidence of recurrence of hyperthyroidism. As most procedures now achieve a low incidence of recurrence of disease, the frequency of hypothyroidism approaches that seen with ^{131}I therapy, and late-onset hypothyroidism, therefore, is less frequently observed.

Ancillary Therapy

Beta-Adrenergic Blocking Agents. Beta-blocking drugs can be useful in the management of hyperthyroid symptoms in the patient being treated with ^{131}I or antithyroid drugs, while awaiting the effects of the definitive therapy. They also play a role in the preparation of patients for thyroid surgery and for managing symptoms while making a diagnosis. The usual starting dose of propranolol (Inderal) is 40 mg orally every 6 hours, and it should be titrated to maintain the resting heart rate at around 70 to 90 bpm. Longer-acting beta blockers such as atenolol (Tenormin), metoprolol (Lopressor), and Inderal-LA offer some advantages over propranolol because of propranolol's short half-life.

Stable Iodine. Large doses of iodine rapidly inhibit thyroidal iodine trapping, thyroglobulin endocytosis, and thyroid hormone synthesis and release. Either Lugol's solution (5% iodine plus 10% potassium iodide) or a saturated solution of potassium iodide (SSKI, approximately 50% KI) can be used with equivalent results. Usual doses are 3 to 5 drops of Lugol's or 1 to 3 drops of SSKI three times daily. Adverse effects include hypersensitivity reactions, manifested as rash, serum sickness–like syndrome, and rarely, angioedema. In prolonged treatment with high doses, iodism can occur with symptoms much like those of the common cold: coryza, sneezing, and sore mouth and throat. Fortunately, these symptoms rapidly abate with discontinuation of the iodine. Occasional patients will develop hypothyroidism with prolonged exposure.

Choice of Therapy

As mentioned, none of the therapeutic options is totally suited to all clinical situations, and each has limitations as well as advantages that must be considered when deciding on a course of treatment. The options should be discussed fully with the patient (and family when appropriate) before arriving at a mutual decision regarding which to choose. Within this framework, most physicians would agree with these statements regarding selection of therapy.

1. The majority of adult patients with Graves' disease can be successfully and permanently treated with ablative ^{131}I therapy, followed by thyroid hormone replacement.

2. Most physicians avoid ^{131}I therapy in children because of the theoretically increased risk of genetic damage. Surgery or antithyroid medications are the major options for these patients.

3. In the reproductive years, some also avoid ^{131}I therapy, although many physicians are now routinely utilizing this form of treatment. If ^{131}I therapy is chosen, it is imperative that the patient be screened for pregnancy before the treatment dose is given and that she use contraception for approximately 6 months thereafter.

4. An elderly patient with unstable cardiac status should be managed with ^{131}I given in doses sufficient to cause hypothyroidism and usually administered only after the euthyroid state has been established with thionamides and beta-blocking agents.

5. [131]I therapy is the treatment of choice for thyrotoxicosis recurring after thyroidectomy.

6. Relapse of hyperthyroidism after an adequate course of antithyroid medications is best managed by either surgical or ^{131}I ablation.

Toxic Uni- or Multinodular Goiter

Solitary thyroid nodules only rarely possess sufficient functional capacity to cause hyperthyroidism. The diagnosis is established by radionuclide scanning of the thyroid showing a "hot" nodule, with suppression of tracer uptake in the remainder of the gland (because of suppressed pituitary TSH secretion). Although the choices of therapy for this syndrome are the same as those for the treatment of Graves' disease noted earlier, some differences in response may be seen. Long-term remissions of the disease generally do not occur with thionamide therapy, and thus, thyrotoxicosis recurs rapidly when the drug is stopped. Toxic nodules less than 5 to 6 cm in diameter can be successfully treated with ^{131}I therapy. Because the normal tissue is suppressed from absence of TSH, the radioiodine is concentrated to a much greater extent by the autonomous nodular cells and thus spares the remaining gland. Therefore, euthyroidism can be achieved with a lower incidence of hypothyroidism, although late occurrence of thyroid failure is seen. However, in very large nodules (greater than 6 cm) [131]I therapy is less successful, likely related to the difficulty in delivering appropriately high doses to the nodule. In these cases, surgery is considered a better choice.

Toxic multinodular goiter (Plummer's disease) occurs most commonly in elderly patients with preexisting goiters and is characterized by the presence of a large, irregular gland. As in the solitary toxic nodule, antithyroid drugs are only a temporary measure of control. Radionuclide scanning shows patchy areas of uptake interspersed with regions of reduced trapping. Because of the inhomogeneous distribution of iodine uptake, ^{131}I therapy is less likely to be effective, especially for very large glands. When ^{131}I is used, multiple and relatively large doses may be needed to achieve euthyroidism. Because these patients frequently have cardiac manifestations of thy-rotoxicosis, rapid control may be desirable; that is best achieved with surgical thyroidectomy. Preoperative beta blockers and thionamides are often used for surgical preparation.

Hyperthyroidism During Pregnancy

It has been estimated that hyperthyroidism complicates 0.2% of pregnancies. When present, thyrotoxicosis causes an increase in the incidence of low birthweight, prematurity, and fetal wastage. By far, the most common cause is Graves' disease. Diagnosis is complicated by the expected increase in T_4 and T_3 levels during normal pregnancy owing to changes in thyroid hormone–binding protein concentrations and by the contraindication to the use of diagnostic or therapeutic ^{131}I during pregnancy. Suppression of the serum level of TSH in modern, sensitive immunoassays and the finding of TSH receptor autoantibodies in the blood can be of considerable diagnostic assistance in questionable cases.

[131]I therapy is contraindicated during pregnancy, leaving surgery or antithyroid drugs as the therapeutic option. Because most obstetricians prefer to avoid general anesthesia and surgery during pregnancy, thionamides are the most commonly employed therapy. Surgery can be reserved for the case of sensitivity to thionamides or medical failure. Patient preparation for surgery is as important during pregnancy as in Graves' disease at other times.

PTU is the thionamide of choice during pregnancy because methimazole has been associated with an unusual scalp disorder, aplasia cutis, that occurs in infants born to mothers treated with the drug during pregnancy. PTU also crosses the placenta more poorly than does methimazole and, as noted later, has less influence on the baby's thyroid.

Thionamides, when given to the mother, cross the placenta and exert inhibitory influences on fetal thyroid function. Thyroid hormone does not as readily cross and the fetus is therefore not exposed to the high maternal T_4 and T_3 levels. When the mother is treated for hyperthyroidism with high doses of thionamides, the fetus may become hypothyroid because of effects of the drug on the fetal thyroid, despite normal hormone levels in the mother. It is therefore desirable to use the lowest dose possible to avoid this complication. We suggest reducing PTU doses to levels sufficient to control hyperthyroid symptoms, but to maintain the serum TSH level at or below the lower limits of normal. In addition, beta-blocking agents can be used for control of thyrotoxic symptoms, as data suggest that they may be safely given to patients during pregnancy.

High maternal levels of TSH receptor antibodies during the third trimester accurately identify patients at highest risk of fetal or neonatal hyperthyroidism. It is important to realize that the currently euthyroid patient (on replacement therapy) who had her thyroid ablated with surgery or ^{131}I previously may still harbor significant levels of these thyroid-stimulating antibodies, and thus may bear a child who will suffer this disorder.

Thyroid Storm

Thyrotoxic crisis is a medical emergency usually occurring in patients with inadequately treated or untreated hyperthyroidism, who are stressed by the occurrence of a significant medical or surgical illness. The mortality rate can be quite high, depending on the nature of the precipitating event and the presence of other underlying diseases. Specific therapy directed at the underlying precipitating factor is obviously important and will not be discussed further here. Supportive measures directed against hyperpyrexia, volume depletion, cardiovascular or respiratory collapse, or other metabolic derangements such as acidosis or adrenal insufficiency are also extremely important.

Treatment of thyroid storm may involve the use of multiple medications and should be initiated as soon as the diagnosis is strongly suspected. Thionamides should be given to limit thyroid hormone production. PTU has the advantage of also inhibiting peripheral conversion of T_4 to T_3. The initial dose of PTU should be from 200 to 300 mg every 4 to 6 hours and must be given orally or by nasogastric tube because no parenteral form of the drug is available. Stable iodine, given orally as SSKI or Lugol's solution (5 to 8 drops every 6 hours) or parenterally as sodium iodide (0.5 to 1 gram every 12 hours) prevents thyroid hormone release but should be given only *after* PTU is given to prevent iodine accumulation. Beta-blocking drugs (propranolol [Inderal], 80 to 120 mg orally every 6 hours, or 2 to 4 mg intravenously every 4 hours) reduce the catecholamine-mediated effects. Finally, systemic corticosteroids (prednisone or equivalent, 40 to 80 mg every 8 hours, tapered rapidly with control of hyperthyroidism) potently inhibit peripheral T_4 to T_3 conversion, stabilize vascular membranes, and protect against possible relative adrenal insufficiency.

THYROID CANCER

method of
WILLIAM H. SNYDER III, M.D.
University of Texas Southwestern Medical Center
Dallas, Texas

The thyroid gland consists of two functionally distinct endocrine components: a large mass of follicular cells that produce thyroid hormone and a small population (less than 1%) of parafollicular or C cells (neural crest origin) that produce calcitonin. The simplest classification of thyroid carcinomas distinguishes those of follicular cell origin (papillary, follicular, and anaplastic) from those of parafollicular cell origin (medullary carcinoma). Lymphomas account for a small portion of thyroid tumors. Papillary, follicular, and Hürthle cell (variant of follicular cell with unknown

function, oxyphil cell) tumors are differentiated thyroid cancers (DTC) and account for 80% of thyroid malignancies. A clinically useful classification of thyroid cancer is listed in Table 1. Although the other types of thyroid cancer are summarized in Table 1, most of this discussion is devoted to differentiated thyroid cancer.

EVALUATION OF THYROID NODULES

The differential diagnosis of thyroid nodules is a problem, because most thyroid diseases are manifested by the formation of nodules. Benign thyroid nodules are common, thyroid cancer is uncommon, and the two are often indistinguishable by noninvasive means. The various modalities available for the evaluation of thyroid nodules include clinical examination, ultrasound, thyroid-stimulating hormone (TSH) suppression, radionucleotide imaging, and fine-needle aspiration (FNA) cytology.

Clinical features supporting the diagnosis of thyroid cancer include a family history of this disease, especially the medullary variety; a history of cervical irradiation; a single or prominent nodule, especially if it is firm or fixed or has undergone rapid painless enlargement; hoarseness; and the presence of suspicious cervical or supraclavicular lymphadenopathy. Additional features increasing the suspicion that a given nodule may be malignant are age less than 30 years and male gender. Clinical examination demonstrates obvious thyroid cancer in the minority of patients; such patients merit thyroidectomies for definitive diagnosis and treatment. The preoperative evaluation should include a chest radiograph to evaluate the possibility of pulmonary metastases and may include FNA to expedite operative treatment.

Most thyroid nodules are in the clinical categories of "possibly malignant" or "probably benign" and require further evaluation. Ultrasound allows accurate measurement of the size of the gland, the number and size of nodules, and whether they are solid, cystic, or mixed. This information may be selectively useful in evaluating thyroid nodules, but no specific sonographic criteria distinguish benign from malignant nodules. Radionucleotide scanning, with radioactive iodine (^{131}I or ^{123}I) or ^{99m}Tc pertechnetate, has been widely used to classify the functional status of thyroid nodules. Because malignant tissue traps or organifies iodine poorly, such lesions usually appear as cold areas on a scan. The difficulties with using scans to differentiate benign from malignant lesions are (1) most benign nodules are also hypofunctional; (2) peripheral nodules or those near the isthmus are poorly outlined; and (3) functioning

TABLE 1. **Classification of Thyroid Cancer**

Differentiated
Papillary
Minimal (occult: <1.0 cm)
Intrathyroidal (encapsulated)
Extrathyroidal
Follicular variant
Follicular ("pure")
Minimally invasive
Extensively invasive
Hürthle cell
Medullary
Anaplastic
Lymphoma
Other (sarcoma, metastatic, etc.)

normal tissue may hide an underlying nonfunctioning nodule. Nucleotide scanning has a very limited role in the evaluation of thyroid nodules. Suppression of TSH with levothyroxine has long been used to differentiate benign from malignant nodules. This is based on the concept that neoplastic lesions are more likely to be autonomous and that non-neoplastic lesions will decrease in size with TSH suppression. Carefully controlled studies demonstrate this approach to be ineffective, because the size of benign nodules is often not altered.

FNA has been used increasingly in the evaluation of thyroid nodules. An experienced cytopathologist is required; such training is now included in residency programs. Inaccuracies may result from sampling error and are more likely in lesions smaller than 1 cm or larger than 4 cm, particularly if they are cystic, because the fluid removed is not representative of the epithelial component. If a satisfactory aspirate is obtained, four cytologic results are possible: benign (abundant colloid and benign follicular cells), suspicious (follicular neoplasm), positive for malignant disease, or indeterminate. More than 60% of aspirates are benign, 5% are malignant, and the remainder are in the suspicious or indeterminate group. A malignant diagnosis has a false-positive rate of 2%, and a benign diagnosis has a false-negative rate of less than 5%. The difficulty in evaluating suspicious lesions reflects the cytologic inability to differentiate benign from malignant follicular and Hürthle cell neoplasms. The routine use of FNA has halved the number of patients undergoing operations for nodular thyroid disease and doubled the incidence of malignant disease detected in excised nodules. The use of FNA in the evaluation of thyroid nodules is depicted in Figure 1.

Isotope scintigraphy after the cytologic diagnosis of follicular neoplasm may demonstrate increased iodine uptake in the nodule, indicating benignity and making operative excision unnecessary. Unfortunately, very few of such lesions are hot, and I use this study infrequently.

In summary, recommendations for the diagnosis/management of thyroid nodules are as follows:

1. Patients with thyroid nodules that have obvious clinical indications of malignancy should undergo thyroidectomy. A preoperative FNA may be performed to expedite the operative procedure, but negative or indeterminate results should not alter the plans for operation.

2. FNA should be performed during the initial evaluation of patients with clinically benign thyroid nodules.

3. Repeat FNA is used liberally to re-evaluate patients with initially indeterminate or benign aspirates.

TREATMENT OF DIFFERENTIATED THYROID CANCER

Operative Treatment

Surgery is the initial treatment for essentially all patients with DTC, but controversy continues concerning the appropriate operation. Some authorities favor lobectomy and isthmusectomy for most patients and consider more extensive resections only in those with obviously advanced disease. Others favor more extensive resections—either near-total or total thyroidectomies—in most patients with the diagnosis of thyroid cancer. A middle ground is the routine performance of an ipsilateral total lobectomy and a contralateral subtotal lobectomy.

The difference between subtotal and near-total lobectomy is not finite, but in general, the former implies leaving a rim of posterior gland about the size of the thumb tip (1 to 2 grams), and the latter is used to describe an intended total resection in which a small amount (less than 1 gram) of tissue is left to avoid devascularizing parathyroid tissue. Lymphadenectomies are limited to the excision of involved nodes or to modified neck dissections, sparing the sternocleidomastoid muscle and, if possible, the internal jugular vein. Radical neck dissections are per-

Figure 1. The use of fine-needle aspiration (FNA) in the evaluation of thyroid nodules. *Abbreviation*: TFTs = thyroid function tests.

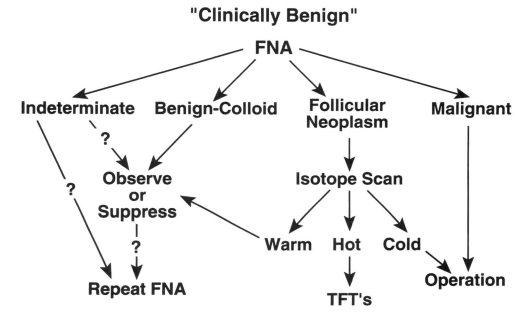

THYROID NODULE

"Clinically Benign"

formed only in patients with extensive disease and adjacent tissue invasion.

The generally accepted principles of thyroidectomy for thyroid cancer are (1) the tumor should be completely resected, with a margin of normal tissue; (2) limited resections are sufficient for occult papillary carcinomas; and (3) more complete resections are indicated for patients with extrathyroidal papillary, invasive follicular, and Hürthle cell cancers and those with bilobar lesions or with extensive lymphatic or distant metastases.

The rationale for limited resections is this: there is a reduced risk of complications (recurrent laryngeal nerve injury and hypoparathyroidism); occult foci of DTC are seldom clinically important; even total thyroidectomy leaves some residual thyroid tissue; contralateral recurrence can be safely treated by lobectomy if the lobe was originally left undisturbed; and enhanced survival has not been proved to result from total or near-total thyroidectomy.

The rationale for total thyroidectomy is this: all intraglandular malignancy is removed; the risks of recurrence and of anaplastic transformation are decreased; the detection and treatment of recurrence and metastatic disease are more feasible in the athyroid patient; and the risk of complications is low with an experienced thyroid surgeon. In general, these goals are accomplished by an ipsilateral total and a contralateral subtotal lobectomy with subsequent radioiodine ablation of the thyroid remnant, as deemed indicated.

A reasonable operative approach is to base the extent of resection on an evaluation of the patient's risk for subsequent recurrence of, or death from, DTC. With this approach, unilateral excision of the total thyroid lobe and isthmus is performed in patients deemed to have low risks, and contralateral subtotal or total lobectomies are added in patients whose risks are projected to be high. The determination of risk in patients with thyroid cancer is based on large retrospective studies. Cady evaluated the outcome of 310 patients treated for papillary and follicular thyroid cancer between 1961 and 1980. Low risk was defined as men less than 40 years and women less than 50 years of age and older patients whose tumors were locally contained and less than 5 cm in diameter without distant metastases. Eighty-nine percent of the patients were low risk; 5% had recurrent disease and 1.8% died. All other patients (11%) were considered high risk; 55% developed recurrences and 46% died. These factors (age, sex, tumor size, local invasion, and distant metastases) are known to the surgeon at the time of operation and provide a basis for the decision regarding extent of resection.

In a retrospective study at the Mayo Clinic, 806 patients with papillary carcinoma were followed 14,200 patient-years. Using a scoring system composed of patient age, histologic grade, and extent and size of the tumor, 86% of the patients were low risk and 14% were high risk. The 25-year mortalities were 2% in the low-risk and 56% in the high-risk

groups. Unilateral (lobectomy) or bilateral (ipsilateral lobectomy and contralateral subtotal, near-total, or total lobectomy) operations were performed based on clinical characteristics and surgeon preference. Based on extent of operation, there was no significant difference in the mortality rate in the low-risk group, but the difference almost reached significance in the high-risk group (65% for unilateral vs. 35% for bilateral). There was no significant difference in the mortality rates in the high-risk group based on the extent of the bilateral operation performed. These and other similar retrospecitve analyses lend support to the use of patient and tumor factors in the decision regarding the extent of thyroidectomy indicated in a given patient.

In my opinion, the optimal operation for most carcinomas of the thyroid is bilateral thyroidectomy. However, this optimum must be balanced by the increased potential for recurrent laryngeal nerve injury and hypoparathyroidism with more extensive thyroidectomy. These risks relate largely to the experience and expertise of the operating surgeon, and it is his or her responsibility to consider this realistically. Occult and well-differentiated intrathyroidal papillary carcinoma without cervical lymph node metastasis and minimally invasive follicular carcinoma are adequately treated by total ipsilateral lobectomy and isthmusectomy. A more radical operation for such lesions requires confident visualization and preservation of at least one viable parathyroid gland and the recurrent laryngeal nerve on the ipsilateral side. With these criteria fulfilled, it seems reasonable to proceed with a contralateral resection.

For patients with metastatic disease or with extrathyroidal papillary, extensively invasive follicular, or Hürthle cell carcinomas, the evidence supporting the advantages of total or near-total thyroidectomy is more conclusive, and this is the optimal operation for such lesions. If question exists concerning the viability of parathyroid tissue or injury to the recurrent laryngeal nerve after the ipsilateral resection, a contralateral subtotal lobectomy is performed.

Postoperative Management

The available components of postoperative care of patients with DTC are TSH suppression with levothyroxine (T_4), radioactive iodine (RAI) ablation of thyroid remnants, and surveillance including physical examinations, chest radiographs, serum thyroglobulin (Tg) assays, and diagnostic total body RAI scans. Cervical ultrasonography and computed tomography scans of the neck or chest are used selectively. The extent of adjunctive treatment and intensity of follow-up are determined by the postoperative estimation of risk and the extent of resection performed. The frequency of follow-up is every 3 months for 1 year, every 6 months for 2 or 3 years, and in patients without evidence of disease, every 5 years for life.

The use of serum Tg determinations and RAI scanning for surveillance requires complete thyroid ablation, either operatively or with a combination of operation and RAI thyroid remnant ablation. Ablation may be considered a therapeutic maneuver as well as an aid to surveillance. For DTC patients with nonoccult or multifocal primary lesions, local or vascular invasion, or involved neck nodes, RAI ablation reduces the risk of recurrence. Although RAI ablation of an entire thyroid lobe is possible, it is an ineffective use of RAI, and I favor completion thyroidectomy (contralateral lobectomy) in patients in whom the need to ablate the contralateral lobe is determined postoperatively.

RAI remnant ablation may be performed on an outpatient basis, with 29.9 mCi of ^{131}I, or on an inpatient basis, with 100 to 150 mCi. Complete ablation of small thyroid remnants can be accomplished in 70 to 80% of patients with the smaller dose and in 80 to 90% with the larger dose. Residual malignant tissue is more likely to be sterilized by the larger dose. In general, the smaller outpatient dose is chosen for patients with limited disease and the larger inpatient dose for those with more extensive disease. A total body scan to demonstrate the site(s) of uptake is obtained a week after the RAI dose, to allow time for dissipation of background activity. Levothyroxine is started or resumed after the scan has been completed.

Although the data supporting the efficacy of TSH suppression are largely anecdotal, the risk and cost are relatively low, and essentially all patients are so treated. TSH is monitored using the "sensitive" assay, performed 4 to 6 weeks after initiation or change of T_4 dose, and the goal is a clinically euthyroid patient with a low or undetectable serum TSH and normal or only slightly elevated serum T_4. The starting T_4 (levothyroxine [Synthroid]) dose is 0.1 mg per day for smaller and older patients and 0.15 mg per day for larger and younger patients.

Surveillance is most effectively performed in athyroid patients, in whom scans and Tg levels are sensitive and specific. Anti-Tg antibodies are measured initially, because their presence renders Tg assays invalid. Serum Tg is most sensitive in the detection of metastatic DTC if measured off T_4. However, serum Tg elevation (more than 10 ng per dL) on T_4 reliably predicts active disease. About 75% of DTC metastases trap RAI, and almost all produce Tg. Iodine scans and serum Tg levels are the laboratory mainstays of postoperative surveillance.

Treatment of Metastasis

Distant metastases are initially present in 4% of papillary and 16% of follicular cancer patients. In patients believed free of DTC after initial treatment, thyroid bed, nodal, or distant recurrences are found in 6%, 9%, and 6%, respectively. Local and remote recurrences decrease survival; the effect of nodal disease is variable. Cervical recurrences are resected when feasible and treated with RAI when not. Lung and bone are the most common sites of remote metastases. Surgical or RAI extirpation of residual thyroid is necessary before metastases can be diagnosed by, or treated with, RAI. Pulmonary metastases found by scan with negative plain radiographs have the best RAI cure rate; the use of Tg assay adds to early diagnosis of these lesions. Complete response to RAI is more likely with pulmonary than osseous metastases. Side effects to RAI are largely dose-related and are infrequent in patients receiving total doses of less than 500 mCi. The use of external beam radiotherapy is limited to unresectable local or remote disease that does not concentrate radioactive iodine.

MEDULLARY CARCINOMA OF THE THYROID

Medullary thyroid carcinoma (MTC) is derived from parafollicular cells, produces calcitonin, and is often associated with the multiple endocrine neoplasia (MEN) Type II syndrome. Hereditary forms of this tumor include MEN IIa (MTC, hyperparathyroidism, and pheochromocytoma), MEN IIb (MTC, multiple mucosal neuromas, pheochromocytoma, and a marfanoid body habitus), and familial MTC without associated endocrinopathies. MTC comprises 10 to 15% of thyroid malignancies, is bilateral in the familial form, and metastasizes to cervical lymph nodes, lung, bone, and liver.

Basal and stimulated (pentagastrin and/or calcium infusions) calcitonin assays have been the basis for surveillance of family members, as early operations greatly enhance successful treatment. Recent discovery of the gene mutation responsible for familial MTC and reliable genetic testing on peripheral blood samples have allowed accurate prediction of patients at risk for the disease. Such testing is indicated in first-degree relatives of known MEN II patients and in patients found to have MTC that may be an index familial case. Genetic testing and concurrent counseling are recommended to begin about 5 years of age. A positive test in kindred members is an indication for total thyroidectomy. Subsequent follow-up and testing of uninvolved family members is unnecessary.

Total thyroidectomy with dissection of the central neck nodes from the hyoid cartilage to the innominate vein and lateral node sampling is the appropriate operative procedure for patients with MTC. Formal radical neck dissection of involved lateral cervical nodes is recommended. The 5-year survival is 90% in patients with negative nodes and 65% in those with positive nodes; this falls to 85% and 40%, respectively, at 10 years.

ANAPLASTIC CARCINOMA OF THE THYROID

Anaplastic carcinoma of the thyroid is one of the most aggressive neoplasms known, and survival is measured in months. It occurs most often in older individuals and accounts for about 10% of thyroid cancers. Symptoms of a rapidly growing mass, dyspnea, hoarseness, pain, dysphagia, cough, and weight loss prompt medical care. Distant metastases are present in one-third of patients at the time of initial presentation. Complete resection is desirable but is very seldom possible; operative treatment is usually limited to biopsy or to tracheostomy to alleviate airway compromise. Very limited success has been achieved with radiation and various chemotherapeutic regimens.

LYMPHOMA OF THE THYROID

Lymphomas comprise less than 5% of thyroid malignancies. They typically present in middle-aged to older-aged women as a rapidly enlarging (usually painless), firm thyroid mass. Pressure symptoms, including stridor, shortness of breath, and dysphagia are common. The duration of symptoms is usually short (weeks to months). A thyroid mass is essentially always palpable. FNA is often not diagnostic, and core needle (TruCut) biopsy is usually required for differentiation from anaplastic lesions and to obtain T and B cell markers.

Thyroidectomy is indicated only in those patients whose disease is confined to the thyroid gland, about one-third of patients. Patients with extrathyroidal disease are treated with radiotherapy, often combined with chemotherapy. Adjuvant therapy also may improve the cure rate in patients undergoing resection of intrathyroidal disease, but resection does not benefit those patients with extrathyroidal disease. The overall 5-year survival in a recent large series was 50%. It was 38% in those with extrathyroidal disease and 86% for those in whom the tumor was confined to the thyroid gland.

PHEOCHROMOCYTOMA

method of
PETER STEIN, M.D.
Medical College of Georgia
Augusta, Georgia

and

HENRY R. BLACK, M.D.
Rush-Presbyterian–St. Luke's Medical Center
Chicago, Illinois

Pheochromocytoma is an unusual yet important disease. This tumor probably accounts for hypertension in less than 1 of 1000 hypertensive patients, hence a generalist physician will see few of these patients in a career. Nonetheless, awareness of this disease and how it presents is essential, since diagnosis leads to cure and failure to recognize this disorder can lead to significant complications or even death. Indeed, although pheochromocytomas are usually histologically benign, they are often metabolically malignant. Since many patients without pheochromocytoma will have symptoms that suggest they have the disease, understanding how to pursue this diagnosis in a cost-effective manner is essential.

Physiology and Blood Pressure Regulation

Hemodynamic profiles of patients with pheochromocytoma have shown that increased peripheral vascular resistance underlies the elevation of blood pressure. Several observations provide insight into the mechanisms of this rise in vascular tone. First, catecholamine levels do not necessarily correlate with blood pressure; and second, the blood pressure–lowering effects of centrally acting sympatholytic agents remain intact, as do the circadian variations in blood pressure. These observations suggest that the increased blood pressure results, at least partly, from increased release of catecholamines at sympathetic nerve terminals. Nonetheless, circumstances that lead to direct catecholamine release, such as rises in intra-abdominal pressure, ischemic necrosis of a tumor, or surgical manipulation of a tumor, clearly cause dramatic blood pressure elevations. Vascular tone and thus hypertension appear to be mediated both by circulating catecholamines and by sympathetic neuronal release of catecholamines.

Clinical Presentation

Pheochromocytoma can present in a wide variety of ways, but usually with a characteristic triad of symptoms: headache, diaphoresis, and palpitations occurring typically in an episodic manner (Table 1). The basis for these symptoms is the overproduction of catecholamines with activation of alpha- and beta-adrenergic receptors, resulting in severe hypertension and often tachycardia. The headache is often of rapid onset over minutes, may be frontal or circumferential in location, and typically occurs at the time of the rapid rise in blood pressure. Although the pain may be aching or of modest intensity, it is frequently described as severe, pressure-like or explosive in nature. Pallor may accompany the headache, as well as nausea, vomiting, and forceful heartbeating or palpitations. With such paroxysms, a wide variety of symptoms have been reported, including blurring of vision, dyspnea, chest or abdominal pain, tremulousness, paresthesias, throat tightness, and even seizures. Often the patient reports weakness or even prostration with an episode, and as the episode remits, the patient may feel drained and may then become flushed or feel warm.

Episodes may last minutes or, less frequently, hours and

TABLE 1. **Symptoms in Patients with Pheochromocytoma**

Symptom	Range (%)
Headache	80–96
Diaphoresis	67–74
Palpitations	62–70
Paroxysms	82–86
Pallor	42–43
Nervousness	22–43
Tremulousness	29–31
Nausea/vomiting	10–42
Weakness or fatigue	26–40
Chest pain	19–22
Abdominal pain	16–22
Dyspnea	10–19
Flushing or warmth	8–18
Throat tightness	8
Dizziness	5–8
Paresthesias/arm pain	4–16
Raynaud's phenomenon	5

may be precipitated by a range of factors such as those that increase abdominal pressure—coughing, laughing, sneezing, or even abdominal palpation. Pharmacologic precipitants such as decongestants and alcohol are also important to recognize, yet many episodes occur without clear precipitants. During the episode, blood pressure increases dramatically, often with diastolic pressures that can range from 120 to 160 mm Hg or even as high as 200 mm Hg. Classically, the pulse pressure is small, reflecting the intense vasoconstriction during the paroxysm.

Although this description is classic as well as common, the physician must be aware that some patients may have only part of this picture, or come to medical attention because of a variety of other complaints or problems. Pheochromocytoma, for example, can present as malignant hypertension, unexplained cardiomyopathy, psychiatric disorders, fever, hypotension, or an acute abdomen. And patients with pheochromocytoma may be seen initially with a complication of their severe hypertension, such as a myocardial infarction, intracranial hemorrhage or stroke, or congestive heart failure. Autopsy series of patients with undiagnosed pheochromocytoma report a high proportion of deaths related to vascular events. Some patients with a pheochromocytoma will not come to medical attention until a stressful situation, such as parturition, anesthesia, or surgery, precipitates a dramatic pressor response or markedly labile hypertension.

A pheochromocytoma crisis is yet another presentation. In this instance, the tumor appears to have acute, dramatic release of catecholamines, perhaps related to ischemic necrosis or hemorrhage. In such patients, severe hypertension or hypotension, extreme pyrexia, pulmonary edema, and confusion or coma may be noted, which progresses to subsequent multiorgan failure and, often, death.

Finally, symptoms may be minimal or absent in some patients with a pheochromocytoma. Such patients may come to medical attention with the discovery of an abdominal or adrenal mass by imaging studies done for other purposes. If surgery is performed, the pathology, to the physician's dismay, reveals a pheochromocytoma. Patients at risk for pheochromocytoma, such as those with neurofibromatosis or a multiple endocrine neoplasia (MEN) II syndrome (Table 2), may also be discovered to have an abnormality by routine screening studies like imaging or biochemical testing before symptoms are reported.

In most series, hypertension is present in more than 90% of patients with a pheochromocytoma, and the hypertension may be of relatively recent onset. Elevated blood pressure may be persistent or paroxysmal. In patients with sustained hypertension, ambulatory monitoring often reveals dramatic lability, often with reversal of usual diurnal variation. Orthostatic hypotension, in association with supine hypertension, should bring pheochromocytoma to mind.

Clinical Diagnosis

Despite the range of clinical features, many patients, perhaps even most, are first seen with some variation of

TABLE 2. Associated Syndromes of Pheochromocytoma

Neurofibromatosis
Von Hippel–Lindau syndrome
Multiple endocrine neoplasia IIA, IIB
Family history of pheochromocytoma

TABLE 3. Clinical Epidemiology: Definitions

Pretest likelihood: Also called "prevalence," the chances that a patient has a disease in question, based on epidemiology, history, examination, and prior testing available.

Sensitivity is the true positive rate, or the number of patients who have a disease and a positive test, divided by all with the disease who had the test.

Specificity is the true negative rate, the number of individuals free of disease who have a negative test, divided by all those free of disease who were tested.

Positive predictive value indicates the likelihood of disease in a patient who has a positive test and is determined by dividing the number of patients with the disease who have a positive test by all patients with a positive test.

Negative predictive value indicates the likelihood of being free of disease if a test is negative and is determined by dividing all patients with a negative test who are free of disease by all patients with a negative test.

the typical symptomatic triad of episodic symptoms associated with severe and often labile hypertension. Considering the diagnosis in this circumstance should not be difficult. On the other hand, many hypertensive patients have symptoms such as headache and palpitations that might suggest a pheochromocytoma. Indeed, in one series, slightly more than 1 in 20 essential hypertensive patients had the entire triad of symptoms. Thus, although symptoms may be useful in suggesting the diagnosis, they are not specific. How useful is the presence of symptoms in "screening" for the diagnosis? That is, do asymptomatic hypertensives need further evaluation? The right answer to this question is difficult. In many series, the majority of pheochromocytoma patients had symptoms or some suggestive finding. In a series in France, 10 of 11 pheochromocytoma patients had the entire triad of symptoms. Other series, however, report characteristic symptoms less frequently. Series from autopsy cases show that symptoms may have been present in only slightly more than half of patients. Clearly, these discrepancies reflect a referral bias: The diagnosis is less likely to be made in patients with only hypertension, and much more likely to be made in patients with classic symptoms. Yet it may also be the case that patients with more severe disease will have more symptoms and are more likely to be diagnosed.

The tenets of modern clinical epidemiology suggest that we can use our assessment of the clinical likelihood of a disease to interpret subsequent testing (Table 3). Estimating the probability or likelihood that a patient has the disease in question, based on the history and examination, is the starting point. In our use of diagnostic testing for rare diseases like pheochromocytoma, we are most interested in predictive values, not sensitivity and specificity. Recall that the latter test characteristics tell us how likely a test will be positive in patients with a disease (sensitivity) or negative in individuals known to be free of disease (specificity). On the other hand, predictive values tell the physician the likelihood or probability of the disease being present, if the test is positive (positive predictive value), or absent, if the test is negative (negative predictive value). Predictive values, however, are based on the sensitivity and specificity and on the probability of the disease before the test is done (the pretest likelihood). If we can estimate the likelihood or probability (which is related to the prevalence) of the disease prior to further laboratory or radiologic testing, we can more effectively interpret the results.

Information about the pretest likelihood, or prevalence, of pheochromocytoma in different clinical settings is somewhat limited, but some general estimates are available (Table 4). Many epidemiologic studies have indicated that in unselected hypertensive patients, pheochromocytomas occur in less than 0.1%. In a referral population to a tertiary care center, the prevalence of pheochromocytoma is higher, probably closer to 0.3%. Among symptomatic patients, a more diverse group, the likelihood is still higher, approaching 5 to 6%. A patient with the classic triad associated with severe labile hypertension of new onset would have a very different likelihood of having a pheochromocytoma than a patient with long-standing hypertension who complains of a headache and occasional palpitations. Although these are both "symptomatic" hypertensives, the former probably has a greater than 50% likelihood, and the latter a less than 1% likelihood of having the tumor. Indeed, in series of patients referred to specialists in which the diagnosis of pheochromocytoma was held to be likely, only about 30 to 50% of patients actually had the disease. Finally, patients with symptoms, hypertension, and a familial syndrome such as those listed earlier have a very high likelihood of having a pheochromocytoma, perhaps 90 to 95%.

The exact pretest likelihood that can be assigned in these various situations has not been well defined using only clinical parameters. For physicians interested in using pretest likelihoods to assess the results of subsequent biochemical testing, we suggest assigning a pretest likelihood in the range of 0.1% to asymptomatic hypertensives, 5% to those modestly symptomatic (symptoms of triad and hypertension but neither severe nor of recent onset), 50% to patients with classic symptoms with typical labile, severe hypertension, and 90% to patients in high-risk groups with symptoms or hypertension. These figures are useful starting points, but until more research on the predictive value of symptoms and signs is done, more exact numbers may not be available.

Biochemical Testing

Before we discuss how to test for pheochromocytoma, it is worth considering whom to test. The strategy of testing all new hypertensives has been shown not to be cost-effective. Since as many as 5% of urine tests in essential hypertensives will be abnormal and only 0.1% of patients will actually have a pheochromocytoma, there would be 50 false-positives for every true-positive collection. Symptomatic hypertensives, however, should have screening testing performed. Patients from the risk groups described, and those who have pressor responses to surgery, parturition, or anesthesia, should also undergo testing.

A wide range of tests has become available in the bio-

TABLE 4. Estimated Pretest Likelihoods from History

Setting	Likelihood of Pheochromocytoma (%)
Asymptomatic hypertensive	0.01–0.1
Symptomatic hypertensive	5–6
Paroxysmal hypertension and classic symptoms (high clinical suspicion)	30–50
New symptoms/hypertension in a patient from a high-risk group	80–90

TABLE 5. Biochemical Testing for Pheochromocytoma

Test	Usual Range of Normal
Plasma catecholamines (total)	<1000 ng/dL
Urinary free catecholamines	<100 μg/24 h
Urinary free norepinephrine	<80 μg/24 h
Urinary free epinephrine	<20 μg/24 h
Vanillylmandelic acid	<6–7 mg/24 h
Metanephrine	<1.1 mg/24 h
Urinary dopamine	<440 μg/24 h

chemical diagnosis of pheochromocytoma, including both blood and urinary assays (Table 5). The plasma assays include those for catecholamines, norepinephrine, and epinephrine. New assays provide accurate results; however, sampling must be done extremely carefully, since needle stick or, indeed, any stress surrounding blood drawing, can increase catecholamine release. Moreover, patients who are hospitalized and symptomatic, such as those with congestive heart failure or myocardial infarction, will have appropriate increases in catecholamines. Thus, plasma testing, although helpful, can result in an unacceptably high number of false-positive tests. In general, plasma catecholamine levels of over 1000 pg/mL are suggestive, whereas levels greater than 1500 to 2000 pg/mL are considered diagnostic. Again, this assumes a nonstressed state with appropriate precautions for sampling. The sensitivity of plasma catecholamines has been variously reported in the literature at anywhere from 50 to 60% to nearly 100%, depending on the cut point and the care with which samples are taken. In most comparisons with 24-hour urine testing, basal plasma catecholamines are less sensitive.

Urine studies include 24-hour collections for free catecholamines (UFC) and for catecholamine metabolites, vanillylmandelic acid (VMA), and metanephrines (MN). MN are the product of partial catecholamine metabolism via catecholamine-o-methyl transferase, whereas VMA is the result of monoamine oxidase and catecholamine-o-methyl transferase, hence a final metabolic product. Only a small portion of catecholamines are secreted unconjugated and unmetabolized, and free catecholamines provide a useful index of total catecholamine production. Over the years, a battle has raged as to which substance to assay for the diagnosis of pheochromocytoma. In the final analysis, all three are useful diagnostically, depending on the institutional methods and experience. Sensitivity of any one of these tests has been reported to vary between 80 and 100%, highest with MN and UFC and lower with VMA. Nonetheless, in institutions with a highly specific VMA assay, where the upper limit of normal is placed at the lower level, sensitivities of close to 100% have been reported.

In the use of urinary testing, a number of caveats must be regarded. Many different assay methods have been applied over the years, from crude spectrophotometric assays to precise high-pressure liquid chromatography (HPLC)–based procedures. Interfering substances, both endogenous and exogenous, such as drugs or foodstuffs, have caused falsely elevated values (Table 6). As assay techniques have been refined, fewer interferences occur. It is important to remember, however, that such interferences can occur as a laboratory artifact, or from effects of the drug in vivo. Monoamine oxidase (MAO) inhibitors, for example, would lower VMA while increasing MN. Tricyclic antidepressants or other chemicals that lead to release of catecholamines

TABLE 6. **Common Drug Interferences with Laboratory Testing for Pheochromocytoma**

VMA	MN	UFC
Decreased Levels		
Aspirin	Radiographic dyes	Methyldopa (Aldomet)
Methyldopa (Aldomet)	Propranolol (Inderal)	Chlorpromazine (Thorazine)
MAO inhibitors		Radiographic dyes
Phenothiazines		Reserpine
Radiographic dyes		
Imipramine (Tofranil)		
Increased Levels		
Caffeine, tea, bananas	Acetaminophen	Methyldopa (Aldomet)
Methocarbamol (Robaxin)	Chlorpromazine	Aspirin
Tetracyclines	Labetalol (Normodyne, Trandate)	Acetaminophen
Levodopa/carbidopa (Sinemet)	Tetracyclines	Chloropromazine
Nitroglycerin	Triamterene (Dyrenium)	Erythromycin
		Labetalol
		Quinidine
		Tetracyclines
		Theophylline
		Methenamine (Mandelamine)

Abbreviations: VMA = vanillylmandelic acid; MN = metanephrines; UFC = urine studies for free catecholamines; MAO = monoamine oxidase.

may lead to a transient rise in UFC. Such effects of therapy must be considered when testing patients for pheochromocytoma. From a practical standpoint, knowledge of the specific techniques applied by the laboratory performing the catecholamine or metabolite assay is essential in the proper preparation of the patient, as well as in the interpretation of the results.

In the interpretation of catecholamine or metabolite plasma or urinary concentrations, the higher the value, the more likely a pheochromocytoma is present. Although as many as 5% (or more, in some series) of essential hypertensives may have elevated values, such values are rarely much above 20 to 50% of the upper limit of normal. When the values are greater than twice the upper limit of normal, the likelihood of a pheochromocytoma dramatically increases. Exceptions to this rule include in vivo or in vitro drug interferences or testing performed in stressed patients. The range of normal that the laboratory reports is established in unstressed outpatients. In practical terms, when the level is dramatically increased in a high-quality assay—for example, VMA greater than 10 to 11 mg per 24 hours, UFC greater than 200 μg per 24 hours—then a pheochromocytoma is quite likely. This does not resolve all diagnostic difficulties, however, since 10 to 20% of patients with a pheochromocytoma will have levels between one and two times the upper limit of normal. The challenge comes in distinguishing symptomatic essential hypertensives from pheochromocytoma patients with modestly elevated urinary testing.

The sensitivity of urine testing can be increased by combining tests. Performing both UFC and a metabolite assay increases sensitivity to greater than 95%. Repeated collections will further increase sensitivity and specificity. Specificity is enhanced, since repeat testing in patients with hypertension who have initially elevated values will often be normal, the so-called regression to the mean. Pheochromocytoma patients can have significant day-to-day variability in urine testing but tend to have persistently elevated values.

For patients who have sustained hypertension or frequent paroxysms, urinary testing tends to have a higher sensitivity, whereas sensitivity is slightly lower in patients with less frequent paroxysms or nonsustained hypertension. Nonetheless, even patients who have less frequent paroxysms usually have elevated urinary catecholamine and metabolite levels, an indication that the correlation between symptoms and production of catecholamines is not tight.

Measurement of specific catecholamines (norepinephrine, epinephrine, dopamine) may also be diagnostically useful. Pheochromocytomas within the adrenal gland, or in the organ of Zuckerkandl at the bifurcation of the aorta, may produce epinephrine as well as norepinephrine, whereas extra-adrenal pheochromocytomas generally produce only norepinephrine. Some pheochromocytoma patients may have normal total UFC but an elevated epinephrine level, hence the diagnosis of adrenal pheochromocytoma is suggested by such an abnormal fractionation.

The proper interpretation of elevated urinary testing can best be illustrated by considering a patient with symptomatic hypertension who has a urinary catecholamine value or metabolite levels that are modestly increased (e.g., 120% of the upper limit of normal). As previously suggested, this patient's pretest likelihood was about 5%. If the sensitivity of the UFC is 90% and the specificity is about 95%, then the likelihood of a pheochromocytoma, given a positive urinary test, is close to 50%. Given a negative test, the likelihood of pheochromocytoma would be less than 1%, which would allow us to stop further testing—unless we considered the pretest likelihood higher. If on the other hand, the UFC is 450 μg per 24 hours, then the diagnosis is extremely likely, approaching certainty. If the patient had been an unselected hypertensive without symptoms whose likelihood of a pheochromocytoma was only 0.1% before testing, the likelihood of a pheochromocytoma with a positive urinary test would have increased to about 2%. Again, if the urinary test was dramatically increased, the likelihood would be much higher, in proportion to the degree of elevation.

Now, consider a patient with typical paroxysmal symptoms associated with new, labile hypertension. We suggested that the pretest likelihood was close to 50%. In this case, an elevated UFC would increase the likelihood to 95%. Moreover, a normal UFC would make the likelihood of a pheochromocytoma about 10%, certainly not low enough to abandon the search for the tumor.

The conclusion to this type of analysis is that the value of testing depends on both the test characteristics (sensitivity and specificity) and the likelihood of the disease before the test is done. The clinical assessment of likelihood is based on (1) the type and severity of symptoms, (2) the presence or absence of other diseases that might explain the symptoms, (3) the type and severity of the hypertension, and (4) the presence or absence of familial risk of pheochromocytoma. As always when using diagnostic testing, a negative test virtually rules out a disease if the pretest likelihood is low, whereas a positive test is suggestive but does not make the definitive diagnosis. When the pretest likelihood is high, a positive test helps rule in a disease, but a negative test does not exclude it.

Stimulation testing, using a variety of agents, was a classic method for diagnosis of a pheochromocytoma. The use of intravenous glucagon is moderately sensitive and specific when using careful criteria; however, most physicians with limited experience avoid this type of testing because significant hypertensive responses can occur. Suppression testing using clonidine has also been investigated and tends to be safer and easier to do. The concept is that the release of catecholamines is autonomous from central sympathetic regulation (even though blood pressure, as reviewed earlier, is not). Hence clonidine, which normally reduces catecholamine release, would fail to do so in a patient with a pheochromocytoma. This test has not been in general use, but experience at a number of institutions suggests that it can be valuable, although both false-positive and false-negative tests have been widely reported.

Radiologic Testing

The emergence of new and accurate imaging studies has made older and more dangerous techniques such as angiography or venous sampling obsolete in the diagnostic approach to patients suspected of harboring a pheochromocytoma (Table 7). An important observation is that clinically symptomatic pheochromocytomas are usually not small, indeed rarely less than 1 to 2 cm. In most series, mean pheochromocytoma size ranges between 3 and 5 cm. Since both computed tomography (CT) and magnetic resonance imaging (MRI) can resolve down to 1 cm, the accuracy of imaging studies is not surprising. Both abdominal CT scan and MRI have a high sensitivity for detecting these tumors. Recall that 98 to 99% of pheochromocytomas are abdominal, whereas about 90% are intra-adrenal. Overall, CT (or MRI) is positive in about 95 to 99% of

TABLE 7. **Imaging Studies for Pheochromocytoma**

Useful
Abdominal CT scan
Abdominal MRI scan
[131]I methyl-iodo-benzylguanidine scan
Sometimes Helpful
Abdominal ultrasound
No Longer Indicated
Abdominal angiography*
IVC venous sampling*

Abbreviations: CT = computed tomography; MRI = magnetic resonance imaging; IVC = inferior vena cava.
*Only indicated in a patient with diagnostic biochemical testing who has negative imaging studies.

patients with a pheochromocytoma, and the sensitivity is close to 100% for intra-adrenal tumors. Extra-adrenal tumors may be detected slightly more often by MRI than by CT scans.

Adrenal adenomas are common in the population, especially in an aging population. CT scanning shows an adrenal nodule in 1 to 2% of normal individuals; in autopsy series, up to 5% will have nodules. Thus, the interpretation of the incidental finding of a nodule must depend on the likelihood that a pheochromocytoma was present before the test was done. If performed in an asymptomatic hypertensive with mildly elevated urinary testing, a negative scan would make pheochromocytoma very unlikely (less than 1%), and a positive scan would increase the likelihood of a pheochromocytoma to about 45%, certainly not confirming the diagnosis. Hence, it is recommended to perform radiologic testing only if clinical and biochemical testing makes the diagnosis likely.

Since false-positive imaging studies are a concern, MRI can provide additional information. A high signal on T_2-weighted images occurs with pheochromocytomas, as well as adrenal metastases and adrenal carcinomas. This finding is not seen with adenomas, the most common cause of adrenal masses on CT imaging. In addition, a protocol designed to look for fat content may prove valuable, as this is present in adenomas but not pheochromocytomas.

Over the past decade, increasing information has become available on the utility of ^{131}I methyl-iodo-benzylguanidine (MIBG) scanning. This radiolabeled guanidine congener is taken up by abnormal sympathetic tissue, including pheochromocytomas and neuroblastomas. Between 80 and 90% of pheochromocytomas take up MIBG and have a positive scan. Equally as important, true false-positive scans are very unusual, making a positive result highly suggestive of a pheochromocytoma. The use of this testing imaging modality in patients with MEN IIA syndrome has shown that this test may become positive early, even before clearly elevated biochemical testing or structural imaging.

In summary, the diagnostic approach starts with a clinical assessment of the likelihood of pheochromocytoma. Biochemical testing using 24-hour urine collections is the next step, followed by radiologic imaging. Patients who are thought to have a high likelihood of a tumor should have repeated testing, even if the initial testing is unrevealing. On the other hand, patients with a low clinical likelihood and negative initial testing probably need little more done. In patients with lower clinical likelihood and positive testing, the degree of elevation of urinary testing is useful. Borderline values increase the likelihood of a pheochromocytoma only marginally, whereas markedly elevated values (more than two times the upper limit of normal) make the diagnosis secure. Radiologic testing can prove valuable both diagnostically and in terms of localization. In a patient in whom there is a lower clinical suspicion and borderline elevated testing, a negative scan makes a pheochromocytoma highly unlikely. The patient should be followed and retested if the clinical pattern changes or symptoms intensify.

TREATMENT

Surgery is the primary therapy for pheochromocytoma, hence, medical management is directed toward stabilizing and preparing the patient for the operating room. In the initial decades of surgical experience with pheochromocytoma, perioperative mortality was high, ranging from 25 to 50%. More recent series have consistently reported rates under 3%. Such dramatic improvements cannot be ascribed to a single new intervention but relate to earlier diagnosis with accurate localization, better preoperative preparation with the introduction of alpha-blocking drugs, improved anesthetic and surgical techniques, invasive hemodynamic monitoring, and improved postoperative care. Since this is an uncommon tumor, centers with experienced teams of surgeons and anesthesiologists will consistently achieve the best outcomes.

Preoperative Preparation

Patients with pheochromocytoma have been shown to have mild-to-modest volume depletion, probably on the basis of high alpha agonist pressor tone and a pressure diuresis. Inadequately or unprepared patients can have dramatic swings in intraoperative blood pressure and arrhythmias. Adequate preoperative preparation provides adrenergic blockade and ensures restoration of euvolemia.

The introduction of alpha-blocking agents appears to have contributed importantly to reductions in perioperative mortality and morbidity. Phenoxybenzamine (Dibenzyline), an orally active alpha$_1$-selective agent, has been shown to reduce perioperative hypotension and, in some studies, hypertension and arrhythmias as well. The increased plasma volume induced by these agents probably contributes to reductions in frequency of intraoperative and postoperative hypotension. Phenoxybenzamine is started at 10 mg twice daily (Table 8) and gradually increased until blood pressure is consistently controlled, with systolic pressures of less than 160 mm Hg and diastolic pressures of less than 90 mm Hg but with orthostatic blood pressure reductions to not less than 80 to 90 mm Hg systolic. Usual doses range from 20 to 60 mg per day, but occasional patients have required doses as high as 200 mg per day. Resistance to phenoxybenzamine has been reported, hence additional antihypertensive agents may occasionally be needed. More highly selective alpha$_1$ blockers such as prazosin (Minipress) have also been successfully used for preoperative preparation with very similar

success rates. Concern has been expressed that failure rates are higher with prazosin, but in our experience outcomes are as good. A first-dose hypotensive effect can occur, hence patients should be supine and carefully observed as this medication is initiated. It has been argued that complete alpha blockade can interfere with the surgeon's search for the tumor, lowering the diagnostic utility of intraoperative rises in blood pressure with palpation of possible tumor sites. However, complete blockade is rarely achieved with usual alpha-blocking doses, hence this concern is largely unfounded. Moreover, preoperative imaging successfully identifies tumor location in the great majority of cases.

Once adequate alpha blockade has been achieved, beta blockers can be safely added, but these should be used only in patients with tachyarrhythmias. The use of beta blockers before alpha blockers must be avoided to prevent paradoxical hypertensive responses from unopposed alpha-agonist activity in the face of diminished beta-vasodilating tone. Selective beta blockers such as metaprolol (Lopressor) are also good choices in these settings. Labetalol (Trandate, Normodyne) has been successfully used in patients with pheochromocytoma; however, it should be noted that this drug has more beta- than alpha-blocking activity, hence it may not provide adequate alpha blockade. Newer selective alpha blockers, such as doxazosin (Cardura) or terazosin (Hytrin), have seen little use in patients with pheochromocytoma; although they are probably effective, limited experience dictates a secondary place for such agents.

Another option that has been successful is the use of metyrosine (Demser). This agent blocks the synthesis of catecholamines and has seen wide use in patients with malignant or unresectable pheochromocytomas. A number of investigators have advocated the combined use of metyrosine and alpha blockade as preoperative preparation. Metyrosine has serious side effects, such as nausea, nightmares, and parkinsonism, and surgical outcomes do not appear to be better with than without routine use of this agent.

Adequate volume repletion preoperatively is an essential component of preoperative preparation. Alpha-blocker therapy and adequate volume replacement result in the repair of volume deficits and greatly improve surgical outcomes. Invasive monitoring may be of use to ensure that plasma volume is normal. Some have argued that all patients should have a Swan-Ganz catheter placed the day before surgery, but others feel that the determination can be made clinically or in the operating room. Certainly patients with underlying cardiac disease should have invasive monitoring before the induction of anesthesia.

The duration of preoperative preparation has not been clearly defined. Traditionally, it had been suggested that patients be treated with pharmacologic agents for at least 7 to 14 days. More recent series looking at outcomes in patients treated for as few as

TABLE 8. **Medical Therapy for Pheochromocytoma**

Medication	Dose Range
Intravenous Therapy	
Nitroprusside (Nipride)	0.5–10 μg/kg/min
Phentolamine (Regitine)	5–10 mg bolus, 0.5–1 mg/min infusion
Oral Therapy	
Labetalol (Transdate, Normodyne)	400–1600 mg/day (bid)
Metyrosine (Demser)	500 mg–4 gm/day
Nifedipine (Procardia)	30–90 mg/day
Phenoxybenzamine (Dibenzyline)	20–120 mg/day (bid)
Prazosin (Minipress)	2–20 mg/day (bid)
Propranolol (Inderal)	40–480 mg/day

4 days before surgery have shown no differences in outcome.

Hypertension in patients with pheochromocytoma can be treated with other antihypertensive agents as well as alpha blockers. Patients with pheochromocytoma have an activated renin-angiotensin axis, probably on the basis of hypovolemia and the direct effects of catecholamines on renin release. Several reports have suggested that angiotensin-converting enzyme (ACE) inhibitors successfully lower blood pressure in pheochromocytoma patients. Similarly, the role of calcium in mediating catecholamine-induced increased vascular tone suggests a potential role for calcium channel blockers. Several reports have, indeed, shown blood pressure–lowering effects. Blood pressure control perioperatively has not been adequate with these agents, hence their use is limited to ancillary rather than primary therapy. Diuretics should be avoided unless objective evidence of volume overload is present.

Intraoperative Management

Careful intraoperative blood pressure control has greatly added to the care of pheochromocytoma patients. Although rapid swings in blood pressure will occur intraoperatively in these patients, if it is appropriately controlled outcomes are good. Hypertension is treated with either phentolamine (Regitine) or nitroprusside (Nipride), whereas hypotension is treated with volume expansion and, usually less often, vasopressors.

In choice of anesthesia, it has been reported that halothane increases arrhythmogenesis in patients with catecholamine cardiomyopathy, hence enflurane or isoflurane has been suggested as a better choice. An anterior operative approach has been considered the standard; however, with improved preoperative localization, a posterior approach has been used by some surgeons. Laparoscopic adrenalectomy has, as yet, had limited application, but this may become an important alternate surgical approach to remove a pheochromocytoma.

Follow-Up After Surgery

Although successful removal of a pheochromocytoma often leads to normalization of blood pressure, several investigators have noted that some patients remain hypertensive, often requiring postoperative antihypertensive therapy. Persistent elevation of blood pressure raises the concern that surgical therapy was incomplete; however, if the preoperative symptoms are gone, urinary or plasma sampling shows normalization, and imaging shows no residual tumor, then residual tumor is most unlikely.

Once a patient has successfully gone through surgical therapy for a pheochromocytoma, regular follow-up is essential. In general, annual examination with careful monitoring of blood pressure and examination of yearly 24-hour urine collections for catecholamines and metabolites is appropriate. If symp-

TABLE 9. **Management Strategy: Overview**

Step 1. Suspect
  Symptomatic hypertensive or severe and labile hypertension
  Risk group
  Severe pressor response to childbirth, anesthesia, surgery
  Adrenal mass

Step 2. Diagnose
  24-hour urinary studies: combined and repeated testing
  Selective use of radiologic studies: CT, MRI, MIBG*

Step 3. Localize
  Abdominal CT scanning, MRI scanning

Step 4. Prepare for Surgery
  Volume repletion
  Alpha-blockade

Step 5. Remove

Step 6. Maintain Long-Term Surveillance for Recurrence

Abbreviations: CT = computed tomography; MRI = magnetic resonance imaging; MIBG = ^{131}I methyl-iodo-benzylguanidine scanning.

toms recur, then earlier evaluation is, of course, warranted. Patients with underlying syndromes associated with pheochromocytoma are at particularly high risk for recurrence. It is important to note that recurrences can occur as early as months after successful surgery to as long as 20 years later.

Pheochromocytoma are unusual, albeit important, tumors. We would suggest that a multistep diagnostic and management strategy be used (Table 9) that begins with suspecting the process and proceeds through diagnosis, localization, and the steps for therapeutic management.

THYROIDITIS*

method of
RICHARD T. KLOOS, M.D., and
JAMES R. BAKER, Jr., M.D.
The University of Michigan Medical Center
Ann Arbor, Michigan

Thyroiditis encompasses diverse inflammatory thyroid conditions that cause a spectrum of illnesses ranging from acute symptomatic infection to insidious chronic autoimmune disease. The clinical presentation of thyroiditis may include pain, goiter, thyroid nodule(s), and hyper- or hypothyroidism. Based on an understanding of the natural history of the thyroiditis syndromes, a cost-effective diagnostic evaluation, that excludes severe illnesses, and treatment plans that may encompass infection control, surgery, symptom management, patient education, and fol-

*Partial support for this manuscript was provided by NIH Grants.

low-up monitoring of thyroid function may be formulated. A classification and framework for evaluation shown in Table 1 includes the well-accepted chronologic headings of acute, subacute, and chronic thyroiditis. Within these headings, however, individual types of thyroiditis may show great variability of symptoms, timing, imaging characteristics, clinical courses, and histology. Further, multiple reports of overlap and cross-over syndromes exist. Given the similarity of therapy for most thyroiditis syndromes, many experienced clinicians proceed with a minimum of diagnostic tests, utilizing only those whose result would alter patient management.

ACUTE THYROIDITIS

Acute thyroiditis (also known as "suppurative" or "pyogenic thyroiditis") is an uncommon, potentially fatal infectious disorder, usually of bacterial origin. About two-thirds of cases involve (in order of decreasing frequency) staphylococci, streptococci, Enterobacteriaceae, *Klebsiella pneumoniae, Escherichia coli,* anaerobes, *Pseudomonas,* and rarely *Nocardia asteroides.* It may also follow a subacute or chronic course when caused by actinomyces, fungi (about 5%), mycobacteria (about 9%), *Pneumocystis carinii* (usually in patients with acquired immune deficiency syndrome [AIDS], receiving inhaled pentamidine prophylaxis), syphilis (about 3%), or parasites (about 15%). The thyroid may be infected hematogenously, by lymphatic extension from a contiguous neck infection, or by penetrating trauma (including fine-needle aspiration [FNA]). A pre-existing thyroid disorder (e.g., nodular goiter) is found in more than 50% of cases. Rarely, no organism can be identified. Immunocompromised patients (including alcoholics and poorly controlled diabetics), children, elderly people, women between the second and the fourth decades of life, and those with anatomic abnormalities (e.g., thyroglossal duct or piriform sinus fistula) are at increased risk.

Patients present with abrupt onset of severe unilateral anterior neck pain (which may radiate to the ear, mandible, or pharyngeal region), fever, diaphoresis, dysphagia, dysphonia, and malaise. Examination typically reveals warm, exquisitely tender, erythematous, localized or diffuse thyroid swelling that may be fluctuant.

Differential diagnosis of acute thyroiditis includes other infections of the anterior neck; hemorrhage into a cyst, thyroid nodule, or tumor necrosis; and painful subacute thyroiditis. Expeditious diagnosis may be established by FNA with cultures and microscopy for organisms and cytology. Special stains and cultures should be performed if an atypical infectious agent is suspected. Blood cultures should be obtained. Other investigations (a left shift on complete blood count [CBC] with differential, normal thyroid-stimulating hormone [TSH], and elevated erythrocyte sedimentation rate [ESR]) may confirm the diagnosis but should not delay the initiation of antibiotic therapy. Thyroid antibodies are usually negative and

their measurement is not indicated. Scintigraphy is usually not warranted but may demonstrate absence of radiotracer accumulation (e.g., a "cold" defect) in the infected area. Computed tomography, magnetic resonance imaging, and ultrasonography may show nonhomogeneous glandular enlargement and abscess formation.

Treatment involves empiric broad-spectrum parenteral antibiotic therapy to cover gram-positive and gram-negative organisms, *Pseudomonas,* and anaerobic bacteria. Therapy is modified based on clinical response and culture results. If a well-formed abscess exists, open surgical drainage or lobectomy is essential. Appropriate management almost always results in complete recovery and preservation of normal thyroid function; however, local pain and tenderness may persist for several weeks. Recurrence suggests an undetected anatomic abnormality.

SUBACUTE THYROIDITIS SYNDROMES

Granulomatous Thyroiditis

Self-limited granulomatous thyroiditis (also known as "giant cell" or "de Quervain's" thyroiditis) is an inflammatory response to a viral infection of the thyroid, which typically presents several days to weeks following an upper respiratory illness (URI). A variety of viruses have been implicated (including adenovirus, influenza, Coxsackie, Epstein-Barr, echovirus, mumps, measles, and enteroviruses), which may explain the seasonal and geographic aggregation of some cases. A minority (less than 20%) of patients have mild, transient evidence of thyroid autoimmunity, including significant antithyroid antibody titers, which is thought to represent an epiphenomenon to local thyroid inflammation. There is a genetic predisposition, including association with HLA B-35 antigen in all ethnic groups. Women are at increased risk relative to men (4.5 : 1), and most present in the second through the fifth decades of life. Subacute thyroiditis is uncommon in elderly people and children, and a pre-existing goiter or other thyroid abnormality is unusual.

Granulomatous thyroiditis typically demonstrates four phases (Figure 1). The initial phase is characterized by a variable prodrome of sore throat or sore neck, low-grade fever (40.0°C or less), malaise, myalgias, arthralgias, fatigue, anorexia, and dysphagia. The hallmark is pain in the thyroid region that may occur gradually or suddenly and is aggravated by turning the head, coughing, or swallowing. Sometimes the pain is unilateral and radiates to the mandible, ear, occiput, or upper chest. Occasionally, referred pain is the major presenting complaint. Absence of pain does not exclude the diagnosis, as some patients present with a diffuse or multinodular goiter or a solitary nodule. Hoarseness and dysphagia may occur. Occasionally, symptoms may have been ongoing for several months. Symptomatic hyperthyroidism lasting 4 to 10 weeks occurs in 50% of cases (representing 5% of all thyrotoxicoses) as a

TABLE 1. **Classification Scheme and Considerations for Thyroiditis**

Type	Prevalence	Pain	Fever	ESR (mm/hr)	Leukocytes	Antithyroid Antibodies	Thyroglobulin	RAIU	Hyperthyroid Phase	Hypothyroid Phase	Therapy	Future Risk of Hypothyroidism
Acute thyroiditis	Uncommon	Yes	Yes	Increased	Increased with left shift	Usually none	Usually normal	Normal	Usually not	Usually not	Antibiotics + surgical	No
Subacute thyroiditides												
Granulomatous	Common	Yes	Yes	Usually >100	Increased without left shift	Mild + transient (10–20%)	Elevated	4 phases; see Fig. 1	50%	20%–30%	Symptomatic	<5%
Painless	Common	Usually none, may be minimal	No	Usually <50	Normal to mild increase	Low titers (25–60%)	Elevated	4 phases; see Fig. 1	Yes	40%	Symptomatic	Up to 50%
Postpartum	Common	Usually none, may be minimal	No	Usually <50	Normal to mild increase	Present in about 85%	Elevated	4 phases; see Fig. 1	Yes	Yes	Symptomatic	20–38%
Drug-induced ¹³¹I acutely	Dependent on dose delivered	Dependent on dose delivered	Dependent on dose delivered	Dependent on dose delivered	Dependent on dose delivered	May develop	Dependent on dose delivered	Low	Possible	Usually persistent	Symptomatic	Yes, dependent on dose delivered
Others	Uncommon	No	No	Normal	Normal	Possible	Usually normal	Low	Possible	Possible	Variable	Uncharacterized
Chronic thyroiditides												
Hashimoto's	Common	Usually none	No	Normal	Normal	Present in 70–80%	Normal	Decreased	Usually not	Usually persistent	Symptomatic	30–40%
Reidel's	Uncommon	No	No	Normal	Normal	Present in >50%	Normal	Normal, decreased if hypothyroid	No	No	Surgical	30–40%

Abbreviations: ESR = erythrocyte sedimentation rate; RAIU = radioactive iodine uptake.

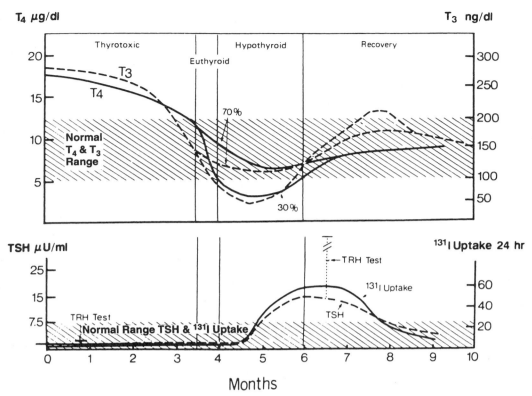

Figure 1. The four phases of subacute thyroiditis. *Abbreviations*: T_4 = thyroxine; T_3 = triiodothyronine; TSH = thyroid-stimulating hormone; TRH = thyrotropin-releasing hormone; ^{131}I = iodine 131. (From Woolf PD: Transient painless thyroiditis with hyperthyroidism: A variant of lymphocytic thyroiditis? Endocr Rev 1(4):412–420, 1980, © The Endocrine Society.)

result of leakage of preformed thyroid hormones from disrupted follicles.

The thyroid is typically mildly to moderately enlarged and may be asymmetrical. The gland is firm or hard, often nodular, and usually exquisitely tender, more so in one lobe. Erythema and warmth of overlying skin and adherence to adjacent structures may be present, but cervical lymphadenopathy is uncommon. In severe cases, obstructive airway or esophageal symptoms may be present. Over the course of several weeks, pain may migrate to previously less affected areas.

The second phase of the illness typically consists of several weeks of euthyroidism with minimal pain and tenderness. This may be followed by a third phase of transient hypothyroidism in 20 to 30% of patients (less than 1% of all hypothyroidism), which may last a few weeks to several months. The final phase consists of an asymptomatic recovery period with normalization of thyroid function, gland size, uptake, and glandular histology. Permanent hypothyroidism occurs in less than 5%. The entire illness usually lasts 2 to 6 months and almost never persists beyond 1 year. Rarely, the disease may become intermittently recurrent and eventually end in permanent hypothyroidism.

The most helpful diagnostic test is an ESR, which is often more than 100 mm per hour in the active phase. A normal ESR during this period argues strongly against the diagnosis. The CBC may reveal a normal leukocyte count or modest leukocytosis (less than 18,000 per μL) without a left shift, and approximately half of patients demonstrate mild anemia, lymphopenia, and thrombocytosis. Early transient liver dysfunction may occur. Serum thyroglobulin values can be useful in equivocal cases; a normal value virtually excludes the diagnosis. Thyroglobulin levels may remain elevated for up to 1 year despite clinical resolution. During the thyrotoxic phase, the radioactive iodine uptake (RAIU) is suppressed (often less than 1 to 5%) as a result of inflammation and destruction of follicular cells and loss of ability to trap iodine. TSH levels may also be suppressed by increased thyroid hormone levels. T_4 to T_3 ratios may be increased (to more than 0.05) owing to release of intrathyroidal T_4 stores. During the hypothyroid phase, the RAIU may become elevated before returning to normal in the fourth phase. Autoantibodies may occur during the hypothyroid phase and return to baseline within 6 months of recovery.

The differential diagnosis of granulomatous thyroiditis includes other inflammatory processes (e.g., pharyngitis and laryngitis), acute hemorrhage into a pre-existing thyroid nodule or cyst, acute onset of Hashimoto's thyroiditis, painless thyroiditis, acute thyroiditis, thyroid malignancy (especially anaplastic thyroid carcinoma or lymphoma), and osseous conditions (spondylosis, spondylarthrosis, cervical ribs, and so on). Hemorrhage and thyroid malignancy typically leave the remainder of the gland unaffected, and thyroid function tests are more likely to be normal, RAIU is not suppressed, and ESR and thyroglobulin levels are not markedly elevated. Fine-needle aspiration may be utilized if other disorders cannot be excluded or the course is atypical. Hyperthyroid painless thyroiditis may be difficult to distinguish from painless granulomatous thyroiditis; however, a normal ESR with elevated antithyroid antibodies suggests the former. Acute suppurative thyroiditis is suggested by a septic focus outside, adjacent to, or within the thyroid; much greater leukocytosis and febrile responses; palpable fluctuance or abscess; and normal RAIU. Hashimoto's disease is usually differentiated by diffuse rather than localized involvement. Some patients with hysteria complain of a ball-like or compressive sensation in the throat (globus hystericus) but do not have localized tenderness nor is the gland enlarged.

There is no established role for thyroid hormone suppression in granulomatous thyroiditis. Rarely, painful recurrences refractory to medical therapy may require subtotal thyroidectomy or radioactive iodine ablation.

Painless Thyroiditis

Painless thyroiditis (also known as "silent," "atypical," or "occult subacute thyroiditis") usually refers to a limited course of lymphocytic thyroiditis with transient hyperthyroidism that may represent early or unusual chronic lymphocytic thyroiditis. It causes 10% of thyrotoxicosis and less than 2% of hypothyroidism. It is characterized by a sudden onset of painless thyroid inflammation and follicle damage with release of thyroid hormone stores and thyroglobulin similar to that of granulomatous thyroiditis. A history of a preceding illness (e.g., URI) is unusual. The histology is similar to that of chronic lymphocytic thyroiditis but less extensive. Painless thyroiditis is also differentiated from chronic lymphocytic thyroiditis by having no definite HLA association. The course of thyroid function tests and RAIU is similar to that of granulomatous and postpartum thyroiditis (see Figure 1). Hypothyroidism lasting 4 to 16 weeks occurs in 40% of patients and resolves completely in 95%. Patients are usually white or Asian, are between 20 and 60 years old, are women (by 2 : 1), and have family histories of autoimmune thyroid disease. Excess iodine intake has been proposed as an initiating factor.

Examination may demonstrate hyperthyroidism. Thyroid pain is rare and mild when present. The gland is firm and may be slightly irregular, with symmetrical enlargement twice normal size occurring in 50 to 60% of patients. Patients are afebrile.

The differential diagnosis includes other causes of hyperthyroidism with suppressed RAIU, including other forms of subacute thyroiditis, functioning metastatic thyroid carcinoma, excess exogenous thyroid hormone usage (thyrotoxicosis factitia), iodine-induced thyrotoxicosis (usually with an underlying abnormal thyroid), and struma ovarii or hyperthyroidism with typically elevated RAIU in patients who have received an acute iodine load. Accidental thyroid hormone ingestion through thyroid-contaminated meat or medication error should be excluded. Surreptitious or accidental intake of excess thyroid hormone is suggested by absence of a goiter, long duration of symptoms, abnormal psychological behavior, absent thyroid antibodies, and low serum thyroglobulin level.

In painless thyroiditis, the ESR tends to be normal or slightly elevated (less than 50 mm per hour). Antithyroid antibodies are present in two-thirds of patients with peak titers during the hypothyroid phase, which resolve in up to 50% of patients. Serum thyroglobulin levels may reach 400 ng per mL, then gradually fall, remaining slightly elevated for up to 24 months, indicating persistent inflammation. Most patients recover completely. However, some studies find long-term abnormalities such as antithyroid antibodies, goiter, or permanent hypothyroidism in about half the patients examined 10 years after diagnosis. Histology of the thyroid up to 36 months after recovery has demonstrated mild lymphocytic thyroiditis in a few patients. Silent thyroiditis may recur in about 10% of patients, for whom some advocate levothyroxine therapy to reduce intrathyroidal hormone stores. Rarely, as in granulomatous thyroiditis, refractory recurrences may require subtotal thyroidectomy or radioactive iodine ablation.

Postpartum Thyroiditis

This refers to lymphocytic thyroiditis, which characteristically occurs 2 to 4 months post partum but may occur any time within 1 year of childbirth. Both autoimmune thyroiditis and Graves' disease tend to improve during pregnancy, only to exacerbate post partum before returning to baseline. Postpartum thyroiditis occurs in 4 to 9% of women and usually recurs with each subsequent pregnancy. Clinical presentations are varied and may include a small goiter or thyroid function abnormalities or a combination. Thyroid function abnormalities and thyroglobulin levels classically follow the same course as that of granulomatous and painless thyroiditis (see Figure 1); however, some patients develop only transient hypothyroidism whereas others develop transient hyperthyroidism before returning to a euthyroid state. Patients usually demonstrate antithyroid antibodies, particularly against thyroid peroxidase. Titers vary over the course of the illness and may aid in the diagnosis. The hyperthyroid phase of postpartum thyroiditis typically demonstrates decreased RAIU, but in a minority the RAIU is elevated, probably due to thyroid-stimulating immunoglobulins as in Graves' disease. Some patients with pre-existing Graves' disease develop postpartum thyroiditis with low RAIU hyperthyroidism followed by hypothyroidism, before returning to a euthyroid or hyperthyroid state. Rarely the hypothyroidism of postpartum thyroiditis does not resolve and requires long-term replacement therapy.

The differential diagnosis of postpartum thyroiditis is similar to that of painless thyroiditis. Women with goiters, Type I diabetes mellitus, or a history of silent thyroiditis should be followed carefully post partum for evidence of thyroiditis, which includes postpartum depression. The most consistent prepartum finding is thyroid peroxidase antibodies; however, only 50% of women with antibodies at 16 weeks' gestation subsequently develop thyroiditis. Because of this, and the relative ease of therapy, screening all pregnant women for antibodies to identify the few at risk for postpartum thyroiditis may not be justified. However, pregnant women with thyroid peroxidase antibodies are at risk for premature parturition, and 16% have an elevated TSH at delivery. Most postpartum thyroiditis is transient, but it carries a 20 to 38% risk of subsequent chronic autoimmune thyroiditis and therefore needs clinical monitoring.

Drug-Induced Thyroiditis

A number of drugs may induce thyroiditis, and this syndrome has become an important diagnosis to differentiate. Iodide-containing drugs or lithium may unmask previously unrecognized autoimmune thyroiditis or hasten its development in predisposed patients, perhaps by enhanced immunogenicity of iodine-rich thyroglobulin. Amiodarone also may cause thyrotoxicosis owing to its iodine content, but a direct toxic effect with follicle disruption also has been postulated. Some patients develop a mild hypothyroid phase, with thyroid tenderness and histologic thyroiditis. Amiodarone-induced hypothyroidism occurs early in therapy, and women with pre-existing antithyroid antibodies taking this drug have a tenfold to twentyfold risk for this side effect.

Alpha-interferon causes thyrotoxicosis, a diffuse nontender goiter, decreased RAIU, hypothyroidism, and a rise in or development of antithyroid antibodies in approximately 12% of patients, which may result from the exacerbation of underlying chronic thyroiditis.

Ionizing radiation (including ^{131}I–sodium iodide therapy) initially induces injury, with hemorrhage, edema, necrosis, and epithelial sloughing. After healing, the gland typically becomes small and firm and may appear nodular. Histologic findings consist of chronic lymphocytic thyroiditis and fibrosis. The incidence of overt hypothyroidism is greatest in the first year after therapy, but cumulative dysfunction continues over years.

Post-Traumatic Thyroiditis

Blunt (e.g., seat belt injury) and surgical trauma may cause transient thyroiditis. Incidental microscopic findings suggest that even clinical palpation of the thyroid may result in mild thyroiditis.

CHRONIC THYROIDITIS
Chronic Lymphocytic (Hashimoto's or Autoimmune) Thyroiditis

Chronic lymphocytic thyroiditis is the most common cause of both thyroiditis and noniatrogenic hypothyroidism. Women account for 95% of cases; 2 to 15% of the female population is affected. The incidence increases with age in women but not in men. There are racial differences in incidence; whites are affected more frequently than blacks or Japanese. The condition results from immune dysregulation leading to production of humoral and cellular immune responses to thyroid antigens, which cause progressive destruction of the thyroid. A genetic predisposition is apparent, since the disease is often familial and is associated with several HLA haplotypes, but the exact mode of inheritance is unknown. The incomplete concordance for thyroid autoimmunity in monozygotic twins suggests that environmental factors are also important. Reports have implicated infections (e.g., *Yersinia enterocolitica*, retroviruses) and stress as potential inciting causes. The prevalence in prepubertal populations is equal in both sexes, compared with female predominance in postpubertal populations, suggesting a role for sex-related factors. Hashimoto's thyroiditis is also more common in Turner's, Noonan's, Klinefelter's, and Down's syndromes. Evidence for an autoimmune predisposition is the strong association of this disorder with other autoimmune diseases, such as Graves' disease, primary adrenal insufficiency, autoimmune oophoritis, Type I diabetes mellitus, systemic lupus erythematosus, Sjögren's syndrome, rheumatoid arthritis, scleroderma, vitiligo, celiac disease, inflammatory bowel disease, myasthenia gravis, and pernicious anemia.

Patients are usually asymptomatic and have symmetrical goiters one and a half to three times the normal size of the gland. The gland is firm and rubbery and has an irregular surface, occasionally appearing asymmetrical or nodular. Cervical lymphadenopathy, dysphagia, thyroid tenderness, and recurrent laryngeal nerve dysfunction are occasionally seen. About 20% of patients present with hypothyroidism, and 5% are hyperthyroid. The latter may be due to release of hormones from damaged follicular cells. However, an overlap syndrome between Graves' and Hashimoto's diseases may exist in some patients, resulting in glandular hyperfunction, the presence of a firm goiter, thyroid-stimulating antibodies, and ophthalmopathy. Hashimoto's disease may also spontaneously remit only to present later with typical Graves' thyrotoxicosis. Alternatively, Graves' disease may evolve into Hashimoto's thyroiditis and eventual hypothyroidism.

Antithyroid antibodies are present in high titer in 70 to 80% of patients. Those directed against the thyroid peroxidase enzyme (previously known as the "microsomal antigen") are most common. In patients without detectable serum antibodies, localized intrathyroidal antibody production has been described, suggesting a similar pathogenesis. Measurement of RAIU is indicated in atypical thyroiditis with hyperthyroidism to exclude hyperthyroid states of high RAIU. Thyroid scanning is indicated for structural questions such as a euthyroid palpable nodule to exclude a "cold" nodule, although FNA of euthyroid nodules may be more cost effective. Thyroid scanning may also be helpful in nodular hyperthyroidism to exclude a "hot" nodule. Most patients with Hashimoto's thyroiditis, however, require only the measurement of serum TSH to assess the need for thyroid hormone replacement therapy.

Invasive Fibrous Thyroiditis (Riedel's Thyroiditis, Riedel's Struma)

This is the rarest form of thyroiditis and has no known cause. It is characterized by replacement of normal thyroid parenchyma with dense fibrous tissue. As the disease progresses, the fibrosis may extend beyond the thyroid capsule into adjacent muscles and soft tissue. Rarely, a systemic fibrosis of retroperitoneum, mediastinum, lungs, periorbital and retro-orbital tissues, lacrimal glands, liver, and biliary tree occurs. Hypoparathyroidism can result from parathyroid destruction. The disease typically manifests in middle-aged women as slowly progressive anterior neck pressure, painless thyroid enlargement, dysphagia, cough, respiratory obstruction, facial puffiness due to superior vena cava obstruction, or vocal cord paralysis due to recurrent laryngeal nerve involvement.

The thyroid is usually rock hard and irregular in shape and size. It may be attached to surrounding structures. Fibrosis can involve only one lobe or diffusely infiltrate the thyroid. Lymphadenopathy is uncommon. Laboratory tests are not helpful for diagnosis; however, hypothyroidism due to loss of thyroid parenchyma occurs in 30 to 40% of cases. Antimicrosomal antibodies occur in over half of patients, and thyroid scans demonstrate decreased uptake in affected areas. Magnetic resonance imaging may demonstrate T_1- and T_2-weighted spin-echo hypointensity.

The major concern is to differentiate Riedel's thyroiditis from primary or metastatic thyroid malignancy. Open biopsy is often necessary for diagnosis and to relieve obstructive symptoms. FNA is inadequate owing to extreme thyroid fibrosis. Therapy with steroids or anti-inflammatory drugs is difficult to evaluate because of the variable course, which may spontaneously remit, progress, or stabilize.

THERAPEUTIC MEASURES FOR THYROIDITIS

Except for antibiotics in acute thyroiditis and surgical decompression for Riedel's thyroiditis, management of the remaining forms of thyroiditis is generally limited to symptomatic therapy and assessment of thyroid function.

Acute Pain Management

Treatment of mild pain includes salicylates and nonsteroidal anti-inflammatory drugs (e.g., ibuprofen [Motrin, Advil], 400 to 800 mg orally every 6 to 8 hours with food). Occasionally, oral glucocorticoids (e.g., prednisone [Meticorten, Deltasone, SK-Prednisone], 40 to 60 mg once per day or in divided doses) for a few weeks may be indicated for relief of pain and swelling, followed by tapering and discontinuation over a month as tolerated. Response is often dramatic, with relief in 24 to 48 hours. If pain and swelling do not resolve in 72 hours, the diagnosis of thyroiditis should be reconsidered. Decreasing thyroid inflammation may hasten return to euthyroidism. Glucocorticoids also decrease peripheral conversion of T_4 to more potent T_3, potentially aiding toxicosis control. Glucocorticoids may transiently decrease TSH secretion, RAIU, and serum T_4 and T_3 (due to decreased serum TBG concentration). TSH and free T_4 levels are not altered by chronic glucocorticoids. Glucocorticoids do not reverse the underlying process, and rebound pain and swelling occur in 10 to 20% of patients while tapering or shortly after discontinuation of therapy. This often requires an additional course of treatment. A rebound of ESR is absent in one-third of such patients.

Transient Hyperthyroidism

Thyrotoxic symptoms are often mild, and reassurance of recovery after 8 to 12 weeks is often all that is necessary. Symptoms may be alleviated with beta-adrenergic blockers (e.g., sustained release propranolol [Inderal L.A.], 80 to 160 mg per day, or atenolol [Tenormin], 50 to 100 mg per day) until thyroid hormone levels normalize. A nonselective beta-adrenergic blocker (e.g., propranolol) is more effective in preventing the rare thyrotoxic periodic paralysis in the susceptible individual. Patients should monitor the pulse rate and contact the physician should the rate be less than 60 beats per minute, or more than 80 beats per minute with continued symptoms of hyperthyroidism. Beta-adrenergic blockers do not effect RAIU. Treatment with antithyroid drugs (e.g., propylthiouracil and methimazole [Tapazole]), which block thyroid hormone synthesis, or super-saturated potassium iodide (SSKI), which acutely inhibits hormone release, is not useful, since the hyperthyroidism is due to leakage of preformed hormones from damaged tissue.

Transient Hypothyroidism

Excessive determinations of thyroid function should be avoided, as they are expensive and most patients recover spontaneously. Empirical therapy for presumptive hypothyroidism is also discouraged. Levothyroxine (Synthroid) therapy is indicated for elevated TSH with significant symptoms of hypothyroidism in doses to relieve symptoms and normalize the TSH 4 to 6 weeks after dosage adjustment. It is prudent to withdraw levothyroxine after several months. This can be done by halving the dose and measuring TSH after 4 to 6 weeks; if this is normal, levothyroxine may be stopped and the TSH determination repeated after 4 to 6 weeks. If hypothyroidism persists for longer than 12 months, it is likely to be permanent. Some argue that maintaining mild TSH elevation may hasten recovery and serve as a marker for remission.

Chronic Hypothyroidism

Lifelong levothyroxine replacement is given for permanent hypothyroidism. Because several of the thyroiditides produce only transient hypothyroidism, it is often reassuring before committing to lifelong therapy to document more than one diagnostic TSH elevation over at least several months, particularly if TSH elevation is modest (20 mU per L or less), if metoclopramide (Reglan) or domperidone (Motilium)* administration has occurred, or if recovery from the euthyroid sick syndrome is possible. Neither a mild elevation of TSH (less than 10 mU per L) nor antithyroid antibodies alone increase the risk of subsequent overt hypothyroidism. Some like to demonstrate deficient thyroid hormone levels before initiating therapy. Owing to the log linear response of TSH in hypothyroidism, it is a more sensitive marker for mild deficiency when the free T_4 remains normal (subclinical hypothyroidism).

One suggested therapeutic goal is to return the TSH to the lower half of the normal range (the normal range is not a normal distribution curve, and most truly normal individuals reside in the lower half of the range) and reduce the associated goiter. The average replacement dosage of levothyroxine (Synthroid, Levoxyl, Levothyroid) necessary to achieve this varies by patient age and weight, ranging from 8 to 10 μg per kg per day in infants to 1.5 to 1.7 μg per kg ideal body weight per day in adults. Full replacement doses may be safely started in young, relatively healthy individuals; however, elderly patients and those with significant cardiovascular diseases should start with doses of 25 to 50 μg per day, increased by 25-μg increments every 6 weeks until TSH values enter the target range. Generic brands of thyroid hormone, thyroid extracts, and T_3-containing preparations may present problems in maintaining stable hormone concentrations. Patients are instructed to make up a forgotten dose by doubling the strength of the next. Noncompliance is suggested when TSH values fluctuate or remain elevated despite reasonable dosage adjustments. Levothyroxine replacement therapy is extremely well toler-

---

*Not yet approved for use in the United States.

ated, but rare patients can have allergies to dye in the tablet, in which case plain tablets (usually 50 μg) may be prescribed. Once a stable dosage is achieved, follow-up TSH may be measured annually and prescriptions given for 3-month supplies.

Although concerns have been raised, no convincing evidence exists to support the contention that levothyroxine therapy in doses to maintain the TSH in the normal range increases the risk of osteoporosis. Dosage adjustments may be required for malabsorption, concomitant drug therapy, and aging. Levothyroxine requirements typically increase 25 to 50% during pregnancy.

Goiter

Levothyroxine therapy may also be indicated in euthyroid patients with prominent diffuse goiter, but shrinkage is less frequent than in those with elevated TSH levels. About 10% of patients presenting with goiter and high antithyroid antibody titers develop hypothyroidism. Treatment is not necessary when the TSH is normal and thyroid enlargement is minimal, unless there is cosmetic concern. Goiters or thyroid nodules that enlarge despite levothyroxine therapy to maintain the TSH in the lower half of the normal range should be considered for FNA biopsy or surgery. The probability of malignancy in a dominant nodule of a multinodular gland is identical to that of an isolated thyroid nodule. Patients should be instructed to seek care immediately should a new nodule be noted. Occasionally, subtotal thyroidectomy is required for benign goiters that continue to grow or cause obstructive symptoms.

General Long-Term Considerations

Little disease-specific follow-up care is indicated for those who spontaneously recover from granulomatous thyroiditis and remain asymptomatic. Patients with a history of painless thyroiditis, postpartum thyroiditis, or Hashimoto's thyroiditis should be followed annually with complete history and physical examinations and a relatively low threshold for TSH determination, given the increased risk for goiter or thyroid failure. In addition, patients with Hashimoto's thyroiditis should have the thyroid gland examined should an enlargement or nodule occur, given the slightly increased risk of thyroid lymphoma.

Section 9

The Urogenital Tract

BACTERIAL INFECTIONS OF THE URINARY TRACT IN MALES

method of
JAMES W. SMITH, M.D.
Department of Veterans Affairs Medical Center
Dallas, Texas

and

STEVEN E. RADEMACHER, M.D.
University of Texas Southwestern Medical School at Dallas
Dallas, Texas

Infections of the urinary tract in males can occur at any level of the urinary tract and at any age. However, invasive infections of the urinary tract are most frequent in the very young (under 3 months of age) or the elderly (greater than 50 years of age). Local infections of the urethra are commonplace in young sexually active men.

The organisms invading the urinary tract represent external colonization of the genital region, with manifestations depending on the organism and its ability to ascend into the urinary tract. Rarely, hematogenous spread to the urinary tract occurs during bacteremic episodes, particularly with *Staphylococcus aureus* or *Candida albicans*. Initiation of infection requires the adherence of the organism to the epithelial cells of the urinary tract.

Organisms acquired during sexual intercourse, such as *Neisseria gonorrhoeae* and *Chlamydia trachomatis*, adhere to the urethral epithelial cells and result in a polymorphonuclear leukocyte response. This manifests clinically as a discharge that may be thick and yellow with *N. gonorrhoeae* or thin to mucoid with *C. trachomatis*. Evaluation of urethral discharge should include a urethral Gram stain for leukocytes and intracellular gram-negative diplococci. If the Gram stain is negative but five or more leukocytes per oil immersion field are present, this represents nongonococcal urethritis. Urinary symptoms and signs could also represent a lower urinary tract infection, so a midstream urine culture may be indicated if no leukocytes are present on uretheral swab.

Older men present with symptoms of dysuria, frequent urination, and occasionally isolated hematuria with their urinary tract infections. It is difficult to localize the infection to the lower urinary tract, prostate, or kidney by clinical symptoms alone. Up to half of elderly men with urinary tract infections have prostate infections as well. Examination of the scrotum should be done, since epididymo-orchitis may be a complication of urinary tract or prostatic infection. Bacterial infection is suspected if the urine leukocyte esterase test and the nitrite test for gram-negative bacteria are positive. Bacterial organisms recovered from urine cultures of men with urinary tract infections are most frequently *Escherichia coli*, with urovirulent strains similar to those found in women and children with upper tract infections. This suggests that a combination of factors leads to urinary tract infection in men, including the inability to empty completely and the ascension of urovirulent organisms from the urethra.

TREATMENT

Therapy depends on distinguishing between gonococcal and chlamydial urethritis. Cultures of urethral discharge from patients with smears that are positive for intracellular diplococci are tested to determine whether the isolate is penicillinase-producing *N. gonorrhoeae* (PPNG). Since PPNG is found throughout the United States, uncomplicated gonococcal infections are best treated with ceftriaxone (Rocephin) 125 mg intramuscularly in a single dose. Alternatively, cefixime (Suprax) 400 mg orally in a single dose can be given, or if the patient is allergic to penicillin, ciprofloxacin (Cipro) 500 mg orally or ofloxacin (Floxin) 400 mg orally can be given as a single dose. Testing for cure is not required with standard treatment for gonococcal infections unless the symptoms persist after treatment. Since many men with gonococcal infection also have chlamydial infection, all patients given the regimens just noted, as well as those with nongonococcal urethritis, should be treated with doxycycline 100 mg orally two times a day for 7 days. Alternative treatments for chlamydial urethritis include azithromycin (Zithromax) 1 gram orally in a single dose, ofloxacin 300 mg orally two times a day for 7 days, or erythromycin base 500 mg orally four times a day for 7 days. *C. trachomatis* may recur in patients who fail to comply with the treatment regimen or who are re-exposed to an untreated sex partner. Recurrent urethritis should be retreated with the initial regimen. In addition, a wet-mount examination of a urethral swab specimen for *Trichmonas vaginalis* should be performed. Another possible cause of recurrent urethritis is tetracycline-resistant *Ureaplasma urealyticum*, which responds to a 14-day course of erythromycin base at a dose of 500 mg orally four times a day.

Men with urinary tract infections and temperatures less than 102° F (39.6° C) can usually be managed as outpatients with trimethoprim-sulfamethoxazole (Bactrim, Septra) one double-strength tablet twice a day for 14 to 21 days. If the patient is allergic to sulfonamides, then quinolones such as ciprofloxacin (Cipro) 500 mg twice daily, ofloxacin (Floxacin) 400 mg twice daily, or lomefloxacin (Maxequin) 400 mg once daily are other effective oral medications that can be used for 14 to 21 days. Oral cephalosporins or penicillin derivatives are rapidly excreted, and they have reduced response rates in comparison with trimethoprim-sulfamethoxazole and quinolones.

Patients with severe upper urinary tract infections and fever greater than 102° F, volume depletion, and/or altered mental status should be hospitalized and treated with intravenous therapy. Intravenous therapy with trimethoprim-sulfamethoxazole 160/800 mg every 12 hours combined with gentamicin 1 mg per kg of patient body weight every 8 to 12 hours, ceftriaxone 1 to 2 grams daily, or ciprofloxacin 200 to 400 mg every 12 hours can be given. If the patient responds and fluid resuscitation is successful, he can be switched to an oral agent on the second or third hospital day. Trimethoprim-sulfamethoxazole or one of the quinolones previously mentioned can be used to complete a 14-day course of therapy. One advantage of 2 to 3 days of parenteral aminoglycoside is that the aminoglycoside persists in the kidney for up to a month after administration, providing continuous synergistic activity with some orally administered agents.

If, however, the patient continues to have fever after 72 hours of therapy, a urine culture should be repeated, and ultrasonography or computed tomography (CT) should be performed to rule out an intrarenal infection such as a phlegmon (nephronia) or a perinephric abscess. A perinephric abscess is more likely to occur in patients who have spinal cord injury, diabetes mellitus, or continuous urinary catheterization. Nephronia occurs in approximately 5 to 10% of those with the clinical diagnosis of pyelonephritis (fever, flank pain, and urinary tract infection). Patients with this intrarenal process generally respond to parenteral antimicrobial therapy continued for more than 2 weeks with some patients requiring up to 6 weeks of parenteral therapy. Patients with multifocal masslike lesions on CT may require percutaneous drainage, since this complication is associated with high mortality rates.

A careful history and physical examination should be done in patients with urinary tract infections to check for possible structural problems that may lead to urinary tract infection, including kidney stones and clinically significant benign prosthetic hypertrophy. If the patient has signs or symptoms of urinary retention, an in-and-out bladder catheterization should be done to check for residual. Other voiding studies, such as an intravenous pyelogram, are not indicated unless evidence of other abnormalities is found during the physical examination or in the history.

After patients respond clinically with a decrease in temperature and symptoms, they can be observed on antimicrobial therapy. A urine culture 2 to 4 weeks after completing therapy can be done to check for recurrence or persistence of infection. If the follow-up urine culture is positive, a 4- to 6-week course of antimicrobial treatment is indicated. However, subsequent courses of therapy for asymptomatic bacteria would not be indicated.

Epididymitis can occur following infection of either the urethra or the urinary tract in sexually active men under 35 years of age, usually with *N. gonorrhoeae* or *C. trachomatis* as the causative organisms. Both urethral discharge and urine with cultures are obtained to determine the causative agent. In men older than 35 years, epididymitis follows urinary tract infection with gram-negative organisms such as *E. coli*. Antimicrobial therapy is determined by the antimicrobial susceptibility of the bacteria recovered from the urinary tract. For patients under 35 years of age, treatment with ceftriaxone 250 mg intramuscularly plus doxycycline 100 mg twice a day for 10 days is indicated; for older men, treatment should include trimethoprim-sulfamethoxazole 160/800 mg twice daily for 14 days or a quinolone. If serious systemic infection is present, a combination of a cephalosporin and aminoglycoside is indicated until the patient responds. In addition, supportive measures, including elevation of the scrotum, are indicated.

BACTERIAL INFECTIONS OF THE URINARY TRACT IN WOMEN

method of
ABDOLLAH IRAVANI, M.D.
Central Florida Medical Research Center
Orlando, Florida

Urinary tract infections (UTIs) are prevalent in women of childbearing age. Approximately 6 to 8% of women between the ages of 20 and 40 years develop UTIs each year. Bacterial pathogens of these infections generally originate from the fecal flora. Initially, potential urinary pathogens contaminate the lower urogenital area and adhere to and colonize the periurethral mucosa. As a result of the interaction of a variety of host factors and bacterial pathogenicity, bacteria ascend the urethra and invade the urinary tract. The most common urinary tract pathogens in women are *Escherichia coli* and *Staphylococcus saprophyticus* (Table 1). Other less common organisms include *Proteus mirabilis*, *Klebsiella pneumoniae*, *Enterobacter* species, enterococci, and *Pseudomonas aeruginosa*. Infections may be confined to the lower tract (cystitis) or involve the upper tract (pyelonephritis) as well. The majority of women of childbearing age have simple, uncomplicated UTIs and structurally and functionally normal urinary tracts.

UTIs are associated with a great risk of renal scarring, chronic renal failure, and hypertension in patients with vesicoureteral reflux, obstructive uropathy, or neurogenic

TABLE 1. **Urinary Pathogens in Women**

Common	Rare
Escherichia coli	*Pseudomonas* spp
Staphylococcus saprophyticus	Enterococcus
Uncommon	*Citrobacter* spp
	Acinetobacter spp
Proteus mirabilis	
Klebsiella pneumoniae	
Enterobacter spp	

bladder. UTIs may result in renal damage and systemic complications during pregnancy or in patients with diabetes mellitus, systemic lupus erythematosus, and sickle cell disorders.

CLINICAL PRESENTATION

The clinical presentation of UTI is variable and not consistent. Dysuria and frequent urination with suprapubic pain and tenderness are clinical indicators of UTI. Patients with pyelonephritis generally present with flank pain and tenderness, fever, chills, and leukocytosis. Approximately 30% of women who have lower UTI symptoms may have asymptomatic upper tract infection as well. Bacteriuria may be found in asymptomatic individuals, whereas dysuria may be experienced by patients with negative urine cultures. Dysuria syndrome or urethral syndrome in patients with negative urine cultures is due to other causes such as infections of the lower urogenital area with *Chylamydia trachomatis, Ureaplasma urealyticum,* genital herpes, *Trichomonas vaginalis,* or *Candida* vaginitis or trauma.

DIAGNOSIS

Diagnosis of UTIs in women is usually based on the presence of clinical symptoms, pyuria, and bacteriuria with 10^4 to 10^5 colony-forming units (cfu) of a bacterium per mL of a clean-catch midstream urine specimen. Semiquantitative urine culture devices such as dip slide (Culturia), roll tube (Bactercult), and small culture plate (Testuria) are low-cost, practical office devices that have facilitated the diagnosis of UTIs. Pyuria 1 or more per high-power field of uncentrifuged urine, 5 to 10 per high-power field of centrifuged urine, and 10 or more per mL³ of urine supports a diagnosis of UTI, but confirmation of UTI cannot be based on the presence of pyuria alone. Pyuria may occur in the absence of UTI for a number of reasons, including contamination of urine with vaginal secretions.

Multistix with nitrate and Multistix with leukocyte esterase are helpful screening devices for UTIs. If both the nitrate and the leukocyte esterase tests are positive, the presence of UTI is highly likely. A positive nitrate test alone may indicate the presence of UTI or bacterial colonization of the urinary bladder. A positive leukocyte esterase test alone may indicate UTI or contamination of urine with vaginal content. Nevertheless, a urine culture provides a definite bacteriologic diagnosis of UTI.

DURATION OF THERAPY AND SELECTION OF ANTIMICROBIAL AGENTS

The duration of antimicrobial therapy ranges from single-dose, short-course (3 to 5 days), or standard (7 to 10 days) regimens for cystitis and uncomplicated UTIs to long-term (10 to 14 days or more) courses for patients with pyelonephritis or more complicated UTIs. Simple, uncomplicated UTIs in women of childbearing age generally respond favorably to single doses or short courses of a variety of antibiotics. Single-dose and short-course antibiotic therapy minimizes the risk of adverse drug effects, the development of vaginal yeast, and the emergence of fecal bacterial resistance. They promote better patient compliance and may be more cost effective.

A large armamentarium of antimicrobial agents is currently available for use in patients with UTI (Table 2). Antimicrobial agents that achieve high urinary concentration in active form generally result in rapid and effective therapeutic response, provided the urinary pathogen is susceptible. Other selection criteria include (1) broad antimicrobial spectrum, (2) once- or twice-a-day dosing, (3) lack of systemic or any body organ toxic effects, (4) good patient tolerance, (5) minimal emergence of fecal bacterial resistance, (6) low incidence of *Candida* vaginitis, and (7) low cost. Antimicrobial therapy should be started with the finding of bacteriuria and pyuria on urinalysis rather than being delayed while the results of urine culture and susceptibility testing are obtained. The following antimicrobial agents are marketed and used for UTIs.

Sulfonamides

Use of sulfonamides has decreased due to a high degree of bacterial resistance, the need for frequent dosing, and the availability of more effective drugs. Over 30% of *E. coli* that causes community-acquired UTIs is resistant to sulfonamides. Oral sulfonamides include sulfisoxazole (Gantrisin) 0.5 to 1.0 grams every 6 hours and sulfamethoxazole (Gantanol) 0.5 to 1.0 grams every 12 hours. Sulfonamides are low in cost. Common side effects are headache, rash, and nausea. They increase the anticoagulant effect of warfarin and may cause phenytoin toxicity.

Trimethoprim

Trimethoprim (Proloprim, Trimpex) is a synthetic bacteriostatic agent that has excellent gastrointestinal tract absorption, high tissue penetration, and urinary excretion as an active form. It is excreted into vaginal fluid and may reduce the colonization of potential urinary pathogens in the genitalia. Trimethoprim is active against most common urinary tract pathogens, but *Pseudomonas* species and enterococci are generally resistant to this drug. Trimethoprim 100 mg twice a day or 200 mg once a day is effective in the treatment of acute uncomplicated UTIs. It is suitable for use in the prophylaxis of recurrent UTIs. Trimethoprim is well tolerated by the majority of patients. The most common adverse reactions are nausea and rash. Trimethoprim decreases the effectiveness of oral contraceptives and may cause digoxin toxicity and potentiate thiazide diuretic effects and hyponatremia.

Trimethoprim-Sulfamethoxazole (TMP–SMX)

Because of the synergistic antibacterial action of trimethoprim and sulfonamides, a fixed combination of trimethoprim 80 mg and sulfamethoxazole 400 mg (Bactrim, Septra) or double-strength tablets is produced. Like trimethoprim, the combination TMP–SMX is active against the majority of common uri-

TABLE 2. **Antimicrobial Agents Used in the Treatment of Urinary Tract Infections in Women**

Agent	Dosage	Times per Day	Comments
Sulfonamides			
Sulfisoxazole (Gantrisin)	0.5–1 gm	4	Poorly effective, low cost
Sulfamethoxazole (Gantanol)	0.5–1 gm	2	
Trimethoprim/sulfamethoxazole (Bactrim DS, Septra DS)	160 mg/800 mg	2	Widely used; frequent adverse effects of rash and headache
Trimethoprim (Proloprim)	100 mg	2	Effective for acute UTI and prophylactic therapy
New quinolones			Highly effective, high cost, sucralfate, antacid, and calcium use decreases absorption
Ciprofloxacin (Cipro)	250–500 mg	2	
Norfloxocin (Noroxin)	400 mg	2	
Lomefloxacin (Maxaquin)	400 mg	1	
Ofloxacin (Floxin)	200–400 mg	2	
Enoxacin (Penetrex)	200–400 mg	2	
Nitrofurantoin	50–100 mg	4	Effective for acute cystitis and prophylactic therapy; nausea and vomiting are common side effects
macrocrystals (Macrodantin)	100 mg	2	
Amoxicillin (Amoxil)	250–500 mg	3	Poorly effective, high incidence of *Candida* vaginitis
Amoxicillin–clavulanate K (Augmentin)	250 mg/125 mg	3	High incidence of diarrhea, vomiting, and *Candida* vaginitis
Cephalosporins			High cost; high incidence of diarrhea, nausea, and *Candida* vaginitis
Cephalexin (Keflex)	250–500 mg	4	
Cefadroxil (Duricef)	250–500 mg	2	
Cefuroxime axetil (Ceftin)	125–250 mg	2	
Cefixime (Suprax)	400 mg	1	
Cefpodoxime proxetil (Vantin)	200 mg	2	
Loracarbef (Lorabid)	200–400 mg	2	

nary pathogens. It is less frequently associated with the emergence of bacterial resistance than either of its components. Nevertheless, the frequency of bacterial resistance to the combination is increasing. TMP–SMX is extensively prescribed for the treatment of UTIs. Common adverse reactions are similar to those occurring with its components. Gastrointestinal disturbances, allergic skin reactions, rashes (including erythema multiforme and Stevens-Johnson syndrome), headaches, and tongue ulcers have been reported with the use of sulfonamides and TMP–SMX. The compound is contraindicated in patients with folate deficiency, during pregnancy and nursing, and in individuals with sensitivity to sulfonamides or trimethoprim. TMP–SMX has drug interactions with oral anticoagulants, oral contraceptives, and phenytoin similar to those of its components.

Aminopenicillins

Aminopenicillins are beta-lactam antibiotics. Ampicillin (Totacillin, Polycillin, Omnipen) 250 to 500 mg every 6 hours, amoxicillin (Amoxil, Polymox, Wymox) 250 to 500 mg every 8 hours, and bacampicillin (Spectrobid) 400 mg every 12 hours are the commonly used aminopenicillins. All these compounds have similar activity against urinary tract pathogens. Amoxicillin and bacampicillin are preferable to ampicillin because of better gastrointestinal absorption, less frequent dosing, and better patient tolerance. Use of aminopenicillins has become considerably limited because of the high prevalence of bacterial resistance. Over 35% of *E. coli* causing community-acquired UTIs are resistant to aminopenicillins. The most common mechanism of bacterial resis-

tance is inactivation of the drug by bacterial beta-lactamases. A fixed combination of amoxicillin 250 mg and the beta-lactamase inhibitor potassium clavulanate 125 mg has been produced (Augmentin). This combination is effective against most bacteria that are resistant to amoxicillin. UTI therapy can be initiated with the combination until the results of bacterial susceptibility testing become available. Aminopenicillins must be avoided in patients with a history of allergy to pencillins. Common adverse reactions include nausea, vomiting, diarrhea, and rashes. *Candida* vaginitis is a common side effect, occurring in up to 16% of patients. Aminopenicillins may decrease the effectiveness of oral contraceptives, aminoglycosides, oral anticoagulants, and beta-adrenergic blockers. They may potentiate cephalosporin nephrotoxicity and fluoroquinolone adverse effects. Concomitant use of antacids decreases oral aminopenicillin absorption.

Cephalosporins

Cephalosporins are beta-lactam antibiotics related to penicillins. Numerous cephalosporins have been developed, each with distinct and unique pharmacologic, pharmacokinetic, and antibacterial properties. Cephalosporins are active in vitro against a wide variety of gram-positive and gram-negative microorganisms. Methicillin-resistant staphylococci are resistant to all cephalosporins.

First-generation cephalosporins include cephalexin (Keflex) 250 or 500 mg three or four times a day and cefadroxil (Duricef, Ultracef) 250 or 500 mg twice a day. They are more active against gram-positive microorganisms than against Enterobacteriaceae.

Bacterial resistance is increasing, and over 30% of *E. coli* causing community-acquired UTIs are resistant to these agents.

Second-generation cephalosporins include cefuroxime axetil (Ceftin) 125 or 250 mg twice a day, cefaclor (Ceclor) 250 or 500 mg three times a day, loracarbef (Lorabid) 200 or 400 mg twice a day, cefprozil (Cefzil) 250 or 500 mg twice a day, and cefpodoxime proxetil (Vantin) 200 mg twice a day. They are beta-lactamase stable and active against both gram-positive and gram-negative microorganisms. They have broader antibacterial activity than their predecessors. Enterococci and *Pseudomonas* species are resistant to first- and second-generation cephalosporins.

The third-generation cephalosporins cefixime (Suprax), ceftriaxone (Rocephin), ceftazidime (Fortaz), and cefotaxime (Claforan) are beta-lactamase stable and highly active against a broad spectrum of gram-negative bacilli, including *Pseudomonas* species (ceftazidime). They are less active against gram-positive cocci, including *S. saprophyticus*. Ceftriaxone has a long half-life, allowing once- or twice-daily dosing. Cefixime has a relatively long plasma half-life, permitting once-daily dosing. Cefixime 400 mg once a day is effective in the treatment of UTIs caused by Enterobacteriaceae. It is not active against *Staphylococcus* species, including *S. saprophyticus*.

Untoward effects of cephalosporins in general include nausea, vomiting, diarrhea, rash, bleeding diathesis, positive direct Coombs' test, and cross-sensitivity reactions in approximately 20% of individuals with allergy to penicillins. Cephalosporins may produce overgrowth of *Clostridium difficile* in the bowel and cause pseudomembranous colitis. *Candida* vaginitis is a common side effect and occurs in up to 16% of patients. Cephalosporins may increase the anticoagulant effect of warfarin (Coumadin), potentiate ethacrynic acid and furosemide nephrotoxicity, and decrease oral contraceptive effect.

Nalidixic Acid

Nalidixic acid (NegGram) is active against common gram-negative urinary tract pathogens. *Pseudomonas* species and gram-positive cocci are resistant to this drug. Cinoxacin (Cinobac) is a derivative of nalidixic acid with a longer plasma half-life and an otherwise similar in vitro antibacterial spectrum. Nalidixic acid is given 1 gram every 6 hours orally, and cinoxacin 250 or 500 mg twice daily orally. Side effects of these agents are relatively common and include visual and sensory neural disturbance, photosensitivity, dizziness, headache, nausea, and rash. They increase oral anticoagulant effects. Currently, the clinical use of nalidixic acid is considerably hampered because of the high incidence of adverse symptoms, the frequent and rapid emergence of bacterial resistance, and the availability of new quinolones.

New Quinolones

New fluoroquinolones are derivatives of nalidixic acid with considerably improved antibacterial activity, pharmacokinetic characteristics, safety profile, and patient tolerance. They are commonly used in the treatment of a wide variety of systemic and urinary tract infections. These agents have a broad spectrum of activity against Enterobacteriaceae, *Pseudomonas* species, and, to a lesser degree, *Staphylococcus* species, including *S. saprophyticus*. There is also some activity against enterococci, although some resistant strains have been reported. Development of resistance to fluorquinolones is rare, but it has been reported for a variety of bacteria, especially *Pseudomonas* species.

New fluoroquinolones are generally absorbed well after oral administration and attain high serum, tissue, and urinary concentrations in active form. Sucralfate, aluminum, calcium, or magnesium antacids and other bivalent compounds decrease their intestinal absorption. Ranitidine (Zantac) may decrease the intestinal absorption of fluoroquinolones such as ciprofloxacin (Cipro) and enoxacin (Penetrex). Fluoroquinolones interfere with methylxanthine metabolism; they also prolong the anticoagulant effect of warfarin (Coumadin) and potentiate cyclosporine nephrotoxicity. Simultaneous administration of new fluoroquinolones and theophylline may result in high serum theophylline levels and severe toxicity. New fluoroquinolones should be taken 1 hour before or 2 hours after meals. They are not recommended for use during pregnancy, in children, or in those with a history of seizure disorders. The commercially available new fluoroquinolones are ciprofloxacin (Cipro) 250 or 500 mg twice daily, norfloxacin (Noroxin) 400 mg twice daily, lomefloxacin (Maxaquin) 400 mg once a day, enoxacin (Penetrex) 200 or 400 mg twice a day, and ofloxacin (Floxin) 200 or 400 mg twice daily. All these agents are highly effective in the therapy of UTIs in women. Ciprofloxacin is also available in parenteral form for intravenous administration in more serious infections. Lomefloxacin, in contrast to the other new quinolones, does not interfere with methylxanthine metabolism and does not cause a rise in serum caffeine or theophylline levels or prolong their bioavailability.

New fluoroquinolones are generally safe and are well tolerated by the majority of patients. Adverse reactions include nausea, vomiting, abdominal pain, dizziness, nervousness, headache, insomnia, anxiety, rash, myalgia, arthralgia, photosensitivity with rash or bullous skin lesions, generalized seizures (rare), and Stevens-Johnson syndrome. Simultaneous use of penicillins may potentiate fluoroquinolones' adverse effects.

Nitrofurantoin

Nitrofurantoin is an antibacterial agent that is absorbed well from the small intestine and is rapidly excreted in the urine without the development of significant blood levels. Nitrofurantoin is active against most common urinary pathogens, including enterococci and *S. saprophyticus*. *Proteus* species and *Pseudomonas* species are resistant to this agent. Nitrofurantoin rarely causes the emergence of bacterial resistance or disturbs bowel bacterial flora. Nitrofurantoin macrocrystals (Macrodantin) 50 to 100 mg orally every 6 hours should be taken after meals to decrease the incidence of nausea and vomiting. Macrobid is a new nitrofurantoin product; the delayed-release 200-mg capsules are taken twice daily.

Nitrofurantoin 50 or 100 mg once daily at bedtime is suitable for the prophylaxis of recurrent UTIs. Common adverse reactions are nausea, vomiting, flatulence, rash, and anorexia. Other adverse reactions are chronic active hepatitis, chronic allergic pneumonitis, anemia, and lupus-like syndrome. The drug is contraindicated in patients with glucose-6-phosphate dehydrogenase deficiency, in patients with less than 50% renal function, and in those at term or during labor and delivery. *Candida* vaginitis is a rare side effect. Antacids decrease intestinal absorption of nitrofurantoin and should be taken 6 hours before or after nitrofurantoin.

Aminoglycosides

Gentamicin (Garamycin), tobramycin (Nebcin), and amikacin (Amikin) are parenteral antibiotics with broad antibacterial activity against gram-negative organisms, including *Pseudomonas* species. Aminoglycosides are useful in doses of 60 to 80 mg intravenously or intramuscularly every 8 hours in patients with more severe or nosocomial infections or in those with multiple antibiotic allergies. More favorable results are reported when the total daily dose of the aminoglycoside is administered as one single dose. Aminoglycosides are well known for their ototoxicity and nephrotoxicity. There is a high risk of nephrotoxicity with concomitant use of amphotericin B, cephalosporins, cisplatin, cyclosporine, and furosemide. Ethacrynic acid, bumetanide, and furosemide highly potentiate the ototoxicity of the aminoglycosides. In patients with renal insufficiency, dosing intervals should be extended according to the degree of renal function, and serum levels should be monitored closely.

SIMPLE, UNCOMPLICATED INFECTIONS

The majority of UTIs in women are simple and uncomplicated infections. They are most often caused by *E. coli* or *S. saprophyticus*. Clinically, these infections present as dysuria and frequent and urgent urination. The length of antibiotic treatment depends on the recent history of UTI, the duration of symptoms, and the degree of pyuria. Patients with 1 to 3 days of symptoms of lower tract infections and mild pyuria (white blood count [WBC] 1 to 5 per high-power field of centrifuged specimen) usually respond well to a single dose (Table 3) or to 3 to 5 days (Table 4) of antibiotic therapy; those with a longer duration of symptoms and heavy pyuria (WBC >5 per high-power field) require 7 to 10 days or longer of therapy.

TMP–SMX is commonly used as the first-choice

TABLE 3. Single-Dose Therapy of Urinary Tract Infections in Women

Antimicrobial Agent	Dosage
Trimethoprim-sulfamethoxazole (Bactrim, Septra)	3 tablets of 160 mg/800 mg PO
Ciprofloxacin (Cipro)	500 mg PO
Amoxicillin (Amoxil, Polymox, Wymox)	3 g PO
Cephalexin (Keflex)	3 g PO
Ceftriaxone (Rocephin)	0.5–1 gm IM
Cefuroxime axetil (Ceftin)	1 g PO

antimicrobial agent for these infections. Alternative drugs include trimethoprim, one of the new quinolones, nitrofurantoin, amoxicillin–potassium clavulanate (Augmentin), or one of the second-generation cephalosporins. In patients with uncomplicated infections, symptoms are usually relieved and urine becomes sterile within 2 days of therapy. Persistence of symptoms and bacteriuria may be due to a variety of reasons, such as upper UTI, bacterial resistance, urinary calculi, obstructive uropathy, or the patient's poor compliance in taking her medication.

ACUTE PYELONEPHRITIS

Acute pyelonephritis is a bacterial infection of the renal parenchyma and pelvis. It is more serious and problematic than lower UTIs. Symptoms include flank pain, fever (temperature >38.5° C), chills, and vomiting. Approximately 30% of women presenting with only symptoms of lower UTI may have covert pyelonephritis. Depending on the severity of the clinical findings and the general condition of the patient, antimicrobial agents may be administered orally or parenterally. In patients who have fever, nausea, and vomiting, a single dose of ceftriaxone (Rocephin) 500 to 1000 mg intramuscularly or intravenously may control the infection, alleviate the symptoms, and improve tolerance to subsequent oral antibiotic therapy. In patients with more severe hyperpyrexia, gastrointestinal symptoms, and dehydration, each of the following antimicrobial agents may be given intravenously with parenteral hydration for 3 to 5 days or until the patient can tolerate oral antibiotic therapy: ceftriaxone (Rocephin) 500 to 1000 mg every 12 hours; ciprofloxacin (Cipro) 200 to 400 mg diluted in

TABLE 4. Three-Day Antibiotic Therapy of Urinary Tract Infections in Women

Antimicrobial Agent	Dosage
Trimethoprim/sulfamethoxazole (Bactrim, Septra)	160 mg/800 mg bid
Trimethoprim (Trimpex, Proloprim)	100 mg bid or 200 mg qd
Ciprofloxacin (Cipro)	500 mg qd or bid or 250 mg bid
Lomefloxacin (Maxaquin)	400 mg qd
Norfloxacin (Noroxin)	400 mg bid
Ofloxacin (Floxin)	200 or 400 mg bid

100 mL intravenous fluid, administered over a 1-hour period every 12 hours; TMP–SMX 160 mg/800 mg (Bactrim, Septra), diluted in 100 to 125 mL of intravenous fluid and administered over a 1-hour period every 12 hours; cefotaxime (Claforan) 500 to 1000 mg every 8 hours; cefuroxime (Zinacef) 750 to 1500 mg every 8 hours; ceftazidime (Fortaz) 1000 mg every 8 to 12 hours. Bacterial susceptibility testing should be performed; based on those results, antibiotic therapy should be continued with an oral agent for a total of 10 to 14 days.

Resolution of symptoms alone is not a reliable indicator of therapeutic success and eradication of the urinary tract pathogen in patients with pyelonephritis. Therefore, it is suggested that urine cultures be repeated 1 and 4 weeks after therapy. In patients with pyelonephritis, a renal sonogram or an intravenous pyelogram is recommended to assess urinary tract anomalies.

RECURRENT URINARY TRACT INFECTIONS

Some women have a propensity to develop recurrent UTIs. The infections recur in 40% of women within 3 months and in 75 to 80% within 2 years after an initial episode of UTI. Over 90% of recurrences are reinfections caused by a different bacterium from the one causing the initial infection. Recurrent UTIs are costly, inconvenient, and an annoying problem for women.

E. coli remains the most common cause of recurrent UTIs. Other Enterobacteriaceae, Pseudomonas aeruginosa, and enterococci are found with a higher proportion in these infections than in simple UTIs. Urinary pathogens of recurrent UTIs commonly reveal multiple antibacterial resistance.

The diagnosis of each episode of recurrent UTI must be established by a positive urinalysis, urine culture, and bacterial susceptibility testing. Due to a high incidence of bacterial resistance to amoxicillin and sulfonamides, these agents are not indicated in treatment of recurrent UTIs. TMP–SMX is widely used in the treatment of recurrent UTIs. Any of the new quinolones is an excellent choice for the treatment of these infections. The length of antibiotic therapy depends on the interval between recurrences, the duration and severity of symptoms, and the degree of pyuria. Single-dose or short-course antibiotic therapy is not appropriate for frequently occurring UTIs. Generally, 7 to 10 days of therapy is indicated.

In most patients with recurrent UTIs, personal hygienic precautions alone are not effective in preventing these infections. Long-term, low-dose continuous or postcoital antimicrobial prophylactic therapy has proved effective, however. Prophylactic therapy is indicated when recurrences occur at frequent, closely spaced intervals—more than four episodes in 12 months. Generally, after the active infection is treated and cleared, a low dose of an antimicrobial agent is taken once daily at bedtime or after coitus

for 3 to 9 months. The antimicrobial agents commonly used for prophylaxis include TMP–SMX 80 mg/400 mg, trimethoprim 100 mg, or nitrofurantoin 100 mg. A complete blood cell count and liver profile tests (aminotransferase enzyme levels) are indicated every 3 months to evaluate the safety of the drug therapy. Sulfonamides and aminopenicillins cause the rapid emergence of bacterial resistance in fecal flora and are not recommended for prophylactic therapy.

A renal sonogram or an intravenous pyelogram is suggested for patients with more than four recurrent UTIs in a 12-month period.

ASYMPTOMATIC BACTERIURIA

Asymptomatic bacteriuria may occur in patients with anatomically and physiologically normal or abnormal urinary tracts. It may clear spontaneously or persist and, in some cases, lead to symptomatic UTI. Since there is a lack of data regarding the natural course and the tissue source of symptomatic bacteriuria, the necessity for treatment has been controversial. Patients with asymptomatic UTIs detected for the first time on a random medical screening require urine culture and treatment with a course of antibiotics. The patient should be observed, and if the infection recurs, radiologic and urologic work-up is warranted. Generally, treatment of asymptomatic UTIs is recommended during pregnancy and in patients with vesicoureteral reflux, renal calculi, obstructive uropathies, renal parenchymal disease, diabetes mellitus, and compromised immune systems. Optimal treatment regimens have not been well-established. However, a 7- to 10-day course of antibiotic therapy and carefully scheduled follow-up urine cultures are essential to confirm eradication of the organisms.

URINARY TRACT INFECTIONS DURING PREGNANCY

Urinary tract infections can be a serious problem during pregnancy. Pregnant women are more prone to develop UTIs than nonpregnant women, largely due to gestational hormonal, physiologic, and mechanical changes. During pregnancy, hydronephrosis, hydroureter, and vesicoureteral reflux may develop, which facilitate pyelonephritis and renal scarring. The incidence of symptomatic UTI in pregnant women is as high as 15%, and the incidence of asymptomatic UTI is as high as 6 to 8%. As many as 20 to 40% of pregnant women with untreated asymptomatic bacteriuria may develop pyelonephritis. Periodic screening for asymptomatic bacteriuria is required during pregnancy. Recommended antimicrobial agents include aminopenicillins, cephalosporins, nitrofurantoin, and sulfonamides. A 7- to 10-day course of therapy usually eradicates the infection. Sulfonamides should not be used during the third trimester because of the risk of kernicterus in the neonate. Nitrofurantoin should not be given during the last month of pregnancy.

COMPLICATED URINARY TRACT INFECTIONS

Some patients who present with symptoms of acute UTI may have structural or functional urinary tract anomalies. These patients usually manifest therapeutic failure and relapses. The presence of significant urologic abnormalities is not common in women of childbearing age and accounts for less than 5% of UTIs. Anatomic, structural, or functional abnormalities that impede urine flow complicate the course of UTI and predispose the patient to chronic or recurrent UTIs. These complicating factors include urethral stricture, bladder diverticuli, urinary calculi, cystocele, and neurogenic bladder. *E. coli* is the leading cause of complicated UTIs, followed by *Proteus, Klebsiella, Providencia,* and *Enterobacter* species.

Management of patients with UTIs and obstructive uropathy may require both antimicrobial therapy and surgical intervention to resolve the obstruction and urinary retention. The choice of antibacterial agent depends on the result of urine culture and susceptibility testing. In complicated infections, bacteriuria may persist or recur at short intervals, necessitating extensive long-term antimicrobial therapy.

BACTERIAL INFECTIONS OF THE URINARY TRACT IN GIRLS

method of
DAVID R. ROTH, M.D., and
JENNIFER M. ABIDARI, M.D.
Baylor College of Medicine
Houston, Texas

After upper respiratory tract infections, urinary tract infections (UTIs) are the most common bacterial infection of childhood. Only during the first 30 days of life does the incidence of UTIs in boys exceed that in girls. After that, girls far outnumber boys in the development of UTIs. During childhood, a girl has an approximately 3% chance of acquiring a symptomatic UTI, and random screening programs have found an incidence of asymptomatic bacteriuria in 1 to 2% of preschool and school-age girls. This incidence peaks during the years of toilet training (ages 2 to 4 years) and then falls to a lower baseline again.

SIGNS AND SYMPTOMS

The signs and symptoms of UTIs in older girls can be communicated by the child and are similar to those in adults: dysuria, frequency, urgency, hematuria, fever, suprapubic discomfort, lethargy, flank pain, and incontinence. However, in the neonate and the baby, signs and symptoms may be much more subtle. A high degree of suspicion for a UTI is appropriate whenever constitutional symptoms occur, such as weight loss, lethargy, nausea, vomiting, and fever, or those referable to the central nervous system (CNS), such as irritability or seizures. In spite of these signs and symptoms, a UTI will be documented in only 20% of these babies and 18% of these girls.

DIAGNOSIS

Whenever a UTI is suspected, it is important to perform a urinalysis. Treatment can be initiated after finding white cells or at least one bacterium per high-power field, which roughly translates into a colony count of 10^6 per mL, corresponding to clinical infection in various studies. A urine culture should then be obtained. The easiest method of obtaining urine for urinalysis or culture is by midstream collection after cleansing of the perineum.

It is important to be aware of the pitfalls of specimen collection in the girl who has not yet been toilet trained. In these, girls' uro-bags, urethral catheterization, or suprapubic aspiration must be utilized. Either of the last two choices give uncontaminated aliquots of urine and are easy to perform. Catheterization is safe at any age and should be done under sterile technique. The initial few drops of urine are discarded to decrease the possibility of urethral contamination from the catheterization. Suprapubic aspiration using a small-gauge needle is simple in an infant since the bladder is an intra-abdominal organ. The bladder should be palpable prior to attempting aspiration; again, this is done using sterile technique. As both methods virtually eliminate all sources of bacterial contamination, any growth is considered pathologic.

A bagged specimen of urine is significant only if there is no growth. There are several sources of false-positive findings when using a bag, including contamination from skin flora or feces and bacterial growth secondary to leaving the bag on the body for longer than 30 minutes. If the bagged specimen shows bacterial growth, the collection should be repeated or an alternative method utilized.

In the toilet-trained girl, a clean midstream aliquot of urine is adequate for the diagnosis of infection in most cases. A pure colony count of more than 10^6 per mL in a clean-catch urine specimen is indicative of a UTI, especially if associated with voiding symptoms. Growths between 10^5 per mL and 10^6 per mL or those with mixed flora may be suggestive but not necessarily diagnostic of a UTI and the examination should be repeated if clinically warranted. Colony counts below 10,000 bacteria per mL on a clean-catch specimen generally do not indicate an infection.

TREATMENT

If the physician feels that a symptomatic infection is present, treatment with antibiotics should be instituted. Amoxicillin is an appropriate choice for the girl who is felt to have a community-acquired infection. If there are any complicating factors such as known urologic abnormalities, prior urologic surgery, multiple UTIs, recent catheterization of the bladder, or recent hospitalization, consideration of an antibiotic with better gram-negative bacterial coverage would be appropriate. Suitable choices include cephalosporins, nitrofurantoin, or trimethoprim-sulfamethoxazole (TMP–SMX) (Bactrim-Septra). Although in adults limited treatments have been utilized with success, no clinical studies in children support courses of antibiotics shorter than 1 week.

Hospitalization should be reserved for those girls who cannot tolerate oral antibiotics, whose urine cultures show organisms resistant to oral antibiotics, who are septic, or who do not respond to oral antibiotic therapy. Initial parenteral therapy includes a third-generation cephalosporin, an aminoglycoside coupled with either ampicillin or a first-generation cephalosporin. Usually hospitalization continues until the child is afebrile for 24 to 48 hours and the bacterial sensitivity results are available. The youngster can then be discharged on either oral antibiotics or, if necessary, home intravenous antibiotics to complete a 10- to 14-day course of treatment.

EVALUATION

Radiologic evaluation is appropriate for all girls with a documented symptomatic UTI in order to identify the anatomic abnormalities that can be found in 20 to 30% of these children. Often the first-documented UTI is not the first infection that the child has had; indeed, over 75% of girls with an initial UTI will have a subsequent infection within 5 years. If the UTI requires hospitalization, an immediate renal ultrasound (RUS) examination should be performed to determine the presence of hydronephrosis, which may make infection more difficult to treat.

Once the UTI is under control, and preferably before discharge, a voiding cystourethrogram (VCUG) or nuclear cystogram (NC) should be obtained. In girls less than 5 years of age who do not require hospitalization, a VCUG or NC to determine the presence of vesicoureteral reflux (VUR) should be obtained after treatment of the infection. If the cystogram is negative, a RUS to rule out urinary obstruction is appropriate. If, on the other hand, the cystogram shows VUR, a technetium-99m dimercaptosuccinic acid (DMSA) nuclear medicine renal scan, which is most accurate for determining the presence of renal scarring, should be performed since scarring is the most significant sequelae of UTI and reflux. If the girl is over 5 years of age and has no prior history of UTIs, the cystogram can be omitted if a RUS is normal. If the RUS shows any abnormalities, further radiologic testing is needed. Cystoscopy, which was often used in the past for the evaluation of UTIs in girls, no longer has a place in the usual work-up of this problem.

Anatomic anomalies can be found in up to 30% of girls with UTIs. By far the most common abnormality is VUR, which is usually treated with prophylactic antibiotics. Less commonly, either upper tract urinary obstruction or duplication anomalies will be discovered. Any abnormal findings of the radiologic investigations should be evaluated by a urologist. If the evaluation is normal, the parents should be counseled that additional infections may be expected and that unless the clinical picture were to change, further work-up is unnecessary.

CHILDHOOD ENURESIS
method of
ROSS M. DECTER, M.D.
The Milton S. Hershey Medical Center
Hershey, Pennsylvania

"Enuresis" is the involuntary voiding of urine. "Diurnal enuresis" means daytime wetting, and "nocturnal enuresis," nighttime wetting. As children become continent, they initially gain daytime control and subsequently become dry at night. Most 5-year-olds are dry in the daytime, but 15 to 20% of them wet at night. Fifteen percent of the children with nocturnal enuresis spontaneously resolve each year, so that by 15 years of age, about 1% of adolescents still wet.

EVALUATION

The evaluation of the enuretic child begins with a history and physical examination. It is important to elicit a description of the child's daytime voiding pattern, including abnormalities of voiding frequency or the urinary stream, a history of urinary tract infections, and any bowel problems. Historical note of other medical and social conditions such as attention deficit disorder (ADD), neurologic events, social upheavals, and a family history of nocturnal enuresis can be revealing. Features of the physical examination suggesting a complicated problem could include the finding of a cutaneous abnormality over the region of the lumbosacral spine, an abnormal rectal tone, a lack of the anocutaneous reflex, or subtle lower extremity abnormalities such as abnormal gait or pes cavus. Detection of these infrequently observed abnormalities mandates a complete neurourologic evaluation. The child with uncomplicated nocturnal enuresis has a normal physical examination, and the only laboratory evaluation necessary is a urinalysis. Some families require reassurance that there is no "physical problem" causing their child's enuresis, and in these instances an ultrasound evaluation of the kidneys and bladder seems reasonable.

ETIOLOGY

It is probable that the etiology of nocturnal enuresis is multifactorial, and more than one factor may be operant in an individual child. A genetic predisposition is a significant risk factor for nocturnal enuresis. In families with a history of bed wetting in both parents, the likelihood of a child wetting is greater than if only one parent wet the bed and much higher than if neither parent manifested nocturnal enuresis. Some contend that there is a maturational lag in the acquisition of nighttime urinary control. Support for this idea comes from the fact that most enuretic children attain dryness in the same sequence as normal children, but in a delayed fashion. Nocturnal enuresis may also be engendered by a variety of social and psychological factors (stress) that cause a developmental delay in the acquisition of nocturnal continence. Enuretic children manifest behavior problems more frequently than nonwetters, but they do not have an increased incidence of true psychopathologic conditions. Disorders of sleep patterns, airway obstruction, and food allergies have all been implicated as causes of nocturnal enuresis. Another physiologic explanation proposes that a nocturnal deficiency in antidiuretic hormone release leads to excess nocturnal urine output and resultant wetting.

MANAGEMENT

The decision to treat depends on the child and the family's perception of the problem. There is no specific age when treatment should begin. We begin therapy when the symptom is perceived as a problem by the child and parent.

Both nonpharmacologic modalities and pharmacologic agents are used to treat nocturnal enuresis. Nonpharmacologic therapies include reassurance, positive reinforcement, and conditioning therapy. Reassurance that there is nothing physically wrong with the child, along with an explanation of the problem and a description of the natural history of the condition may allay anxiety. Many parents then feel comfortable waiting for the problem to remit spontaneously. The use of positive reinforcement or motivational therapy is usually a component of all the treatment approaches. The use of a star calendar seems a simple, reasonable adjunct to the other forms of therapy, but the cure rate for motivational therapy as a solitary modality is unknown. Conditioning therapy is achieved by the use of an alarm device that signals as the child voids. The body-worn alarms that attach to the sleeping garment are perhaps more effective than the sensing pads that lay on the bed. The response rate to these alarms is about 70 to 80%. In order for the alarm to achieve an effect, the child must arise and go to the bathroom when the alarm sounds. This may require involvement of a parent if the child sleeps through the alarm. After the child achieves dryness, which often takes several months, we recommend continued use for a couple of months before stopping the device in order to minimize the relapse rate.

Current pharmacologic therapies include use of the tricyclic antidepressant imipramine (Tofranil) and the antidiuretic hormone desmopressin acetate (DDAVP). The mechanism of action of imipramine in nocturnal enuresis is incompletely understood. It is generally used in a dose of 25 mg given 1 to 2 hours before bed in 6- to 9-year-olds, and 50 to 75 mg in older children. Response rates of up to 50% are reported; however, the relapse rate after the drug is discontinued is significant. Slow tapering of the medication is reported to decrease the relapse rate. Accidental overdose of imipramine can pose serious cardiac risks.

DDAVP administered intranasally in a dose of 10 to 40 micrograms before bed is effective in about 70% of children. The relapse rate is high if the drug is not tapered over a long period of time before it is discontinued. Side effects of DDAVP are infrequently reported. The risk of hyponatremia is low in otherwise healthy children, especially if they are fluid-restricted in the evening. As DDAVP is expensive, this drug is especially attractive for short-term therapy such as sleepovers and camp in children in whom it is effective.

Management of nocturnal enuresis is based on the knowledge that this condition naturally remits in most instances. The therapeutic approach should reassure the patient and child that there is no physical impairment, promote the self-esteem of the child, and employ safe treatment modalities.

URINARY INCONTINENCE

method of
E. ANN GORMLEY, M.D.
Dartmouth-Hitchcock Medical Center
Lebanon, New Hampshire

Urinary incontinence is a significant problem, affecting over 10 million Americans. Patients may not report incontinence because of embarrassment or misconceptions regarding treatment. Since incontinence is often treatable, it behooves the health care professional to identify patients who might benefit from treatment. The treatment varies, depending on the etiology, so the aim of evaluation is to identify the etiology.

ETIOLOGY

Urinary incontinence is generally the result of either bladder or urethral dysfunction (Table 1). Incontinence may also occur as a result of nonurologic causes, which are usually reversible when the underlying problem is treated (Table 2). More uncommon causes of incontinence include urinary fistulas or ectopic ureteral orifices.

Bladder Dysfunction

Bladder dysfunction causes urge or overflow incontinence. Urge incontinence occurs when the bladder pressure is sufficient to overcome the sphincter mechanism. Elevated bladder or detrusor pressure tends to open the bladder neck and urethra. An elevation in detrusor pressure may occur from intermittent bladder contractions (detrusor overactivity) or because of an incremental rise in pressure with increased bladder volume (poor compliance). Detrusor overactivity is termed detrusor instability, unless it is associated with a neurologic disease, when it is then called detrusor hyperreflexia. Detrusor instability is common in elderly people and may be associated with bladder outlet obstruction. Poor bladder compliance results from loss of the viscoelastic features of the bladder or because of a

TABLE 1. **Causes of Incontinence**

Bladder Dysfunction

1. Urge incontinence
   Detrusor overactivity
      Detrusor hyperreflexia
      Detrusor instability
   Poor compliance
2. Overflow incontinence

Urethral Dysfunction

3. Stress incontinence
   Anatomic (Type I or Type II SUI)
   Intrinsic sphincter deficiency (Type III SUI)

Abbreviation: SUI = stress urinary incontinence.
Modified from Raz S, Little NA, Juma S: Female urology. *In* Walsh PC, Retik AB, Stamey TA, Vaughan ED (eds): Campbell's Urology, 6th ed. Philadelphia, WB Saunders Co, 1992, p 2788.

TABLE 2. **Transient Causes of Incontinence (DIAPPERS)**

Cause	Comment
Delirium	Incontinence may be secondary to delirium (acute confusional state) and will often stop when delirium resolves.
Infection	Symptomatic infection may prevent a patient from reaching the toilet in time.
Atrophic vaginitis	Vaginitis may cause the same symptoms of an infection.
Pharmacologic	
Sedatives	Alcohol and long-acting benzodiazepines may cause confusion and secondary incontinence.
Diuretics	A brisk diuresis may overwhelm the bladder's capacity and cause uninhibited detrusor contractions, resulting in urge incontinence.
Anticholinergics	Many nonprescription and prescription medications have anticholinergic properties. Side effects of anticholinergics include urinary retention with associated frequency and overflow incontinence.
Alpha adrenergics	Tone in the bladder neck and proximal sphincter is increased by alpha-adrenergic agonists and can cause urinary retention, particularly in men with prostatism.
Alpha antagonists	Tone in the smooth muscles of the bladder neck and proximal sphincter is decreased with alpha-adrenergic antagonists. Women treated with these drugs for hypertension may develop or have an exacerbation of stress incontinence.
Psychological	Depression may be occasionally associated with incontinence.
Excessive urine production	Excessive intake, diabetes, hypercalcemia, congestive heart failure, and peripheral edema can all lead to polyuria, which can lead to incontinence.
Restricted mobility	Incontinence may be precipitated or aggravated if the patient cannot get to a toilet quickly enough.
Stool impaction	Patients with impacted stool can have urge or overflow urinary incontinence and may also have fecal incontinence.

Modified from Resnick MN: Urinary incontinence in the elderly. Med Grand Rounds 3:281–290, 1984. By permission of Plenum Publishing Corporation.

change in neural regulatory activity. The patient with urge incontinence may appreciate a sudden sensation to void but is then unable to suppress it fully. The amount of leakage is variable, depending on the patient's ability to suppress the contraction. Patients with urge incontinence will often have frequency and nocturia in addition to urgency and urge incontinence. They may also have nocturnal enuresis.

Overflow incontinence occurs at extreme bladder volumes or when the bladder volume reaches the limit of the bladder's viscoelastic properties. The loss of urine is driven by an elevation in detrusor pressure. Overflow incontinence is caused by obstruction or poor bladder contractility, resulting in incomplete bladder emptying. Obstruction is rare in women but can result from severe pelvic prolapse or following surgery for stress incontinence. Patients with overflow incontinence will complain of constant dribbling, and they may also describe extreme frequency.

Urethral Dysfunction

Urethral dysfunction, or stress incontinence, occurs because of either urethral hypermobility or intrinsic sphincter deficiency. Incontinence associated with either minimal or marked urethral hypermobility has been called Type I or Type II stress urinary incontinence. This type of incontinence has also been called anatomic incontinence, since the incontinence is due to malposition of the sphincter unit. Displacement of the proximal urethra below the level of the pelvic floor does not allow for the transmission of abdominal pressure that normally aids in closing the urethra. Anatomic stress urinary incontinence is the most common type of stress incontinence.

Intrinsic sphincter deficiency has been called Type III stress urinary incontinence, and it occurs most commonly after failure of one or more operations for stress incontinence. Other causes of intrinsic sphincter deficiency include myelodysplasia, trauma, and radiation. Ten percent of incontinent females will present with intrinsic sphincter deficiency de novo. The patient with stress incontinence will leak urine with any sudden increase in abdominal pressure. In patients with intrinsic sphincter deficiency, the increase in abdominal pressure required to cause leakage is small, and therefore patients may leak urine with minimal activity.

EVALUATION OF THE INCONTINENT PATIENT

The evaluation of the incontinent patient includes a history and physical and urodynamic examinations. The onset, frequency, severity, and pattern of incontinence should be sought, as well as any associated symptoms such as frequency, dysuria, urgency, or nocturia. Incontinence may be quantified by asking the patient if he or she wears a pad and how often the pad is changed. Obstructive symptoms, such as a feeling of incomplete emptying, hesitancy, straining, or weak stream, may coexist with incontinence, particularly in men and in female patients with previous bladder suspension, cystoceles, or poor detrusor contractility. Response to previous treatments, including drugs, should be noted. Female patients should be asked about symptoms of pelvic prolapse, such as recurrent urinary tract infection, a sensation of vaginal fullness or pressure, or noticing a bulge in the vagina. All incontinent patients should be asked about bowel function and neurologic symptoms. Response to previous treatments, including drugs, should be noted.

Important features of the history include previous gynecologic or urologic procedures, neurologic problems, and past medical problems. A list of the patient's current medications, including use of over-the-counter medications, should be obtained. A knowledge of the patient's social and sexual history may also be important.

Although the history may define the patient's problem, it may be misleading. Urge incontinence may be triggered by activities such as coughing, so that according to the patient's history, he or she would seem to have stress incontinence. A patient who complains only of urge incontinence may also have stress incontinence. Mixed incontinence is very common, with at least 65% of patients with stress incontinence having associated urgency or urge incontinence.

A complete physical examination is performed, with emphasis on a neurologic assessment and the abdominal, pelvic, and rectal examination. In women, the condition of the vaginal mucosa and the degree of urethral mobility is determined. Simple pelvic examination with the patient supine is sufficient to determine whether the urethra moves with straining or coughing. The degree of movement is not as important as the determination of whether movement occurs. The presence of associated vaginal prolapse should also be noted. A cystocele, enterocele, rectocele, or uterine prolapse may contribute to the patient's voiding problems and may have an impact on diagnosis and treatment.

In men, a digital rectal examination is performed to screen for cancer of the prostate and to assess grossly the size of the prostate. The size of the prostate has no relationship to the presence or absence of obstruction but is used to determine the surgical approach if obstruction is diagnosed. The rectal examination in both sexes includes evaluation of sphincter tone and perineal sensation. The bulbocavernosus reflex is elicited to test the integrity of the somatic sacral arc reflex. False-negative results, however, are not uncommon, particularly in women.

A urinalysis is performed to determine whether there is any evidence of hematuria, pyuria, glucosuria, or proteinuria. A urine specimen is sent for cytology if there is hematuria and/or irritative voiding symptoms. The urine is cultured if there is pyuria or bacteriuria. Infection should be treated prior to further investigations or interventions.

A postvoid residual (PVR) should be measured, either with pelvic ultrasound or directly with a catheter. A normal PVR is less than 50 mL, and a PVR in excess of 200 mL is abnormal. A significant PVR urine may reflect either bladder outlet obstruction or poor bladder contractility. The only way to distinguish outlet obstruction from poor contractility is with urodynamic testing.

Urodynamic testing is used to diagnose the patient's incontinence accurately. A cystometrogram assesses bladder behavior during filling. Normally, bladder pressure remains flat during filling. If bladder pressure rises incrementally during filling, a diagnosis of poor compliance is made. When the bladder pressure exceeds the urethral resistance, incontinence results. Sustained bladder pressure of more than 40 cm H_2O impairs ureteral function and ultimately causes upper tract deterioration. Poor bladder compliance in a female patient or in a patient with a neurogenic disorder makes the assessment of bladder neck and urethral function difficult, since the rise in bladder pressure may mimic stress incontinence. Poor compliance and poor urethral function may coexist.

The most common abnormality of bladder function is detrusor overactivity that causes urge incontinence. Detrusor overactivity is defined as the inability to suppress involuntary detrusor contractions during filling. A cystometrogram may fail to demonstrate any detrusor overactivity in a patient who has urge incontinence by history. If these patients undergo ambulatory urodynamic monitoring, involuntary detrusor contractions will be demonstrated to be the cause of their incontinence. Other patients with no history of urge incontinence will have uninhibited detrusor contractions during filling. Any patient with symptoms of urge incontinence by history should be presumed to have urge incontinence. The purpose of urodynamics is not to diagnose detrusor overactivity but to examine compliance, to diagnose stress incontinence, and to rule out obstruction as a cause of either overflow or urge incontinence.

The diagnosis of stress incontinence is best made with measurement of the abdominal pressure required to induce urinary loss (the abdominal leak point pressure), and/or with fluoroscopy. Stress incontinence is diagnosed if there is urethral loss of urine associated with an elevation of abdominal pressure. Abdominal leak point pressure is used to diagnose stress incontinence, since it is abdominal pressure that is the expulsive force in stress incontinence. Measuring the abdominal leak point pressure allows for quantification of the degree of urethral dysfunction. A normal urethra will not leak at any pressure, a mobile urethra will leak at high abdominal pressures (more than 90 cm H_2O), and a poorly functioning intrinsic sphincter will leak at low pressures (less than 60 cm H_2O).

Fluoroscopy may also be used to distinguish between urethral hypermobility and intrinsic sphincter deficiency that is manifest by an open fixed bladder neck at rest. Anatomic incontinence must be distinguished from intrinsic sphincter incontinence since the treatment for each is different.

TREATMENT OF URINARY INCONTINENCE

Urge Incontinence

Patients with urge incontinence need to understand that they leak urine because their bladders contract with little or no warning. The first line of treatment is timed voiding. Often, reminding patients to void every 1 to 2 hours during the day, before they get an urge to void, will result in staying dry. Other behavioral interventions, such as modification of fluid intake or bladder retraining, in which the patient attempts consciously to delay voiding and to increase the interval between voids, may also have a role.

Anticholinergics are the mainstay of medical therapy in achieving continence (Table 3). The side effects of anticholinergics include urinary retention, dry mouth, constipation, nausea, blurred vision, tachycardia, drowsiness, and confusion. They are contraindicated in patients with narrow-angle glaucoma. Anticholinergics are also used to decrease bladder pressure in patients with poor compliance. Anticholinergics are combined with clean intermittent catheterization in patients who have a significant PVR

TABLE 3. **Medical Treatment of Urge Incontinence**

Anticholinergics

Propantheline (Pro-Banthine)
    7.5 to 30 mg PO, three to five times daily

Anticholinergics/Smooth Muscle Relaxants

Oxybutynin (Ditropan)
    2.5 to 5 mg PO, one to three times daily
    May also be used intravesically
Hyoscyamine (Levsin)
    0.125 to 0.375 mg PO, two to four times daily
Dicyclomine hydrochloride (Bentyl)
    10 to 20 mg PO, three times daily

Smooth Muscle Relaxant

Flavoxate (Urispas)
    100 to 200 mg PO, three to four times daily

Anticholinergics/Alpha Agonist

Imipramine (Tofranil)
    10 to 25 mg, once to three times daily

prior to treatment or who develop retention while on anticholinergics.

Patients with intractable detrusor overactivity may require surgical intervention, consisting of bladder denervation or various forms of bladder augmentation.

The primary goal in treating the patient with poor compliance is to treat the high bladder pressure. Sustained bladder pressure of more than 40 cm H_2O impairs ureteral emptying. Complete bladder emptying with clean intermittent catheterization, combined with anticholinergics, will often lower bladder pressure to a safe range. A combination of anticholinergics and alpha agonists may be required in some patients. Bladder augmentation is required when medical management fails.

Overflow Incontinence

Overflow incontinence is treated by emptying the bladder. If the cause of overflow is obstruction, then relieving the obstruction should lead to improved emptying. Anatomic obstruction in men is from either urethral stricture disease or prostatic obstruction. Depending on the severity of urethral stricture disease, the patient may require a urethral dilatation, internal urethrotomy, or a urethroplasty. Prostatic obstruction may be treated in a variety of ways, but transurethral resection remains the "gold standard." If a woman is obstructed from previous surgery or from pelvic prolapse, she may benefit from a urethrolysis or surgical correction of the prolapse. Clean intermittent catheterization is an option in the obstructed patient who does not want or could not tolerate further surgery.

The patient with overflow incontinence secondary to poor detrusor contractility is best treated with clean intermittent catheterization.

Indwelling catheters are not an optimal treatment modality for incontinence. All patients with indwelling catheters will have infected urine that predisposes them to bladder calculi and ultimately to squamous cell carcinoma of the bladder. Any foreign object in the bladder can cause or exacerbate elevated bladder pressure that is associated with hydronephrosis, ureteral obstruction, renal stones, and eventually renal failure.

Stress Incontinence

The amount of incontinence and how it affects the patient will often determine the aggressiveness of treatment. The patient who is severely restricted because of severe leakage with minimal movement may not want to try medical therapy but may opt for surgical treatment, whereas the patient who leaks small amounts infrequently may choose conservative treatment. Pelvic floor exercises can improve anatomic stress urinary incontinence by augmenting closure of the external urethral sphincter and by preventing descent and rotation of the bladder neck and urethra. To benefit from the exercises, women must be taught to do them properly and frequently. The exercises are performed by contracting the levator ani muscles 25 to 200 times per day. Patients should be instructed to alternate sustained contractions (held for 10 seconds) with quick contractions. Any benefit should be seen within 2 to 3 months.

Women who have difficulties doing pelvic floor exercises may benefit from a variety of behavior modification techniques, including weighted vaginal cones or a perineometer. The vaginal cones are a series of tampon-shaped weights that are inserted for 15 minutes twice a day. The patient must contract her pelvic floor muscles in order to retain progressively heavier cones. A perineometer produces a signal as the pelvic floor muscles are contracted as a form of biofeedback.

Estrogen is useful in women with stress incontinence, particularly if they have evidence of atrophic vaginitis. Estrogen "plumps up" the connective tissue and vascular components of the periurethral tissue, allowing for greater coaptation of the tissue. Estrogen also enhances the alpha-agonist response. Conjugated estrogen (Premarin) may be administered orally, 0.3 to 1.25 mg daily, or by dermal patch. Estrogen cream used vaginally, 2 grams or less daily, or applied periurethrally is a good alternative to systemic estrogen. Alpha agonists such as phenylpropanolamine (Entex) or pseudoephedrine (Sudafed) in doses of 25 to 75 mg may be used for the treatment of stress incontinence. The bladder neck and proximal urethra have abundant alpha receptors. Activation of these receptors by alpha agonists leads to an increase in smooth muscle tone. The usual dose is twice daily, but some women who are incontinent with exercise may benefit from taking an alpha agonist 1 hour before exercise. Tricyclic antidepressants, such as imipramine (Tofranil),* have both alpha-agonist and anticholinergic properties. Imipramine is beneficial in patients with mixed (stress and urge) incontinence. The recommended dose is 10 to 25 mg, three times daily.

Surgical therapy for stress incontinence is indicated if medical therapy has not been successful or if the patient does not wish to try medical therapy. The type of surgical therapy depends on the diagnosis (Table 4). Patients who have anatomic stress inconti-

---

*Not FDA-approved for this indication.

TABLE 4. **Surgical Treatment for Stress Incontinence**

Anatomic
Kelly plication
Paravaginal repair
Retropubic suspensions
Burch
Marshall-Marchetti-Krantz
Transvaginal needle suspension (modified Pereyra)
Raz
Stamey
Intrinsic Sphincter Deficiency
Pubovaginal sling
Artificial sphincter
Submucosal injections (collagen, fat)

nence can benefit from a variety of surgical repairs that restore the bladder neck to its normal retropubic position and improve urethral support. Patients with intrinsic sphincter deficiency usually have a well-supported bladder neck. These patients require a procedure that will close or coapt the proximal urethra. A pubovaginal sling is the ideal procedure for the patient with both intrinsic sphincter deficiency and anatomic stress incontinence, as a sling will coapt the proximal urethra and restore the bladder neck to its normal location.

Stress and urge incontinence often coexist. Seventy percent of patients with combined incontinence (stress and urge) will be relieved of urge incontinence following a procedure for stress incontinence. Patients whose urge incontinence does not respond to anticholinergics preoperatively may have a good response to anticholinergics once their stress incontinence is treated.

EPIDIDYMITIS

method of
MARC S. COHEN, M.D.
University of Florida College of Medicine
Gainesville, Florida

Inflammation of the epididymis is usually unilateral and of relatively acute onset. It may affect males of any age, but the causative pathogens and predisposing factors are frequently correlated with the patient's age. The vast majority of epididymitis has been associated with infective etiologies. In prepubertal males, the most common organisms to be isolated are coliforms and *Pseudomonas* species, with underlying congenital, urologic, or neurogenic factors as predisposing causes. In men under the age of 35, epididymitis is usually associated with sexually transmitted pathogens and urethritis. In Western countries, nongonococcal organisms such as *Chlamydia trachomatis* predominate, but *Neisseria gonorrhoeae* and more rarely *Ureaplasma urealyticum* are also recognized. In epididymitis affecting men over 35 years of age, nonsexually transmitted organisms predominate (coliforms, *Pseudomonas* spp) and are more commonly associated with primary genitourinary tract infections or bacterial prostatitis. Infective etiologies secondary to primary infections elsewhere include tuberculosis, mumps, group B coxsackievirus, brucellosis, meningococcal infection, filariasis, and fungal infections. Cytomegalovirus, *Salmonella*, toxoplasmosis, and *Candida albicans* have also been documented in immune-suppressed patients with epididymitis. Urologic instrumentation, particularly chronic indwelling catheters, has been a recognized etiology in all age groups. Noninfectious etiologies include drugs (amiodarone [Cordarone]), vasculitis (Behçet's syndrome), and possibly sterile vasoepididymal reflux (frequently touted as a source of epididymitis but poorly documented or understood).

DIAGNOSIS

The diagnosis of epididymitis in an infant is usually associated with a history suggesting a congenital urinary tract abnormality. A history should include any knowledge of urinary tract infections, hematuria, voiding abnormalities, urinary tract pathology, or instrumentation. The majority of infants have urinalysis or urine culture evidence suggesting infection. In postpubertal or sexually active males, a sexual history to document recent (4- to 6-week) pathogen exposure should be obtained. Evidence of a urethral discharge should be sought. In the absence of an examinable discharge, a urethral swab frequently demonstrates microscopic evidence of a urethritis (Gram's stain is preferable). It is recommended that a culture for *gonorrhea* and a *chlamydial* smear or culture be obtained. In the absence of a sexual history or findings, a voiding history including dysuria or decreased force of stream or a history of previous urinary tract infection, prostatitis, prostatic enlargement, urethral stricture, urologic surgery, or urologic instrumentation can be helpful in establishing an etiology for epididymitis.

On physical examination, the scrotum of the involved testicle may be erythematous and/or edematous. The testicle is usually in a normal position. In early or less acute cases, the point of maximal tenderness is the most dependent portion of the epididymis (globus minor). The epididymis and vas deferens may be obviously or subtly enlarged when compared with the uninvolved, contralateral side. Involvement of the testicle (orchitis) in more advanced cases is not unusual. In many instances, there may be a reactive hydrocele of varying size associated with the inflammatory process, and this may make testicular examination difficult. Bilateral disease in an adult is unusual and could be suggestive of tuberculosis or another systemic etiology. A digital rectal examination in an adult may reveal findings that suggest or help confirm a prostatic source of the epididymitis.

When examining a patient with a painful scrotum or testicle, the physician must differentiate epididymitis from testicular torsion. In children, the incidence of torsion is much higher than that of epididymitis and should be assumed to be the diagnosis until proved otherwise. The use of color-flow Doppler ultrasonography or testicular radionucleotide scanning may be useful in distinguishing torsion from epididymitis. When doubt exists as to which entity is present, the use of these diagnostic aids should not delay definitive treatment (surgical exploration with detorsion, ipsilateral fixation or orchiectomy, contralateral fixation) when testicular torsion is suspected. In all males with an enlarged testicle, but particularly those between 18 and 40 years of age, the possibility of testicular tumor must be considered. Although usually not painful, testicular neoplasm should be considered in patients with testicular enlargement without evidence of infection or in whom testicular enlargement does not respond to antimicrobial and/or anti-inflammatory therapy. Trans-scrotal ultrasonography may be helpful in establishing a diagnosis. Serum tumor markers (human chorionic gonadotropin [beta subunit], alpha-fetoprotein) may also be definitive. When significant concern exists, surgical exploration via an inguinal approach with control of the spermatic cord blood supply is warranted.

TREATMENT

Empirical therapy for epididymitis should be initiated before culture results are available. Patients suspected of having epididymitis secondary to a sexually transmitted pathogen are treated in accordance with the Centers for Disease Control (CDC) protocols with ceftriaxone (Rocephin) 250 mg intramuscularly in a single dose and doxycycline (Vibramycin) 100 mg orally twice a day for 10 days. Alternatively, ofloxacin (Floxin) 300 mg orally twice a day for 10 days is suggested. Sexual partners should be contacted.

Patients with epididymitis related to urinary tract pathogens are best treated by broad-spectrum coverage. In hospitalized patients who require intravenous fluid support, sulfate gentamicin (Garamycin) 5 to 7 grams intravenously in a single dose is employed while awaiting culture results. Alternatively, ceftriaxone (Rocephin) 1 to 2 grams intravenously every 8 hours or cefotaxime (Claforan) 1 to 2 grams intravenously every 8 hours may be utilized. In nonhospitalized patients, particularly those with suspected prostatitis, the use of a fluoroquinolone (ciprofloxacin [Cipro] 500 mg orally twice a day, or ofloxacin [Floxin] 300 mg orally twice a day) provides excellent gram-negative coverage and develops good prostatic tissue antibiotic levels as well. Coverage is continued for at least 10 days in the case of uncomplicated epididymitis. Treatment is recommended for 30 to 50 days in epididymitis associated with prostatitis. Follow-up urinalysis and urine culture are recommended.

The use of bed rest and scrotal support and elevation, particularly in the early stages of infection, may afford some degree of symptomatic improvement. The use of analgesics and anti-inflammatory agents and ice can also be of benefit. Pain usually improves rapidly (24 to 48 hours) with antibiotic support, although epididymal and testicular enlargement may require weeks to resolve. Failure of standard therapy may suggest one of the more unusual pathogens noted previously or may herald abscess formation, which may be found on physical examination or repeat ultrasonographic evaluation. When an abscess is detected, incision and drainage are recommended. Epididymitis may also result in testicular infarction and may contribute in some cases to infertility.

PRIMARY GLOMERULOPATHIES

method of
FERNANDO G. COSIO, M.D., and
JUDITH A. BETTS, M.D.
The Ohio State University
Columbus, Ohio

The term "primary glomerulopathy" refers to a series of renal diseases that mainly affect the glomerulus and are not associated with evidence of a systemic disorder. Glomerular diseases may also be secondary to systemic disorders such as, for example, systemic lupus erythematosus. As our knowledge of glomerular diseases advances, the distinction between primary and secondary glomerulopathies is becoming blurry. For example, recent evidence indicates that some forms of primary glomerulopathy are secondary to systemic disorders that manifest themselves primarily in the kidney. Examples include the association of rapidly progressive glomerulonephritis with Wegener's granulomatosis and the association of membranous nephropathy with chronic systemic viral infections such as hepatitis B and C. Furthermore, the distinction between primary and secondary glomerulopathies cannot be made accurately by kidney biopsy because renal pathologic changes are frequently indistinguishable between both groups of disorders.

GENERAL CLINICAL FEATURES

The approach to patients with a suspected glomerular disease includes the following steps: (1) establish whether on clinical grounds the patient has a glomerular process; (2) search, by clinical and laboratory means, for evidence of a systemic disorder; (3) establish the precise type of glomerular disease as well as its prognosis (these latter determinations will require a kidney biopsy); and (4) based on the diagnosis and prognosis, decide on a form of therapy.

The only pathognomonic feature of a glomerular disease is the presence of proteinuria of more than 2.5 grams per 24 hours and consisting mainly of albumin. However, not all glomerular diseases cause this degree of proteinuria. Other manifestations commonly associated with glomerular diseases are best observed by examination of the urinary sediment, a critical test for evaluating all renal diseases. Thus, glomerular diseases are frequently associated with (1) hematuria, frequently with dysmorphic erythrocyte and/or red blood cell (RBC) casts in the urine sediment. The most characteristic form of dysmorphic RBC is the acanthocyte (familiarly called "RBC with 'Mickey Mouse ears' "), that is, an RBC deformed by herniation of the cell membrane. Although RBC casts are a characteristic feature of a glomerular process, they can be seen, rarely, in other forms of renal diseases not affecting the glomerulus; (2) white blood cell (WBC) casts; indeed, on several occasions we have observed an abundance of WBC casts in the absence of dysmorphic RBCs or RBC casts in patients with biopsy-proved acute glomerular processes, such as rapidly progressive glomerulonephritis.

Clinically, patients with glomerular diseases may present with the classic features of glomerulonephritis or nephrotic syndrome, or a combination of clinical features characteristic of glomerulonephritis and nephrotic syndrome. Furthermore, the routine use of screening urinalyses in general medical practice has increased the frequency of patients with glomerulopathies presenting with asymptomatic urinary findings, such as hematuria and/or proteinuria.

The classic clinical features of glomerulonephritis include sodium and water retention resulting in mild edema and severe hypertension; frequently elevated serum creatinine levels; and urine sediment demonstrating proteinuria, usually of less than 3 grams per 24 hours, and hematuria with RBC casts, dysmorphic RBCs, and WBC casts. An extreme variant of this presentation is exhibited by patients with rapidly progressive glomerulonephritis (RPGN) in whom the features of glomerulonephritis are associated with the rapid development (within weeks) of acute renal failure. Indeed, RPGN may be misdiagnosed as acute tubular necrosis unless the urine sediment is examined carefully.

In patients with nephrotic syndrome, the amount of protein in the urine is always in excess of 3.5 grams per 24 hours, and the proteinuria is associated with hypoalbuminemia (serum albumin less than 3 grams per dL), hyperlipidemia, lipiduria, and peripheral edema. Hypertension may or may not be present in these patients, and the findings in the urinary sediment may range from negative to hematuria and cast formation.

GENERAL THERAPEUTIC CONSIDERATIONS

Treatment of Edema

Peripheral edema may be one of the most debilitating features of a glomerular disease, particularly in patients with nephrotic syndrome. Patients are generally resistant to loop diuretics, such as furosemide (Lasix) or bumetanide (Bumex), most likely because in the urine these drugs are bound to albumin, which inhibits their effects on the loop of Henle. However, a patient's resistance to loop diuretics is unpredictable. Thus, we recommend starting treatment of edema with a relatively low dose of furosemide (Lasix) of 40 mg orally once or twice daily and increasing the dose as necessary. In some patients, doses of furosemide of between 100 and 400 mg or greater twice a day may be necessary. In patients who require doses of more than 160 mg twice daily, we recommend the addition of a second diuretic that affects urinary sodium excretion at a tubular segment different from the loop of Henle. For example, metolazone (Zaroxolyn), 5 mg once or twice a day taken together with furosemide, may result in a brisk diuresis. Spironolactone (Aldactone) may also be considered to enhance the effect of loop diuretics while preventing hypokalemia. However, spironolactone should be used with caution, if at all, in patients with a serum creatinine level of greater than 2 mg per dL.

In patients with edema, oral sodium chloride intake should be reduced to approximately 2 grams per 24 hours. Sodium intake may be monitored by measuring 24-hour urine sodium excretion, which closely reflects the sodium intake. Thus, patients with severe edema should maintain a sodium excretion of approximately 100 mEq per 24 hours (corresponding to approximately 2.2 grams of sodium chloride over the same 24 hours).

Treatment of Hypertension

The treatment of hypertension is critically important in the management of patients with glomerular diseases. The goal in patients with primary glomerulopathy is to maintain an average blood pressure of 125/75. Aside from its deleterious effects on the cardiovascular system, systemic hypertension increases the loss of protein in the urine, and several studies have also shown that systemic hypertension accelerates the progression of glomerular diseases. The treatment of hypertension in most patients should be initiated with diuretics. Indeed, it is difficult to control blood pressure in edematous patients unless a reduction in total body sodium and water content is achieved.

Once diuresis is achieved, we suggest an angiotensin-converting enzyme (ACE) inhibitor, such as captopril (Capoten) or enalapril (Vasotec). ACE inhibitors are the antihypertensive medication of choice because they have an antiproteinuric effect independent of their effect on blood pressure. In addition, ACE inhibitors may slow down the progression of glomerulopathies. ACE inhibitors are not potent antihypertensive medications, particularly in patients who are volume overloaded. However, the following points should be taken into account in deciding on the next choice of antihypertensive medication: Calcium channel blockers are quite effective antihypertensive drugs, although they may worsen peripheral edema. Other vasodilators such as hydralazine (Apresoline) and minoxidil (Loniten) should be avoided in edematous patients because they worsen sodium retention and peripheral edema.

Treatment of Hyperlipidemia

Hyperlipidemia is a frequent and severe complication of patients with glomerulopathies, and the elevation in serum lipids generally correlates with the degree of proteinuria. Thus, therapeutic measures that reduce proteinuria, such as blood pressure control, ACE inhibitors, and dietary protein restriction, will result in reductions in serum lipid levels. Reduction of dietary lipid intake is quite ineffective in controlling this form of secondary hyperlipidemia. Among the antilipid agents, hydroxymethylglutarate coenzyme A (HMG–CoA) reductase inhibitors may be used, and these drugs are reasonably well tolerated. However, in our experience, it is difficult to reduce serum cholesterol concentrations to less than 200 mg per dL in patients with glomerular diseases unless the degree of proteinuria is reduced.

Measures That Slow Progression of Glomerular Diseases

Recently completed national studies have shown that a reduction in dietary protein intake slows the progression of glomerular diseases and reduces urinary protein losses. We therefore recommend a reduction in dietary protein intake to 0.8 gram per kg per day. This amount should be supplemented with 1 gram of dietary protein per each gram of protein lost in the urine. The intake of high-protein diets in patients with proteinuria will result in increased urinary protein excretion and reduced protein synthesis by the liver, thus resulting in negative nitrogen balance. Thus, high-protein intake should be avoided in these patients.

MANAGEMENT OF SPECIFIC FORMS OF PRIMARY GLOMERULOPATHY

Minimal Change Disease

Clinical Features. Minimal change nephrotic syndrome (MCNS) is responsible for 80 to 90% of cases of nephrotic syndrome in children and 20 to 30% in adults. On light microscopy, MCNS glomeruli are seen within normal limits, and it is only by electron microscopy that one can appreciate abnormalities in glomerular epithelial cells, consisting of fusion of epithelial cell foot processes. Patients with MCNS present clinically with an acute onset of nephrotic syndrome infrequently associated with hypertension. The urine sediment most often demonstrates minimal or no abnormalities. In children with MCNS, the kidney function is well preserved. However, in adults, the development of acute nephrotic syndrome may be associated with acute renal failure with rapid elevations of serum creatinine, which may even reach the point of requiring hemodialysis. The glomerular findings and clinical presentation of MCNS may occur in patients treated with nonsteroidal anti-inflammatory drugs (NSAIDs). However, in these patients the urinary sediment demonstrates more white cells, casts, and RBC. By kidney biopsy, patients treated with NSAIDs demonstrated interstitial nephritis in association with MCNS. MCNS has been described in patients with Hodgkin's disease.

Management. MCNS is a disease most often responsive to glucocorticoids. In adults, the diagnosis of MCNS requires a kidney biopsy to rule out other primary glomerulopathies. Steroid treatment should be instituted promptly to avoid the development of acute renal failure and complications of the nephrotic syndrome, such as infections and thrombosis.

TREATMENT OF THE INITIAL EPISODE. In children, the accepted treatment protocol includes prednisone, 60 mg per m² per day for 6 weeks, followed by 40 mg per m² every other day for an additional 6 weeks, and then discontinuation of the therapy. In approximately 80% of children with MCNS, the nephrotic syndrome resolves within 2 weeks of therapy, and approximately 90% of patients respond within 4 weeks. In adults, the response may be slower, and fewer than 90% of the patients respond to steroids within 4 weeks. It is our practice to treat adults with MCNS with a modified course of prednisone consisting of 1 mg per kg per day (not to exceed 80 mg daily) for the first 4 weeks, followed by an abrupt change to 40 mg every other day for an additional 4 weeks. Many variations of these treatment regimens have been proposed in adults, but no randomized studies have tested their effectiveness. Approximately one-third of the patients remain disease-free after the initial course of treatment, one-third have occasional remissions of the disease, and one-third have frequent relapses or become steroid-dependent.

TREATMENT OF MCNS RELAPSES. We recommend treating the first relapse of MCNS as the initial episode. Subsequent relapses can be treated with a shortened course of prednisone consisting of 1 mg per kg daily (not to exceed 80 mg) until the urine is protein-free for a period of 3 days. Then, the patient can be switched to 40 mg of prednisone every other day for an additional 4 weeks. Subsequently, prednisone can be stopped.

TREATMENT OF FREQUENT RELAPSES. In patients with more than one relapse per year, following an 8-week course of steroid therapy as just described, we recommend reducing prednisone over a period of 2 months to determine whether a dose of less than 20 mg every other day can sustain the patient free of proteinuria. If so, that dose of prednisone should be maintained for an additional period of 6 months and then discontinued, to determine whether a relapse will occur. In patients in whom a 6-month course of prednisone fails to achieve a remission-free period and in patients who require more than 20 mg every other day of prednisone to remain disease-free, we recommend a course of alkylating agents. We routinely use cyclophosphamide (Cytoxan) at a dose of 1 to 1.5 mg per kg per day for a period of 8 weeks. Alternatively, chlorambucil (Leukeran),* at a dose of 0.1 to 0.15 mg per kg per day for 8 weeks, may be used. Side effects of these medications and preventive measures for these side effects are discussed later in the section on membranous nephropathy.

TREATMENT OF STEROID-DEPENDENT PATIENTS. Some patients with MCNS, despite treatment with alkylating agents, continue to have frequent relapses and/or continue to be dependent on high doses of prednisone to remain free of proteinuria. If they are dependent on a relatively low dose of glucocorticoid (20 to 30 mg every other day), one may consider the use of levamisole (Ergamisol),* (2.5 mg per kg every other day), an anthelmintic drug that, at least in children, is prednisone sparing and may induce remission of MCNS. It is suggested that the course of levamisole be continued for 6 to 12 months, and simultaneously the dose of prednisone be reduced progressively to reach the minimal dose required to maintain remission. There is increasing experience with the use of cyclosporine (CsA) (Sandimmune)* at a daily dose of less than 5 mg per kg to treat patients with MCNS. In these patients, CsA induces remission of MCNS in 80% of the patients, although relapses are frequent after discontinuation of the drug. Recent reports suggest that doses of CsA of 2 to 3 mg per kg per day for 6 months to 1 year may result in sustained remission of MCNS. However, CsA is expensive, and CsA nephrotoxicity causes permanent damage to the kidney, which initially may not be reflected by an elevation of the serum creatinine. Thus, in our opinion, CsA should be used only in patients with MCNS and debilitating nephrotic syndrome resistant to treatment with prednisone and alkylating agents.

Focal Segmental Glomerulosclerosis

Clinical Features. The diagnosis of focal segmental glomerulosclerosis (FSGS) is based on a kidney biopsy specimen demonstrating glomerular scarring (sclerosis) affecting only some glomeruli (focal lesions) and only some segments of the glomerular tuft (segmental lesion). However, the pathologic lesion of FSGS is nonspecific and may be idiopathic or secondary to other clinical entities. Idiopathic FSGS occurs most often in the second and third decades of life. The patients most frequently present with nephrotic-range proteinuria, frequently in association with hy-

---

*Not FDA-approved for this indication.

pertension, reduced renal function, and an active urinary sediment with dysmorphic RBC and RBC casts. FSGS may be secondary to (1) other glomerulopathies; (2) reduced renal mass—for example, in children FSGS may occur years after renal tissue resection for treatment of Wilms' tumors; (3) vesicoureteral reflux, perhaps due to a reduction of renal mass; and (4) hypertensive nephrosclerosis. The presence of FSGS in association with other glomerulopathies, such as, for example, IgA nephropathy or membranous glomerulonephritis, identifies patients with a poor renal prognosis. The treatment of secondary FSGS should address the primary condition that caused the FSGS.

Management. Idiopathic FSGS is often thought of as an evolutionary step of MCNS. Indeed, an occasional patient with MCNS may demonstrate FSGS on repeat kidney biopsy. However, in contrast to MCNS, FSGS is often resistant to treatment with glucocorticoids. Approximately 25% of patients with FSGS have a complete remission of their nephrotic syndrome following a course of prednisone similar to that described for MCNS. An additional 20 to 30% of patients experience partial remission of proteinuria when treated with prednisone. Prednisone-induced complete or partial remission of FSGS is associated with a good renal prognosis.

No laboratory, clinical, or pathologic characteristic identifies the patient who responds to prednisone. Thus, we strongly recommend a course of prednisone similar to that recommended for the first episode of MCNS in all patients with FSGS. However, we do not recommend prednisone in patients with FSGS, advanced renal insufficiency (serum creatinine greater than 2 mg per dL) *and* advanced interstitial scarring on kidney biopsy. The serum creatinine level should not be used alone to exclude patients for treatment, because an acutely elevated serum creatinine may be the result of the nephrotic syndrome and not reflect advanced histologic renal damage.

Patients who achieve complete remission with the first course of prednisone frequently relapse, and a second course is frequently associated with a partial remission. In patients who achieve partial remission after the first or second course of prednisone, we recommend prednisone on an every-other-day dosage (20 to 30 mg every other day) for a period of 6 months. This aggressive approach is based on the consistent observation in the literature that patients who achieve complete or partial remission of FSGS with treatment have a favorable renal prognosis.

For patients who fail to achieve a reduction of proteinuria with prednisone, we favor the use of cyclophosphamide (Cytoxan) (1 to 1.5 mg per kg per day) or chlorambucil* (0.1 to 0.15 mg per kg per day) for a period of 8 weeks. This therapy rarely achieves an acute reduction of proteinuria; however, in our experience, a progressive reduction in proteinuria for weeks or months after treatment with alkylating agents is frequently detected. The side effects of al-

kylating agents are discussed later in the section on membranous nephropathy.

In patients who do not respond to prednisone or alkylating agents, cyclosporine (CsA),* at doses of less than 5 mg per kg per day in adults, may be considered. CsA may cause a reduction in proteinuria and perhaps have beneficial effects on the evolution of FSGS when used for prolonged periods of time, such as 6 months to 1 year. However, it is clear that CsA may also produce progressive kidney damage with preglomerular vascular damage and progressive interstitial fibrosis, which may not be reflected by elevations of serum creatinine. Thus, we reserve and recommend the use of CsA only in those patients who have failed prednisone and alkylating agent therapy and in whom high-grade proteinuria results in disabling nephrotic syndrome.

Membranous Glomerulopathy

Clinical Features. Membranous glomerulonephropathy (MGN) is a disease resulting from the accumulation of antigen-antibody complexes in the subepithelial portion of the glomerular basement membrane (GBM). Those complexes give the characteristic morphologic feature, by immunofluorescence, of granular deposition of immunoglobulin and complement components in the GBM. By light microscopy, there is no glomerular proliferation, but the GBM appears thickened. The peak incidence of the disease is in the fourth or fifth decade of life, and MGN is the most frequent cause of nephrotic syndrome in adults. Approximately 80% of patients with MGN present with nephrotic syndrome and, characteristically, urinalysis demonstrates heavy proteinuria and mild or no hematuria. RBC casts are rare in the urine. Hypertension is more common in patients with advanced disease, that is, those with heavy proteinuria and elevated serum creatinine on presentation.

Management. When left untreated, 15 to 20% of patients with MGN reach end-stage renal failure within 5 years, and 30% of patients demonstrate a progressive deterioration of kidney function over the same time period. In untreated patients, 25% achieve a complete remission within 2 years, and an additional 25 to 30% of patients have a partial remission with significant reductions in proteinuria. The decision whether and how to treat patients with MGN is based on the following considerations:

IS THE MGN PRIMARY OR SECONDARY?

In as many as 20 to 40% of patients, MGN is secondary to a recognizable agent or disease, such as drugs (e.g., gold, penicillamine); infectious agents (e.g., hepatitis B, hepatitis C); collagen vascular diseases (e.g., systemic lupus erythematosus [SLE]); malignancies (mainly colon, breast, and lung); or other diseases (e.g., thyrotoxicosis, sickle cell anemia). Among those etiologies, the most common associations of MGN are with SLE and malignancy—the latter present in approximately 10% of MGN pa-

---

*Not FDA-approved for this indication.

*Not FDA-approved for this indication.

tients. Thus, it is our recommendation to rule out SLE and to perform a routine survey for the presence of malignancy in all patients with MGN. In patients with secondary MGN, treatment or removal of the primary cause resolves the glomerulopathy.

CLASSIFY THE PATIENT ACCORDING TO PROGNOSTIC FEATURES

TREATMENT OF PATIENTS WITH FAVORABLE PROGNOSTIC FEATURES. Favorable prognostic features include female gender, young, proteinuria of less than 5 grams per 24 hours, normal serum creatinine level on presentation, mild or no hypertension, and minimal interstitial fibrosis by kidney biopsy. We do not recommend the use of immunosuppressant medications in patients with favorable features because their prognosis, if left untreated, is quite good. In addition, there is no evidence that immunosuppressants improve the prognosis in patients with mild MGN. However, these patients should be treated aggressively with the general therapeutic measures described earlier. Furthermore, patients with favorable prognostic markers need to be followed closely, searching for evidence of progressive disease: increasing proteinuria, decreasing creatinine clearance, and so on. We have occasionally encountered patients with proteinuria ranging between 3 and 5 grams per 24 hours but with clinically disabling nephrotic syndrome. Those patients may have very low serum albumin levels and thus, although the total amount of protein in the urine is relatively low, that level of proteinuria indicates a very large clearance rate of protein. Those patients should be considered to have severe MGN.

TREATMENT OF PATIENTS WITH SEVERE MGN. We recommend immunosuppressive therapy for those patients who, on presentation or during subsequent follow-up, have unfavorable prognostic factors (opposite to those just described for patients with mild disease). However, we do not recommend the use of immunosuppressive medications in patients with severe MGN and advanced renal insufficiency—that is, those patients with a chronically elevated serum creatinine level above 3 mg per dL and especially if associated with severe interstitial fibrosis and glomerulosclerosis on kidney biopsy. The reason is that in patients with advanced renal insufficiency, immunosuppressive therapy has little chance of improving the prognosis of MGN, and the treatment may be associated with a higher rate of complications.

Initial studies recommended the use of alternate-day prednisone in a dose of 2 mg per kg. However, two subsequent well-conducted prospective studies demonstrated that prednisone alone does not significantly affect the course of MGN. More encouraging results have been obtained with the use of combinations of prednisone and cytotoxic agents. A prospective, randomized trial demonstrated the beneficial effects of a 6-month course of therapy structured as follows: During months 1, 3, and 5, patients receive methylprednisolone, 1 gram intravenously on the first 3 days of the month and then 0.4 mg per kg of oral prednisone daily. During months 2, 4, and 6, patients receive chlorambucil,* 0.2 mg per kg orally daily. During the chlorambucil months, the prednisone dose should be tapered to 10 to 20 mg orally daily, and the WBC count should be monitored weekly. If the WBC count drops to 5000 or less, the dose of chlorambucil should be reduced to approximately one-third or one-half the original dose.

In our practice, we have modified this treatment protocol as follows: During the first month of therapy, the patient receives oral prednisone, 1 mg per kg daily not to exceed 80 mg per day. The dose of oral prednisone is reduced to 20 mg daily during months 2, 4, and 6 and to 40 mg daily during months 3 and 5. During months 2, 4, and 6, the patient also receives 1 to 1.5 mg per kg of cyclophosphamide daily in the morning. In our experience, cyclophosphamide is associated with fewer gastrointestinal side effects than chlorambucil. During cyclophosphamide treatment, the WBC count should be monitored weekly.

The main concerns in regard to short-term cyclophosphamide treatment include (1) urinary bladder toxicity, which can be successfully prevented if the patient is instructed to take the cyclophosphamide always in the morning, maintain a high fluid intake (including extra glasses of water before going to bed), and empty the bladder frequently, particularly during the morning hours after taking the drug; and (2) gonadal dysfunction, which is more common in men than in women. Irreversible hypogonadism in men is usually associated with the use of at least 200 mg per kg total dose of cyclophosphamide and, indeed, that total dose should not be exceeded using the protocol recommended here.

Immunoglobulin A Nephropathy

Clinical Features. IgA nephropathy, also called "Berger's disease" and "benign recurrent hematuria," is the most common of the primary glomerulopathies in developed countries. The disease usually presents in childhood or young adulthood and males are typically affected earlier and more severely than females. IgA nephropathy is more common in Asians, whites, and Native Americans and is uncommon in African Americans. Patients with IgA nephropathy typically have chronic asymptomatic microscopic hematuria punctuated by episodes of gross hematuria. The gross hematuria is generally painless and characteristically occurs 1 to 3 days after the onset of a mucosal infection, such as an upper respiratory infection, gastroenteritis, or cystitis. Most patients have low-grade proteinuria, but as many as 20% develop the nephrotic syndrome. Rarely, a pattern of rapidly progressing glomerulonephritis with acute renal failure may occur. Additionally, most patients are hypertensive.

Light microscopy studies on renal biopsy tissue show an expanded mesangium with increased cellularity and matrix. The immunofluorescent pattern is diagnostic, with intense, coarsely granular deposits of IgA and frequently C3 in the mesangium.

---

*Not FDA-approved for this indication.

The pathogenesis of the disease is unclear. However, the evidence indicates that patients with IgA nephropathy produce excessive amounts of IgA in response to an antigenic stimulus. Consistent with this observation, serum IgA levels are elevated in about half the patients, and circulating immune complexes containing IgA are detectable as well. It is postulated that in these patients the production of IgA is stimulated by inflammation of the mucosa of the upper respiratory, gastrointestinal, or genitourinary tract, resulting in the formation of IgA-containing immune complexes that deposit in the glomerular mesangium.

Management. Before considering treatment, one must first rule out those diseases that cause a secondary IgA nephropathy by inciting an IgA response. Such disorders include Henoch-Schönlein purpura, chronic liver disease, inflammatory bowel disease, celiac disease, dermatitis herpetiformis, and IgA monoclonal gammopathy. In these secondary types of IgA nephropathy, the renal lesion often improves with treatment of the underlying disease. For primary IgA nephropathy, there are no proven effective immunosuppressive therapies.

Because the pathogenesis of the disease is that of chronic, ongoing antigenic stimulation, short-term trials of steroids, cytotoxic agents, and cyclosporine have not shown benefit. In contrast, recent studies suggest that long-term treatment (1 to 2 years) with alternate-day prednisone (15 to 20 mg orally) may delay the progression of the disease. This latter form of therapy should be considered in patients with IgA nephropathy and unfavorable prognostic markers (discussed later). In patients presenting with nephrotic syndrome, treatment with prednisone, following the regimen described for MCNS, should be considered because there is an association between IgA nephropathy and steroid-responsive MCNS. Phenytoin (Dilantin)* decreases serum IgA concentrations but does not affect the renal histology or the clinical course. Antiplatelet agents and anticoagulants have not shown benefit.

In addition to the general measures used in other glomerular diseases, some benefit may ensue from measures that minimize mucosal antigenic stimulation. "Low-antigen" diets may be useful. For example, it has been suggested that patients can minimize the intake of dietary proteins such as gluten, gliadin, and casein. However, the long-term benefit of these dietary manipulations is unproved. Consuming alcohol may increase the intestinal permeability to antigens; thus excess alcohol should be avoided.

In general, IgA nephropathy carries a good prognosis; however, approximately 20% of patients progress slowly to end-stage renal failure over a period of 10 to 20 years. Adverse prognostic signs include hypertension, heavy proteinuria, crescents or interstitial fibrosis on biopsy, and male gender. Mesangial IgA deposition may recur after renal transplantation but rarely causes significant clinical findings.

Membranoproliferative Glomerulonephritis

Clinical Features. The diagnosis of membranoproliferative glomerulonephritis (MPGN) is based on the pathologic findings of mesangial hypercellularity along with glomerular basement membrane thickening and splitting. MPGN is divided into two types based on the laboratory and biopsy findings. In Type I MPGN, the glomeruli demonstrate deposition of immune complexes mainly in the subendothelial aspect of the GBM. In Type II MPGN, large segments of the GBM are occupied by homogeneous electron-dense material, prompting the name "dense deposit disease." There is little evidence of immune complex formation. Some clinicians recognize a Type III MPGN with the pathologic characteristics of both Type I and Type II. MPGN accounts for about 5% of glomerulopathies, and the disease is more common in whites than in African Americans. Type II is seen more commonly in children and young adults.

Most patients present with asymptomatic subnephrotic proteinuria or microscopic hematuria. In 10 to 20% of cases, patients develop acute glomerulonephritis, particularly in Type II MPGN. Another 10 to 20% present with nephrotic-range proteinuria, together with an active urine sediment, especially Type I MPGN. Serum C3 levels are characteristically low in MPGN. Patients with Type II MPGN may have a serum IgG autoantibody, the C3 nephritic factor, that is directed against the alternative pathway C3 convertase. This autoantibody allows for uncontrolled consumption of complement, resulting in low serum C3 levels. It is unclear whether C3 nephritic factor participates in the pathogenesis of MPGN.

Management. Secondary causes of MPGN should be excluded, especially in Type I MPGN, since treatment in these patients should be directed at the underlying disease process. Common secondary causes include hepatitis B and C, bacterial endocarditis, visceral abscesses, mixed cryoglobulinemia, chronic thrombotic microangiopathies, immunoglobulin light-chain deposition disease, and hematologic malignancies. The treatment of primary MPGN is not very effective. It is controversial whether long-term oral steroid therapy (15 to 20 mg every other day for a year or more) is beneficial, especially in children. Cytotoxic agents are not effective. Treatment with anticoagulants such as warfarin (Coumadin)* and dipyridamole (Persantine)* shows a small benefit but is associated with significant bleeding complications. Antiplatelet therapy with aspirin alone or with dipyridamole may stabilize renal function in the short-term but provides no long-term benefit. Control of hypertension is important in all patients.

MPGN is slowly progressive, leading to end-stage renal failure in half the patients in 10 to 12 years.

---

*Not FDA-approved for this indication.

*Not FDA-approved for this indication.

The prognosis is worst in patients with heavier proteinuria or with MPGN Type II.

Rapidly Progressive Glomerulonephritis

Clinical Features. Rapidly progressive glomerulonephritis (RPGN) is a group of diseases characterized clinically by acute glomerulonephritis and rapidly declining renal function over weeks to months. Many secondary glomerular diseases, such as SLE, and primary glomerular diseases, such as Type II MPGN, can present as an RPGN. In idiopathic RPGN, light microscopic examination of kidney biopsy tissue most often demonstrates the presence of glomerular necrosis and proliferation of visceral epithelial cells forming crescents, thus the term "crescentic glomerulonephritis" that is often used interchangeably (and inappropriately) with the term RPGN.

By immunofluorescent microscopy, idiopathic RPGN can be subdivided into three types: (1) RPGN caused by autoantibodies directed to the GBM (20 to 25% of cases of idiopathic RPGN). Immunofluorescent microscopy demonstrates linear deposition of IgG along the GBM. Two-thirds of the patients have associated pulmonary hemorrhage (Goodpasture's syndrome). (2) RPGN associated with deposition of immune complexes in the glomerulus (20 to 25% of cases of idiopathic RPGN). Immunofluorescent microscopy demonstrates granular deposition of immunoglobulins and complement along the GBM and mesangium. (3) RPGN not associated with deposition of antibodies or immune complexes in the glomerulus, the so-called pauci-immune RPGN (50% of cases of idiopathic RPGN). Immunofluorescent microscopy demonstrates minimal or no deposition of immunoglobulins and complement. This type is associated with the presence of antineutrophil cytoplasmic antibodies (ANCA) in serum, and this disease should be considered as part of the group of ANCA-positive vasculitides that includes Wegener's granulomatosis and microscopic polyarteritis.

Patients with RPGN develop proteinuria, hematuria, hypertension, and acute renal failure. Occasionally the proteinuria is in the nephrotic range. Urinalysis often shows RBC casts and dysmorphic RBCs. In patients with Goodpasture's syndrome, the pulmonary manifestations most commonly precede the renal manifestations of the disease. Patients with immune complex–mediated RPGN frequently have systemic symptoms such as arthralgia and malaise. Finally, patients with pauci-immune RPGN may demonstrate, either on presentation or later, other manifestations of Wegener's granulomatosis such as pulmonary hemorrhage, nasal ulcerations, sinusitis, otitis, and arthritis. Thus, the evidence indicates that all three forms of idiopathic RPGN represent renal manifestations of systemic diseases.

Management. Secondary causes should be sought, particularly in RPGN secondary to immune complexes, because treatment must be directed to the underlying disease. Two principles dictate treatment: (1) The treatment should be started immediately—and indeed we frequently start therapy before the kidney biopsy results are available; and (2) it is critical to determine the type of RPGN by kidney biopsy. Prompt and aggressive immunosuppressive therapy is necessary to prevent rapid progression to irreversible renal failure. Therapy may be initiated with high-dose intravenous corticosteroid for the first 3 to 5 days: for example, methylprednisolone (Solu-Medrol), 15 mg per kg once daily. Others recommend oral high-dose prednisone (1 mg per kg in two divided doses daily). In patients with anti–GBM antibodies and/or Goodpasture's syndrome, the initial therapy should include plasmapheresis three to four times weekly for 2 weeks. It is important to initiate steroid and cytotoxic therapy while the patient is being treated with plasmapheresis.

Following the first few days of treatment, prednisone should be continued at a dose of 1 mg per kg daily for the first month and tapered during the second month (reducing the dose by 10 mg daily every week) until a dose of 30 mg daily is reached. Tapering should then continue with the aim of achieving 20 mg every other day by the fifth month of therapy. For all three forms of idiopathic RPGN, we recommend in addition cyclophosphamide (Cytoxan), 1 to 1.5 mg per kg daily for the first 8 weeks of therapy. In patients with Goodpasture's syndrome or systemic symptoms reminiscent of Wegener's granulomatosis, therapy with alkylating agents should continue for at least 6 months if the systemic symptoms continue. For patients who do not demonstrate symptomatic or laboratory evidence of active systemic disease, it is our practice to discontinue cyclophosphamide after 8 weeks of therapy. However, the patients need to be followed closely (every 2 weeks) to search for evidence of disease recurrence.

Without treatment, patients with RPGN progress to end-stage renal failure within months. However, 60 to 70% of patients respond to treatment, if initiated early. Poor prognostic signs include oliguric acute renal failure, advanced age, more than 75% of crescents on biopsy, and advanced renal insufficiency prior to treatment.

Other Types of Primary Glomerulopathy

Frequently, it is difficult to classify a kidney biopsy into one of the categories just described. This problem is most common in patients who, both clinically and pathologically, present with syndromes that are intermediate between those of MCNS and those of FSGS. The kidney biopsy findings in these patients often are described as *mesangial proliferative glomerulonephritis*, reflecting the presence of almost normal glomeruli with the exception of excessive numbers of mesangial cells. Critical in this diagnosis is the absence of glomerular sclerotic lesions. These pathologic characteristics can be associated with the presence of immunoglobulin M (IgM) in the mesangium *(IgM nephropathy)* or C1q in the same location *(C1q nephropathy)*. Clinically, we have not found these subclassifications particularly useful. Indeed, we recommend managing these patients following the guidelines described for MCNS and FSGS.

ACUTE PYELONEPHRITIS

method of
KEVIN A. AULT, M.D.
University of Kansas Medical Center
Kansas City, Kansas

Acute pyelonephritis is an infection of the renal parenchyma, and the source of the bacteria is usually an ascending infection from the lower urinary tract. The classic signs and symptoms of this disease include fever with shaking chills, flank pain, and associated costovertebral angle tenderness. Rebound, guarding, and tenderness may also be noted on abdominal examination of the affected side. Symptoms of lower tract infection, such as frequency, urgency, and dysuria, can also be present. The presentation may be less dramatic in the very young or elderly patient. Gastrointestinal manifestations include nausea, vomiting, and diarrhea. Gross hematuria may be a presenting complaint. Pyelonephritis is largely a disease of reproductive-age women with some important exceptions, and the differential diagnosis includes appendicitis, pelvic inflammatory disease, cholecystitis, lower lobe pneumonia, and nephrolithiasis. Perinephric abscess, a serious infection involving the soft tissue surrounding the kidney, can also have the same symptoms.

The microbiology of acute pyelonephritis is relatively straightforward. A great majority of infections are caused by a single microbe, usually an enteric gram-negative bacillus. *Escherichia coli* is by far the most common cause. Other important enteric bacteria include *Proteus, Enterobacter,* and *Klebsiella.* These bacteria colonize the perineal skin and gain access to the kidney by ascending infection. Specific virulence factors present in these bacteria allow them to adhere to the uroepithelium. *Staphylococcus saprophyticus* is an important gram-positive coccus that causes urinary tract infections in young women. *Enterococcus,* also gram-positive, can be found in elderly patients. In patients who have been recently hospitalized or examined with instruments, *Serratia* or *Pseudomonas* can be present. The reader should also be aware that tuberculosis may involve the kidney.

Urine culture of patients with pyelonephritis usually yields greater than 10^5 bacteria per mL of urine. Lesser colony counts do not exclude the possibility of significant urinary tract infection. Very high colony counts or multiple microorganisms usually indicate contamination. Careful instructions should be given to the patient regarding specimen collection. Catheterization of the bladder reliably yields specimens for culture. Suprapubic aspiration is a useful technique in pediatric patients. Microscopic examination of the urine shows pyuria and often hematuria. Perhaps the most useful and readily available test is a Gram stain of unspun urine. The presence of bacteria on the Gram stain reliably indicates the presence of 10^5 bacteria on quantitative urine culture.

Treatment

A wide variety of antibiotics are suitable choices for the treatment of pyelonephritis (Tables 1 and 2).

TABLE 1. **Dosages of Antibiotics for Adults**

Antibiotic Agent	Oral	Intravenous
Amoxicillin	500 mg tid	
Cefazolin (Ancef, Kefzol)		500 mg or 1 gm q 8 h
TMP–SMX (Bactrim, Septra)	One DS bid	3 mg/kg as trimethoprim, q 8 h
Ciprofloxacin (Cipro)	250 or 500 mg bid	400 mg q 12 h
Ofloxacin (Floxin)	200 to 400 mg bid	200–400 mg q 12 h
Aztreonam (Azactam)		500 mg or 1 gm q 12 h
Piperacillin (Pipracil)		2–4 gm q 6 hr
Ceftazidime (Fortaz, Tazicef)		1 gm q 12 h
Ticarcillin (Ticar)		3 gm q 6 h
Ticarcillin-potassium clavulanate (Timentin)		3.1 gm q 6 h
Gentamicin		1 mg/kg q 8 h

Abbreviations: TMP–SMX = trimethoprim-sulfamethoxazole; DS = double strength.

Several points should be made. First of all, stable patients without underlying disease or significant nausea and vomiting can be treated as outpatients with careful follow-up. All patients should be treated with 2 weeks of therapy, regardless of the selected agent. Shorter courses of therapy are useful in cystitis; however, a longer duration is required in upper tract infection. Also of note is the fact that 30% of *E. coli* produce beta-lactamase and are subsequently resistant to first-generation penicillins such as amoxicillin and ampicillin. For this reason, first-generation penicillins are not appropriate first-line therapy for pyelonephritis but may be useful after antibiotic sensitivities are available. Cefazolin (Ancef, Kefzol) can be used safely in adults, children, and pregnant women and consequently is a reasonable empirical choice for therapy. The possible exception to this is if gram-positive bacteria are identified on urine Gram stain. This finding could represent *Enterococcus,* and this species is resistant to cephalosporins. The combination of trimethoprim-sulfamethoxazole (TMP–SMX) (Bactrim, Septra) has long been useful for the therapy of urinary tract infections.

Fluoroquinolones such as ciprofloxacin (Cipro) or ofloxacin (Floxin) are useful newer agents and are

TABLE 2. **Dosages of Antibiotics for Children**

Antibiotic Agent	Oral	Intravenous
Amoxicillin	15 mg/kg q 8 h	
Ampicillin		25 mg/kg q 6 h
Cefotaxime (Claforan)		50 mg/kg q 8 h
Cefazolin (Ancef, Kefzol)		20 mg/kg q 8 h
Gentamicin		1–2 mg/kg q 8 h
TMP–SMX (Bactrim, Septra)	5 mg/kg as trimethoprim bid	3 mg/kg as trimethoprim q 8 h
Ticarcillin (Ticar)		50 mg/kg q 6 h

Abbreviation: TMP–SMX = trimethoprim-sulfamethoxazole.

available in both intravenous and oral formulations. Aztreonam (Azactam) is a unique monolactam antibiotic that is highly active against gram-negative bacteria but has no activity against gram-positive organisms. Advanced-generation cephalosporins and penicillins are also potential options. These agents include piperacillin (Pipracil), ceftazidime (Fortaz, Tazicef), and ticarcillin (Ticar). Timentin is the combination of ticarcillin with clavulanate, a beta-lactamase inhibitor. Gentamicin (Garamycin) can be added for additional gram-negative coverage. All the noted antibiotics are excreted by the kidneys, so renal function should be considered, especially when using nephrotoxic agents like aminoglycosides (e.g., gentamicin). Hospitalized patients should be treated with intravenous antibiotics until afebrile for 24 hours. Failure of a patient to respond to therapy should trigger a search for a resistant microorganism or a different diagnosis.

Several clinical settings will modify the work-up and antibiotic therapy. Urinary tract infection will often complicate kidney stones, so special consideration should be given to this item in the differential diagnosis. Staining of urine and/or intravenous pyelogram may be useful. *Proteus* species have especially been associated with nephrolithiasis, and an alkaline pH may be observed on urinalysis. In cases of pyelonephritis with significant complicating medical or urologic conditions, antibiotic therapy should be modified. Examples of such problems include urosepsis, recent hospitalization with instrumentation or surgery of the urinary tract, diabetes, or chronic indwelling Foley catheter. In such cases, broad coverage of potential pathogens should be ensured with an advanced-generation cephalosporin or penicillin with gentamicin. Another special consideration is that patients with human immunodeficiency virus/ acquired immunodeficiency syndrome (HIV/AIDS) appear to be at higher risk of urinary tract infection.

Most isolated cases of pyelonephritis in reproductive-age women do not require further urologic or radiographic studies. However, in women with recurrent disease such studies should be considered. A renal ultrasound and/or an intravenous pyelogram may reveal obstruction or stones in the urinary tract. Children of both sexes should be evaluated with a voiding cystogram to look for vesicoureteral reflux. In men, one would expect a low incidence of pyelonephritis, and imaging studies may reveal underlying abnormalities. Another special circumstance deserves mention: Pyelonephritis is one of the most common infectious complications of pregnancy, and 10% of women with this infection will develop adult respiratory distress syndrome. Asymptomatic bacteriuria is the cause of most cases of pyelonephritis during pregnancy. All pregnant women should be screened with a urine culture early in pregnancy for asymptomatic bacteriuria.

TRAUMA TO THE GENITOURINARY TRACT

method of
WILLIAM GRAHAM GUERRIERO, M.D.
Baylor College of Medicine
Houston, Texas

PRESENTATION AND MECHANISM OF GENITOURINARY INJURY

Genitourinary injury is not usually suspected unless a patient has gross hematuria, but injury can be present without hematuria. Urologic injuries are frequently associated with more life-threatening emergencies and may be overlooked in the initial evaluation. Injury to the genitourinary system should be suspected with any forceful trauma to the body. One should be particularly suspicious when the patient has fallen from a height, been thrown from a moving vehicle, or suffered a crushing injury to the abdomen. Sudden acceleration or deceleration of the body, in addition to causing crush injury to the kidney, may produce intimal disruption of the renal artery or avulsion of the ureter at the ureteropelvic junction. A steering wheel hitting the lower abdomen may produce an intraperitoneal bladder rupture. Fracture of the pelvis is frequently associated with laceration of the bladder, extraperitoneal extravasation of urine from the bladder, or posterior urethral disruption. Injury to the kidney or other portion of the genitourinary system may occur with any penetrating injury of the abdomen, such as gunshot or stab wound, regardless of whether the injury is in the upper or lower portion of the abdomen. Penetrating injuries of the chest can also be associated with injury to the kidney, since the chest cage overlies the outline of the kidney on both the right and left sides.

Initial Evaluation

Initial evaluation of patients with suspected genitourinary injury consists of inspection and palpation of the abdomen and genitalia. The abdomen is palpated for a mass suggestive of a hematoma surrounding the kidney. Unfortunately, a mass in the retroperitoneum that is palpable through the abdomen of a patient suffering injury to the kidney is rarely found, except in those cases with massive rupture of the kidney, aorta, or inferior vena cava. It is more common to see ecchymosis beneath the skin of the flank. The presence of fractures of the lower ribs may suggest that renal injury is present. Fracture of the bony pelvis with associated "absence of the prostate" on rectal examination or an inability to easily pass a Foley catheter into the bladder suggests a posterior urethral disruption. If blood is seen at the urinary meatus, no instrumentation of the urethra should be carried out until the patient has had a urethrogram to demonstrate that urethral injury is not present.

A sample of urine should be obtained from all patients with trauma to determine whether the patient has hematuria. Once the patient has been stabilized, 60 ml of high-density contrast media may be injected into the venous system to obtain an intravenous pyelogram (IVP) in those patients who arrive at the emergency room with microhematuria with shock or gross hematuria alone, or in those patients who have suffered significant blunt trauma to the abdomen or an acceleration-deceleration injury. Currently, it is common to skip the IVP and proceed directly to a computed tomography (CT) scan with contrast in those patients who have suffered blunt trauma. CT visualizes all portions of the abdomen and provides much more information than intravenous pyelography, with better definition of renal injury if present. An adequate IVP, one that visualizes intact renal outlines bilaterally and is associated with prompt excretion of dye into the entire urinary collecting system with visualization of the calices, infundibula, pelvis, and ureters, is satisfactory in most patients. The quality of films obtained by IVP may be enhanced by nephrotomography. The ureters frequently are not well seen, even with a good-quality IVP, as the patient is unprepped and has often had a meal. With blunt trauma, this is not of great consequence, as the ureter is rarely injured with blunt trauma to the abdomen. Patients may have significant urologic injury even with reasonably good IVPs, so if clinical suspicion remains, other imaging studies may be needed.

The extent of renal injury cannot be predicted by the amount of hematuria alone. A number of studies have suggested that when evaluating patients with suspected renal injury, if shock is not present, microhematuria is rarely associated with major renal injury, and usually in these circumstances the patient may be observed without an imaging study of the kidneys with little risk of a missed major renal injury. Patients with shock and microhematuria should be imaged as soon as they are stabilized. Those patients with gross hematuria must have an imaging study of the upper urinary tract. It should also be remembered that patients may have major injuries to the genitourinary system, including ureteral or vascular avulsion, with only microhematuria or no hematuria at all, although this situation is rare. Approximately 60% of patients with blunt renal trauma will have hematuria, and 70 to 80% of those with penetrating injuries will be found to have blood in the urine.

When lower abdominal trauma has occurred and the patient has hematuria, a cystogram is necessary to be sure that the patient has an intact urinary bladder. If the bladder is very distended on IVP and the films are of good quality, one might decide to skip the cystogram. However, if pelvic fracture is present or questionable extravasation is seen near the bladder, a cystogram should be performed to be sure that no bladder rupture has occurred. The cystogram should be done with just enough force to distend the bladder past its normal capacity and should follow the IVP or CT scan. A urethrogram is indicated in those patients who have blood at the urethral meatus or in whom laceration of the anterior or posterior urethra is suspected for any reason. A urethrogram should be obtained prior to the cystogram, and the dye should be injected as slowly as possible to prevent extravasation of dye into urethral veins, which is confusing when one is looking for extravasation. There is no need to mix dense contrast media with K-Y Jelly as has been done in the past, as long as the injection is performed slowly.

Anterior penetrating injury to the abdomen usually necessitates surgical exploration. An exception is in those patients with posterior or flank stab wounds and negative peritoneal lavage. An adequate imaging study must be obtained in patients with penetrating abdominal trauma who are not explored and should be performed in those who are explored to rule out injury to the genitourinary system and demonstrate functioning kidneys. Complete visualization of the urinary tract is frequently not possible in these cases, as ileus is present and the patient may be uncooperative or in shock. One should, at the very least, identify that the patient has two functioning kidneys and note the presence or absence of extravasation prior to going to the operating room. In cases of posterior and flank stab wounds, the surgeon should be concerned that the patient does not have significant persistent hematoma and has an intact renal outline, since these patients may not undergo surgical exploration and are treated expectantly. Cystogram and urethrogram may be necessary in cases of penetrating trauma to the lower abdomen and genitalia. The site of entrance of gunshot and stab wounds should be marked with a metal clip prior to radiographic examination to determine the path of the bullet or knife. One should note whether the bullet has passed completely through the body, as this would suggest injury from a high-velocity weapon. A large bullet on radiograph does not necessarily correlate with significant renal damage; in fact, the presence of the bullet is reassuring and suggests the patient may have a low-velocity injury that will probably require minimal débridement or repair.

Renal Pedicle Injury

The most difficult diagnostic problem in urologic trauma is prompt recognition of renal pedicle injury. A high degree of suspicion is necessary. Anyone sustaining an acceleration or deceleration injury or forceful trauma to the abdomen or chest should have an imaging study with intravenous (IV) contrast to rule out renal pedicle injury. The presence of an apparent solitary kidney or lack of function of a renal segment should be an indication for immediate arteriography. CT scan provides almost as much information as one obtains from arteriography, particularly when the renal artery is injured near its take-off, and is the only study for small children, but segmental renal artery injury usually is best evaluated with arteriography. There is no place for cystoscopy, retrograde pyelography, or delayed IVP films in these patients who failed to visualize, since successful revascularization generally depends on minimal delay after recognition of injury. In most cases, prolonged warm ischemia will prevent salvage of patients with intimal disruption of the renal artery. Postinjury hypertension is common and may be found years after injury.

Other Studies for Renal Trauma

Interest has developed for the use of CT scan for blunt and penetrating renal trauma. CT scan is the most useful test for children or in patients presenting late after renal trauma. Arteriography is rapidly being supplanted by dynamic CT for evaluation of patients with acute blunt renal trauma, when major injury of the kidney is suspected but not proved by IVP. Ultrasound examinations are useful for determining the extent of hematoma present with a renal injury and in following the patient, but they are not particularly helpful in defining the extent of injury of the kidney or other portion of the genitourinary tract. Magnetic resonance imaging (MRI) is not particularly helpful in evaluating patients with renal injury but may provide a good definition when pelvic injury has occurred.

Associated Injuries

Sixty percent of patients with blunt renal trauma and major renal injury will have associated injuries to organs in the abdomen, necessitating abdominal exploration. Ninety percent of patients with penetrating renal injuries will have other associated nongenitourinary injuries, most of which will necessitate abdominal exploration.

CLASSIFICATION OF RENAL TRAUMA

Patients rarely die from renal injury, but renal injury may produce shock or serious long-term sequelae, such as hypertension or abscess formation, or it may produce a urinoma necessitating surgical drainage. With bilateral renal injury or injury to a solitary kidney, the patient may lose significant renal function. It is helpful to separate renal injuries into major and minor categories. Major injuries represent a significant threat to the patient's life or subsequent health, and a minor injury, if untreated, will not result in serious complication for the patient. Minor injuries include renal contusion, disruption of a renal fornix, and shallow cortical laceration. Major injuries include deep cortical lacerations into the urinary collecting system, shattered kidneys, and renal pedicle injury or avulsion injuries of the collecting system.

Not all injuries to the kidney need to be treated surgically. Eighty-five percent fall in the category that one would label as "minor." Only 15% of injuries are major and may require surgical exploration; 5% or less need immediate surgical exploration. Ten percent of renal injuries may need surgical exploration at some time, but a high percentage of these patients may be treated with observation alone. This is possible because the kidney is surrounded by two layers of fascia that contain significant hemorrhage.

TREATMENT

Whether the patient should be treated conservatively or surgically for major renal injuries is hotly debated. Most cases may be observed without surgical treatment. If significant disruption of cortical renal fragments or hemorrhage of greater than 500 ml is found on imaging studies, surgery should be performed at the earliest opportunity if one feels that a surgical procedure would salvage a significant portion of the kidney's renal function, i.e., if one could perform a partial nephrectomy or suture a laceration. If the patient's kidney is shattered, however, and the patient is stable, the only possible surgical procedure may be a nephrectomy. Close observation is desirable in these cases. If the patient has fragments contained by the renal capsule, even if the laceration is deep, the injury may heal with observation alone.

Penetrating injury to the kidney should be explored and débrided, all bleeders ligated, and the defect patched with a pedicle of live fat or simple suture closure. If a low-velocity gunshot wound of the kidney is present but is not actively bleeding, fat is placed in the defect to help prevent hemorrhage. Few cases require partial nephrectomy. All injuries to the kidney should be adequately drained, and if there is concomitant injury to the pancreas or duodenum, one should be liberal with the use of nephrostomy and stent. In addition, attempts should be made to drain the pancreas or duodenum away from the site of renal injury. Only a minimal amount of bed rest is necessary in most cases of renal contusion, but in some cases persistent, significant hematuria may continue. In those patients, bed rest should be continued until the hematuria clears.

Persistent hematuria should make one suspicious that an arteriovenous communication may be present, particularly with penetrating trauma. An arteriogram of the kidneys is indicated. In patients with renal pedicle injury, time is critical. After adequate imaging of the kidney, exploration and attempts to revascularize the kidney should be carried out if the renal injury has existed for less than 24 hours, particularly when there is bilateral nonvisualization of the kidneys. With life-threatening associated injuries, a nephrectomy may sometimes be necessary when the kidney has been lost to arterial occlusion, but in many cases the kidney can just be watched and no therapy offered unless abdominal exploration is necessary.

Options for repair of renal pedicle injury include bypass graft with autologous vein, artery, or synthetic material; simple closure of intimal tears, excision, and reanastomosis; or even autotransplantation. Consider the patient's condition regarding renal ischemia time and ease of repair when making any decision regarding repair versus nephrectomy.

Late Sequelae of Renal Injury

Hypertension may occur at any time up to 10 years after a patient has suffered renal injury. Hypertension is rarely present in patients with minor renal injuries but may occur as a result of constriction of the kidney if the patient has a hematoma of greater than 500 ml or caused by renal pedicle injury, segmental vascular injury, or patchy necrosis of the kidney. The patient may be hypertensive if arteriovenous fistula is present.

Ureteral Injuries

Blunt trauma rarely causes ureteral injury. However, disruption of the ureteropelvic junction or avulsion of the renal collecting system may rarely occur. Penetrating injury of the renal pelvis or ureter is common. Diagnosis is usually made by demonstrating extravasation on IVP, which is present in 90% of cases. Renal pelvic lacerations are major injuries and should be repaired with 4-0 chromic or polyglycolic acid suture material and adequately drained. Stents and nephrostomy tubes may be used as necessary to allow for secondary healing if the patient has an associated pancreatic, duodenal, or left colon injury. Injuries to the right colon or small bowel do not require stenting or diversion for repair, but stenting may be helpful if the repair has to be done under tension. If there is any question of vascular integrity of the ureter, stenting and diversion should be performed. In most cases, however, simple excision of the injured segment with spatulation and anastomosis without a stent or nephrostomy tube is the rule. One should make every effort to débride injured tissue and be sure that adequate blood supply is present at the severed ends of the ureter. The anastomosis should be performed without tension. Wrapping omentum around the ureter after anastomosis may bring blood supply to the ureter and help prevent subsequent stricture.

Iatrogenic injury of the ureter is quite common, particularly in the lower abdomen during gynecologic surgery. Here, as with renal injury, a high degree of suspicion is necessary to confirm the diagnosis early in the postoperative period or in the operating room. The earlier the injury is discovered, the more likely the repair will be successful. This is true in wounds of external violence as well as iatrogenic injury. Injury of the ureter deep in the pelvis is usually best handled with reimplantation of the ureter into the bladder by either a simple reimplant or with an associated bladder hitch or bladder flap. Transureteroureterostomy may be the procedure of choice in the midabdomen or upper pelvis if extensive loss of the ureter has occurred. Most injuries may be repaired with simple reanastomosis. Dismembered pyeloplasty may be necessary if the patient has a disrupted ureteropelvic junction, or if the injury is a penetrating one in the area of the ureteropelvic junction. In some cases, autotransplantation may be necessary. Replacement of the ureter with an ileal segment is usually not necessary.

Bladder injury should be suspected in patients who have pelvic trauma, as 85% of ruptures of the bladder are extraperitoneal and secondary to penetration of the anterior wall of the bladder with a spicule of bone. Fifteen percent of injuries to the bladder are intraperitoneal bladder ruptures. Diagnosis of bladder rupture is by cystogram (both filling and drainage films should be taken). Most bladder injuries can be sutured using 2-0 chromic catgut or polyglycolic acid suture in two layers after adequate débridement of devitalized tissue. The bladder may be contused as well as ruptured, and significant hematuria can occur from bladder contusion with the bladder intact. Simple drainage is indicated in these cases until the hematuria clears.

Urethral Injuries

Anterior urethral injury is diagnosed by urethrogram. Patients usually have blood at the meatus, and catheterization should not be attempted until the urethrogram has confirmed that the urethra is intact. In minor injuries to the anterior urethra, simple drainage of the bladder with a stent in the urethra is all that is necessary to permit healing. Significant injury to the urethra with disruption of more than one-third of the urethral wall should be repaired at the time it is discovered. Injury to the urethra may occur from penetrating trauma, straddle injury, or, in men, fracture of the penis during erection.

Posterior urethral disruption occurs at the junction of the prostate and membranous urethra, or stretching of the urethra may result in rupture just below the membranous diaphragm. These cases are almost always associated with pelvic fracture. Pelvic bleeding causes elevation of the bladder and prostate into the true pelvis. This may be suspected by rectal examination and by IVP. A retrograde urethrogram should be performed to confirm injury. Once posterior

disruption is noted, if there has not been significant displacement of the pubic arch and there is some hope that the bladder and prostate will settle back into the pelvis with time, the patient may be treated by a suprapubic catheter placed into the bladder without a Penrose drain and with no further instrumentation of the urethra. The patient should be re-evaluated 4 to 6 weeks after the injury; if incomplete stricture is present, visual urethrotomy should be attempted or the patient observed with suprapubic catheter drainage for a further period of 2 to 3 months before definitive repair. At that time, a reconstructive procedure of the urethra, which may be as simple as an end-to-end repair or as complicated as a transpubic urethroplasty, should be performed.

Most cases of complete posterior urethral disruption must be managed with exploration and repair 3 to 4 months following the injury. In some cases, the patient is discovered to have a patent urethra at the time of bladder filling and urethrogram at 6 weeks. Removal of the suprapubic catheter should then occur, and no further treatment will be necessary. Minor strictures of the urethra may be treated with dilatation or visual urethrotomy.

At times, injury to the posterior urethra is complex. Displaced pubic fragments must then be elevated and returned to a more normal location so that the bladder and prostate will settle into the pelvis properly. In some cases, placement of a catheter into the bladder is necessary. The use of sutures to pull the bladder and prostate into the deep pelvis may be helpful. Primary repair of posterior urethral disruption in men usually should be discouraged unless the surgeon has great experience with this injury.

Injury to the female urethra is uncommon; when seen, it usually occurs at the bladder neck. Shearing forces avulse the urethra at that point. Injury to the vagina is also commonly associated with this injury. These injuries are usually simple to repair at the time of the initial trauma rather than after 3 to 4 months. When the female urethra is avulsed from the bladder, the bladder rotates anteriorly, and the bladder neck opening is then located in a position 60 to 90 degrees from the access of the urethra, making catheterization impossible.

Injuries to the Genitalia

Penile injury may occur from entrapment by zippers or circular rings (particularly ball bearings) or avulsion by moving machinery. Zipper injuries can be handled by removing the zipper head and parting the zipper. Circular objects that cause paraphimosis sometimes can be removed with adequate lubrication, but these frequently require the old trick of using a string to compress the edema present in the glans penis and removing the object as one would a ring on a finger. Avulsion injuries are more complicated, and a combination of flaps or grafts may be necessary. When penile skin is avulsed, the patient will require immediate skin grafting. Any skin in the distal portion of the penis should be sacrificed, as this will form an encircling, unsightly ring if it is not removed at the time of initial repair. Fracture of the corpus cavernosum of the penis may occur in a patient whose penis is bent during sexual intercourse. Ninety percent of these injuries will heal without surgical treatment, but late surgical treatment may be necessary to correct the deformity.

Avulsion injuries of the scrotum may be frightening when first seen, but if any scrotal skin is present, it can often be stretched to close the defect. If left alone, the scrotal skin will regenerate around the testis. If no scrotal skin is present and the testis is exposed, it may be placed into a thigh pouch and the wound subsequently closed with an abdominal flap or allowed to regenerate, with subsequent placement of the testis into the healed scrotum.

Testis Injuries

Rupture of the tunica albuginea is unusual. The testis may be penetrated as a result of a gunshot wound, lacerated severely with a knife, or ruptured secondary to compression injury. The testis should be explored and the defect closed, attempting to salvage as much testicle as possible. Orchiectomy may be necessary if there is a severe injury.

BENIGN PROSTATIC HYPERPLASIA

method of
WILLIAM D. BELVILLE, M.D.
The University of Michigan Medical Center
Ann Arbor, Michigan

Benign prostatic hyperplasia (BPH) is a very common, directly age-related histologic finding. BPH histopathologic lesions with prostatic enlargement are somewhat less common, occurring in later years. BPH as a cause for bona fide obstructive uropathy is, in contrast, most uncommon. The long-held belief that prostatic enlargement with so-called prostatic symptoms often leads to renal failure if untreated is questionable. In other words, BPH does not equal obstructive uropathy nor is it likely in most cases to inexorably produce a significant clinical problem if left untreated. BPH is not premalignant but commonly coexists with histologic prostatic carcinoma.

PATHOPHYSIOLOGY

BPH is a glandular and stromal proliferation that begins in the periurethral tissue and expands to compress the prostatic capsule and urethra. Current theory suggests that the sheer bulk of the hyperplasia produces a "static" dysfunction while the smooth muscle of the stroma and capsule contributes a "dynamic" component. This smooth muscle is rich in $alpha_1$ receptors. The presence of these alpha receptors allows a blocker-type medical approach to the dynamic component, whereas antiandrogens target the tissue bulk because of the androgen dependence of prostate tissue.

These events are thought to cause obstruction at the bladder neck necessitating high-pressure voiding, which then leads to poor emptying and subsequent loss of the bladder's ability to store urine at low pressure. The process then continues and affects the ureteral pump mechanism at the ureteral vesicle junction with subsequent ureteral failure and hydroureteronephrosis. Today, such hydroureteronephrosis from bulky BPH is most uncommon.

SYMPTOMS

Much attention has recently been given to lower urinary tract symptoms that historically have been called "prostatic." Elaborate symptom score schemas have been developed in an attempt to objectively quantify these subjective complaints. Clinically these symptoms are characterized as "obstructive" or "irritative" (Table 1).

These symptoms can be ascertained by questioning the patient in lay language (Table 2). This method has recently been recommended to assist in the evaluation of the patient with BPH. Although these symptoms and their additive symptom "score" are in everyday use in both clinical practice and research, studies have shown similar symptoms in *aged-matched* women. Such observations place the aging bladder as a key factor in the production of these symptoms. Furthermore, several studies have shown marked improvement in the "symptoms of BPH" by observation alone, whereas others have shown significant placebo effect. Lastly, nocturia, one of the most bothersome symptoms of both sexes, often has little to do with the physiology of micturition but rather the redistribution of bodily fluids when a person is supine.

Although nocturia is often a very bothersome symptom, many elderly men find the irritative symptoms of urgency and urge incontinence the most troublesome. Irritative symptoms without infection should alert the practitioner to rule out bladder carcinoma. Similarly, hematuria, with or without symptoms, requires urologic evaluation.

In addition to serious lower tract abnormality, irritative symptoms are often simply the somatization of stress. Intermittent urinary frequency and urgency without concomitant nocturia usually is not associated with serious organic lesions. Organic lower urinary tract abnormality usually produces symptoms throughout the 24-hour day.

DIAGNOSIS

The diagnosis of BPH can be easily made with a history and a physical examination. A middle-age or older man with symmetrical prostatic enlargement without nodules or induration and a normal urinalysis likely has BPH. The use of prostate ultrasound, although useful for the determination of the exact prostatic volume, is unnecessary in routine cases. Serum prostate-specific antigen (PSA) levels may be helpful to exclude prostatitis or carcinoma, but large overlaps between groups are the rule. Approximately 25% of men with BPH have an elevated

TABLE 1. **Lower Tract Urinary Symptoms**

Obstructive	Irritative
Hesitancy	Dysuria
Straining	Frequency
Slow stream	Urgency
Intermittency	Nocturia
Incomplete emptying	Urge incontinence
Urinary retention	
Postvoid dribbling	

TABLE 2. **AUA Symptom Index**

Questions to be Answered	Not at All	Less than 1 Time in 5	Less than Half the Time	About Half the Time	More than Half the Time	Almost Always
Considering the past month:						
1. How often have you had a sensation of not emptying your bladder completely after you finished urinating?	0	1	2	3	4	5
2. How often have you had to urinate again less than 2 h after you finished urinating?	0	1	2	3	4	5
3. How often have you found you stopped and started again several times when you urinated?	0	1	2	3	4	5
4. How often have you found it difficult to postpone urination?	0	1	2	3	4	5
5. How often have you had a weak urinary stream?	0	1	2	3	4	5
6. How often have you had to push or strain to begin urination?	0	1	2	3	4	5
7. How many times did you most typically get up to urinate from the time you went to bed at night until the time you got up in the morning? Sum of 7 replies equals "AUA Symptom Score" (0–35).	0 (None)	1 (1 time)	2 (2 times)	3 (3 times)	4 (4 times)	5 (≥5 times)

Abbreviation: AUA = American Urologic Association.

Adapted from McConnel JD, Barry MJ, Bruskewitz RC, et al: Benign prostatic hyperplasia: Diagnosis and treatment. Clinical Practice Guideline, No. 8. AHCPR Publication No. 94-0582. Rockville, MD, Agency for Health Care Policy and Research, Public Health Service, U.S. Department of Health and Human Services, February, 1994.

PSA level (>4.0 ng per mL). The PSA test is further hampered by false-negative results especially in early potentially significant carcinomas. This high false-negative rate (approximately 40%) demands a careful family history for prostate carcinoma in young first- or second-degree relatives. A low threshold for prostate biopsy in such individuals is prudent, irrespective of physical examination or PSA level.

Today BPH is a most uncommon cause of the serious sequelae of obstruction, i.e., upper tract stasis, stone, and renal failure; BPH, or prostatism if severe, is viewed as more of a quality-of-life issue. Therefore, the routine diagnostic testing that is appropriate remains somewhat controversial. The deleterious effects on the upper tracts are due to a loss of bladder compliance (the ability to store urine at lower pressure), and *bladder outlet obstruction* can cause a loss in compliance. Compliance can easily be checked by cystometry, but this requires instrumentation. Since symptoms are not related to prostate size and size is not related to obstruction, other approaches are needed. However, most agree that severe and sustained symptoms warrant investigation.

The urinary flow rate at peak flow, if the rate is reduced below 10 mL per second and *if* the results are consistently reproducible, might be a useful screening tool for obstruction. Unfortunately, between the vagaries of voiding in unfamiliar settings and the equivalent result produced by a *weak* detrusor rather than obstruction, a single flow rate alone is often difficult to interpret. Multiple 5-second *home* flow rates at maximum flow help the author understand the interaction of the bladder with its outlet under real conditions. All that is required is a watch and a graduated specimen cup.

Theoretically, before significant bladder compliance is lost from obstruction, the bladder should lose its ability to empty. Postvoid residual urine (PVR), which can easily and accurately be measured noninvasively by ultrasound, may define a clinical situation requiring further investigation. Although considerable variability occurs within individuals, a persistent PVR of greater than 100 mL should alert the clinician. Bothersome symptoms, consistent low peak home flow rates (<10 mL per second), normal bladder capacity, and a significant PVR can be improved by intervention in most cases.

In the unusual case, a simultaneous study of pressure and flow may urodynamically prove the diagnosis of bladder outlet obstruction. In this case, bladder pressure can be plotted graphically against the maximal flow rate to clarify the picture. Unfortunately voiding with invasive pressure monitors in a laboratory setting has its drawbacks. With the exception of recurrent acute urinary retention, however, no modality, be it symptom score or urodynamics, can reliably predict which individual is at great risk for serious complication or when. It is ironic that "silent prostatism" today remains a persistent cause of chonic renal insufficiency and that being asymptomatic, its regular presentation is unlikely to change. Thus the experienced clinician must decide with a knowledgeable patient when or if intervention is appropriate. It has been the author's experience that a patient who is not terribly bothered and who is reassured that he does not have cancer will opt for watchful waiting. Such patients are often even more reassured when told that many individuals their age of both sexes have similar symptoms.

TREATMENT

Within the last 10 years, this country's urologists performed 350,000 to 400,000 prostatectomies per year with an associated cost of nearly $5 billion. This endeavor represented about one-third of their major surgery and a sizable fiscal enterprise. Given this enormous cost (or potential profit) and unfavorable reports from outcome research, the recent attention BPH has received from government and industry is unprecedented. Many less invasive modalities are being used or are under investigation, and drugs for the treatment of BPH have been approved by the Food and Drug Administration (FDA). The common weak thread in much of the drug or device research remains the vagaries of BPH symptoms (nonspecificity and fluctuation) and the aforementioned problems with flow rates done in laboratory settings. Additionally, the variability of PVR, technical problems, patient concerns with invasive urodynamics, and the well-known placebo effect from any medication, as well as an *enormous* placebo effect achieved with urethral instrumentation confound clinical research in BPH. It is estimated that up to one-third of individuals in most of the BPH studies were not obstructed but had primarily poor bladder function.

Before symptom score guidelines, indications for treatment were classified as absolute or relative, and treatment was as simple as reassurance, intermittent self-catherization (ISC), or an operative procedure (Table 3). Today given symptoms as a stand-alone indication, there has been aggressive marketing of "minimally" invasive surgery and medical management. How "minimal" the invasiveness is perceived, however, depends not only on the practitioner's learning curve but, more importantly, on what side of the device the individual resides.

Acute urinary retention requires intervention. We recommend ISC until the bladder is able to resume function. If the retention is repetitive, in a reasonably healthy individual who can be shown to be obstructed, a simple (transurethral prostatic resection [TURP] or open) prostatectomy is recommended. Similarly, recurrent gross hematuria and hydroureteronephrosis with renal insufficiency are best managed by standard, simple prostatectomy. These serious clinical problems were a small percentage of the indications for TURP 20 years ago but likely will become the most accepted indications for intervention to the third-party payers of the future.

There are a multitude of possible interventions for the relative indications or a symptom score of 8 or higher. They include standard therapy, medical therapy, and so-called minimally invasive therapy.

Standard Therapy

Before the realization that TURP was an extraordinary drain on the cost of medical care or, by the observation of unbiased outcome researchers, that the complications were indeed significant. TURP produced, for the most part (80 to 85%), excellent re-

sults. However, if the usual rules of safety with the procedure (1 hour operating time, less than 50 grams of tissue resection) were strictly adhered to, the complication rates were low. However, as optics improved and because of the immediate morbidity of an open prostatectomy, most patients opted for TURP, extending the operating time and producing anticipated complications. These problems included the immediate complication of hemorrhage and excessive irrigation absorption leading to severe hyponatremia and seizures as well as death. Because of excessive urethral trauma from long resection times, urethral stricture disease became more troublesome than the original problem with BPH in some cases. Such all-too-frequent difficulties coupled with the aforementioned extremely high cost led to the development of alternative therapies.

It might seem ironic that TURP spawned such a scenario because it was the high morbidity and mortality associated with open prostatectomies (suprapubic, retropubic, perineal) that was the driving force to improve that situation. Unfortunately it was not the procedures themselves that were problematic; rather it was the associated lack of good anesthesia, fluid and blood bank support, and antibiotics that made these operations too dangerous at their inception. They remain excellent operations today in the appropriately selected patient.

The anticipated results from medical therapy, while statistically significant, reflect only approximately 15 to 25% of the efficacy of standard therapy. Minimally invasive therapies are for the most part too early in their evolution for meaningful contrast of their results.

Medical Therapy

Since eunuchs do not develop BPH and since castration was shown many years ago to have an effect on many individuals with BPH, antiandrogen therapy has undergone extensive research. While theoretically feasible, antiestrogen therapy research has not been fruitful to date, and a recent large multicenter study was aborted.

Antiandrogens. Luteinizing hormone-releasing hormone (LHRH) achieves medical castration within 2 weeks and induces some prostatic involution and reduction in prostate size in most patients. Size alone, however, is not that critical, and the frequency of side effects precludes the use of LHRH. Troublesome hot flashes (greater than 60%) and loss of libido (near 100%) with erectile dysfunction and breast tenderness are regular side effects. The extremely high cost as well as the deleterious effect on PSA surveillance renders this systemic approach unrealistic for treating BPH.

The androgen receptor blocker flutamide (Eulexin)* has undergone extensive testing, but it too was severely limited by side effects despite having efficacy similar to that of LHRH analogues. Although

TABLE 3. **Indications for Intervention**

Absolute	Relative
Acute urinary retention	Symptoms
Recurrent febrile infection	Progressive PVR
Recurrent gross hematuria	Uncomplicated infection
Hydroureteronephrosis	

Abbreviation: PVR = postvoid residual urine.

*Not FDA-approved for this indication.

libido and erectile difficulties were not problematic, gynecomastia (>50%) and significant gastrointestinal disturbances will disallow flutamide to gain favor for the treatment of BPH.

Finasteride (Proscar) is a 5-alpha-reductase inhibitor that blocks the conversion of testosterone to dihydrotestosterone (DHT), the active metabolite at the prostate receptor. The serum testosterone level remains normal, and sexual dysfunction becomes an infrequent complaint. Finasteride is capable of reducing prostate volume, improving symptom score, and improving the maximum urinary flow rate by 1 to 2 mL per second but often requires several months of therapy and probably only really helps that one-third of men whose BPH is hormonally responsive. It produces a durable yet lifelong commitment, with considerable cost, in those helped. Finasteride has an excellent safety profile with minimal side effects. Finasteride also lowers serum PSA levels, but predictably to approximately 50%, which allows the practitioner to extrapolate the untreated value (twice the measured value) for an individual on this drug. Of all the antiandrogens that affect the static (size) fraction of BPH "obstruction," finasteride is the only one that has FDA approval.

Alpha-Adrenergic Blockers. Due to the high-density presence of alpha$_1$ receptors at the bladder neck and prostatic smooth muscle, alpha blockers have been used to address this "dynamic" fraction of the obstruction equation. Nonspecific alpha blockers (e.g., prazosin) have been displaced by the specific long-acting antagonists terazosin (Hytrin) and doxazosin (Cardura). Both have similar efficacy in decreasing smooth muscle tone and improving symptom scores and urinary flow rates. This moderate improvement is seen in a much larger percentage of treated individuals than in those treated with finasteride. Alpha blockers, however, have a much quicker (few weeks for full effect) onset of action but a higher side effect profile, with asthenia, dizziness, and postural hypotension not infrequent reasons for discontinuation. Both terazosin and doxazosin are FDA-approved for the treatment of BPH.

Combination Treatment. Because of the completely different mechanisms of action of antiandrogens and alpha blockers, combination therapy may have some value. At the moment research is underway to test this hypothesis. However, it is unlikely that even combination therapy will approach the objective results of TURP.

Minimally Invasive Therapy

Over the last decade there has been an explosion of less invasive modalities to address bladder neck obstruction (Table 4). Despite excellent results with TURP by skilled hands in correctly selected patients, many other methods have emerged, in an effort to decrease the widespread morbidity of TURP.

Transurethral Incision of the Prostate (TUIP). This brief surgical procedure has produced excellent results in properly selected individuals. A low compli-

TABLE 4. **Minimally Invasive Therapy**

TUIP	Balloons
TUAP	Stents
TULIP	Microwave
VLAP	Focused ultrasound
TUNA	Cryosurgery

Abbreviations: TUIP = transurethral incision of the prostate; TUAP = transurethral ultrasonic aspiration of the prostate; TULIP = transurethral ultrasound-guided laser-induced prostatectomy; VLAP = visual laser ablation of the prostate; TUNA = transurethral needle ablation.

cation rate, short period of catheterization and hospitalization, and maintenance of antegrade ejaculation can be expected. Despite requiring no sophisticated equipment, this modality has not achieved the widespread use it deserves. Reimbursement concerns and a lack of tissue for histologic examination have been implicated in its low utilization rate.

Transurethral Ultrasonic Aspiration of the Prostate (TUAP). Sophisticated equipment allowing endoscopic ultrasonic aspiration of tissues high in water content (BPH, liver, brain) have undergone limited testing recently. Although theoretically sound since tissues with high collagen content (bladder neck, prostate capsule) are spared, this technique has had only limited application to date.

Transurethral Ultrasound-Guided Laser-Induced Prostatectomy (TULIP). TULIP using neodymium:yttrium-aluminum-garnet (Nd:YAG) laser energy has largely been replaced by visual laser ablation of the prostate (VLAP). VLAP requires no ultrasound guidance, and the new side-firing lasers allow Nd:YAG energy to be directed precisely under vision. Although VLAP is said to produce similar results to TURP without complication, the acceptance is not universal. Problems with prolonged catheterization, lack of tissue for histologic interpretation, significant start-up costs, and the learning curve have tempered enthusiasm.

Transurethral Needle Ablation (TUNA). Transurethral needle ablation utilizes high-frequency radio waves to ablate prostatic tissue under direct vision. Proponents say this technique can be performed on outpatients under local anesthesia. Clinical trials are underway. Early results suggest it will share many of the problems associated with VLAP and will require anesthetic support.

Balloons. Balloon dilatation of the prostate was said to achieve rapid resolution of obstruction with minimal morbidity, anesthesia, and hospitalization. There was a rapid disappearance of this modality after a blinded study showed that cystoscopy alone had equal efficacy.

Stents. Intraprostatic stents, or coils to keep the prostatic urethra open, have been tested and shown to be efficacious. Long-term results are rather sparse, as are the limited indications for such intervention. Problems with migration and encrustation as well as the usual learning curve and equipment problems have curtailed widespread acceptance.

Microwave Thermotherapy. Recent studies have

shown symptom scores after thermotherapy to nearly approach those achieved with TURP. Other than the obvious equipment problems, thermotherapy has a unique problem of heat transfer in prostate glands of different water content. Since prostatic tissue heterogeneity is known to occur between different ethnic groups, potential serious problems with thermotherapy are possible.

Focused Ultrasound. Focused ultrasound has great potential applicability. Being able to noninvasively ablate tissue with extracorporeal technology has great appeal. At present the limited availability and experience in the United States precludes recommendation of this technique until it is studied further.

Cryosurgery. Despite being described more than 30 years ago, cryosurgical prostatectomy has not achieved widespread acceptance for the treatment of BPH. The complication rates have been formidable, and efficacy has been questioned. The technique is considered a very poor alternative.

Individual Options

Most individuals, unless severely symptomatic, opt for watchful waiting when comfortably made aware of their very common age-related constellation of symptoms. Should their symptoms be moderately severe and their bother index high, and if they have suitable bladder function, a TURP in good hands remains the "gold standard." For those less bothered, medical alternatives are finasteride, doxazosin, or terazosin. The medical management, however, does not achieve measurable success anywhere near that of standard prostatectomy. The advantages of all the avant-garde modalities over standard TURP done by experienced hands remains to be proved in a controlled fashion. Individual treatment remains individual and given all the opportunities can be tailored to the patient's medical and personal needs.

PROSTATITIS

method of
STACY J. CHILDS, M.D.
Cheyenne Urological, P.C.
Cheyenne, Wyoming

One of the problems encountered in treating prostatitis is deciding what it really is and what causes it. The term broadly implies an inflammation of the prostate, presumably causing symptoms related to the male's perineal area or lower urinary tract. The incidence has been estimated at between 2 and 12% of the adult male population, but the percentages of men having true bacterial prostatitis may be much lower. In fact, of all prostatitis patients, those with a bacterial etiology probably number from 5 to 17%, as opposed to those with nonbacterial prostatitis or prostate pain who equal 85 to 95% of patients presenting with symptoms. Is it a true inflammation or merely a regional symptom complex like the urethral syndrome in women?

The disease is treatable; however, it is helpful to classify the patient into the groups commonly accepted by the urologic community: acute bacterial prostatitis (ABP), chronic bacterial prostatitis (CBP), nonbacterial prostatitis (NBP), and prostatodynia (prostate pain). A managed care approach demands that one attempt to help or cure patients even when the etiology is undetermined and then refer the patient if tests or complicated management are inevitable.

ACUTE BACTERIAL PROSTATITIS

This is the easiest of all of the prostatitis diagnoses to make. The patient may or may not have a history of urinary tract infection but presents with fever, chills, malaise, perineal or lower back pain, and possibly lower urinary tract symptoms such as urinary frequency, dysuria, or decreased stream size. On rectal examination, the prostate is tender, is sometimes warm to touch, and may be swollen and irregular. If the diagnosis is suspected, massage is absolutely contraindicated, as it may cause a septic episode. The gland may have an abscess, and the swelling can actually obstruct the prostatic corridor. In most cases of elevated white blood cell (WBC) count and fever, patients should be hospitalized at least until adequate antimicrobial levels are achieved in the serum. Patients should always be hospitalized if bacteremia or septic episode is suspected.

Treatment must be aggressive and appropriate to the organisms involved. Prostatitis is almost always caused by gram-negative bacilli, the most common of which is *Escherichia coli*. Rarely, abscesses may occur with anaerobes such as *Bacteroides fragilis*. If the patient has impaired micturition, a suprapubic catheter (not a urethral catheter) should be inserted for several days. Most broad-spectrum antimicrobial drugs will easily cross into the inflamed prostate; parenteral choices are aminoglycosides, cephalosporins, or fluoroquinolones (oral or intravenous [IV]), such as ciprofloxacin (Cipro), ofloxacin (Floxin), and lomefloxacin (Maxaquin) or enoxacin (Penetrex). Although 2 weeks of therapy is probably adequate, 4 weeks is preferred to ensure that all bacteria are eliminated from the prostatic bed, limiting the chance of recurrence. If culture data are available, patients can be switched to oral medications and treated as outpatients as soon as fever has abated.

CHRONIC BACTERIAL PROSTATITIS

This disease is extremely rare but not terribly difficult to diagnose. Patients may complain of low back pain, dysuria, perineal discomfort, and possibly burning urination. They will almost always give a history of urinary tract infection or the symptoms thereof. If a patient positive for the human immunodeficiency virus (HIV) presents with these symptoms, true bacterial prostatitis must always be considered. I have treated two such patients.

The classic method of confirming CBP may be impractical for the primary care physician. It consists of the Meares-Stamey technique of collecting the urine specimen in stages. When the patient submits a specimen, the first 10 ml of the voided urine (the VB1) would represent a urethral infection, the next 200 ml of midstream urine (the VB2) would represent a bladder infection, the expressed prostatic secretions (EPS) obtained by massaging the prostate would indicate whether a prostate infection was present, and the last voided specimen after the EPS (the VB3) would also represent a prostate infection as the urine washed out the expressed material from the prostatic corridor. Each of these specimens is plated separately on culture agar and the colony counts compared. If the number of bacteria in the EPS and/or the VB3 appear to be greater than the colony counts in either the VB1 or the VB2, the presumptive diagnosis of true chronic bacterial prostatitis can be made.

As these patients usually do not present in a febrile state, often the diagnosis can be postponed until culture data are available. However, if vigorous massage is done, the risk of making the patient sicker can be avoided by starting antibacterial therapy after collecting the specimens and looking at the EPS under the microscope. Again, organisms are usually common gram-negative bacilli, but gram-positive cocci, such as *Staphylococcus aureus, S. saprophyticus,* and *S. epidermidis,* have been recovered and can be pathogenic in carefully collected specimens. Although a hemacytometer can be used to count the WBCs, it is impractical in a primary care environment. A drop of EPS on a slide that is covered by a cover slip and then viewed with the high-power lens should reveal 10 or greater WBCs per high-power field to indicate significant inflammation. Oval fat bodies (macrophages) are usually present, and bacteria are often seen.

A permanent cure is difficult with CBP. One of the biggest problems has been the lack of currently available antimicrobial choices to diffuse into the prostatic tissue adequately. Erythromycin, clindamycin, carbenicillin, and cephalexin have all been used with limited success. The appearance of the oral fluoroquinolones has been the greatest advance in the treatment of CBP. Ciprofloxacin (Cipro), lomefloxacin, enoxacin (Penetrex), and ofloxacin (Floxin) are the first choice of treatments for this disease and should be continued for a minimum of 1 month and for at least 2 months if the patient has a history of CBP treatment. The patient should be seen and prostate specimens examined at least under the microscope at 1-month intervals. Failure to cure this disease after one round of antibiotics should immediately prompt referral to the urologist for ultrasound, possible biopsies, or endoscopy or other treatment modalities, including transurethral resection as a last resort.

If the patient presents with bacteriuria and prostatitis symptoms, I have attempted to sterilize the urine with nitrofurantoin (Macrodantin) prior to obtaining the appropriate VB1, VB2, EPS, and VB3 cultures. Often, the resulting cultures are negative, however, and the patient is referred to the urologist for this cumbersome technique.

NONBACTERIAL PROSTATITIS

The diagnosis and treatment of this disease is controversial and difficult, to say the least, and extremely variable. Although patients may present with similar symptoms and possibly have an abnormal rectal examination, their cultures are usually negative. Symptoms referable to the musculoskeletal system may be more prominent than dysuria, but orchialgia and suprapubic pain are not uncommon. Examination of the prostatic secretions may show an inflammatory response (just as in CBP) with WBCs and oval fat bodies, but cultures are negative. Attempts to isolate *Chlamydia, Ureaplasma,* and *Mycoplasma* have been successful but these bacteria are extremely sporadic and unpredictable. The possibility of a fastidious organism or of bacteria not expressed by prostate massage being the cause must be considered, however, and most physicians treat this disease as though it is bacterial unless the treatment fails.

Treatment begins with 14 to 21 days of doxycycline (Vibramycin), 100 mg twice daily in those under 35 years old. For those over that age, I prefer either TMP-SMX (trimethoprim-sulfamethoxazole [Bactrim, Septra]) or one of the fluoroquinolone agents (ciprofloxacin [Cipro], enoxacin [Penetrex], lomefloxacin [Maxaquin], or ofloxacin [Floxin]). If the patient does not improve during the first week of therapy, nonsteroidal anti-inflammatory agents such as ibuprofen can be added.

Failure to eliminate the symptoms after 2 to 4 weeks of therapy could mandate the use of a symptom score similar to that of the American Urological Association for evaluating benign prostatic hyperplasia. A score can be modified to the physician's liking but should include at least the items listed in Table 1. Patients with a total score of 4 or so could be presumed to have "prostatitis" and, if previous therapy has failed, an alpha blocker such as terazosin (Hytrin)* or doxazosin (Cardura)* could be tried. A dosage of terazosin, 1 to 10 mg per day, could be titered in an attempt to relieve symptoms if the urethral wall is the possible cause of these symptoms. It is at least possible that reflux of urine into the intraprostatic ducts, because of heightened urethral spasm activity, can cause inflammation from chemical irritation.

If these attempts fail to alleviate symptoms entirely, the patient should be referred to the urologist. Outpatient endoscopy of the lower urinary tract with flexible scopes is now rather easy and almost painless, but the yield of such examinations is limited. If the patient is referred, the urologist will continue seeking the etiologic organism using the Meares-Stamey technique, trying various combinations of pharmaceuticals, and then inevitably cystoscoping the pa-

---

*Not FDA-approved for this indication.

TABLE 1. **Prostatitis Questions: Circle the Number That Best Describes the Symptoms You Are Currently Experiencing**

	No Pain	Occurs Occasionally (Not Every Day)	Usual But Does Not Stop Activity	Incapacitating
Perineal pain/thigh pain: pain in or between legs	0	1	2	3
Orchialgia: painful testicles or scrotal sac	0	1	2	3
Abdominal/inguinal pain/pressure: pain or full feeling in the abdomen	0	1	2	3
Urethral discomfort: pain in penis	0	1	2	3

From Neal D: Use of terazosin in prostatodynia and validation of a symptom score questionnaire. Urology 43:460–465, 1994. Reprinted with permission from Urology.

tient. Surprising facts have emerged, not only from the literature but also from most individual urologists' practices, such as that the avoidance of certain foods can lessen the symptoms of NBP, especially caffeine, alcohol, tobacco, and sometimes citrus juices. The patient can usually tell the doctor which foods aggravate his symptoms.

In addition, almost all patients with CBP will improve on antimicrobial therapy. Double-blind placebo studies with controls are needed for this disease to determine the importance of the placebo effect, which, if low enough, could lead to the implication of nondetected true bacterial prostatitis in this category.

PROSTATODYNIA

Patients not found to have bacteria in their urine, EPS or VB3, with no WBCs in the EPS, are lumped into the category of "prostate pain" or prostatodynia. The patients may present with the same symptoms as in the other categories but with no fever, chills, or signs of systemic infection. The patients do not always present typically. Some may have a fixation on orchialgia, whereas others may have low back pain or perineal aching. Some may complain of urethral burning or severe pain after ejaculation. Many of these patients can relate their pain (especially on questioning) to an occupation or habit such as driving a car for a long time, bicycling, riding on heavy machinery, and so on.

The physical examination can be disappointing. The prostate may or may not feel tender, boggy, or swollen. Rather vigorous massage in an attempt to express fluid, although occasionally quite painful, often brings relief within hours.

The treatment for this disease is not antimicrobials. First-line treatment should include nonsteroidal anti-inflammatory drugs or other non-narcotic analgesics. Low-dose diazepam (Valium)* can be used only temporarily, especially if the buttocks or thighs are greatly involved. If symptoms are not improved within 1 week, a trial of terazosin is wise. Sitz baths are only temporarily palliative. Nevertheless, failure to achieve adequate symptom relief might prompt the physician to refer the patient for psychotherapy. My advice is to refer the patient to a urologist for thorough diagnostic evaluation, and if that fails, let the urologist refer the patient for psychological evaluation.

In the primary care environment, cost-efficient treatment of prostatitis is possible. Selecting the category of diagnosis is important to identify ABP or CBP, because these have well-defined clinical features and treatment methods (Table 2). NBP and prostatodynia deserve a round of treatment by the primary care physician, but failure to adequately relieve symptoms should initiate prompt referral to the urologist. Occasionally, seminal vesiculitis, prostatic abscess, calculi, prostatic carcinoma, or intersti-

---

*Not FDA-approved for this indication.

TABLE 2. **Clinical Features of Different Forms of Prostatitis**

Syndrome	History of Confirmed UTI	Prostate Abnormal on Rectal Examination	Excessive WBCs in EPS	Positive Culture of EPS	Common Causative Agents	Response to Antimicrobials	Impaired Urinary Flow Rate
Acute bacterial prostatitis	Yes	Yes	Yes	Yes	Coliform bacteria	Yes	Yes
Chronic bacterial prostatitis	Yes	±	Yes	Yes	Coliform bacteria	Yes	±
Nonbacterial prostatitis	No	±	Yes	No	None ?Chlamydia ?Ureaplasma	Usually no	±
Prostatodynia	No	No	No	No	None	No	Yes

Abbreviations: UTI = urinary tract infection; WBCs = white blood cells; EPS = expressed prostatic secretion.
From Meares EM Jr: Prostatitis and related disorders. In Walsh PC, Retik AB, Stamey TA, et al (eds): Campbell's Urology, 6th ed. Philadelphia, WB Saunders, 1992.

tial cystitis can be discovered. Failure to recognize these ailments within several months would be truly unfortunate.

ACUTE RENAL FAILURE

method of
MARK S. PALLER, M.D.
University of Minnesota
Minneapolis, Minnesota

Acute renal failure (ARF) is an abrupt decline in renal function occurring over a period of hours to days. This decrease in glomerular filtration rate (GFR) results in retention of nitrogenous metabolic waste products and may also result in abnormalities of sodium, water, acid-base, and potassium balance. ARF complicates the course of approximately 5% of all hospitalized medical-surgical patients. It is far more common in patients requiring intensive care unit treatment. Mortality in patients with ARF severe enough to require hemodialysis is between 30 and 70%. Many forms of ARF are potentially reversible. Therefore, early recognition, diagnosis, and correct management are essential in optimizing the care of these patients.

CLINICAL PRESENTATION

ARF is most often recognized by finding an increase in the serum creatinine or blood urea nitrogen (BUN) levels, or both. The plasma creatinine level is a more reliable marker of renal function than is the BUN. When ARF is first evolving, the rate of change of serum creatinine is a better indicator of the degree of renal function impairment than is the absolute level of serum creatinine. In this non–steady-state situation, in the absence of renal function, creatinine will increase 1 to 2 mg per dL per day. Unusual causes of an increase in creatinine not caused by a decrease in renal function are the drugs cimetidine and trimethoprim, which interfere with tubular secretion of creatinine, and rhabdomyolysis, which results in increased release of creatinine into the bloodstream from damaged muscles. An increase in the BUN is also an indicator of a decrease in GFR under most circumstances. However, the BUN is also affected by dietary protein intake, catabolic state, gastrointestinal tract bleeding, and low urine flow rates (as occurs in volume depletion and congestive heart failure), all resulting in an increase in the BUN in the absence of a reduction in GFR.

A reduction in urine volume is the other indication of ARF. Oliguria has been arbitrarily defined as a urine flow rate of less than 400 mL per day. However, urine output may be normal in as many as 60% of cases of ARF (nonoliguric ARF). Therefore, when urine flow rate is diminished in ARF, both an increase in serum creatinine and diminished urine flow rates develop. However, severe reductions in GFR can occur in the absence of decreased urine volume and will be recognized only by an increase in serum creatinine.

CAUSES OF ACUTE RENAL FAILURE

ARF is best understood by considering how urine is formed. Blood flows to the glomeruli of the kidney (renal blood flow [RBF]) where ultrafiltration of the blood occurs. This plasma ultrafiltrate is modified within the urinary space by reabsorption of those factors to be retained by the body (sodium, water, amino acids, and so on) and secretion of other substances (hydrogen ion, potassium, certain drugs, and so on). The final urine must pass through the intrarenal collecting system, ureters, bladder, and urethra. ARF may be caused by processes involving any of these steps. For simplification, ARF is often categorized as being due to prerenal (or functional) causes, intrinsic renal causes, or postrenal causes. The major causes of ARF are listed in Table 1.

Prerenal Failure

Any cause of diminished renal perfusion can result in ARF. In these circumstances, the kidney parenchyma is normal (in fact, the kidney would perform normally if transplanted into a healthy recipient), and the condition is called "prerenal (or functional) ARF." By far the most common cause of prerenal failure is severe extracellular fluid volume depletion resulting from hemorrhage, diarrhea, diuretics, or burns. Third-space fluid accumulation can also result in a decrease in the effective extracellular fluid volume, as occurs in pancreatitis, sepsis, crush injury, and cirrhosis. Decreased renal perfusion can also be the result of severe heart failure, hypotension, or shock. Renal vasoconstriction severe enough to impair RBF and thus GFR is also seen in the hepatorenal syndrome and with use of the immunosuppressant drug cyclosporine.

Several other commonly used drugs also cause prerenal failure. During volume depletion or the development of renal insufficiency, kidneys respond by increasing the synthesis of vasodilator prostaglandins, which results in afferent arteriolar vasodilatation to maintain or increase RBF and therefore GFR. When patients with renal insufficiency, volume depletion, heart failure, or liver disease take nonsteroidal anti-inflammatory drugs (NSAIDs) or aspirin, these drugs interfere with this compensatory prostaglandin synthesis and may develop prerenal failure. In patients with a severe limitation of RBF (bilateral renal artery stenosis or severe volume depletion), an additional com-

TABLE 1. **Causes of Acute Renal Failure**

Prerenal (Functional)

Hypotension/shock
Extracellular fluid volume depletion (hemorrhage, burns, diarrhea, diuretics)
Third-space fluid accumulation (pancreatitis, sepsis, crush injury, cirrhosis)
Impaired cardiac output (heart failure)
Drugs
    Cyclosporine (Sandimmune)
    Nonsteroidal anti-inflammatory drugs (NSAIDs)
    Angiotensin-converting enzyme inhibitors
Vascular obstruction (renal artery thrombosis, emboli, severe stenosis, or vasculitis)

Intrinsic Renal (Structural)

Acute tubular necrosis
    Ischemic
    Nephrotoxic
Acute interstitial nephritis
Acute glomerulonephritis

Postrenal (Obstructive)

Intrarenal (uric acid, oxalate, methotrexate, or acyclovir crystals)
Extrarenal
    Ureteric obstruction (tumor, stones, tissue, retroperitoneal fibrosis)
    Bladder outlet obstruction (prostatic or urethral)

pensatory change is the intrarenal formation of angiotensin II, which maintains GFR via efferent arteriolar constriction. If such patients receive angiotensin-converting enzyme inhibitors to decrease angiotensin II formation, intraglomerular capillary pressure will not be sustained and renal failure can develop. Vascular obstruction due to thrombosis, emboli, severe stenosis, or vasculitis of the renal arteries is an additional cause of prerenal failure. It is important to note that vascular obstruction must involve both kidneys or a solitary functioning kidney to cause ARF.

In all cases of prerenal failure, if the underlying condition is reversed or the offending drug removed, renal function will rapidly return to normal because by definition the kidney is not structurally damaged. However, prolonged reduction of RBF can lead to ischemic injury of the kidney that is not immediately reversible. Therefore, it is important to diagnose and treat prerenal failure promptly.

Intrinsic Acute Renal Failure

Most cases of ARF are due to intrinsic renal (or structural) causes. Acute tubular necrosis (ATN) makes up the majority of these cases. ATN is the result of ischemic or toxic injury of the kidneys (Table 2). Ischemic injury occurs in the setting of hypotension and shock, sepsis, or prolonged prerenal conditions. Ischemic ATN is a common complication of surgery, particularly cardiac surgery requiring cardiopulmonary bypass, abdominal aortic aneurysm repair, and biliary tract surgery. Nephrotoxins are an equally important cause of ATN. Hospital-acquired ATN is most often a consequence of antibiotic or radiographic contrast agent administration. Aminoglycosides are the antibiotics most frequently causing ATN. Endogenous heme proteins are also nephrotoxins. Hemoglobinuria results from hemolytic reactions, whereas myoglobinuria occurs as a consequence of rhabdomyolysis, which is most often caused by crush injury. Nontraumatic rhabdomyolysis occurs after seizures, cocaine use, alcoholism, strenuous exercise, heat stroke, and infection and with metabolic disorders (hypokalemia, hypophosphatemia). In severely ill patients, ARF is often multifactorial.

ATN must be distinguished from the other intrinsic renal causes of ARF. Acute interstitial nephritis (AIN) is the result of an allergic drug reaction and can sometimes be difficult to distinguish from ATN. The common causes of AIN are listed in Table 3. Acute glomerulonephritis, when severe, may also result in ARF.

Postrenal Failure

Obstruction of the urinary tract is the third category of ARF. The urinary space may be obstructed intrarenally by

TABLE 2. Causes of Acute Tubular Necrosis

Ischemia

Hypotension/shock
Sepsis
Prolonged prerenal conditions

Nephrotoxins

Antibiotics (aminoglycosides, amphotericin B, cephalosporins, tetracycline)
Radiographic contrast agents
Acetaminophen
Cis-platin (Platinol)
Methoxyflurane (Penthrane)
Heavy metals
Organic solvents
Endogenous heme proteins (myoglobin, hemoglobin)

TABLE 3. Causes of Acute Interstitial Nephritis

Beta-lactam antibiotics (methicillin, ampicillin, and so on)	Cimetidine (Tagamet)
Diuretics	Sulfonamides
Allopurinol (Zyloprim)	Rifampin (Rifadin)
Nonsteroidal anti-inflammatory drugs	Phenytoin (Dilantin)

crystals. Uric acid precipitation within the tubules is a consequence of the tumor lysis syndrome resulting in plasma uric acid levels of 15 to 20 mg per dL. The drugs methotrexate and acyclovir can also precipitate within the renal tubules, causing intrarenal obstruction. Extrarenal obstruction is a consequence of either bilateral ureteric obstruction or obstruction of the bladder outlet. In men, prostatic enlargement is the most common cause of obstructive uropathy. In women, pelvic malignancies cause ureteral obstruction. In either gender, stones or renal tissue (necrotic papillae) can cause renal failure if both ureters become obstructed. Retroperitoneal fibrosis and less frequently accidental surgical ligation of the ureters during intra-abdominal or pelvic surgery are the causes of ureteric obstruction.

Clinical Approach to the Patient with Acute Renal Failure

Table 4 suggests the approach to the history, physical examination, and laboratory evaluation of the patient with ARF. In the history, potential causes of extracellular fluid volume depletion should be sought. A history of vomiting,

TABLE 4. Clinical Approach to the Patient with Acute Renal Failure

History

Are there causes of volume depletion (vomiting, diarrhea, blood loss, diuretics, burns)?
Are there symptoms of heart failure?
Are there symptoms of liver failure?
What medications was the patient taking (nephrotoxins, NSAIDs, ACE inhibitors)?

Chart Review

Has the patient's weight fallen or has fluid output exceeded intake?
Have there been hypotensive episodes?
What medications has the patient received (including intraoperatively)?
Did the patient receive radiocontrast medium?

Physical Examination

Is there extracellular fluid volume depletion (orthostatic hypotension, tachycardia, dry mucous membranes and axillae, decreased skin turgor)?
Is there congestive heart failure (rales, S3 heart sound, edema, ↑ central venous pressure)?
Is there evidence for obstructive uropathy (distended bladder, enlarged prostate, pelvic mass)?
Are there skin changes suggesting systemic disease?

Laboratory Evaluation

Urinalysis
Urinary indices
Renal ultrasonography (to exclude obstruction)
Radionuclide renogram (if renal artery occlusion is a possibility)
Kidney biopsy (if acute interstitial nephritis or acute glomerulonephritis is a possibility)

Abbreviations: NSAIDs = nonsteroidal anti-inflammatory drugs; ACE = angiotensin-converting enzyme.

diarrhea, blood loss, diuretic use, or burns suggests a prerenal cause of ARF. Symptoms suggestive of heart failure or liver disease should be sought. The patient should be questioned about the use of NSAIDs or aspirin and the use of angiotensin-converting enzyme inhibitors. Exposure to nephrotoxic drugs or those that might cause AIN should also be assessed (see Tables 2 and 3). Symptoms referable to a systemic disease, including fever, malaise, skin rash, and musculoskeletal complaints, suggest vasculitis or acute glomerulonephritis. Difficulty in voiding; suprapubic, abdominal, or flank pain; or hematuria suggests the possibility of a postrenal cause for ARF.

A careful review of the medical record is often the most revealing diagnostic procedure in patients who have acquired ARF while hospitalized. A review of daily weights or intake and output, when available, is strong documentation for the possibility of extracellular fluid volume depletion. The vital signs records should be reviewed for periods of hypotension. The medication list must be carefully reviewed for potential nephrotoxins and drugs capable of causing AIN. For patients who have undergone operative procedures, it is essential to review the operative record. A review of the anesthesiology record may reveal episodes of hypotension that may have caused ARF but resolved intraoperatively. A large volume of blood loss also suggests transient renal hypoperfusion. Medications given preoperatively or intraoperatively should be evaluated. The possibility that the anesthetic methoxyflurane was used should be considered. Recent radiographic examinations requiring the administration of radiocontrast agents should also be sought. It is important to emphasize that in many cases of ATN multiple potential causes of both renal hypoperfusion and nephrotoxicity can be identified, although no single factor can be definitively blamed for the ARF.

The physical examination should focus on the hemodynamic status of the patient. Evidence of extracellular fluid volume depletion such as orthostatic changes in the pulse and blood pressure, dry mucous membranes and axillae, and decreased skin turgor should be noted. The central venous pressure should be estimated by examination of the neck veins, and evidence for congestive heart failure (pulmonary rales, S3 heart sound, and edema) should be sought. It is sometimes difficult to assess intravascular volume accurately on the basis of the physical examination, and volume depletion cannot be easily excluded. In these cases, invasive monitoring may require the use of a Swan-Ganz catheter to measure left ventricular filling pressure and cardiac output accurately. Physical examination is also useful to detect causes of obstructive renal failure. A distended bladder may be palpable above the symphysis pubis. Intra-abdominal tumors may be palpable or produce abdominal or flank pain. A careful rectal and pelvic examination should always be performed when considering the possibility of obstructive uropathy. The skin should be carefully observed for rashes or other changes that might be compatible with a systemic disease such as vasculitis, allergic drug reaction, or diffuse atheroembolic disease (e.g., livedo reticularis).

URINALYSIS

A careful and complete urinalysis is essential to the accurate diagnosis of the cause of ARF and should be performed by a highly trained technician. Urinalysis is such an important part of the evaluation of the patient with ARF that consulting nephrologists will often perform this test themselves. A normal urinalysis (absence of protein, blood, and white cells by dipstick and the absence of cells or casts in the urine sediment) suggests either a prerenal or a postrenal cause for ARF (Table 5). When abnormalities in the urine sediment are present, microscopic examination can usually differentiate among ATN, AIN, and acute glomerulonephritis. The characteristic urinary sediment in a patient with ATN contains renal tubular epithelial cells and debris derived from necrotic epithelial cells. This debris may be in the form of either amorphous material or numerous dark or "dirty" granular casts. Acute glomerulonephritis is suspected if the dipstick is positive for protein and red blood cells and if examination of the sediment reveals red blood cells, red cell casts, and hyaline casts. In the majority of cases of AIN, the urine sediment will contain polymorphonuclear leukocytes. The presence of eosinophils is more suggestive of AIN. To thoroughly evaluate for the possibility of urinary eosinophils, Hansel's stain should be employed. The finding of dipstick positivity for red cells but their absence in the urinary sediment should suggest the possibility of hemoglobinuria or myoglobinuria as the cause of ATN. In cases of intrarenal obstruction due to crystals, the offending crystal may be noted in the urinary sediment and suggest that possibility.

Often the urinalysis is not diagnostic and the history and physical examination do not adequately differentiate between prerenal and intrinsic ARF. This is not surprising, since a major cause of ARF is ischemia. Therefore, a patient with severe volume depletion and hypotension or with shock may progress from a prerenal state (in which the kidney is hypoperfused but has not sustained irreversible injury) to a state of acute cellular injury (or necrosis) caused by sustained or more severe renal hypoperfusion and oxygen lack. To differentiate between prerenal failure and intrinsic ARF, it is useful to consider how the renal tubule epithelial cells would behave under these two different conditions. In prerenal states, the kidney is underperfused and reacts by maximally reabsorbing filtered salt and water in an attempt to restore extracellular fluid volume. This renal response will occur whether there is true volume depletion or merely perceived volume depletion (as in the case of renal artery obstruction or congestive heart failure). In contrast, when there is tubular cell injury, the ability of the kidney to reabsorb filtered salt and water is impaired. It is helpful to recall that under normal conditions, more than 99% of the filtered salt and water is reabsorbed by the kidney.

A number of urinary tests (or urinary indices) have been

TABLE 5. **Urinary Findings in Acute Renal Failure**

	Urine Sediment	FE$_{Na}$
Prerenal failure	Normal	<1
Intrinsic ARF		
Acute tubular necrosis	Renal tubular epithelial cells, cellular debris, dark granular casts	>1*
Acute interstitial nephritis	Eosiniphils, neutrophils	Not useful*
Acute glomerulonephritis	Proteinuria, hyaline casts, red cells, red cell casts	Not useful*
Postrenal failure	Normal (or red cells or crystals)	Not useful*

*See text for complete explanation.

Abbreviation: FE$_{Na}$ (fractional excretion of sodium) = $U_{Na}/P_{Na} \div U_{Cr}/P_{Cr} \times 100$, where U is the urine concentration and P is the plasma concentration of either sodium (Na) or creatinine (Cr).

employed to differentiate between prerenal and intrinsic renal failure. In prerenal failure, the urine sodium concentration is usually less than 20 mEq per liter, whereas in intrinsic ARF urinary sodium concentration is often more than 40 mEq per liter. An even more useful urinary test to discriminate between prerenal and intrinsic causes of ARF is the fractional excretion of sodium (FE_{Na}). The FE_{Na} is derived from the formula $FE_{Na} = U_{Na}/P_{Na} \div U_{Cr}/P_{Cr} \times 100$, where U is the urine concentration and P is the plasma concentration of either sodium (Na) or creatinine (Cr). In prerenal failure, the FE_{Na} is less than 1%, whereas in ATN it is usually more than 1%. The FE_{Na} has better predictive value in oliguric renal failure than in nonoliguric renal failure, in which it should be used with caution. In some conditions, ATN is associated with an FE_{Na} of less than 1%. This occurs most often with myoglobinuria or radiocontrast injury and suggests that these disorders have a component of profound and contracted renal vasoconstriction. FE_{Na} is less than 1% in patients with acute glomerulonephritis and may also be low in patients with acute obstruction. Therefore, the FE_{Na} should never be used in the absence of a careful urinalysis to exclude acute glomerulonephritis or when obstructive uropathy is a possibility that has not been excluded.

EVALUATION OF POSTRENAL FAILURE

In addition to a careful history and physical examination to consider the possibility of postrenal failure, it may be necessary to perform additional tests to exclude this possibility. This is particularly important when an obvious cause for prerenal or intrinsic renal failure cannot be easily identified or when the possibility of concomitant obstructive uropathy exists. Bladder outlet obstruction is easily evaluated by catheterizing the bladder to determine whether after voiding there is urinary retention of more than 100 mL, suggesting obstruction as the likely cause of renal failure. The most useful noninvasive test to rule out ureteral obstruction is renal ultrasonography. In most cases this is a highly accurate test, although if obstruction is caused by retroperitoneal fibrosis or tumor, the absence of a dilated urinary tract system could be a false-negative result. In these rare cases, computed tomography to evaluate the retroperitoneum and/or retrograde pyelography to definitively rule out ureteral obstruction may be required. However, for most cases, renal ultrasonography is adequate to evaluate the possibility of bilateral ureteral obstruction causing ARF.

OTHER DIAGNOSTIC TESTS

In those patients with a prerenal picture (normal urinalysis, FE_{Na} of less than 1%, no obstruction by renal ultrasonography) who do not have an obvious prerenal condition, renal vascular obstruction should be considered. Radionuclide renogram will demonstrate the presence or absence of perfusion of the kidneys. If renal perfusion is markedly diminished or absent, renal arteriography will better demonstrate the location and possible cause of vascular obstruction (e.g., renal artery stenosis versus thromboembolism).

It may be difficult to differentiate among the causes of intrinsic ARF. In each of the major causes—ATN, AIN, and acute glomerulonephritis—the urinalysis will be abnormal. When the urinalysis is not diagnostic, a kidney biopsy is necessary. For example, when AIN is clinically suspected but the urinalysis does not show eosinophils or substantial numbers of polymorphonuclear leukocytes, then a biopsy

TABLE 6. Major Risk Factors for the Development of Acute Renal Failure

Extracellular fluid volume depletion	Radiocontrast exposure
Congestive heart failure	Septic shock
Aminoglycoside use	Chronic renal insufficiency

would be performed to make the diagnosis. Similarly, in almost all cases of acute glomerulonephritis, a biopsy is necessary to determine the specific disease process.

MANAGEMENT OF ACUTE RENAL FAILURE

Prevention

It is more effective to prevent new cases of ARF than to treat established ARF. Table 6 lists the major risk factors for the development of ARF. Extracellular volume depletion, congestive heart failure, and chronic renal insufficiency are the most serious chronic conditions predisposing to ARF. Prevention of ARF is directed toward risk factor management (Table 7). Extracellular fluid volume depletion should always be corrected in at-risk hospitalized patients. Although it may be difficult to reverse the underlying cardiac condition in patients with congestive heart failure, appropriate use of vasodilators (angiotensin-converting enzyme inhibitors), ionotropic agents (digoxin), and judicious use of diuretics will improve cardiac output and therefore renal perfusion. The use of aminoglycosides should be reserved for life-threatening infection and carefully considered in high-risk patients. Monitoring aminoglycoside blood levels is also useful to avoid excessive dosing and to limit toxicity.

The use of radiocontrast agents should be similarly carefully considered in patients at high risk of developing ARF. When administration of radiocontrast agents is essential for diagnostic tests or therapeutic procedures, particularly in patients with underlying renal insufficiency (plasma creatinine greater than 2 mg per dL), restoration of extracellular fluid volume and maintenance of euvolemia and adequate urine output are essential. Diuretics (either loop-acting diuretics or mannitol) are no longer recommended for prophylactic therapy in patients who are to receive radiocontrast agents. In elderly patients or those with congestive heart failure, diuretics may be necessary to prevent fluid overload, but they should not be administered routinely. A commonly employed

TABLE 7. Preventing Acute Renal Failure: Risk Factor Management

Replace extracellular fluid volume deficits
Treat heart failure (ACE inhibitors, digoxin; avoid excessive reliance on diuretics)
Avoid concomitant use of other nephrotoxins
Avoid agents that cause renal vasoconstriction (nonsteroidal anti-inflammatory drugs)

Abbreviation: ACE = angiotensin-converting enzyme.

protocol to maintain adequate extracellular fluid volume and urine flow for patients receiving radiocontrast media is to administer one-half normal saline at a rate of 125 to 150 mL per hour, beginning 1 hour before the radiographic procedure and continuing for several hours afterward.

Initial Treatment of Acute Renal Failure

In patients with prerenal failure, prompt attention to the underlying condition will rapidly restore renal function to normal and prevent the complications of impaired renal function. Equally as important, reversal of renal hypoperfusion by restoring extracellular fluid volume, treating hypotension, improving cardiac function, and/or stopping administration of vasoconstricting drugs will decrease the chance of the kidney developing structural lesions due to ischemia. Treatment of patients who have already developed structural lesions (ATN) is less satisfactory. In these patients, volume depletion should still be treated and systemic hemodynamics optimized to prevent ongoing renal injury. Patients with rhabdomyolysis, particularly those with crush injury, require aggressive fluid replacement (often in the range of 4 to 20 liters of saline in the first 24 hours). Nephrotoxic agents should be stopped for the same reason. However, once ATN has developed, it generally takes several days to several weeks for healthy renal epithelium to replace the damaged and lost cells and for GFR to return to normal levels.

Patients with ATN and oliguria should be treated with loop-acting diuretics in an attempt to convert them to a nonoliguric state. Successful conversion from oliguria to nonoliguria may not affect the ultimate prognosis of the ATN but will simplify management of the patient by diminishing the need for strict fluid restriction. Diuretics should not be given to the oliguric patient with ATN until extracellular fluid volume deficits have been replaced. Initially, an intravenous (IV) dose of furosemide (Lasix), 80 mg (or bumetanide [Bumex]), 1 mg (or torsemide [Demadex]), 20 mg is tried. If there is no increase in urine output in 30 to 60 minutes, a higher dose should be employed. Because of the risk of ototoxicity with high-dose IV furosemide, either bumetanide (10 mg) or torsemide (100 to 200 mg) is preferable. If urine output does not increase after this second, higher dose of diuretics, additional doses of diuretics should not be employed because of the markedly increased risk of toxicity with repeated doses. Alternatively, some clinicians favor testing a continuous infusion of furosemide (1 mg per kg per hour). A continuous infusion should not be employed for more than a few hours if there is no response.

If there is no response to IV loop-acting diuretics, a brief trial of the vasodilator dopamine in "low dose" or "renal doses" (1 to 3 µg per kg per minute) can also be tested. Dopamine is most likely to be efficacious when there is a component of renal vasoconstriction, such as ATN, due to radiocontrast agents or amphotericin B. Studies of the use of low-dose dopamine to prevent ARF in at-risk patients have been unconvincing and dopamine cannot be recommended for this purpose. If dopamine infusion does not produce a prompt increase in urine volume, its use should not be continued. The benefits of other agents, such as calcium channel blockers or atrial natriuretic peptide (ANP) are still unproved. Several small studies suggest that these agents may be useful to improve urine flow rate and perhaps even produce small improvements in renal function in patients with ATN. Their use cannot be generally recommended, however. Other aspects of the management of the patient with established ARF are discussed later in the context of the complications that arise in patients with severely depressed renal function.

Complications of Acute Renal Failure

Metabolic abnormalities are the most troublesome complications of ARF. Particularly in patients with oliguric ATN, sodium and water balance is difficult to maintain. This becomes an even more important consideration in patients who are receiving large volumes of IV fluids to provide a variety of medications, such as antibiotics, pressor agents, and IV hyperalimentation. A general guideline for patients with ARF is that all IV fluids should be administered in the most concentrated form reasonable to limit the possibility of the patient developing volume overload. Hyperkalemia frequently occurs in patients with ARF and, unless there is evidence for potassium depletion, IV fluids should not contain potassium.

Nutrition is an important consideration in severely ill patients. Patients who are able to eat should be given a diet with a modest sodium restriction. Fluid balance should be carefully monitored in all patients (daily weights are often more accurate than fluid intake and output). Fluids should be given to replace the previous day's losses—urine, gastrointestinal, drainage, plus insensible losses (none for patients on ventilatory support breathing humidified air, 500 mL for most patients, 1000 mL for febrile patients with increased skin losses). In the nonoliguric patient, fluid intake may not have to be restricted. Hyponatremia indicates relative water excess and should be treated with water restriction. Volume overload (jugular venous distention or elevated central venous pressure, rales, and edema) requires restriction of sodium as well as fluids.

Regardless of whether enteral or parenteral nutrition is provided, patients with ARF generally require 25 to 35 kcal per kg per day. The most severely catabolic patients may require as much as 45 kcal per kg per day. Protein requirements are approximately 1 gram per kg per day. Patients not requiring hemodialysis can be mildly restricted to a protein intake of 0.8 gram per kg per day. Those patients already requiring hemodialysis and highly catabolic should be given between 1 and 1.5 grams per kg per day of protein. Larger amounts of protein given as IV amino acids have been tested in small numbers of patients with ARF. Administration of IV nutrients in large quantities requires the administration of excessive fluid and has not been proved beneficial in terms of recovery of renal function or general patient outcomes.

Because many drugs are metabolized by and/or eliminated by the kidney, patients must have their medications carefully reviewed. Many drugs require a significant reduction in dosage (in either dosage amount or dosing frequency) in patients with ARF.

Mild uremic symptoms are common in patients with ARF, but severe problems are usually avoided if patients are properly treated. Neurologic symptoms of lethargy, confusion, and sleep disorder are frequent, whereas seizures and coma are infrequent. Uremic gastrointestinal manifestations are anorexia, nausea, and vomiting. Pleuritis and pericarditis are unusual complications of ARF, whereas volume overload producing hypertension, pulmonary edema, and peripheral edema are frequently encountered. Patients with ARF are at increased risk of developing infection, which is particularly important in patients who have multiple intravascular catheters and wounds.

DIALYSIS THERAPY OF ACUTE RENAL FAILURE

Hemodialysis or other forms of extracorporeal therapy are indicated for patients who develop serious complications owing to the loss of renal function. These include hyperkalemia, severe metabolic acidosis, volume overload resulting in impaired oxygenation (not responsive to IV diuretics), and uremic symptoms (particularly the neurologic or cardiovascular complications of coma, seizures, or pericarditis). Some nephrologists would argue that high BUN and creatinine levels independent of the clinical status are also indications for hemodialysis. Performing hemodialysis for "chemical" indications alone must be balanced against the potential adverse effects of hemodialysis. Hypotension induced by too-vigorous fluid removal during dialysis can result in additional ischemic insults to the already damaged kidney that can potentially impair recovery. Clinical studies have not demonstrated a definitive advantage of aggressive hemodialysis (daily) versus more conservative hemodialysis (three times per week) in patients with ARF who require dialytic therapy. To eliminate adverse consequences of dialysis therapy, these seriously ill patients with ARF should only be treated with biocompatible hemodialysis membranes and bicarbonate dialysate.

In patients in whom volume overload is a greater problem than the other metabolic abnormalities associated with ARF, continuous extracorporeal therapies can be considered. These treatments include continuous arteriovenous hemofiltration (CAVH), continuous arteriovenous hemodiafiltration (CAVHD), and continuous venovenous hemodiafiltration (CVVHD). These procedures are all similar in that highly permeable biocompatible membranes are used to allow removal of large volumes of fluid across the filter. In CAVH, metabolic waste products are removed by convection, whereas with CAVHD and CVVHD, dialysate fluid is also run through the devices so that metabolic waste products can be removed by diffusion as well. Removal of urea is less efficient with these therapies than with intermittent hemodialysis, but during the 24-hour period net removal of fluid is much greater. Continuous treatment has the same limitations of acute hemodialysis, requiring vascular catheterization and systemic heparinization. CVVHD also requires use of a blood pump. A potential advantage is that fluid removal is continuous and can be more carefully controlled to avoid acute hypotension. There are no large-scale studies to suggest that continuous therapies are more effective or beneficial than intermittent acute hemodialysis, and their use often depends on the personal preference of the nephrologist as well as staff familiarity with the procedures in a particular intensive care unit.

PROGNOSIS

Patient survival depends on the severity of the underlying disease and the health of the patient. Table 8 lists those features that adversely affect prognosis in patients with ARF requiring dialysis. As noted earlier, mortality for patients with ARF requiring dialysis ranges between 30 and 70%. In contrast, otherwise well patients who develop ARF following exposure to radiocontrast agents or aminoglycoside antibiotics have a mortality rate of less than 5%. The duration of ARF depends on its cause. Radiocontrast-induced ARF reaches a nadir of renal function a mean of 72 hours after exposure. On the other hand, the median duration of dialysis dependency of patients with ATN complicating aortic aneurysm surgery is 3 weeks, with a range of 2.5 to 5 weeks.

Nonoliguric patients tend to recover renal function more rapidly and tend to require fewer dialysis treatments prior to recovery than do oliguric patients. These patients also tend to be healthier and acquire ARF principally by exposure to antibiotics or radiocontrast agents. It is believed that patients who are spontaneously nonoliguric or are easily converted from oliguria by diuretics have sustained less severe initial renal damage and therefore recover more rapidly. When patients recover from ATN, renal function is generally sufficient to maintain them independent of dialysis. Even so, older patients and those with more severe ATN often do not have complete recovery of renal function and are left with mild-to-moderately diminished GFR.

TABLE 8. **Risk Factors for Poor Survival in Patients with Acute Renal Failure Requiring Hemodialysis**

Hypotension	Sepsis
Need for assisted ventilation	Congestive heart failure
Gastrointestinal tract dysfunction (bleeding, ileus, or obstruction)	Central nervous system dysfunction
	Jaundice

CHRONIC RENAL FAILURE

method of
GLENN M. CHERTOW, M.D., and
J. MICHAEL LAZARUS, M.D.
Harvard Medical School
Boston, Massachusetts

MEASUREMENT OF RENAL FUNCTION AND DIAGNOSIS OF CHRONIC RENAL FAILURE

The most common measure used to estimate kidney function is the serum creatinine. The serum creatinine is a useful, albeit imperfect measure, because of its physical characteristics and handling by the human nephron. Within intact nephrons, creatinine is freely filtered, not reabsorbed, and only minimally secreted. Unlike creatinine, the blood urea nitrogen (BUN) is a relatively poor surrogate for renal function. Many factors may increase the BUN independent of intrinsic renal function, including gastrointestinal bleeding, drugs that promote catabolism (e.g., glucocorticoids, tetracyclines), and impaired renal perfusion (e.g., volume depletion, hepatic cirrhosis).

The creatinine clearance (CrCl) can be determined using the following formula:

$$CrCl \text{ (mL per minute)} = \frac{\text{Urine concentration of creatinine (mg per dL)} \times \text{urine volume (mL per minute)}}{\text{Plasma concentration of creatinine (mg per dL)}}$$

The creatinine clearance closely approximates the glomerular filtration rate (GFR) when the GFR exceeds 50 to 60 mL per minute. However, as renal function deteriorates, the CrCl tends to overestimate GFR because of the relative contribution of secreted creatinine and nonrenal routes of creatinine excretion. In contrast, the urea nitrogen clearance (calculated as in the preceding equation but using urine and serum urea) tends to underestimate GFR because of tubular urea reabsorption. The average of the creatinine and urea clearances is reasonably accurate when the GFR falls below 20 mL per minute.

An approximation of CrCl can be obtained using the Cockcroft-Gault formula:

$$CrCl \text{ (mL per minute)} = \frac{(140\text{-age} \times \text{ideal body weight} (\times 0.85 \text{ if female})}{\text{Serum creatinine} \times 72}$$

Additional methods of assessing renal function are outlined in Table 1.

The urinalysis is an important diagnostic tool that is rapid, inexpensive, and relatively easy to perform. Urine dipsticks can detect modest degrees of hematuria, pyuria, and proteinuria and are often the first clue to the presence of acute or chronic renal disease. A microscopic analysis may provide insight into the severity and/or duration of renal disease. Radiographic studies are also helpful. The abdominal plain film and intravenous urogram are useful

TABLE 1. Methods Used to Estimate Renal Function

Serum creatinine
Blood urea nitrogen
Cockcroft-Gault equation
24-hour urine collection for creatinine and/or urea nitrogen
DTPA renal scan
Radiolabeled iothalamate clearance

Abbreviation: DTPA = diethylenetriaminepenta-acetic acid.

TABLE 2. Most Common Causes of Chronic Renal Failure and End-Stage Renal Disease

Glomerulonephritis/glomerulosclerosis/glomerulopathy
  Diabetic nephropathy
  Hypertensive nephrosclerosis
  Primary renal
    Focal segmental glomerular sclerosis
    Membranous nephropathy
    IgA nephropathy
  Systemic disease
    Systemic lupus erythematosus
    Human immunodeficiency virus–associated nephropathy
    Vasculitis
Tubulointerstitial disease
  Chronic pyelonephritis
  Papillary necrosis/analgesic nephropathy
  Interstitial nephritis
  Multiple myeloma
Hereditary renal disease
  Polycystic kidney disease
  Hereditary nephritis (Alport's disease)
  Vesicoureteral reflux
Decreased renal perfusion/vascular disease
  Renovascular disease
  Atheroembolic disease
  Renal infarction
  Cyclosporine nephrotoxicity
Urinary tract obstruction
  Prostate/bladder pathology
  Retroperitoneal fibrosis/lymphadenopathy
  Irreversible ureteral obstruction
Nephrectomy or partial nephrectomy for malignancy
Renal transplant failure

in the work-up of nephrolithiasis but are rarely sufficient in the patient with renal insufficiency. Rather, renal ultrasound is the preferred diagnostic screening study. Ultrasound can be used to assess kidney structure (e.g., the presence of cysts, hydronephrosis), size (e.g., reduced size with long-standing disease), and integrity (i.e., echogenicity). Occasionally, computed tomography, magnetic resonance imaging, and nuclear medicine studies are used in the diagnosis of chronic renal failure (CRF), particularly when associated with hypertension and vascular disease.

CAUSES OF CHRONIC RENAL FAILURE

The most common causes of CRF are outlined in Table 2. Although many patients progress to end-stage renal disease (ESRD) without a definitive diagnosis, it is important to investigate the cause(s) of CRF, as associated complications may develop in future years.

Conditions associated with prerenal failure, owing to frank volume depletion (e.g., blood loss, gastrointestinal fluid loss, overzealous use of diuretic agents) or to reduced renal perfusion (e.g., congestive heart failure, hepatic cirrhosis, renovascular disease), are the most common causes of acute renal failure in hospitalized adults. However, with the possible exception of renovascular disease, these pathophysiologic states are relatively uncommon causes of CRF and ESRD (i.e., they are reversible). Likewise, postrenal failure, i.e., urinary tract obstruction, infrequently causes CRF or ESRD unless it remains undiagnosed and is bilateral, severe, and prolonged. Rather, the great majority of cases of CRF or ESRD are due to intrinsic renal diseases, which can be broadly categorized as predominantly glomerular or tubulointerstitial in origin.

Glomerular diseases, including diabetic nephropathy

and hypertensive nephrosclerosis, account for the majority of cases of CRF that progress to ESRD. Glomerular diseases can be broadly categorized as nephrotic or nephritic. The term "nephrotic" refers to the loss of large (greater than 3 to 5 grams per day) quantities of protein (usually albumin) in the urine. When full-blown, the nephrotic syndrome includes edema owing to salt and water retention, hypoalbuminemia, hypercholesterolemia, and occasionally a predisposition to venous thrombosis. In contrast, the term "nephritic" refers to the presence of hematuria, hypertension, and mild-to-moderate proteinuria, usually with associated loss of renal function. Several of the glomerular diseases are associated with systemic disease, such as bacterial endocarditis, systemic lupus erythematosus, and vasculitis; others are primary, often idiopathic, and somewhat less aggressive, such as membranous or IgA nephropathy. Among the glomerular diseases, systemic lupus erythematosus, focal segmental glomerulosclerosis (FGS), and human immunodeficiency virus (HIV)–associated nephropathy are associated with frequent progression to ESRD. Although diabetic nephropathy and hypertensive nephrosclerosis are common causes of ESRD, it is important to recognize that some patients with diabetes and/or hypertension with renal failure suffer from other conditions, such as atherosclerotic vascular disease, that may be the actual cause of renal failure, and that among all persons with diabetes and/or hypertension, advanced renal failure develops in the minority.

Tubulointerstitial diseases are somewhat less common, but important, causes of CRF, particularly among women. Chronic pyelonephritis, mostly when associated with reflux nephropathy or other congenital abnormalities, can result in a substantial loss of renal function. In this case, CRF results from the effects of repeated infections leading to scarring and loss of functional renal mass. Papillary necrosis may occur in the setting of diabetes mellitus or sickle cell anemia or as a result of prolonged exposure to nonsteroidal anti-inflammatory drugs (NSAIDs), so-called analgesic nephropathy. Acute interstitial nephritis is usually due to drug exposure. Antibiotics (e.g., penicillins, cephalosporins, sulfonamides) are the most common culprits. Although anecdotal reports have suggested a benefit of glucocorticoids, empirical therapy is usually ill-advised, especially in the setting of an underlying infection. Renal function usually improves after withdrawal of the offending agent, although some degree of CRF develops in 20 to 40% of patients.

COMPLICATIONS OF CHRONIC RENAL FAILURE

Fluid, Electrolytes, and Hypertension

Several characteristic fluid and electrolyte abnormalities manifest during the course of CRF, although they vary widely depending on the primary disease. Owing in part to reduced functional renal mass, hypertension and edema often occur as a consequence of sodium retention. Diabetic renal disease and many forms of glomerulonephritis are associated with this phenomenon. Ironically, arterial vasodilators prescribed for hypertension (e.g., nifedipine [Procardia], prazosin [Minipress], hydralazine [Apresoline], minoxidil [Loniten]) often contribute to further salt and water retention. The addition of a diuretic agent to an antihypertensive regimen consisting of sympatholytics or vasodilators is often required to achieve adequate blood pressure control in individuals with CRF. It is important to manage hypertension aggressively in the presence of renal insufficiency, as uncontrolled hypertension can accelerate the loss of renal function, particularly among hypertensive African Americans.

Hyponatremia may accompany fluid retention, especially with nephrotic syndrome and hypoalbuminemia, or with concurrent cardiac or hepatic failure. In contrast, patients with interstitial renal disease less frequently develop fluid retention or hyponatremia because of an associated disruption in tubular reabsorptive function, owing to tubular inflammation or fibrosis.

Mild hyperkalemia (5 to 6 mEq per liter) is extremely common among patients with advanced renal failure. However, life-threatening hyperkalemia (more than 7 mEq per liter) rarely occurs until the GFR drops below 5 to 10 mL per minute. Hyperkalemia is diet-dependent (potassium is abundant in many fruits and vegetables) and is more common among diabetics and patients taking certain drugs (Table 3). Hyperkalemia can almost always be controlled with withdrawal of offending agents and other conservative measures, including the administration of a cation exchange resin (sodium polystyrene sulfonate [Kayexalate]), insulin and glucose, sodium bicarbonate, and/or beta$_2$-adrenergic receptor agonists. Frequently coincident with hyperkalemia, metabolic acidosis usually results from insufficient ammoniagenesis and an accumulation of organic and inorganic acids.

CRF associated with hypokalemia is rare but can be seen in association with certain nephrotoxic agents, including amphotericin B (Fungizone), *cis*-platin (Platinol), and aminoglycosides, excessive doses of loop or thiazide diuretics, or rarely, in association with hypouricemia, glycosuria and aminoaciduria (the Fanconi syndrome). Similarly, CRF associated with metabolic alkalosis is uncommon; if it is observed, one should carefully rule out excessive vomiting, overzealous diuretic use, or excessive base ingestion, as in the milk-alkali syndrome.

Disorders of calcium, phosphorus, and parathyroid hormone (PTH) are almost universally present as the GFR drops below 25 mL per minute. Phosphorus tends to accumulate with worsening renal function. Hyperphosphatemia itself drops the serum calcium, as does the reduced intestinal absorption of calcium

TABLE 3. **Drugs Associated with Hyperkalemia**

Salt substitutes
Potassium-sparing diuretic agents
Spironolactone (Aldactone)
Amiloride (Midamor)
Triamterene (Dyrenium)
Angiotensin-converting enzyme inhibitors
Nonsteroidal anti-inflammatory drugs
Beta-adrenergic antagonists
Cyclosporine (Sandimmune)
Heparin
Digoxin

owing to vitamin D deficiency. PTH secretion is regulated by calcium (increased with decreased serum calcium), phosphate (increased with increased serum phosphate), and 1,25-OH vitamin D (increased with decreased serum 1,25-OH vitamin D). Although hyperparathyroidism tends to increase the serum calcium toward the normal range, it does so at the expense of bone integrity. This vicious circle of calcium dysmetabolism and secondary hyperparathyroidism results in osteitis fibrosa cystica, the most common form of bone disease in patients with renal failure. Aluminum overload may also be present in the ESRD patient, owing to increased aluminum intake (in the form of phosphate binders) and reduced excretion and may result in a unique form of bone disease (aluminum osteomalacia).

Stepwise management of calcium metabolism includes modest dietary phosphate restriction (e.g., dairy products, especially cheeses, beans, animal proteins) and calcium supplementation with or just after meals. Calcium carbonate (Tums E-X and others) and calcium acetate (PhosLo) are beneficial in that they bind dietary phosphate and provide calcium for systemic absorption. Additionally, these agents provide a small quantity of base equivalents without the additional administration of sodium, such as with sodium bicarbonate. Calcium citrate (Citracal) should be avoided, as citrate markedly enhances the intestinal absorption of aluminum. Likewise, aluminum-based products (e.g., aluminum hydroxide [Amphogel], sucralfate [Carafate]) should be avoided if at all possible. After hyperphosphatemia has been controlled, a vitamin D analogue may be added to improve intestinal absorption of calcium and to directly inhibit PTH secretion.

Hematologic Effects

Anemia and platelet dysfunction are the most common hematologic effects of reduced renal function. The anemia associated with advanced renal failure is usually normocytic and normochromic in type and caused by a reduction in the production of erythropoietin, a growth factor produced within the kidney. However, the usual causes of anemia should not be ignored in patients with renal failure. Gastrointestinal blood loss, owing to peptic ulcer disease, gastritis, esophagitis, malignancy, hemolysis (autoimmune vs. other), and/or nutrient deficiencies (e.g., iron, folate, vitamin B_{12}) is more common among persons with CRF than in the general population and is usually responsive to appropriate therapeutic measures. Aluminum toxicity may result in a microcytic, hypochromic anemia; fortunately, this complication is now rare with diminished administration of aluminum-based phosphate binders.

The anemia associated with reduced erythropoietin production rarely occurs until the GFR drops below 10 to 15 mL per minute. However, this reduction in erythropoietin production is highly variable among individuals and renal diagnoses. For instance, individuals with polycystic kidney disease are less likely to develop severe anemia, presumably owing to the effects of cyst compression on renal tissue, resulting in local ischemia and a relative excess of erythropoietin production. Furthermore, it is important to recognize that, like the reticulocyte count, a level of circulating erythropoietin within the normal range indicates a suboptimal and distinctly abnormal response in a patient with anemia.

Hemostasis can be impaired with severe reductions in GFR (5 to 10 mL per minute). CRF does not appear to affect the clotting cascade, and the prothrombin time and partial thromboplastin time are usually normal except with severe malnutrition or coexistent liver disease. Rather, the hemostatic defect involves platelet dysfunction, which can be diagnosed by an abnormal bleeding time, often exceeding 10 minutes (normal 5 to 7 minutes). Prior to performing any invasive procedure on a patient with renal failure, including renal biopsy, a bleeding time should be assessed. The patient should be off all aspirin products for 1 week and off NSAIDs for several days. If the bleeding time is abnormal, administration of desmopressin acetate (DDAVP), cryoprecipitate, erythropoietin (Epogen) and/or transfusion, or conjugated estrogens (Premarin), or the initiation of dialysis may be needed to improve hemostasis.

Erythropoietin therapy has resulted in the maintenance of adequate hematocrits in most dialysis patients without the need for blood transfusions and has been shown to improve quality of life. Iron stores must be sufficient to support erythropoiesis. Administration of subcutaneous erythropoeitin (Epogen, 2000 to 4000 U once or twice weekly) to individuals with CRF has also been effective.

Gastrointestinal Effects

The most common gastrointestinal manifestations of uremia are nausea and vomiting. These symptoms are attributable to uremia, but other causes of nausea and vomiting, such as myocardial ischemia, diabetic gastropathy, peptic ulcer disease, and other primary gastrointestinal diseases, should be investigated if dialysis does not lead to resolution. Inflammation and edema of the gastrointestinal tract are also relatively common. These changes cause blood loss, altered drug and nutrient availability, and excess absorption of the intracellular constituents of blood, such as nitrogen (derived from hemoglobin), potassium, and phosphorus.

Dialysis markedly improves the nausea and vomiting of uremia. H_2 receptor antagonists, such as ranitidine (Zantac), can be used to reduce dyspepsia. Alternatively, calcium carbonate (Tums E-X and others) can be used, as long as hypercalcemia is not present. Over-the-counter antacids containing magnesium and aluminum (Mylanta) should be avoided.

Serositis

Serositis, or inflammation of the epithelial surfaces of internal organs with altered serosal porosity, can occur with severe reductions in renal function (GFR, 5 to 10 mL per minute). The most frequent manifestations are pericarditis, pleuritis, and enteritis (serositis involving the heart, lung, and gastrointestinal tract, respectively). Uremic pericarditis can be life-threatening. If combined with a bleeding diathesis, hemorrhagic pericarditis can develop; at the extreme this could result in pericardial tamponade. All patients with advanced azotemia should be carefully examined for the presence of a pericardial friction rub. Typically, a three-component rub can be heard best with the patient leaning forward. Intestinal serositis can contribute to nausea and vomiting as well as to hemorrhagic gastritis, esophagitis, and ascites. A pleural rub or pleural effusion should be carefully evaluated. An infectious (e.g., bacterial, especially *Staphylococcus* sp, or mycobacterial, e.g., tuberculous), malignant (e.g., lung or breast carcinoma), or autoimmune (e.g., systemic lupus erythematosus, rheumatoid arthritis) cause should be excluded in all patients.

Central Nervous System Effects

The internist or nephrologist is often asked to evaluate a hospitalized patient with CRF or ESRD and altered mental status. However, unless the GFR is markedly reduced (below 5 mL per minute), an altered mental state is much more commonly due to other causes, such as medication (e.g., benzodiazepines, ethanol, narcotic analgesics, anticholinergic [including antihistaminic] drugs), infection, cerebrovascular disease, hypoxemia, and/or underlying mental illness. Uremia rarely causes seizures, except when accompanied by profound hypocalcemia (less than 5 to 6 mg per dL). The characteristic encephalopathy of uremia is a gradual reduction in mental alertness and attention capacity, extending from lethargy to stupor, and finally at end-stage to coma. The central nervous system manifestations of uremia typically respond quite rapidly to the institution of dialysis.

Dementia in patients with CRF is most often due to strokes secondary to cerebrovascular disease or severe systemic hypertension and/or Alzheimer's disease. "Dialysis dementia" refers to a specific condition associated with severe aluminum poisoning. The recognition of this syndrome, improved water quality control, and the decreased use of aluminum-based phosphate binders have markedly reduced the incidence. "Dialysis disequilibrium" refers to a distinct syndrome associated with the rapid removal of urea and other extracellular solutes with dialysis initiation after the chronic progression of renal failure. Clinically, the syndrome is characterized by headache, confusion, and occasionally seizures and is presumably caused by acute cerebral edema (owing to the removal of extracellular osmolar equivalents). Gradual solute removal with diminished blood and dialysate flow rates can usually prevent the occurrence of dialysis disequilibrium. If more aggressive dialysis is otherwise indicated, an osmotically active

substance, such as mannitol and/or phenytoin (Dilantin), for anticonvulsant prophylaxis can be administered.

Peripheral neuropathy associated with CRF can affect any or all of the sensory, motor, or autonomic nervous systems. Neuropathy can be particularly disabling in individuals with concurrent diabetic or alcohol-associated neuropathy and may or may not improve with dialysis therapy. Common complications of neuropathy in CRF patients include pain typically involving the lower extremities, altered sensation leading to unrecognized trauma, and orthostatic hypotension. Although tricyclic antidepressant agents such as amitriptyline (Elavil) may be successful in reducing pain and disability, these drugs may exacerbate autonomic nervous dysfunction and/or contribute to fatigue and are often poorly tolerated.

General Effects

Additional associated signs and symptoms of uremia are outlined in Table 4.

METHODS OF RENAL REPLACEMENT THERAPY

It is advisable to refer the patient with chronic renal insufficiency (GFR of approximately 50) to a nephrologist well before renal replacement therapy is required. Adequate blood pressure control and attention to various hormonal and metabolic disturbances may ameliorate some of the long-term complications of chronic renal disease and attenuate the progression of renal failure. Several clinical criteria mandate the prompt institution of renal replacement therapy in persons with advanced CRF (Table 5). However, the provision of dialysis under urgent cir-

TABLE 4. **General Effects of Uremia**

Pruritus
Fatigue
Weight loss
Malnutrition
Sleep disturbance (altered day-night cycle, central sleep apnea)
Depression
Musculoskeletal complaints
Nitrogenous fetor
Hair loss

TABLE 5. **Absolute Indications for Initiation of Chronic Renal Replacement Therapy**

Volume overload refractory to sodium restriction and diuretic therapy
Hyperkalemia refractory to dietary restriction and intestinal binders
Uremia
  Pericarditis/serositis
  Encephalopathy/neuropathy
  Bleeding diathesis
  Severe nausea and vomiting
Malnutrition associated with foregoing

cumstances places the patient at undue and unnecessary risk; it is best to prepare an individual carefully and deliberately for what will become a major change in lifestyle, employing either dialysis or transplantation. Sufficient time should be allowed for patient self-examination and discussion with family and friends regarding treatment options. Likewise, the creation of a native arteriovenous fistula or placement of an artificial arteriovenous graft requires several weeks to months to heal and optimally mature. Although no strict laboratory criteria define uremia, a BUN greater than 150 mg per dL and a serum creatinine greater than 12 to 15 mg per dL are often associated with the development of advanced uremic symptoms. Diabetic patients and elderly persons may become symptomatic with less dramatic elevations of serum chemistries.

No one modality can be considered superior in all respects; each method of renal replacement carries its own advantages and disadvantages. It is imperative that the nephrologist assist the patient and family in medical decision making and allow for individualization of care, considering additional issues such as quality of life and emotional and social role function.

Hemodialysis

Hemodialysis is the most common form of renal replacement therapy. Most persons undergo treatment at outpatient centers; fewer are dialyzed at hospital-affiliated units; and a small number dialyze at home with the assistance of a nurse or family member. The procedure is performed as follows. A vascular access (usually a native arteriovenous fistula or polytetrafluoroethylene graft) is needed to provide the obligate blood flows (approximately 350 to 400 mL per minute) required to cleanse the blood efficiently. The clearance of solutes associated with uremia, such as urea nitrogen, creatinine, and other unmeasured or unknown solutes, is achieved primarily by diffusion across a semipermeable membrane, as well as by convection, i.e., solute transfer with ultrafiltration or fluid removal. Whereas low-molecular-weight solutes are very efficiently cleared by diffusion, larger solutes—the so-called middle molecules—are cleared more efficiently by convection. Depending on the size, permeability, and other characteristics of the dialyzer (artificial kidney), increases in blood flow and dialysate flow increase solute clearance.

A typical hemodialysis prescription includes 3 to 5 hours of therapy three times weekly, with blood flows of 300 to 400 mL per minute and dialysate flows of 500 to 800 mL per minute. The dialysate, or fluid against which the blood is bathed, can be individualized to fit the needs of the particular patient. Typically, it is composed of the following electrolytes (concentrations): sodium (138 to 145 mEq per liter), potassium (0 to 4 mEq per liter), chloride (100 to 110 mEq per liter), bicarbonate (35 to 45 mEq per liter), calcium (1.5 to 3.5 mEq per liter), magnesium (1.5

mEq per liter), and glucose (2 grams per liter). An anticoagulant, usually heparin, is required to prevent clotting of blood within the hollow fibers of the dialyzer. The dialysis machine, or delivery system, is not in contact with the blood or dialysate. Rather, its pumps, controls, and safety devices provide precision to the hemodialysis procedure by ensuring proper dialysate composition and temperature and by monitoring the transmembrane pressure required to perform ultrafiltration, or net fluid removal. Complications commonly observed in hemodialysis are listed in Table 6.

Peritoneal Dialysis

Like hemodialysis, peritoneal dialysis is achieved by diffusion, using a semipermeable membrane—in this case the peritoneum rather than the dialyzer. Peritoneal dialysis is less commonly employed than hemodialysis in the United States (approximately 15% of patients), although the fraction of patients who choose peritoneal dialysis varies widely from center to center and among physicians. In addition, a substantial fraction of patients initiated on peritoneal dialysis switch to hemodialysis as residual renal function deteriorates or if recurrent peritonitis renders the peritoneum ineffective as a dialysis membrane. The technique failure rate due to all causes is approximately 50% at 3 years.

Peritoneal dialysis is delivered in one of three major ways. Continuous ambulatory peritoneal dialysis (CAPD) is provided by four to six fluid exchanges throughout the day. Generally these exchanges (2 to 3 liters) are instilled into the peritoneal cavity through a surgically placed Silastic catheter and drained every 3 to 4 hours during waking hours; a 2-liter bag is instilled overnight to provide additional solute clearance. Continuous cyclical peritoneal dialysis (CCPD) utilizes a machine that automatically performs fluid exchanges during the night. Patients on CCPD may retain a dry abdomen during waking hours but receive better dialysis with 1 to 2 liters to

TABLE 6. **Common Complications of Dialysis**

Hemodialysis
  Hypotension
  Arrhythmia
  Catheter-related or endovascular infection
  Hemorrhage
  Pyrogen reaction
  Hypoxemia
  Leukopenia
  Catabolism
  Dialysis disequilibrium

Peritoneal Dialysis
  Peritonitis
  Ultrafiltration failure
  Hyperglycemia
  Hypertriglyceridemia
  Weight gain
  Elevated intra-abdominal pressure
  Constipation

dwell during the daytime. Both continuous techniques must be performed daily and require responsible patients with a strong desire for self-care. Intermittent peritoneal dialysis (IPD) or frequent exchanges on alternate days or thrice weekly may be employed short-term, for instance, during hospitalization. However, IPD rarely provides adequate time-averaged clearance unless substantial residual renal function remains.

Among the peritoneal dialysis regimens, CCPD may be more convenient for some patients, particularly those with children or whose work precludes the ability to perform sterile exchanges. However, the absence of around-the-clock clearance limits dialysis efficiency, particularly for middle molecules. Likewise, because the fluid is instilled while the patient is supine, large volume exchanges (over 2.5 liters) are often poorly tolerated. For all peritoneal dialysis regimens, an increase in the frequency and/or volume of peritoneal exchanges usually results in increased solute clearance. The percentage of dextrose in the peritoneal dialysate in large part determines the ultrafiltration rate—the higher the concentration of dextrose (1.5, 2.5, or 4.25%), the greater the quantity and rate of ultrafiltration.

Peritoneal dialysis exerts important effects on the nutritional status of the patient with ESRD. The instillation and absorption of glucose result in the delivery of 400 to 500 kcal per day, which may augment nutrition in patients with poor appetite but may worsen pre-existent hypertriglyceridemia, particularly among diabetic patients. In contrast, the loss of protein through the peritoneum can contribute to protein malnutrition (discussed later).

Unlike hemodialysis, a reliable measure of delivered dialysis dose in peritoneal dialysis has not been validated. A peritoneal equilibrium test can be used to assess the transport properties of the membrane and does correlate somewhat with dialysis adequacy.

Peritonitis is the most important complication of peritoneal dialysis. It is most often caused by a break in sterile technique and usually (80 to 90%) is associated with the introduction of bacteria colonizing the pericatheter skin (e.g., *Staphylococcus epidermidis, S. aureus, Streptococcus* spp). Peritonitis may also be caused by enteric gram-negative rods, hydrophilic gram-negative rods (e.g., *Pseudomonas* spp), mycobacteria, or fungi. Antimicrobial agents can be administered systemically or directly into the peritoneal cavity. Most cases of peritonitis can be resolved without interruption of dialysis or impairment of peritoneal function. However, repeated gram-negative infections or fungal peritonitis usually require removal of the indwelling catheter. Additional complications of peritoneal dialysis are listed in Table 6.

Transplantation

Kidney transplantation, a third option in renal replacement, is considered by most patients and nephrologists to be the treatment of choice for ESRD. Its major advantages are freedom from long-term dialysis, more complete reversal of uremia and nephroendocrine functions, and an overall reduction in health care costs. However, transplantation is better considered a trade-off rather than a panacea for ESRD, as the agents used to combat rejection have many important short- and long-term adverse effects (Table 7).

Most allografts are derived from cadaver donors. The waiting time ranges from 3 months to years, depending largely on blood type, human leukocyte antigen (HLA) matching, and donor organ availability. In contrast, related-donor transplantation can be performed with a healthy, immunologically compatible, willing family member at almost any time, even before the initiation of dialysis. The short-term outcome of renal transplantation has gradually improved: 80 to 85% of all cadaveric kidneys and more than 90% of living-related kidneys transplanted are functional at the end of a year. Unfortunately, the long-term "survival" of allografts has remained modest (7 years for cadaveric allografts, 14 years for living-related allografts), presumably due to recurrence of underlying disease, poor adherence to immunosuppressive therapy, cyclosporine nephrotoxicity, hyperfiltration-induced (i.e., nonimmunologic damage to remnant nephrons) injury, and financial and other psychosocial constraints. In addition, the sup-

TABLE 7. **Immunosuppressive Drugs Used in Renal Transplantation**

Drug	Major Side Effects	Cost
Cyclosporine (Sandimmune)	Infection Hypertension Hyperkalemia Hyperuricemia and gout Renal dysfunction Lymphoid malignancy Hirsutism Gingival hypertrophy	Very high
Azathioprine (Imuran)	Infection Squamous cell carcinoma of skin Leukopenia	High

Prednisone or
  methylprednisolone
	Infection
	Hypertension
	Fluid retention
	Hyperglycemia and
	  diabetes
	Osteoporosis
	Cataracts
	Hirsutism
	Depression
		Low

Muromonab-CD3
  (Orthoclone OKT3)*
	Infection
	Lymphoid malignancy
	Aseptic meningitis
	Capillary leak
	  syndrome
		Extremely
		high

Lymphocyte immune
  globulin (antithymocyte
  globulin [ATG]) (Atgam)*
	Infection
	Lymphoid malignancy
	Hypersensitivity
		Extremely
		high

*Used for acute rejection or induction therapy.

ply of donor organs has remained stable over several years, whereas the number of eligible potential recipients rises with the treated incidence of ESRD.

NUTRITION AND CHRONIC RENAL FAILURE

The roles of dietary protein and other nutrients in CRF have been investigated intensely in the past decade. Long ago it was recognized that dietary protein intake was associated with uremic symptoms in persons in advanced kidney failure. Before the advent of renal replacement therapy (pre-1950s), uremia was often managed with diets consisting of minimal protein, such as rice, certain vegetables, and fruit juice. Indeed, the reduction in dietary protein intake reduced nausea, vomiting, and some other uremic symptoms. Although life was prolonged for some patients who followed these dietary modifications, many others developed severe protein malnutrition. Later, similar diets supplemented with small quantities of proteins of high biologic value were shown to result in far less protein catabolism. Meanwhile, several investigators suggested that the restriction of dietary protein (and phosphorus) might attenuate the progression of various types of renal disease. Soon after, the administration of low-protein diets became commonplace among patients with CRF and ESRD.

Only recently, however, has the importance of malnutrition been highlighted in several well-designed studies in dialysis patients. A striking association has been demonstrated between mortality and diminished levels of serum albumin (a proxy for visceral protein mass) and creatinine (after adjustment for dialysis intensity, a proxy for somatic protein mass). In addition, results of a prospective trial of protein restriction in patients with chronic renal insufficiency (the Modification of Diet in Renal Disease Study) showed only modest overall benefit in terms of rate of progression of renal failure among patients on a low-protein (or very-low-protein) diet. Although some benefit of protein restriction cannot be excluded, it is advisable to exercise caution with this therapeutic modality. Indeed, attention to blood pressure control may be equally if not more effective and has fewer potential hazards. If protein restriction is prescribed, nutritional status should be carefully monitored. Several methods of nutritional assessment are serial measurements of body weight, anthropometry, serum chemistries (e.g., albumin, transferrin, total lymphocyte count), and functional assessment (e.g., exercise tolerance).

MALIGNANT TUMORS OF THE UROGENITAL TRACT

method of
JOSEPH A. SMITH, JR., M.D.
Vanderbilt University Medical Center
Nashville, Tennessee

PROSTATE CARCINOMA

Adenocarcinoma of the prostate is the most common cancer in men in the United States and the second leading cause of death from cancer. Although prostate cancer is being diagnosed more often in younger men, the incidence of the disease is relatively low in men under the age of 50 but increases progressively with advancing age. Carcinoma of the prostate will be diagnosed clinically in almost 10% of men in the United States, and nearly 3% will die from it. However, autopsy studies show that the pathologic incidence of the disease greatly exceeds the rate of clinical recognition. Thus, prostate cancer remains clinically occult in the majority of men but develops into a cause of considerable morbidity or death in others. The inability to predict the clinical course with accuracy in an individual patient contributes to the controversy and dilemma regarding treatment of prostatic cancer.

Detection and Diagnosis

Early-stage prostatic cancer is asymptomatic. Bladder outlet obstruction, hematuria, perineal pain, or ureteral obstruction appear with locally advanced disease. Metastatic carcinoma of the prostate usually presents with bone pain, although weakness, weight loss, and anorexia may also be observed.

The issue of whether prostate cancer screening should be performed on a population-wide basis is controversial. There are concerns that some of the cancers detected through screening may be clinically unimportant, and their diagnosis may subject an individual to the potential side effects of therapeutic intervention. Most studies have shown, however, that the cancers detected through screening are of a clinically significant volume, distinguishing them from the very small volume cancers detected incidentally in autopsy series. Since up to 10 years may elapse between diagnosis and clinically significant disease progression or death, prostate cancer screening generally is not recommended in men who have less than a 10-year life expectancy.

Newer methods for the screening and detection of prostate cancer, particularly the use of prostate-specific antigen (PSA), have increased the ability of screening techniques to detect prostate cancer. PSA is an enzyme whose physiologic function is to lyse semen. Normally, a small amount of PSA is found in the serum. Normal levels vary according to the method of measurement, but values of less than 4.0 ng per mL are usually considered normal.

PSA levels are increased by pathologic conditions of the prostate. However, PSA is not prostate cancer specific. Prostatitis, prostatic infarct, and prostatic trauma or manipulation (such as urethral catheterization) may elevate PSA levels. The most common cause of PSA elevation is benign prostatic hyperplasia (BPH). PSA's lack of specificity in detecting prostate cancer adds to the controversy regarding screening. Overall, around one-fourth of men with modestly elevated PSA levels are found to have carcinoma of the prostate on biopsy.

PSA levels rise gradually with increasing age, probably because of volume increases in the prostate. Also, the amount of PSA per volume of measurable prostate tissue can be calculated. Age indexing or calculation of PSA density is recommended by some as a means of increasing the specificity of PSA screening. Longitudinal follow-up with annual PSA determinations can also be used. Depending on a number of factors, annual changes of greater than 0.75 ng per mL are considered significant.

Digital palpation of the prostate remains an important method for detecting prostate cancer. Induration, nodularity, or asymmetry of the prostate should be considered with a high index of suspicion for carcinoma. Prostate cancer may be detected by digital rectal examination in the face of a normal serum PSA level.

Transrectal ultrasonography is the best imaging modality for the prostate. Prostate cancer typically is seen as a hypoechoic area, most often located in the peripheral zone of the prostate. Transrectal ultrasonography has proved to be too nonspecific for use in general screening, but it is used to direct prostate biopsies.

When prostate carcinoma is suspected because of either an elevated PSA level or a palpable abnormality, prostate biopsy is indicated. This can be digitally guided, but most often it is performed with transrectal ultrasonography. A spring-loaded biopsy gun is directed transrectally to the area of suspicion. In situations in which there is no palpable abnormality or identifiable lesion on ultrasound, random biopsies of both lobes of the prostate are obtained. Biopsy is performed without anesthesia and has a less than 1% risk of infection if broad-spectrum antibiotics are given beforehand.

Staging

Carcinoma of the prostate is graded according to the individual cellular characteristics and the architectural pattern of the cancer. Prognosis and tumor size are linked to the degree of differentiation. Poorly differentiated tumors are more aggressive and usually either locally extensive or metastatic at the time of diagnosis.

Local extent of the tumor is judged primarily by digital palpation (Table 1). Although this is a relatively insensitive staging method, no imaging modalities have proved to be superior. Transrectal ultrasonography may provide complementary information

TABLE 1. **TNM Staging System for Prostate Cancer**

Stage	Description
T1a	Incidentally detected tumor, ≤5% of resected tissue
T1b	Incidentally detected tumor, >5% of resected tissue
T1c	Impalpable tumor, detected by needle biopsy (usually because of elevated prostate-specific antigen level)
T2a	Tumor confined to prostate, <50% of lobe involved
T2b	Tumor confined to prostate, >50% of lobe involved but not both lobes
T2c	Tumor confined to prostate, involves both lobes
T3a	Unilateral extension through prostate capsule
T3b	Bilateral extension through prostate capsule
T3c	Tumor invades seminal vesicle(s)
T4a	Tumor invades bladder neck, external sphincter, or rectum
T4b	Tumor invades levator muscles and/or is fixed to pelvic wall
N1	Metastasis to lymph node, ≤2 cm in greatest diameter
N2	Metastasis to lymph node, >2 cm but ≤5 cm in greatest diameter
N3	Metastasis to lymph node(s), >5 cm in greatest diameter

but has not proved to be superior to digital rectal palpation. PSA levels can provide indirect staging information. Tumors confined within the prostatic capsule usually have a PSA level of less than 20 ng per mL. Computed tomography (CT) scanning provides little additional information about local extent. Endorectal magnetic resonance imaging (MRI) coils are being investigated for staging the local extent of prostate cancer.

The first site of disease beyond the prostate is usually the pelvic lymph nodes. Pelvic CT scanning, however, is rarely useful, except in patients with very high PSA levels or obvious extracapsular extension. Laparoscopic lymph node dissection is performed as a staging maneuver in some patients.

The most common site of distant metastatic disease is bone, usually the axial skeleton. Radionuclide bone scan is the most sensitive method for detecting bone metastasis. Bone scans rarely show metastatic disease in untreated patients with a PSA of less than 10 ng per mL (Hybritech method) but should be obtained in all symptomatic men or those with higher PSA levels.

Treatment

Localized Disease

The appropriate treatment of patients with carcinoma of the prostate, especially in early stages, remains a subject of great controversy. In part, this is due to the variable natural history of the disease and the inability to predict the prognosis for individual patients. The treatment options relate directly to the stage of the disease at the time of diagnosis and are also dependent on the age and health of the individual.

SURVEILLANCE

A withholding of active intervention (sometimes termed "surveillance" or "watchful waiting") is recommended by some, even in the face of a known diagnosis of carcinoma of the prostate. This philosophy is prompted by the recognition that the cancer may be slowly progressive and not a cause of death or significant morbidity for up to 10 years. Studies from Scandinavia have shown that watchful waiting is appropriate in some individuals, especially those with small volume, well-differentiated tumors and a life expectancy otherwise of less than 10 years.

Most clinicians agree that watchful waiting is appropriate in most men 75 years of age or older. For younger men in otherwise good health, however, active intervention may be indicated. Up to one-third of younger men with at least moderately differentiated tumors may die from prostate cancer within 10 years if left untreated.

A number of factors must be weighed in considering a watchful waiting approach. Patient age, health status, and family history must all be considered. Tumor factors such as size, grade, and serum PSA levels provide some prognostic information. Nonetheless, the wishes of an informed patient are paramount, as there is uncertainty about the significance of a particular tumor in any individual.

RADICAL PROSTATECTOMY

Radical prostatectomy is a surgical procedure that involves removal of the entire prostate with its enveloping fascial layers and the seminal vesicles. The operation can be performed from a retropubic approach through a lower midline abdominal incision or through a perineal incision. The operative mortality is less than 1%, and few patients require homologous blood transfusion.

Modifications and refinement in surgical technique have decreased complications and side effects associated with radical prostatectomy. Sexual potency can be preserved in some men by preservation of the neurovascular bundle. The success of this maneuver is proportionate to patient age and sexual function preoperatively. Patients with palpable tumor nodules near the prostatic apex are not good candidates for a nerve-sparing approach because of a risk of positive surgical margins in the area of the neurovascular bundle.

Regaining urinary control is a gradual process that occurs over several months after radical prostatectomy. A few patients are left with severe incontinence and may seek additional treatment for this, such as collagen injection or implantation of an artificial urethral sphincter. Up to 15 or 20% of patients have mild stress urinary incontinence after radical prostatectomy, but a substantial majority regain total urinary control.

Long-term results after radical prostatectomy are excellent for men with tumors pathologically confined to the prostate. A significant percentage of patients with large palpable tumors or high PSA levels, however, are understaged clinically and are proved histologically to have positive surgical margins. The value of postoperative irradiation in this setting is uncertain.

After radical prostatectomy, PSA levels should be near zero. Any detectable PSA in the serum is considered biochemical evidence of residual disease (either in the prostatic fossa or at distant sites). Although many years may elapse until the development of clinically recognizable disease, treatment failure is ultimately anticipated in patients with detectable PSA levels after radical prostatectomy. Adjuvant hormonal therapy is sometimes used in this setting.

EXTERNAL IRRADIATION

External irradiation delivered to the prostate and periprostatic region is a treatment alternative for patients with apparently localized carcinoma of the prostate. There are no good prospective studies comparing the results of radical prostatectomy and those of external irradiation in patients with carcinoma of the prostate. Survival studies with up to 10-year follow-up suggest little difference in results. However, concerns have been expressed about a positive biopsy rate in over half of men after external beam irradiation therapy.

After external beam irradiation, 5 to 10% of patients experience some degree of cystitis, proctitis, or urethral stricture. Sexual potency declines gradually after external beam irradiation and ultimately is preserved in around the same percentage of men in whom it is preserved after nerve-sparing radical prostatectomy.

PSA levels can be used to follow patients after external beam irradiation, but with less sensitivity than after radical prostatectomy. PSA should decline to at least the normal range after external beam irradiation. Any subsequent rise or a failure to reach normal levels is evidence of treatment failure.

CRYOTHERAPY

Cryosurgery involves freezing the prostate with a transurethral probe. The ice ball can be monitored with a transrectal ultrasound probe. The procedure must be considered investigational, and there are no long-term results on the therapeutic success of cryotherapy.

Metastatic Disease

The most common site of distant metastasis for carcinoma of the prostate is bone, usually the axial skeleton. Soft tissue disease in the absence of bone metastasis is relatively unusual. Bone pain is a common presenting symptom in men with metastatic prostate cancer.

For over 50 years, endocrine manipulation with the intent of androgen deprivation has been the primary form of treatment for metastatic prostate cancer. The goal of therapy is to deprive the cancer cells of androgens. Testicular production of testosterone is the dominant androgen in men. Serum testosterone levels are suppressed rapidly after a surgical bilateral orchiectomy. Alternatively, medical therapy may be used. Orally administered estrogens effectively lower testosterone levels but are associated with cardiovascular side effects.

The most common medical therapy used for the suppression of testicular androgens is the administration of a depot preparation of a luteinizing hormone-releasing hormone (LHRH) analogue. During the first week after the administration of LHRH analogues, serum testosterone levels are increased. Subsequently, there is a rapid and profound suppression of testosterone to the castrate range. LHRH analogues are administered on a monthly basis via a depot injection.

The side effects of LHRH analogues are limited to the consequences of serum testosterone suppression. Accordingly, decreased libido and impotence develop. In addition, almost two-thirds of men have vasomotor hot flashes. Similar side effects are seen after orchiectomy. Hot flashes can be suppressed by the administration of low-dose oral progesterone agents.

A small amount of circulating androgens in men is of adrenal origin. The contribution of these androgens to the growth and development of carcinoma of the prostate has been a subject of controversy. However, it appears that the addition of an antiandrogen to either bilateral orchiectomy or an LHRH analogue extends the duration of response for a few months. This effect may be observed particularly in patients with minimal amounts of metastatic cancer.

In the United States, the only antiandrogen approved by the Food and Drug Administration is flutamide (Eulexin). The drug is administered in three divided daily doses of 250 mg each. Some degree of gynecomastia is common in patients taking flutamide, and diarrhea may develop in up to 20% of men.

After hormonal therapy, both subjective and objective evidence of disease response occurs. Serum PSA levels decrease, and disease-related symptoms improve or are eliminated. Unfortunately, however, the duration of response is usually only 18 to 24 months. Once disease progression occurs, there is no treatment that has been shown to have a favorable effect on survival. Various investigational protocols are being pursued, but the primary aim of treatment should be palliation. External irradiation is effective for isolated areas of metastatic bone pain. In men with diffuse osseous metastases and bone pain, intravenous administration of strontium-89 chloride (Metastron) can provide effective palliation.

UROTHELIAL TUMORS—TRANSITIONAL CELL CARCINOMA

Transitional cells line the urothelium from the renal calices to the prostatic urethra. Transitional cell carcinoma may occur at any of these points and is often a "field charge" tumor that affects different areas simultaneously or in sequence.

Detection and Diagnosis

The most common presenting sign or symptom in patients with transitional cell carcinoma is gross painless hematuria. Flank pain may occur in patients with upper tract tumors associated with the passage of blood clots. Irritative voiding symptoms such as urinary frequency and urgency are sometimes seen in patients with bladder involvement.

Since malignant cells are sloughed readily, cytopathologic examination of the urine is often capable of detecting malignant cells. The diagnosis is confirmed by endoscopic visualization of tumors in the bladder and by transurethral resection or biopsy. For upper tract tumors, the diagnosis is usually made based on a typical appearance of a filling defect on intravenous pyelography and direct visualization by ureteroscopy.

CARCINOMA OF THE RENAL PELVIS

Transitional cell carcinoma may occur in the renal pelvis or the caliceal system. Except in situations in which there is a solitary kidney or compromised renal function in the opposite kidney, nephroureterectomy is the preferred treatment. In patients with solitary kidneys, a conservative approach is warranted. If feasible, partial nephrectomy is performed. Alternatively, neodymium:YAG laser treatment or electrocautery fulguration can be performed. For low-stage, low-grade tumors, the prognosis after treatment is excellent. High-grade tumors are associated with a poor prognosis. After nephroureterectomy for renal pelvic transitional cell carcinoma, there is an approximately 5% incidence of an asynchronous tumor in the opposite kidney.

URETERAL CARCINOMA

Transitional cell carcinoma of the ureter most often involves the distal one-third. Traditionally, nephroureterectomy has been the treatment for these lesions. Increasingly, more conservative approaches are being used when the tumor is in the distal ureter. Distal ureterectomy with reimplantation of the ureter into the bladder using either a psoas hitch or a Boari flap allows preservation of the ipsilateral kidney. Endoscopic management through ureteroscopes is sometimes feasible. When more conservative approaches are used for proximal ureteral tumors, tumor recurrence in the ureter distal to the lesion is frequent. Consistent with a theory of "field change" as well as with tumor cell implantation, there is a high incidence of subsequent tumor within the bladder, especially near the ipsilateral trigone, in patients with a history of carcinoma of the ureter.

BLADDER CANCER

There are over 50,000 new cases of bladder cancer diagnosed annually in the United States. The male/female ratio is approximately 3:1. Certain chemical carcinogens have been definitely associated with bladder cancer, especially beta naphthalene and certain dyes. Chronic bladder irritation from indwelling Foley catheters or infection with schistosomiasis is associated with squamous cell carcinoma of the bladder. Finally, there is a definite and strong association with cigarette smoking.

Approximately 80% of bladder cancers occur in a superficial, low-grade, low-stage form (Table 2). Patients with superficial bladder cancer are treated by transurethral electrocautery resection or neodymium:YAG laser photocoagulation. Laser therapy offers some practical advantages for patients, but both treatments are equally effective in eliminating visible tumors. After either electrocautery resection or laser treatment, there is a greater than 50% recurrence rate. Because of the high recurrence rate, patients must undergo close surveillance after treatment of tumors. In general, cystoscopy and cytologic examination of the urine are performed every 3 months for 1 year, then every 6 months for another year, and then yearly unless tumor recurs. Most recurrences are superficial. However, there is a 15% incidence of progression in grade or stage in patients who initially present with superficial tumors.

Intravesical chemotherapy or immunotherapy is capable of decreasing the recurrence rate of superficial bladder cancer. Treatment should be given to any patient with recurrent tumors, multiple tumors at the time of diagnosis, tumors larger than 4 cm in size, or dysplasia or carcinoma in situ in adjacent areas of the bladder. Thiotepa is the most frequently used chemotherapeutic agent and is given intravesically in doses of 30 mg weekly for 6 weeks. The white blood cell count should be monitored, since intravascular absorption and myelosuppression may occur in as many as 10% of patients. Mitomycin C (Mutamycin) 40 mg intravesically weekly for 6 weeks is also active against superficial bladder cancer but is quite expensive. Bacille Calmette-Guérin (BCG), an attenuated strain of *Mycobacterium tuberculosis*, is the most effective intravesical agent for the prophylactic treatment of superficial bladder cancer. The exact mechanism of action is uncertain, but local immunologic response within the bladder is likely. Tuberculosis skin tests (intermediate purified protein derivative) may convert to positive in patients after intravesical BCG therapy, and bladder biopsies often show granuloma formation in the bladder wall. Therapy is usually well tolerated, although irritative voiding symptoms are common, and fever and malaise

may be seen on the day of drug administration. Systemic infections with BCG develop in a small percentage of patients and manifest as granulomatous hepatitis, pulmonary disease, or prostatitis. Systemic antituberculous therapy is indicated in this situation. When BCG is used in a prophylactic manner after the removal of existing bladder tumors, approximately 80% of patients have no evidence of recurrence. In addition, BCG is the most effective intravesical treatment for carcinoma in situ of the bladder.

Transitional cell carcinoma that invades the detrusor muscle is usually high grade and not manageable by transurethral resection. Partial cystectomy with removal of only the involved segment of the bladder is indicated in the unusual situation in which the remainder of the bladder is normal and the tumor is located in a mobile portion of the bladder wall. Most often, the tumor involves the bladder trigone or there is an antecedent history of tumors in other portions of the bladder. Radical cystectomy is the most proven form of therapy for muscle-invasive transitional cell carcinoma of the bladder. In men, this includes removal of the prostate and seminal vesicles; in women, the uterus, fallopian tubes, ovaries, and anterior portion of the vagina are removed along with the bladder. Pelvic lymph node dissection should be performed in all patients. Approximately one-fourth of patients with invasive bladder cancer have histologic nodal metastasis, and a distinct minority of these patients are cured by surgery alone. Randomized studies have shown no benefit of preoperative pelvic irradiation. After bladder removal, urinary reconstruction can be via a continent reservoir or an ileal conduit. An ileal conduit transports urine to the skin and requires a collection device. Continent cutaneous reservoirs are usually constructed with either right colon or small bowel. The patient performs self-catheterization every 4 to 5 hours but otherwise has a small and easily covered stoma. Orthotopic placement of continent reservoirs can be performed, and many patients find this preferable. The reservoir of either large or small bowel is anastomosed directly to the urethra after bladder removal. Continence is via the intact external urethral sphincter. Most often, continence is excellent after orthotopic placement of a neobladder. Continent cutaneous or orthotopic reservoirs have decreased some of the concerns associated with quality of life following cystectomy.

As an alternative to cystectomy, radiation therapy can be curative in some patients. Methods of bladder preservation using radiation plus chemotherapy are being explored. In general, however, radiation is reserved for patients who refuse or who are not candidates for radical surgery, since the cure rates are less than with bladder removal, and radiation does not prevent the formation of new tumors.

METASTATIC DISEASE

Each year, approximately 10,000 people die in the United States from metastatic transitional cell carci-

TABLE 2. **TNM Staging System for Bladder Cancer**

Stage	Description
Ta	Noninvasive papillary carcinoma
TIS	Carcinoma in situ: flat tumor
T1	Tumor invades subepithelial connective tissue
T2	Tumor invades inner half of superficial muscle
T3a	Tumor invades deep muscle
T3b	Tumor invades perivesical fat
T4a	Tumor invades prostate, uterus, or vagina
T4b	Tumor invades pelvic or abdominal wall
N1	Metastasis to single node, ≤2 cm in greatest diameter
N2	Metastasis to single node, between 2 and 5 cm in greatest diameter
N3	Metastasis to node(s), >5 cm in greatest diameter

noma, usually with the bladder as the primary site. Lung, liver, and bone are the primary sites of distant metastatic disease, but local pelvic recurrence or involvement of retroperitoneal lymph nodes is not uncommon. Cisplatin and methotrexate are the most active single cytotoxic agents for metastatic transitional cell carcinoma. The best reported response rates have occurred using a combination of methotrexate, vincristine (Oncovin), doxorubicin (Adriamycin), and cisplatin (Platinol), the so-called M-VAC regimen. The regimen is toxic and requires adequate renal function. The role of adjuvant chemotherapy either before or after radical surgery is being explored. However, there may be a survival advantage for patients with poor prognostic parameters and for patients who receive early chemotherapy.

TESTICULAR CARCINOMA

Germ cell tumors of the testis are the most common malignancy in men between the ages of 25 and 39 years. Less commonly, juvenile embryonal cell carcinoma is seen in young children, and there is a somewhat increased incidence of seminoma in men in the sixth decade of life. Testicular tumors are quite uncommon in blacks. A history of cryptorchidism introduces an increased risk for the development of testicular cancer.

The presentation is most often as a hard, sometimes irregular mass intrinsic to the testis. The tumors are typically asymptomatic and nontender, but pain may occur when there is hemorrhage within the tumor or associated epididymitis. In general, inguinal exploration of the testis should be performed whenever physical examination raises suspicions of tumor. Inguinal orchiectomy with removal of the entire spermatic cord to the level of the internal inguinal ring should be performed in all patients with testicular carcinoma.

Local recurrence is unusual unless there has been violation of the scrotal sac. The first echelon of metastatic disease is to the retroperitoneal lymph nodes near the origin of the spermatic vessels. CT scanning is the best single staging procedure for the detection of retroperitoneal nodal disease. A chest radiograph is obtained in all patients, since lungs are the most common site of disease beyond the retroperitoneum. Serum levels of alpha$_1$-fetoprotein are diagnostic of nonseminomatous elements.

Seminoma

Seminoma is the most common single histologic variety of testis tumor. Its natural history and response to treatment are different from those of nonseminomatous tumors. Most patients have clinical Stage I disease at the time of presentation, with no evidence of residual tumor after orchiectomy. Although a substantial majority of these patients will have no recurrence without further treatment, retroperitoneal irradiation provides a cure rate of over 95% with low morbidity. Radiation is delivered to the retroperitoneal nodes and ipsilateral pelvic nodes. Supradiaphragmatic irradiation is not indicated in this group. Excellent cure rates are also achieved with radiation in patients with small volume retroperitoneal disease. When retroperitoneal nodes exceed 5 cm in size or when there is evidence of disease outside the retroperitoneum, chemotherapy should be used. Various cisplatin-based regimens of chemotherapy have been shown to be active against seminoma. Often, the same combinations that are used against nonseminomatous tumors are employed for seminoma, with response rates that equal or exceed those for nonseminomatous lesions.

Nonseminomatous Tumors

Nonseminomatous tumors include a variety of histologic types, including embryonal cell carcinoma and teratocarcinoma as well as tumors with mixed elements. Pure choriocarcinoma accounts for less than 1% of testis tumors, is associated with a poor prognosis, and should be treated with aggressive combination chemotherapy. Treatment for other nonseminomatous testis tumors depends on the stage at the time of diagnosis. Because of the inaccuracies of clinical staging, retroperitoneal lymph node dissection is recommended for patients with Stage I disease. If the retroperitoneal lymph nodes are histologically normal, no further treatment is needed, and recurrence rates are under 10%. In patients with microscopic involvement of the retroperitoneal lymph nodes, two courses of cisplatin-based chemotherapy provide cure rates of over 95%. Alternatively, careful follow-up can be used, with chemotherapy salvage for patients whose tumors recur. If a technique that preserves the sympathetic nerves responsible for ejaculation is used, fewer than 10% of patients are rendered infertile because of retroperitoneal lymphadenectomy. However, there is an overall increased incidence of infertility in men with testis tumors because of abnormalities in the semen pattern. Some patients can be observed carefully without lymphadenectomy. Although no randomized studies are available, cure rates approach those obtained in patients treated with lymphadenectomy. However, this approach applies only to a minority of patients with testis tumors. To be considered for such a protocol, a patient should have a primary tumor that does not invade the epididymis or spermatic cord, an unequivocally normal CT scan of the retroperitoneum, a normal chest radiograph, and normal serum levels of alpha$_1$-fetoprotein and human chorionic gonadotropin-beta. Furthermore, the patient must be both willing and able to comply with a stringent follow-up regimen. Physical examination, chest radiograph, and blood studies should be obtained monthly for 2 years and a CT scan at least every 3 months. Approximately 25% of the tumors can be expected to recur and require treatment.

Chemotherapy should be used initially in patients with metastatic disease beyond the retroperitoneum or in those with retroperitoneal lymph nodes that are greater than 5 cm in size. Excellent response rates are observed, and over 70% of patients with metastatic disease can be cured. Combination treatment with cisplatin, etoposide (VePesid), and vinblastine (Velban) is used most often. In patients who have not undergone lymphadenectomy, a residual retroperitoneal mass is often evident. Fibrosis is found after surgical removal in approximately 40% of patients, and another 20% have residual malignant elements. In the other 40% of patients, mature teratoma is identified. Teratoma must be resected completely, because subsequent enlargement may compromise adjacent organs, or malignant degeneration may occur. No further treatment is indicated if a mature teratoma is resected completely, but additional chemotherapy should be used if malignant elements are present.

TUMORS OF THE KIDNEY

Over 90% of tumors that arise from the renal parenchyma are malignant. Sarcomas or metastatic tumors to the kidney are seen occasionally. However, the substantial majority of kidney tumors are renal cell carcinomas in adults and Wilms' tumors in children.

Renal Cell Carcinoma

Renal cell carcinomas arise from the proximal tubular epithelium and are adenocarcinomas. These tumors are commonly referred to as hypernephromas. The classic triad of symptoms associated with hypernephroma—flank pain, a palpable mass, and hematuria—is seen rarely. Increasingly, renal cell carcinomas are being detected incidentally on abdominal imaging studies performed for evaluation of other organs. Because they may produce no symptoms and the kidney is not readily palpable on physical examination, renal cell carcinomas may attain great size before they are detected. Lung, bone, and brain are the most common sites of metastatic disease, but renal cell carcinomas are notorious for having unusual patterns of metastasis. Tumor-associated findings such as anemia, erythrocytosis, liver function abnormalities, and hypercalcemia are not uncommon. The diagnosis of renal cell carcinoma is most often based on a characteristic CT scan appearance. Occasionally, a benign angiomyolipoma of the kidney is mistaken for a renal cell carcinoma, but a CT scan showing fat within the tumor is diagnostic of angiomyolipoma. Oncocytomas are benign tumors but cannot be distinguished reliably from renal cell carcinoma by CT scan or other diagnostic methods. Arteriography was used frequently in the past but is rarely indicated now for either diagnosing or staging renal cell cancers. Percutaneous needle biopsy of renal masses is not usually rewarding. A diagnosis based on radiographic findings provides sufficient clinical accuracy, and a biopsy showing only benign elements does not exclude the presence of a renal cell carcinoma.

Radical nephrectomy is the treatment of choice for renal cell carcinomas when there is a normal contralateral kidney. Gerota's fascia and its contents are removed en bloc, including the kidney, the perirenal fat, and the ipsilateral adrenal gland. Lymphadenectomy provides prognostic information but is probably of little therapeutic value. Prognosis for tumors confined within the renal capsule is fairly good, with a 70% 5-year survival. If the tumor penetrates into the perirenal fat, 5-year survival after radical nephrectomy is around 50%. Radical surgery is rarely curative in patients with positive regional lymph nodes. In patients with solitary kidneys or in situations in which there is compromised function of the contralateral kidney, parenchymal sparing procedures are indicated. For polar lesions, partial nephrectomy with a margin of normal kidney is indicated.

Some 10 to 15% of renal cell cancers invade the renal vein or inferior vena cava. In the absence of distant metastatic disease, surgical removal can provide surprisingly good cure rates if regional lymph nodes are not simultaneously involved. Cardiac bypass and complete circulatory arrest have been used for some tumors that extend into the right atrium. Most often, the caval thrombus does not actually invade the wall of the inferior vena cava and can be extracted through a vena cavotomy.

Metastatic renal cell carcinoma is one of the most resistant tumors to chemotherapy. No cytotoxic agent has been identified that produces satisfactory response rates or that has been shown to improve survival. Hormonal therapy, often medroxyprogesterone acetate (Depo-Provera) 10 mg intramuscularly once a week, is sometimes used but is probably ineffective. Removal of the primary tumor in patients with known metastatic disease usually is not indicated unless there is pain or recurrent bleeding. Although spontaneous regression of metastatic disease after removal of the primary lesion has been documented, it occurs in fewer than 1% of patients. Interferons generally provide around a 15% response rate without any evidence that survival is improved. Some response has been reported for a combination of lymphokine-activated killer cells (LAK) and interleukin-2. Other biologic response modifiers are being investigated.

TUMORS OF THE PENIS

Squamous cell carcinoma of the penis is the most common cancer in some countries but accounts for less than 1% of tumors in men in the United States. Squamous cell carcinoma of the penis is exceedingly rare in men who underwent neonatal circumcision. The disease is most often seen in the sixth or seventh decade of life but may occur earlier. The primary lesion usually involves the glans penis or prepuce. Typically, the tumors are painless, and patients may not present until the lesion has attained a large size. Secondary infection with purulence and drainage is common. A biopsy is used to establish the diagnosis.

The first site of metastatic disease is the inguinal lymph nodes. Palpable lymph nodes at the time of presentation may be reactive, but fine-needle aspiration can help distinguish this tumor from metastatic disease. In the presence of abnormal lymph nodes, inguinal lymphadenectomy should be performed. When the nodes are normal palpably, a limited dissection and sentinel node biopsy are performed if the primary tumor is high grade and infiltrative. Although a negative sentinel node biopsy does not ensure negative lymph nodes elsewhere, this approach is preferable to observation alone. The primary morbidity of inguinal lymphadenectomy—skin flap necrosis and lower extremity edema—can be prevented by avoiding excessive thinning of the skin flap and dissection of the lymphatic channels lateral to and behind the femoral vessels. Lymphadenectomy can be curative in almost half of patients who have metastasis limited to the inguinal lymph nodes. Pelvic node involvement or distant disease is associated with a very poor prognosis. Cisplatin, methotrexate, and bleomycin are the most frequently used cytotoxic drugs, but none has been shown to increase survival.

Extensive primary tumors with involvement of the proximal corpora cavernosa may require total penectomy and perineal urethrotomy. Usually, the primary lesion can be excised with an adequate margin if partial penectomy is performed approximately 2 cm proximal to the glans penis. For minimally infiltrative tumors, a neodymium:YAG laser provides excellent local control rates, with functional and cosmetic results that are superior to those obtained with partial penectomy.

ADRENAL TUMORS

Adrenal cortical carcinomas are tumors that arise from the adrenal cortex. The majority of these tumors are hormonally functional and may produce Cushing's syndrome from excessive glucocorticoids or virilization from excessive androgen production. When the tumors do not retain endocrine function, they may remain asymptomatic until they attain great size.

Aggressive surgical resection should be performed for adrenal carcinomas. This may require ipsilateral nephrectomy, but the prognosis for unresectable or metastatic adrenal carcinoma is dismal. Mitotane (Lysodren) is an insecticide that has shown some activity against metastatic adrenal carcinoma. However, the drug has severe side effects and has not been shown to improve survival. In patients with steroid-producing cancers, periodic steroid excretion tests can be used for postoperative monitoring, since recurrent tumors may be detected by a rising steroid excretion.

Pheochromocytomas may arise anywhere along the sympathetic chain in the retroperitoneum or the mediastinum. However, the most common intra-abdominal location is the adrenal medulla. Only 10% of pheochromocytomas are malignant, and histologic features of the primary tumor are unreliable in determining whether the lesions are malignant. Most often, the diagnosis of malignancy is based on the presence of nodal metastasis or metastatic disease. Aggressive surgical resection is indicated, but the prognosis for malignant pheochromocytomas is poor.

URETHRAL STRICTURE

method of
ROY WITHERINGTON, M.D.
Medical College of Georgia
Augusta, Georgia

Urethral strictures may result from either infection or trauma. Postinfective strictures are common, involve the anterior urethra, can be treated in many ways, and frequently recur. Post-traumatic strictures involve either the prostatomembranous or the bulbous urethra and respond well to excision and reanastomosis. A tentative diagnosis can be made when a small flexible catheter will not pass into the bladder, and diagnosis can be confirmed by urethrography. When a urethral stricture is associated with either inflammation or trauma, preliminary suprapubic cystostomy is indicated to allow the reaction to subside and the scar to mature. A properly planned approach to management requires a knowledge of location, cause, extent, and severity of the lesion.

MANAGEMENT

General Methods

Urethral Dilatation. Urethral dilatation is still the "gold standard," and most patients can be managed on a long-term basis by simple dilatation. It is imperative that progressive dilatation rather than forceful tearing be accomplished. Tears heal by scarring, and stricture can be worsened by overzealous treatment. Tight strictures are best managed using filiforms and Phillips followers (either catheters or bougies). After passage of a small follower (No. 8 French), progressively larger followers are passed until resistance is met. The instrument is removed, and voiding is usually much improved. Repeat dilatation is performed at 7- to 10-day intervals, and each time the urethra can usually be dilated to a larger diameter. LeFort sounds can be substituted for Phillips followers after the first or second session. Once dilated to Nos. 22 to 24 French, Van Buren sounds can be used instead of filiforms and followers or LeFort sounds. When the urethral diameter reaches Nos. 26 to 28 French, dilatations are required less frequently. Patients with urinary retention and particularly dense strictures that cannot initially be dilated beyond Nos. 8 to 10 French can be managed by leaving an indwelling catheter-type follower. The follower is held in place by two silk sutures that are tied around it just distal to the meatus and carefully taped to the penis. After 2 to 3 days, progressive dilatation can be accomplished with ease. Once the lumen of the urethra is enlarged to Nos. 16 to 18

French, placement of a small Foley catheter can accomplish soft dilatation. The catheter can be changed to a larger size every 2 to 3 days until the desired urethral caliber is reached. Successful long-term management depends on careful atraumatic dilatation every 3 to 6 months. Many patients can be taught to dilate their own strictures by periodically passing either a catheter or a sound.

Internal Urethrotomy. Incision of urethral strictures can be accomplished by either a blind or a visual technique. Blind urethrotomy is done using an Otis urethrotome. The device is No. 16 French in diameter and therefore cannot be used initially to treat tight strictures. The shaft of the instrument is made larger by turning a proximally positioned wheel, and changes in size can be read from a calibrated dial on the instrument. A dull knife blade is inserted on the top of the shaft and, when properly introduced, is hidden at the distal end. Once the instrument has been inserted and enlarged to the point where it is snug within the urethra, the knife is quickly drawn through the stricture to produce a clean dorsal cut. The urethra can be enlarged to any desired diameter, usually Nos. 28 to 30 French, by repeated cuts. Proper use requires that overzealous stretching not occur prior to making any cuts. A Teflon-coated latex catheter that must be No. 2 French smaller than the size of the incised urethra is left indwelling for 3 weeks to allow epithelium to grow across the incised area and to enlarge the urethral lumen. Visual urethrotomy necessitates a distal urethral lumen of fairly large caliber to permit introduction of the urethrotome. This device has a sharp blade and is most often used to incise short strictures. The stricture is visualized and either a small ureteral catheter or a guidewire is passed through it to maintain access and orientation. The blade is extended, and clean cuts are made through the stricture in one or more locations to enlarge the diameter to Nos. 26 to 30 French. This method of management is best for clean iris diaphragm–type strictures; extensive, tight strictures often cannot be treated in this way. If the stricture is short and not very fibrotic, post-treatment catheterization may not be necessary. When extensive incisions are made, a short period of catheterization for both hemostasis and diversion of urine is wise. Following urethrotomy, residual stricture is usually present and can be managed by either periodic dilatations or repeat internal urethrotomy.

Open Surgical Techniques

Patch Graft Urethroplasty. Strictures in the distal bulbous and pendulous urethra can be managed by patch graft urethroplasty. A ventral incision is made through the stricture, and it is extended at least 1 to 1.5 cm proximally and distally into normal urethra. A free full-thickness graft of distal prepuce is harvested, tailored to fit, and sewn into the defect over a stenting catheter. All subdermal tissue is excised, and epidermis is placed toward the lumen.

With particularly severe segmental strictures, it may be necessary to excise the strictured area and to interpose a tubularized graft. The stenting catheter is left indwelling for 10 to 14 days. Pedicle island grafts of penile or scrotal skin can be substituted for free patch grafts in many instances. Long-term results of both free and pedicle graft urethroplasties appear to be good.

Excision of Stricture with Urethrourethrostomy. Short post-traumatic bulbous and prostatomembranous urethral strictures can be easily managed by excision and accurate spatulated urethrourethrostomy over a stenting catheter. The stent is left indwelling for 10 to 14 days.

Multistaged Procedures. These techniques initially externalize the strictured area when adjacent penile or scrotal skin is sewn directly to the ventrally incised urethra (first stage). The externalized area is allowed to become soft and pliable prior to urethral reconstruction (second stage). The strip of epithelium used for urethral reconstruction must be wide enough to produce a tube of adequate caliber, and a small fenestrated catheter is left in the urethra to act as an internal drain. The multistage techniques can be applied to strictures located anywhere from the prostatomembranous junction to the distal penis. They are most often used for proximal bulbous strictures.

Suprapubic cystostomy at the time of urethroplasty or urethral reconstruction by any technique is wise, so that proximal urinary diversion can be accomplished should there be extravasation from the repair site following removal of the urethral stent.

Treatment of Stricture by Location

Meatal Strictures. Simple postinfective meatal strictures can be managed by dorsal or ventral meatotomy. Dorsal meatotomy using the Otis urethrotome results in a good cosmetic result and an absence of splayed stream. Following dorsal meatotomy, a catheter must be left indwelling for a few days to allow hemostasis to occur. Then, self-dilatation to maintain the caliber of the meatus is necessary until healing is complete. Ventral meatotomy is accomplished by incision of the ventral meatal area and suture approximation of skin to urethral epithelium. With ventral meatotomy, the cosmetic result is not good, and splaying of the urinary stream often occurs. Meatal stricture secondary to balanitis xerotica obliterans is best managed by meatoplasty. Here, the strictured area is incised ventrally until normal urethra is encountered. A U-shaped skin flap is created on the ventral surface of the penis near the frenulum, which is sewn into the urethral meatus to enlarge its caliber. The cosmetic result is not pleasing, but the functional result is usually quite acceptable.

Pendulous Urethral Strictures. These may be managed by periodic dilatations, internal urethrotomy, either patch graft or pedicle graft urethroplasty, and multistaged urethroplasty. The multistaged technique is particularly applicable to dense pan-urethral postinfective strictures.

Bulbous Urethral Strictures. Post-traumatic bulbous urethral stricture is best treated by excision and accurate spatulated urethrourethrostomy. Distal bulbous postinfective strictures can be managed by periodic dilatations and by either patch graft or pedicle island graft urethroplasty. A very proximal bulbous postinfective stricture can be managed by periodic dilatations but should not be managed by patch graft urethroplasty, because the lesion is adjacent to the active part of the urethra (sphincter). This stricture is best managed by a two-stage procedure. A popular technique is to use a posteriorly based perineal skin flap where the tip extends onto the scrotum. The urethra is incised proximally and distally at least 1 to 1.5 cm from the stricture, and the flap is sewn in place. The externalized area is carefully observed over the next 6 months, and if either granulation tissue or synechiae appear, they are destroyed. The externalized urethra is allowed to become soft and pliable. Adequate stomal caliber (Nos. 28 to 30 French) must be ensured before second-stage urethroplasty is accomplished.

Prostatomembranous Urethral Strictures. These nearly always follow trauma and are best handled by excision and accurate spatulated urethrourethrostomy. With short strictures, a transperineal approach gives excellent results. Long or complex strictures with associated fistulas, sinuses, diverticula, and bone spicules within the urethra are best managed by a combined retropubic and perineal approach. The combined approach allows appropriate treatment of associated lesions, accurate urethral anastomosis, and placement of a pedicle graft of omentum around the repair site, which lends blood supply, fills dead space, and prevents excessive postoperative fibrosis. Short prostatomembranous strictures can sometimes be managed satisfactorily by transurethral incision and periodic dilatations.

NEPHROLITHIASIS

method of
DEAN G. ASSIMOS, M.D.
The Bowman Gray School of Medicine of Wake Forest University
Winston-Salem, North Carolina

Renal and ureteral calculi may cause a number of symptoms and signs, including flank, abdominal, groin, and scrotal pain; urinary frequency and urgency; microscopic or gross hematuria; and urinary tract infection. Nephrolithiasis affects males more commonly, is less common in African Americans, and usually manifests between ages 30 and 50 years. Stone formation is a multifactorial phenomenon influenced by increased excretion of constituent ions, supersaturation of stone-forming salts, crystal retention, deficits in urinary inhibitors, urinary pH, genetic composition, the environment, diet, and undefined intranephronal

events. Approximately 70% of patients with nephrolithiasis have calcium oxalate calculi. Mixed calcium, calcium phosphate, struvite (magnesium ammonium phosphate–calcium carbonate), uric acid, cystine, matrix, xanthine, 2,8-dihydroxyadenine, and triamterene calculi occur less frequently.

The diagnosis is usually established with intravenous pyelography, which defines the size and anatomic position of the stone. Retrograde pyelography may be required if intravenous pyelography is not confirmatory and in patients with contrast allergy or renal dysfunction. Uric acid calculi are frequently radiolucent, and ultrasonography or uninfused computed tomography (CT) may be employed for identification in these cases. Sometimes the aforementioned studies are inconclusive, and endoscopy of the ureter and renal collecting system (ureterorenoscopy) using rigid or flexible instruments is performed to establish the diagnosis.

Most patients have ureteral calculi, which are typically small and pass spontaneously. Stone size may be utilized to predict the chances of spontaneous passage. Stones with a maximal width of 5 mm have a greater than 50% chance of passing spontaneously, whereas this rarely occurs in patients with calculi 7 mm or greater. Patients who are trying to pass ureteral calculi are given oral analgesics and are instructed to strain their urine. They should be evaluated every 2 to 3 weeks with a kidney, ureter, and bladder x-ray and renal ultrasonography to determine whether the stone is migrating distally and to assess for hydronephrosis. If the stone is not making progress in descent or if the patient develops unremitting colic, has signs of sepsis, or is in danger of permanent renal dysfunction, urologic consultation should be obtained. Patients with asymptomatic nonstruvite calyceal calculi usually do not require stone removal unless required by vocation (e.g., commercial airline pilots). Most patients requiring treatment can be managed with extracorporeal shock wave lithotripsy (ESWL) or ureteroscopic techniques. Percutaneous nephrostolithotomy is employed in individuals harboring large renal calculi (>2.5 cm). Open surgery is rarely needed and is reserved for those failing the aforementioned minimally invasive procedures, individuals with extremely large staghorn calculi, associated collecting system obstruction requiring open surgical correction, and certain patients with extreme morbid obesity.

Approximately 50% of first-time calcium stone formers form another stone within 10 years. The interval to recurrence tends to decrease with each new stone formed. Therefore, it is certainly justifiable to evaluate and recommend medical therapy for patients with recurrences, especially those with short stone-free intervals (less than 2 years). Patients with a solitary kidney or with renal insufficiency are at greater risk of stone-related morbidity and may benefit from such therapy after the formation of only one stone, whereas others may require it because of their vocation (e.g., commercial airline pilots).

PATIENT EVALUATION

The minimal work-up of a first-time stone former includes stone analysis, urine culture, and a serum chemistry panel. A serum parathyroid hormone (PTH) level is obtained in patients with hypercalcemia. While on their regular diet, recurrent stone formers collect two 24-hour urine specimens that are analyzed for calcium, creatinine, uric acid, oxalate, magnesium, phosphorus, sodium, and citrate levels. In addition, a cystine screen (cyanide-nitroprusside test) is done. If it is positive, a quantitative urinary amino acid analysis is performed. A fasting urinary pH level is also obtained. If it is above 6, an ammonium chloride acid load test is done to assess for renal tubular acidosis. Individuals with hypercalciuria (>300 mg in adult males; >250 mg in adult females) undergo further testing. After 1 week of a low-calcium (400 mg) and restricted-sodium (100 mEq) diet, they collect another 24-hour urine specimen for similar testing. At the end of this week, calcium load testing is also performed. Urine is collected after a 12-hour fast and after a 1-gram oral calcium gluconate load. Patients with renal leak hypercalciuria have a form of secondary hyperparathyroidism and remain hypercalciuric during low-calcium intake, fasting, and calcium loading. Individuals with Type I absorptive hypercalciuria remain hypercalciuric while on a low-calcium diet but revert to a normal calciuric state during fasting. In contrast, patients with Type II absorptive hypercalciuria have normal urinary calcium levels while on a low-calcium diet and during fasting. In both types of absorptive hypercalciuria, there is a marked increase in calcium excretion after the calcium load.

GENERAL TREATMENT

Hydration is one of the most effective and morbidity-free treatments that benefits all stone-forming patients. Adults are urged to increase their urine output to 2 to 3 liters daily, with special emphasis given to increased hydration before bedtime. Patients are instructed to drink at least 8 to 10 ounces of fluid hourly while awake. Despite the simplicity of this therapy, many individuals are noncompliant. Having such individuals monitor their urinary specific gravity by dipstick testing may involve them more actively in their therapy. Patients are instructed to check their specific gravity early and later in the day and to drink enough fluid to keep it below 1.015. Individuals with calcium stones are advised to limit their intake of sodium and animal protein, which decreases calcium and uric acid excretion while enhancing citrate excretion—changes that benefit such stone formers. These measures are not associated with adverse metabolic sequelae, unlike indiscriminate calcium restriction, which may cause hyperoxaluria.

SPECIFIC TREATMENT
Calcium Stones

Renal Leak Hypercalciuria

Thiazide diuretic therapy is the treatment of choice for patients with renal leak hypercalciuria. Thiazides decrease urinary calcium excretion by increasing calcium reabsorption in the early portion of the distal convoluted tubule and by promoting calcium reabsorption in the proximal tubule. Various types can be used, including hydrochlorothiazide 25 to 50 mg twice daily, trichlormethiazide 1 to 2 mg twice daily, bendroflumethiazide (Naturetin) 2.5 mg twice daily, and chlorthalidone (Hygroton) 25 mg twice daily. Indapamide (Lozol) 2.5 mg daily, a nonthiazide diuretic with similar hypocalciuric effects, may also be employed. Thiazide preparations that contain triamter-

ene should not be used, because triamterene may crystallize and form stones. Sodium intake should be limited to increase the hypocalciuric action of the thiazide. Adverse side effects of thiazides include hypokalemia, hyperglycemia, hyperuricemia, hypercalcemia, hypercholesterolemia, hypertriglyceridemia, rash, and interstitial nephritis. A recent study demonstrated that changes in lipid profiles in recurrent stone formers receiving thiazide therapy are probably clinically insignificant. Thiazide therapy is contraindicated in untreated primary hyperparathyroidism. Periodic serum chemistry panels and 24-hour urinary calcium levels are monitored to detect electrolyte disturbances and to ensure that calcium excretion is decreasing. Hypokalemia requires correction because it results in lower renal excretion of citrate, an inhibitor of crystallization of stone-forming calcium salts. Potassium supplementation with potassium chloride or potassium citrate can be used. Potassium citrate is preferred because it also increases urinary citrate.

Type I Absorptive Hypercalciuria

There are three therapeutic options for these patients: thiazide diuretics, cellulose sodium phosphate, and wheat or rice bran. A disadvantage of thiazide diuretics is that, with time, some patients become refractory to their hypocalciuric action. Bone density may also increase with thiazide treatment, but this is inconsequential. This approach might be best for children or individuals with osteoporosis. When taken with meals, cellulose sodium phosphate (Calcibind) 5 grams two or three times per day for adults binds both calcium and magnesium, which decreases their gastrointestinal absorption and limits urinary excretion of these ions. This agent may also promote increased oxalate and phosphorus excretion. Magnesium 1 to 1.5 grams twice daily between meals prevents hypomagnesemia. Moderate dietary restriction of calcium, oxalate, and sodium is also recommended. Cellulose sodium phosphate is contraindicated in patients with primary or secondary hyperparathyroidism, hypomagnesemia, bone disease, hypocalcemia, and hyperoxaluria. It is not recommended for pediatric or pregnant patients. Every 6 months during therapy, a complete blood count should be performed, and the levels of urinary calcium, magnesium, sodium, and oxalate and the levels of serum PTH, calcium, magnesium, alkaline phosphatase, copper, zinc, and iron should be assessed. Increasing dietary fiber with wheat or rice bran promotes decreased calcium excretion by a number of mechanisms, including binding of calcium to phytic acid (a component of bran), decreasing intestinal transit time, and direct complexation with bran. Concomitant dietary oxalate restriction is advised to prevent hyperoxaluria.

Type II Absorptive Hypercalciuria

Moderate dietary calcium restriction (600 to 800 mg per day) combined with limited sodium intake (100 mEq per day) may control hypercalciuria in these patients. This diet provides less calcium to complex with oxalate in the gut. Therefore, dietary oxalate restriction should also be imposed to prevent hyperoxaluria.

Renal Phosphate Leak

In these individuals, the renal phosphate leak causes hypophosphatemia, which stimulates the synthesis of calcitriol. This promotes calcium absorption from the gut and mobilization of calcium from bone, which results in hypercalciuria. These patients are treated with neutral orthophosphates (Neutra-Phos) 500 mg three times daily. Orthophosphates are contraindicated in patients with an active urinary tract infection, struvite calculi, or renal failure. Diarrhea is the most common side effect of orthophosphate therapy.

Hyperuricosuria

Hyperuricosuria promotes calcium oxalate stone formation through a variety of mechanisms, including epitaxy, heterogeneous nucleation, and binding of crystallization inhibitors. Decreasing the urinary uric acid level helps retard calcium oxalate stone formation in such individuals. This can sometimes be accomplished by limiting purine and animal protein intake. If dietary restriction is unsuccessful, allopurinol (Zyloprim) 100 to 300 mg per day is recommended. Adverse side effects of allopurinol include fever, rash, acute gouty arthritis, xanthine stone formation, and Stevens-Johnson syndrome.

Hypocitraturia

Low urinary citrate levels are encountered in a variety of calcium stone–forming patients, including those with distal renal tubular acidosis, those with chronic diarrhea, and those receiving thiazide therapy. Citrate lowers the urinary saturation of calcium oxalate by complexing calcium. Citrate also inhibits nucleation and crystallization of stone-forming calcium salts. Hypocitraturia can be corrected with oral potassium citrate 10 to 20 mEq three times daily, either as a liquid or as a tablet. The liquid preparation is preferable for patients with rapid gastrointestinal transit, such as those with diarrhea. Potassium citrate is contraindicated in patients with hyperkalemia, peptic ulcer disease, decreased gastrointestinal transit time, renal insufficiency, active urinary tract infection, or struvite stones. Adverse side effects are mainly gastrointestinal. Sodium citrate or sodium bicarbonate may be utilized for patients unable to consume potassium citrate. Patients with distal renal tubular acidosis typically have calcium phosphate calculi. Causative factors include hypocitraturia and hypercalciuria generated by the acidosis and a higher urinary pH, which promotes calcium phosphate crystallization.

Primary Hyperparathyroidism

Less than 1% of stone patients have primary hyperparathyroidism. Calcium oxalate stones are the most common type, but calcium phosphate and mixed calcium stones may also occur. Stone formation is attributed to increased calcium excretion, but other factors may be contributory. Surgical removal of the diseased parathyroid gland or glands usually eradicates stone activity. However, if stone problems persist, a search for other metabolic abnormalities is recommended.

Enteric Hyperoxaluria

Enteric hyperoxaluria results from small bowel malabsorption due to surgical resection; intrinsic pathology, such as Crohn's disease or ulcerative colitis; other causes of malabsorption, including pancreatic insufficiency, nontropical sprue, and biliary cirrhosis; and jejunoileal bypass. This increases the delivery of fatty acids and bile acids to the large colon, which enhances oxalate transport in this bowel segment. Fat malabsorption promotes saponification of enteric calcium and magnesium, which provides more free oxalate for absorption. Dietary fat and oxalate should be limited. Calcium citrate (Citracal) or calcium carbonate (Os-Cal) 0.25 to 1 gram four times daily with meals should be administered. Magnesium supplementation may be substituted for or added to this regimen. Cholestyramine (Questran),* an agent that binds fatty acids, bile acids, and oxalate, may be added (1 to 4 grams with meals) if the former are not effective. These patients usually have hypocitraturia, which should also be treated.

Primary Hyperoxaluria

There are two types of primary hyperoxaluria that result from deficits in hepatic enzymes involved in oxalate metabolism. Patients with these disorders have calculous disease at an early age and frequently develop interstitial nephritis and eventual renal failure. Initial management includes increased fluid intake, pyridoxine supplementation, and therapy for any other identified metabolic abnormalities.

Idiopathic Hyperoxaluria

Idiopathic hyperoxaluria is the most common type. Pyridoxine (vitamin B_6) 50 to 250 mg per day may decrease oxalate excretion. Dietary oxalate restriction should be considered, since some of these patients hyperabsorb oxalate. Foods to limit include spinach, peanuts, almonds, pecans, chocolate, and tea. Supplemental ascorbic acid consumption should be avoided, as this may enhance oxalate excretion.

Infectious Stones

Infectious stones form as a result of urinary tract infection with certain organisms, including *Proteus, Klebsiella, Pseudomonas,* and staphylococcal species. These urease-producing bacteria hydrolyze urea and generate high levels of bicarbonate and ammonia, which promotes formation of struvite and carbonate apatite stones. Total stone removal and prevention of recurrent infection are the two most important

---

*Not FDA-approved for this indication.

therapeutic goals. These stones can destroy the kidneys if left untreated. Individuals with residual postoperative stone fragments and patients who are prone to stone recurrence, such as those with neurogenic bladder or urinary diversion, may benefit from treatment with acetohydroxamic acid (Lithostat), a urease inhibitor, 250 mg three times daily. Acteohydroxamic acid is contraindicated in patients with moderate to severe renal insufficiency or anemia, as well as during pregnancy. Adverse reactions include hemolytic anemia, bone marrow suppression, gastrointestinal problems, thrombophlebitis, and disseminated intravascular coagulation.

Uric Acid Stones

Dehydration and low urinary pH are the usual causes of uric acid stones. Patients are encouraged to consume more fluid and less purines and animal protein. The solubility of uric acid is markedly increased at urinary pH values of 6.5 to 7.0, which can be achieved with sodium bicarbonate, potassium citrate, or sodium citrate therapy. Patients should monitor their urinary pH levels to ensure adequate alkalinization. Overalkalinization (pH 7.5 or higher) is discouraged, because this might promote formation of calcium phosphate stones. Some individuals are also hyperuricosuric and may benefit from allopurinol 100 to 300 mg per day. The preceding measures should prevent recurrent uric acid lithiasis and may cause dissolution of existing calculi.

Cystine Stones

Conventional treatment of cystine stones attempts to lower the concentration of cystine below the solubility limit of 300 mg per liter and to increase its solubility by urinary alkalinization to a pH greater than 7.0. Good oral hydration during the day and night is imperative. Sodium bicarbonate, potassium citrate, or sodium citrate therapy should achieve appropriate urinary alkalinization. Unresponsive patients can be treated with sulfhydryl medications such as penicillamine (Cuprimine) or tiopronin (Thiola). These agents may induce dissolution of cystine stones. The mechanism is based on a thiol-disulfide exchange reaction in which cystine reacts with the sulfhydryl groups of these medications to form a disulfide compound and cysteine, which are both highly soluble. Many patients do not comply with penicillamine therapy because of its many side effects, which include epidermolysis, rash, loss of taste and smell, fever, nephrotic syndrome, arthralgia, and pancytopenia. The side effects of tiopronin are less severe, which makes it a better treatment choice.

Section 10

The Sexually Transmitted Diseases

CHANCROID

method of
MARK TYNDALL, M.D.
University of Nairobi
Nairobi, Kenya

Chancroid is a sexually transmitted infection caused by *Haemophilus ducreyi*, which produces painful and destructive genital ulceration. Areas in which chancroid is endemic are characterized by poverty, prostitution, substance abuse, uncircumcised men, and limited access to treatment. Outbreaks are common during periods of war and other societal disruptions. Chancroid is essentially without long-term consequences or systemic involvement, but the substantial association between chancroid and the transmission of human immunodeficiency virus (HIV) has dramatically increased scientific and public health interest.

In endemic areas, the epidemiologic pattern of heterosexual transmission indicates that a relatively small group of women working as prostitutes transmits the infection to a larger group of men. Many of these women have minimal symptoms and do not actively seek treatment. In contrast, men who become infected usually develop severe symptoms, and the pain and appearance of the ulcer result in cessation of sexual activity and a desire to seek treatment. Therefore, control strategies should be focused on providing medical services and screening for women who sell sex and access to effective treatment for the men who frequent them. Promotion of barrier contraceptives and economic alternatives to prostitution are other necessary components of control programs.

Initial manifestations of chancroid consist of a tender papule that becomes pustular, ulcerated, and eroded within 48 hours. The period from exposure to clinical disease is 4 to 10 days. At the time of presentation, most patients have single or multiple painful ulcers with ragged edges and a purulent base. In uncircumcised men, the ulcers are usually confined to the mucosal area beneath the foreskin. These ulcers take longer to heal and respond less well to conventional treatment. Susceptibility to both chancroid and HIV infection appears to be enhanced in men who are not circumcised.

Inguinal lymphadenopathy associated with chancroid is common, with about 30% of cases progressing to form fluctuant inguinal node masses, known as buboes. In most cases, buboes are unilateral and resolve spontaneously; however, in a minority of cases, they can rupture, forming deep draining abscesses.

In most settings, the diagnosis of chancroid relies on clinical and epidemiologic criteria. Although culture media are available, *H. ducreyi* is a fastidious gram-negative bacillus that is difficult to isolate. In the most experienced labs, culture isolation from clinically suspicious lesions is about 70%. Other infectious causes of genital ulceration include syphilis, herpes, lymphogranuloma venereum, and donovanosis. Knowledge of the incidence of these pathogens in a particular geographic area helps guide treatment decisions. In most cases, empirical therapy for genital ulcers should include treatment for primary syphilis.

TREATMENT

The treatment of chancroid has become complicated due to both the emergence of resistance to antimicrobial therapy and concurrent infection with HIV. Although new alternative treatments exist, these agents are generally expensive and largely unavailable in developing countries, where they are most needed.

The standard treatment for chancroid remains erythromycin 500 mg orally four times daily for 7 days. In resource-poor settings, variations on this dosage regimen may be just as effective; they include 500 mg orally three times a day for 7 days, 500 mg orally four times a day for 5 days, or even 250 mg orally three times a day for 7 days.

Ceftriaxone (Rocephin) as a single 250-mg intramuscular dose has been effective in most studies, although recent experience in Kenya has shown high failure rates. The inconvenience of intramuscular administration and the high cost also limit its use.

Trimethoprim-sulfamethoxazole (Bactrim, Septra) has also been an effective treatment. However, resistance to both agents has developed during recent years, and this combination is no longer effective in most settings.

Quinolone antibiotics provide effective oral therapy. Ciprofloxacin (Cipro) 500 mg orally twice a day for 3 days is the recommended dosage, although, based on limited experience, 500 mg as a single oral dose appears to be effective. Fleroxacin* 400 mg orally is also effective as a single-dose treatment. High cost and lack of availability remain the major obstacles to widespread use.

Ampicillin-clavulanic acid (Augmentin) 500 mg/125 mg three times daily for 7 days has been used successfully, although the cost of this regimen may be prohibitive. Shorter-course therapy has not been adequately evaluated.

---

*Not available in the United States.

Azithromycin (Zithromax) 1 gram orally as a single dose is a recent addition to the treatment of chancroid. It is effective and well tolerated, but high cost and unavailability limit its use in developing countries.

The single-dose treatment regimens currently available should not be given to individuals known to be HIV positive or used empirically in populations known to have high HIV prevalence. However, since the effectiveness of single-dose treatment appears to be limited by inadequate duration or concentration of drug at the site of infection rather than microbial resistance, longer treatment with any of the single-dose agents may be appropriate for HIV-positive individuals. Further studies are needed to determine optimal duration of treatment with these drugs.

In addition to those with HIV infection, men who are uncircumcised experience higher rates of treatment failure. In our experience in Kenya, uncircumcised men who are HIV positive may require prolonged therapy, and in some cases, the ulcers have been unresponsive to any of the treatments given. Such individuals generally have severely suppressed immune systems.

Buboes that become fluctuant should be drained in order to prevent rupture. Aspiration should be approached from the superior aspect of the bubo through normal skin at the margin of the inflammation, using a large-bore needle. Some patients may require repeated aspirations, as the pus reaccumulates. Delayed resolution of the bubo following healing of the ulcer is not an indication for additional antimicrobial treatment, as the bubo pus is usually sterile.

Measures to control the transmission of chancroid should include the treatment of sexual contacts. Unfortunately, the populations most affected by chancroid are often those that are hardest to reach. Another approach to chancroid control includes mass treatment programs targeted at high-risk groups. This strategy requires further study.

GONORRHEA

method of
FRANKLYN N. JUDSON, M.D.
Denver Public Health Department
Denver, Colorado

Gonorrhea is an ancient disease, and descriptions of illness resembling it can be found in the writings of the Chinese emperor Huang Ti in 2637 B.C., as well as in later Hebrew, Egyptian, and Greek literature. The causative bacterium was first described in 1879 by Albert Ludwig Neisser in stained smears of exudates from acute cases of purulent urethritis and ophthalmia neonatorum, and first cultivated in 1882 by Leistikow. Humans are the only natural host for the species *Neisseria gonorrhoeae*.

EPIDEMIOLOGY

In many developed countries, gonorrhea incidence increased dramatically from the early 1960s into the mid-1970s, plateaued, and then fell steadily during the 1980s and into the 1990s. The decline has been attributed to fear of acquired immune deficiency disease (AIDS) and successful health education efforts, which resulted in a reduction in gonorrhea incidence of more than 95% in homosexual men and of 50% in heterosexual men and women. Nonetheless, the prevalence and incidence of infection remain high in the urban underclasses of North America, particularly where sex is exchanged for drugs, and the World Health Organization has estimated that 35 million cases of gonorrhea occurred in 1990, second only to *Chlamydia trachomatis* among bacterial sexually transmitted infections. As a leading cause of salpingitis, acquired infertility, and neonatal blindness, the gonococcus continues to inflict significant morbidity on a global basis. Finally, gonorrhea has proved to be one of the best single measures of recent unsafe sexual behavior and, therefore, of related human immunodeficiency virus (HIV) epidemic trends.

DISEASE SPECTRUM

Neisseria gonorrhoeae is capable of infecting or colonizing a very wide range of columnar or transitional epithelial mucous membranes. These include the urethras of men and women, a variety of genital glands such as Tyson's in men and Bartholin's in women, the uterine cervical canal and tubes, the epididymis, the anal canal and distal rectum, the conjunctiva, and the pharynx. Although more than 95% of urethral infections in men become symptomatic within an average incubation period of 2 to 5 days, a large majority of cervical infections are not associated with specific symptoms, and most anorectal and pharyngeal infections in men and women are completely asymptomatic. Salpingitis is thought to follow untreated cervical infection in 5 to 15% of cases. Blood-borne dissemination of *N. gonorrhoeae* has become very uncommon, occurring in much less than 1% of infections. Most disseminated infections present as the arthritis-dermatitis syndrome; endocarditis and meningitis are exceedingly rare.

TREATMENT CONSIDERATIONS
Antimicrobial Resistance

Treatment success correlates closely with the minimum concentration of the antibiotic needed to inhibit the pretreatment isolate of *N. gonorrhoeae*. This is important because during the modern antibiotic era the gonococcus has demonstrated great genetic resiliency in acquiring a large number of resistance mechanisms. They have come to be further classified according to whether the genetic locus is on a plasmid (e.g., penicillinase-producing *N. gonorrhoeae*, or PPNG; tetracycline-resistant *N. gonorrhoeae*, or TRNG) or a chromosome (e.g., chromosomally mediated resistant *N. gonorrhoeae* [CMRNG], resistant to penicillin, tetracycline, spectinomycin, and/or others). In the United States 1 to 15% of all recent isolates have been PPNG, and 25% exhibit at least one type of resistance. Thus, in the absence of good evidence to the contrary, it should be assumed that infection is caused by a resistant strain.

Effective Antimicrobial Agents

During the past decade a number of new antimicrobial agents have been approved for single-dose

TABLE 1. **Treatment of Gonococcal Infections**

Type of Infection	Recommended Regimen
Uncomplicated urethral, cervical, rectal, or pharyngeal	Ceftriaxone (Rocephin), 125 mg IM in single dose *or* Cefixime (Suprax), 400 mg PO in single dose *or* Ciprofloxacin (Cipro), 500 mg PO in single dose *or* Ofloxacin (Floxin), 400 mg PO in single dose *plus* Regimen effective against possible co-infection with *Chlamydia trachomatis*, such as doxycycline 100 mg PO bid for 7 days
Conjunctivitis (adults)	Administer single 1-gm dose of ceftriaxone IM and lavage infected eye once with saline solution
Bacteremia or arthritis	Ceftriaxone 1 gm IM or IV every 24 h until 24–48 h after improvement, then switch to cefixime 400 mg PO bid to complete 7 days of therapy
Meningitis or endocarditis	After taking cultures, initiate therapy with 1–2 gm of ceftriaxone q 12 h and consult expert
Pelvic inflammatory disease	
Inpatient	Cefoxitin (Mefoxin) 2 gm IV q 6 h *or* cefotetan 2 gm IV q 12 h *plus* Doxycycline 100 mg IV *or* PO q 12 h continued for at least 48 h after clinical improvement; then switch to doxycycline alone 100 mg PO bid to complete 14 days of therapy
Outpatient	Cefoxitin 2 gm IM *plus* probenecid, 1 gm orally in single dose, *or* ceftriaxone 250 mg IM *or* other parenteral third-generation cephalosporin (e.g., ceftizoxime, or cefotaxime [Claforan]) *plus* Doxycycline 100 mg PO bid for　14 days
Epididymitis (<35 years of age)	Ceftriaxone 250 mg IM in single dose *plus* Doxycycline 100 mg PO bid for 10 days
Neonatal	
Conjunctivitis	Ceftriaxone 125 mg IM in single dose plus saline irrigation
Arthritis, septicemia, and/or meningitis	Consult expert
Infants and children	Consult expert; consider sexual abuse

From CDC 1993 Sexually Transmitted Diseases. MMWR *42*:1–102, 1993.

treatment of uncomplicated urethral, cervical, anorectal, and, to a less confident extent, pharyngeal infections (Table 1). They include the "third generation" cephalosporins ceftriaxone (Rocephin), 125 or 250 mg intramuscularly, and cefixime (Suprax), 400 mg orally; and the fluorinated quinolones ofloxacin (Floxin), 400 mg orally, and ciprofloxacin (Cipro) 500 mg orally. Each of these agents usually is fully active against PPNG, TRNG, and CMRNG and achieves greater than 98% cure rates for anogenital infection. Ceftriaxone, even in the 125-mg dose, has the best overall therapeutic profile; however, it is more expensive and has not been marketed in vials of less than 250 mg. Although ciprofloxacin, ofloxacin, and other fluorinated quinolones are less expensive and provide convenient, oral dosing, this class has been associated with central nervous system toxicity (usually not of consequence with single-dose treatment of healthy young adults), phototoxicity, and the emergence of bacterial resistance. Also quinolones are contraindicated for pregnant or nursing women and for persons 17 years of age or less owing to cartilage damage observed in studies of young animals. To ensure treatment compliance in uncomplicated infection, single-dose, care-provider-administered therapy is desirable.

Pelvic Inflammatory Disease

The fraction of acute pelvic inflammatory disease that is caused by the gonococcus varies with the prevalence of *N. gonorrhoeae* in local populations and can range from less than 10 to more than 50%. It is also important to realize that even with experienced physicians, a clinical diagnosis of pelvic inflammatory disease in a typical outpatient setting is laparoscopically confirmed as salpingitis in no more than 50 to 60% of women. These diagnostic limitations combined with a lack of controlled efficacy trials using bacterial sterilization of the uterine tubes and control of inflammation and scar tissue as outcome measures make selection of a recommended treatment regimen problematic. With this in mind, experts have selected regimens that are probably quite effective in eradicating *N. gonorrhoeae* and *C. trachomatis*, and of lesser or unknown efficiency in controlling abscess-associated infections caused by secondarily invading vaginal anaerobes and Enterobacteriaceae.

Although there is no evidence that hospitalization per se leads to a better outcome, it may be necessary when there is vomiting and dehydration, diagnostic uncertainty, or suspected abscess. Concern over compliance with self-administered therapy should not be a reason to hospitalize, as there are several less expensive ways to accomplish compliance including directly observed therapy in the home and/or clinic.

Pregnancy

Tetracycline- and quinolone-class antibiotics are contraindicated in pregnancy. For chlamydial coverage, erythromycin (but not the estolate form) 500 mg orally four times a day can be substituted for doxycycline 100 mg orally two times a day. For women with a history of allergy to beta-lactam drugs, especially immediate or accelerated reactions, spectinomycin 2 grams intramuscularly in a single dose can be used to treat uncomplicated anogenital gonorrhea.

Co-Existing Chlamydial Infections

Although co-existing chlamydial infection has been reported in up to 50% of women with gonorrhea, recent rates seem to be closer to 10 to 15% in men and 20 to 25% in women. Nonetheless, until universal sensitive testing for *Chlamydia* is available, co-therapy with 7 days of tetracycline or erythromycin is the single most cost-effective approach to *Chlamydia* control. In addition, dual treatment may further reduce the possibility of treatment failure and selection for antibiotic resistance.

Tests for Other Sexually Transmitted Diseases

Because gonorrhea, syphilis, and HIV infections share most of the same risk behaviors and are highly prevalent in poor, urban ethnic minorities, the diagnosis of one infection should lead to a search for others. Therefore, all patients with gonorrhea should have a serologic test for syphilis and should be offered confidential counseling and testing for HIV infection.

Follow-Up

As a result of the extremely high cure rates with the recommended regimens, patients need not return for a test of cure unless symptoms persist. These uncommon cases should be cultured for *N. gonorrhoeae* and any isolates tested for antimicrobial susceptibility. The possibility of reinfection or a different infectious cause should also be considered.

In the author's opinion, single doses of ceftriaxone and/or 7-day courses of either doxycycline or erythromycin are highly likely to cure the occasional co-infection with incubating syphilis. As a result, no further follow-up is indicated for patients who were seronegative for syphilis at the time they were treated for gonorrhea with one of these regimens.

Sex Partners

Sexual partners, especially women, should be notified of exposure to gonorrhea and offered evaluation and treatment. In our Denver sexually transmitted diseases (STD) clinic nearly 50% of the women diagnosed with gonorrhea sought treatment only after notification by a patient. If the patient is unwilling or unable to ensure that partners seek care, this responsibility falls to the physician along with state or local disease intervention specialists. Priority efforts should be directed at the most recent partners.

Sexual Abuse or Assault

Whenever sexual abuse (e.g., any preadolescent child with gonorrhea) or sexual assault is suspected, it is essential that a qualified response team be confidentially notified and that cultures be obtained so that any *Neisseria* isolates can be further tested to verify that they belong to the species *N. gonorrhoeae*. Most noncultural test results do not stand up in court.

RECOMMENDED TREATMENT REGIMENS

Table 1 is a selected compilation of recommended regimens for gonorrhea published by the Centers for Disease Control and Prevention (CDC). This publication is available through CDC and state STD and HIV prevention programs and can be consulted for further information on infrequently needed alternative regimens, unusual conditions in adults, infections of infants and children, and opthalmia neonatorum prophylaxis.

NONGONOCOCCAL URETHRITIS IN MEN

method of
STEPHEN R. TABET, M.D., M.P.H., and
CONNIE CELUM, M.D., M.P.H.
University of Washington School of Medicine
Seattle, Washington

EPIDEMIOLOGY

Nongonococcal urethritis (NGU), also known as "nonspecific urethritis," is a common sexually transmitted disease in North America, more common than gonococcal urethritis. *Chlamydia trachomatis* (CT) has been reported to cause NGU in about 30 to 50% of patients, but in some clinical settings, the proportion of NGU associated with CT is decreasing. *Ureaplasma urealyticum* may be a causative agent of NGU, but its role remains controversial because of its high prevalence in asymptomatic men. Recent evidence suggests that *Mycoplasma genitalium*, a fastidious organism, may be associated with NGU in men, particularly in persistent or recurrent NGU. Studies have documented other less common causes of NGU, including meningococcus, *Haemophilus*, *Trichomonas vaginalis*, and herpes simplex virus, but all these pathogens together are responsible for only a small percentage of cases of NGU. In at least 30% of cases of NGU in heterosexual men and the majority of cases in homosexual men, an infectious cause cannot be identified. Further studies are needed to elucidate pathogens in these culture-negative cases of NGU, as well as to investigate the possible association of insertive oral sex with NGU.

DIAGNOSIS

The incubation period of NGU averages 2 to 3 weeks but can vary from 1 to 6 weeks. The major signs and symptoms are urethral discharge, urethral itching, and dysuria (but not urinary frequency). On an individual basis, NGU is often indistinguishable from urethritis due to *Neisseria gonorrhoeae* (GC). Studies have shown that men with gonococcal urethritis are more likely to develop acute symptoms usually within 5 days after infection, with profuse and purulent discharge, and to seek medical attention sooner than men with NGU. These aspects of signs and symptoms can be helpful in suggesting a diagnosis, but urethral Gram's stain and GC cultures are important since there is overlap in clinical manifestations of different causes of urethritis. A significant proportion of men with NGU remain either mildly symptomatic or asymptomatic, for which laboratory tests are useful in confirming the diagnosis of urethritis.

The presumptive diagnosis of NGU is made after excluding the diagnosis of gonococcal urethritis by microscopic examination (looking for gram-negative intracellular diplococci) and the presence of at least two of the following:

1. Symptoms: Urethral discharge and/or dysuria;
2. Physical examination: Presence of urethral discharge, either spontaneous or after milking the urethra;
3. Laboratory documentation of urethral inflammation: Urethral Gram's stain showing five or more polymorphonuclear leukocytes per 1000 × field (oil immersion) in at least three fields in areas of maximal cellular concentration. If Gram's stain is nondiagnostic in the presence of signs or symptoms of urethritis, a leukocyte esterase test is performed on 15 mL of first-void urine; a positive leukocyte esterase test (1+ or greater) suggests urethritis.

To determine the microbiologic cause of urethritis, a test for GC and CT should be performed. The "gold standard" for diagnosis of GC and CT has been culture. Recent advances in DNA detection, such as polymerase and ligase chain reaction (PCR and LCR), have indicated 15 to 20% higher sensitivity of PCR and LCR for CT than culture of urethral samples. The PCR and LCR assays are comparably sensitive on first-void urine samples. If urethral cultures are being performed, the CT sample should be obtained from columnar epithelial cells, which requires insertion of a Dacron swab approximately 2 cm into the urethra. GC cultures can be obtained from urethral discharge, if present, or from a urethral swab, which is plated directly onto modified Thayer-Martin media or sent to the laboratory in an appropriate transport medium.

TREATMENT

The recommended treatment for an initial episode of NGU with no episode in the previous 6 weeks is doxycycline (Vibramycin), 100 mg orally twice daily for 7 days. Alternative regimens include erythromycin stearate or base, 500 mg orally four times daily, or enteric-coated erythromycin base, 666 mg orally three times daily, each for 7 days. Azithromycin (Zithromax), 1 gram taken orally as a single dose, is as effective as a 7-day course of doxycycline for CT urethritis and possibly nonchlamydial urethritis. The single-dose regimen of azithromycin is especially attractive for patients unlikely to comply with a multi-dose regimen. The patient should be strongly advised to abstain from sexual activity for 1 week, and it is essential to evaluate and treat sexual contacts.

Persistent or recurrent NGU should first be confirmed by physical and laboratory examination, ascertaining that the patient was compliant with medical therapy and that reexposure to an untreated partner has not occurred (e.g., by inquiring about sexual activity since the last visit and whether the partner was treated). Patients with persistent urethritis while on therapy should have first-void urine and urethral swab specimens tested for *T. vaginalis* (by wet mount and culture) and then should be retreated with erythromycin or doxycycline. If the patient does not respond or is not able to tolerate doxycycline or erythromycin, ofloxacin (Floxin), 300 mg twice daily for 7 days, can be used. If the patient has *T. vaginalis* or is a contact of a person with trichomonas, he should be treated with metronidazole (Flagyl), 2 grams orally as a single dose. Patients with persistent urethral symptoms after several courses of antibiotics (especially in the absence of objective findings of urethritis) may have prostate gland disease, urethral stricture, herpes simplex infection, intraurethral condyloma, or other less common disorders and should be referred to a sexually transmitted disease (STD) specialist or urologist.

GRANULOMA INGUINALE
(Donovanosis)

method of
TED ROSEN, M.D.
Baylor College of Medicine
Houston, Texas

Granuloma inguinale (GI) is a disorder generally accepted to be due to the sexual transmission of an obligate intracellular, pleomorphic gram-negative bacillus, *Calymmatobacterium granulomatis*. This disease primarily occurs in endemic foci in both tropical and subtropical areas of the world, most prominently in South Africa and southeast India. Other significant foci occur in Australia and New Guinea, the Caribbean (particularly Grenada) and eastern sections of South America, Vietnam and portions of Japan, and Zambia. Most of 100 or so patients seen annually in the United States are reported from the southern and southeastern states.

Following an incubation period of 1 to 12 weeks (average, 2 to 3 weeks), papules or small nodules appear. Lesions rapidly erode to form painless ulcers with sharp, raised, and rolled borders and clean, friable, "beefy-red" bases. Multiple lesions may coalesce, and lesions are prone to inexorable extension that may lead to mutilating tissue destruction. Rare clinical manifestations include soft, erythematous papules with granulation tissue–like surfaces (nodular variant) and large, vegetating masses that resemble condyloma acuminatum (hypertrophic variant). Lesions favor the prepuce and coronal sulcus in men and the labia in women. Perianal lesions can occur in either sex, and the vagina or cervix may rarely be involved in women. True inguinal lymphadenopathy does not occur, and systemic complaints are notably uncommon.

Diagnosis is based on a characteristic clinical picture in conjunction with direct visualization of the causative bacteria (Donovan's bodies). Tissue crush smears or biopsy specimens are examined after staining with Giemsa, Wright's, Leishman's, or Warthin-Starry silver stains for the presence of pathognomonic bipolar-staining bacilli within histiocytes. Cultural isolation remains impractical. Although several complement-fixation studies and skin tests have been developed, they are not yet established diagnostic tools.

TREATMENT

Although instances of resistance have been reported, tetracycline remains the drug of choice because of overall safety and low expense. Tetracycline (Sumycin, Achromycin) is administered in an oral dose of 500 mg four times daily until healing occurs. An equally efficacious first-line treatment consists of double-strength co-trimoxazole (Bactrim) given as 1 tablet, twice daily. Chloramphenicol (Chloromycetin) in an oral dose of 500 mg every 8 hours is quite effective but carries the risk of potentially fatal blood dyscrasia. Parenteral aminoglycosides such as gentamicin (Garamycin) are reserved for recalcitrant cases. Pregnant women are treated with 500 mg of erythromycin (PCE, Ery-Tab) taken four times daily; response is slower with this regimen. Late sequelae, such as massive tissue destruction, strictures, and fistulas, may require surgical reconstruction.

Patients with GI should be screened for concomitant sexually transmitted diseases as well as for human immunodeficiency virus (HIV) infection. Known sexual contacts should be examined, although strictly prophylactic treatment is not recommended.

LYMPHOGRANULOMA VENEREUM

method of
TED ROSEN, M.D.
Baylor College of Medicine
Houston, Texas

Lymphogranuloma venereum (LGV) is a sexually transmitted disease caused by serotypes L1, L2, or L3 of *Chlamydia trachomatis*. These serovars are more virulent and invasive than the other chlamydial subtypes. Although a lack of reliable epidemiologic data makes accurate determination of prevalence and incidence difficult, the disorder is clearly endemic in portions of Africa, Southeast Asia, India, the Caribbean, and South America. About 500 to 1000 cases are encountered in the United States annually.

LGV is classically divided into three stages. The first stage consists of a small, painless, ulcerated papule that appears after an incubation period of 3 to 30 days. This transient lesion heals in 1 week or less and goes unnoticed in the majority of patients. Primary anorectal infection,

however, is characterized by acute proctocolitis manifested by rectal pain, tenesmus, mucopurulent discharge, and bloody diarrhea. The second stage, which appears 2 to 6 weeks later, demonstrates painful regional lymphadenitis, low-grade fever, and constitutional symptoms (anorexia, malaise, myalgia, and arthralgia). In men, the "groove sign," consisting of inguinal and femoral adenopathy separated by Poupart's ligament, strongly suggests LGV. In women, primary lesions often occur at anatomic sites that drain into deep iliac or perirectal nodes; lower abdominal or back pain may be presenting symptoms. The late stage of untreated LGV consists of various combinations of perirectal abscesses, chronic anogenital ulcerations or fistulas, lymphatic fibrosis and genital elephantiasis, and anogenital stricture formation.

Diagnosis is based on a compatible clinical picture accompanied by an LGV complement-fixation (CF) titer of 1 : 64 or greater. Although serologic testing is only genus-specific, CF titers due to routine chlamydial urethritis, cervicitis, or conjunctivitis are rarely over 1 : 16. Recovery and serotyping of chlamydia from anogenital ulcers or lymph node aspirates is ideal; however, culture remains technically difficult and expensive, with recovery rates in LGV rarely exceeding 50%. Histologic examination of affected lymph nodes demonstrates stellate microabscesses surrounded by histiocytes. Histologic examination of affected rectal tissue demonstrates granulomatous inflammation that may be confused with inflammatory bowel disease. Tissue nucleic acid probes and fluorescent monoclonal antibody stains are currently in development.

TREATMENT

The recommended therapy for LGV is either doxycycline (Vibramycin, Monodox), in an oral dose of 100 mg twice daily, or tetracycline (Achromycin, Sumycin), in an oral dose of 500 mg four times daily. Two to 3 weeks of treatment is recommended. Acceptable alternatives include erythromycin (PCE, Ery-Tab) and sulfisoxazole (Gantrisin), in an oral dose of 500 mg four times daily. Fluctuant lymph nodes should be aspirated and obvious abscesses incised and drained. Late sequelae may require surgical correction.

Patients with LGV should be screened for other sexually transmitted diseases as well as for human immunodeficiency virus (HIV) infection. Known sexual contacts should be examined, and if LGV is not found, they should be given a prophylactic 7-day course of doxycycline, tetracycline, erythromycin, or sulfisoxazole in doses comparable to the aforementioned.

SYPHILIS

method of
CHARLES B. HICKS, M.D.
Duke University Medical Center
Durham, North Carolina

The dramatic increase in reported cases of syphilis that was noted in the late 1980s and early 1990s ended as suddenly as it began. The number of cases of early syphilis reported to the Centers for Disease Control and Prevention (CDC) for 1993 was 25,875, a total similar to that noted in the mid-1980s; provisional totals for 1994 are slightly less. Despite the decline in numbers of new cases, considerable controversy and concern persists regarding the proper management of patients infected with *Treponema pallidum*, the causative organism of syphilis. Such factors as early central nervous system (CNS) involvement, co-infection with the human immunodeficiency virus (HIV), and the adequacy of standard doses of penicillin make management of the patient with syphilis a challenge for the clinician.

A major difficulty in diagnosing syphilis and assessing the response of infected persons to therapy is the inability to culture *T. pallidum* in vitro. Because of this problem, the diagnosis is generally based on clinical grounds and confirmed by indirect methods such as serologic examination or, less commonly, dark-field microscopy. The response to treatment is most often assessed by following serologic titers after therapy. It is well recognized that there may be considerable variability in serologic responses from patient to patient, with such things as previous episodes of syphilis, the duration of infection before treatment, the stage of syphilis, and HIV co-infection all having an important influence on the rapidity with which antibody titers fall. As a consequence of these factors, it has been extremely difficult to assess systematically the various treatment regimens that have been recommended for various stages of syphilis. The treatment guidelines discussed here are therefore based in large measure on clinical experience and the consensus recommendations of subject matter experts as compiled in the CDC's 1993 Sexually Transmitted Diseases Treatment Guidelines.

TREATMENT

Principles

The treatment of syphilis was revolutionized by the introduction of penicillin into clinical practice and the demonstration of its efficacy in this disease by Mahoney in the 1940s. In contrast to *Neisseria gonorrhoeae*, *T. pallidum* has not developed resistance to penicillin, and it remains exquisitely sensitive to this antimicrobial. The clinical value of penicillin has been established by years of successful use, and it is the mainstay of therapy for all stages of syphilis.

Because the replication cycle of *T. pallidum* is relatively long and the mechanism of action of penicillin requires actively dividing organisms, it is important that the duration of therapy be sufficient to kill all the treponemes present. Early on, this was accomplished by the use of repeated doses of penicillin, but this approach has been superseded by depot preparations such as benzathine penicillin, which slowly release the drug from intramuscular injection sites. For syphilis outside the CNS, this appears to be quite efficacious, but the blood-brain barrier imposes a serious obstacle to this approach for CNS infection.

In considering the issue of CNS syphilis (or neurosyphilis), it is important to remember that invasion of the CNS by *T. pallidum* occurs early and frequently in the course of syphilis. It is clear, however, that this frequent involvement of the CNS in early

syphilis does not invariably lead to subsequent clinical neurosyphilis. Indeed, most patients with evidence of early CNS invasion probably do not go on to clinical neurosyphilis later, and the circumstances under which CNS invasion ultimately leads to clinically important neurologic disease are not well understood. This issue is very relevant to the treatment of early syphilis since benzathine penicillin as it is commonly used does not result in measurable levels of penicillin in the cerebrospinal fluid (CSF). The inability to culture *T. pallidum* makes the diagnosis of neurologic involvement and neurosyphilis especially problematic.

Despite the frequent invasion of the CNS in early syphilis, clinical experience has shown that in normal hosts the use of a single dose of benzathine penicillin for primary and secondary syphilis is not associated with unacceptably high neurologic relapse rates. Numerous small series and case reports, however, suggest that this may not be the case in immunocompromised patients, especially those with HIV infection. These findings have been interpreted as indicating that the contribution of the host immune response may be crucial to the ultimate outcome in patients with syphilis. For this reason, it is important that HIV-infected patients with syphilis be managed with particular care, often with more intensive treatment regimens.

In penicillin-allergic patients, alternative treatments such as tetracycline, erythromycin, and chloramphenicol have often been used. In general, these are less effective, and every effort should be made to use penicillin regimens if at all possible, especially in neurosyphilis. Newer agents such as ceftriaxone and azithromycin have relatively good activity against *T. pallidum* and may ultimately prove to be of benefit. At present, however, they are not well-established treatments for syphilis and should not be used as first-line agents.

Treatment of Early Syphilis

"Early syphilis" refers to primary, secondary, and early latent syphilis (generally defined as the first year after infection is acquired). It is the period during which the disease is infectious, and it is generally more likely to be cured with shorter-duration therapy. Treatments recommended for patients with early syphilis also apply to patients with incubating syphilis. A crucial determinant in the management of patients with early syphilis is whether the patient is also co-infected with HIV. Every effort should be made to ascertain the HIV status of any patient with syphilis. If this information is unavailable, it may be prudent to treat such patients with the more intensive regimens suggested for immunocompromised HIV-infected persons.

HIV-Seronegative Patients

For immunocompetent patients with early syphilis, a single 2.4 million U intramuscular dose of benzathine penicillin (given as 1.2 million U in each buttock) is generally accepted as the treatment of choice. Although this regimen has never been subjected to a controlled clinical trial, it is well established as highly efficacious with a greater than 95% cure rate. Patients who are penicillin-allergic should be treated with doxycycline, 100 mg orally twice daily for 14 days.

HIV-Infected Patients

Accumulating evidence suggests that HIV-infected patients with syphilis may not respond to therapy as well as patients who are HIV-seronegative do. This may be particularly true for patients with more advanced HIV disease. There is insufficient information to know the frequency with which treatment failure occurs or at what level of immunosuppression it may be a greater risk. Patients with early stages of HIV disease are probably more like HIV-seronegative patients, and those with early syphilis are likely to respond to single-dose benzathine penicillin as recommended earlier. Patients who are more immunocompromised appear to be at greater risk of failing standard treatment regimens with the subsequent development of neurologic disease and/or ocular syphilis. As such, they may benefit from more intensive therapy, although this is unproved. Decisions as to what constitutes appropriate therapy must be individualized, but it is important not to undertreat what should in most instances be a readily curable disease.

Otherwise asymptomatic HIV-infected patients with incubating, primary, and secondary syphilis whose immune status is relatively intact (e.g., with CD4 counts >400 per mm³) may be treated with benzathine penicillin as recommended for HIV-seronegative patients. Patients with symptomatic HIV disease and/or low CD4 counts should receive a more intensive course of therapy. Options include multiple doses of intramuscular benzathine penicillin (i.e., 7.2 million U given in three weekly 2.4 million–U doses) or single-dose benzathine penicillin supplemented with oral therapy (for specific oral regimens, see Table 1). If the latter approach is chosen, it must be discussed thoroughly with the patient in order to improve compliance. In most instances it is surprisingly well tolerated.

All HIV-infected patients with latent syphilis, regardless of its duration, should undergo lumbar puncture with examination of the CSF to assess for CNS involvement. This applies to all HIV-infected patients with any degree of immunosuppression. Patients with normal CSF may be treated with three weekly doses of intramuscular benzathine penicillin G, each dose being 2.4 million U. If there is a reactive CSF Venereal Disease Research Laboratory (VDRL) test or an unexplained CSF pleocytosis, a treatment regimen appropriate for neurosyphilis is necessary. The appropriate course for patients whose only CSF abnormality is an elevated protein level is less clear, but a neurosyphilis regimen or a more intensive regimen as described previously for immunocompromised patients with early syphilis is suggested. If CSF examination cannot be performed, treatment with a neurosyphilis regimen is the safest course,

but if this is not possible, the intensive regimen mentioned earlier may be substituted if post-treatment follow-up is assured.

Post-Treatment Follow-Up

Careful follow-up after treatment is important in any patient with syphilis, but it is particularly important in HIV-infected persons with syphilis. Clinical examination and serologic testing should be repeated at 3 and 6 months after treatment for early syphilis. Exactly what constitutes an adequate response to therapy is a matter of considerable debate, but a fall in the nontreponemal test (rapid plasma reagin [RPR], VDRL) titer after therapy should be seen. Follow-up tests should be done with the same methodology as was used in the original diagnostic test, preferably by the same laboratory. In patients with a relatively high pretreatment titer (e.g., 1:16 or greater), a fourfold decline should occur within 3 to 6 months. In other patients, a fall in titer should occur relatively promptly, especially in primary and secondary syphilis, but it may not be seen for as long as a year in some instances. If no response is noted or if the titer should show a sustained fourfold increase, examination of the CSF is essential, and appropriate retreatment should be given based on CSF results. Those with normal CSF should be retreated with the regimen recommended for late latent syphilis. If the CSF is abnormal, a neurosyphilis treatment regimen is recommended.

Treatment of Late Syphilis

In its later stages, syphilis may be asymptomatic (a condition termed "late latent syphilis"), or may cause symptomatic disease involving the cardiovascular system, the CNS, or virtually any organ of the body as gummatous syphilis. The latter term refers to a relatively indolent form of syphilis in which granulomatous-like lesions are seen, most often in bones, skin, and mucocutaneous tissues. Cardiovascular syphilis most commonly produces aneurysmal dilatation of the ascending aorta. Both these conditions are now quite rare. The majority of cases of late syphilis diagnosed today are either asymptomatic infection (typically diagnosed when serologic testing for syphilis is done for any of a number of reasons) or neurosyphilis, which may be asymptomatic or cause a variety of neurologic manifestations. The treatment for all types of late syphilis other than neurosyphilis is the same: three weekly doses of intramuscular benzathine penicillin G, each dose being 2.4 million U, for a total of 7.2 million U.

The distinction between late latent syphilis and asymptomatic neurosyphilis may be quite difficult. Lumbar puncture is essential for any patient in whom neurosyphilis is suspected; the CSF should be examined for cell count, protein level, and VDRL reactivity. Lumbar puncture is also recommended in any patient with latent syphilis for whom the date of acquisition of infection is not clearly established as being less than 1 year previously. All HIV-infected

TABLE 1. **Treatment of Syphilis***

Stage of Infection	Standard Regimens	Penicillin-Allergic Patients†
Early syphilis‡		
HIV –	Benzathine penicillin G, 2.4 million U IM, single dose	Doxycycline, 100 mg PO bid for 14 days
HIV +, >400 CD4 cells§	Benzathine penicillin G, 2.4 million U IM, single dose	Doxycycline, 100 mg PO bid for 14 days
HIV +, symptomatic, and/or <400 CD4 cells§	Benzathine penicillin G, 7.2 million U IM, over 3 weeks,	Penicillin desensitization, then same regimens as for those without penicillin allergy
	or	
	Benzathine penicillin G, 2.4 million U IM, single dose, plus either oral regimen A or B‖	
Latent syphilis, HIV +, (any CD4 count)		
Normal CSF	Benzathine penicillin G, 7.2 million U IM, over 3 weeks	Penicillin desensitization, then same regimens as for those without penicillin allergy
Abnormal CSF (see text)	Treat for neurosyphilis	Treat for neurosyphilis
Late syphilis		
Late latent syphilis, latent syphilis of unknown duration, cardiovascular syphilis, gummatous syphilis¶	Benzathine penicillin G, 7.2 million U IM, over 3 weeks	Doxycycline, 100 mg PO bid for 28 days
Neurosyphilis	Aqueous crystalline penicillin G, 3–4 million U, IV every 4 h, for 10–14 days	Penicillin desensitization, then same regimens as for those without penicillin allergy
	or	
	Procaine penicillin G, 2.4 million U, IM per day, plus probenecid, 500 mg PO, 4 times daily, both for 10–14 days	
Syphilis in pregnancy	Same treatment as for nonpregnant patients, by stage of syphilis	Penicillin desensitization, then same regimens as for those without penicillin allergy
Congenital syphilis**	Aqueous crystalline penicillin G, 50,000 U/kg IV q 12 h during the first 7 days of life, then q 8 h thereafter, for 10–14 days,	Penicillin desensitization, then same regimens as for those without penicillin allergy
	or	
	Procaine penicillin G, 50,000 U/kg, IM daily for 10–14 days††	

*Recommendations are based on clinical experience and consensus of subject matter experts.
†Data on nonpenicillin treatment regimens is extremely limited.
‡"Early syphilis" refers to primary and secondary syphilis, incubating syphilis, and latent syphilis known to be of less than 1 year in duration.
§Regimens recommended for HIV-infected patients are those of the author.
‖Regimen A = amoxicillin, 2 gm plus probenecid, 500 mg both given orally tid for 10 days.
 Regimen B = doxycycline, 200 mg orally bid for 21 days.
¶Patients with late latent syphilis, or with latent syphilis of unknown duration should have a CSF examination to assess for the presence of asymptomatic neurosyphilis.
**Regimens recommended are for neonates.
††Only recommended for infants without active disease, with normal CSF, and with treponemal titers less than or equal to maternal values.
Abbreviations: HIV = human immunodeficiency virus; CSF = cerebrospinal fluid.

patients with latent syphilis of any duration should undergo CSF examination, irrespective of the degree of HIV-induced immunosuppression. Although the CSF examination is particularly crucial in HIV-infected persons with latent syphilis, it should also be strongly considered in all persons with latent syphilis that is not known to be of less than 1 year's duration. As discussed earlier, a reactive CSF VDRL is diagnostic of neurosyphilis, and an otherwise unexplained CSF pleocytosis is presumptive evidence for this diagnosis. Patients with normal CSF parameters have latent syphilis and may be treated with three weekly intramuscular doses of benzathine penicillin G as described earlier.

Neurosyphilis

The variety of neurologic manifestations that may be a consequence of neurosyphilis is quite extensive, helping to earn this infection its reputation as the "great imitator." Thus any patient who has a reactive syphilis serologic test and an otherwise unexplained neurologic syndrome should be strongly suspected of having neurosyphilis. Lumbar puncture is indicated in all such patients, and those with abnormal CSF (as discussed earlier) should be treated for neurosyphilis. Similarly, patients with latent syphilis who undergo lumbar puncture and are found to have abnormal CSF should be considered to have neurosyphilis and treated as such. Additionally, syphilis involving the eye or ear should be considered CNS disease and managed with regimens appropriate for neurosyphilis. Indications for CSF examination are listed in Table 2.

The treatment of neurosyphilis is problematic, but the consequences of incomplete treatment may be severe. Thus, the use of the most effective possible therapy is essential. The requirement that the drug used traverse the blood-brain barrier in order to achieve adequate levels in the CNS makes the design of neurosyphilis treatment regimens difficult. Only intravenous penicillin has been shown to achieve consistently satisfactory CNS penetration. Accordingly, all patients with neurosyphilis should optimally receive intravenous penicillin. Patients allergic to penicillin should undergo desensitization under the supervision of a physician experienced in the use of penicillin-desensitization regimens.

The preferred regimen for the treatment of neurosyphilis is intravenous aqueous crystalline penicillin G, 3 to 4 million U given every 4 hours for 10 to 14 days. Every effort should be made to treat patients with intravenous penicillin, but if this is not possible, the alternative is procaine penicillin G, 2.4 million U intramuscularly, given daily for 10 to 14 days. This must be accompanied by probenecid (Benemid), 500 mg orally four times daily for the entire length of treatment.

After completing treatment for neurosyphilis, patients must be followed carefully to ensure an adequate response, usually with the CSF examination

being repeated at 6-month intervals. This is particularly important for HIV-infected persons since they have been shown to have a particularly high failure rate, even with intravenous penicillin. The best indicator of a satisfactory response is a significant improvement in the CSF pleocytosis 6 months after treatment with normalization of the CSF white cell count by 2 years after treatment. Reductions in the CSF VDRL titer and protein level are also often seen, but they are less reliable markers of a satisfactory response.

Treatment of Syphilis During Pregnancy

The increase in cases of syphilis in the late 1980s occurred predominantly in heterosexuals and as such included a marked increase in cases in women. Not surprisingly, there was an associated increase in cases of congenital syphilis in the children of these women. It is extremely important that such infections be avoided if at all possible—all pregnant women should have syphilis serologic testing during the early stages of pregnancy, and this testing should be repeated late in pregnancy and at delivery if the patient comes from a high-risk setting.

The treatment of syphilis in pregnant women does not differ from that used in nonpregnant patients except that doxycycline should not be used. Penicillin regimens should be used for virtually all patients since erythromycin-based treatment has been associated with a significant risk of failure and the subsequent development of congenital syphilis in the infants of women so treated. Women allergic to penicillin should be desensitized and treated with penicillin.

Pregnant women treated for syphilis during the second half of pregnancy are at risk for premature labor and fetal distress after treatment. This is particularly a risk for women who experience a Jarisch-Herxheimer reaction (constitutional symptoms that may include headache, fever, myalgias, and apparent worsening of specific syphilis manifestations, occurring a few hours after treatment). Women should be advised to seek medical attention if they note a change in fetal movements or experience contractions after treatment for syphilis. It is important to remember that the benefits of treatment far outweigh these risks, and all pregnant women with syphilis must be treated. As with all patients, HIV testing is strongly encouraged for pregnant women with syphilis.

Treatment of Congenital Syphilis

The management of congenital syphilis can be a relatively complicated matter that is usually best handled by physicians experienced in the management of this condition. A complete discussion of this topic is beyond the scope of this article. It is important that all infants born to women diagnosed with syphilis during pregnancy be carefully assessed for the presence of congenital syphilis. As emphasized in the CDC's 1993 Sexually Transmitted Dis-

TABLE 2. **Indications for Cerebrospinal Fluid Examination in Syphilis**

1. Neurologic, auditory, or ocular signs or symptoms in any patient with reactive syphilis serologic test
2. Latent syphilis of any duration in HIV-infected patients
3. Late latent syphilis in any patient
4. Inadequate serologic response to treatment (sustained fourfold rise in nontreponemal titer, failure of initially high nontreponemal titer to fall within 3–6 months of treatment)
5. Clinical failure after treatment
6. Infants born to syphilis-seropositive women who
   a. Have untreated syphilis
   b. Were treated for syphilis with a nonpenicillin regimen
   c. Were treated for syphilis within 1 month of delivery
   d. Did not have at least a fourfold decline in nontreponemal titer after treatment
   e. Did not have a well-documented history of treatment for syphilis
   f. Did not have sufficient follow-up after treatment for syphilis before pregnancy to ensure satisfactory response

eases Treatment Guidelines, "No infant should leave the hospital without the serologic status of the infant's mother having been documented at least once during pregnancy. Serologic testing should be performed at delivery in communities and populations at risk for congenital syphilis. Serologic tests can be nonreactive among infants infected late during their mother's pregnancy."

The clinical evaluation of infants at risk for congenital syphilis includes physical examination, syphilis serologic testing, CSF examination, long bone x-ray examination, and examination of the placenta and amniotic cord for evidence of treponemal infection. If congenital syphilis is diagnosed, it is usually treated with aqueous crystalline penicillin G, 100,000 to 150,000 U per kg per day (administered as 50,000 U per kg intravenously every 12 hours during the first 7 days of life and every 8 hours thereafter) for 10 to 14 days, or alternatively, pro-

caine penicillin G, 50,000 U per kg intramuscularly in a single dose daily for 10 to 14 days. The procaine penicillin regimen is recommended only for infants without evidence of active disease, with normal CSF, and with nontreponemal test (RPR, VDRL) titers less than or equal to maternal values.

As with all patients with syphilis, careful follow-up is essential in cases of congenital syphilis. It is recommended that such patients be seen every 2 to 3 months after treatment. Nontreponemal serologic titers (RPR or VDRL) should decline by 3 months and should be nonreactive by 6 months. If a CSF pleocytosis was detected before treatment, follow-up CSF examination should be done every 6 months until the cell count is normal. Retreatment is recommended for infants whose CSF cell count is still abnormal after 2 years, whose CSF–VDRL is still reactive at 6 months, or if a downward trend is not present at each examination.

Diseases of Allergy

ANAPHYLAXIS AND SERUM SICKNESS

method of
RODERICK ROBINSON, M.D., and
HENRY G. HERROD, M.D.
University of Tennessee
Memphis, Tennessee

Anaphylaxis is a potentially fatal, acute symptom complex resulting from the release of chemical mediators from tissue mast cells and blood basophils into the circulatory system. The term was first used in the early twentieth century to distinguish this reaction from prophylaxis. Clinical symptoms of anaphylaxis can range from mild cutaneous manifestations such as generalized erythema, urticaria, and angioedema to life-threatening hypotension and cardiac arrhythmias. Classic anaphylaxis is an immunologic reaction involving IgE and the release of chemical mediators. Anaphylactoid reactions have the same clinical manifestations as classic anaphylaxis but are not caused by the IgE-mediated release of chemical mediators from mast cells and basophils. Increasingly, the term anaphylaxis is used to denote the symptom complex, whether it is IgE-mediated or not. There are numerous inciting agents that can produce anaphylaxis and, with its broader definition, there are a variety of pathophysiologic mechanisms that produce the symptoms.

Serum sickness results in a different symptom complex. Clinical symptoms such as urticaria, fever, lymphadenopathy, and joint pain typically occur 6 to 21 days after exposure to an inciting antigen. True serum sickness is uncommon today. Serum sickness occurs as a result of immune complexes involving IgG, IgM, or both binding with antigens. These complexes activate the complement system, which results in localized inflammatory tissue damage.

PATHOPHYSIOLOGY

Classic anaphylaxis is an IgE-mediated reaction to a foreign antigen. The list of antigens associated with IgE-mediated anaphylaxis is extensive and includes antibiotics, foreign proteins, therapeutic agents such as estradiol, and foods (Table 1). In these reactions, exposure to an antigen results in the production of specific IgE antibodies that bind to mast cells and basophils through IgE receptors on the surface of these cells. Upon re-exposure, the antigen can bind and cross-link the IgE antibodies on these cells. This leads to degranulation and release of chemical mediators such as histamine, leukotrienes, prostaglandins, kallikrein, platelet-activating factor, and chemotactic factors. These mediators produce the clinical symptoms of anaphylaxis by causing vasodilation, increased vascular permeability, and smooth muscle contraction.

Non-IgE-mediated anaphylactic reactions result in similar symptoms and may be due to one of several mechanisms. One of these mechanisms is the activation of the complement system, resulting in the formation of the anaphylatoxins C3a and C5a. Another mechanism is through the direct action of certain agents on mast cells and basophils. Agents implicated in these anaphylactic reactions include hyperosmolar radiocontrast media, opiates, and some muscle relaxants. There are still other situations in which the mechanism for anaphylactic reactions is not clearly understood. These reactions include systemic reactions that may be associated with exercise or with no obvious inciting agents. The distinction between anaphylaxis due to IgE-mediated events and non-IgE-mediated reactions has little clinical meaning, because the symptom complex and the treatment are the same.

CAUSATIVE AGENTS

There are hundreds of agents that can cause anaphylactic reactions (see Table 1). The most common are drugs, insect stings, foods, and food substances. Penicillin remains one of the most common drugs that causes anaphylaxis. Of the patients who have died from penicillin anaphylaxis, 75% had no history of previous reaction to penicillin. Deaths are more common with parenterally administered penicillin than that given orally. It is estimated that between 2 and 7% of patients allergic to penicillin (by history and skin testing) are allergic to cephalosporins as well; therefore, these patients should not receive this class of antibiotics.

Food and food substances are also a common cause of anaphylaxis. Legumes (peanuts, peas, soybeans, and beans), nuts, fish, shellfish, cow's milk, and eggs are the most common food allergens. Stings or bites by an insect in the order Hymenoptera, which includes fire ants, hornets, yellow jackets, wasps, and honey bees, may produce anaphylaxis. All patients who experience true anaphylaxis caused by one of these insects should undergo allergy testing to document sensitivity to venom and receive immunotherapy for the incriminating venom. Rubber products are implicated in an increasing number of cases of anaphylaxis. There are documented reports of anaphylaxis during

TABLE 1. **Agents That Can Cause Anaphylaxis**

IgE-Mediated

Drugs
    Antibiotics—penicillins, cephalosporins, nitrofurantoin
    Other drugs—estradiol, methylprednisolone, thiopental, cisplatin
Foreign proteins—insulin, asparaginase, fire ant venom, latex
Foods—milk, egg whites, shellfish, nuts, legumes

Non-IgE-Mediated

Immune complex–mediated—blood products
Modulators of arachidonic acid metabolism—tartrazine, nonsteroidal anti-inflammatory agents
Direct histamine-releasing agents—radiocontrast media, pentamidine, dextran, opiates

surgical and radiologic procedures that is caused by latex objects such as gloves or catheters. Medical personnel, people with a history of pruritus from latex exposure, and spina bifida patients are at highest risk for latex anaphylaxis. Food-induced anaphylaxis in persons allergic to latex has recently been reported.

CLINICAL MANIFESTATIONS

Anaphylactic reactions can occur within seconds to minutes after exposure to the responsible agent, and most reactions occur within 1 hour of exposure. In some patients, the onset of symptoms may be delayed for several hours, especially when foods are the inciting agent. The severity of an individual's response is dependent on the rate, amount, and site of mediator release as well as personal risk facts such as asthma, cardiac disease, or use of medications that cause beta blockade. The most commonly affected organ systems are the skin, respiratory tract, gastrointestinal tract, and cardiovascular system (Table 2).

Skin manifestations are frequently the first indications of anaphylaxis. Erythema; nasal, eye, and genital pruritus; urticaria; and angioedema can all be signs of an impending fatal anaphylactic reaction. Respiratory symptoms include dyspnea, tachypnea, and wheezing; in cases of massive mediator release, laryngospasm, bronchospasm, and epiglottitis can cause upper airway obstruction, with resultant stridor or suffocation. Gastrointestinal manifestations include nausea, vomiting, cramping abdominal pain, and diarrhea. Other signs include hypotension, cardiac arrhythmias, syncope, and uterine cramping. Most cases of fatal anaphylaxis occur as a result of respiratory complications. Cardiovascular dysfunction accounts for other fatal cases. Some patients can experience a recurrence of symptoms up to 8 hours after the initial reaction. These recurrences may be caused by partial therapy. Persistent anaphylaxis may last 5 to 32 hours and occurs in up to one-fourth of patients.

When the signs and symptoms of anaphylaxis occur within minutes of exposure to a known causative agent, it is not difficult to make the diagnosis of anaphylaxis. But when the precipitating event is not known, the diagnosis can be confused with other medical emergencies that mimic anaphylaxis clinically (Table 3). Vasovagal episodes are commonly mistaken for anaphylaxis. These episodes are usually preceded by a stressful or frightening event and are characterized by sweating, pallor, hypotension, and bradycardia. Vasovagal reactions can usually be dis-

TABLE 3. **Medical Conditions That May Mimic Anaphylaxis**

| Vasovagal response |
| Primary cardiac collapse |
| Stroke |
| Foreign body aspiration |
| Systemic mastocytosis |
| Scombroid poisoning |
| Hereditary angioedema |
| Carcinoid syndrome |
| Pheochromocytoma |

tinguished from anaphylaxis by lack of pruritus, urticaria, and bronchospasm.

TREATMENT

Immediate assessment and treatment of anaphylaxis are critical because it is a potentially life-threatening event (Table 4). This assessment includes a rapid evaluation of recent events, the severity of the clinical manifestations, the rate of progression of symptoms, and a medical history. Management of acute anaphylaxis should begin with the ABCs (airway, breathing, circulation) of emergency management. If necessary, the patient should be given high-flow oxygen by face mask and placed in Trendelenburg's position.

After initial rapid assessment, aqueous epinephrine should be administered, which causes the inhibition of mediator release, restores vasomotor tone, and relaxes bronchial smooth muscle. Many deaths from anaphylaxis could be prevented if epinephrine were given at the first sign of symptoms. If the agent causing anaphylaxis has been injected into an extremity (e.g., insect sting, drug injection), continued absorption of the agent can be decreased by the use of a tourniquet proximal to the site of injury. Epinephrine can also be given subcutaneously near the injection site to help retard systemic absorption of the offending agent.

Although not effective in the acute management of anaphylaxis, antihistamines and corticosteroids are

TABLE 2. **Clinical Manifestations of Anaphylaxis**

Organ System	Symptoms
Respiratory tract	Stridor, hoarseness, cough, dyspnea, wheezing, respiratory arrest
Cardiovascular system	Tachycardia, hypotension, arrhythmias, coronary artery spasm
Gastrointestinal tract	Nausea, vomiting, cramping, diarrhea
Skin	Erythema, pruritus, urticaria, angioedema
Eye	Conjunctival injection, pruritus
Nose	Rhinorrhea, sneezing, congestion, pruritus
Mouth	Lip swelling, tongue swelling

TABLE 4. **Management of Anaphylaxis**

1. Secure and maintain airway; administer oxygen at 4–6 L/min
2. Subcutaneous administration of epinephrine 1:1000 repeated every 10–15 min at a dose of 0.01 mL/kg to a maximum of 0.3 mL
3. If inciting event is injection into an extremity (e.g., insect sting), tourniquet should be placed proximal to injection site; local injection of epinephrine 0.01 mL/kg or 0.1 to 0.2 mL subcutaneously around site may be helpful
4. Antihistamines: H_1, e.g., diphenhydramine (Benadryl) 1 mg/kg up to 50 mg IM or IV slowly over 4–6 h; H_2, e.g., cimetidine (Tagamet) 4 mg/kg or ranitidine (Zantac) 12.5 to 50 mg IV every 6–8 h (use of H_2 blockers remains controversial)
5. Corticosteroid administration: IV hydrocortisone 5–10 mg/kg up to 500 mg every 4–6 h
6. Frequently monitor vital signs
7. Persistent hypotension or signs of vascular collapse should be treated with normal saline or colloids

commonly used to help control later events. The early use of antihistamines blocks histamine effects such as cardiac arrhythmias and helps control the pruritus and skin manifestations. Also, the use of H_2 antihistamines such as ranitidine (Zantac),* in conjunction with H_1 antihistamines such as diphenhydramine (Benadryl), may be beneficial in treating hypotension. Corticosteroids, such as hydrocortisone, may prevent a protracted course of anaphylaxis and decrease the magnitude of late sequelae.

Following the initial interventions, the patient's condition should be reassessed in order to determine the next course of therapy. Hypotension can occur after the administration of subcutaneous epinephrine secondary to an increase in capillary permeability as well as a vasodilation and decreased arteriolar tone. In such cases, normal saline or an equivalent colloid may be used as a rapid infusion. The patient's response, urine output, cardiovascular status, age, and weight should be used as guidelines for the total amount of fluid to be given. Usually, a total of 3 liters can be given rapidly to an adult without ill effects. The infusion rate should be adjusted to maintain a systolic blood pressure of at least 80 to 100 mmHg. If hypotension persists, administration of norepinephrine (2 mg in 500 mL normal saline at 8 to 12 μg per minute) or dopamine (250 mg in 250 mL administered at 2 to 20 μg per kg per minute) should be undertaken to maintain blood pressure.

The use of antiarrhythmic agents is indicated in the presence of cardiac arrhythmias and shock resulting from a combination of the chemical mediators, hypoxia, hypotension, and epinephrine. Resistance to epinephrine may be seen in patients with a history of cardiac disease and in patients taking beta-blocking agents. In those patients, glucagon 0.5 to 1 mg as an intravenous bolus can help overcome this resistance, but it must be used very carefully, since glucagon can potentiate hypertension. If bronchospasm is present, administration of an inhaled beta agonist or intravenous aminophylline should be used as if treating status asthmaticus. Patients with severe anaphylaxis should be observed for a minimum of 6 to 8 hours because of the possibility of a protracted course or recurrence of symptoms.

PREVENTION

The key to preventing the recurrence of anaphylaxis is identification of the triggering agent. Once the causative agent is identified, the treatment of choice is avoidance. If avoidance of the agent is impossible, other measures of prevention are available. Venom immunotherapy should be offered to all patients with documented Hymenoptera anaphylaxis. This therapy has been shown to prevent anaphylaxis in greater than 95% of treated patients. In situations in which a known anaphylactic agent is required for therapy, desensitization protocols are available. This situation is most likely to occur when drugs such as

---

*Not FDA-approved for this indication.

TABLE 5. **Premedication for Radiocontrast Media Reaction**

1. Prednisone 50 mg PO 13, 7, and 1 h before procedure
2. Diphenhydramine (Benadryl) 50 mg IM 1 h before procedure
3. Ephedrine 25 mg PO 1 h before procedure; this should not be used in patients with cardiovascular disease
4. Discontinuation of beta blockers if the patient is taking them

---

penicillin or other antibiotics to which a patient is sensitive have to be administered because of a lack of suitable alternative medications.

All patients with a history of anaphylaxis should wear a medical identification bracelet (Medic Alert). They should also be equipped with and educated in the use of self-administered epinephrine such as EpiPen (Center Lab, Port Washington, NY) or the AnaKit/AnaGuard (Hollister Stier, Spokane, WA). If an exposure occurs, the patient should be able to use this form of epinephrine immediately and go directly to a medical facility for evaluation. Parents of children with a history of anaphylaxis should provide schools and camps with instructions on when and how to administer epinephrine.

Host sensitivity to potential anaphylactic inducing agents should be determined if a patient is likely to be exposed. Such sensitivity can be determined using either skin testing or radioallergosorbent tests (RAST). Skin testing has the potential to induce anaphylaxis, so it should be done only under carefully controlled conditions by a trained individual with resuscitation equipment available.

Patients with anaphylactic reactions to contrast media should be pretreated as indicated in Table 5 if imaging studies requiring contrast media are necessary. Such pretreatment can greatly reduce the likelihood of reactions. Patients with exercise-induced anaphylaxis should wait 4 to 6 hours after eating to exercise and should not exercise alone.

SERUM SICKNESS

Serum sickness is a syndrome that occurs secondary to deposition of circulating immune complexes. It was first described in the early 1900s in association with the use of antiserum derived from animals, which was used in the treatment of various infectious diseases. Currently, drugs are the most common causes of serum sickness (Table 6). The disease is usually milder in children and more severe in adults.

TABLE 6. **Common Causes of Serum Sickness**

Antibiotics
   Penicillin
   Cephalosporins
   Sulfonamides
Blood products
Other
   Hydantoins
   Naproxen
   Propranolol

Symptoms are not present when the inciting antigen is first introduced but occur after a latent period of 1 to 2 weeks. Immune complexes consisting of the inciting antigen and antibody may be deposited in various tissues. Such complexes may activate the complement system with release of anaphylatoxins such as C3a and C5a. These complement fragments act as mediators that can increase vascular permeability and are chemotactic for phagocytic cells. As these phagocytic cells try to engulf the immune complexes, they may release proteolytic enzymes, which can cause tissue damage. The resulting inflammation can lead to vasculitis. As the immune response continues and antibody excess develops, complexes are ultimately taken up by phagocytes, and symptoms eventually resolve. A spectrum of clinical findings can occur. Cutaneous eruptions are seen in more than 90% of all patients and include urticaria, maculopapular or purpuric lesions, and erythema multiforme. A characteristic purpuric or erythematous band at the junctions of the palmar and plantar skin of the hands and feet has been described. Most patients with serum sickness experience fever and malaise. Some may experience peripheral edema and arthritis or arthralgia. In severe cases, peripheral neuritis, glomerulonephritis, and, rarely, a Guillian-Barré–like syndrome occurs. Fortunately, most serum sickness reactions are mild and resolve spontaneously within 2 to 3 weeks.

If the agent causing serum sickness can be identified, exposure to the agent should be stopped and subsequently avoided. Treatment goals are usually directed at symptomatic relief. During the acute phase, the patient should receive antihistamines such as diphenhydramine (Benadryl) 50 mg every 4 hours (1.25 mg per kg in children) or hydroxyzine (Atarax, Vistaril) 25 mg every 4 hours (0.3 mg per kg in children), which have proved to be of value in treating pruritus and urticaria. If fever and arthralgia are present, nonsteroidal anti-inflammatory agents (aspirin in adults and acetaminophen in children) may be used. Prednisone is useful at a dose of 1 to 2 mg per kg per day (maximal dose 60 mg), tapering over 5 to 7 days and followed by a smaller daily morning dose for an additional week. In more severe cases, prednisone may be required for longer periods.

The diagnosis of serum sickness is usually made on the basis of the typical symptom complex, although certain laboratory findings are helpful. Total hemolytic complement (CH_{50}) and the specific complement components C3 and C4 may be decreased, the erythrocyte sedimentation rate is usually elevated, and there may be peripheral eosinophilia with leukocytosis or leukopenia, proteinuria, hematuria, and electrocardiographic changes. Circulating immune complexes may also be detected by using C1q binding assays or Raji cell immunoassays. If symptoms last longer than 3 weeks, re-evaluation of the diagnosis is indicated because of the many clinical similarities between serum sickness and other inflammatory diseases.

ASTHMA IN ADULTS AND ADOLESCENTS

method of
DEBORAH ORTEGA–CARR, M.D.
University of Wisconsin
Madison, Wisconsin

and

ROBERT K. BUSH, M.D.
William S. Middleton Veterans Affairs Hospital
Madison, Wisconsin

Asthma prevalence and morbidity have increased over the last decade. New insights into the pathophysiology of asthma have changed the definition of asthma as well as its modes of treatment. We now define asthma as a chronic disease characterized by airway hyperresponsiveness, recurrent and usually reversible airflow obstruction, and symptoms of wheezing and breathlessness. Each of these components must be addressed in the overall management of asthma, in both the acute and the chronic setting. The National Asthma Education Program (NAEP) has developed guidelines for asthma management that include patient education on the basic principles of the disease and effective methods of asthma monitoring. NAEP recommendations also stress reducing or avoiding asthma triggers, particularly through environmental allergen control. Furthermore, pharmacologic intervention, aimed at both obstruction and inflammation, is now felt to be essential for optimal control.

PRECIPITATING OR AGGRAVATING FACTORS

Recent research has shown that asthma is a complex interaction of many cell processes and that the events that trigger or initiate these processes are multiple and varied. Two major triggers are allergens and viral infections. Although these two factors may be especially important in the pediatric population, they can provoke asthma symptoms in all age groups.

Allergens and Asthma

Allergens play a significant role in asthma pathogenesis in many patients. Up to 85% of asthma patients have positive skin test reactions to common aeroallergens. House dust mites are important in the development of allergic asthma; other pertinent indoor allergens include animal danders, particularly cat, and possibly insects, such as cockroaches. Fungal spores and pollens have also been associated with asthma exacerbations.

In patients with allergic asthma, inhalation of antigen first triggers immediate bronchoconstriction. In roughly half of the subjects with asthma, this challenge also provokes a delayed response 4 to 8 hours later, which is characterized by persistent airflow obstruction, airway inflammation, and bronchial hyperresponsiveness.

Viral Infections and Asthma

Viral infections also provoke and alter asthmatic responses. Viral respiratory illnesses may produce their effects by causing epithelial damage, producing specific IgE

TABLE 1. **Occupational Allergens**

Agriculture	Animal proteins: domestic animals, insects, ascarids
	Plant proteins: cereal grains, cottonseed, tobacco leaf
Food processing	Animal proteins: seafood
	Plant proteins: coffee dust, soy dust, cocoa dust, psyllium, flour
	Plant enzymes: papain, pectinase, flavorings
Woodworking (forestry, carpentry, wood manufacturing)	Wood dusts: boxwood, mahogany, oak, redwood, western red cedar (plicatic acid)
Animal handlers (laboratory workers, veterinarians, pet shop owners)	Animal proteins: dander, saliva, urine
	Avian proteins
Pharmaceutical industry	Drugs: antibiotics (penicillin), proteolytic enzymes (trypsin, pancreatin)
Manufacturing (automobile assembly, paint, foundry, polyurethane foam, plating, plastics including epoxy resins)	Chemicals: toluene diisocyanate, diphenylmethane diisocyanate, platinum, nickel phthalic anhydride, trimetallic anhydride, tetrachlorophthalic anhydride

against respiratory viral antigens, and enhancing mediator release. Besides aggravating asthma, viral upper respiratory infections cause increased airway responsiveness that may persist for weeks beyond the infection, producing chronic symptoms of wheezing.

Additional Precipitating or Aggravating Factors

Other precipitating or aggravating factors include exposure to occupational chemicals (Table 1) and irritants such as cigarette smoke. Drugs that can precipitate an asthma attack include aspirin and cross-reactive nonsteroidal anti-inflammatory agents. The intensity of these reactions is variable and may be associated with naso-ocular symptoms. In certain subsets of asthma patients, particularly those with rhinosinusitis and nasal polyps, the prevalence of asthma sensitivity may approach 30 to 40%. The nonsteroidal anti-inflammatory agents that inhibit cyclooxygenase are most cross-reactive with aspirin; acetaminophen and salsalate, which are weak inhibitors of cyclooxygenase, are much less cross-reactive. Sulfiting agents, such as the bisulfites and metabisulfites of sodium and potassium, are antimicrobial agents and oxidants used as preservatives in various foods and medications. These agents can also precipitate attacks of asthma.

Strenuous exercise results in airway obstruction in nearly all asthmatics. The problem is clinically important in at least two-thirds of adolescents with asthma because it interferes with school and recreational activities. The mechanisms by which exercise causes bronchial obstruction are unknown, but a fall in temperature of the intrathoracic airway is a critical inciting event. Exercise-induced asthma usually begins after 6 to 10 minutes of exercise or after exercise is completed. In half of the patients, repetition of exercise within 1 hour elicits progressively smaller changes in peak expiratory flow and forced expiratory flow in 1 second (FEV_1). Swimming and activities that involve brief intervals of strenuous activity interspersed with rest are best tolerated. The use of prophylactic drug therapy prior to exercise generally provides adequate protection for the patient. This prophylaxis usually consists of 2 puffs of a beta$_2$-agonist inhaler such as albuterol (Proventil, Ventolin) immediately prior to exercise. If patients continue to have symptoms during exercise, 2 puffs of cromolyn sodium (Intal) or nedocromil sodium (Tilade) can be added 15 minutes prior to exercise.

Any associated problems that may contribute to asthma symptoms should be identified. Coexistent illness, such as congestive heart failure with pulmonary edema, can also cause wheezing. Gastroesophageal reflux can induce cough and bronchospasm. Medications such as methylxanthines,

in asthmatic patients, may decrease gastroesophageal sphincter tone and worsen gastroesophageal reflux, which in turn can provoke asthma.

Sinusitis and asthma frequently coexist, and several studies have reported a high (40 to 60%) incidence of sinusitis among patients with asthma. Also, patients with refractory asthma show relief of symptoms when the concurrent sinusitis is appropriately treated. The mechanisms by which sinusitis affects asthma are not yet clear but may involve the dripping of mediators from the sinuses to the lower airways or the presence of eosinophils acting as a common effector cell for both the upper and the lower airways.

DIAGNOSIS/CLASSIFICATION

The diagnosis of asthma is based on the clinical history and examination, as well as the demonstration of reversible airflow obstruction. Clinical complaints include cough, wheezing, and chest tightness. The pattern of symptoms may also be helpful. Patients who cough or wheeze after certain exposures, or who wheeze with exposure to cold air or exercise, may be more likely to have asthma. In addition, patients whose symptoms interrupt their activity or their sleep often have more significant disease.

Airway reversibility is usually determined by pulmonary function testing. Baseline spirometry is performed; then the patient receives either nebulized isoproterenol or 2 puffs of a beta$_2$-agonist bronchodilator (albuterol, pirbuterol, terbutaline, or metaproterenol) by metered-dose inhaler. An improvement in the FEV_1 of at least 15% is considered significant.

The methacholine inhalation challenge may be employed as an additional diagnostic tool. This test is usually performed in a pulmonary function laboratory and should only be used on individuals with normal baseline pulmonary function. A positive methacholine challenge, however, does not identify asthma specifically; rather, it merely indicates the presence of airway hyperresponsiveness, which can be present in other situations such as cigarette smoking, chronic obstructive pulmonary disease (COPD), and postviral infection. Other challenge methods include exercise or cold air. The diagnostic work-up for asthma must include the clinical evaluation as well as these objective measures.

In the asthmatic patient with significant obstruction and airway inflammation (FEV_1 < 70% of predicted), bronchodilator administration may not reveal a significant reversible component. In these patients, reversible airflow obstruction is best evaluated by pulmonary function testing before and after a short trial of oral corticosteroid, such as

TABLE 2. **Classification of Asthma**

Mild	Moderate	Severe
<2 episodes per week	>1–2 episodes per week	Continuous symptoms Limited exercise and activity
Rare or absent nocturnal symptoms	Frequent nocturnal symptoms	Frequent exacerbations requiring excessive beta$_2$-agonist use
Normal FEV$_1$ between episodes	Exacerbations lasting >24 hours, FEV$_1$ 60–80% of baseline	Emergency room evaluations and hospitalizations Highly variable FEV$_1$ <60% of baseline

Abbreviation: FEV$_1$ = forced expiratory volume in 1 s.

prednisone, 30 mg per day for 5 to 7 days, followed by prednisone, 10 mg per day for an additional 5 to 7 days.

TREATMENT

The NAEP has developed a clinical classification of asthmatic patients (Table 2) that we use to guide therapy. It is important to identify and avoid triggering agents, especially in allergic and occupational asthma. Dust mite control measures, especially in sleeping areas, can reduce symptoms. If it is impossible to remove a pet from the home, it should, at minimum, be kept from the bedroom at all times.

Medications to relieve symptoms of airflow obstruction as well as inflammation are vital for adequate control. Inhaled (beta$_2$-agonist) medications (Table 3) are the most effective bronchodilators and can quickly relieve airway obstruction. Anti-inflammatory agents include inhaled corticosteroids (Table 4), cromolyn sodium, and nedocromil sodium. These medications should be used in a stepwise fashion based on the NAEP guidelines. For a patient with mild asthma, therapy should consist of an inhaled (beta$_2$-agonist) medication as needed and pretreatment with 2 to 4 puffs of an inhaled beta$_2$ agonist (Proventil, Ventolin, Maxair, Brethaire) with or without 2 puffs of cromolyn sodium or nedocromil prior to exercise or contact with other triggers. Cromolyn or nedocromil may give additional protection from exercise- or allergen-induced bronchospasm.

For the patient with moderate asthma, chronic anti-inflammatory therapy (e.g., with an inhaled corticosteroid or inhaled cromolyn/nedocromil) is required. Inhaled corticosteroids have been shown both to relieve symptoms and to improve pulmonary function measurements and also to allow for decreased use of supplemental medication. Inhaled corticoste-

roids may be used at a dosage of 4 puffs twice a day, which may improve patient compliance. Inhaled beta$_2$ agonists should be continued on an as-needed basis for chronically symptomatic asthmatics. Should these measures not achieve optimal control, adding sustained-release theophylline (400 mg at bedtime or 200 to 300 mg twice daily) can be considered or, alternatively, using a long-acting beta$_2$ agonist such as salmeterol (Serevent) 2 puffs twice daily. Patients with acute symptoms or a marked change in status require a short course of oral corticosteroids followed by continuation of inhaled corticosteroids, possibly at a higher dose. A typical dosing schedule for a course of oral prednisone is 30 to 40 mg daily given in divided doses (two to three times a day) for 1 week, followed by 10 to 15 mg daily for an additional week.

Assessment by an asthma specialist should be considered if symptoms are not controlled by these measures, if pulmonary function tests continue to show marked variability, or if frequent courses of oral corticosteroids are required to control symptoms. Asthma specialists and particularly allergists may also be helpful in identifying allergic or environmental triggers.

Patients with severe asthma require high doses of inhaled corticosteroids (8 to 16 puffs per day). Despite this, these patients often receive frequent short courses of oral corticosteroids for repeated exacerbations and may even require prolonged courses of daily prednisone for control. The lowest effective dose of prednisone should be used in these circumstances, and alternate-day dosing with corticosteroids may produce fewer side effects. For patients with continued nocturnal symptoms, the addition of sustained-release theophylline (Uniphyl), 400 to 800 mg at supper, or the use of salmeteral, 2 puffs at bedtime, may offer additional relief. Peak serum concentrations of

TABLE 3. **Beta$_2$ Agonists**

Drug	Trade Name	Dose	Special Characteristics
Metaproterenol	Alupent	2 puffs q 4–6 h as needed	Less beta$_2$ selective than others, may have more systemic effects
Albuterol	Proventil, Ventolin	2 puffs q 4–6 h as needed	Beta$_2$ selective
Pirbuterol	Maxair	2 puffs q 4–6 h as needed	Beta$_2$ selective, may produce less muscle tremor in some patients
Terbutaline	Brethaire	2 puffs q 4–6 h as needed	Beta$_2$ selective, bronchodilator of choice in pregnancy
Salmeterol	Serevent	2 puffs bid	Slow-onset, prolonged duration of action

TABLE 4. **Anti-Inflammatory Medications**

Drug	Trade Name	Dose/Actuation (µg)	Recommended Adult Dosage
Beclomethasone dipropionate	Beclovent, Vanceril	42	2–4 puffs, 3–4 times daily
Flunisolide	AeroBid	250	2–4 puffs, 2–4 times daily*
Triamcinolone acetonide	Azmacort	100	2–4 puffs, 3–4 times daily
Cromolyn sodium	Intal	800	2 puffs, 4 times daily
Nedocromil sodium	Tilade	1750	2 puffs, 2–4 times daily

*Exceeds dosage recommended by the manufacturer.

theophylline should be monitored and kept optimally in the 8 to 15 mg per liter range. Inhaled beta$_2$ agonists and theophylline are usually the most effective bronchodilators in asthma, and often both are required in severe asthma. For patients with severe asthma and COPD, ipratropium bromide (Atrovent) may also offer some benefit. High-potency inhaled corticosteroids (budesonide,* fluticasone*) are under investigation and show promise for asthma therapy.

Acute Asthma

An acute exacerbation of asthma is an urgent medical problem. The best strategy for management is early recognition, evaluation, and treatment to prevent deterioration and to abort further exacerbation and respiratory compromise. Each patient should have a "plan of action" to follow for acute asthma exacerbations.

The intensity of the acute attack and its outcome are influenced by several factors, including the patient's age (with elderly patients having the greatest risk); the duration of the current episode; a history of previous life-threatening asthma exacerbations requiring hospitalization, intubation, and intensive care or of complications secondary to hypoxia; recent and frequent emergency room visits; and either systemic corticosteroid usage or recent withdrawal from corticosteroids.

The first line of therapy in this setting is repetitive inhalation of beta$_2$ agonists. Subcutaneous epinephrine (0.3 ml of 1 : 1000) may be administered on an emergency basis as well as repeated treatments with nebulized beta$_2$ agonists (as frequently as every 20 minutes for the first hour). Methylprednisolone, 1 to 2 mg per kg intravenously, should be administered if no immediate response is noted to beta$_2$-agonist therapy. As discussed previously, patients with acute exacerbations require 1 to 2 weeks of oral corticosteroids after discharge from the emergency room.

GENERAL CONSIDERATIONS

Asthma is a chronic disease with various presentations. Management must encompass modalities such as patient education, continued reassessment, and specific therapeutic intervention for successful long-term control.

Patient education should include the basic patho-

physiology of asthma, identification and avoidance of specific triggers, and methods of objective monitoring with peak flowmeters. Baseline values of peak flow measurement can be obtained over a 2-week period; then peak flow values are obtained during symptomatic episodes. These measurements can be helpful in devising a plan of action for acute exacerbations. Patients may receive individual instructions on the adjustment of their medications (such as instituting a short course of prednisone, 30 mg per day for 5 to 7 days followed by 10 mg per day for 5 to 7 days) should peak flows fall to less than 70% of baseline with associated symptoms. Patients must also be instructed to contact a physician immediately for management of acute symptoms. Any emergency evaluation should be followed by a subsequent visit to the clinician's office for a reevaluation of overall asthma control.

Patients with moderate-to-severe asthma require close follow-up and frequent assessment of pulmonary function. These patients should also receive influenza vaccine every fall (except egg-allergic patients).

Inhaler technique should be continually reviewed on follow-up visits in all patients. In addition, compliance must be reassessed and factors that may affect compliance (e.g., socioeconomic or psychosocial) should be discussed.

ASTHMA IN CHILDREN

method of
ROBERT C. STRUNK, M.D., and
THOMAS F. SMITH, M.D.
Washington University School of Medicine
St. Louis, Missouri

Asthma is the most common chronic illness in childhood. In spite of increased knowledge of pathophysiology and treatment of this disease, both the prevalence of asthma and the morbidity and mortality due to asthma are increasing. These trends are in contrast to the achievable expectation that children with asthma can lead full lives without limitations.

Asthma is a disease that continues to defy specific definition. From an epidemiologist's view, asthma is cough and/or wheeze without a cold; from an asthmatologist's view, it is reversible airway obstruction involving airway inflammation characterized by bronchospasm, delayed

*Investigational drug in the United States.

phase reactions, and bronchial hyperresponsiveness, for which allergens play a central role; and from a pathologist's view, it is chronic eosinophilic desquamative bronchiolitis. The National Heart, Lung, and Blood Institute of the National Institutes of Health recently defined asthma as: (1) airway obstruction that is reversible (but not completely so in some patients), either spontaneously or with treatment; (2) airway inflammation; and (3) airway responsiveness to a variety of stimuli.

The presence of eosinophils in asthmatic sputum and airway mucosa has been known for decades. More recently, the importance of lymphocytes in the development of eosinophilic airway inflammation has been recognized. Studies of basic pathophysiology of asthmatic airway inflammation, along with prospective clinical studies of patients with asthma, have emphasized the importance of environmental factors in the course of the disease and the usefulness of anti-inflammatory medications to control symptoms that cannot be prevented by environmental modification. The fundamental role of allergy in childhood asthma has been increasingly recognized, in that most children with moderate and severe asthma have positive skin tests by 14 years of age, the prevalence of asthma in populations is strongly associated with elevations of total serum IgE, and the prevalence and severity of asthma are associated with the presence and extent of indoor allergens (dust mite, cat, and cockroach).

DIAGNOSIS OF ASTHMA

The first priority is to diagnose asthma among the diseases that present with recurrent cough and wheeze, particularly in patients under the age of 5 years. There is no pathognomonic test for asthma. Asthma is a "reactive airway disease." Clinical features of reactivity, such as improvement in symptoms or increase in pulmonary function with bronchodilator treatment, should be observed. However, there are many diseases other than asthma that present with airway reactivity, particularly in young children (Table 1). Recognition of and intervention in some of these diseases can significantly change the course of the illness, such as the presence of an airway foreign body, anatomic abnormalities with compression of the larger airways (e.g., vascular ring, mediastinal mass), lesions that compress smaller airways (e.g., cystic adenomatoid malformation, tuberculosis), and congestive heart failure. It also is important to recognize cystic fibrosis and bronchopulmonary dysplasia as diseases associated with airway reactiv-

ity, as they both require specialized forms of therapy in addition to therapy for cough and wheeze. A chest radiograph should be obtained at the time of diagnosis in children with significant disease; to diagnose asthma, the radiograph should be normal except for hyperinflation and peribronchial cuffing.

In our opinion, use of the term "bronchiolitis" should be restricted to the first episode of wheezing in a child under 1 year of age precipitated by a viral respiratory tract infection (most often respiratory syncytial virus). A second wheezing episode should be considered evidence of a reactive airway disease. Elimination of exposure to cigarette smoke is essential in these children. If asthma is diagnosed, elimination of environmental allergens may improve the overall course of the disease. Elimination of allergens is particularly important for children with a family history of asthma or other atopic disease. This was most impressively put forward by Sporik and coworkers, who demonstrated that children with a family history of asthma had an earlier onset of asthma; higher prevalence of asthma at 11 years of age; and more severe asthma, as indicated by regular medication requirement, if they had a high concentration of mites in their bedroom dust as infants. In addition, early treatment of subsequent exacerbations of chest symptoms with bronchodilators and anti-inflammatory agents can decrease the severity of these episodes and even decrease the total number of episodes.

EDUCATION ABOUT ASTHMA TO DEVELOP PARTNERSHIP IN ASTHMA MANAGEMENT

An asthma education curriculum should include information about the pathophysiology of the disease process; precipitating factors (triggers), particularly the role of allergens and irritants in the environment; early warning signs of asthma for the child; the importance of controlling environmental allergens and irritants; types, uses, and side effects of medications; and expectations of treatment (i.e., children with asthma can lead full lives without limitation). In the educational process, specific plans for chronic and acute care of asthma symptoms are developed, with input from the child, the family, and the physician. The overall goal is to establish open communication among patient, caregivers, and the medical team. Plans for care must be developed with input from the patient and family so that they will have a stake in the plan and be encouraged to participate in it. The ultimate goals of the educational process are to develop a partnership between patient and physician and to give patient and family motivation, skill, and confidence to control the asthma.

There are a number of mechanisms and materials available to educate children and families about asthma. Involvement in asthma support groups is an excellent mechanism, and asthma education sessions are often provided by local chapters of the American Lung Association or the Asthma and Allergy Foundation of America. Education is an ongoing process, and the principles learned in the initial education, whether provided in a group or individually, must be reinforced at each visit for regular and acute care.

TABLE 1. **Differential Diagnoses of Recurrent Cough and Wheeze**

Diagnosis	Work-Up
Foreign body	History, chest fluoroscopy
Anatomic abnormality obstructing large airway (e.g., vascular ring, mediastinal mass)	Barium swallow
Anatomic abnormality obstructing smaller airway(s) (e.g., cystic adenomatoid malformation, tuberculosis)	Chest x-ray, skin test
Recurrent aspiration	Barium swallow
Congestive heart failure	Chest x-ray, physical examination
Bronchopulmonary dysplasia	History, chest x-ray
Cystic fibrosis	Sweat test
Bronchiolitis obliterans	Chest x-ray, history

ASSESS AND MONITOR ASTHMA SEVERITY WITH OBJECTIVE MEASURES OF LUNG FUNCTION

Monitoring of lung function, preferably by spirometry but acceptably by peak flowmeter, at the time of initial presentation and at each follow-up visit provides an opportunity to assess severity and determine the accuracy of the child's perception of and accuracy in reporting the severity of airway obstruction. Testing with a bronchodilator provides the opportunity to teach about signs of asthma to increase accuracy of reporting or to discover a child's tendency to disregard perceived obstruction (i.e., the child is aware of the feeling of the obstruction but does not want to discuss it or have others know that the feeling is there).

Monitoring of pulmonary function is essential in the hospital-based management of exacerbations. The value of the peak expiratory flow (PEF) obtained in the emergency department, compared with the child's best value, quantitates the degree of obstruction and is useful in making decisions about hospital admission. The physical examination is particularly insensitive to level of obstruction during the period of improvement from acute symptoms. For example, once the subjective symptoms and objective signs of asthma are completely resolved, decreases in pulmonary function are often as much as 50% from pre-exacerbation baseline values. Quantitation of the remaining degree of obstruction is necessary to manage medication in the days to weeks after an exacerbation.

Home PEF monitoring should be considered for patients who take medications daily. Such monitoring can facilitate communication between the family and physician during acute asthma symptoms, i.e., the severity of the asthma can be quantitated. It is important to remember that the peak flow is like any other test and is only as good as the meter and the patient's effort in using it. If there is a discrepancy between the PEF and the patient's status, inaccuracy in the test result must be considered as a possibility.

IDENTIFY AND CONTROL ASTHMA TRIGGERS

Identification and control of factors that induce airway inflammation or cause acute increases in airflow obstruction are fundamentally important in the management of asthma. Avoidance or control of these factors—asthma triggers—can reduce symptoms. It is most important to avoid those triggers that cause airway inflammation—allergens, irritants, pharmacologic agents, and viral infections—if possible. It is also important to prevent or control symptoms caused by triggers that do not increase airway inflammation, such as exercise, cold air, and emotions; these triggers should not be avoided, however.

Allergy plays a central role in asthma in childhood, and environmental aeroallergens are a major cause of airway hyperreactivity. As indicated earlier, environmental control may affect the severity and even the likelihood of developing asthma in susceptible children. Reduction of house dust mite allergen exposure decreases asthma symptoms and airway hyper-reactivity in mite-allergic children, and it is reasonable to assume that this applies to other environmental allergens as well. It is important to emphasize to the patient and his or her parents that environmental control measures can reduce the need for, or at least the level of, pharmacologic treatment to control symptoms.

Routine environmental control measures are directed against exposure to house dust mites, warm-blooded pets, cockroaches, indoor molds, outdoor allergens that come into the house through open windows, and irritants such as tobacco smoke and smoke from wood-burning stoves and fireplaces. House dust mite control measures are listed in Table 2. We recommend routine mite precautions for all children with asthma who live in climates where there are house dust mites. In particular, mite-proof encasings on all mattresses and pillows and hot-cycle washing of bedding and stuffed animals are simple, effective measures that are easy to institute. Removal of warm-blooded animals from the patient's home environment is also important; all warm-blooded pets produce dander, urine, and saliva that contain potent allergens that circulate freely through the house and accumulate in carpeting and upholstered furniture. Weekly washing of pets may reduce the allergen load somewhat, but it is unclear whether the reduction is sufficient to be of clinical benefit. It may take months after the pet has left for allergen levels to decrease sufficiently to detect any benefit. Avoidance of cockroach exposure may require professional extermination of roaches. Although outdoor pollens and molds are impossible to avoid completely, exposure to these may be reduced by using air conditioners and by closing windows and doors during peak pollen and mold seasons. Avoiding indoor irritants such as tobacco and wood smoke, household sprays, and other air pollutants is important, because exposure to these may worsen asthma. Exposure to tobacco smoke has been linked to the development of asthma. We believe that it is mandatory that no one smoke in the asthmatic child's home or car.

TABLE 2. **House Dust Mite Control Measures**

Routine

Encase the mattress and box springs in an allergen-nonpermeable cover
Either encase the pillow or wash it weekly
Wash all bedding weekly in water of 130° F (55° C)
Avoid sleeping or lying on furniture upholstered with fabric
Reduce indoor humidity to less than 50%

Heroic

Remove carpets that are laid on concrete
Remove carpets from the bedroom
Use chemical agents to kill mites (acaricides such as benzyl benzoate) or to reduce mite allergen levels in the house (3% tannic acid)

Exercise is a common precipitating factor in asthma that deserves special mention. Exercise avoidance commonly occurs. Asthmatic children learn to sit on the sidelines rather than wheeze, parents stop play at the first sign of symptoms, and physical education teachers discourage asthmatic children from participating in sports. Exercise-induced asthma is best approached by treating the asthma rather than by avoiding exercise. In addition, medicines such as albuterol, cromolyn, and nedocromil can be used prophylactically to block exercise-induced asthma and allow full participation. The numerous Olympic athletes with asthma testify to this possibility.

Some medications may exacerbate asthma. Aspirin and other nonsteroidal anti-inflammation agents can cause severe episodes of asthma in sensitive patients. Beta blockers also may worsen asthma and should generally be avoided in asthma patients or used only under close medical supervision.

The role of specific immunotherapy in asthma is under ongoing investigation. Controlled studies have shown that specific immunotherapy with appropriately selected extracts and safe administration of doses may be effective in asthma management. Use of immunotherapy for asthma patients requires caution, however, because of the risk of causing a severe exacerbation of asthma from an immunotherapy injection. Before an injection is given, the patient should be asymptomatic and the FEV_1 (forced expiratory volume in 1 second) should be at least 70% predicted. We do not recommend immunotherapy as an alternative to allergen avoidance.

ESTABLISH MEDICATION PLANS FOR CHRONIC MANAGEMENT

Chronic management should permit control of the child's asthma, as defined in Figure 1. Control is achieved by a stepwise approach in which the number and frequency of medications are increased with increasing asthma severity, as outlined in Figure 1. Dosages for therapy with the various medications are presented in Table 3. Moving to the next step is warranted when control is not achieved (see step-up in Figure 1). The goal is to control asthma with the least possible medication given on the least frequent dosing schedule. Clinicians must judge whether to increase treatment in a gradual, stepwise manner or to give maximum treatment initially, including using oral glucocorticoids, to achieve control. In either case, once control is sustained, a stepwise reduction in therapy can be considered and is needed to identify the minimum therapy required to maintain control. This is particularly important for children who experience episodic increases in asthma severity, for example, during the winter because of viral respiratory infections or during a pollen season. For these children, the level of therapy may need to be increased during their usual season of increased symptoms but should then be decreased after the season is over, as long as asthma control is maintained.

TABLE 3. Dosages for Therapy in Childhood Asthma

Beta₂ Agonists for Rescue Therapy

Inhaled

Examples: Albuterol, metaproterenol, bitolterol, terbutaline, pirbuterol

MODE OF ADMINISTRATION

MDI	2 puffs q 4–6 h
Dry powder inhaler	1 capsule q 4–6 h
Nebulizer solution*	Albuterol, 5 mg/mL; 0.1–0.15 mg/kg in 2 mL of saline q 4–6 h; maximum, 5.0 mg
	Metaproterenol 50 mg/mL; 0.25–0.50 mg/kg in 2 mL of saline q 4–6 h; maximum, 15.0 mg

Oral

LIQUIDS

Albuterol	0.1–0.15 mg/kg q 4–6 h
Metaproterenol	0.3–0.5 mg/kg q 4–6 h
TABLETS	2- or 4-mg tablet, q 4–6 h
Metaproterenol	10- or 20-mg tablet q 4–6 h
Terbutaline	2.5- or 5.0-mg tablet q 4–6 h

Beta₂ Agonists for Maintenance Therapy

Salmeterol (Serevent) MDI	21 μg/puff; 2 puffs bid
Albuterol	4-mg sustained-release tablet q 12 h

Cromolyn Sodium (Intal)

MDI	1 mg/puff; 2 puffs qid
Dry powder inhaler	20 mg/capsule; 1 capsule qid
Nebulizer solution	20 mg/2 mL ampule; 1 ampule qid

Nedocromil Sodium (Tilade)

MDI	2 mg/puff; 2 puffs bid–qid

Theophylline

Liquid Tablets, capsules Sustained-release tablets, capsules	Dosage to achieve serum concentration of 5–15 μg/mL

Corticosteroids

Inhaled†

Beclomethasone (Beclovent, Vanceril)	42 μg/puff; 2–4 puffs bid–qid
Triamcinolone (Azmacort)	100 μg/puff; 2–4 puffs bid–qid
Flunisolide (AeroBid)	250 μg/puff; 2–4 puffs bid

Oral‡

LIQUIDS

Prednisone	5 mg/5 mL
Prednisolone	5 mg/5 mL
	15 mg/5 mL

TABLETS

Prednisone	1, 2.5, 5, 10, 20, 25, 50 mg
Prednisolone	5 mg
Methylprednisolone	2, 4, 8, 16, 24, 32 mg

*Premixed solutions are available. It is suggested that the per kg dosage recommendations be followed.

†Consider use of spacer devices to minimize local adverse effects.

‡For acute exacerbations, doses of 1–2 mg/kg in single or divided doses are used initially and are then modified. Reassess in 3 days, as only a short burst may be needed. There is no need to taper a short (3- to 5-day) course of therapy. If therapy extends beyond this period, it may be appropriate to taper the dosage. For chronic dosage, the lowest possible alternate-day morning dosage should be established.

Abbreviation: MDI = metered-dose inhaler.

From National Institutes of Health, U.S. Department of Health and Human Services: Executive Summary: Guidelines for the Diagnosis and Management of Asthma. Washington, DC, U.S. Government Printing Office, 1991.

Step-Up: Progression to the next higher step is indicated when control cannot be achieved at the current step and there is assurance that medication is used correctly. If PEFR ≤60% predicted or personal best, consider a burst of oral corticosteroids and then proceed.

Step-Down: Reduction in therapy is considered when the outcome for therapy has been achieved and sustained for several weeks or even months at the current step. Reduction in therapy is also needed to identify the minimal therapy required to maintain control.

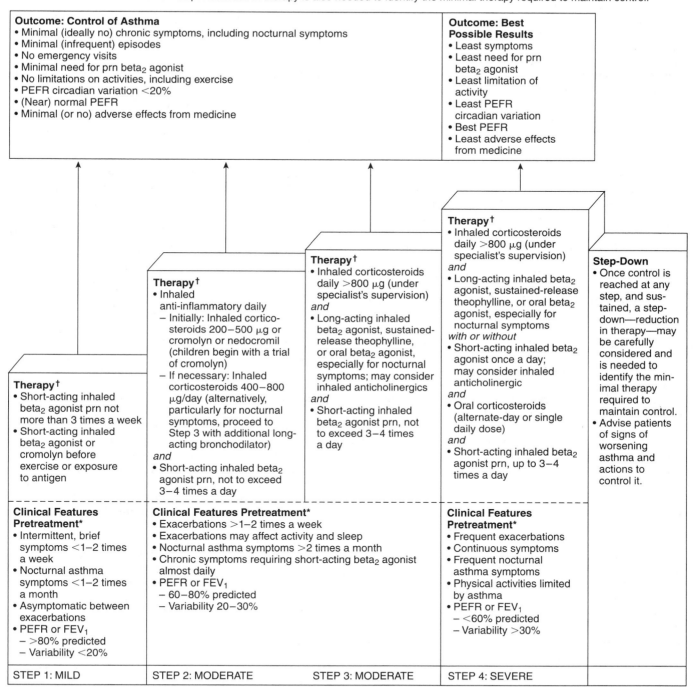

Outcome: Control of Asthma
- Minimal (ideally no) chronic symptoms, including nocturnal symptoms
- Minimal (infrequent) episodes
- No emergency visits
- Minimal need for prn beta$_2$ agonist
- No limitations on activities, including exercise
- PEFR circadian variation <20%
- (Near) normal PEFR
- Minimal (or no) adverse effects from medicine

Outcome: Best Possible Results
- Least symptoms
- Least need for prn beta$_2$ agonist
- Least limitation of activity
- Least PEFR circadian variation
- Best PEFR
- Least adverse effects from medicine

Therapy†
- Inhaled corticosteroids daily >800 μg (under specialist's supervision) *and*
- Long-acting inhaled beta$_2$ agonist, sustained-release theophylline, or oral beta$_2$ agonist, especially for nocturnal symptoms *with or without*
- Short-acting inhaled beta$_2$ agonist once a day; may consider inhaled anticholinergic *and*
- Oral corticosteroids (alternate-day or single daily dose) *and*
- Short-acting inhaled beta$_2$ agonist prn, up to 3–4 times a day

Step-Down
- Once control is reached at any step, and sustained, a step-down—reduction in therapy—may be carefully considered and is needed to identify the minimal therapy required to maintain control.
- Advise patients of signs of worsening asthma and actions to control it.

Therapy†
- Inhaled corticosteroids daily >800 μg (under specialist's supervision) *and*
- Long-acting inhaled beta$_2$ agonist, sustained-release theophylline, or oral beta$_2$ agonist, especially for nocturnal symptoms; may consider inhaled anticholinergics *and*
- Short-acting inhaled beta$_2$ agonist prn, not to exceed 3–4 times a day

Therapy†
- Inhaled anti-inflammatory daily
  - Initially: Inhaled corticosteroids 200–500 μg or cromolyn or nedocromil (children begin with a trial of cromolyn)
  - If necessary: Inhaled corticosteroids 400–800 μg/day (alternatively, particularly for nocturnal symptoms, proceed to Step 3 with additional long-acting bronchodilator) *and*
- Short-acting inhaled beta$_2$ agonist prn, not to exceed 3–4 times a day

Therapy†
- Short-acting inhaled beta$_2$ agonist prn not more than 3 times a week
- Short-acting inhaled beta$_2$ agonist or cromolyn before exercise or exposure to antigen

Clinical Features Pretreatment*
- Intermittent, brief symptoms <1–2 times a week
- Nocturnal asthma symptoms <1–2 times a month
- Asymptomatic between exacerbations
- PEFR or FEV$_1$
  - >80% predicted
  - Variability <20%

Clinical Features Pretreatment*
- Exacerbations >1–2 times a week
- Exacerbations may affect activity and sleep
- Nocturnal asthma symptoms >2 times a month
- Chronic symptoms requiring short-acting beta$_2$ agonist almost daily
- PEFR or FEV$_1$
  - 60–80% predicted
  - Variability 20–30%

Clinical Features Pretreatment*
- Frequent exacerbations
- Continuous symptoms
- Frequent nocturnal asthma symptoms
- Physical activities limited by asthma
- PEFR or FEV$_1$
  - <60% predicted
  - Variability >30%

STEP 1: MILD | STEP 2: MODERATE | STEP 3: MODERATE | STEP 4: SEVERE

*One or more features may be present to be assigned a grade of severity; an individual should usually be assigned to the most severe grade in which any feature occurs.
†All therapy must include patient education about prevention (including environmental control where appropriate) as well as control of symptoms.

Figure 1. Chronic management of asthma: stepwise approach to asthma therapy. *Abbreviations*: PEFR = peak expiratory flow rate; FEV$_1$ = forced expiratory volume in 1 s. (From International Consensus Report on Diagnosis and Treatment of Asthma. Bethesda, MD, National Heart, Lung, and Blood Institute, National Institutes of Health, 1992.)

Children who have mild, intermittent asthma may be treated with a short-acting beta$_2$ agonist as needed for symptomatic or "rescue" therapy (Step 1). Need for treatment with a beta$_2$ agonist more than 2 to 3 times per week indicates a level of asthma that warrants anti-inflammatory therapy (Step 2). Increasing use indicates deteriorating control. Aerosol or inhaled therapy with a beta$_2$ agonist produces better bronchodilation than oral therapy and causes fewer systemic adverse effects (such as cardiovascular stimulation or skeletal muscle tremor).

Children with moderate asthma should receive inhaled anti-inflammatory therapy on a daily basis, using cromolyn, nedocromil, or a glucocorticoid. Cromolyn sodium (Intal) is a nonsteroidal, topically active agent that has been shown to be beneficial in the management of chronic asthma in children and adults. A 4- to 6-week trial may be needed to determine efficacy in an individual patient. Adverse effects are rare. Cromolyn must be given at least three times per day to be effective. Nedocromil sodium (Tilade) is another nonsteroidal, topically active agent. It is more potent than cromolyn in vitro, and a benefit may be seen sooner than with cromolyn. Treatment is not associated with any significant adverse effects. A minority of patients complain of its taste, which may be ameliorated by use of a spacer. Nedocromil is probably effective with twice-a-day dosing.

Inhaled glucocorticosteroids are the most effective anti-inflammatory treatment for asthma. Glucocorticoids reduce nonspecific airway responsiveness and improve symptoms and lung function. Although they do not block acute challenges such as allergen or exercise provocation, they will decrease the response to these over time. Beclomethasone (Beclovent, Vanceril), triamcinolone (Azmacort), and flunisolide (AeroBid) are currently available in the United States; all are roughly equivalent in safety and efficacy. They can be given twice a day. A spacer device can reduce oropharyngeal adverse effects and systemic absorption.

If the child's asthma is not controlled by Step 2 measures, then an additional increase in therapy (Step 3) is warranted and input from an asthma specialist indicated. Increasing the dose of inhaled glucocorticoid should be considered, but doses above 800 μg per day may result in systemic adverse effects. The addition of cromolyn or nedocromil to regular inhaled corticosteroid may be useful in children with exercise- or allergen-induced asthma. Addition of the long-acting, inhaled beta$_2$ agonist salmeterol (Serevent) or oral sustained-release theophylline may be considered, particularly to control nocturnal symptoms. Salmeterol also may be especially useful in children with exercise-induced asthma because of its long duration of action: a morning dose may prevent asthma from exercise for at least 12 hours, including during or after school.

Complete control as described in Figure 1 may not be possible in children with severe asthma. Therapy may require multiple daily medicines (Step 4). Such children should be followed in consultation with an asthma specialist.

ESTABLISH PLANS FOR MANAGING ACUTE EXACERBATIONS

An asthma management zone system has been suggested to help patients monitor the disease, identify the earliest possible signs that control of asthma is deteriorating, and act quickly to regain control. The zones are based on a traffic light system to make it easier for the patient to use and remember. Patient and parent understanding of the zones will be improved if there is a written treatment plan that includes PEF values, medicines, and doses to be used.

The *Green Zone* (no symptoms and PEF >80% of best recorded value, or "personal best") indicates that asthma is under control (as described in Figure 1).

The *Yellow Zone* indicates that asthma is not under adequate control. The child may be having asthma symptoms, and the PEF is 50 to 80% of personal best. Doses of a short-acting beta$_2$ agonist ("rescue medicine") can be given as often as every 4 hours to control symptoms and bring the PEF back into the Green Zone. Need for rescue medicine every 4 hours for 24 hours or more often than every 4 hours, symptoms severe enough to limit activity for 48 hours, or increasingly severe symptoms suggest that a short course of oral glucocorticoid (e.g., prednisone 2 mg per kg per day for 2 days, then 1 mg per kg per day for 2 days) should be given. Frequent fluctuations into the Yellow Zone (e.g., symptoms or use of rescue medicine more than two times a day or more than 2 days a week) may indicate the need to increase the level of maintenance therapy by one step.

The *Red Zone* indicates a medical alert. Asthma symptoms are present at rest or interfere with activity. PEF is below 50% of personal best. Rescue medicine should be given immediately. If PEF remains below 50% in spite of rescue bronchodilator, immediate medical attention is needed, preferably in a hospital-based emergency department. If PEF improves into the Yellow Zone, then the previously outlined strategy should be followed.

Office or emergency department management and hospital-based management of acute exacerbations of asthma are suggested in Figures 2 and 3. In either situation, treatments are designed to relieve airway obstruction, relieve hypoxemia, and restore lung function to normal as soon as possible. The primary therapies are repetitive administration of the rescue bronchodilator and early use of glucocorticoids. If a child is seen in the office or emergency department for an acute exacerbation of asthma, whatever therapy prescribed beforehand was not adequate (because of either inadequate therapy or inadequate adherence), and it is highly likely that the outpatient plan needs to be changed. It is important to identify the reason for the exacerbation and to review and adjust the Green Zone therapy and patient adherence to the medication plan and environmental control measures.

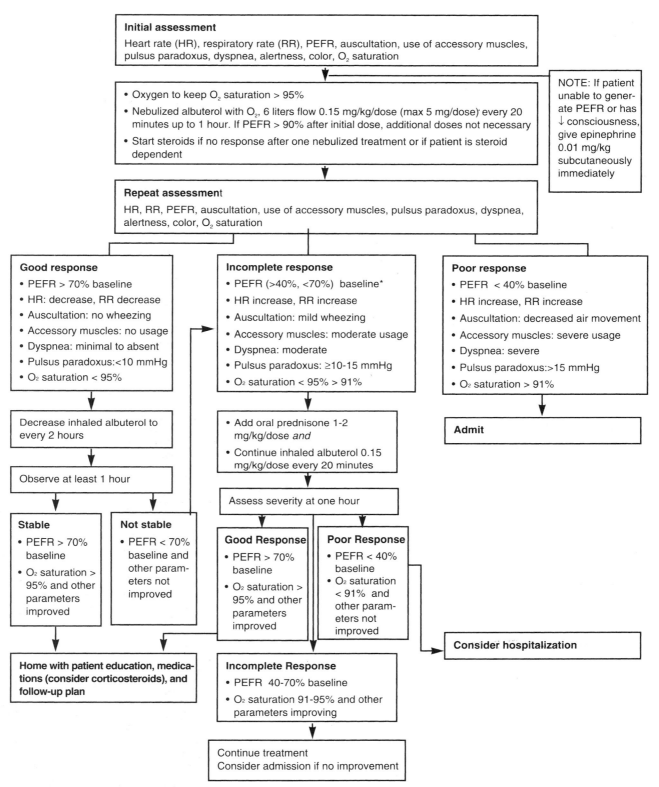

Initial assessment
Heart rate (HR), respiratory rate (RR), PEFR, auscultation, use of accessory muscles, pulsus paradoxus, dyspnea, alertness, color, O₂ saturation

- Oxygen to keep O₂ saturation > 95%
- Nebulized albuterol with O₂, 6 liters flow 0.15 mg/kg/dose (max 5 mg/dose) every 20 minutes up to 1 hour. If PEFR > 90% after initial dose, additional doses not necessary
- Start steroids if no response after one nebulized treatment or if patient is steroid dependent

NOTE: If patient unable to generate PEFR or has ↓ consciousness, give epinephrine 0.01 mg/kg subcutaneously immediately

Repeat assessment
HR, RR, PEFR, auscultation, use of accessory muscles, pulsus paradoxus, dyspnea, alertness, color, O₂ saturation

Good response
- PEFR > 70% baseline
- HR: decrease, RR decrease
- Auscultation: no wheezing
- Accessory muscles: no usage
- Dyspnea: minimal to absent
- Pulsus paradoxus:<10 mmHg
- O₂ saturation < 95%

Incomplete response
- PEFR (>40%, <70%) baseline*
- HR increase, RR increase
- Auscultation: mild wheezing
- Accessory muscles: moderate usage
- Dyspnea: moderate
- Pulsus paradoxus: ≥10-15 mmHg
- O₂ saturation < 95% > 91%

Poor response
- PEFR < 40% baseline
- HR increase, RR increase
- Auscultation: decreased air movement
- Accessory muscles: severe usage
- Dyspnea: severe
- Pulsus paradoxus:>15 mmHg
- O₂ saturation > 91%

Decrease inhaled albuterol to every 2 hours

- Add oral prednisone 1-2 mg/kg/dose *and*
- Continue inhaled albuterol 0.15 mg/kg/dose every 20 minutes

Admit

Observe at least 1 hour

Assess severity at one hour

Stable
- PEFR > 70% baseline
- O₂ saturation > 95% and other parameters improved

Not stable
- PEFR < 70% baseline and other parameters not improved

Good Response
- PEFR > 70% baseline
- O₂ saturation > 95% and other parameters improved

Poor Response
- PEFR < 40% baseline
- O₂ saturation < 91% and other parameters not improved

Consider hospitalization

Home with patient education, medications (consider corticosteroids), and follow-up plan

Incomplete Response
- PEFR 40-70% baseline
- O₂ saturation 91-95% and other parameters improving

Continue treatment
Consider admission if no improvement

NOTE: Therapies are often available in a physician's office. However, most acutely severe exacerbations of asthma require a complete course of therapy in an Emergency Department.

*PEFR % baseline refers to the norm for the individual, established by the clinician. This may be % predicted based on standardized norms or the patient's personal best.

Figure 2. Acute exacerbations of asthma in children: Emergency department management. *Abbreviation*: PEFR = peak expiratory flow rate. (From National Institutes of Health, U.S. Department of Health and Human Services: Executive Summary: Guidelines for the Diagnosis and Management of Asthma. Washington, DC, U.S. Government Printing Office, 1991.)

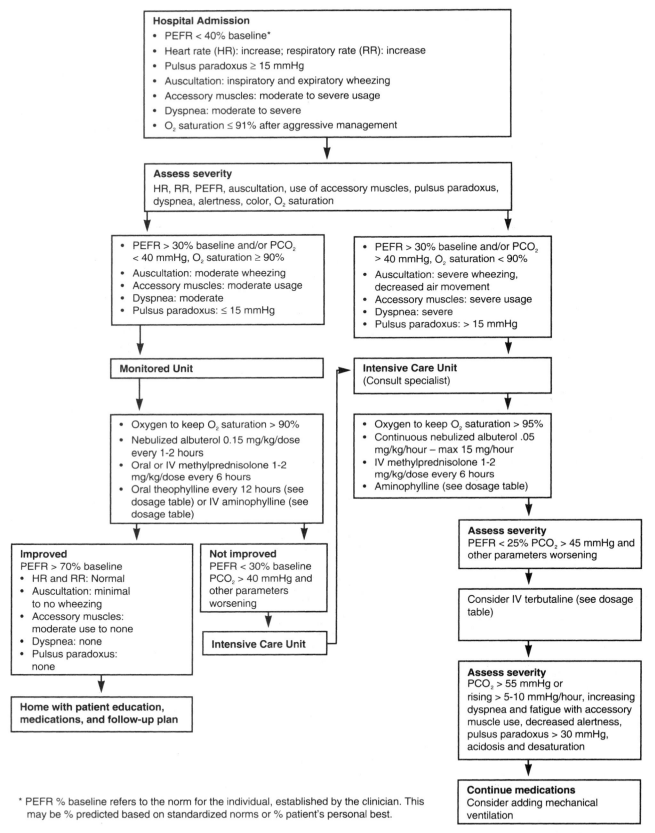

Figure 3. Acute exacerbations of asthma in children: Hospital management. *Abbreviation*: PEFR = peak expiratory flow rate. (From National Institutes of Health, U.S. Department of Health and Human Services: Executive Summary: Guidelines for the Diagnosis and Management of Asthma. Washington, DC, U.S. Government Printing Office, 1991.)

Full recovery from asthma exacerbations is usually gradual; it may take days or weeks for lung function to return to normal and longer for airway hyperreactivity to decrease. Symptoms may not be accurate indicators of lung function or lung healing. An increased level of treatment should be continued until objective measures of lung function return to the patient's personal best; the level can then be decreased incrementally to ensure that control of asthma is maintained.

Certain patients are at high risk of asthma-related death. These include patients with a history of intubation for asthma, those experiencing psychological problems in the child and/or family that result in poor communication during exacerbations and noncompliance with the medication plan, patients recently withdrawn from systemic corticosteroids, and those hospitalized for asthma in the past year. These patients require particularly close monitoring and prompt care.

PROVIDE REGULAR FOLLOW-UP CARE

The National Asthma Education Program Guidelines for the Diagnosis and Management of Asthma (from the National Heart, Lung, and Blood Institute of the National Institutes of Health) recommend that patients with asthma be "monitored continually." While control of asthma is being achieved, variability in peak flow within 24-hour periods and continued presence of symptoms indicate a need to re-evaluate medication use, environmental aggravators and efforts to control them, and the presence of concomitant upper respiratory disease. Once control is established, regular follow-up visits, at least every 3 months, continue to be essential. These visits are used to monitor and review treatment plans, medications, and management techniques. When control is sustained, reduction (step-down) in therapy can be considered. Pulmonary function needs to be measured objectively (such as with spirometry or peak flowmeter) throughout this process.

If an exacerbation results in the need for emergency care or hospitalization, re-evaluation must be scheduled within 7 days to ensure complete resolution of the exacerbation and to review the long-term management plan. Such discussions provide an opportunity to review difficulties in the plan that allowed the asthma to reach a degree of severity requiring emergency care.

PROBLEMS AND PITFALLS

Psychological effects of asthma can be significant and alter the effectiveness of medical care. Children with serious asthma demonstrate psychological symptoms more frequently than healthy peers. The correlation between severity of asthma and intensity of psychological problems is not absolute, however; children with mild asthma can have severe dysfunction, and some children with severe disease can be well adjusted. Depression is probably seen more frequently in children with severe asthma. Young children can also manifest psychological difficulties as sleep disturbances, fearfulness, depressed mood, oppositionality, and negative interactions with caregivers.

Making a diagnosis of asthma remains a challenge. The approach outlined earlier will provide clarity in most situations. A tendency to avoid the diagnosis of asthma in patients under the age of 2 years continues, making environmental control and planning for therapeutic changes early in the course of exacerbations unavailable. Another tendency is to diagnose pneumonia in a young child with previous cough or wheeze who presents with chest symptoms and an infiltrate (which is often due to atelectasis).

The long-term outcome of asthma may not be as good as previously considered. For decades, physicians have told parents that their child was likely to "outgrow" asthma. New studies indicate that although asthma improves in many children during the adolescent years, asthma symptoms return in later adulthood in up to 50% of individuals. Factors associated with remission in adolescence are infrequent attacks and normal FEV_1. Factors associated with relapse are smoking, any wheezing, productive cough at times other than colds, airway hyperreactivity, and allergy (allergic rhinitis, eczema, positive skin tests). For adolescent patients, advice should include to continue follow-up care with a physician, avoid exposure to precipitating factors (do not buy a cat, and continue to avoid cigarette smoke), and consider possible irritant exposure when selecting a job.

ALLERGIC RHINITIS CAUSED BY INHALANT FACTORS

method of
JONATHAN CORREN, M.D., and
GARY S. RACHELEFSKY, M.D.
University of California, Los Angeles, School of Medicine
Los Angeles, California

Allergic rhinitis is the most common of all allergic diseases and has been estimated to affect up to 15% of the population in the United States. Although allergic rhinitis can develop at any age, two-thirds of patients report the onset of symptoms before age 30 years. Symptoms of nasal allergy vary widely, but in many cases they are of sufficient severity to result in significant loss of time from school and the workplace. Allergic rhinitis is also strongly associated with chronic and recurrent sinusitis, otitis media, and bronchial asthma, and there is growing evidence that treatment of rhinitis may improve control of these other disorders.

DIAGNOSIS

Appropriate therapy for allergic rhinitis requires differentiation of this syndrome from other forms of chronic rhinitis (Table 1). A thorough history and physical examination are frequently all that is required to make an initial diagnosis and begin therapy.

History

Allergic rhinitis typically presents with symptoms of intermittent nasal congestion, clear rhinorrhea, sneezing, and itching of the nose, palate, and/or ears. A significant number of patients also report tearing, redness, and itching of the eyes, usually when nasal symptoms are most active. Nasal and ocular pruritus are among the most helpful symptoms in differentiating allergic from other forms of chronic rhinitis. In severe cases, mucous membranes of the eustachian tubes, middle ears, and sinuses may become involved, causing ear fullness or popping, muffled hearing, and facial pressure. Significant postnasal drainage may result in sore throat and chronic cough. Malaise and fatigue may be prominent, usually in patients with florid nasal symptoms during the height of the pollen season.

In seasonal allergic rhinitis (pollinosis or hay fever), this constellation of symptoms occurs during a predictable, defined season, depending on which allergens the patient has become sensitized to. This temporal pattern is a key feature in distinguishing seasonal allergic from other forms of rhinitis. In perennial allergic rhinitis, however, aeroallergens are present in the environment throughout the year (e.g., house dust mite and animal proteins), causing symptoms to vary little between seasons and making differentiation from other types of rhinitis more difficult. Additionally, patients with perennial allergic rhinitis (particularly due to dust mites) tend to be more affected by persistent nasal congestion and rhinorrhea and less by ocular symptoms, making it difficult to discriminate allergic from nonallergic causes.

Physical Examination

Inspection of the face often reveals periorbital darkening, or "allergic shiners," owing to chronic venous pooling. Children frequently rub their noses upward in response to itching (allergic salute), which may produce a persistent horizontal crease across the nose. The conjunctivae commonly appear mildly injected, with either watery or gelatinous exudate present. Both the allergic salute and the ocular findings are helpful in differentiating allergy from other causes of rhinitis.

Anterior rhinoscopy with a nasal speculum allows visualization of the anterior one-third of the nasal airway. Patients with allergic rhinitis typically have pale, swollen inferior and middle turbinates and clear discharge. Very red, irritated mucosa and thick, discolored secretions should raise suspicions regarding other causes of rhinitis. When severe mucosal edema is present, it may be helpful to spray the nose with a topical decongestant, such as

TABLE 1. **Differential Diagnosis of Chronic Rhinitis**

Allergic rhinitis
Vasomotor rhinitis
Nonallergic rhinitis with eosinophilia
Rhinitis medicamentosa
Chronic sinusitis
Nasal polyps
Anatomic obstructive lesions (e.g., septal deviation, adenoidal hypertrophy)

oxymetazoline (Afrin), in order to visualize structures located more posteriorly. Better visualization of the nasal cavity may allow the examiner to detect a variety of obstructive abnormalities, including posterior deviation of the septum, septal spurs, and polyps.

Laboratory Testing

If the diagnosis has not been made from the history and physical findings, cytologic examination of nasal scrapings can be helpful. Significant eosinophilia in nasal secretions (greater than five eosinophils per high-power field) is an excellent clue to the presence of allergy. Although the detection of nasal eosinophilia is suggestive of allergic rhinitis, it is not diagnostic since eosinophils are also found in NARES (nonallergic rhinitis with eosinophilia). Large numbers of neutrophils without eosinophils should alert the clinician to the possibility of chronic bacterial rhinosinusitis.

Principal indications for allergy skin testing or in vitro measures of specific IgE (e.g., radioallergosorbent testing [RAST]) are determination of allergic sensitivities prior to institution of aggressive allergen avoidance measures or allergy immunotherapy. Assays for specific IgE are not necessary in patients who respond well to and tolerate empirical medical therapy for rhinitis. Skin or in vitro testing must be done in the context of the patient's geographic location and specific home environment in order to include all relevant allergens. Skin testing is the preferred method of investigation because of greater sensitivity, broader variety of available antigens, and lower cost. In most situations, prick or puncture tests are sufficient to assess specific sensitivities in allergic rhinitis, and intradermal testing should be reserved for special circumstances. In vitro allergy testing should be employed in patients who suffer from widespread dermatitis or dermatographism, who have poorly reactive skin (as seen in some young infants and elderly patients), who cannot withhold antihistamines, or who have recently taken astemizole (which suppresses responses for several weeks). Results often vary greatly among laboratories performing these assays, making interpretation difficult. Assessment of total serum IgE is an inadequate screening test, since many patients with normal or low levels of IgE may have strongly positive response to a small but highly relevant group of allergens on allergy skin or RAST testing.

TREATMENT

Allergen Avoidance Measures

Avoidance of aeroallergens is an effective, nonpharmacologic method for treating allergic rhinitis. These measures will ultimately limit long-term expense and potential adverse effects of medications. Since environmental control measures may be inconvenient and expensive to implement, allergy testing should be performed to confirm allergic sensitivities.

Outdoor Aeroallergens. For patients with strictly seasonal rhinitis caused by exposure to plant pollens, avoidance of outdoor activity during peak pollen hours (early afternoon) may be helpful. For patients who are allergic to grass pollen, wearing a surgical-type mask while mowing the lawn or gardening may help avert symptoms. Keeping the windows closed throughout the day is important, and use of an air conditioner prevents airborne pollen from entering the home. HEPA (high-efficiency particulate air) filters placed in the home also reduce indoor pollen counts.

Indoor Aeroallergens. For patients with perennial symptoms, the most common source of allergen sensitization is the house dust mite. Large reservoirs of these microscopic insects are usually found in bedding, mattresses, and carpeting. Down-filled pillows and comforters and wool blankets should be eliminated. Washing of all sheets, mattress pads, pillow cases, and blankets every 1 to 2 weeks in hot (>130° F) water effectively kills these organisms. Specially constructed mattress covers are available that act as a barrier between the interior of the mattress and the patient. Carpeting can be treated with a commercially prepared tannic acid spray, which denatures allergenic mite proteins. If these measures do not result in satisfactory improvement, patients can consider removing the carpeting from the bedroom, providing there are hardwood or linoleum floors underneath. Vacuuming with conventional vacuum cleaners does not significantly reduce mite numbers in carpeting and often increases the number of airborne mite allergens for short periods of time. Available acaricides have been demonstrated to provide only minimal benefit to mite-allergic patients.

Domestic pets are an important source of allergen exposure in many atopic patients. The first and most important step in allergen avoidance is removal of the animal from the home environment. Since patients are often reluctant to do this, other less drastic methods of environmental control can be recommended. The animal should be kept out of the bedroom at all times and central air vents to the bedroom should be kept closed. Following removal of the pet from the bedroom, consideration should be given to removing upholstered furniture and carpeting. An HEPA filter reduces the quantity of airborne animal allergens. Finally, the pet should be washed every 1 to 2 weeks, preferably by someone other than the allergic patient. The patient should be informed that it may take several weeks to months for indoor levels of animal dander to return to low levels.

Indoor fungi, such as *Aspergillus* and *Penicillium* species, are usually found in homes that have experienced water damage. Leaky roofs and ceilings, flooded basements, damaged plumbing, and wet crawl spaces are common sites of mold growth within homes. The only effective way to reduce indoor levels of fungal spores is repair of water-damaged areas. For damp spaces where mold growth is a potential problem, a high-intensity heat lamp can be turned on for 1 to 2 hours. Although most indoor plants do not elevate household levels of mold spores, wicker basket planters should be avoided.

Medications

Antihistamines. Antihistamines are frequently used as first-line therapy for patients with allergic rhinitis (Table 2). These medications effectively re-

TABLE 2. Commonly Used Antihistamines

Antihistamine	Sedation	Dose
Diphenhydramine (Benadryl)	Strong	25–50 mg qid
Tripelennamine (PBZ)	Moderate	25–50 mg qid
Chlorpheniramine (Chlor-Trimeton)	Moderate	4 mg qid
Brompheniramine (Dimetane)	Moderate	4 mg qid
Clemastine (Tavist)	Mild	1.34–2.68 mg bid
Terfenadine (Seldane)	None	60 mg bid
Astemizole (Hismanal)	None	10 mg qd
Loratadine (Claritin)	None	10 mg qd

duce rhinorrhea, sneezing, and nasal and ocular pruritus but have little effect on nasal congestion. Antihistamines are effective when taken occasionally for intermittent symptoms, although they work best when administered before the onset of symptoms.

Patients often treat their symptoms with a variety of classic antihistamines that are available over the counter. These drugs have several possible central nervous system side effects, the most common of which is sedation. The sedative effect often attenuates with continued use over a period of 1 to 2 weeks, but if sedation persists, taking the antihistamine at bedtime only (e.g., chlorpheniramine, 4 to 8 mg) is clinically effective and significantly minimizes daytime sleepiness. An equally important adverse effect is prolongation of voluntary reaction time, the extent of which cannot be gauged by the degree of sedation. Classic antihistamines also have anticholinergic effects, including dryness of the mouth and eyes, blurred vision, and urinary retention. These drugs should be used cautiously in older patients, particularly elderly men, and should be strictly avoided in patients with histories of symptomatic prostatic hypertrophy, bladder neck obstruction, and narrow-angle glaucoma.

Newer antihistamines have clinical efficacy equal to or greater than that of the classic antihistamines but without central nervous system or anticholinergic side effects. Presently, all three of the currently available nonsedating antihistamines are approved for use in patients older than 12 years of age. Because of long drug half-lives, loratadine (Claritin) and astemizole (Hismanal) have the advantage of once-daily dosing. Whereas loratadine has a relatively rapid onset of action, astemizole often requires several hours or longer to control symptoms. Terfenadine (Seldane) and astemizole have been noted to cause prolongation of the QT interval when taken in the following situations: larger than prescribed doses; with concomitant administration of ketoconazole, itraconazole, erythromycin, clarithromycin, or troleandomycin; and in patients with severe hepatic dysfunction. In association with QT interval prolongation, there have been rare reports of cardiovascular adverse events, including torsades de pointes, other ventricular arrhythmias, cardiac arrest, and death. Neither QT prolongation nor cardiovascular events have yet been linked to loratadine, even with high blood levels.

Decongestants. Alpha-adrenergic agonists are potent vasoconstrictors that are available in both topical and systemic forms. These medications significantly reduce nasal swelling and rhinorrhea but do not affect other symptoms of allergic rhinitis. Topical preparations include oxymetazoline (Afrin) and phenylephrine nasal sprays (Neo-Synephrine). In patients with severe nasal congestion, these medications enhance the penetration of other topical drugs, such as nasal cromolyn (Nasalcrom) and corticosteroids. Use should be limited to 3 to 5 days to avoid rebound nasal congestion and rhinitis medicamentosa.

Oral decongestants, such as pseudoephedrine and phenylpropanolamine, are also effective in relieving nasal blockage and do not cause rebound nasal swelling after prolonged periods of use. They are most often combined with antihistamines for treatment of allergic rhinitis (e.g., Drixoral) and are superior in clinical efficacy to either drug used alone. Oral decongestants frequently cause nervousness and insomnia and should not be taken during the evening hours in susceptible patients. Although these drugs do not usually cause significant changes in blood pressure, they should be used with caution in patients with hypertension.

Cromolyn Sodium. Cromolyn sodium, given as a 4% topical nasal spray (Nasalcrom), appears to work by stabilizing mast cells and by direct anti-inflammatory effects on granulocytes. It is comparable to oral antihistamines in controlling symptoms of seasonal and perennial allergic rhinitis and is only partially effective in reducing nasal congestion. Nasal cromolyn needs to be used on a prophylactic basis, 1 spray per nostril three to four times per day. Cromolyn is not effective when taken on an as-needed basis. Except for mild, transient stinging, nasal cromolyn is well tolerated by most patients and is particularly useful in children who cannot tolerate classic antihistamines and decongestants.

Corticosteroids. Corticosteroid nasal sprays are an extremely effective form of therapy for allergic rhinitis. When started before allergen exposure, these medications reduce mast cell mediator release (e.g., histamine, prostaglandin D_2) and retard eosinophil influx into nasal tissue. They have been approved for use in seasonal and perennial rhinitis in patients over 6 years of age. Unlike many other available treatments for nasal allergy, topical corticosteroids are effective in controlling nasal congestion. Although these drugs are most beneficial when used on a regular schedule, there is recent evidence suggesting that they may also be helpful when used on an as-needed basis. In addition to controlling allergic rhinitis, nasal corticosteroids appear to reduce lower airway symptoms in patients with concomitant bronchial asthma. Principal side effects include transient stinging, occasional mild epistaxis, nasal dryness, and pharyngeal irritation. Stinging and dryness may be lessened by switching from an aerosol to one of the aqueous preparations or by using a saline nasal spray before administering the corticosteroid. Epi-

staxis will usually resolve by stopping the spray for 2 to 3 days and applying a topical ointment, such as boric acid (Borofax), to the nasal septum. With long-term use, there do not appear to be any significant local effects on the nasal mucosa and septal perforations have been reported only on rare occasions.

The six available formulations, including beclomethasone (Vancenase, Beconase), triamcinolone (Nasacort), flunisolide (Nasalide), budesonide (Rhinocort), dexamethasone (Dexacort), and fluticasone (Flonase), are comparable in efficacy (Table 3). The most important difference among these products is the type of vehicle used. Vancenase and Beconase are available in both aerosol and aqueous preparations, whereas Nasacort and Rhinocort are available as aerosols only, Flonase as an aqueous preparation only, and Nasalide as a solution containing propylene and polyethylene glycol. Deciding among these preparations is largely a matter of individual patient choice, although the majority of patients in our experience prefer the aqueous or aerosol formulations over solutions containing glycol.

In patients who have very severe nasal swelling, a 3- to 5-day course of oral corticosteroids (e.g., prednisone, 0.5 mg/kg in three divided doses, maximum 30 to 40 mg per day) may be helpful prior to starting topical anti-inflammatory therapy. Because of the risk of severe complications (e.g., osteoporosis), long-term oral or injectable corticosteroid therapy should be avoided in allergic rhinitis.

Anticholinergic Agents. An aerosol preparation of ipratroprium bromide (Atrovent)* has been demonstrated to reduce watery nasal secretions. An infant feeding nipple with an enlarged hole can be attached to the holder of the metered-dose inhaler for nasal use. Ipratroprium bromide has little effect on nasal congestion, sneezing, and pruritus and is best used as a supplemental medication when rhinorrhea has not responded to other measures. An initial starting dose is 1 puff per nostril twice daily, which may be increased to 2 puffs per nostril three times daily, as tolerated. As might be expected, the principal side effect is mucosal dryness, which can be reduced by adjusting the dose. There appears to be no significant systemic absorption at these doses given nasally.

Immunotherapy

Allergy immunotherapy (hyposensitization therapy) should be considered in patients who do not respond to allergen avoidance or medications, who have significant adverse side effects from medications, or who have difficulty adhering to a complex regimen of multiple drugs. Since immunotherapy has also been shown to be effective in allergic asthma, patients with concomitant rhinitis and asthma should be strongly considered as candidates for immunotherapy. Several placebo-controlled studies have documented efficacy with a variety of allergens,

---

*Not FDA-approved for this indication.

TABLE 3. **Intranasal Corticosteroids**

Preparation	Trade Name	Vehicle	Dose*
Beclomethasone	Vancenase, Beconase	Freon/alcohol	1–2 puffs bid
	Vancenase AQ, Beconase AQ	Aqueous	1–2 sprays bid
Flunisolide	Nasalide	Polyethylene glycol	2 sprays bid
Triamcinolone	Nasacort	Freon	2–4 puffs qd
Budesonide	Rhinocort	Freon	2 puffs bid or 4 puffs qd
Fluticasone	Flonase	Aqueous	1–2 puffs qd
Dexamethasone	Dexacort	Freon	1–2 puffs bid

*Dose per nostril.

including dust mite, cat dander, and multiple grass, tree, and weed pollens. Approximately 80% of patients will experience symptomatic improvement after 1 to 2 years, and therapy should be continued for a total of 4 to 5 years. Although the beneficial effects of hyposensitization persist for several years in some patients, in others it may be lost once the injections are stopped. These patients should be evaluated for the development of new sensitivities and may require immunotherapy on a long-term basis. Although the mechanisms by which immunotherapy works are still unclear, it has been documented to reduce mast cell mediator release, eosinophil infiltration, and circulating levels of specific IgE.

The success of immunotherapy depends on accurate confirmation of allergic sensitivities with skin or in vitro testing and a history suggestive of clinical worsening after allergen exposure. The cumulative dose of extract is also important: low-dose immunotherapy has been shown to be no more effective than placebo. As the dose of extract is increased, local reactions are common and systemic reactions can occasionally occur. For this reason, it is important that immunotherapy be administered by practitioners who are skilled in adjusting the dose of immunotherapy and treating untoward reactions.

At present, effective allergy immunotherapy is available only by injection (subcutaneous route). Recent research has shown mixed results for other methods of extract delivery, including both the intranasal and the oral routes.

ALLERGIC REACTIONS TO DRUGS

method of
MICHAEL SCHATZ, M.D., and
MICHAEL MELLON, M.D.
Kaiser-Permanente Medical Center
San Diego, California

and

ROY PATTERSON, M.D.
Northwestern University Medical School
Chicago, Illinois

Currently, 15 to 30% of all hospitalized patients experience an adverse reaction that is an unintended or unde-

sired consequence of drug therapy. These reactions may be classified as shown in Table 1. *Allergic drug reactions* occur in a small percentage of the population receiving the drug and can occur with low dosages of the drug. Usually there has been no reaction on initial exposure to the drug, and a latent (sensitization) period typically occurs during which the drug is taken with no adverse effect. Patients who have histories of multiple-drug reactions tend to have reactions to unrelated drugs, but atopic patients do not appear to be at increased risk for drug allergy.

MECHANISMS AND PATTERNS OF ALLERGIC DRUG REACTIONS

Allergic drug reactions may occur as a result of a number of immunologic mechanisms (Table 2). Most drugs are low-molecular-weight compounds, so the drug or a reactive metabolite must combine with tissue, plasma proteins, or cells to become antigenic. In addition, some drugs appear to cause *anaphylactoid* reactions—clinical manifestations of anaphylaxis apparently due to the direct (nonimmunologic) release of mediators. This type of reaction can be seen with the administration of radiographic contrast media, opiates, and some intravenous anesthetics.

Clinical manifestations of allergic drug reactions may be classified by organ system (Table 3). Cutaneous symptoms are the most common manifestations of drug allergy, especially maculopapular or morbilliform eruptions. Features suggesting a drug etiology to a maculopapular eruption include acute onset, symmetrical distribution, predominantly truncal involvement, and definite pruritus. Although a maculopapular eruption may be associated with little morbidity, it can progress to exfoliative dermatitis, visceral damage, and death. In addition, a maculopapular eruption can be associated with fever or manifestations of drug allergy in other organ systems.

CLINICAL APPROACH TO DRUG ALLERGY

Current Reaction

When the clinical manifestations are compatible with an allergic drug reaction (Table 3), the history is the most important tool in identifying the responsible drug. All drugs taken by the patient must be identified and suspected, although drugs most frequently responsible for the clinical syndrome (see the *Physicians' Desk Reference*) and drugs most recently started should be especially considered. Although peripheral eosinophilia may accompany an allergic drug reaction, it is not specific or sensitive enough to be diagnostic. No skin tests or in vitro tests are

TABLE 1. **Classification of Adverse Drug Reactions**

Type of Reaction	Definition	Example
Overdosage	Toxic pharmacologic effects that are dose-related	Respiratory depression with sedatives
Side effects	Therapeutically undesirable but unavoidable pharmacologic actions with normal dosages	Tachycardia with epinephrine injection
Secondary effects	Events only indirectly related to the primary pharmacologic action of the drug	Vaginal yeast infection with broad-spectrum antibiotics
Drug interaction	One drug alters the normal physiology of the host, which affects the pharmacokinetics or pharmacodynamics of another drug	Theophylline toxicity in patients simultaneously treated with erythromycin
Intolerance	Production of a characteristic pharmacologic effect of a drug by small doses	Nausea with theophylline
Idiosyncrasy	A qualitatively abnormal response to a drug that is different from its pharmacologic effects and that does not involve an immune mechanism	Primaquine-induced hemolytic anemia in a G6PD-deficient patient
Allergy	A qualitatively abnormal response to a drug that is different from its pharmacologic effect and proved or presumed to be due to an immunologic mechanism	Penicillin-induced anaphylaxis

Abbreviation: G6PD = glucose-6-phosphate dehydrogenase.

appropriate for the diagnosis of an ongoing drug reaction. The presumptive diagnosis is made by resolution of symptoms and signs on discontinuation of the presumed responsible drug. If the patient is on multiple, potentially responsible medications, all medications should be discontinued or switched to non–cross-reacting medications. Necessary drugs least likely to have caused the reaction may be cautiously introduced after resolution of the reaction.

Discontinuation of the responsible drug is the most important treatment of an ongoing reaction. If symptomatic therapy of a cutaneous reaction is required, antihistamines (e.g., hydroxyzine 25 mg every 6 hours) usually suffice. Corticosteroids (e.g., prednisone 40 to 60 mg or more daily for 3 to 5 days and taper over the next 7 to 10 days) are indicated for severe cutaneous reactions and serum sickness and will hasten recovery from hematologic, vasculitic, hepatic, renal, and pulmonary reactions. Treatment of anaphylaxis is described in the article "Anaphylaxis and Serum Sickness."

History of Prior Reaction and Current Indication

Ideally, patients should avoid all drugs and cross-reacting agents to which they have experienced a prior reaction, and in most cases, an alternative medication can be found. However, readministration of a

necessary drug that has previously caused a reaction may be appropriate when (1) there are no acceptable substitutes for treating a life-threatening illness or (2) the history of allergic reaction is equivocal or remote enough that current sensitivity is questionable. In these circumstances, several techniques may be utilized to identify current sensitivity and/or to increase the safety of drug administration.

1. Immediate skin testing. High-molecular-weight drugs, such as vaccines, antisera, and insulin, are complete antigens and can be used as reliable skin test materials. Most other drugs are low-molecular-weight compounds for which reactive metabolites or suitable drug-protein complexes have not been identified, and skin testing with these drugs is not useful. Exceptions to this general rule include penicillin and, apparently, induction agents, muscle relaxants, and local anesthetics (see later).

2. Incremental challenge testing. When skin tests are negative or not available, incremental challenge testing may be utilized: small initial doses (1:1,000,000 to 1:1000 of the final dose) by the recommended route are followed by incremental increases (usually by a factor of 10 every 15 to 60 minutes) until a reversible reaction occurs or a therapeutic dose is achieved. Incremental challenge testing should be performed under the supervision of a physician experienced in the procedure and with

TABLE 2. **Immunologic Classification of Allergic Drug Reactions**

Type*	Immune Reactants	Clinical Examples
I. Anaphylactic	Specific IgE	Anaphylaxis, urticaria, angioedema
II. Cytotoxic	IgG or IgM antibody against cell-surface antigens; complement	Anemia, thrombocytopenia, nephritis
III. Immune complex	Immune complexes; complement	Serum sickness, systemic lupus erythematosus syndrome, vasculitis
IV. Cell-mediated	Lymphocytes	Contact dermatitis, organ damage

*Gell and Coombs classification.
Modified from Mellon MH, Schatz M, Patterson R: Drug allergy. *In* Manual of Allergy and Immunology, 3rd ed. Lawlor GJ, Fischer TJ, Adelman DC (eds). Boston, Little, Brown, 1995, p. 264. Published by Little, Brown and Company.

TABLE 3. **Organ System Patterns of Allergic Drug Reactions**

Organ System	Type	Probable Mechanism*
Multisystem	Anaphylaxis	I
	Serum sickness	III
	Fever	?III, ?IV
	Vasculitis	III, IV
Cutaneous	Urticaria/angioedema	I, ?III
	Maculopapular, morbilliform	IV
	Contact dermatitis	IV
	Photosensitivity eruptions	IV
	Fixed drug eruption	?IV
	Toxic epidermal necrolysis	IV
	Erythema multiforme (including Stevens-Johnson)	IV
	Erythema nodosum	?
	Purpura	?
	Exfoliative dermatitis	IV
Hematologic	Eosinophilia	?
	Coombs-positive hemolytic anemia	II
	Thrombocytopenia	II
	Neutropenia	II
	Lymphadenopathy	?
Pulmonary	Asthma	Nonimmunologic (aspirin)
	Pulmonary infiltrates with eosinophilia	?
	Pulmonary edema	?
	Interstitial pneumonitis/fibrosis	IV
Hepatic	Hepatocellular (acute, chronic)	?IV
	Cholestatic jaundice	?
Renal	Interstitial nephritis	?II, ?IV
	Nephrotic syndrome	?
Cardiac	Myocarditis	?
Neurologic	Encephalomyelitis	?IV
	Myasthenic syndrome	II

*Gell and Coombs classification (see Table 2).

Modified from Mellon MH, Schatz M, Patterson R: Drug allergy. *In* Manual of Allergy and Immunology, 3rd ed. Lawlor GJ, Fischer TJ, Adelman DC (eds). Boston, Little, Brown, 1995, pp. 267–268. Published by Little, Brown and Company.

TABLE 4. **Clinical Approach to Patients with Histories of Reactions to Specific Drugs**

Drug	Mechanism*	Skin Testing†	Incremental Challenge Testing†	Desensitization†‡	Pretreatment§
Aspirin (rhinitis, asthma)‖	Unknown	No	Yes. *Caution!*¶	Yes.** *Caution!*¶	—
General anesthetics	Type I, may be anaphylactoid as well	Induction agents Muscle relaxants Latex	—	No	Yes
Heterologous antisera (anaphylaxis)††	Type I	Yes (all patients)	—	Yes. *Caution!*¶	—
Insulin	Type I	Yes	—	Yes	—
Local anesthetics	Rarely (if ever) Type I	Empirically useful	Yes	—	—
MMR vaccine	Type I	Yes	—	Yes	—
Penicillin (urticaria, angioedema, anaphylaxis)‖	Type I	Major determinant (penicilloyl polylysine) and penicillin G‡‡	—	Yes. *Caution!*¶	—
Radiographic contrast media	Anaphylactoid	No	—	—	Yes§§
Sulfonamides	Unknown	No	Yes. *Caution!*¶	Yes. *Caution!*¶	—
Tetanus (urticaria, anaphylaxis)	Type I	Yes	—	Yes	—

*See Table 2.

†For detailed protocols, see Patterson R, Deswarte RD, Greenberger PA, et al: Drug allergy protocols for management of drug allergies. Allergy Proc *15*:249–264, 1994; Mellon MH, Schatz M, Patterson R: Drug allergies. *In* Lawlor GJ, Fisher TJ, Adelman DC (eds): Manual of Allergy and Immunology, 3rd ed. Boston, Little, Brown, 1995, pp. 273–289.

‡When sensitivity demonstrated but drug essential for life-threatening illness and no suitable alternatives.

§Prednisone 50 mg PO 13 h, 7 h, and 1 h prior to the procedure; diphenhydramine 50 mg PO 1 h prior to the procedure.

‖See text for additional information.

¶Reactions during this procedure may be particularly severe and potentially fatal.

**The authors use aspirin desensitization only when aspirin is essential for antithrombotic therapy.

††Serum sickness may occur with negative skin tests and usually occurs following desensitization.

‡‡Inclusion of other minor determinants (penicilloate and penilloate) is preferable, but these reagents are not generally available.

§§Nonionic radiographic contrast media should be administered.

Abbreviation: MMR = measles-mumps-rubella.

personnel and facilities immediately available for treatment of anaphylaxis.

3. Desensitization. Desensitization resembles incremental challenge testing but is utilized when sensitivity is demonstrated but readministration is essential. The goal is neutralization of immune reactants by the drug allergen. The protocol utilized depends on the specific drug, the urgency of the therapy, and the prior reaction. This is a dangerous procedure and must be approached with extreme caution (see later).

4. Pretreatment. For anaphylactoid reactions, pretreatment with antihistamines and corticosteroids has been empirically shown to reduce subsequent reactions. Pretreatment is *not* generally recommended during incremental challenge testing or desensitization because it may mask early, mild reactions but not prevent severe ones.

SPECIFIC DRUGS

The clinical approach to patients with histories of reactions to specific drugs is summarized in Table 4. In addition to rhinitis and asthma, *aspirin* or other nonsteroidal anti-inflammatory drugs (NSAIDs) may occasionally cause urticaria or anaphylaxis that is apparently IgE-mediated and due to the specific NSAID used. In this case, if an NSAID is essential, a chemically non–cross-reacting drug could be carefully administered by incremental challenge testing. NSAIDs may also aggravate chronic urticaria, and avoidance is the only satisfactory approach.

Penicillins represent the most common cause of drug-induced hypersensitivity. Immediate type reactions (urticaria/angioedema, anaphylaxis) are IgE-mediated, may be predicted by skin tests, and may require desensitization. Late reactions are more common, usually present as morbilliform rashes or fever, are not IgE-mediated, cannot be confirmed or excluded by skin tests, and are not amenable to desensitization. Cross-reactivity among certain beta-lactam antibiotics (including semisynthetic penicillins and imipenem) appears high, but in vitro data and clinical experience do not suggest clinically important cross-reactivity between penicillins and currently available cephalosporins. However, if cephalosporins are to be administered to a patient with a history of *anaphylaxis* to penicillin, incremental challenge testing is prudent. There is no in vitro or clinical evidence of cross-reactivity between penicillin and aztreonam (Azactam).

ALLERGIC REACTIONS TO INSECT STINGS

method of
MARIA SOTO-AGUILAR, M.D., and
RICHARD D. deSHAZO, M.D.
College of Medicine, University of South Alabama
Mobile, Alabama

Flying insects of the order Hymenoptera (Figure 1) cause the majority of allergic reactions to insects in humans. These insects include yellow jackets, wasps, white and yellow hornets, commonly grouped as vespids, and honeybees and bumblebees. In the southwestern and southeastern United States, respectively, the hybrid African-Brazilian africanized bee and the imported fire ant have expanded their habitat, are known for their pugnacious disposition, and are the source of increasing morbidity.

Anaphylactic reactions after insect stings occur in 0.4 to 4% of the general population per year in the United States and result in 30 to 50 deaths per year. Established predisposing factors for anaphylactic reactions include male sex, with a 2 : 1 male/female predominance, and age under 20 years. From 33 to 40% of insect sting–allergic patients have other allergic conditions. The risk of death from anaphylaxis is enhanced in men over 30 years of age, and the risk of anaphylaxis is higher in family members of beekeepers.

Patients who experience allergic reactions to insect stings frequently seek medical advice. Fortunately, many of the patient management issues discussed here have been clarified by a series of recent investigations of insect allergy in both the United States and Europe.

CLASSIFICATION OF STING REACTIONS

Reactions to insect stings occur either from the pharmacologic and enzymatic properties of the venom or from immunologic responses to specific venom proteins. These reactions may be characterized as "usual" or "unusual" (Table 1). Histamine and other vasoactive components of the venom of these insects more often than not induce immediate wheal and flare dermal reactions at the sting sites, usually within 15 minutes.

The interaction of venom and venom-specific immunoglobulin E (IgE) on mast cells may result in both immediate or late allergic reactions including biphasic dermal reactions and/or anaphylaxis. *Anaphylaxis* is characterized by combinations of cutaneous erythema, generalized pruritus, urticaria, angioedema, airways obstruction, hypotension, syncope, diarrhea, or cardiac arrhythmia in patients sensitized by previous stings. Biphasic (immediate and late) dermal reactions occur when wheal and flare reactions evolve into erythematous, indurated, *large local reactions*, which peak in size 6 to 12 hours later and may persist for up to 48 hours. Individuals with such biphasic reactions appear to be at no greater risk for anaphylaxis on a subsequent sting than individuals with isolated wheal and flare reactions. Some late dermal reactions may occur without previous wheal and flare reactions, but these are unusual.

A number of unusual reactions to insect stings have also been reported (see Table 1). *Toxic reactions* occur after massive stings and reflect pharmacologic responses to venom constituents. The other reactions appear to be im-

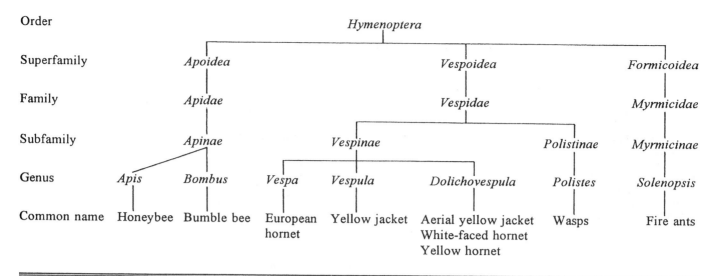

Figure 1. Taxonomy of Hymenoptera that are clinically significant. (Modified from Mueller UR: Insect Sting Allergy. Stuttgart and New York: Gustav Fischer, 1990.)

munologically mediated, primarily by venom-specific IgG antibody. *Cutaneous infection* can develop after fire ant and wasp stings and lead to septicemia.

MANAGEMENT OF INSECT STING REACTIONS

Isolated *immediate reactions* to insect stings should be cleansed with an antibacterial soap and treated symptomatically with the indirect application of ice to the site, and a rapid-acting oral antihistamine such as diphenhydramine, chlorpheniramine, or terfenadine (Seldane). A topical antihistamine such as 5% doxepin (Zonalon) may also be helpful. In individuals stung by honeybees, the stinger and venom sack should be removed with a knife blade. Removal with fingers or tweezers may result in injection of more venom.

The pruritus of *large local reactions* also responds to antihistamines. Local reactions involving the extremities may be severe enough to compromise the

TABLE 1. Insect Sting Reactions Reported in the Medical Literature

Timing	Type of Reaction
Usual	
Immediate (<2 h)	Wheal and flare dermal reactions
	Anaphylaxis
Late (biphasic, peaks at 6–12 h)	Large local (late dermal)
	Anaphylaxis
Unusual	Toxic
	Serum sickness
	Vasculitis
	Nephrosis
	Peripheral neuropathy
	Cerebrovascular accidents
	Transverse myelitis
	Encephalopathy
	Infection

vascular supply to distal tissues. In such cases elevation, treatment with topical, oral, or parenteral glucocorticoids, or fasciotomy may be necessary.

Although many individuals experience *generalized urticaria* as the only manifestation of anaphylaxis after insect stings, it is impossible to determine when generalized urticaria will progress to anaphylactic shock. Therefore, all patients with generalized urticaria should be treated for anaphylaxis. Successful treatment of anaphylaxis is dependent on the early administration of appropriate doses of epinephrine in order to maintain airway patency and oxygenation and prevent the loss of intravascular volume and attendant hypotension (Figure 2). The concomitant administration of oral or intravenous rapid-acting antihistamines also appears to be useful. In patients with bronchospasm, inhaled bronchodilators such as albuterol appear to be safer than intravenous aminophylline, which may induce cardiac arrhythmia. Intravenous glucagon should be strongly considered in individuals on beta blockers whose hypotension does not respond to epinephrine. Up to 25% of patients experience *recurrent anaphylaxis* 6 to 12 hours after the initial episode. Corticosteroids should be strongly considered in all patients with anaphylaxis to prevent or attenuate such late-phase anaphylactic reactions. Since anaphylaxis may recur even after adequate initial treatment, overnight hospitalization should be considered for individuals with severe reactions, those who are unaccompanied at home, or those who live distant from medical facilities.

Finally, all patients with anaphylactic reactions to insect stings should be encouraged to carry self-injectable epinephrine. This is available as EpiPen (0.3 mg), or EpiPen Jr. (0.15 mg) (Center Laboratories, 35 Channel Drive, Port Washington, NY 11050), in a pressure-sensitive, spring-loaded device with a concealed needle. Individuals should be carefully taught how to use this device, as it is frequently

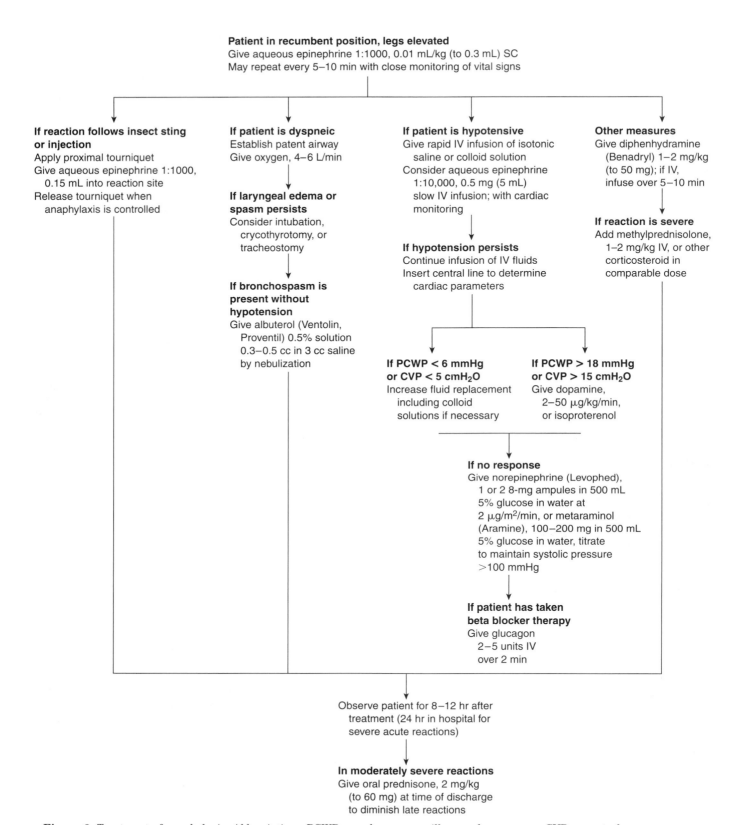

Figure 2. Treatment of anaphylaxis. *Abbreviations*: PCWP = pulmonary capillary wedge pressure; CVP = central venous pressure. (Modified from Soto-Aguilar MC, deShazo RD, Waring NP: Anaphylaxis: Why it happens and what to do about it. Postgrad Med 82:154–174, 1987.)

misused otherwise. Epinephrine is also available in a kit with a preloaded syringe with two doses of 0.3 mL of 1:1000 aqueous epinephrine, a tourniquet, and a chewable antihistamine (Ana-Kit, Hollister-Stier Laboratories Miles, Inc., 400 Morgan Lane, West Haven, CT 06516).

PREVENTION

Although avoidance of stinging insects is not always possible, a number of common sense measures are useful in this regard and are outlined in Table 2. Individuals with previous anaphylaxis to insects should wear a medical alert bracelet (Medic Alert Foundation, Turlock, CA 953801), carry epinephrine to be used immediately after a sting, and be instructed to seek immediate medical attention. Beta blockers should be avoided in such patients, including beta blocker eye drops.

Patients with anaphylactic reactions to insects should be referred to an allergist for evaluation and possible *immunotherapy*. Patients are selected for immunotherapy on the basis of history and results of skin testing with standardized concentrations of commercially available honeybee, yellow jacket, wasp, yellow hornet, and white-faced hornet venom. In patients in whom skin testing is not possible, for instance in those with eczema, in vitro assessment of venom-specific IgE is possible using the radioallergosorbent test (RAST). This test is less sensitive than skin tests and more expensive. Adults and children with severe anaphylactic reactions and positive venom skin tests are routinely treated. Adults with generalized urticaria and angioedema are also candidates. Children who experience urticaria without other evidence of anaphylaxis are not at risk for more severe reactions on resting, and therefore are not treated. Patients with local dermal reactions or unusual reactions to stings are also not treated.

Immunotherapy to flying insects is administered in a progressive fashion from dilute concentrations (0.01 µg/mL) up to a concentration of 100 (µg/mL) of

TABLE 2. **Avoidance Measures for Insect Sting–Allergic Patients**

1. Avoid wearing brightly colored clothes (light brown, white, green, khaki, and neutral colors are better), flower prints, and perfumes or scented cosmetics.
2. Do not walk barefoot or wear sandals when out of doors; wear long pants when walking on grass; wear long sleeves, gloves, and hat when gardening.
3. Stay away from open flowers and over-ripe, fallen fruit.
4. Maintain good sanitation; wrap and cover garbage.
5. If eating outdoors, avoid open canned drinks.
6. Do not disturb fallen logs or trees (nesting vespids).
7. Avoid sudden movements when bee or vespid comes near.
8. Have professional exterminator remove all hives and nests around home; treat for fire ants if appropriate.
9. Have insecticides available if insects are detected in home. Insect repellents do not necessarily prevent insect stings.
10. Carry emergency kit containing antihistamines and epinephrine.

insect venom. This therapy is continued for a period of 3 to 5 years, whereupon in most cases it can be discontinued with long-term protection against further anaphylaxis.

IMPORTED FIRE ANTS

Fire ants were introduced into the United States through the port of Mobile, Alabama, in the 1930s. Their habitat now includes much of Florida, South Carolina, Georgia, Alabama, Louisiana, and Mississippi, and they have been noted to be present in North Carolina, Tennessee, Arkansas, Oklahoma, Texas, and Puerto Rico. Fire ants build mounds in yards, playgrounds, and open fields in concentrations as high as 200 colonies per acre and are not only highly aggressive hunters but also easily provoked to sting. Thus, 30 to 60% of the population in urban areas infested by ants are stung each year.

In stinging, the ant attaches itself to the skin using its mandibles, arches its body, and injects up to 0.11 µL of venom through a stinger located in a distal abdomen. The ant then rotates its body around the mandibles and stings repeatedly. The venom induces an immediate and severe burning sensation at the site of the sting followed by itching that may last for many days. Topical corticosteroids or rapidly absorbed antihistamines provide symptomatic relief of the itching. All individuals who are stung experience a local *wheal and flare reaction* that lasts up to an hour followed at the same site by a unique lesion termed a *sterile pustule*. The epidermis covering the pustule sloughs off over a period of 48 to 72 hours, and healing takes place at the base of the lesion as it is covered with new epidermis. The pustule results from the cytotoxic activity of unique piperidine alkaloids, which make up 95% of fire ant venom. No treatment has been convincingly shown to prevent or facilitate the resolution of these lesions. If pustules become excoriated and superinfected, pyoderma or even sepsis can result, a special problem in diabetic patients.

Between 17 and 56% of patients have biphasic *large local reactions* at the site of fire ant stings. Treatment of these was discussed previously. Local reactions respond to immunotherapy, but it is rarely required.

Isolated urticaria and *angioedema* are estimated to occur in 16% of fire ant stings and life-threatening *anaphylaxis* occurs in 0.6 to 4% of stings. Thus, fire ant stings are the most common cause of anaphylaxis in the Gulf South. More than 32 deaths due to fire ant stings have been reported. The risk of repeat anaphylaxis appears to be high, and the ability to avoid fire ants in indigenous areas is limited. Thus, patients with anaphylaxis to fire ants should be referred to a specialist for allergy skin testing and consideration for immunotherapy.

Less common reactions to imported fire ant stings include focal or generalized *seizures* and peripheral *neuropathy*, reactions that have also been reported after vespid stings. With the increasing density of fire ants, reports of home infestation have become more common, and fire ant attacks of neonates and bed-bound patients have occurred.

Purified fire ant venom is not yet commercially available. Fortunately, substantial although variable amounts of venom are present in fire ant whole-body extracts, which is not the case with flying insects. The effectiveness of fire ant whole-body extract for diagnostic testing and immunotherapy has been supported in uncontrolled trials. Treatment consists of weekly subcutaneous injections of fire ant whole-body extracts given in a stepwise fashion from dilute to 1:10 dilutions. Maintenance injections are given monthly for 3 to 5 years. Systemic reaction rates to stings in patients on maintenance therapy have been reported to be about 2%. Many patients eventually become skin test–negative so that immunotherapy may be discontinued.

Diseases of the Skin

ACNE VULGARIS AND ROSACEA

method of
SHARON S. RAIMER, M.D.
University of Texas Medical Branch
Galveston, Texas

Acne affects most teenagers to some degree and frequently persists or develops in individuals in their twenties, thirties, and occasionally beyond. Even though the development of acne is an almost expected occurrence with the onset of puberty, inflammatory lesions are tender and unsightly; they may be devastating to adolescents' self-esteem and can result in disfiguring scarring. Acne thus warrants treatment. The pathogenesis of acne is not completely understood, but certain events appear to be important in its development. Hormonal stimulation occurring near the time of puberty causes sebaceous glands to enlarge and produce more sebum. Keratinous obstruction of the follicular outlet may lead to the accumulation of sebum and keratin, resulting in the formation of open (blackheads) and closed (whiteheads) comedones. *Propionibacterium acnes* may then colonize trapped sebum, inciting an inflammatory reaction that results in inflammatory papules, pustules, and nodules. Therapy is directed toward diminishing outlet obstructions, diminishing the number of *P. acnes* bacteria, reducing the inflammatory reaction, and occasionally, in females, reducing oil gland size and sebum production with hormone therapy.

A combination of topical and systemic agents may be needed to clear acne. Presently, there is no evidence that diet has a role in the pathogenesis of acne. Even though acne is not caused by a lack of washing, cleansing the face twice daily is helpful to remove oil and surface debris. Specific acne cleansers are not necessary, but chlorhexidine (Hibiclens) is effective against *P. acnes* and may be useful when inflammatory lesions are present. Picking of lesions increases the chances of scarring and should be avoided. Patients should be aware that stress can cause acne to flare, and therapy may need to be increased during times of unavoidable stress.

TOPICAL THERAPY OF ACNE

The most commonly used topical agents are benzoyl peroxide, topical antibiotics, and tretinoin. Older preparations such as those containing sulfur, resorcinol, and salicylic acid are occasionally useful.

Benzoyl Peroxide

Benzoyl peroxide is available in over-the-counter products and by prescription, most commonly as gels in strengths of 2.5, 5, and 10%. Some preparations are less drying than others, with water-based products generally being less drying than those containing alcohol or acetone. Benzoyl peroxide affects follicular keratinization and *P. acnes* bacteria; thus, it is useful for treating both comedonal and inflammatory acne. This drug has been known to help prevent resistance of *P. acnes* to erythromycin and tetracycline in patients consistently on these antibiotics and to help rid patients of resistant organisms resulting from previous treatment.

Benzoyl peroxide should be applied lightly once or twice daily to the entire area of involvement. Mild irritation may occur, particularly with initial use. A severe reaction or one persisting for more than 1 or 2 days after discontinuing the medication likely represents a contact dermatitis to benzoyl peroxide, and future use should be avoided. Patients should be aware that benzoyl peroxide may bleach clothing. For this reason, use on the trunk is usually restricted to nighttime application.

Topical Antibiotics

Topical antibiotics exert their effect on *P. acnes* bacteria and thus are useful for treating inflammatory acne. They may be used as single agents or in combination with other medications such as benzoyl peroxide or tretinoin. The two major drugs in use are clindamycin (Cleocin T), available in solution, gel, and lotion forms, and erythromycin (A/T/S, EryDerm, Erycette, Staticin, T-Stat), available in solutions, gels, and saturated swabs. Resistance may develop with prolonged use of these medications. A combination product (Benzamycin) containing 5% benzoyl peroxide and 3% erythromycin has been shown to be somewhat superior to either agent used singly, but it must be kept refrigerated and is moderately expensive.

Topical Tretinoin

Tretinoin acts primarily on the abnormal follicular keratinization and is the most effective topical agent in the treatment of comedones. With time, tretinoin appears to help prevent the development of inflammatory lesions; however, it may initially aggravate these lesions. Therefore, I do not use this medication for severe inflammatory acne until improvement has been obtained with other treatments. Tretinoin (Retin-A) is available in three different vehicles and a variety of concentrations. The mildest preparations are the 0.01% gel and the 0.025% and 0.05% creams. The gel is generally preferred for acne patients, but the cream may be used if the skin is dry. Treatment should be initiated with the mild preparations, which are also effective for maintenance therapy in the majority of patients. Occasionally, patients need to be advanced to intermediate-strength preparations—the 0.025% gel or the 0.1% cream. Use of the strongest preparation, a 0.05% solution, is rarely indicated.

The initial irritation generally experienced by users of tretinoin can usually be avoided if the patient is instructed to apply the medication very sparingly and not to rub it into the skin. Initially, patients should begin with less than nightly applications of tretinoin and then work up to nightly applications over a 2- to 3-week period. Because tretinoin is expensive and less effective on the trunk, its use is generally confined to the face.

SYSTEMIC THERAPY FOR ACNE

Systemic Antibiotics

Oral antibiotics act on the bacteria involved in acne and may also have an anti-inflammatory effect. Typically, twice-daily therapy is initiated for the first 2 months. If the acne is well controlled at that point, antibiotics may be tapered over the next several months while maintaining topical therapy. If significant improvement has not occurred after 6 to 8 weeks of therapy, an alternative antibiotic should be tried.

Some patients require long-term antibiotic therapy, and bacterial resistance to a specific antibiotic can develop. Changing to an alternative drug is often useful.

Tetracycline is the antibiotic most frequently employed. It is inexpensive and usually well tolerated. For most patients, the usual starting dose is 500 mg twice daily. Patients should be instructed to take the medication on an empty stomach, because food (particularly dairy products) interferes with its absorption. Side effects from tetracycline are uncommon. Vaginal candidiasis may develop in women, particularly those on birth control pills. Tetracycline has also been implicated in reducing the efficacy of birth control pills, but this has not been proved. Photosensitivity rarely occurs during tetracycline use.

Erythromycin is the second most frequently employed antibiotic. It is somewhat more expensive than tetracycline but still moderately priced. The standard starting dose is 500 mg twice daily or its equivalent. Gastrointestinal side effects are more frequent than with tetracycline, but if this is a problem, many erythromycin preparations can be taken with meals, because food interferes much less with their absorption than with the absorption of tetracycline.

If tetracycline and erythromycin fail, alternative antibiotics can be considered. Doxycycline (Vibramycin) and minocycline (Minocin) 100 to 200 mg daily may be somewhat more effective than tetracycline, but doxycycline occasionally causes photosensitivity and minocycline is very expensive. Trimetho-prim-sulfamethoxazole (Bactrim) is efficacious, but side effects are of concern, including rashes and rare cases of agranulocytosis.

Retinoids

The development of isotretinoin (Accutane) revolutionized the treatment of severe, therapy-resistant acne. This agent profoundly shrinks sebaceous glands and reduces follicular hyperkeratinization. Other therapies primarily control the acne process until the patient "outgrows it," but Accutane induces long-term (sometimes indefinite) remissions in many patients. Its use is restricted to nodular acne, severe papulopustular acne, scarring acne, and debilitating acne in patients who have not responded to the treatment modalities previously discussed. The drug is prescribed in a dose of 1 mg per kg daily for 20 weeks. During the first month, some patients notice a flare-up of their disease. This reaction can sometimes be alleviated by treating the patient with systemic erythromycin until improvement occurs. The tetracyclines should not be used with retinoids, as this may increase the incidence of pseudotumor cerebri.

Side effects are numerous. Of most concern is the teratogenic effects of this and all other retinoids. Therefore, it must be used with great caution in women of childbearing age. The manufacturer of the drug provides an informational kit that includes consent forms for women contemplating this therapy. They must employ effective birth control measures, and a pregnancy test must be performed before initiating therapy and at monthly intervals thereafter. It is critical that physicians and patients who use Accutane be fully aware of its teratogenic risk and carefully follow the guidelines outlined for its use in women.

Other frequent side effects associated with the use of Accutane include chapped lips, red and dry skin, dry eyes (therefore, contact lenses may be contraindicated), and dryness of the nose, sometimes accompanied by nosebleeds. Less frequently, patients may develop severe headaches due to pseudotumor cerebri, muscle or joint aching, fatigue, hair loss, and a multitude of other reactions. Because retinoids can increase plasma triglycerides, blood levels should be checked initially and 4 to 6 weeks into therapy. Further monitoring is needed only if levels are above normal. Liver function studies should be obtained before therapy. If normal, further monitoring is generally not required.

Accutane is taken for 20 weeks, after which most patients are clear of acne, and many remain so for an indefinite period. Those who relapse do so slowly over the course of many months to years. Relapses are usually milder than the initial condition and can usually be managed with standard therapy. Accutane is quite expensive.

Hormone Therapy

Women with acne who wish to take oral contraceptives may benefit from one in which the progestin component has low androgenic potential, since androgens stimulate sebum production and tend to aggravate acne. Two new progestins with low androgenicity, desogestrel (Desogen, Ortho-Cept) and norgestinate (Ortho-Cyclen, Ortho Tri-Cyclen), are now available. Women with acne who also have hirsutism and irregular menses may need to be evaluated for androgen excess.

TREATMENT OF ROSACEA

Rosacea is an acneiform condition that most commonly affects middle-aged patients. It is characterized by papules and pustules often occurring on a background of erythema and telangiectasia of facial skin. The process tends to affect mainly the middle third of the face, from forehead to chin. Comedones are not typically present. Seborrheic dermatitis is frequently present in patients with rosacea. Some patients with rosacea develop the thickened skin and enlarged sebaceous glands of rhinophyma.

Topical Therapy

Topical metronidazole (MetroGel) applied twice daily is the most effective topical therapy for rosacea. It is applied for several months and then tapered. Preparations containing sulfur such as Novacet may be beneficial but can cause irritation. Topical erythromycin or topical clindamycin (Cleocin) is sometimes helpful. The seborrheic dermatitis that frequently accompanies rosacea generally responds to 1% hydrocortisone cream. Recurrences of rosacea are common, and retreatment can be instituted safely.

Systemic Therapy

As in acne vulgaris, systemic antibiotics are effective in treating rosacea. Lower dosages can often be employed—for example, tetracycline or erythromycin in a dose of 250 mg twice daily. After the first month, the dosage can often be lowered and the drug ultimately discontinued. Recurrences are common, and repeated courses of antibiotics may be needed. Antibiotics are also helpful in treating the blepharitis and keratitis that are occasionally associated with rosacea.

Rosacea that fails to respond to the above measures may be treated with low-dose (0.5 mg per kg) Accutane for a 20-week course. Results are usually good, but recurrences are common.

Surgical Therapy

Medical treatment has a limited effect on erythema and no impact on telangiectasia. If desired, telangiectasia can be treated with electrosurgery or laser therapy. Rhinophyma may be shaved with an electric loop followed later by dermabrasion if needed, or excess tissue may be removed by laser.

DISEASES OF THE HAIR
method of
JERRY SHAPIRO, M.D.
University of British Columbia
Vancouver, Canada

Diseases of the hair most commonly involve hair loss (alopecia), and this discussion is restricted to that topic.

ALOPECIA

There are a number of potential etiologic factors in alopecia. Endocrine abnormalities, genetic factors, systemic illness, drugs, psychological abnormalities, diet, trauma, infections, and structural hair defects may all cause hair loss. Evaluation of the patient must be thorough and include history, physical examination, and appropriate laboratory work-up.

History is of utmost importance in focusing on the correct diagnosis (Table 1). The duration of hair loss, family history, location of hair loss (diffuse vs. patterned), drug intake history, hair care habits (bleaching, back brushing, permanent waving), and other aspects of physical development such as coincidental acne and abnormal menstrual cycles are all important clues in determining the correct diagnosis. It is important to determine whether the hair falls out from the roots or breaks off along the shaft. This will establish the appropriate differential diagnosis (Table 2).

Clinical examination of all hair-bearing areas should be performed. Checking for inflammation, infection, and scarring (loss of the hair follicle) is of utmost importance. The differential diagnosis of hair loss is based on whether the hair loss is scarred or not (Table 3).

Regarding laboratory testing, nonscarring alopecia may require a complete blood count, thyroid-stimulating hormone, serum iron and ferritin, antinuclear antibodies, and Venereal Disease Research Laboratories. In women with androgenetic alopecia and other virilizing signs, an androgen work-up for free testosterone, androstenedione, and dehydroepiandrosterone (DHEAS) is advised. Scarring alopecias are difficult to differentiate from one another clinically and almost always require a 4-mm scalp biopsy for determination of the correct diagnosis.

TABLE 1. **Hair Loss History Questionnaire**

Is the hair coming out by the roots, or is it breaking?
Increased shedding or increased thinning?
Age of onset
Drugs
Menses, pregnancy, menopause
Past health
Family history
Hair care, hair cosmetics
Diet

TABLE 2. **Differential Diagnosis**

Hair Coming Out by Roots	Hair Breaking
Telogen effluvium	Tinea capitis
Androgenetic alopecia	Structural hair shaft abnormalities
Alopecia areata	
Drugs	Breakage due to improper use of hair care cosmetics
	Anagen arrest

TABLE 3. **Causes of Alopecia**

Nonscarring	Scarring
Androgenetic alopecia	Discoid lupus erythematosus
Telogen effluvium	Lichen planus
Alopecia areata	Pseudopelade
Tinea capitis	Severe fungal, viral, or bacterial infection
Hair breakage	

Androgenetic Alopecia

Most cases of hair loss are due to androgenetic alopecia (AGA). Fifty percent of men by age 50 years and 40% of women by menopause have some degree of AGA. Hair loss is gradual, with miniaturization of genetically programmed hair follicles. Uptake, metabolism, and conversion of testosterone to dihydrotestosterone by 5-alpha-reductase is increased in balding hair follicles. AGA presents differently in men as compared with women. In men with AGA, depending on severity, hair loss occurs in the frontotemporal regions and on the vertex of the scalp. In female AGA patients, it is more diffuse and located centroparietally. The frontal hairline is usually intact in women.

Treatment is either medical or surgical. The only proven medication with an indication for AGA is topical minoxidil (Rogaine). Its success for cosmetically acceptable regrowth is approximately 10% in men. In women, 50% show minimal regrowth and 13% moderate regrowth. Treatment is lifelong. Seven percent of patients may experience some irritation (burning, itching, redness) from the minoxidil solution. The 5% minoxidil solution has greater efficacy than the 2% minoxidil solution (Rogaine). The higher concentration will probably be available in the United States shortly. In women, the use of a systemic antiandrogen such as spironolactone (Aldactone)* 50 to 200 mg per day, cyproterone acetate (Androcur), or flutamide (Eulexin)* may have some benefit in reducing the amount of hair thinning. Regarding future possibilities for the treatment of AGA, an oral 5-alpha-reductase inhibitor has shown some promise in men.

Hair transplantation of permanent hairs from the back and sides of the scalp to balding areas in the front is a successful procedure but usually requires three to four sessions over 2 years to fill in an area with adequate density. The advent of mini- and micrografting has revolutionized hair transplantation into a more natural-looking process, eliminating clumping or tufting. Donor harvesting with strips rather than plugs has made the donor site more cosmetically acceptable. Hair transplantation is useful not only in men but also in women.

Telogen Effluvium

Excessive shedding of normal club hairs can be brought about by a number of stresses: parturition,

*Not FDA-approved for this indication.

febrile illness, psychological stress, crash diets, drugs (Table 4). These factors may cause termination of the growing phase (anagen) of the hair follicles and transformation into the resting phase (telogen), causing a telogen fallout 2 to 4 months later. The normal average scalp has 100,000 hairs. Approximately 90% are in anagen, 10% in telogen. Normal average daily hair fallout is 100 hairs. With telogen effluvium, the anagen/telogen ratio may be shifted to 70% anagen, 30% telogen, with average daily shedding of 300 hairs. Treatment is finding out the cause and correcting it.

Alopecia Areata

Alopecia areata (AA) is considered an autoimmune disease that affects 1% of the population. It usually presents with an oval patch or multiple confluent patches of asymptomatic nonscarring alopecia. Twenty percent of cases may proceed to alopecia totalis, affecting the entire scalp. One percent may go on to alopecia universalis, affecting all body hairs, including eyebrows and eyelashes. The disease frequently resolves spontaneously within 1 year. Recurrences, however, are common. Severe disease has less of a tendency to resolve on its own, especially in children or atopic individuals. Frequently, fingernails may show dystrophic changes such as pitting, ridging, and thinning of the nail plate. Treatment depends on the extent of disease and the age of the patient. For small patchy disease, intralesional corticosteroid is the treatment of choice. Triamcinolone acetonide (Kenalog) suspension 5 mg per mL is injected with a 30-gauge needle directly into the patches with tiny injections of 0.1 mL each spread over affected areas. The total amount should not exceed 10 mg of triamcinolone acetonide per visit. Injections are repeated every 4 to 6 weeks. Other options include topical minoxidil, anthralin, and steroid. For more extensive disease, the use of a contact allergen (diphencyprone) is the treatment of choice,

TABLE 4. **Causes of Telogen Effluvium**

High fever
Childbirth
Severe infection
Severe chronic illness
Severe psychological stress
Major surgery
Hypo- or hyperthyroidism
Crash diets; inadequate protein
Drugs

with some studies showing 40% success rates. Diphencyprone is difficult to obtain in the United States but is more readily available in Europe and Canada. Other treatment options include psoralens and ultraviolet A radiation (PUVA) and the use of systemic steroids. The use of systemic steroids is controversial, since steroids have a high side effect profile and patients may have to be on the drug for a long time. Usually when the systemic steroid is discontinued, hair shedding occurs. I rarely use systemic steroids.

Patients with AA require encouragement and emotional support. Many cities now have support groups, which are invaluable to a large number of patients. The National Alopecia Areata Foundation, 710 C Street #11, San Rafael, California 94901–3853, is an excellent resource for patients.

Trichotillomania

A compulsion to repetitively pull or pluck one's hair is trichotillomania. It gives rise to an unnatural pattern of hair loss. Clinical diagnosis can sometimes be quite difficult and may require a scalp biopsy for diagnostic confirmation. Examination of the distal hair shaft for bizarre twisting and fracture will increase the physician's index of suspicion. Fewer than 5% of such patients have deep-seated psychological disorders. Most cases resolve spontaneously. In severe cases, clomipramine may be prescribed.

Tinea Capitis

Cases of tinea capitis may be inflammatory or noninflammatory. The etiologic organisms depend on geographic area. In North America, they are *Trichophyton tonsurans* and *Microsporum canis*. Diagnosis is made clinically as well as by potassium hydroxide scraping, mycologic culture, and Wood's light examination. Hair infected by *M. canis* fluoresces under Wood's light; hair infected by *T. tonsurans* does not. Treatment is systemic with griseofulvin (Fulvicin) or ketoconazole (Nizoral) for 6 to 8 weeks. Itraconazole (Sporanox)* and an allylamine such as terbinafine (Lamisil)* may also be used in the treatment of tinea capitis.

Hair Shaft Abnormalities

If a patient complains of hair breakage rather than the hair falling out at the roots, one may be dealing with a shaft problem. Microscopic examination of the actual shafts (hair mount) may be necessary to make the diagnosis. The most common cause of a hair shaft abnormality or hair fragility is trichorrhexis nodosa, with nodelike swellings through which the shaft readily fractures. This usually appears as a result of trauma.

Scarring Alopecia

Localized areas of scarring alopecia of the scalp may result from bacterial, viral, and fungal infec-

---

*Not FDA-approved for this indication.

tions. More importantly, lesions of discoid lupus erythematosus, lichen planus, and pseudopelade present with this scarring picture. An accurate diagnosis is necessary to determine the treatment, and biopsy is usually necessary to determine the cause. Evidence of cutaneous disease elsewhere on the skin, oral or genital mucous membranes, and nails should be looked for carefully. Treatment of discoid lupus erythematosus of the scalp includes intralesional corticosteroid and, if severe, antimalarials or retinoids.

CANCER OF THE SKIN

method of
SCOTT W. FOSKO, M.D.
*Saint Louis University Health Sciences Center
St. Louis, Missouri*

The incidence of nonmelanoma skin cancer (NMSC), primarily basal cell carcinoma (BCC) and squamous cell carcinoma (SCC), continues to increase, especially in elderly people. The lifetime risk of an individual born in 1994 of developing a BCC is estimated to be 28 to 33% and for SCC 7 to 11%. It is projected that 900,000 to more than 1.2 million individuals in the United States will develop an NMSC in 1994. Fortunately, NMSCs are quite curable, if caught at an early stage.

ETIOLOGY

NMSC is most commonly seen in individuals of light pigmentation, especially those with a fair complexion, blond hair, blue eyes, a tendency to sunburn and freckle easily, and an inability to tan. Having had an NMSC also predisposes one to develop additional skin cancers. It has been well demonstrated that ultraviolet radiation is associated with SCC, as well as with BCC, but less so. Genetic defects of altered DNA repair from solar radiation damage also predispose one to cutaneous carcinomas (e.g., xeroderma pigmentosum and nevoid basal cell nevus syndrome patients). Alteration in the tumor suppressor gene *p53* has demonstrated conflicting results in its role in NMSC development. As with cervical neoplasia, various serotypes of human papillomavirus (5, 16, 18) have been associated with certain SCCs. In addition, immune surveillance deficits as seen with individuals on immune suppressive therapy, as with organ transplant patients, show an increased incidence of SCC greater than that of BCC.

DIAGNOSIS

Basal Cell Carcinoma

BCC accounts for 80% of cutaneous carcinomas and most commonly occurs on sun-exposed parts of the body, but may occur anywhere. On the face, the nose is the most commonly involved site, followed by the cheek and forehead. This tumor originates from the basal cell layer of the epidermis. There are several subtypes, with the noduloulcerative type most common. The classic clinical presentation is that of a pearly, translucent papule with telangiectasias within it. At times the border of the lesion can be raised and rolled. Ulceration may occur. A bleeding, nonhealing "sore" is often the patient's presenting complaint. The other subtypes can be more subtle in their clinical features, with slight scaling and brown pigmentation. The morpheaform BCC is the most difficult subtype to diagnose; it may present as a subtle change in the texture of the skin with a white, scarlike appearance and slight firmness with palpation. When an individual presents with "an enlarging scar," this may indeed be a morpheaform BCC. Morpheaform BCCs can be quite extensive, despite their subtle clinical features, and often are the most challenging to manage and treat successfully.

BCC rarely metastasizes (less than 1% of all BCCs) but does so usually in the setting of a tumor of long-standing duration and prior treatments, especially radiation therapy. Lymph node and lung involvement are the most common distal sites.

Basal Cell Carcinoma in Young Adults

It has been shown in several studies that young individuals (median age of 28.3 years) may present with BCCs of a more aggressive clinical subtype. Some studies have shown women to be more predisposed to this than men. The central face region (nose) is a frequent site for this aggressive subtype in women, with the forehead and temples the sites seen in men. Tanning salon use is being shown to be associated with BCC development in young individuals.

Squamous Cell Carcinoma

SCC is even more commonly seen in a sun-exposed distribution, with the head and neck region, followed by the backs of the hands, the most frequent sites of involvement. Mucous membranes can be involved. SCC most characteristically presents as a raised, scaly, red to flesh-colored papule, patch, or plaque that may evolve into a nodule or tumor. The in situ, or frequently referred to as "Bowen's subtype" of SCC, may present as a flat, reddish-brown, slightly scaly patch or thin plaque. The epidermal keratinocyte is the cell of origin for SCC. Approximately 4% of SCCs will have metastasized at the time of presentation, with regional lymph nodes the most common site of initial spread. SCCs of the lower lip, ear, or dorsum of the hands or those originating in scars, leg ulcers, or chronic osteomyelitis sinus tracts have a greater propensity to metastasize. Lesion size and certain histopathologic features are also correlated with metastatic potential. A thorough lymph node examination and selective use of computed tomography should be part of the evaluation.

TREATMENT

Treatment of NMSC falls into two categories. The first is *field therapy*. This modality treats the obvious clinically involved tissue, as well as an area of clinically noninvolved tissue. With this modality, tissue is usually not sent for histopathologic margin assessment. Such treatment modalities include curettage and electrodesiccation, cryosurgery, radiation treatment, and intralesional interferon. The second category of treatment is *margin-controlled excision* with either conventional excision or Mohs' cutaneous micrographic technique. In the appropriate clinical setting, each treatment modality can be very successful, with nearly 90 to 95% 5-year cure rates approached. The type and subtype of neoplasm, location of the

neoplasm, and known histologic features should guide selection of therapy. A representative biopsy is imperative in directing proper therapy. Neoplasms that are large (greater than 2 cm), in the *central facial region* involving the nose, lips, eyelids and ears, occur in individuals who are *immune suppressed*, and those individuals with *recurrent* neoplasms are at high risk for recurrence with conventional modalities, especially field therapy. This high-risk subgroup of patients should be treated with Mohs' cutaneous micrographic surgical technique.

Field Therapy

Cryosurgery

Cryosurgery uses liquid nitrogen, which freezes the skin and subcutaneous tissue to $-196°$ C. An appropriate margin of uninvolved tissue must be treated. As the depth of freezing cannot be visualized, a thermocouple assists in accurately recording the depth of freezing. This treatment modality results in a chronically oozing wound that may take 4 to 8 weeks to heal completely. Cosmetic results can be acceptable, with a hypopigmented scar the most common outcome. Success rates as high as 96% have been reported in the literature. This modality is best used for well-defined BCCs and SCCs, and not for recurrent or infiltrative tumors.

Curettage and Electrodesiccation

This is a biphasic treatment modality. First, a sharp curette is used to remove the tumor. Then electrosurgery is performed with electrodesiccation of the curetted base. The charred base is then curetted and electrodesiccated for a total of three cycles. The wound heals by second intention over 4 to 6 weeks and results in a hypopigmented scar. This modality demonstrates high cure rates of 90%. It also is best used for well-defined, nodular, and superficial BCCs smaller than 1 cm. Tumors of the central face have a much higher failure rate with this technique, with one study showing residual tumor in 40% of tumors treated by curettage and electrodesiccation for three cycles.

Radiation Therapy

Radiation has proved helpful in treating BCCs and SCCs that are unresectable or in patients who are poor surgical candidates. High 5-year cure rates (approximately 90%) have been demonstrated. Previously, orthovoltage had been the primary radiation source, but more recently, electron beam has become the treatment of choice for cutaneous neoplasms. Electron beams are more selective to the cutaneous layers, and less morbidity is possible to deeper and surrounding tissue, which may result in less long-term side effects. Treatment regimens vary, but usually involve several fractionated daily treatments over 2 to 6 weeks. Cosmetic results can be quite acceptable; however, as seen with orthovoltage-treated patients, delayed chronic radiation damage may create undesirable outcomes cosmetically.

Intralesional Interferon-Alfa

This recently developed immunotherapy has proved effective for small, especially superficial, NMSCs. It requires two to three times weekly injections for several weeks. Flulike side effects are usually well tolerated by the patient. Again, high-risk neoplasms, especially of the central face, appear to be less responsive to this treatment.

Margin-Controlled Excision

Excisional Surgery

This is the most common method of managing NMSC. The tumor is visually defined and a "normal" margin of tissue is chosen, ranging from 4 to 6 mm, based on tumor characteristics. Histopathology (with or without frozen-section review) of the excised tissue determines tissue margin status. Routine histopathology reviews less than 1% of the actual tissue margin and is the major pitfall of this technique, especially for infiltrative, poorly differentiated, or recurrent tumors. Five-year cure rates range from 80 to 90%. Higher failure rates occur with "high-risk" tumors.

Mohs' Micrographic Surgery

Mohs' surgery was developed by Dr. Frederic E. Mohs in the early 1930s. This technique involves fresh tissue surgical excision and immediate processing of the tissue in such a way that virtually 100% of the surgical margin is evaluated before the surgical wound is repaired. Mohs' surgery allows precise subclinical tumor extension to be mapped out and surgically removed, while uninvolved nearby tissue is conserved. The technique is quite helpful in areas where excessive tissue is not available for wide margin excision, such as the eyelids, nose, lips, and ears. BCCs and SCCs are the most commonly treated NMSCs, but other rare cutaneous tumors also benefit from this approach. Mohs' surgery has evolved into the treatment of choice for both recurrent BCCs and those clinically and histologically (morpheaform) high-risk tumors as well as aggressive SCCs. This surgical technique provides 5-year cure rates of 99% for primary BCC, 95% for recurrent BCC (as opposed to 50% 5-year cure rates for other conventional modalities), and 90 to 95% for SCC. This technique is usually performed on an outpatient basis under local anesthetic.

Investigational Treatments

Photodynamic Therapy

This is an evolving treatment modality for multiple cutaneous neoplasms, as well as selected metastatic cancers to the skin. It involves the administration of a systemic photosensitizing agent, which is absorbed by the tumor, followed by tumor exposure to a selective wavelength of light, usually provided by a laser. This modality is currently being evaluated and fur-ther developed. It has shown to be quite effective for superficial tumors, but fails when tumors are deeply invasive and of the central facial region. The newest area of investigation uses a topically applied photosensitizer to minimize the risk of systemic photosensitivity.

5-Fluorouracil

Topical 5-fluorouracil (5-FU) (Efudex, Fluoroplex) is shown to treat actinic keratosis, a pre-SCC lesion. Intralesional injections of SCC and BCC are being investigated. As with intralesional interferon, this may prove effective for selected NMSCs.

PROGNOSIS

Overall, the prognosis for the treatment of BCCs and SCCs is excellent. It is possible to achieve a nearly 100% cure rate if an appropriate treatment is selected early, based on the tumor type, location, clinical, and histologic features. In areas of high risk, it is strongly recommended that a treatment modality with margin control be employed. For recurrent NMSC, Mohs' surgery should be done.

PREVENTION

Studies have shown that the use of synthetic oral retinoids (isotretinoin [Accutane]* and etretinate [Tegison]*) can prevent the development of new NMSCs, but this effect is lost once the medication is discontinued. This can be helpful in immune suppressed individuals or those with genetic defects. Retinoids are not without significant side effects and must be used with caution.

More importantly, it is imperative that patient education be provided at the time of diagnosis of cutaneous neoplasms. It has been estimated that 80% of an individual's ultraviolet exposure occurs by 18 years of age. Therefore, the educational effort should be directed not only at the patient but also at any of the patient's family members, and especially their children. Day care centers should also be educated. Sun habits should be reviewed and it should be cautioned that excessive sun exposure be avoided. Peak sun exposure time is between 10 A.M. and 3 P.M. The use of a sunscreen with a sun-protection factor of at least 15 should be used on a regular basis to minimize ultraviolet damage. The use of sun-protective hats and clothing may be more convenient and more easily accepted by patients. Self-examination and regular physician visits should also be emphasized.

*Not FDA-approved for this indication.

MYCOSIS FUNGOIDES

method of
RICHARD T. HOPPE, M.D.
Stanford University Medical Center
Stanford, California

Mycosis fungoides (MF) is a cutaneous lymphoma and neoplasm of helper T cell origin. It has a variable but often long clinical course. MF is an uncommon malignancy, accounting for only 2 to 3% of cases of non-Hodgkin's lymphoma; only about 500 to 600 new cases and 100 to 200 deaths are reported each year in the United States. It is most common in older males. The median age of onset is about 60 years, and the male/female ratio is 2 : 1. The etiology of MF is unclear. Chemical exposure, chronic antigen stimulation, and viral causes have been proposed, but careful epidemiologic studies have failed to confirm these associations. In some instances, components of the human T cell lymphotropic virus Type I (HTLV-I) genome have been isolated from the DNA of peripheral blood cells of patients with MF, but there is no solid epidemiologic support for HTLV-I as an etiologic agent.

DIAGNOSIS

The diagnosis of MF is often difficult, especially when it presents in the earliest phase of skin involvement. Symptoms may be present for as long as 10 years before a firm diagnosis can be established. The typical light microscopic features of MF include a polymorphous upper dermal infiltrate that is intimate with the epidermis and has atypical mononuclear cells. These atypical mononuclear cells have hyperconvoluted ("cerebriform") nuclei, and monoclonal antibody staining reveals that they have the phenotypic characteristics of helper T cells (CD4+). These cells must be present in the epidermis as either scattered individual cells or small clusters (Pautrier's microabscesses) in order to establish a definitive diagnosis. Sequential biopsies are indicated when the diagnosis of MF is suspected clinically but biopsy results are only suggestive.

CLINICAL APPEARANCE

The characteristics of the cutaneous lesions of MF are variable. Some patients present with poikilodermatous patches characterized by variable atrophy and telangiectasia. Other patients display well-demarcated erythematous scaling patches or infiltrated plaques. Lesions may regress partially or completely, even without treatment. The disease often appears initially in the bathing trunk distribution, including the lower abdomen, upper thighs, and buttocks, but the pattern of disease may vary markedly among individuals. The lesions are usually pruritic, and itching is often the main presenting complaint. Some patients present with or develop exophytic or ulcerating tumors, which may become secondarily infected.

Occasionally, patients present with generalized erythroderma, often accompanied by marked skin atrophy. There may be profound hyperkeratosis of the palms and soles. Some patients may be found to have abnormal cells circulating in the peripheral blood, identical to those found in the dermal and epidermal infiltrates. Palpable lymphadenopathy and splenomegaly may be present as well, and this constellation of findings is referred to as the "Sézary syndrome." These patients usually have severe generalized pruritus and exfoliation.

STAGING

In staging MF, the most important considerations are the extent of skin involvement, lymphadenopathy, and the presence of visceral disease. Table 1 summarizes the TNMB (tumor, node, metastases, blood) staging system for MF. Skin involvement characterized as limited plaque (T1) implies patches or plaques involving less than 10% of the total skin surface. Generalized plaque disease (T2) involves more than 10% of the skin surface. Tumorous involvement (T3) implies frank cutaneous tumors, and erythroderma (T4) indicates total skin erythema.

Staging studies completed in these patients include a thorough history and physical examination, with careful mapping of cutaneous lesions. Examination of the skin should also include careful evaluation of the scalp, palms, soles, fingernails, and toenails. Lateral and posteroanterior chest radiographs, a complete blood cell count (including Sézary cell preparation), and serum chemistry studies are indicated both to rule out extracutaneous involvement by MF and to evaluate for the presence of other pathology. Patients with palpable lymphadenopathy undergo a lymph node biopsy. If this shows involvement by MF, other staging studies should follow to determine the extent of extracutaneous disease. Most commonly, computed tomography (CT) scanning of the abdomen and pelvis is performed at this point. If any of these studies suggest visceral involvement, biopsy documentation is warranted, since other cancers are common in patients of this age group and may account for abnormal findings. The most common site of identifiable extracutaneous MF is the lymph nodes, and the most common visceral sites are the lungs and liver.

TREATMENT
Cutaneous Therapy

The curative potential of treatment of MF is controversial. However, most patients are symptomatic

TABLE 1. **TNMB Staging System for Mycosis Fungoides**

Stage	Description
T1	Limited plaque; patches or plaques covering less than 10% of the total skin surface
T2	Generalized plaque; patches or plaques covering 10% or more of the total skin surface
T3	Tumorous; one or more cutaneous tumors
T4	Erythroderma; total skin erythema, with or without cutaneous tumors
N0	No palpable lymph nodes
N1	Palpable lymph nodes; if a biopsy is done, light microscopic appearance of specimen may be consistent with reactive changes or dermatopathic lymphadenitis but not with actual involvement by mycosis fungoides (MF)
N2	Palpable lymph nodes that have been biopsied; specimen reveals MF microscopically
M0	No evidence of visceral involvement
M1	Visceral involvement present; should be documented by biopsy
B0	No evidence of peripheral blood involvement
B1	≥5% atypical cells in peripheral blood

N Stage	T Stage*			
	T1	*T2*	*T3*	*T4*
N0	IA	IB	IIB	IIA
N1	IIA	IIA	IIB	IIIB
N2	IVA	IVA	IVA	IVA

*Any T, N with an M = 1 is Stage IVB.

owing to pruritus or are handicapped by the cosmetic effects of the disease, and treatment with palliative intent is almost always indicated. At the time of initial diagnosis, it is reasonable to employ aggressive topical therapy in order to clear the skin. Some patients achieve complete skin clearance, maintain that response for variable periods of time, and occasionally remain disease free. More important, data indicate that when disease on the skin can be kept at a minimal level, the likelihood that extracutaneous disease will develop is exceedingly small. The treatments utilized for newly diagnosed patients include topical chemotherapy with nitrogen mustard, photochemotherapy with psoralens and ultraviolet A (PUVA) radiation, and total skin electron beam therapy.

Topical nitrogen mustard* may be utilized either in an aqueous solution or in an ointment base in a concentration of 10 to 20 mg per dL. Patients initiate treatment to the entire cutaneous surface, sparing only the eyelids. Intertriginous areas are treated sparingly. If the disease is only regional, the total skin application is reduced to generous regional coverage after 1 to 2 months of treatment. Cutaneous lesions may be slow to respond to this therapy, and complete response, if it occurs, may require more than 6 months of daily treatment. Maintenance therapy is continued for a variable period following complete skin clearance, usually 6 to 12 months. The disease may recur when treatment is discontinued. The main potential complication of this therapy is a hypersensitivity reaction, which may be managed by reducing the concentration of the preparation.

Therapy with PUVA consists of oral methoxsalen (Oxsoralen) followed by exposure to long-wavelength ultraviolet A (UVA) light. The psoralens intercalate with DNA and, on exposure to UVA, form cross-links that inhibit DNA replication. Generally, three treatments per week are given until moderate clearing has been achieved. Thereafter, maintenance programs are initiated at a frequency of two treatments per week, gradually tapering to as infrequently as once every 4 to 6 weeks. Generally, if treatment is discontinued completely, the disease recurs. The main potential hazard of PUVA therapy is the increased risk of developing squamoproliferative lesions after long-term use.

Total skin electron beam therapy provides the greatest likelihood of skin clearance. Electrons are a form of ionizing irradiation that penetrates to a specific depth, depending on their energy. Electrons of appropriate energy penetrate the skin for only several millimeters, and special techniques of treatment permit irradiation of the entire skin. Treatments are administered 4 days a week for about 9 weeks (total dose 30 to 36 Gy). About 80% of patients achieve complete skin clearance with this treatment; however, in 50 to 75% of patients, the disease recurs. Often, only minimal disease is present at this time, and it can be treated effectively with topical nitrogen

mustard, PUVA, or spot radiation therapy. The side effects of total skin electron beam therapy are more marked than those that occur with topical nitrogen mustard or PUVA. Temporary loss of hair and sweat gland function and long-term skin dryness are common.

Recommendations for Cutaneous Treatment. In patients who present with the limited plaque phase of skin involvement, treatment with topical nitrogen mustard* is a reasonable first-line therapy. Although the time to skin clearance may be prolonged, as many as 50% of patients will achieve a complete response. Even in those who do not achieve a complete response, there is usually a significant improvement in disease and resolution of most symptoms. If the disease fails to respond to topical nitrogen mustard or progresses during therapy, initiation of PUVA or total skin electron beam therapy is appropriate. Patients who present with generalized plaque disease with only a minimally infiltrative component and who have a long history of disease without recent progression may be treated in a similar fashion. However, if there are very infiltrated plaques or recent progression of disease, total skin electron beam therapy is the preferable treatment option. The majority of patients treated in this fashion achieve a complete response. However, since subsequent relapse is common, it is reasonable to institute a program of maintenance treatment with topical nitrogen mustard immediately following the completion of electron beam therapy.

Patients who present with tumorous involvement are treated initially with total skin electron beam therapy. In addition, supplemental small-field irradiation with low-energy x-rays to individual tumor lesions is indicated. After completion of irradiation, topical nitrogen mustard is used as a maintenance therapy.

Patients who present with erythroderma are difficult to manage inasmuch as their skin is often atrophic and very sensitive to any type of therapy. Low-exposure PUVA therapy can be successful in achieving gradual skin clearance. If either topical nitrogen mustard or electron beam therapy is utilized, the concentration or daily dose of these agents must be reduced. Some patients may benefit from interferon-alpha or extracorporeal photopheresis.

Palliative Management of Skin Lesions. Frequently, despite the use of total skin therapies, individual lesions develop that are refractory and symptomatic. Local topical measures that may be helpful in this setting include topical corticosteroids, small-field irradiation with either low-energy x-rays or electrons, or more intensive localized treatment with higher concentrations of nitrogen mustard (e.g., 50 mg per dL).

Management of Extracutaneous Disease

The median survival of patients who develop extracutaneous disease is only 1 to 2 years. Patients with

*Not FDA-approved for this indication.

*Not FDA-approved for this indication.

TABLE 2. **Five- and Ten-Year Survival After Treatment for Mycosis Fungoides**

Stage (No. of Patients)	5-Year Survival (%)	10-Year Survival (%)
Limited plaque (101)	95	87
Generalized plaque (175)	74	57
Tumorous (97)	41	25
Erythroderma (77)	45	29
Extracutaneous disease (51)	18	5

disease that is apparently limited to lymph nodes, as well as those with other extracutaneous disease sites, have a similarly poor prognosis. Systemic therapies, although occasionally achieving good partial responses, seldom achieve complete responses, and remissions are generally brief. When extracutaneous sites are clinically localized (e.g., localized adenopathy), local field megavoltage irradiation can achieve a good palliative and symptomatic response. Generalized systemic disease is usually treated with combination chemotherapy using agents such as cyclophosphamide (Cytoxan), doxorubicin (Adriamycin), vincristine (Oncovin), and prednisone (the CHOP protocol). Some patients benefit from treatment with interferon-alpha. Investigational therapies, including anti–T cell monoclonal antibodies, toxin-linked antibodies, and high-dose therapy with peripheral stem cell rescue, are all reasonable treatment approaches in this group of patients.

An uncommon form of systemic disease is the Sézary syndrome. Sézary syndrome is incurable, but treatment is required for relief of symptoms (e.g., pruritus). Daily treatment with chlorambucil (Leukeran) and prednisone, with monitoring of the white blood cell count, is often successful in achieving palliative responses. PUVA may be added to help control the cutaneous manifestations of disease. When the disease becomes resistant to this approach, more intensive chemotherapy programs or investigational treatment programs may be initiated, but the response is unpredictable. Patients who have erythroderma in the absence of peripheral blood involvement may be candidates for treatment with extracorporeal photopheresis.

PROGNOSIS

Prognosis is related to the extent of skin involvement, the presence of extracutaneous disease, the type of therapy administered, and other factors such as age and intercurrent disease. The median survival of large groups of patients is greater than 10 years but is dependent on the initial extent of disease and the treatment programs utilized. Table 2 summarizes our results of treatment at Stanford employing the principles of treatment outlined above.

PAPULOSQUAMOUS DISEASES
method of
MICHAEL ZANOLLI, M.D., and
MICHEL McDONALD, M.D.
Vanderbilt University Medical Center
Nashville, Tennessee

The papulosquamous diseases are a varied group of disorders that share a clinical presentation of raised lesions described as papules or plaques with overlying scale.

PSORIASIS

Psoriasis is an inflammatory disease of the skin that affects approximately 1.5% of the population. The mean age of onset is between 20 and 30 years and the course is chronic, with intermittent exacerbations. In patients with psoriasis, involved areas of skin demonstrate excessive cellular proliferation of epidermal cells. The pathogenesis and etiology, however, have not been completely elucidated, despite the major advancements that have been made in the understanding of the disease process in the past 10 years.

Clinical Types of Psoriasis

There are distinct clinical variants of psoriasis vulgaris: plaque, guttate, erythrodermic, and pustular. Plaque-type psoriasis is the most common form. The clinical presentation of plaque-type psoriasis is characterized by variably sized well-demarcated erythematous plaques with an overlying thick, adherent silvery-white scale most frequently located on the extensor surfaces of the elbows and knees. The scalp, umbilicus, and intergluteal cleft are also frequent sites of involvement. Bilateral symmetrical involvement is a consistent feature of psoriasis.

Guttate psoriasis is characterized by smaller papules of 1 to 2 cm with an acute eruptive onset. The trunk is the predominant site of involvement. Psoriatic erthroderma presents as generalized intense erythema. Pustular psoriasis has three subsets—generalized, localized, and hand and foot—that share the presentation of sterile pustules ranging from 2 to 3 mm in diameter.

Areas of involvement other than the skin include the nails, which may demonstrate pits of the nail plate as well as onychodystrophy in 30 to 50% of patients with psoriasis. The joints may also be affected with an inflammatory process, and up to 15 to 20% of patients with psoriasis have joint complaints. Demonstrable psoriatic arthritis is less frequent but is a source of increased morbidity and presents most commonly with a peripheral asymmetrical oligoarthritis involving the hands and feet. Depending on genetically determined factors, the arthritis associated with psoriasis may also take the form of a spondyloarthritis or a rheumatoid factor–negative symmetrical polyarthritis.

Treatment of Psoriasis

The approach to the treatment of psoriasis encompasses the need not only to treat the physical characteristics of the disease but also to determine the psychological impact it has on the patient. Consequently, the provider of care must assess the extent to which this disease alters the daily activities of the patient and take this into account when counseling the patient about the disease process and available treatments. The other major consideration is the balance between the risks and the benefits of treatment. It must be remembered that the tendency to express the disease is an inherited trait, most likely from multiple genes, and the available treatments do not remove this tendency but merely treat the symptoms of the disease. The goal of the health care provider is to bring the psoriasis into remission or an inactive state, which may mean leaving residual lesions on selected areas of the body rather than proceeding to more aggressive treatment. Whenever factors that are known to provoke the activity of psoriasis are present, such as streptococcal infection, alcohol excess, certain drugs (e.g., lithium), or excessive stress, they should be addressed appropriately.

The treatments for psoriasis are divided into three main categories: topical, ultraviolet light, and systemic. These may be used as monotherapy or in combination, depending on the severity of the disease, the potential risks for side effects, and the overall health of the patient.

Topical Therapy

Topical corticosteroids are the most common form of therapy for psoriasis in the United States. The potency of the particular compound used is dependent on the location on the body and the severity of the psoriasis. In general, the thicker plaques present on the trunk or extremities require application of the superpotent class (Class I) of corticosteroids for a 2-week period, followed by the use of these drugs 2 days a week to help maintain the response achieved. An alternative is to use a less potent class of topical corticosteroids after the initial 2-week induction period.

Parts of the body that are more susceptible to the skin atrophy associated with the use of corticosteroids are the face, groin, axilla, and genital areas. In these locations, the use of superpotent topical corticosteroids should be avoided, and a less potent class of compound should be used.

Tar preparations are still of value in the treatment of psoriasis, especially when used for the treatment of mild scalp psoriasis in the form of shampoos and on limited plaque-type psoriasis of the skin. Patients are sometimes reluctant to accept tar treatments because of the smell and staining properties of these compounds. The use of crude coal tar in an emollient base is still an essential part of the Goeckerman therapy for resistant psoriasis when used in combination with ultraviolet B (UVB) light.

Anthralin compounds have never been used to the same degree in the United States as they are in Europe—especially the United Kingdom. This chemical is known to have beneficial effects on psoriasis, and it is especially useful for the treatment of well-marginated thick plaque psoriasis. Patients must be educated as to the proper use of the medication to avoid skin irritation and possible burning. The other major consideration with anthralin therapy is the staining properties of all anthralin preparations resulting from oxidation of the anthralin chemical.

The most recent advancement in the treatment of mild to moderate psoriasis has been the development of vitamin D_3 analogues for topical application which diminishes the problem of hypervitaminosis D_3. Calcipotriene (Dovonex) has been shown to be as effective as medium-to-potent topical steroids in the treatment of psoriasis. One of the additional benefits is that there does not appear to be any atrophigenic potential with its use. The main side effect, which occurs in approximately 10% of patients who use this treatment, is mild irritation of the skin at the site of its use. This is especially prominent on the face and body folds. The total amount of this product to be applied to the skin is limited to 100 grams per week in patients with normal renal function to avoid possible calcium metabolism alterations and hypercalcemia.

Phototherapy

UVB light is one of the primary treatments of moderate-to-severe psoriasis and is effective in clearing 70 to 80% of patients with plaque-type psoriasis. The use of erythemogenic doses of UVB has a more beneficial effect than less aggressive treatment regimens. The delivery of therapeutic UVB light is best done under the supervision of a trained dermatologist.

The use of photochemotherapy in the form of psoralens and ultraviolet A radiation (PUVA) treatments is one of the major advancements in the treatment of psoriasis in the past 25 years. This treatment modality is very effective in treating psoriasis, with 85 to 90% of patients having an excellent response. PUVA treatment also requires that the supervising physician be proficient in its delivery and familiar with the potential side effects. The oral dose of the oil emulsion form of methoxsalen is 0.4 to 0.6 mg per kg and must be given 1 to 1½ hours prior to the delivery of the UVA light. The dose of the UVA light is dependent on the skin type of the patient, which is measured by the patient's inherent response to ultraviolet light and his or her ability to tan.

The most significant side effects to be considered with the use of PUVA and UVB therapy are the potential for ocular damage and the long-term risks of developing cutaneous malignancies. There are many textbooks available on the subject of phototherapy for psoriasis and the application of these treatment modalities in other cutaneous diseases.

Systemic Medications

Systemic antibiotic therapy is used to treat recognized infections in patients with exacerbations of their psoriasis, but it is often overlooked as a treatment for the overall disease state. Infections are known to exacerbate the condition, and antibiotic use should be considered part of the management.

Methotrexate is one of the more effective agents utilized for severe, extensive, or debilitating psoriasis. This medication can be delivered orally or given parenterally through a subcutaneous or an intramuscular route. The use of methotrexate should be reserved for patients who are resistant to the less toxic and potentially less dangerous forms of therapy described previously, because even though it can be highly effective, the drug is not curative. If there is normal renal function in an otherwise healthy adult, the usual dose is 15 mg per week in a divided dose taken 1 day a week. The most frequent method of delivery is to give 2.5 to 5 mg every 12 hours for a total of three doses. Once there is an adequate response, which may take 4 to 6 weeks, the dose may be reduced to a maintenance dose of 7.5 to 10 mg per week. Laboratory monitoring for acute effects on the hematopoietic system and for signs of long-term effects on the liver, such as fibrosis or cirrhosis, is essential. Monitoring of the state of the liver is especially important, as psoriasis patients appear to have a greater incidence of hepatic abnormalities than rheumatoid arthritis patients. The single best test for the accurate evaluation of the state of the liver continues to be a liver biopsy to determine any histologic changes that may have taken place. It is recommended that patients without risk factors for methotrexate use have a liver biopsy after receiving 1.5 grams of the medication. Longitudinal laboratory determination, including a complete blood count with platelet count and liver enzymes, should be done every 4 to 8 weeks during therapy.

Systemic retinoid therapy is an important consideration when treating certain forms of psoriasis or when specific locations are involved. The retinoid most commonly used for the treatment of psoriasis is etretinate (Tegison). The efficacy of etretinate is most pronounced with pustular forms of psoriasis when it can be used as a monotherapy. Utilization of retinoids for severe, resistant plaque-type psoriasis can be combined with other treatment modalities such as PUVA or UVB. When retinoids are combined with either form of phototherapy, the total dose and number of treatments necessary to reach a complete response are reduced. The usual dose of etretinate when used alone or in combination therapy is between 0.5 and 1.0 mg per kg per day. Once the desired response is attained, the retinoid dose can be tapered over weeks and then discontinued, depending on the clinical setting.

The side effects of the systemic retinoids are myriad, with the primary consideration being the potent teratogenic properties of this class of compounds. It is imperative that precautions be taken to prevent pregnancy during therapy with retinoids. The long half-life for etretinate, 100 to 120 days, makes this an even more problematic drug for any woman with childbearing potential, and most clinicians seek other

alternatives. In reported cases, there were measurable blood levels of etretinate or metabolites in the serum up to 2 years after discontinuation of therapy due to storage in and slow release from the adipose tissue. Obviously, caution and patient education must be undertaken when using this drug, and the physician should be familiar and comfortable with all the precautions and long-term follow-up needed for its safe and effective use.

Among the other possible immune-suppressing agents that have been used to treat psoriasis, cyclosporine (Sandimmune)* has received the most attention. Only the most severe cases of psoriasis should even be considered for treatment with this agent because of the possible side effects associated with its use, such as nephrotoxicity. However, there are cases in which cyclosporine can be considered in the context of short-term use, with long-term maintenance being accomplished with a less hazardous form of therapy such as PUVA. The usual dose of cyclosporine for the treatment of psoriasis is 3 mg per kg per day, and this should be adjusted, depending on the response to therapy.

LICHEN PLANUS

Lichen planus is an inflammatory disease of unknown cause that affects less than 1% of the population. It is characterized by small, polygon-shaped, flat-topped, smooth papules that are erythematous to violaceous in color. The sites of predilection are the flexor surfaces of the forearms and wrists as well as the neck, thighs, and shins. These papules are characteristically intensely pruritic. The scalp may be involved, progressing to a scarring alopecia in some cases.

Lichen planus also involves the mucous membranes in about 66% of cases. Classically, it presents as a reticulated white patch with fine lines called "Wickham's striae." The buccal mucosa is the most frequently involved site, but it may occur in any area of the oral or genital mucosa.

Drug-induced lichen planus can be associated with a number of different medications, including angiotensin-converting enzyme inhibitors, antimalarials, thiazide diuretics, and the antibiotics streptomycin and tetracycline (Table 1). It is essential that any diagnosis of a lichen planus type of skin change be accompanied by a previous drug history and discon-

---

*Not FDA-approved for this indication.

TABLE 1. **Drugs Associated with Lichen Planus–Like Eruption**

Captopril (Capoten)	Tetracycline
Enalapril (Vasotec)	Streptomycin
Gold	Penicillamine
Phenothiazine derivatives	Thiazides
Quinacrine	Chlorpropamide (Diabinese)
Chloroquine (Aralen)	Tolazamide (Tolinase)
Quinidine	

tinuation of any drugs associated with the development of a lichen planus–type reaction.

Treatment of Lichen Planus

Therapy for lichen planus must take into consideration that approximately 66% of patients will undergo spontaneous remission within 1 year.

The initial therapeutic modality most frequently used for lichen planus is topical corticosteroids. Class I or II topical corticosteroids are required to cause regression of plaques. Intralesional corticosteroids such as triamcinolone at a strength of 5 to 10 mg per mL are effective treatment for lesions on the trunk or extremities. For extensive or generalized disease, a 2- to 4-week course of oral prednisone beginning at 40 mg per day followed by a tapering of the dose can be instituted to control the eruption. Intramuscular corticosteroids may also be of use in the active stage of the disease.

Antihistamines such as hydroxyzine may be helpful in ameliorating the intense pruritus that many patients experience. PUVA has also been reported to be efficacious in the treatment of generalized symptomatic lichen planus. Involvement of the oral or genital mucosa can be treated with topical corticosteroids, but mid- or low-potency agents should be used in these regions.

PITYRIASIS ROSEA

Pityriasis rosea has a characteristic clinical presentation and a suspected infectious cause, although no specific infectious agent has yet been identified. Classically, patients have a prodrome of nausea, anorexia, fever, and arthralgias. Within 2 days to 3 weeks, an initial plaque—called the "herald patch"—may appear in 50% of patients. The herald patch is characterized as the largest of the skin lesions with a salmon color and oval shape and a peripheral collarette of scale. It may occur anywhere on the skin but is most frequently found on the trunk. This is followed by smaller salmon-colored oval plaques with collarettes of scale, most commonly on the abdomen and trunk in a "fir-tree" distribution. These are mildly pruritic in up to 75% of patients. The total duration of the eruption ranges from 4 to 16 weeks.

Treatment of Pityriasis Rosea

As pityriasis rosea is self-limited, often no therapy is necessary. Emollients in addition to midpotency topical corticosteroids may be helpful in ameliorating any mild symptoms. If the patient is experiencing significant pruritus or extensive involvement, 5 to 10 erythemogenic doses of UVB therapy can improve the symptoms considerably and shorten the overall duration of the disease.

SEBORRHEIC DERMATITIS

Seborrheic dermatitis is a common cutaneous disease with a characteristic appearance. The yeast *Malassezia furfur* is known to be present in increased numbers in active lesions, and their eradication causes the disease expression to subside.

Clinically, seborrheic dermatitis may present in infancy as thick, greasy, yellow to white scales and crusts on a mildly erythematous base. Characteristically, the scalp is involved as well as the intertriginous regions. The face, neck, chest, and extremities may also be involved in extensive disease.

In adolescents and adults, the disease presents as pink to erythematous plaques with thin, white, greasy scales. Classic sites of distribution are the scalp, eyebrows, nasolabial folds, postauricular regions, external auditory canals, and central chest.

Treatment of Seborrheic Dermatitis

Mild seborrheic dermatitis responds to treatment with antifungal medications that have activity against yeast. The use of ketoconazole (Nizoral) in the form of shampoo or cream usually obtains a satisfactory response within 2 weeks. The initial response may be accelerated with concomitant Class V or VI topical corticosteroids, and their use should then be tapered to avoid atrophy in the central facial area.

Intermittent use of shampoos inhibiting the growth of the *M. furfur* yeast, such as those containing ketoconazole, selenium sulfide, and zinc pyrithione, is usually enough to maintain good results.

PITYRIASIS RUBRA PILARIS

Pityriasis rubra pilaris is a rare cutaneous disease that may be either inherited or acquired. Initially, the lesions are hyperkeratotic follicular papules with underlying orange erythema. Classically, these first present on the scalp and face and eventually progress downward. The erythema then expands to involve skin between the hair follicles. Characteristically, within large plaques of orange erythema there are "islands" of normal skin. The palms and soles develop thick hyperkeratosis. At this later stage, the initial hyperkeratotic follicular papules are less conspicuous in areas of diffuse erythema but tend to remain perceptible on the dorsal digits, providing insight into the diagnosis.

The acquired type of pityriasis rubra pilaris in adults has a fluctuating course, with an 80% chance of spontaneous resolution within 3 years. The childhood presentation of the familial type of pityriasis rubra pilaris does not remit, but the clinical features are partially responsive to therapy.

Treatment of Pityriasis Rubra Pilaris

Both topical and oral medications have been used in the treatment of pityriasis rubra pilaris. Keratolytics such as propylene glycol and lactic acid aid in controlling the symptoms of dry scaling skin, but these agents usually do not cause regression of the lesions. Oral vitamin A at a dosage of 1×10^6 IU per day for 2 weeks has been demonstrated to be helpful.

Systemic retinoid therapy at a dosage of 1 to 2 mg per kg per day for 1 to 2 months has also demonstrated beneficial effects by decreasing the duration of disease activity. Methotrexate in low doses of 2.5 to 5 mg every 2 to 3 days has been shown to help alleviate the symptoms of skin disease. With any of these systemic treatments, there are potentially serious side effects. These agents are best given by physicians who are familiar with the side effects as well as with the type of monitoring patients require while receiving therapy.

PITYRIASIS LICHENOIDES

Pityriasis lichenoides can be separated into a self-limited variant—pityriasis lichenoides acuta, or Mucha-Habermann disease—and a more persistent variant called pityriasis lichenoides chronica. Pityriasis lichenoides acuta presents as a generalized eruption of pink to light brown papules with overlying thin scales usually less than 1 cm in size. This disease characteristically displays individual lesions in various stages of activity, from early erythematous papules to older lesions with a central scale crust, which may leave a residual scar. Pityriasis lichenoides chronica presents as recurrent crops of pink to erythematous papules with thin overlying scales. Crusting or scarring is not part of the clinical presentation, and the individual plaques tend to be larger than in the acute form. Histopathologic specimens are necessary to accurately confirm the clinical diagnosis. Both forms usually present on the trunk and proximal extremities.

Treatment of Pityriasis Lichenoides

Pityriasis lichenoides acuta may be treated with oral antibiotics such as erythromycin or tetracycline in combination with topical corticosteroids. Both demonstrate variable results. However, the best results for both acute and chronic forms are obtained with PUVA. Methotrexate in low doses of 5 to 7.5 mg per week has also been reported to be effective in recalcitrant cases.

PARAPSORIASIS

The term "parapsoriasis" encompasses large plaque parapsoriasis and small plaque parapsoriasis. Large plaque parapsoriasis is characterized by well-demarcated erythematous to light brown plaques with a surface described as "cigarette-paper wrinkling." The plaques vary in size from 5 cm to greater than 10 cm. The sites of predilection are the lower trunk, buttocks, and thighs, or a bathing trunk distribution. The breasts are also commonly involved in women. It is estimated that large plaque parapsoriasis may progress to cutaneous T cell lymphoma in 5 to 10% of patients. At the present time, there is no means of accurately predicting which patients are at risk. Therefore, patients with this clinical and histologic diagnosis are treated as if they have the potential for developing cutaneous T cell lymphoma.

Small plaque parapsoriasis presents as round erythematous plaques with fine scales less than 5 cm in diameter. The plaques are usually well demarcated and appear parallel to one another. The most common sites of involvement are the trunk and proximal extremities. Small plaque parapsoriasis does not appear to have the same malignant potential as the large plaque variety. Clinicopathologic correlation of biopsies from multiple sites is usually needed to arrive at an accurate diagnosis.

Treatment of Parapsoriasis

A range of treatment modalities for parapsoriasis is available, depending on the extent of the disease. Mid- to high-potency topical corticosteroids applied twice daily may cause temporary regression of localized plaques, which recur after discontinuance of treatment. Ultraviolet radiation with either UVB or PUVA is the treatment of choice to obtain long-term remission. The highest rates of remission are accomplished with PUVA therapy. Topical nitrogen mustard is also efficacious.

Small plaque parapsoriasis generally does not require the same degree of aggressive therapy. Both topical corticosteroids and phototherapy have been used. With either of type of parapsoriasis, the patient should be examined at 6- to 12-month intervals to evaluate for recurrence or progression of the disease.

CUTANEOUS T CELL LYMPHOMA

Cutaneous T cell lymphoma or mycosis fungoides is a malignant neoplasm that originates from a clonal T cell population in the skin. There are four main presentations, and a pathologic determination, often aided by immunohistochemical markers for malignant cells, is mandatory for an accurate diagnosis.

1. Patch stage mycosis fungoides is characterized by well-demarcated erythematous macules with overlying fine scale, most commonly on unexposed areas.

2. Plaque stage may progress from the patch stage or may arise spontaneously. There are well-demarcated erythematous to violaceous plaques with thick overlying scale, which can present on any area of the skin.

3. Tumor stage is characterized by erythematous to violaceous nodules that most commonly arise on the face and in the body folds. These nodules may ulcerate and become secondarily infected.

4. Erythroderma stage, or Sézary syndrome, can arise as progression from pre-existing disease or de novo. There is diffuse, intense erythema with overlying white scale and concomitant fever, chills, and often disturbances in temperature regulation. A markedly thickened epithelium of the hands and feet known as "tylosis" may accompany this form of disease.

Treatment of Cutaneous T Cell Lymphoma

Patch and plaque stage disease may be treated by several different modalities alone or in combination. These include topical nitrogen mustard, PUVA, total skin electron beam radiotherapy, and single-drug chemotherapy in extensive disease. Extracorporeal photopheresis has been shown to be therapeutic for the erythrodermic varient and in some cases of plaque stage disease. Tumor stage and Sézary syndrome require systemic chemotherapy alone or in combination with the other modalities listed previously.

SYPHILIS

The clinical presentation of syphilis is classified into primary, secondary, and tertiary stages. Secondary syphilis must be considered in the differential diagnosis of any of the papulosquamous disorders. The lesions are circular erythematous papules or plaques, often indurated with overlying light scale. The scale may present as a ring on the outer edge of the papule. These can present on the trunk, abdomen, and extremities. Involvement of the palms and soles is characteristic of syphilis, as is the presence of mucous patches on the oral mucosa, which occur in only a minority of cases. Lymphadenopathy is also frequently present, and the patient should be examined for the presence of epitrochlear node enlargement.

Treatment of Syphilis

There are several therapeutic regimens listed by the Centers for Disease Control and Prevention (CDC) to treat secondary syphilis. If the patient has had syphilis for more than 1 year or for an indeterminate period, the recommendation is benzathine penicillin 2.4 million U intramuscularly for 3 consecutive weeks, given 1 week apart. The alternatives are doxycycline 100 mg twice a day for 4 weeks or tetracycline 500 mg four times a day for 4 weeks. The course is different for patients known to have syphilis for less than 1 year, patients with neurosyphilis, pregnant patients, and neonates. The reader is advised to refer to the latest CDC guidelines regarding the treatment of syphilis.

CONNECTIVE TISSUE DISORDERS

method of
JOHN H. KLIPPEL, M.D., and
MARK F. GOURLEY, M.D.
*National Institute of Arthritis and
Musculoskeletal and Skin Diseases
National Institutes of Health
Bethesda, Maryland*

The term "connective tissue disorders" is used to describe a group of related idiopathic chronic inflammatory syndromes in which abnormalities of the immune system are thought to be central in pathogenesis. The four classic connective tissue disorders are systemic lupus erythematosus, scleroderma (systemic sclerosis), inflammatory myopathy, and Sjögren's syndrome. The diseases differ substantially in the organ systems affected and the types of immune abnormalities found. Clinically, however, they share in common a great heterogeneity of clinical expression and disease severity ranging from mild inconsequential illness to severe, life-threatening disease.

SYSTEMIC LUPUS ERYTHEMATOSUS

Systemic lupus erythematosus (SLE) is the most common of the connective tissue disease syndromes and is characterized by the development of antinuclear antibodies and the involvement of multiple organ systems. The clinical spectrum ranges from a relatively benign chronic disease process with rash, arthritis, and fatigue to a very severe and life-threatening illness with renal failure and irreversible central nervous system damage. A large differential diagnosis must be considered in patients with a positive antinuclear antibody and suspected SLE (Table 1). Differentiating lupus from related rheumatic or connective tissue diseases may be particularly difficult early in the disease course; the detection of serologic abnormalities relatively unique to SLE, such as antibodies to Sm (Smith antigen) or double-stranded DNA or depressed levels of serum complement, are valuable in such circumstances. Common clinical and laboratory findings that occur in patients with SLE are displayed in Table 2; a subset of these

TABLE 1. **Disease States Associated with a Positive Antinuclear Antibody**

Connective tissue/rheumatic diseases	Rheumatoid arthritis, lupus, inflammatory myopathies, scleroderma, Sjögren's syndrome, mixed connective tissue disease
Drug-induced lupus	Procainamide, hydralazine, phenylhydantoin, penicillamine, chlorpromazine, many others
Hematologic disorders	Autoimmune hemolytic anemia, autoimmune thrombocytopenic purpura
Skin diseases	Psoriasis, pemphigus vulgaris, lichen planus, porphyria
Pulmonary diseases	Idiopathic pulmonary fibrosis, asbestosis, primary pulmonary hypertension
Hepatic diseases	Autoimmune hepatitis, primary biliary cirrhosis, chronic viral hepatitis, alcoholic liver disease
Infectious diseases	Parasitic diseases, chronic bacterial diseases (particularly SBE), viral diseases
Endocrine disorders	Diabetes mellitus, autoimmune thyroiditis, Graves' disease
Neurologic diseases	Multiple sclerosis, subacute sensory neuropathy

Abbreviation: SBE = subacute bacterial endocarditis.

TABLE 2. **Clinical and Laboratory Findings in Systemic Lupus Erythematosus***

Constitutional	*Musculoskeletal*
Fever	**Arthritis**/arthralgia
Fatigue	Subcutaneous nodules
Anorexia	Myositis
Weight loss	Osteonecrosis
Myalgias	Deforming arthropathy
	(Jaccoud's)
Mucocutaneous	*Cardiopulmonary*
Photosensitivity	**Pleuritis/pericarditis**
Malar rash	Endocarditis (Libman-Sacks)
Discoid rash	Pneumonitis
Oral/nasal ulcers	Raynaud's phenomenon
Alopecia	Thrombophlebitis
Xerostomia/xerophthalmia	
Renal	*Neurologic/Psychiatric*
Active urine sediment	**Seizures**
(nephritis)	Stroke syndromes
Proteinuria (nephropathy)	Movement disorders
Renal vein thrombosis	**Psychosis**
Hematology	*Immunologic Studies*
Lymphopenia or leukopenia	**Antinuclear antibody**
Anemia/**hemolytic anemia**	**Positive LE cells**
Thrombocytopenia	**Anti-DNA and anti-Sm**
False-positive STS	Antiphospholipid antibodies
Increased PTT	Depressed serum complement
	levels

*Criteria for classification of SLE developed by the American College of Rheumatology are indicated in bold print (Tan EM, Cohen AS, Fries JF, et al: The 1982 revised criteria for the classification of systemic lupus erythematosus. Arthritis Rheum 25:1271–1277, 1982). Diagnosis of SLE requires presence of four criteria during any period of observation.

Abbreviations: LE = lupus erythematosus; PTT = partial thromboplastin time; Sm = Smith antigen; STS = serologic test for syphilis.

features has been established as criteria for the classification of the disease by the American College of Rheumatology and serves to aid in diagnosis.

Treatment

Skin Rashes

The cutaneous manifestations of lupus may be divided into acute, subacute, and chronic varieties. Whereas the acute rashes are typically intermittent and nonscarring, both subacute and chronic lesions have a tendency to produce permanent atrophy of the involved skin with hypo- and hyperpigmentary changes. The most commonly recognized expressions of acute lupus are the erythematous maculopapular rash over the malar regions (butterfly rash) and between the interphalangeal joints of the fingers; however, a similar rash may appear on the trunk or upper extremities. Two types of subacute lupus have been described—annular and psoriasiform. These too have a tendency to involve mainly the face and trunk. The most common form of chronic cutaneous lupus is discoid lupus, a highly disfiguring lesion that most commonly affects the face, scalp, ears, and upper extremities.

Most lupus rashes are photosensitive, and patients should be advised to avoid intense sun exposure and use sunscreens. Topical applications of corticosteroid preparations are helpful in most patients. Potent fluorinated corticosteroid preparations such as 0.05% fluocinonide (Lidex), 0.05% betamethasone dipropionate (Diprolene), or 0.05% clobetasol proprionate (Temovate) are particularly effective but should be used with caution and never for more than 1 week to minimize cutaneous side effects, including atrophy and the formation of telangiectases. Discoid lesions may be injected directly with long-acting triamcinolone suspensions (Kenalog, Aristocort). Antimalarial drugs, particularly hydroxychloroquine (Plaquenil) in doses of 200 to 400 mg daily, are recommended in patients with generalized lupus rashes or rashes that fail to respond fully to topical corticosteroids. Options for drug therapy for patients with rashes refractory to topical corticosteroids and hydroxychloroquine include antimalarial combinations (hydroxychloroquine, chloroquine, quinacrine), dapsone, retinoids (Accutane, Tegison), azathioprine (Imuran), and low-dose oral corticosteroids.

Musculoskeletal Disease

Most lupus patients develop joint complaints during the course of their disease. The two most common patterns of arthritis are a symmetrical polyarthritis that resembles rheumatoid arthritis and a migratory oligoarthritis. The finding of a persistent monoarthritis, particularly of the knees or hips, suggests osteonecrosis (avascular necrosis) or less commonly septic arthritis. About 10% of lupus patients develop a deforming arthropathy of the hands (Jaccoud's arthropathy). The deformities are fully reducible, and bone erosions are not evident on radiographs of the hands, findings that are helpful in distinguishing the disease from rheumatoid arthritis.

The arthritis of SLE typically responds well to full-dose nonsteroidal anti-inflammatory drug (NSAID) therapy with drugs like naproxen (Naprosyn) or sulindac (Clinoril); in patients with chronic arthritis, low-dose prednisone (5 to 10 mg daily), hydroxychloroquine (Plaquenil), 200 to 400 mg daily, or oral weekly methotrexate (Myotrex) (7.5 to 10 mg weekly) may be needed to control joint symptoms. Early physical therapy is important in patients with Jaccoud's arthropathy to prevent progression of the malalignments and minimize functional disability. Options for the medical management of patients with osteonecrosis are limited; patients should be referred to an experienced physical therapist for recommendations to reduce forces across the joint surfaces. Decompression core biopsy should be considered in patients with very early, extensive involvement detected on magnetic resonance imaging scans only. Patients with advanced osteonecrosis are candidates for total joint replacements.

Hematologic Disorders

Hematologic manifestations of lupus include anemia, leukopenia, and thrombocytopenia, which typically respond to moderate-dose oral prednisone (20 to 30 mg daily). Acute hemolytic anemia or aplastic anemia and severe thrombocytopenia with platelet counts of less than 50,000 per mm³ are fortunately rare but serious complications that require aggressive treatment with high-dose corticosteroids combined with intravenous cyclophosphamide (Cytoxan) (see "Renal Involvement"). Additional treatment options that should be considered include dapsone, immune globulin, and splenectomy.

Renal Involvement

In most patients the presence of lupus nephritis or lupus nephropathy is first detected on routine screening studies with the finding of abnormalities on urinalysis or elevations of the blood urea nitrogen (BUN) or serum creatinine. The extent of the evaluation depends largely on the type and degree of abnormality found. For example, the finding of mild proteinuria on dipstick (trace to 1 +) and occasional red or white blood cells may resolve entirely on its own and can generally be safely followed without any change in therapy. On the other hand, the finding of higher levels of proteinuria; greater numbers of cellular elements, particularly cellular casts, in the spun urinary sediment; or clinical signs of renal disease such as peripheral edema or hypertension are clear indications of the need for a thorough evaluation and drug treatment. In lupus patients with impairments of renal function, it is important to exclude other causes such as NSAID-induced renal changes before ascribing the loss of function to lupus per se.

The intensity of drug therapy in lupus nephritis-nephropathy is determined by factors related to the prognosis and severity of the renal disease. In general, a renal biopsy is required to determine whether proliferative changes are mild (mesangial or focal proliferative nephritis) or severe (diffuse proliferative nephritis) or whether membranous or membrano-proliferative nephropathy is present. From a prognostic standpoint, the biopsy is particularly helpful in documenting glomerular sclerosis or tubulointerstitial disease, so-called chronicity features associated with an increased risk of end-stage renal failure (ESRF).

In all patients with lupus nephritis-nephropathy, it is extremely important to control hypertension aggressively, use diuretics for fluid overload states, and treat hyperlipidemia with diet or drug interventions. Corticosteroids, typically oral prednisone in doses of 0.5 to 1.0 mg per kg given in the morning, are the mainstay of initial drug therapy in all types of lupus renal disease. Bolus intravenous methylprenisolone (Solu-Medrol) (15 mg per kg or 1 gram) is often given at the start of oral prednisone therapy as a way to control kidney inflammation more rapidly, particularly in patients who are massively nephrotic or have an extremely active urinary sediment with red blood cell casts. The dose of oral prednisone is gradually reduced after 1 month; tapering varies greatly, depending on how well the patient has responded and whether residual symptoms of lupus are present.

In patients with diffuse proliferative glomerulonephritis, studies have clearly shown that bolus intra-venous cyclophosphamide (Cytoxan)* (0.75 to 1.0 gram per meter²) reduces the risk of ESRF. The bolus cyclophosphamide is given monthly for a period of 6 months. The decision of whether to stop cyclophosphamide treatment at that point or change to a maintenance 3-month regimen is difficult and depends largely on how well the patient has responded to treatment.

The role of prednisone and bolus cyclophosphamide in patients with lupus membranous nephropathy is less clear. In general, patients with nephrotic-range proteinuria or evidence of loss of renal function should be treated the same way as patients with diffuse proliferative nephritis, whereas conservative prednisone treatment should be used in the remainder of lupus membranous patients. Lupus patients who develop ESRF are treated with hemo- or peritoneal dialysis and become candidates for renal transplantation.

Neurologic or Psychiatric Disease

The range of potential neurologic or psychiatric manifestations in patients with lupus is extensive. Clinical findings of central nervous system involvement predominate: most common are seizures, stroke syndromes, and transverse myelopathies. Minor psychiatric disorders such as depression or disturbances of mental function are frequent, yet in many patients it is often difficult to be absolutely certain that these disorders are secondary to underlying lupus, as opposed to the stresses associated with chronic illness. Furthermore, the evaluation of patients with neurologic or psychiatric illnesses is complicated by the frequent failure to detect any abnormalities on routine testing with lumbar puncture, electroencephalograms, and magnetic resonance or computed tomography (CT) scans.

Management of these patients is complex without good therapeutic studies to guide treatment. Attention to standard neurologic practices, including anticonvulsant therapy for patients with seizures, anticoagulants for transient ischemic episodes, and acute and chronic stroke care, is important. Aggressive drug management with high-dose corticosteroids or bolus intravenous cyclophosphamide as used in lupus nephritis is indicated in acute settings in which vasculitis can be documented. Thrombotic thrombocytopenic purpura is a rare but important cause of neurologic disease in lupus patients and represents the only clear, unequivocal indication for plasmapheresis.

SCLERODERMA

"Scleroderma" describes various syndromes characterized by fibrosis of the skin and visceral organs (Table 3). The most common form, idiopathic scleroderma (systemic sclerosis), is divided into diffuse and limited subsets based on the extent of skin involvement. In diffuse scleroderma, a rapidly progressive,

---

*Not FDA-approved for this indication.

TABLE 3. Classification of Scleroderma Syndromes

Idiopathic scleroderma
  Diffuse
  Limited

Chemically induced scleroderma
  Toxic oil syndrome
  Eosinophilia myalgia syndrome (L-tryptophan)
  Vinyl chloride disease
  Bleomycin-induced fibrosis
  Trichloroethylene-induced fibrosis

Localized scleroderma
  Morphea
  Linear scleroderma
  Eosinophilic fasciitis

Pseudoscleroderma
  Graft-versus-host disease
  Porphyria cutanea tarda
  Amyloidosis
  Carcinoid
  Acromegaly

generalized skin thickening affects the distal and proximal extremities and trunk. In contrast, the skin thickening in limited scleroderma is confined to the distal extremities and face. Limited scleroderma is often referred to as the "CREST syndrome" for typical clinical findings of calcinosis, Raynaud's, esophageal dysmotility, sclerodactyly, and telangiectasia. Diffuse and limited forms of idiopathic scleroderma differ slightly in the frequencies with which visceral organs are involved, the types of autoantibodies that develop, and prognosis (Table 4).

Treatment

Skin and Calcinosis

Skin changes are first noted in the fingers in most patients. The skin goes through phases of early edema in which it is swollen, shiny, and taut, followed by a slowly progressive hardening; both hypo- and hyperpigmention may be seen. Pruritus is a frequent complaint and is usually benefited by lanolin skin lotions. Ulcerations on the tips of the fingers from minor trauma are a common nagging problem in many patients. Regular soaking of the ulcers in an antiseptic solution, topical application of an antibiotic ointment such as bacitracin, and use of occlusive dressing are helpful; however, it may take many weeks before ulcers fully heal. Joint contractures as a result of fibrotic changes within tendon sheaths should be aggressively treated with physical therapy. Drug therapy for the skin disease of scleroderma is largely unsatisfactory—patients with progressive, diffuse scleroderma should be treated with D-penicillamine (Cuprimine, Depen) starting at 250 mg daily and increasing by 250 mg monthly to a maximal daily dose of 1000 mg.

Treatment options for subcutaneous calcium deposits that develop on the hands and in periarticular tissues along bony eminences are limited. NSAIDs or chronic oral colchicine (0.6 mg three times a day)

may be helpful in suppressing inflammatory changes around the deposits; diltiazem (Cardizem),* warfarin,* and diphosphonates may have a role in patients with severe, progressive calcinosis. Calcific deposits frequently ulcerate, causing a white, chalky drainage and secondary infection typically with staphylococcal species that requires antibiotic treatment. Surgical excision and drainage of large deposits should be reserved for patients with massive accumulations because of problems with wound healing and the high likelihood of recurrence.

Raynaud's Phenomenon

All patients with scleroderma suffer from Raynaud's phenomenon. Mild symptoms are generally easily controlled with attention to practical measures such as adjusting the thermostat upward, avoiding exposure to the cold, dressing warmly, and using insulated mittens or gloves. Smokers need to be reminded of the importance of stopping smoking. Battery-operated or chemical hand and foot warmers sold in sporting goods stores may help some patients. Warming hands in tepid water is usually an effective way to abort an attack.

Drug therapy should be reserved for patients with severe symptoms. Calcium channel blocking agents are often effective, particularly nifedipine in the slow-release form (Procardia XL).* However, in many patients the dosage needed to improve symptoms is associated with intolerable vasodilatory side effects such as headaches, flushing, dizziness, palpitations, or fluid retention. Other drug approaches helpful in patients with recalcitrant Raynaud's include pra-

*Not FDA-approved for this indication.

TABLE 4. Comparison of Diffuse and Limited Idiopathic Scleroderma

	Diffuse (%)	Limited (CREST) (%)
Skin findings		
Telangiectasias	30	90
Calcinosis	5	50
Raynaud's	90	99
Musculoskeletal		
Arthralgias/arthritis	95	95
Tendon friction rubs	70	5
Myopathy	40	10
Gastrointestinal		
Esophageal hypomotility	80	80
Pulmonary		
Pulmonary fibrosis	70	30
Pulmonary hypertension	5	25
Renal crisis	20	0
Antinuclear antibodies	95	95
Anticentromere antibody	5	50
Antitopoisomerase I (Scl-70)	40	10
Cumulative survival		
5-year	70	90
10-year	50	75

Abbreviation: CREST = calcinosis, Raynaud's phenomenon, esophageal dysmotility disorders, sclerodactyly, and telangiectasia; Scl-70 = scleroderma 70 antigen.

zosin (Minipress)* or nitroglycerin* preparations as either a paste (Nitro-Bid 2% ointment) or transdermal patches (Minitran or Nitro-Dur).

Gastrointestinal Involvement

Gastrointestinal complaints are extremely common in patients with scleroderma. Dysphagia and symptoms of gastroesophageal reflux require attention to simple practical measures such as elevating the head of the bed, avoiding alcohol and caffeinated beverages, and eating frequent small meals. Reflux esophagitis is managed with antacids, proton-pump inhibitors such as omeprazole (Prilosec) or H_2 receptor antagonists cimetidine (Tagamet) or ranitidine (Zantac), and sucralfate (Carafate) used as a thick slurry prior to meals and at bedtime. In patients with esophageal strictures, periodic dilatation may be necessary. Reduction of fiber and fat content of the diet helps minimize abdominal symptoms from dysmotility of the small bowel. Advanced involvement of the bowel by scleroderma can lead to malabsorption and the need for oral liquid supplements or intravenous hyperalimentation. Bacterial overgrowth may contribute to abdominal symptoms, including malnutrition, and should be treated with short, rotating courses of broad-spectrum antibiotics such as ampicillin, tetracycline, or ciprofloxacin (Cipro).

Pulmonary Involvement

Several different types of lung pathologies are seen in patients with scleroderma, including diffuse inflammatory alveolitis, interstitial fibrosis, and pulmonary hypertension. In addition, scleroderma patients are at increased risk for the development of lung cancer. General measures of pulmonary care are important and include prevention of aspiration through the use of antireflux regimens, bronchodilators in patients with wheezing, yearly influenza vaccinations and early treatment of respiratory infections, and strongly encouraging smokers to stop. Bronchoalveolar lavage or high-resolution CT scans should be used to identify patients with inflammatory alveolitis who should be treated with a combination of prednisone at a dose of 30 to 40 mg daily and intravenous bolus cyclophosphamide (Cytoxan) in doses of 750 to 1000 mg. There is no evidence that any drug therapy influences the course of interstitial pulmonary fibrosis or pulmonary hypertension. Oxygen supplementation and other supportive measures should be used as needed; in patients with advanced, end-stage disease, lung or heart-lung transplantation should be considered.

Renal Crisis

Renal crisis with malignant hypertension, microangiopathic hemolytic anemia, thrombocytopenia, and rapidly progressive renal failure is a serious, life-threatening complication of scleroderma. Prompt and aggressive treatment of the hypertension using angiotensin-converting enzyme (ACE) inhibitors is

*Not FDA-approved for this indication.

critical. There is *no* role for corticosteroids, plasmapheresis, or immunosuppressive drugs in scleroderma renal crisis. Intravenous enalapril (Vasotec IV injection) or short-acting oral ACE inhibitors (Capoten or Lotensin) may be used to acutely titrate the blood pressure to normal levels. Minoxidil (Loniten) is indicated in patients who fail to respond to ACE inhibitors in maximal dosage. Blood transfusions and diuretics may be used to manage symptoms of congestive heart failure. Patients who progress to ESRF should be treated with hemodialysis (or peritoneal dialysis), and the experience with renal transplantation in these patients has been promising.

INFLAMMATORY MYOPATHIES

The inflammatory myopathies consist of a group of chronic inflammatory muscle diseases characterized by immune-mediated injury to skeletal muscle tissues. Two major forms are recognized: polymyositis and dermatomyositis, which differ clinically only on the basis of whether rashes are found. A third variant, termed "inclusion body myositis," has slightly different clinical features and unique findings on electron microscopy of muscle biopsy sections showing microtubular or filamentous inclusions. The inflammatory myopathies may develop in patients with other connective diseases (mixed or overlap syndromes). Moreover, an extensive differential diagnosis must be considered in patients with proximal muscle weakness and suspected inflammatory myopathies (Table 5).

Routine studies helpful in the evaluation of patients with suspected inflammatory myopathies include measurement of levels of various enzymes in the serum, electromyography, and muscle biopsy. Levels of creatinine kinase and aldolase are sensitive markers of muscle inflammation; in addition, many patients have elevations of lactate dehydrogenase

TABLE 5. **Differential Diagnosis of Inflammatory Myopathies**

Drug- and toxin-induced	Corticosteroids, colchicine, cimetidine, zidovudine (AZT), lovastatin, D-penicillamine, chloroquine, alcohol, heroin, cocaine
Endocrinopathies	Hyper- and hypothyroidism, acromegaly, Cushing's syndrome, Addison's disease
Electrolyte disturbances	Hypokalemia, hypercalcemia, hypocalcemia, hypomagnesemia
Neurologic diseases	Myasthenia gravis, amyotrophic lateral sclerosis, muscular dystrophy, Guillain-Barré syndrome, periodic paralysis
Infections	Viruses (influenza, coxsackie, human immunodeficiency virus, adenovirus, hepatitis B, rubella), toxoplasmosis, trichina, rickettsial, bacterial toxins (staphylococcal, streptococcal, clostridial)

(LDH), serum glutamic-oxaloacetic transaminase (SGOT), and serum glutamic-pyruvic transaminase (SGPT) and mistakenly undergo assessments for liver disease. The electromyogram is helpful in discriminating between pure neurologic and myopathic disorders. However, muscle biopsy remains the only means to establish the diagnosis with certainty.

Treatment

Muscle Weakness

Patients with inflammatory muscle disorders typically present with complaints of weakness of the proximal muscles of the upper and lower extremities. Most commonly these involve difficulties in performing simple daily functions like rising from a chair, climbing stairs, dressing, or grooming. The weakness may be of abrupt or insidious onset. Other muscle groups commonly affected include the neck flexors (the patient is unable to lift the head against gravity), muscles of the oropharynx or esophagus (dysphagia), and diaphragmatic and intercostal muscles (dyspnea). Involvement of distal muscles is a late finding; impairment of distal muscles early in the disease course suggests inclusion body myositis. Ocular and facial muscles are essentially never involved in the inflammatory myopathies.

Therapy should be initiated with high-dose corticosteroids, typically oral prednisone in doses of 1 mg per kg daily. The response to corticosteroids is often slow, and several weeks of therapy are generally required before muscle strength begins to improve. In patients with very severe, acute disease, particularly those in whom constitutional signs such as fever, anorexia, and weight loss are prominent, intravenous bolus methylprednisolone (Solu-Medrol) in doses of 1 gram or 15 mg per kg often provides more immediate benefit. Methotrexate, either orally in doses of 7.5 to 25 mg weekly or intramuscularly in doses of 0.2 to 0.3 mg per kg weekly, and/or azathioprine (Imuran) is recommended in patients who fail to respond completely to corticosteroids within 4 weeks. Treatment failures with combined corticosteroid and antimetabolite drugs are a problem—preliminary studies suggest there may be a role for gamma globulin or cyclosporine (Sandimmune) in such patients. Patients with inclusion body myositis tend to respond poorly to drug therapy.

Rashes

Several distinctive rashes occur in patients with dermatomyositis. The rashes may rarely develop in the absence of frank myositis, so-called dermatomyositis sine myositis. Scaly violaceous patches (Gottron's papules) form over the extensor surfaces of joints, most commonly over the knuckles, elbows, and knees. The radial surfaces and pads of the fingers may become dry and cracked, with black pigmentary changes (mechanics' hands). Erythematous, often photosensitive, rashes occur on the neck, shoulder, upper chest (V sign or shawl sign), and malar region of the face. The facial rash can easily be confused with the butterfly rash of SLE; crossing of the nasolabial fold is a helpful physical finding that occurs in dermatomyositis. The upper eyelids may become edematous and develop a purplish (heliotrope) hue. Subcutaneous calcifications may develop within muscle planes, particularly in childhood-onset dermatomyositis, that may ulcerate, drain, and become secondarily infected.

In most patients, specific therapy directed at the skin disease is not required, and rashes improve as the muscle inflammation comes under control. Hydroxychloroquine (Plaquenil) in doses of 200 to 400 mg daily should be considered in patients with severe or progressive skin disease, particularly of the erythematous, photosensitive variety. There are no satisfactory treatments for calcinosis (see "Skin and Calcinosis" under "Scleroderma").

Pulmonary Disease

Dyspnea in patients with inflammatory muscle disease has several different causes. Myositis of the diaphragm or intercostal muscles directly interferes with the mechanics of respiration, dysfunction of the pharyngeal muscles may result in aspirations, and involvement of the myocardium or cardiac conduction system leads to congestive heart failure. Pulmonary involvement secondary to muscular factors improves as the inflammatory muscle disease comes under control. Interstitial alveolitis and progressive fibrosis occur in a subset of patients with antibodies to transfer RNA synthetases; the most common antibody found is directed against histadyl t-RNAase (Jo-1). Therapy of interstitial lung disease in inflammatory myopathies is identical to that described for scleroderma (see "Pulmonary Involvement" under "Scleroderma").

SJÖGREN'S SYNDROME

Sjögren's syndrome is a chronic, immune-mediated inflammatory disease of the exocrine glands. In most patients, the presenting complaint is dryness, typically of the eyes (xerophthalmia) or mouth (xerostomia). Tenderness or swelling of the parotid glands may also be seen. Sjögren's syndrome is divided into primary and secondary forms based on whether another rheumatic disorder is present, such as rheumatoid arthritis, SLE, systemic sclerosis, or polymyositis. Sjögren's syndrome must be differentiated from a number of other disorders that affect the salivary glands (Table 6).

Studies used to evaluate patients with suspected Sjögren's syndrome include biopsy of the minor salivary glands of the lip, functional tests of ocular or oral glands, and tests for autoantibodies. Minor salivary gland biopsy is the only reliable method to diagnose the disease with certainty. The typical pathologic finding consists of focal aggregates of lymphocytes, plasma cells, and macrophages adjacent to and replacing the normal acini. Larger foci often exhibit formation of germinal centers.

TABLE 6. **Diseases Associated with Parotid Enlargement**

Viral infections (mumps, human immunodeficiency virus, Epstein-Barr, others)
Sarcoidosis
Amyloidosis
Hyperlipoproteinemia
Endocrine disorders (acromegaly, diabetes mellitus, hypogonadism)
Chronic pancreatitis
Alcoholism/hepatic cirrhosis
Uremia
Tumors, especially lymphoma

Schirmer's tear test is used to evaluate tear secretion by the lacrimal glands. Keratoconjunctivitis sicca, the sequela of decreased tear secretion, is diagnosed using rose bengal staining of the corneal epithelium. Rose bengal is an aniline dye that stains the devitalized or damaged epithelium of both the cornea and the conjunctiva. Slit-lamp examination after rose bengal staining shows a punctate or filamentary keratitis. Autoantibodies are commonly detected in patients with Sjögren's syndrome, in particular rheumatoid factors, antinuclear antibodies, and antibodies to extractable nuclear antigens, in particular autoantibodies termed "Ro (SS-A)" and "La (SS-B)." These autoantibodies are not specific for Sjögren's syndrome but may be found in other autoimmune diseases, especially SLE.

Treatment

The treatment of patients with Sjögren's syndrome is mainly symptomatic, with the goal of keeping mucosal surfaces moist. Lubrication of dry eyes with artificial tears should be done as often as necessary. A variety of preparations (Liquifilm Tears, Tears Plus, Refresh, and Hypotears) are available that differ primarily in viscosity and preservative. The thicker, more viscous drops require less frequent application, although they can cause blurring and leave residue on the lashes. Less viscous drops require more frequent applications. Soft contact lenses may help protect the cornea, especially in the presence of filamentary keratitis. However, the lenses themselves require wetting, and patients must be followed very carefully because of the increased risk of infection. Avoidance of windy and/or low humidity environments is helpful. Cigarette smoking and drugs with anticholinergic side effects such as phenothiazines, tricyclic antidepressants, antispasmodics, and antiparkinson agents should be avoided whenever possible.

Treatment of xerostomia is difficult. Most patients learn on their own the importance of taking small sips of water frequently and carrying bottles of water with them at all times. Stimulation of salivary flow by chewing sugar-free gum or using lozenges is often helpful. Patients should be instructed to avoid dry food, smoking, or the use of drugs with anticholinergic side effects that serve to decrease the salivary flow. Periodontal disease and tooth decay are serious problems in xerostomia, and patients should be reminded of the importance of regularly brushing the teeth after meals. Topical treatment of the teeth with stannous fluoride enhances dental mineralization and retards damage to tooth surfaces. In rapidly progressive dental disease, the fluoride can be directly applied to the teeth from plastic trays that are used at night. Vaginal dryness is treated with lubricant jellies, and dry skin with moisturizing lotions.

Systemic corticosteroids (oral prednisone, 0.5 to 1 mg per kg daily) and immunosuppressive drugs such as oral or intravenous cyclophosphamide (Cytoxan)* are used for severe extraglandular disease, including interstitial pneumonitis, glomerulonephritis, vasculitis, and peripheral neuropathy. Sjögren's patients are at increased risk for the development of lymphoma, and treatment depends on the histologic type, location, and extension. Decisions regarding chemotherapy and/or radiation should be guided by experienced oncologists.

*Not FDA-approved for this indication.

CUTANEOUS VASCULITIS

method of
THOMAS E. FLEMING, M.D., and
CRAIG A. ELMETS, M.D.
Case Western Reserve University
Cleveland, Ohio

The term "vasculitis" refers to a diverse group of diseases in which blood vessels are the principal target of an inflammatory response. Often, this is the result of immunologic hypersensitivity in which antigen-antibody complexes accumulate within the vessel wall, and vessels are inadvertently damaged in the body's attempt to eliminate the inciting factors. Inflammatory damage to the vasculature results in thrombosis and hemorrhage, which, in turn, can compromise the functions of affected organs. The skin is frequently involved in vasculitis, and at times it is the only target organ for these syndromes. This, coupled with its accessibility for biopsy procedures and for close and repetitive observation, makes the skin an especially important tissue for the evaluation and management of many of the vasculitides. The importance of prompt recognition and appropriate management of the cutaneous manifestations cannot be overemphasized, since early intervention may prevent many of the more serious cutaneous and systemic manifestations of these disorders.

There is considerable overlap in the clinical, histologic, and immunologic manifestations of the vasculitides, and the causative agents that commonly cause these diseases are unknown. Consequently, there is no uniformly accepted classification scheme for this group of disorders. Those in general use today have differentiated vasculitis on the basis of (1) size and type of vessels involved, (2) distribution of organs affected, (3) histologic features of the process, and (4) abnormalities of certain laboratory parameters. Table 1 lists one classification scheme for the more common types of vasculitis.

EVALUATION

It is important to point out that large differences exist in the treatment of the various forms of vasculitis. Therefore, a thorough and complete evaluation to establish the diagnosis precisely, to determine the cause, and to define the extent to which other organs are involved is essential for optimizing therapy. In addition to a comprehensive history and physical examination, histologic analysis of evolving cutaneous lesions, or at times other organs, is crucial for delineating the precise form of vasculitis. Early evolving lesions are much more informative than are well-established ones. Specimens should be examined using routine histologic procedures and immunofluorescent techniques. Histopathologic specimens should include medium-sized vessels to distinguish small from medium-sized vessel vasculitis and should contain sufficient material to adequately characterize the nature of the inflammatory infiltrate. Direct immunofluorescent biopsies of skin for the demonstration of immunoglobulins and complement, if positive, are helpful in distinguishing IgA-associated cutaneous vasculitides and Henoch-Schönlein pupura (in which deposition of IgA predominates in the vessels) from other forms of vasculitis in which IgG or IgM deposition is more common.

Laboratory studies should include complete blood count with differential and platelets, urinalysis, blood urea nitrogen (BUN) and creatinine, liver function tests, hepatitis B surface antigen, erythrocyte sedimentation rate, tests for occult fecal blood, antinuclear antibodies, rheumatoid factor, cryoglobulins, complement components C3 and C4, streptozyme, throat culture, and chest roentgenogram. Antineutrophil cytoplasmic antibody (ANCA) is another important diagnostic study. This serologic test is positive in Wegener's granulomatosis but may also be found in other forms of vasculitis, in particular polyarteritis nodosa. In the appropriate clinical setting, it may be important to

TABLE 1. **Classification of Vasculitis**

Leukocytoclastic vasculitis (hypersensitivity angiitis)
    Urticarial vasculitis
    Henoch-Schönlein purpura
    Essential mixed cryoglobulinemia
    Serum sickness
    Erythema elevatum diutinum
    Secondary to
        Infection
        Drugs, medications, and chemicals
        Connective tissue diseases
        Malignancy
        Other causes
    Idiopathic
Systemic necrotizing vasculitis
    Polyarteritis nodosa
    Allergic angiitis and granulomatosis of Churg-Strauss
    Polyangiitis overlap syndrome
Wegener's granulomatosis
Giant cell arteritis*
Takayasu arteritis*
Buerger's disease*
Behçet's disease
Kawasaki disease
Miscellaneous vasculitides

*Not covered in this article.

obtain blood for serum protein electrophoresis and serum immunoelectrophoresis as well.

TREATMENT

Leukocytoclastic Vasculitis (Hypersensitivity Angiitis)

This condition is composed of vasculitic syndromes involving small vessels. Urticarial vasculitis, Henoch-Schönlein purpura, cryoglobulinemia, serum sickness, erythema elevatum diutinum, and secondary syndromes associated with connective tissue disease, infection, drug, or malignancy are all types of leukocytoclastic vasculitis. Clinically, cutaneous manifestations predominate, although joint, kidney, gastrointestinal tract, lung, central and peripheral nervous system, and heart may also be targets. In the skin, dependent areas of the body, in particular the lower legs, are most commonly affected. The most characteristic cutaneous manifestation of leukocytoclastic vasculitis is palpable purpura, consisting of non-blanchable, slightly elevated erythematous papules. However, lesions may also take the form of nodules, ulcers, hemorrhagic bullae, vesicles, or urticaria. Occasionally, gangrenous changes may develop in the digits where there is little collateral circulation. This results from ischemia due to thromboses and vessel wall damage caused by the inflammation.

When a cause has been determined, leukocytoclastic vasculitis will resolve when the underlying disorder has been treated or the causative agent removed. Thus, a careful search for causative factors should be undertaken. However, consideration should be given to the fact that in 40 to 60% of cases, no causative agent can be found. Generally, treatment should be conservative, since most cases are self-limited. Leg elevation and reduction in the level of normal activities should be recommended to the patient. Topical steroids have little role in the management of vasculitis. In patients with mild disease of recent onset, nonsteroidal anti-inflammatory agents are often tried but rarely result in significant improvement when used alone. H_1 and H_2 antihistamines have not been found to be particularly effective, and their role is largely limited to providing symptomatic relief of any associated pruritus. The one exception to this is in urticarial vasculitis, a form of leukocytoclastic vasculitis in which persistent urticarial lesions predominate. In that disease, antihistamines do seem to have a therapeutic role.

Colchicine* is recommended as a first-line agent in leukocytoclastic vasculitis. It attenuates the inflammatory response but does not appear to influence formation of circulating immune complexes. Most patients will have at least a partial response to 0.6 mg twice daily and should begin to respond within 1 to 2 weeks. Gastrointestinal complaints—diarrhea, nausea, and vomiting—are the most common side effects, but are infrequent unless higher doses are used. Colchicine is contraindicated for women of

*Not FDA-approved for this indication.

childbearing age unless contraception is reasonably ensured. It has also been shown to cause azoospermia in men. Rarely, bone marrow suppression has been reported, so patients on long-term therapy should have complete blood counts monitored every 3 to 4 months.

Dapsone* is also commonly employed in mild to moderate cases of leukocytoclastic vasculitis and is particularly effective for erythema elevatum diutinum, an uncommon form that results in tender red to violaceous papules and plaques distributed symmetrically over extensor surfaces of the distal extremities. Like colchicine, dapsone exerts its therapeutic effect by inhibiting the inflammatory response. Most patients with leukocytoclastic vasculitis respond to doses of 100 to 150 mg per day. Larger doses (200 to 300 mg per day) may be necessary to achieve a therapeutic response in some patients, but higher doses are associated with a greater incidence of hemolysis, methemoglobinemia, leukopenia, peripheral neuropathy, and hepatitis, which are the main side effects of the drug. Dapsone is contraindicated in patients with an inherited deficiency of glucose-6-phosphate dehydrogenase (G6PD), because it predisposes them to hemolytic anemia. Accordingly, all patients should be screened for G6PD deficiency prior to initiation of therapy. Agranulocytosis and other blood dyscrasias occur rarely. Complete blood counts should be monitored weekly during the first month of therapy, monthly for the next 6 months, and semimonthly thereafter. Liver function tests should be monitored periodically as well.

Another therapeutic option in mild to moderate vasculitis is low-dose methotrexate (Rheumatrex). An oral regimen of 7.5 to 15 mg per week tapered over several months has been shown efficacious in both rheumatoid and urticarial vasculitis. A combination that has been used successfully to treat erythema elevatum diutinum is tetracycline, 250 mg four times daily, and niacinamide, 100 mg three times daily.

When cutaneous involvement is severe, such as incipient gangrenous changes in the digits, or when there is significant involvement of other organ systems, participation of physicians experienced in the management of severe vasculitis is warranted. Systemic corticosteroids are generally indicated. Therapy with oral prednisone is usually initiated at a dose of 40 to 60 mg per day, but this may need to be increased if no response occurs. Attempts should be made to taper the steroids as rapidly as possible to prevent long-term complications of this medication, which include immunosuppression, osteoporosis, diabetes mellitus, hypertension, glaucoma, and cataracts.

In severe cases, immunosuppressive agents may also be added to the regimen. The therapeutic effect of these agents may not be observed for 4 to 6 weeks after therapy is begun. Cyclophosphamide (Cytoxan)* at 2 mg per kg and azathioprine (Imuran)* in doses ranging from 100 to 200 mg daily are most frequently employed. The main complications of cyclophosphamide therapy include lymphocytopenia, granulocytopenia, thrombocytopenia, and hemorrhagic cystitis. The incidence of hemorrhagic cystitis can be reduced by maintaining a high fluid intake. Prolonged cyclophosphamide therapy has been associated with an increased incidence of malignancies. Azathioprine also produces lymphocytopenia, granulocytopenia, and thrombocytopenia but is not associated with hemorrhagic cystitis. It may, however, be toxic to the liver and pancreas. Patients on all forms of immunosuppressive therapy for vasculitis should be monitored closely to avoid excessive reductions in their blood counts. Individuals treated with azathioprine should additionally be monitored for abnormalities in liver function tests.

Systemic Necrotizing Vasculitis

Systemic necrotizing vasculitides (polyarteritis nodosa, allergic angiitis and granulomatosis of Churg-Strauss, and polyangiitis overlap syndrome) involve medium-sized vessels with or without small vessel involvement. Histologically, there is an acute inflammatory infiltrate. Cutaneous lesions typically take the form of dermal and subcutaneous nodules, ulcers, and livedo reticularis. Purpura, papules, bullae, and urticaria may also occur in these patients. Systemic involvement is the rule, although polyarteritis nodosa localized to the skin and isolated to other single organs has been described. The disease has been associated with infection with hepatitis B and human immunodeficiency virus (HIV), hyposensitization therapy, collagen vascular diseases, intravenous administration of amphetamines, and serous otitis media.

For patients without significant systemic involvement, therapy should be initiated with systemic corticosteroids alone. The usual dose of prednisone is 1 mg per kg daily. The patient should be maintained on this dose for 1 to 2 months and, depending on the response, should be converted to alternate-day therapy for several months. The dose should be tapered to the lowest amount required to maintain control of the disease. If there is no improvement within 1 week or if there are signs of severe systemic involvement, it is important to add cyclophosphamide* to the regimen. The usual dose is 2 mg per kg daily. Cytotoxic drugs such as cyclophosphamide should be administered only by physicians experienced with the use of these agents. In addition, given the potential for end-organ dysfunction and possible side effects of cytotoxic therapy, a multidisciplinary team approach is essential in the management of these patients. Patients placed on these drugs should be monitored for potential complications as described earlier.

---

*Not FDA-approved for this indication.

*Not FDA-approved for this indication.

Plasmapheresis has been employed for recalcitrant vasculitis unresponsive to other measures. Its role in the management of vasculitis should be considered only when all other therapeutic modalities fail.

Wegener's Granulomatosis

Wegener's granulomatosis is a necrotizing granulomatous vasculitis of the small vessels that primarily involves the upper respiratory tract, lungs, and kidneys. Cutaneous lesions are present in 40 to 50% of patients and may take the form of papules and plaques with ulcerations, urticarial lesions, purpura, and subcutaneous nodules.

Wegener's granulomatosis is a serious disease that requires aggressive therapy. The mortality rate is greater than 90% in patients in whom the disease is untreated. Fortunately, the combination of prednisone and cyclophosphamide* will induce remissions in more than 90% of patients. Controlled clinical trials have clearly demonstrated the superiority of combined therapy with cyclophosphamide and prednisone over treatment with prednisone alone. Therapy should be initiated with prednisone at a dose of 1 mg per kg per day and with cyclophosphamide at 2 to 4 mg per kg daily. As with the more severe cases of systemic necrotizing vasculitis, experience with cyclophosphamide and a multidisciplinary team approach are essential. Special attention should be paid to the pulmonary and renal complications of the disease.

When patients are unable to tolerate standard doses of cyclophosphamide, pulse cyclophosphamide therapy has been used successfully. Preliminary results with methotrexate have also been promising.

Behçet's Disease

Behçet's disease is characterized by a symptom complex of oral aphthae and two of the following: genital ulcers, arthritis, posterior uveitis, cutaneous pustular vasculitis, and meningoencephalitis. The cutaneous lesions begin as a leukocytoclastic vasculitis and evolve into a lymphocytic vasculitis.

Patients with mucocutaneous complications of the disease are often treated with topical steroids such as desoximetasone 0.25% (Topicort) cream or ointment for cutaneous lesions and triamcinolone in Orabase (Kenalog in Orabase) for oral involvement. Intralesional triamcinolone (3 mg per mL) is also commonly employed. Topical anesthetic agents are often applied for symptomatic relief of oral ulcerations. In cases unresponsive to topical and intralesional steroids, colchicine* (0.6 mg two to three times daily) may be used to treat the disease. Dapsone* in doses similar to those employed for leukocytoclastic vasculitis (see earlier) is an alternative therapeutic option.

Ocular and neurologic complications are the major sources of morbidity and are associated with a poorer prognosis. Thus, more aggressive therapy is warranted. Management, in general, should include physicians skilled in the care of ophthalmic and/or neurologic complications. Treatment options include systemic prednisone therapy alone or in combination with cytotoxic agents (azathioprine, cyclophosphamide, chlorambucil [Leukeran]*) or cyclosporine (Sandimmune).*

Kawasaki Disease

Kawasaki disease, or mucocutaneous lymph node syndrome, is primarily a disease of children under the age of 5 years, although the disease has been reported in young adults as well. The diagnostic criteria include fever of 5 days' duration or greater without another cause and four or more of the following criteria: bilateral nonexudative conjunctival congestion, oropharyngeal changes (reddening or fissuring of the lips, injection of the oropharyngeal mucosa, "strawberry" tongue), erythema of the palms and soles, hand or foot edema, periungual desquamation, a polymorphous exanthem, and nonsuppurative cervical lymphadenopathy. The disease can also be diagnosed with less than four of these criteria when coronary artery aneurysms are demonstrated on two-dimensional echocardiography or coronary angiography. The disease is classified as a vasculitis because the characteristic histopathologic feature in many of the organs involved is a vasculitis of small vessels and of the intima and vasovasorum of larger arteries. The mucocutaneous lesions, however, do not appear to be vasculitic in origin, at least from a histopathologic standpoint.

Kawasaki disease is usually a self-limited process. However, 1 to 2% of patients develop severe involvement of the coronary arteries, which at times leads to myocardial infarction. The goal of therapy is to prevent or minimize this potentially devastating complication. Aspirin (80 to 100 mg per kg daily) is the mainstay of treatment. The objective is to attain a blood salicylate level of 20 to 25 mg per dL. In this dose range, aspirin also provides symptomatic relief for the joint pains, malaise, and fever. It has been recommended that aspirin be continued after defervescence at a dose range of 3 to 5 mg per kg because of its antiplatelet effects.

Several studies have shown that the addition of high-dose intravenous gamma globulin* (Gamimune N, Gammagard, intravenous Sandoglobulin, 400 mg per kg daily for 4 days) will further reduce the incidence of coronary artery abnormalities. There is no role for the use of corticosteroids in Kawasaki disease, and their use may actually increase the risk of cardiac complications.

Treatment of the mucocutaneous manifestations is largely symptomatic, with emollients (e.g., Moisturel cream or lotion, Eucerin lotion) and mild to moderate topical steroid preparations (desonide cream 0.05% [DesOwen, Tridesilon], triamcinolone cream 0.025%

---

*Not FDA-approved for this indication.

*Not FDA-approved for this indication.

[Kenalog], mometasone furoate [Elocon]). Antihistamines, such as diphenhydramine (Benadryl) and hydroxyzine (Atarax) work well for control of pruritus.

POLYARTERITIS NODOSA AND CUTANEOUS POLYARTERITIS NODOSA

method of
KAREN A. HEIDELBERG, M.D.
Mayo Graduate School of Medicine
Rochester, Minnesota

and

W. P. DANIEL SU, M.D.
Mayo Clinic and Mayo Foundation
Rochester, Minnesota

POLYARTERITIS NODOSA

Polyarteritis nodosa (PAN) is a necrotizing vasculitis of small and medium-sized arteries that can be life-threatening. This disease can affect any organ system, although the lung and spleen are usually spared. The incidence of polyarteritis nodosa is unknown; however, it is most commonly reported in middle-aged men. The cause of PAN is not well understood. Reports of the disease developing after an infectious process such as hepatitis B, streptococcal infections, and otitis media support the suggestion of an immune complex process.

Presentation

Patients with PAN can present with nonspecific symptoms and signs, making diagnosis difficult and often delaying it. The most commonly involved organs and organ systems are the kidneys, heart, liver, gastrointestinal tract, testes, and peripheral and central nervous systems. The skin is involved in 20 to 40% of cases. In addition to the clinical manifestations caused by organ involvement, nonspecific constitutional symptoms often occur. Clinical manifestations of the disease often include renal failure and hypertension owing to renal involvement. Congestive heart failure, myocardial infarction, and pericarditis may occur as a result of cardiac involvement. Nausea, vomiting, and abdominal pain are not uncommon with gastrointestinal tract involvement. Finally, patients often present with symptoms of mononeuritis multiplex, which indicates involvement of the nervous system. The cutaneous findings associated with the disease are variable; however, they are most commonly found on the lower extremity. Patients often present with painful nodules and ulcerations on a background of livedo reticularis. Palpable purpura is also seen.

Diagnosis

There are no diagnostic serologic tests for PAN. Diagnosis is based on the finding of inflammation and destruction of medium-sized muscular arteries on biopsy of involved organs. If tissue is not easily accessible from involved organs, visceral angiography should be considered. Aneurysmal dilatation in medium-sized arteries is characteristic of PAN. It is unusual to find changes on angiography without signs and symptoms of visceral involvement. Associated laboratory findings correlate with the underlying features of the disease; however, they are not diagnostic. As expected, patients often have an elevated erythrocyte sedimentation rate, leukocytosis, thrombocytosis, anemia, and decreased levels of albumin. In addition, patients present with laboratory findings suggestive of visceral organ involvement, that is, elevated results of liver function tests and abnormal results of urinalysis. Eosinophilia is usually not found in PAN; if present, it should suggest an alternative diagnosis.

Treatment

PAN should be diagnosed as early as possible and treated aggressively. Management of PAN depends on the extent of the disease and the rate of progression at the time of diagnosis. Initial management for limited nonprogressive disease includes high doses of corticosteroids. The initial dose is 60 mg of prednisone or 100 mg of hydrocortisone per day in divided doses. This dose should be continued for approximately 3 to 6 months. As the clinical status improves and the sedimentation rate normalizes, the dose can be slowly tapered. The dose should be reduced by 5 to 10 mg every 2 weeks until 15 mg per day is reached. At that time, a slower taper can be started. Too rapid a taper results in flaring of the disease. Long-term therapy should be continued with the lowest possible dose of prednisone. Patients generally do not do well with every-other-day dosing or once-a-day dosing of prednisone unless they have limited disease. Combination therapy with corticosteroids and platonin, a photosensitive dye, has been reported to have good results in a pediatric patient with PAN.

Patients with extensive disease and evidence of progression may require the addition of a steroid-sparing agent. Cyclophosphamide (Cytoxan)* or azathioprine (Imuran) can be selected. In combination, prednisone should be given at a dose of 60 mg per day in divided doses. After approximately 1 month, the prednisone can be given every other day at the same dose, followed by tapering and discontinuation over a 6-month period. Cyclophosphamide is given at a dose of 1 to 2 mg per kg per day. The dose should be adjusted to maintain a neutrophil count at 1500 per µL. Cyclophosphamide should be continued for 1 year after complete remission of the disease. At that time, the medication can be slowly tapered. Azathio-

---

*Not FDA-approved for this indication.

prine can be given at the same dosage as cyclophosphamide.

Clinicians who prescribe cyclophosphamide and azathioprine should be aware of their potential side effects. Patients treated with cyclophosphamide should have a hematologic profile monitored regularly. Urine should be examined on a regular basis to rule out hemorrhagic cystitis. Patients being treated with azathioprine should have a complete blood cell count, including platelets, weekly during the first month of treatment, twice a month during the second and third months of treatment, and then on a monthly basis.

CUTANEOUS POLYARTERITIS NODOSA

Cutaneous polyarteritis nodosa (C-PAN) is a distinct clinical entity. This disease, unlike its systemic counterpart, has no visceral lesions and has a benign clinical course. Although there is no visceral involvement, extracutaneous manifestations occur. These include arthralgias, arthritis, and neuropathy. Clinically, patients have painful nodules on the lower extremities that are often complicated by ulcerations. The patients experience periods of exacerbations and remissions of the disease. This course has been noted in some patients with or without treatment. As with classic PAN, C-PAN is diagnosed with biopsy of the involved area.

Treatment of the disease depends on the severity of symptoms. Initial management can be conservative, with local management of the ulcers and medication for adequate pain control (salicylates). This therapy is sometimes sufficient. If conservative measures are inadequate, patients generally respond to oral prednisone, 40 to 60 mg a day in divided doses. As the clinical symptoms improve, the dose can be slowly tapered to the lowest necessary dose for disease control. It is usually necessary to continue corticosteroid therapy for 3 to 6 months. Sulfapyridine*, in dosages of 500 mg four times a day, or dapsone,† 100 to 150 mg per day, also has given excellent results in the treatment of C-PAN.

Several patients have been noted to have elevated antistreptolysin titers, and disease flares have been associated with streptococcal infections. These patients have responded well to treatment with penicillin G. Successful treatment has been reported with pentoxifylline (Trental)† at a dosage of 400 mg three times a day, and this is gradually tapered after a clinical response is observed. Some patients with C-PAN may require only nicotinic acid,† 300 mg per day in divided doses, to achieve remission. However, occasionally, patients may be resistant to therapy and require a combination of systemic corticosteroids and dapsone or sulfapyridine or other immunosuppressive agent.

---

*Investigational drug in the United States.
†Not FDA-approved for this indication.

DISEASES OF THE NAILS

method of
ANTONELLA TOSTI, M.D., and
BIANCA MARIA PIRACCINI, M.D.
University of Bologna
Bologna, Italy

The nail unit consists of four specialized epithelia: the nail matrix, the nail bed, the proximal nail fold, and the hyponychium. The nail matrix is a germinative epithelial structure that gives rise to a fully keratinized multilayered sheet of cornified cells: the nail plate. In longitudinal sections the nail matrix consists of a proximal and a distal region. Because the vertical axes of nail matrix cells are oriented diagonally and distally, proximal nail matrix keratinocytes produce the upper portion of the nail plate. The lower portion of the nail plate derives from distal nail matrix keratinocytes. Replacement of a fingernail usually requires about 6 months, and replacement of a toenail requires 12 to 18 months. The peculiar kinetics of nail matrix keratinization explain why diseases of the proximal nail matrix result in nail plate surface abnormalities whereas diseases of the distal matrix result in abnormalities of the ventral nail plate or the nail free edge or both.

Nail plate corneocytes are tightly connected by desmosomes and complex digitations.

The nail plate is a rectangular, translucent, and transparent structure that appears pink because of the vessels of the underlying nail bed. The proximal part of the nail plate of the fingernails, especially the thumbs, shows a whitish, opaque, half-moon-shaped area, the lunula, that corresponds to the visible portion of the distal nail matrix. The shape of the lunula determines the shape of the free edge of the plate. The nail plate is firmly attached to the nail bed, which partially contributes to nail formation along its length. The longitudinal orientation of the capillary vessels in the nail bed explains the linear pattern of the nail bed hemorrhages. Proximally and laterally the nail plate is surrounded by the nail folds. The horny layer of the proximal nail fold forms the cuticle, which intimately adheres to the underlying nail plate and prevents its separation from the proximal nail fold. Distally the nail bed continues with the hyponychium, which marks the separation of the nail plate from the digit. The nail plate grows continuously and uniformly throughout life. Average nail growth is faster in fingernails (3 mm per month) than in toenails (1 to 1.5 mm per month).

BRITTLE NAILS

Nail brittleness causes several clinical symptoms including splitting, softening, lamellar exfoliation, and onychorrhexis.

Brittle nails are a common complaint. They are often an idiopathic condition but can also be a symptom of a large number of dermatologic nail disorders. Although brittle nails have been linked with many internal diseases, the high frequency of nail fragility in the general population makes it difficult to prove the validity of any such association. Environmental and occupational factors that produce a progressive dehydration of the nail plate play an important role in the development of idiopathic nail brittleness. Management of brittle nails requires preventive and protective measures to avoid nail plate dehydration. Patients should wear cotton gloves under rubber gloves during household chores, avoid frequent hand-washing, and keep their nails short. Nail varnishes may be protective, but the use of nail varnish removers should be avoided because it exacerbates brittleness.

Local therapies are useful in the treatment of nail brittleness. Application of hydrophilic petrolatum (Aquaphor) on wet nails at bedtime helps to retain the moisture in the nail plate. Regular application of topical preparations containing hydrophilic substances such as hyaluronic acid, alpha-hydroxy acids, and proteoglycans may favor nail plate rehydration.

An oral treatment with biotin,* 2.5 mg per day for several months, can be useful because it may improve the synthesis of the lipid molecules that produce binding between nail plate corneocytes. A solution of 5% aluminum chloride in propylene glycol and water may improve soft nails. This solution should be applied daily.

ACUTE PARONYCHIA

Acute paronychia is usually caused by *Staphylococcus aureus*, although other bacteria and herpes simplex virus may occasionally be responsible. A minor trauma commonly precedes the development of the infection. The affected digit shows an acute inflammation with erythema, swelling, pus formation, and pain. Whenever possible cultures should be taken. Treatment includes local medications with antiseptics, the administration of systemic antibiotics, and incision and drainage of the abscess.

Acute digital ischemia may present with a clinical picture that closely resembles that of acute paronychia. In ischemia, however, the affected digit is cold.

CHRONIC PARONYCHIA

Chronic paronychia is an inflammatory disorder of the proximal nail fold typically affecting patients whose hands are continually exposed to a wet environment and multiple microtraumas that favor cuticle damage. When the cuticle is damaged or lost, the epidermal barrier of the proximal nail fold is destroyed and the proximal nail fold is suddenly exposed to a large number of environmental hazards. Irritants and allergens may easily penetrate the proximal nail fold and produce a contact dermatitis that is responsible for the chronic inflammation. An immediate hypersensitivity reaction to food ingredients is commonly observed. Clinically the proximal and lateral nail folds show mild erythema and swelling. The cuticle is lost and the ventral portion of the proximal nail fold becomes separated from the nail plate. With time the nail fold retracts and becomes thickened and rounded. The nail plate frequently shows transverse grooves and discoloration of the

---

*Not FDA-approved for this indication.

lateral margins. Onychomadesis may be the result of a severe inflammatory exacerbation. The course of chronic paronychia is frequently interspersed with self-limited episodes of painful acute inflammation due to secondary *Candida* and bacterial infections.

Patients with chronic paronychia should avoid a wet environment, chronic microtrauma, and contact with irritants or allergens.

High-potency topical steroids (clobetasol propionate 0.05% [Temovate ointment]) once a day at bedtime are an effective first-line therapy. If *Candida* is present a topical imidazole derivative should be applied in the morning. Topical antifungals alone and systemic antifungals are not useful. In severe cases systemic steroids (prednisone 20 mg per day) can be given for a few days to obtain a prompt reduction of inflammation and pain.

Acute exacerbations of chronic paronychia do not necessitate antibiotic treatment because they subside spontaneously in a few days. Complete recovery from the condition usually requires several weeks, and treatment should be continued until the cuticle has regrown. Recurrences are frequent because the barrier function of the proximal nail fold may be impaired for months or even years after an episode of chronic paronychia.

ONYCHOLYSIS

Onycholysis is the detachment of the nail plate from the nail bed. Starting from the central or lateral portion of the nail plate free margin, onycholysis progresses proximally and can even involve the whole nail. The onycholytic area looks whitish because of the presence of air under the detached nail plate. It may occasionally show a greenish or brown discoloration due to colonization of the onycholytic space by chromogenic bacteria (*Pseudomonas aeruginosa*), molds, or yeasts. Onycholysis may be idiopathic or represent a symptom of numerous diseases such as psoriasis, onychomycosis, contact dermatitis, or drug reactions. The pathogenesis of idiopathic onycholysis is still unknown. A water-borne environment facilitates the development of this condition, which is much more frequent in homemakers. We found Zaias's suggestion of using a hair dryer to dry the subungual area after immersion in water very useful. The detached nails should be cut away, and this procedure should be repeated until the nail plate grows attached. A symptomatic treatment with a topical antiseptic solution (thymol 4% in chloroform) or a topical imidazole derivative can be prescribed. *Pseudomonas* colonization can be treated with sodium hypochlorite solution (Milton's solution) or 2% acetic acid.

ONYCHOMYCOSIS

The term "onychomycosis" describes the infection of the nail by fungus. Almost all cases of onychomycosis, however, result from a dermatophytic invasion of the nail; onychomycosis due to nondermatophytic molds or yeasts is rare.

Dermatophytes may be responsible for three different types of onychomycosis: white superficial onychomycosis, distal subungual onychomycosis, and proximal subungual onychomycosis.

In white superficial onychomycosis, dermatophytes colonize the most superficial layers of the nail plate without penetrating it. For this reason white superficial onychomycosis is easily cured by any topical antifungal after scraping the affected nail plate surface.

Treatment of distal subungual onychomycosis and proximal subungual onychomycosis requires the administration of a systemic antifungal. Griseofulvin (Grifulvin V) 1 to 2 grams per day should be administered for 6 months in fingernail onychomycosis and up to 12 months in toenail onychomycosis. About 50% of toenail infections, however, fail to respond to griseofulvin, and recurrences are frequently observed even in patients who have had a complete cure.

In the last few years, three new systemic antimycotics have been introduced on the market: fluconazole, itraconazole, and terbinafine. All these drugs have been shown to reach the distal nail soon after the therapy is started and to persist in the nail plate for a long time (2 to 6 months) after interruption of treatment. The persistence of high post-treatment drug levels in the nail permits shorter therapies with a lower incidence of relapses and side effects. Partial nail avulsion and concomitant treatment with a topical antifungal agent further reduce relapses and the duration of treatment.

Fluconazole (Diflucan)* and itraconazole (Sporanox)* are triazole derivatives with broad-spectrum fungistatic activity. Fluconazole 150 mg given once weekly or 100 mg every other day for 3 to 6 months has been successfully tried in a limited number of patients.

Itraconazole is effective at dosages of 200 mg per day for 2 (fingernail infections) or 3 to 4 months (toenail infections). The drug should be administered with a fat meal to improve its absorption. Concurrent intake of antacids and H_2 blockers reduces itraconazole absorption. Itraconazole interferes with the clearance of terfenadine, calcium channel blockers, and cyclosporin A.

Terbinafine (Lamisil)† is an allylamine derivative with primary fungicidal properties against dermatophytes. Recommended dosages are 250 mg per day for 2 (fingernail infections) or 3 to 4 months (toenail infections). Terbinafine absorption is not affected by the ingestion of food, but the drug delays gastric emptying. About 5% of patients receiving the drug experience nausea, fullness, or dyspepsia.

Both itraconazole and terbinafine are also effective when given as intermittent or pulse therapy. Intermittent itraconazole is given at a dosage of 400 mg daily for 1 week every month for 2 (fingernail infec-

tions) or 3 to 4 months (toenail infections). Intermittent terbinafine is administered at a dose of 500 mg daily for 1 week every month for 2 (fingernail infections) or 3 to 4 months (toenail infections). Patients should be followed for 4 to 8 months after discontinuation of treatment to confirm the efficacy of treatment.

Accelerated nail growth has been reported during and after itraconazole treatment.

Both itraconazole and terbinafine are very well tolerated. Most adverse reactions are of mild severity: gastrointestinal disturbances, pruritus, skin rashes, headache. A transitory loss of taste is not rare during terbinafine treatment. Symptomatic or asymptomatic hepatic damage is very rare with both drugs, and laboratory monitoring of patients during treatment is not mandatory.

In our experience a complete cure of toenail onychomycosis is more frequently obtained using continuous than intermittent therapy, the percentage of patients who are completely cured being around 75% with continuous and 50% with intermittent treatment.

Recurrences can be prevented by the regular application of topical antifungals on the previous affected nails, soles, and toe webs. When distal subungual onychomycosis involves only the distal two-thirds of a few nails, a topical therapy with 5% amorolfine nail lacquer (Loceryl),* 8% ciclopirox nail solution, or bifonazole 1% in 40% urea ointment* may be prescribed as an alternative to systemic antifungals. Data about the efficacy of these new topical drugs are, however, still scarce. Although they have been reported to be effective in a proportion of patients, further studies are needed for a final judgment. Amorolfine 5% nail lacquer has the advantage of requiring weekly instead of daily application.

Onychomycosis due to nondermatophytic molds is usually resistant to systemic antimycotics. Chemical avulsion of the affected nail can be useful in some cases.

Onychomycosis of chronic mucocutaneous candidiasis can be treated with ketoconazole (Nizoral), 400 mg daily, or itraconazole, 200 mg daily, the latter being safer from side effects.

PSORIASIS

Because the treatment of nail psoriasis is always disappointing, before a therapy is started the individual problems of every patient, and in particular the degree of discomfort that results from the nail lesions, should be considered. Reassuring the patient is probably the best approach for isolated nail pitting, oily patches, mild onycholysis, and splinter hemorrhages. However, diffuse onycholysis, subungual hyperkeratosis, and severe nail plate surface abnormalities may require a therapeutic approach.

Local therapy of nail psoriasis is scarcely effective and only rarely induces a complete remission of the

*Not FDA-approved for this indication.
†Not available in the United States.

*Not available in the United States.

disease. Topical steroids or combinations of topical steroids with salicylic acid or retinoic acid, or both, are widely prescribed. Their efficacy is poor, even when they are applied with occlusive dressing after chemical or mechanical avulsion of the onycholytic nail plate. Long-term application of topical steroids may result in a marked atrophy of the soft tissues of the digits or even in focal resorption of the distal phalanges. When onycholysis and subungual hyperkeratosis are prominent symptoms, topical calcipotriol (Dovonex) can be useful.

Intralesional injections of triamcinolone acetonide (Kenalog)* 2.5 mg per mL, have been proved effective in some cases of nail matrix psoriasis. However, routine use of this therapy is not recommended because of the pain caused by the injections, the local side effects (subungual hematoma, reversible atrophy, and hypopigmentation on the injection site), and relapses of the nail abnormalities after discontinuation of the therapy.

A systemic treatment with steroids, methotrexate, or cyclosporin A (Sandimmune)* can resolve the nail changes, but we recommend its use only when nail psoriasis is associated with widespread disease or psoriatic arthritis.

Retinoids are only of little value in the treatment of nail psoriasis. The administration of etretinate (Tigason) can even worsen the nail changes as a result of the development of nail brittleness, pyogenic pseudogranuloma, and chronic paronychia. Oral photochemotherapy is scarcely effective because of poor penetration of the ultraviolet A light (UVA) through the proximal nail fold and nail plate. Pustular psoriasis of the nail unit usually fails to respond to conventional topical treatments. Retinoids, systemic steroids, psoralen plus UVA (PUVA), and cyclosporine can arrest the development of pustular lesions and avoid permanent scarring of the nail apparatus.

LICHEN PLANUS

Specific nail involvement occurs in about 10% of patients with lichen planus, and permanent damage of at least one nail occurs in approximately 4% of patients. Most commonly, the nail changes consist of thinning, longitudinal ridging, and distal splitting of the nail plate. The severity of the disease may vary in degree from nail to nail and within the same nail. Onycholysis and subungual hyperkeratosis can also be seen. Erythematous patches in the lunula are occasionally present. Definitive destruction of the nail matrix is responsible for pterygium and onychoatrophy.

Systemic steroids are effective in treating nail lichen planus and in preventing destruction of the nail matrix. Oral prednisone, 0.5 mg per kg every other day for 2 to 8 weeks, or intramuscular triamcinolone acetonide, 0.5 mg per kg every month for 2 to 3 months, usually produces recovery of the nail abnormalities. Intralesional injections of triamcinolone

acetonide, 2.5 mg per mL, represent a possible, though painful, alternative when the disease is limited to a few fingernails. Mild relapses are frequently observed, but recurrences are usually responsive to therapy.

ALOPECIA AREATA (TWENTY NAIL DYSTROPHY)

Alopecia areata has been associated with a large number of nail changes including diffuse or localized color changes, nail plate surface abnormalities, and onychomadesis. Most commonly, alopecia areata of the nails produces a regular and superficial pitting that is due to focal involvement of the proximal nail matrix. A chronic and diffuse involvement of the nail apparatus causes twenty nail dystrophy (trachyonychia), which may occasionally be the only symptom of the disease. The nail plate surface is opaque, lusterless, and rough because of excessive longitudinal striation. The nail changes do not necessarily involve all twenty nails and may occasionally be limited to a few digits.

Trachyonychia is absolutely a benign condition that never causes nail scarring; the nail changes usually regress spontaneously in a few years. No treatment is recommended.

NAIL PIGMENTATION

The term "melanonychia" describes a brown-black discoloration of the nail plate. Longitudinal melanonychia may be caused by a focal activation of the nail matrix melanocytes or by nail matrix nevus or melanoma. Focal hyperactivity of the nail matrix melanocytes is usual in blacks and common in Japanese, but it is rare in whites. It may be seen in a large number of nail disorders or systemic conditions. It can also be a side effect of numerous drugs including cancer therapeutic agents and zidovudine (AZT).

Differential diagnosis between benign longitudinal melanonychia and melanoma may be impossible on a clinical basis.

Nail pigmentation due to drugs or systemic disorders is usually reversible after discontinuation of the drug or resolution of the associated disease.

YELLOW NAIL SYNDROME

The term "yellow nail syndrome" describes the association of slowly growing yellow nails with primary lymphedema and respiratory tract involvement. Nails are pale yellow to yellow-green, thickened, opaque, and excessively curved from side to side. Onycholysis is frequent. The nail changes may improve spontaneously or after resolution of the associated systemic disease. Oral vitamin E*† at dosages of 600 to 1200 IU daily for 6 to 18 months induces a complete clearing of the nail changes in some pa-

---

*Not FDA-approved for this indication.

---

*Not FDA-approved for this indication.
†Exceeds dosage recommended by the manufacturer.

tients. Although the mechanism of action of vitamin E in yellow nail syndrome is still unknown, antioxidant properties of alpha-tocoferol may account for its efficacy.

A 5% solution of vitamin E*† in dimethyl sulfoxide produced marked clinical improvement in a double-blind controlled study. The efficacy of topical vitamin E, however, still needs confirmation.

Itraconazole may improve yellow nail syndrome by enhancing nail growth.

INGROWN NAILS

Ingrown nails, which more commonly affect the great toe of young adults, are a common complaint. Hyperhidrosis, congenital malalignment, improper cutting of toenails, and unsatisfactory footwear all contribute to the development of this painful condition. The condition starts when spicules breaking off from the lateral edge of the nail plate penetrate into the tissues of lateral nail fold. In this phase the inflammatory reaction produces pain, redness, and swelling. Treatment is conservative and includes extraction of the embedded spicules and introduction of a package of nonabsorbent cotton (soaked in a disinfectant) under the corner of the nail to prevent further penetration of the lateral nail fold. This dressing should be replaced daily. In advanced stages, the lateral edge of the nail plate is enclosed in an overgrowth of granulation tissue that, with time, may become epithelialized. Although the application of high-potency steroids or cryosurgery may reduce the granulation tissue, surgical or chemical (phenol) partial matricectomy is necessary in most cases.

WARTS

Periungual and subungual warts are usually difficult to treat and frequently recur.

Routine treatments include cryosurgery, electrocautery and desiccation, CO_2 laser, and topical anti-wart solutions containing salicylic and lactic acids. Intralesional injections of bleomycin (Blenoxane)* have been successfully used to treat viral warts for many years. The powder should be diluted with saline to a concentration of 1 U per mL. This solution can be stored at $-20°$ C in glass for several months. Part of this solution should be further diluted to 0.1 to 0.5 U per mL and injected into multiple loci of the warts. Patients with vascular impairment and women of childbearing age should not be treated because the drug has been reported to produce Raynaud's disease and to be systemically absorbed.

A bifurcate vaccination needle can be used to introduce bleomycin (1 U per mL sterile saline solution) into warts using the multiple puncture technique suggested by Shelley.‡ After local anesthesia, the

bleomycin solution is dropped onto the wart, which is then punctured with a disposable bifurcated needle (Allergy Laboratory of Ohio, Inc.) approximately 40 times per 5-mm^2 area of the wart. No medications are required. Three weeks after treatment, the eschar can be pared away and the area examined for residual warts, which can be reinjected. This technique minimizes the amount of bleomycin introduced into the skin and avoids introduction of the drug into the dermis. Topical immunotherapy with strong topical sensitizers (squaric acid dibutylester [SADBE],* diphenylcyclopropenone) is an effective and painless method of treatment for multiple warts. We use SADBE or diphenylcyclopropenone 2% in acetone for sensitization. After 21 days, weekly applications are carried out with dilutions from 0.001 to 1% according to the patient's response. Complete cure usually requires 3 to 4 months.

Multiple warts can also be treated with cimetidine (Tagamet)†‡ 750 to 1200 mg daily for 3 to 4 months. The efficacy of the drug is possibly related to its immunomodulatory effects.

MYXOID CYSTS

Myxoid cysts are common benign tumors of the nail unit, most frequently affecting elderly women.

The cyst, which is usually located on the dorsal aspect of the distal phalanx, has a viscous, gelatinous content. Cysts localized in the proximal nail fold may compress the nail matrix and produce longitudinal depressions or grooves in the nail plate. The cysts frequently communicate with the distal phalangeal joint through a tract that pumps synovial fluid into the cysts.

Treatments of myxoid cysts include surgical excision, intralesional injections of triamcinolone acetonide (3 to 5 mg per mL), or sclerosing agents (1–3% solution of sodium tetradecyl sulfate [Sotradecol]* after evacuation of the cyst content with a sterile needle. Cryosurgery is effective but painful and is associated with considerable morbidity. Two 30-second freezes separated by 4 minutes of thaw time are usually necessary. Before freezing, it is advisable to express the cyst content and ask the patient to remove rings.

Unfortunately recurrence rates are high with any of the available treatments, and cysts frequently recur even after surgery if the tract leading from the cyst to the joint capsule is not dissected.

ONYCHOGRYPHOSIS

Chemical avulsion of the overgrowing nail plate is useful in onychogryphosis and provides considerable relief of the patient's discomfort. For chemical nail

---

*Not FDA-approved for this indication.
†Not available in the United States.
‡Shelley WB, Shelley ED: Intralesional bleomycin sulfate therapy for warts. Arch Dermatol 127:234–236, 1991.

---

*Not available in the United States.
†Not FDA-approved for this indication.
‡Orlow SJ, Paller A: Cimetidine therapy for multiple viral warts in children. J Am Acad Dermatol 28:794–796, 1993.

avulsion we usually use 40% urea in 60% white petrolatum.

Before the ointment is applied on the nail plate surface, the periungual skin should be covered with a plastic tape to avoid maceration. The urea ointment is then applied on the nail and covered with a plastic wrap. The medication is fixed to the digit with plastic tape and maintained in place for 7 to 10 days. At this time, the softened nail plate can easily be cut off using a nail clipper.

Chemical nail avulsion can also be successfully used to remove onychomycotic nails as well as thickened psoriatic nails.

NAIL BITING AND ONYCHOTILLOMANIA

Frequent application of distasteful topical preparations on the nail and periungual skin can discourage patients from biting and chewing their fingernails. Possible alternatives include:

1% clindamycin (Cleocin T)
Quaternary ammonium derivatives
4% quinine sulfate in petrolatum

Patients with severe onychophagia or onychotillomania can be helped in interrupting their habit by daily bandaging of the injured fingers with Micropore.

KELOIDS

method of
W. THOMAS LAWRENCE, M.P.H., M.D.
University of North Carolina
Chapel Hill, North Carolina

Keloids and hypertrophic scars are the end products of excessive wound healing. Wound healing is the body's biologic response to injury, and it generally results in the appropriate quantity of scar to heal a wound. Occasionally, for unknown reasons, the response may be more vigorous than is required for healing, and a keloid or a hypertrophic scar is produced.

There is no histologic or biochemical method to differentiate keloids from hypertrophic scars. They are differentiated on the basis of their gross appearance. Hypertrophic scars are raised scars confined to the limits of the original wound, whereas keloids are raised scars that extend beyond the boundaries of the wound that initiated them. Although the differentiation of keloids and hypertrophic scars is generally clear, often it is less obvious which type of lesion is represented.

The precise incidence of keloids is not known. They occur more commonly in some populations than others and are seen in 5 to 15% of individuals in high-risk populations. Darker-skinned individuals are at greater risk to develop both keloids and hypertrophic scars than are light-skinned individuals. People between the ages of 2 and 40 years are most likely to get hypertrophic scars or keloids. Excessive scarring is more common in the deltoid and sternal areas, where the skin is tight, than in other parts of the body. Hypertrophic scars differ from keloids in that they generally develop soon after a wound is created and sometimes improve with time, whereas keloids develop up to a year after wounding and rarely spontaneously recede. Hypertrophic scars more commonly develop across flexion surfaces.

ETIOLOGY AND BIOLOGY

The etiology of keloids and hypertrophic scars is unknown. The propensity to develop keloids is higher in some families, although no specific form of inheritance has been reliably demonstrated. Exposure to excessive skin tension, relative ischemia in the wound owing to the proliferation of perivascular cells, various hormonal abnormalities, autoimmune responses to any of a large number of substances, and infectious agents have all been postulated to be causative. No theory can reliably explain all cases that develop, suggesting a multifactorial etiology.

When keloids develop, the early phases of wound healing are normal. The pathology develops because collagen synthesis occurs more actively and persists for a longer period of time than in wounds that heal with normal scars. There is increasing evidence that keloid fibroblasts respond more actively to the stimulation of cytokines than fibroblasts from normal dermis. There may also be less functional collagenase in keloids owing to an increase in collagenase inhibitors such as alpha globulins. The result of increased synthesis and decreased collagen breakdown is whorls of excess collagen.

TREATMENT

Patients with keloids often seek treatment to alleviate the cosmetic deformity as well as the itching and pain associated with the keloid. Smaller keloids are amenable to intralesional injections of triamcinolone (Kenalog). Up to 3 mL of 40 mg per mL triamcinolone may be administered at 3-week intervals, with a 50 to 100% response rate. Skin atrophy and depigmentation can occur, however, particularly with repeated injections. Pressure, topical silicone gel, and radiation are several of the additional methods that have been successful as single-treatment modalities for smaller lesions. Larger keloids usually will not completely respond to nonsurgical treatment. If a keloid is surgically excised and no adjunctive treatment is given, approximately two-thirds will recur. Other ablative modalities, including lasers of various types and cryosurgery, have been used, although none has clearly demonstrated superiority to more traditional excisional methods.

Multiple adjunctive modalities have been combined with surgery, including pressure, radiation, intralesional triamcinolone, oral pentoxifylline, and topical Silastic gel. The great disparity in published results makes it difficult to state definitively that one combination of treatments is superior to another. No treatment is successful 100% of the time, however. Adjunctive radiation provides at least a theoretical risk of contributing to the development of skin cancers in the distant future. For that reason, many prefer to avoid radiation, or at least reserve it for the most recalcitrant keloids.

No available method can prevent keloids. Unnecessary incisions should be avoided in keloid-prone individuals. Incisions in high-risk individuals have been injected with triamcinolone or radiated prophylactically; although the approaches are reasonable, no study has proved that these modalities limit the development of keloids or hypertrophic scars.

WARTS
(Verruca Vulgaris)

method of
KAREN E. ZANOL, M.D.
University Hospital and Clinics
Columbia, Missouri

Warts are caused by human papillomavirus infection. They are common among children and young adults, with an incidence of 7 to 10% in this population. Although we have multiple treatment options, none has been shown to eradicate the virus, and persistence of virus in a subclinical state probably accounts for the high rate of recurrence. Long-term cure rates for any treatment modality rarely exceed the expected rate of natural resolution.

Warts are generally asymptomatic but may become painful in an area subject to trauma such as the sole of the foot. Two-thirds of all warts resolve spontaneously within 2 years without any treatment, but most patients desire treatment owing to impatience and perceived disfigurement. Choice of treatment modality depends on the age of the patient and the size, location, and number of the warts.

Diagnosis is usually straightforward; however, plantar warts may be difficult to distinguish from calluses or clavi (corns) without paring. Warts have visible thrombosed capillaries or pinpoint areas of bleeding after paring with a No. 15 blade. Clavi show only a central core of translucent skin.

Diagnosis should be questioned and a biopsy taken when a solitary wart does not respond to treatment. Squamous cell carcinoma or even melanoma can appear very much like verrucae, especially on the fingers and soles of the feet.

Wart resolution seems ultimately dependent on the function of the cellular immune system. The treatment of verrucae in patients with impaired cellular immunity can be challenging.

STANDARD THERAPY

Keratolytics

Topical application of keratolytic preparations is inexpensive and effective but requires daily applications over a period of 6 to 12 weeks. A preparation containing 17% salicylic acid, with or without 17% lactic acid, is applied to warts daily after soaking and paring. The best time for treatment is immediately after bathing when the thickened stratum corneum overlying the wart may be easily removed with a pumice stone or callus file. Salicylic acid is also available in a 40% plaster (Mediplast) that is applied directly to the wart and left on overnight. The primary difficulty with this therapy is getting the medicated patch to stay in place. If it slips away from the wart, surrounding healthy skin is irritated.

Topical keratolytics, used properly over 12 weeks, result in cure rates of 70 to 80% of hand warts and 80% of simple plantar warts. This is a very popular method of treatment in children, as it is less painful than most other treatments. It does, however, require a motivated parent and child to accomplish.

Cryotherapy

Freezing warts with liquid nitrogen is the most common method of office-based wart removal currently in use. It is reliably effective in 70 to 80% of patients, relatively well tolerated, and generally free of serious complications when used carefully. It is favored over other, more destructive modalities such as electrocautery and surgery because cryotherapy is less likely to result in permanent scarring. Liquid nitrogen can be applied using a cotton swab or a spray device. If a cotton-tipped applicator is used, the swab is dipped into a Styrofoam cup containing liquid nitrogen. A new swab is used for each application because papillomavirus can survive in liquid nitrogen and can be transmitted on the swab. The wart and a 1- to 2-mm margin of surrounding skin are frozen with a 30- to 45-second freeze-to-thaw time, either once or twice depending on the thickness of the wart. This is associated with immediate burning, stinging pain that lasts about 5 minutes. Dull, throbbing pain may continue for several hours but this is usually easily relieved by over-the-counter analgesics. Patients are warned about blister formation that may become hemorrhagic. Infection is extremely unusual. Patients are instructed to leave the blister intact. If it is very painful it may be drained, but the roof should be left in place as a natural dressing. The most common complication is hypopigmentation.

Particular caution is warranted when freezing over the digital nerves or nail matrices. These structures can be damaged if freezing is too aggressive. Cryotherapy is contraindicated in patients with conditions associated with cold intolerance such as Raynaud's disease.

Cure rates with cryotherapy drop if the interval between treatments is too long. Treating every 3 weeks until normal skin markings return is optimal. Patients may be asked to use keratolytics between treatments to potentiate therapy.

RESISTANT WARTS

Immunotherapy

Dinitrochlorobenzene (DNCB) is a potent contact sensitizer that is quite effective in treating resistant or widespread warts. It is particularly helpful when extensive periungual warts are present and there is increased risk of inducing permanent nail dystrophy or excessive pain with cryotherapy. The patient is sensitized on normal skin of the same limb as the warts, usually forearms or medial ankles, with 2% DNCB. Most patients will develop an allergic contact dermatitis in the area of application. When sensitization is successful, the chemical is applied directly to the warts on subsequent visits spaced 3 to 4 weeks apart. Warts disappear over an average of four to six treatments. This treatment is well tolerated by children with multiple warts. It is not painful, but bothersome allergic contact dermatitis may occur around warts. Patients are given topical steroids to have on hand should this become a problem.

Although this is an effective, well-tolerated procedure, multiple office visits are generally required. Another source of concern has centered around the fact that the chemical has a positive Ames test for mutagenicity. There is no evidence that DNCB constitutes any real danger, but this concern has led many to reserve its use for particularly resistant or widespread wart disease. Contact immunotherapy may also be accomplished with other chemicals such as diphenylcyclopropenone and squaric acid. These chemicals have a negative Ames test but cure rates are somewhat lower.

Bleomycin

Bleomycin (Blenoxane)* is an antibiotic type of chemotherapeutic agent injected in small quantities into resistant warts. Bleomycin sulfate at 0.5 to 1.0 U per mL is injected directly into the wart with a 30-gauge needle or is introduced with multiple punctures of a bifurcated vaccination needle after topical application. This treatment is highly effective and wart resolution is usually accomplished in one to three treatments. Because patients commonly experience significant pain on injection, we reconstitute bleomycin in 1% lidocaine. The total volume of the injection varies with wart size and is limited to 2 to 3 mL per visit. Because serious complications such as persistent Raynaud's disease and localized tissue necrosis may result, it is recommended that this technique be used by experts experienced in its application.

Carbon Dioxide Laser

The CO_2 laser has been used in the treatment of resistant warts. It offers a great degree of precision in tissue destruction and enjoys excellent short-term cure rates. Unfortunately, the long-term follow-up studies available show no fewer recurrences with laser therapy than with other destructive techniques. It is also expensive and permanent scarring is very common, particularly after treatment of hand warts. Careful protective equipment is required because intact human papillomavirus DNA has been recovered from the CO_2 laser plume during wart treatment.

FLAT WARTS

Because flat warts are indeed almost flat, it is easy to damage surrounding normal skin with conventional wart treatments and a different approach is needed. Tretinoin (Retin-A) cream 0.05% or 0.1% ap-

*Not FDA-approved for this indication.

plied daily will induce the mild inflammatory reaction needed to clear flat warts. Use of sunscreen is very important during treatment, as ultraviolet light exposure reliably spreads flat warts. If response has been poor after 6 to 10 weeks of tretinoin cream and sunscreen, daily application of 1 to 2% 5-fluorouracil cream can be added. Excessive irritation is the primary complication of topical 5-fluorouracil cream but persistent hyperpigmentation has also been reported. Very light application of liquid nitrogen to flat warts may also be considered in resistant cases.

ADDITIONAL THERAPIES

Cantharidin

Cantharidin (Cantharone) is a chemical derived from the blister beetle. It causes a bulla just under the epidermis and is generally painless to apply. It is applied in the office after paring, and treatment requires several office visits. The most problematic complication of this therapy is the formation of a ring of new warts surrounding the original wart.

Trichloroacetic Acid

Trichloroacetic acid in varying concentrations, usually 10 to 50%, causes tissue destruction on application and can be used for wart treatment. Penetration is difficult to control, however, and ulceration, pain, and scarring are common.

Suggestion

No discussion of the treatment of common warts would be complete without mention of the great power of suggestion. Studies suggest it is more helpful with children than with adults and explains the effectiveness of folk remedies. It can be used with any wart treatment by simply telling the patient that his or her warts will be gone after a specified period of treatment.

CONDYLOMATA ACUMINATA
(Genital Warts)

method of
KENNETH F. TROFATTER, JR., M.D., PH.D.
University of Tennessee Medical Center
Knoxville, Tennessee

Anogenital human papillomavirus (HPV) infections are among the most prevalent sexually transmitted diseases. The most recognizable manifestation of HPV infection is condylomata acuminata (genital warts); however, HPVs also play a role in the etiology of dysplastic and neoplastic conditions throughout the anogenital tract. Conservative estimates indicate that condylomata account for more than 2 million provider encounters, including 250,000 to 500,000 new patient visits, annually in the United States. Furthermore, at least 2 to 3% of women have abnormal Papanicolaou smears attributed to HPVs. Clearly, the economic burden imposed on the health care system by these viruses is enormous.

HPVs are highly contagious, with primary infectivity rates at least 60 to 70%. Infectious virus particles must reach the basal epithelium to establish infection, and this requires disruption of the superficial epithelium such as occurs during coitus. Casual contact and fomites may account for a small percentage of clinically significant infections. Following HPV infection, there is a "latency period" of about 4 to 12 weeks (range, 2 weeks to many years) before clinical manifestations develop. Presentation is commonly with exophytic lesion characteristic of condylomata acuminata. These are often pleomorphic, with gross and histopathologic features variably dependent on HPV type, site of infection, skin type, host response, age of the lesion, and numerous other factors such as tobacco use, pregnancy, concomitant infections, hormonal status, associated medical conditions, and immune suppression. Multiple sites of overt involvement are often found, particularly in women, and this usually represents only a small portion of the tissues infected with the virus. Common presenting complaints include genital and perianal pruritus, irritation, burning, pain, dyspareunia, postcoital bleeding, and copious, often chronic and unresponsive, vaginal discharge.

In patients who develop condylomata acuminata, spontaneous and inducible remission is common during the first 9 to 12 months. Disappearance of overt lesions is correlated with a marked decrease in infectivity, but resolution of lesions does not represent "cure" from HPV colonization. Remission seems to depend on the development and maintenance of an adequate and specific immune response to the virus. Indeed, factors associated with immune suppression, particularly of cell-mediated immunity, are correlated with more extensive disease, fewer spontaneous remissions, more frequent recurrences, resistance to therapy, and increased risk for dysplastic and invasive neoplastic sequelae. Despite common teaching, reinfection from the same sexual partner is probably not an important cause of recurrences.

More than 70 different HPV types have been identified, and about one-fourth of these have been implicated in anogenital disease. Molecular biologic characteristics of different HPVs have made it possible to group them as to those usually associated with "benign" conditions (HPV-6, -11, -42, -43, -44, and so on) and those more likely to be found in higher-grade dysplastic and neoplastic disease (HPV-16, -18, -31, -33, -35 and so on). The HPV-6/11 group is responsible for about 80% of genital disease, and infection is manifest primarily as condylomata. When associated with epithelial dysplasia, these viruses usually cause low-grade lesions with little risk for progression. The HPV-16/18 group is responsible for only 20% of anogenital disease but more than 50% of all dysplasia, and greater than 90% of all high-grade dysplasia of the cervix, vulva, anus, and penis. Although these viruses can cause exophytic lesions, they are often associated with macular or maculopapular disease. It must be emphasized that any of these HPVs may cause condylomata, and as many as 33% of patients will be colonized by more than one HPV type. Therefore, regardless of the appearance of disease, the apparent areas of involvement, and even the suspected HPV type grouping, reliable management decisions and follow-up cannot be based on these observations alone. Indeed, even microscopically, the complete spectrum of condylomata, dysplasia, and invasive carcinoma can be found at times in contiguous areas.

TREATMENT

Currently, there is no specific therapy for HPV infection. Remission, or "successful" therapy (i.e., elimination of gross lesions, minimizing infectivity, and preventing disease progression) probably depends on the development and maintenance of a specific immune response, regardless of therapeutic approach. Successful treatment, even with extensive involvement, can often be achieved with topical or other medical therapy early in the course of disease (less than 9 to 12 months). However, with chronic infections or when dysplastic or invasive conditions are present, surgical therapy, or a combined surgical/medical approach, is often necessary. Adjuncts to therapy include treating partners, discouraging smoking, diagnosing and treating underlying medical problems such as diabetes and thyroid disease, treating associated sexually transmitted diseases, and providing education, reassurance, and support. Common treatment modalities are presented next and general guidelines for their use given.

Podophyllin

Podophyllin compounds have antiproliferative, antimitotic, and intense local inflammatory activity. The inflammatory reaction probably enhances the immune response to HPV, occasionally resulting in improvement of lesions outside the treatment area. Unpurified podophyllin preparations are inexpensive and can be highly effective when dealing with early, extensive condylomata. To maximize response, the following approach is suggested: Clean areas to be treated with 5% acetic acid and dry; apply podophyllin (20 to 25%) (Podocon 25, Podofin), in benzoin; dry for 2 to 3 minutes; apply second coat of podophyllin; wash treated areas with plain soap and water in no more than 3 to 4 hours. Using this protocol, treatment is not repeated for at least 10 days. If remission does not occur with this regimen within one to four cycles, another treatment approach is usually necessary. Podophyllin can have hepatic, renal, and neural toxicity; therefore, the patient should receive counseling regarding potential side effects. Initial manifestations of systemic toxicity include nausea, vomiting, abdominal pain, and diarrhea.

Recently, podofilox, a purified podophyllotoxin derivative (Condylox) has become available for patient use on external lesions. This is applied twice daily for 3 days then not used for at least 4 days, and the cycle is repeated as needed. It generally causes less severe local reactions and pain than unpurified podophyllin compounds and has minimal systemic toxicity.

Overall response rates for podophyllin preparations are in the range of 30 to 90%; recurrences occur in about 33% of patients. Because of increased systemic absorption, podophyllin should be used very cautiously on mucosal surfaces. Podophyllin preparations are contraindicated for use in pregnancy.

Cantharidin

Although not widely employed for genital lesions, cantharidin (Cantharone 0.7%) may be used when podophyllin is contraindicated. Cantharidin is an extract from a South American beetle that causes a blistering reaction limited to the epithelium. Like podophyllin, it induces an intense inflammatory reaction that may enhance the development of a specific immune response to HPV. After cleaning the treatment area with 5% acetic acid, cantharidin should be applied sparingly to external lesions, allowed to dry, covered with an absorbent pad, and then washed off within 1 hour. It has no systemic toxicity when applied to the skin. The major local side effects are pruritus, irritation, and pain. Complete healing without scarring usually ensues within 7 to 14 days, and 3 to 4 weeks are recommended between treatments.

5-Fluorouracil

Another compound with both antiproliferative and local inflammatory activity is the pyrimidine antagonist 5-fluorouracil (5-FU). Alone, 5-FU is not recommended for the primary management of condylomata, but it may be useful when combined with ablative modalities. Application regimens are highly variable and depend to some extent on the sensitivity of the individual patient. For external therapy, 5-FU (Efudex) (2 or 5% solution or cream) is usually applied daily until erythema or desquamation develops, then not used again until healing ensues. On keratinized epithelia, major side effects include pain, swelling, pruritus, scaling, soreness, and occasionally scarring and hyperpigmentation. Systemic toxicity is rare. 5-FU was originally popularized for the management of vaginal mucosal disease, but this use is now discouraged. Severe local responses can result in chronically inflamed, poorly healed vaginal lesions and, occasionally, strictures and vaginal agglutination. Actual efficacy of 5-FU in management of condylomata is unknown, owing to a lack of controlled clinical trials. As with podophyllin, 5-FU is contraindicated for use in pregnancy.

Ablative Therapy

With limited internal and external lesions of any age, application of trichloroacetic acid (TCA), cryotherapy, electrosurgery, and even local excision are reasonable approaches with comparable clearance and recurrence rates. Of these, TCA (Tri-Chlor) is particularly convenient for treating more extensive external and anogenital mucosal condylomata because it can be rapidly applied. Indeed, since it can be used to treat diffuse vaginal disease with minimal discomfort and is not absorbed systemically, TCA has become the treatment of choice for pregnant women. Results can be optimized if the treatment areas are first cleansed with 5% acetic acid and TCA is applied directly to the lesion and in a 1-to-2mm margin around its base. There is no need to wash TCA off once it has been applied. Pain associated with application of TCA is moderate but transient. Treated tissues blanch, ulcerate over several days, then usually heal within 10 to 14 days. Scarring rarely occurs if 3 or 4 weeks pass between treatments.

Laser Surgery. One of the most popular ablative techniques used today for the management of condylomata is carbon dioxide laser surgery. Although it is highly effective and relatively safe when used by a skilled operator, it can be counterproductive or even dangerous in inexperienced hands. Furthermore, compared with topical therapy and other ablative techniques, laser surgery is expensive. For these reasons, it is suggested that it be reserved for patients who have failed topical therapy or who have chronic disease or significant dysplasia. Several guidelines are worth mentioning: (1) The operator should become thoroughly familiar with the characteristics of the epidermis and dermis at various depths. Awareness of these "surgical planes" helps fit the operation to the severity of the disease, maximize efficacy, and minimize complications: (2) To minimize thermal injury, chill surgical areas with iced saline, learn to operate with high-power outputs (25 to 100 watts) and high-power densities (750 to 2000 watts per cm), using a pulsed wave and partially defocused beam, and finally recool the surgical area at the end of the procedure; and (3) use a good evacuation system. HPV DNA has been found in laser plumes and is potentially infectious.

Interferon

Interferons have antiviral, antiproliferative, and immunomodulatory properties that justified their use in clinical trials for management of condylomata. Although efficacy has been demonstrated for both intralesional therapy and systemic therapy, in most instances interferons offer no advantage over the therapeutic modalities already mentioned. Precluding their widespread acceptance, interferons are relatively expensive and inconvenient to use, requiring frequent office visits and multiple injections. Furthermore, they have untoward, albeit self-limited, dose-dependent side effects, including fever, chills, headache, malaise, nausea, vomiting, myalgia, elevated liver function tests, leukopenia, and thrombocytopenia. Currently, several natural and recombinant interferon-alpha preparations are available, and the following guidelines are suggested for their use.

Intralesional Therapy. Despite rare occurrences of laboratory abnormalities with intralesional therapy, obtain baseline urine analysis, complete blood count, and blood chemistries to include creatinine, blood urea nitrogen (BUN), uric acid, electrolytes, and liver function tests. Premedicate with acetaminophen (650 mg) or ibuprofen (600 to 800 mg). Using a small (30-gauge) needle, inject individual warts, intradermally, with interferon alpha (interferon alfa-2a* [Roferon A], interferon alfa-2b [Intron A], or in-

---

*Not FDA approved for this indication.

terferon alpha-n3 [Alferon N]), 0.25 to 1 million units (MIU), depending on lesion size, twice or thrice weekly for 3 to 4 weeks. In extensive or recalcitrant disease, doses up to 6 MIU per day can often be given with acceptable levels of patient tolerance. A drug-free interval of at least 1 month between treatment courses is advised; since improvement may continue during this period and preclude the need for additional therapy.

Parenteral Therapy. Obtain baseline laboratory studies and premedicate as just noted. Inject 2 to 3 MIU of interferon (or, up to 3 MIU per/m^2) intramuscularly or subcutaneously, either thrice weekly or every other day. With extensive or recalcitrant disease, a schedule of daily injections for 2 weeks, followed by a thrice-weekly or every-other-day regimen, may be used. Usually, the patient or a family member can be taught to perform the injections, reducing the frequency of office visits. Initially, plan a course of therapy to last 4 to 6 weeks. Continue therapy for at least 1 week after the resolution of lesions. Wait at least 1 month between treatment courses. Under most circumstances, the relapse rate is low if complete resolution of disease is obtained. Certain conditions associated with immunosuppression or chronic HPV infection (e.g., juvenile laryngeal papillomatosis) are associated with high relapse rates and require prolonged treatment courses to maintain remission.

Regional Therapy. When extensive disease is present or diffuse subclinical disease is felt to be contributing to intolerable symptoms, as is found in cases of recalcitrant pruritus or vulvodynia, regional therapy can be tried. Baseline laboratory studies and premedication are done as noted. Generally, 4 to 6 MIU of interferon is administered intradermally, dividing the dose into 6 to 8 injection sites without attention to specific lesions, twice or thrice weekly for 4 to 6 weeks.

Combination Therapy

In the most severe infections, particularly in immune suppressed individuals, combination therapy may be the key to disease control. For example, podophyllin or ablative therapy followed by intermittent use of 5-FU or interferon may increase remission rates and prolong the intervals to recurrence.

NEVI

method of
LOREN E. GOLITZ, M.D.
University of Colorado School of Medicine
Denver, Colorado

Melanocytic nevi are one of the most common benign neoplasms of humans. Their importance lies in their potential to transform into malignant melanoma or in the perception that they are a cosmetic problem. The normal epidermal melanocyte migrates from the neural crest in early fetal life and eventually resides in the basal layer of the epidermis. Melanin pigment produced by melanocytes accounts for the variation in skin color among individuals and serves to protect the skin from the damaging effects of ultraviolet light. Normally, about every tenth cell in the basal layer is a melanocyte. Melanocytic nevi represent focal proliferations of melanocytes to produce collections (nests) of nevus cells. Nevus cells lack the dendrites of melanocytes but retain the ability to produce melanin pigment. Melanocytic nevi can be classified into acquired and congenital forms. Acquired melanocytic nevi account for 99% of all nevi and have a number of distinctive variants, including halo nevi, Spitz' nevi, and dysplastic nevi.

ACQUIRED MELANOCYTIC NEVI

Common acquired melanocytic nevi appear in infancy as minute tan macules that slowly enlarge and darken in color. They increase in size and number during the first 3 decades of life, with the average peak number being about 15 nevi. During puberty and pregnancy, nevi may enlarge and become darker in color. After middle age, nevi decrease in number, and some individuals over 70 years of age may be completely free of nevi.

Common acquired melanocytic nevi are classified as junctional, intradermal, or compound, depending on whether the nests of nevus cells are located at the junction of the epidermis and dermis, within the dermis, or at both sites, respectively. Junctional nevi are more common in childhood and are flat or slightly elevated lesions. They are usually less than 6 mm in diameter, are uniformly pigmented, and have smooth borders and a round-to-oval shape. Compound nevi are the most common form of melanocytic nevi in adults. They are usually raised and often are papillomatous, cerebriform, or pedunculated. Compound nevi typically have a uniform tan to medium brown color. Intradermal nevi are often dome-shaped or papillomatous and are usually lighter in color than junctional or compound nevi. Color change or rapid growth of nevi other than that expected during puberty or pregnancy should arouse suspicion of the transformation of a melanocytic nevus to melanoma. The colors red, white, blue, or gray rarely occur in benign nevi, and their occurrence should cause the clinician to consider surgical excision. Table 1 lists nine reasons to excise an acquired melanocytic nevus.

Variants of Acquired Melanocytic Nevi

Halo nevi typically occur on the back or chest during the second or third decades of life. They may be solitary or multiple. Ordinary brown raised compound nevi develop a white halo that is 1 to 4 mm wide. Over a period of months, the central nevus becomes flat and loses its pigmentation, leaving a round or oval white macule. Eventually, the white macule repigments and the skin appears normal.

TABLE 1. **Nine Reasons to Excise an Acquired Melanocytic Nevus**

Unexpected, rapid growth
Sudden darkening in color
Red, white, blue, gray color hues
Asymmetry
Notched or scalloped margins
Ulceration
Pruritus
Irritation by clothing
Cosmetic reasons

Histologically, halo nevi show a dense lymphocytic inflammation and mild atypia of the nevus cells. If a halo nevus is excised, it is important to inform the pathologist that a halo was present clinically to minimize the possibility of the overdiagnosis of the lesion as a melanoma. Inflammation identical to that seen with a halo nevus occasionally occurs in lesions without a clinical halo. Inflammation is one mechanism by which the number of melanocytic nevi decrease with age. Halos may occur with malignant melanomas. It has been said that everything with a halo is neither holy nor benign.

Spitz' nevi (spindle and epithelioid cell nevi) are an uncommon form of acquired melanocytic nevus that are important because they share many histologic features with malignant melanoma. About two-thirds of Spitz' nevi occur in the first 2 decades of life, and they become progressively less common with increasing age. A typical Spitz nevus is pink-to-red in color, dome-shaped, and less than 6 mm in diameter. The onset and growth are often rapid. Spitz' nevi in children are most often located on the head, whereas they are more common on the extremities of adults. Some lesions may be darkly pigmented, and rarely they may be multiple and grouped. Spitz' nevi are benign but, especially in adults, may cause the pathologist considerable difficulty in distinguishing them from melanoma.

Dysplastic nevi are variants of acquired melanocytic nevi that are usually evident by age 20 years, but they may continue to develop throughout an individual's life. They are usually larger (0.5 to 1.5 cm) than ordinary nevi and show irregular or fuzzy borders and a haphazard display of several shades of brown. Dysplastic nevi may occur anywhere on the body, and, unlike ordinary nevi, they commonly occur on sun-protected areas such as the breasts and buttocks. The diagnosis of a dysplastic nevus should be confirmed by a biopsy, which will show architectural disorder and focal cytologic atypia of nevus cells. About 25% of nevi that clinically appear dysplastic fail to show histologic atypia.

Dysplastic nevi were originally described in families in which at least two members had melanoma and in which other members had large, atypical nevi. These nevi have been shown to be inherited as an autosomal dominant trait and are associated with a single gene on the short arm of chromosome 1. Subsequently, sporadic dysplastic nevi were found to occur in the general population. The risk for developing melanoma in individuals with dysplastic nevi can be separated into two categories: (1) a slightly increased prospective risk for melanoma in individuals with no family or personal history of melanoma, and (2) a high prospective risk for melanoma in individuals with a personal or family history of melanoma.

CONGENITAL MELANOCYTIC NEVI

Only 1% of newborn infants have a congenital melanocytic nevus, and fewer than 10% of congenital nevi are larger than 3 to 4 cm in diameter. Nevi larger than 10 cm in diameter occur in less than 1 in 20,000 births. Congenital nevi are arbitrarily classified as small (less than 1.5 cm in diameter), medium (1.5 to 20.0 cm in diameter), or large (over 20.0 cm in diameter). The importance of large congenital nevi lies in their 6 to 7% lifetime incidence for the development of melanoma and in their significant cosmetic manifestations. The incidence of malignant degeneration in small and medium-sized congenital nevi appears to be increased but is less well defined.

Small congenital nevi are slightly to moderately raised and tend to be darker brown or black compared with acquired nevi. They increase in size in proportion to body growth and tend to fade slightly in color with age. Large congenital nevi may cover large areas of the body and have been referred to as "bathing trunk nevi" or "garment nevi," depending on their location. Most are raised and dark brown but they may vary from light tan to jet black. Larger lesions may have a pebbly or nodular surface. Most congenital nevi have some coarse, pigmented hairs. Larger nevi may have one or more black nodules, which should be biopsied. Approximately 50% of melanomas that develop in giant congenital nevi do so in the first decade of life.

TREATMENT

Nevi are usually biopsied or excised because of concern about their transformation to melanoma; their irritation by clothing, jewelry, or shaving; or for cosmetic reasons (see Table 1). All nevi that are biopsied or excised should be sent to the laboratory for histologic examination. Nevi should not be frozen with liquid nitrogen or treated by laser without histologic documentation of their benign nature. It is not acceptable to submit multiple nevi in the same container unless each is properly identified, such as with colored ink. If the clinician has a concern about the malignant potential of a pigmented lesion because of an atypical clinical appearance, this information should be clearly communicated to the pathologist. The great majority of melanocytic nevi are easy to diagnose accurately histologically; however, a small percent represent one of the most difficult problems faced by a pathologist. In these cases, it may be prudent to request consultation by a pathologist or dermatologist with special qualification in dermatopathology.

Melanocytic nevi that are uniformly colored and symmetrical, with smooth margins and no history of recent change, do not require treatment. Since the average person has 15 or more nevi, it is not practical nor medically warranted to attempt to remove all nevi. However, if the patient has a personal or family history of melanoma or has one or more nevi that are large and irregularly shaped with color variation, consideration should be given to biopsy or removal.

The most effective way to remove an acquired melanocytic nevus is by elliptical excision, which requires closure with sutures. In exophytic lesions that appear completely benign, a tangential shave excision may be easier, and suturing is not required. Occasionally, a small, 1- to 2-mm nevus may be completely removed with a 3- to 4-mm punch biopsy. The defect heals better if closed with a suture. Again, histologic confirmation of the diagnosis is important.

The therapy of congenital melanocytic nevi is a greater problem and is controversial. In my opinion, small (1.5 cm or less) congenital nevi that can be easily removed should be surgically excised within the first decade of life. The nevi appear to have a small but significant risk of transforming into melanoma after the first decade of life, and removal can be performed under local anesthesia with minimal risk. Medium and large congenital melanocytic nevi are felt to carry a 6 to 7% lifetime risk of melanoma.

This is significantly higher than the approximately 1% lifetime risk for melanoma in an otherwise normal infant born today.

There is no clear consensus on whether all large, congenital melanocytic nevi should be removed. The surgery usually requires one or multiple procedures under general anesthesia. The resultant skin grafts often leave a cosmetic result that is not ideal. Dermabrasion and deep shave excisions of large congenital nevi do reduce the number of melanocytes and the dark clinical color but have not been proved effective in reducing the potential for malignant degeneration. Expansion of tissue with a subcutaneous balloon catheter may allow some medium and large nevi to be excised and closed primarily.

There has been no prospective, controlled study to show that prophylactic removal of giant congenital melanocytic nevi is effective in reducing the mortality from melanoma. In 1983, the National Institutes of Health sponsored a consensus panel that made the following conclusions: (1) the management of congenital melanocytic nevi depends primarily on their size and the perceived risk of melanoma, (2) there are insufficient data at present to recommend prophylactic excision of all congenital nevi, (3) patients should be examined periodically, first by their parents and then by self-examination, and (4) if the nevus changes, it should be evaluated by a physician, and biopsied if deemed appropriate.

MALIGNANT MELANOMA

method of
JAMES S. ECONOMOU, M.D., Ph.D.
UCLA Medical Center
Los Angeles, California

Melanoma is the eighth most common malignancy, and its incidence has increased at a striking rate. The lifetime risk among whites is expected to be 1 in 90 by the year 2000. In 1994, there were 32,000 new cases diagnosed in the United States, with 6900 deaths (22%).

Melanomas arise from melanocytes, melanin-containing dendritic cells located at the dermal-epidermal junction of the skin. A fair complexion, tendency to sunburn, red or fair hair, and blue eyes are associated with increased risk. Exposure to ultraviolet B radiation (290 to 320 nm) is considered a major cause. There is a clear familial predisposition in individuals with dysplastic nevus syndrome. The potential roles of genetic alterations and tumor suppressor genes are being actively studied.

There are four major melanoma growth patterns. Superficial spreading melanoma constitutes the majority (70%) and usually arises from a pre-existing nevus. It may evolve slowly over a period of years before rapid change. These melanomas are characterized by irregular borders and areas of depigmented regression and commonly arise in women on the lower extremities. Nodular melanomas (15 to 30%) are more biologically aggressive, arise de novo (not from nevus), and are more common on the head, neck, and trunk of men. These tumors may resemble blood blisters; a small percentage (5%) are amelanotic, which can delay clinical diagnosis. Lentigo maligna melanomas (4 to 10%) arise in sun-damaged skin on the face and neck of older patients. They are generally large, flat lesions that grow slowly and tend not to metastasize. Acral-lentiginous melanomas (2 to 8%) occur on the palms, soles, and nail beds and tend to predominate in individuals of African, Asian, and Hispanic descent.

Any cutaneous pigmented lesion with clinical features suggestive of melanoma—change in size, pigmentation, border irregularity, or ulceration—should be biopsied. Small lesions require full-thickness excisional biopsy. Larger lesions may be evaluated using a punch biopsy. Shave biopsies should never be performed. The immunohistochemical markers S-100 and HMB-45 may be used to aid in diagnosis. Accurate microstaging is critical in designing treatment and estimating prognosis. Breslow thickness (measured with an optical micrometer) is a more objective and accurate predictor of prognosis than Clark's level (degree of dermal invasion). Other independent prognostic variables include gender (women fare better than men), anatomic site (extremity better, head and neck poorer), superficial ulceration (poor), satellites (poor), and histology (lentigo better).

The American Joint Commission on Cancer (AJCC) melanoma staging system considers both tumor thickness and the presence of regional or systemic metastases. Stage I (up to 1.5 mm) and Stage II (>1.5 mm) do not have evidence of regional metastatic disease (N0). The estimated 15-year survival for these patients stratified for melanoma thickness is: less than 0.76 mm, greater than 95%; 0.76 to 1.49 mm, 80 to 85%; 1.50 to 2.49 mm, 60 to 70%; 2.50 to 3.99 mm, 50 to 60%; 4.00 to 7.99 mm, 40 to 50%; and more than 8.0 mm, 30%. Patients with Stage III disease (clinical nodal involvement) have a poorer overall prognosis (15 to 40%), which varies as a direct function of the number of nodes involved. Stage IV disseminated disease carries a very poor prognosis.

There is little controversy that narrower surgical margins are adequate for thin and intermediate thickness lesions. For in situ lesions (noninvasive), a 0.5-cm margin is adequate. Melanomas less than 1.0 mm in depth may be treated with a 1-cm margin of excision. Intermediate thickness (1 to 4 mm) lesions can be treated with a 2-cm margin without increased risk of local recurrence or survival. Thick melanomas (>4 mm) have not been studied in a randomized trial, but a 3-cm margin provides local control in 80 to 90% of patients.

Regional lymph nodes are the most common metastatic site of malignant melanoma. There is good evidence that melanoma can metastasize in a temporal sequence (primary to regional nodes to systemic sites) and that addressing nodal disease at an early microscopic stage confers greater survival advantage. The older strategy of elective lymph node dissection in clinically negative, high-risk patients is controversial, and the evidence that it confers significant survival advantage is not convincing. This issue is largely moot with the advent of intraoperative lymphatic mapping and microstaging. This new technique employs a lymphatic dye injected intradermally at the melanoma biopsy site. Within minutes, the dye enters draining lymphatic channels and stains the sentinel lymph node in the regional lymph node basin. This sentinel lymph node is the first and most likely site of micrometastatic disease and can be identified and biopsied in a minor procedure. The presence of micrometastases identifies patients requiring lymphadenectomy. In several large studies, the absence of melanoma micrometastases in the sentinel node correlated closely with their absence in all other nodes in that basin. This approach allows accurate staging of patients with a minor procedure and reliably identifies the majority of patients requiring regional lymphadenectomy.

Regional hyperthermic isolated limb perfusion is reserved for patients with extensive in transit or recurrent disease limited to an extremity. Melphalan is the most active agent, and complete response rates of 40% have been reported.

Melanoma can metastasize to any organ or tissue. The most active single chemotherapeutic agent, dacarbazine (DTIC), can produce 15 to 25% response rates of generally short duration. Modern combination regimens employ DTIC, carmustine (BCNU), cisplatin (Platinol), and tamoxifen (Nolvadex), with response rates as high as 55% reported. Biologic therapy using interleukin-2 (IL-2) and interferon-alfa (IFN-α) can produce dramatic responses in a small percentage of patients. Adoptive immunotherapy using IL-2–supported lymphokine-activated killer (LAK) cells does not improve response rates above those observed with IL-2 alone. Tumor-infiltrating lymphocyte (TIL) adoptive immunotherapy is investigational, as are various gene therapy strategies currently being tested clinically. Autologous or allogeneic melanoma vaccine treatment of metastatic disease has been uniformly disappointing.

There is emerging evidence from cooperative trials that IFN-α is active in an adjuvant setting. Interim analysis of prospective randomized trials showed a significant impact on disease-free survival in high-risk patients. There is no evidence supporting a role for adjuvant chemotherapy or vaccine therapy.

Radiation is important in managing metastatic brain disease, spinal cord compression, and symptomatic bone disease. Radiotherapy following lymphadenectomy for clinically involved nodes reduces the regional recurrence rate.

PREMALIGNANT SKIN LESIONS

method of
HEIDI C. MANGELSDORF, M.D., and
BARRY LESHIN, M.D.
Wake Forest University Medical Center
Winston-Salem, North Carolina

A "premalignant lesion" can be defined as one that has a tendency to develop into a malignancy. In addition to truly premalignant lesions, this article describes in situ (intraepidermal) cutaneous malignancies and conditions that predispose individuals to develop skin cancers (Table 1).

Cumulative sun exposure is the cause of most cutaneous malignancies. These lesions tend to occur in those with fair skin (skin types I and II by Fitzpatrick's classification of skin type [Table 2]). Individuals at risk for such malignancies should be educated with regard to sun protection and recognition of suspicious lesions. In addition, close follow-up by a physician is optimal.

ACTINIC KERATOSIS

Actinic keratoses (AKs) (also called "solar keratoses," "senile keratoses") are the most common precancerous lesions, and they typically arise on chronically sun-exposed areas in individuals with skin types I and II. These lesions most commonly arise on the face, hands, and forearms. Diffuse AKs of the lower lip is known as "actinic cheilitis."

Although most prevalent in elderly people, AKs may develop in individuals living in sunny climates as early as the teenage years. Historically, men have had a higher incidence than women owing to occupational exposure to ultraviolet radiation (UVR), but recreational exposure has led to an increased incidence in women.

Clinically, AKs are scaly macules with an erythematous or hyperpigmented appearance, and are often

TABLE 1. **"Premalignant" Skin Lesions and Conditions**

Lesion or Condition	Associated Carcinoma
Actinic keratosis	SCC
Arsenical or chemical keratoses	SCC
Bowen's disease (in situ SCC)	SCC
Chronic radiodermatitis	BCC, SCC, melanoma
Scar	BCC, SCC, melanoma
Atypical mole	Melanoma
Congenital nevus (large)	Melanoma
Lentigo maligna (in situ melanoma)	Melanoma
Bowenoid papulosis	SCC (rare)
Albinism, xeroderma pigmentosa	BCC, SCC, melanoma
Basal cell nevus syndrome	BCC
Immune suppression	BCC, SCC, melanoma
Porokeratosis	BCC, SCC (rare)
Nevus sebaceus of Jadassohn	BCC
Chronic ulcers	SCC

Abbreviations: SCC = squamous cell carcinoma; BCC = basal cell carcinoma.

TABLE 2. **Fitzpatrick's Classification of Skin Type**

Skin Type	Reaction to Sun	Skin Color
I	Always burn	White/freckled
II	Usually burn	White
III	Sometimes burn	White to olive
IV	Rarely burn	Brown
V	Very rarely burn	Dark brown
VI	Never burn	Black

multiple. Visualization of AKs may be difficult on a background of photodamaged skin, and gentle palpation of the sun-exposed skin is a valuable aide to examination.

Hyperkeratotic, projectile nodules, referred to as "cutaneous horns," may overlie an AK. However, such horns may arise from a bonafide malignancy, and therefore biopsy is warranted.

Keratoses arising from chemical exposure or by physical means behave in a similar fashion to AKs. These include arsenical, hydrocarbon, thermal, chronic radiation, and chronic cicatrix keratoses.

Squamous cell carcinoma (SCC) develops in less than 1% of patients with AKs. Basal cell carcinoma (BCC) is also common in individuals with AKs, but the carcinoma does not develop from a pre-existing AK. These two lesions share the common risk factor of long-term sun exposure.

The differential diagnosis for AKs includes Bowen's disease, seborrheic keratosis, superficial BCC, eczema, and chronic cutaneous lupus erythematosus. If there is a palpable dermal component, a shave biopsy should be performed to evaluate for malignancy.

AKs may be prevented and have been shown to regress with regular sun protection. Most sun exposure occurs during childhood with 75% of lifetime UVR exposure occurring before 18 years of age, indicating the importance of protection during these years. Adequate sun protection includes using a sunscreen with a sun protection factor (SPF) of 15 or greater, wearing a hat and sun-protective clothing, and avoiding sun exposure between the hours of 10 A.M. and 2 P.M., especially in areas of low latitude.

Multiple treatment modalities are available for AKs. Cryotherapy to individual lesions with liquid nitrogen is one of the most common. Liquid nitrogen is applied with a spray or cotton swab for 5 to 10 seconds to typical AKs and slightly longer for hypertrophic AKs. Freeze times longer than 10 to 15 seconds often result in hypopigmentation.

Chemexfoliation with topical 5-fluorouracil (5-FU) (Efudex) is frequently used to treat multiple AKs. One or 2% 5-FU is used to treat the face and lips, and 5% 5-FU is used to treat the scalp, neck, extremities, and trunk twice daily for 3 to 8 weeks, depending on the site being treated. 5-FU is available as a cream (1%, 5%) or solution (1%, 2%, 5%). The solution is more active than the cream with equivalent concentrations of medication. Application of 5-FU should be to an entire area, not just to individual lesions. Inflammation of clinically apparent and subclinical lesions may be severe, and concurrent application of a medium-strength topical corticosteroid should reduce the severity of the irritation. Sunlight intensifies the cutaneous reaction, so treatment is often performed during the winter months. Tretinoin (Retin-A) 0.05% cream has been used as pretreatment for 2 to 3 weeks or in combination with 5-FU for refractory lesions. Other treatment modalities for AKs include dermabrasion and medium-depth chemical peel.

BOWEN'S DISEASE

Bowen's disease, or cutaneous SCC in situ, occurs most frequently on sun-exposed skin and affects predominantly older individuals. Prior chronic arsenic exposure may be implicated in Bowen's disease on nonexposed sites, the source often being ingestion of inorganic arsenic in well water or medications for asthma or psoriasis. Bowen's disease on the glans penis is known as erythroplasia of Queyrat, and occurs exclusively in uncircumcised males. Overall, 3 to 5% of Bowen's disease evolves into invasive SCC.

Clinically, Bowen's disease is a solitary, well-demarcated, erythematous, scaly plaque. The differential diagnosis includes tinea corporis, nummular eczema, psoriasis, and superficial BCC. A shave biopsy of the thickest part of the plaque should be performed to confirm the diagnosis.

Bowen's disease related to arsenic exposure is associated with the internal malignancies connected with arsenic exposure. Otherwise, current literature indicates that Bowen's disease should not be considered a marker of internal malignancy.

Therapeutic modalities include excision, cryotherapy with liquid nitrogen, curettage and electrodesiccation, 5-FU, and radiotherapy. Performing a full–dermal thickness excisional biopsy affords the advantage of removing any deep follicular involvement. This approach also allows for histologic evaluation of resection margins and assessment for potential invasiveness of the neoplasm.

MELANOCYTIC LESIONS

The lifetime risk of malignant melanoma is 1% among white populations, and has been increasing for decades. Melanoma may arise in a pre-existing nevus; however, 67% of melanomas are not associated with a precursor lesion. Atypical moles and congenital nevi may be markers for individuals at increased risk for developing invasive melanoma.

Atypical nevi, previously referred to as "dysplastic nevi," have certain clinical and histologic criteria. Atypical mole syndrome is characterized by increased number and size of nevi. The lifetime risk of melanoma approaches 100% in individuals with atypical mole syndrome and a family history of melanoma in two or more relatives. Recent studies suggest that the presence of atypical moles, or many typical nevi, slightly increases the risk of melanoma.

Removal of all nevi is not warranted, but consideration should be given to histologic evaluation of the most clinically atypical lesions.

Large congenital nevi (often defined as greater than 20 cm) have a 5 to 10% lifetime risk of melanoma. Small (less than 1.5 cm) and intermediate congenital nevi may have a slightly increased risk for malignant transformation, but this risk is not well defined. Removal of intermediate and large congenital nevi is usually recommended.

Lentigo maligna is melanoma in situ on sun-damaged skin. Evolution to invasive melanoma may occur, making early recognition and treatment paramount. It is recommended that melanoma in situ be excised with a 5-mm margin of normal skin.

CHRONIC RADIODERMATITIS

Chronic radiodermatitis occurs in areas of the skin previously exposed to ionizing radiation. Half a century ago, patients with acne vulgaris and atopic dermatitis were frequently treated with superficial x-rays. Such individuals have been noted to develop cutaneous malignant neoplasms in the irradiated fields later in life. The mean latency time to development of a cutaneous malignancy is 25 years. Neoplasms reported in areas of radiodermatitis include radiation keratosis, BCC, SCC, and melanoma. Areas of skin affected by chronic scarring also have an increased frequency of malignancy. SCC is well documented in burn scars and has a high rate of metastasis (20 to 30%).

Previously irradiated skin may appear atrophic with altered pigmentation and prominent telangiectasias. Destruction of adenexal components gives the skin a dry appearance, and there is loss of skin elasticity.

Treatment includes regular follow-up to assess for cutaneous malignancies. Emollients may decrease the associated discomfort at the involved sites.

HUMAN PAPILLOMAVIRUS

Bowenoid papulosis (BP) is characterized by the presence of multiple, reddish-brown papules on the mucocutaneous genital region of young adults. The lesions are often confused with genital warts clinically.

Histologically, BP is identical to Bowen's disease. However, there is a high frequency of spontaneous regression, and transformation to invasive SCC is rarely seen. Multiple human papillomavirus (HPV) types have been identified in lesions of BP, including HPV 16, 18, and 31. Female patients with BP, or consorts of male BP patients, with these HPV genotypes may have an increased incidence of cervical neoplasia.

Close clinical follow-up is indicated, including gynecologic evaluation. Treatment modalities used for genital warts are appropriate.

GENODERMATOSES

Albinism is an autosomal recessive trait with absent or decreased levels of tyrosinase resulting in skin that completely or partially lacks pigment. Without the protection of melanin, affected individuals are at greatly increased risk for BCC, SCC, and malignant melanoma. Photodamage and cutaneous malignancies appear in early childhood. Xeroderma pigmentosum is an autosomal recessive genodermatosis characterized by defective DNA repair and a marked tendency to develop cutaneous malignant neoplasms.

Nevoid BCC syndrome is a rare, autosomal dominantly inherited disorder of unknown cause. BCC develops prior to 20 years of age and is associated with palmar pits, mandibular cysts, partial agenesis of the corpus callosum, bifid ribs, and hypertelorism.

IMMUNE SUPPRESSION

Individuals who are chronically immune suppressed, either iatrogenically (e.g., organ transplant recipients) or by an underlying malignancy (e.g., chronic lymphocytic leukemia), are at increased risk for developing cutaneous malignancies. SCC (including the keratoacanthomatous type) is the most common malignancy associated with immunosuppression. HPV may play a role in such settings. Other cutaneous malignancies with an increased incidence in immune suppressed individuals include BCC, malignant melanoma, and Kaposi's sarcoma. AKs also develop with increased frequency in the immune suppressed individual. Malignancies developing in this setting may be aggressive and require appropriate surgical management.

MISCELLANEOUS

Nevus sebaceus of Jadassohn is a neoplasm with an increased number of several cutaneous tissue elements and has been reported to develop into BCC in up to 10% of patients. The most common location is the scalp, where it appears as a yellow patch of alopecia at birth. During puberty, the lesion becomes raised, and may develop a verrucous appearance. Complete local excision is the treatment of choice, but lesions in cosmetically sensitive areas may be followed clinically.

Porokeratoses, the most common being disseminated superficial actinic porokeratosis (DSAP), are a group of disorders that share a common histologic pattern. The primary lesion is an erythematous, scaly, slightly atrophic macule with a characteristic raised rim of epidermis. DSAP is characterized by multiple lesions typically on the lower extremities of older females. Rarely, BCC, Bowen's disease, and SCC may occur in porokeratoses. Treatment and follow-up as indicated for AKs is appropriate.

Chronic ulcers may develop SCC, and consideration should be given to biopsy to assess for malignancy. SCC has been reported in association with ulcerative lesions of lichen planus, discoid lupus erythematosus, lichen sclerosis et atrophicus, chronic osteomyelitis, hidradenitis suppurativa, epidermolysis bullosa dystrophica, granuloma inguinale, lymphogranuloma venereum, and lupus vulgaris.

BACTERIAL DISEASES OF THE SKIN*

method of
RICHARD F. EDLICH, M.D., PH.D.,
SUN M. PARK, M.D., and
DIETER H. M. GRÖESCHEL, M.D., PH.D.
University of Virginia
Charlottesville, Virginia

In considering common bacterial diseases of the skin, rather distinct clinical responses to a variety of bacterial infections have been identified. In these cases, it is the specific site of infection and the attendant inflammatory responses that provide the characteristic clinical picture.

IMPETIGO

There are two classic forms of impetigo: the nonbullous and the bullous forms. Nonbullous impetigo is the most common pediatric skin infection; however, it can occur at any age. It starts in a traumatized area (a scratch or insect bite). It occurs primarily in exposed anatomic sites, such as the face and extremities. Adults living in close quarters, as well as those with an increased risk of bruising, are especially prone to nonbullous impetigo. This form of impetigo is usually noted in the summer in temperate climates, and it may be endemic year-round in warm climates. Factors implicated in this disease include warm ambient temperature, humidity, crowding, skin bruising, and poor hygiene.

The typical lesion usually begins as an erythematous papule that becomes a unilocular vesicle measuring less than 0.5 mm in diameter, situated between the stratum corneum and stratum granulosum and often located near the opening of a hair follicle. When the subcorneal vesicle becomes pustular, it ruptures, releasing a yellow, cloudy fluid and leaving a weeping bed. The seropurulent fluid dries, forming a yellow, golden crust that is the hallmark of the disease process.

These lesions rarely elicit pain, and usually are not accompanied by fever or systemic signs (malaise or anorexia). This asymptomatic nature accounts for the frequent delay in seeking medical attention. Without treatment, the condition often remains stable or becomes slowly progressive over a period of weeks. Occasionally, it may progress to ulcer formation. Regional lymphadenitis, cellulitis, and septicemia become evident in a small percentage of patients, who always seek treatment for these complications

rather than the primary problem, nonbullous impetigo. When a nephritogenic strain of group A streptococci is present, acute glomerulonephritis may follow. Postinfectious glomerulonephritis may occur in a sporadic form or in outbreaks. Although 95% of such patients with nephritis recover, progressive renal failure occasionally is encountered. The average time between the onset of impetigo and the development of nephritis is 20 days. Treatment of nonbullous impetigo probably does not decrease the chance of an individual's developing acute glomerulonephritis, but the successful treatment of these lesions may prevent spread to others and thereby reduce the general incidence of glomerulonephritis.

Nonbullous impetigo is caused by *Staphylococcus aureus*, group A streptococci, or both. Because it is difficult to distinguish on clinical examination between a streptococcal or staphylococcal cause, Gram's stain and culture of the vesicle fluid or weeping bed are recommended. *S. aureus* is the sole pathogen recovered most often. *S. aureus* alone or in combination with group A streptococci is found in over 80% of the patients. *S. aureus* is encountered at all ages, whereas group A streptococci are not frequently observed before the age of 1 and 2 years but are noted in older children.

Treatment

Treatment of this condition must include intervention against the pathogen and improvements in the hygiene and living conditions of the patient. A fundamental tenet in the treatment of impetigo is to débride the crust (scab) from the wound surface. This scab is an accumulation of extravasated blood proteins, including fibrin, that surround the bacteria and protect them from host defenses as well as from topical and systemic antibiotics. The scab also serves as a culture medium that encourages bacterial growth to concentrations greater than 10^8 bacteria per gram of tissue. Disruption and removal of the crust are accomplished by aggressive wound cleansing. The lesions are scrubbed with a coarse mesh gauze sponge (Type VIII) soaked in a soap to prevent reaccumulation of crusts. The pain encountered in this mechanical scrub can be lessened considerably by the use of a nontoxic surfactant, poloxamer 188 (Shur-Clens), as the wound cleanser. Wound cleansing must be complemented by antibiotic treatment.

If the lesions are not widespread, topical mupirocin, applied three times daily, is the treatment of choice. A beta-lactamase–resistant antibiotic drug is indicated if there is widespread disease. Erythromycin should not be used if there is widespread erythromycin resistance in the community. Impetigo should respond to these treatments in 7 days. If the results of treatment are not satisfactory, antibiotic resistance of the pathogen or poor patient compliance should be suspected, necessitating reculturing the wound. If poor compliance is confirmed, daily intramuscular ceftriaxone should be implemented.

Because this condition is commonly found under

*Our clinical studies have been supported by a grant from the Texaco Foundation, White Plains, New York.

conditions of poor hygiene and overcrowding, improvements in the patient's living conditions, personal hygiene, and general health are an integral part of our treatment regimen. The patient should shower twice daily with soap, using a clean washcloth and towel. The patient should be instructed to use only his or her towels and washcloths, which are not to be used by other family members. Daily washing of the patient's own clothing and bed linen is also advised. Reduction in minor skin trauma through control of biting insects appears to be important in preventing infection. Efforts are also made to identify the source of infection, focusing on members of the immediate family or friends who are simultaneously ill with a skin pyoderma.

Bullous impetigo is the less common form of impetigo. It occurs in infants and is characterized by rapid progression of vesicles to the formation of bullae measuring larger than 5 mm in diameter in previously untraumatized skin. These lesions frequently occur in the axilla, with satellite lesions soon appearing that may cover large portions of the body. The bullae are flaccid and transparent. In the neonate, this disease is so extensive that it is called pemphigus neonatorum. This type of infection is highly contagious, leading to epidemics in the nursery. When the large intraepidermal blebs rupture, the seropurulent discharge dries, forming a thin crust. As the lesions spread peripherally by autoinoculation, central healing of the denuded vesicles usually occurs without scarring. Cellulitis and lymphangitis are rarely encountered.

Bullous impetigo is caused exclusively by staphylococci and is seldom superinfected by streptococci. The bacteriocin produced by this strain of staphylococcus inhibits the growth of streptococci and may account for their absence. This organism also produces an exfoliative toxin that may cause the bulla formation. Treatment of this condition must include meticulous wound care complemented by the intravenous administration of a beta-lactamase–resistant penicillin (oxacillin [Bactocill, Prostaphlin] or nafcillin [Nafcil, Unipen]).

FOLLICULITIS

Folliculitis is a pyoderma located within a hair follicle. S. aureus is the most frequent pathogen. Less common pathogens are coliform bacteria and streptococci. This infection is classified according to its depth of penetration as either superficial or deep. The superficial type is a form of impetigo (Bockhardt's impetigo) in which the pustule is located at the opening of the hair follicle, often surrounded by a rim of erythema. Rupture of a pustule leads to crust formation and, in some cases, to the development of another superficial follicular abscess. The lesions usually heal within several days and only rarely persist to become furuncles. The location of the superficial folliculitis varies according to the age of the patient. The infection appears often in the scalp of children.

In the adult, the scalp, beard, or an extremity may be involved.

This superficial folliculitis may extend beyond the confines of the hair follicles, resulting in several types of deep folliculitis. A furuncle or boil is the most common skin lesion of deep folliculitis. It occurs particularly in regions subject to friction and perspiration (face, neck, axillae, and buttocks). Chronic carriers of S. aureus are especially prone to this disease. The systemic host factors that predispose an individual to furuncles include obesity, blood dyscrasia, defects in neutrophil function, immune globulin deficiency states, and treatments with corticosteroids and cytotoxic agents. The infection in a furuncle spreads along multiple tracts into the subcutaneous tissue. It starts as a tender red nodule, usually located at the nape of the neck, in the axilla, or on the buttock. As the nodule enlarges, it becomes tender and fluctuant, and eventually ruptures, discharging creamy, yellow pus and a core of necrotic debris from multiple draining sinuses with interconnecting tracts. Keratin plugs filling dilated follicular infundibula are characteristic features of furuncles. Accumulation of keratin may be due to overproduction, possibly stimulated by sweat or sebum or the result of decreased shedding of keratin. Carbuncles are aggregates of interconnecting furuncles that drain through multiple openings of the skin. A carbuncle is a larger, more serious inflammatory lesion with a deeper base. The involved area is red and indurated, and multiple pustules soon appear on the surface, eventually draining externally around multiple hair follicles. Sycosis barbae (barber's itch), a less common form of deep folliculitis, occurs in the bearded area of the face. If the condition is left untreated, it may progress to the deep chronic cicatricial form of sycosis barbae called "lupoid sycosis."

Acne keloidalis is a chronic folliculitis of the posterior neck and occipital scalp of young black men. It is exhibited clinically by follicular papules that coalesce into firm plaques and nodules. Hair can be seen perforating the papules. Ingrown hairs are not seen. Successful treatment of this condition involves complete removal of the scarred skin with its hair follicles.

In most cases, superficial and deep folliculitis are minor problems. After the lesions rupture, the redness and edema disappear in several days. Recurrence of these lesions does, however, occur in some patients over a period that may last several years. Bacteremia is a rare but clinically significant consequence of this type of pyoderma. Folliculitis around the lips and nose may spread to the cavernous sinus via the emissary veins.

Treatment

Treatment of folliculitis must include searching for and avoiding any predisposing factors that encourage its development. Plucking hair (e.g., eyebrows, upper lips) should be discouraged. Shaving should be performed with razors with recessed blades or electric

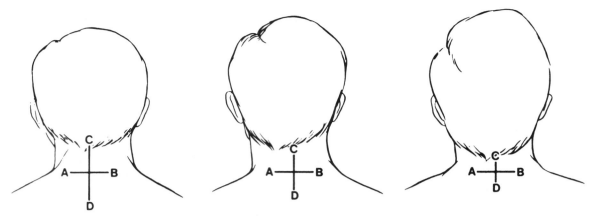

Figure 1. As the neck flexes (left) and extends (right), the distance between points C and D changes considerably, whereas the distance between points A and B remains relatively unchanged. Incisions for drainage of carbuncles located in the posterior neck should be placed in the direction of points A and B, which are perpendicular to the dynamic skin tensions.

clippers that avoid nicking the injured skin. The skin should be kept dry, providing a climate that is not conducive to bacterial growth. Frictional forces from surfaces such as a tight collar should be avoided.

Treatment of a small, isolated pyoderma of a hair follicle can be initiated with warm skin compresses until the lesion ruptures. In these cases, antimicrobial therapy is not needed. When the pyoderma involves multiple hair follicles, surgical intervention complemented by antimicrobial prophylaxis is recommended. Because the skin around a carbuncle is exquisitely sensitive, a regional nerve block of the site with a local anesthetic (1% lidocaine) is recommended. In skin that is not easily susceptible to this anesthetic technique, infiltration anesthesia via a No. 27 needle through the skin around the carbuncle is necessary. Surgical drainage of the carbuncle must be accomplished with an incision that will heal with the most esthetically pleasing scar. This goal can be accomplished by designing the incision so that its long axis is perpendicular to the dynamic tensions of the skin.

The ultimate appearance of the planned incision can be predicted by rather simple practical measurements. At the ends of the planned incision, mark points A and B, and then mark points C and D to be perpendicular to and equidistant from points A and B (Figure 1). Measure first the distance between points A and B and then the distance between C and D, both before and after flexion or extension of the neck or contraction of the muscles of facial expression. The dynamic skin tensions will be in the direction of the greatest changes in dimension. If the long axis of the incision is perpendicular to the direction of dynamic skin tensions, it will heal with a narrow scar that does not interfere with function and has an esthetically pleasing appearance.

After deepening the incision into the pyoderma, the necrotic debris and exudate must then be evacuated using 0.9% saline irrigation delivered to the infected site under low pressure (Asepto syringe, 1 pound per square inch). Undermining the skin edges may be necessary to open and expose subcutaneous tracts of the carbuncle. The wound is then packed with a 1-inch-wide gauze pack (Type 1). One day after surgery, the gauze is removed to permit cleansing with 0.9% saline that is again delivered to the wound using an Asepto syringe, after which the wound is packed with sterile gauze. Daily wound care is repeated until the cavity becomes filled with granulation tissue and the wound edges close by contraction. Without this meticulous care, wound repair may be accomplished by epithelial cells that migrate into the interstices of the wound, resulting in epithelialized sinus tracts. These sinusoidal tracts provide a moist environment for the growth of bacteria that may lead to the development of recurrent pyoderma.

Immediately before surgical intervention, antibiotic treatment is initiated with either a beta-lactamase–resistant antibiotic (cloxacillin [Tegopen] or dicloxacillin [Dynapen], 25 to 50 mg per kg of body weight per day in four divided doses given orally every 6 hours) or a cephalosporin (cephalexin [Keflex] or cephradine [Velosef], same dose as for cloxacillin) if not contraindicated in patients who are allergic to penicillin. If a cephalosporin is contraindicated, clindamycin (Cleocin) or a quinolone may be used. Antimicrobial therapy should be continued until the inflammation has disappeared. The antimicrobial sensitivity of the pathogen must be checked to ensure that this antibiotic regimen is indeed appropriate.

Management of patients with recurrent episodes of carbuncles is a challenging problem. In addition to treatment of the localized infection, careful evaluation for any predisposing systemic illnesses or local factors is essential. Pyogenic infections in other family members or friends must be considered. The following skin care measures must be initiated in an effort to reduce the numbers of *S. aureus* on the patient's clothes and bed linen. Local use of antibiotic ointment containing mupirocin* in the nasal vestibule has been suggested to reduce the nasal carriage of *S. aureus* and thereby limit the dispersal of these bacteria to other regions of the body. Thrice-daily

---

*Not FDA-approved for this indication.

treatment must be continued for at least 3 months, because recurrence of carbuncles is very frequent after short courses of topical antibiotic treatment. Draining lesions should be covered with sterile dressings to prevent autoinoculation. After each dressing change, the dressings should be wrapped in a plastic bag and promptly disposed of. Although immunization with staphylococcal vaccines of various types would also appear to be reasonable in such cases, it has not been successful in the prevention of recurrent infections.

Surgery occasionally is warranted as prophylaxis against recurrent infections. The indication for surgery is the presence of epithelialized tracts that are sequelae of wound repair of the drained carbuncle. These tracts extend deep into the subcutaneous tissue and harbor prodigious numbers of bacteria. Their serpiginous course can be traced by passing a probe coated with methylene blue dye through their orifices on the surface of the skin. The staining of the tracts with the blue dye facilitates their identification when wide surgical excision of the scarred tissue is accomplished.

The development of epithelialized sinus tracts after drainage is also encountered in hidradenitis suppurativa. This is an extremely troublesome infection of blocked hair follicles occurring in the axillary, perianal, and genital regions. Use of antiperspirants appears to predispose an individual to its development. After repeated applications, they form an occlusive cover over the skin that blocks the hair follicles. Initial lesions appear as small red nodules at the site of obstructed hair follicles. When the nodules become fluctuant and drain, they form irregular sinus tracts that predispose the patient to further infections. In the presence of these blind-ended sinuses, radical excision of the involved tissue is necessary.

CELLULITIS

Cellulitis is an acute inflammatory reaction involving the skin and underlying subcutaneous tissue. It usually starts as erysipelas and may advance to lymphangitis, lymphadenitis, or gangrene. Erysipelas is a superficial, acute, expanding infection of the skin, usually of the face and head, characterized by its reddened, brawny, edematous appearance.

Periorbital cellulitis is a distinct clinical entity that is usually secondary to an infection of a contiguous structure (e.g., paranasal sinusitis, osteomyelitis, conjunctivitis, dental infections). Infected thrombi are sometimes evident in associated lymphatics and veins that may extend posteriorly from the orbital cellulitis to involve the cavernous sinus. Inflammatory exudate accumulates within the bony orbit, resulting in proptosis and painful ophthalmoplegia. The diagnosis of periorbital cellulitis is made when an abscess cavity is noted on computed tomography or when pus is drained from the orbit or subperiosteal space at the time of surgery. Immediate treatment of this condition may prevent life-threatening complications, such as cavernous sinus thrombosis, meningitis, and brain abscess.

Treatment

In general, antimicrobial prophylaxis is the cornerstone of treatment of cellulitis. The selection of the appropriate antibiotic is based on the results of Gram's stain, which are confirmed by the culture and antibiotic sensitivity tests. Cellulitis occurring in the absence of a break in the skin is usually due to *Streptococcus pyogenes* (Group A streptococci) and should be treated with penicillin G, 1 to 2 million Units intravenously every 2 to 3 hours. Patients allergic to penicillin may be treated with cefazolin (Ancef, Kefzol), 75 to 80 mg per kg of body weight per day, given intravenously in four divided doses. Because of the cross-sensitivity in penicillin-allergic and cephalosporin-allergic patients, one might prefer to use vancomycin (Vancocin). In patients between the ages of 3 and 24 months with cellulitis in whom Gram's stain reveals gram-negative rods, *Haemophilus influenzae* should be suspected as the pathogen, and ampicillin,* 200 to 250 mg per kg of body weight per day, should be administered intravenously in six divided doses. With the recent emergence of beta-lactamase-producing, ampicillin-resistant strains, a cephalosporin (cefuroxime or cefotaxime) is very useful in these cases. In the penicillin-allergic patient, trimethoprim-sulfamethoxazole is a useful alternative agent. When Gram's stain reveals a mixture of gram-positive and gram-negative organisms, a combination of a cephalosporin, an aminoglycoside, and clindamycin should be used. As an alternative, imipenem may be used as a single agent. For the penicillin-allergic patient, vancomycin may be used with an aminoglycoside and clindamycin.

A prompt response to antimicrobial therapy is usually seen within 72 hours. In conjunction with antimicrobial treatment, immobilization and elevation of the injured extremity are mandatory. Cool, sterile saline soaks decrease the local pain and are particularly helpful in the presence of bullae. In periorbital cellulitis, it is important to determine the primary site of infection so that the appropriate surgical therapy can be instituted. For example, pus-filled maxillary sinuses should be subjected to immediate drainage.

Cellulitis occasionally progresses to gangrene, after the vessels of the skin thrombose. The occurrence of gangrene usually indicates the presence of a mixed bacterial infection. The location of these gangrenous changes has led physicians to coin a variety of names for this clinical entity such as Fournier's gangrene, necrotizing fasciitis and myositis.

Fournier's gangrene is streptococcal cellulitis of the scrotum and penis. It occurs spontaneously in most cases and has no apparent portal of entry. Anatomically, the subcutaneous tissues down to and including Colles' and Scarpa's fasciae are involved in

---

*Exceeds dosage recommended by the manufacturer.

the infectious process. The distribution of the cellulitis throughout the tissues of the penis, scrotum, and anterior abdominal wall mimics the dissection of urine between Colles' and Buck's fasciae, which occurs following transection of the urethra. Consequently, extension of the cellulitis into the thigh does not often occur because of the attachment of Colles' fascia along the inguinal ligament.

Necrotizing fasciitis is a severe infection involving the subcutaneous soft tissues as well as the superficial and often deep fascia. Sites of predilection for this infection are the extremities, the abdominal wall, perianal area, and the groin. The portal of entry is often a site of trauma (e.g., laceration, abrasion, insect bite, and burns) or a laparotomy performed in the presence of peritoneal contamination. Patients with diabetes mellitus, alcoholism, and parenteral drug abuse are predisposed to this infection. The affected area is exquisitely tender and painful and has shiny, erythematous, and edematous overlying skin. Within 3 to 5 days, the skin may become insensitive, signaling the development of thrombosis of the small blood vessels and damage of the superficial nerves. This development of anesthesia may antedate the occurrence of skin bullae and accompanying gangrene.

Necrotizing fasciitis is caused by two distinct bacteriologic entities. The first is a mixed bacterial infection involving at least one anaerobic species (most commonly *Bacteroides* and *Peptostreptococcus*) in combination with one or more facultative anaerobic species such as *Streptococcus* (other than Group A). In the second entity, Group A streptococci, either alone or in combination with other species, are isolated. In this latter entity, the Group A streptococci have been coined by the press as "flesh-eating" bacteria. Distinguishing necrotizing fasciitis from spontaneous gas gangrene due to *Clostridium* species may be difficult, although the presence of crepitus or gas in tissue would favor clostridial infection.

The cornerstone of treatment of gangrene is immediate débridement in conjunction with appropriate antibiotic therapy. Patients with gangrene of the skin are often hypermetabolic and require considerable nutritional support. If this requirement is left unsatisfied, the caloric demand leads to weight loss and impaired resistance to infection. The nutritional needs of these patients must be calculated and supplied by the enteral route, if possible. If enteral feeding is impossible, intravenous alimentation techniques must be used to achieve caloric and nitrogen balance.

VIRAL DISEASES OF THE SKIN

method of
PAUL F. ROCKLEY, M.D., and
VINCENZO F. GIANNELLI, M.D.
Washington Hospital Center
Washington, D.C.

Five families of viruses can affect the skin or the neighboring mucous membranes: herpesviruses, poxviruses, picornaviruses, retroviruses, and papovaviruses. This section focuses on the clinical manifestations and therapy of the first four of these virus families.

HERPESVIRUSES

Herpesviruses affect millions of Americans each year. The seven members of the herpesvirus family that are frequently associated with human disease include (1) herpes simplex virus 1 (HSV 1), causing most cases of orofacial herpes; (2) herpes simplex virus 2 (HSV 2), causing most cases of genital herpes; (3) varicella-zoster virus (VZV), the cause of both chickenpox and shingles; (4) Epstein-Barr virus (EBV), the cause of both infectious mononucleosis and oral hairy leukoplakia; (5) cytomegalovirus (CMV), which is associated with congenital anomalies in infants and immunosuppressive disease in adults; (6) herpesvirus 6, the cause of roseola in children; and (7) herpesvirus 7, a newly described family member.

Herpes Simplex Viruses

HSVs can infect any site on the body. HSV 1 tends to cause infections above the waist (face, eye, brain), whereas HSV 2 usually infects sites below the waist (genital area, sacrum, buttocks). However, these closely related viral types produce clinically indistinguishable lesions. Furthermore, some cases of orofacial and genital herpes are associated with HSV 2 and HSV 1, respectively.

Transmission of HSV can occur via direct contact with active lesions or result from exposure to asymptomatically shed virus at orogenital sites. The majority of people who are infected with HSV 1 or HSV 2 remain asymptomatic for an extended period of time. A true primary infection is the initial exposure to either type of HSV. Since many people have been infected with HSV 1 or HSV 2 by the time they reach adulthood, most patients' first symptomatic episode is not a true primary infection. During a primary infection with either type of HSV, the virus replicates at the infected cutaneous or mucosal site. Viral replication produces severe discomfort, followed sequentially by erythema, blisters, ulcers, and then crusts. In the absence of therapy, these lesions heal within 4 weeks. About one-half of the people experiencing primary episodes also complain about systemic symptoms, including neuralgia, headache, myalgia, malaise, and fever.

Following the primary infection, HSV travels in a

retrograde direction along sensory nerve fibers and establishes latency in sensory ganglia. Viral reactivation can be triggered by emotional or physical stressors such as febrile illnesses, intense sunlight exposure, or menstruation. HSV replication within sensory ganglia leads to anterograde viral transport back to the skin and mucous membranes. Recurrent infections are usually less severe than primary infections. Recurrences can be clinically obvious, or they may consist of asymptomatic viral shedding. Most clinically evident outbreaks progress from a prodrome of burning or itching to skin lesions localized to the site of previous infection. In the absence of antiviral therapy, these lesions often heal within 2 weeks. Recurrent genital infections are more commonly caused by HSV 2 than by HSV 1, whereas orofacial HSV 1 infections recur more often than orofacial HSV 2 infections.

Most mucocutaneous HSV infections resolve without sequelae. Complications are more likely to occur in untreated patients. Genital HSV infection in pregnancy can lead to congenital defects or fetal death. Recurrent ocular infections can result in corneal blindness. Airway obstruction owing to herpetic tracheobronchitis has been described in elderly patients. HSV encephalitis can cause neurologic deficits or even death.

Treatment

Antiviral therapy reduces the frequency and severity of HSV infections. Outbreaks can be prevented if therapy is initiated promptly during the prodromal phase or if daily suppressive therapy is administered to patients who have more than six recurrences per year. Episodic therapy shortens the duration of viral shedding, relieves symptoms, and reduces the time to healing. The safest and most efficacious antiherpes drug is acyclovir (Zovirax), which is available in topical, oral, and intravenous formulations (Table 1).

Acyclovir is preferentially taken up by virus-infected cells and phosphorylated to its active form by viral thymidine kinase. Intravenous acyclovir, 5 mg per kg every 8 hours for 7 to 10 days, is indicated for severe initial episodes or recurrences, complicated disease, and infections unresponsive to oral therapy. Oral acyclovir, 200 mg five times daily for 5 to 10 days, is indicated for mild initial episodes and most recurrences. Two to four 200-mg capsules per day are recommended for prophylaxis in patients with severe or frequent recurrences.

Acyclovir-resistant HSV infections can result from mutant HSV strains with either a relative deficiency of thymidine kinase or alterations in thymidine kinase or viral DNA polymerase. These resistant strains are being increasingly recognized in chronic ulcerative infections of patients with acquired immune deficiency syndrome (AIDS) and leukemia, and in bone marrow transplant recipients. Acyclovir-resistant HSV infections can frequently be managed by increasing the dose of intravenous acyclovir to 10 mg per kg every 8 hours for 7 to 10 days, followed by oral acyclovir, 800 mg five times daily until all lesions

TABLE 1. **Therapy of Viral Diseases of the Skin***

Antiviral Agent	Route of Administration	Dosage/Duration	Indication (Disease/Host)
Acyclovir (Zovirax)	Topical	5% ointment qid × 7 days	Minor initial or recurrent HSV episodes; less effective than PO or IV routes
	Oral	200 mg 5 times a day × 10 days	Mild-mod initial HSV episode—nl host
		200 mg 5 times a day × 5 days	Mild-mod recurrent HSV episode—nl host
		400 mg bid up to 12 months	Suppression of sev or frequent HSV—nl host
		200–400 mg 5 times a /day × 10 days	Mild-mod initial or recurrent HSV episode—ic host
		≥400 mg bid up to 12 months	Suppression of sev or frequent HSV—ic host
		20 mg/kg qid × 5 days (maximal dose, 800 mg qid)	Mod-sev primary varicella—nl child under 12 yr old
			Mild-sev primary varicella—nl adult
		800 mg 5 times a day × 7–10 days	Mild-sev herpes zoster—nl host
	Intravenous	5 mg/kg q 8 h × 5 days	Sev initial or recurrent HSV episode—nl host
		5 mg/kg q 8 h × 7–10 days	Sev initial or recurrent HSV episode—ic host
		250 mg/m² q 8 h × 7–10 days	Sev initial or recurrent HSV episode—ic child under 12 yrs old
		10 mg/kg q 8 h × 7–10 days	Mild-sev primary varicella—ic host 12 yr of age or older; Mild-sev herpes zoster—ic host; Acyclovir-resistant HSV—ic host
		500 mg/m² q 8 h × 7–10 days	Mild-sev primary varicella—ic child under 12 yr old
Famciclovir (Famvir)	Oral	500 mg tid × 7 days	Mild-sev nonophthalmic herpes zoster—nl adult
Foscarnet (Foscavir)	Intravenous	40 mg/kg q 8 h × 2–4 wk	Acyclovir-resistant HSV† or VZV—ic host
		60 mg/kg q 8 h × 2 wk	Ganciclovir-resistant CMV—ic host
Ganciclovir (Cytovene)	Intravenous	5 mg/kg q 12 h × 2–3 wk	CMV ulceration

*Dosages are for adults with normal renal function unless otherwise noted.
†Not FDA-approved for this indication.
Abbreviations: HSV = herpes simplex virus; ic = immunocompromised; mod = moderate; nl = normal; sev = severe; VZV = varicella-zoster virus; CMV = cytomegalovirus.

are healed. Alternatively, foscarnet (Foscavir)* can be used to treat acyclovir-resistant HSV. Foscarnet inhibits viral DNA polymerase activity directly, and thus it is an effective agent against thymidine kinase–deficient or altered HSV. The major side effects of foscarnet are nephrotoxicity, electrolyte alterations, and seizures. Foscarnet is administered intravenously at a dose of 40 mg per kg thrice daily for 2 to 4 weeks or until all acyclovir-resistant lesions are healed.

Varicella-Zoster Virus

VZV causes two distinct disorders, primary varicella (chickenpox) and herpes zoster (shingles). Chickenpox is acquired by inhalation of infectious respiratory secretions or by direct contact with skin lesions. The skin lesions that initially appear on the face and trunk begin as small red macules and progress rapidly over 12 to 14 hours through stages to papules, vesicles, pustules, and crust formation. Since the eruption appears as successive crops of rapidly evolving lesions, a characteristic feature of chickenpox is the simultaneous presence of lesions in all stages of development in the same anatomic area. In immunocompetent children, chickenpox is generally a mild disease and resolves in 2 to 3 weeks with symptomatic treatment. In contrast, some adults and immunocompromised children suffer significant morbidity and mortality in the absence of antiviral therapy.

After the skin lesions of chickenpox resolve, VZV establishes latency in sensory ganglia of cranial nerves and/or spinal nerves. Reactivation of latent VZV can later lead to viral replication and migration along sensory nerves, producing dermatomal pain and skin lesions characteristic of shingles. Shingles affects 10 to 20% of the population at some time during their lives. Shingles is more common in elderly people and in individuals with impairment of cell-mediated immunity (CMI). The unilateral dermatomal eruption of shingles progresses sequentially from erythematous macules and papules to vesicles, pustules, crusts, and healing within 4 weeks in the absence of therapy.

Since shingles represents a reactivation of latent VZV infection, this disease can affect anyone with a history of a VZV infection. Although a nonimmune individual can develop chickenpox after exposure to the skin lesions of a patient with acute zoster, there is no evidence that a person can develop shingles as a result of close contact with patients having either chickenpox or shingles.

Elderly patients and immunocompromised individuals are more likely to suffer complications of shingles. The most common and most debilitating complication is postherpetic neuralgia (PHN), defined as pain lasting more than 1 month after the onset of skin lesions, or pain persisting after all crusts are lost. Ophthalmic zoster can result in visual impairment or even blindness. Facial and auditory nerve involvement can lead to loss of taste and hearing, respectively. Direct extension of infection from sensory ganglia to anterior horn cells can produce motor paralysis. Rarely, hematogenous dissemination can lead to visceral involvement.

Treatment

Acyclovir is indicated for children or adults with moderate to severe VZV infections. Mild cases of chickenpox or shingles in immunocompetent individuals may not require antiviral therapy. The treatment of choice for most cases of chickenpox or shingles in otherwise healthy adults is acyclovir, 800 mg orally five times daily for 7 to 10 days. In 1994, oral famciclovir (Famvir), 500 mg three times daily for 7 days, received U.S. Food and Drug Administration (FDA) approval as an alternative therapy for nonophthalmic shingles in immunocompetent adults (see Table 1). Both acyclovir and famciclovir have similar clinical efficacy when they are administered within 72 hours of the onset of cutaneous lesions. In adults who are severely immunocompromised or unable to take oral medication, the recommended therapy is intravenous acyclovir, 10 mg per kg every 8 hours for 7 to 10 days. Acyclovir-resistant VZV infections can be treated with intravenous foscarnet,* 40 mg per kg thrice daily for 2 to 4 weeks or until all lesions are healed.

The major reason for treating shingles is to prevent complications, especially PHN. Acyclovir and famciclovir have limited success in reducing the incidence of PHN. Although the use of corticosteroids for preventing PHN remains controversial, some patients may benefit from short-term systemic or intralesional therapy. Patients experiencing PHN can be treated with analgesics, antidepressants, anticonvulsants, tranquilizers, substance P inhibitors (capsaicin [Zostrix]), regional anesthetics (local, epidural, and sympathetic), and transcutaneous electrical nerve stimulation (TENS). Surgical options for crippling PHN refractory to medical therapy include rhizotomy, cordotomy, or dorsal root entry zone operations. A VZV vaccine is currently available for prophylaxis in immunocompromised children, and it is expected to receive FDA approval for general use in healthy children in 1995.

Epstein-Barr Virus

EBV is the cause of both infectious mononucleosis (IM) and oral hairy leukoplakia (OHL). These infections are transmitted by direct contact, usually intimate but not necessarily sexual. Primary EBV infection is often subclinical in children, but it usually results in IM during adolescence and adulthood. Classic IM is characterized by fever, sore throat, tender lymphadenopathy, and organomegaly. Cutaneous and mucous membrane lesions are present in about one-fourth of patients with IM. A macular or

---

*Not FDA-approved for this indication.

*Not FDA-approved for this indication.

morbilliform eruption frequently occurs on the trunk and upper extremities. The mucous membrane lesions consist of distinctive pinhead-sized petechiae, 5 to 20 in number, at the junction of the soft and hard palate. Whereas immunocompetent individuals generally experience a single episode of mild EBV disease, reactivation of EBV can cause severe or chronic disease in persons who have high rates of viral shedding, such as organ transplant recipients and human immunodeficiency virus (HIV)–infected patients.

OHL is a clinically benign form of EBV infection in which a poorly demarcated, corrugated white plaque is seen on the lateral aspects of the tongue of immunodeficient patients, especially those with AIDS.

Treatment

No specific therapy exists for acute uncomplicated IM, but none is needed since most cases resolve in 4 to 6 weeks. IM complicated by streptococcal pharyngitis should be treated with penicillin or erythromycin rather than ampicillin or amoxicillin. The latter two drugs have been strongly associated with morbilliform eruptions in EBV patients. Systemic corticosteroid therapy is reserved for life-threatening complications, such as airway obstruction owing to severe pharyngeal inflammation and edema. Systemic antiviral therapy can suppress EBV replication in IM patients as well as induce remission in OHL patients. However, viral replication and relapse of disease invariably occurs on discontinuation of antiviral medication. Thus, antiviral therapy provides little or no clinical benefit in most EBV infections.

Cytomegalovirus

CMV is transmitted during close contact with infected individuals, most commonly through exposure to body secretions or leukocyte-containing blood products. The risk of CMV infection is increased in infants of infected mothers, children and workers in day care centers, blood transfusion recipients, and immunocompromised patients. CMV infection is most often subclinical and asymptomatic. In patients with clinically apparent disease, cutaneous lesions are rare and nonspecific. In immunocompetent hosts, primary infection infrequently manifests as a mononucleosis-like syndrome with a short-lived rubelliform or morbilliform eruption. Severe CMV infections in neonates or immunocompromised patients can cause visceral disease and neurologic damage, resulting in significant morbidity and mortality. A rare cutaneous manifestation of advanced congenital infection is a generalized, purpuric papular and nodular eruption with "blueberry muffin" lesions. A prominent cutaneous feature of CMV infection in immunocompromised patients is ulceration, especially in the perianal area.

Treatment

Most CMV infections do not require specific therapy. Ganciclovir (Cytovene), a nucleoside analogue of acyclovir that does not require viral thymidine kinase for activation, and foscarnet have been successfully used to treat active viral disease. Interferon-alfa,* CMV immune globulin (CMV–IGIV [Cyto-Gam]),* and live attenuated vaccines† hold promise in the prevention of serious CMV infections in at-risk individuals.

Herpesvirus 6

Herpesvirus 6 is the causative agent of roseola infantum (exanthema subitum, sixth disease). Roseola is a common cause of high fever in infants between 6 and 36 months of age. As the prodromal fever drops by the fourth day, a morbilliform eruption consisting of rose-colored discrete macules may suddenly appear on the neck, trunk, and buttocks. The face and extremities occasionally become involved, but the mucous membranes are spared. Periorbital edema may precede the eruption, which fades after 1 or 2 days.

Treatment

No specific therapy is needed as the eruption completely resolves within 2 days.

Herpesvirus 7

Herpesvirus 7 has been associated with a variety of conditions; however, its role in human disease has not been established.

Poxviruses

Molluscum contagiosum is characterized by multiple, discrete, smooth, dome-shaped, umbilicated, 2- to 6-mm papules. It is commonly seen as a nonsexually transmitted disease on any area of the skin or mucous membranes in children and as a sexually transmitted disease on the genitalia of adults. Widespread lesions are frequently present in individuals with impaired CMI, particularly patients with AIDS.

Orf and milker's nodules are two rare diseases caused by parapoxviruses. Orf, or ecthyma contagiosum, is acquired by farmers and veterinarians from direct contact with virus-infected sheep or goats or virus-containing objects. Milker's nodules are transmitted to cattle handlers and slaughterhouse workers from direct contact with infected cows. Both diseases are manifested by painful nodules and plaques localized to the distal upper extremities.

Treatment

Molluscum contagiosum is best treated by light electrocautery or liquid nitrogen with or without curettage. Alternative therapeutic modalities include topical application of cantharidin collodion (Cantharone), tretinoin (Retin-A) gel, podofilox (Condylox), or trichloroacetic acid. These simple destructive thera-

---

*Not FDA-approved for this indication.
†Investigational drug in the United States.

pies are less efficacious in AIDS patients with extensive involvement. AIDS patients frequently require repeated treatments, and they may benefit from combining cytodestruction with the antiviral effects of systemic interferon or cimetidine hydrochloride (Tagamet).

Orf and milker's nodules are treated symptomatically. These diseases spontaneously resolve in 4 to 6 weeks.

Picornaviruses

Enterovirus members of the Picornaviridae that cause febrile exanthems and enanthems include 30 types of coxsackievirus and 33 types of echovirus. These viruses replicate in the gastrointestinal tract so that spread is by the oral-oral and fecal-oral routes. Summertime epidemics often cause subclinical or mild disease in children. Coxsackievirus types A16, A4–7, A9, A10, B1–3, and B5 or enterovirus 71 cause hand-foot-and-mouth disease, a distinctive disorder characterized by small, gray, round or oval vesicles on the hard palate, tongue, and buccal mucosa. These oral lesions rapidly ulcerate and are accompanied by similar lesions on the hands and feet. Coxsackie A2–6, A8, and A10 viruses cause herpangina, which appears as gray-white papules, vesicles, and ulcers on the anterior fauces, tonsillar pillars, soft palate, and uvula. Echo 16 virus causes the "Boston exanthem," which consists of a generalized morbilliform eruption and punched-out ulcers on the soft palate and tonsillar pillars. Echo 9 viral exanthems occur as a rubelliform or morbilliform eruption with petechiae mimicking meningococcemia.

Treatment

No specific therapy is available or necessary as most picornavirus infections resolve completely within 1 to 2 weeks.

Retroviruses

Retroviruses that cause or are associated with cutaneous findings include human T cell leukemia/lymphoma virus Type I (HTLV-I) and human immunodeficiency viruses (HIV-1 and HIV-2). Retroviruses are transmitted by sexual contact with an infected person, via exposure to infected blood products, and perinatally from an infected mother to her child. HTLV-I infection is characterized by the acute onset of cutaneous infiltrates, lymphadenopathy, hepatosplenomegaly, hypercalcemia with or without lytic bone lesions, and interstitial pulmonary infiltrates. Two-thirds of HTLV-I–infected patients develop skin lesions resembling mycosis fungoides, such as papules, nodules, tumors, erythematous patches, or erythroderma.

Two to 4 months after acquiring primary HIV-1 (or HIV-2) infection, up to 50% of patients develop a self-limited mononucleosis-type syndrome that may be accompanied by an asymptomatic, erythematous, macular, or urticarial eruption of the trunk and face.

In addition, a chronic, pruritic eruption consisting of discrete, skin-colored, 2- to 5-mm papules on the head, neck, and upper trunk may occur early in the course of HIV infection. In contrast to these early-stage eruptions that can be ascribed to HIV, most skin conditions are attributable to declining CD4 cell counts and thus occur during the late stages of HIV infection. Skin biopsy and culture are often helpful in establishing the diagnosis of cutaneous viral infections complicating late-stage HIV disease. Chronic or extensive mucocutaneous HSV infections may serve as AIDS-defining illnesses as well as cofactors in the acquisition or progression of HIV-related disease.

Treatment

No one who has developed AIDS has recovered. Most AIDS patients die from opportunistic infection, central nervous system disease, wasting, or malignancy within 2 years of diagnosis. Antiretroviral therapy can prolong survival by slowing the progression of disease, reducing the incidence of opportunistic infection, and delaying the onset of AIDS-defining illness. Although most skin diseases are not life-threatening, it is important to treat skin conditions to improve the quality of life of HIV-infected individuals. The therapy of herpetic and poxvirus infections complicating HIV disease has been discussed previously.

Combination chemotherapy has produced brief remissions in some HTLV-1–infected patients, but relapses are frequently unresponsive to therapy.

PARASITIC DISEASES OF THE SKIN

method of
FUAD S. FARAH, M.D.
State University of New York—HSC Syracuse
Syracuse, New York

Although more common in tropical areas, parasitic diseases of the skin can occur in nonendemic areas. The increasing mobility of the world population and the ease, speed, and increase in worldwide travel have decreased the geographic limitations. It has become necessary for the modern physician to be acquainted with diseases not so common in his or her own environment.

PROTOZOAN INFECTIONS

Amebiasis

The protozoa are single-cell organisms, represented by *Entamoeba histolytica*, that invade the human intestine and may occasionally affect other tissues such as liver and lung, producing abscesses in these locations. Extraintestinal lesions are prone to secondary infections. The skin is involved by direct extension from the colon, hepatic abscess, surgical intervention, or direct contact with infected material. Asymptomatic patients who pass cysts in stools are treated with a single drug that is active in the intestine only. The drug of choice is iodoquinol (Yodoxin), 650 mg three times daily for 20 days. Alternative choices are diloxanide furoate (Furamide),* 500 mg three times daily for 10 days, or paromomycin (Humatin), 25 to 30 mg in three doses for 7 days. For symptomatic patients, the drug of choice is metronidazole (Flagyl), 750 mg three times daily for 10 days, followed by iodoquinol or paromomycin with aforementioned dosages. In severe cases, dehydroemetine (Mebadin),* may be considered at a dose of 1 to 1.5 mg per kg per day (maximum, 90 mg) intramuscularly for up to 5 days. Emetine could be used instead of dehydroemetine, but it is associated with multiple organ toxicity, the most serious of which is cardiovascular. The dose should not exceed 60 mg daily for 10 days. Chloroquine phosphate, 1.0 grams per day for 2 days, followed by 0.5 gram per day for 2 to 3 weeks is also effective. Pediatric dosages should be adjusted accordingly.

Flagellate Protozoa

The flagellates *Giardia* and *Trichomonas* inhabit the gastrointestinal and genitourinary tracts, respectively, and do not involve the skin. They do respond to metronidazole, 250 mg three times daily for 5 days, or quinacrine HCl (Atabrine), 100 mg three times daily for 5 days.

The trypanosomes are flagellated protozoa widely distributed around the equator, resulting in African trypanosomiasis and American trypanosomiasis. The latter ranges from the United States to Argentina.

African Trypanosomiasis

Trypanosoma gambiense is transmitted by the bites of infected *Glossina palpalis* and other flies to its natural host, the human. *T. rhodesiense*, morphologically similar to *T. gambiense*, is transmitted primarily by infected *G. morsitans* flies and infects mainly wild animals, such as antelopes. These zoonoses cause acute and fulminant infections in humans. Often there are no cutaneous lesions, but at times the fly bite is followed by a red nodule surrounded by a white halo (trypanosome chancre), which is seen in Europeans but not in Africans. It is accompanied by lymphangitis, lymphadenopathy, and constitutional symptoms. There may be a pruritic exanthem similar to that of erythema multiforme. Erythema nodosum sometimes occurs, as well as erythema and edema of the eyelids.

Treatment should be initiated early with suramin,* in a 100 to 200 mg test dose intravenously, followed by 1.0 gram weekly for 5 weeks thereafter. Pentamidine isothionate (Pentam 300), 4 mg per kg per day or every other day for 10 doses, is also used. Suramin does not penetrate the central nervous system. It has many untoward effects and is contraindicated in patients with liver or kidney disease.

American Trypanosomiasis

Also known as Chagas' disease, this is caused by *T. cruzi* transmitted by blood-sucking insects called kissing bugs. In the blood, it is a flagellate with an undulating membrane that invades the reticuloendothelial tissues and assumes the Leishman-Donovan form. Clinically, the lesion appears at the site of inoculation within 5 days. The portal of entry is through the conjunctiva (80%). Conjunctivitis, edema, and swelling of the lacrimal glands occur. If inoculation is through the skin, a cutaneous adenopathy complex follows (chagoma). A cutaneous exanthem appears, resembling erythema multiforme. Myocarditis almost always occurs in the chronic forms.

Treatment is not satisfactory. Nifurtimox (Lampit),* 8 to 10 mg per kg per day in four divided doses for 120 days, is given, and also benznidazole,† 5 to 7 mg per kg for 30 to 120 days.

Leishmaniasis

Leishmania organisms produce a wide spectrum of clinical disease. Systemic infections involve the reticuloendothelial tissues, and there is a cutaneous involvement without systemic manifestations. In the middle of the spectrum is mucocutaneous leishmaniasis, with cutaneous involvement and metastatic mucous membrane infection. The disease is transmitted by several phlebotomine sandflies. The hosts' immunologic status can greatly modify the clinical outcome. Table 1 summarizes the *Leishmania* spectrum.

The cutaneous leishmaniasis lesion (oriental sore) is a single or multiple, well-demarcated, granulomatous ulcer that is often secondarily infected and usually heals in about 1 year with a characteristic scar. It is autoinoculable.

American leishmaniasis (mucocutaneous leishmaniasis) is manifested as a cutaneous ulcer similar to the oriental sore or as mucocutaneous lesions of the nose and pharynx. The condition persists for years if untreated and might result in death because of secondary infection.

Treatment for cutaneous leishmaniasis includes the application of heat to the localized lesion, cryotherapy, or even surgical excision. Antibiotics should be used to control secondary infection. Sodium stibogluconate (Pentostam)* is the treatment of choice for large or multiple lesions, in a dose of 10 mg per kg per day, not to exceed 600 mg, intramuscularly or intravenously, for 20 days. It may be repeated in a month's time. Ketoconazole has been used effectively.

Mucocutaneous leishmaniasis is treated similarly with sodium stibogluconate,* 20 mg per kg per day (maximum, 800 mg), intramuscularly or intravenously, for 20 days. It may be repeated until there is a response. Amphotericin B (Fungizone), 0.25 to 1.0 mg per kg per day by slow infusion daily or every other day for up to 8 weeks, may be used. Ketoconazole has also been tried.

---

*Investigational drug in the United States.

*Investigational drug in the United States.
†Not available in the United States.

TABLE 1. **Leishmaniasis**

Clinical Disease	Species	Main Geographic Location
Visceral, dermal, leishmanoid	*L. donovani donovani*	India
	L. d. infantum	Middle East, Mediterranean, Russia and the former republics
	L. d. sinensis	China
Visceral, mucocutaneous	*L. d. nilotica*	Africa (Sudan and Ethiopia)
Cutaneous	*L. tropica major*	Middle East, Mediterranean, China, India
	L. t. minor	Middle East, Mediterranean
Cutaneous and DCL	*L. t. aethiopica*	Ethiopia
	L. mexicana mexicana	Mexico and Central America
	L. m. amazonensis	Brazil and South America
DCL, cutaneous	*L. m. pifanoi*	Brazil and Central America
Cutaneous and mucocutaneous	*L. viannia braziliensis*	Brazil and Central America
	L. v. panamensis	Central America

Abbreviation: DCL = diffuse cutaneous leishmaniasis.

HELMINTHIC INFECTIONS

Platyhelminths (Flatworms)

Schistosomiasis

Schistosoma, the cause of schistosomiasis, also known as bilharziasis, has a complex life cycle. The disease depends on the penetration of the cercariae into the intact skin, reaching the portal vein. The skin may have a schistosomal dermatitis, which is a papular pruritic eruption not different from cercarial dermatitis due to nonhuman schistosomes. Urticarial reactions are especially associated with *S. japonicum* infestations. Paragenital granulomas might occur, as well as ectopic cutaneous lesions, especially on the trunk. Treatment is most effective with praziquantel (Biltricide), 20 mg per kg once. Antimony potassium or sodium tartrate and Niridazole have also been used.

Cercarial Dermatitis

This papular pruritic inflammatory eruption, known commonly as "swimmer's itch," is incited by the entry of cercariae into the human skin. Both freshwater and marine forms of schistosomes are responsible. Urticarial reactions may occur. Treatment is symptomatic with antipruritic agents. The cercariae do not live in the human skin, and the lesions subside spontaneously.

Sparganosis

This condition is found worldwide but is most common in the Orient. It follows ingestion of procercoid larvae (sparganum) of *Spirometra mansonoides* found in drinking water or in raw or lightly cooked muscles of the host (snakes, birds, frogs, and mammals). The painful, edematous lesions appear in the muscle or subcutaneous tissues, and they last indefinitely. The worm may migrate from one area to another. The treatment is surgical. Arsenicals have been said to be effective.

Echinococcosis

Hydatid disease is caused by *Echinococcus granulosus* (of dogs) or *E. multilocularis* (of wild animals) that parasitize humans in the larval stage. The skin is occasionally involved with soft, flocculent, subcutaneous cysts of various sizes. They are not painful. Urticaria may be a common and prominent complication. Treatment is surgical when feasible. Medications used are mebendazole (Vermox), 100 mg twice daily for 3 to 5 days, or praziquantel, 20 to 25 mg per kg thrice daily for 1 to 2 days.

Cysticercosis

The larval forms (cysticerci) of *Taenia solium* (pork tapeworm) produce human intestinal infestation. Poor sanitary habits lead to the ingestion of cysticerci, and the larvae are found in various organs but are predominantly subcutaneous. A nonspecific inflammation with ultimate fibrosis and calcification is seen. The treatment is surgical and with mebendazole or niclosamide (Niclocide), 2 grams per day for 7 days.

Nematodes (Roundworms)

Larva Migrans

Creeping eruption is caused by various nematodes for which humans are an abnormal final host. When the larvae migrate to involve the viscera, the condition is referred to as visceral larva migrans, in contrast to cutaneous larva migrans. Many species are involved, including members of Strongyloidea, Rhabdiasoidea, Spiruroidea, Trichuroidea, Dracunculoidea, and Filarioidea. Most produce similar reactions in the skin, beginning with a nonspecific pruritic eruption at the site of penetration. Migration of the larvae is manifested by a wandering, linear, thin, raised, tunnel-like lesion 2 to 3 mm wide containing serous material. It becomes dry and crusted. Migration is usually slow; when fast, it is referred to as larva currens. Urticaria, eosinophilia, hepatomegaly, pneumonitis, and hyperglobulinemia may follow.

The condition is limited, since the human is a "dead-end" host. The natural duration of the disease is about 4 weeks in the majority of cases. Treatment is with thiabendazole (Mintezol), 25 to 50 mg per kg for 2 to 4 days. Topical thiabendazole is also effective. Freezing the advancing edge of the lesion to produce sloughing of the epidermis and exposure of the parasite is an option.

Trichinosis

Trichinosis results from the ingestion of poorly cooked or raw meat (pork, bear, wild pig) that is infected with *Trichinella spiralis*. The larvae are deposited in the human intestine and migrate till the adult stage, when the female deposits mobile embryos in human tissues. These enter the circulation where they cause intense inflammation, but encystment occurs only in muscle. The skin is pruritic and urticarial; macular, papular, or petechial eruption develops. Splinter hemorrhages may be seen. Eosinophilia develops, along with an acute illness.

Treatment with thiabendazole, 50 mg per kg per day for 7 days, is effective in the early stages but not in older infections.

Tissue Nematodes

Dracunculosis

Common in the Middle East in areas with a scarcity of water (Arabia, Iran, Pakistan), *Dracunculus* is known as the guinea or Medina worm. *D. medinensis* is the causative agent. The gravid female travels to the skin mostly of the lower extremities, where it discharges large numbers of larvae upon contact with water. Severe systemic symptoms appear, including urticaria, erythematous rashes, malaise, and fever. The skin ruptures, allowing the worm's uterus to extrude and discharge the larvae. Secondary infection is not uncommon.

Treatment is with metronidazole, 750 mg three times daily for 10 days. Mebendazole, 100 mg, is repeated after 2 weeks.

Filariasis

This is caused by nematodes of the family Filarioidea, which is of worldwide distribution, mostly in tropical and subtropical areas. *Wuchereria bancrofti* and *Brugia malayi* produce a similar picture. Lymphangitis and lymphadenitis develop, at times accompanied by fever, leading ultimately to fibrosis and obstruction of the lymphatics, resulting in elephantiasis of the affected parts, the genitalia, and the lower extremities.

Treatment is with diethylcarbamazine (Benocide),

50 mg orally on day 1, 50 mg three times daily on day 2, and 100 mg three times daily on day 3; then 2 mg per kg three times daily on days 4 to 21. Surgical intervention may be successful in reducing the elephantiasis.

Loiasis

Loa loa is transmitted by a blood-sucking fly that feeds on infected humans or monkeys. After a year, the adult worm wanders around the viscera; in the subcutaneous tissue it causes distinctive swellings to develop rapidly, which may be painful. They last for a few days and never suppurate. The worm is visible when it is in the conjunctiva. Treatment is with diethylcarbamazine, as for filariasis.

Onchocerciasis

Onchocerca volvulus is transmitted by a black fly vector in tropical areas. The microfilariae reside in the subcutaneous tissue and lymphatics of the skin and in some instances in the eye. Clinically, granulomatous dermal nodules appear mostly on exposed parts of the body. The 3- to 35-mm nodules calcify. In the eye, they lead to blindness. Pruritus may be an early symptom, along with an exanthem that could be generalized. Pruritus leads to chronic lichenification. Hypo- and hyperpigmentation may develop.

The treatment is designed to kill the adult worm and the microfilariae. Diethylcarbamazine kills the microfilariae and is initially given as 0.5 to 1.0 mg per kg per day for 3 days, followed by 3 mg and 4 mg per kg for the second and third week, respectively. Suramin kills the adult worm; it is given intravenously as a 10% solution, 1.0 gram per week for 5 to 6 weeks. It is toxic to the kidneys.

Intestinal Nematodes Infecting Humans Through Eggs

Enterobiasis

Infection with *Enterobius (Oxyuris) vermicularis* is the most common helminthic infection of humans and is worldwide in distribution, affecting 30% of children and 16% of adults. Humans are the only hosts. It is seen most frequently in whites and is more common in cool and temperate zones. *E. vermicularis* lives in the cecum, and the gravid female migrates to the anal area to deposit its eggs. Perianal and perineal pruritus is most common, especially at night. Occasionally vulvovaginitis might develop.

Treatment with mebendazole, 100 mg twice daily for 3 days, is effective, along with good personal hygiene.

FUNGAL DISEASES OF THE SKIN

method of
JACK L. LESHER, JR., M.D.
Medical College of Georgia
Augusta, Georgia

OVERVIEW OF ANTIFUNGAL AGENTS

This discussion of treatment of fungal problems of the skin presupposes that the clinician has confirmed the diagnosis with potassium hydroxide examination and/or culture of lesional material.

Quite a number of over the counter antifungal preparations are available, in a number of different vehicles. Tinea cruris and tinea pedis may respond to tolnaftate (Aftate, Tinactin, or Zeasorb-AF), or undecylenic acid and its derivatives (Cruex, Desenex). Tinea corporis, or more severe cases of tinea cruris or tinea pedis, may respond to clotrimazole (Lotrimin-AF or Mycelex) or miconazole (Micatin). Vaginal preparations of clotrimazole and miconazole are also available over the counter for treating vulvovaginal candidiasis.

Topical prescription antifungals include econazole (Spectazole), ketoconazole (Nizoral), sulconazole (Exelderm), and oxiconazole (Oxistat). These azoles, along with the over-the-counter agents clotrimazole and miconazole, are effective in tinea corporis, tinea cruris, and tinea pedis, as well as cutaneous candidiasis. Another group of broad-spectrum antifungals is the allylamines naftifine (Naftin) and terbinafine (Lamisil). Ciclopirox olamine (Loprox) is also broad-spectrum. These latter agents are used primarily for dermatophyte infections, although they have some activity against yeasts as well. While in general the mycologic cure rate for all these topical antifungals is very similar, it seems that the fungicidal nature of the allylamines does confer some advantage to them—specifically, shorter treatment courses and less likelihood of relapse. Infections may respond faster to these allylamines as well. The main side effect from all these topical agents is occasional burning and irritation. Those with sulfite sensitivity should avoid Nizoral cream.

The major oral medication for treating dermatophyte infections is griseofulvin. This agent is not effective against yeasts such as *Candida* or *Pityrosporum*. The usual dosage of griseofulvin microsize is 10 to 15 mg per kg per day, which in most adults is approximately 1000 mg daily, in divided doses with meals. The main drug interactions with griseofulvin are warfarin (griseofulvin producing increased levels) and barbiturates (which can decrease griseofulvin levels). Griseofulvin may have a disulfiram-like reaction, and patients should be advised to stop alcohol intake while on griseofulvin. The drug may also aggravate lupus erythematosus, and it may interfere with the efficacy of birth control pills.

Ketoconazole (Nizoral) is an imidazole broad-spectrum antifungal that is occasionally used orally in dermatophytoses, candidiasis, and pityriasis versicolor. Dosage schedules vary, but the average dose of ketoconazole is 200 mg daily for these infections. The newer triazole antifungals fluconazole (Diflucan) and itraconazole (Sporanox) are still being investigated for use in superficial fungal infections of the skin. The average daily dose for these agents is 100 mg (higher for onychomycosis). Particularly with ketoconazole, one must be aware of potential hepatotoxicity, and periodic monitoring of liver function tests is recommended, especially for courses greater than 2 weeks. I check liver function studies periodically with all oral azoles. All these azole antifungals may have potential drug interactions, particularly with warfarin, phenytoin, and cyclosporine. Azoles may alter metabolism of terfenadine (Seldane) and astemizole (Hismanal), leading to increased levels of these antihistamines with a potential for cardiac dysrhythmia, so concomitant use of these drugs is contraindicated.

The new allylamine antifungal, terbinafine (Lamisil), is currently being investigated for oral use in superficial fungal infections. Initial studies have demonstrated that this drug should be extremely effective against dermatophytes, less useful for candidiasis, and not good orally for pityriasis versicolor. This drug demonstrates a good safety profile.

SPECIFIC FUNGAL INFECTIONS

Dermatophyte Infections

Any of the topical antifungals previously described is appropriate therapy for tinea corporis. Treatment should be continued for at least a week after apparent clearing of the problem. Infection in family members should also be sought and treated. Widespread or severe tinea corporis may need treatment with oral agents, with griseofulvin microsize being my drug of first choice. This should be used for at least 2 weeks, or until the time of clearing. The other azoles, as just described, are also effective.

Noninflammatory tinea cruris generally responds to a variety of topical antifungals. Again, treatment is continued once or twice daily at least to the time of clearing, or preferably for about a week after apparent resolution. Occasionally, in a severely inflamed infection, oral antifungal drugs must be used. I prefer not to use a combination medication such as betamethasone/clotrimazole (Lotrisone), which contains a potent topical corticosteroid. Tub soaks two to three times daily may be necessary with inflamed or exudative types of tinea cruris. Hydrocortisone 1% cream twice daily for a few days can improve inflammation.

Tinea pedis is sometimes referred to as "athlete's foot," and it is probably the most common fungal infection. There is a rare bullous or pustular variant that may require treatment with oral antifungals such as griseofulvin, but generally tinea pedis responds to a topical antifungal. Most of the topical antifungals previously described are effective. Some of the over-the-counter antifungal powders may be useful in controlling perspiration and odor. Patients must be cautioned to dry their feet thoroughly after bathing and use absorbent cotton socks. Frequent shoe changes are recommended. Clinicians should be aware of the so-called "one hand–two feet" syndrome, in which fungal infection occurs on one palm (tinea manuum) accompanied by bilateral tinea pedis.

One of the most challenging dermatophyte infections to treat is tinea capitis. In the United States, this fungal infection of the scalp is generally due to the organism *Trichophyton tonsurans*. Often the appearance mimics seborrheic dermatitis, with diffuse scalp scaling and some associated hair breakage. Another type of tinea capitis is kerion formation, which is an inflammatory, boggy, exudative mass that develops as a result of a localized immune reaction to the fungus. Griseofulvin remains the treatment of choice for tinea capitis, and I prefer microsize griseofulvin in the dose of 10 to 15 mg per kg per day, although higher doses (up to 20 mg per kg per day) may be necessary if the infection is not responding. The issue of obtaining screening laboratory tests for individuals on griseofulvin is controversial. Treatment will need to be continued for at least 2 to 3 months. The patient should also be given medicated shampoos. I try to keep patients home from school for at least the first few days of treatment. Family members should be cautioned not to share hats, combs, and so on. Sometimes the infection fails to respond to griseofulvin, in which case I turn to my second choice drug, itraconazole, at a dose of 100 mg per day. If kerion is present, concomitant oral antibiotics may be given, in addition to soaks.

Tinea unguium (a type of onychomycosis) is generally caused by *Trichophyton* organisms. I prefer to treat only fingernail infections and discourage treatment of toenail onychomycosis as it is so prone to recur. Treatment requires a long-term commitment on the part of the patient. Topical agents have rarely been effective for mild, limited onychomycotic infections, and, although I might use them adjunctively, I prefer use of an oral agent. Griseofulvin has been the mainstay of therapy for years, but it must be used 6 months or more. I have come to depend increasingly on the newer agent itraconazole (Sporanox) for treating fingernail onychomycosis. The exact treatment regimen is still under investigation; however, many experts in this field are suggesting that intermittent courses of itraconazole may be effective (for example, 200 mg daily for 1 week each month, over a 4-month cycle). Fluconazole is another oral azole antifungal agent that is being investigated for use in tinea unguium. The new agent terbinafine likewise should be useful orally for tinea unguium.

Candidal Infections

Oral candidiasis, or thrush, is very common, particularly in children and immunocompromised patients. This generally responds to nystatin (Mycostatin) in oral suspension and troches, or clotrimazole (Mycelex) troches. In patients with acquired immune deficiency syndrome (AIDS), oral agents such as fluconazole are generally necessary.

Although vulvovaginal candidiasis will often respond to topical therapy, this can be messy and unpleasant for patients, and one may use oral agents such as fluconazole (Diflucan) in short courses.

In candidal intertrigo, there are pustules along the leading edge of an erythematous plaque. These infections may require compresses or tub soaks. These usually respond to topical antifungals, again used for at least 1 to 2 weeks or until time of clearing. Affected areas should be "air dried" as much as possible.

Chronic paronychia is a persistent and recurrent problem of the proximal fingernail folds that is due primarily to *Candida* infection. This is often seen in patients who have their hands in water frequently, and decreasing water exposure is important to help control the problem. I like to use a liquid antifungal, such as ciclopirox olamine (Loprox) solution, or sulconazole (Exelderm) solution, applied to the affected nail fold two to three times daily. Also, it sometimes helps to use a topical corticosteroid lotion such as mometasone furoate (Elocon) once daily in this area to help decrease the associated inflammation.

In the unusual disorder of chronic mucocutaneous candidiasis, primary candidal invasion of all nails occurs. These patients will require long-term treatment with an oral antifungal such as ketoconazole, itraconazole, or fluconazole.

Pityriasis Versicolor

Pityriasis (tinea) versicolor is a very common infection, seen particularly during the summer months and especially in the southern part of the United States. This often presents as hypopigmented macules and patches involving primarily the trunk and proximal extremities. The potassium hydroxide (KOH) preparation is helpful in diagnosis, and it generally reveals the stubby hyphae and yeasts ("spaghetti and meatballs") typical of *Pityrosporum orbiculare*.

Generally I use topical treatment with selenium sulfide lotion (Selsun) applied for 20 minutes to the affected areas, and then washed off, daily for 3 days. Alternatively, the medication may be left on overnight and washed off in the morning, and this is repeated in about 1 week. Particularly for patients living in hot, humid environments, I recommend use of a keratolytic soap such as the Sastid or ZNP bar, once or twice weekly, especially during the spring, summer, and fall months. Although topical antifungals may be used, this can be expensive because of the wide area of involvement. Some experts have advocated use of oral antifungals such as ketoconazole. There is controversy as to the best regimen, but I favor use of 400 mg of ketoconazole on one day with this dose repeated 1 week later. Recurrences are common, however.

DISEASES OF THE MOUTH

method of
DENIS P. LYNCH, D.D.S., PH.D.
The University of Tennessee, Memphis
Memphis, Tennessee

DEVELOPMENTAL DISTURBANCES

Lip Pits. Commissural lip pits are developmental anomalies associated with the formation of minor salivary glands. Surgical excision of the pit and associated salivary gland may be indicated for esthetic reasons; however, they are otherwise of no clinical significance.

Cleft Lip and Cleft Palate. Clefting of the upper lip and palate occurs in 1 in 800 births. Untreated infants experience difficulty in nursing and speech development. Surgical intervention is indicated, with multiple reconstructive procedures periodically throughout childhood.

Fordyce's Granules. These ectopic sebaceous glands appear as whitish-yellow papules on the buccal mucosa in approximately two-thirds of the population. Coalescing papules may form prominent plaques. Occasionally, Fordyce's granules are present on the vermilion borders of the lips. They are of no clinical significance.

Leukoedema. This condition represents a variation of normal buccal mucosa. It is characterized by a translucent, milky-white cast of the buccal mucosa, which disappears when the cheek is stretched. Leukoedema is prevalent in African Americans.

Tori and Exostoses. Tori are bony protuberances, most commonly found on the lingual surface of the mandible (torus mandibularis) and the midline of the hard palate (torus palatinus). They are prone to trauma but do not require surgical removal unless they interfere with the construction of dental prostheses. Exostoses are similar lesions found on the maxillary buccal alveolar bone.

Hairy Tongue. This condition results from elongation of the filiform papillae on the dorsal surface of the tongue; these papillae retain oral debris, chromophilic microorganisms, and *Candida albicans*. Most cases of hairy tongue are asymptomatic; however, a tickling sensation on the palate may occur during swallowing. It is treated by regular brushing of the dorsal surface of the tongue with a toothbrush.

Fissured Tongue. This condition has been associated with both nutritional deficiencies and dehydration; however, the vast majority of cases are idiopathic and of no clinical significance.

Glossitis Areata Migrans. Geographic tongue is characterized by multiple, irregular, depapillated, erythematous areas on the dorsal tongue, which are surrounded by serpiginous, whitish-yellow borders. The locations of the lesions change over time. Geographic tongue is normally asymptomatic; however, superimposed candidiasis may result in stomatopyrosis. Such superinfections are easily treated with nystatin pastilles (Mycostatin) or clotrimazole troches (Mycelex), one every 4 hours for 2 weeks.

Ankyloglossia. This condition results from an over-attachment of the lingual frenum ("tongue-tied") and may interfere with nursing and speech development. The condition is easily treated surgically.

Hemangioma. This congenital malformation is most often found in the body of the tongue but may also be present in the lips and buccal mucosa, as a reddish or violaceous mass. These lesions should not be confused with oral varices, which are commonly found on the ventral surface of the tongue. The significance of hemangiomas is proportional to their size, i.e., small lesions that do not pose any functional or esthetic problems do not require any treatment. Larger lesions may be treated with laser surgery, cryosurgery, embolization, or sclerosing agents.

Lymphangioma. Congenital macroglossia is most frequently caused by lymphangiomas. Unlike hemangiomas, these lesions are often of normal color, with a bluish hue apparent in more superficial lesions. The dorsal surface of the tongue often exhibits multiple nodules, representing lymphangiomatous infiltration of normal papillae. Treatment of lymphangiomas is similar to that of hemangiomas.

Developmental Disturbances of Teeth. A variety of developmental disorders may affect the teeth. Inherited disorders, such as amelogenesis imperfecta and dentinogenesis imperfecta, affect the structural integrity of the enamel and dentin, with increased susceptibility to dental caries and discoloration, respectively. Congenitally missing teeth (partial anodontia) are most often idiopathic, e.g., maxillary lateral incisors, but may be associated with a variety of syndromes, e.g., ectodermal dysplasia. Gemination and fusion of teeth will also result in alterations of both the number and shape of teeth. Solitary or segmental dilaceration of teeth results from trauma to the developing tooth buds. Discoloration of teeth may be iatrogenic, e.g., tetracycline staining, or associated with systemic disease, e.g., porphyria.

Developmental Cysts. These cysts result either from the inclusion of epithelial rests trapped in the process of jaw formation or from residual odontogenic epithelium that undergoes cystic degeneration. Fissural cysts may be found at any embryonic fusion line. Odontogenic rests of Serres may result in gingival cysts. Dental follicles that surround developing teeth may result in the formation of follicular (dentigerous) cysts. These lesions have the capacity for significant expansion and local destruction and are treated surgically. Eruption "cysts" represent enlarged, often fibrotic, dental follicles that impede normal tooth eruption. Such lesions appear as fluid-filled sacs that surround the crowns of erupting teeth. They are treated by incision or deroofing of the follicle to permit continued normal tooth eruption.

BENIGN AND MALIGNANT NEOPLASMS

Leukoplakia and Erythroplakia. Leukoplakia literally means a "white patch," which cannot be removed or characterized clinically or histopathologically as any other specific disease. The term carries no implication as to the malignant potential of the lesion. Erythroplakia is similar to leukoplakia, except that the lesion is red rather than white. Frequently, the two conditions are seen concurrently. Leukoplakia may be found on all mucosal surfaces of the mouth but is seen most frequently on the tongue, buccal mucosa, floor of the mouth, and labial mucosa as a well-defined white area. Approximately 20% of oral leukoplakias have atypical epithelial changes.

Leukoplakia can have a variety of causes, e.g., prominent, sharp cusps of teeth or defective restorations. External agents, such as tobacco use and alcohol consumption, are prominent etiologic factors. With rare exception, e.g., obvious local factors, leukoplakias should be biopsied to rule out underlying dysplasia or carcinoma. Excision is the treatment of choice for those leukoplakias in which premalignant changes can be identified. Recently, chemotherapeutic agents, e.g., beta-carotene and other vitamin A analogues, have been successfully used to alter epithelial cell differentiation and maturation.

Unlike leukoplakia, erythroplakia has a much higher incidence of dysplastic changes. These lesions appear as velvety red patches, often combined with areas of leukoplakia (erythroleukoplakia or speckled leukoplakia). All erythroplakic lesions should be biopsied, even in the presence of obvious local factors. Local excision of erythroplakia is preferred, although partial excision with close follow-up may be necessary, due to the location of the lesion.

Squamous Carcinoma. These lesions are the most common oral cancer in humans, with an incidence of approximately 30,000 new cases annually in the United States. Approximately one-third of these patients will eventually die of their disease or its complications. Squamous carcinoma is most commonly found in middle-aged men; however, the incidence in women and younger individuals is increasing. The vermilion border of the lower lip and lateral border of the tongue are most commonly affected. Long-term survival is directly proportional to the location of the malignancy, with vermilion border lesions having the best prognosis and those at the base of the tongue having the worst.

Squamous carcinoma is often asymptomatic, presenting as an area of leukoplakia or erythroplakia. As the disease progresses, the lesions become indurated, ulcerated, and either endophytic or exophytic, with metastases to the cervical lymph nodes. Size, location, and metastases are all important factors in the staging of the disease and the predicted prognosis. Aggressive surgical excision, with regional lymph node dissection where indicated, is the therapy of choice for squamous carcinoma. Radiation therapy is also used for combined therapy and treatment of recurrent disease. Chemotherapy has a limited role, except in the treatment of widespread metastatic disease.

Verrucous Carcinoma. This lesion is most commonly associated with the use of smokeless tobacco; however, human papillomavirus has also been implicated in its etiology. Unlike squamous carcinoma, lesions are usually exophytic and warty-appearing. Verrucous carcinoma is locally destructive, with little metastatic potential.

Melanoma. Oral melanomas most often arise in the palate and maxillary alveolar ridge. Lesions vary from a flat, slowly enlarging area of pigmentation to a rapidly proliferating, exophytic mass. Despite aggressive resection and adjunctive radiation and chemotherapy, the prognosis for oral melanoma is poor.

Fibroma and Lipoma. These lesions are two of the most common benign mesenchymal neoplasms found in the oral cavity. They consist of proliferations of connective tissue and fat cells, respectively. Many fibromas are actually thought to represent non-neoplastic proliferations of fibrous connective tissue, i.e., fibrous hyperplasias, rather than true neoplasms.

The lesions are asymptomatic, soft-to-firm, well-circumscribed masses. Superficial lipomas are white to yellow in color, whereas fibromas are tan to pink. More superficial lesions are dome-shaped; however, deeper lesions may only be detected by palpation. Small lesions may require no treatment, provided they are reassessed periodically. Larger lesions are treated by surgical excision.

Kaposi's Sarcoma. This lesion was considered highly unusual in the oral cavity until the onset of the human immunodeficiency virus (HIV) epidemic. Kaposi's sarcoma is the most common malignancy in HIV-positive individuals. One-third of acquired immune deficiency syndrome (AIDS) patients with Kaposi's sarcoma have lesions present in the head and neck. Kaposi's sarcoma can occur on any oral mucosal surface. The gingiva and palate are the most frequent sites. The majority of lesions are bluish-purple and frequently asymptomatic. Large lesions respond favorably to local injection of both sclerosing agents, e.g., sodium tetradecyl sulfate (Sotradecol) and chemotherapeutic agents, e.g., vinblastine sulfate (Velban).

Leukemia. Of the various categories of leukemias, monocytic leukemia is the most likely to exhibit oral manifestations. Secondary thrombocytopenia results in palatal petechiae and spontaneous gingival hemorrhages. Neutropenic ulcerations are common, as is superinfection with *Candida albicans* and persistent recurrent herpes simplex virus (HSV-1) lesions. Alveolar bone destruction with loosening of teeth is common. In addition to antimicrobial therapy, proper oral hygiene is essential in the management of the opportunistic oral infections.

SALIVARY GLAND DISEASE

Xerostomia. The most common form of salivary dysfunction is xerostomia. This condition usually results from medications that secondarily suppress salivary gland function, e.g., anticholinergics, antidepressants, and antihypertensives. The lips and cheeks often stick to the teeth, and dysphagia is common. Frequently there is a generalized erythema of the mucosa due to a superimposed candidiasis. Sjögren's syndrome is an autoimmune disease characterized by xerophthalmia, xerostomia, and rheumatoid arthritis. In the late stages of the disease there is a characteristic enlargement of the major salivary glands, especially the parotids.

Oral hygiene is extremely important in xerostomia, as affected patients are unduly susceptible to dental caries. Topical fluoride therapy, e.g., acidulated 0.4% stannous fluoride gel (Gel-Kam) or neutral 1% sodium fluoride gel (Thera-Flur-N) applied once daily in a fluoride tray for 5 minutes is very effective in preventing dental caries. Iatrogenic xerostomia is best handled by adjustment of the causative medication. In some cases, however, the xerostomia must be treated symptomatically with artificial saliva (Xerolube, Salivart) and sialogogues, e.g., sugar-free lemon drops. Residual functional salivary gland tissue also responds well to pilocarpine hydrochloride solution or urecholine tablets (Bethanechol), 25 mg thrice daily.

Sialolith. Salivary gland stones can be found in all of the major, as well as minor, salivary glands. The submandibular glands are most frequently affected. Patients most frequently complain of unilateral pain in the region of the affected gland, especially at mealtime. Often there is a visible swelling, which, combined with an inability to express saliva from the gland, is a strong indication of the existence of a sialolith. Frequently, sialoliths can be seen near the orifice of Wharton's or Stensen's ducts and may be manually expressed from the duct. When this is not possible, the duct can be incised and the stone removed. If the stone is located deep within the gland, the surgical removal becomes more technically involved.

Pleomorphic Adenoma. Benign mixed tumors are the most common salivary gland neoplasm, comprising over 90% of benign and 50% of all salivary gland neoplasms. They present as painless, slow-growing, firm masses, most commonly on the hard palate. Surgical excision is curative.

Malignant Salivary Gland Neoplasms. These malignancies include mucoepidermoid carcinoma and adenoid cystic carcinoma, which comprise over one-half of all salivary gland malignancies. Both these lesions present initially as asymptomatic swellings, often followed by ulceration. Pain is a common feature of advanced adenoid cystic carcinoma. Mucoepidermoid carcinomas are most commonly found in the parotid, followed by the palate, and are the most common salivary gland malignancy in children. Adenoid cystic carcinomas are most commonly found in the palate. They tend to recur locally and result in distant metastases, with a poor long-term survival rate.

ODONTOGENIC CYSTS AND TUMORS

Dentigerous Cyst. This lesion is the most common odontogenic cyst and is usually associated with the crown of an unerupted third molar or maxillary cuspid. Left untreated, these lesions can cause significant local destruction.

Ameloblastoma. This is the best-known of the odontogenic tumors, and it arises from the epithelial portion of the developing tooth. It is most commonly found in the posterior mandible of adults, usually in the fourth decade of life. Early lesions are clinically undetectable; however, late-stage lesions often cause significant mandibular expansion. Ameloblastomas, while benign, are locally aggressive and can cause significant destruction of the jaws. Aggressive surgery, e.g., en bloc resection, is the treatment of choice.

Other odontogenic tumors include calcifying epithelial odontogenic tumor, ameloblastic fibroma, odontogenic myxoma, odontoma, and cementoblastoma. All these lesions are benign but may cause problems if not removed surgically.

BACTERIAL INFECTIONS

Dental Caries. Dental caries is a multifactorial infectious disease that depends on the relationship between cariogenic bacteria, e.g., *Streptococcus mutans*, an appropriate dietary substrate, e.g., fermentable carbohydrate, and a susceptible host. The fermentation of dietary carbohydrates by *S. mutans* results in the formation of an adherent film (plaque), in which bacteria produce acids that demineralize tooth enamel and dentin. Prevention strategies include reduction of fermentable carbohydrates in the diet (reduced sugar consumption), mechanical removal of bacteria and food debris (tooth-brushing and flossing), and chemical strengthening of the enamel (water fluoridation).

Dental caries begins as a whitish area of demineralization on the occlusal or interproximal surfaces of the teeth. The lesions subsequently become detectable radiographically, later followed by clinical cavitation. Untreated dental caries can result in pulpal and periapical disease, including abscess, granuloma, and cyst formation. Such lesions are easily treated with endodontic (root canal) therapy; however, untreated lesions can serve as a focus of infection and may cause significant local destruction of bone.

Periodontal Disease. Chronic inflammatory periodontal disease is the most significant dental disease of adults. Like dental caries, periodontal disease is a bacterial infection that is preventable through proper oral hygiene. The earliest clinical indication of periodontal disease is a reversible inflammation of the gingiva, i.e., gingivitis, which resolves with the institution of appropriate oral hygiene. Progression of the disease involves the underlying supporting and investing structures of the teeth, i.e., periodontium, and results in both the recession of the soft tissues and irreversible destruction of the underlying bone.

Advanced periodontal disease is treated primarily by surgery to make infected areas more self-cleansing. Antibiotic therapy is indicated for refractory cases, both systemically, utilizing amoxicillin (Augmentin), 250 mg every 8 hours, and metronidazole (Flagyl), 250 mg thrice daily for 2 weeks, as well as locally, with tetracycline-impregnated fibers placed in the gingival sulcus (Actisite). Antimicrobial therapy with 0.12% chlorhexidine gluconate rinses (Peridex and PerioGard), 0.5 oz twice daily, is also useful in selected cases.

Other forms of periodontal disease, e.g., acute necrotizing ulcerative gingivitis (trench mouth), linear gingival erythema, and necrotizing periodontitis associated with HIV infection, are well-known but less common in occurrence. Treatment considerations are, in general, the same as with chronic inflammatory periodontal disease.

Tuberculosis. The recent resurgence of disseminated tuberculosis has resulted in an increase of reported oral lesions. Such lesions present as painless, indurated ulcers, most commonly on the tongue.

Syphilis. Primary lesions (chancres) are shallow, asymptomatic ulcers covered by pseudomembrane and surrounded by an erythematous halo, resulting from direct contact with an infected lesion. Untreated chancres resolve spontaneously. Secondary lesions (mucous patches) appear approximately 6 weeks after the disappearance of an untreated chancre. Unlike with chancres, the mucous patches of secondary syphilis do not result from direct contact; i.e., oral-genital contact is not a prerequisite for the appearance of oral mucous patches. The lesions present as yellowish-white plaques that can be removed to reveal an erythematous, often eroded, base. Lesions of tertiary syphilis (gummas) have been reported in the tongue and palate; however, they are exceedingly rare due to intervention and treatment of primary and secondary lesions. They appear as an ulcerating granulomatous mass, which, in the palate, can destroy bone and result in an oral-nasal or oral-antral fistula.

Gonorrhea. Gonorrhea is the most common sexually transmitted disease, with increasing reports of oral infections secondary to oral-genital contact. The clinical signs and symptoms of oral gonorrhea are nonspecific and may mimic any of a variety of bacterial infections from pharyngitis to parotitis.

FUNGAL INFECTIONS

Candidiasis. *C. albicans* is found normally in one-third of the healthy population and over 90% of denture wearers. Predisposing conditions for candidiasis include diabetes mellitus, broad-spectrum antibiotic use, corticosteroid use, and immunosuppression secondary to HIV infection. Candidiasis is the most common oral fungal infection and has several distinct, but overlapping, clinical presentations.

Pseudomembranous candidiasis (thrush) is the best-recognized form of the infection and is characterized by white, curdlike plaques with an underlying erythematous, often eroded, mucosal base. Erythematous candidiasis presents as a diffuse mucosal erythema, without any visible fungal colonies. Hyperplastic candidiasis (candidal leukoplakia) is a unique form of candidiasis in which the organism invades the epithelium to stimulate an epithelial hyperplasia.

The diagnosis of oral candidiasis is relatively straightforward, utilizing potassium hydroxide (KOH) digestion with dark-field or phase-contrast microscopy, histopathologic staining (Gram's, Gomori's methenamine silver), latex agglutination (CandidaSure), in-office culture (Oracult), or traditional mycologic culture techniques. Hyperplastic candidiasis may require an incisional biopsy for definitive diagnosis, as the organisms are primarily interepithelial rather than superficial.

Oral candidiasis is easily treated in most cases. Topical antifungals include nystatin (Mycostatin) pastilles and clotrimazole (Mycelex) troches, one every 4 hours for 2 weeks. Systemic antifungals such as ketoconazole (Nizoral), 200 mg daily for 2 weeks, fluconazole (Diflucan), 100 mg daily for 2 weeks, and itraconazole (Sporanox), 200 mg daily for 2 weeks, have all proved to be effective, especially for refractory infections.

Median Rhomboid Glossitis. This unique form of candidiasis appears as an asymptomatic, diamond-shaped, erythematous, depapillated area on the dorsal surface of the tongue at the junction of the anterior two-thirds and posterior one-third of the tongue. This localized candidiasis responds to antimycotic therapy but returns upon cessation of therapy. It does not evolve into any other form of candidiasis. For this reason, no treatment is indicated.

Angular Cheilitis. Angular cheilitis, or perlèche, presents as a bilateral maceration of the commissures of the lips. The great majority of the lesions are due to a focal candidal infection, with ariboflavinosis and decreased vertical dimension of the jaws serving only as predisposing factors. Once the predisposing factors have been attended to, e.g., nutritional therapy or construction of new dental prostheses, angular cheilitis is easily treated with any of a variety of topical antifungal creams, e.g., 100,000 U per gram of nystatin (Mycostatin), 1% clotrimazole (Mycelex-G), or 2% miconazole (Monistat-7) applied every 6 hours for 2 weeks.

VIRAL INFECTIONS

Herpes Simplex, Type 1. Primary herpes simplex, Type 1 (HSV-1) infections are symptomatic in less than 20% of infected individuals. Such cases are characterized by fever, malaise, cervical lymphadenopathy, and a vesicular eruption of the vermilion borders of the lips and all oral mucosal surfaces. The lesions resolve uneventfully within 14 days; however, the virus remains dormant in the peripheral nerves.

A number of factors can reactivate HSV-1, including sunlight, trauma, immunosuppression, and hormonal imbalances. Reactivated virus travels down nerve trunks and results in a cluster of small vesicles on the vermilion border, attached gingiva adjacent to the teeth, or the hard palate.

Primary HSV-1 can be treated with systemic acyclovir (Zovirax), 200 mg every 3 hours for 10 days. Recurrent lesions have been reported to respond to topical 5% acyclovir applied every 2 hours during the prodromal stage, although the ointment form is poorly absorbed through skin and is difficult to apply to oral mucosa. Systemic acyclovir is also effective but only if taken in the prodromal stage of the recurrent infection. Lip balms, lotions, and gels with ultraviolet light blockers, e.g., para-amino benzoic acid (PreSun), are effective in preventing vermilion border lesions.

Oral Hairy Leukoplakia. Oral hairy leukoplakia is an epithelial hyperplasia, secondary to Epstein-Barr virus replication, first described in HIV-positive homosexual men and subsequently in hemophiliacs and transfusion recipients. It is not a specific sign of HIV infection but rather a manifestation of generalized immunosuppression. The majority of lesions occur on the lateral surfaces of the tongue as a corrugated leukoplakia. Lesions on the ventral tongue have a more plaque-type appearance, whereas those on the dorsal tongue are more "hairy." A biopsy is necessary for diagnosis. The lesions will resolve with the administration of oral antiviral agents, e.g., acyclovir (Zovirax), desciclovir,* dihydroxy-propoxy-methyl-guanine (DHPG), and azidothymidine (Zidovudine); however, they return when the medication is discontinued. Vitamin A has been used topically, as has podophyllin resin, with variable results.

Human Papillomavirus. Of the over 60 types of human papillomavirus (HPV), less than 1 dozen have been associated with lesions of the oral mucosa. Of greatest interest is the recently discovered association of HPV-16 and -18 with dysplastic and neoplastic conditions of oral mucosal epithelium.

Oral warts (squamous papillomas and verruca vulgaris) are most commonly found on the vermilion borders of the lips, the hard and soft palates, and the uvula. They have been associated with HPV-2, -6, -11, and -29. Squamous papillomas are normally small, solitary, asymptomatic, pedunculated, exophytic lesions, whereas verruca vulgaris lesions are often sessile. Both lesions are asymptomatic unless secondarily traumatized. HPV-6 and -11 are associated with oral condylomata acuminata, which present as multiple, small, sessile masses, which may coalesce to form larger exophytic masses. Focal epithelial hyperplasia is associated with HPV-13 and -32 and is characterized by widespread, pink soft tissue masses, which may be either dome-shaped or papular.

Solitary lesions are normally treated with conservative surgical excision. Electrodesiccation, cryosurgery, and laser ablation have also been used. Recently, podophyllin resin and interferon have been used experimentally with success.

PHYSICAL AND CHEMICAL INJURIES

Pyogenic Granuloma, Peripheral Ossifying Fibroma, and Peripheral Giant Cell Granuloma. These are all reactive, blastomatoid lesions with a putative etiology of chronic irritation and subsequent inflammation. Pyogenic granulomas are often referred to as "pregnancy tumors" because of their in-

creased incidence in pregnant women. The lesions are thought to occur secondary to retained subgingival food debris or dental calculus (tartar), which act as a focus of chronic irritation. They most commonly occur on the gingiva as rapidly growing, erythematous, exophytic masses that bleed easily upon manipulation. Small lesions may be treated with a thorough dental prophylaxis, which is followed by involution and resolution of the lesion. Long-standing lesions require surgical removal.

Peripheral ossifying fibromas frequently occur on the buccal and labial gingiva of children and teenagers as erythematous, exophytic masses, often with a secondarily ulcerated surface. These lesions are less prone to hemorrhage upon manipulation and are often firmer than pyogenic granulomas. Surgical excision is the treatment of choice.

Peripheral giant cell granulomas resemble pyogenic granulomas. Incomplete excision of these lesions often leads to recurrence.

Mucocele. Trauma to the lower lip, especially in children, often damages the ducts of minor salivary glands, resulting in an occlusion of the duct and formation of a mucocele. This lesion appears as an asymptomatic, translucent, fluid (saliva)-filled soft tissue mass on the mucosal surface of the lower lip, which frequently ruptures and reforms. They are treated with surgical excision of both the mucocele and the associated minor salivary gland. Analogous lesions occurring in the submandibular and sublingual glands are called ranulas.

Fluorosis. Excess fluoride in the drinking water can result in mottling of the enamel. Fluorosis is commonly seen in northern Texas and southern Oklahoma, where endemic water fluoride concentrations exceed the ideal 1.0 ppm. Fluorosis is primarily an esthetic problem, which may respond well to bleaching.

Tetracycline Staining. Tetracycline has a great affinity for developing teeth and bone and, as such, is contraindicated in children, due to its deposition in dentin. Affected children have dark brown to gray teeth that are resistant to bleaching.

Attrition, Abrasion, and Erosion. Attrition is the physiologic process of tooth wear and a normal result of aging. Bruxism is a pathologic process of tooth wear, due to improper occlusion or jaw relationships. Abrasion is the wearing away of tooth structure by physical substances, such as abrasive toothpastes and hard toothbrushes. Erosion is the chemical dissolution of tooth substance. This is most commonly seen in individuals with unique dietary habits, e.g., lemon sucking, and behavioral disturbances, e.g., bulimia.

Chemical Burn. Patients will occasionally place aspirin at the site of a painful oral lesion. The low pH of aspirin results in a mucosal slough with attendant pain and discomfort. The lesion presents as a friable, white, often shaggy plaque that is easily removed to reveal an eroded epithelial base. The diagnosis is made on the basis of history.

Traumatic Ulcer. These lesions are erythematous,

*Not available in the United States.

tender, and occasionally indurated, often with regional lymphadenopathy. They can be treated with occlusive dressings (Orabase, Orabase with benzocaine, Zilactin, Zilactin-B, or ZilaDent). Topical corticosteroids are also effective, e.g., 0.05% fluocinonide (Lidex) gel, applied every 4 hours, often in combination with an occlusive dressing. In the absence of a chronic irritant, the lesions should heal within 2 weeks. Persistent lesions should be biopsied.

Drug-Induced Gingival Hyperplasia. A number of medications, including immunosuppressives, e.g., cyclosporine (Sandimmune), antiseizure drugs, e.g., phenytoin (Dilantin), and calcium channel blockers, e.g., diltiazem (Cardizem) and nifedipine (Procardia), result in significant fibrous hyperplasia of the gingiva. Late-stage lesions require surgical intervention; however, a dramatic decrease in such side effects can be achieved with the use of a 0.12% chlorhexidine gluconate rinse (Peridex and PerioGard), 0.5 oz twice daily, in conjunction with proper oral hygiene.

Amalgam Tattoo. The most common pigmented oral mucosal lesion is an amalgam tattoo (focal argyrosis). This lesion results from the implantation of dental amalgam in the oral mucosa during the restoration of the teeth. The lesions are pigmented, flat, and asymptomatic but may increase in size over time. The amalgam present in the lesion is rarely visible radiographically. The lesions may occur in locations distant from the site of the dental restoration. In the absence of radiographic evidence of the presence of submucosal amalgam, a biopsy is necessary to confirm the diagnosis to rule out other significant pigmented lesions, e.g., melanoma. No further treatment is necessary.

MUCOCUTANEOUS DISEASE

Recurrent Aphthous Ulcers and Behçet's Syndrome. Recurrent aphthous ulcers are the most common oral ulcers. The specific etiology is unclear; however, there is no evidence that recurrent aphthous ulcers result from any infectious agent. The lesions present as shallow ulcers, covered by pseudomembrane and surrounded by an erythematous halo. In contrast to major aphthous ulcers, minor aphthae are smaller and shallower and heal rapidly without scar formation. Recurrent aphthous ulcers are best treated with topical corticosteroids, e.g., 0.05% fluocinonide (Lidex) gel or 0.05% clobetasol propionate (Temovate) ointment applied every 6 hours, often followed by an occlusive dressing (ZilaDent), for up to 10 days. Behçet's syndrome consists of a triad of oral, ocular, and genital ulcers.

Lichen Planus. This disorder is the most common of the mucocutaneous diseases and occurs most commonly in perimenopausal females. Oral lesions are more common than cutaneous lesions and present as lacelike striations (Wickham's striae), leukoplakia, erythema, mucosal atrophy, and, occasionally, bullae. Gingival manifestations of the disease are easily confused with chronic inflammatory periodontal disease. Wickham's striae are not always present and,

when present, may be confused with the radiating striations associated with oral mucosal lesions of lupus erythematosus.

Asymptomatic lesions of oral lichen planus do not require any therapeutic intervention. Symptomatic lesions respond well to topical 0.05% fluocinonide (Lidex) gel and 0.05% clobetasol propionate (Temovate) ointment applied every 4 hours. Severe lesions may require systemic prednisone, up to 80 mg daily, occasionally in conjunction with azathioprine (Imuran), 50 mg twice daily. Several reports of malignant degeneration of oral lichen planus have been reported; however, the actual malignant potential, if any, remains unclear.

Lupus Erythematosus. Lupus erythematosus is an autoimmune disease that ranges in severity from the discoid (mucocutaneous) form to systemic lupus erythematosus, which involves multiple organ systems. Oral lesions have been reported in all forms and are characterized by punctate leukoplakia, mucosal atrophy, and radiating striations. A biopsy is mandatory for diagnosis.

Most oral lesions of lupus erythematosus are symptomatic; however, an overlying candidiasis often contributes to the stomatopyrosis and stomatodynia. Asymptomatic lesions require no treatment; however, topical 0.05% fluocinonide (Lidex) gel and 0.05% clobetasol propionate (Temovate) ointment, applied every 4 hours, are useful in decreasing any associated discomfort. There is a well-described tendency for malignant degeneration in lupus erythematous lesions of the vermilion borders of the lips; therefore, routine follow-up of otherwise asymptomatic lesions is indicated.

Erythema Multiforme and Stevens-Johnson Syndrome. These two related conditions are thought to represent an exaggerated hypersensitivity reaction to various antigens. The most common precipitating event for erythema multiforme is an otherwise uncomplicated episode of recurrent HSV-1 infection. Oral lesions can occur in the absence of pathognomonic target or bull's-eye lesions on the skin and mimic primary HSV-1 infection.

Oral lesions begin as large, fluid-filled, often bloody bullae of the vermilion borders and oral mucosa. The lesions rapidly rupture, resulting in large, crusted lip lesions and widespread oral ulcers. The histopathologic features of the disease are often inconclusive, and a biopsy of oral lesions is of little diagnostic value. Topical anesthetics (lidocaine 2% [Xylocaine Viscous]) are useful for temporary pain relief at mealtime; however, systemic corticosteroids are usually necessary to control the acute phase of the disease.

Pemphigus Vulgaris. Of all of the different types of pemphigus, vulgaris is the most severe form and the most likely one to exhibit oral manifestations, often before any cutaneous lesions are apparent. Vesicles may appear on any oral mucosal surface, but they rapidly rupture, resulting in widespread ulceration. Oral lesions of pemphigus vulgaris may respond to topical corticosteroid therapy, e.g., 0.05%

fluocinonide (Lidex) gel and 0.05% clobetasol propionate (Temovate) ointment applied topically every 4 hours; however, systemic prednisone or other corticosteroid analogues are frequently necessary. Azathioprine (Imuran), 50 mg twice daily, is a useful adjunct, especially in patients who cannot tolerate large doses of systemic corticosteroids.

Cicatricial Pemphigoid. Cicatricial pemphigoid is an autoimmune vesiculobullous disease most frequently seen in middle-aged women. Ocular lesions (symblepharons) and genital mucosal manifestations are seen less frequently than oral lesions. Cutaneous lesions are uncommon. Oral lesions commonly affect the gingiva and may mimic chronic inflammatory periodontal disease. A biopsy is necessary for diagnosis. The oral mucosal lesions of cicatricial pemphigoid respond well to topical corticosteroids. Gingival lesions are especially responsive to topical 0.05% fluocinonide (Lidex) gel and 0.05% clobetasol propionate (Temovate) ointment under an occlusive vinyl stent. Widespread lesions can also be treated with systemic corticosteroids (prednisone), 80 mg daily, or dapsone USP, 25 to 50 mg daily.

VENOUS STASIS ULCERATIONS

method of
JAMES H. STEWART, M.D.
Mayo Clinic Jacksonville
Jacksonville, Florida

Ulcerations from venous disease are termed "venous stasis ulcerations," "venous ulcers," or "varicose ulcers." They represent the end-stage skin changes of chronic venous insufficiency (CVI), also called "stasis dermatitis," "liposclerosis," or "lipodermatosclerosis."

NORMAL VENOUS PHYSIOLOGY

When a person is supine, the principal driving force for venous return is the dynamic pressure from cardiac systole. Each systole generates 12 to 15 mm Hg of dynamic venous pressure; during diastole, right-sided heart pressures encourage venous return. During inspiration, the downward force of the diaphragm increases pressure on the peritoneal cavity and inferior vena cava, decreasing venous return from the lower extremities. Expiration reverses these factors, allowing increased venous return from the legs. When one is upright, the calf muscle pump is the force returning venous blood to the heart, because other factors are inadequate against the effects of gravity (hydrostatic pressure).

The "muscle pump" is the term for the effects of calf muscle contractions forcing blood toward the heart as the deep veins are compressed. During walking, an external pressure on the deep veins of 200 mm Hg or more is generated. This pumps venous blood proximally against the hydrostatic pressure. With each calf muscle contraction, deep venous valves open upward from the brief relative increase in venous pressure, followed by a reduction in venous pressure to 0 to 30 mm Hg with muscle relaxation and valve closure. Perforator valves close, preventing flow to the superficial veins. The ambulatory venous pressure thus normally drops with exercise, slowly rising again with rest as the deep venous blood volume is refilled from arterial inflow and superficial vein drainage into the deep system. Excessive venous pooling is prevented by the one-way venous valves (which remain mostly closed when a person is upright).

VENOUS PATHOPHYSIOLOGY

When a person is upright, the hydrostatic pressure transmitted downward should cause venous valve closure. Non-closure (incompetence) of the valves may result from scarring after a deep venous thrombosis (DVT), vein dilatation, inherited valvular defects, trauma, or degeneration. Incompetent valves, venous outflow obstruction, and calf muscle weakness result in muscle pump dysfunction. Subsequent venous hypertension leads to dilatation and elongation of distal vessels and a transudate depositing fibrin around the capillaries, adversely affecting nutrition and oxygenation of surrounding tissue. Swelling, brown pigmentation, varicose veins, and ulceration may then follow.

Typically, venous leg ulcers begin years after a DVT, preceded by other, more benign, skin changes. In many, a preceding history of DVT may not be apparent, and the lesions may be from primary deep venous insufficiency. Lastly, some practitioners feel that many venous ulcers result from superficial venous disease alone; however, this condition is either almost nonexistent, or there is a great regional variation in its incidence. If a careful history is taken, many of these patients will be found to have had events suspicious for DVT. In others, deep venous insufficiency (DVI) is noted by proper vascular laboratory testing. In general, primary varicose veins, i.e., in the absence of DVI, are infrequently of more than cosmetic concern.

CLINICAL FEATURES

Heaviness or aching is often described by persons with DVI, relieved promptly by leg elevation. Typically, there is little discomfort even with ulcerations, which are mostly found on the medial aspect of the lower leg just above the malleolus (over perforator veins). Less often they are located more laterally or proximally. If other characteristic changes of chronic venous insufficiency are not found, the etiology is in question. Well-defined margins, a moist pink or yellow-pink base, and drainage of significant amounts of clear, straw-colored fluid are the rule. A biopsy from the ulcer margin is recommended if the type of ulcer remains uncertain after physical examination and vascular laboratory testing. Alternatively, a treatment trial is also appropriate, when suspected, since 90% of chronic leg ulcers are venous ulcers.

DIFFERENTIAL DIAGNOSIS

Other chronic ulcers of the lower legs are less common; nevertheless, the most common skin lesions mistaken for venous ulcers include neoplastic skin lesions, cutaneous forms of vasculitis, wounds from trauma, and primary infectious lesions. Ischemic ulcers have a quite different appearance, being generally dry, necrotic, and painful and most often involving the toes or any distal pressure point. Neurotrophic ulcers form from repeated focal trauma in the setting of a sensory neuropathy, with ulcerations at sites of pressure, especially near the metatarsal heads. The surrounding callus, concomitant neurologic condition, and typical locations make these quite unlike venous ulcers.

VASCULAR LABORATORY TESTING

Vascular laboratory testing is helpful when the type of ulcer is unclear and to differentiate between deep and superficial venous insufficiency. Although continuous-wave (hand-held) Doppler testing and the duplex venous ultrasonography test for reverse flow (incompetence) in specific veins suggest venous reflux if positive, physiologic testing of the calf muscle pump function gives more definitive and convincing information. These tests involve plethysmographic (volume) measurement of the leg with calf muscle exercise. The photoplethysmograph (PPG) and light reflection rheography (LRR) machines are easy to operate and use light reflection to determine the volume of blood in superficial vessels and its change with forced flexion and extension of the ankle. Calf exercise empties the distal vessels of blood, with the normal time for a return to baseline after rest of greater than 20 seconds; shorter times indicate venous filling from venous reflux across incompetent valves in addition to that from arterial inflow. Repeating an abnormal test after placement of a superficial vein occluder on the ankle and calf helps localize the involvement to the deep or superficial venous systems. If available, the air-plethysmograph (APG) accurately depicts the function of venous valves and the calf muscle pump, adding to the results of PPG testing. Venous outflow obstruction, quantitation of venous insufficiency, and the effects of stockings are also evaluated with this method.

TREATMENT

The goal of treatment is to heal the ulceration quickly, simply, without great expense, and without the patient becoming an invalid. Although no regimen is clearly the best, certain aspects of care are paramount. John J. Cranley, M.D., has emphasized that healing occurs invariably if the limb can be kept above the level of the heart or if sufficient compression is applied to the limb of the ambulatory patient. To avoid the debilitating effects of prolonged bed rest, these two measures are ideally combined.

Elastic support aids venous return by allowing the muscle pump to work on both deep and superficial veins despite incompetent valves. The external pressure helps prevent edema formation and limit wound drainage. This may involve an elastic wrap, an Unna boot, or one of the compressive devices, but it is best accomplished with elastic support stockings that apply graduated compression. Knee-high stockings with 30 to 40 mm Hg of compression may be slipped over a thin dressing (longer stockings are difficult to apply and keep in place). Compliance is high if initial instructions are given on the application technique and their benefit explained. The Unna boot (a wrapped paste bandage) is of historical importance but is best avoided, because it allows no access to the ulcers, causes maceration, becomes foul-smelling, and requires a caregiver for weekly applications. With elastic stockings, the patient may remain active, maintaining the bulk and strength of the calf muscles. Edema reduction and decreased wound drainage are further aided by elevation of the leg at or above the level of the heart for 30 to 60 minutes two to three times daily. Keeping a written record

of the leg elevation has been suggested to improve compliance.

The wound dressing of choice for venous ulcers remains controversial, and there is little help in the literature to guide the clinician. On the other hand, the selection is limited if desired characteristics of dressings include simplicity, low cost, nonadherence to the ulcer, comfort, prevention of ulcer drying, good absorption, avoidance of maceration, wound accessibility, and allowances of external compression (Table 1).

Calcium alginate dressings are well suited, because they can be easily removed and maintain a moist environment (possibly by forming a gel) better than dry gauze without apparent wound trauma; however, both are simple and effective. Some nonstick gauze dressings are desirable, depending on their construction; they may cause problems with maceration if the transudate is not able to pass through easily to overlying dry gauze. Occlusive dressings (including hydrocolloid and foam types) have become well known because of their ease of application. They offer a moist environment and require little maintenance but may cause maceration, can hide infection, are frequently difficult to remove, and may leak retained drainage when compressed under elastic garments. These seem to be best utilized for the treatment of early, dry, or nearly healed ulcers, or over an eschar, to speed its removal.

The recommended regimen for venous ulcer management is very similar to the "Oregon Protocol" described in recent literature. The ulcer is cleansed without soaking, using a washcloth, a gentle soaping, and water to remove dried wound drainage. After rinsing, a dry gauze pad, a nonstick, porous dressing or alginate dressing is placed on the ulcer and covered with a thin layer of dry gauze pads. The dressing is secured with a knee-high nylon stocking, avoiding the use of tape and excessive gauze wrappings. A knee-high elastic stocking is then slipped over the nylon. The nylon is always worn, whereas the elastic stocking is removed at night. Dressings are changed daily or every other day if no significant drainage is noted on the overlying gauze (Table 2).

At office visits spaced every 1 to 3 weeks, this process is reinforced. No topical solutions, creams, or ointments are applied to the ulcer except with special conditions (see later). These may retard granulation tissue or lead to local (contact) or generalized hyper-

TABLE 1. **Dressing Types**

Gauze Dressings
    Dry gauze pads
    Nonstick gauze (Adaptic, Telfa, Vaseline gauze)
    Impregnated gauze (Unna boot)

Occlusive Dressings
    Calcium alginate (AlgiDERM, Algisorb,
        Kaltostat, Sorbsan)
    Hydrocolloid (Actiderm, DuoDERM, Restore)
    Foam (Epigard, LYOfoam, Mitraflex)

TABLE 2. **Venous Ulcer Regimen**

Change the dressing daily (or every other day if little drainage)

Cleanse with mild soap, water, and washcloth; rinse well

Apply dry gauze, a porous, nonstick dressing, or calcium alginate dressing and cover with 3–4 dry gauze pads

Secure with a knee-high nylon stocking

Wear 30–40 mm Hg graduated elastic stockings during the daytime, remove at night

Elevate the legs above the heart for 30 min two to three times daily

Perform daily toe and heel raises to strengthen the calf muscles

sensitivity reactions and may sensitize the patient to the use of oral or parenteral agents. If débridement is needed after washing, for removal of dried secretions or nonviable tissue, this may be achieved with little trauma using a tongue blade or occasionally a No. 15 scalpel. At each visit, the wound should be measured and written instructions given to the patient if there is a change in wound care. Home care nursing may help initiate and instruct in the care of the ulcer(s) and monitor for progress. Admission to the hospital is indicated if there is a need for surgery or for intravenous antibiotics.

Special Conditions

For significant edema, pneumatic extremity pumping is performed to properly fit the patient for elastic stockings at the first visit. If this is not available, elevation and elastic wrapping of the leg at a morning visit may allow fitting. Diuretics are ill advised, but intermittent use may be unavoidable for initially severe edema.

Concomitant arterial disease slows healing; however, unless it is severe, the treatment regimen is unchanged, except that the ideal compression may be less than usual, and it is important that the stockings be removed when the patient is supine. In the presence of severe arterial disease, nonhealing ulcers are an indication for arterial revascularization.

Cellulitis is not a frequent complication of venous ulcers, and culturing a noninflamed ulcer is more likely to result in unwanted information about numerous resident bacteria. Antibiotics are not recommended unless there are signs of cellulitis, including pain, a change in drainage, surrounding skin erythema, lymphangitis, or systemic signs such as fever, chills, or malaise. Even in this setting, cultures obtained are seldom helpful unless purulent material is obtained without contamination from resident flora. Hospitalization is favored if there are systemic signs or with presumed poor compliance.

Simple colonization with resident skin flora and organisms resulting from the ulcer milieu appears seldom to be detrimental to wound healing. On occasion, a pathogenic bacterium may become dominant,

harming the granulation tissue and producing a foul-smelling, discolored drainage, without cellulitis. Therapeutic measures for this include more frequent cleansing and dressing changes or application of diluted antiseptics such as sodium hypochlorite (one-quarter-strength Dakin's solution); povidone-iodine (one-tenth-strength Betadine); sodium chloride; 0.25 to 0.5% acetic acid; 3% boric acid; or gentian violet. Unfortunately, these tend to be at least mildly caustic, and their use is limited owing to tissue toxicity, staining, or odor. Topical antibiotics (bacitracin, mupirocin, neomycin, polymyxin B, silver sulfadiazine, and so on) are probably more harmful than beneficial in this setting.

Maceration from persistent moisture under occlusive dressings slows healing. Therapeutic measures include the use of dry gauze dressings moistened only at changing times or nonstick, porous dressings covered by dry gauze. Sometimes exposure of the surrounding skin to air for 15 to 20 minutes at each dressing change is helpful. Increased elevation of the leg or applying more compression (or light compression even at night) should decrease the amount of wound drainage. Finally, a moisture-repellent cream or ointment may be applied around the ulcer.

Hypertrophic granulation tissue infrequently develops with venous ulcers, producing a protruding sore. This responds well to silver nitrate stick applications. Poor granulation tissue is more challenging and is marked by an ulcer base lined with yellow or gray material not removed by cleansing. In the absence of infection, débridement surgically or chemically is indicated. One chemical method is to apply 10% benzoyl peroxide dressings for a few days, using care to shield the surrounding skin.

Inflammation of the lower leg from either venous stasis or contact dermatitis generally responds well to 0.025% triamcinolone cream especially if a tap water–wet dressing is then applied. Avoidance of all other topical applications may aid in healing; however, patch testing may be beneficial if clearing does not follow. Generalized skin rashes from venous stasis dermatitis or sensitization from topical agents should respond to the aforementioned treatment, adding a course of oral glucocorticoid drugs and antipruritic agents if necessary.

Atrophie blanche (livedoid vasculitis) is manifested by hypopigmented, recurrent, painful, and irregularly shaped regions of ulceration or scarring on the ankle or foot. The pearly white color persists after healing. Clearly related to deep venous insufficiency, it has also been noted in the literature with other conditions. The areas involved show evidence of ischemia and are quite tender. Many treatments have been studied with varying success, including compression and leg elevation, topical or injected corticosteroids, and antithrombotic agents. Currently, there is no consensus regarding treatment.

Surgical Treatment

The role of surgical therapy, except for skin grafting, remains controversial in the setting of deep venous insufficiency. For the rare case of venous ulcers from superficial venous insufficiency, surgical treatment is potentially curative. In general, surgical results are difficult to interpret, since much, if not all, of the benefit may be from the extended bed rest and postoperative insistence on elastic compression stockings. With a good medical regimen, treatment failures should be infrequent, especially if there is compliance with adequate compression. Skin grafting is best reserved for larger ulcers that show little or no improvement with the medical regimen, since treatment time may be shortened dramatically. For best results, postoperative bed rest and lifelong elastic compression are needed. Extensive débridement is occasionally recommended for a deeper ulcer without a granulating base. Treatment of the concomitant varicose veins has been advocated by some; however, except with primary superficial venous disease, the benefit is questionable and a new wound is created. Single or combination procedures with stripping, ligation, stab avulsion, and sclerotherapy find supporters in the literature. Venous reconstructions, including transpositions, venous segment transfers, valve transplantation, and valvuloplasty, remain experimental, with variable short-term and relatively unknown long-term results.

Alternative Therapies

Many therapeutic strategies to augment healing have been studied. Treatments with whirlpool (termed hydrotherapy) and hyperbaric oxygen have advocates but are without convincing results. Pentoxyfylline (Trental) offers apparent benefit in some studies, and further development of autologous growth factors remains promising.

PRESSURE ULCERS

method of
BRUCE A. FERRELL, M.D., and
MUHAMMAD GHADAI, M.D.
Sepulveda Veterans Affairs Medical Center
Sepulveda, California

Pressure ulcers are a common and serious problem, especially among those patients who are bed-bound, chairbound, or unable to reposition themselves. These lesions usually occur as a result of ischemia and necrosis in the skin and underlying tissues, caused by unrelieved pressure or shearing forces over bony prominences. Other known risk factors for their development include immobility, incontinence (moisture), malnutrition, and sensory impairment. Pressure ulcers remain a difficult problem because they occur most often in frail or elderly persons with multiple confounding medical problems, and in those with scant resources for prevention and management. Indeed, the cost of pressure ulcer prevention and management has been estimated as high as $4000 to $40,000 per ulcer.

PREVENTION

In 1992, the Agency for Health Care Policy and Research released clinical practice guidelines for the prediction and prevention of pressure ulcers in adults. These guidelines have become the "gold standard" of care in most facilities. Table 1 lists the major goals recommended by this expert panel based on research evidence, consensus, and expert opinion. The panel also made more than 50 specific suggestions for the systematic screening of pressure ulcer risk as well as suggestions for routine skin care, use of pressure-reducing support surfaces, and content for educational programs.

TREATMENT OF PRESSURE ULCERS

Healing pressure ulcers expeditiously requires successful management of risk factors as well as careful management of underlying disease. Morbidity and mortality are usually related more to underlying disease than to ulcer complications. For some, such as terminal patients or those with limited treatment goals, alternative approaches might be appropriate to avoid deterioration of an ulcer rather than risky or costly interventions aimed at complete cure.

Pressure reduction is the single most important aspect of treatment. Relief can be accomplished by mobilizing the patient as much as possible, frequently turning or repositioning the patient (every 2 hours), and using pressure-reducing cushions and mattresses. Only air-fluidized beds (Clinitron) and low-air-loss beds (Kinair) have been shown in randomized trials to speed healing compared with conventional alternating air mattresses or foam mattresses and 2-hour turning.

Infection (e.g., cellulitis, osteomyelitis, and sepsis) is the most common complication. All wounds will colonize with skin flora; therefore, routine wound cultures are not helpful. Cultures (wound and blood) are most helpful in patients with fever, spreading cellulitis, osteomyelitis, or poorly healing wounds with persistent drainage. Topical antibiotics only select for only the more virulent organisms. Topical antiseptics may reduce bacterial counts but are toxic to proliferating fibroblasts and epithelial cells. Sys-

TABLE 1. **Summary of the Agency for Health Care Policy and Research Clinical Practice Guidelines for Prediction and Prevention of Pressure Ulcers in Adults**

1. Identify at-risk individuals needing prevention and the specific factors placing them at risk.
2. Maintain and improve tissue tolerance to pressure in order to prevent injury.
3. Protect against adverse effects of external mechanical forces: pressure, friction, and shear.
4. Reduce the incidence of pressure ulcers through educational programs.

Adapted from Panel on Prediction and Prevention of Pressure Ulcers in Adults: Pressure Ulcers in Adults: Prediction and Prevention. Clinical Practice Guideline, Number 3. AHCPR Publication No. 92-0047. Rockville, MD, Agency for Health Care Policy and Research, Public Health Service, U.S. Department of Health and Human Services, 1992.

temic antibiotics should be reserved for those with spreading cellulitis, osteomyelitis, or sepsis.

Débridement of necrotic tissue is essential to control infection and prepare wound beds for granulation tissue. Surgical débridement may be required for complicated wounds, but most can be débrided at the bedside using abrasive cleaning and frequent dressing changes over a few days. Enzymatic agents may help liquefy proteinaceous material for easier removal.

Dressings serve barrier functions against wound contamination. Granulating tissue (fibroblasts and epithelial cells) require moisture and ambient oxygen. Dressings that are impermeable to oxygen and moisture retard healing, macerate the skin, and are a source of bacterial overgrowth. Saline-soaked gauze dressings are appropriate for most wounds.

Nutritional support is essential, including the use of enteral or parenteral hyperalimentation in patients whose appetite or disability impairs adequate intake. A multivitamin and mineral supplement is probably reasonable. Administration of vitamin C and zinc, even in the absence of a deficiency state, may be of benefit.

Surgical intervention may be appropriate for those patients with deep ulcers who can tolerate the necessary anesthetic procedures. Excision of the entire ulcer and rotation of myocutaneous skin flap procedures are highly successful, but high recurrence rates have been reported in patients who remain immobile and at high risk.

ATOPIC DERMATITIS

method of
ALFONS L. KROL, M.D.
University of Alberta
Edmonton, Alberta, Canada

"Atopic dermatitis" (AD) is the term used by Weisz and Sulzberger to describe an inherited skin disorder with a characteristic distribution, associated xerosis, and a propensity to produce excessive amounts of IgE (reagins) antibodies in response to a variety of common environmental antigens. The term "atopy" was originally used by Coca in 1923 to describe the genetically transmitted hyperreactivity of patients with hay fever and asthma. Hill and Sulzberger used the term "atopic dermatitis" to describe the cutaneous disorder that many of these patients presented with. In some areas of Europe, AD is still referred to as "Besnier's prurigo."

Although clinical criteria and identifying characteristics of atopic dermatitis have been established and accepted, no one feature is pathognomonic of the disease. The most characteristic and common feature of the disease is pruritus. This in turn leads to relentless rubbing and scratching of the skin, producing lichenification (thickening of the skin with an increase in the normal skin markings), which is the next most characteristic feature of the disorder. Recent studies have suggested the incidence AD is increasing. The prevalence rate of AD in studies conducted following the Second World War was 5%. This figure rose to 12% by 1970. The cause of this increasing prevalence is unknown. Approximately 70% of patients with AD will have a family history of associated disorders including asthma, hay fever, and urticaria.

AD is often the initial manifestation of an atopic diathesis. It may present in the first few days or weeks of life, manifesting in over 80% of patients by the end of the first year. Onset of the disease after the age of 5 years is distinctly uncommon. Late onset may indicate mild disease that remitted in childhood, only to recur at a later stage in the patient's life. Three clinically distinct phases are recognized that may overlap or be separated by variable periods of remission: (1) The infantile phase from birth to 2 years of age; (2) the childhood phase from age 2 years to puberty; and (3) the adult phase following puberty.

The infantile phase is characterized by involvement of the cheeks and scalp, as well as the extensor aspects of the limbs. The skin is generally quite dry with ill-defined erythematous scaly patches to more well-defined discoid lesions with superficial crusting and excoriations present. Scaling on the scalp in young infants may be misdiagnosed as seborrheic dermatitis, which may, on occasion, coexist with AD. The diaper area is often spared and may be the most normal-appearing area of skin in young infants with AD.

In the childhood phase, flexural involvement becomes most prominent. This is typically noted in the antecubital and popliteal fossae, the lateral neck, lower portion of the retroauricular folds, wrists, and ankles. The dorsum of the hands and feet may be involved. The morphology of the lesions varies with the chronicity of the process, initially being erythematous and ill defined, becoming more lichenified with time. If the eruption persists beyond puberty, involvement of the face, lateral neck, and upper body again becomes prominent often with persistent lesions in the flexures. Pigmentary changes may occur in all patients owing to the inflammatory process, and are most marked in darker-skinned patients. This dyspigmentation generally resolves on its own after several months.

The prognosis of the disease for the majority of patients is excellent with gradual improvement throughout childhood, and partial or complete remission in most patients as they approach puberty. Persistent disease in adulthood often manifests as nonspecific hand dermatitis and a tendency to recurrent facial or eyelid dermatitis. A small minority of patients will have persistent severe disease throughout their lives. The diagnosis of AD is usually evident in a patient with a typical presentation. Eczematous lesions with associated intense itch are also the hallmark of other disorders including scabies or other infestations, allergic contact dermatitis, or autosensitization reactions associated with tinea infections that may mimic AD or may develop in patients with AD.

TREATMENT

General Measures

The treatment of AD, particularly in infancy and early childhood, should be a straightforward process in the majority of patients with compliance to a standardized regimen. The physician must have the confidence and cooperation of the parents and later the patient, emphasizing that he or she can provide not a cure but, rather, good control of AD. The initial visit is most important when evaluating these patients to ensure the parents have a clear understanding of the nature of the disease and the specific measures required to control it. The management of severe AD will be a challenge to any physician's therapeutic skill and patience. In young infants and children, treatments must be carried out by the parents. As the child begins school and matures, responsibility for treatments should be gradually given to the patient.

Bathing, particularly in young infants with AD, should be carried out once daily for no more than 10 minutes without the use of soap. Use of a bland emollient such as petrolatum applied immediately after the bath is an excellent method of maintaining hydration of the skin and alleviating xerosis. In northern climates, because of low winter temperatures and centrally heated houses that produce low ambient humidity, AD tends to worsen. At the other extreme, as many of these patients tend to itch when sweating, particularly during the childhood and adult phase, summer exacerbations may occur. Fever from any cause may produce a flare of AD.

Because these patients have a lowered threshold to stimuli that produce itch, clothing is important. Wool fibers contain innumerable tiny harpoons on their endings, making this fabric impossible to wear for the majority of patients with AD. Cotton clothing is the least irritating fabric, and although pure cotton is preferable, most patients will tolerate polyester-cotton blends that are at least 50 to 70% cotton. Occlusive synthetic fabrics such as nylon should be avoided.

The role of aeroallergens such as house dust mite antigen and animal danders is controversial. Recent studies in Europe suggest these may contribute to exacerbations of AD in some patients, and that an attempt at reduction of exposure to these in the home environment may be useful in patients with severe AD when conservative measures have failed to control the disease process.

The role of food is even more controversial, and the literature is full of inconsistent and inconclusive studies without adequate controls. Both skin testing and radioallergosorbent test (RAST) antibody measurement to specific foods have failed to provide clear information on the value or role of dietary therapy. My own personal approach is to keep an open mind to the possibility of foods exacerbating AD, and if the parents feel a particular food is consistently exacerbating AD to withdraw it for a trial period. The American Task Force on Pediatric Dermatology recommends not instituting dietary management if the patient shows a limited dermatitis that responds to basic therapy; it also emphasizes that severe and prolonged dietary restriction should not be introduced without full consideration of its impact on the patient's general health. Excessively restrictive diets have led to malnutrition and rickets in some children.

Specific Measures

Topical Treatment

The goals of therapy are to reduce the inflammation, alleviate xerosis, and control itch. In young in-

fants and children with mild disease, this is accomplished with 1% hydrocortisone ointment applied two to three times daily. On the trunk and limbs, if the disease fails to respond to 1% hydrocortisone ointment, then a mid-potency corticosteroid ointment such as betamethasone valerate (Valisone) 0.1% or 0.05% or mometasone furoate (Elocon) 0.1% ointment may be applied three times daily until improvement occurs, and in most patients is required for 10 to 14 days.

At this point it is preferable to return to bland emollient treatments with petrolatum to lubricate the skin, thus allowing a rest period from use of the steroid. The majority of patients with AD will respond to this intermittent cyclical routine of topical steroid use followed by a definite rest period lasting up to 7 days or longer. This type of regimen reduces the risk of steroid side effects and lessens the incidence of tachyphylaxis. Ointments are preferred over creams, particularly in children, as preservatives in cream bases, particularly propylene glycol, may cause irritation and stinging when applied, lessening compliance. In the scalp, a nonalcohol-based corticosteroid lotion such as Desonide (Des Owen) 0.05% lotion applied thinly two to three times a day is helpful. If scaling of the scalp is severe or associated cradle cap occurs, a bland cleansing shampoo such as Ionil (salicylic acid and benzalkonium chloride) is helpful.

Plain petrolatum is the most effective and simplest emollient, and is best applied to moist skin following a short bath. Petrolatum is well tolerated in northern climates on a year-round basis, although in extremely hot and humid weather, a lighter water-based cream may be preferable to minimize sweat retention and miliaria. Urea-containing moisturizers will sting when applied to open areas of skin, and should be applied only after a hydrating bath and only during periods of remission of the active dermatitis. They should not be applied to the face. Prolonged bathing, sponging the skin to clean it, showering, and using bubble bath and soap should be avoided in children with AD. As the child approaches puberty and in adults with AD, a bland soap such as unscented Dove may be used in the axillae and groin regions. Tar preparations such as 5 to 10% liquor carbonis detergens (LCD) are useful in patients with chronic, thick, lichenified lesions on the limbs. Short, controlled application of more potent fluorinated steroids such as fluocinonide (Lidex) 0.01 to 0.05% or amcinonide (Cyclocort) 0.1% ointment twice daily for brief periods to resistant areas on the limbs or trunk may be required. When more potent steroids are needed, the amount prescribed and used by the patient must be strictly controlled and closely monitored to avoid unwanted local or systemic side effects.

In most patients, control of the inflammation and xerosis will subsequently result in diminished itch. Severely affected infants may have relentless pruritus, requiring use of antihistamines such as hydroxyzine hydrochloride (Atarax), which is given as an initial dosage of 1 to 2 mg per kg per day divided into three or four doses orally in infants under 1 year of age, and increasing to 2 to 4 mg per kg in older children. In school-age children, the drowsiness this agent produces may limit its effectiveness or desirability during the day, in which case a nonsedating antihistamine such as cetirizine (Reactine) may be given at an initial dosage of 5 mg orally every morning, increasing to 10 mg daily as required.

Secondary infection, particularly with *Staphylococcus aureus* or beta-hemolytic streptococci, may occur during exacerbation of AD, and when localized, this responds well to topical antibiotic therapy with mupirocin (Bactroban) ointment. When secondary impetiginization of lesions is extensive, appropriate oral antibiotic therapy should be given. There is controversy as to whether patients with AD are more prone to develop viral infections such as warts and molluscum contagiosum. Recent population-based studies suggest that the incidence of these viral infections is not increased in AD.

Eczema herpeticum is a well-recognized complication of AD owing to dissemination of the herpes simplex virus over a large skin surface area in an atopic patient. Depending on the severity of involvement, this process may be mild to severe with accompanying constitutional symptoms including fever, headache, malaise, and regional or generalized lymphadenopathy. It is often initially confused with secondary bacterial infection, but in the majority of cases, a contact source of recent herpes simplex virus infection, often in a family member, can be elicited. Eczema herpeticum responds dramatically to oral acyclovir therapy at a dosage of 10 to 15 mg per kg per day in three divided doses for children and 200 mg five times daily orally for adults.

Systemic Therapy

In severe AD, the physician may be confronted with an infant or child whose disease is unremitting despite compliance to an appropriate regimen of topical therapy. Systemic corticosteroids will often produce dramatic short-term results in these patients. Oral prednisone is given at a dosage of 1 mg per kg per day tapered over 14 days. Rebound flare of the disease usually occurs and the use of systemic steroids in children is rarely indicated. Chronic use of oral steroids in AD cannot be justified in view of their well-known serious side effects. A preferable alternative to oral corticosteroids in children is admission to hospital for a brief period in which the disease often improves with continued supervised topical treatment; this simultaneously provides welcome rest for distraught parents.

Older children and adolescents may respond well to phototherapy with ultraviolet B light. Atherton showed long-term remissions in patients treated with oral psoralen with ultraviolet A light (PUVA). Not all patients will respond to this therapy, and the heat produced in the ultraviolet treatment unit may worsen some patients.

Recent advances in the understanding of the immune mechanisms involved in the pathogenesis of AD, particularly the role of cytokines, has shown that immune suppressive therapy with cyclosporine and immunomodulation therapy with interferon-gamma may produce substantial remission of AD. Small clinical trials have been completed with encouraging results; however, this therapy must still be considered experimental.

Oral therapy with a decoction of 12 Chinese herbs in a standardized preparation was shown to be effective in a short double-blind trial conducted by Sheehan and Atherton. One-year follow-up of these children showed continued benefit in approximately 50% of the patients with a high withdrawal rate owing to the unpalatability of the preparation. Two patients developed significant liver function abnormalities during treatment.

Patients and parents of patients with chronic disorders such as AD may in frustration seek out alternative or unconventional therapies and start or continue them with or without the physician's knowledge. Many of these therapies may be harmless; however, increasing reports of liver or renal toxicity of certain herbal products emphasizes the need to inform our patients of their potential adverse effects.

ERYTHEMA MULTIFORME

method of
NEIL H. SHEAR, M.D.
University of Toronto Medical School
North York, Ontario, Canada

Despite its name, erythema multiforme describes a specific clinical syndrome with specific pathologic features. The term "erythema multiforme" refers to a reaction pattern in the skin that is characterized by the presence of target lesions and blistering of the mucous membranes. The pathologic term "erythema multiforme" refers to a lymphocytic infiltrate in the skin that causes keratinocyte necrosis. The classification of erythema multiforme has been in flux over the past few years, and the differentiating features are of major clinical importance (Table 1). The three major clinical syndromes are

1. Erythema multiforme (EM) minor
2. EM major, Stevens-Johnson syndrome (SJS), and toxic epidermal necrolysis (TEN)
3. Pure plaque–type TEN

ERYTHEMA MULTIFORME MINOR

EM minor is an acute, and sometimes recurrent, condition that is characterized by classic three-ringed target lesions on the extremities. These have a dusky center with an edematous, light-colored second ring, surrounded by erythema. These lesions are raised, but there is no major blistering at the center, nor is there skin detachment. These patients may have a fever and often have no symptoms other than skin findings. EM minor may follow herpes simplex virus or mycoplasma infection. There are many other infections and inciting causes. This syndrome usually is not a reaction to drugs. EM minor may occur without an obvious cause and often is termed idiopathic.

TABLE 1. **The Clinical Spectrum of Erythema Multiforme**

| Disease | Skin | | Mucosa | Systemic Findings | Common Causes | |
	Targets	Blistering			Infections	Drugs
EM minor	3-ring, acral	No	Minimal, if at all	No	HSV, mycoplasma	Not usually
EM major	2- or 3-ring generalized	Minimal	Usually	Yes*	As above	Sulfonamides, AEDs, NSAIDs
SJS	2-ring generalized	Yes Small lesions	Usually	Yes*	As above	As above
TEN	2-ring, generalized	Small and large sheets of detached skin	Usually	Yes*	Not usually	As above
TEN–plaque type	No	Large sheets of detached skin	Usually	Yes*	Not usually	As above

*Systemic findings most commonly are fever and lymphadenopathy. Presence of hepatitis, nephritis, hematologic toxicity, atypical lymphocytosis, pneumonitis, or pharyngitis may be part of a systemic hypersensitivity drug reaction.

Abbreviations: EM = erythema multiforme; HSV = herpes simplex virus; AEDs = antiepileptic drugs (phenytoin, phenobarbital, carbamazepine, lamotrigine, valproic acid); NSAIDs = nonsteroidal anti-inflammatory drugs (especially piroxicam and related drugs); SJS = Stevens-Johnson syndrome; TEN = toxic epidermal necrolysis.

ERYTHEMA MULTIFORME MAJOR, STEVENS-JOHNSON SYNDROME, AND TOXIC EPIDERMAL NECROLYSIS

The second clinical group is characterized by the presence of target lesions, blistering, and detachment on the skin and mucous membranes. The targets are not the well-structured three-ring targets of EM minor, but rather flat or raised two-ring targets with a dark, red or purple center surrounded by a flat flare of erythema. The blisters may be small, localized areas that can coalesce into large sheets of detached skin. The erythema that precedes the blistering is often painful to touch. This is a helpful and relatively specific feature. Mucous membranes have blistering and denudement of the mucosa with hemorrhagic crust formation. The most common membranes involved are the lips and oral mucosa first, followed by the conjunctiva and genitalia. Conjunctival involvement may lead to scarring and loss of vision.

To differentiate among these severe types of erythema multiforme is clinically helpful. It aids in the determination of cause and in prognostication. All these conditions have some type of target lesion, blistering, and mucosal involvement. It is not helpful to worry about the number of mucosal sites involved. The differentiation is based more on the extent of epidermal detachment. In EM major there is often a fair amount of skin involvement with erythema; however, the actual skin detachment is minor. In TEN one can expect more than 30% of the body to be affected by skin detachment, and this condition has a fatality rate approaching 25%. EM major and SJS are usually self-limited conditions. These diseases may lead to long-term sequelae, such as conjunctival scarring with loss of vision and pigmentary changes of the skin.

EM major and SJS follow infections such as herpes simplex virus and mycoplasma infection. They are also associated with a multitude of drugs, but the most common drugs implicated are sulfonamide antibiotics, antiepileptic drugs, and nonsteroidal anti-inflammatory drugs (NSAIDs) (especially piroxicam-related medications). Antiepileptic drugs include phenytoin, phenobarbital, carbamazepine, lamotrigine, and valproic acid. Patients who start with EM major do not necessarily progress to SJS or TEN.

PLAQUE TOXIC EPIDERMAL NECROLYSIS

The third type of condition, TEN of the plaque type, does not usually have targets associated with it, but localized large sheets of detached skin. This condition may be relatively well tolerated or may be life-threatening. The presence of mucosal involvement is not necessary for the diagnosis of this condition. It is generally drug-induced.

SYSTEMIC ASSOCIATIONS

EM minor is not associated with systemic findings; however, EM major and its accompanying conditions are. The systemic findings may simply be fever and lymphadenopathy; however, one should look for the presence of hepatitis; nephritis; hematologic toxicity (from neutropenia to agranulocytosis to aplastic anemia); atypical lymphocytes; pneumonitis; or pharyngitis. Systemic involvement might suggest an underlying infection but may also be part of a systemic hypersensitivity reaction to a drug. The delay of onset from the initiation of drug therapy to the development of EM major, SJS, or TEN is usually from 3 to 6 weeks.

INVESTIGATION

The first step in the investigation of these eruptions is to determine the *diagnosis*. This may require the exclusion of other skin diseases, and to this end a skin biopsy for routine histologic and immunofluorescence studies, may be very helpful. Blistering conditions such as staphylococcal scalded skin syndrome would show a very different histologic picture from that of EM or TEN. Blistering disease like bullous lupus erythematosus, bullous pemphigoid, and pemphigus vulgaris would also be different on histologic and immunofluorescence studies.

To help determine the cause of the reaction, it is important to look at a history of drug exposure and prior infection. Recurrent episodes suggest a recurrent infection such as herpes simplex virus or recurring drug use, such as intermittent NSAID therapy.

The severe reactions require a search for systemic involvement. This is important in the management of the patient and may help in determining the cause.

TREATMENT

EM minor requires symptomatic therapy. This condition usually is not itchy. Extreme itching is suggestive of an annular urticaria rather than EM.

Therapy with drugs that are suspected as the cause of the reaction should be stopped. There is a possibility of cross-reaction among the aromatic anticonvulsants (phenytoin, phenobarbital, and carbamazepine). Therefore, if one of these drugs is suspected, an alternative drug, not from this group, should be chosen.

Treatment of mucosal involvement requires the control of inflammation. In eyes and mouth, topical corticosteroids are very helpful. Patients may develop secondary candidal infections in the mouth with potent corticosteroid therapy (e.g., clobetasol propionate ointment) and may require adjunctive therapy for candidal infection (e.g., nystatin rinses, ketoconazole).

Pain can be controlled with systemic medication as well as topical anesthetics such as lidocaine (Xylocaine) or benzocaine. Attention to oral hygiene is helpful to prevent secondary infection and ultimately decreases the discomfort of the patient.

For patients with skin detachment greater than 15% of the body surface area, management may be best in a burn unit. Attention to fluid balance and electrolyte levels is important. The most common topical antimicrobial in use is silver sulfadiazine. This is contraindicated in patients who have had sulfonamide-induced disease. For them polymyxin B–bacitracin (Polysporin) may be used.

The prophylactic use of systemic antibiotics in TEN is not uniformly recommended. Our experience is that most patients end up needing this, and a patient who has severe neutropenia should be treated as a febrile neutropenic patient according to local guidelines.

The use of systemic corticosteroids for each of these conditions is controversial. For minor disease, systemic corticosteroid therapy is not needed at all. If eye involvement is severe, then systemic corticosteroids may help to prevent scarring and ultimately blindness. The usual doses of steroids are 40 to 60 mg of prednisone per day or equivalent. Some specialists argue that systemic steroid therapy for EM major, SJS, or TEN leads to secondary infections and prolongs the course. Patients who are transferred to burn units almost never receive corticosteroids. This decision is extremely controversial and should be made in consultation with local experts.

For recurrent EM major, the problem is usually secondary to herpes simplex virus infection, and patients may be troubled with severe pain and blistering in the mouth and eyes. In this case, acyclovir has been found to be very useful either as a short course of 5 days at the first sign of viral disease or as a suppressive, prophylactic daily regimen. In patients in whom acyclovir does not work, dapsone, prednisone, and azathioprine have been used. Acyclovir is the drug of choice.

BULLOUS DISEASES

method of
DIYA F. MUTASIM, M.D.
University of Cincinnati Medical Center
Cincinnati, Ohio

Bullous diseases are a wide group of disorders in which blistering of the skin and/or mucous membranes occurs. Other lesions that are usually seen in addition to blisters include erythematous patches or wheals (early, prebullous phase) and erosions (resulting from the rupture of blisters). There are several ways of classifying this large group of disorders. One convenient method of classification divides these disorders into autoimmune, mechanical, metabolic, and allergic types (Table 1). The autoimmune bullous diseases are discussed here. Some of the remaining bullous diseases are discussed elsewhere in this book.

The complete laboratory evaluation of patients with bullous diseases includes histopathology and direct and indirect immunofluorescence (Table 2).

PRINCIPLES OF THERAPY OF AUTOIMMUNE BULLOUS DISEASES

Many of the autoimmune bullous diseases have severe morbidity and high mortality if untreated. This generally results from loss of fluids and electrolytes, secondary bacterial infections, and decreased food intake in patients with severe oral involvement. Accordingly, most patients with bullous diseases are treated aggressively to induce a clinical remission. The majority of these diseases are mediated by antibodies that bind specific adhesion molecules that normally maintain cell-cell and cell-matrix adhesion. Through various mechanisms, the binding of these antibodies to the adhesion molecules leads to the disruption of cell-cell adhesion (the pemphigus group of diseases) or cell-matrix adhesion (the remaining autoimmune bullous diseases). In some of these diseases, particularly those in the pemphigus group, binding of antibodies to the adhesion molecules ap-

TABLE 1. **Classification of Bullous Diseases**

Autoimmune
Pemphigus
Pemphigoid
Epidermolysis bullosa acquisita
Dermatitis herpetiformis
Linear IgA disease

Mechanical (Epidermolysis Bullosa)
Epidermolytic
Junctional
Dermolytic

Metabolic
Porphyria
Diabetic bullae
Bullous amyloidosis

Allergic
Bullous erythema multiforme
Toxic epidermal necrolysis
Bullous drug eruption
Acute allergic contact dermatitis

TABLE 2. **Laboratory Evaluation of Patients with Bullous Diseases**

Histopathology: punch or shave biopsy of small, very early vesicle, including adjacent skin
Direct immunofluorescence: punch or shave biopsy of normal-appearing skin immediately adjacent to a blister or erythematous plaque
Indirect immunofluorescence: serum or blood

pears to induce loss of cell-cell adhesion (acantholysis) without the direct involvement of other components of the humoral or cellular immune system. In other bullous diseases, particularly pemphigoid and dermatitis herpetiformis, the binding of antibodies to their target molecules leads to the influx of inflammatory cells (neutrophils and eosinophils) that subsequently release hydrolytic enzymes that digest the cell-matrix adhesion, resulting in blister formation.

It is obvious that drugs used in the therapy of these diseases should have effects that are immune suppressive or anti-inflammatory, or both. Immune-suppressive medications are aimed at inducing a clinical and immunologic remission, whereas anti-inflammatory medications are aimed at suppressing clinical disease.

Anti-inflammatory medications (with potentially fewer side effects) are usually used in lifelong diseases (such as dermatitis herpetiformis) and in mild cases (such as limited bullous pemphigoid). Immune-suppressive medications are usually reserved for the potentially severe cases, particularly with pemphigus.

Because of the potentially serious side effects of many medications used in the treatment of bullous diseases, it is important to define the goals of treatment clearly to the patient. Although many patients desire to have no lesions whatsoever, it is important to remember that this is not a realistic goal; it would necessitate high doses for prolonged periods, with all the subsequent hazards of such therapy. It is reasonable to allow the presence of a few lesions, especially in areas that do not interfere with the patient's eating or other daily activities. Finally, it is important to remember that many of these diseases are rare. Accordingly, there are no large studies that address in a controlled manner the efficacy of the various medications used. The information that follows is based on the author's personal experience and reviews of the available studies and case reports in the literature.

PEMPHIGUS VULGARIS

Clinical Manifestations and Diagnosis

Pemphigus vulgaris affects predominantly individuals in the third to fifth decades of life, with no sex predilection. In most patients, the initial lesions appear in the mouth. Vesicles and bullae rupture rapidly leading to painful, persistent erosions that may affect the pharynx and larynx. Other mucous membrane involvement is rather rare. Following a period of time that varies from a few months to a few years, patients develop vesicles and bullae over the scalp and face. As the disease progresses, lesions occur over the neck and upper trunk. As the vesicles and bullae rupture, painful erosions that are very slow to heal persist and are prone to secondary bacterial infection. Histologic examination of a vesicle reveals acantholysis above the epidermal basal layer. Direct immunofluorescence of normal-appearing perilesional skin adjacent to a blister or erosion reveals deposition of IgG around the epidermal (and epithelial) cell surface in 100% of cases. Complement components are often present, but with less intensity. Indirect immunofluorescence reveals circulating IgG antibodies in the sera of most patients with active disease. These antibodies bind the epidermal (or epithelial) cell surface of many stratified squamous epithelia (especially monkey esophagus). These antibodies are directed against a molecule within the epidermal and epithelial desmosomes (desmoglein 3). Until 5 decades ago, pemphigus vulgaris had a very high mortality rate because of the relentless progression of the disease, resulting in dehydration and sepsis.

Therapy

Animal model studies, as well as other experimental evidence, confirm the direct role of IgG antibodies in the induction of skin lesions of pemphigus vulgaris. Patients with higher levels of antibodies (higher titers on indirect immunofluorescence) tend to have more severe disease. The treatment of pemphigus vulgaris aims at inducing an immunologic remission (clearance of the antibodies) that usually leads to clinical disease remission. The autoimmune phenomenon in pemphigus vulgaris is "aggressive," necessitating intensive immune suppression in order to induce a remission. This disease is best managed by someone with special interest and expertise in the area of autoimmune bullous diseases.

The choice of therapy depends only slightly on the severity of the disease at presentation. Many patients with only limited oral disease need as much intensive therapy to induce a remission as patients with extensive skin involvement. Unless there is an absolute contraindication, the initial therapy for pemphigus vulgaris is systemic corticosteroids. The most frequently used agent is prednisone. The starting dose is 1 mg per kg per day in one to three doses. Most patients obtain a complete or almost complete clinical remission within 4 to 8 weeks. The dose is then decreased by 10 to 20 mg every 2 to 4 weeks. When the dose is 40 mg daily, the patient is changed to an every-other-day schedule. This is accomplished by keeping the first day's dose at 40 mg and decreasing the second day's dose by 5 to 10 mg every 2 to 4 weeks. When the patient is taking 40 mg every other day, the dose is tapered by 5 mg every 2 to 4 weeks. If there is no significant recurrence, the patient is usually maintained on 5 to 7.5 mg of prednisone daily or every other day for several years.

Other immune-suppressive drugs are used in the treatment of pemphigus vulgaris if prednisone fails to induce a remission or if the patient develops serious corticosteroid complications. These include high blood pressure, elevated blood sugar, osteoporosis, weight gain, aseptic necrosis of the bone, and increased susceptibility to infections. The most commonly used steroid-sparing agents are cyclophosphamide (Cytoxan)* and azathioprine (Imuran).* Less frequently used drugs include chlorambucil (Leukeran),* methotrexate,* and cyclosporin A (Sandimmune).*

Cyclophosphamide is usually used at a dose of 1 to 2 mg per kg per day, whereas azathioprine is used at a dose of 2 to 3 mg per kg per day. Cyclophosphamide seems to suppress the immune response in pemphigus vulgaris more effectively than does azathioprine. This appears to be the result of the preferential cytotoxic effect of cyclophosphamide on proliferative plasma cells. Its major side effects include a predictable leukopenia, hemorrhagic cystitis, and an increased risk of malignancy, especially lymphoma and leukemia. Cyclophosphamide may induce sterility in young patients with childbearing potential. The effects of cyclophosphamide on the bone marrow and urinary bladder must be monitored closely (initially every week, then slowly decreased to every 2 to 4 weeks). Although it is slightly less effective than cyclophosphamide, azathioprine appears to be more widely used as a steroid-sparing agent in the treatment of pemphigus vulgaris. It is less toxic than cyclophosphamide and therefore needs much less frequent monitoring. It is indicated in young individuals in whom it is more desirable to use a less toxic agent to reduce the risk of sterility and the lifetime risk of malignancy. It is also indicated in patients who cannot tolerate cyclophosphamide.

Chlorambucil may be a useful alternative to cyclophosphamide in patients who develop hemorrhagic cystitis. Its side effects include bone marrow suppression and carcinogenic potential. Methotrexate was used as a steroid-sparing agent before newer, more effective immune-suppressive agents became available. It is generally less effective than other agents. Cyclosporin A has been used with success in some patients with pemphigus vulgaris. Its potentially serious side effects (nephrotoxicity and hypertension) preclude using it routinely.

Gold therapy (intramuscular as well as oral) has long been reported to be beneficial for some patients with pemphigus vulgaris. The response to gold, however, is rather unpredictable and is generally not marked. The incidence of hypersensitivity reactions in various organs (skin, kidney, and lung) is rather high. At present, gold is used only sporadically as a third-line agent.

Plasmapheresis has been used in the treatment of pemphigus vulgaris with variable results. Plasmapheresis produces a relatively abrupt disappearance of the pathogenic serum antibodies. This often results in clinical improvement. If plasmapheresis is used as the mainstay of therapy, however, acute flares may occur. This is usually secondary to the rebound rise in antibody levels, since antibody production is under feedback inhibition. It is most effective to use plasmapheresis in conjunction with oral corticosteroids and other immune-suppressive agents such as cyclophosphamide. Plasmapheresis is usually reserved for patients with extensive or life-threatening disease.

PEMPHIGUS FOLIACEUS

Clinical Manifestations and Diagnosis

Pemphigus foliaceus affects individuals in all age groups, but, compared with pemphigus vulgaris, it occurs with increased frequency in the older age group. Blisters favor the head and upper trunk area and almost never affect mucous membranes. Blisters are more superficial than those in pemphigus vulgaris and, accordingly, rupture easily. This results in the frequent lack of intact blisters in this disease. Instead, lesions are dominated by features of superficial desquamation and fine crusting. Histologic examination reveals acantholysis in the superficial layers of the epidermis. Direct and indirect immunofluorescence reveals results similar to those in pemphigus vulgaris. The antibodies, however, bind to a different desmosomal molecule involved in cell-cell adhesion (desmoglein 1). Like pemphigus vulgaris, this disease tends to be chronic. Because of the lack of oral involvement as well as the superficial nature of the lesions, pemphigus foliaceus has much less morbidity compared with pemphigus vulgaris and almost no mortality.

Therapy

The aim of therapy in the management of patients with pemphigus foliaceus is similar to that in pemphigus vulgaris, that is, to prevent the immune system from producing the pathogenic antibodies. This is usually accomplished using the same drugs as in pemphigus vulgaris. The autoimmune response in pemphigus foliaceus, however, appears to be less aggressive than that in pemphigus vulgaris. Patients usually respond to oral corticosteroids. The starting dose is usually prednisone 0.5 to 1 mg per kg per day, with a tapering schedule similar to that in pemphigus vulgaris. It is less common to need steroid-sparing agents, but the drugs that are used in this disease are similar to those used in pemphigus vulgaris.

PARANEOPLASTIC PEMPHIGUS

Clinical Manifestations and Diagnosis

Paraneoplastic pemphigus is a recently described entity in which patients develop a blistering disorder

---

*Not FDA-approved for this indication.

of the skin and mucous membranes in the presence of an underlying malignancy. Most individuals have lymphoproliferative disorders such as non-Hodgkin's lymphoma, chronic lymphocytic leukemia, Castleman's tumor, thymoma, or Waldenström's macroglobulinemia. The clinical appearance of the lesions is most similar to that of pemphigus vulgaris, with particular involvement of mucous membranes. There is, however, overlap with the clinical manifestations of other autoimmune blistering disorders such as bullous pemphigoid and erythema multiforme. Histologic examination reveals changes similar to those of pemphigus vulgaris in addition to changes of erythema multiforme (lymphocytic infiltration of the dermal-epidermal junction as well as necrosis of lower epidermal cells). Direct immunofluorescence of perilesional skin reveals deposition of IgG around the epidermal cell surface and frequently deposition of IgG and complement components along the basement membrane area. Indirect immunofluorescence reveals antibodies that bind the cell surface of stratified squamous epithelium, similar to pemphigus vulgaris and pemphigus foliaceus. Unlike the antibodies in the latter two diseases, antibodies in the sera of patients with paraneoplastic pemphigus also bind transitional epithelium of urinary bladder, respiratory epithelium, intestinal epithelium, and other nonepithelial tissues such as heart and liver. These antibodies recognize desmosomal proteins that are not unique to stratified squamous epithelia. The initial patients reported with paraneoplastic pemphigus had a poor prognosis. The severity of the mucosal and skin disease paralleled that of the underlying malignancy. It appears that if a remission of the underlying malignancy is induced, a remission of the mucocutaneous disease is likely. The high rate of mortality in this disease is attributed to multiple factors, including sepsis, gastrointestinal bleeding, respiratory failure, and multiorgan failure. Patients with underlying benign tumors such as thymoma or Castleman's tumor may obtain a complete remission after excision of the tumor.

Therapy

There are two arms to the management of patients with paraneoplastic pemphigus. The first is to treat the underlying neoplasm. The second is to suppress the immune response from producing the pathogenic antibodies. This is usually accomplished by agents similar to those used in pemphigus vulgaris. The response of lesions in paraneoplastic pemphigus, however, is less dramatic than that in pemphigus vulgaris.

BULLOUS PEMPHIGOID

Clinical Manifestations and Diagnosis

Bullous pemphigoid is a relatively common bullous disease that affects predominantly the elderly. In its classic presentation, large bullae occur on the neck and flexural areas of the axillae and groin. Bullae are tense and tend to contain clear fluid. Following rupture of the bullae, superficial erosions tend to heal spontaneously as other bullae continue to appear. Occasionally, mild, transient involvement of mucous membranes may be seen. Histologic examination of an early blister reveals a split at the dermal-epidermal junction, with underlying inflammatory infiltrate that is variable in intensity and usually rich in eosinophils. Direct immunofluorescence of perilesional skin reveals deposition of C3 and IgG along the dermal-epidermal junction. Indirect immunofluorescence reveals antibodies in the patients' sera that bind the basement membrane of stratified squamous epithelium. These IgG antibodies bind proteins within the basal cell hemidesmosomes. There is strong evidence that these antibodies are pathogenic.

In addition to the classic presentation of bullous pemphigoid, patients may occasionally present with localized lesions, especially over the head and neck area or on the lower legs. Herpes (pemphigoid) gestationis is a form of pemphigoid that occurs in pregnant women and resolves after delivery.

Therapy

Similar to other bullous diseases, pemphigoid is a disorder that results from an abnormal immune response (antibodies) and that has prominent inflammatory features (cellular infiltrate). Therapies for pemphigoid should suppress inflammation and/or the immune response. Before a therapy is chosen, variables that relate to the disease (extent of involvement and symptoms) and to the patient (age; other illnesses such as diabetes, hypertension, or tuberculosis) must be considered. The goal of therapy is to heal the lesions and prevent new lesions from appearing. If therapy fails, an elderly patient with extensive erosions may develop complications such as fluid loss, electrolyte imbalance, bacterial colonization with potential sepsis, scarring, and decubitus ulcers.

Potent topical steroids should be considered and favored in the management of patients with localized disease, since this variant of pemphigoid responds very well to such therapy. Most patients with generalized bullous pemphigoid require systemic therapy. The most commonly used systemic agents are the corticosteroids. Prednisone is the most commonly used corticosteroid and is sufficient in the majority of cases. Depending on the extent of disease and the weight of the patient, the starting daily dose is 40 to 80 mg. Unlike pemphigus vulgaris, bullous pemphigoid requires higher doses of prednisone only rarely. A clinical response is usually obtained within 2 to 4 weeks and is indicated by healing of existing lesions and cessation of new blister formation. The prednisone dose is then gradually decreased by 10 mg every 2 weeks initially and by 2.5 to 5 mg later. When the daily dose is 30 to 40 mg, shifting to an every-other-day schedule is encouraged to decrease the potential for long-term corticosteroid side effects. This is usually accomplished by decreasing the second day's dose by 5 to 10 mg every 1 to 2 weeks. Once the second day's dose is nil, the first day's dose may be tapered slowly. If the patient develops a disease flare during the tapering phase, the dose may be increased by 10 to 20 mg for 2 to 3 weeks and then tapered more slowly. In the majority of patients, prednisone can be completely discontinued after 6 to 9 months of therapy.

Immune-suppressive therapy with chemotherapeutic agents should be considered for patients who require high maintenance doses of corticosteroid, patients who develop corticosteroid side effects, and patients whose disease does not respond completely to corticosteroid therapy. The most commonly used immune-suppressive agents are azathioprine, cyclophosphamide, methotrexate, and recently cyclosporin A. Azathioprine is commonly used in a dose of 1 to 3 mg per kg per day. Cyclophosphamide is used in a dose of 1 to 2 mg per kg per day. Methotrexate is used less frequently and is probably less effective. Cyclosporin A is used in a dose of 6 mg per kg per day (in two equal doses). The side effects of each of these medications were discussed earlier under the therapy for pemphigus vulgaris.

Dapsone* has been used effectively in a few cases. Dapsone is usually started at 25 to 50 mg daily and increased by 25-mg increments every week until a beneficial effect is obtained. Patients should be monitored appropriately for potential side effects, including bone marrow suppression, hemolysis, liver and renal toxicity, and peripheral neuropathy. Plasmapheresis has been reported to be effective in the management of patients with bullous pemphigoid. The rationale for this therapy is the removal of pathogenic antibodies from the circulation. The procedure, however, is costly, time consuming, and of only temporary benefit.

The most recently investigated therapy for bullous pemphigoid is the use of tetracycline* with or without niacinamide. The rationale for the use of antibiotics such as tetracycline (or erythromycin) is to take advantage of their anti-inflammatory properties. The mechanism of the anti-inflammatory and immune-modulating properties of these medications is poorly understood. Initial case reports suggested a moderate beneficial effect of tetracycline with or without niacinamide. A recent study compared the effectiveness of the combination of tetracycline and niacinamide versus that of prednisone in the treatment of several patients with generalized bullous pemphigoid. The combination of the two medications was as effective as prednisone. Tetracycline is given in a dose of 500 mg four times daily and niacinamide in a dose of 500 mg three times daily. If patients develop side effects with tetracycline, minocycline (Minocin)* 100 mg twice daily can be used with equal success. The advantage of therapy with these medications is obvious in a population that is elderly and often

sickly. The use of tetracycline and niacinamide may be beneficial in two situations. In mild cases, the combination alone may lead to a complete clinical remission. In more extensive cases, the addition of this combination to prednisone may have a steroid-sparing effect.

CICATRICIAL PEMPHIGOID

Clinical Manifestations and Diagnosis

Cicatricial pemphigoid is a chronic blistering disease of the mucous membranes and occasionally the skin. Most patients with cicatricial pemphigoid are elderly (mean age of 66 years). Patients most often present with mucosal involvement. The relative frequency of involvement of each of the mucosal surfaces varies among different reports, likely reflecting patient selection bias for a disease that may present to numerous medical specialties, including ophthalmology, oral surgery and dentistry, dermatology, and primary care. Oral and ocular involvement occurs consistently, with oral involvement occurring in almost 100% of patients in select series and ocular involvement occurring in 70%. Other mucosal surfaces that may be involved include the pharynx, nasal mucosa, larynx, esophagus, genital mucosa, and rectum. Skin involvement occurs in approximately 25% of patients. Severity of involvement of one mucous membrane does not correlate with severity or presence of involvement in other mucous membranes.

Regardless of the affected site, the initial lesions are vesicles and bullae that rupture and consistently recur at the same site. This is usually accompanied by acute and chronic inflammation of the affected sites. If untreated, lesions of cicatricial pemphigoid tend to be associated with a high degree of scarring that leads to high disease morbidity. Complications include loss of vision and strictures in affected mucous membranes, such as the esophagus.

The immunofluorescence findings in cicatricial pemphigoid are similar to those in bullous pemphigoid. The frequency of positive indirect immunofluorescence, however, is very low compared with that in bullous pemphigoid.

Therapy

Therapy of cicatricial pemphigoid depends on the disease extent and severity. In limited oral disease, topical therapy with local anesthetic agents and local corticosteroids in addition to appropriate oral hygiene may suffice. The corticosteroid can be applied under occlusion with a prosthetic device or injected intralesionally. Patients with extensive oral involvement or ocular involvement need systemic therapy. Dapsone* has been reported to be effective in some patients with cicatricial pemphigoid. The response of oral lesions appears to be faster than that of ocular

---

*Not FDA-approved for this indication.

*Not FDA-approved for this indication.

lesions. Dapsone is especially effective in treating the early, superficial, erosive lesions in the oral cavity. The dose and monitoring are similar to those in bullous pemphigoid. In more severe cases and in those who do not respond adequately to dapsone, systemic corticosteroids, usually in addition to immune-suppressive drugs such as azathioprine and cyclophosphamide, are indicated. The rationale for such aggressive therapy in a localized disease is to prevent potential complications, especially in the eyes. The response to therapy is slower than that seen in patients with bullous pemphigoid. Prednisone is used in a dose of 1 mg per kg per day, and cyclophosphamide in a dose of 1 to 2 mg per kg per day. Prednisone is given for approximately 6 months, whereas cyclophosphamide is continued for 18 to 24 months. Azathioprine in a dose of 2 to 3 mg per kg per day appears to be less effective than cyclophosphamide.

Patients with severe ocular scarring may benefit from cryotherapy ablation of scar tissue. Ocular surgery is contraindicated during the active phase of the disease, since it may cause explosive flares of the disease, resulting in corneal ulceration and loss of vision. Similarly, resection of laryngeal or esophageal stenosis in the presence of active disease may lead to worsening of the strictures.

EPIDERMOLYSIS BULLOSA ACQUISITA

Clinical Manifestations and Diagnosis

Epidermolysis bullosa acquisita is a bullous disease of adults that has a variable clinical spectrum. There are two common clinical types of the disease: inflammatory and noninflammatory. The noninflammatory type presents with skin fragility and trauma-induced blisters over the hands and feet and, to a lesser extent, elsewhere on the skin surface. As the disease progresses, healing of individual erosions is associated with the appearance of multiple milia. The inflammatory type presents in a pattern similar to that in bullous pemphigoid. Histologic examination of a vesicle usually reveals a subepidermal blister with an underlying inflammatory infiltrate of variable intensity (very mild in the noninflammatory type, and relatively dense and rich in neutrophils in the inflammatory type). Direct immunofluorescence of perilesional skin reveals deposition of multiple immune globulin classes as well as complement components along the dermal-epidermal junction. Indirect immunofluorescence reveals antibodies in the sera that are directed against collagen VII molecules, which constitute the anchoring fibrils of the sublamina densa zone of the dermal-epidermal junction. The course of this disease tends to be chronic. There is a variant of the disease with lesions limited to mucous membranes (similar to cicatricial pemphigoid).

Therapy

The goals and rationale for therapy as well as the drugs used in the treatment of epidermolysis bullosa acquisita are similar to those for bullous pemphigoid. Some patients respond rapidly and favorably. Because this disease is mediated by neutrophils, dapsone has a particularly significant steroid-sparing effect. A group of patients appears to have a disease that is resistant to conventional therapy. In these patients, other immune-suppressive drugs, including azathioprine, cyclophosphamide, methotrexate, and gold, have been used with variable success. Cyclosporin A, however, has been associated with consistent, successful results. It is given in a dose of 6 mg per kg per day in two equally divided doses. After inducing a clinical remission, the dose can be decreased slowly to 3 mg per kg per day.

DERMATITIS HERPETIFORMIS

Clinical Manifestations and Diagnosis

Dermatitis herpetiformis is a rather uncommon bullous disease with a mean age of onset in the fourth decade. Lesions classically involve the elbows, knees, buttocks, scalp, and face. The eruption is extremely pruritic. Primary lesions consist of grouped, erythematous, edematous, papulovesicles and papulopustules that are only rarely seen intact because they are very rapidly excoriated. Occasionally, urticarial and bullous lesions are seen. Eighty percent of patients have histologic evidence of gluten-sensitive enteropathy, similar to that seen in celiac disease. Only 10% of patients, however, have symptomatic intestinal disease. Histologic evaluation of an early papulovesicle reveals neutrophilic microabscesses in the dermal papillae that ultimately coalesce to form a subepidermal vesicle or pustule. Direct immunofluorescence of perilesional skin is diagnostic and reveals granular deposition of IgA in dermal papillae and, to a lesser degree, along the dermal-epidermal junction. The IgA appears to be deposited on microfibrillar components of elastin in the upper dermis. Indirect immunofluorescence fails to reveal circulating antibodies against skin components. Approximately 40% of patients have IgA-containing circulating immune complexes. The pathogenetic mechanisms responsible for IgA deposition in the skin are not clear. One theory proposes that gluten antigens gain access through the gut to the local lymphatics, where sensitization takes place. Gluten proteins then bind dimeric IgA, and complexes circulate in the serum until trapped by a specific antigen in the skin (possibly gluten receptor).

Therapy

Dermatitis herpetiformis is a lifelong disease. The goal of therapy is to suppress the clinical manifestations of the disease, that is, pruritus and lesions. Most patients need lifelong therapy. A gluten-free diet may lead to clearance of the lesions in 12 to 36 months and may decrease or rarely eliminate the requirement for drug therapy. Since skin lesions are induced by the influx of neutrophils to the dermal papillae, drugs that interfere with neutrophil chemotaxis are expected to be helpful in the management of patients. Dapsone is the most studied and most effective of these medications. Although dapsone has no effect on the deposition of IgA in the skin and no direct effect on the immune response, its clinical usefulness served as a therapeutic test, before immunofluorescence tests became available, to confirm the diagnosis of this disease. Patients respond dramatically to an adequate dose of dapsone within 24 to 48 hours. The pruritus subsides, followed by remission of the lesions. Most patients remain in remission as long as they are maintained on an adequate dose of dapsone. This dose varies among patients from 25 mg to 200 mg daily. Some patients require a slow increase in the dapsone dose over years to decades. In other patients, the requirement may actually decrease. Patients are usually kept on dapsone for life. Monitoring for the acute and chronic side effects of dapsone is therefore very important.

Sulfapyridine* in a dose of 2 to 4 grams daily in divided doses appears to have a similar effect in patients who are intolerant to dapsone. It is important to maintain generous oral intake of fluids to avoid crystallization of the drug in the urinary tract.

Curiously, dermatitis herpetiformis has a minimal response to topical steroids as well as to systemic anti-inflammatory agents, including corticosteroids.

LINEAR IgA DISEASE

Clinical Manifestations and Diagnosis

Linear IgA disease occurs in two forms, the adult form and the childhood form, otherwise known as chronic bullous disease of childhood. This disease affects all age groups and presents with a variably pruritic eruption that is clinically similar to dermatitis herpetiformis and/or bullous pemphigoid. Histologic examination of a vesicle reveals a subepidermal blister with a relatively dense mixed infiltrate in the superficial dermis that is composed of neutrophils and eosinophils. Direct immunofluorescence of perilesional skin reveals continuous linear deposition of IgA along the epidermal basement membrane. The pattern of fluorescence is similar to that of bullous pemphigoid. Indirect immunofluorescence reveals circulating IgA antibodies against components of the dermal-epidermal junction. The course of the disease is variable, but, unlike dermatitis herpetiformis, it tends to be self-limited, lasting several months to a few years.

Therapy

The clinical and immunologic profiles of this disease share features with both dermatitis herpetiformis and bullous pemphigoid. Most patients with linear IgA disease respond to dapsone in doses similar to those for dermatitis herpetiformis. In resistant

cases or in cases of intolerance to dapsone, systemic corticosteroids are usually helpful. It is important to remember that not infrequently this disease is induced by a systemic drug. Considering a drug etiology and discontinuing the drug are helpful in selected cases.

CONTACT DERMATITIS

method of
WILLIAM L. EPSTEIN, M.D.
University of California San Francisco
San Francisco, California

Contact dermatitis is a common skin condition having several modes of presentation that, taken together, constitute approximately 10% of a clinical dermatologist's practice.

ACUTE CONTACT DERMATITIS

When the cause is an irritant, the clinical diagnosis is usually self-evident. Although this sort of injury can occur in the home or during recreational activity, it is more common as an occupational hazard. In work places, such as caustic plants and biochemistry laboratories, where this poses a significant, potential emergency, showers are available to quickly wash off the offending chemical and minimize the degree of injury. Office treatment of this dermatitis is simply supportive. One should make certain no residual chemical is left, and the damaged area is treated with cool soaks. Depending on the extent of injury, the patient may be advised to rest at home for a day or two until the area begins to heal. The use of nonsteroidal anti-inflammatory drugs, sedatives, and analgesics may be indicated in patients with extensive chemical burns, but there is no benefit from the use of systemic or topical corticosteroids. Fortunately, these lesions tend to heal quickly, and the problem is rapidly resolved.

Allergic contact dermatitis is a different matter. This is a form of cell-mediated immunity and, as such, has a delayed onset (2 to 7 days after exposure) and presents as erythema, edema, vesiculation, intense pruritus, and in extreme cases, bullae. Except for poison oak/poison ivy dermatitis, most patients are unaware of the cause, at least during the initial bout.

In mild-to-moderate cases seen 2 to 4 days after onset of the eruption, therapy should be conservative, with the prospect of self-healing in 7 to 10 days. Treatment includes cool soaks of water or Burow's solution (aluminum acetate) (1 : 40), tepid baths (starch and soda, Aveeno), and shake lotions (calamine lotion without additives). Topical antihistamines in the acute phase may induce contact sensitization. Systemically, aspirin in large doses (0.65 gram [10 grains] every 3 to 4 hours) or antihista-

*Investigational drug in the United States.

TABLE 1. **Relative Potency of Some Topical Corticosteroids***

Potent	Moderate	Mild
Betamethasone dipropionate (Diprosone)	Amcinonide (Cyclocort)	Desonide (DesOwen)
Clobetasol propionate (Temovate)	Halcinonide (Halog)	Hydrocortisone salts (Hytone)
Diflorasone diacetate (Florone)	Mometasone furorate (Elocon)	
Fluocinonide (Lidex)	Triamcinolone acetonide (Kenalog)	
Halobetasol propionate (Ultravate)		

*Topical corticosteroids are generally classified into seven categories of potency according to chemical structure, concentration, and base. Gels and optimized bases give better results than creams and lotions. Only mild corticosteroid preparations are recommended for use on the face and in intertriginous areas owing to untoward response after continual, frequent, or unmonitored use by patients.

mines in sedative doses may reduce pruritus. A hypnotic at bedtime (chloral hydrate, 0.5 to 0.2 gram [7.5 to 30 grains]) is required occasionally. If edema becomes noticeable, as often happens when the dermatitis occurs on the face or genitalia, I use systemic corticosteroids (see further on). In the healing stages, when the skin is dry and scaly, pruritus is best controlled by use of topical corticosteroids. A list of topical corticosteroids and their relative potency appears in Table 1.

Acute contact dermatitis from plants in a very sensitive person should be considered a dermatologic emergency requiring timely and aggressive therapy. In this situation, the dermatitis begins within hours of exposure to the plant and is associated with erythema and marked edema. Definitive therapy requires the use of large doses of systemic corticosteroids. I have best results with adrenocorticotropic hormone (ACTH) gel, 80 U given intramuscularly as soon as the patient is seen, followed by a second injection 8 to 10 hours later. If the disease effervesces in 2 or 3 days, another injection of 80 U of ACTH gel is given. A modified regimen calls for 20 tablets of the physician's favored corticosteroid (most dermatologists choose prednisone). My choice is dexamethasone 0/75 mg, four tablets given five times during the day. This is repeated on 2 consecutive days and then abruptly stopped. Again, the patient is seen 2 days later and, if necessary, given 20 tablets (4 tablets five times daily) to ingest. Usually, this is sufficient to result in healing. An alternative favored by many is to give 80 mg of prednisone for the first few days and then reduce the dose over a period of 2 weeks, with alternate-day therapy at the end.

During the first few days of severe acute allergic contact dermatitis, it is best to have the patient rest at home. Hospitalization is not indicated because of the possibility of secondary infection, expense, and the restrictions of managed care programs.

CHRONIC CONTACT DERMATITIS

Chronic contact dermatitis presents an entirely different problem, and different strategies are needed. The main approach is the judicious use of topical corticosteroids. When the disease affects areas such as the face, hands, and intertriginous areas, one must be careful not to use fluorinated steroids for prolonged periods. Corticosteroid gels are not recom-

mended because of the possibility of systemic effects from absorbed drug. I frequently use triamcinolone acetonide (Kenalog) alone or with occlusion at bedtime for a week, switching as healing begins to the less potent corticosteroids such as hydrocortisone or desonide (see Table 1).

Systemic antihistamines may also be indicated, but these are not nearly as effective antipruritics as hydroxyzine (Atarax) and the tricyclic antidepressants,* such as doxepin (Sinequan), which can be given in small doses throughout the day or to tolerance. Topical use of doxepin (Zonalon)* has become popular, but this can give systemic effects.

An important consideration is the use of emollients, and these should be tailored to the acceptance of the patient. Some prefer greasy preparations, such as ointments or oils, whereas others like a cream or lotion base. One should not be too rigid in prescribing these preparations. It is more important that the patient feel comfortable and obtain subjective relief from whatever topical agent is used. Sometimes, with chronic contact dermatitis, particularly on the hands and feet, the involved areas become markedly thickened and hyperkeratotic. This calls for keratolytic agents, such as salicylic acid (Keralyt gel) and urea, and propitious use of tars. However, these formulations may produce additional irritation and aggravate the situation. Another common occurrence is the appearance of deep, painful fissures. Our preferred treatment is the use of Castellani's paint, with or without added phenol. Sometimes use of an instant glue gives relief, but it also can be irritating.

Alternative therapy includes the use of grenz rays for chronic hand eczema. Oral methoxsalen (Oxsoralen) plus long-wavelength ultraviolet light therapy (PUVA) is another therapy of merit, especially for localized dermatitis on the hands and feet. This is a nonspecific treatment for chronic dermatitis.

PREVENTION

One of the most satisfying aspects of caring for patients with contact dermatitis is that once the allergen or irritant is recognized, it is possible to devise protocols and procedures whereby the patient is either protected against or avoids the contactant. Space allows discussion of only two of the most im-

---

*Not FDA-approved for this indication.

portant allergens. Nickel sensitivity occurs in about 10% of women and 1 to 2% of men. It manifests usually as jewelry dermatitis and often can be prevented by spraying the jewelry with clear plastic or by putting a potent topical corticosteroid on the area where jewelry is to be worn, giving protection for about 6 hours. In persistent cases with unusual presentations, a nickel spot test using dimethylglyoxime can be used to discover where at home or in the work place nickel is being contacted (available through Westwood Squibb Pharmaceutical). When all attempts to prevent recurrent dermatitis fail, the patient should be examined by an expert for other metal sensitivities, such as chromium, cobalt, or the esoteric ones, palladium and gold.

Poison ivy and poison oak sensitivity occur in approximately 50% of North Americans. Very sensitive patients should be advised to stay completely out of areas infested with these weeds. However, mild to moderately sensitive people may be able to reduce the risk of dermatitis by learning to recognize what the plants look like, wearing protective clothing, and decontaminating themselves after exposure. Decontamination is best accomplished by use of an organic solvent, such as isopropyl alcohol, in copious amounts applied to areas such as the face, arms, and exposed sites, followed by thorough rinsing with plain water. All clothing, including boots, should be washed before entering the home. Previously, it was possible to hyposensitize these patients by feeding them the poison oak/ivy antigen, urushiol, by mouth in small increasing doses over a long period of time. However, in 1993 the U.S. Food and Drug Administration mandated that these products be removed from the market until they are better standardized.

SKIN DISEASES OF PREGNANCY

method of
NEIL J. KORMAN, Ph.D., M.D.
Case Western Reserve University
Cleveland, Ohio

A variety of skin diseases may occur during pregnancy. Patients may present with an exacerbation of a skin disease that was present prior to pregnancy, a coincidentally acquired skin disease, or a skin disease specifically related to pregnancy. The specific dermatoses of pregnancy discussed here—herpes gestationis (HG) and pruritic urticarial papules and plaques of pregnancy (PUPPP)—are relatively rare. Pregnant patients are more likely to have skin disorders that are unrelated to pregnancy. It is therefore important to consider more common diagnoses such as drug eruption, erythema multiforme, contact dermatitis, and insect bites in the evaluation of a pregnant patient with a skin disorder. If one of the specific dermatoses of pregnancy is being considered, it is important to obtain tissue for histologic and immunopathologic evaluation. These studies are best performed under the guidance of a specialist, because the interpretation will be facilitated by

their submission to laboratories with this specific expertise.

HERPES GESTATIONIS

HG is an uncommon pruritic, nonviral disease of young women that occurs during or shortly after pregnancy. This disorder has no relationship to herpesvirus infection. Unfortunately, the name "herpes," which was used historically to describe any skin disease characterized by the formation of grouped vesicles, has remained associated with this disease. Some have proposed changing the name of this disease to "pemphigoid gestationis" owing to its similarities to bullous pemphigoid, an autoimmune blistering disease of the elderly. HG has a reported incidence of approximately 1 per 50,000 births in North American whites and an even lower incidence in blacks. Typical HG lesions include urticarial papules and plaques with polycyclic wheals that evolve into vesicles and bullae. This evolution usually takes approximately 4 weeks. Lesions start periumbilically in most patients and later spread, involving larger areas of the abdomen, buttocks, and extremities. In more severe cases, there may be lesions involving the palms, soles, chest, and back. Lesions in HG are almost invariably pruritic and frequently interfere with the patient's daily comfort level and ability to sleep. Some infants born to affected mothers have similar skin lesions, but these usually last for only a few weeks and typically do not require any therapeutic intervention.

The disease may begin during any trimester of pregnancy as well as post partum, but the most common time of onset is the second or third trimester. It is important to evaluate patients carefully soon after delivery not only because HG can present at this time but also because severe disease exacerbations may occur in patients who were previously well controlled. Although HG usually resolves within weeks to months of parturition, patients may have recurrences in subsequent pregnancies. Exacerbations of disease may rarely occur between pregnancies, particularly after menstruation or ingestion of oral contraceptives or other hormonal stimuli.

An important but controversial point is whether HG is associated with any increased risk of fetal morbidity or mortality. Widely varying results derive from different studies, with one showing completely normal outcomes, one revealing an increased risk of small for gestational age infants, and one demonstrating an increased risk of prematurity and stillbirths. These differences may be related to several factors, including reporting bias. Given this information, the most prudent recommendation is to have HG patients managed jointly by both a dermatologist and an obstetrician experienced in high-risk management, with the delivery occurring in a facility equipped with a neonatal intensive care unit.

Definitive diagnosis of HG is made by skin biopsy. Histologic examination of a blister reveals a subepidermal blister with eosinophils similar to the findings observed in bullous pemphigoid. Since these histopathologic findings do not adequately differentiate HG from other eruptions of pregnancy, direct immunofluorescence microscopy of perilesional skin is necessary. This study reveals linear deposits of C3 at the basement membrane in all patients, along with linear deposits of IgG in some patients.

The goal of treatment in HG is to control pruritus, suppress new lesion formation, and care for sites of blisters and erosions. Some patients with mild disease respond to potent topical corticosteroids such as 0.05% fluocinonide (Lidex) three to five times daily along with the administration of oral antihistamines such as diphenhydramine (Benadryl) 25 to 50 mg every 4 to 6 hours. However, the majority of patients with HG require treatment with moderate doses of systemic glucocorticosteroids (oral prednisone 20 to 60 mg daily) throughout much of their pregnancy. These patients should be treated with a single morning dose of prednisone and incremental tapering as tolerated, usually by 5 mg every 1 to 2 weeks. If a postpartum flare of disease occurs, prednisone should be restarted (or increased) at a dosage of 20 to 40 mg every morning. Systemic corticosteroids should be used with care during pregnancy, but extensive experience with their use in pregnant asthmatic patients suggests relatively low risks if the patients are properly monitored. When systemic corticosteroids are used during pregnancy, the newborn should be monitored for signs of adrenal insufficiency. Individual moist weeping or eroded bullous lesions of HG should be treated with wet compresses of either saline or 1:40 Burow solution (Domeboro) three to four times daily for 10 to 20 minutes to promote drying and débridement. Bullae should be left intact to promote skin protection and re-epithelialization. Skin lesions should be evaluated for signs of infection and should be promptly treated with antibiotics if necessary.

PRURITIC URTICARIAL PAPULES AND PLAQUES OF PREGNANCY

PUPPP is a common, highly pruritic eruption that usually occurs late in the third trimester in women who are pregnant for the first time. Although there are no data on the exact incidence of PUPPP, it is seen more commonly than HG. PUPPP is characterized by the onset of red, blanchable urticarial papules and plaques that usually occur on the abdominal striae, lower abdomen, buttocks, and thighs and may later coalesce into large urticarial plaques. The lesions are exceedingly pruritic, often interfering with daily activities and sleep, but skin excoriations are extremely rare. PUPPP usually responds readily to treatment and also remits after delivery. The disease does not tend to flare post partum, recur in future pregnancies, or develop on ingestion of oral contraceptives or other hormones. PUPPP is not associated with any increased risk of fetal morbidity or mortality and has no related systemic symptoms or laboratory abnormalities.

Biopsies of involved skin from patients with PUPPP reveal a superficial or mid-dermal perivascular lymphohistiocytic infiltrate, along with occasional eosinophils and dermal edema. These histologic findings are relatively consistent, although they are not completely diagnostic. Direct immunofluorescence studies that are negative help differentiate PUPPP from HG, which has a characteristic pattern, as described earlier.

Treatment of PUPPP is aimed at symptom control, since patients promptly clear at delivery. The majority of patients achieve excellent control with potent topical corticosteroids such as 0.05% fluocinonide (Lidex) three to five times daily. Oral antihistamines such as diphenhydramine (Benadryl) 25 to 50 mg every 4 to 6 hours are often added to the treatment regimen. Once the eruption is controlled, the frequency of topical steroid treatment can be decreased, and a less potent topical steroid can be substituted. This treatment regimen controls the large majority of patients, but selected patients with severe involvement may require treatment with systemic corticosteroids. In these cases, 20 to 40 mg of prednisone each morning results in rapid control of the skin eruption and the associated pruritus. A rapid taper of the prednisone—5 mg at 3- to 4-day intervals—can usually be accomplished.

PRURITUS ANI AND VULVAE

method of
SHARON ZELLIS, D.O.
Philadelphia College of Osteopathic Medicine
Philadelphia, Pennsylvania

and

STEPHANIE H. PINCUS, M.D.
State University of New York at Buffalo
Buffalo, New York

Anogenital pruritus is a frequent and distressing complaint. It may reflect a primary skin disorder or a systemic condition. A thorough assessment is essential prior to initiating empirical therapy. The likelihood of an underlying irritant, allergic, inflammatory, infectious, or neoplastic process must be considered (Table 1). Idiopathic pruritus ani and vulvae implies persistent itching in the absence of a specific identifiable factor.

A rational approach to the therapeutic management of individuals with anogenital pruritus must first focus on prior exacerbating factors, duration, and characteristics of symptoms. A complete cutaneous examination with attention to the oral mucosa, scalp, and nails may provide diagnostic clues suggestive of a coexisting condition such as seborrheic dermatitis, atopic dermatitis, lichen planus, or psoriasis that may involve anogenital skin. Primary anogenital pathology may be evident on close inspection, and a pelvic examination should be performed if indicated. Microscopic examination or cultures will accurately diagnose an infectious etiology. Skin biopsy is reserved for features suspicious of a premalignant or neoplastic condition and for individuals with recalcitrant pruritus despite appropriate therapy.

TABLE 1. **Causative Factors in Anogenital Pruritus**

Dermatoses
   Irritant dermatitis
   Allergic contact dermatitis
   Psoriasis
   Lichen planus
   Lichen sclerosus

Infectious agents
   Fungal—*Candida*
   Infestations—scabies, pediculosis pubis, pinworms
   Viral—condylomata, herpes
   Bacterial infection, local abscess

Premalignant conditions
   Extramammary Paget's disease
   Bowen's disease

Systemic disease
   Diabetes
   Thyroid disease

Anatomic disorders
   Anal fissure, fistula, papilloma
   Rectal prolapse
   Prolapsed hemorrhoids

Dietary factors

TREATMENT

Successful management of patients with anogenital pruritus is predicated on correctly identifying causative factors. Once a diagnosis of idiopathic pruritus is entertained, the institution of general measures to interrupt the itch-scratch cycle is crucial.

Proper perineal hygiene is essential. Cleansing after urination and defecation should be performed by using plain water and unscented white toilet tissue and patting the area dry. Residual fecal material may be very irritating. Soap should be used sparingly and adequately removed. Talcum powder should be discouraged because of its irritant potential. Frequent and vigorous bathing is unnecessary, and it may result in excessive drying of the skin, thus leading to further itching.

Modification of environmental exposures can minimize anogenital contact with potential sensitizers (Table 2). Undergarments should be laundered through a double-rinse cycle, and fabric softeners should be avoided. Menstruating women with pruritus vulvae tend to tolerate unscented tampons over sanitary napkins during their cycle.

Excessive sweating can contribute to symptoms of

TABLE 2. **Common Sensitizers in Anogenital Pruritus**

Topical medications
   Neomycin
   Ethylenediamines
   Diphenhydramine

Rubber condoms, diaphragms

Fragrant soaps, toilet tissue, sanitary napkins, and
   fabric softeners

Dye

Nickel

anogenital pruritus. Therefore, loose cotton undergarments are suggested. In addition, tight-fitting outerwear should be discouraged. Finally, cleansing after vigorous exercise is recommended.

Alteration of dietary habits may be of particular benefit to individuals with pruritus ani. Coffee and alcohol propagate incremental sphincter relaxation and soilage, and therefore avoidance of these beverages may be advantageous.

Symptomatic relief may be obtained from short courses of low-potency nonfluorinated hydrocortisone cream (1 to 2.5%) applied twice daily. A trial of oral antihistamines may also prove beneficial in disrupting the itch-scratch cycle. Agents with sedative properties such as hydroxyzine (Atarax) or diphenhydramine (Benadryl), beginning at dosages of 10 to 25 mg each evening with subsequent titration, are recommended. Night-time doses of tricyclic antidepressants such as amitriptyline (Elavil) and doxepin (Sinequan), beginning with 10 to 25 mg, appear effective. Their ability to treat subclinical depression, which may be associated with this disorder, may also be important.

Combinations of hydrocortisone with topical nonsensitizing anesthetics (Pramosone) are especially useful, and they can be applied four to six times per day. Conditions such as severe contact dermatitis or psoriasis may benefit from limited courses of more potent fluorinated steroids, such as triamcinolone or betamethasone valerate. Potent and ultrapotent steroids are best avoided. A therapeutic trial with topical antifungals (Spectazole, Nizoral) is often warranted.

URTICARIA

method of
JERE D. GUIN, M.D.
University of Arkansas
Little Rock, Arkansas

Urticaria represents a complex of conditions that is characterized by whealing. Angioedema is a deeper form of swelling that may or may not be associated with hives. The approach to treatment is determined by the form of urticaria present. Classifications vary in complexity, but the conditions affecting most patients fit into the category of acute, chronic, physical or contact urticaria, or urticarial vasculitis.

EVALUATION

Acute and chronic urticarias may or may not be associated with dermographism or angioedema, and they are distinguished by having more or less than a certain duration, usually 6 to 8 weeks. Physical urticarias are easily recognized by their location, pattern, history, and frequently, by a characteristic lesion, such as the linear whealing in dermographism, or the 3- to 5-mm wheals with a large flare seen in cholinergic urticaria. Often, these conditions can be confirmed by relatively simple tests. Contact urticaria is common, but it often goes unrecognized because it is not presented for medical treatment.

Urticarial vasculitis is a special case. It represents an immune complex vasculitis involving complement consumption. A diligent search for an underlying problem is indicated in patients with this condition (especially for hepatitis B and C, infectious mononucleosis, and rheumatologic diseases), and its treatment is very different from that of most other conditions appearing as urticaria. Lesions often persist for 1 to 3 days, leaving a discolored, scaly, or purpuric mark; frequently, the lesions burn or sting rather than itch. Other symptoms found include arthralgias, gastrointestinal complaints, fever, adenopathy, erythema multiforme-like lesions, and neuralgic disorders. Laboratory abnormalities include an elevated erythrocyte sedimentation rate and a depressed complement level in most patients and a histologic appearance of vasculitis in a high percentage of patients. The latter may be the most reliable laboratory criterion, but no one finding is absolute.

The history in acute and chronic urticaria should concentrate especially on medications being taken, and in cases of the chronic type, the physician should tactfully and empathically look for emotional stress. One should also identify previous therapy and vasodilating influences. Treatment of chronic urticaria is both challenging and time consuming, but it should not be considered hopeless. Searches for a specific cause are indicated, although as few as 10% may be positive if one eliminates emotional causes and physical urticarias, in patients in whom the cause is obvious and the eruption is identifiable. A more aggressive approach is probably indicated for persons who are unresponsive to treatment. A history of a prior urticarial reaction to penicillin indicates the need for a trial of avoidance of dairy products, which may be contaminated with penicillin. Internal disease, parasitic infestation, malignancy, or a focus of infection may rarely be found as an underlying cause in a specific patient, but work-ups for problems should be ordered on a case-by-case basis, because extensive testing for routine screening has been shown not to be cost effective. In my experience, when a cause for chronic urticaria is found, it is most commonly a drug and often occurs after a totally negative history on a number of earlier occasions.

In chronic urticaria, certain dietary ingredients, although not obvious to the patient, may represent a source of aggravation. Use of a printed questionnaire in taking the history allows the patient to mark the various foods containing salicylates, benzoates, and azo dyes (especially FD&C Yellow No. 5). In patients who demonstrate an immediate skin test reaction to yeast, it may also help to look for foods containing yeast and perhaps tyramine; this can also be accomplished with the same printed form. Such dietary factors probably do not represent a source of allergy but are probably pharmacologically aggravating.

Identifying the presence (or absence) of emotional stress can also be helpful in chronic urticaria. This requires tact and empathy on the part of the physician, and it is best done personally in a quiet environment, where an unhurried and sympathetic attitude to the patient's plight demonstrates genuine care and concern for what is often an impressively stressful situation. Formal psychological testing may help prove that stress is present, but this is not usually necessary. Developing a relationship of trust and understanding is helpful in another way. Compliance with the routine required of patients with chronic urticaria is difficult at best, and the patient is much more likely to be compliant if the physician is perceived as being genuinely involved.

ACUTE URTICARIA

It is obvious that a known cause should be eliminated whenever possible. Although diet can be important as a source of allergy in acute urticaria, patients with acute urticaria due to food allergy are not often a problem because the patient generally identifies the offending food. Treatment of adults with oral cyproheptadine (Periactin), 4 mg four times daily, or hydroxyzine (Atarax), 10 to 25 mg three or four times daily, is helpful in controlling symptoms. Intramuscular or intravenous diphenhydramine (Benadryl), 50 mg, can be helpful in severe reactions. In patients in whom a known cause can be found and eliminated (as in an urticarial drug reaction), one might consider a course of oral corticosteroid therapy for those without contraindications. The initial dosage depends on the severity of the condition, but a typical course might comprise an initial dose of 30 to 40 mg of prednisone by mouth daily after breakfast, tapered over a 10- to 14-day period.

Severe laryngeal edema or other life-threatening situations may require subcutaneous or intramuscular administration of 0.3 to 0.5 mL of 1:1000 epinephrine. Intravenous use, which is limited to severe anaphylaxis with signs of shock, requires dilution to 1:10,000 concentration, administering 0.25 to 0.5 mL at a time and repeating the dosage if no response is obtained. One should be wary of inducing hypertension in patients on certain beta blockers. Maintenance of the airway may require intubation or even tracheostomy, and maintaining an intravenous saline drip has been recommended for patients with severe reactions.

CHRONIC URTICARIA

Adults are typically treated with oral cyproheptadine (Periactin), 4 mg four times daily, or hydroxyzine (Atarax), 10 to 25 mg three or four times daily, or both, with drowsiness being a limiting factor. For persons who are extremely sensitive to the sedative effect or who are intolerant to anticholinergic effects of antihistamines, terfenadine (Seldane), 60 mg twice daily; astemizole (Hismanal), 10 mg daily; or loratadine (Claritin), 10 mg daily, by mouth can often be substituted. With the first two drugs, one must exclude persons with hepatic disease and those who are on treatment with macrolide antibiotics (e.g., erythromycin), ketoconazole (Nizoral), or itraconazole (Sporanox). Unresponsive patients sometimes improve with either oral doxepin (Sinequan) or amitriptyline (Elavil), 10 mg three times daily, but an effective dose may be a bit higher. These agents are much better antihistamines than most other tricyclic antidepressants; so for patients who already are taking another such medication, it may be helpful to substitute doxepin. Addition of an H_2 blocker theoretically should reduce the effect of histamine on blood vessels but may adversely affect mast cells, which form histamine and other inflammatory mediators. This may explain the conflicting reports on the effectiveness of such treatment in chronic urticaria.

The calcium channel blocker nifedipine (Procardia)* reportedly helps some resistant cases. Treatment is started with a single dose, increasing to 10 mg three times daily, avoiding H_2 blockers and monitoring for hypotension.

Elimination of vasodilating factors such as heat, exercise, and alcohol, and the avoidance of nonspecific histamine-releasing agents such as opiates are indicated. Exposure to salicylates and certain azo dyes, especially FD&C Yellow No. 5 (tartrazine), tends to aggravate the problem, especially in more severe cases and at higher levels of challenge. FD&C Yellow No. 6, found in many antihistamines, can also be a problem. Diet lists of foods high in salicylate content are available, and foods and drugs that contain tartrazine must by law be labeled as containing FD&C Yellow No. 5. Patients demonstrating an immediate skin test reaction to yeast are said to be more likely to benefit from a yeast-free diet because many foods containing yeast are high in tyramine as well.

URTICARIAL VASCULITIS

Urticarial vasculitis is frequently associated with an underlying cause, including medications, hepatitis B, mononucleosis, and a variety of rheumatologic conditions. There are uncontrolled reports of benefit with oral colchicine, 0.6 mg twice daily; dapsone, 100 mg daily; indomethacin (Indocin), 75 to 200 mg daily in divided doses; or hydroxychloroquine (Plaquenil), 200 mg twice daily. I have seen good results with colchicine. The minimal effective dose of prednisone is likely to be high, so another agent seems preferable for initial treatment.

PHYSICAL URTICARIAS

Dermographism can usually be adequately controlled with low doses of cyproheptadine or hydroxyzine, along with avoidance of unnecessary trauma and vasodilating factors, especially heat. For an adult, one might start with cyproheptadine, 2 to 4 mg four times daily, or hydroxyzine, 10 mg three or four times daily by mouth, and adjust the dosage to the patient's response. In some cases, 2 to 4 mg daily of oral cyproheptadine is adequate for maintenance. Treatment is directed toward preventing the response to injury. The duration of the eruption is short, so one cannot wait until the eruption appears to treat it. Effectiveness of treatment can be measured by controlled stroking of skin of the upper back.

Some cases of cold urticaria may require a serologic test for syphilis and a test for cryoproteins to rule out symptomatic cold urticaria, but the most common cause is essential acquired cold urticaria, which can be treated in adults with avoidance of cold and the administration of oral cyproheptadine (Periactin), 4 mg four times daily. When a patient is known to have an IgE-mediated urticaria, elimination of exposure (in the case of penicillin allergy, avoidance of dairy products) is sometimes associated with clearing. Control here can be measured with change in response to a 5-minute application of an ice cube in a plastic bag.

Recommended treatment for cholinergic urticaria involves administration of oral hydroxyzine, 25 mg three times daily and avoidance of sweating. Aquagenic pruritus reportedly improves with antihistamines and doses of ultraviolet B radiation (UVB) sufficient to cause erythema, and graduated exposure to ultraviolet A radiation (UVA), UVB, and psoralen with UVA light (PUVA) plus antihistamines raises the threshold in at least some patients with solar urticaria.

Acute treatment of hereditary angioedema sometimes requires maintenance of an airway and intravascular volume. Some advocate intravenous C1-esterase inhibitor, human* (C1-INH) concentrate (where available) for acute attacks. Long-term treatment is with oral anabolic steroid therapy, especially danazol (Danocrine), 200 mg twice or three times daily, tapered to 200 mg daily or alternate days according to the patient's response. An alternative drug is stanozolol (Winstrol), 2 mg three times daily initially, reduced to 2 mg daily. The maintenance dose is individualized, but there is a high incidence of flares when less than 2 mg is administered daily. Hepatic dysfunction can be a complication. About 50% of women treated with 2 mg daily have an androgenic effect; 20% will show this effect at 0.5 mg daily, a dose that is not adequate to prevent episodes in most patients. Both drugs alter menses but are not effective as contraceptives, so birth control is required in sexually active females. Patients with delayed pressure urticaria and nonhereditary angioedema associated with lymphoproliferative disease may also respond to this treatment approach, but those with acquired angioedema without lymphoproliferative disease (with antibodies to C1-INH) may not respond, and corticosteroids have been recommended.

CONTACT URTICARIA

Contact urticaria may be immunologic or nonimmunologic, but treatment of the latter in most cases is not a problem, because most patients do well by avoiding the offending substance. The mediators for contact urticaria vary, and antihistamines are helpful for some agents but not others. Nonsteroidal antiinflammatory agents benefit nonimmunologic contact urticaria from several mediators, but have less effect on nonimmunologic contact urticaria from cinnamaldehyde. Antihistamines do not markedly reduce non-

---

*Not FDA-approved for this indication.

*Investigational drug in the USA.

immunologic contact urticaria from these three mediators but may reduce severity of the condition from many other mediators.

Immunologic contact urticaria to latex gloves and other rubber objects has become a widespread problem in health care workers and their patients. Contact with many protein materials and certain medications can cause whealing, eczema, and even anaphylaxis requiring immediate treatment as with acute urticaria.

Contact urticaria comprises a diverse group of immediate "urticarial" reactions, and it includes reactions following exposure to certain plants and animals, such as nettles, jellyfish, and caterpillars. Pretreatment with topical corticosteroid also helps in prevention but does not totally eliminate the reaction. For most patients with contact urticaria, avoidance of the cause is the most important treatment.

PIGMENTARY DISORDERS

method of
ANNE-SOPHIE J. GADENNE, M.D., and
JAMES J. NORDLUND, M.D.
University of Cincinnati Medical Center
Cincinnati, Ohio

The four pigments that are primarily responsible for skin color are oxygenated hemoglobin, reduced hemoglobin, carotenoids, and melanin. Of these, melanin is the major determinant of skin color. Disorders of pigmentation can be caused by at least three mechanisms: (1) an enhanced or diminished production of melanin by the melanocyte, (2) an increase or decrease in the number of melanocytes, or (3) an abnormal location of melanin and/or melanocytes within the dermis. The clinical result is either decreased pigment (hypopigmentation) or increased pigment (hyperpigmentation).

HYPERPIGMENTATION

Ultraviolet Light–Induced Hyperpigmentation (Suntan)

Etiology

The constitutive or baseline skin color is genetically determined. It is independent of extrinsic factors such as exposure to sunlight. Facultative skin color is the inducible darkening of the skin that most often follows exposure to ultraviolet (UV) radiation. Suntan results from two different mechanisms. Longwave UV light (Type A [UVA], 320 to 400 nm, or "black light") causes immediate darkening of pigment. This occurs within 15 to 30 minutes after exposure and disappears within hours. It is probably caused by an oxidative change in the pre-existing melanin molecules. UVA can also induce an increase in melanin synthesis but does so more slowly than other spectra of UV light.

Shortwave ultraviolet light (Type B [UVB], 290 to 320 nm) produces sunburn as well as delayed tanning. Delayed tanning is often much darker than the immediate type and is caused by the proliferation of melanocytes as well as enhanced production of melanin. It takes 3 to 4 days to develop and lasts for many weeks.

Both longwave and shortwave UV light contribute to photoaging, and it is likely that both increase the risk of skin cancers. However, the role of UVA in the cause of skin cancer is under intensive study, and definitive conclusions about its role in cancer are not yet possible. Both types of UV light are responsible for the mottled hyperpigmentation and the wrinkling that are observed on heavily exposed areas of the skin such as the face, neck, and dorsum of the hands. Exposure to UV radiation in tanning parlors also hastens the processes of photoaging and wrinkling. If UVA is involved in causing skin cancer, then exposure to UVA in tanning parlors increases the risk of developing skin cancers.

Treatment

The patient must recognize that sun-induced pigmentation can be reversed only by avoiding exposure of the skin to all forms of UV light. There are many physical sun blocks that reflect UV light and protect the skin as well. Clothing such as beachwear or hats, which can be very elegant, are excellent protectants. Other chemical sun blocks such as zinc oxide, calamine, talc, titanium dioxide, and kaolin are opaque and are effective sun shields. These products must be applied in a thick coat.

Chemical sunscreens function in a different way. They absorb UV light, especially in the shortwave range (UVB, 290 to 320 nm). The most common chemical sunscreens contain para-aminobenzoic acid (PABA), the esters of PABA, and salicylates. Other chemicals, like the benzophenone derivatives, anthralinates, and cinnamates, absorb UVB and offer additional absorption in the UVA (320 to 350 nm) range.

Two factors should be considered when choosing a sunscreen: the sun protection factor (SPF) and the substantivity. The SPF is the ratio of the minimal sunburn (UVB) dose of sunlight on chemically protected skin compared with that on unprotected skin. In midsummer (June 21) the average unprotected person burns after 15 to 20 minutes of direct sun exposure to the sun at noontime. A sunscreen with SPF 2 absorbs one-half of the UVB striking the skin. Therefore it takes twice as long to burn the treated skin (30 to 40 minutes of exposure on June 21). An SPF of 15 to 20 (which requires 15 to 20 times more UVB to burn the skin) is considered to be adequate protection against UVB radiation.

The substantivity of the sunscreen is its ability to withstand removal from the skin by sweating or water immersion. Table 1 gives examples of current commercially available sunscreens with SPFs equal to or greater than 15 that also have good to excellent water and sweat resistance. Ideally, all sunscreens should be reapplied after prolonged swimming or heavy sweating. Only one sunscreen (UVA Guard) protects against the entire UVB and UVA spectra.

TABLE 1. **Partial List of Combination Sunscreens with Sun Protection Factor Equal to or Greater than 15 That Have Good-to-Excellent Substantivity**

Brand Name Sunscreens (SPF)	Active Ingredients
Total Eclipse lotion (15)	Benzophenones, PABA, 2-phenylbenzamidazole-5 sulfonic acid
PreSun (15)	Benzophenones, PABA
Sundown (15) (waterproof sunblock)	Benzophenones, cinnamates, salicylates, titanium dioxide
Banana Boat (15) (sunblock)	Benzophenones, cinnamates, salicylates
Almay lotion (15) (waterproof)	Benzophenones, cinnamates, salicylates
Bain de Soleil (15) (waterproof sunblock)	Benzophenones, cinnamates, octocrylene, titanium dioxide
Ti-Screen lotion (16)	Titanium dioxide
Shade UVAGuard (15)	Parsol

Abbreviations: SPF = sun protection factor; PABA = para-aminobenzoic acid.

Special protective wear for children and adults is now available with an SPF of 15 (Solumbra, Frog-Wear). These clothes are made of synthetic, lightweight, breathable fabric available in many forms including pants, shorts, T-shirts, sweatshirts, and accessories. Children younger than 6 months of age should not be directly exposed to sunlight for more than short periods. Children 6 months of age and older should be trained to use, during the summer months, sunscreens with an SPF of at least 15 or special clothing as mentioned above.

Postinflammatory Hyperpigmentation

Etiology

A variety of inflammatory conditions and infections (Table 2) cause hyperpigmentation of the skin, usually called "postinflammatory hyperpigmentation." The dyschromia follows the pattern and distribution of the original disease, but its intensity is not necessarily related to the degree of the previous inflammation. Postinflammatory hyperpigmentation is common and rather persistent in darkly pigmented people. It is caused by stimulation of melanocytes to produce excessive amounts of melanin. If the melanin remains in the epidermis, the color of the skin appears to be deep tan to dark brown. Often the inflammation is associated with disruption of the dermal-epidermal barrier. Melanin is then deposited

TABLE 2. **Some Common Causes of Postinflammatory Hyperpigmentation**

Exanthems	Acne
Drug eruptions	Tinea versicolor
Lichen planus	Cutaneous lupus
Atopic dermatitis	Psoriasis
Trauma, burns	Lichen simplex chronicus
Herpes zoster	Pityriasis rosea
Ashy dermatosis	Fixed drug eruption

in the upper dermis. When brown melanin is located in the dermis, its color appears to be slate gray or bluish.

Treatment

Epidermal forms of hyperpigmentation may respond to treatment with bleaching agents. Dermal hyperpigmentation does not respond to any medical treatment and usually is permanent. Modern lasers such as the neodymium:yttrium-aluminum-garnet (Nd:Yag) laser can remove dermal pigment. It is important, therefore, to determine whether the pigmentation has mainly an epidermal or a dermal component. Examination of the patient with a Wood lamp (black light) in a totally dark room can facilitate this evaluation. Epidermal melanin turns almost black when viewed with the Wood's lamp. In contrast, dermal pigmentation, when observed with a Wood lamp, is not visible to the examiner, and the blemishes on the patient's skin disappear.

There are several topical therapies for hyperpigmentation (Table 3). Prevention of further hyperpigmentation is paramount. Optimal management of the primary skin problem is essential.

Melasma

Etiology

Melasma (mask of pregnancy) is a common patchy, irregular, tan to brown pigmentation that is usually located on the face of women. It occurs in women who are taking oral contraceptives or who are pregnant. It usually fades slowly after the termination of either event and is exacerbated by exposure to sunlight. It also occurs in women who are not taking birth control pills or whose last pregnancy occurred many years earlier. Occasionally, it occurs in men. Melasma is caused by increased epidermal melanization, although in some patients there is a moderate amount of dermal pigment as well. In these latter

TABLE 3. **Some Bleaching Agents for Hyperpigmentation (Applied Two or Three Times Daily)**

Over-the-counter preparations
  Eldopaque cream with opaque base (2% hydroquinone + sunblock)
  Eldoquin (2% hydroquinone)
  Esotérica cream (2% hydroquinone)
  Artra (2% hydroquinone + sunscreen)
  Ambi cream (2% hydroquinone)
Prescription preparations
  Eldopaque-Forte with opaque base (4% hydroquinone + sunblock)
  Solaquin Forte (4% hydroquinone + sunscreen)
  Melanex solution (3% hydroquinone)
Combination of medications
  Hydroquinone 4% and salicylic acid 2% cream
  Hydroquinone 2 or 4%, hydrocortisone 2%, and tretinoin cream 0.05% applied sequentially
  Hydroquinone 4%, tretinoin 0.1%, and dexamethasone 0.1% applied sequentially

individuals, treatment can never return the skin entirely to its normal appearance.

Treatment

The epidermal hyperpigmentation of melasma may be significantly attenuated by daily application of tretinoin (Retin A) 0.1% cream and 4% hydroquinone preparation on the affected areas. Tretinoin is a vitamin A derivative that may cause considerable irritation if applied excessively or on moist skin. A "pea" size amount is adequate for the entire face.

Freckles (Ephelides)

Freckles first appear in childhood in individuals who have fair complexions and who are genetically of Celtic or northern European ancestry. Freckles fade in the winter and become more prominent after exposure to sunlight. Middle-aged and older adults usually lose some or all of their freckles.

Solar Lentigines

Solar or senile lentigines are dark brown macules, usually 1 to 3 mm in diameter, that occur on the chronically sun-exposed surfaces of elderly individuals, especially on the dorsum of the hands or on the face. They are commonly misnamed as "liver spots." In contrast to freckles and melasma, they do not fade in the winter but persist throughout the calendar year. They must be distinguished from lentigo maligna or seborrheic keratoses.

Treatment

Patients with these sun-induced pigmentary disorders must avoid further exposure to sunlight. Sunscreens or sunblocks help to prevent further pigmentary abnormalities.

Various bleaching medications are available, either as single agents or in combinations (see Table 3). There is considerable individual variation in the response to treatment, but most patients respond to one of the combination preparations. Most bleaching medications must be applied conscientiously, often for 6 to 12 months, to achieve optimal results.

Hydroquinone suppresses pigmentation, probably by blocking the activity of tyrosinase, the enzyme that is primarily involved in melanin synthesis. Side effects from hydroquinone are rare but include mild skin irritation. At higher concentrations, colloid milia, dermal pigmentation, or both have been reported. The addition of a low-potency, nonfluorinated corticosteroid cream increases the effectiveness of the hydroquinone and possibly reduces the frequency of skin irritation. Caution must be exercised when prescribing corticosteroids for prolonged periods.

On the face, steroids can cause telangectasia, atrophy, or acneiform lesions. The more potent fluorinated corticosteroids should not be used on the face except under special circumstances. On the arms and trunk, potent topical steroids can cause striae. These are irreversible. Tretinoin cream can also be used in conjunction with hydroquinone and/or mild (Class IV) corticosteroids to decrease epidermal hyperpigmentation. There has been a great deal of interest in the use of tretinoin alone to remove pigmentation associated specifically with photoaging. Tretinoin can be very irritating to the skin and can cause erythema, desquamation, and soreness. To minimize the side effects, the following approach is suggested. Therapy should be initiated with 0.025 or 0.05% tretinoin applied at bedtime twice weekly for 1 month, three times weekly for the second month, followed by nightly applications. Thereafter the concentration of the cream can be increased to 0.1% as tolerated by the patient.

Monobenzyl ether of hydroquinone (monobenzone) (Benoquin) should never be used to treat disorders of hyperpigmentation. It is always contraindicated because in some individuals it causes destruction of melanocytes and leaves permanent disfiguring white spots. It is used only for complete depigmentation of patients with extensive vitiligo.

There are methods for treating localized pigmented spots like freckles or solar lentigines. Gentle freezing with liquid nitrogen can decrease the amount of color. Melanocytes are particularly susceptible to destruction by this treatment. One must avoid causing necrosis of the skin or blistering. Dark-skinned patients should not have lesions frozen except in special circumstances because of the risk of permanent depigmentation.

Laser therapy is another modality effective in removing freckles and solar lentigines. The physician should be well acquainted with and thoroughly trained in the use of lasers to avoid undesirable complications. Such complications include darkening of the treated areas, hypopigmentation, and infections. Several different types of lasers are now available. Side effects include the high price of the treatment and a stinglike sensation for each laser pulse applied.

Systemic Causes of Hyperpigmentation

Etiology

Generalized hyperpigmentation is associated with many systemic disorders. Usually the color is due to melanin; for example, in Addison's disease. Metabolic, nutritional, or endocrine disorders should be considered in patients with widespread or diffuse hyperpigmentation. Generalized hyperpigmentation can also be caused by drugs or heavy metals. A partial list of these disorders and drugs is given in Table 4.

Minocycline (Minocin) is often given for the treatment of acne in dosages ranging from 50 to 100 mg twice daily. There is an increased risk of developing bluish hyperpigmentation of pre-existing scars, gingiva, or sun-exposed skin on the tibial surfaces in patients who have been taking the drug for a prolonged period of time. This hyperpigmentation is usually but not always reversible.

TABLE 4. **Some Systemic Causes of Hyperpigmentation**

Metabolic Conditions	Drugs and Heavy Metals
Hemochromatosis	Mercury
Porphyria cutanea tarda	Silver
Addison's disease	Arsenic
Vitamin B_{12} deficiency	Gold
Pellagra	Antimalarial agents
Scleroderma	Minocycline
Acanthosis nigricans	Phenothiazines
Pregnancy	Carotinemia

Treatment

Treatment of hyperpigmentation caused by systemic disorders is directed at correcting the underlying disease or discontinuing the medication.

HYPOPIGMENTATION

Vitiligo

Etiology

Vitiligo is a common acquired depigmenting disorder that occurs in about 1% of the general population. It is characterized by white (depigmented) patches on the skin. Only about 5% of affected individuals have a positive (primary family) history of vitiligo. About 15% of patients with vitiligo have thyroid disease, and 5% have diabetes mellitus. These prevalence rates are similar to those of the population at large. Rarely the patient with vitiligo has Addison's disease, pernicious anemia, or other endocrine disorders.

There are two types of vitiligo. In the generalized form, the white patches are spread symmetrically over the body. In the second form, segmental vitiligo, the patches are limited to localized areas (e.g., one-half of the face, an entire arm, or one leg). Segmental vitiligo usually does not follow dermatomes. In either type of vitiligo, the white patches generally appear spontaneously without a pre-existing rash. The depigmented areas are completely devoid of epidermal melanin and melanocytes. The cause of vitiligo is not known. Although it is commonly assumed to be an autoimmune disease, depigmentary disorders in several animal models that resemble human vitiligo suggest that the disorder may have several causes, including a biochemical basis.

Treatment

The physician should be aware of the strong psychosocial impact that vitiligo has on the patient and should be prepared to provide reassurance, explanation, and appropriate referral to support groups, consultants, or psychiatrists as needed. For most people, vitiligo is a devastating disfigurement.

For certain individuals, the use of cosmetics or stains to conceal the more apparent vitiligo is all that is desired. Cabot, Covermark, Dermablend, and Clinique Continuous Coverage are several opaque-type makeups that some patients find helpful. Vitadye and Dy-O-Derm are quick tan preparations. Both are stains that contain dihydroxyacetone. They are less acceptable because they tint the skin an orange-brown hue. Patients may need assistance from trained personnel in developing the skill to apply cosmetics or dyes.

Judicious use of broad-spectrum sunscreens is recommended for three reasons. First, the areas of vitiligo burn more easily when exposed to sunlight. Second, injury like sunburn extends the depigmentation, a process called "isomorphic response." Third, exposure to sunlight induces darkening of the surrounding normal-appearing skin and causes accentuation of the cosmetic disfigurement.

Repigmentation requires regrowth of melanocytes into the white epidermis. Unfortunately melanocytes do not migrate more than a few millimeters from the edge of the lesion. Thus successful repigmentation requires the presence of hair bulbs from which melanocytes can be stimulated to migrate into the surrounding white skin. Skin on the dorsa of the hands or distal to the ankles cannot repigment because this skin lacks a sufficient number of hair bulbs.

The most effective treatment for vitiligo is photochemotherapy. It requires a motivated patient who is committed to prolonged therapy. It is intended for patients older than 10 years of age who are neither pregnant nor lactating. There must be no history of a photosensitivity disorder. If a collagen vascular disorder is suspected, an antinuclear antibody level and other evaluations should be obtained before photochemotherapy is started. Psoralens (Oxsoralen-Ultra, Trisoralen) are potent photosensitizers in combination with UVA (PUVA). PUVA therapy for vitiligo takes 6 to 24 months and must be given optimally (i.e., three times a week at correct dosages). The patient must be given careful instructions in the proper use of protective glasses that block out UVA to prevent damage to the retina and lens. Physicians prescribing PUVA should have special training in the correct use of this medication.

Topical PUVA is intended for treatment of limited areas of vitiligo. Skin treated with a topical psoralen is extremely sensitive to sunlight and UVA. Even inadvertent exposure of the treated skin to sunlight through car windows for a few minutes can cause painful second-degree burns. Topical psoralen should be used only by physicians thoroughly acquainted with its safe use.

Topical steroid creams like hydrocortisone 2.5% or desonide (DesOwen) 0.05% applied only once daily often are successful for treating vitiligo. The medication must be applied for 6 to 12 months. The patient should be observed carefully to prevent damage to the skin from the steroids. Caution must be used when applying steroids around the eyes. Patients with vitiligo probably should have a baseline eye examination that is repeated yearly if they are receiving PUVA or applying steroids near the eyes.

For patients with extensive vitiligo (more than 50%), careful consideration should be given to total depigmentation of the remaining pigmented skin. This is accomplished by the application of 20% monobenzyl ether of hydroquinone (monobenzone) twice daily. The medication is applied until depigmentation is complete. This medication causes irreversible destruction of melanocytes. This procedure should be done only after the patient gives informed consent. Patients need to understand that the depigmentation is permanent and makes them ineligible for repigmentation. They will always be sensitive to sunlight. However, the cosmetic result is outstanding. The physician should be thoroughly acquainted with uses of this drug.

Postinflammatory Hypopigmentation

Etiology

Many of the same inflammatory disorders or infections that cause postinflammatory hyperpigmentation can also cause hypopigmentation. The most common of these are eczema, atopic dermatitis, tinea versicolor, secondary syphilis, chickenpox, and psoriasis. Pityriasis alba is a mild form of dermatitis that is common in children. It is characterized by hypopigmented patches with fine scales. Although most commonly noted on the face, it can also affect the arms, thighs, or trunk.

Treatment

Unlike postinflammatory hyperpigmentation, most instances of postinflammatory hypopigmentation resolve slowly over time. Hydrocortisone 2.5% in a cream or lotion applied twice daily might accelerate repigmentation, although the response is slow.

OCCUPATIONAL DERMATOSES

method of
JAMES S. TAYLOR, M.D.
Cleveland Clinic Foundation
Cleveland, Ohio

Occupational skin disorders are the second most common cause of all reported work illnesses, despite the fact that they are almost fully preventable. No industry, whatever its size, scope, or location, is immune to their occurrence. Occupational skin diseases are produced from old chemicals in processes both old and new, new chemicals in new processes, and a wide variety of biologic, mechanical, and physical agents. The major categories of work-related skin disorders are contact dermatitis (allergic, irritant, and photosensitivity), acne and follicular eruptions, and pigmentary abnormalities. Accurate diagnosis is imperative in patients with putative occupational skin disorders. Diagnostic procedures in addition to history and physical examination include skin scrapings for fungi, viruses, parasites, and fiberglass; cul-

tures for microorganisms; skin biopsy; and tests for allergy (patch, photopatch, or prick). Physicians treating these conditions should have some knowledge of their individual state's workers' compensation regulations.

CONTACT DERMATITIS

In this category are most occupational dermatoses. They may be caused by a number of the hundreds of thousands of chemicals used in industry. About 80% of cases of contact dermatitis are produced by irritants, 20% by allergens, and a small percentage, which are often overlooked, by photosensitivity. Most affected are the hands, but any part of the body may be involved. High-risk occupations include those dealing with wet work and chemical exposure, such as food processing, homemaking, cosmetology, health care, metal working, and chemical manufacturing.

Treatment of Acute Contact Dermatitis

1. Avoid contact with the offending agent. This may require several days away from work or temporary transfer to another job.

2. Avoid contact with potential aggravating factors such as excessive soap and water, alcohol, thimerosal, and sensitizers, such as topically applied antihistamines, antibiotics (neomycin or nitrofurazone), and anesthetics ("caine" preparations). Other contributing factors to be avoided are heat, friction, and radiant energy.

3. Apply cool, wet compresses to weeping and blistered areas for 15 minutes, two to three times daily. Isotonic saline solution may be used. With commercial preparations of Burow's solution (Bluboro powder or Domeboro powder or tablets), 1 packet or tablet per 500 mL (pint) of water makes approximately a 1:40 dilution. Make certain the mixture is completely dissolved before it is applied. A soft cloth such as Kerlix gauze; an old, clean, thin white handkerchief; or a towel is immersed in the solution. The cloth is wrung slightly and applied to the affected area of the skin. When the cloth begins to dry, remove it completely and resoak it in the solution before reapplying. Do not pour the solution directly on the dressing; a fresh solution should be prepared before each treatment.

As an alternative, the patient may soak the affected part, such as a hand or a foot, directly in the solution for the same period of time.

For severe, generalized involvement, especially with secondary infection, hospitalization may be necessary. Compresses may be applied to all affected areas of the body, and in some cases, baths with use of an agent such as Aveeno Oilated Bath may be preferable.

Treatment should be continued for no more than a few days (usually 3 to 4) to avoid excessive drying of the skin.

4. Immediately following the compresses, soaks, or baths, apply a topical corticosteroid spray (triamcino-

lone acetonide [Kenalog] spray or betamethasone dipropionate [Diprosone] aerosol). A 2- or 3-second spray to each affected area is sufficient with the container held at a distance of 6 inches from the skin. One of the many topical corticosteroid creams such as betamethasone valerate (Valisone), triamcinolone, or fluocinolone acetonide (Synalar) may be used when the acute dermatitis is not extensively vesicular. Avoid ointments in the acute stages.

5. Do not apply fluorinated topical corticosteroids to the face for more than 2 weeks; prolonged use may produce severe steroid rosacea.

6. Oral antihistamines such as cyproheptadine (Periactin), hydroxyzine (Atarax), or diphenhydramine (Benadryl) help relieve itching. It is imperative that persons be warned not to drive or operate dangerous machinery while taking these antihistamines.

7. Systemic use of corticosteroids is indicated in patients with severe, localized dermatitis, such as a vesiculobullous eruption of the hands or feet, or with severe, generalized dermatitis. An injection of 1 mL of triamcinolone acetonide suspension (Kenalog-40 injection) may be given, or oral corticosteroids such as prednisone (Deltasone), 30 to 60 mg daily in two or three divided doses, are begun initially and tapered over 10 to 30 days.

Treatment of Subacute and Chronic Contact Dermatitis

1. Avoid the same elements as outlined in items 1, 2, and 5 in the previous section.

2. Do not use compresses or soak.

3. Use a topical corticosteroid cream or ointment two to three times daily and continue treatment for 2 to 3 weeks after the skin appears normal.

4. Administer oral antihistamines as in item 6 in the previous section.

5. The author wishes to emphasize that frequently recurring cases of acute contact dermatitis should be considered chronic, and frequent use (more than once every 3 months) of short courses of systemic corticosteroids should be avoided. In these patients, a tireless search for precipitating and aggravating factors is necessary (see "Ancillary Measures for Diagnosis and Treatment" later).

Treatment of Secondarily Infected Contact Dermatitis

In the author's experience, this is a rare condition. A low-grade bacterial infection such as that from a coagulase-positive *Staphylococcus* may occur. In patients with this condition, compresses or soaks with povidone-iodine (Betadine solution) are helpful. Bacterial cultures should be made, and antibiotic therapy such as erythromycin stearate (Erythrocin), 250 mg three to four times daily for 10 days, is initiated. As the infection resolves, topical corticosteroid therapy may be reinstituted. Acute cellulitis with accompanying chills, fever, and lymphangitis requires more aggressive and closely supervised antibiotic therapy; hospitalization may be necessary.

ANCILLARY MEASURES FOR DIAGNOSIS AND TREATMENT

Resources to Identify Causative Agent(s)

It is imperative that the causative agent(s) be identified in every patient. Unless this is accomplished, treatment may be doomed to failure and the patient will experience recurrences of the dermatosis. A careful job description and work history should be obtained to determine all the patient's past and present industrial contacts. Inquiry into exposures from second jobs, hobbies, and household contacts is essential, as is the presence of predisposing factors such as atopy, prior skin disease, or use of harsh cleansers or solvents to clean the skin. In this regard, the author has found it most helpful to consult standard texts on occupational and contact dermatitis. In addition, two other resources are helpful:

1. Division of Technical Services, National Institute for Occupational Safety and Health, United States Public Health Service, 4676 Columbia Parkway, Cincinnati, OH, 45226, AC, 800-356-4674.

2. The patient's employer (with the consent of the patient), such as the plant manager, the industrial research department, the plant physician, the nurse, the safety officer, the industrial hygienist, the toxicologist, or the personnel manager.

Together, these resources may provide lists of chemicals contacted in various occupations (material safety data sheets should be requested), information on cutaneous and systemic toxicity of chemicals, suggested patch-testing concentrations, and information on sources of products and processes containing a particular chemical. Knowledge of chemicals used is extremely important, because a worker may be exposed to the same chemical at home and at work (e.g., rubber, metal, chromates, dyes, plastic resins), or at several sources at work.

Diagnostic Patch Testing

Patch testing, when properly performed and correctly interpreted, is unquestionably of great value in identifying the causative agent(s) of allergic contact dermatitis. Initial testing is usually conducted with the most frequent contact allergens (nickel, chromates, rubber, medicaments, preservatives, dyes, and resins). Other materials found at home or work may also have to be tested *in appropriate concentrations* to distinguish occupational and nonoccupational factors. Patch testing should be employed only by physicians experienced with this technique. Pre-employment patch testing generally should be avoided. The same recommendations and precautions apply to photopatch testing, which is used to diagnose photoallergic contact dermatitis.

Preventive Measures

It is impossible to separate treatment from prevention. Personal protective measures such as gloves, masks, and clothing may be required when they can be worn safely. Barrier or protective creams should be used only as a last resort and should not be applied to inflamed skin. Environmental controls such as good housekeeping, local exhaust ventilation, process isolation, engineering controls, and removal of physical and chemical hazards are the most important preventive measures.

FIBERGLASS DERMATITIS

This special form of pruritic papular, eczematous, and occasionally, purpuric dermatitis is produced by mechanical irritation from glass fibers. Body folds and areas touched by tight-fitting clothing are common sites of involvement. Hardening usually occurs after several weeks of exposure.

Treatment

1. Limit further exposure to fiberglass by environmental control.
2. Wear loose-fitting clothing, which is changed daily.
3. Clean skin frequently.
4. Use topical corticosteroid creams (see "Contact Dermatitis" earlier).
5. Lightly apply a thin coating of talcum powder.
6. Workers with dermographism or urticaria should not work with fiberglass.

OIL ACNE

Today most cutting fluids are synthetic or semisynthetic types that typically cause contact dermatitis (for treatment, see "Contact Dermatitis" earlier). However, exposure to insoluble, straight cutting fluids may produce folliculitis (so-called oil boils) in areas uncommon for acne vulgaris, usually on the extremities.

Treatment

1. Avoid contact with oils and grease.
2. Change work clothing daily.
3. Cleanse the skin frequently with soap and water.
4. Avoid cleansing the skin with fabric waste, which is intended only for cleaning machines and tools.
5. Use local acne medications (benzoyl peroxide 5% gel [Panoxyl 5] or tretinoin cream 0.025% to 0.1% [Retin-A]).
6. Bacterial culture and appropriate oral antibiotics (e.g., tetracycline, 250 mg four times daily, or minocycline, 100 mg two times daily) are indicated in severe cases.

CHLORACNE

This extremely refractory form of industrial acne is produced by exposure to various polyhalogenated aromatic compounds, such as naphthalenes, biphenyls, dibenzofurans, and phenol and aniline herbicide intermediates.

Treatment

1. Chemical exposure should be absolutely avoided through a totally enclosed manufacturing process.
2. Possible systemic toxicity should be appraised, including liver, kidney, neurologic, and porphyrin studies.
3. Work clothing should be laundered at work.
4. Double locker rooms (clean and dirty) with adequate shower facilities should be provided.
5. Barrier creams should not be used.
6. Optimal control is obtained by preventing formation of the toxic chloracnegen by altering the chemical synthesis pathway.
7. Isotretinoin (Accutane), 0.5 to 1 mg/kg/day, may be indicated in severe cases for a course of up to 20 weeks. This drug should be administered only by those experienced in its use and in strict accordance with current prescribing instructions. It is a potent teratogen with other potentially significant side effects.

PIGMENTATION DISORDERS

Staining

A number of chemicals stain the skin by direct external contact. The stain usually responds to attempts at cleansing, avoidance of chemical exposure, and the passage of time.

Hyperpigmentation

Exposure to tar, pitch, and chemicals such as psoralens in combination with ultraviolet light may produce increased pigmentation of the skin. Protective clothing and sunscreens may be helpful. Hydroquinone (Eldopaque-Forte), applied twice daily for up to 3 months, may reduce the pigmentation. In resistant cases, tretinoin cream 0.025% (Retin-A), initially applied once every 3 days, increasing to once daily as tolerated for up to 3 months, may help.

Hypopigmentation

Exposure to paratertiary butyl phenol or catechol, or paratertiary amyl phenol (found in some germicidal disinfectants, oils, plastics, paints, or resins) and certain other chemicals may produce occupational leukoderma. Treatment involves avoiding chemical exposure and using dihydroxyacetone-containing stains for the skin (Vitadye, Dyo Derm). Photochemotherapy with oral psoralen (8-methoxypsoralen [Oxsoralen-Ultra]) and psoralen plus ultraviolet A light (PUVA) may occasionally be effective in the treatment of this form of leukoderma.

OTHER OCCUPATIONAL DERMATOSES

Microbial infections (sporotrichosis), granulomatous reactions (foreign bodies), ulcerations (chrome), neoplasms (tar, pitch), and repeated mechanical trauma (calluses, blisters, and vibration white finger) may occasionally occur. In addition, patients with tight-building syndrome and alleged multiple chemical sensitivity syndrome may present with nonspecific skin complaints that are difficult to evaluate. There is a wide spectrum of other occupational dermatoses, and therapy depends on their cause. The hallmarks for the successful treatment of occupational dermatoses are identifying the causative agent(s), prescribing therapy early, and preventing further exposure.

SUNBURN

method of
CHERYL F. ROSEN, M.D.
Women's College Hospital
Toronto, Ontario, Canada

Sunburn is an acute, erythematous response to sunlight exposure. The ultraviolet (UV) radiation component of sunlight produces this effect. UV radiation forms part of the spectrum of electromagnetic radiation, with wavelengths between x-rays and visible light. It has been arbitrarily divided into three portions—ultraviolet A (UVA), ultraviolet B (UVB), and ultraviolet C (UVC). Only UVA (320 to 400 nm) and UVB (290 to 320 nm) reach the earth's surface. Of the total solar radiant energy that reaches the earth, approximately 3 to 5% is UV. Stratospheric ozone completely absorbs UVC (200 to 290 nm), absorbing UVB to a lesser extent. People may be exposed to UVC from artificial sources of radiation, such as germicidal lamps. It is of note that window glass absorbs all UVB radiation, but transmits UVA.

An artificial source of UVA available in the community is found in tanning salons. People who wish to become tanned are exposed to fluorescent sources of UV, primarily UVA. The American Academy of Dermatology and the Canadian Dermatology Association have issued statements that condemn the use of artificial UVA for cosmetic purposes.

Sunburn can be painful. The affected areas of skin may feel warm and may be tender, itchy, or painful. With a sufficiently intense exposure, the skin may be edematous, and vesicles and bullae can be seen. Sunburn may be accompanied by fever, chills, and malaise.

Histology study shows vasodilatation and edema. Dyskeratotic "sunburn cells" are noted within the epidemis after UVB exposure. In the dermis there may be perivascular accumulation of neutrophils and lymphocytes, as well as endothelial damage.

Arachidonate metabolism appears to be involved in the production of sunburn. Levels of arachidonic acid and its cyclooxygenase (prostaglandin D_2, prostaglandin E_2, and 6-oxo-prostaglandin $F_{1\alpha}$) and lipooxygenase products are elevated in association with the onset of erythema. The increase in prostaglandins may be mediated by histamine released from dermal mast cells.

The dose of radiation required to cause sunburning varies from person to person, based on the constitutive level of pigmentation and other factors. The dose of UVA to produce erythema in human skin is 1000 times greater than that required for UVB-induced erythema. A minimal erythema dose (MED) can be determined for an individual. This is the amount of solar irradiation (or UVA or UVB alone) that can induce clearly visible erythema at a particular timepoint, usually 24 hours. The MED is used in sunscreen testing as the sun protection factor (SPF) measures the ratio of the MED in sunscreen-protected skin to the MED in unprotected skin. Thus, a product with an SPF of 15 would increase the dose required to induce erythema by 15 times. The average MED, the qualitative nature of the erythema, and the time course (onset of erythema, time to peak erythema, time to resolution) differ for UVB and UVA. UVB-induced erythema appears 3 to 5 hours after exposure, peaks at 12 to 24 hours, and fades by 72 hours. With UVA, the erythema peaks at 8 hours and can persist 24 to 48 hours, depending on the dose.

It is important to remember that damage to the skin can occur at doses below 1 MED. That is, the prevention of sunburn does not mean that other harmful effects of UV radiation, such as DNA damage, have not occurred.

A childhood history of painful or blistering sunburns is associated with an increased risk of melanoma. Skin that burns easily and an increased duration of sunburn erythema are associated with an increased risk of basal cell and squamous cell carcinoma.

PREVENTION AND TREATMENT

Prevention is the main approach to dealing with sunburn. Public education concerning sun avoidance, particularly between the hours of 11:00 A.M. and 2:00 P.M., is very important. Shade-seeking behavior and protective clothing are part of a program of sun protection. Sunscreens contain compounds that reflect and/or absorb UV radiation. SPF values refer primarily to UVB protection, and an SPF of 15 or greater is recommended. At the present time there is no standard for assessing the degree of UVA protection. A person must read the product label to determine whether the sunscreen contains a benzophenone, such as oxybenzone, or Parsol 1789, which are UVA absorbers. Since the use of a sunscreen prevents sunburn, people may be staying outdoors longer and thus may actually be exposed to greater amounts of UV radiation. They must be cautioned to use sunscreens appropriately; sunscreens should be used during sun exposure but should not be used to increase the length of time spent out in the sun.

Once sunburn has occurred, symptomatic treatment can be used. Cool compresses may be soothing. Topical steroids may be helpful. Aspirin and nonsteroidal anti-inflammatory agents may also be of use, along with systemic steroids for more severe sunburn.

The Nervous System

BRAIN ABSCESS

method of
BRIAN WISPELWEY, M.D., and
W. MICHAEL SCHELD, M.D.
University of Virginia School of Medicine
Charlottesville, Virginia

Brain abscess is a focal suppuration within the brain parenchyma. The incidence is estimated to be 1 in 10,000 hospital admissions, and in large autopsy series, brain abscess was reported to occur in 0.18 to 1.3% of all patients. Brain abscesses occur more commonly in males, with a median age of 30 to 45 years. The age distribution varies with etiology; abscesses secondary to otitis media have a bimodal distribution, with peaks in the pediatric age group and in persons over 40 years of age, whereas paranasal sinusitis occurs most commonly in patients aged 10 to 30 years.

PATHOGENESIS

There are four clinical settings associated with the development of a brain abscess (Table 1). Brain abscesses are located most commonly in the frontal or temporal area, followed in frequency by frontoparietal, parietal, cerebellar, and occipital. The location of a brain abscess may provide important information about the underlying predisposing factor. Brain stem abscesses or the presence of multiple abscesses most commonly indicates hematogenous dissemination from a distant site. Frontal or temporal abscesses are more commonly related to infection in the associated contiguous space.

It is postulated that brain abscess may develop from a contiguous site either by direct extension through adjacent osteitis or osteomyelitis or via retrograde thrombophlebitis of the diploic or emissary veins. In otogenic infections, spread may also occur through existing channels such as the internal auditory canal or the vestibular or cochlear aqueducts. However, these proposed mechanisms do not entirely explain the pathogenesis of brain abscess, including the mechanism by which organisms cross an intact dura.

Brain abscesses secondary to hematogenous dissemination have several characteristics in common: distant focus of infection (often in the chest), middle cerebral artery distribution, and location at gray-white junction. They are poorly encapsulated and are associated with high mortality.

Brain abscesses rarely occur in the setting of bacteremia if the blood-brain barrier is intact. For example, brain abscess rarely complicates infective endocarditis (9 brain abscesses in 218 cases), although this entity is defined by sustained bacteremia.

ETIOLOGY

The organisms isolated from brain abscesses are outlined in Table 2. Thirty to 60% of pyogenic abscesses are mixed infections caused by a combination of streptococci, anaerobes, and members of Enterobacteriaceae. Conversely, *Staphylococcus aureus* is frequently isolated in pure culture.

In addition to bacterial pathogens, yeasts and dimorphic fungi have been implicated as causes of a minority of brain abscesses, typically in immunocompromised patients. Protozoa and helminths should also be considered in the appropriate epidemiologic setting.

Immunocompromised patients are susceptible to a wider

TABLE 1. Clinical Settings Associated with Brain Abscess

Spread from a Contiguous Focus
Otitis media, mastoiditis—40% of all brain abscesses
Sinusitis—frontal
Dental infections (<10%)—typically with molar infections; abscesses usually frontal, but may be temporal
Meningitis—rarely complicated by brain abscess (but must be considered in neonates with *Citrobacter diversus* meningitis, 70% of whom develop brain abscess)
Hematogenous Spread from a Distant Focus
Empyema
Lung abscess
Bronchiectasis
Cystic fibrosis
Wound infections
Pelvic infections
Intra-abdominal sepsis
Trauma
Penetrating head trauma—brain abscess develops in ≈3% (more common after gunshot wounds)
Neurosurgical procedures—complicated by brain abscess in only 6 to 17 per 10,000 clean neurosurgical procedures
Cryptogenic
Asymptomatic pulmonary arteriovenous malformations
Cyanotic congenital heart disease—present in 5–10% of brain absceses and is the most common predisposing factor in some pediatric series

TABLE 2. Etiologic Organisms in Brain Abscess

Organism	Percentage of Cases
Streptococci (including *S. anginosus*)	60–70
Bacteroides and *Prevotella* spp	20–40
Enterobacteria	23–33
Staphylococcus aureus	10–15
Fungi, yeasts*	10–15
Streptococcus pneumoniae	<1
Haemophilus influenzae	<1
Protozoa, helminths† (varies geographically)	<1

Aspergillus, Mucor, Candida, cryptococci, agents of coccidioidomycoses, *Cladosporium trichoides, Pseudallescheria boydii.*
†*Entamoeba histolytica,* schistosomes, agents of paragonimiasis and cysticercosis.

array of pathogens. Patients with defects in cell-mediated immunity may develop brain abscesses with *Toxoplasma gondii, Nocardia asteroides, Cryptococcus neoformans*, mycobacteria, and *Listeria monocytogenes* in addition to the pathogens outlined previously. Neutrophil defects are associated with an increased incidence of infections due to members of Enterobacteriaceae, *Pseudomonas*, and fungi. Patients with AIDS may develop focal central nervous system (CNS) lesions due to a variety of pathogens (Table 3).

CLINICAL MANIFESTATIONS

The clinical course of patients with brain abscess varies dramatically. In approximately 75% of patients, symptoms are present for less than 2 weeks. The prominent symptoms are secondary to mass effect, not infection. Headache is the most common symptom and may be hemicranial or generalized. Varying degrees of altered mental status are present in the majority of patients.

Brain abscesses in certain locations may present with additional symptoms. For example, cerebellar abscesses are often associated with nystagmus, ataxia, vomiting, and dysmetria. Frontal lobe abscesses present with headache, drowsiness, inattention, and decline in mental function. Temporal lobe abscesses are associated with early ipsilateral headache and, if in the dominant hemisphere, aphasia. Intrasellar abscesses simulate pituitary tumors. Brain stem abscesses often present with facial weakness, headache, fever, hemiparesis, dysphagia, and vomiting.

LABORATORY

Most laboratory tests are not diagnostic for brain abscess. Lumbar puncture is contraindicated in patients with known or suspected brain abscess. Not only are cerebrospinal fluid findings nonspecific, but patients may herniate after the procedure. In one series, 41 of 140 patients deteriorated within 48 hours after lumbar puncture, and 25 died. Similar results have been reported in other studies.

Imaging studies are most useful in making a diagnosis of brain abscess. A computed tomography (CT) scan can be

TABLE 3. Etiology of Parenchymal Central Nervous System Lesions in Patients with AIDS

Toxoplasma gondii: most common focal lesion; occurs in ≈10% of all AIDS patients; >1 lesion seen on MRI with surrounding edema, mass effect, and ring enhancement; most common location is the basal ganglia; majority Toxo IgG(+)
1° CNS Lymphoma: occurs in ≈2% of AIDS patients; the lymphoma is B cell in origin; lesions are hyper- or isodense on CT, with edema, mass effect, and variable enhancement
Progressive Multifocal Leukoencephalopathy: occurs in 2–5% of AIDS patients; lesions occur at gray-white junction and adjacent white matter; on imaging, lesions are hypodense without mass effect
Less Common:
  *Cryptococcus neoformans**
  *Histoplasma capsulatum**
  *Coccidioides immitis**
  Other fungi—*Aspergillus, Candida, Mucor;* agents of syphilis*
  *Mycobacterium tuberculosis**
  Mycobacterium avium complex
  Cytomegalovirus†
  Metastatic malignancy (notably Kaposi's sarcoma)
  Acanthamoeba
  Bacterial brain abscess—*Listeria, Nocardia, Salmonella*

*More commonly presents as meningitis.
†More commonly presents as encephalitis.
Abbreviation: CNS = central nervous system.

used to evaluate all cranial structures. It can detect edema, hydrocephalus, shift, or imminent ventricular rupture. A brain abscess appears as a hypodense center with an outlying uniform ring of enhancement, surrounded by a variable hypodense region of brain edema. Contrast enhancement is essential. Although CT is very sensitive for detecting brain abscess, the findings are not specific, particularly in early disease. Magnetic resonance imaging (MRI) is rapidly becoming the diagnostic procedure of choice. It appears to be more sensitive for detecting cerebral edema and early changes associated with brain abscess. MRI is more accurate in differentiating the central necrosis of brain abscess from other fluid accumulations. Gadolinium enhancement provides additional information about brain abscess structure.

GENERAL APPROACH TO MANAGEMENT

The major distinction in treating focal CNS lesions is whether the patient has cerebritis or a brain abscess. Cerebritis is an area of low density on imaging studies surrounded by ring enhancement that does not decay on contrasted scans 60 minutes later. An encapsulated abscess is one in which there is a faint ring on unenhanced scans that is more pronounced on enhanced images and decays on delayed CT. It represents the early stages of a focal CNS infection. The difference is important, because cerebritis can be cured with antibiotics alone, without the subsequent development of an abscess.

There were 67 cases of brain abscess reportedly cured by medical therapy alone from 1975 to 1985: The initial diagnosis and resolution of the abscess were documented by CT, patients were treated with parenteral antibiotics for more than 8 weeks, and there was lack of surgical or histopathologic evidence of encapsulation. It is possible that these results actually signify successful treatment of cerebritis rather than abscess. In addition, several patients underwent diagnostic aspirations, which may bias the results toward a more favorable outcome. (A diagnostic aspiration is frequently therapeutic.)

APPROACH TO PATIENTS WITH SUSPECTED BRAIN ABSCESS

Patients who present with altered consciousness, focal CNS signs, or seizures are usually candidates for contrast-enhanced CT or MRI. In hospitals where these imaging techniques are not available, a 99mTc brain scan can be employed. Lumbar puncture is usually postponed until a space-occupying CNS lesion is excluded. If rapid clinical progression is occurring, blood cultures for bacteria and fungi may be done and empirical antimicrobial therapy begun prior to neuroimaging. In every case, management should be done in conjunction with a neurosurgeon. A probable focus in the paranasal sinus or middle ear should prompt consultation with an otolaryngologist as well. Empirical treatment depends on the presence or absence of immune suppression, particularly AIDS.

Patients with a lesion on CT or MRI consistent with bacterial brain abscess are begun on empirical antibiotic therapy, even if urgent neurosurgical intervention is indicated. The most frequently recommended regimen for adults is to begin with penicillin G 4 million U intravenously every 4 hours plus metronidazole (Flagyl), 7.5 mg per kg (often rounded out to 500 mg) every 6 hours. Chloramphenicol is less frequently utilized. Cefotaxime (Claforan) 2 grams intravenously every 4 to 6 hours is an acceptable and perhaps favored replacement for penicillin in this regimen, based on recent preliminary information. Antibiotic therapy should not preclude efforts to isolate the organism by aerobic and anaerobic culture of surgical material obtained later. Additional antibiotics may be necessary, depending on the eventual microbiology (Table 4).

Most patients require surgery as part of their management. If the patient remains stable and the abscess is accessible, aspiration (CT guided, if possible) is desirable to make a specific bacteriologic diagnosis and narrow the antimicrobial regimen. Although this delay may render cultures negative, aspiration during the cerebritis stage may be dangerous, with resultant hemorrhage. Certain poor prognostic parameters, clinical or radiographic, may necessitate earlier aspiration. If the lesion appears encapsulated by CT scan criteria, antibiotic treatment can be started and aspiration (for diagnosis and drainage) performed without delay. Subsequent management is dependent on clinical and radiographic (CT) parameters. Later neurologic deterioration or failure of the abscess to decrease in size as detected by CT scan is an indication for further surgery, often excision, if feasible. The duration of microbial therapy remains unsettled. Many authorities treat parenterally for approximately 4 to 6 weeks. Duration cannot be determined by resolution of all CT or MRI abnormalities. A cured brain abscess may continue to appear as nodular contrast enhancement on CT scans for 4 to 10 weeks—even up to 6 months—after completion of successful therapy. No empirical regimen consisting solely of oral agents is recommended, even in the later stages of therapy.

PATIENTS WITH AIDS

Patients with advanced HIV infection or AIDS and who have CNS lesions on MRI or contrast-enhanced CT consistent with toxoplasmosis are usually begun on empirical therapy with pyrimethamine (Daraprim) and sulfadiazine. Pyrimethamine is given to adults as a single loading dose of 75 to 100 mg, followed by 25 to 50 mg daily. Folinic acid 10 mg daily is given to decrease bone marrow suppression from pyrimethamine. Sulfadiazine is given 1 gram orally every 6 hours. If sulfadiazine is not available, clindamycin is an acceptable substitute (600 mg intravenously every 6 hours). Low-grade fever and a gradual onset also prompt this approach. The limitation of empirical therapy is that radiologic distinction between toxoplasmosis and other lesions is not accurate. Progressive deterioration, an atypical CT or MRI, or failure to show clinical and imaging improvement during 2 weeks of therapy generally prompts biopsy or aspiration. Some physicians also use a negative *Toxoplasma* serology to prompt early neurosurgical intervention. Patients taking trimethoprim-sulfamethoxazole prophylaxis for pneumocystosis may be at a lower risk of toxoplasmosis and are therefore more likely to have an alternative diagnosis.

OTHER IMMUNE-SUPPRESSED PATIENTS

The range of etiologic agents for brain abscess is so broad in these patients that empirical therapy has limited value. Early neurosurgical intervention is usually indicated.

CORTICOSTEROIDS

Corticosteroids may be lifesaving in certain settings, including when there is rapid neurologic deterioration associated with an increase in intracranial pressure. The role of corticosteroids in the treatment of brain abscess remains controversial. Concerns include the possibility of delayed antibiotic entry into CNS, delayed healing, and alteration in CT scan appearance as inflammation decreases.

PROGNOSIS

There are several factors associated with a poor prognosis. Characteristics such as patient age, large abscess size, and presence of metastatic lesions also influence outcome. Neurologic sequelae occur in 30 to 55% of patients, and in 17% of these, such sequelae can be incapacitating. Seizures result in a variable percentage of patients (35 to >90%).

The introduction of improved imaging studies and stereotactic guided aspiration has made a dramatic impact on the outcome in patients with brain abscesses. The current approach to diagnosis and treatment results in 0 to 24% mortality in different series.

TABLE 4. **Antimicrobial Therapy**

Antimicrobial Agent	Total Daily Dose
Cefotaxime (Claforan)	8–12 gm
Ceftazidime (Fortaz, Tazidime)	6–12 gm
Chloramphenicol	4–6 gm
Metronidazole (Flagyl)	30 mg/kg
Nafcillin (Unipen)	9–12 gm
Penicillin G	24 million U
Vancomycin	2 gm

ALZHEIMER'S DISEASE

method of
MARIO F. MENDEZ, M.D., PH.D.
University of California at Los Angeles
Los Angeles, California

Alzheimer's disease (AD) is a devastating illness and the most common cause of dementia. Although it can strike in middle-age or younger, AD is predominantly a disease of elderly people. AD affects about 5% of people over 65 years of age, and the incidence raises exponentially after age 70 years. Over 4 million Americans are currently afflicted with this disorder, and the numbers may reach 14 million by the year 2050 in proportion to the increasing mean age of the U.S. population. Moreover, AD is the fourth leading cause of death for adults, taking more than 100,000 lives annually, and costing $90 billion per year.

The definitive diagnosis of AD requires clinicopathologic correlation. The neuropathologic markers of AD are increased numbers of neurofibrillary tangles and neuritic plaques, particularly in the cerebral cortex, more than expected for the patient's age. The neurofibrillary tangles are intracellular bundles of paired filaments, including abnormally phosphorylated tau proteins. The neuritic plaques are extracellular structures containing a central amyloid core surrounded by abnormal dendrites and axons. This beta/A4 amyloid is a product of amyloid precursor protein whose gene lies on chromosome 21.

In recent years, much research has elucidated the neurobiology of AD. There are multiple deficiencies in neurotransmitter systems, especially in the cholinergic system necessary for memory. Acetylcholine is up to 85% depleted in the cortex of AD patients, and there are neurofibrillary tangles in the nucleus basalis of Meynert, the source of most of this acetylcholine. The familial risk for AD is approximately four times greater than for the general population. Most patients with strongly familial AD appear to have an unknown defect on chromosome 14, and a few AD families have mutations of the amyloid precursor protein gene on chromosome 21. Although the vast majority of AD patients do not have defects on chromosomes 14 or 21, they are often homozygous for the chromosome 19 allele for apolipoprotein-E (apoE) $_\epsilon$4. This plasma protein binds to neurofibrillary tangles and neuritic plaques and may be a significant risk factor for AD.

Other purported risk factors for AD are low education and a history of prior head trauma. Exposure to toxins such as aluminum remains unproved as a cause for AD. An infectious or inflammatory theory for AD is suggested by inflammatory changes in and around plaques. Finally, some authorities believe that everyone is susceptible to this disorder, if they live long enough, and that AD results from an accelerated rate of neuronal loss.

DIAGNOSIS OF DEMENTIA

Dementia is an acquired impairment in multiple areas of intellectual function not due to delirium. There is a compromise in three or more of these cognitive areas: memory, language, visuospatial skills, emotion or personality, executive abilities, and the manipulation of information (e.g., calculations). Alternatively, the American Psychiatric Association's *Diagnostic and Statistical Manual,* fourth edition (DSM–IV), criteria require the presence of memory loss plus an aphasia, agnosia, or apraxia, or a disturbance in executive functions. In addition, the DSM–IV criteria specify that these cognitive impairments are a clear decline from a previous level of functioning, are severe enough to interfere with social or occupational activities, and are not due to delirium.

Dementia is a syndrome with many potential causes. Among those patients with dementia, over 50% have AD, about 20% have vascular dementia, another 10% have mixed AD plus vascular dementia, and the remaining 10 to 20% have other causes (Table 1). A complete history, mental status and neurologic examinations, neuroimaging studies, and laboratory data can clarify the cause of the dementia—for example, the presence of cerebrovascular risk factors suggests vascular dementia, and the presence of movement disorders suggests neurodegenerative conditions such as Parkinson's disease or Huntington's disease. A high index of suspicion is needed for psychiatric "pseudodementias." Multiple cognitive deficits due to depression can be very difficult to distinguish from other dementias. The diagnosis of AD is possible only after all of these disorders are excluded.

Delirium, age-associated memory impairment (AAMI), and an isolated amnesia can masquerade as dementia in the elderly. Older people are highly susceptible to delirium, a condition that affects attention and the registration of new information. AAMI is a mild memory loss characterized by a retrieval difficulty that improves with recognition and cuing. This "age-appropriate" memory loss is exemplified by the scoring of the Wechsler Memory Scale—Revised; the norms for people 70 to 74 years old are up to 50% lower than for those 25 to 34 years old. The diagnosis of AAMI requires documentation of an otherwise adequate intellectual background and the absence of dementia or a causative medical or psychiatric condition. Finally, amnesia, or an inability to learn new information, is often the first symptom of a dementia syndrome, but it also occurs as an isolated manifestation of focal lesions in limbic structures.

DIAGNOSIS OF ALZHEIMER'S DISEASE

There is as yet no definitive clinical test for AD. The diagnosis of AD is based on the presence of dementia, a progressive course, and the completion of a work-up for other causes of dementia (Table 2). A minimal laboratory

TABLE 1. **Differential Diagnosis of Dementia**

Alzheimer's disease
Frontotemporal degenerations such as Pick's disease
Other neurodegenerative diseases
Hydrocephalus
Toxic-metabolic disorders
  Anoxia and hypoglycemia
  Hepatic failure and hepatocerebral degeneration
  Renal failure and dialysis dementia
  Vitamin B_{12}, thiamine, folate, niacin, and other deficiencies
  Thyroid, parathyroid, adrenal, and other endocrinopathies
  Medications, alcohol, cocaine, other recreational drugs
  Heavy metals, organophosphates, other industrial toxins
Infections such as acquired immune deficiency syndrome (AIDS), neurosyphilis, and Creutzfeldt-Jakob disease
Psychiatric disease, especially depression
Miscellaneous conditions
  Trauma
  Neoplastic
  Epilepsy-related
  Demyelinating disease
  Inherited adult-onset biochemical disorders

TABLE 2. **NINCDS–ADRDA Criteria for the Diagnosis of "Clinically Probable" Alzheimer's Disease**

1. Dementia established by clinical examination and documented by mental status scales and confirmed by neuropsychological testing.
2. Deficits in more than one cognitive area such as memory, attention, language, personality, visuospatial functions, and executive functions.
3. The cognitive deterioration is progressive.
4. The cognitive deterioration occurs in the presence of a clear sensorium, i.e., in the absence of delirium.
5. Age of onset between 40 and 90 years of age; most are older than 65 years of age.
6. Absence of systemic or other illnesses that affect the brain and that can produce dementia.

Abbreviations: NINCDS = National Institute of Neurological and Communicative Disorders and Stroke; ADRDA = Alzheimer's Disease and Related Disorders Association.

evaluation includes routine chemistries and blood counts, blood studies for vitamin B_{12} deficiency or thyroid abnormalities, syphilis serology, and a brain scan. Functional brain imaging techniques such as positron emission tomography and single-photon emission tomography are useful but not definitive, and investigators are still evaluating the sensitivity of AD patients to tropicamide eye drops and other recently proposed tests.

AD progresses through three general clinical stages to death in 8 to 12 years. The first symptom of AD is usually an inability to incorporate new knowledge despite continued ability to retain old, established memories. A second early cognitive impairment is an inability to retrieve words. Visuospatial impairment is a third early finding in AD patients and is manifested as an inability to orient themselves in their surroundings or to make drawings and other constructions. In the middle stage, early memory and word-finding difficulty are replaced by prominent amnesia, aphasia, and apraxia. The aphasia is a transcortical sensory one with comprehension difficulty and empty speech but with relatively preserved repetition. In the last stage, patients are "globally" demented, emaciated, and susceptible to the intercurrent illnesses that bring death.

In addition to cognitive deficits, behavioral disturbances cause great distress and are the most frequent reason for the hospitalization of AD patients. AD patients are predisposed to agitation, aggressive behaviors, hallucinations, and delusions. They may incorrectly feel that people are stealing from them (the delusion of theft), that a deceased relative continues to interact with them, that an intruder is living in their home (phantom boarder syndrome), or that their caregiver or guardian is an impostor or has been replaced by a malevolent double (Capgras syndrome). Many AD patients are depressed, but this depression can go undetected if it is masked by cognitive impairments or other behavioral difficulties.

TREATMENT

Treatable aspects of AD include the functional aspects, cognitive impairment, behavioral disturbances, and caregiver needs. Foremost, it is necessary to determine whether the patient has an adequate support structure. AD is a process of gradual, progressive loss of abilities, and family members, caregivers, or guardians must be available to compensate for the patient's losses as they occur—for example, activities of daily living (e.g., driving, buying groceries, preparing meals, doing laundry, and basic functions such as walking safely and maintaining personal hygiene) are progressively impaired. Clinicians also need to determine the safety and adequacy of the patient's home situation. When patients cannot safely be left alone in their homes, they may need to be transferred to more supervised environments. Eventually, many AD patients require complete care in nursing homes or other institutions.

Drug Treatment of Cognitive Symptoms

Although there is no curative medication for AD, drug therapy can provide transient improvement of memory and other cognitive impairments. To date, only ergoloid mesylates (Hydergine) and tacrine (Cognex) have been specifically approved for the treatment of dementia. Although a recent meta-analysis of ergoloid mesylates suggests some improvement with this medication, its effects are still unclear. On the other hand, tacrine has resulted in modest improvement or a decreased rate of decline in about one-third to one-half of patients with mild-to-moderate AD. This constitutes an increase in three points on the Mini-Mental State Examination or about a 1-year stay in deterioration. The starting dose of 10 mg four times a day is gradually increased to 40 mg four times a day, or the highest dose tolerated, with weekly monitoring of liver function tests (LFTs). About one-half of patients develop elevated LFT values, usually in the mild range, and many patients complain of nausea, vomiting, diarrhea, headache, myalgia, and ataxia from tacrine. Drug therapy for AD is a very active area of research, and other medications may be available in the near future (Table 3).

Drug Treatment of Behavioral Symptoms

Psychiatric medications are helpful for the delusions, agitation, and other behavioral symptoms of AD patients. The drugs discussed here are used in a trial-and-error fashion, at the lowest possible dose, in divided doses, and with routine, recommended

TABLE 3. **Investigational Drug Therapies for Alzheimer's Disease**

Acetylcholinesterase inhibitors	Cholinergic precursors
Muscarinic receptor agonists	Indirect cholinergic enhancers
Serotoninergic/other aminergic agents	Estrogens
Psychoactive drugs	Psychostimulants
Ergoloid mesylates (Hydergine)	Circulatory drugs
	Vinca alkaloids
Nootropic agents	ApoE binding to amyloid preventers
Beta-amyloid expression preventers	Calcium channel blockers
Anti-inflammatory drugs	Selegiline (Eldepryl)
Sabeluzole	Angiotensin-converting enzyme
Acetyl-L-carnitine	Nerve growth factor
Excitatory amino acids	Phosphatidylserine
GM_1 gangliosides	

monitoring for side effects in elderly patients. Potentially effective drug therapies for the delusions of AD patients include haloperidol (Haldol; 0.5 to 3 mg), molindone (Moban; 5 to 40 mg), and the newer antipsychotic agents such as clozapine (Clozaril; 12.5 to 100 mg) and risperidone (Risperdal; 0.5 to 2 mg). Agitation may respond to haloperidol,* thioridazine (Mellaril; 10 to 150 mg), propranolol (Inderal; 80 to 240 mg),* trazodone (Desyrel; 50 to 400 mg),* or carbamazepine (Tegretol; 200 to 1200 mg).* Anxiety may also respond to lorazepam (Ativan; 0.5 to 6 mg) or buspirone (BuSpar; 15 to 30 mg). Useful antidepressants include nortriptyline (Aventyl, Pamelor; 50 to 100 mg) and the selective serotonin receptor inhibitors such as fluoxetine (Prozac; 10 to 80 mg) and sertraline (Zoloft; 50 to 200 mg).

Nonpharmacologic Management

The memory difficulty may be helped with behavioral techniques. During the early stages, memory aids such as keeping a notebook and a diary are often useful. Instructions can be simplified and frequently repeated. When patients are more impaired, orienting techniques will become important. These include reminders of the day, time, and current activities and periodic reorientation to the environment and situation. A large calendar and a large digital clock are recommended.

Occasionally, external prompts such as associating colors or large signs with certain rooms in the house (e.g., the bathroom or bedroom) are helpful. It is important to maintain the patient's routine. The patient should be encouraged to use old knowledge and maintain usual activities, because these will be preserved for a long time. In some AD patients, reminiscences of past life are especially reassuring.

Behavioral strategies for the management of agitation, wandering, and delusions are possible. Agitation, suspiciousness, and noncompliance among AD patients can result from misperceptions and misinterpretations. In addition to careful explanations and clarifications for the patients, one can decrease the possibility of misperceptions by maintaining a familiar, constant, and accepting environment. Minimize unnecessary stimuli such as too frequent visitors or too much environmental noise, and encourage a regular day-night cycle. Good management for a major emotional reaction includes avoiding direct confrontation, diverting the patient's attention, and removing any precipitating factors.

Driving is a special problem in the management of patients with AD. AD patients have more accidents than comparable elderly or middle-aged individuals. Some states, such as California, require that patients who receive the diagnosis of AD be reported to the state for purposes of reevaluating their driving privileges. Recent studies, however, indicate that AD patients in the first 2 to 3 years of their disease have fewer accidents per year than young people (16 to 24 years old), and most AD patients cease driving on their own. In any case, frequent assessment with driver's tests are indicated.

Finally, the management of patients with AD also involves the care of the caregivers. They are subject to a tremendous strain, particularly after years of coping with the patient's cognitive, behavioral, functional, and psychosocial losses. Clinicians and others teach patients and caregivers about the disease, alleviate concerns or misconceptions about dementia, and inform about what the future might hold. One very good mechanism for this is through the support groups sponsored by the Alzheimer's Association. In addition, the Alzheimer's Association can provide lists of local day care, respite care, home health care, nursing homes, and other community resources. It may be necessary to determine the financial situation of the patient and family. The average long-term care of an AD patient costs $18,000 to $30,000 per year, a financial burden that can leave patients and families in an impoverished state.

INTRACEREBRAL HEMORRHAGE

method of
KAREN L. FURIE, M.D., and
EDWARD FELDMANN, M.D.
Brown University School of Medicine
Providence, Rhode Island

The treatment of intracerebral hemorrhage is contingent on the cause and location of the hematoma. The causes of nontraumatic intracerebral hemorrhage are hypertension, aneurysm, arteriovenous malformation, coagulopathy, tumor, amyloid angiopathy, sympathomimetics, and vasculitis. Medical therapy may be diagnosis-specific, as for hemorrhages due to hypertension or coagulopathies, but the principles of supportive medical care apply to hemorrhages of any cause. The role of surgery is controversial. Its efficacy depends on the location of the hematoma and the clinical status of the patient.

GENERAL MEDICAL CARE

Initial management of the patient with intracerebral hemorrhage is directed at correction of hemodynamic and ventilatory disorders. If necessary to protect the airway or maintain oxygenation, intubation should be performed by experienced personnel. This helps avoid transient elevations of intracranial pressure (ICP), which could cause herniation, or of systemic blood pressure, which could result in extension of the hemorrhage. The use of local laryngeal anesthetic has been advocated to facilitate nontraumatic tube placement. Sphygmomanometry and electrocardiography should be performed to identify hypotension, cardiac arrhythmias, or myocardial ischemia that requires immediate treatment.

Decubitus ulcers can be prevented with frequent repositioning of the patient. Sedentary patients should receive either subcutaneous heparin (5000

---

*Not FDA-approved for this indication.

units every 12 hours) or pneumatic compression boots to prevent deep vein thrombosis. Incontinent or immobile patients require either a condom or a Foley catheter.

A nasogastric tube for medications and feedings is indicated in patients who cannot protect their airway owing to dysphagia or somnolence. If there is a question of swallowing competence, the patient should not receive oral medications or feedings until a barium swallow can be obtained. Large hemorrhages with subsequent intracranial hypertension increase the risk of hypergastrinemia and stress ulcers. Although unproved, patients with intracerebral hemorrhages may benefit from prophylactic H_2 blockers, such as ranitidine (Zantac) 50 mg intravenously every 8 hours. There is no evidence that one specific H_2 blocker is superior to another in this setting.

The syndrome of inappropriate antidiuretic hormone secretion (SIADH) is a common complication of intracerebral hemorrhage. Patients should have serum sodium checked daily in the acute period. Fluid intake and output should be carefully recorded. SIADH can be managed with fluid restriction as an initial measure. If the sodium fails to correct, demeclocycline (Declomycin), 150 mg by mouth four times a day, can be initiated.

HYPERTENSION

Hypertension is reportedly associated with up to 90% of intracerebral hemorrhages. Proper blood pressure management is crucial in the care of patients with intracerebral hemorrhage, since there are risks associated with either overly aggressive or inadequate therapy.

An "ischemic penumbra" is viable brain tissue adjacent to an area of injury that is threatened by vascular compromise and the chemical and immune responses to an infarction or hemorrhage. An intracerebral hematoma can elevate ICP, thus increasing the necessary perfusion pressure. Normal cerebral vessels adapt to changes in blood pressure, P_{CO_2}, and pH, but autoregulation may be deranged in patients with atherosclerotic disease or hypertension. Since autoregulatory mechanisms are often not functioning in the ischemic tissue, perfusion of these areas becomes more sensitive to changes in systemic blood pressure. Thus, if blood pressure is lowered drastically, the threatened areas may progress to infarction. Conversely, uncontrolled hypertension after an initial intracerebral hemorrhage can lead to rebleeding.

It is recommended that for elevated blood pressure, such as systolic pressure over 195 mm Hg or diastolic pressure greater than 130 mm Hg, mean arterial blood pressure should be reduced by no more than 25%. Cerebral perfusion pressure can be calculated as the difference between the mean arterial pressure and the ICP. If the ICP is being measured by an intracranial monitor, the cerebral perfusion pressure should be maintained at 50 to 60 mm Hg.

Numerous antihypertensive agents are available. Intravenous administration is preferable in most patients because of more rapid onset of action and increased bioavailability. Intravenous antihypertensive agents should be titrated to the desired mean arterial pressure measured by an intra-arterial monitor. Vasodilators such as nitroprusside, hydralazine, or verapamil are effective but not ideal because of concomitant elevations in ICP as a result of vasodilatation. There have been no trials comparing the efficacy of beta blockers, calcium channel blockers, or angiotensin-converting enzyme (ACE) inhibitors in this setting. There is a theoretical advantage to beta blockers such as labetalol or ACE inhibitors owing to the relative preservation of cerebral perfusion pressure in the face of lowered mean arterial pressure in animal models.

COAGULATION DISORDERS

Coagulopathies are responsible for approximately 10% of all intracerebral hemorrhages. Therapeutic anticoagulation is the most common coagulopathy causing intracerebral hemorrhage. Some hemorrhages are the result of a primary hematologic abnormality, such as a factor deficiency or platelet abnormality. Screening blood tests should include prothrombin and thromboplastin times, platelet count, and bleeding time. Hematologic causes of intracerebral hemorrhage with their specific treatments are presented in Table 1.

Coagulation disorders that present with intracerebral hemorrhage require rapid correction. Antiplatelet agents (aspirin, ticlopidine [Ticlid], dipyridamole [Persantine]) and anticoagulation (heparin, coumadin) should be discontinued. The effects of heparin can be reversed with protamine sulfate. Each milligram of protamine neutralizes 90 to 115 units of heparin. Protamine should be injected intravenously over 10 minutes, in doses not exceeding 50 mg. Cou-

TABLE 1. **Hematologic Causes of Intracerebral Hemorrhage and Their Treatment**

Hematologic Disorders	Treatment
Factor VII, VIII, IX, X, XIII deficiencies	Factor replacement for Factors VIII, IX; fresh-frozen plasma
Thrombocytopenia	
Thrombotic thrombocytopenic purpura	Plasma exchange, steroid therapy or splenectomy; heparin contraindicated
Idiopathic thrombocytopenic purpura	Methylprednisolone or gamma globulin; platelet transfusions
Von Willebrand's disease	Cryoprecipitate before surgery and after trauma or hemorrhage; DDAVP for quantitative deficiencies
Disseminated intravascular coagulation	Correct underlying condition; replace factors and blood products

Abbreviation: DDAVP = 1-deamino-(8-D-arginine)-vasopressin.

madin can be rapidly reversed with 2 to 4 units of fresh-frozen plasma (FFP). Vitamin K, 10 mg subcutaneously daily, will permanently reverse the effect of coumadin, but it does not correct the coagulopathy immediately. Factor deficiencies can be treated with FFP, each unit of FFP raising the clotting factor level by 2 to 3%. Platelet deficiencies can be corrected with platelet transfusions, each unit raising the platelet count by 5000 per μL. Treatment seeks to achieve a minimal platelet count of 50,000 per μL.

ELEVATED INTRACRANIAL PRESSURE

Elevated ICP is a potentially life-threatening complication of intracerebral hemorrhage. The symptoms of intracranial hypertension are decreased level of alertness, headache, diplopia, and when severe, coma. Clinical suspicion can be confirmed by a computed tomography (CT) scan of the head, which may reveal edema around the hemorrhage causing mass effect and shift, diffuse intracerebral edema, or ventriculomegaly resulting from communicating hydrocephalus.

ICP monitors allow for more precise pressure control. There are no firm indications for their placement. An assortment of devices can be used to measure ICP. Fiberoptic monitors that can be placed in the subdural space, brain parenchyma, or ventricles are the most accurate. A ventriculostomy is indicated if there is intraventricular extension of hemorrhage and hydrocephalus. This allows for ICP monitoring as well as cerebrospinal fluid drainage.

Medical management of elevated ICP includes immediate intubation and hyperventilation to a PCO_2 of 25 to 30 mm Hg, the administration of furosemide (Lasix) (0.5 mg per kg intravenously), and mannitol (Osmitrol) (1 gram per kg bolus intravenously). Isotonic fluids should be restricted to two-thirds of the routine maintenance rate. Patients with hemodynamic instability should have a Swan-Ganz catheter placed to monitor venous and arterial pressures.

SEIZURES

Seizures occur in approximately 13% of patients at onset of intracerebral hemorrhage. They can be life-threatening owing to subsequent aspiration, elevation of ICP, or hyperthermia. Phenytoin (Dilantin) is recommended in the acute setting because it can be administered intravenously with relatively little risk of cardiopulmonary collapse. Patients should be on cardiac and blood pressure monitors because of the potential for arrhythmias and hypotension, with rapid loading of phenytoin. A loading dose of 15 mg per kg should be administered as quickly as possible without exceeding the maximal rate of 50 mg per minute. If the patient continues to have seizures, additional doses of phenytoin can be administered in 300- to 500-mg increments to a total of 2 grams.

Phenobarbital is an alternative agent; it can be administered intravenously. It can be used in pa-

tients with phenytoin allergy or intolerance, or as a second drug in those who continue to have seizures after receiving a full dose of phenytoin. Phenobarbital can cause respiratory depression; therefore, patients receiving high doses should be intubated. The intravenous loading dose of phenobarbital is 10 to 20 mg per kg, infused at a maximal rate of 100 mg per minute.

Patients should be maintained on anticonvulsants throughout the acute hospitalization. The decision to continue treatment may be determined by the frequency of subsequent seizures and the electroencephalogram, but most patients will require long-term anticonvulsant therapy.

The use of prophylactic anticonvulsants after intracerebral hemorrhage is controversial. In patients with head trauma and in postcraniotomy patients, the use of prophylactic anticonvulsants reduces the incidence of acute seizures but does not affect the development of a chronic seizure disorder. Intracerebral hemorrhage patients at greater risk of seizure, such as those with lobar hemorrhages involving the cortex, may benefit from prophylactic anticonvulsant therapy acutely to prevent the complications associated with seizures. Long-term anticonvulsant treatment is not indicated.

SURGICAL MANAGEMENT

The rationale for surgical intervention is based on the belief that removing the hematoma will prevent herniation, reduce vasogenic edema, diminish ischemia caused by reduced perfusion pressure, and facilitate pathologic diagnosis.

The clinical status of the patient can be used to exclude those unlikely to benefit from surgery. Patients in coma at the time of presentation are generally deemed poor surgical candidates. The exception to this rule, however, is cerebellar hemorrhage in which the poor clinical status may be reversible with surgical decompression. One study advocated the microsurgical evacuation of caudate hemorrhages within 7 hours of the ictus if the patient was semicomatose and without evidence of brain stem compression.

The location of hemorrhage often determines whether surgical evacuation is possible. Lobar hemorrhages are superficial and therefore most accessible to aspiration. Surgical evacuation of supratentorial hemorrhages has been shown to reduce mortality but not severe neurologic morbidity. The issue of whether subcortical hemorrhages are amenable to surgery is controversial. Thalamic hemorrhages that extend into the internal capsule or subthalamus may have a better outcome with stereotactic surgery compared with the best medical therapy. Evacuation of putaminal hemorrhage in patients with clinical deterioration due to mass effect may preserve life but not functionability. Overall, there is insufficient evidence to support the routine evacuation of subcortical hemorrhages. Surgery can preserve life, but the residual deficits may be profound.

Cerebellar hemorrhages have a grave prognosis because of the risk of brain stem compression or hydrocephalus owing to obstruction of the fourth ventricle or the aqueduct. Cerebellar hemorrhages are often evacuated emergently to prevent herniation. The criteria used in deciding which cerebellar hemorrhage patients will benefit from surgery are discussed later.

Surgical evacuation may be desirable if a pathologic diagnosis is required or an identifiable source of bleeding, such as an aneurysm, arteriovenous malformation, or tumor, is detected. Nonhypertensive patients over age 65 years with lobar hemorrhage in whom cerebral amyloid angiopathy is suspected have a relatively low risk of complications from diagnostic stereotactic biopsy performed to exclude other sources of bleeding. Prior to surgery, a cerebral angiogram or magnetic resonance imaging study is usually performed to exclude an aneurysm or arteriovenous malformation.

The size of the hemorrhage may influence the decision to proceed with surgery. Large lobar hemorrhages exerting mass effect should be removed. Cerebellar hematomas over 3 cm in diameter should be surgically evacuated emergently. Smaller cerebellar hemorrhages can be managed medically unless there is neurologic deterioration, indicating a need for surgery.

The neurosurgical management of intracerebral hemorrhage has been revolutionized by stereotactic aspiration and endoscopic surgery. Utilizing CT guidance, the hematoma can be stereotactically located and aspirated with a needle inserted through a burr hole. The removal of organized clot may be facilitated by fibrinolytic instillation and mechanical aspiration. Endoscopic surgery allows fiberoptic visualization of potential bleeding sites, allowing for cautery, without having to perform a craniotomy. One study of endoscopic surgery demonstrated improved survival and neurologic recovery in patients younger than 60 years of age who underwent evacuation of lobar hematomas.

FOCAL ISCHEMIC CEREBROVASCULAR DISEASE

method of
MARC I. CHIMOWITZ, M.B., CH.B.
Emory University School of Medicine
Atlanta, Georgia

EPIDEMIOLOGY

Stroke is a major health care problem throughout the world. In 1991, approximately 500,000 patients suffered a stroke in the United States, of whom 150,000 died. This makes stroke the third leading cause of death in the United States following coronary artery disease and cancer. The annual cost of stroke due to health care expenses

and lost productivity in the United States in 1994 has been estimated at $20 billion.

Eighty percent of strokes are caused by cerebral ischemia, and 20% are caused by intracerebral hemorrhage (intraparenchymal or subarachnoid). The focus of this chapter is on the diagnosis and treatment of focal ischemic stroke.

Ischemic stroke may be caused by a variety of vascular abnormalities. Common examples of these include atherosclerotic occlusive disease of the major extracranial or intracranial arteries, embolism from a variety of cardiac sources, and lipohyalinosis or atherosclerosis of small arteries that penetrate the brain substance ("small vessel disease"). Less common causes of ischemic stroke include nonatherosclerotic vasculopathies (e.g., dissection, arteritis, fibromuscular dysplasia, moyamoya disease), migraine, antiphospholipid antibody syndrome, procoagulant states, and sickle cell disease. The cause of ischemic stroke is cryptogenic in up to 40% of patients in some series.

The major risk factors for ischemic stroke are age (the risk doubles in each successive decade after age 55), hypertension (fivefold risk), male sex (25% higher risk than in females), smoking (three- to fourfold risk), diabetes, heavy alcohol use, and hyperlipidemia (less well established than with coronary artery disease).

CLINICAL AND BRAIN IMAGING DIAGNOSIS

Patients with acute ischemic stroke should be evaluated urgently because they have a high risk of recurrent stroke and frequently develop neurologic and medical complications (e.g., cerebral edema with raised intracranial pressure, seizures, aspiration pneumonia, myocardial ischemia or arrhythmias, deep vein thrombosis, pulmonary embolism).

The goals of the diagnostic evaluation are to determine the cause of stroke so that specific therapy can be instituted to prevent recurrent stroke and to detect complications so that these can be treated. Examples of cause-specific therapies to prevent recurrent stroke are carotid endarterectomy for carotid occlusive disease and anticoagulation for cardioembolism (e.g., stroke associated with atrial fibrillation or acute myocardial infarction).

The following clinical data are useful for determining the cause of ischemic stroke: vascular risk factor profiles; the characteristics of previous transient ischemic attacks (TIAs); the onset and subsequent course of the neurologic deficit; the nature of the neurologic deficit; associated features like headache and bruits, and features of infarction on computed tomography (CT) or magnetic resonance imaging (MRI) of the brain.

Vascular Risk Factors

Stroke in the elderly is likely to be caused by atherosclerotic large artery disease, small vessel disease, or cardioembolism. Stroke in young patients is uncommon, and the cause is cryptogenic in up to 50% of these patients. African Americans have a higher prevalence of hypertension, which increases the likelihood of atherosclerotic large artery disease and small vessel disease. The location of atherosclerotic large artery disease depends on race—the extracranial internal carotid artery is typically involved in whites, whereas the carotid siphon or middle cerebral artery is the usual location in African Americans and Chinese.

Although hypertension, diabetes, smoking, and hyperlipidemia are established risk factors for large artery atherosclerotic cerebrovascular disease, they are also direct risk factors for small vessel cerebrovascular disease and indirect risk factors for cardioembolic stroke. For example, patients with one or more of these conditions are at increased risk of nonvalvular atrial fibrillation and myocardial infarction, which in turn are common causes of cardioembolic stroke. Patients with mitral stenosis, a prosthetic heart valve, or atrial fibrillation are obviously predisposed to cardioembolic stroke. However, other causes of stroke also occur more frequently in some of these patients compared with control populations. For example, the frequency of carotid stenosis with more than 50% occlusion is significantly higher in patients with nonvalvular atrial fibrillation than in age-matched patients without atrial fibrillation.

Transient Ischemic Attacks

From a clinical standpoint it is vitally important to determine the cause of TIAs because early recognition of certain vascular lesions (e.g., carotid occlusive disease) offers an opportunity for stroke prevention. Most of the major etiologic subtypes of cerebrovascular occlusive disease may cause TIAs, but the characteristics of the TIAs differ depending on the cause. About 50 to 75% of patients who have stroke because of carotid occlusive disease have preceding TIAs. These usually consist of recurrent, brief (<10 minutes) episodes of ipsilateral transient monocular blindness, contralateral hand weakness, or disturbed speech. The TIAs frequently occur over a period of weeks to months. In patients with cardioembolic stroke, TIAs rarely precede the infarction and usually last longer than 1 hour. Approximately 20% of patients who have stroke because of small vessel disease have preceding TIAs. These TIAs often occur in a flurry within 1 week of the stroke.

Temporal Profile of Neurologic Deficit

Strokes caused by large artery occlusive disease and small vessel disease frequently are present on awaking, whereas cardioembolism typically occurs during daily activities. The hallmark of an embolic mechanism (cardiac or artery to artery) is maximal neurologic deficit at onset. Approximately 80% of patients with cardioembolic stroke have a maximal deficit at onset, whereas 30 to 45% of patients with large artery disease or small vessel disease have a maximal deficit at onset. Other temporal profiles that are common with large or small vessel occlusive disease, and rarely associated with embolism, are a stuttering or stepwise course, a smoothly progressive course, or a fluctuant course.

The Nature of the Neurologic Deficit

The findings on neurologic examination are important, not only for stroke localization, but also for making inferences about the cause of stroke. Some neurologic signs enable the exclusion of certain causes of stroke from the differential diagnosis (e.g., aphasia or hemianopia essentially excludes small vessel disease), whereas other signs increase the likelihood of a specific cause of stroke. Examples of neurologic syndromes that favor specific causes of ischemic stroke are Wernicke's aphasia and top of the basilar syndromes, which favor an embolic mechanism; lateral medullary syndrome, which is invariably caused by occlusive disease of the vertebral artery; and pure motor hemiparesis and pure sensory stroke, which are usually caused by subcortical infarction caused by small vessel disease.

Associated Features like Bruits and Headaches

The presence of a carotid bruit usually implies that carotid occlusive disease is present; however, it does not necessarily imply that carotid disease is the cause of the patient's symptoms. For example, in a patient with hypertension, pure motor hemiparesis, and a small infarct in the internal capsule, the presence of a carotid bruit ipsilateral to the capsular lesion may signify the coexistence of small vessel disease and asymptomatic carotid stenosis. Indeed hypertension is the most important risk factor for both small vessel disease and carotid stenosis. On the other hand, in a patient who has been experiencing recurrent episodes of right hand weakness and numbness, the presence of a carotid bruit on the left greatly increases the likelihood that the symptoms are caused by carotid occlusive disease. The absence of a carotid bruit in a patient experiencing typical carotid territory TIAs should not argue against a diagnosis of carotid occlusive disease, since low flow through a tight stenosis may not produce a bruit. Furthermore the carotid artery may be occluded. In the latter case, a contralateral orbital bruit may be heard because of increased flow through the contralateral internal carotid artery.

Headache is a relatively common accompaniment of stroke caused by atherosclerotic large artery occlusive disease, nonatherosclerotic large artery disease (e.g., dissection), and cardioembolism but is relatively uncommon in patients with stroke caused by small vessel disease.

Features of Infarction on Computed Tomography or Magnetic Resonance Imaging

Several features of an infarct visualized on CT or MRI are useful for making inferences about the cause of stroke. These include the size, shape, and location of the infarct. Additionally, the number of infarcts is important. A subcortical lesion of 2 cm or greater rules out disease of a single penetrating artery (small vessel disease) as a possible cause, whereas a subcortical lesion of 1.5 cm or less (often termed a "lacunar infarction") is highly predictive of an occlusion of a single penetrating artery. Cardioembolism is associated with hemorrhagic infarction on CT in up to 40% of cases, which is substantially higher than the rates of hemorrhagic infarction associated with other causes of ischemic stroke. The probable explanation for the high rate of hemorrhagic infarction associated with cardioembolism is that reperfusion after spontaneous lysis of the embolus leads to bleeding from vessels injured by the preceding ischemia.

Comma-shaped lesions of 2 to 5 cm involving the internal capsule and caudate, putamen, or globus pallidus are called "striatocapsular infarcts." These lesions have also been termed "giant lacunae," an incorrect term since it suggests that the penetrating arteries are directly involved in the pathologic process. In fact, striatocapsular infarcts are usually caused by occlusive disease of, or cardioembolism to, the middle cerebral artery proximal to or at the origins of the lateral lenticulostriate arteries. Wedge-shaped cortical infarcts, particularly in the distribution of the middle cerebral artery, are usually caused by an embolic mechanism (either cardioembolism or artery-to-artery embolism), whereas irregular, patchy infarcts in the border zones between the middle cerebral artery and the anterior cerebral artery or posterior cerebral artery are typically caused by low flow from carotid occlusive disease or global hypoperfusion. Multiple cortical infarcts in different vascular territories are most suggestive of cardioembolism; however, rarer causes are diffuse atherosclerosis, coagulopathy, or vasculitis.

DIAGNOSTIC VASCULAR STUDIES

Over the last 2 decades the development of sophisticated technology such as echocardiography, carotid ultrasound, transcranial Doppler ultrasound (TCD), and magnetic resonance angiography (MRA) has enabled clinicians to determine the cause of stroke in a majority of patients. Echocardiography enables the identification of cardiac lesions predisposing to embolism. These include mitral stenosis, left ventricular aneurysm or dyskinesia, atrial or ventricular clot, valvular vegetations, myxomas, and interatrial shunts. Transesophageal echocardiography (TEE), a relatively recent innovation, is substantially more sensitive and specific for detecting left atrial appendage clot, right-to-left interatrial shunts, atrial septal aneurysms, and valvular vegetations than conventional transthoracic echocardiography. Additionally in patients with sluggish flow in the left atrium (e.g., patients with atrial fibrillation or mitral stenosis), TEE may detect left atrial spontaneous echo contrast (red cell microaggregates), which may be a precursor of thrombus.

Duplex carotid ultrasound is a useful screening test for detecting carotid occlusive disease (sensitivity, 90%; specificity, 90%). The development of TCD has enabled the measurement of blood flow velocities in all the major cerebral arteries. This technique has enabled the noninvasive detection of stenoses of the major intracranial arteries with a sensitivity of 75 to 85% and a specificity of 95%.

An exciting new development is the use of MRA for imaging the cerebral vessels noninvasively. This technique produces angiographic-like images of the cerebral arteries without the use of contrast media. This technique has a sensitivity of 90 to 95% and a specificity of 99% for detecting extracranial or intracranial occlusive lesions but is not reliable for estimating the degree of stenosis accurately. Therefore, intra-arterial angiography remains the "gold standard" for estimating the degree of stenosis of extracranial and intracranial arteries.

TREATMENT

Therapeutic options for managing patients with acute ischemic stroke are numerous, but none have been shown to be effective in prospective randomized studies. These options include the use of antiplatelet agents; anticoagulation with heparin; hemodilution; and calcium channel blockers. Newer therapies that hold promise and are currently being evaluated in controlled trials include thrombolytic agents; neuroprotective agents such as free radical scavengers and glutamate antagonists; and antibodies to leukocytes that irreversibly block the microcirculation after acute ischemic stroke.

Regardless of the choice of pharmacologic therapy for the treatment of acute stroke, the management should always include the avoidance of hypotension, hyperglycemia (avoidance of dextrose-containing intravenous fluids), hypoxemia, and infections. Elevated blood pressure should not be treated in the acute stroke setting unless the mean arterial blood pressure exceeds 130 mmHg or the systolic pressure exceeds 220 mmHg. In this setting, parenteral therapy with sodium nitroprusside or labetalol is preferred to oral therapy. Accumulating evidence suggests that patients with acute stroke have a better outcome if managed in an acute stroke unit rather than a general ward. The use of anticoagulation in the setting of acute ischemic stroke is controversial. I use intravenous heparin (maintaining the partial thromboplastin time at 1.2 to 1.5 times normal) while the diagnostic evaluation is proceeding if the suspected cause of stroke is cardioembolism or large artery occlusive disease, the patient has no contraindication to anticoagulation, the patient's deficit is minor or moderate in severity (i.e., the patient has "a lot more to lose"), and there is no evidence of hemorrhage on the CT scan of the brain. At the very least, all patients with hemiparesis should receive subcutaneous heparin for prophylaxis against deep venous thrombosis (which develops in at least one-third of these patients). If subcutaneous heparin is contraindicated, aspirin should be used in addition to alternating pressure stockings.

Most of the important achievements in the treatment of ischemic stroke over the past 2 decades have occurred because of the development of effective primary and secondary therapies for stroke prevention. The primary prevention of stroke involves the early recognition and treatment of vascular risk factors that predispose to the development of cerebrovascular disease. There are convincing data showing that the control of these risk factors, especially hypertension, has been the major factor contributing to the decline in mortality and incidence of stroke over the last 20 years.

The last 2 decades have also seen important progress in the area of secondary stroke prevention, i.e., the use of therapies such as antiplatelet agents, anticoagulants, and carotid endarterectomy to prevent stroke in patients with established cerebrovascular disease. This success, in large part, has been due to our increasing reliance on large, randomized, controlled, multicenter studies to prove the efficacy of a particular therapy. The initial trials focused on the efficacy of different antiplatelet therapies for preventing stroke in patients presenting with TIA or minor stroke. A thorough search for the cause of the qualifying TIA or stroke was not mandatory in these studies, but patients with an obvious cardioembolic source were excluded. It is likely, therefore, that patients enrolled in these early multicenter studies (performed in the late 1970s and early 1980s) had heterogeneous vascular disorders such as extracranial large artery atherosclerotic disease, intracranial large artery atherosclerotic disease, small vessel disease, inobvious cardioembolic sources, and prothrombotic states. These studies established that aspirin (1300 mg per day) was significantly more effective than placebo for lowering the risk of ischemic stroke in this heterogeneous group of patients. Subsequent studies have also indicated that low-dose aspirin (75 to 325 mg per day) is also effective for lowering the risk of stroke in patients with TIA or minor stroke; however, the debate continues as to whether low-dose aspirin is as efficacious as high-dose aspirin.

Ticlopidine hydrochloride (Ticlid), another antiplatelet agent, is also effective for lowering the risk of stroke in patients with TIA or minor stroke from noncardioembolic causes. In the only study that compared ticlopidine (250 mg bid) with aspirin (1300 mg per day), the relative risk of stroke was 21% lower in patients treated with ticlopidine. Since ticlopidine causes neutropenia or thrombocytopenia in approximately 1% of patients within 3 months of initiating therapy, it is necessary to check complete blood counts every 2 weeks for the first 3 months of therapy. If neutropenia or thrombocytopenia occur, withdrawal of ticlopidine results in normalization of the neutrophil and platelet count. Diarrhea is the most common side effect of ticlopidine, occurring in 6% of patients.

Recent stroke-prevention trials have focused on patients with specific vascular abnormalities, e.g., extracranial carotid occlusive disease or nonvalvular atrial fibrillation. Multicenter trials of patients with symptomatic carotid stenosis (i.e., patients with ocular or hemisphere TIA or minor stroke ipsilateral to carotid stenosis) have established that carotid endarterectomy and aspirin therapy (at least 325 mg daily) reduces the relative risk of ipsilateral stroke compared with aspirin therapy alone by 65% in patients with 70% or more carotid stenosis measured by angiography. These trials have also established that carotid endarterectomy is not effective for treating patients with less than 30% carotid stenosis and ipsilateral symptoms. Studies to determine whether endarterectomy and aspirin therapy is more effective than aspirin therapy alone in patients with moderate carotid stenosis (30 to 69%) and ipsilateral symptoms are ongoing.

Within the past year, the Asymptomatic Carotid Atherosclerosis Study (ACAS) has established that carotid endarterectomy, in addition to medical therapy (aspirin and aggressive management of modifiable risk factors), is also significantly more effective than medical therapy alone for the prevention of ipsilateral stroke in patients with *asymptomatic* carotid stenosis greater than 60%. In that study, Kaplan-Meier projections showed that the risk of ipsilateral stroke over 5 years was 4.8% for patients treated surgically compared with 10.6% for patients treated medically. This represents an absolute risk reduction of 5.8% over a 5-year period (or approximately 1.1% per year for 5 years). Of note, however, is that the success of the operation is dependent on surgeons performing the procedure with a perioperative morbidity and mortality of less than 3%. Since the absolute risk reduction in stroke from endarterectomy in asymptomatic patients is relatively low, the decision to recommend medical or surgical therapy in this setting remains difficult. Factors that favor a surgical approach in my opinion are high-grade stenosis ($\geq$80%), young patient (i.e., less than 65 years), ulceration associated with stenosis, and the absence of conditions that may increase surgical risk (e.g., coronary artery disease).

Over the past 5 years, several multicenter studies have evaluated the efficacy of warfarin or aspirin for stroke prevention in patients with nonvalvular atrial fibrillation. The weight of evidence from these trials suggests that patients younger than 65 with lone atrial fibrillation (i.e., patients without identifiable vascular risk factors) should be treated with aspirin alone because the risk of stroke in these patients is low ($\leq$1% per year). The most effective dose of aspirin has not been established, but most of the trials used 300 to 325 mg per day. For high-risk patients younger than 65 years (i.e., patients with a history of hypertension, diabetes, congestive heart failure, TIA, or stroke) and all patients 65 to 75 years of age, warfarin therapy (target international normalized ratio [INR] of 2.0 to 3.0) appears warranted based on the weight of the evidence. In patients older than 75 years, warfarin should probably only be used in patients at high risk of thromboembolism (i.e., those with previous TIA or stroke; left atrial spontaneous contrast or thrombus at TEE; or congestive heart failure) because of the higher risk of major hemorrhagic complications in this age group. Elderly patients without these risk factors should be treated with aspirin.

Warfarin is considered first-line therapy for stroke prevention in patients with TIA or stroke attributed to the following cardiac conditions: mitral stenosis, valvular or nonvalvular atrial fibrillation, cardiomyopathy, acute myocardial infarction, and left atrial or ventricular thrombus. The treatment of patients with TIA or minor stroke caused by atherosclerotic occlusive disease of a major intracranial artery is empirical. Therapeutic choices include antiplatelet therapy (aspirin or ticlopidine) or warfarin. A recent retrospective study suggests that warfarin may lower the risk of stroke, myocardial infarction, or vascular death by 45% in these patients. The role of angioplasty for the treatment of atherosclerotic intracranial disease is under investigation.

REHABILITATION OF THE STROKE PATIENT

method of
ELLIOT J. ROTH, M.D.
Northwestern University Medical School
Chicago, Illinois

Stroke is the most common cause of serious physical disability that requires hospitalization. The techniques applied in stroke rehabilitation programs serve as prototype practices for rehabilitation methods in the care of patients with other physical disabilities. Although stroke causes substantial impairment in its survivors, there is evidence that rehabilitation can reduce the level of stroke-related disability.

Stroke rehabilitation consists of not only a set of tasks but also a philosophy of care. The major purpose of rehabilitation is to restore the patient to maximal physical and psychosocial functioning. Because the therapeutic program involves returning as much control to the patient as possible, it is essential that the patient and family are involved in the processes of setting goals, planning treatment, and implementing clinical activities. Motivation and determination are critical because stroke rehabilitation is done *with* the patient, rather than *to* the patient.

Therapeutic exercise regimens are the most prominent components of the program, but many rehabilitation activities extend beyond the specific therapy or treatment sessions. Psychological counseling, patient and family education, social advocacy, recruiting community resources, and optimizing medical status are also considered stroke rehabilitation activities. The five major functions of stroke rehabilitation are

1. Prevention, recognition, management, and reducing the impact of co-morbid illness and intercurrent medical complications
2. Training the patient to restore maximal functional independence
3. Facilitating psychosocial coping and adaptation of the patient and family
4. Promoting the resumption of prior life roles and reintegration into home, family, recreational, vocational, and community activities; and ultimately
5. Enhancing quality of life

The ultimate goal of the rehabilitation effort is long-term, safe, independent, energy-efficient, pleasurable, and high-quality functioning in the community.

Stroke causes substantial impairments in the areas of motor control, strength, sensation, swallowing, cognition, communication, emotional control, and social functioning. The vocational and economic implications of stroke, and the impact of stroke on the family system, are enormous.

The multidimensional nature of the problems of stroke patients requires that rehabilitation care be provided by a specialized and experienced interdisciplinary team of professionals from a variety of specialties. Typical members of this team include not only the rehabilitation physician but also the rehabilitation nurse, psychologist, social worker, physical therapist, occupational therapist, speech-language therapist, vocational rehabilitation specialists, therapeutic recreation specialist, orthotist, chaplain, and others.

Not all the gains that are made during formal rehabilitation programs are the direct results of specific rehabilitation interventions. Patients can and do experience natural recovery of motor control, cognition, language, swallowing, and other areas of neurologic functioning, usually in relatively predictable stereotypic patterns. Neurologic recovery occurs by a number of mechanisms, including resolution of local harmful factors (such as reduction of local edema, resorption of local toxins, improved local circulation, and recovery of partially damaged ischemic neurons), and neuroplasticity, which is the ability of the nervous system to modify its structural and functional organization in response to injury, most likely by collateral sprouting of new synaptic connections and unmasking of previously latent functional pathways. Whereas most of the natural recovery occurs during the first 3 to 6 months, some patients demonstrate late improvement.

Rehabilitation starts on the first day. Early interventions focus on prevention of complications and initiation of activation techniques. Physical activities should begin as soon as it is medically safe for the patient to be upright. Sitting in bed or a chair is often both preventive and therapeutic. Training patients in the performance of specific functional techniques for bedside activities of daily living, such as dressing and transferring, can be initiated early. Ambulation training can be performed as soon as feasible. Education and counseling, both of which are ongoing activities, can be very effective when started early in the poststroke course. Although it is difficult to prove, there is some evidence that early activation of the poststroke patient results in improved functional outcomes. Evaluation for continuing with more formal and ongoing rehabilitation also takes place during the early stages. The decision for continuing rehabilitation is based on the specific functional, medical, and psychosocial needs of the patient.

Stroke rarely occurs in isolation; most stroke patients have many other associated medical conditions. These problems include preexisting medical illnesses that require ongoing care following stroke (such as hypertension and diabetes), secondary intercurrent poststroke complications (some of which are preventable, such as deep venous thrombosis and pneumonia), or poststroke acute exacerbations or manifestations of preexisting chronic diseases (such as angina in patients with ischemic heart disease). Other common problems include physiologic deconditioning, bladder and bowel dysfunction, falls with injuries, and painful states (especially hemiplegic shoulder pain). Management of these conditions sometimes comprises major portions of the rehabilitation effort. Some stroke patients are even more disabled by the associated co-morbid medical conditions, such as heart disease, than by the stroke itself.

Therapeutic exercise programs designed to enhance both sensorimotor functioning and the ability of the patient to perform daily activities are among the most important interventions that are used during stroke rehabilitation programs. Interventions begin with establishing proper positioning in the supine, sitting, and standing postures, performance of and training in passive and active range of motion exercises, balance training, and, ultimately, progressive resistive exercises and endurance training. The major focus of most rehabilitation programs is training patients in the performance of compensatory methods to allow them to carry out specific self-care tasks, mobility skills, and advanced or instrumental activities of daily living. The patient is taught and encouraged to make use of residual abilities to develop new ways of achieving old goals and performing routine tasks such as dressing, bathing, toileting, transferring, and walking.

Several neuromuscular facilitation exercise approaches have been developed and used in the care of stroke patients. These methods employ techniques that facilitate or inhibit motor activity in specific ways as means of enhancing motor control in patients with stroke. Relatively newer behavioral approaches have been developed recently; these include kinesthetic, positional, and electromyographic biofeedback and "forced use" exercises (see next paragraph). Biofeedback technology makes the patient consciously aware of joint position or of the presence or absence of muscle activity by using external auditory or visual representation of internal activity. The efficacy of biofeedback therapy is still under investigation, but at this time it is considered an adjunctive therapy to standard voluntary exercise techniques.

Whereas most typical therapeutic exercise programs focus on compensatory functional training as a way to assist the patient in achieving independence in the community, it is important to note that most of these activities emphasize use of residual strengths and abilities. An alternative approach has been proposed, the forced use method, that emphasizes the importance of using the weak limb and preventing or overcoming "learned nonuse." Another technique, functional electrical stimulation of muscles that lack voluntary control, may help facilitate movement or compensate for lack of voluntary muscle activity.

Assistive devices such as canes or walkers, adaptive equipment such as dressing sticks or reachers, and other durable medical equipment including wheelchairs and bathbenches assist the stroke patient in achieving maximal independence. Resting hand splints are usually used to prevent deformity and to maintain the hemiplegic wrist in a slightly extended position. Ankle-foot orthoses support the foot in a way that minimizes footdrop and facilitates an optimal gait pattern.

Training of family members and other caregivers in the performance of specific care techniques constitutes a major additional focus of the rehabilitation effort. This training includes methods to prevent complications, perform physical functions, and encourage the patient to perform any activities he or she is capable of.

Additional focused procedures are employed by the stroke rehabilitation team to manage various aspects of cognitive and communicative problems, including dysarthria, aphasia, and cognitive dysfunction. Goals of therapy are to improve the patient's ability to speak, understand, read, and write and to assist patients in developing alternative strategies that compensate for or circumvent speech and language problems that are not directly remediable. A number of specific aphasia therapy strategies have been developed. One of these, Melodic Intonation Therapy, utilizes noninjured functioning neural pathways in the nondominant hemisphere that carry musical information. Other techniques rely on encouraging verbalizations and oral reading, and encouraging any vocalizations as a step toward developing more meaningful verbal communication. Dysarthria exer-

cise methods include sensory stimulation procedures, oromotor speech muscle strengthening exercises, and retraining of articulatory patterns. Alternative forms of communication and augmentative devices may be used, especially communication boards and electronic devices.

A major factor that affects both the extent of the patient's participation in the rehabilitation program and the level of outcome that can be achieved from the program is the patient's motivation level. The amount of family support probably also affects the potential level of outcome achieved. Counseling, education, and behavioral methods are often helpful to improve psychological and social functioning. Poststroke depression occurs in between one-third and two-thirds of stroke patients, from a combination of organic and reactive causes. Treatment consists of psychotherapy, psychosocial support, milieu therapy, and medications. Sexual dysfunction is also common and is most likely related to psychological factors (e.g., fear, anxiety, depression, discomfort) rather than being organic, although spasticity, pain, and sensory deficits may pose problems for some patients. Issues related to self-esteem, affection, and relationships should be emphasized, as should specific practical suggestions on positioning, timing, and techniques.

For most patients, physical performance, functional capabilities, psychologic and social functioning, and quality of life are considerably better after rehabilitation and during long-term care than at the onset of the stroke. A substantial proportion of stroke survivors achieve independence in their ability to complete mobility (as many as 80%) and self-care tasks (as high as 70%), but social and vocational outcomes are not as favorable (approximately 70% have reduced vocational function and 60% have reduced socialization outside the home). The implications of these data are enormous. For example, most stroke patients are able to walk, but very few walk outside their home or participate in community activities. These findings indicate the need for changes in societal and community barriers to socialization and employment of the disabled.

Rehabilitation is a lifelong process. The emphasis on education, mobilization, activity, independence, coping, family involvement, and especially quality of life should be incorporated into the patient's lifestyle, even long after completion of the formal rehabilitation program.

Although there is a paucity of literature on the efficacy of stroke rehabilitation and existing experimental data have methodologic flaws, there is evidence from several studies and extensive clinical experience to indicate that directed stroke rehabilitation efforts enhance functional ability over and above the extent to which natural recovery results in improved function.

EPILEPSY IN ADOLESCENTS AND ADULTS

method of
MARCIO SOTERO, M.D.
Harvard Medical School
Boston, Massachusetts

and

MOHAMAD MIKATI, M.D.
American University of Beirut
Beirut, Lebanon

Epilepsy is a disorder defined by the occurrence of recurrent seizures (at least two) unprovoked by any known proximate insult. Seizures are characterized by episodes of central nervous system (CNS) dysfunction associated with specific electrographic discharges that result in abnormal, increased, or decreased movements and/or sensations, with or without alteration of consciousness. When the manifestations of seizures are movements, they often are rhythmic (clonic convulsions). At times, only a change in the patient's behavior is seen. In some cases, an arrest of ongoing activities is noticed, during which the person may have abnormal sensations or experience a loss of consciousness. The incidence of epilepsy in patients 10 to 19 years old ranges from 37 to 58 per 100,000 per year. The incidence in the adult population aged 20 to 39 years is 23 to 44 per 100,000; it drops to 12 to 37 per 100,000 in the age group 40 to 59. Above the age of 60 years, the incidence increases to 50 to 92 per 100,000. There are numerous causes of seizures (Table 1), but some of them may be more common in specific age groups. In many cases, an identifiable cause cannot be determined. The most common identifiable etiologic factors for seizures in the second decade of life are trauma, CNS infection, and CNS malformations (e.g., hamartomas). Seizures beginning in the third and fourth decades are usually associated with trauma, neoplasia, and, less commonly, cerebrovascular and degenerative diseases. In the fifth and sixth decades, cerebrovascular and degenerative diseases are the most frequent causes, followed by trauma. During the seventh decade and beyond, cerebrovascular disease is by far the most common cause of seizures, followed by degenerative diseases and tumors.

DIAGNOSIS

Knowledge of the disorders that could mimic seizures (Table 2), of the international classification of epileptic seizures (Table 3), and of the epileptic syndromes that

TABLE 1. **Causes of Epilepsy and Seizures in Adolescents and Adults and Potential Etiologies (or Contributing Factors)**

Vascular

Ischemic
  Obstructive cerebrovascular disease or stroke, embolic and
    thrombotic (tissue hypoxia)
  Hypoxic-ischemic (excitatory amino acid release?)
    Cardiorespiratory arrest
    Distant perinatal hypoxic-ischemic insult
    Strangulation
Intraparenchymal and superficial hemorrhages
Venous infarct (venous obstruction, usually with hemorrhage)
Microangiopathic (thrombotic thrombocytopenic) purpura
Hypertensive encephalopathy (vasodilatation/vasospasm?)
Aneurysm (mass effect, subarachnoid hemorrhage, vasospasm)
Arteriovenous malformation (ischemia and compression of the
  surrounding brain parenchyma, hemorrhage)
Cavernous angioma (hemorrhage)
Vasculitis (e.g., systemic lupus erythematosus)

Intoxication

Carbon monoxide poisoning (tissue hypoxia)
Cholinesterase inhibitors
Cocaine/amphetamine
Iron
Isoniazid (vitamin B_6 depletion)
Lead
Lithium
Nitrous oxide anesthesia
Phenytoin (high free levels)
Strychnine
Theophylline (very high levels)

Drug Withdrawal

Alcohol
Benzodiazepines
Barbiturates
Phenytoin
Meperidine

Infectious

Meningoencephalitis, abscess (parenchymal inflammation, infarct)

Infectious *Continued*

Viral (herpes simplex, enterovirus)
Bacterial
Parasites (cysticercosis, malaria, toxoplasmosis)
Fungal *(Cryptococcus)*

Head Trauma

Acute (ischemia, hemorrhage, excitatory amino acid release?)
Chronic (gliotic scar)
  Postnatal
  Perinatal

Mesial Temporal Lobe Sclerosis (Causes Simple and Complex Partial Seizures)

Neoplastic

Primary brain tumors (compression, hemorrhage)
  Glial tumors (astrocytoma, glioblastoma multiforme,
    oligodendroglioma)
  Neural tumors (ganglioglioma, neurocytoma)
  Primary central nervous system lymphoma
Metastasis

Metabolic/Endocrinologic

Hypoglycemia/hyperglycemia
Thyrotoxic states
Pyridoxine deficiency (poor intake, use of isoniazid)
Electrolyte imbalance
  Hyponatremia
  Hypocalcemia/hypomagnesemia

Degenerative

Alzheimer's dementia
Jakob-Creutzfeldt disease
Others

Idiopathic or Primary Epilepsy Syndromes

Childhood absence epilepsy persisting into adolescence/
  adulthood
Juvenile absence epilepsy
Juvenile myoclonic epilepsy
Generalized tonic-clonic seizures on awakening

TABLE 2. **Paroxysmal Events That Mimic Seizures in Adolescents and Adults**

Cardiac
    Arrhythmias, sick sinus syndrome
    Complete heart block/syncope
    Vasovagal syncope
Hyperventilation syndrome
Migraine
Movement disorders (e.g., paroxysmal choreoathetosis)
Nonepileptic seizures
    Due to conversion disorder
    Due to malingering
Nonepileptic myoclonus (brain stem related)
Non-REM parasomnias (e.g., somnambulism)
Narcolepsy
Stroke, transient ischemic attacks
Vertigo

Abbreviation: REM = rapid eye movement.

occur in adults and adolescents is essential for the proper diagnosis and management of patients with epilepsy.

Classification of Seizures

Generalized seizures have bilateral clinical and electrographic manifestations. Partial seizures have a unilateral onset that is usually focal. If a seizure has a unilateral onset and later becomes bilateral, it is called secondarily generalized. Primary generalized seizures start bilaterally. Simple partial seizures cause no impairment of consciousness, but complex partial seizures are associated with loss of awareness and lack of memory of what happened during the event.

Generalized tonic-clonic seizures (grand mal seizures), the most widely known type of generalized seizure, are characterized by bilateral tonic contractions of the upper and lower extremities, followed by rhythmic jerks of the limbs. One must be aware that bystanders and relatives frequently get to the patient and observe him or her seconds or even minutes after the seizure onset. Owing to this fact, patients with secondarily generalized partial seizures (see the discussion later) are commonly described as having "grand mal attacks" and may be erroneously labeled as having primary generalized seizures.

Tonic seizures are characterized by bilateral upper and lower extremity contractions that are sustained for a few seconds to minutes. If the patient is standing, the seizure often causes him or her to fall. These seizures usually indicate involvement of the premotor cortex either from the onset, as part of a generalized discharge, or secondary to spread of ictal activity to that region.

Atonic seizures are characterized by a sudden loss of tone, usually involving the axial muscles. If mostly the neck muscles are involved, then just a head drop is seen. When trunk and leg muscles are involved, the patient falls down and the seizure is called a "drop attack." At times, the patient may have a myoclonic jerk followed by a loss of postural tone (myoclonic-atonic seizure).

Myoclonic seizures are sudden and fast muscle contractions involving either one limb (focal myoclonus) or most of the body (massive myoclonus).

Absence seizures are generalized from the onset. They are characterized by the sudden onset of decreased responsiveness or loss of consciousness, often accompanied by rhythmic blinking with a frequency of 3 Hz. The electroencephalogram (EEG) shows a 3-Hz spike and wave discharges during the episode. These seizures are commonly referred to as typical absences or "petit mal." Many patients and their relatives refer to other types of seizures as "petit mal," but on further questioning, one usually finds that these events are, in reality, partial seizures (see the discussion later). In trying to distinguish partial seizures from absences, keep in mind that the latter are usually short (10 to 15 seconds). The former usually last longer than 1 minute and are frequently preceded by an aura and followed by postictal confusion. Atypical absences are characterized by their association with a variable degree of decreased responsiveness, usually with partially preserved awareness and with the occurrence of some tonic stiffening or loss of tone during the seizure. The EEG shows slow (1 to 2.5 Hz) spike and wave discharges during the event.

Partial seizures originating from the temporal lobe usually manifest themselves initially with an aura, which may consist of a visceral sensation, a strange smell (e.g., burning rubber), a strange taste (e.g., metallic taste), or even unprovoked fear. Stereotyped and repetitive movements of the arms or orofacial muscles, which are called automatisms, are often the next manifestation and are commonly accompanied by loss of consciousness (complex partial seizures). Experiential manifestations can also be seen in these patients, such as déjà vu (a feeling of going through a situation identical to one lived in the past) and jamais vu (a feeling of unfamiliarity with an otherwise customary situation and environment). At times, patients may go on

TABLE 3. **International Classification of Epileptic Seizures**

Partial (Focal, Local) Seizures

Simple partial seizures (consciousness not impaired)
    With motor symptoms
    With somatosensory symptoms
    With autonomic symptoms
    With psychic symptoms
Complex partial seizures (with impairment of consciousness)
    Beginning as simple partial seizures and progressing to
        impairment of consciousness:
        With no other features
        With automatisms
    With impairment of consciousness at onset:
        With no other features
        With features as seen in simple partial seizures (see above)
        With automatisms
Partial seizures evolving to secondarily generalized seizures
    Simple partial seizures evolving to generalized seizures
    Complex partial seizures evolving to generalized seizures
    Simple partial seizures evolving to complex partial seizures
        then to generalized seizures

Generalized Seizures

Absence seizures (typical or atypical)
Tonic seizures
Atonic seizures (astatic seizures)
Clonic seizures
Tonic-clonic seizures
Myoclonic seizures

Unclassified Seizures

This category includes seizures that cannot be classified in the above groups owing to lack of complete data or for any other reason. This group includes the "subtle" neonatal seizures (swimming, bicycling, and chewing movements).

Modified from the Commission on Classification and Terminology of the International League Against Epilepsy: Proposal for revised clinical and electroencephalographic classification of epileptic seizures. Epilepsia 22:489–501, 1981.

to experience a secondary generalized tonic-clonic seizure. Partial seizures of frontal lobe origin are often very peculiar. Bilateral motor manifestations are common and often occur even if the seizure discharge does not spread to the contralateral hemisphere. Bilateral arm elevation, fencing posture, and symmetrical tonic arm posturing are often seen. Bicycling movements, hyperventilation, pelvic thrusting, or sexual automatisms can also occur. This combination of manifestations, plus the fact that these patients may have bilateral motor involvement with partial or complete preservation of consciousness, can lead to the erroneous diagnosis of "pseudoseizures." Other clues for localization of partial seizures include visual hallucinations (usually unformed) in occipital lobe seizures. These often develop into complex partial seizures (similar to those described earlier) after the discharge spreads to the temporal lobe. Prominent somatosensory auras are seen in parietal lobe seizures, which tend to show a tonic component after the discharge spreads to the frontal lobe.

Pseudoseizures are conversion reactions that may be confused with seizures. The description of the clinical event often includes limb flailing, head side-to-side turning, and pelvic thrusting. Although pseudoseizures often occur in patients with epilepsy, those clinical features, the personality profile, the lack of a postictal period, and the ability to induce and stop some spells by suggestion are aids in establishing the diagnosis of pseudoseizures.

Epileptic Syndromes Commonly Seen in Adults and Adolescents

In juvenile absence epilepsy, males and females are equally affected, and the onset is usually around age 15 years (range, 10 to 40 years). The patients tend to have fewer absence seizure episodes a day than do patients with childhood absence (petit mal) epilepsy. The majority of patients also have generalized tonic-clonic (GTC) seizures. The prognosis of juvenile absence epilepsy is usually very good, even in patients with GTC seizures or myoclonic seizures. The EEG shows 3.5- to 4-Hz generalized spike and wave or polyspike and wave discharges occurring in bursts. Photosensitivity is only rarely seen. Juvenile absence epilepsy has to be distinguished from petit mal epilepsy (pyknoepilepsy), which only rarely persists into adulthood. In petit mal epilepsy, the age of onset is in childhood, and seizures are associated with 3-Hz spike wave discharges.

Juvenile myoclonic epilepsy usually starts between 12 and 18 years of age, but onset before age 10 and after age 30 can occur. Most patients have myoclonic jerks of the upper extremities and, less frequently, the lower extremities. GTC seizures are present in more than 90% of patients; they often occur upon awakening and are often preceded by myoclonic jerks. Although commonly described as GTC seizures, these are frequently clonic-tonic-clonic seizures. Absences can be seen in 10 to 20% of patients. All seizures tend to be worsened by sleep deprivation and possibly by hyperventilation. The EEG shows a typical pattern of generalized polyspike and wave discharges with a 4- to 6-Hz frequency. In patients with absences, 3- to 4-Hz spike and wave discharges are seen. Asymmetrical bursts and even focal spikes can be present. Photosensitivity is seen in about one-third of the patients in various studies; eye closure may also precipitate EEG discharges. Although most patients achieve seizure control with therapy, subsequent antiepileptic drug withdrawal is associated with a high rate of seizure relapse.

Epilepsy with GTC seizures on awakening is an epileptic syndrome with an age of onset between 10 and 25 years. Sleep deprivation and use of alcohol are common seizure precipitants in patients with this syndrome. The seizures tend to occur in the first 2 hours after waking (including daytime sleep) or later in the evening when patients are "relaxing." The EEG commonly shows generalized spike and wave discharges and photosensitivity.

In Lennox-Gastaut syndrome, patients commonly start having seizures when they are between 3 and 8 years of age, but the seizures usually persist throughout adolescence and early adulthood. Multiple seizure types are seen in this syndrome. Tonic seizures and atypical absences are the most prominent seizure types, but atonic, myoclonic, and tonic-clonic seizures are also frequently seen. The EEG usually shows slow (1 to 2.5 Hz) spike and wave discharges during the awake state and fast discharges during sleep, which sometimes coincides with the tonic seizures.

Other less common epileptic syndromes occurring in adults and adolescents include reading epilepsy and some progressive myoclonic epilepsies. Reading epilepsy is characterized by bilateral contraction of muscles involved in speech that could be either tonic or myoclonic. This clinical manifestation appears during either silent reading or reading aloud, but more promptly during the latter. Often a generalized seizure ensues if the patient tries to continue to read. Progressive myoclonic epilepsies are a rather heterogeneous group of diseases characterized by myoclonic seizures with variable degrees of intellectual and motor deterioration. These diseases may present during the second decade of life or, more rarely, beyond age 20 years. A few examples of these syndromes include Baltic myoclonus, or Unverricht-Lundborg disease (slow mental deterioration, Nordic ancestry); sialidosis type I, or cherry-red-spot-myoclonus syndrome (ataxia, cherry red spot on funduscopy, visual loss, neuropathy, sialidase deficiency); and MERRF, or myoclonic epilepsy with ragged red fibers (ataxia, hearing loss, myopathy with ragged red fibers on biopsy).

Patients with partial or secondarily generalized seizures originating from specific lobes have frontal lobe, temporal lobe, parietal lobe, or occipital lobe epilepsy. These represent the most common types of epilepsy in adults and are often caused by specific anatomic lesions (e.g., tumor, arteriovenous malformation, or mesial temporal sclerosis). In many of these patients, seizures are easily controlled with medications, but in others, the seizures become intractable, often requiring surgical resection. The prognosis of patients with the preceding syndromes also depends on the underlying etiology. Other patients, usually with GTC seizures without specific localizing findings, are encountered in daily clinical practice, and the conditions of many are difficult to classify into specific syndromes. Follow-up of such patients often clarifies the clinical picture and the epileptic syndrome.

ACUTE MANAGEMENT AND EVALUATION

The causes of seizures are many (see Table 1), so a focused evaluation is necessary to maximize the chances of finding a cause. While evaluating a patient after the first seizure, one must keep in mind the subject's age and the circumstances around the time of the seizure (e.g., accident, precipitating factor). The past medical history can yield clues, such as in patients with a cardiac valve prosthesis (embolic stroke), lung or breast carcinoma (CNS metastasis), or diabetes (hypoglycemic seizure). Individuals who ingest large quantities of alcohol on a daily basis may have withdrawal seizures due to a sudden cessation of or even reduction in alcoholic beverage consumption. This usually happens when the patient is unable to obtain alcohol, such as during hospitalization for an acute medical illness.

All patients presenting with focal seizures, meningeal signs, and fever, and some patients presenting with seizures without an apparent cause, should have a lumbar puncture to rule out meningitis or encephalitis as a cause of their seizures. In this situation, one should first rule out increased intracranial pressure (papilledema, vomiting, headaches, decreased level of consciousness, bradycardia, hypertension) to avoid inducing transtentorial herniation. When in doubt, obtain a head computed tomography scan first. Toxic metabolic conditions frequently cause seizures. The treating physician should be familiar with the "standard" toxicologic testing of the particular institution. Great variability is seen in the types of substances tested. One should not forget about electrolyte (including calcium) imbalance as a cause of seizures, mostly in patients with medical problems or in those taking medications. An electrocardiogram may be helpful by showing an increased QT_C interval or QRS duration, such as in tricyclic antidepressant intoxication (not diagnostic, but helpful in the face of known depression and seizures). Increased QT_C duration can be seen in patients with hypocalcemia and may be a more reliable indicator of free serum calcium than total serum calcium is. Neuroimaging is mandatory in patients presenting with partial seizures or secondary generalized seizures. Because the onset of a seizure may not be witnessed, a focal onset can be missed.

The treatment of status epilepticus is beyond the scope of this article, but the general guidelines for the treatment of acute seizures are summarized in Table 4. If serum glucose is low, then 20 to 50% glucose should be given intravenously. When a quick glucose assay (e.g., Dextrostix) is not available, empirical treatment with glucose is an acceptable alternative until serum glucose can be measured. Treatment with glucose may acutely precipitate thiamine deficiency in patients with low levels of that vitamin. It is therefore a good practice to give thiamine before administering glucose. Thiamine 100 mg intravenously should be given to virtually all adult patients presenting with acute seizures of unknown etiology. One should always be aware of the time elapsed from the onset of the seizure, since treatment of the patient is dictated by this time factor. Seizures that have been going on for a long time deserve more aggressive treatment. This is especially true when there is poor or no response to the initial standard treatment.

INITIATION AND MAINTENANCE OF ANTIEPILEPTIC DRUGS

Some general rules apply to the initiation and maintenance of almost all antiepileptic drugs (AEDs)

TABLE 4. **Treatment of Acute Seizures**

Preliminary Steps	
First priority—ABCs:	Ensure airway patency, breathing, circulation
	Monitor electrocardiogram, vital signs, oxygenation continuously
Start an IV line:	Draw blood for SMA-20, calcium, arterial blood gases, complete blood count, antiepileptic drug levels, and so forth
	Thiamine 100 mg IV
	50% glucose 20–50 mL IV
	Start treatment if: Seizure going on for more than 5 min
	Patient has been seizing for unknown period of time

Treatment (pay attention to the time since the onset of the seizure)

First step (5–30 min):	Diazepam (Valium) 5–20 mg IV slowly (2 mg/min) or lorazepam (Ativan)* 2–4 mg IV slowly, then phenytoin (Dilantin) 18 mg/kg up to 1000 mg IV over 30 min (do not dilute in D5W)
	Be ready to intubate the patient at any time
Second step:	Phenobarbital 3–20 mg/kg up to 700 mg IV, usually given in 200-mg increments, or midazolam (Versed)* IV drip: loading dose, 0.1–0.2 mg/kg; infusion rate, 0.1–0.2 mg/kg/h
Third step:	Pentobarbital anesthesia* (patient already intubated): loading dose, 3–7 mg/kg (may repeat 5 mg/kg); maintenance, 0.5–3.0 mg/kg/h
	Monitor EEG, keep in burst-suppression pattern with 4–6 bursts per minute
	Monitor blood pressure closely

*Not FDA-approved for this indication.
Abbreviations: SMA-20 = Sequential Multiple Analyzer-20; EEG = electroencephalogram.

(Table 5). When starting an AED, it is often advisable to increase the dose gradually so that the medication will be better tolerated. Increase the dose until the seizures are controlled (details following) or until signs of toxicity or intolerance are noted. Monotherapy is the desirable situation because of the lower chance of side effects and better compliance with one medication. A few patients, however, may require polytherapy. Anticipate possible changes in the AED serum levels every time a new drug is started. Try to gather all available information (history, examination, and complementary tests) before starting an AED. After the occurrence of a known acute insult associated with seizures, try using a nonsedating drug such as phenytoin (Dilantin) to avoid disturbing follow-up neurologic assessments. Most physicians do not start treatment until after the second unprovoked seizure, since between a third and a half of patients will have only a single seizure, even after a 5-year follow-up.

Carbamazepine (Tegretol)

Carbamazepine is useful for patients with partial and secondary generalized seizures. Although it can

TABLE 5. **Characteristics of Antiepileptic Drugs**

Drug	Elimination Half-Life	Adult Dosage (mg)	Serum Level Range (μg/mL)	Type of Seizure
Phenytoin (Dilantin)	12–24 h	300–400	10–20	GTC, PS
Carbamazepine (Tegretol)	12–24 h	600–1200	8–12	GTC, PS
Phenobarbital	2–6 days	90–150	20–40	GTC, PS
Primidone (Mysoline)	12 h	500–750	4–10	GTC, PS
Valproic acid (Depakene, Depakote)	5–15 h	1000–3000	50–100	GTC, PS, ABS, MYO
Ethosuximide (Zarontin)	30–60 h	750–2000	40–100	ABS
Methsuximide (Celontin)	30–40 h*	900–1200	20–40*	ABS, PS
Clonazepam (Klonopin)	30–40 h	1.5–5	20–80†	ABS, MYO
Gabapentin (Neurontin)	5–9 h	900–1800	—†	GTC, PS
Lamotrigine (Lamictal)	25 h	150–500	—†	GTC, PS

*Active metabolite (N-desmethyl)-2-methyl-2-phenylsuccinimide. Methsuximide is usually limited to adjunctive therapy in otherwise intractable patients.
†Serum levels are not very useful or not yet established.
Abbreviations: GTC = generalized tonic-clonic seizures; PS = partial seizures; ABS = absence seizures; MYO = myoclonic seizures.

also be efficacious against primary generalized seizures, patients with spike and wave discharges and with prior absence seizures may experience worsening of their seizures. The usual adult dosage is 600 to 1200 mg per day divided in three doses. When this drug is given orally, the bioavailability is around 80%. Peak plasma concentrations after ingestion of the tablet are achieved in 4 to 8 hours. The main metabolite is carbamazepine epoxide, which shares some of the anticonvulsant actions of the parent drug and can contribute to the occurrence of adverse events. The half-life of the drug after a single dose is 18 to 55 hours and is 12 to 24 hours after chronic use (15 days or more) owing to self-induced increased clearance. The main pathways by which the drug is biotransformed and excreted are hepatic glucuronidation and epoxidation with hydroxylation. After that, the drug is mostly (75%) excreted in the urine. About one-third of carbamazepine is bound to protein. Phenobarbital and phenytoin may decrease carbamazepine serum levels, but dextropropoxyphene, acetazolamide, desipramine, and cimetidine can increase them.

Patients often complain of being tired and drowsy in the first few weeks after the initiation of carbamazepine therapy, but this effect tends to go away with time. Initiating patients on a low dose such as 100 or 200 mg a day and increasing it slowly over 1 to 3 weeks will minimize these side effects. These symptoms plus blurred or double vision and headaches may occur intermittently as a manifestation of peak serum level effects. In this case, readjustment of the dose (e.g., giving smaller amounts of the drug more frequently) usually abolishes the problem. Carbamazepine has an antidiuretic hormone–like action that may cause significant hyponatremia, especially with concomitant use of phenobarbital or valproic acid. Comedication with phenytoin or lithium may counteract this antidiuretic effect. Nystagmus (horizontal or vertical), dry mouth, glossitis, and peripheral neuropathy may be seen occasionally. Intoxication produces dizziness, ataxia, confusion, choreiform movements, and double or blurred vision. Rashes are common (about 5% of the cases). Rarely, severe dermatologic

reactions such as Stevens-Johnson syndrome occur. Severe idiosyncratic reactions are very rare but may be fatal; they include hepatic and bone marrow failure. These hematologic problems are more common during the first 2 months of treatment and include thrombocytopenia, agranulocytosis, aplastic anemia, and pancytopenia. These severe reactions should not be confused with a mild and nonprogressive leukopenia seen in up to 10% of the patients taking this drug. Hepatic problems are more common in adults. Cardiac toxicity can be seen in patients taking carbamazepine. In older patients, bradycardia and slow atrioventricular conduction are potential problems. Children may manifest cardiac toxicity by tachycardia, especially in the presence of volatile anesthetics.

Measurement of total cell blood count and liver function tests should be done before and usually 2, 4, and 6 weeks after the initiation of therapy. Even though subsequent periodic monitoring (e.g., every 3 to 4 months) of these test results has been recommended for patients taking carbamazepine and other AEDs, the value of this monitoring has been challenged. Education of patients, parents, and spouses about new or unusual signs and symptoms may be more important than such periodic measurements. The treating physician should be notified immediately if pallor, weakness, petechiae, fever, and infection (especially sore throat) are noted during AED therapy.

Phenytoin (Dilantin)

Phenytoin can be useful against both partial (simple and complex) and generalized seizures. Tonic seizures in patients with Lennox-Gastaut syndrome may respond, at least partially, to phenytoin. Its most convenient features are that it can be given intravenously and causes relatively little sedation. These features make phenytoin the drug of choice for the treatment of patients with acute prolonged convulsions or post-traumatic seizures. When this drug is given orally, the bioavailability is around 90%. The half-life of phenytoin is dependent on the serum concentration, being longer with higher levels. The fraction bound to protein varies from 70 to 90%. Patients with hyperbilirubinemia or hypoalbuminemia and those on concurrent valproic acid therapy usually have an increased free fraction of the drug. The excretion of this drug is variable and can be saturated. Gradual increases in the dose by a fixed amount (e.g., 15% of the total dose) may cause a large increase in the serum level of the drug at some point (Figure 1). Febrile illnesses may increase the clearance of phenytoin and cause low serum levels and loss of seizure control. Occasionally, patients may tolerate and need serum levels between 20 and 25 μg per mL for proper seizure control. Free serum levels are helpful in patients taking concurrent valproic acid and in cases of liver failure. The therapeutic range of free phenytoin levels is 1.0 to 2.0 μg per mL. The usual dose for an adult is 300 to 400 mg per day. The loading dose intravenously is 18 mg per kg (up to 1000 mg), usually given over 20 minutes. *Intravenous phenytoin should never be given faster than 50 mg per minute.* Fast infusions of this drug may cause significant hypotension. This medication should not be diluted in 5% dextrose in water, since it may precipitate. The loading dose can also be divided in three and given orally every 3 or 4 hours. Phenytoin should not be given intramuscularly, since this route has been associated with crystal formation, which may cause muscle necrosis. In nonemergency situations, initiation of the maintenance dose without loading is usually acceptable.

The side effects of phenytoin include rash due to allergy (usually accompanied by eosinophilia), coarsening of facial features, hirsutism, megaloblastic anemia (folate deficiency), hepatitis, nephritis, thyroiditis, and a lupus-like syndrome. Lymph node enlargement may be seen with variable severity, ranging from asymptomatic, palpable cervical nodes to a prominent lymphoma-like syndrome. Gingival hyperplasia can also occur, although aggressive oral hygiene such as multiple daily flossing and regular visits to an oral hygienist may minimize this compli-

cation. Peripheral neuropathy may also be seen in patients who have been taking this drug for many years. Toxic levels of phenytoin (usually about 20 μg per mL) may cause nystagmus, dysarthria, ataxia, lethargy, mental changes, and paradoxic exacerbation of seizures, usually associated with total levels above 30 μg per mL. Severe reactions are rare and include Stevens-Johnson syndrome, aplastic anemia, agranulocytosis, and thrombocytopenia.

The drug interactions of phenytoin are multiple. Serum concentrations of primidone, valproic acid, carbamazepine, and ethosuximide are decreased by phenytoin. The interaction with phenobarbital is more complex and unpredictable, but usually phenytoin concentrations remain stable after phenobarbital is added. Significant increases in the serum concentration of phenytoin may be seen with the concomitant use of carbamazepine, anticoagulants (dicoumarol), cimetidine (Tagamet), disulfiram (Antabuse), and certain antibiotics (sulfonamides, chloramphenicol, isoniazid). Agents such as rifampin, alcohol, folic acid, vinblastine, and cisplatin can cause reductions in the phenytoin serum level. Phenytoin increases the biodegradation of many drugs, which may lead to a reduction in or loss of their therapeutic effect. Among these medications are anticoagulants, oral contraceptives, antiarrhythmic agents (digoxin, quinidine, disopyramide), antibiotics (chloramphenicol, rifampin, doxycycline), immune suppressants (cyclosporine and corticosteroids), and opiate analgesics. Preparations containing the acid phenytoin (Dilantin suspension and 50-mg chewable tablets [Infatabs]) contain approximately 8% more of the drug than those containing the sodium phenytoin (Dilantin 30- and 100-mg capsules). The latter capsule preparations can be given once every 24 hours.

Valproic Acid (Depakene, Depakote)

Valproic acid is useful in the treatment of both generalized and partial seizures. It is usually slightly less effective and has more side effects than carbamazepine when used for the treatment of partial seizures. Patients with absence and myoclonic seizures usually respond well to this medication. It is the drug of choice for patients who have both absence and generalized seizures and for those with juvenile myoclonic epilepsy. It has also been considered by many to be the drug of choice for myoclonic epilepsies in general. Patients with Lennox-Gastaut syndrome usually have some improvement in most of their seizure types when they use valproic acid, although permanent seizure control is rarely achieved. Valproic acid is available in a tablet form and as a liquid preparation. It has a half-life of around 15 hours. The liquid form is more quickly absorbed and excreted, which often requires dosing three or four times a day to maintain steady therapeutic serum levels. Divalproex sodium (Depakote) is another form of this medication with slower absorption, which permits dosing two or three times a day and fewer fluctuations in the serum concentrations. It is available

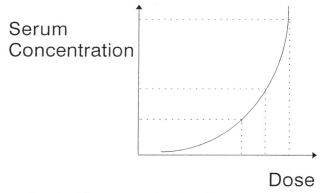

Gradual increases in the dose may at some point cause a large increase in serum concentration of phenytoin due to the saturation (=zero order) kinetics of this drug.

Figure 1. Phenytoin pharmacokinetics.

in 125-mg sprinkle capsules and 125-, 250-, and 500-mg enteric coated tablets). When this drug is given orally, the bioavailability is close to 100%. The usual range for serum levels of valproic acid varies from 50 to 100 μg per mL, and at times up to 150 μg per mL. The lower levels (50 to 70) are associated with a high proportion of protein binding (up to 90%). Conversely, higher serum levels (above 80) have been associated with lower protein binding (60 to 80%) of the drug. Some patients may require serum levels around 150 μg per mL to maintain adequate seizure control, but the incidence of side effects is higher at those concentrations, and closer monitoring of the patient is warranted. Increases in free fatty acids after meals may cause displacement of the bound fraction of the drug, with a subsequent increase in the free levels of valproic acid. This is one of the reasons for the daily fluctuations in levels of this drug. The usual adult oral dose of valproic acid is 1000 to 2000 mg per day. A main interaction of valproic acid with other AEDs occurs with the hepatic enzyme–inducing AEDs such as phenytoin, carbamazepine, and phenobarbital, causing an increase in the biodegradation of valproic acid. Thus, patients on both valproic acid and those other drugs require an increased valproic acid dosage to keep the same serum levels.

Side effects of valproic acid include tremor, nausea, hair loss, weight gain, transient elevation of serum transaminases, hyperammonemia, and low platelets. The tremor may be dose related and often improves with a lowering of the dosage. Nausea and gastrointestinal upset may improve by using the enteric coated form (Depakote). Among the more serious reactions to this drug are pancreatitis and severe hepatotoxicity (both can be fatal). Although liver failure can occur in any age group, adult patients on monotherapy are less often affected (children less than 2 years old on polytherapy are the most frequently affected). Patients with inborn errors of metabolism are at particular risk for liver toxicity. Other situations that are associated with a higher incidence of these severe reactions are polypharmacy (including multiple AEDs) and acute infections. One should be very careful with patients on valproic acid (or divalproex sodium) who are acutely ill with nausea or vomiting. These patients deserve a thorough evaluation that often includes testing for serum ammonia, amylase, and liver function. Less commonly, skin rashes occur. Macrocytic anemia, thrombocytopenia, and significant bone marrow toxicity can also be seen. These are usually dose dependent. In some patients, valproic acid may alter platelet function (aggregation), and this drug should be used with extreme caution (if at all) in patients who are going to undergo major surgery. Use of valproic acid during pregnancy is associated with an increased risk of neural tube defects in the offspring (see the later section on the use of AEDs during pregnancy).

Ethosuximide (Zarontin)

Most neurologists consider ethosuximide the drug of choice for absence seizures when this is the only type of seizure the patient is having. This drug may occasionally be effective against some myoclonic or atonic seizures. Partial and generalized tonic-clonic seizures do not respond to ethosuximide treatment. Oral absorption of this drug is almost complete, and peak plasma concentrations occur in 1 to 4 hours. Protein binding is negligible, and 90% of the drug is metabolized in the liver, with the rest being excreted unchanged in the urine. The half-life is 50 to 60 hours in adults. Therapeutic serum concentrations are between 40 and 100 μg per mL, but some patients may require and tolerate higher levels. Drowsiness and gastrointestinal upset (nausea, hiccups, vomiting, and anorexia) are common side effects. Patients are usually started on 500 mg a day and have the dose increased by increments of 250 mg per day. Drug interactions are uncommon, probably owing, in part, to the low protein binding.

Barbiturates

Although phenobarbital and primidone (Mysoline) are frequently used in infants, teenagers and adults do not tolerate these drugs as well as they do carbamazepine and phenytoin. Sedation and decreased mental concentration are common complaints. Occasionally, patients taking these medications since early childhood continue to tolerate them rather well. Their main advantage is their low cost. Both phenobarbital and primidone are protective against partial and generalized tonic-clonic seizures. The usual adult oral dose of phenobarbital is 90 to 240 mg per day, and the therapeutic serum concentration is 20 to 40 μg per mL. Primidone is partly metabolized into phenobarbital, so serum concentrations of both drugs should be checked during primidone therapy. The usual adult oral dose of primidone is 500 to 750 mg per day, and the therapeutic serum concentration range is 4 to 10 μg per mL.

Clonazepam

Clonazepam (Klonopin) is useful in the treatment of myoclonic, photosensitive, and atonic seizures. In juvenile myoclonic epilepsy, clonazepam is helpful in the treatment of the morning myoclonus but less so for the generalized clonic-tonic-clonic seizures. Clonazepam is also used as adjunctive treatment in patients with partial seizures. The bioavailability of clonazepam is close to 100%. After oral administration, peak serum concentrations occur in 1 to 4 hours. The half-life is around 30 hours (range, 20 to 50). The usual starting dose for adults is 0.5 mg three times a day (1.5 mg per day). This dose should be increased by 0.5 mg every 3 days until seizure control or side effects are obtained. Common side effects include sedation and drowsiness, which are seen in half of patients. Slow dose increases may minimize this problem. Personality changes are noted in about a third of patients, and ataxia is seen with similar frequency at higher doses. Neurologically impaired patients commonly have excessive drooling, which in some cases (if poor swallowing is present) may lead to an increased incidence of respiratory tract infection. Clorazepate dipotassium is another benzodiazepine that is helpful as adjunctive therapy for partial seizures. It tends to produce fewer side effects than clonazepam.

Gabapentin (Neurontin)

Gabapentin has recently been approved in the United States for use as an add-on drug in adolescent and adult patients with refractory partial epilepsy. It is ineffective against typical absence seizures. It is absorbed in the gut with the help of a carrier (L-amino acid transporter system). The bioavailability of gabapentin is about 60% with doses of 300 to 600 mg three times a day but may be lower at higher doses. Peak serum concentrations are achieved in 2 to 4 hours. The half-life is 5 to 9 hours. The excretion is almost exclusively renal. Patients with impaired renal function should have their doses corrected according to their creatinine clearance. No metabolites have been detected so far. The usual dose for adults is 900 to 1800 mg per day. Higher doses have occasionally been used without major complications. Gabapentin has very little protein binding and almost no interaction with other drugs. Common side effects include drowsiness, fatigue, dizziness, ataxia, nystagmus, and, less frequently, behavioral changes, tremor, and double vision.

Lamotrigine (Lamictal)

Lamotrigine has also recently been approved as adjunctive therapy in patients over 16 years of age with partial seizures. It reportedly has potential efficacy in absence and myoclonic seizures as well. Its half-life is about 25 hours, but it is prolonged (more than doubled) by valproic acid and shortened by co-medication with enzyme-inducing AEDs. The usual adult dosage is 300 to 500 mg per day given in two daily doses, but lower doses are used for patients on concurrent valproic acid (up to 150 mg per day). Common side effects include rashes, which occur most commonly during co-medication with valproic acid, as well as ataxia, diplopia, blurred vision, dizziness, nausea, and headache. Severe allergic skin reactions occur rarely.

Felbamate (Felbatol)

The use of felbamate has recently been restricted because of the associated increased incidence of aplastic anemia and hepatotoxicity. It had been approved for therapy of partial seizures and for seizures occurring in Lennox-Gastaut syndrome. Few patients remain on the drug, and those who do should be monitored very closely with repeated blood studies, as specified in the package insert. The usual adult dosage is 2400 to 3600 mg per day divided into three daily doses. Common adverse effects include insomnia, weight loss, behavior problems, and frequent drug interactions. Felbamate increases phenytoin, valproic acid, and carbamazepine epoxide levels and reduces carbamazepine levels. Its metabolism is reduced by valproic acid and enhanced by phenytoin and carbamazepine.

STOPPING AEDs

Usually, patients should be seizure free while taking their AEDs for at least 2 years before one starts decreasing the dose. A normal EEG, a normal neurologic examination, and good seizure control may help predict successful weaning from AEDs. Some epileptic syndromes are associated with a high incidence of seizure recurrence after stopping AEDs, despite good control with medications (e.g., juvenile myoclonic epilepsy).

THE USE OF AEDs DURING PREGNANCY

Most AEDs have been associated with some teratogenic effects, but the possibility of having seizures during pregnancy should be considered a significant risk factor for both mother and fetus. Ideally, the pregnancy should be planned ahead of time. If appropriate, and if a woman has been seizure free for more than 2 years, an attempt should be made to reduce and then stop the medication. If that fails, one may at least establish the lowest effective concentration of the AED for this patient and keep her in that range during the pregnancy. In many cases, however, this is not feasible. When medication must be continued, monotherapy is preferable to polytherapy.

Since most of the teratogenic effects take place in the first trimester, patients who do not come for advice until the second or third trimester should not have their anticonvulsant medications stopped then. Use of valproic acid during pregnancy is associated with a 1 to 2% risk of neural tube defects in the offspring. Patients taking carbamazepine may also have an increased risk of neural tube defects in the offspring (probably about 1%). Any pregnant woman taking valproic acid or carbamazepine or both should have ultrasonography at 16 weeks of gestation and have periodic serum alpha-fetoprotein checks. A fetal anticonvulsant syndrome has been described, with the babies showing hypoplastic nails, short distal phalanges, and hypertelorism. This effect is not unique to phenytoin, since similar findings occur with intrauterine exposure to carbamazepine. Treatment with folic acid started before or as soon as possible after conception (0.5 to 2 mg per day) may significantly reduce the risk of neural tube defects.

Many pharmacokinetic changes take place during pregnancy. Usually there is decreased absorption, increased volume of distribution, and increased rate of biodegradation. Owing to these changes, one should check pregnant patients' levels and, if needed, make adjustments in their dosages more frequently (at least every month) than before pregnancy. Two weeks prior to delivery, patients should be started on vitamin K orally 20 mg per day. Immediately after birth, the neonate should receive vitamin K 1 mg intramuscularly to prevent hemorrhagic disease of the newborn.

Ideally, counseling about the potential risks should occur before conception. It is also important to counsel all women of childbearing potential with epilepsy about the interactions of AEDs and contraceptives. Carbamazepine, phenytoin, and barbiturates may decrease oral contraceptive levels, causing breakthrough bleeding and unwanted pregnancies. Valproic acid does not have this problem but may be associated with a higher risk of polycystic ovary disease.

USE OF AEDs IN THE ELDERLY

Elderly patients are often more sensitive to the adverse effects of AEDs because of their age, the numerous other medications they may be taking, and their need for smaller doses owing to a gradually decreasing rate of drug metabolism and excretion with increasing age. Particular attention must be paid to blood levels and to interactions with other drugs these patients might be taking, such as anticoagulants, antacids, and antibiotics (e.g., cimetidine and erythromycin, which can increase carbamazepine levels). Clear instructions should be given, and the patient's compliance and ability to follow through with the instructions should be monitored.

ACKNOWLEDGMENT

We thank Nemat Harmoush for typing the manuscript.

EPILEPSY IN INFANTS AND CHILDREN

method of
FRITZ E. DREIFUSS, M.B.
University of Virginia School of Medicine
Charlottesville, Virginia

The goals of epilepsy management include the elimination and prevention of seizures.

ELIMINATION OF SEIZURES

Seizures are the symptom of an underlying brain disturbance that manifests itself by causing repetitive electrical discharge of aggregates of nerve cells. The most effective means of eliminating seizures are those that eliminate the underlying cause. These include the reversal of hypoglycemia; the correction of other metabolic disturbances, including those of amino acid metabolism; the removal of tumors, abscesses, or toxins; and the restoration of energy metabolism. Individual seizures are expressed according to the origin, rapidity, and direction of spread of the electrical discharges. In childhood, more than half of the cases are of unknown etiology and frequently occur on the basis of a genetic predisposition. In most instances, epilepsy must still be treated symptomatically, and the mainstay of therapy continues to be the administration of antiepileptic medications.

Uncontrolled seizures may be responsible for further neuronal impairment and may ultimately lead to intractability through mechanisms that cause changes in neuronal circuits by altering synaptic connectivity. In addition, uncontrolled seizures may impair a patient's social, psychological, vocational, and recreational quality of life.

There are three major decision points in the evaluation of a child with seizures. The first is to determine whether the seizure represents epilepsy or a paroxysmal nonepileptic event. These are not always easy to distinguish and include shuddering or sleep myoclonus in infants, breath holding or self-stimulation, esophageal reflux, paroxysmal vertigo in basilar migraine, hyperventilation, paroxysmal sleep disorders, cardiac or vasovagal syncope, and paroxysmal movement disorders such as tics or choreoathetosis in older children.

The second decision involves identifying the type of seizure. Because epileptic seizures are etiologically diverse, because different types of seizures involve different mechanisms of propagation and excitation, and because the development of antiepileptic drugs has been toward specific drugs for specific seizure types, accurate identification and classification are important in seizure management. In fact, accurate seizure identification is a sine qua non for the initiation of appropriate therapy.

The third cardinal point is the determination of which syndrome the seizures represent. This determination is basic to the formulation of a prognosis, on which management strategy hinges. For example, in a benign febrile seizure situation or with benign childhood partial seizures, a more conservative course may be adopted, whereas in partial complex seizures due to mesial temporal sclerosis, a more aggressive approach is called for, including consideration of the surgical option. Equal in importance to the institution and maintenance of therapy is the consideration of when to terminate therapy after an appropriate seizure-free period. This decision depends to a large extent on the nature of the underlying epilepsy and its prognosis, which determines the benefit/risk ratio in maintaining therapy or curtailing it.

In classifying epileptic seizures, it is important to distinguish between seizures that are primarily generalized and those that are basically partial seizures, with or without secondary generalization, because these require different medications. It may be difficult to distinguish between absence seizures and complex partial seizures, but the distinction is imperative to avoid the use of inappropriate medications. Since all medications have a potential for unwanted side effects, mistakes should be avoided. The choice of a specific drug is determined by its potential efficacy and its relative freedom from side effects (Tables 1 and 2). Whichever drug is used, the patient and

TABLE 1. **Classification of Epileptic Syndromes and Their Drugs of Choice**

Syndrome	Drug
Idiopathic Epilepsies	
With partial seizures	Carbamazepine, valproate*
With generalized seizures	
Childhood absence	Ethosuximide, valproate
Juvenile absence	Valproate
Juvenile myoclonic epilepsy	Valproate, phenytoin
Myoclonic absence	Valproate plus ethosuximide
Symptomatic Epilepsies	
With partial seizures (lesional)	Carbamazepine, phenytoin, valproate,* vigabatrin,† gabapentin,‡ lamotrigine‡
With generalized seizures	
West's syndrome	ACTH, prednisone, valproate, lamotrigine*‡
West's syndrome in tuberous sclerosis	Vigabatrin,† valproate*
Lennox-Gastaut syndrome	Felbamate (but see side-effect profile), lamotrigine,‡ valproate, clonazepam
With known metabolic disorders	Pyridoxine, biotin, diets, steroids, benzodiazepines as appropriate
Neonatal seizures	Phenobarbital plus eliminate cause
Febrile convulsions	Intermittent rectal diazepam,* long-term phenobarbital (but note side-effect profile)
Reflex epilepsies	Valproate,* benzodiazepines

*Not FDA-approved for this indication.
†Not available in the United States.
‡FDA approval restricted to use as add-on drug.

family must be educated about the importance of compliance, the need for occasional therapeutic blood level determinations, and the recognition of both dose-related and idiosyncratic side effects. Drugs should be gradually introduced to lessen the incidence of side effects. Monotherapy should be the therapeutic aim, but substitution of another drug may be mandated by failure of the first drug. The first drug is then slowly withdrawn as the second drug is introduced. Occasionally, more than one drug may be necessary, but if polytherapy is used, knowledge of potential drug interactions is essential. If possible, the drugs should be complementary and have different modes of action. Drug doses and side effects are summarized in Table 3.

MANAGEMENT OF INDIVIDUAL EPILEPTIC SYNDROMES

Epileptic syndromes are concatenations of factors, including seizure type, etiology, precipitating factors, age of onset, severity and chronicity, diurnal and circadian cycling, family history, and prognosis. Childhood epilepsy syndromes may be classified according to age. Thus, one may recognize neonatal seizure syndromes, infantile spasms, the syndrome of febrile convulsions, Lennox-Gastaut syndrome, childhood petit mal, benign childhood partial seizures, juvenile myoclonic epilepsy, epilepsia partialis continua, and the reflex epilepsies, as well as etiologically identifiable diseases such as the lipidoses, progressive myoclonic epilepsy, and other storage diseases presenting with seizures, as well as the mitochondrial encephalomyopathies. Most of the childhood epilepsy syndromes can be divided into primary or idiopathic epilepsy that occurs on a genetic basis, and secondary or lesional or symptomatic epilepsy. The primary or idiopathic epilepsies are unassociated with underlying pathology, and there is usually no abnormal neurologic finding other than the occurrence of seizures. The conditions are often self-limited and responsive to medication. Symptomatic epilepsies are frequently associated with other neurologic and developmental abnormalities; the seizures are frequently difficult to control and persist despite treatment. The progressive epilepsies are of the symptomatic variety.

TABLE 2. **Classification of Epileptic Seizures and Their Drugs of Choice**

Seizure	Drug
Partial	
Simple partial	Carbamazepine, phenytoin, valproate,* vigabatrin,† gabapentin,‡ lamotrigine‡
Complex partial	Carbamazepine, phenytoin, valproate,* vigabatrin,† primidone, gabapentin,‡ lamotrigine‡
Partial, secondarily generalized	Carbamazepine, phenytoin, valproate,* phenobarbital, gabapentin,‡ lamotrigine‡
Generalized	
Absence	Ethosuximide, valproate
Myoclonic	Valproate,* clonazepam, lamotrigine,* felbamate, pyridoxine
Atonic	Valproate,* lamotrigine,* felbamate, corticosteroids
Tonic, clonic, or tonic-clonic	Valproate,* cabamazepine, phenytoin, barbiturates

*Not FDA-approved for this indication.
†Not available in the United States.
‡FDA approval restricted to add-on drug.

TABLE 3. **Drug Therapy in the Management of Seizures**

Drug	Dosage* Starting	Dosage* Maintenance	Blood Level	Side Effects	Precautions
Carbamazepine (Tegretol)	5 mg/kg/day	10–25 mg/kg/day	5–12 µg/mL	Dose related: diplopia, drowsiness, vertigo, headache, diarrhea, inappropriate antidiuretic hormone, leukopenia Idiosyncratic: aplastic anemia, hepatotoxicity, arrhythmia, teratogenicity	Blood counts and SGOT monthly for 6 mo, then every 4 mo; warn of possible interactions with birth control medications in adolescents and adults and erythromycin
Clonazepam (Klonopin)	0.05 mg/kg/day	0.2 mg/kg/day	13–73 µg/mL	Dose related: drowsiness, hypotonia, increased secretions, behavior problems, tolerance	Begin with low dose; extreme caution on withdrawal
Ethosuximide (Zarontin)	20–25 mg/kg/day	20–25 mg/kg/day	40–100 µg/mL	Dose related: drowsiness, headache, hiccup, nausea Idiosyncratic: aplastic anemia, erythema multiforme, Stevens-Johnson syndrome, SLE	Blood counts monthly; report skin, joint, mucous membrane symptoms, sore throat
Felbamate (Felbatol)	15 mg/kg/day	45–60 mg/kg/day	50–100 µg/mL suggested	Dose related: headache, insomnia, anorexia, fatigue, vomiting, weight loss, fever Idiosyncratic: rash, aplastic anemia, hepatic failure	Blood counts, including platelets and reticulocytes, every 2 wk; liver function every 2–4 wk; recommended only after careful benefit/risk analysis
Gabapentin† (Neurontin)	Not available	Over 12 years, 900–1800 mg/day	Unknown	Somnolence, ataxia, fatigue	Except for cimetidine, few drug interactions; approved as add-on therapy in partial seizures
Lamotrigine† (Lamictal)	12.5 mg/day if co-medication with valproate; 25 mg/day with P-450 inducers	Over 16 years of age up to 200 mg/day if co-medication with valproate; 200–400 mg/day with P-450 inducers	Unknown	Dose related: skin rash, drowsiness; half-life greatly prolonged in presence of valproate	Keep dosage low and introduction slow to avoid skin rash; in presence of valproate, clearance is reduced and high blood levels result
Phenytoin (Dilantin)	4–8 mg/kg/day Status epilepticus: 1–2 mg/kg/min, up to 25 mg/kg total	4–8 mg/kg/day; max 300 mg —	10–20 µg/mL	Dose related: dizziness, ataxia, diplopia, gingival hyperplasia, hirsutism, coarse facies, folate deficiency, cerebellar dysfunction Idiosyncratic: skin rashes, exfoliation, Stevens-Johnson syndrome, SLE, pseudolymphoma, teratogenicity, hepatotoxicity	Animal blood counts, oral hygiene; warn of possible effects on birth control medications
Primidone (Mysoline)	1–2 mg/kg/day	10–25 mg/kg/day	5–12 µg/mL	Dose related: sedation, vertigo, behavior disturbances Idiosyncratic: skin rash, fever	Begin with very small dose; avoid in school-age children if possible; use caution on withdrawal
Phenobarbital (Luminal)	Neonate: 10–20 mg/kg/day Child: 3–4 mg/kg/day Status epilepticus: 20 mg/kg IV	3–4 mg/kg/day 5 mg/kg/day —	10–40 µg/mL	Dose related: sedation, short attention, irritability, hyperactivity, poor school performance Idiosyncratic: skin rash, exfoliation, fever	
Divalproex sodium (Depakene, Depakote)	15 mg/kg/day	Up to 60 mg/kg/day	50–100 µg/mL trough level	Dose related: drowsiness, gastrointestinal disturbance, alopecia, weight gain, tremor, SGOT elevation, hearing loss, thrombocytopenia Idiosyncratic: leukopenia, hepatic necrosis, pancreatitis, teratogenicity	Complete blood count, platelets, SGOT, SGPT every 2 wk for 2 mo, then every mo for 1 yr; caution in small children on polytherapy and especially in cases of metabolic encephalopathy

*All doses are for a child, unless otherwise indicated.

†Not yet FDA-approved for children under 12 years old.

Abbreviations: SGOT = serum glutamic-oxaloacetic transaminase; SGPT = serum glutamate pyruvate transaminase; SLE = systemic lupus erythematosus.

Originally adapted from Dreifuss FE: In Porter R and Morselli PL (eds): Butterworths International Medical Reviews in Neurology, vol. 5. Epilepsies. London, Butterworth, 1985.

Neonatal Seizures

Neonatal seizures frequently have an identifiable etiology. Many are the result of prematurity or birth trauma, including intracranial hemorrhage, infection, and metabolic disorders or developmental malformations. Occasionally, the seizures are benign, self-limited, and familial. Rapid diagnosis and immediate removal of the underlying remediable causes are essential. Hypoglycemia is treated with intravenous 25% glucose 2 to 4 mL per kg. Hypocalcemia is managed with intravenous 5% calcium gluconate 200 mg per kg while the child's heart rate is monitored. Hypomagnesemia is treated with 0.2 mL per kg of 50% magnesium sulfate intramuscularly. Because pyridoxine deficiency may cause continuing seizures, pyridoxine 100 mg can be given intravenously during electroencephalography; this is a relatively rare cause of neonatal convulsions, however.

Specific anticonvulsant treatment is undertaken while awaiting definitive therapy or if the cause cannot be ascertained or seizures persist. In neonates, the drug of choice is phenobarbital, which may be given intravenously in two divided doses to a total of 20 mg per kg. Subsequent oral phenobarbital therapy is used to maintain satisfactory blood levels. Phenytoin (Dilantin) may also be used but must be given intravenously very slowly—no more than 1 to 2 mg per kg per minute up to 20 mg/kg—because of the danger of cardiac arrhythmia. The phenobarbital maintenance dose is 3 mg per kg per day; phenytoin's is 6 mg per kg per day. With either drug, frequent blood levels must be obtained. Duration of therapy depends on the underlying etiology and is usually just a few weeks, although in the case of an ongoing process, impaired development, or persistent electroencephalogram (EEG) abnormality, long-term therapy may be needed. In the case of benign neonatal convulsions, treatment is usually stopped within 2 weeks.

Infantile Spasms

Infantile spasms are the manifestation of an early childhood epilepsy syndrome characterized by myoclonic or tonic flexion or extension spasms that are usually bilateral and often occur in clusters. The associated EEG pattern is hypsarrhythmia, although the actual EEG during spasms may be electrodecremental. The idiopathic variety known as West's syndrome is characterized by normal development up to the onset of spasms, usually between 4 months and 1 year of age. With the onset of the attacks, neurologic development stagnates, but with appropriate treatment, it may revert to normal. Symptomatic infantile spasms may begin in the postnatal period, when they are usually associated with severe brain disease, anoxia, congenital malformations, or metabolic abnormalities. Infantile spasms may be due to tuberous sclerosis. Occasionally, the spasms are unilateral or show some focality, which may be the result of an underlying focal develop-

mental anomaly. The treatment of choice is intramuscular adrenocorticotropic hormone (ACTH), and it is believed that early treatment is associated with a better prognosis. The dosage is 30 to 40 U of ACTH daily for 4 to 6 weeks. If this is not successful or if spasms recommence, valproic acid (Depakene, Depakote) 30 to 60 mg per kg or clonazepam 0.05 to 0.2 mg per kg may be used. Nitrazepam* is an effective benzodiazepine, but it is not approved for use in the United States and may be hazardous because of increased bronchial secretions and inhibition of pharyngeal sphincter closure, which may result in aspiration. Side effects of ACTH include hypertension, cushingoid changes, and interference with immunity. It is contraindicated if the spasms are secondary to cytomegalovirus. Elective immunizations should be avoided during the time of administration. If valproate is used, liver function should be carefully monitored.

In symptomatic spasms due to focal brain dysfunction, surgical removal of dysmorphic brain may result in marked improvement. In the absence of amelioration, the syndrome may merge into Lennox-Gastaut syndrome, and the emergent seizure is treated accordingly.

Febrile Convulsions

Febrile convulsions are common, occurring in approximately 50 per 1000 children between the ages of 6 months and 5 years. In each case, intracranial infection or other causes must be excluded. Idiopathic febrile seizures are not associated with a major risk of subsequent epilepsy, but if they recur frequently, they should be treated. The risk of a recurrent seizure with fever is approximately 30%, and after a second seizure, 50%. Major risk factors predisposing to recurrence or the development of nonfebrile seizures include a family history of epilepsy, abnormal neurologic development prior to the onset of febrile seizures, prolonged seizures (longer than 15 minutes), an element of focality, or clusters of seizures. Among high-risk children, long-term prophylaxis should be considered. The drug of choice continues to be phenobarbital, with the aim of reaching blood levels between 15 and 30 μg per mL until a 2-year seizure-free interval has been attained. Rapidly gaining in popularity is the rectal administration of diazepam (Valium) or lorazepam (Ativan) at the onset of fever in children with recurrent febrile convulsions. Intermittent therapy with rectal benzodiazepines is deservedly popular because it is safe and effective and avoids the side effects of phenobarbital—namely, hyperactivity—and possible interference with cognitive development.

Lennox-Gastaut Syndrome

Lennox-Gastaut syndrome is characterized by astatic myoclonic seizures, atypical absence, and

---

*Not available in the United States.

axial tonic seizures, as well as localization-related attacks. This is usually a severe disorder characterized by developmental delay and extreme intractability to most medication regimens. A relatively benign form of astatic myoclonic epilepsy may respond to valproate therapy, and this is always the drug of first choice. In the benign variant, the interictal EEG usually shows relatively little disturbance, and the spike wave discharges are well formed and faster than 3 cycles per second; in Lennox-Gastaut syndrome, the interictal EEG is considerably disrupted, with significant slowing interspersed with slow spike waves and, during sleep, with rapid high-voltage discharges. Akinetic drop attacks are quite frequent and damaging. Anticonvulsant drugs are frequently given in combination, including benzodiazepines and a major anticonvulsant such as valproate. Felbamate (Felbatol) up to 60 mg per kg was found to be the most successful treatment but has been virtually abandoned because of the risk of aplastic anemia and hepatopathy with prolonged use. Lamotrigine (Lamictal) is reportedly useful in this syndrome, but it is not yet approved in the United States for use in children. In Europe, clobazam (Frisium)* is a popular benzodiazepine with less tendency than the other benzodiazepines to encourage the development of tolerance. As a last resort, a 3:1 ketogenic diet may be tried. In this diet, three-fourths of the caloric intake is derived from fat. When a ketogenic diet is used, anticonvulsant drugs should not be dispensed in a carbohydrate vehicle such as sweetened syrups.

Pyknoleptic Petit Mal

Pyknoleptic petit mal is characterized by childhood absence seizures occurring frequently each day (pyknoleptic means crowding of seizures). Each seizure has a sudden onset and consists of interruption of ongoing activities, a blank stare, and, frequently, a brief outward rotation of the eyes. In addition, there may be mild clonic components, changes in postural tone, automatisms, or autonomic components. The ictal EEG usually consists of regular and symmetrical 3-cycle-per-second spike and wave complexes. In "atypical absence," there may also be astatic myoclonic components as in Lennox-Gastaut syndrome. Absence may occur in the form of status or "spike wave stupor," which is characterized by continuing absence activity for hours or even days with stuporous, confused, or dazed behavior. The treatment of choice is ethosuximide (Zarontin) monotherapy 10 to 30 mg per kg, with an effective blood level of 40 to 100 µg per mL. The principal side effects include gastrointestinal disturbance, hiccups, drowsiness, and headache. Idiosyncratic side effects include erythema multiforme, blood dyscrasia, and systemic lupus erythematosus. The other drug of choice, particularly when other seizure types occur in addition to absence, is divalproex sodium (Depakote), which is ranked second only because of the potential seri-

ousness of idiosyncratic hepatic and pancreatic side effects. It is given in a dose of 30 to 60 mg per kg, with an expected trough blood level of 50 to 100 µg per mL. In the case of the syndrome of myoclonic absence, a combination of ethosuximide and valproate may be more successful than either drug alone. Sensitive anticonvulsants should be avoided because these tend to potentiate absence seizures, as does carbamazepine. If generalized tonic-clonic seizures emerge, valproate becomes the drug of choice for the treatment of both conditions. Clonazepam (Klonopin) is also effective in a dose of 0.05 to 0.2 mg per kg, with a therapeutic blood level between 13 and 72 ng per mL. The side effects and the development of tolerance have reduced its popularity, however. The treatment of choice for absence status is the intravenous use of diazepam (Valium) or lorazepam (Ativan) followed by valproate. The pyknoleptic petit mal syndrome has a good prognosis for spontaneous resolution in adolescence, and treatment is frequently discontinued after a 2-year seizure-free interval.

Rolandic Epilepsy

Rolandic epilepsy is a benign form of partial seizure associated with a centrotemporal spike EEG abnormality. A stereotypical focal childhood attack responds well to most anticonvulsant drugs. Either carbamazepine (Tegretol) or valproate may be used, although some pediatric epileptologists recommend no treatment for this usually self-limited condition. Because the prognosis is never certain, and because of the anxiety induced by the attacks, the author prefers to administer carbamazepine, aiming for a therapeutic blood level of 8 to 12 µg per mL. Usually by the time the child is 13 years old the attacks go into spontaneous remission.

Juvenile Myoclonic Epilepsy

Juvenile myoclonic epilepsy occurs in childhood and adolescence and is characterized by frequent myoclonic jerks, usually occurring in the morning, interspersed with generalized tonic-clonic seizures. Frequently, there is also juvenile absence, which differs from childhood absence in that it does not respond as well to medication and is nonpyknoleptic, occurring much more randomly and infrequently. Sleep deprivation is a common precipitating factor, and strobe lights may produce photosensitive seizures. The drug of choice is valproate. Discontinuation of the medication frequently leads to a recurrence of seizures; thus, therapy should be long term.

Reflex Seizures

Reflex seizures include those seizures regularly induced by external stimuli, such as flashing lights, certain sounds, or certain proprioceptive stimuli. Reading epilepsy, musicogenic epilepsy, and kinesiogenic epilepsy are examples of reflex epilepsies. The

---

*Not available in the United States.

majority of these respond well to valproate monotherapy, but benzodiazepines are also effective.

Epilepsies Characterized by Partial Seizures

In both simple partial seizures and complex partial seizures, the drugs of choice include carbamazepine (Tegretol), phenytoin (Dilantin), phenobarbital, and primidone (Mysoline). In a large trial, the latter drug proved to be less satisfactory by virtue of its poorly tolerated side effects. Serious side effects are infrequent with both carbamazepine and phenytoin, which are relatively benign in children in relation to central nervous system toxicity. Phenytoin continues to be a popular drug in the treatment of most forms of seizures, including partial seizures, but it is becoming less popular than carbamazepine because of the prevalence of side effects during long-term therapy. It does have the advantage of requiring only once-daily administration, which improves compliance, and it is relatively inexpensive—an increasingly important economic consideration. Transient leukopenia is common, but persistent leukopenia should lead to reduction or discontinuation of this drug.

Partial seizures are frequently difficult to control, particularly complex partial seizures, and especially those associated with mesial temporal sclerosis. Polytherapy is therefore used more frequently than in other forms of childhood epilepsy. A satisfactory second drug is gabapentin (Neurontin). Although this drug has not been officially approved for use in children, it is increasing in popularity because of its relative lack of side effects and lack of interaction with other medications. Felbamate (Felbatol) was also found to be useful, but its use had to be curtailed as previously noted because of the possibility of aplastic anemia and hepatopathy. Lamotrigine has been found to be useful in partial seizures. Divalproex sodium (Depakote) and clorazepate (Tranxene) are frequently used for adjunctive therapy, and the GABA re-uptake inhibitor Tiagabine,* at present an experimental drug, appears to hold promise in the alleviation of partial seizures.

Epilepsies Characterized by Generalized Tonic-Clonic Seizures

The drugs used in the treatment of partial seizures are also generally employed in the management of generalized tonic-clonic seizures, but the order in which the drugs are used may depend on the setting in which the seizures occur. When there are concomitant absence seizures, valproic acid or divalproex sodium (Depakene, Depakote) is the drug of choice, as one is dealing with primary generalized epilepsy. Under other circumstances, particularly when the tonic-clonic seizures are secondary generalized episodes, carbamazepine or phenytoin might be pre-

*Investigational drug in the United States.

ferred. The prognosis of primary generalized epilepsy is considerably better than if the epilepsy were symptomatic of an underlying cerebral lesion, as evidenced by concomitant neurologic dysfunction such as intellectual impairment or the presence of abnormal neurologic findings, or if other seizure types were also present. Under those circumstances, more than one drug might have to be given, leading to the potential complications inherent in drug interactions; gabapentin (Neurontin) may be a preferred additive drug.

Status Epilepticus

Status epilepticus is defined as recurrent seizures without intervening recovery and becomes operative usually after 30 minutes of uninterrupted seizure activity. This represents a medical emergency because of the threat to life and to continued integrity of brain function posed by anoxia, hypoglycemia, increasing acidosis, and, of course, the disorders leading to the status epilepticus in the first place. A treatment plan must include maintenance of vital functions, including airway, oxygenation, and blood pressure. An intravenous line should be placed to provide venous access for blood studies of glucose, electrolytes, and anticonvulsant levels, and for the administration of glucose and anticonvulsant drugs. In children, glucose is administered as 50% dextrose and water, 1 gram per kg. Pharmacologic management includes the administration of a benzodiazepine and/or phenytoin or phenobarbital intravenously. The preferred benzodiazepine is lorazepam (Ativan), although diazepam (Valium) may also be used in a previously untreated patient, followed by a longer-acting drug such as phenytoin. In a patient previously treated with barbiturates, diazepam may cause respiratory and cardiovascular depression, and phenytoin or more phenobarbital might be preferred. Diazepam is administered in a dose of 0.25 to 0.4 mg per kg over 2 minutes, with a maximum injection of 5 to 10 mg. Lorazepam is given in a dose of 0.05 to 0.2 mg per kg. Either benzodiazepine is followed by a longer-acting drug, usually phenytoin, at 20 mg per kg intravenously at a rate of 1 to 2 mg per kg per minute. Alternatively, phenobarbital may be administered 5 to 10 mg per kg at 30 mg per minute; this may be repeated to a maximum of 25 mg per kg. All intravenous anticonvulsants can cause apnea and hypertension, and patients should be carefully monitored in an intensive care unit. If seizures are not controlled by these medications, general anesthesia may have to be used, although an intravenous midazolam drip may be a temporalizing expedient. Partial status, or epilepsia partialis continua, may be treated similarly but constitutes considerably less of an emergency. It represents the expression of a severe focal underlying lesion, and management should be directed toward the underlying cause. In a child, this condition is usually a manifestation of a progressive, intractable underlying process with a poor prognosis.

GENERAL CONSIDERATIONS IN THE MANAGEMENT OF CHILDREN WITH EPILEPSY

Efforts should be made to prevent children from developing psychosocial problems as a result of epilepsy by giving attention to those factors that influence a person's coping style. These include factors inherent in the epilepsy, such as age of onset, site of lesion, and nature and dose of medications employed, as well as the child's underlying personality, family support, and innate mechanisms for coping with stress. By and large, children should be encouraged to become independent despite the burden of epilepsy and not to be unduly restricted or shielded from competition and exploratory activities, which are necessary for the attainment of independence and confidence. Threatening situations such as operation of a bicycle or motor vehicle, solo bathing, and contact sports in which head injury is a frequent and predictable consequence should be avoided, however. Most athletic activities can be engaged in, and supervised swimming is usually not contraindicated.

THE ROLE OF NEW ANTIEPILEPTIC DRUGS

Pharmacologic research in the past decade has resulted in the appearance of new drugs. In the European community, Canada, and Latin America, vigabatrin (Sabril)* has been found to be useful in partial seizures and in the treatment of infantile spasms, particularly those associated with tuberous sclerosis. Lamotrigine (Lamictal) is rapidly gaining favor in the management of intractable childhood epilepsies such as Lennox-Gastaut syndrome. Clobazam† is a widely used benzodiazepine with a record of assuaging seizures by more than 50% in approximately 50% of children given this drug.

In the United States, the use of felbamate, which showed much promise, has been severely curtailed by the appearance of aplastic anemia and occasional hepatopathy in enough patients to present a severe disincentive to its use, except under special circumstances. Gabapentin (Neurontin) has been approved as an add-on drug, and studies are under way to ascertain whether it will fulfill its promise as a freestanding antiepileptic agent. Tiagabine,† zonisamide,† and topiramate† are under active investigation. A recent conference emphasized the need for the participation of children in drug testing, as the special needs of children with specific epilepsy syndromes are of particular urgency, in view of the vulnerability of the developing nervous system.

THE PLACE OF EPILEPSY SURGERY IN THE MANAGEMENT OF CHILDHOOD SEIZURES

The success of epilepsy surgery in improving the lot of patients with intractable seizures has encour-

---

*Not available in the United States.
†Investigational drug in the United States.

aged its use in younger and younger age groups, where the early curtailment of an intractable seizure disorder can improve the quality of life immensely. The standard temporal lobectomy for the treatment of intractable complex partial seizures; focal cortical excision for dysplastic cortex; and hemispherectomy for hemimegalencephaly, intractable seizures in association with severe infantile hemiplegia, and epilepsia partialis continua have been a great boon. Corpus callosotomy continues to be somewhat controversial but is a palliative procedure for severe drop attacks. Removal of tuberous sclerosis lesions such as tubers and giant cell astrocytomas, as well as subpial transection in patients with Landau-Kleffner syndrome, is still largely experimental.

GILLES DE LA TOURETTE SYNDROME

method of
ANN BERGIN, M.B., and
HARVEY S. SINGER, M.D.
*Johns Hopkins University School of Medicine
Baltimore, Maryland*

OVERVIEW

Gilles de la Tourette syndrome (TS) is a chronic neurologic disorder characterized by the presence of involuntary motor and phonic tics and is often associated with comorbid neuropsychiatric problems. The disorder occurs worldwide and is estimated to have a prevalence of about 1 to 10 per 10,000 children. TS is more common in males than in females (more than 4:1), and the mean age of onset of symptoms is typically between 6 and 7 years. There is a hereditary influence that has not been clearly elucidated. Some studies have suggested an autosomal dominant trait with variable penetrance, whereas others have postulated a polygenic inheritance. Tics are manifest as sudden, involuntary, brief, stereotyped and repetitive movements or vocalizations. The movements may be simple, such as an eye blink, shoulder shrug, or face twitch, or more complex coordinated actions, such as jumping, gesturing, or spinning. Similarly, vocal tics may be as simple as a sniff or throat-clearing sound, or more complex with repeated words and phrases, echolalia, and the rarer coprolalia. The frequency, intensity, and form of tics wax and wane. Tics typically become more obvious in situations of stress, anxiety, and fatigue but are usually less noticeable (although not absent) during periods of relaxation and sleep. Neurologic examination and neuroradiologic studies are typically normal. The natural history of TS is highly variable. In general, about two-thirds have improvement or resolution of their tics in late adolescence or early adulthood. There are no reliable features that allow prognostication in either the short or long term for individual patients. Tic manifestations may interfere significantly with social adjustment and psychosocial development. In addition to impairment by tics, many affected individuals are also afflicted by comorbid conditions, including attention deficit hyperactivity disorder (ADHD), obsessive-compulsive disorder (OCD), learning difficulties, and other psychopathologic conditions.

DIAGNOSIS

The Tourette Syndrome Classification Study Group's diagnostic criteria for TS differ from those for Tourette's "disorder," as outlined by the *Diagnostic and Statistical Manual of Mental Disorders,* fourth edition (DSM-IV). In the former, the criteria for TS are (1) the presence of multiple motor tics and at least one vocal tic (not necessarily concurrently), (2) a waxing and waning course with tics evolving in a progressive manner, (3) the presence of tic symptoms for at least 1 year, (4) the onset of symptoms before 21 years of age, (5) the absence of precipitating illness (e.g., encephalitis, stroke, or degenerative disease) or medication, and (6) the observation of tics by a knowledgeable individual. The DSM-IV criteria for Tourette's "disorder" add an "impairment" criterion requiring that "marked distress or significant impairment in social, occupational or other important areas of functioning" be present. In addition, the age of onset has been lowered to before 18 years, and there should be no tic-free interval of greater than 3 months. Controversy exists as to the wisdom of adding a subjective impairment requirement to the diagnostic criteria.

TREATMENT

Decision regarding treatment for an individual patient requires an initial comprehensive evaluation including an analysis of tics, the documentation of co-morbid conditions, and an assessment of their severity and any resulting impairment. Therapeutic priorities should be established. The mere presence of tics is not a sufficient reason for drug treatment. Since none of the available pharmacotherapies for tics are curative and all are associated with the potential for side effects, therapy should be reserved for those symptoms that are functionally disabling for the patient. Patients with mild tics may be counseled and observed for the progression of symptoms. Psychological impact should be determined by specific inquiries concerning the effect of tics on peer relationships, interactions with teachers or family members, interference with school work or job performance, or the capacity to engage in and enjoy normal social activities. These areas may also be disrupted by the presence of co-morbid conditions, such as deficits in the ability to maintain attention, control impulses, or regulate activities; problems with obsessive thoughts and compulsive rituals; or specific learning disabilities. Since no single treatment is effective against all potential causes, therapy should be directed at the symptom causing the greatest degree of psychosocial disruption.

Tics

The decision to treat tics depends on the social and psychological impact of the movements and/or vocalizations on school and work performance or peer and family relationships. Before prescribing medication it is often helpful to enlist the aid of school personnel in implementing approaches designed to assist the child and the child's peers adjust to this disorder. Strategies such as education of the other students, extra break periods to allow "release" of tics, provision of a refuge area for the child if the tics become severe, and the waiving of time limitations on tests may all relieve stress sufficiently to reduce both the frequency of tics and their social impact. These measures alone may be adequate to obviate the need for medication in the milder cases, thus avoiding exposure to the potential side effects of drugs. In situations in which medication is indicated, the goal is not to suppress movements entirely but to reduce them to the point at which they no longer cause a significant psychosocial disturbance. Medications are initiated at low doses and increased gradually. Patients started on pharmacotherapy are followed periodically to evaluate the efficacy of treatment, and to monitor for side effects. After several months of successful treatment, medications are tapered during a nonstressful time (e.g., summer vacation months) and patients are observed for re-emergence of symptoms. Treatment is reinstituted only if the recurrent movements and/or vocalizations are functionally disabling.

Our first line of pharmacotherapy in children with milder TS or those with other behavioral problems is clonidine (Catapres).* This alpha$_2$-adrenergic receptor agonist acts selectively at the presynaptic level when used in lower doses (4 to 5 micrograms per kg per day). Higher doses (7 to 15 micrograms per kg per day), which additionally act postsynaptically, may not be as effective in controlling symptoms. Clonidine is started at a low dose of 0.05 mg per day (one-half tablet) and increased by increments of 0.05 mg at 5- to 7-day intervals to a maximum of 0.4 mg per day. For treatment of tics alone, we have found a twice-daily dose regimen to be adequate. However, for treating ADHD, the daily dose is divided into four-times-daily doses. Clonidine is also available as a transdermal patch, but we have not found this a useful route of administration, owing to the occurrence of local skin reactions and difficulties keeping the patch on active children. The beneficial effect of clonidine may be delayed for a number of weeks. The main side effect is sedation, which frequently improves with time. Dry mouth, itchy eyes, postural hypotension, and headache are reported rarely. Tics may intensify if the drug is withdrawn abruptly: therefore, a taper is needed when therapy is ending, or before a change of medication is undertaken.

For patients whose tics fail to improve, or in whom unacceptable side effects occur, our next drug is a neuroleptic, which is introduced after the clonidine has been withdrawn. The neuroleptics as a group interfere with dopaminergic neurotransmission at the D$_2$ receptor. They are about 70 to 80% effective in suppressing tics. A variety of neuroleptic agents have been used. Although haloperidol (Haldol) was the first agent of this type used, our preferred sequence is to start with pimozide (Orap) and progress, if necessary to fluphenazine (Prolixin), and then to haloperidol. This approach is based on our personal

---

*Not FDA-approved for this indication.

experience of how these drugs are tolerated by patients. The side-effect profile is common to all neuroleptics, and the most frequent problems include sedation, weight gain, dysphoria, movement abnormalities (acute dystonic reactions, bradykinesia, and akathisia), depression, and poor school performance, with or without school phobia. Children, either on stable doses or being withdrawn from neuroleptics, have suffered from tardive or withdrawal dyskinesia. We do not routinely use anticholinergic agents (Cogentin or Artane) with the neuroleptic drugs, preferring to wait until they are indicated in the small number of patients who manifest movement abnormalities.

Pimozide is a diphenylbutylpiperidine distinct from haloperidol and phenothiazines. Before starting therapy with this agent we obtain an electrocardiogram (ECG) because of the potential of the medication to prolong the QT interval. Pimozide should not be used if the QT interval is abnormal before therapy. The medication is started at a dose of 1 mg per day (one-half tablet) at bedtime and is increased, if necessary, in 1-mg increments at 5- to 7-day intervals. Our maximum daily dose is about 10 mg per day in children and 20 mg per day in adults. Although pimozide has a long half-life, we use a twice-daily dosage to reduce sedative side effects.

If pimozide is ineffective we switch to fluphenazine after withdrawal of pimozide. This drug is an equal antagonist at both D_1 and D_2 dopaminergic receptors. Medication is started at a dose of 1 mg at bedtime and is increased in a similar manner to pimozide, increasing by 1 mg every 5 to 7 days, while following the patient for a therapeutic response or side effects.

Haloperidol is a butyrophenone and represents our third choice of neuroleptic agent for tic control. Its tic-suppressing effect is seen with quite low doses. Patients are started on 0.5 mg per day and increased gradually at 5- to 7-day intervals. Most patients respond to doses in the range of 1 to 5 mg per day. Phenothiazines such as thioridazine (Mellaril)* and trifluoperazine (Stelazine)* are occasionally used for the control of tics.

A newer neuroleptic agent, risperidone (Risperidal), has been shown in preliminary studies to have tic-suppressing capabilities. Risperidone, a benzisoxazole derivative, has both serotonin- and dopamine-blocking activity. The medication is started at 0.5 mg per day at night and increased as tolerated at 5-day intervals to a maximum of 2.5 mg per day in two divided doses. Side effects include fatigue, acute dystonic reactions, weight gain, and transient photophobia.

Several other agents, including clonazepam (Klonopin), reserpine, tetrabenazine,† calcium channel blockers, and opiate antagonists have been advocated, but their efficacy remains questionable and requires further investigation.

Nonpharmacologic therapies also have a role in our management of tics. We recommend behavioral therapies, particularly relaxation therapy, as the sole therapy in motivated patients with mild tics, and as adjunctive therapy with medication in those with stressful life situations or in whom increasing the medication dose may result in excessive side effects. "Relaxation training" is a generic term that describes a variety of different procedures, including progressive muscle relaxation, tensing and releasing muscle groups, deep breathing, visual imagery, audiogenic training, repeating statements suggesting a relaxed state, and learning to produce postures and activities characteristic of a relaxed person. Whether it works by directly affecting the tic disorder or indirectly by helping the patient deal more effectively with the stress level is unclear.

Attention Deficit Hyperactivity Disorder

As in all children with ADHD, a variety of behavioral and educational approaches should be implemented before pharmacotherapy is considered. The treating physician should work with school authorities to achieve a program providing moderate structure and flexibility. We often advocate the use of assignment sheets, preferential seating, classroom breaks, changes of tasks, color coding of text and notebooks, shortened classroom and homework assignments, and, if appropriate, the use of computers.

Although psychostimulant medications are generally regarded as the treatment of choice for ADHD, their use in children with TS is controversial because of the potential to provoke or intensify tics. Hence in the child with tics and ADHD, we currently begin with a trial of clonidine as described above. Because clonidine dosages may be an important factor, we utilize this medication in the range of 4 to 5 micrograms per kg per day, given in four daily doses (average dose is 0.05 mg four times daily). If ADHD symptoms are not well controlled, we switch to another medication. In the patient who is not receiving a tic-suppressing agent, we begin a trial with desipramine hydrochloride (Norpramin).* Before initiating desipramine therapy, we require a normal baseline ECG or approval by a cardiologist in questionable situations. Desipramine therapy is initiated at a dose not exceeding 25 mg and is gradually increased on a weekly basis, if necessary, to a maximum dose of 3 mg per kg. Follow-up ECGs are obtained. If both clonidine and desipramine are ineffective in a patient not receiving a tic-suppressing medication, a brief trial with a central stimulant (methylphenidate [Ritalin]) is initiated (see later). If the child improves and tics are not exacerbated, methylphenidate therapy is maintained, whereas if the ADHD improves, but tics worsen, the drug is withdrawn and further trials with either another stimulant (pemoline [Cylert]) or an alternative medication (nortriptyline [Pamelor], selegiline [Eldepryl])* are begun.

---

*Not FDA-approved for this indication.
†Not available in the United States.

*Not FDA-approved for this indication.

Another common scenario occurs with a child who is already being treated with tic-suppressing medication but is having problems with ADHD. In this instance, if the patient's tics are being well controlled with the administration of either clonidine or a neuroleptic, then methylphenidate is added for the target symptom of ADHD. Our starting dose is 5 mg in the morning before the child leaves for school. After 1 week of treatment, if the desired therapeutic effect has not been achieved, the dose is increased by an additional 5 mg. On a dose-per-kilogram basis, our initial dose is in the range of 0.3 mg per kg with increases to about 0.6 mg per kg. In those instances in which ADHD symptoms become worse in the afternoon, an additional dose of medication may be administered 3 to 4 hours after the first dose. If symptoms persist after several weeks, the medication is changed by utilizing other pharmacotherapies for ADHD (described earlier).

Obsessive-Compulsive Disorder

In TS patients with severely disabling obsessive-compulsive symptoms, additional therapeutic and behavioral modification techniques should be considered. Several antidepressant medications that are selective serotonin re-uptake inhibitors (SSRIs), including fluoxetine (Prozac), clomipramine (Anafranil), and sertraline (Zoloft),* may be beneficial. Fluoxetine is generally our initial drug because it tends to be better tolerated, producing less sedation and appetite suppression. In older children and adults we begin with 20 mg each morning, recognizing that older individuals may require doses up to 60 mg per day. Fluoxetine has been used in conjunction with clonidine and pimozide.

Other Behavior Disorders

Argumentativeness, disruptive behavior, temper tantrums, conduct disorder, anxiety, and depression are relatively common problems encountered in patients with TS. In many individuals these difficulties are co-mingled with ADHD and OCD, providing a complex challenge for the family and physician. In our experience some behavior disturbances improve or at least become more acceptable after pharmacotherapy directed at accompanying associated problems. We are also impressed at how symptoms of childhood depression are often intertwined and manifested by inattentiveness and agitated behaviors. Appropriate interventions may include counseling for the family unit, behavior modification, educational intervention, and psychiatric referral. A multidisciplinary team approach is strongly advocated.

SUMMARY

The physician caring for individuals with TS should be prepared to address a variety of issues, in addition to the diagnosis and therapy of tics. Initial goals are to clarify each of the patient's problems, to determine whether the major source of stress is related to tics or associated behaviors, and to develop an individualized multimodal treatment program. Discussing the treatment of co-morbid symptoms as separate entities from tics has enabled families and health care specialists to focus on individual needs more effectively. The nonprofit Tourette Syndrome Association, 40-42 Bell Boulevard, Bayside, New York 11361-9596, telephone number 718-224-2999, is a highly recommended source of information.

HEADACHE

method of
ROBERT S. KUNKEL, M.D.
Cleveland Clinic
Cleveland, Ohio

Headache is certainly one of the most common complaints seen in the physician's office. The vast majority of headaches are not due to any serious disease and are not related to structural or organic conditions. Although many patients with chronic headache continue to expect a "cure" by their physician, in reality a cure of chronic headache is very rare. Headache due to infection or some other disease may often be curable, but the chronic primary headache syndromes such as migraine, cluster, and tension-type headache are not curable but are usually controllable. Helping the person with chronic headache involves much time and patience on the part of the treating physician.

Migraine, cluster, and tension-type headaches are called "primary headache syndromes" because there is no known anatomic or structural abnormality. Although the pathophysiology is poorly understood, it is now felt that these headaches involve the central nervous system as well as peripheral mechanisms involving the blood vessels, nerves, mucous membranes, and muscles. Many people feel that chronic headache can best be classified as a headache continuum with typical migraine on one end and tension-type on the other. Cluster headache has enough unique features to separate it from this theory. There is no doubt that many patients have headaches that are hard to classify as to whether they are indeed tension-type or migraine, but I believe that in the majority of patients, one can make a diagnosis of either tension-type headache or migraine from the history. Many patients seen in headache clinics have a mixed headache pattern with both migraine and tension-type headache. These headaches often overlap and blend together, and it may be difficult to separate when one headache begins and the other ends.

CLASSIFICATION

A simple classification of headache divides headaches into vascular types, muscle tension–type, and traction and inflammatory headaches. Traction and inflammatory headaches account for the headaches due to diseases that cause distortion, compression, or inflammation of the intracranial structures and inflammation of the pericranial tissues. Migraine and cluster headaches are felt to be of a vascular nature, although the central nervous system is undoubtedly the source of the initiation of each attack. There is

---

*Not FDA-approved for this indication.

increasing evidence that tension-type headache is also likely due to a central nervous system disorder, although there are many patients in whom muscle spasms of the neck and scalp muscles play a prominent role in the pain. Tension-type headache is usually not disabling and often responds to simple over-the-counter medications. Correcting stress or learning relaxation techniques may also be helpful.

In 1988, the International Headache Society (IHS) proposed a new classification of headache. Table 1 lists the major headings of this very complex and detailed classification—a hierarchical type in which headaches can be classified according to as much detail as desired. There are several varieties of migraine and variants of cluster headache. Tension-type headache is classified as to whether evidence of muscle spasm or tension is present and whether the headache is episodic or of a chronic nature, which by definition means that headache is present more than 15 days a month.

The IHS classification is very helpful for those doing research in headache because each category is followed by specific diagnostic criteria. By fulfilling these criteria one will have a uniform sample of headache patients of any specific type, and therefore research should be more reproducible.

One of the classifications of headache that has not been proposed before is that due to the use or abuse of chemical agents or drugs. Of increasing importance in the management of chronic headache is that many persons suffering from chronic headache take excessive amounts of daily analgesics and many of these compounds also contain caffeine. Frequent ergotamine use can cause rebound vascular-type headache, and the daily intake of analgesic compounds, particularly those containing caffeine, can lead to chronic headache resulting from dependency on these substances. Chronic use of analgesics may cause depletion of endorphins and therefore may perpetuate pain sensation.

The first three headache types are the primary headache syndromes and the remaining categories are those due to diseases or structural abnormalities.

In the evaluation and diagnosis of the cause of a headache problem, the history and physical examination are most important. Rarely do diagnostic tests disclose an unsuspected cause if the physician has taken a thorough history and done a good physical and neurologic examination. Any headache of recent onset warrants diagnostic testing. Other "red flags" that may warrant imaging or other testing are a change in one's headache pattern or the development of new symptoms. Migraine headache is not uncommonly associated with neurologic symptoms and at least one imaging study should be done on all patients with migraine who have neurologic abnormalities. Occasionally an arteriovenous malformation of the brain can mimic migraine.

HEADACHES DUE TO DISEASE

Headaches due to organic origin are usually of rather recent onset. The headache due to a mass lesion in the brain is generally accompanied by neurologic abnormalities. It is rare for a brain tumor to present with only headache as a symptom. Usually neurologic symptoms and signs are present. Inflammatory conditions involving any of the areas of the head should be readily apparent from the history and be evident on physical examination.

In someone older than 50 years of age, tic douloureux (trigeminal neuralgia) and temporal arteritis are conditions usually amenable to treatment. Anyone having a new onset of headache after age 50 years should be evaluated for temporal arteritis. Tic douloureux presents such a typical pattern with trigger points about the face that the diagnosis is generally readily apparent. Temporal arteritis, however, can present with any type of headache, and early in the course, the fatigue and visual symptoms are rare. It is important to make this diagnosis to prevent visual loss. The sedimentation rate is almost always elevated in temporal arteritis. Mild anemia and low-grade fever may be present as well.

Post-traumatic headache can present as either a tension-type headache or a more typical migraine-type of headache. Usually the history of a head injury is obtained. Flexion-extension injuries of the neck, which are so common in motor vehicle accidents, can lead to neck pain and general headache.

Treatment of Organic Headache

Infection of the sinuses, ears, or dental structures should be treated with proper antibiotics. Brain neoplasms or subdural hematomas need to be treated surgically. Tic douloureux is usually treated medically. Carbamazepine (Tegretol) is the preferred medication and is usually started with a dose of 200 mg a day, which is then gradually increased up to a total of 1200 mg a day in divided doses. Side effects of carbamazepine include nausea, dizziness, and ataxia. Rarely, leukopenia will occur; routine blood checks are warranted in a patient receiving this medication. Phenytoin (Dilantin)* in a dosage of 300 to 400 mg a day may also be useful in the medical management of trigeminal neuralgia. Other medications that are

TABLE 1. **1988 International Headache Society Classification (Major Categories)**

1. Migraine
   Migraine without aura
   Migraine with aura
2. Tension-type headache
   Episodic tension-type headache
   Chronic tension-type headache
3. Cluster headache
4. Miscellaneous headache without structural lesion
5. Headache associated with head trauma
6. Headache associated with vascular disorders
7. Headache associated with nonvascular intracranial disorders
8. Headache associated with substances or their withdrawal
9. Headache associated with noncephalic infection
10. Headache associated with metabolic disorder
11. Headache or facial pain associated with disorder of cranium, neck, eyes, ears, nose, sinuses, teeth, mouth, or other facial or cranial structures
12. Cranial neuralgias, nerve trunk pain, and deafferentation pain
13. Headache not classifiable

Reprinted from Classification and diagnostic criteria for headache disorders, cranial neuralgias and facial pain by Oleson J from Cephalalgia, 1988, Vol. 8, Suppl. 7, p. 1, by permission of Scandinavian University Press.

*Not FDA-approved for this indication.

less effective but that at times may be helpful include clonazepam (Klonopin)* and baclofen (Lioresal).*

If treatment with any of the medications fails, the patient should be referred to neurosurgery and one of the surgical procedures for this condition may be indicated. Radiofrequency or glycerol lesioning of the trigeminal ganglion in Meckel's cave may be tried. Posterior fossa decompression of the trigeminal nerve root (Jennetta's procedure) can be performed but it requires a craniotomy with the increased risk of morbidity.

Temporal arteritis should be diagnosed promptly. It should be suspected if there is an elevated sedimentation rate. The diagnosis is confirmed with a temporal artery biopsy. Prednisone 60 to 80 mg daily should be started at once and slowly tapered. Patients often have to be on corticosteroid treatment for several months or even a few years. Prednisone should be tapered over a few months to the lowest dose that keeps the sedimentation rate within the normal range. If this condition is not promptly treated, 30 to 50% of persons with temporal arteritis will suffer some permanent visual deficit. Other neurologic deficits can occur from temporal arteritis.

TENSION–TYPE (MUSCLE CONTRACTION) HEADACHE

Tension-type headache, which has been previously known as muscle contraction or tension headache, is the most common type. The IHS classification splits tension-type headache into "episodic," meaning that headache is present less than 15 days a month, and "chronic" tension-type headache, which implies headache is present on more than half the days.

A term used frequently in the United States, "chronic daily headache," is not in the IHS classification. Chronic daily headache is often a useful term for those patients who have headaches on a daily basis that at times may be of a tension type and at other times seem to be more migrainous. In the IHS classification, this person would be diagnosed as having two headaches—tension-type and migraine. People suffering with tension-type headache usually describe their discomfort as a feeling of pressure or tightness in the head. A feeling of a tight band around the head is the classic description. Others will feel that the skin is too tight. Tension-type headache is usually bilateral but at times is localized. The neck and shoulders are often tight and tense. The ongoing debate as to whether the pain actually arises in the scalp muscles is due to the fact that some electromyography (EMG) studies have failed to show any increased amount of muscle tension in the scalp muscles, whereas in other persons with the same description of symptoms EMG studies do show increased levels of muscle tension. There is a question as to whether EMG studies on the superficial scalp muscles are reliable because of the different techniques used and because of the fact that patients

with migraine often have more evidence of excessive muscle contraction than do persons complaining of typical tension-type headache.

Depression is often present in people with chronic tension-type headache and many persons cannot identify any specific stress or tension factors. As mentioned previously, the daily use of analgesics and caffeine-containing compounds is often a problem in patients with chronic tension-type headache and management may be quite difficult until these compounds are removed from daily use.

Some conditions can lead to chronic tension-type headache—diseases of the temporomandibular joint and cervical spine and chronic infection or inflammation in structures of the head. Reflex muscle spasm can cause pain owing to injury or irritation.

The temporomandibular joint syndrome, which has also been called myofascial pain dysfunction syndrome, is of much interest to anyone dealing with headache patients, including dentists. In the past, specific causes such as bite problems and disease of the temporomandibular joint have been overdiagnosed. Many patients have undergone extensive surgery and restorative dental work with no relief. The majority of patients with pain in and about the muscles and ligaments of the temporomandibular joint suffer from stress and tension and the muscle pain is caused from excessive clenching or grinding of the teeth. This is called "bruxism." These patients respond to muscle relaxation, heat, relaxation exercises, and stress reduction techniques.

Treatment of Tension-Type Headache

The treatment of tension-type headache can be difficult. The episodic tension-type headache is usually well treated with simple analgesics. People with episodic tension-type headache generally do not come to the physician for help. It is important that one explain to the patient that even though there is no organic disease present, the pain is usually real and rarely due to an underlying psychiatric problem. A thorough history and physical examination are essential to reassure patients as to the lack of any underlying disease. Many patients find relief by following an active physical therapy program, especially if there is evidence of spasm in the neck and shoulder muscles or poor posture. Range-of-motion exercises and postural improvement exercises done on a regular daily basis by these patients are often beneficial. The use of hot packs or a hot shower followed by massage can also be helpful, but this needs to be done on a regular daily basis and not once or twice a week at some provider's office. Occasionally cervical traction may be indicated, especially if there is evidence of some underlying degenerative disk disease in the neck.

In addition to an active exercise program for the neck and shoulders, biofeedback and relaxation training may be helpful for many patients with chronic tension-type headache. Patients who are successful with biofeedback are motivated enough to

---

*Not FDA-approved for this indication.

practice these techniques daily and to work them into their daily life. Many patients unfortunately hope that biofeedback techniques will be a quick cure for their pain and are unwilling to spend the time and effort involved in practicing these techniques. Younger people seem to do better with biofeedback training.

In the pharmacologic management of chronic tension-type headache, tranquilizers and pain relievers, which may cause dependency and addiction, should be avoided if at all possible. By far the most common problems seen in headache clinics are patients who are dependent on daily doses of compounds containing barbiturates and caffeine. For prophylactic treatment of chronic tension-type headache, the medication of choice is one of the tricyclic antidepressant (TCA) compounds. Amitriptyline (Elavil),* doxepin (Sinequan, Adapin),* and nortriptyline (Pamelor)* are the three most commonly used TCAs. These are generally given in a single bedtime dose and the dosage needed for headache is usually less than what is needed for the treatment of depression. Many patients experience relief of headache with 10 to 50 mg of amitriptyline, doxepin, or nortriptyline at bedtime. Cyclobenzaprine (Flexeril),* another TCA, can also be used in a dosage of 10 mg one to three times daily. It is very sedating and many patients cannot tolerate it during the day. Ten to 20 mg may be useful in a single bedtime dose. All of these TCAs produce unpleasant side effects, such as dryness of the mouth, constipation, sedation, and increased appetite. They should not be used in patients with narrow-angle glaucoma or prostatism. Cardiac arrhythmias may also limit their use. This is generally not a severe problem. Trazodone (Desyrel)* may be helpful in causing sleep and lacks the unpleasant anticholinergic effects of the TCAs.

The new antidepressants, called "selective serotonin reuptake inhibitors," such as fluoxetine (Prozac),* sertraline (Zoloft),* and paroxetine (Paxil),* along with venlafaxine (Effexor)* and nefazodone (Serzone), are better tolerated in that they lack the anticholinergic side effects of the TCAs and usually do not increase appetite. In fact they may be helpful as anorexics. Unfortunately they do not seem to be nearly as effective in the treatment of chronic head pain as the TCAs. In a patient suffering depression, of which the headache may be a manifestation, this group of medications may be very useful.

Nonsteroidal anti-inflammatory drugs (NSAIDs) can also be useful in treating patients with chronic tension-type headache. They have an analgesic effect and do not seem to be habituating. However, long-term use of these agents is frequently associated with gastrointestinal problems and patients on these medications for a long time must be closely monitored for any renal or hepatic dysfunction. Naproxen (Naprosyn) or flurbiprofen (Ansaid) are most commonly used on a regular daily basis. At times they can be used along with the TCAs with good benefit.

Tranquilizers and analgesics for the most part need to be avoided in patients with chronic tension-type headache because of the habituation problem. It is very difficult to make any progress in improving pain as long as the patient is dependent on a large amount of analgesics and/or caffeine. Many patients take caffeine-containing compounds every 3 to 4 hours to keep their headache under control. A good clue to the fact that patients may be dependent and habituated to caffeine or analgesics is that they awaken every morning with a headache, and only those compounds containing caffeine or barbiturates are helpful in relieving the discomfort. The head pain recurs several hours after dosing. One must get patients off their daily analgesics before progress can be made in controlling their headache.

There are times when one might want to use an anxiolytic such as diazepam (Valium)* on a temporary basis. Diazepam is a very good muscle relaxant as well as a tranquilizer. One should set some guidelines, however, and use it only for a short period of time to relieve obvious muscle spasm. Buspirone (BuSpar)* is an antianxiety agent that lacks dependency potential and can be safely used for longer periods of time.

Persons with chronic daily headache in which there may be a migrainous component often respond to a combination of a TCA and a beta blocker such as propranolol (Inderal) or nadolol (Corgard).* The fatigue that occasionally occurs with these beta blockers may be intolerable, particularly if they are taken along with a very sedating TCA.

MIGRAINE HEADACHE

Migraine is an inherited disorder in which the intracranial and extracranial vessels seem to be extraordinarily sensitive to various stimuli. It is felt that the basic disorder in migraine is a cyclical dysfunction of central neuro-autoregulation. The underlying pathophysiology is at this time poorly understood. Migraine is a complex syndrome in which hormonal changes, various humoral factors including platelet agglutination, and alterations in vasoactive amines all play a role in the initiation of the migraine attack.

Migraine is an intermittent disorder in which there is usually a pulsating, throbbing headache on one side of the head that is accompanied by nausea and/or vomiting, photophobia, phonophobia, and disability. Typically the pain is worsened with activity and one usually retreats to a dark, quiet room during the attack. Anorexia and/or nausea and vomiting are the most common symptoms of migraine other than headache. The headache is usually unilateral but can occur bilaterally. A few patients can have migrainous symptoms without much headache, but in the majority of patients the headache is the most prominent symptom. Other symptoms accompanying the migraine attack include chills and sweating, diar-

---

*Not FDA-approved for this indication.

*Not FDA-approved for this indication.

rhea, and sensitivity to odors. Many women note that there is a menstrual relationship to their headache in that the headaches are worse around their periods and often remit during pregnancy. After menopause, migraine may greatly improve.

The most common type of migraine is called "migraine without aura," which used to be known as common migraine. Perhaps 80 to 85% of patients with migraine suffer from this type of headache. By definition, this migraine attack is not preceded by a distinct visual or neurologic aura. The remaining 15 to 20% of patients with migraine have "migraine with aura" (classic migraine) that is preceded by visual or neurologic symptoms lasting 15 to 60 minutes. By definition, in the IHS classification the headache must follow the aura within 1 hour.

It is not well appreciated that there are several other variations of migraine. Basilar migraine (basilar artery migraine, vertebrobasilar migraine), ophthalmoplegic migraine, and hemiplegic migraine are not common but do occur and need to be differentiated from other neurologic problems. Basilar migraine is the most common of these three variants; it is accompanied by neurologic symptoms emanating from the areas supplied by the posterior cerebral circulation. Patients with basilar migraine have diplopia, ataxia, hearing changes, speech abnormalities, and often a posteriorly located headache.

Often not well recognized are migraine symptoms that occur in the absence of a headache. These used to be called migraine equivalents or acephalgic migraine. The term used in the IHS classification is "migraine aura without headache." These symptoms can be quite disturbing and frightening. They usually occur in a patient who has had migraine or who has a strong family history of migraine. These symptoms need to be differentiated from transient neurologic ischemic symptoms. In addition to the visual and neurologic symptoms occurring without headache, occasional attacks of periodic nausea and vomiting, vertigo, and mental confusion can be manifestations of migraine without headache. These variants of migraine should be considered in anyone who has recurring neurologic or visual symptoms with no evidence of neurologic disease on testing.

Treatment of Migraine

The treatment of migraine begins when the diagnosis is made and an explanation is given to the patient as to what this condition actually is. Migraine rarely leads to any permanent neurologic sequelae. In rare instances a cerebral infarct will occur during a migraine attack. When this occurs, it usually does not lead to permanent neurologic deficits but the symptoms may linger for several weeks.

Although patients with migraine are severely disabled at times, in general this is a benign condition. An important first step in managing migraine is to help the migraine sufferer identify various trigger factors that may play a role in bringing on attacks. Patients with migraine need to avoid excessive fa-

tigue and tiredness and should eat on a fairly regular basis. Variable living habits seem to make a patient prone to migraine attacks. Skipping meals can be a trigger in many patients. An attempt should be made to identify other trigger mechanisms such as dietary, biochemical, or emotional factors. Weather changes with low-pressure fronts seem to set off migraine in many patients. Such weather changes are of course unavoidable. Allergies rarely play a role in triggering migraine but certain dietary substances can provoke attacks through their chemical action. It is very helpful to have a patient keep a diary in which she or he records foods ingested in the 24 hours prior to the onset of the migraine attack. About 10% of patients with migraine can identify food substances that trigger attacks. Table 2 lists food substances that have been reported to trigger migraine attacks.

Estrogens, when used in a cyclical nature, may also provoke migraine headache attacks. This does not seem to occur as frequently now that oral contraceptives contain lower doses. The fluctuation of estrogen in the body seems to be the most common hormonal trigger. Postmenopausal women should take estrogen on a regular daily basis and not skip days. If the uterus is intact, then progesterone needs to be taken on either a cyclical basis or a daily basis.

In addition to estrogens, other medications may aggravate migraine headaches. The vasodilating drugs used for the treatment of coronary artery disease and high blood pressure can aggravate migraine. Nitrates, hydralazine, prazosin (Minipress), and the calcium channel blockers, particularly nifedipine (Procardia), can induce or aggravate migraine. Other medications that can aggravate migraine include reserpine, indomethacin (Indocin), and the aminophylline compounds. Daily use of analgesic compounds containing caffeine and frequent use of ergotamine tartrate can also be factors in the frequency and severity of attacks.

Although attacks can be reduced by identifying certain trigger factors, most patients require pharmacologic treatment for migraine. Almost all patients need to take an abortive medication at the time of the attack. The physician needs to decide whether the headaches are frequent or severe enough to warrant treatment with daily prophylactic medication. In general, if migraine occurs more than 3 times monthly, daily prophylactic medication should be considered. Occasionally less frequent migraine may require prophylactic therapy if the attacks are uncon-

TABLE 2. **Food Substances That May Trigger Migraine**

Chocolate	Yogurt
Aged cheese	Freshly baked bread
Red wine	Monosodium glutamate
Alcohol	Preservatives in meat
Vinegar	Pickled herring
Onions	Chicken livers
Bananas	Excessive salt
Citrus fruits	Aspartame (Nutrasweet)

trolled with abortive medication or the headaches are quite prolonged in duration.

At times the physician might consider prescribing intermittent prophylactic therapy. This is often useful in a woman who has her only migraine attack during her menstrual period. When the menstrual period occurs on a very regular schedule, it is often beneficial to treat that person with a prophylactic drug started a few days before the period is due. The use of the estrogen patch has occasionally been helpful when used for a period of 10 days around the menstrual period. A combination of belladonna extract, ergotamine, and phenobarbital (Bellergal-S) has also been used intermittently at the time of the period with occasionally good results. The NSAIDs such as naproxen (Naprosyn) or flurbiprofen (Ansaid) can at times be very beneficial and can be used intermittently, starting a few days before the onset of menses. In women who have a lot of fluid retention, the use of a diuretic for a few days before the period often modifies the severity of the menstrually related migraine attack.

The aim of any prophylactic therapy is to reduce the severity and frequency of migraine attacks. It is unreasonable to assume that migraine can be completely controlled, but often the use of any of the prophylactic agents described later in this article can give very satisfactory results, with many patients having very few migraine attacks.

Prophylactic Treatment of Migraine (Table 3)

Beta-Blocking Agents. Propranolol (Inderal, Inderal-LA) and timolol (Blocadren) are the only two beta blockers approved by the Food and Drug Administration (FDA) in the United States for the prophylactic treatment of migraine. Propranolol is the most widely used preventive agent for migraine in the United States. Other commonly used beta blockers include nadolol (Corgard),* metoprolol (Lopressor),* and atenolol (Tenormin).* All these agents have been reported to be beneficial in the prophylaxis of migraine. The usual doses are listed in Table 3. Severe tiredness and fatigue are the most common side effects and occur perhaps in about 10% of users. None of these beta-blocking agents should be used in an individual who has severe heart failure or heart block. Allergic asthma is also a contraindication, although occasionally the selective beta blockers such as atenolol and metoprolol may be used with extreme caution. Beta blockers should also be used with caution in patients with labile diabetes and those with severe peripheral vascular disease.

The beneficial effects of the beta-adrenergic blocking drugs are not well understood. They have many effects in the body. The prevention of dilatation of arteries may be important but effects on platelet aggregation and stabilization of cell membranes are undoubtedly also important. In addition to the side effect of fatigue, gastrointestinal disturbances, in-

TABLE 3. **Drugs Used for the Prophylaxis of Migraine**

Preparation	Daily Dosage (mg)
Beta Blockers	
Propranolol (Inderal, Inderal LA)*	80–240
Metoprolol (Lopressor, Toprol XL)	50–100
Nadolol (Corgard)	40–120
Atenolol (Tenormin)	50–100
Timolol (Blocadren)*	10–20
Calcium Channel Blockers	
Verapamil (Calan, Isoptin, Verelan)	120–480
Diltiazem (Cardizem, Dilacor XR)	120–480
Nimodipine (Nimotop)	90–120
Nicardipine (Cardene)	40–80
Flunarizine (Sibelium, not in U.S.)	10–30
Nonsteroidal Anti-Inflammatory Drugs	
Naproxen (Naprosyn)	500–1000
Flurbiprofen (Ansaid)	100–200
Ibuprofen (Motrin, Rufen)	400–2400
Fenoprofen (Nalfon)	800–1600
Antidepressant Medications	
Amitriptyline (Elavil, Endep)	10–100
Doxepin (Sinequan, Adapin)	10–100
Nortriptyline (Pamelor)	10–100
Protriptyline (Vivactil)	10–40
Fluoxetine (Prozac)	20–60
Sertraline (Zoloft)	50–100
Phenelzine (Nardil)	30–60
Anticonvulsants	
Divalproex (Depakote)	500–1500
Phenytoin (Dilantin)	100–300
Serotonin Antagonists	
Methysergide (Sansert)*	4–8
Cyproheptadine (Periactin)	8–16
Alpha-Adrenergic Agonists	
Clonidine (Catapres)	0.2–0.4
Guanabenz (Wytensin)	8–16

*Approved by the FDA as effective for migraine prophylaxis.

somnia, and deepening of an underlying depression can occasionally occur with use of these medicines.

As can be seen by the dosages listed in Table 3, the dose range of effectiveness is quite variable. One should start with a low dose and gradually increase the dosage until a beneficial effect is obtained or until side effects or bradycardia become prevalent. Many times physicians give up on these prophylactic agents before increasing the dose to an effective level. One needs to be patient and to continually increase the dosage to obtain maximal benefit.

As with any prophylactic agent, once headache frequency and severity are well controlled for several months, attempts should be made to lower the daily dosage. Many patients can get along with a lower dose once the attacks are controlled.

Calcium Channel Blockers. Verapamil (Calan, Isoptin, Verelan)* is fairly effective in reducing the number of migraine attacks. The calcium channel blockers have not been approved by the FDA nor are they listed as antimigraine agents by the manufacturer. Diltiazem (Cardizem, Dilacor)* can also be useful in preventing migraine and may cause less

---

*Not FDA-approved for this indication.

*Not FDA-approved for this indication.

constipation than does verapamil. Nimodipine (Nimotop)* has been reported to be effective in migraine but in practice does not seem to be very beneficial. It is very costly to use and needs to be taken several times a day. Likewise nicardipine (Cardene)* will occasionally be helpful but is not used very often.

Nifedipine (Procardia)* is used by some to prevent migraine but should usually be avoided because it induces vascular headache in 20 to 25% of those patients who are put on this drug. It is a very potent dilator of vessels and often aggravates the underlying migraine situation.

Calcium channel blockers inhibit the movement of calcium ions into the smooth muscle cells of the arterioles. It is felt that by blocking calcium entry into the smooth muscles, vascular spasm is controlled. It is assumed that this phenomenon plays a major role in the effectiveness of these agents in controlling migraine, although there are undoubtedly other effects that also play a beneficial role. Side effects of verapamil include constipation and occasionally fluid retention. On rare occasions even verapamil tends to exacerbate the underlying migraine by causing more throbbing in the head.

The doses used are shown in Table 3. Most persons will use the long-acting form of verapamil at a dose of 180 to 240 mg as a start. The maximal benefit from the use of verapamil in migraine may not occur for 6 to 8 weeks. Both the migraine sufferer and the physician must be very patient in its use.

Nonsteroidal Anti-Inflammatory Drugs. Many NSAIDs are on the market and many have been used with good beneficial effects in migraine. Some have a long duration of action and need to be taken only once or twice a day whereas others need to be taken three times a day. Naproxen (Naprosyn) and flurbiprofen (Ansaid) are the most commonly used prophylactic NSAIDs in migraine. The usual dose is twice a day but they can be used three times daily. Indomethacin (Indocin) has been used most widely for treatment of exercise-induced migraine. It rarely has a role in the daily prevention of ordinary migraine.

The beneficial effects of the NSAIDs are probably mediated through their antiprostaglandin activity. They must be used with caution in persons complaining of gastrointestinal disease and in those with chronic renal disease. Elderly persons with borderline renal function need to be treated very cautiously with NSAIDs. These drugs are contraindicated in persons with peptic ulcer disease. Side effects include fluid retention and gastric discomfort.

Antidepressant Medications. The TCAs are widely used for the treatment of both tension-type headache and migraine. The therapeutic effect probably occurs through their action on neurotransmitters such as serotonin and noradrenaline. Amitriptyline (Elavil, Endep),* doxepin (Sinequan, Adapin),* and nortriptyline (Pamelor)* are the most widely used TCAs for the treatment of migraine just as they are for the tension-type headache. They should be given at bedtime only and the dosage ranges from 10 to 100 mg. Serotonin reuptake inhibitors such as fluoxetine (Prozac)* and sertraline (Zoloft)* can also be used in migraine and have fewer side effects than the TCAs. As in tension-type headache, they are probably slightly less effective on the actual migraine headache.

Phenelzine (Nardil)* is a monoamine oxidase (MAO) inhibitor that is used with variable success in the treatment of migraine that has not responded to other medications. When using an MAO one must instruct the patient as to specific dietary and medication restrictions. The MAO inhibitors should not be used in persons with severe liver disease, congestive heart failure, or hypertension. Many over-the-counter drugs that have vasoconstrictive effects need to be avoided, as does meperidine (Demerol). The MAO inhibitors can be used with extreme caution in combination with low doses of the TCAs. The usual dose of phenelzine is 15 mg three or four times daily.

Anticonvulsants. Although phenytoin (Dilantin)* has been used on and off for many years, it has not been very effective in controlling migraine. Valproate (Depakote, Depakene)* has been found to be effective in the prophylactic treatment of migraine and occasionally of chronic headache. Valproate is an anticonvulsant that increases brain levels of gamma-aminobutyric acid (GABA). Its effect in migraine may be through its action on serotonergic transmission. The effective dose is usually between 500 and 1000 mg per day in divided doses. Doses up to 2000 mg have been used. The drug should be started at 250 mg a day and slowly increased to reduce the side effect of nausea that often will limit its use.

Nausea is the most common side effect but fatigue, tremor, and hair loss can also occur. The hair loss is temporary but patients should be warned about this possibility. Although hepatotoxicity has been reported in infants, this is not a problem in healthy adults.

The effects of valproate on migraine may not occur for many weeks. It is another prophylactic migraine agent that needs to be used for several weeks or even months before maximal benefit may be achieved, and it is important to discuss this with the patient.

Serotonin Antagonists. Methysergide (Sansert) is undoubtedly the most effective prophylactic agent for migraine available in the United States. However, it is not used very frequently for migraine because of the potential side effect of fibrotic reactions in various areas of the body. The development of fibrosis seems to be dose-related and rarely occurs when methysergide is used on an intermittent basis. The patient should take a drug holiday every 4 to 6 months for a period of 4 to 6 weeks. It is used with excellent results in cluster headache.

Methysergide should not be used in patients who have cardiovascular disease, hypertension, or peptic ulcer disease. The most common side effects are mus-

---

*Not FDA-approved for this indication.

*Not FDA-approved for this indication.

cle cramps, abdominal discomfort, and mental aberrations such as hallucinations.

The usual dosage of methysergide is 2 mg two to four times daily. Careful monitoring of the patient for the development of heart murmurs or bruits over peripheral arteries is essential. If the drug is stopped every 6 months, I do not think routine intravenous pyelograms need to be done, which has been advocated in the past to pick up early changes of retroperitoneal fibrosis.

In migraine, methysergide can be used for the intermittent prophylactic treatment of migraine around the menstrual period. A few people have cycles in which their migraine attacks are quite frequent and methysergide can be used intermittently for those patients just as it would be used in treating cluster headache attacks during the active cycle.

Cyproheptadine (Periactin) is an antiserotonin and antihistaminic that is useful in the treatment of migraine in children. It does not work as well in adults and is often accompanied by drowsiness and increased appetite. Children, however, seem to tolerate this drug very well and the usual dose is 4 mg one to four times daily.

Other Agents. Several drugs, although not usually effective, can at times be helpful in reducing the severity and frequency of migraine attacks. The alpha-stimulating antihypertensives such as clonidine (Catapres)* and guanabenz (Wytensin)* are at times helpful. Their use in treating migraine has diminished in recent years with the discovery of the effectiveness of calcium channel blockers. Alpha-stimulating antihypertensives are fairly well tolerated, although side effects such as fatigue, dryness of the mouth, and drowsiness may occur. The doses listed in Table 3 are used in divided doses twice daily.

Bellergal-S is a compound that contains phenobarbital, ergotamine tartrate, and alkaloids of belladonna. It may be fairly effective in controlling mild migraine attacks. Side effects are rare but it can induce drowsiness. One-half tablet may be quite effective in children who have frequent migraine attacks. It is also used fairly often for the intermittent prophylactic treatment of menstruation-related migraine.

Bellergal-S does contain ergotamine tartrate and one must be cautious about using ergotamine tartrate on a regular daily basis in order to avoid ergotamine-rebound headaches. This is rarely a problem, probably because of the low amount of ergotamine contained in the preparation. Lithium carbonate, which is so helpful in controlling cluster headache, is occasionally beneficial in migraine. It is usually used in migraine headaches that tend to occur in cycles or bunches. It may be effective for controlling menstruation-related migraine. The usual dosage is 300 mg three times daily. If one is on lithium carbonate for any length of time, blood levels need to be monitored, as do thyroid and renal function.

Antiplatelet agents have been tried in the prophylaxis of migraine because of the demonstration of platelet aggregation at the onset of many migraine attacks. However, the antiplatelet agents do not seem to be very effective. Double-blind studies have not shown them to be much more effective than placebo.

Abortive Therapy of Migraine (Table 4)

Abortive therapy is used for the treatment of acute migraine attacks. Even if a patient is on a daily prophylactic medication she or he will need to take an acute abortive agent when the attack occurs. Many patients do not want to take daily medication and want only abortive therapy. In general if the headaches occur more frequently than three to four times a month, prophylactic therapy should be offered in addition to the acute abortive therapy.

Vasoconstrictive Agents. Ergotamine tartrate has been used for many years in the treatment of migraine and still remains one of the most effective abortive agents for the acute attack. Unfortunately about 50% of patients who use ergotamine tartrate become quite nauseated and ill with the medication. In the United States, ergotamine tartrate is combined with caffeine in just about every formulation. It is available as an oral tablet and as a rectal suppository. Its main effect in aborting the migraine attack is felt to be its vasoconstrictive action. Ergotamine tartrate is contraindicated in persons with cardiovascular disease, hypertension, or chronic infection and those who are pregnant.

If ergotamine tartrate is taken orally, two tablets should be taken at once followed by one tablet in 1/2 hour if needed. At times one tablet will be enough. It is important that ergotamine be taken as early as possible during the migraine attack. If it is taken prior to the severe gastrointestinal distress that many patients with migraine get, it can often abort the attack. In those patients who are quite nauseated or who may have trouble with vomiting, the suppository form should be considered. One suppository is used at the onset of the headache, followed by another suppository in an hour or so. Many patients find that one-third or one-half of a suppository is adequate dosage since it is readily absorbed.

Dihydroergotamine (D.H.E. 45) is a parenteral form of ergotamine that can be given subcutaneously, intramuscularly, or intravenously. Many patients can be taught to give themselves an injection at the onset of the headache. Its real place in migraine has been with a protocol using it repetitively intravenously for 2 or 3 days to break up a prolonged migraine siege. Dihydroergotamine does not cause nausea or gastrointestinal upset as often as ergotamine tartrate and in general is better tolerated, although it is not effective orally.

Dihydroergotamine has been developed as a nasal spray* and this has proved to be quite effective and well accepted by patients. It is hoped that this will be available for use very soon.

---

*Not FDA-approved for this indication.

*Not yet approved for use in the United States.

TABLE 4. **Abortive Therapy for Acute Migraine Attacks**

Preparation	Dosing Schedule
Vasoconstrictive Agents	
Ergotamine tartrate (Cafergot, Wigraine)	
Oral	2 tablets at onset; 1 every ½ hour × 3 prn
Rectal	1 suppository at onset; 1 in 1 h prn
Sumatriptan (Imitrex)	
Subcutaneous	6 mg; may repeat within 24 h if headache recurs
Oral	25–50 mg; may repeat if necessary
Dihydroergotamine	
Parenteral (D.H.E. 45)	1 mg at onset intramuscularly; repeat up to 3 mg/day prn
	0.5 mg intravenously; repeat every 6–8 h × prn
Intranasal	1 spray each nostril; repeat in 15 min
Isometheptene (Midrin, Isocom)	2 at onset; 2 in 1 h and repeat 1–2 every 3 h prn
Nonsteroidal Anti-Inflammatory Drugs	
Meclofenamate (Meclomen)	2 at onset; 1 or 2 in 1 h prn
Ketorolac (Toradol)	
Oral (10 mg)	1 or 2 every 4 prn
Intramuscular (60 mg)	60 mg IM at onset of headache
Naproxen sodium (Anaprox DS)	1 or 2 at onset; repeat 1 in 2–3 h prn
Ibuprofen (Motrin, Rufen)	400–800 mg every 3–4 h prn
Corticosteroids	
Methylprednisolone (Medrol)	
Oral	Medrol Dosepak
Intramuscular	80 mg Depo-Medrol IM
Dexamethasone (Decadron)	
Oral	1.5 mg bid × 2 days
Intramuscular	8–16 mg Decadron-LA IM
Antiemetics	
Metoclopramide (Reglan)	10–20 mg prior to abortive drug
Phenothiazine	Variable; oral, rectal, parenteral

Isometheptene (Midrin, Isocom) is a mild vasoconstrictive agent. It is combined with acetaminophen and dichloralphenazone, a mild nonbarbiturate sedative. It is not as effective as ergotamine tartrate but is much better tolerated and produces very few side effects. At the very onset of migraine two capsules should be taken at once followed by one or two capsules in 1 hour. This can be repeated in 3 or 4 hours if necessary (limit of five capsules in 12 hours).

Recently, the introduction of sumatriptan (Imitrex) has been an important addition to the agents available for the treatment of acute migraine attacks. This can be given 6 mg subcutaneously by an autoinjector. Patients very quickly learn how to use this injector and the medication comes prepackaged in a syringe that is easily inserted into the injector and administered.

Many patients get an unpleasant burning sensation in the upper chest and neck area following the injection. This is transient. Occasionally a constriction or pressure effect is also felt in the neck and throat, which is sometimes quite disturbing but again is very transient. This constriction is not due to coronary artery spasm and is felt to be probably related to esophageal constriction. Sumatriptan not only stops the pain of migraine but also usually aborts the commonly associated symptoms such as nausea, photophobia, and phonophobia.

A 6-mg dose is administered at the onset of migraine. Seventy to 75% of patients will be free of headache within 1 hour. In those patients in whom the headache may recur within 24 hours, a second dose may be used. It does not seem to be helpful to repeat a dose within 1 hour if the initial dose does not stop the headache.

An oral form of sumatriptan is available. Because of its poor absorption, the oral tablets contain 25 and 50 mg of sumatriptan. One tablet is taken at once and this may be repeated if needed. The oral form should be better tolerated by those who experience the unpleasant constriction or burning immediately following the injectable form, but it will be slower acting.

Anti-Inflammatory Agents. Rapid-acting anti-inflammatory agents are often quite effective in aborting migraine attacks. They probably work through their antiprostaglandin and analgesic effects. Meclofenamate (Meclomen) is probably the most rapid-acting of this group and is often associated with fewer gastrointestinal symptoms. Occasionally diarrhea will occur. Two capsules are taken at once followed by two capsules in 1 hour if needed.

Ketorolac (Toradol) 10 mg at onset and 10 mg in 4 hours if needed is often helpful. Ketorolac also comes in an injectable form in which one would use 60 mg intramuscularly at the onset of the migraine attack. Naproxen sodium (Anaprox, Anaprox DS, Aleve) is a more rapid-acting form of naproxen (Naprosyn). One or two tablets are taken at onset followed by another tablet or two in a few hours.

Corticosteroids. Although corticosteroids should not be used very frequently, they are quite effective in aborting acute migraine attacks. Their use should be limited to about once a month. Either oral forms or intramuscular forms may be used. In a patient without severe nausea and vomiting, oral methylprednisolone (Medrol) in the form of a Medrol Dosepak can be used. Another effective regimen is dexamethasone (Decadron) 1.5 mg twice daily for 2 days.

If the patient is quite ill with nausea and vomiting, the intramuscular route is preferred. Depo-Medrol 80 mg or 8 to 16 mg of Decadron LA intramuscularly is often effective. Although these agents do not work very promptly, usually the headache is controlled within 24 hours.

Antiemetics. Because nausea and vomiting are so common during the migraine attack, antinauseants are often indicated. Not only will the symptoms of nausea and vomiting be reduced but these drugs will allow patients to take oral agents that may otherwise be vomited.

The phenothiazines, such as prochlorperazine (Compazine) and hydroxyzine (Vistaril), are very effective in controlling nausea and vomiting. They also have a sedative effect, which can be helpful. These medicines can be used by the oral, rectal, or parenteral route. Intravenous prochlorperazine has been reported to be helpful in stopping acute migraine attacks by itself.

Metoclopramide (Reglan) is an antinauseant that has been found to be very effective as an adjunctive aid in controlling nausea and promoting absorption of orally administered medication. Metoclopramide works on the gastric musculature and relaxes the pylorus. Very early on in the headache, 10 to 20 mg should be taken, following which a vasoconstrictive or analgesic agent may be used for relief of the pain.

Migraine Status. Occasional attacks of migraine linger for days and are nonresponsive to medications already discussed. In these situations long-acting steroids such as methylprednisolone (Depo-Medrol) 80 mg or dexamethasone (Decadron-LA) 12 mg can be given intramuscularly. If this does not break the attack then the dyhydroergotamine (D.H.E. 45) protocol should be considered. Although this can be accomplished to some degree on an outpatient basis, the patient is usually admitted for 3 days and 1 mg of dihydroergotamine is administered every 8 hours for a total of eight to ten doses. Generally an antinauseant is given prior to the intravenous bolus of dihydroergotamine. Corticosteroids can be used along with the dihydroergotamine.

This intravenous use of dihydroergotamine can be used to break up a migraine status or to control rebound headaches when the physician is trying to get a patient off a dependency on ergotamine tartrate or analgesics.

Nonpharmacologic Therapy. Biofeedback can be an alternative to pharmacologic management of migraine. Patients undergoing biofeedback training must be motivated to practice their techniques. This method of treatment works better in younger individuals and is particularly effective in children. In some patients who can tell when their headache is coming on, the attack may be aborted by biofeedback techniques. For the most part, however, it is used as a prophylactic adjunct to help reduce the stress and anxiety that may trigger or accompany the migraine attacks.

Migraine Aura Without Headache

Patients may suffer visual or neurologic symptoms of migraine without any headache being present. This may be a diagnostic problem when the attack occurs for the first or second time, but if these attacks are repetitive without any permanent neurologic sequelae, it is unlikely that these symptoms are due to any structural vascular abnormality and migraine needs to be considered. If these symptoms occur quite frequently, one of the prophylactic agents used for migraine should be instituted. Usually calcium channel blockers such as verapamil are the most effective in controlling the auras that occur without headache.

At times the auras may be quite disturbing, but if they do not occur frequently, one may not wish to use daily preventive medications. The use of sublingual nitroglycerine or sublingual nifedipine (Procardia)* at the onset of the aura symptoms often quickly aborts and clears the symptoms. Ordinarily these vasodilating agents cause headache in a patient with migraine, but if used very early in the aura, they rarely bring on an attack of migraine headache.

CLUSTER HEADACHE

Cluster headache is a periodic condition occurring mostly in males. Like migraine, it is a headache that involves both the central nervous system and the blood vessels of the head. This is a cyclical condition that is probably triggered by disturbances in the hypothalamus. There is good evidence of marked increase blood flow and dilatation of cerebral vessels during each individual attack. Parasympathetic overactivity and sympathetic underactivity account for some of the striking symptoms that accompany the severe pain of cluster headache. The cluster headache attacks are short, usually lasting less than 2 hours. They generally occur daily for a period of several weeks or months, following which the patient goes into a remission during which he or she is free of headaches for several months or even years. Some persons have several attacks in a 24-hour period. The attacks of cluster headache are almost exclusively unilateral and the pain is very intense. Autonomic symptoms such as redness and tearing of the ipsilateral eye and nasal stuffiness on the same side often accompany the painful attack. Unlike the pain of migraine, which is usually pulsatile in nature, the pain of cluster headache is generally of a steady burning nature, located in and around the eye, al-

---

*Not FDA-approved for this indication.

though the pain often does extend back into the sub-occipital area.

A small number of persons experience chronic cluster headache in which the attacks are typical of the acute episodic cluster pattern but periods of remission are not present. These are perhaps the most difficult headache patients to treat, since the pain is so severe and the headache has become chronic because of the failure of medication to induce remission. Addiction to narcotics is very common in patients with chronic cluster headache.

Treatment of Cluster Headache (Table 5)

Prophylactic Therapy of Cluster Headache

Prophylactic treatment of cluster headache is the preferred method. The attacks of pain are so quick and short that acute abortive agents are often not effective quickly enough. When a patient starts having a cluster headache, it is important to get that person on daily prophylactic agent. Verapamil is safe and well tolerated and can be used in persons with hypertension, ulcer disease, and cardiovascular disease, often present in these patients. Usually 240 to 720 mg daily is used. Unfortunately verapamil may take several weeks to be effective and one may want to use a quicker-acting agent, although side effects may be more prevalent.

A good combination is to start with prednisone 10 mg four times a day and verapamil. The prednisone is then tapered down by 10 mg each week and discontinued. The verapamil should be continued until the patient is free of headache for several weeks, following which it should be discontinued. Patients with peptic ulcer disease should not be put on corticosteroids such as prednisone.

Methysergide (Sansert) is a very effective treatment for cluster headache. If not contraindicated, it can be very useful. It is fairly expensive and verapamil has replaced methysergide as the therapeutic drug of choice. However, methysergide does work very quickly and should have the cluster headache

TABLE 5. **Therapy of Cluster Headache**

Prophylactic Therapy
Verapamil (Calan, Isoptin, Verelan)
Prednisone
Lithium carbonate
Methysergide (Sansert)
Divalproex (Depakote)
Nonsteroidal anti-inflammatory drugs

Abortive Therapy
Ergotamine tartrate
Dihydroergotamine (D.H.E. 45)
Sumatriptan (Imitrex)
Oxygen
Analgesics
Capsaicin (Zostrix)

Surgical Therapy
Radiofrequency lesion of trigeminal nerve
Glycerol lesion of trigeminal nerve
Posterior fossa decompression

under control within a few days. Methysergide can be used with either prednisone or verapamil. It should not be used longer than 4 months without a drug holiday. Since most cluster headache bouts do not last longer than a few weeks or months, treatment with methysergide is quite safe in patients with cluster headache.

The fourth effective drug that is used often is lithium carbonate.* It can be very effective, although it may take a few weeks to control the attacks. Generally 300 mg three times a day is used. Occasionally the dose will have to go higher, which can be monitored with blood levels.

Divalproex (Depakote)* 500 to 1500 mg in divided doses has been reported to be effective in cluster headache prophylaxis. Since we are just beginning to use this, experience has not been extensive in cluster headache. Occasionally the anti-inflammatory drugs such as naproxen (Naprosyn) or indomethacin (Indocin) can be helpful in controlling cluster attacks. Ergotamine tartrate 1 or 2 mg two or four times a day is also very effective and patients with cluster headache do not seem to get in an ergotamine-rebound situation. Ergotamine tartrate on a daily basis can be used with prednisone.

Histamine desensitization, which was administered subcutaneously in the past, has been found by some to be effective when used intravenously in a concentrated course. Generally it is given daily for 10 days with increasing doses being used. Other preventive medications such as lithium carbonate, prednisone, or verapamil are often given in conjunction with histamine desensitization, usually on an inpatient basis.

Abortive Therapy of Cluster Headache

As mentioned earlier, the most effective way to treat cluster headache is by putting the patient on a daily prophylactic medication or combination of medications. Ergotamine tartrate or an injection of sumatriptan (Imitrex) or dihydroergotamine (D.H.E. 45) can quickly stop an acute attack. Since many patients have two or three attacks a day, injection of these vasoconstrictive agents may not be practical.

Oxygen in 100% concentration given by mask at a rate of 7 liters a minute may shorten the attack of cluster headache in about 50% of patients. If the patient is having most of the attacks at night, an oxygen tank at the bedside may be very helpful. Oxygen should be used for no longer than 10 minutes per hour, since at high concentrations oxygen is a very potent vasoconstrictor and can cause pulmonary vascular constriction and subsequent fibrosis. The oxygen will be effective within 5 to 10 minutes and the patient gains nothing by continuing to use it for this period.

Various analgesics may be helpful. People have tried using intranasal capsaicin as either liquid drops or an ointment. The results are variable. The treatment itself is quite uncomfortable but after us-

*Not FDA-approved for this indication.

ing this daily for a few days, substance P in the nerve endings of the nasal mucosa seems to be depleted and the drug becomes better tolerated. Whether this will prove helpful is uncertain but currently most physicians have given up its use.

Surgical Treatment

For years, various surgical procedures have been attempted to control cluster headache in those patients who are unresponsive to the various pharmacologic agents mentioned previously. Section of the trigeminal nerve and the greater superficial petrosal nerve have been done in the past. Long-term results have been discouraging, although initially many patients have relief for a short period of time. Section of the vidian nerve ganglion has also been tried. More recently surgical therapy for chronic cluster headache has been attempted using either radiofrequency or glycerol on the trigeminal ganglion. Radiofrequency lesions, to be effective, need to be accompanied by facial numbness and this may lead to increased morbidity because of corneal anesthesia. The instillation of glycerol into Meckel's cave surrounding the gasserian ganglion may control cluster headaches in perhaps 30% of patients. Unfortunately the attacks tend to recur after a few weeks or a few months. This procedure can be repeated several times if necessary.

At times following the recurrence of headache after a surgical procedure the prophylactic medicines that were ineffective prior to the surgery are found to be effective.

It is my opinion that glycerol instillation or the radiofrequency lesion, whichever is preferred by the neurosurgeon doing the procedure, should be tried in those few patients who have failed to respond to any of the available prophylactic medications. By definition chronic cluster headache is a headache present for at least a year with no remission longer than 1 week. These patients have failed all available pharmacologic treatment.

MIXED HEADACHE

"Mixed headache" or "chronic daily headache" is a term used to describe headache patterns having more than one component. Generally "mixed headache" is used to describe a combination of tension-type and migraine headaches. These patients are usually dependent on large amounts of analgesics and/or caffeine. Some patients can separate the migraine from the tension component, but most cannot. As mentioned in the previous discussion on classification, this category is not included in the IHS classification.

Patients with mixed headaches are very difficult to treat because of the use and abuse of chronic medications. The physician must make every effort to detoxify them from caffeine and daily analgesics. Biofeedback may be helpful in these patients once they are off medications.

The most effective pharmacologic agents are the TCAs, as mentioned in the discussion on tension-type headache. The most effective treatment would be the TCAs combined with biofeedback, relaxation training, and often psychotherapy as indicated.

EPISODIC VERTIGO

method of
TIMOTHY C. HAIN, M.D.
Northwestern University
Chicago, Illinois

"Vertigo" is the sensation of rotational motion, and "episodic vertigo" denotes a vertigo that recurs in spells. Causes of episodic vertigo fall into three broad categories. *Otologic disturbances* include disorders of the inner ear such as benign paroxysmal vertigo and vestibular neuritis. Treatment of these disorders is often specific and effective. *Central nervous system disturbances* include entities such as migraine or stroke. Treatment of these disorders is often less effective, and considerable effort must usually be devoted to the prevention of recurrence. *Vertigo of uncertain origin* is, unfortunately, the most common "diagnosis." Management of patients in this category is necessarily empirical.

OTOLOGIC VERTIGO

Otologic disturbances (inner ear disease) account for most cases of episodic vertigo. Table 1 lists commonly encountered causes. There are five subcategories.

TABLE 1. **Common Causes of Otologic Vertigo**

Benign paroxysmal positional vertigo (BPPV)
    Classic form involving posterior canal
    Lateral canal form
Unilateral vestibular paresis or disturbance
    Labyrinthitis
    Vestibular neuritis
    Herpes zoster
    Syphilis and Lyme disease
    Mass lesions
        Acoustic neurinoma
        Meningioma
        Cholesteatoma
    Neurovascular compression
Meniere's disease
    Classic form
    Labyrinthine concussion
    Autoimmune form
Middle ear dysfunction
    Otosclerosis
    Eustachian tube malfunction
    TMJ dysfunction
    Otitis media
Fistula and other sources of pressure sensitivity
    Classic fistula
        Barotrauma, cholesteatoma, stapes surgery, Mondini malformation, syphilis
    Hypermobile stapes footplate
    Vestibular fibrosis
    Vestibular atelectasis
    Meniere's disease with pressure sensitivity
    Alternobaric vertigo

Benign Paroxysmal Positional Vertigo

Benign paroxysmal positional vertigo (BPPV) is the most common type of otologic vertigo. There has been dramatic improvement in the last 5 years in our management of BPPV.

BPPV is diagnosed by combining a history of positional vertigo with a typical nystagmus pattern (a burst of upbeating or torsional nystagmus) that appears on positional testing. Symptoms are precipitated by movement or position change of the head or body. Getting out of bed or rolling over in bed are the most common "problem" motions. A burst of nystagmus can often be provoked by placing the head in positions in which the posterior canal is made vertical.

It is currently thought that BPPV is caused by the presence of free otoconia within the semicircular canals, dislodged from the otolith organs by trauma, infection, or degeneration (Figure 1). Patients may be told that they have "ear rocks." The otoconial debris can move about by changes of head position, causing vertigo and nystagmus as they tumble through the semicircular canals. The duration of symptoms is brief, since dizziness occurs only while the debris shifts position.

Physical treatments based on manipulation of the head are the most effective treatment for BPPV. These maneuvers reposition the otolithic debris to an insensitive location within the inner ear. I use one or both of two maneuvers, the "Epley maneuver," and the "Brandt-Daroff exercises," in most patients.

The Epley maneuver as shown in Figure 2 (also known as the "canalith repositioning procedure," or CRP) is ordinarily my first treatment of BPPV. The maneuver is optimally performed on an adjustable examination table with side rails, putting the patient's head where the feet would ordinarily go. The table is adjusted so that there is a 20-degree angle between the head and trunk when the patient is lying down. The procedure can also be performed on a hospital bed, with the patient lying crossways on the bed. I occasionally premedicate anxious pa-

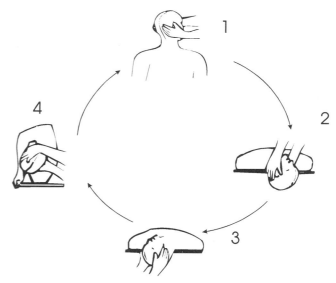

Figure 2. Epley's maneuver for office treatment of BPPV.

tients, or those who became very nauseated during Dix-Hallpike testing. Any of the vestibular suppressants in Table 2 will work, but the scopolamine patch (Transderm Scōp) is particularly convenient.

The Epley maneuver is performed as follows:

1. Start with the patient's head upright (Position 1 in Fig. 2).
2. Proceed into a Dix-Hallpike–provoking position (Position 2 in Figure 2). Wait until nystagmus stops. Then apply a hand-held massager to the mastoid region of the down ear. Wait another 30 seconds.
3. Turn the patient's head to the opposite side (Dix-Hallpike position, Position 3 in Figure 2). It is very important that the head be dependent (below horizontal) at this step. Wait another 30 seconds after nystagmus (if any) stops. Ideally, one sees a nystagmus similar to that of Step 2, beating toward the up ear. Use the massager again, on the same side as in Step 2.
4. Have the patient roll into the side-lying position, keeping the head-on-neck position as in Step 3, to obtain a 180-degree position with respect to Position 2 (Position 4 in Figure 2). Wait for nystagmus, if any, to stop. Apply massager, and then wait another 30 seconds. Again, one hopes to see a nystagmus beating toward the up ear.
5. Return the patient rapidly to a sitting position (Position 1), keeping the head-on-neck position the same as in Step 4 until the patient is entirely upright. Incline the head slightly forward, and wait 1 minute.
6. Repeat Steps 2 to 5 two more times. Stop if there is no dizziness or nystagmus at this point. If dizziness or nystagmus still occurs, keep repeating steps 2 to 5 to a maximum of six maneuvers completed. As each cycle takes roughly 3 minutes, this could take 20 minutes.

The patient sleeps semirecumbent (45-degree angle) for 2 days, usually using a lounge chair or

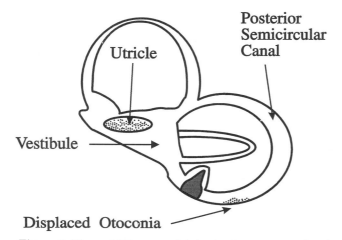

Figure 1. "Ear rock" theory explaining benign paroxysmal positional vertigo (BPPV).

TABLE 2. **Vestibular Suppressants, Arranged in Order of Preference**

Drug	Dose†	Adverse Reactions and Precautions	Pharmacologic Class
Meclizine (Antivert, Bonine)	25–50 mg q 4–6 h	Sedating Precautions in prostatic enlargement	Antihistamine, anticholinergic
Lorazepam (Ativan)*	0.5 mg bid	Mildly sedating Drug dependency	Benzodiazepine
Clonazepam (Klonopin)*	0.5 mg bid	Mildly sedating Drug dependency	Benzodiazepine
Scopolamine (Transderm Scōp)	0.5 mg patch q 3 days	Topical allergy with chronic use Precautions in glaucoma, tachyarrhythmias, prostatic enlargement	Anticholinergic
Dimenhydrinate (Dramamine)	50 mg q 4–6 h	Same as meclizine	Antihistamine, anticholinergic
Diazepam (Valium)*	2–10 mg (1 dose) given acutely PO, IM, or IV	Sedating Respiratory depressant Drug dependency Precaution in glaucoma	Benzodiazepine

*Not FDA-approved for this indication.
†Doses are all those used routinely for adults and are generally not appropriate for children.

couch. The patient avoids provoking positions for 1 week. I also advise the patients to sleep with the bad ear up and to use two pillows. Repeat examination and treatment are given at a 1-week follow-up visit. The patient is given the Vestibular Disorders Association handout on BPPV (Portland, Oregon). Most authors report an 80% or better cure rate at 1 week.

Occasionally, the Epley maneuver converts a classic "BPPV"-type positional nystagmus into a direction-changing horizontal nystagmus, which beats downward with respect to the dependent ear. This phenomenon, called "canal conversion," appears when debris has moved out of the posterior canal into the lateral canal ("lateral canal BPPV"). These patients uniformly do well.

For patients who fail the Epley maneuver, have recurrence, or in whom I am uncertain as to the side to treat, I proceed to the Brandt-Daroff exercises. In these exercises (Figure 3), patients repeatedly bring on their vertigo by going from the sitting to alternating side-lying positions. Five repetitions are performed three times per day for 2 weeks. This procedure helps more than 90% of patients with BPPV.

The main disadvantage of these exercises is the requirement that the vertigo be induced repeatedly over several weeks.

If the Brandt-Daroff exercises are ineffective in eliminating positional vertigo and the symptoms have persisted for a year or longer, a surgical procedure may be considered. Posterior canal plugging is presently the procedure of choice. However, because of the tendency of patients to improve spontaneously and also because the physical treatments of BPPV work so well when patients do not spontaneously improve, very few patients are referred for surgery.

Although drug treatment is not nearly as effective as the physical treatments described above, mild antiemetics such as meclizine (Antivert, Bonine) are helpful in patients with BPPV whose vertiginous spells are followed by nausea.

Vestibular Neuritis and Other Unilateral Vestibulopathies

Vestibular neuritis is a self-limited condition that presents with vertigo, nausea, ataxia, and nystag-

Figure 3. Brandt-Daroff maneuver for home treatment of BPPV.

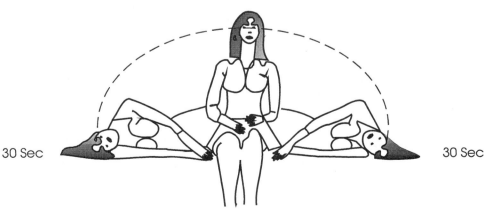

TABLE 3. **Antiemetics (Alphabetical Order)**

Drug	Usual Dose (Adults)*	Adverse Reactions	Pharmacologic Class
Droperidol (Inapsine)	2.5 or 5 mg, sublingually or IM q 12 h	Sedating Hypotension Extrapyramidal	Neuroleptic
Meclizine (Antivert, Bonine)	12.5–25 mg q 4–6 h PO	Sedating Precautions in glaucoma, prostate enlargement	Antihistamine and anticholinergic
Metoclopramide (Reglan)	10 mg PO tid or 10 mg IM	Restlessness or drowsiness Extrapyramidal	Dopamine antagonist
Prochlorperazine (Compazine)	5 or 10 mg IM or PO q 6–12 h or 25 mg rectal q 12 h	Sedating Extrapyramidal	Phenothiazine
Promethazine (Phenergan)	25 mg PO q 6–8 h or 25 mg rectal q 12 h or 12.5 mg IM q 6–8 h	Sedating Extrapyramidal	Phenothiazine
Trimethobenzamide (Tigan)	250 mg PO tid or 200 mg IM tid	Sedating Extrapyramidal	Similar to phenothiazine
Thiethylperazine (Torecan)	10 mg PO, up to tid or 2 mL IM, up to tid	Sedating Extrapyramidal	Phenothiazine

*Doses are all those used routinely for adults and are generally *not* appropriate for children.

mus. Most cases of vestibular neuritis are monophasic; however, in some cases there are multiple recurrences. Hearing is not impaired; when there are similar symptoms with hearing affected, the syndrome is termed "labyrinthitis." Vestibular neuritis is thought to be caused by a viral infection of the vestibular portion of the eighth cranial nerve. Extremely similar presentations are found in herpes zoster oticus (a rash is present in addition to vestibular and hearing disruption) and rarely in Lyme disease.

Severe distress associated with constant vertigo, nausea, and malaise usually lasts 2 or 3 days, and less intense symptoms ordinarily persist for 1 or 2 weeks. The treatment strategy involves the sparing use of antiemetics and vestibular suppressants as necessary (Table 3; see also Table 2). In the first few days of the illness, patients usually severely restrict their activities, as rapid head movements and activities such as sitting up or turning over in bed may cause increased vertigo. Vestibular suppressants and antiemetics are commonly used at this point, prescribed as suppositories if necessary. By the third day, it is usually possible to greatly reduce the usage of vestibular suppressants, and the patient should be encouraged to increase activity as tolerated.

Approximately 10% of patients may take as long as 2 months to improve substantially. These patients usually have a significant fixed vestibular paresis combined with central dysfunction that slows their compensation. For example, patients with alcoholic cerebellar degeneration or persons of advanced age may recover much more slowly. Such patients often benefit from visual-vestibular exercises. *Vestibular exercises* may be given out to patients in the form of a handout (Table 4). These exercises are done three times daily, moving from the easier procedures to more difficult ones as recovery ensues. Specialized physical therapy programs are also available in which individualized therapy can be offered and supervision provided when appropriate. Finally, numerous avocational activities serve well to promote vestibular compensation. Depending on the abilities and interests of your patients, you might prescribe golf, bowling, racquetball, bicycling, or even t'ai chi!

TABLE 4. **Vestibular Rehabilitation Exercises**

A. In bed—sitting up if possible
  1. Do eye movements–at first slowly, then quickly
    (at least 5 minutes).
    a. Up and down
    b. From side to side
    c. Focusing on finger moving from 3 to 1 ft away from face
  2. Do head movements at first slowly, then move quickly
    (5 minutes).
    a. Bending forward and backward
    b. Turning from side to side
B. Sitting
Repeat 1 and 2. For head movement exercise, watch card taped to wall and attempt to keep letters in focus ("gaze stabilization" exercises).
  3. Do shoulder shrugging and circling (to keep from tightening neck up).
  4. Bend forward and pick up objects from ground.
C. Standing
Repeat 1–4
  5. Change from sitting to standing with eyes open and shut.
  6. Throw small ball from hand to hand (above eye level).
  7. Throw small ball from hand to hand under knee level.
  8. Change from sitting to standing and back to sitting, with turn around in between.
D. Walking
  9. Walk across room with eyes open and eyes closed. If possible practice in pedestrian traffic situation (such as mall), first with traffic, then against traffic.
  10. Practice making sudden turns (whole body) while walking.
  11. Practice walking while head is moving from side to side, as if in museum ("museum walking").
  12. Participate in any game involving stooping and stretching such as bowling, volleyball, basketball.

There are numerous other potential causes of unilateral vestibular paresis, but practically, they are encountered extremely rarely. *Acoustic neuromas* and other cerebellopontine angle tumors are infrequent sources of dizziness—because acoustics grow very slowly, hearing impairment rather than dizziness is usually the presenting symptom. *Neurovascular compression* of the eighth nerve is discussed in the section "Central Vertigo."

Meniere's Disease

Meniere's disease is discussed in detail elsewhere, but it is the archetype of episodic vertigo. Vertigo related to Meniere's disease is ordinarily separated from other forms of episodic vertigo by means of hearing symptoms, particularly including a fluctuating low-frequency sensorineural hearing impairment. Vestibular suppressants and antiemetics are used in a way similar to that described for vestibular neuritis. Variants of Meniere's disease include a form that follows head injury (labyrinthine concussion or delayed endolymphatic hydrops), and a bilateral form attributed to autoantibodies or genetic predisposition.

Middle Ear Disturbances

Middle ear disease is an infrequent cause of vertigo, episodic or otherwise. Examples of middle ear disease associated with episodic vertigo include cerumen impaction, eustachian tube dysfunction, and temporomandibular joint (TMJ) dysfunction. In most instances, the mechanism by which these entities cause vertigo or ataxia is unclear.

Cerumen impaction or its removal is an uncommon cause of vertigo. Patients with unilateral wax impaction may develop an "alternobaric vertigo," related to the pressure differential that can develop between the ears. The treatment is wax disimpaction. Occasionally, patients have vertigo after cerumen removal. These cases usually sort out into one of three categories: (1) vertigo due to the caloric effect of syringing of the ear, (2) BPPV associated with the supine positioning used for removal, or (3) perilymph fistula-like symptoms, presumably due to a mobilization of the stapes footplate due to forceful manipulation of the tympanic membrane.

Eustachian tube malfunction typically presents with popping, clicking, or snapping in the ears; otalgia; and a fullness that may be relieved by swallowing or yawning. These patients often complain of a mild and vague dizziness that fluctuates with their aural fullness and is attributed to "alternobaric vertigo" as above. Decongestants and intranasal steroids are routinely used in this situation, although generally with little effect. Although ventilation tubes may reduce symptoms, it is generally thought that this is unduly aggressive.

TMJ dysfunction, with crepitus, pain, or clicking over the TMJ, is more highly prevalent in patients with dizziness and/or headaches than in the general population, and there is also a significant association between TMJ dysfunction and vertigo. Severe vertigo is reported by 20% of the TMJ population, compared with between 3.5 and 7.5% of controls. The cause of these symptoms is presently uncertain. Usual treatment includes referral back to the patient's dentist for a "night guard," or plastic insert worn at night to reduce bruxism. Amitriptyline* taken in a dose of 25 mg at bedtime is also sometimes helpful.

Fistula and Related Conditions

Patients with *perilymphatic fistula* (PLF) present with episodic vertigo, ataxia, and pressure sensitivity, generally after an episode of barotrauma. A typical symptom complex is vague dizziness that starts about 15 minutes after getting out of bed, aural fullness, and dizziness when the patient blows his or her nose. Commonly, symptoms are inseparable from those of Meniere's disease. Surgical exploration of the middle ear is appropriate for patients with a history of barotrauma and/or clear pressure sensitivity. Many of these patients respond to a benzodiazepine, such as lorazepam (Ativan),* 0.5 mg, twice a day.

There are several other uncommon causes of episodic vertigo that also have pressure sensitivity. Otologic conditions include hypermobility of the stapes footplate, the "too long stapes prosthesis" syndrome, which may follow otosclerosis surgery, and vestibulofibrosis. In all these conditions, episodes of vertigo are provoked by belching, coughing, straining, nose blowing, or loud noises. The mechanism is jostling of the utricle or saccule by the stapes, through the oval window. Referral to an otologic surgeon for insertion of a ventilation tube or a destructive procedure is the treatment. Vertigo induced by straining is also found in the Arnold-Chiari malformation (see the next section).

CENTRAL VERTIGO

Central vertigo is unusual. In the emergency room setting or otolaryngology clinic, a central vertigo is diagnosed in less than 5% of cases. Central vertigo is largely caused by vascular disorders (Table 5). Stroke and transient ischemic attack account for one-third of cases. Vertigo attributed to vertebrobasilar migraine causes another 15% of cases. A large number of individual miscellaneous neurologic disorders such as seizures, multiple sclerosis, and the Arnold-Chiari malformation make up the remainder. Because of the diverse causes of central vertigo, the management of these patients is usually specific, and space does not permit a detailed discussion, but several common presentations bear some comment.

Headache and episodic vertigo is an extremely common presentation. These patients are usually women in the 30- to 40-year age group, in whom the incidence of migraine peaks in the general popula-

---

*Not FDA-approved for this indication.

TABLE 5. **Most Common Causes of Central Vertigo**

Stroke and transient ischemic attack (TIA)
Cerebellar
AICA distribution
PICA distribution
Vertebrobasilar migraine
Usual adult form
Childhood variant (benign paroxysmal vertigo of childhood)
Seizure (temporal lobe)
Multiple sclerosis, postinfectious demyelinations
Arnold-Chiari malformation, basilar impression
Tumors of eighth nerve, brain stem, or cerebellum
Paraneoplastic cerebellar degeneration
Neurovascular compression

Abbreviations: AICA = anterior inferior cerebellar artery; PICA = posterior inferior cerebellar artery.

tion. This is also a common symptom complex after head injury and is also a common presentation of the Arnold-Chiari malformation. When vertebrobasilar migraine is suspected, a prophylactic drug should be tried. A sustained-release preparation of verapamil (Calan SR, Isoptin SR, Verelan)* 180 mg every morning is often effective. A trial of amitriptyline* can be made if the patient does not tolerate verapamil. Amitriptyline is favored over newer antidepressant medications because of its anticholinergic activity. Beta blockers* form a third line of treatment.

Another common presentation is that of the patient with *"quick spins,"* usually combining dizziness, head trauma, and an abnormal electroencephalogram (EEG). These patients relate a history of one or two spins, in which the world goes by once or twice in a second. Spells may recur 20 or more times per day. Carbamazepine (Tegretol),* in therapeutic doses for epilepsy (200 mg three times a day), is tried in such patients, especially if symptoms have been persistent over months and they have not responded to vestibular-suppressant medication. A variant of quick spins is "episodic tilts." Again, these patients often respond to carbamazepine, although the EEG is nearly always normal. Many of these patients have ectatic vertebral and basilar arteries, which may be causing symptoms by compression of the vestibular nerve or the root entry zone of the eighth nerve in the medulla.

Another common and often frustrating presentation is that of the patient with a *known structural lesion of the brain stem or cerebellum,* in whom you would like to reduce symptoms of vertigo or ataxia. Meclizine 25 mg twice a day is occasionally successful. Benzodiazepines, such as lorazepam,* clonazepam (Klonopin),* and diazepam (Valium),* are frequently helpful (see Table 2 for doses), but one must be wary of psychological addiction and physical dependence. Physical therapy emphasizing the effective use of appliances such as canes, walkers, and footwear is often useful.

VERTIGO OF UNKNOWN CAUSE

Table 6 enumerates conditions that share the unifying feature of a lack of abnormality on otologic and

*Not FDA-approved for this indication.

neurologic examination. Regardless of whether one is practicing in the emergency room or otolaryngology or neurology clinic, variants of unlocalizable diagnoses such as "unknown diagnosis," "psychogenic vertigo," "hyperventilation syndrome," "post-traumatic vertigo," and "nonspecific" dizziness are the most common single "cause" of dizziness reported. In this situation, it is often suggested that symptoms are psychogenic, and some authors indicate that as many as 50% of all dizzy patients have a "functional" source of complaints.

The work-up should include a thorough neurologic, otologic, and audiometric examination. All patients with positional symptoms are given a trial of the Brandt-Daroff exercises. If this is not the case, or exercises are ineffective, then electronystagmographic (ENG) and MRI studies of the head are often recommended. When all results are normal, the patient is gently advised to consult with a psychiatrist or psychologist. It is often helpful to couch the recommendation in terms of "In this way, we will probably establish that you have a clean bill of psychiatric health," or to point out that it is results that really count, and if the vertigo is psychogenic, it is best just to get on with it.

In parallel with the psychiatric evaluation, we usually empirically try several drug treatments. First the patient is asked to log the symptoms on a calendar. Next, for patients already taking medication, we withdraw drugs that could affect the vestibular system, recording symptoms for 2 weeks or more. This strategy may identify persons with ataxia caused by medication. One must be careful not to eliminate a medication critical to the patient's well-being.

Several drugs are then tried. Meclizine (12.5 mg, as much as three times daily) may be prescribed on an as-needed basis. If meclizine is already being used and is ineffective, it may be replaced by a small dose of lorazepam. Clonazepam* can be used in a similar fashion. It is generally difficult to exclude mild Meniere's disease, and salt restriction (no added salt) and a diuretic such as triamterene plus hydrochlorothiazide (Dyazide)* 1 tablet every morning may be

*Not FDA-approved for this indication.

TABLE 6. **Diagnoses Made in Patients with Vertigo Without Objective Findings**

Vertigo of "unknown cause" or "nonspecific vertigo"
Post-traumatic vertigo
Labyrinthine concussion
Hyperventilation syndrome
Disequilibrium of the elderly
Matutinal vertigo
Psychiatric disturbances
Psychogenic vertigo
Phobic postural vertigo
Agoraphobia
Anxiety and panic
Major depression
Malingering
Somatization disorder

tried. A trial of migraine prophylaxis with sustained-release verapamil* (180 mg each morning) is sometimes helpful in patients with dizziness and headaches or patients with the diagnosis of "vestibular Meniere's." A long-acting antihistamine such as astemizole (Hismanal) may also be tried for several weeks.

If patients do not respond to the above regimen, they are followed at 3- to 6-month intervals and undergo yearly audiometric screenings. The ongoing follow-up is important for several reasons. Occasionally the symptoms of persons with small acoustic neurinomas or early Meniere's disease evolve into an identifiable clinical presentation. Certain intermittent conditions, such as BPPV, may take several examinations before the characteristic positional nystagmus is discovered and definitive treatment can be initiated. Finally, the ongoing process of follow-up allays patient anxiety.

---

*Not FDA-approved for this indication.

MENIERE'S DISEASE

method of
DERALD E. BRACKMANN, M.D.*
University of Southern California School of Medicine
Los Angeles, California

Meniere's disease is a common disorder of the inner ear characterized by episodic vertigo, fluctuating hearing loss, tinnitus, and ear pressure. It afflicts between 2 and 5 million Americans. Meniere's disease is a specific disorder of the membranous inner ear characterized by endolymphatic hydrops. It should be differentiated from other diseases that produce hearing loss or vertigo. Other varieties of Meniere's disease include *cochlear hydrops*, characterized by fluctuating hearing loss, tinnitus, and ear pressure without vertigo, and *vestibular hydrops*, in which there is episodic vertigo without hearing loss or tinnitus.

The mechanism of production of endolymphatic hydrops is unknown. The most commonly accepted theory is that there is a malfunction of the resorptive mechanism in the endolymphatic sac.

EVALUATION

All patients with vertigo, tinnitus, or hearing impairment should undergo a thorough neurologic evaluation to eliminate the possibility of an acoustic tumor and to identify other syndromes that may mimic Meniere's disease. A thorough history and examination, including a neurotologic examination, should be performed. Audiometric tests should be done. The classic finding is a low-frequency sensorineural hearing impairment with moderate impairment of speech discrimination. Auditory brain stem response audiometry is done to screen for an acoustic tumor. If the

---

*From the House Ear Clinic, Inc., Los Angeles, sponsored by a grant from the House Ear Institute, an affiliate of the University of Southern California School of Medicine, Los Angeles, California.

test results are abnormal or the symptoms are not classic, magnetic resonance imaging with gadolinium enhancement is done to exclude an acoustic neuroma.

Electronystagmography should be performed; a normal or moderately reduced vestibular response on the affected side is expected.

Blood tests include a fluorescent treponemal antibody (FTA) absorption test to exclude the possibility of syphilis of the inner ear, which may mimic Meniere's disease. A sedimentation rate is obtained as a screening test for autoimmune inner ear disease. If it is positive, other tests for autoimmune disease are obtained. Abnormal results of any of these tests indicate a condition requiring appropriate treatment. When all results are negative, the diagnosis of idiopathic Meniere's disease is established.

TREATMENT

The goal of treatment of Meniere's disease is to control or even eliminate the episodes of vertigo. A secondary goal is to prevent the sensorineural hearing impairment that occurs in progressive Meniere's disease. Preservation of hearing is important in Meniere's disease, because disease develops in the other ear in 30 to 50% of patients who are followed for 10 years or more.

Medical Therapy

The majority of patients with Meniere's disease are treated by medical and dietary measures. Different treatments are necessary for acute attacks and for the long-term management of these patients.

Management of the Acute Attack

In the early stages of Meniere's disease, patients usually experience a prodrome of increased aural pressure and tinnitus prior to the definitive attack of vertigo. With the attack of vertigo, hearing decreases, and nystagmus is apparent on examination. The patient is often nauseated and may vomit. During the acute attack, any movement exacerbates symptoms, and bed rest is recommended. A severe attack of Meniere's disease usually lasts no more than 2 to 3 hours, and only supportive therapy is required. If the patient is not vomiting, I recommend meclizine (Antivert) 25 mg every 4 hours. If the patient cannot take oral medications, I prescribe a 25-mg prochlorperazine (Compazine) suppository. Occasionally, if the attack is prolonged, intravenous fluids may be necessary to maintain hydration; diazepam (Valium) 5 to 10 mg slowly titrated intravenously is effective in relieving the acute attack. Diazepam is a very effective vestibular suppressant, but because of its addictive properties, I avoid its use for long-term management.

In more advanced stages of Meniere's disease, patients may have severe attacks of vertigo with very little warning. This presents a severe risk to the patient, and surgical therapy is often necessary for the management of these attacks.

Long-Term Medical Management

There are no medications that have proved effective in controlling endolymphatic hydrops. Nevertheless, all agree that a trial of medical management should be given before resorting to surgical therapy. A variety of medications have been used for Meniere's disease, including niacin, Lipoflavonoid vitamin supplement, propantheline bromide (Pro-Banthine), diphenhydramine hydrochloride (Benadryl), and histamine by the sublingual, subcutaneous, and intravenous routes. Vasodilating medications, diuretics, and a low-salt diet are frequently prescribed. I try to avoid the use of tranquilizers for the long-term management of Meniere's disease. Corticosteroids are occasionally prescribed during periods of exacerbation of symptoms. My specific medical management is as follows:

1. *Low-salt diet.* Patients are instructed to add no salt to their food, use no salt in cooking, and avoid foods high in sodium content, such as preserved foods.

2. *Diuretics.* Hydrochlorothiazide (HydroDIURIL) 50 mg each morning is prescribed, along with a potassium supplement. It is necessary to monitor serum potassium levels periodically. Diuretics are given in an attempt to reduce systemic fluid volume and secondarily to reduce intralabyrinthine fluid and thus endolymphatic pressure.

3. *Vasodilators.* A vasodilating medication, such as papaverine hydrochloride (Pavabid) 150 mg twice daily or cyclandelate (Cyclospasmol) 200 mg three times a day, is prescribed. There is no proof that systemic vasodilators improve inner ear circulation. Recent studies, however, have shown that circulation to the endolymphatic sac is derived from extracranial circulation, and vasodilators may be beneficial in increasing endolymph resorption.

4. *Meclizine.* Meclizine (Antivert) 12.5 to 25 mg three times a day is often effective for patients with instability and may also reduce the incidence of definitive attacks.

5. *Cawthorne positional exercises.* This program of positional exercises is effective in reducing chronic vestibular dysfunction.

6. *Avoidance of caffeine, alcohol, tobacco, and stress.* Although these factors do not cause Meniere's disease, they can make patients susceptible to attacks and seem to bring on exacerbations.

7. *Reassurance.* Meniere's disease is a frightening, disabling disorder. Patients often feel that they are doomed to a sedentary life by the episodic vertigo. Reassurance that something can be done to relieve these symptoms is an important part of therapy.

Surgical Treatment

Despite an intensive medical regimen, some patients continue to experience vertiginous attacks frequently enough to cause disability. Surgical therapy should be considered for these patients. Once the surgical options are explained, the patient is left with the decision whether to continue with medical management or to undergo a surgical procedure. Many factors enter into the decision. Some patients are not greatly bothered by an occasional attack of vertigo, but for others, even an occasional spell is disabling. Table 1 outlines the recommended surgical management. If any hearing remains in the diseased ear, the first operation is an endolymphatic sac procedure. Occasionally, in a patient with far advanced Meniere's disease, I recommend a selective vestibular nerve section and at the same time perform an endolymphatic sac procedure. If no hearing remains in the diseased ear, a destructive procedure is recommended. In the elderly, this is a transcanal labyrinthectomy; in the young, this is a translabyrinthine vestibular nerve section. More extensive surgery is recommended for younger patients because the transcanal procedure fails to control unsteadiness in certain cases. This has been found to be due to the formation of a traumatic neuroma in the vestibule that produces constant unsteadiness.

Occasionally, I recommend a cochleosacculotomy for elderly patients. The specific indication for this procedure is an older patient with poor hearing and good vestibular function (the reasons for this are noted later).

If the initial endolymphatic sac procedure fails to relieve vertigo, a selective denervation procedure is recommended unless there is no hearing remaining in the ear, in which case a destructive procedure is performed.

The question is often raised as to how poor the hearing should be before one considers a destructive procedure. I believe that any residual hearing is worth preserving in Meniere's disease, because of the disease's tendency to become bilateral. I therefore recommend a destructive procedure only for patients who have profound hearing impairment with no speech discrimination ability. Otherwise, I recommend a procedure that spares the hearing.

Endolymphatic Mastoid Shunt

The endolymphatic sac procedure is performed under general anesthesia. A complete, simple mastoidectomy is performed through a postauricular incision. Mastoid air cells are removed to expose the endolymphatic sac, which lies in the posterior fossa dura. Bone is removed from about the sac, which is then opened, and a sheet of thin polymeric silicone (Silastic) is placed within the lumen of the sac. Ap-

TABLE 1. **Surgical Management of Meniere's Disease**

Status	Procedure
Following Medical Treatment Failure	
Hearing good	Endolymphatic shunt
Hearing poor, elderly, good vestibular function	Cochleosacculotomy
No useful hearing (elderly)	Transcanal labyrinthectomy
No useful hearing (young)	Translabyrinthine nerve section
Following Endolymphatic Shunt Failure	
Hearing remains	Retrolabyrinthine vestibular nerve section
No useful hearing (elderly)	Transcanal labyrinthectomy
No useful hearing (young)	Translabyrinthine nerve section

proximately 1 hour is required to complete the procedure, and the patient is hospitalized for 1 day.

The morbidity associated with this procedure is very low. Less than 1% of patients experience further loss of hearing, which is the only risk of the procedure other than the risk of the general anesthetic. Fifty percent of patients are relieved of definitive spells of vertigo, and another 25% are markedly improved. Because of this low morbidity and simplicity, I recommend this as the primary procedure for patients with disabling Meniere's disease who are unresponsive to medical therapy.

Cochleosacculotomy

Cochleosacculotomy is a drainage procedure in which a small hook is placed into the inner ear through the middle ear. The operation is performed with the patient under local anesthesia. In my experience, this procedure is associated with a high incidence of hearing impairment, so I reserve it for patients who already have severe hearing loss. It does not produce acute vertigo and is therefore useful in elderly patients who have good balance function and in whom a sudden destruction of the balance function might result in disability and unsteadiness. Patients are hospitalized for 1 day, and recovery is rapid. Approximately 75% of patients are relieved of definitive attacks of vertigo, but hearing loss results in over 80% of patients.

Retrolabyrinthine Vestibular Nerve Section

For patients in whom vertigo is not controlled by an endolymphatic sac procedure and in whom useful hearing remains, I recommend a retrolabyrinthine vestibular nerve section. In this procedure, the posterior fossa is entered through the mastoid, and the vestibular nerve is sectioned between the brain stem and the internal auditory canal. The vestibular nerve is separated from the acoustic nerve and divided. Two hours are required, and the patient is hospitalized for 5 to 6 days.

More than 95% of patients are relieved of their balance disorder with this surgery. There is a 5% risk of sensorineural hearing impairment and a 2% risk of total hearing loss in the operated ear. Other than hearing loss, the morbidity associated with the procedure is low. I have not had any patient with facial paralysis, and the incidence of infection is less than 1%.

Destructive Procedures

If a patient has no remaining useful hearing, the most certain way of relieving vertigo is to perform a destructive procedure.

TRANSCANAL LABYRINTHECTOMY

Transcanal labyrinthectomy is performed through the ear canal using general anesthesia. The eardrum is raised, and the bone over the inner ear is removed with a small drill. All the contents of the inner ear are then removed. This results in a total loss of hearing and vestibular function in the involved ear.

The patient is hospitalized for approximately 3 days, depending on the degree of vertigo postoperatively. There is a period of unsteadiness that may last for several weeks, with the patient showing gradual improvement. Vestibular exercises are beneficial during this time to speed recovery.

A certain number of patients have disabling unsteadiness in the postoperative period. This has been shown to be due to the formation of a neuroma in the vestibule. Because of this possibility, I reserve this operation for elderly patients. In others, I recommend a translabyrinthine vestibular nerve section in which the entire vestibular nerve and ganglion are removed.

TRANSLABYRINTHINE VESTIBULAR NERVE SECTION

A translabyrinthine vestibular nerve section is the most certain way to completely ablate labyrinthine function. It is the recommended procedure in the majority of patients who have nonuseful hearing. The only exception would be a patient in poor general health who presents increased risk for prolonged general anesthesia.

A mastoidectomy is completed, and all the semicircular canals are removed. The internal auditory canal is then opened, and the vestibular nerve, along with Scarpa's ganglion, is removed. If the patient has tinnitus, the cochlear nerve is also removed. Approximately 50% of patients experience improvement of tinnitus following this procedure. The patient is hospitalized for approximately 5 days, depending on the amount of unsteadiness experienced postoperatively. Over 95% of patients are relieved of their balance problems. The disadvantage is the inevitable loss of hearing that occurs. This procedure is therefore reserved for those patients who have no remaining hearing in the diseased ear.

BILATERAL MENIERE'S DISEASE

As previously mentioned, bilateral Meniere's disease eventually develops in 30 to 50% of patients. Therefore, preservation of hearing is a major goal of treatment. When a procedure has been employed that has removed vestibular function from one ear and disabling attacks of vertigo develop from the other ear, I use streptomycin therapy for ablation of vestibular function. Patients are given 20 grams of streptomycin sulfate intramuscularly over a 2-week period, with careful monitoring of auditory and vestibular function. This results in depression of vestibular function in the remaining ear. If vestibular function remains with that dosage, more streptomycin can be given to the point of vestibular ablation, with preservation of hearing function.

VIRAL MENINGITIS AND ENCEPHALITIS

method of
C. ALAN ANDERSON, M.D., and
DONALD H. GILDEN, M.D.
University of Colorado School of Medicine
Denver, Colorado

Viral infections of the central nervous system (CNS) can be conveniently classified into four general types, each with different clinical features and outcomes. The four types are aseptic meningitis, viral encephalitis, postinfectious encephalomyelitis, and chronic progressive encephalitis.

ASEPTIC MENINGITIS

Aseptic meningitis is the most common form of CNS viral infection and is characterized by headache, fever, and stiff neck and is occasionally accompanied by irritability, lethargy, photophobia, nausea, vomiting, myalgias, and neck or back pain. Physical examination reveals fever, signs of meningeal irritation, and the absence of mental status changes or focal neurologic deficits. The most common causative agents are the enteroviruses (coxsackievirus and echovirus), herpes simplex virus (HSV) type 2, the arboviruses (California and St. Louis), mumps, and lymphocytic choriomeningitis (LCM) virus. Less common agents include human immunodeficiency virus (HIV), varicella-zoster virus, cytomegalovirus (CMV), and Epstein-Barr virus (EBV). Clinical clues for identifying the causative agent include seasonal prevalence and associated symptoms and signs. Enterovirus and arbovirus infections are more common in the summer and early fall. LCM infection is more common in the fall and winter, and mumps is more common in the spring. LCM is associated with arthritis, adenopathy, and leukopenia. CMV and EBV produce jaundice, leukopenia or atypical lymphocytosis, and lymphadenopathy. Mumps virus causes parotitis and infects other glands; an elevated serum amylase suggests subclinical pancreatitis. Exposure to mice and hamsters is a risk factor for LCM infection. Confirmation of the causative agent is by isolation of the virus from cerebrospinal fluid (CSF), feces, urine, or throat washings or by demonstration of intrathecal antibody production or a fourfold rise in specific antibody titers in acute and convalescent sera. However, these confirmatory studies take days to weeks to perform and are rarely helpful in acute management decisions. Identification of specific viruses by polymerase chain reaction (PCR) techniques holds promise as a rapid means of diagnosis. By PCR, it is possible to amplify specific fragments of DNA (e.g., viral) using synthetic DNA primers that bind to complementary DNA sequences in the test sample. This provides a highly sensitive, specific test for the detection and identification of even trace amounts of viral nucleic acids. Since viral DNA or RNA is not normally found in the CSF, its presence is strong presumptive evidence of a disease state.

Patients with viral meningitis must be distinguished from those with other causes of aseptic meningitis, such as partially treated bacterial meningitis, parameningeal foci of infection, CNS vasculitis, granulomatous meningitis (tuberculosis, syphilis, fungal toxoplasmosis, sarcoidosis, and *Brucella*), and *Listeria* meningitis. These conditions should be considered in patients with known systemic illness, immune suppression, or malignancy. A history of recent antibiotic use is common in patients with partially treated bacterial infection of the CNS. The granulomatous infections have a predilection for the basilar meninges and often produce cranial nerve palsies, focal deficit, and hydrocephalus. Depression of CSF glucose, marked elevation of CSF protein, or the persistence of polymorphonuclear leukocytes (PMNs) in the CSF suggests an etiology other than viral.

Management of a patient presenting with the clinical symptoms and signs of meningitis begins with a prompt evaluation to exclude nonviral causes. The key step is examination of the CSF. The typical profile is a normal to slightly increased opening pressure, clear fluid with an average of 30 to 300 white blood cells per mL (with a range of 10 to 2000 cells), and a greater number of lymphocytes than PMNs, although PMNs may predominate in the first 24 to 48 hours of the infection. The CSF protein is usually slightly elevated but rarely exceeds 100 mg per dL. The CSF glucose is usually normal (except in some cases of mumps or LCM). Gram's stains, acid-fast preparations, and bacterial and fungal cultures are negative.

If there is any suspicion of increased intracranial pressure, an imaging study of the brain should be done before the lumbar puncture. Noncontrasted computed tomography (CT) is usually adequate. If there is any delay in scanning or performing the lumbar puncture, broad-spectrum parenteral antibiotics should be given. If CSF results are equivocal in excluding a bacterial etiology, antibiotics should be continued until cultures are negative. Repeat examination of the CSF is often helpful.

Viral meningitis is treated symptomatically with rest, hydration, antiemetics, analgesics, and antipyretics. Most patients recover within 2 weeks, although a small percentage have fatigue and headache persisting weeks to months after the infection has cleared. Deterioration in a patient should prompt a repeat CSF examination and consideration of empirical treatment for fungal infection, tuberculosis, or other nonviral etiologies.

VIRAL ENCEPHALITIS

The second most common form of viral infection of the CNS is viral encephalitis, representing viral invasion of the brain parenchyma. Patients with encephalitis present with the meningeal and constitutional symptoms mentioned earlier, plus alterations in the patient's state of consciousness, visual field deficits, cranial nerve deficits, hemiparesis, hemisensory loss, and focal and generalized seizures. Personality changes, language and memory disturbances, and psychotic features are frequent. Viral encephalitis must be distinguished from nonviral conditions that can present a similar clinical picture. These include bacterial infections (Lyme disease, tuberculosis, syphilis, listeriosis, mycoplasmosis), fungal infections (coccidioidomycosis, cryptococcosis, nocardiosis), parasitic infections (toxoplasmosis, cysticercosis), brain abscess, subdural hematoma or abscess, brain tumor, CNS vasculitis, and toxic or metabolic encephalopathies.

Viral encephalitis may be epidemic or sporadic. Causes of epidemic viral encephalitis include the arboviruses, enteroviruses, mumps, and LCM virus. The arboviruses are RNA viruses transmitted by mosquitos (arthropod borne), with a peak incidence in the warm summer months. This group includes St. Louis, eastern and western equine, Japanese, and California encephalitides. Eastern equine encephalitis is associated with high mortality and morbidity, but the rest of the arboviruses have a milder course. The enteroviruses include coxsackie- and echoviruses and cause encephalitis during the summer and early fall. Serious sequelae are rare. Mumps encephalitis is more common in the winter and spring. LCM is more common in the fall and winter. Sporadic cases of encephalitis are associated with HSV-1, rabies, and EBV.

HSV-1

The most common cause of serious sporadic acute viral encephalitis is HSV-1. Because of HSV-1's predilection for the medial temporal lobe and the orbital surface of the frontal lobe, focal neurologic signs are prominent, as well as mental status changes; language, memory, and behavioral problems; hemiparesis; and seizures. Mortality in untreated HSV-1 encephalitis is 60 to 70%. Treatment with acyclovir reduces mortality to 25 to 30%. Early treatment is associated with a more favorable outcome. Consequently, early identification and treatment are critical.

CSF examination, brain imaging, and electroencephalography (EEG) should be performed as soon as the diagnosis is suspected. Brain imaging should precede lumbar puncture if elevated intracranial pressure is suspected. CT of the brain shows hypodense lesions in the medial temporal lobes. Fifty percent or more of scans show contrast enhancement of the temporal lesions. The majority have evidence of edema and mass effect. Magnetic resonance imaging (MRI), which is more sensitive than CT scanning, typically shows decreased signal on T1-weighted images and increased signal on T2-weighted images. MRI changes are more extensive and are seen earlier than those revealed by CT. EEG during the first few days of illness shows generalized or focal slowing, predominantly over the involved temporal region. Within days, periodic sharp and slow wave complexes at intervals of 2 to 3 seconds develop. The CSF is abnormal in 90 to 95% of patients and reveals an elevated opening pressure, a lymphocytic pleocytosis, and elevated protein. In contrast to other viral infections of the CNS, about 20% of patients with HSV-1 encephalitis have red blood cells and xanthochromia in their CSF, reflecting the hemorrhagic nature of the brain lesions caused by HSV-1. Rarely, hypoglycorrhachia occurs. Increased antibody titers to HSV-1 can be found in the serum and CSF but may not appear until 2 or more weeks after the onset of symptoms. HSV-1 is very difficult to isolate from CSF, so cultures are rarely helpful. In a small percentage of patients with HSV-1 encephalitis, the CSF and CT scan may be normal for 3 to 4 days or more into the illness. MRI and EEG are more sensitive, and negative studies provide strong evidence against HSV-1 infection.

HSV-1 DNA from the CSF of patients with HSV encephalitis can be amplified by PCR techniques. The presence of HSV DNA in the CSF is strong presumptive evidence for infection and is sufficient for diagnosis in immunocompetent individuals, although the reliability of PCR in identifying the causative agent in immunocompromised patients requires further study. Until recently, brain biopsy has been the diagnostic method of choice for HSV encephalitis. With the availability of PCR analysis of CSF, brain biopsy should be reserved for cases in which the diagnosis is uncertain and there is a high likelihood of another treatable illness.

Specific Therapy. Early treatment of HSV encephalitis with acyclovir (Zovirax) is associated with decreased mortality and morbidity and should be started as soon as the diagnosis is suspected. Such treatment 1 to 2 days before brain biopsy will not compromise pathologic or virologic identification of HSV-1 encephalitis. Acyclovir is given intravenously 30 mg per kg per day in three divided doses for 10 to 14 days. It is generally well tolerated. Side effects include occasional gastrointestinal disturbances, reversible renal dysfunction, and a rare drug-induced encephalopathy. Relapses after acyclovir therapy have been reported and should be treated at the higher dose of 15 mg per kg every 8 hours for 21 days.* Relapse should also prompt a search for another disease process.

Seizures. Initial seizures are treated with diazepam (Valium) 2 mg per minute intravenously, for a maximum total dose of 15 to 20 mg, or lorazepam (Ativan) 2 mg per minute intravenously, for a maximum total dose of 5 to 10 mg, followed by a loading dose of phenytoin (Dilantin) 18 to 20 mg per kg given intravenously no faster than 50 mg per minute. Maintenance doses of phenytoin average 300 to 400 mg per day in divided doses. Therapy is guided by blood levels, side effects, and absence of seizures. Anticonvulsants should be continued for several months after the acute illness.

Cerebral Edema. Cerebral edema may be the

---

*Exceeds dosage recommended by the manufacturer.

most frequent cause of death from HSV encephalitis. Edema is treated by intubation and hyperventilation to bring the partial pressure of carbon dioxide to 25 mmol per liter. This reduces increased intracranial pressure (ICP) by causing constriction of the intracranial vasculature. After 24 to 48 hours, hyperventilation is less effective. Dexamethasone should be administered intravenously at an initial dose of 10 mg, then 4 to 8 mg every 4 to 5 hours for the next 3 days. The benefit in managing increased ICP is greater than the risk of steroids potentiating virus infection. Total fluid intake should be reduced to one-half to two-thirds of maintenance, and the patient's head should be elevated to 30 degrees. Incipient herniation may be managed with osmotic diuretics. Mannitol is given in repeated doses of 0.25 to 2 grams per kg. The serum osmolality should be monitored closely and kept below 310 mOsm per liter. Mannitol's effectiveness decreases with repeated use, and rebound increases in ICP may occur.

General Supportive Measures. The patient should get bed rest. Isolation procedures should be followed until the cause of the illness is established. The patient's airway should be protected by repeated suctioning and, in some cases, endotracheal intubation or tracheostomy. Nutritional support is important, but only conscious patients with intact brain stem function should be given oral feedings. All others should be fed by parenteral or nasogastric techniques. Patients should be watched closely for secondary infections, especially of the urinary tract and lungs. Passive range-of-motion exercises and the use of foot boards or Styrofoam boots will minimize contractures. Frequent turning decreases the risk of bed sores. Patients with encephalitis may develop an inappropriate secretion of antidiuretic hormone and become water intoxicated, which can lead to deepening coma and sometimes seizures. Serum and urine electrolytes and urine output should be monitored frequently. Treatment consists of fluid restriction and, rarely, administration of hypertonic saline solution. Headache is a frequent problem and is treated with acetaminophen, ibuprofen, codeine, and, occasionally, meperidine (50 mg every 4 to 5 hours). Fever is treated with acetaminophen. Most viruses are thermolabile, and modest temperature elevation may serve as a natural defense mechanism.

Rabies

Rabies is caused by a rhabdovirus that is maintained in an animal reservoir. In the United States, it is most common in wildlife (raccoons, skunks, foxes, coyotes, and bats). Transmission to humans is nearly always by animal bite, with rare cases transmitted by inhalation and cornea transplant. Virus in animal saliva is inoculated into the wound and reaches the CNS by retrograde axonal transport in peripheral nerves. The incubation period depends on the location of the bite and severity of exposure, and is usually between 2 weeks and 3 months.

Prodromal symptoms of fever, headache, malaise, abdominal pain, sore throat, and pain and paresthesias at the inoculation site lead to one of two clinical syndromes. Between 85 and 90% of patients develop "furious" rabies, with agitation, confusion, aggressiveness, and psychosis. Focal and generalized seizures are common. Severe pharyngeal muscle spasms occur with attempts to swallow, producing hydrophobia. Between 10 and 15% of patients develop "dumb" or paralytic rabies, with a progressive flaccid paralysis similar to the Guillain-Barré syndrome. Cranial nerves are predominantly affected, producing ptosis, ophthalmoparesis, hearing loss, and dysphagia. With either form, the acute phase may last several days to 2 weeks. Patients who survive the acute phase progress to coma. There are only isolated reports of recovery.

People who are likely to be exposed should be vaccinated. Treatment after exposure begins with washing the wound with soap and water. Human rabies immune globulin (HRIG) 20 IU per kg is given, with half the dose administered intramuscularly in the deltoid muscle and the other half infiltrated around the wound site. Human diploid cell vaccine is started with the HRIG, and 1 mL is given intramuscularly on days 0, 3, 7, 14, and 28. If the biting animal is not captured and examined for rabies infection, the decision to start treatment is based on the nature and circumstances of the bite, the species of the biting animal, and the prevalence of rabies in the region. Treatment started after the onset of symptoms is ineffective.

POSTINFECTIOUS ENCEPHALOMYELITIS

The third type of viral encephalitis consists of the postinfectious encephalopathies associated with the exanthematous childhood diseases such as measles and chickenpox. The neurologic features are identical to those that may follow vaccination with live or inactivated virus. Pertinent symptoms and signs include headache, fever, stiff neck, mental changes, and focal neurologic deficit, which usually occur 7 to 14 days after virus infection, although they may also occur at the time of the rash. Because postinfectious encephalomyelitis is highly inflammatory and associated with brain edema, patients are treated with corticosteroids. Methylprednisolone is given 1 gram per day intravenously for 3 to 5 days, followed by oral prednisone 1 mg per kg per day for 7 days. The prednisone is then tapered over 7 to 10 days. Patients with more severe illness, or those who worsen during the course of treatment, may need larger doses or longer duration of treatment.

CHRONIC PROGRESSIVE ENCEPHALITIS

The fourth type of viral meningoencephalitis includes chronic forms of encephalitis of proven viral cause. Examples are subacute sclerosing panencephalitis (SSPE), caused by measles and rubella virus, and progressive multifocal leukoencephalopathy, caused by JC, a human papovavirus. These disorders are characterized by slowly progressive neurologic deterioration occurring over a period of many months or years. Mental changes occur early. Focal neurologic deficits are common, and myoclonic seizures are frequent in the later stages of SSPE. There is no specific treatment.

REYE'S SYNDROME

method of
JOEL A. THOMPSON, M.D.
Primary Children's Medical Center
Salt Lake City, Utah

In 1963, Reye and coworkers described a disease entity termed "encephalopathy and fatty degeneration of the viscera." Since 1981, there has been a decreasing incidence of Reye's syndrome (RS) in children 0 to 10 years of age and a stable to increased incidence in children over 10 years old. The decreased incidence of RS in younger children has been linked by some U.S. investigators to diminished use of salicylates in the context of varicella and influenza-like respiratory illnesses. Although Japanese and Australian data do not support a link between RS and salicylate use, as do some U.S. data, the use of salicylates in children in the context of varicella and influenza-like illnesses remains contraindicated.

An increasing number of RS-like illnesses are now attributed to inborn errors of metabolism (urea cycle disorders, organic acidurias, and defects of fatty acid oxidation), perhaps accounting for part of the decreased incidence of RS in younger children.

DIAGNOSIS

The diagnosis of RS is one of exclusion but is strongly suspected in any child with an antecedent viral infection, particularly varicella or influenza, who appears to be recovering and then develops unexplained pernicious vomiting followed by deterioration in level of consciousness over a period of minutes to hours. The diagnosis is supported by laboratory studies showing, at a minimum, a threefold elevation of alanine aminotransferase (ALT) or aspartate aminotransferase (AST). Most children demonstrate hyperammonemia, hypophosphatemia, and prolongation of the prothrombin and partial thromboplastin times. Alternative diagnoses producing simultaneous hepatopathy and encephalopathy, including sepsis, meningitis, encephalitis, poisoning, acute liver failure, and inborn errors of metabo-

lism, need to be excluded historically and by appropriate laboratory studies.

PHYSIOLOGIC BASIS FOR THERAPY

RS is presumably a temporary viral-induced disturbance in the function of most mitochondria-borne enzymes, resulting in a complex disturbance of carbohydrate, lipid, and protein metabolism. Accumulation of ammonia, free fatty acids, and lactic acid as well as other metabolic by-products results in a progressive encephalopathy. Hypoglycemia, diminished production of high-energy phosphate compounds and clotting factors, and secondary carnitine deficiency are also noted. Preventive therapy is specifically and empirically aimed at preventing catabolism of carbohydrates, proteins, and lipids, which results in the accumulation of toxic products. Glucose is the mainstay of metabolic therapy. Hyperglycemia reduces gluconeogenesis and lipolysis and reduces the generation of ammonia and free fatty acids. Hyperglycemia may also promote sufficient brain levels of glucose.

THERAPEUTIC APPROACH

Assessment of Severity

A staging system is utilized to evaluate disease severity (Table 1) and determine the intensity of therapeutic support (Table 2).

Therapeutic Components

Supportive Care (All Stages)

Unpredictable, rapid progression of RS makes admission to a hospital with pediatric intensive care and neurosurgical capabilities advisable. Careful attention should be given to the physical protection of delirious patients, but sedation is not recommended because it may impair the assessment of level of consciousness. Vital signs and neurologic status should be assessed at frequent intervals by individuals capable of determining their significance.

Metabolic Management (All Stages)

Meticulous metabolic management dictates hourly serum glucose determinations. Serum electrolytes, AST, ALT, ammonia, phosphate, and osmolarity should be obtained at 4-hour intervals. After the first 24 hours, the frequency of laboratory studies may be decreased.

Glucose. The serum glucose is maintained at 200 to 300 mg per dL for at least 24 hours. A central

TABLE 1. **Staging Reye's Syndrome**

Parameter	Stage I	Stage II	Stage III	Stage IV	Stage V
Level of consciousness	Lethargy; follows verbal commands	Combative/stupor; verbalizes inappropriately	Coma	Coma	Coma
Posture	Normal	Normal	Decorticate	Decerebrate	Flaccid
Response to pain	Purposeful	Purposeful/nonpurposeful	Decorticate	Decerebrate	None
Pupillary reaction	Brisk	Sluggish	Sluggish	Sluggish	None
Oculocephalic reflex (doll's eyes)	Normal	Conjugate deviation	Conjugate deviation	Inconsistent or absent	None

TABLE 2. **Summary of Therapy for Reye's Syndrome**

Stage	Therapy
I and II	Hospitalization; IV fluids; meticulous management of glucose, fluid, and electrolyte balance
III, IV, and V	Intensive care support; mechanical ventilation; continuous monitoring of intracranial pressure; treatment of increased intracranial pressure with osmotic agents or barbiturate coma

venous line is usually necessary to allow continuous infusion of hypertonic solutions. An initial bolus of 50% glucose at 1 mL per kg intravenously should be given on diagnosis, and, if the hourly serum glucose is less than 200 mg per dL, a bolus of 25% glucose at 1 mL per kg intravenously should be given, with coincident upward adjustment in the strength of the hypertonic glucose maintenance solution.

Fluid and Electrolyte Therapy. Most patients with RS are dehydrated and hyperosmolar. Fluid therapy is aimed at maintenance of sufficient vascular volume to avoid shock and ensure adequate urine output (1 mL per kg per hour). It is important to give fluids that will not precipitously drop serum osmolarity and induce cerebral edema. Most patients can be maintained with fluid volumes of two-thirds to full maintenance if serum osmolarities are carefully monitored along with intake and output. Proper fluid management usually necessitates use of a urinary catheter, nasogastric tube, central venous line, and arterial line, particularly in patients in Stage III or deeper.

Hyperammonemia. This is most effectively managed by maintaining a high serum glucose and preventing catabolic production of ammonia. Neomycin enemas (25 to 50 mg per kg per dose) and lactulose may be helpful, but hemodialysis and exchange transfusions are rarely indicated.

Hypophosphatemia. This may be corrected by giving potassium phosphate instead of potassium chloride in the maintenance intravenous solution and titrating this against the serum phosphate. Avoid high serum phosphate levels.

Clotting Abnormalities. Prolonged prothrombin and partial thromboplastin times indicate clotting abnormalities, which are treated with vitamin K (AquaMEPHYTON) 1 mg intravenously or 5 mg intramuscularly. Fresh frozen plasma, 10 mL per kg, may be necessary in patients with actual hemorrhage. On rare occasions, thrombocytopenia occurs and may require treatment with platelet transfusions.

Carnitine Deficiency. Carnitine serves an important function in fatty acid oxidation. Secondary deficiency of carnitine in RS makes supplementation with intravenous L-carnitine advisable in the acute stages.

Intracranial Pressure (Stages III–V)

Patients in Stage III or deeper may have increased intracranial pressure, which requires careful monitoring to prevent transtentorial herniation and cerebral ischemia. Intracranial pressure is monitored utilizing a fiberoptic intraparenchymal monitor. Pressures greater than 20 mmHg for longer than 5 minutes or a cerebral perfusion pressure (mean arterial pressure minus intracranial pressure) of less than 40 mmHg dictates therapy for increased intracranial pressure.

METHODS OF PRESSURE CONTROL

Head inclination by 30 degrees improves venous return from the brain. Be careful not to turn the head, thus compressing the jugular venous system.

Hyperventilation reduces the PCO_2 and causes cerebral vasoconstriction, which reduces cerebral blood volume. This is best accomplished by paralyzing the patient with pancuronium bromide (Pavulon) 0.1 mg per kg and utilizing a mechanical ventilator. A PCO_2 of 22 mmHg is optimal. Increasing the PO_2 to 100 to 125 mmHg will also cause cerebral vasoconstriction and lower the intracranial pressure but is not as effective as reducing PCO_2. Avoid a high PO_2, which may cause pulmonary oxygen toxicity.

Osmotherapy with mannitol is effective in decreasing intracranial pressure, assuming that renal function is intact. Mannitol (20% solution) may be given by intravenous push at a dosage of 0.5 to 1.0 gram per kg every 4 hours as long as the osmolarity does not exceed 330 mOsm per liter and the patient is not hypotensive. Intracranial pressure is very responsive to serum osmolarity, and it is important not to increase volumes of maintenance fluid following a dose of mannitol unless the patient is in shock, since this will drop osmolarity and increase intracranial pressure.

Barbiturate coma reduces intracranial pressure by causing cerebral vasoconstriction. It may also be of benefit by reducing the cerebral metabolic rate. We have not found barbiturates to be more effective than the previously listed methods for controlling intracranial pressure, although they may have an infrequent role in the control of refractory pressure. Barbiturates fix and dilate the pupils, removing all major parameters for assessment of neurologic function. They can cause cardiac arrhythmia and hypotension.

If barbiturates are used, a loading dose of pentobarbital 3 to 6 mg per kg is given, followed by a maintenance dose of 1 to 3 mg per kg every hour. Optimal therapeutic effect is attained by maintaining a burst suppression pattern on continuous electroencephalogram (EEG) monitoring with a suppression phase of no longer than 20 to 30 seconds. Serum pentobarbital levels should not exceed 5.0 μg per mL.

COMPLICATIONS OF REYE'S SYNDROME

Autonomic collapse, manifested by a sudden drop of blood pressure and loss of cerebral autoregulation, is usually fatal and may occur either early in the course of the illness or later as the patient begins to awaken. This is to be distinguished from hypotension resulting from barbiturate coma or volume contraction from osmotherapy. Although volume expanders such as Plasmanate at 10 mL per kg and vasopressors may help remedy the problem, they are often ineffective.

Uncontrollable increased intracranial pressure is an infrequent but usually fatal complication, commonly reflecting severe underlying cerebral injury.

Hemorrhage is an infrequent complication and usually involves the gastrointestinal tract. Blood loss in the gastrointestinal tract may also aggravate hyperammonemia.

Hypoglycemia is more common in children under 5 years of age and usually occurs early in the course of the illness, resulting in additional encephalopathy, which often proves fatal.

Seizures are an indication of hypoglycemia if they occur early in the course of the illness. They may occur later as a preterminal event, reflecting severe encephalopathy. Correction of hypoglycemia and therapy with phenytoin (Dilantin) in a loading dose of 15 mg per kg may be indicated.

Pancreatitis and renal failure are very rare occurrences with RS and are treated symptomatically.

PROGNOSIS

The mortality rate in children who do not progress beyond Stage III is often no greater than 10%. Failure to recognize hypoglycemia, late diagnosis (Stages IV and V), and inadequate therapy increase the mortality substantially. Presentation with a serum ammonia of greater than 400 mg per dL suggests a poor outcome.

MULTIPLE SCLEROSIS

method of
R. PHILIP KINKEL, M.D., and
RICHARD A. RUDICK, M.D.
Cleveland Clinic Foundation
Cleveland, Ohio

Multiple sclerosis (MS) is the most common cause of nontraumatic neurologic disability afflicting young adults in the United States, with an estimated 250,000 to 350,000 patients with established diagnoses. In temperate zones of North America and Europe, the prevalence may reach 0.1 to 0.3% of the population, making this disorder common enough to be seen regularly in most primary care and neurology practices. The chronic and protean nature of MS and its variability over time make management extremely challenging.

DIAGNOSIS

In an era of increasing reliance on sophisticated diagnostic technology, it is important to remember that the diagnosis of MS is based on clinical features, frequently but not always supplemented by diagnostic testing. In many ways, the diagnostic process used in a possible MS case is similar to that used to diagnose common rheumatic conditions such as systemic lupus erythematosus (SLE) and rheumatoid arthritis (RA). Making an MS diagnosis based on magnetic resonance imaging (MRI) findings alone is as inappropriate as establishing a diagnosis of SLE or RA based on elevated antinuclear antibodies or rheumatoid factor titers. The diagnosis of MS requires certain essential clinical features. Since inflammatory demyelination, the underlying pathologic process in MS, can disrupt virtually any central nervous system (CNS) pathway, the diagnosis of MS is an inherently complex process requiring, at a minimum, the consultative services of a neurologist.

A basic diagnostic requirement is the presence, over time, of multiple areas of clinically evident CNS demyelination in the absence of an alternative diagnosis capable of presenting in that fashion. Laboratory tests such as MRI, spinal fluid analysis, and sensory evoked potentials play a major role in confirming the diagnosis and eliminating other diagnostic possibilities.

There is one point in the illness when it is absolutely impossible to establish a diagnosis with certainty. This is after the first episode of demyelination resulting in neurologic symptoms. Initial symptoms commonly include optic neuritis, partial transverse myelitis, and various brain stem syndromes. The diagnosis of MS cannot be rendered at this time, since the clinical course has not fulfilled the requirement of multiple areas of CNS involvement at different points in time. Diagnostic testing with MRI scanning allows the practitioner to exclude alternative causes and to assess the short-term risk of the individual experiencing recurrent demyelination, which may at that time lead to a clinical diagnosis of MS. Even in patients who have clearly experienced recurrent neurologic symptoms over time, we frequently find it necessary to observe further before establishing a diagnosis of MS. We cannot overemphasize the profound psychological, vocational, economic, and social impact of an MS diagnosis on an individual and his or her family. Therefore, the diagnosis should not be made prematurely, and patients should be educated and counseled about diagnostic uncertainty early in the disease. When uncertainty in the MS diagnosis exists, this should be discussed directly with the patient in a nonpaternalistic fashion. Education and follow-up plans should be made and the patient given free access to the practitioner if future problems should develop. Those patients unable to cope with an uncertain diagnosis, even after appropriate education, frequently give a history of maladaptive coping to stresses and uncertainties in their lives. Such individuals may benefit from psychotherapy, either individually or in a group setting.

Although establishing a diagnosis is beyond the scope of this book, it is useful to discuss two common diagnostic errors. The first error is in diagnosing MS in patients with no definable neurologic disease. It is quite common for us to see patients who have acquired a diagnosis of MS because of nonspecific neurologic symptoms such as general weakness, fatigue, or tingling, at times supplemented by minimal changes on the MRI. By far the most common syndrome in this group of patients is recurrent paresthesias (usually described as pins and needles) in the extremities without any discernible abnormalities on neurologic examination. The condition is so frequent that it is sometimes labeled "benign paresthesias." We have followed a number of patients with this condition for many years. Although some eventually develop MS, the majority never develop any neurologic illness. In some cases, a somatization disorder becomes apparent over time. It is difficult to remove an incorrect diagnosis in such a patient, but it is important to do so for his or her overall health and well-being.

The second type of error is making an MS diagnosis in a patient who has some other neurologic disease. We have listed a number of "red flags" that should alert physicians to the possibility of an alternative diagnosis (Table 1). When any one of these red flags exists, a thorough evaluation should be undertaken to exclude alternative etiologies. Even in the absence of alternative etiologies, the diagnosis of MS should always be considered tentative as long as the red flag exists.

EDUCATION AND COUNSELING

As with other chronic illnesses of uncertain etiology and prognosis, education and counseling may be not only therapeutic but also the main treatment required. This is especially true in early cases of MS, prior to the onset of any significant or persistent disability. All too often, patients at this stage of the illness are inappropriately reassured by being told that they have "benign MS" or are given no significant information except to "call if new problems develop." So many health care resources are brought to bear on establishing a diagnosis that little time remains to address the questions and concerns of patients and their families. This, in turn, leads to frustration and a breakdown in communication between the patient and the health care provider.

What follows is a list of commonly encountered questions with suggested explanations. Neither the list nor the responses are meant to be an exhaustive compendium of information for practitioners. Instead, they are meant to be used as a starting point in the education process.

What Is Multiple Sclerosis?

Accumulating evidence suggests that MS (literally translated as multiple scars) is the result of organ-specific autoimmunity initiated and perpetuated by immune dysregulation in a genetically susceptible host. The inflammatory or autoimmune target in MS appears to be some component or components of the myelin sheath that wraps around CNS axons. The peripheral nervous system is *not* involved by the MS process, but peripheral nerve rootlets and cranial nerves are commonly affected where they exit from the CNS. Pathologically, acute MS lesions are characterized by perivascular cuffs of intense inflammation in the white matter of the CNS surrounded by a zone of macrophage

TABLE 2. **Essential Clinical Features of Multiple Sclerosis**

Peak age of onset is 18 to 35 years (any age possible)
More common in females (approximately two-thirds)
More common in temperate climates
Demyelination can cause motor, sensory, visual, bowel, bladder, cognitive, affective, and autonomic disturbances
Relapsing-remitting course at onset in 80% of cases
Progressive course from onset more common in older-onset patients (>40 years)
65% of patients disabled 15 years after onset

infiltration and demyelination with relatively preserved axon processes. During acute episodes of demyelination (i.e., when a new lesion is formed or an older lesion enlarges), breakdown of the blood-brain barrier occurs, which can be detected with gadolinium (Gd)–enhanced MRI scanning. Since Gd enhancement persists for a few weeks, Gd–enhanced MRI helps in determining the activity of the disease at a given point in time. As the inflammatory process subsides, gliosis or scarring ensues. New inflammatory lesions can occur unpredictably in adjacent or totally different areas of the CNS, even during the recovery of recent inflammatory lesions.

The essential features of the disease are given in Table 2. The plethora of symptoms and signs is a testament to the importance of CNS myelin in the conduction of electrical impulses throughout the CNS. When myelin is stripped away from axons, electrical impulses are blocked, slowed, or produce aberrant signals. In the case of motor system involvement, this can produce weakness, exertional fatigue, or paroxysmal muscle contractions. Of course, the same mechanisms can affect virtually any centrally mediated neural system, creating a variety of symptoms that are at times difficult to explain. Nevertheless, certain syndromes listed in Table 3 are so commonly encountered as to be considered strongly suggestive of MS in the correct clinical setting.

Two additional points about the disease process should be emphasized. First, not all MS lesions produce symptoms

TABLE 1. **Red Flags Casting Doubt on the Diagnosis of Multiple Sclerosis**

Absence of eye findings reflecting optic nerve or oculomotor dysfunction
Absence of remission, particularly in a patient younger than 30 years of age
Localized disease, particularly posterior fossa, craniocervical junction, or spinal cord
Atypical clinical features, particularly absence of sensory findings, reflexes, or bladder involvement
Normal MRI scan
Normal cerebrospinal fluid examination

Abbreviation: MRI = magnetic resonance imaging.
Modified from Rudick RA, Schiffer RB, Schwetz K, Herndon RM: Multiple sclerosis: The problem of misdiagnosis. Arch Neurol 43:578–583, 1986. Copyright 1986, American Medical Association.

TABLE 3. **Characteristic Clinical Syndromes in Multiple Sclerosis**

Optic neuritis: acute, unilateral (rarely bilateral) loss of central vision with pain on eye movement and an afferent pupillary defect
Partial transverse myelitis: ascending numbness and/or paresthesias with hyper-reflexia and, frequently, a "tight-band" sensation at the level of spinal cord involvement; variable motor, bowel, and bladder involvement
Acute brain stem syndromes: commonly a unilateral or bilateral internuclear ophthalmoplegia; variable additional presentations
Trigeminal neuralgia: MS until proved otherwise in patients <40 years old
Lhermitte's phenomenon: electrical or shocklike sensations down the spine and/or into the limbs with forward neck flexion
Useless hand syndrome: clumsy unilateral hand and arm movements with relatively preserved strength and primary sensation (i.e., light touch and pinprick) but variable loss of joint position sensation and an inability to recognize objects placed in the hand
Tonic spasms: paroxysmal, painful, unilateral dystonic muscle contractions with a flexion posture of the upper extremity and an extension posture of the lower extremity, if the latter is involved

or signs. Many lesions occur in areas of the CNS that are clinically silent. For instance, serial MRI studies have demonstrated that the majority of new lesions—even early in the course of the disease, during clinical remissions, when patients are asymptomatic—occur in these silent areas. Therefore, the absence of symptoms cannot be taken as evidence that the disease is in remission. Second, early in the disease process, the CNS is capable of recovery following inflammatory demyelination. This contributes to the dramatic recovery often seen even with severe attacks. However, with recurrent inflammatory demyelination, recovery becomes less complete.

What Can I Expect to Happen to Me?

Unlike most debilitating diseases of young adults, life expectancy after MS onset is only a few years short of normal. Recent studies suggest that most of the variance is explained by suicides. Not unexpectedly, the majority of patients tend to develop considerable disability over time. Twenty to 30% of patients are unable to walk unassisted or conduct normal work activities 5 years after the onset of disease. The number of patients so disabled increases to 50% at 15 years, and 80% at 30 years. Approximately 20% of patients in whom MS can be diagnosed with certainty experience a truly benign course, defined as the absence of significant disability 10 or more years from symptom onset.

A hallmark of MS is the unpredictable course of the disease. It is not possible early in the disease to determine the rate at which an individual patient will develop disability or the pattern of clinical features. Seventy to 80% of patients with MS beginning between the ages of 20 and 40 years experience an exacerbating-remitting course during the early years of their disease. Each exacerbation is characterized by a rapid decline in neurologic function; each remission is characterized by spontaneous improvement that ranges from complete recovery to only slight improvement. When recovery is complete early in the disease, there may be no persisting symptoms between exacerbations. The average patient experiences approximately two exacerbations every 3 years. After a variable period of time and following a variable number of exacerbations, MS patients tend to develop less clear attacks and a more or less steadily progressive course. Acute exacerbations may be superimposed on this steady worsening. This stage of the illness, termed secondary progressive MS, occurs in about 50% of patients within 10 to 15 years after onset. In 10 to 15% of patients with onset between the ages of 20 and 30 years, a progressive course occurs from the onset (i.e., primary progressive MS) without exacerbations. In its most common form, this consists of a progressive myelopathy. The primary progressive form of MS is age dependent, occurring more commonly in older patients. The risk of this form of the disease is over 50% in patients with MS onset after the age of 40. Clinical, genetic, imaging, and histopathologic differences between exacerbating-remitting and primary progressive MS suggest that there may be etiologic differences between the two types.

Because of its unpredictable nature, MS patients may experience long intervals of stability after periods of progressive decline or may even go decades between exacerbations. Generally speaking, the course of MS during the first 5 to 10 years after symptom onset can be used as a guide to the eventual course. Favorable prognostic signs after the first 5 years of MS include predominance of sensory involvement with relatively little motor impairment, long intervals between attacks, substantial or complete recovery between attacks, and minimal disease on brain MRI. Unfavorable prognostic signs include prominent motor and cerebellar involvement, frequent attacks, poor recovery between attacks or a progressive course, and heavy involvement on brain MRI. Even with these guidelines, however, predictions cannot be made in individual cases with great accuracy; predictions should be made to reassure patients who appear to have more benign MS and to explain and justify more aggressive medical management for patients who appear to have a worse prognosis.

What Makes My Illness Better, and What Makes It Worse?

Most patients and their families harbor certain beliefs about the effects of certain behaviors on MS. These beliefs vary a great deal among patients and families but generally represent a need to gain some measure of control over the illness. Patients do not generally articulate these beliefs and rarely have insight into their need for more control over the disease. We encourage patients to verbalize what they think will improve or worsen their MS. If possible, active control measures should be directed toward healthy behaviors such as proper eating, exercise, and stress management. We discourage only beliefs that result in behavior that could have detrimental consequences, such as seeking dangerous or expensive alternative therapies without proven value. Many patients regain a sense of control by instituting a fitness program, improving their diet, reducing their weight, and eliminating negative behaviors such as smoking and alcohol and drug abuse.

Most patients also believe that certain events or activities precipitate MS disease activity. These beliefs are often held with surprising conviction. The most common of these is the belief that stress precipitates MS worsening or exacerbations. According to a survey in our center, over two-thirds of our patients believe that stress makes MS worse. Although the evidence on this relationship is mixed and by no means conclusive, we often use the perceived relationship to recommend stress management to patients. Furthermore, patients selectively remember events just preceding exacerbations. For example, a patient experiencing an exacerbation shortly after a divorce or a minor car accident is likely to assign a causal relationship. Patients often believe that inoculations or vaccinations precipitate MS disease activity. There is no evidence for this. We currently recommend that patients who are wheelchair-restricted or residing in nursing homes and patients at high risk for influenza (e.g., day care or health care workers) receive yearly influenza vaccinations. The precipitants that are recognized should be discussed with patients. Rigorous studies have established viral illnesses, usually of the upper respiratory tract, as known precipitants of exacerbations. Other febrile illnesses, particularly urinary tract infections (UTIs), commonly aggravate MS symptoms or precipitate significant new disease activity. Consequently, significant infection should be treated aggressively in MS patients, and UTIs should be specifically ruled out in an MS patient experiencing a decline in function. Recurrent UTIs should be prevented by eliminating the cause (e.g., calculi, poor hygiene, poor catheter technique, chronic urinary retention). Similarly, chronically infected decubital ulcers should be treated aggressively and the cause (e.g., poor nutrition, contractures, and excessive pressure from immobility) managed.

Patients should be counseled that increased core body temperature, from either infection or hot weather, can have a profoundly detrimental effect on MS symptoms. Most but not all patients are heat sensitive. Each individual patient should be advised about the relationship between body temperature and MS symptoms, but it is generally not necessary for MS patients to avoid all heat exposure. Most but not all MS patients can tolerate warm or hot showers, a day on the beach, or aerobic exercise. Few MS patients with moderate or severe disability, however, tolerate significant fever. Even in heat-sensitive patients, there is little evidence that heat worsens the course of MS or provokes new disease activity. Moderation and common sense are the only requirements.

Can I Have Children?

Most studies have found that women with MS have normal fertility, normal pregnancies, and normal babies. There is little evidence to suggest that pregnancy accelerates disease progression, and women with MS who wish to have children should be encouraged. However, numerous studies suggest that pregnant women with MS experience fewer exacerbations during pregnancy and have a higher risk of exacerbation in the first 4 to 6 months post partum. We advise women with mild to moderate disability to plan pregnancies on the basis of issues other than MS. The pregnancy should be planned to avoid the use of potentially teratogenic medications, such as interferon-beta (Betaseron), during any portion of the pregnancy. Pregnancy, labor, and delivery management should be routine. There is no reason to avoid epidural anesthesia. Breast-feeding should be supported if this is the wish of the patient. We advise breast-feeding mothers to avoid exhaustion by pumping their breasts at night and sleeping while other family members feed the infants by bottle.

Will Any of My Family Get MS?

We inform our MS patients that the lifetime risk of MS in a first-degree relative (e.g., child or sibling) is 3 to 5%. Although 30 to 50 times greater than the risk in the general population, this is still a small risk. Dizygotic twins have an identical MS concordance rate as nontwin siblings; monozygotic twins have a 40% concordance rate.

SYMPTOMATIC TREATMENT

Spasticity

A cardinal clinical feature of MS is the upper motor neuron (UMN) syndrome, which results in a characteristic pattern of motor dysfunction, of which spasticity is a main component. Spasticity is defined clinically as a velocity-dependent increase in muscle tone; this sign is closely associated with other components of the UMN syndrome: loss of dexterity and weakness, hyperactive reflexes, clonus, spasms, and extensor plantar responses. Spasticity in MS is usually of spinal cord origin and affects predominantly the lower extremities and trunk. Problems range from easy fatigability, loss of dexterity, and difficulty with stressed gait maneuvers such as running or hopping to stiffness, pain, severe weakness, involuntary spasms, and eventually contractures. The spastic gait appears stiff with short steps and, at times, scissoring of the legs. Stiffness is enhanced by more rapid ambulation, frequently causing a bouncing or jiggling appearance. Spasticity is more directly evaluated by passively stretching muscle groups with the patient seated or supine, which produces a "catch," or resistance to further movement, after the limb is displaced. In mild cases, this catch can be demonstrated only with rapid rates of passive movement across a joint (usually flexion and extension of the knee, but any muscle group can be tested). In severe cases, slow movements for a very short distance may provoke a catch, as well as involuntary spasms or clonus.

The management of spasticity must involve a comprehensive approach. Medication alone is often inadequate to prevent the complications of contractures, joint malalignment, and pain, and the functional consequences of spasticity vary from patient to patient. For example, spasticity may be beneficial in certain cases by allowing severely weak patients to ambulate. Therefore, treatment of spasticity must be tailored to the patient's impairment and disability. Most patients benefit from evaluation and treatment by a physical therapist experienced in this field, and patients with significant upper extremity spasticity or mobility problems (usually wheelchair dependent) should also be assessed by an occupational therapist. Physician and therapist should outline the goals of treatment and communicate this to the patient or caregivers. It is generally useful to reduce pain when possible and to treat infections, both of which exacerbate spasticity. Proper positioning also helps reduce spasticity. Simple measures such as flexion at hips and knees during sleep can reduce spasticity significantly. Examples of common therapeutic goals include alleviating knee pain from a spastic footdrop, improving perineal hygiene by eliminating hip adductor spasticity, decreasing nocturnal leg spasms, and reducing contractures in a bedridden patient.

Medications are considered adjuncts to physical measures. Antispastic drugs fall into four categories: gamma-aminobutyric acid (GABA) agonists, benzodiazepines, skeletal muscle relaxants, and alpha$_2$ agonists. Baclofen (Lioresal), the only selective GABA-B agonist available, is usually the drug of first choice. The therapeutic window for this medication is wide, and the optimal dose must be individually determined. We usually begin treatment at 5 mg three times a day and instruct the patient to increase the dose by 5- to 10-mg increments every 3 days as needed. Mild cases may respond to doses ranging from 5 mg three times a day to 10 mg four times a day. Moderate spasticity usally requires 10 to 20 mg four times a day. More severe cases may require in excess of 200 mg per day,* if tolerated. The principal limitations of baclofen are the unmasking of underlying weakness as spastic muscle tone is reduced and confusion, especially in cognitively impaired individuals. All patients should be instructed not to suddenly discontinue baclofen, as this may precipitate withdrawal seizures.

Benzodiazepines, principally diazepam (Valium), are frequently used in conjunction with baclofen. Because benzodiazepines potentiate the central effects

---

*Exceeds dosage recommended by the manufacturer.

of baclofen, adding small doses of diazepam to baclofen may augment the antispastic effect without sedation. We generally use diazepam in patients who are unable to tolerate therapeutic doses of baclofen or who have painful or disabling spasms. We begin by adjusting the baclofen dose to a tolerable level and then add diazepam at a dose of 2 mg two to three times a day. Diazepam can be increased gradually by increments of 4 mg per week. If side effects become troublesome, the dose is temporarily decreased before attempting a more gradual dose increase. Beneficial responses are usually observed at doses of less than 20 mg per day. Rare cases may require doses ranging from 40 to 60 mg per day. Diazepam monotherapy should be reserved for patients who are unable to tolerate low doses of baclofen or for those patients with prominent nocturnal spasms. For the latter indication, a dose of 5 to 20 mg at bedtime is usually effective. Single doses of diazepam at bedtime are frequently well tolerated, even in patients with severe forebrain disease.

Dantrolene (Dantrium) is usually reserved as a third-line agent in nonambulatory patients because of its potential hepatotoxicity and tendency to aggravate muscle weakness. Dantrolene acts on skeletal muscles by producing a dose-dependent reduction in myofibril contraction. Therapy is initiated at 25 mg given at bedtime and gradually increased to a maximum dose of 100 mg four times a day. As a single bedtime dose, dantrolene is well tolerated and effectively controls nocturnal cramps and spasms in patients who are unable to obtain relief with baclofen or diazepam. As the dose is increased and spread throughout the day, patients predictably develop diarrhea, anorexia, nausea, and sometimes vomiting. Some patients don't tolerate effective doses, since gastrointestinal side effects are dose dependent. Dantrolene may cause toxic hepatitis. The incidence of this potentially fatal complication increases with doses above 400 mg per day and is more common in women and patients over age 35. Because of this complication, we monitor transaminase levels throughout the course of therapy and discontinue dantrolene in patients with serum glutamic-oxaloacetic transaminase (SGOT) levels greater than two times the upper limit of normal.

Noradrenergic alpha$_2$ agonists act within the spinal cord to enhance noradrenergic-mediated polysynaptic inhibition. In addition to demonstrated effects on spasticity and spasms, these drugs exert antinociceptive effects mediated by alpha$_2$ receptors in the dorsal horn of the spinal cord. Experience with the use of these drugs for spasticity is limited in the United States. Tizanidine,* an alpha$_2$ agonist with fewer cardiovascular effects than clonidine, has been marketed in Europe and Canada but is not currently approved for use in the United States. Investigators claim similar effects on spasticity and flexor spasms as observed with baclofen, without the negative effect of increased weakness. One of us (RPK) has used

clonidine (Catapres) in a limited number of MS patients, either as monotherapy or in combination with baclofen. From our limited experience, it appears that combination therapy (clonidine 0.05 mg twice a day to 0.1 mg three times a day with low-dose baclofen) reduces spasms without the sedation and confusion commonly observed with high doses of baclofen or diazepam. Also, symptomatic hypotension does not appear to be a problem if the dose if titrated slowly or if long-acting clonidine patches (Catapres-TTS 0.1 to 0.3 applied once a week) are used. Clonidine is particularly advantageous in patients with coexisting hypertension or detrusor sphincter dyssynergia.

The management of severe spasticity and flexor spasms in wheelchair-restricted or bedridden MS patients is difficult, since these patients tolerate high doses of baclofen or diazepam poorly due to cognitive or bulbar dysfunction. Without adequate spasticity management, caregiving, especially perineal hygiene and positioning of limbs, is difficult and contractures develop rapidly. This may result in skin breakdown and frequent UTIs, which further aggravate spasticity and spasms. Baclofen may be infused into the lumbar subarachnoid space at a continuous rate via an implantable, externally programmable pump that was recently approved by the U.S. Food and Drug Administration (FDA). Intrathecal baclofen dramatically reduces spasticity and spasms in most severe cases that are refractory to oral antispastic drugs. Side effects from intrathecal baclofen are minimal, since it is concentrated in the thoracolumbar spinal fluid. Implantation of a pump and use of intrathecal baclofen should be done at centers with experience in the procedure to optimize outcome.

Bladder Dysfunction

Eighty percent of MS patients experience significant bladder dysfunction at some point in their illness. Fifty percent of mildly affected MS patients demonstrate abnormalities that are amenable to treatment early in their disease course. Bladder dysfunction results in restricted social, vocational, and leisure activities, disruption of sleep, UTI, kidney and bladder stone formation, and renal disease, and it interferes with normal sexual activities. There are three common categories of neurogenic bladder dysfunction observed in MS patients: (1) failure to store urine (small-capacity or irritable bladder), (2) failure to empty urine (large-capacity, atonic bladder or failure to relax the urinary sphincter), and (3) combined failure to store and failure to empty urine (usually due to an irritable bladder and inability to relax the urinary sphincter—termed "detrusor sphincter dyssynergia" [DSD]). An accurate diagnosis cannot be made by history alone. Bladder management strategies are most effective when the underlying bladder pathophysiology has been fully defined. All three categories of bladder dysfunction may produce urgency and frequency, nocturia, and urge incontinence. Similarly, hesitancy may imply an inability to relax the urinary sphincter or poor bladder contrac-

---

*Not yet approved for use in the United States.

TABLE 4. **Management of Bladder Dysfunction**

	Failure to Store	Failure to Empty	Combined*
Void volume	<200 mL	<200 mL	100–300 mL
Postvoid residual volume	<100 mL	>300 mL	100–300 mL
Treatment	1. Anticholinergics: oxybutynin (Ditropan) 2.5 mg bid to 5.0 tid *or* propantheline (Pro-Banthīne) 15 mg tid to 30 mg qid *or* hyoscyamine (Levsin) (time release) 0.375 mg bid to tid 2. If ineffective, urodynamic testing	1. Intermittent catheterization 4–6 times per day 2. If ineffective, add an anticholinergic 3. If ineffective, urodynamic testing	1. Alpha-adrenergic blocker (also use intermittent catheterization if postvoid residual volume >200 mL): terazosin (Hytrin) 1 mg qhs *or* clonidine (Catapres) 0.05–0.1 mg bid† *or* imipramine (Tofranil) 10–25 mg tid 2. If ineffective, add an anticholinergic 3. If ineffective, urodynamic testing

*Combined failure to store and failure to empty is a complex management problem that benefits from early urodynamic testing to guide therapy.
†May also use clonidine patches (transdermal therapeutic system [TTS] 0.1–0.3 mg) applied weekly.

tions. Therefore, a history of bladder symptoms in an MS patient requires testing. The initial evaluation consists of a urinalysis. If the urinalysis shows evidence of infection, a culture should be obtained and appropriate antibiotics initiated. If symptoms do not clear after a course of antibiotics or no infection is found, a measurement of voided volume and postvoid urinary residual volume should be obtained. Optimally, this measurement should be made when the bladder is full and when the patient experiences the usual urge to void. Table 4 outlines our management approach based on this testing. If the postvoid residual volume is high, one cannot distinguish a hypotonic bladder from DSD or from mechanical outlet obstruction. However, one can empirically manage a patient with high residual volume. Initially, management should be directed at DSD, since this is much more common in MS patients than bladder hypotonia. Both scenarios require intermittent self-catheterization (ISC) at least temporarily. If initial management strategies fail or the patient is reluctant to perform ISC, urodynamic studies will be necessary.

Patients with significant symptoms should cut down on caffeinated beverages, but fluid restriction should be discouraged. Patients should be encouraged to acidify their urine with cranberry juice daily to avoid UTIs. Patients with frequent UTIs despite good hygiene and catheterization technique require a complete urologic evaluation. Prophylactic antibiotics should be avoided unless all other measures fail. It has been our experience that suprapubic catheters, at least in women, do not prevent UTIs. Our experience in men is too limited to form an opinion.

Severe cases of nocturia that are unresponsive to evening fluid restriction, anticholinergic medications, and ISC at bedtime usually respond to desmopressin acetate nasal spray (DDAVP) 0.1 to 0.2 mL (10 to 20 μg) given at bedtime. DDAVP is well tolerated and rarely results in a significant drop in serum sodium levels. Nevertheless, sodium levels should be monitored weekly for 2 weeks and then every 3 months.

Bowel Dysfunction

Constipation is common in MS patients. The etiology is multifactorial, with poor dietary habits, immobility, fluid restriction, and concurrent medications (e.g., anticholinergics) contributing significantly. Table 5 outlines our approach to constipation; laxatives should be avoided. Bowel incontinence is relatively rare in mild to moderately affected MS patients. The same bowel regimen described in Table 5 may establish regular bowel movements and reduce bowel incontinence. Addition of an anticholinergic medication, particularly hyoscyamine (Levsin), may decrease excessive bowel motility. Patients should be counseled to defecate at regular intervals, preferably 30 to 60 minutes after eating, when the gastrocolic reflex occurs.

Sexual Dysfunction

Sexual dysfunction is common even in mild cases and does not invariably coexist with bladder or bowel problems. Most MS patients do not spontaneously

TABLE 5. **Management of Constipation**

Eliminate unnecessary medications or substitute medications less inclined to cause constipation
Maintain fluid intake >2 L/day, add bulk-forming agents (bran or psyllium), increase physical activity
Regular planned defecation 30 to 60 min after eating
Add stool softeners (docusate sodium) or mild oral laxatives (milk of magnesia or docusate sodium plus casanthranol)
Glycerin or bisacodyl suppositories 30 min prior to planned defecation
Fleet enema at time of planned defecation
Manual disimpaction

report sexual dysfunction, but many will readily report it with gentle direct questioning. Erectile dysfunction is the most common problem in men. Women commonly experience decreased libido, decreased perineal sensation, and decreased lubrication. The problem is most commonly multifactorial. Demyelination in the lower spinal cord may contribute to symptoms, but psychological factors such as depression and marital discord, as well as the effects of medications, need to be considered. Regardless of the cause, sexual dysfunction is best managed by a comprehensive sexual dysfunction clinic.

Tremor and Ataxia

Cerebellar tremor and ataxia are among the most disabling physical symptoms of MS, but they respond poorly to drug therapy. Therefore, pharmacotherapy should always be buttressed by a rehabilitation approach. Occupational therapists can provide adaptive equipment to help maintain independence, and physical therapists can assist in gait training. Patients with a predominantly ataxic gait should be equipped with a four-wheel rollator-type walker for safe ambulation. Many drugs have been advocated as treatment for intention tremors in MS. In our experience, clonazepam (Klonopin) is the most effective and warrants a trial in most significantly affected patients. Before initiating treatment, a simple trial of wrist weights should be tried. If that is ineffective or only partially effective, we begin clonazepam at a dose of 0.5 mg given at bedtime. Morning and afternoon doses are gradually added over 10 to 14 days. Thereafter, the daily dose is increased by 0.5 mg every 5 days, always beginning with the evening dose. The dose is gradually increased to an end point of effective control or unacceptable sedation. Rarely do patients tolerate doses in excess of 6 mg per day. Patients should be cautioned to discontinue clonazepam slowly.

Carefully selected patients may benefit from stereotactic ablation of the ventrolateral thalamic nucleus. This ablative procedure reduces the amplitude of tremor in the contralateral arm; complications include contralateral weakness, cortical deficits such as contralateral neglect, and aphasia. Therefore, stereotactic thalamotomy should be done only in neurosurgical centers with demonstrated experience. We have performed this procedure in 15 MS patients during the past 6 years. In most cases, tremor was dramatically decreased or eliminated. Most of the patients developed some degree of weakness in the contralateral limbs, and ambulatory patients found it more difficult to walk. We currently restrict the procedure to nonambulatory patients who have been stable for at least 6 months, who have not responded to an adequate trial of clonazepam, who have severe tremor in both arms that precludes independent function, and who have no significant bulbar or cognitive dysfunction.

Fatigue

Classically, MS-related fatigue is described as a feeling of exhaustion that comes on with exertion, usually late in the day. The pathophysiology is unclear, since patients can display significant fatigue in the absence of demonstrable motor dysfunction. Patients should first be evaluated for specific causes of fatigue that are amenable to specific treatments, including coexisting medical conditions such as thyroid disease or anemia, primary or secondary sleep disorders (the latter includes frequent awakening due to nocturia), depression, and aggravating medications. If no alternative etiology can be found, the patient may benefit from amantadine (Symmetrel)* 100 mg in the morning and early afternoon. Pemoline (Cylert)* 18.75 to 37.5 mg in the morning and early afternoon is effective for some patients who do not respond to amantadine. Patients who respond to either drug frequently develop tolerance after a variable interval of time. This can be avoided by taking the medication only on weekdays. In those patients who require the medication 7 days a week, a drug holiday for 1 to 2 weeks can restore the effectiveness of the drug. Patients should be re-evaluated for alternative causes of fatigue, especially depression. Medical management should be supplemented with a regular exercise program to enhance aerobic capacity and endurance.

Heat Sensitivity

MS symptoms frequently worsen or recur in the heat, and increased ambient temperature may lead to exhaustion. This arises from conduction failure in partially demyelinated axons. Air conditioning may be required for almost all environments during the summer. If troublesome neurologic symptoms occur due to overheating, we advise cool showers or baths until the symptoms subside. Fevers from infections should be treated promptly with antipyretics and, if necessary, cooling blankets. Some individuals who are dramatically heat sensitive or have occupations that preclude air conditioning (e.g., factory or construction workers) benefit from custom-fitted cooling vests. The local chapter of the National MS Society should be able to provide information about available vendors.

Pain Syndromes

Pain syndromes are very common in MS patients and can be separated into four broad categories: neuralgia, pain from meningeal irritation, centrally mediated dysesthesias, and secondary musculoskeletal pain. The dorsal root entry zone of virtually any peripheral or cranial sensory nerve can become irritated by an MS plaque, creating neuralgia. This sharp, lancinating pain occurs spontaneously or is triggered by certain movements or tactile stimulation

---

*Not FDA-approved for this indication.

within the distribution of the affected nerve. Trigeminal neuralgia is a classic example, but glossopharyngeal neuralgia and occipital neuralgia are quite common. MS plaques in the cervical spinal cord may produce a pseudoradicular pain that can be difficult to differentiate from spondylitic radiculopathy. In addition to paroxysmal neuralgic pain, MS patients may experience constant, severe, aching pain in the same sensory distribution as the neuralgia. At times, this type of pain is more difficult to treat than the neuralgia. For neuralgia, we begin treatment with carbamazepine (Tegretol) at a dose of 100 to 200 mg twice daily. The dose is titrated to pain relief or until unacceptable toxicity occurs. For patients who do not respond to or cannot tolerate carbamazepine, phenytoin (Dilantin),* amitriptyline,* and baclofen monotherapy are alternatives. Recent reports suggest that misoprostol (Cytotec)* at a dose of 200 mg three times a day is effective in relieving refractory, atypical facial pain and trigeminal neuralgia. This medication must be avoided in pregnant women. Patients who do not respond to medications frequently respond to percutaneous rhizotomy.

Pain from meningeal irritation frequently occurs during episodes of optic neuritis or transverse myelitis in which the pain-sensitive dura is stretched or inflamed by involvement of adjacent optic nerve or spinal cord, respectively. As this usually occurs during acute episodes of inflammation, we treat this pain with high-dose intravenous corticosteroids (see section on MS exacerbations).

Spontaneous dysesthesias, usually of a burning quality, are common and difficult to treat. At times, dysesthesia is accompanied by temperature and vasomotor changes in the limb, suggesting sympathetically mediated pain. Unfortunately, local blocks to sympathetic ganglia are usually not effective. Tricyclic antidepressants and carbamazepine are the most effective drugs for dysesthesias. Doses should be increased gradually to allow patients time to develop tolerance to side effects. Doses of 150 to 250 mg per day of amitriptyline are commonly required. We have had no success with mexiletine (Mexitil).* Occasional patients with severe, refractory pain may require perphenazine (Trilafon)* or fluphenazine (Prolixin)* in combination with amitriptyline, although the risk of tardive dyskinesia should be considered.

Musculoskeletal pain, frequently in the lumbar spine, hips, knees, or shoulders, is common in patients with abnormal gait, poor sitting posture, or weakness in the upper extremities. Treatment must be directed at the underlying cause. Lumbar back pain in ambulatory patients should initially be treated with exercise to strengthen the paraspinal and abdominal muscles. Some patients who are too weak to benefit from exercise may benefit from an elastic lumbar corset. Gait training may improve posture and pain in selected patients. Nonsteroidal anti-inflammatory drugs, with or without a transcutaneous electrical nerve stimulation (TENS) unit, may

relieve pain enough for patients to undergo physical therapy. Narcotics should be avoided except for short courses to control acute exacerbations of pain. Wheelchair-bound patients with lumbar pain may benefit from a lumbar roll or other types of lumbar support. In many cases, custom cushions for the wheelchair are effective in relieving pain.

Knee and hip pain are common in patients with a spastic gait, especially with a footdrop. Custom-fitted ankle-foot orthotic (AFO) devices not only improve ambulation but also relieve pain in the majority of patients. If a well-fitted AFO fails to relieve knee pain, the addition of a Swedish knee cage or Don Joy brace will further alleviate hyperextension at the knee joint. Unfortunately, patients who hyperextend at the knee to compensate for weak knee extensor muscles may not be able to walk with a knee brace that prevents hyperextension.

Frozen shoulders from acute or chronic tendinitis are common in wheelchair-dependent or bedridden MS patients. This must be treated aggressively to preserve residual upper extremity function. Patients should receive intra-articular infiltration with a glucocorticoid combined with an anesthetic to allow aggressive physical therapy. Stretching exercises should be continued indefinitely to prevent further recurrences.

Paroxysmal Motor Symptoms

Paroxysmal motor phenomena are common in MS. The classic type has been variously described as "tonic spasms" or "tonic seizures"—the latter term deriving from the superficial resemblance to focal motor seizures. During a spasm, one arm is forcibly contorted in a dystonic flexion posture while the ipsilateral leg is unaffected or forcibly extended. These spasms last seconds, occur repeatedly, and are frequently painful. Carbamazepine (Tegretol) is remarkably effective at controlling these spasms, even at subtherapeutic, anticonvulsant doses. We begin with 100 to 200 mg twice daily and increase rapidly to 200 to 400 mg twice daily. For minor symptoms without pain, the dose can be increased more slowly. Patients who are unable to tolerate carbamazepine may respond to phenytoin (Dilantin) or, rarely, baclofen. We usually continue treatment for 6 months and then gradually taper the medication. The spasms do not usually require long-term treatment.

Other forms of paroxysmal motor phenomena are less common in MS patients. Hemifacial spasm—a forceful, grimacing contortion of one side of the face—responds to the same treatments as tonic spasms. Rarely, patients describe "drop attacks" in which their legs suddenly go out from underneath them with no warning. Since this complaint is so rare, it is unclear whether this phenomenon represents bilateral tonic extensor spasms of the leg.

True seizures occur in 5% of MS patients, usually late in the course of the disease. A diagnostic evaluation to exclude alternative etiologies, including MRI scanning with and without contrast and, sometimes,

---

*Not FDA-approved for this indication.

cerebrospinal fluid analysis, should be performed after the first seizure. Seizures should be treated in the same manner as other symptomatic seizure disorders.

Vertigo, Nystagmus, Oscillopsia

Vertigo or dizziness may be disabling in MS patients. Acute vertigo is usually observed in the setting of a brain stem exacerbation. Treatment consists of intravenous corticosteroids combined with a 1- to 2-week course of a vestibular suppressant. We prefer diazepam (Valium) at a dose of 2 to 5 mg three times a day, although higher doses are often required. Residual vestibular symptoms may respond to vestibular rehabilitation exercises. Chronic, ill-defined dizziness is much more difficult to treat. Vestibular testing may be helpful in clarifying the underlying pathophysiology. Alternative diagnoses such as Meniere's disease, benign positional vertigo, or cerebellopontine angle tumor are sometimes found.

Abnormal eye movements, such as nystagmus, may degrade vision and create an illusory motion of the visual environment termed oscillopsia. Pharmacotherapy is generally ineffective, but patients may benefit from optical stabilization devices, available at specialized neuro-opthalmic centers. Effective treatment can have a profoundly beneficial effect on the patient's quality of life.

Affective Disorders and Emotional Distress

Emotional distress is common in MS and tends to occur in response to a perceived loss or threat. Although this can occur at any time, it is most common at diagnosis, when symptoms become persistent rather than intermittent, and with the development of significant disability. It is often difficult to identify major depression in MS patients. Symptoms may overlap with certain MS-related symptoms such as fatigue, diminished attention and concentration, and pain. We have a very low threshold for exploring emotional issues, referring patients to a psychologist and treating with antidepressants. For patients with prominent sleep disturbances or anxiety, we prefer tricyclic antidepressants with sedative properties, such as amitriptyline (Elavil). The anticholinergic effects may also improve urinary urgency and nocturia. For patients with prominent sleep disturbances who are unable to tolerate prominent anticholinergic effects, we prefer trazodone (Desyrel) or desipramine (Norpramin) as a single bedtime dose. For patients with prominent fatigue, we prefer serotonin uptake inhibitors such as fluoxetine (Prozac) 20 mg every morning. Bipolar disorders are 15 times more common in MS patients than in the general population. In rare cases, an organic bipolar disorder is triggered by disease involving the mesial temporal lobes. Treatment is no different from that used to treat bipolar disorders in the general population. Emotional lability, so-called pathologic laughing and cry-

ing, is less common than depression but equally disabling. This tends to occur with extensive frontal lobe white matter disease. It is usually controllable with low doses of amitriptyline (25 to 75 mg at bedtime).

Cognitive Impairment

MS-related cognitive impairment can be demonstrated in approximately 40% of patients. Such impairment is generally circumscribed rather than global; recent memory and information processing are most commonly affected. Cognitive impairment may have a devastating impact on everyday function, including activities at school, work, and home. It is important to consider the possibility of cognitive impairment in an MS patient who is having difficulty with any of his or her roles if the severity of motor or visual impairment is inadequate to explain the problems. Neuropsychological testing is required to determine the extent and type of cognitive impairment. Although there is currently no specific drug treatment for cognitive impairment, it is important to accurately diagnose the problem for vocational and educational planning.

DISEASE-SPECIFIC TREATMENT

Treatment of Exacerbations

Corticotropin and high-dose intravenous methylprednisolone have been documented in controlled trials to hasten recovery from acute exacerbations of MS. Recent evidence suggests that high-dose intravenous methylprednisolone may have a more rapid onset of action and may be more effective over time than other steroid preparations. Furthermore, conventional doses of oral prednisone alone (1 mg per kg per day) in a study of optic neuritis were associated with an increased recurrence rate of optic neuritis in the same or opposite eye. The similarities between monosymptomatic optic neuritis and exacerbations in established MS should make physicians pause before prescribing conventional doses of oral prednisone alone in MS patients. Our current practice is to treat only those patients experiencing demonstrable functional impairment from exacerbations. Physicians should resist the temptation to treat patients with corticosteroids for symptom fluctuations without functional consequences. All patients should be seen and evaluated for alternative causes of neurologic decline, particularly UTIs. For significant attacks, we use intravenous methylprednisolone 500 or 1000 mg per day for 3 days. This is followed by a short course of oral prednisone beginning at 60 mg every morning and tapering by 20 mg every 4 days. If clear deterioration occurs during the prednisone taper, the dose is increased to 60 mg per day and tapered over 6 weeks. Prednisone tapers of longer duration should be avoided if possible. This protocol has been well tolerated and safely administered in the outpatient setting. Patients are hospitalized if they have concurrent medical conditions requiring close monitoring during intravenous methylprednisolone treatment, such as diabetes, severe hypertension, or coronary artery disease. Patients are also hospitalized for severe exacerbations resulting in the loss of independent function (e.g., ambulatory patients no longer able to walk).

Common side effects include a metallic taste during the infusion; gastrointestinal upset or, rarely, ulcers; insomnia; flushing; a temporary increase in blood pressure; fluid retention; weight gain; easy bruising; muscle pains (usually during the prednisone taper); and hiccups. We commonly prescribe ranitidine (Zantac) or another H_2 blocker as a single bedtime dose during the entire 15 days of steroid treatment. Patients with insomnia should be given appropriate sedation with a short-acting hypnotic. Diuretics should be avoided because of the risk of electrolyte imbalances. Edema is best managed with tight stockings, fluid restriction, and leg elevation. Rarely, patients experience significant depression, mania, or psychosis during or after treatment with corticosteroids. Premedication with trazodone, lithium, or an antipsychotic drug is usually effective at preventing recurrent episodes with repeated steroid courses.

Interferon-Beta

The recent approval of interferon-beta-1b (IFN-β-1b [Betaseron]) for the treatment of ambulatory, relapsing-remitting MS patients represents a milestone in MS therapeutics. For the first time, an experimental therapy has progressed from the confines of controlled clinical trials to the practice of every physician caring for MS patients. Although the exact mechanism of action is unclear, it appears that the immunomodulatory properties of this recombinant human cytokine are at least partly responsible for the observed benefits. The benefits observed with IFN-β-1b have now been confirmed and extended by the results of the interferon-beta-1a (IFN-β-1a) trial in relapsing-remitting MS. Both products reduced the frequency of exacerbations by one-third and significantly reduced the development of new lesions by MRI scan. More importantly, the IFN-β-1a trial demonstrated a 40% reduction in the rate of disease progression (i.e., the development of permanent new impairments). Since IFN-β-1b is the only product currently approved by the FDA, the following discussion is confined to this product.

Current FDA guidelines restrict the use of IFN-β-1b to ambulatory patients with relapsing-remitting (sometimes referred to as exacerbating-remitting) disease. Further indications are unknown at this time, since no other patient populations have been studied. Specifically excluded from this indication are chronic progressive and wheelchair-dependent MS patients. The ideal candidate has active, relapsing-remitting disease with one or more exacerbations per year and a relatively short duration of disease (less than 10 years). The decision to start IFN-β-1b should be made only after consulting with a neurologist,

preferably one with experience using this medication. Patients must be well educated about the potential risks and benefits, injection techniques, and strategies to minimize side effects. Table 6 outlines our protocol for initiating treatment.

The major side effect of IFN-β-1b therapy is the "flulike syndrome." This usually begins 4 to 8 hours after a subcutaneous injection and may persist until the next day. One or more of the following symptoms may occur with this syndrome: fever, chills, myalgia, anorexia, insomnia, weight loss, and fatigue. Although 60% of patients experience some flulike symptoms at the onset of therapy, only 10% have persistent symptoms after 2 months of treatment. In most cases, symptoms are controlled with acetaminophen (Tylenol) or a nonsteroidal anti-inflammatory agent (see Table 6). If severe flulike symptoms occur with the first injection, we frequently decrease the dose 50% for the next month before resuming a full dose. This allows the patient time to develop tolerance to this adverse effect. Injection site reactions are a more common and persistent early side effect. The skin reactions are commonly painful or pruritic but respond well to icing, antihistamines, and topical corticosteroids. Additional side effects include elevated serum transaminase levels, neutropenia, leukopenia, anemia, palpitations, and menstrual irregularities. Rarely do these side effects necessitate drug discontinuation. If they are significant, we always reduce the dose or hold the medication until an evaluation for alternative etiologies is completed. If the problem clears, treatment is cautiously restarted. Neurobehavioral side effects, including irritability, anxiety, depression, suicidal ideation, paranoid ideation, and delirium, are particularly disturbing and a frequent cause of drug discontinuation. Depression is best managed with serotonin uptake inhibitors (e.g., fluoxetine) and a temporary reduction in dosage. Patients should be closely monitored and treatment dis-

TABLE 6. **Betaseron Protocol**

Determine whether referral to neurologist is indicated.

Register patient with Berlex Laboratories (1-800-788-1467).

Patient fills out packet of information sent by Berlex. This will determine whether he or she is eligible for the indigent patient program or the support program (both financial assistance programs). Patient reviews educational material.

At this point, the patient requires education about side effects and self-injection technique. The local MS Society should be able to provide locations for this education in the community.

CBC, SGOT, and SGPT done at baseline, then every month for 3 months, then every 6 months.

Premedicate with acetaminophen 650 mg at the time of injections and 4 h later. If ineffective, use ibuprofen 400 mg. If patient has difficulty sleeping, add diphenhydramine (50 mg) to the bedtime dose of acetaminophen.

Injections should be given in the early evening—8 mIU (1.0 mL) SC every other day. Patient needs instruction on rotating injection sites.

If significant side effects occur, consider temporarily holding injections or decreasing to half the dose for 1 month.

Abbreviations: CBC = complete blood count; SGOT = serum glutamic-oxaloacetic transaminase; SGPT = serum glutamate pyruvate transaminase.

continued if a prompt response to treatment does not occur.

Experimental Therapies

Recent advances in immunology, molecular biology, neuroimaging, and clinical trial methodology have revolutionized our approach to therapeutic research in MS. Most investigators would agree that global immune suppression with therapies such as high-dose intravenous cyclophosphamide (Cytoxan)* is still useful in cases of rapidly progressing MS. Unfortunately, the benefits are modest and transient, and significant toxicity precludes long-term treatment. Biopharmaceuticals now allow us to focus on therapies with acceptable toxicity targeted at specific components of the immune system. Conventional drugs are still under investigation to answer some remaining questions. First, can monthly or bimonthly pulses of intravenous methylprednisolone slow the progression of unstable MS? Second, what is the role of more specific immune suppressants, such as the lymphotoxic drug cladribine (Leustatin)*? Third, what is the role of conventional drugs used to treat other inflammatory disorders, such as sulfasalazine (Azulfidine)* and methotrexate*? A recent clinical trial of low-dose weekly oral methotrexate in chronic progressive MS patients demonstrated a significant slowing of the disease process without any significant toxicity. This needs to be confirmed and the indications clarified by studies currently in progress. Until a truly effective treatment for MS is found, all treatments should be considered experimental. Patients should be referred to a neurologist with expertise in this field prior to instituting any disease-modifying treatments.

---

*Not FDA-approved for this indication.

MYASTHENIA GRAVIS

method of
JAMES F. HOWARD, JR., M.D.
The University of North Carolina at Chapel Hill
Chapel Hill, North Carolina

CLINICAL FEATURES

Myasthenia gravis (MG) is the most common primary disorder of neuromuscular transmission. The usual cause is an acquired immunologic abnormality directed against the postsynaptic acetylcholine receptor (AChR) complex, but some cases result from genetic abnormalities producing a structural abnormality at the neuromuscular junction. The prevalence of MG in the United States is estimated at 14 per 100,000 people, with approximately 36,000 cases. However, MG is probably underdiagnosed, and the prevalence is probably higher. The most common age at onset is the second and third decades in women and the seventh and eighth decades in men.

Ocular motor disturbances, ptosis or diplopia, are the initial symptom of MG in two-thirds of patients; almost all have both symptoms within 2 years. Oropharyngeal muscle weakness—difficulty in chewing, swallowing, or talking—is the initial symptom in one-sixth of patients and limb weakness in only 10%. Initial weakness is rarely limited to single muscle groups such as neck or finger extensors or hip flexors. The severity of the weakness fluctuates during the day, usually being least in the morning and worse as the day progresses, especially after prolonged use of affected muscles. Ocular symptoms typically become worse while reading, watching television, or driving, especially in bright sunlight, and many patients find that dark glasses reduce diplopia and also hide drooping eyelids. It is of note that weakness of the orbicularis oculi muscle is found in virtually all patients with MG. Jaw muscle weakness typically becomes worse during prolonged chewing, especially tough meats, lettuce, or chewy candy.

DIAGNOSIS

The clinical diagnosis of MG is based on the characteristic picture of fluctuating weakness: improvement with rest only to have the weakness return with the resumption of activity. The diagnosis is confirmed by the demonstration of abnormal synaptic transmission, by improvement with acetylcholinesterase (AChE) inhibitors, by electrophysiologic abnormalities (decremental response to repetitive nerve testing [RNS] or increased jitter and blocking on single-fiber electromyography [SFEMG]), and by the demonstration of antibodies directed against the AChR complex.

Weakness caused by abnormal neuromuscular transmission characteristically improves after intravenous administration of edrophonium chloride, an AChE inhibitor. With the exception of the ocular and pharyngeal muscles, the examiner must rely on the patient to exert maximal effort before and after drug administration to assess its effect. For this reason, the test is most reliable when the patient has ptosis or nasal speech. Improved strength after edrophonium administration is not unique to MG. It may also be seen in motor neuron disease, rapidly progressive motor neuropathies, and lesions of the oculomotor nerves. The ideal dose of edrophonium cannot be predetermined. A single fixed dose, such as 10 mg, may be too much in some patients and cause increased weakness. An incremental dosing schedule is recommended. Two milligrams are injected intravenously and the response monitored for 60 seconds. Subsequent injections are 3 and 5 mg. If improvement is seen within 60 seconds after any dose, no further injections are given. Ten milligrams of edrophonium does not weaken normal muscle, and the occurrence of weakness after edrophonium indicates an abnormality of neuromuscular transmission. The total dose of edrophonium in children is 0.15 mg per kg administered incrementally. Subcutaneous administration can be used in neonates and infants, but the response may be delayed for 2 to 5 minutes.

An Ambu bag and oral suctioning equipment should be available when giving edrophonium since some people are supersensitive to even small dosages and may stop breathing or have excessive secretions that may interfere with respiration. Blind or double-blind edrophonium testing to improve objectivity is of questionable value and is not needed when the end point is well defined, such as relief of ptosis.

Not all patients will respond to intravenous edrophonium. Some may respond to intramuscular neostigmine, because of the longer duration of action. Intramuscular neostigmine is particularly useful in infants and children whose response to intravenous edrophonium may be too brief for adequate observation. In some patients, a therapeutic trial of daily oral pyridostigmine may produce improvement that cannot be appreciated after a single dose of edrophonium or neostigmine.

Seventy-six percent of patients with acquired generalized myasthenia and 54% with ocular myasthenia have serum antibodies that bind human AChR. The serum concentration of AChR antibody varies widely among patients with similar degrees of weakness and cannot predict the severity of disease in individual patients. Approximately 10% of patients who do not have binding antibodies have other antibodies that modulate the turnover of AChR in tissue culture. An elevated concentration of AChR-binding antibodies in a patient with compatible clinical features confirms the diagnosis of MG, but normal antibody concentrations do not exclude the diagnosis. Repeat studies are appropriate when initial values are normal.

The failure of the muscle fiber to depolarize sufficiently for the end-plate potential (EPP) to reach action potential (AP) threshold is the basis of the clinical electrodiagnostic abnormalities in patients with MG. The resulting impulse blocking accounts for the decremental responses seen in RNS studies and the impulse blocking seen with SFEMG. In addition, the time variability of when the EPP reaches AP threshold accounts for the neuromuscular jitter seen in the latter technique. The RNS test is the most frequently used electrodiagnostic test of neuromuscular transmission. The decrementing response to RNS is seen more often in proximal muscles than in hand muscles. A significant decrement to RNS in either a hand or shoulder muscle is seen in 70% of patients with generalized myasthenia but in less than 50% of patients with ocular MG. SFEMG is the most sensitive clinical test of neuromuscular transmission and shows increased jitter in some muscles in nearly all patients with MG. Increased jitter is a nonspecific sign of abnormal neuromuscular transmission and can be seen in other motor unit diseases, and conventional needle EMG must be performed to exclude neuronopathy, neuropathy, or myopathy. Normal jitter in a weak muscle excludes abnormal neuromuscular transmission as the cause of weakness.

Radiographic imaging of the anterior mediastinum is necessary in all patients diagnosed with MG to exclude a thymoma. All patients should be screened for associated autoimmune disorders, including vitamin B_{12} deficiency, thyroid disease, and collagen vascular disease.

TREATMENT

There has never been a large, controlled, clinical trial for any medical or surgical modality used to treat MG. All recommended regimens are empirical, and experts disagree on treatments of choice. Treatment decisions must be individualized and based on knowledge of the natural history of disease in each patient and the predicted response to a specific form of therapy. Treatment goals will be different for each patient and must be established according to the severity of disease, the patient's age and sex, and the degree of functional impairment. The response to any form of treatment may be difficult to assess because the severity of symptoms fluctuates. Spontaneous improvement, even remissions, occurs without specific therapy, especially during the early stages of the disease. The treatment strategies for MG are listed in Table 1.

Enhancement of Neuromuscular Transmission

Acetylcholinesterase Inhibitors

AChE inhibitors slow the enzymatic hydrolysis of acetylcholine (ACh) at cholinergic synapses, so that ACh accumulates at the neuromuscular junction and its effect is prolonged. AChE inhibitors may produce significant improvement in some patients and little to none in others. These drugs produce a differential response—that is, different muscles respond differently; with any dose, certain muscles get stronger, others do not change, and still others become weaker. Strength rarely returns to normal.

Pyridostigmine bromide (Mestinon) and neostigmine bromide (Prostigmin) are the most commonly used AChE inhibitors. Pyridostigmine is preferred because it has a lower frequency of gastrointestinal side effects. The initial oral dose in adults is 30 to 60 mg every 6 to 8 hours. The equivalent dose of neostigmine is 7.5 to 15 mg. In infants and children, the initial oral dose of pyridostigmine is 1.0 mg per kg and of neostigmine, 0.3 mg per kg. Equivalent dosages of these drugs are listed in Table 2. Pyridostigmine is available as a syrup (60 mg per 5 mL) for children or for nasogastric tube administration in patients with impaired swallowing. A timed-release tablet of pyridostigmine (Mestinon Timespan, 180 mg) has been used as a bedtime dose for patients who are too weak to swallow in the morning. However, its absorption is erratic, leading to possible overdosage and underdosage, and it should not be used during waking hours. Even at night, it is preferable for the patient to awaken at the appropriate dosing interval and take the regular tablet.

No fixed dosage schedule will suit all patients. The need for AChE inhibitors varies from day to day and during the same day in response to a number of factors, including infection, menstruation, emotional stress, and hot weather. Different muscles respond

TABLE 1. **Treatment Strategies for Myasthenia Gravis**

Enhancement of neuromuscular transmission
  Acetylcholinesterase inhibitors
  Aminopyridines
  Ephedrine

Immune suppression
  Corticosteroids
  Cytotoxic drugs
    Azathioprine (Imuran)
    Cyclosporine (Sandimmune)
    Cyclophosphamide (Cytoxan)

"Debulking" patient of circulating immune factors
  Plasma exchange
  Intravenous immunoglobulin

Removal of site of break in immune tolerance
  Thymectomy

TABLE 2. **Equivalent Doses of Acetylcholinesterase Inhibitor Drugs**

	Route and Dosage (in mg)			
	Oral	IM	IV	Elixir
Neostigmine bromide (Prostigmin)	15			
Neostigmine methylsulfate (Prostigmin)	1.5	0.5		
Pyridostigmine bromide (Mestinon)	60	2.0	0.7	60 mg/5 mL
(Mestinon Timespan)	90–180			
Ambenonium chloride (Mytelase)	7.5			

Note: Values are approximations only. Appropriate dosages should be determined for each patient based on the clinical response.

differently, and with any dose, certain muscles get stronger, others do not change, and still others become weaker. Therefore the drug schedule should be titrated to produce an optimal response in muscles causing the greatest disability. Ideally, the effect of each dose should last until time for the next, without significant underdosing or overdosing at any time. In practice, this is not possible. Attempts to eliminate all weakness by increasing the dose or shortening the interval cause overdosage at the time of peak effect. The goal is to keep the dose low enough to provide definite improvement 30 to 45 minutes later, and expect the effect to wear off before the next one is given. This minimizes the possibility that the dose will be increased to the point of causing cholinergic weakness.

Adverse effects of AChE inhibitors result from ACh accumulation at nicotinic receptors of skeletal muscle and at muscarinic receptors on smooth muscle and autonomic glands. Central nervous system side effects are rarely seen with the doses used to treat MG. Acute overdosage may cause fasciculations and increased weakness, including respiratory muscles, apnea, and even ventilatory failure. The practice of giving edrophonium when pyridostigmine has its maximal effect, to determine whether the patient will respond to greater dosages of AChE inhibitors, can be dangerous and may precipitate a cholinergic crisis. There is no readily available "antidote" for nicotinic receptor toxicity, and the patient must be supported through this crisis.

Gastrointestinal complaints are common: queasiness, loose stools, nausea, vomiting, abdominal cramps, and diarrhea. Increased bronchial and oral secretions are a serious problem in patients with swallowing or respiratory insufficiency. Symptoms of muscarinic overdosage may indicate that nicotinic overdosage (weakness) is also occurring. Gastrointestinal side effects can be suppressed with loperamide, propantheline, glycopyrrolate, and diphenoxylate. Bromism, presenting as acute psychosis, is a rare complication in patients taking large amounts of pyridostigmine bromide. The diagnosis of bromide intoxication can be suspected by the discrepancy between the serum sodium and chloride levels and confirmed by direct measurement of the serum bromide level. Some patients are allergic to bromide and develop a rash even at modest doses.

Immune Suppression of the Patient

Corticosteroids

Marked improvement or complete relief of symptoms occurs in more than 75% of patients treated with prednisone, and some improvement occurs in most of the rest. Much of the improvement occurs in the first 6 to 8 weeks, but it may take several months to reach maximal improvement. The severity of disease does not predict the ultimate improvement. The best responses occur in patients with recent onset of symptoms, but patients with chronic disease may also respond. Patients with thymoma have an excellent response to prednisone before or after removal of the tumor.

The most predictable response to prednisone occurs when treatment begins with a daily dose of 1.5 to 2 mg per kg per day. This dose is given until sustained improvement occurs, which is often within 2 weeks, and is then switched to an alternate-day schedule, beginning with 100 to 120 mg. This dose is gradually decreased over many months to the lowest dose necessary to maintain improvement, which is usually less than 20 mg every other day. The rate of decrease must be individualized: patients who have a prompt, complete response to prednisone can reduce the alternate-day dose by 20 mg each month until the dose is 60 mg, then by 10 mg each month until the dose is 20 mg every other day, then by 5 mg every 3 months to a minimal dose of 10 mg every other day. Most patients who respond well to prednisone become weak if the drug is stopped but maintain strength on very low dosages (5 to 10 mg every other day). For this reason, it is recommended not to reduce the dose further than this. Others recommend discontinuing prednisone if the patient is doing well after 2 years. In our experience, weakness ultimately returns if this is done.

About one-third of patients become weaker temporarily after starting prednisone, usually within the first 7 to 10 days, and lasting for up to 6 days. This worsening can usually be managed with AChE inhibitors. In patients with oropharyngeal weakness or respiratory insufficiency, the use of plasma exchange before beginning prednisone may prevent or reduce the severity of steroid-induced exacerbations and produce a more rapid response. Because initial high-dose prednisone may exacerbate weakness, patients with oropharyngeal, respiratory, or significant generalized involvement should be hospitalized to start treatment. Once improvement begins, further exacerbations are unusual. Treatment can be started at low dose to minimize exacerbations; the dose is then slowly increased until improvement occurs. Exacerbations may also occur with this approach, and the response is less predictable. The preceding prednisone regimen can be used for both generalized and purely ocular myasthenia. An alternative approach in treating ocular myasthenia is to begin with 5 or 10 mg of daily prednisone and increase the dose 5 mg every 3 to 4 weeks until improvement begins. The dose is then kept constant until maximal improvement is achieved and then tapered over 4 to 6 months to a maintenance dose of 5 to 10 mg every other day.

The major disadvantages of chronic corticosteroid therapy are the side effects. Hypercorticism occurs in about half of patients treated with the suggested regimen. The severity and frequency of adverse reactions increase when high daily doses are continued for more than 1 month. Fortunately, this is rarely necessary, especially if plasma exchange is begun at the same time as prednisone. Most side effects begin resolving as prednisone is tapered and become minimal at dosages of less than 20 mg every other day. Side effects are minimized when patients use a low-fat, low-sodium diet and take supplemental calcium and vitamin D. Patients with peptic ulcer disease or symptoms of gastritis need H_2 antagonists.

Immune Suppressive Drugs

Azathioprine (Imuran)* improves myasthenic weakness in most patients, but the effect is delayed by 4 to 8 months. The initial dose is 50 mg per day, which is increased in 50 mg per day increments every 7 days to a total of 2 to 3 mg per kg per day. Once improvement begins, it is maintained for as long as the drug is given, but symptoms recur 2 to 3 months after the drug is discontinued or the dose is reduced below therapeutic levels. Patients in whom corticosteroids fail may respond to azathioprine, and the reverse is also true. Some respond better to treatment with both drugs than to either alone. Because the response to azathioprine is delayed, both drugs may be started simultaneously with the intent of rapidly tapering prednisone when azathioprine becomes effective.

Approximately one-third of patients have mild dose-dependent side effects that may require dose reductions but do not require stopping treatment. Gastrointestinal irritation can be minimized by using divided doses after meals or by dose reduction. Leukopenia and even pancytopenia can occur any time during treatment. The blood count must be monitored every week during the first month, each month for a year, and every 3 to 6 months thereafter. If the peripheral white blood cell (WBC) count falls below 3000 cells per mm³, the dose should be temporarily reduced and then gradually increased after the count rises above 3000 cells per mm³. Counts below 1000 WBC per mm³ require that the drug be temporarily discontinued. Serum transaminase concentrations may be slightly elevated, but clinical liver toxicity is rare. Treatment should be discontinued if transaminase levels exceed twice the upper limit of normal, and the drug is restarted at lower dosages when normal values are obtained. Rare cases of azathio-

prine-induced pancreatitis are reported, but the cost effectiveness of monitoring serum amylase concentrations is not established. A severe allergic reaction with flulike symptoms and rash may occur within 2 weeks after starting treatment; this requires that the drug be stopped. Because azathioprine is potentially mutagenic, women of childbearing age should practice adequate contraception.

Cyclosporine (Sandimmune)* inhibits T lymphocyte–dependent immune responses and is sometimes beneficial in treating MG. Treatment is started with 5 to 6 mg per kg per day, in two divided doses taken 12 hours apart. Serum concentrations of cyclosporine and creatinine should be measured monthly and the dose adjusted to produce a trough serum cyclosporine concentration of 75 to 150 ng per mL and a serum creatinine concentration of less than 150% of pretreatment values. The needed dose decreases after tissue saturation is achieved. Simultaneous treatment with 10 to 20 mg of prednisone every other day is often better than cyclosporine alone. Most patients with MG improve 1 to 2 months after starting cyclosporine, and improvement is maintained as long as therapeutic doses are given. Maximal improvement is achieved 6 months or longer after starting treatment. After achieving the maximal response, the dose is gradually reduced to the minimum that maintains improvement. Renal toxicity and hypertension, the important adverse reactions of cyclosporine, are usually avoided or managed using the regimen provided. Many drugs interfere with cyclosporine metabolism and should be avoided or used with caution.

Cyclophosphamide (Cytoxan)* has been used intravenously and orally for the treatment of MG. The intravenous dose is 200 mg per day for 5 days, and the oral dose is 150 to 200 mg per day to a total of 5 to 10 grams as required to relieve symptoms. More than half of patients become asymptomatic after 1 year. Alopecia is common, whereas leukopenia, nausea, vomiting, anorexia, and discoloration of the nails and skin occur less frequently.

Life-threatening infections are an important risk in immune suppressed patients, but this risk appears limited to patients with invasive thymoma or patients receiving three or more immune suppressive drugs. The long-term risk of malignancy is not established, but there are no substantive reports of an increased incidence of malignancy in patients with MG receiving immune suppression.

Removal of the Site of Break in Tolerance

Thymectomy

Thymectomy is recommended for most patients with MG. Most reports do not correlate the severity of weakness before surgery and the timing or degree of improvement after thymectomy. The maximal favorable response generally occurs 2 to 5 years after

---

*Not FDA-approved for this indication.

*Not FDA-approved for this indication.

surgery. However, the response is relatively unpredictable, and significant impairment may continue for months or years after surgery. Sometimes, improvement is only appreciated in retrospect. The best responses to thymectomy are in young people early in the course of their disease, but improvement can occur even after 30 years of symptoms. Patients with disease onset after the age of 60 years rarely show substantial improvement from thymectomy. Patients with thymomas do not respond as well to thymectomy as do patients without thymoma.

The preferred surgical approach is a sternotomy. Transcervical and endoscopic approaches have less postoperative morbidity but do not allow sufficient exposure for total thymus removal. In our experience, the operative morbidity from transthoracic thymectomy is very low when patients are optimally prepared with plasma exchange or immune suppression and skilled postoperative management is provided. Extubation is usually accomplished within hours after surgery and patients may be discharged home as early as the third or fourth postoperative day. Repeat thymectomy provides significant improvement in some patients with chronic, refractory disease and should be considered when there is concern that all thymic tissue was not removed at prior surgery and when a good response to the original surgery is followed by later relapse.

"Debulking" of Circulating Immune Factors

Plasma Exchange

Plasma exchange (PLEX) is used as a short-term intervention for patients with sudden worsening of myasthenic symptoms, to rapidly improve strength before surgery, and as a chronic intermittent treatment for patients who are refractory to all other treatments. The need for PLEX and its frequency of use are determined by the clinical response in the individual patient. Almost all patients with acquired MG improve temporarily following PLEX. A typical PLEX protocol is to remove 2 to 3 liters of plasma three times a week until improvement plateaus, usually after five to six exchanges. Improvement begins within 48 hours of the first exchange. Maximal improvement may be reached as early as after the first exchange or as late as the fourteenth. Improvement lasts for weeks or months, and then the effect is lost unless the exchange is followed by thymectomy or immune suppressive therapy. Most patients who respond to the first PLEX will respond again to subsequent courses. Repeated exchanges do not have a cumulative benefit.

Adverse reactions to PLEX include transitory cardiac arrhythmias, nausea, lightheadedness, chills, visual obscurations, and pedal edema. Other reactions occur in specific situations: thromboses, thrombophlebitis, and subacute bacterial endocarditis when arteriovenous shunts or grafts are placed for vascular access, an influenza-like illness in patients with reduced immunoglobulin levels, and severe bacterial and systemic cytomegalovirus infections in patients being treated with cyclophosphamide. Hypertensive patients being treated with angiotensin-converting enzyme (ACE) inhibitors may experience hypotension during plasma exchange, and these drugs should be withheld for the 24 hours prior to each procedure.

Intravenous Immune Globulin

Many patients will have significant improvement in strength with high-dose (2 grams per kg infused over 2 to 5 days) intravenous immune globulin (IVIG). The most likely mechanisms of action are down-regulation of antibodies directed against AChR and the introduction of anti-idiotypic antibodies. The indications for IVIG are similar to those for PLEX. IVIG may prove to be an effective alternative to plasma exchange, particularly in patients with poor vascular access. Improvement occurs in 50 to 100% of patients, usually beginning within 1 week and lasting for several weeks or months. The common side effects of IVIG are related to the rate of infusion and include headaches, chills, and fever. These reactions can be reduced by giving acetaminophen or aspirin with diphenhydramine (Benadryl) before each infusion. Severe reactions such as alopecia, aseptic meningitis, leukopenia, and retinal necrosis are rare. Renal failure may occur in patients with impaired renal function. Vascular-like headaches are often sufficiently severe to limit the use of IVIG, but these headaches can be managed by giving intravenous dihydroergotamine before and immediately after the IVIG. IVIG is contraindicated in patients with selective IgA deficiency as they may develop anaphylaxis to the IgA in immune globulin preparations. Immunoglobulin levels are obtained in all patients prior to starting IVIG therapy in order to detect such conditions. Human immunodeficiency virus is not known to be transmitted by IVIG, but transmission of hepatitis C by IVIG has been reported.

Miscellaneous Treatments

Ephedrine can be useful in patients with congenital myasthenia and in patients with acquired myasthenia in whom AChE inhibitors alone are not effective. Many patients report increased fatigue or weakness when their serum potassium level is low or low normal. This is more likely in those patients receiving prednisone therapy or those who are taking diuretics for other disorders. Serum potassium levels should be kept in the mid-4 range to minimize these complaints. Splenectomy, splenic radiation, and total body irradiation have been used in a small number of patients who failed all other forms of immunotherapy. The results are variable, and these modalities are not typically used. The aminopyridines facilitate neurotransmitter release at central and peripheral synapses. 3,4-Diaminopyridine (DAP)* and 4-aminopyridine (4-AP)* may produce significant improve-

---

*Investigational drug in the United States.

ment in acquired MG and congenital myasthenic syndromes, especially in combination with pyridostigmine. Confusion and seizures are the limiting side effects of 4-AP. DAP has similar, less central, toxicity but is not commercially available at this time.

ASSOCIATION OF MYASTHENIA GRAVIS WITH OTHER DISEASES
Treatment of Associated Diseases

The effect of concomitant diseases and their treatment on myasthenic symptoms is an important consideration. MG is often associated with other immune-mediated diseases, especially hyperthyroidism, pernicious anemia, rheumatoid arthritis, and systemic lupus erythematosus. Thyroid disease should be vigorously treated; both hypo- and hyperthyroidism adversely affect myasthenic weakness. Intercurrent infections require immediate attention because they exacerbate MG and can be life-threatening in patients who are immune suppressed.

Annual immunization against influenza is recommended for all patients with MG, and immunization against pneumococcus is recommended before starting prednisone or other immune suppressive drugs. Inactivated polio vaccine rather than attenuated live oral polio vaccine should be used in people who are immunocompromised and in children who have household contacts with immunocompromised individuals. The Centers for Disease Control and Prevention states that those patients taking less than 2 mg per kg per day of prednisone or alternate-day prednisone are not at risk.

TREATMENT PLAN
Ocular Myasthenia Gravis

Most patients are started on AChE inhibitors. If the response is unsatisfactory, prednisone is added, in either incrementing doses or high daily doses. The development of weakness in muscles other than the ocular or periocular muscles directs patients to the generalized myasthenia protocol.

Generalized Myasthenia Gravis, Onset Before 60 Years of Age

Thymectomy is recommended in all patients. High-dose daily prednisone or plasma exchange is used in patients with oropharyngeal, respiratory, or significant generalized muscle weakness to minimize the risks of surgery. If disabling weakness recurs or persists after thymectomy, or if there is not continual improvement 12 months after surgery, immune suppression with high-dose daily prednisone, azathioprine, or cyclosporine is recommended, as discussed earlier.

Generalized Myasthenia Gravis, Onset After 60 Years of Age

Life expectancy and concurrent illness are important considerations in developing a treatment plan. The initial treatment is usually with AChE inhibitors. If the response is unsatisfactory, azathioprine can be used in patients who can tolerate a delay before responding. If treatment with azathioprine is unsatisfactory, high-dose daily prednisone is added, or cyclosporine is substituted for azathioprine. High-dose daily prednisone is used as the first drug, with or without plasma exchange, in patients who need a rapid response. Azathioprine is added to prednisone if the response to prednisone alone is not satisfactory or unacceptable weakness develops as the prednisone dose is reduced.

Juvenile Myasthenia Gravis

The onset of immune-mediated MG before 20 years of age is referred to as juvenile myasthenia gravis (JMG). The pathophysiology is the same in children and adults. Twenty percent of children with MG, and almost 50% of those with onset before puberty, are seronegative. Treatment decisions in children with autoimmune MG are made more difficult because the rate of spontaneous remission is high, but the response to early thymectomy in the first year of symptoms is good. AChE inhibitors alone are recommended in prepubertal children who are not disabled by weakness. If these drugs do not prevent disability or progressive weakness, thymectomy with or without immune suppression should be considered. Removal of the thymus in infants or children does not have deleterious effects on subsequent immunologic development. Children with postpubertal onset of disease are treated the same as adults.

Seronegative Myasthenia Gravis

One-quarter of patients with acquired, immune-mediated MG do not have detectable serum antibodies against AChR. Seronegative patients are more likely than seropositive patients to be male and to have milder disease, ocular MG, fewer thymomas, less frequent thymic hyperplasia, and more frequent thymic atrophy. In seronegative patients, the diagnosis is based on the clinical presentation, the response to AChE inhibitors, and EMG findings. Genetic myasthenia must be considered in all childhood-onset seronegative MG. The treatment of seronegative acquired MG is the same as for seropositive patients. The absence of AChR antibodies does not mean that an unsatisfactory response to immune suppression, plasma exchange, or thymectomy is expected.

Thymoma

Thymectomy is indicated in all patients with thymoma. Patients are pretreated with high-dose daily prednisone, with or without plasma exchange, until maximal improvement is attained. Postoperative radiation is used if tumor resection is incomplete or if the tumor has spread beyond the thymic capsule. Medical treatment is then the same as for patients without thymoma. Diagnosis should not be made by needle biopsy of the mass because of the possibility of seeding the mediastinum with tumor cells. Rather, sternotomy with en bloc resection is preferred. Elderly patients with small tumors, who are not good candidates for surgery because of other health problems, can be managed medically while tumor size is monitored radiographically.

SPECIAL SITUATIONS

Myasthenic and Cholinergic Crisis

Myasthenic crisis is respiratory failure from disease. Patients in myasthenic crisis who previously had well-compensated respiratory function usually have a definable precipitating event, such as infection, surgery, or rapid tapering of immune suppressive drugs. Cholinergic crisis is respiratory failure from overdosage of AChE inhibitors. It was more common before the introduction of immune suppressive therapy when very large dosages of AChE inhibitors were used. Respiratory failure of any cause is a medical emergency and requires prompt intubation and ventilatory support. In theory, it should be easy to determine whether a patient is weak because of too little or too much AChE inhibitor, but in practice this is often difficult. Administration of edrophonium should distinguish overdose from underdose, but its use in crisis is dangerous unless the patient is already intubated and ventilated, and an apprehensive patient cannot cooperate with the test. Further, edrophonium may make some muscles stronger and others weaker. The safest approach to crisis is to admit the patient to an intensive care unit, discontinue all AChE inhibitors, and ventilate the patient. AChE inhibitors should be resumed at low doses and slowly increased as needed.

Respiratory assistance is needed when the patient cannot maintain an inspiratory force of more than -20 cm H_2O, a tidal volume of 4 to 5 mL per kg body weight, and a maximal breathing capacity three times the tidal volume, or when the forced vital capacity is less than 15 mL per kg body weight. A mask and breathing bag can be used in an emergency situation, but tracheal intubation should be done quickly with a low-pressure, high-compliance, cuffed endotracheal tube. A volume-controlled respirator set to provide tidal volumes of 400 to 500 mL and automatic sighing every 10 to 15 minutes is preferred. The pressure of the tube cuff should be checked frequently and the tube position verified daily by chest radiographs. Assisted respiration is used when the patient's own respiratory efforts can trigger the respirator. An oxygen-enriched atmosphere is used only when arterial blood oxygen values fall below 70 mm Hg. The inspired gas must be humidified to at least 80% at 37° C to prevent drying of the tracheobronchial tree. Tracheal secretions should be removed periodically, using aseptic aspiration techniques. Low-pressure, high-compliance endotracheal tubes may be tolerated for long periods of time and usually obviate the need for tracheostomy.

Weaning from the respirator should be started for 2 or 3 minutes at a time and increased as tolerated. Extubation should be considered when the patient has an inspiratory pressure of greater than -20 cm H_2O and an expiratory pressure of greater than 35 to 40 cm H_2O. The tidal volume should exceed 5 mL per kg, which usually corresponds to a vital capacity of at least 1000 mL. If the patient complains of fatigue or shortness of breath, extubation should be deferred even if these values and the results of blood gas measurements are normal. Following extubation, the patient should be observed for a period of at least 12 to 24 hours in an intensive care setting for muscle fatigue and respiratory failure.

Anesthetic Management

The stress of surgery and some drugs used perioperatively may worsen myasthenic weakness. Local or spinal anesthesia is preferred over inhalation anesthesia. Neuromuscular blocking agents should be used sparingly, if at all. Adequate muscle relaxation can usually be produced by inhalation anesthetic agents alone. The required dosage of depolarizing blocking agents may be greater than needed in nonmyasthenic patients, but low dosages of nondepolarizing agents cause pronounced and long-lasting blockade that requires prolonged postoperative assisted respiration.

Pregnancy

Myasthenic women may improve, worsen, or remain unchanged during pregnancy. Worsening during the first trimester is more common in first pregnancies, whereas third-trimester worsening and postpartum exacerbations are more common in subsequent pregnancies. Therapeutic abortion is rarely, if ever, needed because of MG. The use of intravenous AChE inhibitors is contraindicated during pregnancy because they may produce uterine contractions. Although pregnancy is not usually recommended in patients treated with corticosteroids, adverse outcomes in children born to myasthenic mothers taking even high doses throughout pregnancy are not reported. Cytotoxic drugs should be avoided during pregnancy because of their potential mutagenic effects. Labor and delivery are usually normal, and cesarean section is needed only for obstetric indications. Reginal anesthesia is preferred for delivery or cesarean section. Magnesium sulfate should not be used to manage preeclampsia because of its neuromuscular blocking effects. Barbiturates usually provide adequate treatment. Breast-feeding is not a problem, despite the theoretical risk of passing maternal AChR antibodies to the newborn infant.

The serum concentration of AChR antibodies in the mother and her newborn baby is similar. It is also likely that the fetuses of affected mothers have an elevated concentration of AChR antibodies. Decreased fetal movement suggests the diagnosis of intrauterine myasthenia. Affected neonates may have arthrogryposis multiplex congenita because of decreased intrauterine movement, and decreased fetal movement is considered an indication for plasma exchange or IVIG.

Transient Neonatal Myasthenia

A transient form of MG affects 10 to 20% of newborn infants whose mothers have immune-mediated MG. The severity of symptoms in the neonate does not correlate with the severity of symptoms in the mother. Affected neonates are hypotonic and feed poorly during the first 3 days. Symptoms usually last less than 2 weeks but may continue for as long as 3 months. Myasthenia does not recur later on. All children of myasthenic mothers should be assessed for transient neonatal MG. The diagnosis is confirmed by edrophonium, characteristic electrodiagnostic studies, or antibodies to the AChR. Affected neonates require symptomatic treatment with AChE inhibitors if swallowing or breathing is impaired. Plasma exchange should be considered in neonates with respiratory weakness.

Penicillamine-Induced Myasthenia Gravis

D-Penicillamine (Cuprimine) is used to treat rheumatoid arthritis, Wilson's disease, and cystinuria. Patients treated with D-penicillamine for several months may develop a myasthenic syndrome that disappears when the drug is stopped. D-Penicillamine–induced myasthenia is usually mild and often restricted to the ocular muscles. The diagnosis is often difficult because weakness may not be recognized when there is severe arthritis. The diagnosis is established by the response to AChE inhibitors, characteristic EMG abnormalities, and an elevated concentration of serum AChR antibodies. The myasthenic response induced by D-penicillamine usually remits within 1 year after the drug is stopped. AChE inhibitors usually relieve the symptoms. If myasthenic symptoms persist after D-penicillamine is stopped, the patient should be treated for acquired MG.

DRUGS THAT ADVERSELY AFFECT MYASTHENIA GRAVIS

Patients with disorders of neuromuscular transmission may experience worsening of their strength following the administration of a variety of therapeutic agents. In all instances there is a further reduction in the safety factor of neuromuscular transmission. With the exceptions of D-penicillamine and botulinum A toxin, no drugs are absolutely contraindicated in patients with MG. Avoidance of drugs that are known to impair neuromuscular transmission is desirable, but this is not always possible. In such instances they must be used with caution, and a thorough knowledge by the physician of the deleterious side effects can minimize their potential danger. It is useful to place a list of potentially hazardous

TABLE 3. **Drug Alert for Patients with Myasthenia Gravis**

1. D-Penicillamine and botulinum toxin A should *never* be used in myasthenic patients.
2. The following drugs produce worsening of myasthenic weakness in most patients who receive them. Use with caution and monitor patient for exacerbation of myasthenic symptoms:
   Neuromuscular blocking agents: both depolarizing and competitive agents
   Quinine, quinidine, or procainamide
   Aminoglycoside antibiotics: particularly gentamicin, kanamycin, neomycin, or streptomycin
   Erythromycin
   Beta blockers: oral as well as ocular preparations; particularly propranolol (Inderal) or timolol (Blocadren)
   Calcium channel blockers
3. Many other drugs are reported to exacerbate the weakness in some patients with myasthenia gravis.
4. All patients with myasthenia gravis should be observed for increased weakness whenever a new medication is started.

drugs on the front of the hospital chart and for these patients to carry a Drug Alert card in their wallets (Table 3). Competitive neuromuscular blocking agents, such as pancuronium and D-tubocurarine have an exaggerated and prolonged response in patients with MG. Depolarizing blocking agents such as succinylcholine have similar effects on myasthenic weakness. Many antibiotics, particularly the aminoglycosides and erythromycin, may also potentiate myasthenic weakness. If corticosteroids are needed to treat concomitant illness, the potential adverse and beneficial effects on MG must be anticipated and explained to the patient.

The occurrence of glaucoma, coronary artery or peripheral vascular disease, and hypertension is common in the aging myasthenic population. Treatment of these disorders is problematic for the patient with MG. Unwittingly, these patients are often given beta or calcium channel blockers or quinidine by their physicians, who do not recognize that these drugs have the potential for markedly worsening myasthenic weakness. Alternative treatments should be used, but if necessary, the patient must be monitored closely for any change in the clinical examination.

TRIGEMINAL NEURALGIA

method of
JOSHUA B. BEDERSON, M.D.
Mt. Sinai Medical Center
New York, New York

Trigeminal neuralgia is a dramatic clinical syndrome with a stereotypical presentation and several effective treatments. Patients experience intense, lancinating facial pain that is disabling during the attack but have a striking lack of symptoms between attacks. The pain is strictly unilateral, most commonly involving the second trigeminal division (V2), and may spread to involve V1 or V3 over a period of months or years. Painful attacks are frequently triggered by chewing, drinking hot or cold liquids, brushing the teeth, talking, or shaving. A history of dental work on the affected side is common, usually having been performed in a vain attempt to diagnose and treat the pain.

Painful episodes are intermittent in trigeminal neuralgia and may be separated by "remissions" lasting weeks or months. Although patients usually report no abnormalities between attacks, careful neurologic examination may disclose mild sensory disturbances in the affected division. Rarely, patients with true trigeminal neuralgia report mild pain between attacks. Many patients describe a gradual progression of both the intensity and the frequency of attacks over a period of years. Women are affected more frequently than men, and the condition is more common in the elderly.

The cause of trigeminal neuralgia is thought to be altered conduction within the proximal trigeminal nerve root near its entry to the brain stem. The most common etiology (in approximately 90% of patients) is compressive demyelination by an ectatic blood vessel, but tumor or arteriovenous malformation can also be causative. As many as 5% of patients with multiple sclerosis present with trigeminal neuralgia, presumably due to demyelination of the proximal nerve root.

An initial excellent response to carbamazepine (Tegretol) is supportive evidence of the correct diagnosis. In contrast, certain aspects of the history should raise the suspicion of an alternative diagnosis. These include age less than 40 years, the presence of a significant sensory abnormality between attacks, any other cranial nerve involvement, bilateral pain, or significant pain between attacks.

MEDICAL THERAPY

All patients with a suspected diagnosis of trigeminal neuralgia should undergo magnetic resonance imaging (MRI) to rule out a lesion in the cerebellopontine angle. The mainstay of medical treatment is carbamazepine, which is usually initiated at 200 mg twice daily and increased, to a maximum of 1200 mg per day, until pain is relieved or side effects (drowsiness, confusion, ataxia, allergic reactions) are seen. Baseline and intermittent blood counts and liver function tests are required to detect idiosyncratic reactions and bone marrow toxicity. The majority of patients with trigeminal neuralgia respond to medication and require lifelong treatment. Some patients who obtain protracted relief can eventually be weaned from the medication without pain recurrence. A number of patients gradually develop recurrent pain despite escalating doses. These patients, and those who fail the initial trial, can be treated with other drugs, including phenytoin (Dilantin),* usually started at 100 mg three times daily; baclofen (Lioresal),* usually started at 10 to 20 mg per day; clonazepam (Klonopin),* usually started at 0.5 to 1.0 mg per day; or pimozide (Orap),* usually started at 4 to 10 mg per day. These drugs are generally less effective than carbamazepine and are typically increased until pain is relieved or side effects are seen. Newer, unproven treatments include gaba-

pentin, an antiepileptic medication, and stereotaxic radiosurgical lesioning of the trigeminal ganglion.

SURGICAL THERAPY

Surgical treatments of trigeminal neuralgia are used in patients who have unacceptable side effects of medical treatment or persistent or recurrent pain despite increased doses of medication. The procedures can be classified as either open (microvascular decompression) or percutaneous (ablative).

Microvascular Decompression

The majority of cases of trigeminal neuralgia are caused by acquired vascular compression and can be effectively treated by microneurosurgical vascular decompression of the nerve root. The procedure is performed under general anesthesia, requires a small retromastoid craniectomy, and consists of displacing the offending vascular loop and interposing a small Teflon pledget between vessel and nerve. It has an approximate 90% initial success rate and the lowest recurrence rate (less than 10% at 5 years) of any procedure used to treat trigeminal neuralgia. Because it is an open procedure, it carries a small risk of serious complications. Microvascular decompression is a nonablative technique that does not destroy nerve fibers or cause associated sensory loss. It can be performed when pain has recurred after a percutaneous ablative procedure, but the success rate may be lower in this situation. These factors plus its high cure rate make microvascular decompression the initial procedure of choice in all patients who are surgical candidates. In a small percentage of patients, no vascular compression is found at surgery. In this group, a partial sensory rhizotomy (nerve section) or one of the percutaneous ablative techniques can be performed.

Percutaneous Ablative Techniques

The percutaneous approaches include radiofrequency lesion (rhizolysis), injection of a neurotoxin (glycerol), and balloon compression of the gasserian ganglion. In comparison with microvascular decompression, these techniques are less invasive, require shorter hospitalization, and have less major morbidity or mortality. Although they have a higher pain recurrence rate than microvascular decompression, they can often be repeated with similar good initial results. However, because they depend on the destruction of nerve fibers, pain relief is associated with sensory loss. When too much destruction occurs, corneal anesthesia or painful paresthesias result, which can be as disabling as the original pain. In addition, there is evidence that neuroablative procedures increase the complication rate and decrease the success rate of open procedures. Therefore, we recommend that the percutaneous neuroablative procedures be used as a second line of treatment in patients who are frail or elderly and poor candidates

---

*Not FDA-approved for this indication.

for general anesthesia or who have failed microvascular decompression.

Percutaneous Radiofrequency Rhizolysis

Radiofrequency rhizolysis produces a thermal injury of the gasserian ganglion via a needle that is placed radiographically through the cheek and foramen ovale. Needle placement is performed with the patient under intravenous sedation, which is adjusted to maintain comfort while the lesion is made. The initial success rate is high (approximately 80%), but the recurrence rate is also high (30 to 40%), requiring additional treatments.

Percutaneous Glycerol Rhizolysis

This procedure uses the neurotoxin anhydrous glycerol instead of heat to produce a trigeminal injury. Like the radiofrequency lesion, it has a good initial success rate and a high pain recurrence rate. Glycerol injection can be used in patients with first-division trigeminal neuralgia who cannot tolerate anesthesia and microvascular decompression.

Percutaneous Balloon Compression

This technique relies on inflation of a balloon to compress the gasserian ganglion and produce trigeminal injury. Although it is a newer technique than the other percutaneous approaches, results appear to be similar, with high initial success rates and high recurrence rates.

OPTIC NEURITIS

method of
R. MITCHELL NEWMAN, M.D., and
LANNING B. KLINE, M.D.

Eye Foundation Hospital
Birmingham, Alabama

The term "optic neuritis" denotes primary inflammation of the optic nerve, including that accompanying demyelinating disease or contiguous spread of inflammation from meninges, orbital tissues, or paranasal sinuses. Optic neuritis has an incidence of 3.5 new cases per 100,000 population per year in North America. It occurs three times as frequently in females as in males and five to six times as frequently in whites as in nonwhites. Peak age of onset is between 20 and 50 years.

It is important to realize that the diagnosis of optic neuritis is based on clinical criteria. The critical elements in establishing the correct diagnosis are a detailed history and accurate examination.

CLINICAL CHARACTERISTICS

A course of typical optic neuritis begins with the rapid onset of visual loss, which progresses over 1 to 2 weeks before gradually improving over the next 6 to 12 weeks. The degree of visual loss during an attack is highly variable, ranging from minimal impairment of Snellen acuity to no light perception. Tenderness of the globe and periorbital pain may precede or accompany the visual loss and are characteristically precipitated or aggravated by eye movement.

In addition to reduced visual acuity, patients with optic neuritis may report other visual complaints, such as phosphenes. These are positive visual phenomena, seen as flashes or sparks of light, often accompanying eye movements. Other complaints include difficulty with contrast sensitivity and depth perception.

In addition to visual acuity, other objective parameters of visual function are disturbed during an attack of optic neuritis. Deficits in color vision are common, tested with either Ishihara pseudoisochromatic color plates or simple comparison of color saturation and intensity between the involved eye and the normal eye. A relative afferent pupillary defect (Marcus Gunn) can be demonstrated with the swinging flashlight test. Visual field examination typically reveals a central scotoma but may also show altitudinal or arcuate defects. On funduscopic examination, the optic disk is swollen (papillitis) in one-third of patients and is normal in two-thirds (retrobulbar neuritis). Occasionally, other funduscopic features such as vitreous cells or sheathing around peripheral retinal vessels are seen. These findings are suggestive of an intraocular inflammatory process and should prompt a search for an associated systemic disorder such as sarcoidosis or syphilis.

The visual prognosis of patients experiencing optic neuritis is excellent. Most visual improvement occurs within the first 2 weeks following an attack, and 95% of patients attain acuity of 20/40 or better at 1 year. Following recovery, patients frequently complain of persistent defects in depth perception, brightness of vision, and color saturation. Some describe visual blurring with activities that raise body temperature, known as Uhthoff's sign. This complaint is highly suggestive of multiple sclerosis.

OPTIC NEURITIS TREATMENT TRIAL

A national collaborative study, the Optic Neuritis Treatment Trial (ONTT), assessed the potential for therapy of optic neuritis. A total of 457 patients were included in the study; 77% were women, and the mean age was 32 years. Patients were randomized to three clinical treatment arms: oral prednisone 1 mg per kg per day for 14 days; intravenous methylprednisolone 1000 mg per day for 3 days, followed by oral prednisone 1 mg per kg per day for 11 days; and oral placebo for 14 days. Although patients treated with intravenous methylprednisolone did show faster recovery of visual acuity at 6 months, especially in eyes with initially poor visual acuity, by 1 year, visual outcome did not vary among the three groups. The regimen of oral prednisone alone not only failed to improve vision but was also associated with an increased rate of new attacks of optic neuritis in both the initially affected eye and the other eye. Thus, the ONTT demonstrated that there is currently no effective therapy for optic neuritis.

RELATIONSHIP OF OPTIC NEURITIS TO MULTIPLE SCLEROSIS

There is a strong association between optic neuritis and multiple sclerosis. Up to one-third of patients who experience optic neuritis have a previous history of or neurologic findings consistent with multiple sclerosis. A related clinical question arises as to the frequency with which multiple sclerosis follows an attack of monosymptomatic optic neuritis. In untreated adults followed up to 4 years in the ONTT, 4% with normal magnetic resonance imaging (MRI) brain scans developed multiple sclerosis, whereas 30% of patients with abnormal MRI studies developed demyelinating disease. In assessing this and other reports, it appears that at least half of those who develop multiple sclerosis show clinical signs of the disease within 3 years of an attack of optic neuritis; thereafter, 2 to 7% per year continue to develop the disease.

OPTIC NEURITIS IN CHILDREN

In children, optic neuritis commonly occurs with a viral illness such as chickenpox, measles, or mumps. Optic nerve involvement develops either concomitantly with the viral illness, believed to be due to direct central nervous system infection, or 1 to 3 weeks later as a postinfectious (immunologic) phenomenon. Optic neuritis is more likely to be bilateral and simultaneous in children and is frequently accompanied by exudative macular star formation (neuroretinitis). In addition, it appears to be a less frequent harbinger of multiple sclerosis when it occurs in children as compared with adults.

PATIENT EVALUATION AND DIFFERENTIAL DIAGNOSIS

Additional tests obtained on all patients entering the ONTT included antinuclear antibodies, fluorescent treponemal antibody absorption test (FTA-ABS), chest radiograph, and MRI brain scan. These studies were of no value in establishing the correct diagnosis of optic neuritis, nor did they provide any prognostic data to help determine visual recovery.

Which patient should be categorized as having "atypical" optic neuritis and be evaluated for a systemic disorder other than multiple sclerosis? Four criteria provide guidance: (1) optic neuritis in a patient outside the 20- to 50-year age span; (2) bilateral, simultaneous optic neuritis, particularly in adults; (3) progressive visual loss beyond 2 to 3 weeks after onset; and (4) optic neuritis accompanied by abnormalities in the patient's history or examination that cannot be attributed to multiple sclerosis.

Table 1 summarizes the majority of settings in which optic neuritis occurs. Although it is not an exhaustive list, it covers those conditions practitioners most frequently encounter in clinical practice.

TABLE 1. **Causes of Optic Neuritis**

Demyelinating

Multiple sclerosis
Devic's disease
Adrenoleukodystrophy (Schilder's disease)

Infectious

Viral: paraviral, postviral, postvaccination
Fungal: histoplasmosis, cryptococcosis, aspergillosis, mucormycosis
Bacterial: sinusitis
Spirochetal: syphilis, Lyme disease

Associated with Intraocular Inflammation

Infection: nematode, zoster, toxoplasmosis
Acute multifocal placoid pigment epitheliopathy
Birdshot chorioretinopathy

Associated with Systemic Disease

Sarcoidosis
Guillain-Barré syndrome
Wegener's granulomatosis
Connective tissue disease: systemic lupus erythematosus, "autoimmune"
Behçet's disease
Paraneoplastic syndrome

TREATMENT

The ONTT clearly demonstrated that there is no effective long-term benefit of systemic corticosteroid use in the recovery of vision from optic neuritis. Unexpectedly, the study found that the group receiving the intravenous regimen of steroids had a lower rate of development of multiple sclerosis (7.5%) within the first 2 years of follow-up than did the placebo (16.7%) or prednisone (14.7%) groups. However, by 3 years of follow-up this "protective effect" could no longer be demonstrated. Further, the ONTT found that cranial MRI is a powerful predictor of the 2-year risk of multiple sclerosis. Patients with two or more typical white matter lesions had a 2-year risk of multiple sclerosis of 36%, whereas patients with normal scans had a risk of 3%.

Therefore, it seems appropriate to obtain a cranial MRI scan on all patients experiencing acute optic neuritis. Subjects with abnormal scans consistent with multiple sclerosis should be considered for treatment with intravenous steroids to retard the development of multiple sclerosis during the next 2 years. Treatment with intravenous steroids should be considered in all patients with acute optic neuritis, whether the cranial MRI scan is abnormal or not, as this medical regimen can lead to a more rapid improvement of visual function when compared with untreated patients. However, when treatment decisions are made, the fact should always be kept in mind that at 1 year following the onset of optic neuritis, the final visual outcome remains the same whether or not the patient received intravenous steroid therapy.

GLAUCOMA

method of
JEFFREY W. KALENAK, M.D.
Medical College of Wisconsin
Milwaukee, Wisconsin

The glaucomas are a group of diseases rather than a single disease process. The range of diseases is characterized by diverse clinical and pathologic manifestations. Genetic linkage analysis in glaucomas, still in its infancy, has already begun to identify different genetic loci for different types of glaucoma. The common clinical findings ("final common pathway") are progressive, acquired damage to the optic nerve head associated with characteristic defects of the visual field. Total blindness is possible and irreversible. Elevated intraocular pressure (IOP), considered to be the most important risk factor for the glaucomas, may or may not be present.

The traditional classification has separated the glaucomas into primary (idiopathic) and secondary types, and into open-angle and angle-closure types. Primary open-angle glaucoma (POAG), in particular, is the form of glaucoma in which we have failed to identify the pathophysiologic events that lead to elevated IOP and optic nerve damage. With the secondary glaucomas, we recognize a predisposing condition that leads to the typical clinical findings.

On a population basis, POAG is the most common form of glaucoma. Acute primary angle-closure glaucoma (PACG) requires immediate recognition and emergency treatment. These will be reviewed here. Secondary, congenital, and developmental glaucomas are beyond the scope of this discussion.

PRIMARY OPEN-ANGLE GLAUCOMA

POAG is the most common form of glaucoma in the United States. At least 2.25 million Americans 40 years of age or older have POAG. The prevalence of POAG increases with age and differs among races. Recent epidemiologic studies indicate the prevalence of POAG in the United States to be approximately 1.3% among whites 40 years of age and older and 4.7% among blacks in the same age group. POAG is

the third leading cause of blindness among white Americans and the leading cause of blindness among black Americans.

The most important risk factor for developing POAG is elevated IOP (more than 21 mm Hg). Other important risk factors include increasing age, a family history of the disease, and vertical enlargement of the central cup of the optic nerve head at initial examination. Additional risk factors include black race, diabetes mellitus, and myopia. There are no symptoms of POAG in most persons. Therefore, persons with known risk factors should have eye examinations at routine intervals. In the absence of symptoms, individuals should undergo a comprehensive eye examination, including checking for glaucoma, every 1 to 2 years for those 65 years of age or older, and every 2 to 4 years for those between the ages of

TABLE 1. **Drugs Available to Treat Primary Open-Angle Glaucoma**

Class	Drug	Form	Common Dosage and Concentration	Action	Systemic Side Effects	Ocular Side Effects
Beta-adrenergic antagonists Nonselective	Timolol (Betimol) Timolol (Timoptic-XE) Levobunolol (Betagan)	Solution Solution Solution	bid (0.25, 0.5%) daily (0.25, 0.5%) daily or bid (0.25, 0.5%)	Supress aqueous production	Bradycardia, arrhythmia, heart block, congestive heart failure, fatigue, depression, headache, rash, bronchospasm; masks hypoglycemia, impotence	Burning, stinging, blepharoconjunctivitis, decreased corneal sensation
	Metipranolol (OptiPranolol)	Solution	bid (0.3%)			
	Carteolol (Ocupress)	Solution	bid (1%)			
Beta₁ cardio-selective	Betaxolol (Betoptic) Betaxolol (Betoptic S)	Solution Suspension	bid (0.5%) bid (0.25%)	Suppress aqueous production	Same as above, less reactive airway distress	Same as above
Cholinergic drugs	Pilocarpine (many brands)	Solution	qid (0.5, 1, 2, 3, 4, and 6%)	Improve aqueous outflow	Salivation, syncope, arrhythmia, gastrointestinal cramping, vomiting, diarrhea, asthma, urinary frequency, sweating	Burning, stinging, conjunctival hyperemia, blurring of vision, miosis, headache, retinal detachment
	Pilocarpine Pilocarpine (Ocuset Pilo-20 or -40)	Gel Controlled-release insert	qhs (4%) q 5–7 days			
	Carbachol (Isopto Carbachol)	Solution	tid (0.75, 1.5, 3%)			
	Echothiophate (Phospholine Iodide)	Solution	bid (0.125, 0.25%)			Same as above, also cataract
Alpha₂ agonists	Apraclonidine (Lopidine)	Solution	bid or tid (0.5%)	Suppress aqueous production	Headache, asthenia, dry mouth, dry nose, taste perversion	Conjunctival hyperemia, allergic lid reaction, pruritus, tearing, ocular discomfort, blurred vision
Epinephrine compounds	Epinephrine (Epifrin, others)	Solution	bid (0.25, 0.5, 1, 2%)	Decrease aqueous inflow, improve aqueous outflow	Systemic hypertension	Stinging, browache, conjunctival hyperemia, adrenochrome deposits, allergic lid reaction
	Dipivefrin (Propine)	Solution	bid (0.1%)			
Carbonic anhydrase inhibitors	Acetazolamide (Diamox)	Tablet	Orally qid (125, 250 mg)	Suppress aqueous production	Sulfonamide reactions, including Stevens-Johnson syndrome, blood dyscrasias, urolithiasis, metabolic acidosis, paresthesias, fatigue, anorexia	
		Capsule	Orally bid (500 mg)			
	Methazolamide (Neptazane)	Tablet	Orally bid (25, 50 mg)			
	Dorzolamide (Trusopt)	Solution	tid (2%)			Burning, stinging, conjunctival hyperemia, pruritus, allergic lid reaction

Modified from Wilson MR, Bacharach J: Glaucoma. *In* Rakel RE (ed): Conn's Current Therapy 1994. Philadelphia, WB Saunders, 1994.

40 and 64 years. Because black Americans have a higher prevalence, younger age of onset, and more aggressive course of the disease, blacks between the ages of 20 and 39 years should have a comprehensive examination every 3 to 5 years.

Current methods of screening populations for POAG are inadequate. Neither testing the IOP nor examining the optic nerve head yields a useful combination of sensitivity and specificity. For example, at least one-half of individuals with POAG will be missed by glaucoma screenings that use IOP measurements alone (cutoff at 21 mm Hg). Therefore, routine eye examinations take on greater importance.

The diagnosis of POAG is based on glaucomatous optic nerve atrophy associated with typical visual field defects. The visual field should be tested with formal perimetry. The IOP may or may not be elevated. The symptoms usually are none, although persons with very advanced stages of the disease may complain of reduced vision or "tunnel" vision. Detailed examination of the optic nerve head usually reveals an enlarged area of central cupping. Notching and generalized pallor of the rim of the optic nerve head are often seen. Splinter hemorrhages at the margin of the optic disk may occur but may not be observed because of their transient nature. Asymmetry in the size or contour of the central cups is highly suggestive of unilateral glaucomatous damage.

The visual field deficits are not noticed by patients with early-to-moderate stages of POAG. These characteristic defects can only be elicited by careful visual field testing. In an advanced stage, a patient may retain only a central island of visual field yet have 20/20 Snellen visual acuity. In the end stages, the central island of vision is abolished, and the patient will lose central visual acuity permanently.

Treatment

Unfortunately, there is no treatment that can restore lost optic nerve axons or function. Therefore, treatment is directed at reducing one risk factor, IOP. The clinician considers the degree of glaucomatous damage and estimates a therapeutic goal or "target IOP." As initial therapy, several classes of topical and oral drugs are prescribed (Table 1) to attempt to achieve the target IOP. Argon laser trabeculoplasty

is usually the next mode of treatment. It may lower IOP as well as an additional good drug, but its effect may not be long-lasting in many patients.

Surgical treatment is usually recommended when the disease continues to advance despite medical and laser therapy. The most common operation, trabeculectomy, creates a fistula between the anterior chamber and the subconjunctival space. This bypasses the obstruction to aqueous outflow. The ongoing Collaborative Initial Glaucoma Treatment Study seeks to determine whether initial medical therapy or initial trabeculectomy offers greater benefit to patients with this chronic disease. Episcleral fibrosis and scarring are the main causes of failure following trabeculectomy. Therefore, in eyes felt to be at high risk of surgical failure, topical antimetabolites, such as 5-fluorouracil or mitomycin-C (Mutamycin),* may be used to inhibit scar formation. Alternatively, these high-risk eyes may receive implantation of a tube-shunt device to shunt aqueous humor posteriorly to a reservoir. Procedures to ablate the ciliary body, in order to decrease the rate of aqueous production, may be reserved for the treatment of refractory cases.

PRIMARY ANGLE-CLOSURE GLAUCOMA

Although PACG accounts for only about 10% of cases of glaucoma in the United States, it is the predominant form of glaucoma among Eskimos and many Asian populations. The configuration of the eye is the main predisposing factor to PACG. That is, eyes with small, crowded anterior segments, such as in hyperopia (farsightedness), are at higher risk of PACG. Additional risk factors include increasing age, female sex, and a positive family history of angle-closure.

The hallmark of PACG is closure of the anterior chamber angle (and drainage apparatus) because of pupillary block. Pupillary block is a resistance to the flow of aqueous humor from the posterior chamber to the anterior chamber, resulting in forward bowing of the iris toward the angle. The subtypes of PACG include acute, chronic, and subacute (intermittent).

Acute PACG results from sudden closure of the

---

*This use of 5-fluorouracil and mitomycin-C is not listed in the manufacturers' official directives.

TABLE 2. **Initial Medical Treatment for Primary Angle-Closure Glaucoma**

Class	Example	Dose
Carbonic anhydrase inhibitor	Acetazolamide (Diamox)	500 mg PO or IV
Beta-adrenergic antagonist	Timolol 0.5% (Timoptic)	1 drop
Alpha₂ agonist	Apraclonidine 0.5% (Iopidine)	1 drop
Osmotic agent	Isosorbide 45%, or	1.5 gr/kg PO
	mannitol 20%	1–2 gr/kg IV over 30–60 min
Topical corticosteroid	Prednisolone acetate 1% (Pred Forte)	1 drop q 30 min × 2, then q 1 h
Cholinergic agent	Pilocarpine 1% or 2%	1 drop q 15 min × 2
	Pilocarpine 0.5%	1 drop to fellow eye

Modified from Wilson MR, Bacharach J: Glaucoma. In Rakel RE (ed): Conn's Current Therapy 1994. Philadelphia, WB Saunders, 1994.

anterior chamber angle, which causes a rapid rise of IOP to dangerously high levels, often to 60 mm Hg or higher. The symptoms may include pain around the eye, blurred or foggy vision, and colored haloes around lights. Nausea and vomiting may accompany an attack, sometimes predominating and leading a clinician to misdiagnose a gastrointestinal disorder. Signs usually include conjunctival injection, corneal edema, and a sluggishly reactive or fixed, mid-dilated pupil.

Because of the extremely high IOP, substantial damage to the optic nerve may occur in a short time. Therefore, acute PACG is an emergency, and immediate referral must be made to an ophthalmologist. Initial management employs medical therapy to reduce the IOP (Table 2). Definitive treatment requires laser iridotomy to resolve the pupillary block. The fellow, uninvolved eye should have laser iridotomy prophylactically at the same time because of its risk of acute angle-closure. If treated early, acute PACG can be resolved with minimal damage to the optic nerve.

Subacute or intermittent PACG is less dramatic and typically not an emergency. Patients may report intermittent but self-limited episodes of discomfort or pain, blurred vision, and/or haloes around lights. During an episode, the IOP is high and the angle is at least partially closed. Between episodes, the IOP is normal and the angle is not closed. Subacute PACG may progress to acute or chronic PACG. Therefore, eyes with this condition should be treated with laser iridotomy.

Chronic PACG is characterized by slowly progressive closure of the anterior chamber angle. Symptoms are usually absent, much as in POAG. Laser iridotomy is recommended. Diagnosis and treatment are best relegated to the ophthalmologist.

ACUTE FACIAL PARALYSIS

method of
KEDAR K. ADOUR, M.D.
Kaiser Permanente Medical Center
Oakland, California

Before the advent of sophisticated techniques and technology, clinicians relied on history and physical signs and symptoms to diagnose disease and formulate hypotheses regarding pathophysiology. So it was in 1907, when J. Ramsay Hunt introduced a new facial paralysis syndrome with aural complications termed "herpes zoster oticus" and postulated that it was a type of geniculate ganglionitis. This concept was challenged by leading neurologists, and only 1 year later, Hunt recognized that other cranial nerves were affected and suggested subcategories of his new syndrome. In 1967, Blackley correctly suggested that the obsession with facial nerve palsy obscured the true extent of the disease and that the proper term for this condition should be "herpes zoster cephalicus." This suggestion has been confirmed, and ironically, the known clinical manifestations of herpes zoster cephalicus have been instrumental in clarifying the pathophysiology of Bell's palsy.

CLASSIFICATION OF FACIAL PARALYSIS

Herpes zoster (varicella-zoster virus [VZV]) facial paralysis is simply a more florid form of Bell's palsy, which is probably caused by reactivated herpes simplex virus (HSV). Both diseases are best described as mononeuritis multiplex because they can present in mononeuritic or polyneuritic form. Both affect the cranial nerves (Table 1); the difference is one of severity. VZV is more likely than HSV to cause complete clinical paralysis, complete electrical denervation, and incomplete recovery, with the late complication of contracture with synkinesis.

During gadolinium-enhanced magnetic resonance imaging (MRI), considerable enhancement of the geniculate ganglion was observed in 37 of 46 (88.1%) Bell's palsy patients and in 6 of 6 (100%) Ramsay Hunt syndrome patients. Paradoxically, no difference exists between the two diseases in facial enhancement intensity or pattern. In patients with internal auditory symptoms such as vertigo and tinnitus, not only the facial nerve but also the vestibular and cochlear nerves were enhanced.

Auditory testing can suggest cochlear and retrocochlear pathology, which is consistent with pathologic findings at autopsy and with MRI findings. Mononeuritis multiplex facial paralysis with sensorineural hearing loss statistically portends, and probably is pathognomonic of, VZV. Recovery from hearing loss is problematic and incomplete at best. In the VZV form of mononeuritis multiplex, balance problems are severe and are often incapacitating in the elderly.

Electrical testing has shown that, in HSV infection, the major damage to the facial nerve occurs within 10 days, but in VZV infection, this damage does not occur until 2 to 3 weeks after the onset of paralysis. This association is consistent with what has been discovered about VZV nerve destruction through studies done with animals. Therefore, prognosis for recovery of facial function can be made within 10 to 14 days after the onset of paralysis in Bell's palsy but cannot be made until 3 weeks after the onset of paralysis in VZV infection.

We calculate that, in the United States, a new case of VZV-induced Ramsay Hunt syndrome occurs every 52 minutes (5 per 100,000 population per year) compared with a new case of Bell's palsy every 10 minutes (20 per 100,000 population per year) (Figure 1). The age-corrected incidence figure for VZV cranial neuritis is almost identical to the figure that Hope-Simpson postulated for VZV infection in the general population.

TABLE 1. **Cranial Nerves Affected in Bell's Palsy and Varicella-Zoster Virus (VZV) Facial Palsy**

Cranial Nerve		Bell's Palsy, % (n = 48)	VZV, % (n = 47)
V	(sensory)	25	36
V	(motor)	4	11
VIII	(vestibular)	42	36
VIII	(cochlear)	29	26
IX	(sensory)	35	23
X	(superior laryngeal)	19	19

Adapted from Adour KK, Hilsinger RL Jr, Callan EJ: Facial paralysis and Bell's palsy: A protocol for differential diagnosis. Am J Otol (Suppl): 68–73, Nov 1985.

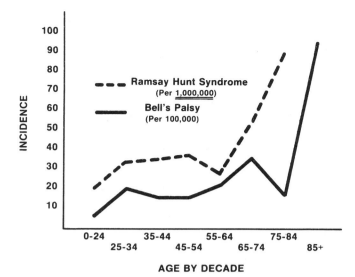

Figure 1. Age-corrected incidence of Ramsay Hunt syndrome (varicella-zoster virus infection) and Bell's palsy (herpes simplex virus infection) in Kaiser Permanente Medical Care Program health plan population in Northern California. (From Robillard RB, Hilsinger RL Jr, Adour KK: Ramsay Hunt facial paralysis: Clinical analyses of 185 patients. Otolaryngol Head Neck Surg 95[3Pt1]:292–297, 1986.)

DIAGNOSIS

An accurate medical history and a complete physical examination often yield sufficient information to provide the diagnosis or suggest which diagnostic tests are needed. The physical examination should exclude a diagnosis of lesions that can mimic Bell's palsy. The clinician should document four points: (1) all facial nerve branches are diffusely affected, (2) otoscopic examination findings are normal, (3) no skin blebs or blisters are evident (as in herpes zoster), and (4) no ipsilateral parotid masses are evident. These points distinguish idiopathic Bell's palsy from non-HSV infection, tumor, trauma, and stroke.

The distinction between central and peripheral lesions is not well defined. For clarification, a central lesion is probable when forehead function is spared, voluntary and emotional facial muscle motions are unequal, ipsilateral motor weakness is found in the arm or leg, or dysarthria or confusion is noted. Mononeuritis multiplex facial paralysis, which accounts for 90 to 95% of all cases, is considered peripheral, although inflammation is often present from the brain stem to the stylomastoid foramen.

Symptoms and Signs

Determining whether the onset of paralysis is acute or progressive is crucial. Acute cases include those in which paralysis reaches maximal severity within 2 weeks of onset. Cases of Bell's palsy are similar in history, natural course, and outcome. Onset of paralysis is often preceded by a viral syndrome. Symptoms and signs during the early phase of facial paralysis include facial numbness, epiphora, dysgeusia (aberrant taste), hyperacusis (dysacusis), and decreased tearing (Table 2). Facial numbness is diagnostic of trigeminal nerve disease because no somatosensory fibers have been found in the facial nerve. The pain is usually retroauricular, which indicates inflammation of the second or third cranial nerve, but can and does radiate into the face (fifth cranial nerve) or into the neck and arm (fourth, fifth, and sixth cranial nerves). Dysgeusia suggests dysfunction of the geniculate ganglion, which contains the cell bodies of the chorda tympani nerve and is probably the site of reactivation of the HSV. These symptoms are usually unilateral but can be contralateral. The hyperacusis is better labeled dysacusis because it reflects intolerance to noise and not more acute hearing. Dysacusis is not related to stapedial muscle paralysis but probably represents loss of inhibitory nerve impulses to the cochlea. After evaluating more than 4000 patients with all forms of facial paralysis, we have concluded on the basis of statistical calculation that dysgeusia or dysacusis in a patient with acute facial paralysis is sufficient for definitive diagnosis of HSV or VZV mononeuritis multiplex.

Physical Findings

Physical findings always include inflammation of the fungiform papillae, almost always include hypesthesia of the fifth cranial nerve and the second cervical nerve, and occasionally include inflammation of the circumvallate papillae of the tongue and hypesthesia of the ninth cranial nerve. Motor paralysis of branches of the vagus nerve is seen as a unilateral shift of the palate or as a shortening of one vocal cord with rotation of the posterior larynx to the affected side. Thus, Bell's palsy can be diagnosed when

TABLE 2. **Statistical Difference in Presenting Signs and Symptoms in Patients with Ramsay Hunt Syndrome (VZV Infection) and Bell's Palsy (HSV Infection)**

Symptom	Ramsay Hunt Syndrome (VZV), % (n = 102)	Bell's Palsy (HSV), % (n = 772)	Statistical Significance
Pain	100	55	p = .001
Dysgeusia	67	57	NS
Epiphora absent*	55	67	p = .001
Hyperacusis	52	30	p = .001
Decreased tears (by history)	43	22	p = .001
Decreased tears (by test results)	42	24	p = .001
Fifth cranial nerve palsy absent*	34	52	p = .001
Vertigo	11	1	p = .001
Hearing loss and tinnitus	21	0	p = .001

*More frequent in Bell's palsy.
Abbreviations: VZV = varicella-zoster virus; HSV = herpes simplex virus; NS = not significant.
From Robillard RB, Hilsinger RL Jr, Adour KK: Ramsay Hunt facial paralysis: Clinical analyses of 185 patients. Otolaryngol Head Neck Surg 95(3Pt1):292–297, 1986.

facial paralysis is peripheral in origin, when systemic disease is not evident, when the onset is acute, and when concomitant sensory cranial polyneuritis is evident. No further diagnostic tests are needed.

The VZV form of facial paralysis is differentiated from the HSV form by increased severity of symptoms, presence of auricular vesicles (Ramsay Hunt syndrome), and a rising titer of antibody to VZV. HSV may produce segmental, focal lesions that resemble herpes zoster, and VZV reactivation is known to occur without the pathognomonic vesicles (zoster sine herpete). In one study, in which VZV serum complement fixation titers were used, of the 892 patients with "Bell's palsy," 73 (8.2%) were diagnosed as having zoster sine herpete. A "zoster-like form" of Bell's palsy without the vesicles or antibodies diagnostic of VZV has been noted. Patients with this syndrome have a higher risk of nerve degeneration and poor outcome. The classic vesicular eruption on the pinna is not always present. If vesicles appear, they can appear before, during, or after facial paralysis.

Exclusion Criteria

The diagnosis of HSV (Bell's palsy) and VZV facial paralysis mononeuritis multiplex should not be made when:

1. Partial facial paralysis does not resolve in 3 to 6 weeks, is accompanied by electrical evidence of nerve degeneration, or is accompanied by ipsilateral hearing loss.

2. Any facial paralysis is accompanied by evidence of chronic otitis media or history of previous ear surgery.

3. Total facial paralysis is followed by no return of facial motion within 4 months. Even with total loss of nerve excitability, nerve regeneration ensues and results in midfacial contracture with synkinesis in 99% of all cases of Bell's palsy or Ramsay Hunt syndrome. The earliest sign of regeneration is return of the stapedial reflex; the next earliest sign is mouth motion with voluntary forced closure of the eyes (synkinesis).

4. Any facial paralysis with electrical evidence of nerve degeneration resolves without midfacial contracture with synkinesis (facial nerve degeneration with regeneration after HSV or VZV paralysis is followed by midfacial contracture with synkinesis).

5. Facial paralysis progresses during weeks or months (damage to the nerve is complete by day 14 in Bell's palsy and by day 21 in Ramsay Hunt syndrome).

6. Recurrent ipsilateral facial paralysis is accompanied by recovery and electrical evidence of nerve degeneration but not by contracture with synkinesis within 4 months.

TREATMENT

Discussing diagnosis and prognosis with the patient is essential to treatment. Protecting the eye is paramount. Dark glasses should be worn during the day, artificial tears instilled at the slightest evidence of drying, and a bland eye ointment used during sleep. Taping the eye closed is not recommended, but early exposure keratitis may require patching or, rarely, tarsorrhaphy.

When Bell's palsy was recognized as a virally induced, immune-mediated disease probably caused by HSV-1, we compared the efficacy of prednisone and acyclovir (Zovirax) with that of prednisone and placebo in treating patients with Bell's palsy. Treatment with prednisone-acyclovir or prednisone-placebo was

given for 10 days. Prednisone-acyclovir's greater effectiveness in producing complete return of volitional muscle motion and in preventing electrical degeneration was statistically significant. We concluded that prednisone-acyclovir is the proper treatment for Bell's palsy and that surgical decompression should be abandoned.

Corticosteroid agents remain the best treatment for inflammatory, virally induced, immune-mediated disease. Because mononeuritis multiplex can progress from a mild, incomplete paresis to a severe, complete paralysis, all patients should be treated with corticosteroid agents. Predicting which patients will progress to the severe form of the disease is impossible. If treatment is delayed until severity is determined, irreversible nerve damage may occur. Patients should receive both prednisone and acyclovir, and treatment should be tailored to the degree of disease severity. For adults, a daily total of 1 mg per kg of body weight of prednisone, taken in divided doses in the morning and evening, is suggested for treating both Bell's palsy and Ramsay Hunt syndrome. Acyclovir 200 to 400 mg orally five times daily is given for Bell's palsy. Because absorption of acyclovir from the gut is poor, the dose should be increased to 800 mg five times daily for Ramsay Hunt syndrome; intravenous treatment should be considered. Newer forms of acyclovir are being tested and may be effective when taken three times daily.

The patient should be seen on the fifth or sixth day after the onset of paralysis. If paralysis is incomplete, prednisone can be tapered to zero over the next 5 days, and acyclovir can be discontinued. If there is any question about severity or progression, the full dose of prednisone and acyclovir should be continued for 10 days, and the prednisone should then be tapered to zero over the next 5 days.

No reliable, widely available test for early identification of VZV infection currently exists. Because VZV carries a considerably poorer prognosis than does HSV, patients infected with VZV require longer follow-up, longer treatment, and greater emotional support. Early treatment with prednisone-acyclovir should offer better recovery.

Until early diagnosis is feasible, all therapeutic decisions must be made on a clinical basis. As in the past, reliance on history and physical examination is crucial in selecting patients for aggressive treatment. If a patient complains of concomitant severe pain or experiences sensorineural hearing loss, consider the diagnosis to be VZV rather than Bell's palsy (HSV) and treat the patient aggressively.

When reviewing the literature, question the validity of any results of treatment of Bell's palsy when the number of patients who show electrical evidence of nerve degeneration does not equal the number of patients who show contracture with synkinesis.

Electrotherapy is of no benefit and may be harmful. Experimental research has shown that electrical stimulation of denervated muscle retards ingrowth of neurofibrils to the motor end-plates.

Surgical facial nerve decompression is unnecessary

and harmful in treating virally induced neuritis and facial paralysis attributable to acute otitis media.

PROGNOSIS

Predicting prognosis is an integral part of therapy. Any practitioner who elects to evaluate patients with facial paralysis should have electrical tests available. Percutaneous nerve excitability tests are simple, reproducible, inexpensive, and reliable prognostic indicators. Elaborate electrical tests such as electroneurography, evoked electromyography, and strength-duration curves were used when facial nerve decompression was the standard treatment for viral facial paralysis and are therefore not recommended.

ACKNOWLEDGMENT

The Medical Editing Department, Kaiser Foundation Research Institute, provided editorial assistance.

PARKINSON'S DISEASE

method of
ROBERT L. RODNITZKY, M.D.
University of Iowa College of Medicine
Iowa City, Iowa

Parkinson's disease (PD) is a common neurologic disorder that is most prevalent in elderly patients, although it can occur over a wide range of ages. There are no practical and reliable diagnostic tests for PD; rather, the diagnosis is established on clinical grounds alone. The characteristic features of rest tremor, bradykinesia, rigidity, and impairment of postural reflexes allow the diagnosis to be made. It must be kept in mind, however, that not all these features are present in each patient with PD. On the other hand, a variety of different conditions, often referred to collectively as the "Parkinson's Plus syndromes," mimic PD in that they are associated with one or more of these clinical signs, most often akinesia and rigidity. These syndromes include other neurologic signs and symptoms not typically found in PD, allowing the distinction to be made among the disorders. Among the conditions classified as Parkinson's Plus are such disorders as progressive supranuclear palsy, multiple system atrophy, and corticobasal ganglionic degeneration, to name only a few. Acquired conditions such as arteriosclerosis and normal-pressure hydrocephalus can also result in parkinsonism.

It is important to distinguish these other forms of parkinsonism from PD because of their differences in response to treatment and prognosis. For example, the symptoms of PD are usually remarkably relieved by levodopa, whereas the parkinsonian component of progressive supranuclear palsy is often much less improved by this therapy. In terms of prognosis, there is usually a more rapid rate of progression to severe disability in progressive supranuclear palsy than in PD.

The number of medical and surgical options for treating PD has increased substantially since the introduction of levodopa, the most important therapy, just over 25 years ago. Understanding when each of these treatment modalities should be instituted in a given patient and appreciating how they can be combined allows their full potential to be realized.

TREATMENT OF EARLY AND MILD PARKINSON'S DISEASE

An accurate assessment of disease-related disability is extremely important in deciding whether and what form of therapy should be instituted in a given patient. In early PD there may be sufficient signs or symptoms to allow a clinical diagnosis to be made, but there may not yet be real disability. When evaluating disability in PD it is important to explore the various facets of the patient's life on which neurologic dysfunction could have an impact. Occupational disability with threatened loss of employment is the most important form of disability for most patients and is the circumstance that most urgently calls for therapeutic intervention. Social disability is characterized by withdrawal from church or community affairs or from involvement in recreational activities. Cosmetic disability is usually the result of embarrassment or self-consciousness over a resting tremor or an expressionless facial appearance. If the manifestations of PD are causing clear disability in any of these realms and having a negative impact on the patient's daily routine, symptomatic therapy should be started. Neuroprotective therapy, discussed later, can be considered even in the absence of disability.

If disability is present but is relatively mild, therapy with levodopa or dopamine agonist drugs can be reserved for use later in the course of the illness. In such mildly affected patients there are three considerations for initial therapy: selegiline (Eldepryl), amantadine (Symmetrel), or anticholinergic agents such as trihexyphenidyl (Artane) or benztropine (Cogentin).

Selegiline is a selective inhibitor of the enzyme monoamine oxidase-B (MAO-B). Unlike with nonselective MAO inhibitors, which also inhibit the A form of the enzyme, there is little risk of a hypertensive crisis when the drug is taken along with tyramine-containing foods (the "cheese" effect) in the recommended dosage of 5 mg twice daily. This agent has been shown to significantly delay the need for more potent dopaminergic drugs when used in patients with early and mild PD. It is not yet clear whether this beneficial effect results from the drug's mild dopaminergic action and relief of PD symptoms or from a primary neuroprotective effect that delays the further degeneration of dopaminergic neurons. It is possible that it has both effects. Whichever mechanism is operative, its ability to delay the appearance of severely disabling symptoms makes selegiline an excellent choice for initial therapy in patients with mild disability. Because of its putative neuroprotective action, this agent should also be considered even in patients who have no disability. The usual dosage is 5 mg twice daily, morning and noon. Dosages administered later in the day may result in insomnia.

Although no dietary restrictions are necessary in

patients taking this selective MAO-B inhibitor, there are some potentially serious drug interactions. Severe central nervous system toxicity and autonomic reactions, some of which have been fatal, have been reported in a small number of patients taking selegiline while also receiving either tricyclic antidepressants or selective serotonin re-uptake inhibitors. Selegiline should therefore be discontinued at least 14 days before starting drugs belonging to either of these classes of antidepressant.

Amantadine was originally introduced as an antiviral agent and later found to ameliorate the symptoms of PD as well. It has mild dopaminergic properties. This agent mildly benefits all the cardinal clinical features of PD and is an appropriate choice for initial treatment of mild parkinsonian symptoms, especially when tremor is not the predominant manifestation. The usual dosage is 100 mg twice daily. For some patients, the benefit of this agent begins to wane after only 2 or 3 months of therapy, and in most there is a noticeable reduction in effect by 1 year. Caution should be exercised in prescribing this agent for elderly PD patients because of its propensity to cause confusion and hallucinations in this patient group. Less serious but relatively frequent side effects include livedo reticularis and ankle edema, neither of which require discontinuance of the drug.

Anticholinergic drugs are also mildly effective in treating the symptoms of PD. These agents are especially useful for relieving tremor and should strongly be considered as the first therapy in patients whose major disability stems from this symptom. The two most commonly used anticholinergic agents are trihexyphenidyl (Artane) and benztropine (Cogentin). These drugs have the potential to produce noticeable peripheral anticholinergic side effects, including visual blurring, dry mouth, constipation, and urinary retention. Even more distressing are the central anticholinergic side effects, such as memory impairment, confusion, and hallucinations. Cognitive and behavioral side effects such as these are particularly likely to occur in elderly patients or those suffering from dementia. Accordingly, anticholinergic drugs should not be used in the presence of dementia and only very cautiously and in very low dosage in the elderly.

The peripheral anticholinergic side effects can be minimized by using a low initial dosage followed by a very slow upward titration. Trihexyphenidyl should be started at a dosage of 1 mg twice daily and increased by no more than 1 mg per day per week until there is improvement or a dosage of 2 mg three times daily is reached. Benztropine can be started at 0.5 mg daily and slowly titrated to as much as 1 mg twice daily. Anticholinergic drugs should not be discontinued precipitously because of the risk of rebound worsening of the symptoms of PD.

TREATMENT OF MODERATELY ADVANCED PARKINSON'S DISEASE

This group of patients has definite and significant disability that is beyond the scope of efficacy of anticholinergics, amantadine, or selegiline alone. Treatment with a primary dopaminergic agent is indicated in these patients, and in most instances levodopa is the drug of choice. The decision to begin levodopa therapy has major long-term implications. Within 5 years of beginning levodopa therapy, approximately 50% of patients will have developed complications consisting of daily fluctuations in response to the medication, abnormal involuntary movements, or both. It is not yet clear whether the development of these complications is due to the amount and duration of levodopa therapy or relates to the natural progression of the underlying disease process. Until these questions are answered, it is prudent not to initiate levodopa therapy prematurely and, once initiated, to keep the dosage at the lowest level consistent with a satisfactory clinical response.

Levodopa is administered in a combination tablet (Sinemet), which also contains carbidopa, an inhibitor of the enzyme dopa decarboxylase. By inhibiting this enzyme and preventing the metabolism of levodopa to dopamine outside the blood-brain barrier, carbidopa reduces peripheral dopaminergic side effects, most notably nausea. To achieve optimal protection against levodopa side effects, most patients require a daily dosage of at least 60 mg of carbidopa, and some require as much as 150 mg. In devising the initial dosage of carbidopa/levodopa, these carbidopa dosing requirements should be kept in mind. It is difficult to achieve a daily dosage of 60 mg or more of carbidopa when using the 10/100 dosage form of carbidopa/levodopa. Consequently, this dosage form should not be chosen for initiation of levodopa therapy. Patients receiving adequate amounts of levodopa in the combination tablet but still experiencing nausea may benefit from taking an additional 50 to 75 mg of supplemental carbidopa each day. Carbidopa tablets (Lodosyn) are not yet available at pharmacies, but can be obtained by special request from the pharmaceutical manufacturer (Dupont Pharma).

Patients occasionally experience nausea and other side effects of levodopa that are so bothersome that they are extremely hesitant to embark on another trial of this preparation. In this circumstance, it is worthwhile attempting to "prime" the patient with carbidopa alone for 5 to 7 days in a dosage of 25 mg four times daily before attempting to reintroduce daily treatment with carbidopa/levodopa tablets.

Carbidopa/levodopa is marketed in both standard release (Sinemet) and sustained-release (Sinemet CR) formulations. Either form can be utilized for initial treatment. The standard carbidopa/levodopa is slightly less expensive and is available in generic form, whereas the CR preparation offers the convenience of fewer daily doses. Sinemet CR also has a very important potential advantage. Recent research suggests that response fluctuations and dyskinesias that develop after long-term levodopa therapy may be in part due to the pulsatile stimulation of dopamine receptors related to the periodicity of levodopa ingestion. On the other hand, continuous stimulation of these receptors diminishes these complications. It is postulated, but not yet proved, that the sustained-release formulation may therefore reduce the potential for development of long-term complications of levodopa therapy since it results in more constant plasma levodopa levels throughout the day.

The initial dosage of sustained-release carbidopa/levodopa is 25/100 mg twice daily, in the morning and midafternoon. After 7 to 10 days the dosage will need to be increased to 50/200 twice daily in most patients. Efficacy on this dosage should be evaluated after 4 weeks, and if clinically indicated, the dose can be further increased. Sustained-release carbidopa/levodopa has a slower onset of action than the standard formulation. This prolonged latency to effect is most noticeable with the first dosage of the day. For patients bothered by this delay, one-half to one tablet of standard carbidopa/levodopa 25/100 can be added to the first dosage in the morning. If the sustained-release preparation is not effective or not tolerated, standard carbidopa/levodopa 25/100 can be prescribed instead in a dosage of one-half tablet three times daily and then increased, if needed, after 7 to 10 days, to one tablet three times daily. Again, there should be consideration of further upward titration if, after 4 weeks, there is still suboptimal clinical response.

In patients for whom there is inefficient symptom control despite a levodopa dosage as high as 600 to 800 mg daily, it is best to consider adding a dopamine agonist such as bromocriptine or pergolide (as discussed later) rather than adding still more levodopa at this point. Absence of any response to levodopa raises the question as to whether the patient is suffering from a form of parkinsonism other than PD.

Patients who were previously placed on selegiline can remain on it after levodopa is begun for its possible neuroprotective effect and for its levodopa-sparing potential. Those on anticholinergics or amantadine should continue these agents only if there is clear evidence that they are still receiving benefit.

FLUCTUATIONS IN THE RESPONSE TO MEDICATIONS

Initially, most patients with PD respond favorably to therapy with levodopa and the response remains constant throughout the day. With time however, many begin to note an increasingly shorter duration of benefit from each single dosage so that symptoms of PD re-emerge before the next dosage takes effect—a phenomenon referred to as "wearing off." Less commonly, particularly in the more advanced stages of the illness, periodic loss of efficacy occurs without obvious relationship to the timing of levodopa dosages, the so-called "on-off" or "random off" effect. Both wearing off and random off episodes can begin suddenly, especially the latter.

The treatment of both types of response fluctuations is very similar, but much more success can be anticipated in ameliorating wearing off than random off episodes. The management of response fluctuations includes the following strategies:

Shortening the Interdose Interval of Carbidopa/Levodopa

Patients who notice return of symptoms just before the next dosage of carbidopa/levodopa may benefit from taking dosages more frequently. Sustained-release carbidopa/levodopa is seldom administered more often than every 3.5 hours, and the standard preparation is rarely required more often than every 2 hours. Requirement of a dosing frequency in excess of this suggests that other strategies will need to be employed to treat wearing off.

Addition of Selegiline

This agent prolongs and enhances the central effect of dopamine and is therefore of benefit in treating wearing off. For patients not already receiving it, it can be added to either standard or sustained-release carbidopa/levodopa in a dosage of 5 mg twice daily. Some patients experience enhanced levodopa side effects, consisting of confusion, hypotension, or involuntary movements, when selegiline is combined with levodopa. If this occurs, a trial on a lower dosage of 5 mg daily can be considered.

Sustained-Release Levodopa

This preparation, marketed as Sinemet CR, has much slower dissolution properties than standard Sinemet has, resulting in a slower fall in plasma levodopa levels after each dosage. Therefore, changing from standard to the CR form of Sinemet can be expected to improve wearing off. When this changeover is made, the interdose interval will usually need to be increased by approximately 50%. Also, the total daily dose of levodopa will usually need to be increased by 10 to 20% since the bioavailability of levodopa in the sustained-release formulation is approximately 80% of that from the standard preparation. Even with these initial adjustments, further titration in timing and amount of dosage will be required for many patients based on their initial clinical response. As mentioned previously, the first daily dosage may need to be supplemented with a small amount of standard carbidopa/levodopa for patients noting a very slow onset of effect. It is important to advise patients not to chew the CR tablets, as that destroys their sustained-release property.

Addition of a Dopamine Agonist

Dopamine agonists are useful as supplemental therapy in patients not adequately relieved of symptoms despite a daily dosage of 600 to 800 mg of levodopa, and also as a means of treating patients experiencing response fluctuations on levodopa. It has been suggested that these agents can be used for the initial therapy of PD, thus forestalling the use of levodopa. There are an increasing number of proponents of this strategy. Those who do not favor this approach point out the very long induction period required for these agents and emphasize their relatively lower clinical efficacy and slightly higher side effect profile compared with levodopa. There is little controversy over the usefulness of dopamine agonists in patients who are experiencing response fluctuations while on carbidopa/levodopa. Both currently available agonists, pergolide and bromocriptine, have a longer efficacy half-life than levodopa has. Additionally, these drugs are less susceptible than levodopa to changes in gastrointestinal absorption or transit across the blood-brain barrier, thereby providing a more stable base of dopaminergic effect.

In patients experiencing response fluctuations, bromocriptine can be added to levodopa in an initial dosage of 1.25 mg once or twice daily. The dosage is then gradually increased at the rate of 1.25 to 2.5 mg per week, depending on tolerance. The ultimate effective dose when used in conjunction with levodopa is usually between 10 and 30 mg per day. Pergolide is introduced at a dosage of 0.05 mg per day and increased very slowly, at first by 0.05 mg every 3 days and then, when higher dosages are reached, by 0.25 mg every 3 days. The usual effective daily dose is between 1.5 and 5 mg and the average daily dosage is approximately 2.5 mg. With either of these drugs, the early appearance of side effects such as nausea, sedation, or hypotension suggests that a still slower titration be used. As the dosage of the dopamine agonist begins to approach therapeutic level, the dosage of levodopa should be reduced by 10 to 25%, if possible, to lessen the likelihood of dose-related side effects such as dyskinesias and hallucinations.

Dietary Adjustments

Both the rate of gastric emptying and the level of diet-derived amino acids in the plasma can have a significant impact on the efficacy of levodopa. Levodopa is absorbed in the small bowel, so it is important that it pass through the stomach rapidly and efficiently. Because gastric emptying is more rapid when the stomach is empty, patients suffering from wearing off should be instructed to take their levodopa at least 15 to 20 minutes before a meal. In patients who experience nausea after taking levodopa on an empty stomach, this strategy may not be practical. These patients should try taking their levodopa with a small, low-protein snack rather than with a meal.

Ingested levodopa competes for absorption in the small bowel with dietary large neutral amino acids and also competes with circulating amino acids for entry into the brain across the blood-brain barrier. The latter competition is especially important in determining the effectiveness of a given dosage of levodopa. A variety of dietary strategies can be employed to ameliorate this potentially negative effect of amino acids. Such adjustments in dietary habits are especially important in patients who discern a definite lessening of levodopa effect after protein-containing meals. As the first measure, the patient should be advised to spread daily protein intake evenly across all three meals of the day, avoiding meals with a very high protein content. If this is ineffective, the next step is to institute a low-protein diet that allows almost no protein at all during the daytime, but packages almost all the daily protein requirement into the evening meal. On this program, some patients note definite improvement in the levodopa effect during the day but are noticeably slower after the evening meal. To be effective, these dietary plans require considerable instruction. They are not practical for patients who have not demonstrated a high level of compliance in the past. Many patients read about protein redistribution or protein restriction diets in informational pamphlets and inappropriately place themselves on such a plan. These dietary restrictions are not required for those not experiencing complications of levodopa therapy. They are certainly not required in patients on other antiparkinson drugs who are not yet taking levodopa.

Liquid Carbidopa/Levodopa

Delayed gastric emptying and erratic plasma levodopa levels can be partially overcome by administering carbidopa/levodopa in liquid form. As this combination drug is not marketed in a liquid form, patients must learn to prepare it themselves. This is accomplished by adding ground carbidopa/levodopa tablets containing a total of 1000 mg of levodopa to 1000 mL of tap water, along with 2000 mg of abscorbic acid. If needed, a ratio of 2 mg of levodopa per 1 mL of water can be used. The daily dosage of levodopa is then divided into hourly doses of the liquid preparation. Titration of the amount of each dose and the interval between dosages can then be carried out according to the patient's response. A fresh solution must be made every 24 hours and a supply of the liquid preparation must be carried by the patient throughout the day, leading to considerable inconvenience. However, the compliant patient may be rewarded with fewer and less severe fluctuations and possibly less prominent dyskinesias.

DYSKINESIAS

Dyskinesias are involuntary movements that occur in two major forms—chorea and dystonia. Choreiform dyskinesias are characterized by arrhythmic writhing or flinging movements of the extremities, undulating movements of the trunk, or head bobbing. They usually appear at the time of peak levodopa effect, near the middle of the interdose interval, and are accordingly referred to as "peak dose dyskinesias." Several strategies can be employed to control this complication. The initial attempt should be a modest reduction in levodopa dosage, hoping not to seriously diminish the beneficial effects of levodopa at the same time. Some patients who experience peak dose dyskinesias on standard carbidopa/levodopa fare better on sustained-release carbidopa/levodopa because plasma levodopa peaks are lower on this preparation. If these approaches fail, replacement of 20 to 40% of the daily levodopa dosage with a dopamine agonist is another useful strategy that can result in lower plasma levodopa peaks. Additionally, dopamine agonists have less potential than levodopa to cause dyskinesias. One additional option for treating peak dose dyskinesias is a trial on liquid Sinemet, described earlier.

Diphasic dyskinesias are choreodystonic movements that occur at the beginning and end of the interdose interval, just when the levodopa effect is beginning and again when it is starting to decline. This pattern of dyskinesias is more difficult to treat but fortunately is more rare than the peak dose variety. Treatment possibilities include attempting to use more frequent dosages of levodopa, replacing some levodopa with a dopamine agonist, or changing from standard to sustained-release carbidopa/levodopa. All these strategies are aimed at preventing a periodic drop-off in the net effect of the dopaminergic agents in use.

Dystonic dyskinesias occasionally appear as a result of PD itself, but more commonly they are a side effect related to dopaminergic treatment. These involuntary movements are slower and more sustained than chorea. Although dystonic dyskinesias occasionally occur in conjunction with the peak effect of levodopa, they are much more common at the end of the interdose interval when the levodopa effect is wearing off. Accordingly, all the aforementioned strategies to combat wearing off are potentially useful in treating end-of-dose dystonia. Among these strategies, the addition of a dopamine agonist is especially useful. If tolerated, small dosages of anticholinergic drugs (trihexyphenidyl or benztropine) may also benefit dystonia in PD.

Early morning dystonia, occurring after an entire night without dopaminergic medication, is a particularly bothersome and painful form of end-of-dose dystonia. Patients note severe uncomfortable dystonic spasms, often of one or both feet, upon first awakening in the morning. This can be treated by prescribing a bedtime dosage of a long-acting dopaminergic agent, such as bromocriptine, pergolide, or sustained-release carbidopa/levodopa. Similarly, a bedtime dosage of baclofen (Lioresal) may be effective. Lastly, the simple expedient of awaking 1 hour earlier than usual, taking a dose of carbidopa/levodopa, and then returning to bed may be effective for some patients.

FREEZING

Freezing is a form of response fluctuation that merits special discussion. It is characterized by sudden inability to initiate or continue a repetitive motor activity. The most common motor activity affected in this manner is walking. Patients find it impossible to take the first step or, if already under way, they note that a real or imagined obstacle, such as a narrow doorway, causes their feet to "freeze" in one spot. Freezing episodes that occur mainly during the time when antiparkinson medications have obviously worn off may respond to therapies that promote more "on" time. Basically, one can utilize the same strategies used for treating wearing off as discussed earlier. Freezing that occurs in the midst of a period when the patient otherwise appears to be enjoying good

benefit from medication, i.e., when the patient is "on," does not respond well to further addition of antiparkinson drugs. In this circumstance, patients can be taught a variety of "tricks" to unfreeze. Walking to a cadence or a rhythm is a useful means of preventing freezing when approaching a doorway or other obstacle. Once a patient is frozen, stepping over an object on the floor such as the handle of an inverted cane can be a very effective means of initiating the first step.

DEPRESSION AND PSYCHOSIS

A variety of behavioral symptoms can occur in PD patients. The most common is depression, which in recent studies has been found to be present in approximately 50% of patients. Depression often responds to the tricyclic antidepressants, such as amitriptyline (Elavil) or nortriptyline (Pamelor). The anticholinergic properties of these drugs may not be well tolerated by patients with orthostatic hypotention or dementia. Accordingly, for some patients the latter agent will be preferable because of its lower anticholinergic effect. Selective serotonin re-uptake inhibitors such as fluoxetine (Prozac), sertraline (Zoloft), or paroxetine (Paxil) are also useful in these patients. There have been a few reported instances of worsening of PD symptoms in patients receiving these serotonergic agents, but other studies have suggested that this adverse reaction is rare. In patients refractory to antidepressant agents, electroconvulsive therapy is effective. This therapy also transiently improves the motoric symptoms of PD. Neither tricyclic antidepressants nor selective serotonin re-uptake inhibitors should be administered to patients receiving selegiline, as a potentially fatal interaction has been reported.

When psychosis occurs, it is usually in advanced patients receiving several antiparkinson drugs. This complication is characterized by delusional or paranoid thoughts and by visual hallucinations. Extremely vivid dreams may be an early sign of psychosis. These symptoms are usually the result of one or more antiparkinson medications; therefore the initial treatment should consist of reduction and withdrawal of potentially offending agents. The magnitude of medication withdrawal has to be balanced against the risk of serious exacerbation of the underlying parkinsonian symptoms. Virtually all the antiparkinson drugs have some potential to cause or exacerbate psychosis. The less efficacious drug should be withdrawn first. Accordingly, selegiline, amantadine, anticholinergics, and dopamine agonists should be withdrawn in that order. If psychosis persists, a downward titration of levodopa should be tried, assuming the patient's clinical state will allow it. Withdrawal of anticholinergic drugs should be carried out over 1 to 2 weeks, if possible, to avoid rebound worsening of parkinsonism. Withdrawal of dopamine agonists or reduction of levodopa should be done in a similarly gradual fashion since neuroleptic malignant syndrome has been associated with precipitous reduction of dopaminergic agents.

If drug reduction to the extent possible has not relieved psychotic symptoms, the use of antipsychotic drug therapy is indicated. The neuroleptic drugs thioridazine (Mellaril), molindone (Moban), and risperidone (Risperdal) have relatively low potential for inducing extrapyramidal side effects and can be used in low dosage without great risk of exacerbating the signs of parkinsonism. A dosage of 20 to 30 mg per day for thioridazine or 0.5 to 1 mg per day for risperidone is appropriate for this purpose. If hallucinations are largely nocturnal, these neuroleptic agents can be administered at bedtime. For patients not responding to any of these approaches, the novel neuroleptic agent clozapine (Clozaril) can be used. This agent is very effective in relieving psychotic symptoms in PD and carries no risk of exacerbating the underlying illness. However, the association of clozapine with agranulocytosis and the requirement to perform weekly blood counts on patients receiving the drug inhibits its use except in refractory psychosis.

ADDITIONAL NONMOTORIC SYMPTOMS

Constipation

This is a very common problem in PD owing to a combination of drug effects, immobility, advanced age, and a direct effect of the illness on bowel motility. Patients with severe constipation should avoid anticholinergic drugs, maintain adequate hydration, and incorporate extra fiber into their diet. The regular use of a stool softener is recommended. The prokinetic drug cisapride (Propulsid) enhances colonic transit and can be used to improve constipation in PD. Because it is a cholinergic drug it carries a small risk of exacerbating PD symptoms.

Orthostatic Hypotension

Symptomatic orthostatic hypotension can result from primary involvement of the autonomic nervous system in PD as well as from the effect of antiparkinson drugs, especially levodopa and dopamine agonists. Severe orthostatic hypotension early in the course of the illness raises the possibility that the patient does not have PD but rather is suffering from multiple system atrophy, one of the Parkinson's Plus syndromes. The first step in managing orthostatic hypotension is encouraging fluid and sodium intake if there are no cardiac or renal system abnormalities that would contraindicate this strategy. Graduated compression stockings worn during the day and extending to at least the midthigh are useful as long as the patient has the ability or the assistance to get them on and off. If these measures fail, pharmacologic therapy can be started with indomethacin (Indocin), 25 mg three times daily. This agent presumably works by inhibiting the synthesis of prostaglandins that promote vasodilatation. Fludrocortisone (Florinef) is more effective than indomethacin, but its use requires greater caution since it can result in recumbent hypertension or significant fluid retention. This agent is begun in a dose of 0.1 mg daily and titrated upward as needed to as much as 0.5 mg daily. The alpha-adrenergic drug midodrine (Midamine)* has proved to be effective for orthostatic hypotension in several studies at a dosage of 5 to 10 mg four times daily; however, it has not yet been approved for general use.

Sialorrhea

Excessive drooling is a major problem for some patients with advanced PD. An anticholinergic antiparkinson drug such as trihexphenidyl can be used to treat this symptom provided there are no contraindications such as dementia, constipation, or urinary retention. The peripherally acting anticholinergic drug propantheline (Pro-Banthīne) is also useful in a dosage of 15 to 30 mg three times daily. This agent cannot cause confusion or exacerbate dementia like the centrally active antiparkinson anticholinergics, but it can worsen constipation and inhibit bladder emptying.

SURGICAL THERAPIES FOR PARKINSON'S DISEASE

Transplantation of fetal mesencephalic tissue into the brain of PD patients has been carried out at several centers throughout the world. This procedure is still experimental and is not widely available. A controlled study that seeks to objectively determine the efficacy of this procedure is currently under way. Uncontrolled studies have indicated that some transplanted cells survive in the host brain and elaborate dopamine. These studies have suggested that PD symptoms are generally improved by this procedure, and the net requirement of antiparkinson medication is reduced.

Implantation of a stimulator in the thalamus or stereotactic lesioning of the thalamus has been shown to be useful in relieving the tremor of PD. Stimulation therapy is still experimental but may prove to be an improvement over stereotactic lesioning, since the stimulator can be turned on and off at will and can be applied to both sides of the brain with less risk of serious complications than is the case with bilateral lesioning. Another stereotactic procedure, posteroventral pallidotomy, is gaining increasing acceptance. Unlike thalamotomy, which largely improves tremor, this operation has the potential to improve rigidity, bradykinesia, and impaired postural reflexes as well. Modern intraoperative stimulation and recording techniques have significantly reduced the incidence of inadvertent lesioning of the adjacent optic tract, accounting for greatly improved outcomes compared to previous experience with this procedure.

---

*Investigational drug in the United States.

PERIPHERAL NEUROPATHIES

method of
ROBERT W. SHIELDS, JR., M.D.
Cleveland Clinic Foundation
Cleveland, Ohio

The peripheral nervous system may be affected by a wide range of disorders. Clinical symptoms and signs are related to the pathophysiology of the disorder and the fiber types that are affected. Thus, a combination of sensory, motor, and autonomic dysfunction may occur. Peripheral nerve disorders may evolve in a rather acute and abrupt fashion or may follow a subacute or more chronic course. Most polyneuropathies are generalized and relatively symmetrical, whereas others may be focal and asymmetrical. There are many methods of classifying peripheral nerve disorders. The classification illustrated in Table 1 divides peripheral nerve disorders into very basic clinical syndromes of acute and chronic polyneuropathies. This is useful in approaching the differential diagnosis of peripheral nerve disorders and identifying those for which specific treatment is necessary.

In the strictest sense, all peripheral nerve disorders are treatable. However, there are relatively few peripheral nerve disorders in which specific therapy has a significant impact on the current neurologic deficits and the ultimate prognosis. These "treatable" peripheral nerve disorders are emphasized in this review.

GENERAL MEASURES

Regardless of the specific cause of the peripheral nerve disorder, there are general therapeutic measures that may be applied to all patients. Motor weakness tends to involve muscles in a distal-to-proximal gradient with the lower extremities more affected than the upper extremities. Significant lower extremity weakness typically produces gait disorders, most commonly a steppage gait from footdrop. This often causes the toes to catch on uneven surfaces and may result in falls and injuries. Patients with footdrop may benefit from an ankle-foot orthosis

TABLE 1. **Classification of Generalized Peripheral Polyneuropathies**

I. Acute polyneuropathies
  1. Guillain-Barré Syndrome (GBS)
  2. Porphyric neuropathy
  3. Metal neuropathy
II. Chronic polyneuropathies
  1. Chronic inflammatory demyelinating polyneuropathy (CIDP)
  2. Diabetic polyneuropathy
  3. Alcoholic and nutritional polyneuropathies
  4. Uremic polyneuropathy
  5. Paraneoplastic neuropathies
  6. Myeloma or dysproteinemia
  7. Drugs or toxins
  8. Amyloidosis
  9. Endocrine neuropathies
  10. Infectious polyneuropathies
  11. Sarcoid neuropathy
  12. Vasculitic neuropathies
  13. Heredofamilial neuropathies

(AFO). Wrist and finger braces are helpful in preventing stretching of the extensor tendons that may occur in wrist-finger drop. In general, physical therapy measures, including stretching and passive range of motion exercises, may be helpful in preventing contractures, maintaining mobility, and preserving function. Various aids to ambulation, including canes and walkers, assist the patient in maintaining independent ambulation and preventing falls and injuries. Occupational therapy may optimize fine motor functions, especially with the aid of various devices and appliances, such as large-handled utensils. Sensory loss can impart a sensory ataxia that may also benefit from devices such as canes or walkers. The management of pain is discussed in the section dealing with small fiber neuropathies.

ACUTE GENERALIZED SENSORIMOTOR POLYNEUROPATHIES

Guillain-Barré Syndrome

Guillain-Barré syndrome (GBS) is by far the most common and important of the acute polyneuropathies. GBS is an inflammatory demyelinating immune-mediated disorder of the peripheral nervous system. GBS typically evolves over several days up to 1 to 2 weeks or so. It is characterized by generalized and relatively symmetrical weakness involving distal and proximal muscles. Sensory symptoms of tingling, aching, or pain are typically present but not prominent. GBS can produce generalized severe weakness with respiratory failure over a period of several days. Autonomic dysfunction consisting of hypertension fluctuating with hypotension, tachycardia, bradycardia, and urinary retention may occur as well. Cranial nerve involvement including facial diplegia and dysphagia may also be observed. GBS often follows an infectious illness, typically a nonspecific viral infection. However, prior infection with *Campylobacter jejuni,* a gram-negative rod that causes diarrhea, has been documented in up to 60% of patients with GBS. GBS may also be associated with infectious mononucleosis, viral hepatitis, and human immunodeficiency virus (HIV) infection.

Patients with GBS display generalized weakness, areflexia, and variable degrees of sensory loss. Electrodiagnostic studies often document signs of an acquired segmental demyelinating polyneuropathy consisting of focal and asymmetrical conduction block, slowing of conduction velocities, prolonged distal latencies, and dispersion of the responses. Examination of the cerebral spinal fluid (CSF) classically displays increased protein with acellular fluid, so-called cytoalbuminologic dissociation. However, elevation of the CSF protein level may not be present initially and, in fact, may increase over the ensuing 2 to 3 weeks after the onset of symptoms.

GBS is a very distinctive clinical entity, and diagnosis is usually not difficult. However, it is important to distinguish GBS from spinal cord compression, especially when GBS has spared the cranial nerves. The cardinal features of spinal cord disease including a sensory level, retained or heightened tendon reflexes, and Babinski's signs helps to differentiate these two entities. Needless to say, neuroimaging of the spinal cord to exclude myelopathy from external compression and other causes should be considered if there is any question regarding the presence of myelopathy.

Patients with GBS should be admitted to the hospital for close monitoring of pulmonary and autonomic function, general supportive care, and specific treatment against the immune-mediated process. It is critical that the pulmonary status be monitored frequently, especially in patients who are demonstrating a rapid evolution of generalized weakness. The forced vital capacity (FVC) and arterial blood gas (ABG) levels should be tested initially for baseline measurements. The FVC should be assessed frequently as the patient's clinical status requires. If the FVC is reduced to 12 to 15 mL per kg or if the PO_2 is less than 70 mmHg on room air, then intubation must be considered. Although these guidelines are helpful in identifying patients in need of intubation, it is equally important to take into account the rapidity of the decline in pulmonary function. It is imperative that patients with progressive pulmonary failure be intubated as an elective procedure rather than waiting until intubation becomes an emergency. In addition, patients with bulbar paralysis who have prominent dysphagia, and difficulty maintaining a patent airway may also require intubation. Autonomic dysfunction should be managed symptomatically, but most often the dysautonomia responds to specific treatment of the GBS. However, conventional means of treating hypotension with increasing fluids may be necessary. Second- or third-degree atrioventricular (AV) block and severe bradycardias should prompt consideration for a temporary demand pacemaker.

Patients with GBS should receive vigorous respiratory toilet and chest physiotherapy to prevent atelectasis and secondary pneumonia. Patients should be turned frequently to retard the development of bed sores and ulcerations, and careful physical and occupational therapy should be directed to maintaining flexibility of the joints and preventing contractures. The use of wrist splints and foot boards may be helpful for patients with wrist- and footdrop, respectively. Subcutaneous heparin at 5000 U twice daily should be administered to prevent the development of deep vein thrombophlebitis and secondary pulmonary embolism.

The specific treatment against the immune-mediated process in GBS incorporates the use of plasma-exchange treatments. The efficacy of plasmapheresis in GBS has been established by several controlled randomized and carefully monitored trials. These trials have indicated that plasmapheresis is effective, especially if initiated early. There is compelling evidence that plasmapheresis reduces the time spent in the hospital, the time spent on a respirator, and the time before the patient is able to ambulate. Ideally, plasmapheresis should be initiated within the first week of illness or certainly before the second week. Plasmapheresis is usually administered in a series of three to five treatments in which 3 to 3.5 liters are exchanged per treatment. In most plasmapheresis units, albumin and saline, as opposed to fresh-frozen plasma, are used as replacement fluids. This reduces the risk of hepatitis and other infectious disorders that can result from the use of fresh-frozen plasma. Although relapses may occur after a course of plasmapheresis, they are relatively uncommon and tend to respond to additional plasmapheresis treatments. Plasmapheresis is a relatively safe procedure for most patients; however, the presence of severe cardiac dysautonomia may be a relative or absolute contraindication to its use.

There is mounting evidence that intravenous immune globulin (IVIG)* is effective in the treatment of GBS. Although the precise role of IVIG in the treatment of GBS still needs further clarification, IVIG represents a reasonable alternative to plasmapheresis in patients who are at increased risk for complications from plasmapheresis because of cardiac dysautonomia or in circumstances in which plasmapheresis is not available. Treatment is usually initiated with 400 mg of gamma globulin per kg of body weight given intravenously each day for 5 consecutive days. Relapses may be more frequent after IVIG therapy than after plasmapheresis. IVIG carries additional risks of cerebral ischemia and renal failure. In addition, patients may experience headache and other general constitutional symptoms during the infusions. A contraindication to IVIG is the presence of immunoglobulin A (IgA) deficiency associated with IgA antibodies. In this circumstance, IVIG treatment may induce severe anaphylaxis. The use of corticosteroids for the treatment of GBS appears to be ineffective and is generally not recommended.

GBS carries a reasonably good prognosis for a good functional recovery. Nearly 80% of patients have a full recovery, with the remaining 20% having mild to moderate residual deficits.

Porphyric Neuropathy

Porphyric neuropathy may be the product of acute intermittent porphyria, variegate porphyria, or coproporphyria. These porphyrias represent very rare autosomal dominantly inherited disorders of heme synthesis. Porphyric neuropathy typically presents with acute attacks of a predominantly motor neuropathy often associated with dysautonomia, abdominal pain, psychosis, convulsions, and delirium. On occasion, some patients present with truncal sensory levels and cranial nerve involvement. Attacks of porphyric neuropathy are usually precipitated by drugs that induce the hepatic microsomal cytochrome P-450 system. A wide variety of drugs including barbiturates

---

*Not FDA-approved for this indication.

and various anticonvulsants can precipitate attacks. Thus, the primary therapeutic objective in patients with porphyria is to prevent attacks by avoiding these drugs. Management of patients in the midst of acute porphyric neuropathy includes intravenous glucose administration, up to 500 grams over 24 hours. Hematin (Panhematin) at a dose of 2 to 5 mg per kg per day administered intravenously over 30 to 60 minutes for 3 to 14 days is typically helpful in controlling the attack. Patients may be treated with chlorpromazine (Thorazine) for agitation and anxiety and meperidine (Demerol) or morphine for pain.

Acute Metal Neuropathy

Acute polyneuropathy may also be the product of heavy metal intoxication. Acute exposure to arsenic typically results in abdominal pain, nausea, vomiting, diarrhea, delirium, psychosis, and a progressive sensorimotor polyneuropathy. Treatment is often initiated with British antilewisite (BAL) or with D-penicillamine (Cuprimine, Depen). BAL may be administered by intramuscular injection at a dosage of 2.5 mg per kg four times daily for 2 days, two times on day 3, and once daily for 10 days. D-Penicillamine may be given orally at 250 mg four times daily while monitoring 24-hour urinary arsenic excretion. Treatment is continued until arsenic excretion falls below 25 mg per 24 hours. Acute intoxication with thallium produces a similar clinical picture. In addition, thallium produces alopecia and sometimes a movement disorder. Treatment with BAL, potassium salts, and Prussian blue has been recommended, but definitive evidence of efficacy is lacking. The key to the treatment of heavy metal intoxication is to recognize the clinical syndrome, confirm the diagnosis, and avoid re-exposure.

CHRONIC POLYNEUROPATHIES
Chronic Inflammatory Demyelinating Polyneuropathy

Chronic inflammatory demyelinating polyneuropathy (CIDP) is an immune-mediated sensorimotor polyneuropathy that typically produces prominent motor symptoms in a symmetrical fashion, sometimes with prominent proximal muscle involvement. In approximately two-thirds of patients, the course is slow and monophasic, whereas in the other third the course may be recurrent and relapsing. A relatively small percentage of patients may experience cranial nerve involvement and autonomic dysfunction. Typically, patients demonstrate weakness, hypo- or areflexia, and sensory loss. The CSF examination reveals a moderate elevation of protein levels without pleocytosis. However, in approximately 10% of patients the CSF protein levels may be normal. Results of sural nerve biopsy typically reveal inflammation, active and chronic demyelination, and some elements of axon loss. However, in some series almost 25% of patients may have an essentially nor-

mal sural nerve biopsy. Possibly the most valuable diagnostic aid in evaluating a patient for CIDP is the electrodiagnostic examination. Because CIDP represents an acquired demyelinating neuropathy, nerve conduction studies usually show typical features of segmental demyelination such as slowing of nerve conduction velocity, dispersion of responses, prolongation of distal latencies, and conduction block. These changes may be generalized but are usually distributed in a somewhat focal and asymmetrical fashion, which distinguishes CIDP from the chronic hereditary forms of demyelinating polyneuropathy.

CIDP is regarded as an idiopathic immune-mediated polyneuropathy. However, there are disorders essentially indistinguishable from CIDP that are the product of underlying medical disorders. CIDP-like neuropathies may be the product of multiple myeloma, osteosclerotic myeloma (POEMS syndrome: polyneuropathy, organomegaly, endocrinopathy, M protein, skin changes) and monoclonal gammopathy of uncertain significance (MGUS). Thus, in all patients with suspected CIDP it is important to search for an M protein in the serum and urine with serum and urine protein immunoelectrophoresis. Because some patients with osteosclerotic myeloma do not have an associated M protein, it is important to perform skeletal surveys to rule out the possibility of an osteosclerotic lesion. A CIDP-like polyneuropathy may also occur in the setting of HIV infection.

The treatment of CIDP must be individualized for each patient, keeping in mind the patient's clinical symptoms and the risks and potential benefits of the therapies. Clearly, patients with minimal symptoms may not require any treatment. However, in patients with a significant deficit and a progressive course, therapy is essential. For ambulatory patients with relatively mild to moderate clinical deficits, corticosteroid therapy may be initiated with prednisone (Deltasone) at a dose of 60 mg orally per day until a clinical response occurs and the patient plateaus. This usually occurs within 3 months of treatment. Once a clinical plateau is achieved, the prednisone therapy may be tapered slowly, usually by no more than 2.5 to 5 mg per week. Before a potentially chronic course of corticosteroid therapy is begun it is essential that patients have a purified protein derivative (tuberculin) (PPD) skin test to exclude the possibility of an occult tuberculosis infection. Furthermore, calcium supplementation, using approximately 1 gram of calcium orally per day as well as vitamin D supplementation of 50,000 U orally twice weekly is often recommended to prevent osteoporosis. During high-dose steroid therapy, the use of a histamine receptor blocking drug such as ranitidine (Zantac)* 150 mg orally at bedtime may be helpful in preventing steroid-associated peptic ulcer disease.

For patients with more substantial clinical weakness, especially those patients who are nonambulatory, treatment should begin with plasmapheresis. Plasmapheresis is usually administered twice weekly

---

*Not FDA-approved for this indication.

for 3 weeks then once weekly for 3 additional treatments. Guidelines for plasmapheresis are similar to those for GBS. Most patients, if not all, show some clinical improvement with plasmapheresis. However, most relapse once the therapy is discontinued. If a patient responds to plasmapheresis and does not require an additional treatment for 6 weeks or longer, management may consist of infrequent periodic plasmapheresis treatments. Most patients require the addition of corticosteroid treatment to maintain their response and avoid frequent plasmapheresis therapies. In this circumstance, prednisone is used as outlined above.

Evidence is mounting that IVIG* is efficacious in the treatment of CIDP and that it represents a compelling alternative to the more traditional approach of corticosteroids and plasmapheresis. IVIG may be administered intravenously at 400 mg per kg per day for 5 consecutive days. IVIG may then be repeated at intervals required to maintain clinical improvement. A "taper" of IVIG is accomplished by reducing the total dosage rather than increasing the interval between dosing. Similar guidelines for IVIG treatment are adhered to as indicated in the discussion regarding IVIG therapy of GBS. Specifically, patients should be screened for IgA deficiency, as IVIG may produce anaphylactic reactions in patients with low IgA levels. Furthermore, acute renal failure may occur during the course of IVIG treatment, particularly in patients with pre-existing renal disease. IVIG appears to have a distinct advantage over corticosteroids and plasmapheresis in that the clinical response appears sooner and subsequent IVIG treatments may be performed at longer intervals than plasmapheresis treatments.

Prognosis for patients with CIDP is generally favorable in that over two-thirds of patients have a good functional recovery and remain ambulatory and able to work despite mild persistent deficits. Ultimately, however, the prognosis is the product of the chronicity of the neuropathy and the presence of axonal degeneration versus segmental demyelination. Patients with rather severe axon loss are not likely to show dramatic or significant improvement in their deficits although progression of the neuropathy is halted and slow, modest recovery may ensue. Patients with predominantly demyelinating changes and significant conduction block may show rather dramatic and rapid improvement in their clinical deficits.

Diabetic Neuropathies

Diabetes can produce a wide range of peripheral nerve disorders (Table 2). The most common of the diabetic neuropathies is the generalized sensorimotor polyneuropathy of diabetes (GSMP-DM). The presence and severity of the GSMP-DM is usually related to the duration and severity of the hyperglycemia. However, this form of diabetic neuropathy can occur

*Not FDA-approved for this indication.

TABLE 2. **Diabetic Neuropathies**

Generalized sensorimotor polyneuropathy
Autonomic neuropathy
Small fiber neuropathy
Polyradiculopathy
   Diabetic amyotrophy
   Thoracoabdominal neuropathy
Mononeuritis multiplex
Mononeuropathies—compression and entrapment
Cranial neuropathies

as a presenting symptom of occult diabetes, and occasionally significant sensorimotor abnormalities are encountered in patients with only mild degrees of hyperglycemia. Most patients with GSMP-DM are essentially asymptomatic or have only minimal sensory symptoms; however, mild to moderate motor weakness, including footdrop, can occur. Pain may also be a prominent symptom. This is discussed in the section dealing with small fiber neuropathies. Autonomic neuropathy is also a frequent accompaniment of GSMP-DM.

The clinical features of GSMP-DM are rather nonspecific, and thus the differential diagnosis includes a wide variety of sensorimotor polyneuropathies. One must keep in mind that the mere occurrence of a chronic sensorimotor polyneuropathy in a diabetic patient does not automatically indicate that the polyneuropathy is caused by the diabetes. A careful evaluation for other causes, especially more treatable causes of chronic sensorimotor polyneuropathy, should be undertaken before arriving at a diagnosis of GSMP-DM.

Traditionally, optimal glycemic control has been the foundation of the treatment of GSMP-DM. The results of the Diabetes Control and Complications Trial have confirmed the long-held belief that optimal and aggressive glycemic control can have a beneficial effect on the development and the progression of GSMP-DM.

Another important type of diabetic neuropathy is diabetic polyradiculopathy. This is a term that is applied to a number of diabetic neuropathy syndromes, the most common of which is diabetic amyotrophy syndrome. In this syndrome, patients typically develop unilateral proximal thigh pain and weakness in the L2–3 myotomes. The disorder generally occurs in patients over the age of 65 years, many of whom have relatively mild diabetes of short duration. The pain usually subsides after several weeks, although in some patients it may last for several months. The weakness, however, typically persists for many months. There is often a profound weight loss, sometimes approaching 10% of body weight or greater. The disorder is self-limited, with spontaneous improvement generally within 1 year of onset. In some patients the disorder is bilateral but not simultaneous. Less commonly, a painless syndrome of bilateral and symmetrical lumbar radiculopathy involving the L2–3 myotomes may occur. A syndrome involving one or more of the lower thoracic roots, typically causing severe pain over the abdomen, has been referred to as "thoracoabdominal neuropathy of diabetes." Less commonly, the cervical roots may be affected by a similar process. It is important to exclude disorders of the spine before diagnosing diabetic polyradiculopathy. Treatment consists of aggressive physical therapy as well as measures to control pain (see the discussion in the small fiber neuropathy section).

Diabetic mononeuropathies may occur because of the increased susceptibility of nerves to compression or entrapment at common sites such as the median nerve at the wrist (carpal tunnel syndrome), the ulnar nerve at the elbow, the peroneal nerve at the fibular head, the lateral femoral cutaneous nerve at the inguinal ligament (meralgia paresthetica), and the radial nerve at the spiral groove (Saturday night palsy). A syndrome of mononeuritis multiplex may occur in diabetic patients, presumably on the basis of acute ischemic mechanisms. This must be differentiated from vasculitic mononeuropathies. Management of mononeuropathies is the same as for patients who are nondiabetic and is discussed in the section on mononeuropathies and nerve entrapments.

Isolated cranial neuropathies affecting the third, sixth, and occasionally the fourth cranial nerves appear to occur with increased frequency in patients with diabetes. These are typically self-limited disorders of presumed vascular cause. The most common cranial neuropathy is the oculomotor or third-nerve neuropathy of diabetes. This typically affects patients over the age of 50 years and develops in an abrupt fashion with pain. The clinical examination discloses evidence of oculomotor palsy with sparing of pupillary fibers. Pupillary sparing has been attributed to ischemia occurring in the central zone of the third nerve, sparing the peripherally located parasympathetic pupilloconstrictor fibers. The differential diagnosis includes mass lesions causing third-nerve compression including aneurysms of the posterior communicating artery. The evaluation of patients with diabetic oculomotor neuropathy usually requires brain imaging and occasionally lumbar puncture and angiography. Prognosis is good and no specific intervention is necessary. Prisms may be needed in those patients with residual diplopia.

Alcoholic and Nutritional Polyneuropathies

A generalized, predominantly sensory polyneuropathy is a common complication of chronic alcoholism. Although there is some evidence that alcohol may act as a toxin on peripheral nerves, the preponderance of evidence suggests that the associated nutritional deficiency that occurs in chronic alcoholism is the principal mechanism of nerve injury in alcoholic polyneuropathy. It is generally accepted that alcoholic or nutritional polyneuropathy is caused by a deficiency of various B vitamins. Most patients have a history of poor nutrition with significant weight loss before the onset of their symptoms. Pain and other sensory symptoms are the typical clinical features, but severe and sometimes rapidly evolving motor weakness can occur. Diagnosis depends on the recognition of alcoholism and poor nutrition as potential etiologic factors and the exclusion of other causes. Treatment consists of the institution of proper nutrition. Vitamin supplements, particularly with multiple B-complex vitamins, may be effective.

A sensory and sometimes painful polyneuropathy can result from vitamin B_6 deficiency, often encountered in patients treated with isoniazid or hydralazine. Daily supplemental vitamin B_6 at doses of 50 mg orally prevents further progression of the polyneuropathy.

Vitamin B_{12} deficiency typically produces the syndrome of subacute combined degeneration of the spinal cord. The paresthesias typically encountered in this disorder are believed to be due to spinal cord disease, although peripheral neuropathy is believed to occur as well. Vitamin B_{12} deficiency most often occurs as a result of pernicious anemia but can occur after gastrectomy, as a result of blind loop syndrome, or in the setting of severe dietary restrictions, particularly in strict vegetarians. Vitamin B_{12} 100 μg intramuscularly per day for 5 days per week for 2 weeks, then twice weekly for 4 weeks, and then once monthly thereafter, provides adequate replacement treatment for vitamin B_{12} deficiency. The institution of vitamin B_{12} treatment prevents further progression of the spinal cord syndrome and neuropathy, but symptoms that were present for 3 months or longer are likely to persist despite treatment. Rarely, vitamin E deficiency may be a product of malabsorption and produce a spinocerebellar degeneration along with a neuropathy involving the dorsal root ganglia. Vitamin E deficiency can be confirmed by a low serum level. Patients respond to vitamin E supplementation, usually initiated with large oral doses of 1 to 4 grams per day.

Uremic Polyneuropathy

It is estimated that approximately 60% of patients with chronic renal failure before the initiation of dialysis have some clinical or laboratory features of underlying sensorimotor polyneuropathy. The incidence and severity of uremic polyneuropathy appear to be related to the severity and duration of the chronic renal failure. Uremic polyneuropathy is predominantly a sensory polyneuropathy, although prominent motor involvement, sometimes with rapid evolution, may occur. This typically occurs in the setting of sepsis and other acute illness. Uremic neuropathy responds to hemodialysis or chronic peritoneal dialysis but may progress slightly despite treatment. A more dramatic response is often achieved after successful renal transplantation.

Paraneoplastic Neuropathies

A variety of sensorimotor polyneuropathies have been attributed to the remote effects of malignancy. These are typically chronic or subacute disorders that may precede or follow detection of the underlying malignancy. Diagnosis is established by excluding other causes of polyneuropathy and documenting the presence of the malignancy. Although treatment of the malignancy may result in improvement in the neuropathy in most patients, in some the neuropathy may progress or worsen despite adequate treatment. A pure sensory neuropathy syndrome may also result as a consequence of malignancy, typically in small cell cancer of the lung. This disorder is characterized by pure sensory loss beginning asymmetrically in the upper extremities and then involving the lower extremities. Sensory ataxia may be prominent. This neuropathy is often associated with anti-Hu autoantibodies. There is little tendency for this type of neuropathy to respond to treatment of the underlying tumor.

Myeloma and Dysproteinemias

A variety of peripheral nerve disorders may be seen in patients with myeloma and dysproteinemias. Polyneuropathy is a rare complication of multiple myeloma. It may present as a nonspecific generalized sensorimotor deficit with axon loss or occasionally segmental demyelinating features on electrodiagnostic testing. Treatment of the multiple myeloma typically does not result in improvement in the polyneuropathy. Polyneuropathy is a cardinal feature of the POEMS syndrome associated with osteosclerotic myeloma. This polyneuropathy may resemble that of CIDP. A skeletal survey will disclose evidence of one or more osteosclerotic lesions. The polyneuropathy typically responds to radiation treatment of the osteosclerotic lesions, but patients with more widespread lesions may require chemotherapy, usually consisting of melphalan (Alkeran) and prednisone (Deltasone). Polyneuropathy is not an uncommon complication of MGUS. These polyneuropathies may be axon loss in type but may also resemble CIDP. Before attributing a polyneuropathy to MGUS, it is critical that other disorders such as multiple myeloma, osteosclerotic myeloma, lymphoma, and amyloidosis have been excluded. If the polyneuropathy associated with MGUS is clinically significant, treatment may be initiated using the same guidelines as for CIDP. There is some evidence that plasma-exchange therapy is less effective for polyneuropathy associated with an IgM M protein than for that associated with IgG and IgA M proteins.

Drugs and Toxins

A wide variety of drugs (Table 3) and industrial toxins (Table 4) can cause polyneuropathies. The most important components of therapy are to identify the offending agent, to exclude other causes of polyneuropathy, and to eliminate exposure to the drug or toxin.

Amyloidosis

A variety of amyloid disorders including primary systemic amyloidosis as well as secondary amy-

TABLE 3. **Drug-Induced Polyneuropathies**

Drug	Clinical Features
I. Antibiotics	
Chloramphenicol (Chloromycetin)	Sensory, optic neuropathy
Isoniazid (INH)	Sensory, vitamin B_6 deficiency
Metronidazole (Flagyl)	Sensory
Nitrofurantoin (Macrodantin)	Sensorimotor, subacute
Suramin	Sensorimotor
2′,3′-Dideoxyinosine (didanosine)	Sensory
2′,3′-Dideoxycytidine (zalcitabine)	Sensory
2′,3′-Didehydro-3′-deoxythymidine (stavudine)	Sensory
II. Cardiovascular	
Amiodarone (Cordarone)	Sensorimotor, optic neuropathy
Hydralazine (Apresoline)	Sensory, vitamin B_6 deficiency
Perhexiline	Sensorimotor, papilledema
III. Rheumatologic	
Chloroquine (Aralen)	Sensory, myopathy
Colchicine	Sensory, myopathy
Gold (Myochrysine)	Sensorimotor
IV. Chemotherapeutic	
Cisplatin (Platinol)	Sensorimotor, ototoxicity
Cytarabine (Cytosar-U)	Sensory
Procarbazine (Matulane)	Sensorimotor
Vinblastine (Velban)	Sensorimotor
Vincristine (Oncovin)	Sensorimotor
Paclitaxel (Taxol)	Sensorimotor
V. Miscellaneous	
Almitrine	Sensory
Dapsone	Motor
Disulfiram (Antabuse)	Sensory
Phenytoin (Dilantin)	Sensorimotor
Pyridoxine (vitamin B_6)	Sensory, ataxia

TABLE 4. **Polyneuropathies Caused by Industrial Toxins**

Toxin	Industry	Clinical Features
Acrylamide	Flocculators, grouting agents	Sensorimotor, ataxia
Allyl chloride	Resin, pesticides	Sensory
Carbon disulfide	Rayon, cellophane	Sensorimotor
Dimethylaminopropionitrile	Polyurethane	Sensory, sacral dermatomes, urologic dysfunction
Ethylene oxide	Gas sterilization	Sensorimotor, ataxia
Hexacarbons	Solvents	Sensorimotor, coasting
Methylbromide	Fumigant, refrigerant, insecticide, fire extinguisher	Sensorimotor
Organophosphorus esters	Insecticides, plastics, petroleum additives	Sensorimotor, cholinergic symptoms
Trichloroethylene	Dry cleaning, degreaser, rubber	Cranial neuropathies

Data from Schaumburg HH, Berger AR: Human toxic neuropathy due to industrial agents. *In* Dyck PJ, Thomas PK, Griffin JW, et al (eds): Peripheral Neuropathy. Philadelphia, WB Saunders Co, 1993, pp 1533–1548.

loidosis and familial amyloidosis can produce amyloid neuropathy. Amyloid neuropathy is typically a generalized sensorimotor polyneuropathy with prominent or early sensory symptoms, sometimes conforming to a small fiber neuropathy syndrome. In addition, amyloid neuropathy typically involves the autonomic nervous system. Prognosis, however, is usually dictated by cardiac and renal involvement. There is no satisfactory primary therapy for amyloidosis.

Endocrine Neuropathies

A mild predominantly sensory polyneuropathy often associated with carpal tunnel syndrome may be encountered in patients with hypothyroidism and acromegaly. Treatment of these endocrine polyneuropathies consists of correcting the endocrine disturbance.

Infectious Polyneuropathies

Lyme disease, a disorder caused by the tick-transmitted spirochete *Borrelia burgdorferi,* can affect various components of the peripheral nervous system. Typically, Lyme disease causes a painful polyradiculitis; individual mononeuritis or mononeuritis multiplex syndrome; cranial neuritis; or generalized polyneuritis, often in the setting of a lymphocytic meningitis or meningoencephalitis. These neurologic syndromes typically follow an annular erythematous skin lesion, erythema migrans, which occurs within a few days to up to 1 month after the tick bite and may last for approximately 1 month. During this early stage of the illness, generalized systemic symptoms of malaise, fever, and adenopathy may occur. In stages 2 and 3, the peripheral and central nervous systems may be affected. Diagnosis of Lyme disease peripheral neuropathy syndromes can be made with a history of erythema migrans; serum and CSF immunoreactivity against *B. burgdorferi;* other organ involvement typical of Lyme disease; and seroconversion or a fourfold rise in titer of antibody between acute and convalescent sera. There are a variety of

options for the treatment of peripheral nervous system involvement in Lyme disease including treatment with penicillin G 20 to 24 million U intravenously per day for 10 to 14 days or ceftriaxone (Rocephin) 50 to 80 mg per kg per day intravenously for 2 to 4 weeks. Other regimens using cefotaxime (Claforan) and doxycycline (Vibramycin) have also been described.

Various peripheral nerve syndromes have been described in the context of HIV infection including syndromes indistinguishable from GBS and CIDP. Therapeutic approaches are similar to those for patients with GBS and CIDP without HIV infection. Generalized sensorimotor polyneuropathy or a predominately sensory polyneuropathy may also occur with HIV infection. Treatment for these more chronic generalized polyneuropathies is symptomatic. Cytomegalovirus (CMV) can produce an acute polyradiculoneuropathy in HIV patients that typically begins as a rapidly progressive cauda equina syndrome that can eventually spread to involve the upper extremity and occasionally cranial nerves. The CSF shows a pleocytosis with elevated protein and low sugar levels. CMV may be cultured from the blood, urine, or CSF. Recognition of this particular syndrome is important as patients may be treated with ganciclovir (Cytovene), which may stabilize the process and be associated with modest improvement.

Sarcoid Neuropathy

Sarcoidosis is a systemic disease that can produce a variety of peripheral nerve syndromes, including cranial mononeuropathies, multiple mononeuropathies, radiculopathy, GBS-like syndrome, and chronic sensorimotor polyneuropathy. Treatment is directed at the underlying systemic disease and typically involves corticosteroids. GBS-like syndrome may be treated according to guidelines for idiopathic GBS.

Vasculitic Neuropathies

There are a variety of disorders associated with vasculitis that may affect peripheral nerves. Many of these disorders, including polyarteritis nodosa, Churg-Strauss syndrome, Wegener's granulomatosis, giant cell arteritis, systemic lupus erythematosus, and rheumatoid arthritis, may produce a mononeuritis multiplex syndrome or occasionally a distal sensorimotor polyneuropathy. Peripheral neuropathies associated with Sjögren's syndrome may include a distal sensorimotor polyneuropathy, a trigeminal sensory neuropathy, or a pure sensory neuronopathy syndrome. Scleroderma may produce a trigeminal neuropathy or, very rarely, a sensorimotor polyneuropathy. The treatment of neuropathies associated with these disorders is directed at the underlying disorder. In most cases, this includes corticosteroid therapy and/or cytotoxic drugs.

Heredofamilial Neuropathies

Most of the heredofamilial neuropathies produce a rather chronic syndrome of sensorimotor polyneuropathy. The most common of these is Charcot-Marie-Tooth disease. Treatment is symptomatic.

There are two hereditary neuropathies that require specific treatment. Refsum's disease is a rare, autosomal recessive disorder of lipid metabolism that is associated with the accumulation of phytanic acid in various tissues. Refsum's disease typically produces cardinal features of retinitis pigmentosa, peripheral neuropathy, and cerebellar ataxia. Treatment consists of dietary restriction of phytanic acid and periodic plasmapheresis treatments for very high serum phytanic acid levels.

Abetalipoproteinemia is a rare, autosomal recessive lipid disorder that produces a syndrome of spinocerebellar degeneration, retinitis pigmentosa, polyneuropathy, mental retardation, and acanthocytosis. Progression of the neuromuscular involvement can be prevented with vitamin E supplementation, 1 to 2 grams orally per day for infants and 5 to 10 grams orally per day for older children and adults.

Small Fiber Neuropathies or Painful Neuropathy

"Small fiber neuropathy" (SFN) is a term referring to generalized polyneuropathies in which small-diameter myelinated (A delta group) and unmyelinated (C group) fibers are affected exclusively or to a much greater extent than the larger-diameter myelinated fibers. These small fiber types subserve sensory modalities of thermal sensation and pain, as well as autonomic functions. Thus, SFN typically produces symptoms and signs of pain, numbness, tingling, and other unpleasant spontaneous sensations as well as autonomic dysfunction. Most SFNs are in fact not pure neuropathies affecting only small fibers but represent neuropathies with predominant involvement of small fibers. Also, many generalized sensorimotor polyneuropathies may begin as "SFNs" but later evolve into a process affecting both small and large fiber types.

The typical symptoms of SFN include spontaneous sensations of prickling, tingling, or burning. Severe pain is also a typical feature of SFN. The pain is sometimes described as jabbing and lancinating but may also be dull, aching, or burning. Typically, the pain is worse at night and frequently interferes with sleep. The natural history of most painful SFNs is that as the neuropathy progresses over time, the painful component subsides and is replaced by numbness. Clinical examination often discloses loss of pain and thermal sensation in a distal-to-proximal gradient. Vibratory and proprioceptive functions may be relatively preserved. Although widespread autonomic dysfunction is usually not typical early in the course of most SFNs, reduced sweating in the feet or vasomotor instability with cold, pale feet or red, warm feet may be observed.

A wide variety of disorders may produce SFN (Table 5). Clearly, the most common cause of SFN is diabetes mellitus. However, SFN may be the product of primary systemic amyloidosis; alcoholic or nutritional neuropathy; neuropathies due to drugs and toxins; primary biliary cirrhosis; hypothyroidism; and some rare heredofamilial disorders. Approximately 40 to 50% of patients with SFN do not have a diagnosable cause, and their conditions are thus termed "idiopathic." The evaluation of a patient with SFN includes a search for the diagnosable and treatable causes, especially diabetes, nutritional deficiency, drugs and toxins, and hypothyroidism. Electromyography (EMG) and nerve conduction studies may be normal in SFN as nerve conduction studies and EMG assess the function of large myelinated fibers. Quantitative sensory testing is valuable in the diagnosis of SFN by documenting selective or predominant small sensory fiber dysfunction (abnormal thermal sensation) with relatively preserved large fiber function (vibratory sensation).

The therapy of SFN is initially directed at the underlying diagnosable cause if indeed it is a treatable cause. For example, in diabetic SFN optimal glycemic control may improve or stabilize the poly-

TABLE 5. **Causes of Small Fiber Neuropathy**

Diabetes mellitus
Amyloidosis
    Primary systemic amyloidosis
    Familial amyloidosis Types I, II, III
Alcoholic or nutritional
Drugs or toxins
    Metronidazole (Flagyl)
    Cisplatin (Platinol)
    Isoniazid (INH)
    Disulfiram (Antabuse)
    Metals (gold, arsenic, thallium)
Primary biliary cirrhosis
Hypothyroidism
Heredofamilial
    Hereditary sensory autonomic neuropathy
      (HSAN) Types I, III, IV
    Tangier disease
    Fabry's disease
    Dominantly inherited burning foot neuropathy
Idiopathic

neuropathy. In patients with alcoholic or nutritional polyneuropathy, the institution of proper nutrition and abstinence from alcohol may be beneficial. In toxic or drug-induced SFN, recognizing the toxic cause and removing the patient from continuing exposure is the principal therapeutic intervention. Hypothyroidism associated with SFN is managed by thyroid replacement therapy.

Unfortunately, for most patients with SFN there is no specific therapy that can be addressed to the underlying cause. Thus, treatment is symptomatic and directed at the pain. It is important to educate patients with SFN that it is likely that their pain is self-limited and will gradually improve spontaneously over time, typically over 1 to 2 years. Although minor analgesics are often prescribed for painful SFN, they are usually of limited utility. Some patients find relief from the use of cold compresses or soaks or gentle massage of their feet with moisturizing creams.

Effective management of the painful component of SFN usually requires pharmacotherapy. Capsaicin cream (Zostrix 0.75%) may be helpful for some patients. Although initial applications often provoke increased burning pain, with persistent use this treatment-induced pain subsides. Most patients require several applications per day. This type of therapy may be most effective for patients in whom a relatively small area of the feet and toes is affected by the pain.

A variety of tricyclic antidepressant medications have demonstrated efficacy in the treatment of painful SFN, particularly for constant continuous pain. Amitriptyline (Elavil)* may be very effective, especially in patients with insomnia who require sedation for sleep. However, the anticholinergic side effects of amitriptyline may exaggerate underlying dysautonomia, especially constipation or bladder dysfunction. Amitriptyline may also aggravate orthostatic hypotension. It is usually prudent to begin amitriptyline therapy at very low doses as some patients demonstrate significant improvement with doses as small as 10 or 20 mg orally at bedtime. Increasing to more conventional antidepressant doses of 75 to 150 mg daily may be required. Desipramine (Norpramin)* is an excellent alternative for patients who cannot tolerate the anticholinergic side effects of amitriptyline or in those patients not requiring sedation for sleep. This is a much less sedating drug with a relatively low anticholinergic side-effect profile. It is particularly well tolerated, especially at the higher doses that might be needed to achieve optimal pain control. However, desipramine, like amitriptyline, can exacerbate orthostatic hypotension. Dosing is similar to that of amitriptyline.

Anticonvulsants, especially carbamazepine (Tegretol), have been successfully used for the treatment of painful SFN, particularly for intermittent jabbing or stabbing pain. Carbamazepine may be used in conventional anticonvulsant doses to achieve "thera-

peutic levels." Typically, carbamazepine therapy is initiated at a dose of 200 mg orally twice daily. After 7 to 10 days the serum level is assessed and the dosage is adjusted appropriately. Once adequate serum levels are achieved, a clinical response should be noted. Failure to respond after several weeks of treatment should prompt tapering and discontinuation of the medication.

Mexiletine (Mexitil)* is an oral antiarrhythmic agent, a lidocaine derivative, that has shown efficacy in the treatment of diabetic painful neuropathy. This drug must be used with caution as it has a pro-arrhythmic effect and may also produce side effects of gastrointestinal upset and tremors. Typically, mexiletine therapy is initiated at a dosage of 150 mg orally twice daily for several days and then increased to a dose of 10 mg per kg per day in divided doses.

The serotonin re-uptake inhibitor antidepressants, including fluoxetine (Prozac),* sertraline (Zoloft),* and paroxetine (Paxil),* have demonstrated some efficacy for improving pain in patients with painful polyneuropathy. However, it appears that these drugs improve pain by treating coexisting depressive reactions rather than providing a direct analgesic effect in nondepressed patients.

The use of narcotics is rarely indicated in the management of chronic painful polyneuropathy. Although the use of phenothiazines alone or in conjunction with tricyclic antidepressant drugs has been reported to be effective in the treatment of painful neuropathy, it is difficult to justify the potential side effect of tardive dyskinesia against the limited benefit of these drugs in the management of the painful neuropathy.

MONONEUROPATHY MULTIPLEX SYNDROME

A variety of disorders may produce the syndrome of multiple mononeuropathies. Most of these are related to systemic disorders, especially the vasculitides. Management is directed at the systemic disorder. A relatively uncommon and unique syndrome is that of multifocal motor neuropathy with conduction block (MMNCB). This is a syndrome of essentially pure motor weakness typically beginning in the upper extremities, often asymmetrically and with variable clinical progression. Electrodiagnostic studies document multifocal conduction block of peripheral nerves confined to motor fibers. Typically, the conduction block involves fibers at sites quite atypical for focal compression or entrapment. Some patients with this syndrome have responded to high-dose intravenous cyclophosphamide (Cytoxan)* given at a dosage of 3 grams per square meter of body surface administered in five divided doses over 8 days followed by an oral maintenance dose of 2 mg per kg per day. Clinical improvement may occur within 3 to 6 months after this therapy. More recently, IVIG therapy administered at a dosage of 400 mg per kg of body

---

*Not FDA-approved for this indication.

*Not FDA-approved for this indication.

weight daily for 5 consecutive days has also proved beneficial in these patients. Guidelines for the use of IVIG are discussed under the sections dealing with IVIG treatment for GBS and CIDP.

COMPRESSION AND ENTRAPMENT NEUROPATHIES

A variety of individual peripheral nerves may be damaged by external compression or entrapment at specific anatomic sites. The most common entrapment neuropathy is median nerve entrapment at the wrist beneath the transverse carpal ligament, the carpal tunnel syndrome. This typically produces symptoms of intermittent paresthesia in the hand, particularly with use and often at night, awakening the patient from sleep. Carpal tunnel syndrome is easily diagnosed on clinical grounds. The diagnosis can be confirmed and the degree of compression quantitated by electrodiagnostic studies. Except in severe carpal tunnel syndrome, management is usually initiated with conservative measures such as anti-inflammatory medications, wrist splints, and modification of activities that may have precipitated the entrapment. For patients who do not respond to conservative measures and for those patients with progressive severe entrapment, referral to a surgeon for carpal tunnel release is usually indicated. The ulnar nerve is vulnerable to external compression at the elbow as it passes across the medial epicondyle. It can also be damaged via an entrapment mechanism in the cubital tunnel. Patients typically present with paresthesia or sensory loss in the ulnar nerve distribution. Weakness of ulnar intrinsic hand muscles may occur with more advanced neuropathies. Conservative measures including the use of elbow pads and nonsteroidal anti-inflammatory medications may be helpful. The indication for ulnar nerve transposition surgery is somewhat controversial; however, surgery should be considered in patients with progressive ulnar neuropathy referable to compression or entrapment at the elbow segment. Radial neuropathy at the spiral groove, "Saturday night palsy," is usually the result of acute compression. Typically, this produces wrist- and finger-drop, which may be managed conservatively with the use of wrist and finger splints to prevent stretching of the extensor tendons. Spontaneous improvement is usually the rule. Peroneal neuropathy caused by compression at the fibular head is most common in leg crossers and produces a clinical deficit of footdrop. Management is aimed at preventing further injury by avoidance of leg crossing. Conservative measures including physical therapy and the use of an ankle-foot orthosis (AFO) may be helpful. Prognosis is variable depending on the severity of the nerve compression. The lateral femoral cutaneous nerve of the thigh is vulnerable to entrapment beneath the inguinal ligament (meralgia paresthetica). Patients present with pain, numbness, and paresthesia over the anterolateral thigh. This entrapment neuropathy is often associated with weight gain. Most patients can be managed conservatively with nonsteroidal anti-inflammatory medication and weight reduction if appropriate. Rarely, nerve blocks or surgical therapy will be required.

ACUTE HEAD INJURIES IN ADULTS

method of
PATTI L. PETERSON, M.D.,
DANIEL B. MICHAEL, M.D., Ph.D., and
J. PAUL MUIZELAAR, M.D., Ph.D.
Detroit Neurotrauma Institute
Detroit, Michigan

Acute trauma remains the leading cause of morbidity and mortality for those under the age of 44 years. It is estimated that 7 million people per year sustain head injuries, and of these, half a million are hospitalized. The annual cost, in both direct and indirect costs to society, is believed to be in excess of $83.5 billion. The great majority of traumatic brain injuries (approximately 80%) are mild; the remainder (moderate and severe injuries) are associated with significant mortality (5% and 25%, respectively) and long-term morbidity. Nearly 100,000 patients per year are left with permanent disabilities, and 1 million per year suffer sequelae of their head injuries, including headache, cognitive impairment, and behavioral changes.

The majority of head-injured patients are in the 15 to 29- and 65 to 75-year age ranges, and males are injured two to three times as frequently as females. The most common mechanism of injury is transport related (motor vehicle, motorcycle, pedestrian). The incidence of falls and interpersonal violence varies, depending on the area of the country and season of the year. Over half of those admitted to the hospital with head injury have alcohol in the bloodstream, and other illegal substances (cannabinoids, cocaine, etc.) are frequently found.

PATHOPHYSIOLOGY OF HEAD INJURY

Only recently has it been appreciated that traumatic brain injury is a progressive disorder consisting of two components: primary and secondary injury. The initial, immediate structural damage that occurs is referred to as primary injury; secondary injury results from progressive cellular damage due to the brain's response to the injury. The recognition that traumatic brain injury is a progressive disorder was a critical concept in therapeutic research. The possibility that pharmacotherapy could lessen the extent of secondary injury has led to a number of phase III clinical trials of various drug therapies. Currently, these include an oxygen radical scavenger, polyethylene glycol-superoxide dismutase (PEG–SOD) (Dismutec)* a lipid peroxidation inhibitor, tirilazad mesylate (Freedox)* and the NMDA antagonist CGS-19755 (Selfotel).*

ASSESSMENT OF HEAD INJURY

Head injury can be classified by several methods, including the neurologic examination, neuroimaging, and mechanism of injury. In classic cerebral concussion, there is a

---

*Investigational drug in the United States.

TABLE 1. **Glasgow Coma Scale**

Test	Score
Eye opening	
Spontaneously	4
To verbal command	3
To pain	2
No response	1
Best motor response	
To verbal command	6
Localizes pain	5
Flexion—withdrawal	4
Flexion—abnormal	3
Extension	2
No response	1
Best verbal response	
Oriented and converses	5
Disoriented and converses	4
Inappropriate words	3
Incomprehensible words	2
No response	1
Total score	3–15

transient loss of consciousness associated with fleeting systemic changes, including bradycardia, hypertension, and apnea. The length of post-traumatic amnesia is a good measure of severity of injury. The neurologic examination provides the basis for the Glasgow Coma Scale (GCS), which is a simple, objective means of classifying head injuries as mild (GCS 13 to 15), moderate (GCS 9 to 12), or severe (GCS 3 to 8) (Table 1). The GCS is an objective measure and should be serially repeated in order to identify patients, early in the clinical course, who are deteriorating. Neuroimaging, including skull films and computed tomography (CT) of the brain, can also be used to classify head-injured patients (Table 2) and provides critical information necessary for patient management. Last, the mechanism of injury is an additional means of classifying head-injured patients and bears some prognostic significance. Patients who are victims of motor vehicle accidents and those who sustain penetrating head injuries tend to suffer more severe injuries and require longer periods of hospitalization.

EMERGENCY DEPARTMENT MANAGEMENT

Mild Head Injury

Those patients who do not experience a loss of consciousness or post-traumatic amnesia and have no risk factors for intracranial injury (Table 3) may not require a CT of the brain. Post-traumatic headaches are usually vascular in nature and respond to

TABLE 2. **Neuroimaging of Head Injury**

Skull films
    Skull fracture
Computed tomography of the brain
    Diffuse axonal injury
    Subarachnoid hemorrhage
    Contusion
    Intraparenchymal hemorrhage
    Epidural hematoma
    Subdural hematoma

TABLE 3. **Risk Factors for Intracranial Injury**

Focal neurologic signs on clinical examination
Advanced age
Unreliable clinical examination (e.g., if patient is intoxicated)
Increasing headache, nausea, and vomiting
Clotting disorders or anticoagulant use

oral ibuprofen (Motrin) 400 to 800 mg every 6 hours. These patients can be followed as outpatients on an as-needed basis. Patients with mild head injuries (GCS 13 to 15) who have unremarkable CTs of the brain, no evidence of skull fracture, and no risk factors for intracranial injury may be discharged (ideally to a responsible friend or family member) after a short (3 to 6-hour) period of observation and followed as outpatients. Patients with persistent vomiting usually require a short inpatient stay.

Moderate and Severe Head Injury

When a moderately or severely head-injured patient arrives in the emergency department, the immediate concern should be to correct and prevent those conditions known to exacerbate secondary brain injury (e.g., hypoxia and hypotension). The initial examination is performed and, in a patient with multiple trauma, a priority for assessment and management of all injuries should be established. The ABCs of emergency management are imperative: airway establishment, with the neck and head maintained in a neutral position; breathing—adequate ventilation; and circulation—appropriate fluid resuscitation. The patient should be placed in a cervical collar (if one is not already in place) until a lateral cervical spine film to T1 is obtained, as 2% of comatose patients have significant associated spinal injuries.

Intravenous access and an intra-arterial line for monitoring capability should be established and fluid resuscitation accomplished. The goal of fluid resuscitation is to maintain a minimum systolic blood pressure of 90 mmHg. Isotonic saline is recommended. Packed red blood cells may be given if hypovolemic shock is present. The presence of shock should not be indiscriminately attributed to the head injury. The role of hypertonic saline and colloids in cerebral resuscitation requires further investigation. Appropriate laboratory studies should be performed, including a screen for drugs of abuse. If the patient's blood alcohol level is less than 200 mg per dL, the alcohol should not be assumed to be the cause of the compromised level of consciousness. In a severely injured patient, nasotracheal intubation may be considered unless there are significant facial fractures. The patient should be oxygenated with 100% O_2 until a blood gas analysis confirms adequate oxygenation (minimum P_{O_2} 80 torr). Hyperventilation should not be indiscriminately used in the emergency department management of head-injured patients.

A Foley catheter and nasogastric tube should be

inserted. A 1 gram per kg bolus of mannitol should be administered if the neurologic status of the patient is deteriorating; if not, a lower dosage (0.5 gram per kg) may be given. Intravenous cefazolin (Ancef) is given to patients with open head wounds. Anticonvulsant therapy (intravenous phenytoin [Dilantin] 20 mg per kg) should be administered to all patients with active seizures and those with a GCS of 8 or less. The head of the bed can be elevated 20 degrees with the patient's head maintained in a neutral position to facilitate cerebral venous return. Serial GCS and evaluation of the pupils should be performed. A CT of the brain should be obtained as soon as possible.

INDICATIONS FOR OPERATIVE INTERVENTION

After the patient has been resuscitated in the emergency department and a CT of the brain has been obtained, clinical judgment will indicate whether the patient is directed to the operating room or the intensive care unit. If a neurosurgeon is not available and emergency cerebral decompression is imperative (e.g., in the case of an epidural hematoma), any appropriately trained surgeon can perform a craniotomy or burr holes. A neurosurgeon should be involved in the patient's management as soon as possible.

The indications for surgical intervention include placement of an intracranial monitoring device or removal of a surgically accessible lesion (e.g., subdural hematoma, epidural hematoma, large contusion). Once the decision to operate has been made, a rapid surgical decompression should be carried out. Intraoperative ultrasonography may be useful in identifying an intraparenchymal hematoma or falcial brain shift. Every effort should be made to close the dura and replace the bone flap.

INTENSIVE CARE UNIT MANAGEMENT

The goals of ICU management are to ensure optimal cerebral perfusion and oxygenation, avoid and treat conditions that exacerbate secondary brain injury, identify and promptly manage neurologic deterioration at an early stage, and adequately meet the patient's nutritional needs.

The provision of an adequate supply of glucose and oxygen to the brain is absolutely critical. It is important in head-injured patients to ensure a cerebral perfusion pressure (CPP) greater than 70 mmHg. CPP is defined as the mean arterial pressure (MAP) minus intracranial pressure (ICP). CPP falls if the MAP decreases or the ICP rises.

The normal ICP is 0 to 15 torr and requires treatment in a head-injured patient if it rises above 20 torr. ICP can be monitored with a ventriculostomy catheter (a catheter in the lateral ventricle), a Camino monitor (a fiberoptic probe usually placed in the cerebral parenchyma), or less commonly, a subarach-

noid bolt. Ideally, the monitoring device should be at the level of the head. A ventricular catheter has the advantage of monitoring and treating ICP by cerebrospinal fluid drainage.

The initial management in maximizing CPP is to treat increased ICP. Table 4 summarizes the sequential steps one can take to treat increased ICP. The head should be in a neutral position. The tracheostomy ties should not be fastened too tightly in order to facilitate venous return. Optimal head-body position is usually 30 degrees of elevation, although some patients may experience a decrease in CPP and benefit from a lesser degree of or no elevation of the head of the bed.

Sedation can be accomplished with reversible agents. The following drugs are recommended for the treatment of increased ICP: short-acting narcotics (intravenous morphine sulfate 0.05 to 0.1 mg per kg every 1 to 2 hours as needed), which can be reversed with a narcotic antagonist (intravenous naloxone [Narcan] 0.1 to 0.2 mg every 2 to 3 minutes); benzodiazepines (intravenous lorazepam [Ativan] 1 to 2 mg every 1 to 2 hours as needed), which can be reversed with intravenous flumazenil (Romazicon) 0.2 mg repeated every 30 to 60 seconds to a maximum dose of 3 mg; or intravenous propofol (Diprivan) 5 to 50 μg per kg per minute in 5-minute intervals, the effect of which can be reversed in 30 to 60 minutes by stopping the infusion. Since the patient is intubated and ventilated, there is no need to worry about respiratory depression.

If a ventricular catheter has been placed, cerebrospinal fluid can be intermittently or continuously drained. Nondepolarizing neuromuscular blocking agents (intravenous pancuronium [Pavulon] or vecuronium [Norcuron] 0.1 mg per kg) can be used but are recognized to increase the incidence of pneumonia. Clinical judgment in each particular case will indicate whether paralysis is of potential benefit. Hyperosmolar agents such as mannitol can be used to treat increased ICP and increase cerebral blood flow (by decreasing blood viscosity). Repeated boluses of mannitol can be administered, but it is necessary to monitor the serum osmolality and ICP response to therapy. If the osmolality rises above 320 mOsm, mannitol should not be administered, as acute tubular necrosis and renal failure may occur. Although hyperventilation is effective in producing a rapid decrease in ICP, its routine use has become increasingly controversial. Hyperventilation is known to have a limited duration of efficacy (less than 24 hours) and

TABLE 4. **Treatment of Increased Intracranial Pressure**

Head-body positioning
Sedation
Ventricular drainage
Paralysis
Mannitol
Hyperventilation
Artificial coma

can result in and exacerbate cerebral ischemia and deleteriously affect outcome. Hyperventilation should not be routinely used in ICU management of increased ICP. If it is used, its efficacy should be measured by the response of ICP and cerebral oxygenation monitoring.

When all else fails, artificial coma can be induced to decrease cerebral metabolic demands. This can be accomplished with intravenous pentobarbital 5 to 10 mg per kg per hour as needed to maintain the plasma level between 3 and 5 mg per dL or the patient in electrical burst suppression. Although the outcome at this stage of therapy is usually poor, some individuals make a remarkable recovery.

Jugular bulb oximetric catheter monitoring to determine the cerebral arteriovenous difference of oxygen (AVDo$_2$) can be used to guide patient management. AVDo$_2$ measures provide a rapid means of assessing the effectiveness of therapeutic measures and identifying compromised cerebral metabolism. Episodes of desaturation are strongly correlated with poor neurologic outcome.

An additional means of improving CPP is to increase MAP. Hemodynamic monitoring with a Swan-Ganz catheter is helpful. MAP can be increased by appropriate fluid resuscitation and use of colloids (albumin). A Starling curve (pulmonary capillary wedge pressure vs. cardiac output) can optimize cardiac response to fluid therapy for each individual patient. The addition of vasopressors (e.g., dopamine) may be necessary.

The metabolic requirements of a patient with a severe head injury are comparable to those of a patient with a 30% burn. The goal of nutrition is to achieve a positive nitrogen balance with a respiratory quotient less than one and to maintain the blood glucose at less than 200 mg per dL. The enteral route is ideal, but a head-injured patient may initially be intolerant to such feedings. Although total parenteral nutrition (TPN) may transiently increase ICP, if no enteral route is available by day 2 or 3, TPN should be initiated. The patient is eventually converted to enteral feeding. The gastrointestinal tract should be protected with an H$_2$ blocker (ranitidine [Zantac], famotidine [Pepcid], antacids, and/or sucralfate [Carafate]). Intragastric pH monitoring is helpful.

COMPLICATIONS OF HEAD INJURY

Acute

Acute complications of head injury include seizure, delayed hemorrhage, cerebrospinal fistula, infection, hyponatremia, and neuroendocrine disorders. Seizures occurring at the time of impact in trivial or mild head injuries (impact seizures) typically do not require long-term anticonvulsant therapy, but early seizures should be treated. The duration of therapy is controversial. Prophylactic administration of anticonvulsants should be continually reassessed.

Delayed traumatic intracranial hemorrhages most notoriously develop in the frontal or temporal lobe in contused areas. Cerebrospinal fluid fistulas, both otorrhea and rhinorrhea, occur with fractures of the skull base and tear of the dura and arachnoid. The great majority respond to nonoperative management, including bed rest with elevation of the head of the bed and lumbar subarachnoid drainage. Meningitis is the most common infectious complication and occurs most often in patients with a skull fracture and dural tear. Prophylactic antibiotics have been shown to increase the incidence of infection with resistant organisms, making their use controversial. The choice of antibiotic therapy in meningitis depends on results of the Gram stain; if it is negative, empirical coverage should be based on the most likely infecting organism.

Hyponatremia after head injury is not uncommon and requires treatment only if the serum sodium concentration falls below 130 mEq per liter. In the majority of head-injured patients, hyponatremia is due to cerebral salt wasting. The syndrome of inappropriate antidiuretic hormone (SIADH) is also a recognized cause of hyponatremia. In SIADH, the extracellular fluid volume is high, and the patient is managed with fluid restriction. In cerebral salt wasting, extracellular fluid volume is low, and hypertonic saline is the treatment of choice. Half of the sodium deficit should be corrected over the first 24 hours in order to avoid the complications of a rapid rise of sodium concentration. In the majority of severely injured patients, diabetes insipidus is usually an ominous occurrence with grave prognostic significance.

Long Term

Long-term neurologic complications of head injury include post-traumatic epilepsy, postconcussion syndrome, and neurobehavioral disorders. Patients with penetrating injuries, depressed skull fractures, severe injuries, and early seizures are at risk for the development of post-traumatic epilepsy. Postconcussion syndrome occurs following mild head injury; it is characterized by cognitive and mood disorders and is of significant medicolegal concern.

Neurobehavioral sequelae occur after moderate and severe injuries and include memory and language dysfunction, attention and problem-solving deficits, and personality changes. Neurobehavioral changes have a tremendous impact on patients and their families.

OUTCOME

Outcome in acute head injury could be improved by a number of strategies, including a more aggressive emphasis on the prevention of injury. There should be greater efforts to educate those at greatest risk regarding the use of helmets for cyclists and seat belts and air bags for occupants of motor vehicles. Improvements in rehabilitation therapies have also improved long-term outcome. The greatest potential for significant improvement in outcome lies in a better understanding of the basic pathophysiology of head injury and the development of effective pharmacotherapy to lessen secondary injury.

ACUTE HEAD INJURIES IN CHILDREN

method of
ANN-CHRISTINE DUHAIME, M.D.
Children's Hospital of Philadelphia
Philadelphia, Pennsylvania

Head injury in children is the single greatest cause of mortality beyond the newborn period and is the single most common cause of acquired disability in the pediatric age group in the United States. Each year, at least 150,000 children suffer head injuries resulting in hospitalization or death, and approximately 10 times that number receive outpatient medical attention. At least 7000 children die, and nearly 30,000 suffer permanent neurologic sequelae annually. No matter how it is analyzed, the cost is enormous. This is particularly notable, since the majority of serious pediatric head injuries are preventable.

CLASSIFICATION OF PEDIATRIC HEAD INJURIES

Head injuries can be classified by severity and by injury type. Although the Glasgow Coma Scale (GCS) is widely used, it is applied with difficulty to preverbal or uncooperative children. Various modifications have been proposed, but to date, none has met widespread acceptance; thus, injuries are still largely classified as mild, moderate, or severe based on the best GCS score obtained after initial resuscitation. More than 80% of head injuries in children are mild, with the remainder nearly evenly divided between moderate and severe injuries.

There are clear correlations between mechanism of injury, injury severity, and injury type in children. The majority of head trauma, especially in young children, occurs from falls, and when this involves heights of 4 feet or less, serious injuries rarely occur. The exception is the occasional epidural hematoma in infancy; this can result from low-height falls in which contact forces applied through the thin skull tear the middle meningeal or other dural artery. Uncomplicated linear skull fractures can also occur from low-height falls in infants and young children but usually require greater forces in older children with thicker skulls. Falls greater than 4 feet may be associated with contusion, subarachnoid hemorrhage, epidural hemorrhage, and more complex skull fractures. Trauma caused by motor vehicle accidents involves significantly greater forces, including rotational deceleration, which may produce the contact injuries already mentioned along with subdural hematoma and diffuse axonal injury. The latter injury types are associated with major morbidity and mortality and account for the majority of severe head injuries. In infancy, these two injury types are produced most commonly in the setting of inflicted injury (the shaking-impact syndrome). In all children, the addition of significant hypoxia or ischemia worsens outcome.

EVALUATION OF A HEAD-INJURED CHILD

A careful history of the mechanism of injury from witnesses or emergency medical personnel is the first step in a guided evaluation of an injured child. How did the child fall? What did he or she hit? Was there crying? Seizure activity? What was the behavior afterward? What time did the injury occur? For more severely injured children, for example, those struck by automobiles, what was the speed of the car? What did the child do immediately after impact? Was apnea apparent? Was extensor posturing noted? Was there early activity or speech followed by deterioration? These questions begin to address both the severity and the type of injury that is likely to be present; the answers guide the aggressiveness of early treatment for complications such as mass lesions or brain swelling.

For the majority of children with minor injuries and mechanisms consistent with milder forces, the initial physical examination consists primarily of observation while the history is obtained. Young children will be most comfortable on the parent's lap. The level of spontaneous activity, symmetry of movement, and cervical mobility should be noted. Palpation of the fontanelle in infants and of the skull for cephalohematomas and fractures should be done, but repeated palpation of tender impact sites is redundant if radiologic evaluation is diagnostic. Ambulatory children should be observed walking, holding the parent's hand if necessary. Painful stimulation is rarely necessary in a child with a minor injury. Sleeping children are most effectively awakened by increasing ambient light, uncovering the child, and sitting the child up.

Children who have a decreased level of consciousness must be assessed for adequacy of airway, breathing, and circulation, with appropriate corrective measures instituted. Here too, however, the history is of great importance in predicting injury severity. For example, an unresponsive child ejected from a car who was posturing at the scene warrants intubation, whereas a child who had an impact seizure after a low-height fall or low-velocity impact who is breathing well spontaneously and is improving may be managed more conservatively. Extreme hyperventilation should be avoided; initial PCO_2 in the middle 30s is appropriate for most children. Circulating volume must be restored, especially since hemorrhage from fractures, visceral injuries, scalp lacerations, and cephalohematomas may be considerable. Volume replacement should be accomplished with fluid that is not hypotonic, as excess free water overload may exacerbate subsequent brain swelling. Marked hypothermia must be corrected, but core temperatures of 35° to 36° C may help protect the brain.

The neck should be immobilized in the field or on arrival at the hospital in any child with a decreased level of consciousness, a mechanism of injury consistent with a significant risk of spinal injury (e.g., significant fall, motor vehicle or sports injury), or complaints of transient or persistent neck pain, weakness, numbness, or other signs or symptoms of possible spinal cord injury. Because ligamentous injuries occur more commonly than bony injuries in children, the spine must be cleared on clinical grounds; "normal" plain spinal films are insufficient in a child who cannot be examined for pain or limitation of movement. Magnetic resonance imaging (MRI) may be useful in disclosing ligamentous hemorrhage or avulsion in some children.

Any child with possible intracranial pathology based on the history or physical findings should undergo a computed tomography (CT) scan (or in some instances, MRI). This is urgent in children who are unresponsive, have clinical signs of increased intracranial pressure, have lateralizing signs (e.g., hemiparesis or dilated pupils), or demonstrate a deteriorating level of consciousness. Skull films are most useful in infants who have sustained low-height falls and appear well clinically; the finding of a fracture may suggest sufficient focal force to warrant a CT scan, especially if the fracture crosses the territory of the middle meningeal artery or a venous sinus, or if the fracture is separated widely. Multiple or stellate fractures in infants point to a possible nonaccidental etiology for the injury.

SPECIFIC INJURIES: PRESENTATION, MANAGEMENT, AND OUTCOME

Concussion

Concussion is defined as a head injury accompanied by loss of consiousness or amnesia for the event. Functionally, the injury affects the brain diffusely, and experimental evidence suggests that some degree of rotational deceleration of the brain is required for a concussion to occur. By convention, the majority of concussive injuries involve unconsciousness lasting for minutes, but loss of consciousness may last up to 6 hours in more severe cases. Unconsciousness for longer than 6 hours is classified functionally as diffuse axonal injury or is related to a coexisting problem, such as hypoxic injury.

Concussion in children occurs most commonly in association with falls or other contact injuries. Although loss of consciousness results from movement of the brain within the skull, the specific contact forces involved in the injury determine whether surface trauma such as skull fractures or contusions also occur in a given patient. This explains why some quite impressive contact injuries, such as open depressed skull fractures or focal penetrating injuries, may occur with no loss of consciousness at all and thus may not be accompanied by postconcussive symptoms.

Many children with concussion sustain a brief loss of consciousness and then appear to recover promptly, with few sequelae. Others may develop symptoms immediately or within a few hours, including headache, nausea and vomiting, confusion, and sleepiness. A CT scan differentiates these children from those with mass lesions. In the vast majority of patients, symptoms resolve within a few days. Children whose symptoms do not resolve or whose symptoms progress require further evaluation, which may include repeat scanning for delayed hemorrhage or swelling. The latter is most often related to hyponatremia or ischemia. Electrolytes must be monitored carefully, since aggressive fluid administration coupled with trauma-related secretion of antidiuretic hormone may combine to predispose to symptomatic hyponatremia, particularly in children with multisystem trauma.

One striking phenomenon that is seen occasionally is postconcussive blindness. This occurs most often from falls against the back of the head. Young children may not be able to articulate their difficulty and present in the emergency room combative and terrified. A history of a fall on the occiput and a carefully tailored examination disclose that although mental status is preserved, the child cannot see. Postconcussive blindness nearly always resolves in 1 to 2 days after the injury with no long-term sequelae. A CT scan and ophthalmic examination differentiate these children from those with more serious problems.

Postconcussive seizures are more common in children than in adults, occurring in about 12% of patients. These have no implication for the later development of epilepsy. Treatment with anticonvulsants is usually not necessary unless the seizures recur or interfere with patient assessment. Anticonvulsants given in the first week after head injury have been shown to reduce the risk of seizures occurring during that time but have no impact on the development of late post-traumatic epilepsy, which is rare after uncomplicated concussion in children.

After the acute recovery from concussion, some children are moody and short-tempered and have difficulty with short-term memory and attention for weeks to as long as a few months after injury. Intermittent blurred vision, ringing in the ears, and dizziness may occur. Although such symptoms may interfere with activities and school performance and require some remedial help, the vast majority resolve within 3 months after the injury. Counseling parents that such symptoms are typical and nearly always resolve is helpful. Concussion does not appear to alter long-term neuropsychological outcome.

Contusion and Laceration

Contusions and lacerations reflect injury to the surface of the brain, usually related to direct contact forces. Neurologic symptoms depend on the function of the involved cortex. Thus, patients with anterior frontal contusions may have few symptoms, whereas those with injuries involving the motor strip or dominant temporal lobe may show weakness or aphasia. Treatment depends on the size and location of the lesion. Although most contusions can be managed nonoperatively, swelling often occurs around the lesion, and evacuation may be necessary to avoid dangerous compression of adjacent structures, particularly in contusions involving the medial temporal lobe. Contusions and lacerations resolve with time and leave a variable region of encephalomalacia and gliosis. Besides any deficit related to damage to eloquent cortex, the major long-term risk is seizures, which may occur years later, although the overall risk is probably less than 5%.

Skull Fracture and Cephalohematoma

Linear fractures of the calvarium occur from contact forces to the head and are of little direct consequence to the brain. However, they may be associated with late sequelae in at least two instances. The first is the so-called growing fracture of infancy. This occurs when the dura is torn at the time of trauma in an infant with a growing head. Presumably, arachnoid is trapped in the fracture and, rather than healing, the fracture enlarges over time; a pulsatile swelling can be felt at the site. This occurs most often in the setting of a fall greater than 4 feet in which the fracture is widely separated; an underlying contusion is often seen on CT scan where the fractured bone has indented the dura and bruised the underlying brain. Follow-up studies reveal an area of encephalomalacia with a cystic fluid collection extending through the fracture site. Treatment is surgical, with repair of the dural defect and cranioplasty with split-thickness autologous bone.

The second instance involves linear fractures of the posterior wall of the frontal sinus in older children, which may predispose to intracranial contamination and abscess formation. Management depends on the degree of disruption of the bone and sinus mucosa and ranges from observation to antibiotics to early surgery and sinus exenteration. A child with a history of recent trauma to this area who presents with headache and fever should undergo intracranial imaging.

Basilar fractures appear clinically as postauricular or periorbital ecchymosis (Battle's or raccoon sign) or with hemotympanum, otorrhea, or rhinorrhea. These fractures may also result in cranial nerve deficits related to disruption or compression. This occurs most commonly with temporal bone fractures in which hearing is impaired. Deficits in smell, visual acuity, extraocular motility, or facial nerve function may also occur with basilar skull fractures. About half of cranial nerve deficits improve spontaneously; in selected cases, cranial nerve decompression is warranted. Dural tears may predispose to meningitis, although most seal within a few days. Use of prophylactic antibiotics is controversial and may predispose to infection with resistant organisms. Persistent leaks are treated with cerebrospinal fluid diversion; occasionally, direct repair is needed.

Depressed fractures are treated surgically if they are open with significant contamination or if unacceptable skull deformity is present. Deficits result from contusion or laceration and depend on the specific region involved.

Cephalohematomas occur commonly at the site of direct impact or fracture. In infants, these can be large enough to result in shock. A common scenario involves an impact injury in which the scalp contour initially looks quite normal, but after a few days a sizable fluctuant collection is noted at the site. This occurs because the initially solid clot has liquefied; it does not represent new injury. The collection usually resolves gradually, although on rare occasions calcification occurs.

Epidural Hematoma

Arterial epidural hematomas result from contact forces that rupture a dural artery, producing a rapidly expanding mass lesion. The inciting injury may be quite minor, especially in infants. Because the primary brain injury is usually mild, patients classically present with a lucid interval followed by deterioration over minutes to hours. If untreated, epidural hematomas can be fatal; however, prompt evacuation

leads to an excellent outcome in the majority of children.

Venous epidural hematomas are commonly found as localized collections underlying a calvarial fracture. In this setting, they are usually small and most often resolve spontaneously. Venous collections resulting from tears of the dural venous sinuses, however, may be sizable and require evacuation, particularly when they involve the posterior fossa. As with arterial collections, delayed deterioration is the usual clinical picture, although the time course may be slower.

Subdural Hematoma

Unlike epidural hematomas, in which the primary injury to the brain itself is often minor, bleeding into the subdural space occurs from angular deceleration forces that also significantly injure the brain itself. The bleeding occurs when the bridging veins, which course from the brain surface to the dural venous sinuses, are torn due to displacement of the brain relative to the skull and adherent dura. This explains why the morbidity and mortality associated with subdural hemorrhage are so high.

Motor vehicle trauma, child abuse, and, less often, significant falls are the usual mechanisms of injury, and children typically become immediately unresponsive. Abnormal posturing and pupillary abnormalities may be seen.

Subdural hematomas are often associated with major brain swelling. Therapy is directed toward controlling increased intracranial pressure, maintaining perfusion, and affording brain protection. Prompt evacuation of significant clots with mass effect is indicated, but very small "smear" subdurals may be managed medically. Intracranial pressure monitoring and adjuncts such as ventricular drainage, osmotherapy, mild or moderate hyperventilation, barbiturates, mild hypothermia, and other neuroprotective strategies may be employed. In some children, areas of infarction become apparent, and this adds to the morbidity. As in other forms of severe head injury, the outcome can be predicted by the initial neurologic status, presence and duration of unresponsiveness, intracranial pressure course, and parenchymal changes seen on serial neuroimages.

Diffuse Axonal Injury

Like subdural hematomas, diffuse axonal injuries also occur from angular acceleration-deceleration and result from similar mechanisms. Patients are immediately unresponsive. Posturing and autonomic dysfunction are common. The diagnosis is made on clinical and radiographic grounds. The acute CT scan may appear normal or show scattered hemorrhages in the deep white matter. MRI provides improved resolution of visible lesions, which can also be found in the corpus callosum, cerebral peduncles, and brain stem. Diffuse axonal injury may coexist with other injury types, depending on the particular forces involved.

When diffuse axonal injury is uncomplicated by major contusions or hypoxia or ischemia, brain swelling is usually less problematic than in subdural hematoma. Nonetheless, intracranial pressure monitoring and careful attention to other physiologic parameters are warranted to maximize cerebral protection.

Recovery from diffuse axonal injury is fairly stereotyped in survivors. The deeper stages of coma give way to a more agitated state prior to the end of coma, which is marked by the resumption of the ability to reliably follow commands. At this stage, rehabilitation can switch from passive to active, and gains in children may be rapid. Long-term deficits include motor, cognitive, and behavioral problems, with memory, attention, and judgment particularly vulnerable. Unlike adults, children may continue to show improvement for 2 or 3 years after injury. However, severely injured children may remain in a persistent vegetative state or show permanent severe disability.

Gunshot Wound

Unfortunately, the incidence of gunshot wounds to the head in children has increased dramatically in the past decade. These injuries cause both focal and diffuse damage to the brain because of direct laceration and shock wave effects. Intracranial pressure is often extremely elevated. Acute management involves measures to control pressure and to decrease infectious complications and includes both medical and surgical interventions. Although there are many anecdotal examples of remarkable recoveries in children with gunshot wounds to the brain, few studies of long-term adult function in these children have been undertaken. Prevention is the best strategy for these morbid injuries.

Shaking-Impact Syndrome

Also known as the shaken baby syndrome, this phenomenon is the single most common cause of serious head injury in children under 2 years of age. Although the exact mechanism remains controversial, most authors agree that this syndrome is not caused by trivial trauma, shaking during play, or other commonly occurring infant activities. Rather, these injuries result from deliberate, severe inflicted trauma that requires extreme force and perhaps head impact.

Most often, infants present with a history of trivial trauma or no history of trauma at all, with symptoms ranging from lethargy and irritability to coma. Subdural and subarachnoid blood is found by CT scan or when a lumbar puncture for sepsis work-up reveals bloody fluid. Hemorrhage most commonly occurs as thin layers over the hemispheres and in the posterior interhemispheric fissure, but larger collections requiring surgical evacuation may also be seen. Retinal hemorrhages are common, and various fractures of the ribs, long-bone metaphyses, and skull may be found. Mortality in children who present in coma approaches 70%. Survivors may show remarkable parenchymal loss as areas of hemispheric hypodensity atrophy. Children with less severe injuries have variable outcomes.

PREVENTION

Although most childhood head injury is mild, because of the large numbers of children who are injured, the individual and public health burden of serious head injury is probably larger than any other single childhood health problem. Prevention is of utmost importance, and all health workers who care for children should advocate the use of auto restraints, bike helmets, and other safety measures to decrease the risk of serious head injury in their patients.

BRAIN TUMORS

method of
N. SCOTT LITOFSKY, M.D., and
LAWRENCE D. RECHT, M.D.
University of Massachusetts Medical Center
Worcester, Massachusetts

Brain tumors represent a heterogeneous group of neoplasms that has different presentations, prognoses, and treatments. Defining a single approach to these lesions can therefore be difficult. To facilitate decision making, we have noted that management issues for all brain tumor patients generally are classifiable into one of three possible categories: (1) symptoms arising from tumor or treatment effects on normal brain, (2) issues concerning correct diagnosis of the lesion, and (3) specific therapeutics of the particular brain tumors. The management of brain tumor symptoms spans the patient's entire clinical course; management decisions here are for the most part histology-independent, depending more on tumor location, the presence of mass effect, patient age, and the particular symptoms encountered. Decisions concerning making the proper diagnosis—specifically, when to operate and how much tumor to remove—are also for the most part histology-independent, being affected mainly by such issues as location and patient age. Only the specific therapy of brain tumor is crucially dependent on tumor histology.

We have found that dealing with brain tumors is much easier if treatment issues are first classified and dealt with. Such an approach facilitates management by non-neurooncologists, because most treatment decisions are related to symptoms and therefore are largely histology-independent. Furthermore, it emphasizes the importance of attending to patient symptoms, the effective treatment of which can markedly improve quality (and sometimes quantity) of life.

SYMPTOMATIC ISSUES
Seizures

Seizures are an important cause of morbidity in the brain tumor patient. In approximately 40% of patients with gliomas, seizure is the earliest manifestation of the disease, and 55% have had at least one spell by the time the tumor is diagnosed. Seizure frequency and pattern may vary as tumor size and pathology change. Status epilepticus is a frequent occurrence and may be a presenting symptom. In addition to the morbidities commonly associated with idiopathic epilepsy, seizures in tumor patients are particularly dangerous because of their propensity to increase intracranial pressure (ICP) in a patient with impaired compliance; this can result in sudden death due to cerebral herniation.

Although surgical resection can provide effective relief in patients with persistent refractory seizures secondary to infiltrative tumors in the temporal or frontal lobes, pharmacologic therapy remains the mainstay of treatment. Pharmacotherapy is unique for brain tumor patients in a number of aspects: (1) Brain tumor patients are frequently receiving other medications that may interact with anticonvulsants. For example, patients on phenytoin (Dilantin) frequently require higher doses of drug when they are on dexamethasone; conversely, when steroids are tapered, serum phenytoin levels may rise to toxic levels. (2) Brain tumor patients frequently receive cranial irradiation therapy (RT) which may predispose to Stevens-Johnson syndrome and erythema multiforme reactions; this is especially common with phenytoin. (3) Patients frequently have other neurologic impairments that can make anticonvulsant side effects more distressing. For example, brain tumor patients are particularly prone to develop shoulder-hand syndrome and diffuse arthralgias that can be discomforting enough to warrant withdrawal of the medication.

Despite these complications, phenytoin is generally the first-line drug. If breakthrough seizures develop or allergic reactions occur, carbamazepine (Tegretol), phenobarbital, or valproate (Depakote) can be substituted. In lower-grade neoplasms, tumor resections can be performed specifically to relieve epilepsy when medical management is ineffective. Patients with brain tumors are prone to develop seizures after intravenous contrast medium for computed tomography (CT) examinations. This tendency can be minimized by preprocedural administration of 5 mg of diazepam intravenously.

Mass Effect

Patients frequently present with symptoms related to mass effect from the tumor. These symptoms can be subdivided into symptoms of elevated ICP and those of focal neurologic deficits.

Brain tumors raise ICP either by the local effects of tumor mass coupled with vasogenic edema or by producing obstruction of cerebrospinal fluid (CSF) pathways leading to the development of hydrocephalus. Elevated ICP may therefore manifest itself in a variety of ways. *Headache* results from distortion of the dural membranes and intracranial blood vessels. The headache typically is described as holocranial

and occurs on arising, because recumbency at night decreases venous drainage of the brain, and mild hypoventilation as the patient is sleeping causes cerebral vasodilatation. Patients may also experience *vomiting,* which is a result of pressure on the area postrema. Nausea may not be present, and the vomiting occurs most often in the morning (along with a headache) and is frequently projectile in nature. Chronically elevated ICP may also produce progressive cognitive abnormalities with resultant changes in personality and behavior or, alternatively, progressive diminution in the level of consciousness.

Medical and mechanical therapies are available that can treat both mechanisms responsible for causing elevated ICP. Patients with brain masses and symptoms or signs of elevated ICP should have the head of the bed elevated at least 30 degrees to increase cerebral venous drainage and reduce intracranial volume. Additionally, limiting fluid intake to 1.5 liters per day may help reduce the amount of edema fluid produced.

Analgesics may make the patient more comfortable. However, patients with large intracranial masses who hypoventilate even mildly may rapidly decompensate because of their limited cerebral compliance; therefore, sedation, with its attendant hypoventilation, should be avoided. Codeine is thus preferable to other narcotic analgesics because it is less sedating. Antiemetics are also helpful to reduce vomiting and improve patient comfort. Trimethobenzamide (Tigan) at a dose of 250 mg every 6 hours orally or 200 mg every 6 hours rectally is preferable to prochlorperazine (Compazine) or promethazine (Phenergan). Phenothiazine agents, while good antiemetics, can reduce the seizure threshold, an effect that should be avoided.

The most serious effect of elevated ICP is cerebral herniation. Management of this neurologic emergency includes patient hyperventilation and the administration of osmotic diuretics and steroids. Hyperventilation requires patient intubation and its effect rapidly attenuates; however, lowering P_{CO_2} will immediately cause cerebral vasoconstriction and decreased intravascular blood volume, effectively reducing ICP and potentially reversing the herniation syndrome. P_{CO_2} should not be lowered to below 25 torr, which may cause cerebral ischemia. Osmotic diuretics such as mannitol are also useful; their onset of action is slower than hyperventilation. An initial dose of 1 gram per kg, followed by 0.25 gm per kg every 4 to 6 hours, reduces the extracellular brain water volume and can control elevated ICP for several days. An initial dose of furosemide (Lasix) at 1 mg per kg can also hasten the response by its vasodilatative effect on the peripheral vasculature.

Glucocorticoids such as dexamethasone (Decadron) or methylprednisolone (Medrol) stabilize cell membranes and reduce vasogenic edema. Since their onset of action requires at least 30 to 60 minutes, they should be used only in conjunction with other modalities if the situation is an emergency. They are particularly useful, however, in the chronic management of elevated ICP. Dexamethasone is most commonly utilized. The initial dose is 10 mg, followed by 4 mg every 6 hours. It may be given either orally or intravenously, the latter route being necessary in urgent cases when the patient is unable to take oral medication.

Mechanical therapy can also be provided by placement of a ventriculostomy. This surgical procedure can be performed relatively rapidly by a neurosurgeon to divert CSF. Such intervention may rapidly reduce ICP and reverse a herniation syndrome, making it the treatment of choice for the deteriorating patient with hydrocephalus. The ventricular catheter can be removed once the CSF pathway is opened by reduction of edema, or by surgical decompression of tumor bulk. If continued CSF diversion is required following these maneuvers, then placement of a permanent ventriculoperitoneal shunt may be necessary.

Patients may develop focal neurologic deficits from mass effect, as well. These symptoms and signs may include hemiparesis from frontal, parietal, or thalamic masses, aphasia from dominant temporal lobe masses, hearing loss from vestibular schwannomas, visual loss from parasellar masses (such as pituitary adenomas, optic nerve and hypothalamic gliomas, and dorsum sella meningiomas), and hypothalamic-pituitary insufficiency from sellar and suprasellar masses.

Treatment for these symptomatic issues is similar to that described for elevated ICP. Dexamethasone is very effective in reducing neural compression by reducing edema and may significantly improve the symptoms. Often, however, surgical decompression of the affected structure by removal of the offending mass is required for improvement. If the symptoms are related to endocrine insufficiency, replacement therapy is the most effective method of improving the clinical condition. In the specific instance of visual loss from a sellar/suprasellar mass with an elevated prolactin level (usually a pituitary prolactinoma), treatment with bromocriptine (Parlodel) may rapidly shrink the tumor and improve vision.

Immediate and Long-Term Symptoms Related to Treatment

In recent years the treatment of patients with brain tumors has become more intensive, resulting in better response and survival rates. These more aggressive therapies are also associated with morbidities that must be distinguished from tumor progression.

Although operative mortality has decreased significantly in recent years, medical and neurologic morbidities of neurosurgical procedures remain problematic. Postoperative infections, including subdural empyema and meningitis, can be significantly reduced by the administration of prophylactic antibiotics. Abscesses are particularly difficult to differentiate from tumor both radiographically and clinically. Fever and high leukocyte count may suggest infection, but they are not invariably present in the patients who are on steroids. Abscess should therefore be a consideration in any patient developing signs of neurologic deterioration postoperatively, especially if imaging studies reveal an enlarging concentric ring lesion.

Shunt malfunctions can also produce symptoms and signs mimicking tumor recurrence; correction will reverse symptoms and afford effective palliation. Therefore, a high index of suspicion for malfunction is required in tumor patients with shunts, and appropriate imaging studies must be performed before attributing clinical worsening to tumor progression.

Radiation and chemotherapy, although mainstays of neuro-oncologic treatment, also may result in early and delayed neurologic side effects that may either mimic tumor recurrence or impair quality of life. External beam irradiation may result in symptomatic worsening either during its acute administration or as a delayed effect occurring from weeks to months after its completion. The early reactions are related to cerebral edema and usually respond to steroid administration. The delayed effects are more serious and usually represent a form of cerebral radionecrosis. This latter development is often indistinguishable in conventional imaging studies and clinical manifestations from tumor recurrence and represents a difficult diagnostic and therapeutic problem. We have found thallium-201, single photon emission computed tomography (SPECT) scans particularly useful in helping differentiate necrosis from recurrence; if decreased uptake in the area of imaging abnormality is noted, then necrosis is the more likely diagnosis. Often however, biopsy is the only way to make the diagnosis. Surgical excision is sometimes required for symptomatic relief. No medical treatments are very effective, although recent reports of improvement after therapeutic anticoagulation are promising.

A number of more subtle long-term complications also arise in irradiated patients. Endocrine deficiency is a common occurrence. This generally results from the effects of irradiation (and possibly chemotherapy) on the hypothalamus and pituitary. A decrease in gonadotropin hormones is most common, and patients will frequently develop either amenorrhea or impotence. Thyroid dysfunction is also a common occurrence, and patients should be periodically screened for this problem.

A more vexing long-term complication of treatment is a deterioration in cognitive capabilities. Both very young and very old patients are particularly vulnerable to this development. Furthermore, the effects occur more frequently with higher total and fractionated doses of radiation and are probably aggravated by the addition of chemotherapy. The underlying pathologic process probably represents a leukoencephalopathy that is reflected by increased white matter abnormalities on magnetic resonance imaging (MRI). A gradual deterioration in cognitive abilities coupled with other signs of white matter dysfunction, especially gait dysfunction, characterize the disorder.

Unfortunately, no effective treatments exist for this problem.

Deep Venous Thrombosis and Pulmonary Embolism

Deep venous thrombosis (DVT) and pulmonary embolism (PE) occur frequently in the brain tumor patient and present a difficult management problem. Patient immobilization and release of tissue thromboplastin from the brain tumor make peripheral venous thrombosis especially common in brain tumor patients, with incidence figures as high as 33%. Thrombosis can occur at any time of the disease, although it is more likely to develop in the first 6 weeks after craniotomy.

Patients with brain tumors who develop leg swelling or pain should be screened for DVT with impedance plethysmography. Patients who develop sudden shortness of breath or an encephalopathy of uncertain etiology should be evaluated for PE with radionuclide lung scanning. In those in whom DVT or PE is documented, treatment is indicated. The optimal therapy remains uncertain because of the risk of anticoagulating a patient with a brain tumor who has recently undergone craniotomy. Placement of a Greenfield filter or other type of vena caval interruption procedure has been advocated as a safer alternative to anticoagulation in the immediate postoperative period (i.e., within 4 weeks). However, the documented long-term morbidities of this procedure make it a less desirable choice for other patients, especially since anticoagulation is relatively safe with a very low incidence of intracranial hemorrhage.

Although they are liberally used in patients with malignant brain tumors, steroids are not without serious long-term complications. Myopathy, glucose intolerance, osteoporosis, avascular necrosis of the hips, and mental status changes can all result from their usage. Unfortunately, these problems often develop in a patient who needs the symptomatic benefit that steroids can provide. In these situations, *oral glycerol* (Osmoglyn), a potent osmotic diuretic that can achieve the same benefits as mannitol, can be substituted. Although the medication may be quite unpalatable for many patients, most patients will tolerate it when it is mixed with orange juice. Frequently, its addition will allow a reduction in or even discontinuation of glucocorticoid dosage.

DIAGNOSTIC ISSUES

Sometimes a definitive diagnosis of a brain lesion can be made on imaging and clinical criteria alone, such as when a cancer patient develops multiple enhancing lesions in the setting of progressive systemic disease. Often, however, establishing a definitive diagnosis is essential for planning specific therapy. Since tissue is required for a definitive diagnosis, a surgical procedure can be designed to make a tissue diagnosis as well as to decompress the lesion and improve symptoms. In some instances, however, diagnosis should be made by biopsy only, without specific therapeutic benefit to the patient.

Obviously, an adequate diagnostic work-up must be done before an appropriate surgical procedure can be performed. Patients between 20 and 40 years of age with parenchymal lesions are at risk for human immunodeficiency virus (HIV) related central nervous system (CNS) masses. If the patient is HIV-positive, stereotactic biopsy can establish whether the lesion(s) is related to an opportunistic infection or CNS lymphoma. Conversely, patients over the age of 40 years are more likely to have metastatic lesions. Therefore, screening tests consisting of a rectal examination with stool guaiac, urinalysis, skin and breast examinations, complete blood count (CBC), and chest radiograph may suggest a primary focus. If a primary lesion is identified, resection of a single parenchymal metastatic lesion will result in an improved prognosis. For multiple lesions, empiric radiation therapy is usual if a primary lesion is identified, and stereotactic biopsy can confirm the pathology if no primary lesion is found.

Most patients with newly diagnosed mass lesions do undergo some type of surgical procedure for either diagnostic or therapeutic purposes. Open craniotomy is necessary if therapeutic decompression (and acquisition of pathologic material) is desired. In most instances, this operation requires administration of general anesthesia. Some masses, such as meningiomas and metastatic neoplasms, have well-defined planes between themselves and the brain; these lesions can often be grossly totally removed. Other lesions, such as anaplastic astrocytoma and glioblastoma multiforme, send macro- or microscopic infiltrating fingers of tumor out from their tumor bulk; they can never be completely resected, but they can be significantly decompressed to reduce mass effect. If craniotomy is not felt to be indicated, then stereotactic biopsy is the preferable means of acquiring tissue for diagnostic purposes. This procedure can be performed under local anesthetic using CT or MRI guidance with minimal risk.

The choice of which surgical approach to use depends on a number of factors, including neuroimaging appearance, whether symptoms of mass effect are present, and patient age. Extra-axial lesions are well suited for surgical excision since these can often be totally removed. Lesions that are exerting significant mass effect on imaging studies are also suitable for surgical decompression if they do not involve eloquent cortical or subcortical structures. Stereotactic approaches are usually not appropriate for hemorrhagic lesions, which are probably better handled by craniotomy. On the other hand, those lesions involving the deep nuclear structures of the thalamus, basal ganglia, and brain stem are usually not amenable to surgical decompression, even if they have significant mass effect. If multiple lesions are present, stereotactic biopsy is likewise preferred.

The patient's age is an important determinant of surgical approach. For many childhood tumors, children have a more favorable prognosis with more radical excision of the mass. Therefore, if the lesion is in a surgically accessible location, craniotomy for resection is preferable. On the other hand, very elderly patients may not tolerate craniotomy well. Unless the lesion has significant mass effect, stereotactic biopsy is indicated.

SPECIFIC THERAPEUTIC ISSUES

A tumor's histology becomes particularly important when considering specific therapies such as radiation, chemo-, immune, and endocrine therapies that are administered specifically to eradicate tumor or control its growth. Even in this particular area of treatment, however, other factors must be taken into account. For example, in making the decision whether to administer radiation therapy, patient age must be taken into account because of the high incidence of deleterious effects that occur in the very young and very old patients.

The following brief survey will orient the physician to some of the more common brain tumors encountered. Since these are relatively rare events for which many clinical investigations are ongoing, we advise that whenever possible patients should be evaluated in settings where multidisciplinary (i.e., neurosurgery, radiation therapy, oncology) input is available.

Brain Metastasis

In patients older than 40 years, brain metastasis is the most common cause of brain tumor. Lung and breast cancers are the most frequent primary tumors; although most brain metastases develop late in the clinical course when systemic cancer is obvious, they may also be evident at time of presentation and not uncommonly may herald the diagnosis. For this reason, newly diagnosed brain tumor patients should have at least a chest radiograph (CT scan of the chest in patients with a smoking history), mammogram, urinalysis, and CT scan of the abdomen in patients in whom there is a suspicion of an intra-abdominal or retroperitoneal lesion prior to neurosurgical intervention.

The prognosis of patients with intracranial metastasis from systemic cancer is poor, with median survivals being less than 6 months. However, certain patients, especially those with no evidence of systemic disease at the time of neurologic presentation, may do much better.

From a therapeutic standpoint, brain metastases are approached differently depending on whether they are single or multiple. MRI most accurately determines the number of intracranial lesions. In patients with two or more lesions, whole brain radiation therapy, generally consisting of 10 fractions of 300 cGy per fraction, is the treatment of choice. Because of the long-term neurologic side effects of this high fractionation scheme, it has been our practice to administer an equivalent total dosage using only 200 cGy per dose in those patients who are deemed to be capable of a longer-term survival. In addition, if one larger lesion, especially in the posterior fossa, is causing significant neurologic deficits unresponsive to dexamethasone, surgical decompression may rapidly improve symptoms.

Management of single intracranial metastatic lesions depends on their location and the patient's symptoms. If the patient has a lesion in noneloquent brain or has significant symptoms of mass effect, then surgical resection followed by radiation therapy provides the best long-term care. On the other hand, if the patient has minimal neurologic signs and the lesion is in or adjacent to eloquent brain, radiation therapy alone will eliminate possible neurologic deficits related to surgery. Considering many recent studies documenting better outcomes in surgically treated patients, it has been our approach to consider all patients with single lesions, stable or inactive systemic disease, and reasonable performance status for surgical resection unless a contraindication exists.

High-Grade Gliomas

High-grade or malignant gliomas are the most commonly encountered primary brain tumors. They affect mostly middle-aged adults although they can occur at any age. The most malignant tumor of this group is the glioblastoma multiforme (GBM), characterized pathologically by the presence of endothelial proliferation and tissue necrosis. Anaplastic astrocytomas are distinguished from glioblastomas by the absence of necrosis. A number of factors affect prognosis: patient age (younger most favorable), the presence of necrosis on pathologic section (unfavorable), and postoperative performance status are the most frequently associated ones.

Unfortunately, these tumors are incurable, and treatment is geared toward maximal palliation. Debulking of as much tumor as deemed safe, combined with postoperative external beam radiation therapy to maximal brain tolerance (approximately 60 cGy), is associated with median time to tumor progression in patients with GBM of less than a year. Increasing the radiation dosage has minimal added effect and increases toxicity, as do newer radiation therapy modalities such as stereotactic radiosurgery. The addition of chemotherapy, administered either as a single agent or in combination, modestly increases survival, mainly by increasing the number of longer-term survivors. Patients with anaplastic astrocytomas have slightly better prognoses, and 5-year survivals, although uncommon, do occur.

Although chemotherapy is generally associated with at best a modest efficacy, recent reports indicate that a particular subtype of malignant glioma, the aggressive oligodendroglioma, may be particularly chemosensitive to a combination of procarbazine (Matulane), CCNU (lomustine [CeeNu]), and vincristine (Oncovin). A number of other experimental chemo- and immune therapies are currently being evaluated, but none so far has proved superior to the standard conventional approach of surgery, external beam irradiation, and single-agent chemotherapy.

Low-Grade Gliomas

Although gliomas represent a continuum of tumor types, it has been clinically useful to separate them into higher (i.e., malignant) and lower grades; however, it is important to remember that although clinically less aggressive, the low-grade tumors also are often incurable and represent low-grade malignancies rather than benign tumors. The most common tumor type is the diffuse fibrillary astrocytoma; oligodendroglioma and mixed tumor types are other important tumor types.

These tumors tend to occur at younger ages, usually between 20 and 50 years. They tend to arise in the cerebral hemispheres and present with a seizure or seizures. They pose a particularly difficult clinical problem when they produce an isolated seizure in an otherwise young, healthy patient whose imaging studies reveal an unenhancing supratentorial lesion without mass effect, since it is unclear whether early intervention results in improved patient outcome.

Unfortunately, although at the outset these tumors frequently behave very indolently, at some point (usually within 7 to 8 years), they begin to behave more like their malignant counterparts. It is not clear whether early irradiation postpones this event or prolongs survival, although a number of retrospective series suggest this. It has been our practice to approach each case individually and make clinical decisions based on the potential for complete resection, patient age (the older the patient, the sooner the tumor will become more aggressive so we tend not to postpone treatment), and patient and physician preference.

Central Nervous System Lymphomas

Primary CNS lymphomas were once considered rare, but their incidence is increasing, especially in the acquired immune deficiency syndrome (AIDS) population but also in the elderly. These tumors are identical in histology to non-Hodgkin's lymphomas that occur systemically. They tend to be multifocal and occur in deep periventricular locations; however, it is impossible to distinguish these tumors from GBM preoperatively.

Owing to their oncolytic actions versus lymphomas, the administration of glucocorticoids may result in a complete disappearance of the lesion; when this occurs, it strongly suggests lymphoma as a diagnosis. On the other hand, because it obscures the ability to make the diagnosis, it is recommended that at least a biopsy be obtained if possible before the long-term administration of steroids in patients in whom lymphoma is suspected.

Stereotactic biopsy is indicated to make the diagnosis; retrospective data indicate that more extensive surgery may be associated with a poorer outcome. Radiotherapy affords long-term palliation, but the median survival of these patients is still only slightly greater than a year. A number of reports demonstrate that these tumors are sensitive to chemotherapy; effective regimens include high-dose methotrexate and more intensive therapies. We thus routinely administer chemotherapy preirradiation to newly diagnosed, non-immune suppressed patients with CNS lymphoma.

In patients with AIDS and CNS lymphoma, irradiation offers effective palliation; although survival is not appreciably increased, the pattern of disease is changed, and patients generally succumb to other complications of their disease. Chemotherapy has not proved particularly effective in this cohort of patients, although ongoing studies continue.

Meningiomas

Meningiomas are extraparenchymal tumors that arise from leptomeningeal tissue and produce symptoms by compressing contiguous neural structures. They are benign in the sense that they can be cured if totally removed; if this is not possible, however, further tumor growth can occur, which can produce further neurologic deficits or death. Thus, the goal of surgery is total resection of the tumor and its dural attachment without damaging surrounding neural and vascular structures. This may not be possible if the tumor has invaded the skull base or is attached to neural or vascular structures that would cause unacceptable neurologic morbidity if the tumor were completely removed. In these instances, the goal of surgery should be to remove as much of the tumor bulk as possible.

If a complete resection can be performed, no further therapy is necessary. When only partial removals are accomplished, radiation therapy focused on the residual component of tumor can be just as effective in preventing recurrence as "complete" excision in the long term. By using a focused form of radiation, the complications of radiation therapy on normal brain can be minimized. No truly effective chemotherapeutic agent has been identified for adjuvant therapy. RU486 (mifepristone) the "birth control" pill, has been shown to have some efficacy in some cases, but further study is necessary before this agent or others become part of the standard care.

Not all meningiomas require therapy. In many patients, lesions are discovered incidentally during evaluation of unrelated symptoms. In these cases, close follow-up with serial imaging every 6 months to a year can establish a growth pattern of the lesion. Surgical removal is indicated when progressive growth is documented or symptoms or signs develop.

Medulloblastoma

Medulloblastomas are primitive neuroectodermal tumors that arise most frequently in the cerebellum. They represent the most common malignant brain tumor of childhood. They affect mainly young children or adolescents; occurrence after 20 years of age is much less frequent. Until the early 1970s, fewer than one-third of patients with medulloblastomas survived 5 years after treatment. Owing to several factors including earlier diagnosis, safer anesthesia, advances in surgical techniques, improved postoperative care, and more effective use of radiotherapy, 5-year disease-free survival rates approaching 50% are common.

Generally, patients can be characterized into those of average risk (no disseminated disease, no marked hydrocephalus, total or near-total resection, and age greater than 4 years) and poor risk (some combination of disseminated disease, hydrocephalus or tumor infiltration of the brain stem, a less than total resection, or age less than 4 years). Medulloblastomas, unlike most other brain tumors, have a high likelihood of disseminating to other CNS sites early in the course of illness, and over 30% of patients will have either CSF cytologic or imaging evidence of lepto-

meningeal disease at diagnosis (which can be asymptomatic). Therefore, every newly diagnosed patient should have MRI of the spine, lumbar puncture for cytology, and bone marrow examination as part of their staging work-up.

Since many patients develop tumor outside the primary tumor site after local radiotherapy, the entire neuraxis is usually irradiated to improve long-term disease control. Conventionally, 36 cGy are given to brain and spine and an additional 20 cGy administered to the local disease site. Children with poor risk indicators may benefit from chemotherapy; other children do not. The optimal chemotherapy regimens for both initial and recurrent disease are currently being studied in prospective trials.

Section 14

The Locomotor System

RHEUMATOID ARTHRITIS

method of
JAMES L. McGUIRE, M.D., and
ELAINE LAMBERT, M.D.
Stanford University Medical Center
Stanford, California

Rheumatoid arthritis (RA) is a chronic systemic disease that typically presents in women in their fourth and fifth decades. Recent epidemiologic studies have suggested improved outcomes, in part relating to aggressive therapy with so-called disease-modifying antirheumatic drugs (DMARDs). Moreover, the longer a patient with rheumatoid arthritis takes DMARDs over the course of the disease, the better the activity of daily living (ADL). These principles and a managed care economic environment have reemphasized the role of primary care physicians in the early diagnosis and the early initiation of treatment, including DMARD therapy.

In the past, the role of the rheumatologist was to initiate and monitor DMARDs, such as gold and cytotoxic agents, in addition to performing arthrocentesis and joint injections with corticosteroids. The overall therapeutic plan has been termed "the pyramid" to emphasize the stepwise progression of additive drugs and interventions as appropriate for the severity of persistent disease activity not controlled at the lower tiers of the pyramid. Some investigators have suggested inverting the pyramid to provide the maximal therapy early in the disease course in an effort to produce a complete remission before the establishment of the proliferative synovial lesion. Nevertheless, the pyramid, as described in Figure 1, is the standard integrated plan for both primary care physicians and rheumatologists with the main issue relating to the timing of advancement to the next therapeutic level.

Several epidemiologic studies have directly affected current therapeutic consensus. (1) The understanding that progressive disability and even death occurred more frequently than previously reported resulted in earlier use of DMARDs in the course of RA. (2) The rates and potential mortality of upper gastrointestinal (GI) bleeding caused by nonsteroidal anti-inflammatory drugs (NSAIDs) resulted in both more aggressive efforts to protect the stomach during NSAID use and the elucidation of risk factors for this problem. (3) The understanding that certain human leukocyte antigen (HLA) genes, especially HLA-DR4 and its subtypes, are associated with more severe outcomes in RA influenced treatment plans. The development of the early aggressive treatment schemes based in part on the presence of these "severity" genes is currently being evaluated. (4) The role of estrogen-containing birth control pills in the prevention of RA and the amelioration of disease severity has been debated in moderately large epidemiologic studies. Although not yet conclusive, these studies do give the clinician confidence in using estrogen in RA for both birth control and osteoporosis prevention. (5) Formal education and ADL appear to influence mortality rates. Although little can be done about the former, the latter provides further justification for aggressive and early therapy for RA. A physician philosophy to keep the patient maximally active and involved in a full range of life's activity is probably wise.

Early treatment relies on early diagnosis. Rheumatoid arthritis is classically a symmetrical arthritis that typically has bony erosions in and around joints on plain radiographs. Patients with established disease typically test positive for the rheumatoid factor. However, these characteristics of RA are often a function of the duration of the disease, especially in severe cases. At the earliest presentation, the arthritis is often asymmetrical, beginning in a single joint before involving the contralateral side. The radiograph of the joint rarely demonstrates erosions before 1 year of active disease. Moreover, the rheumatoid factor is positive in approximately 50% of patients at presentation with conversion to positivity in 80% of cases with persistent disease.

If the primary care physician is expected to initiate potentially aggressive therapy with DMARDs, the early and sometimes atypical features of RA must be emphasized and distinguished from other arthritis, such as the more common osteoarthritis and transient viral arthritis. Additionally, a woman with arthritis of the hands who is rheumatoid factor–negative but has a positive antinuclear antibody (ANA) may have either systemic lupus erythematosus (SLE) or early RA. RA, even when asymmetrical, has the usual pattern of joint involvement observed in more advanced disease. In the hands, the proximal interphalangeal (PIP) joints, metacarpophalangeal (MCP) joints, and wrists are affected, sparing until late in the disease the distal interphalangeal (DIP) joints, which are typically involved in early osteoarthritis. The distribution of joint involvement in SLE is similar to that of RA.

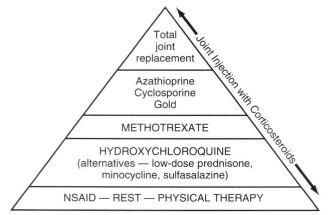

Figure 1. The pyramid of therapeutic options in rheumatoid arthritis.

TABLE 1. **Disease-Modifying Antirheumatic Drugs (DMARDs)**

Name of Drug	Maintenance Usual Dose	Monitoring Selected for Side Effects
Hydroxychloroquine (Plaquenil)	200 bid PO	Eye check q 6–12 months
Methotrexate (Rheumatrex)	10 mg weekly PO	LFTs, CBC, creatinine levels
Prednisone	5 mg q A.M. PO	Bone density, blood sugar level
Gold Salts (Solganal)	50 mg IM monthly	CBC for platelets, urinalysis for protein
Sulfasalazine (Azulfidine)	1 gm bid PO	CBC, rash
Cyclosporine (Sandimmune)	3 mg/kg/day PO	Creatinine, cyclosporine blood levels
Azathioprine (Imuran)	50 mg bid PO	CBC
Minocycline (Minocin)	200 mg daily PO	Rash, upset stomach

Before using a DMARD, please consult hospital formulary or Physicians' Desk Reference (PDR) for full adverse effect profile and dosing regimen. *Abbreviations:* LFT = liver function test; CBC = complete blood count.

DIFFERENTIAL DIAGNOSIS

Two additional historical factors may be helpful in making the early diagnosis of RA. First, the age of presentation of rheumatic diseases often clusters around a decade. RA typically appears in the fourth and fifth decades, whereas SLE presents earlier, in the second and third decades of life. Second, morning stiffness lasting more than 1 hour is typical of RA and is extremely rare in osteoarthritis. Fibromyalgia can present in women in the fifth decade with morning stiffness and myalgia but no joint swelling or laboratory abnormalities suggestive of a connective tissue disease. The disorder should be easily distinguished from RA. In a similar fashion, polymyalgia rheumatica has severe morning stiffness and an elevated erythrocyte sedimentation rate (ESR), but almost exclusively presents after the age of 55 years.

THERAPEUTIC PYRAMID APPROACH TO THERAPY

The confidence in the diagnosis translates into a more aggressive approach within the therapeutic pyramid. When the diagnosis is not secure, a more cautious approach with NSAIDs alone is appropriate. In general, NSAIDs are administered alone for 1 to 2 months. If symptoms in a patient with just a few active joints have not resolved on NSAIDs, it is appropriate for a primary care physician to start a first-line DMARD (Table 1). The antimalarial hydroxychloroquine (Plaquenil) would be a typical agent at 200 mg twice a day (or 5 to 7 mg per kg per day). Other medications could include sulfasalazine (Azulfidine),* low-dose prednisone, or methotrexate (MTX) (Rheumatrex), but for various reasons, including a lack of familiarity, these agents are usually prescribed in concert with rheumatologic consultation. Historical interest in using antibiotics to treat the presumptive infection that triggers RA has led to recent interest in the use of minocycline (Minocin),* which may have additional immunomodulatory properties.

METHOTREXATE

Most rheumatologists would advise adding MTX to the hydroxychloroquine if the arthritis is not completely controlled by 3 or 4 months. This would have been the traditional positioning of gold therapy, which has largely been supplanted by MTX, which has proved over the last decade to be both effective and well tolerated. MTX is usually given in weekly doses of 7.5 to 15 mg on a single day of the week and may be given orally, subcutaneously, or intramuscularly. Monitoring by blood work would include a complete blood cell count (CBC), liver function tests (LFTs), and tests for creatinine levels. This should be done every 1 to 2 months throughout the entire course of MTX therapy. A liver biopsy should be considered after 3 to 5 years of continuous weekly MTX therapy, especially if minor abnormalities have been noted. Prescreening of patients to be treated with MTX with hepatitis B and C antibodies and chest x-ray films (because of the rare side effect of MTX-induced pneumonitis) and having the patient eliminate ethanol usage greatly reduces the incidence of hepatotoxicity. Morbid obesity, diabetes, and renal insufficiency (creatinine level >2 mg per day) are other contraindications to the use of MTX. Other side effects include oral ulcers, abdominal distress, and flulike symptoms after the weekly dose. Many clinicians give daily folic acid 1 mg per day orally to prevent the gastrointestinal symptoms. The folate dose does not seem to diminish the efficacy of the MTX. The suggested dose of MTX is rarely associated with cytopenias. This toxicity may be more likely if renal insufficiency is present. In summary, the popularity of MTX relates to the sustained efficacy over years, the speed of the initial response (often within several weeks), and the relatively safe profile alone or in combination with hydroxychloroquine.

CORTICOSTEROIDS

Corticosteroid therapy has a long history in RA. The emergence of corticosteroids resulted in the first dramatic therapeutic trials in RA. Unfortunately, the high dose of these steroids used in the early 1950s resulted in a wide variety of predictable side effects that all but stopped their use in this disease. In the last decade, low-dose prednisone, in morning dosages of 5 to 7 mg, has been very popular with rheumatologists, presumably as a DMARD rather than for the relatively weak anti-inflammatory properties at this

---
*Not FDA-approved for this indication.

dose. Nevertheless, some patients have a dramatic response to low-dose prednisone and seem exquisitely sensitive even to minimal tapering of the steroid dose. Prednisone should be used cautiously by primary care physicians. Dose escalations for maximal anti-inflammatory effects, especially in the evening, can cause suppression of the hypothalamic-pituitary-adrenal (HPA) axis. These changes in dosing are often done by the patients on their own, and therefore prednisone should be given only to patients with an excellent history of drug compliance.

Corticosteroids are usually given intra-articularly for the control of one or two inflamed joints in which the inflammation is out of proportion to the overall disease activity. Most primary care physicians are comfortable with the injection of the knees and occasionally the shoulders. The duration of response varies with each preparation. For intra-articular injection, most clinicians use a longer-acting preparation such as triamcinolone hexacetonide (Aristospan) or methylprednisolone acetate (Depo-Medrol), which can be expected to control inflammation locally for a month or longer. Most rheumatologists feel comfortable with injecting a variety of smaller joints including the hands and feet, and this can provide dramatic functional improvement.

NONSTEROIDAL ANTI–INFLAMMATORY DRUGS

NSAIDs have been a central component of the foundations of the pyramid along with physical therapy, occupational therapy, and rest. NSAIDs have traditionally meant salicylates, which still remain an inexpensive alternative for the control of inflammation and pain. Compliance with salicylate therapy has been variable because of the absolute number of pills that need to be taken three to four times a day to achieve an anti-inflammatory effect. Other NSAIDs have become extremely popular, especially with the advent of once-a-day medications that appear to have relatively low rates of gastrointestinal irritation. NSAIDs have a variety of effects but especially inhibit prostaglandin synthesis. Prostaglandins promote inflammation and stimulate bone resorption within a joint. Therefore, the synthesis of prostaglandins should potentially decrease both pain and bony destruction. On the other hand, prostaglandins are beneficial to the stomach mucosa and kidney. A prostaglandin blockade by NSAIDs can lead to gastric ulceration and reduced renal blood flow. Risk factors for gastric ulceration and bleeding from NSAIDs include advanced age, rheumatoid arthritis, previous NSAID-induced ulceration, and possibly prednisone use. Many physicians now use a prostaglandin analogue, misoprostol (Cytotec), for gastric and small bowel protection during chronic NSAID therapy for high-risk groups. Misoprostol 200 μg is usually given twice a day, along with food and/or the NSAID itself, depending on the dosing frequency of the NSAID.

The choice of NSAIDs other than salicylates is often difficult. The following guidelines may help. First, all NSAIDs taken at maximal doses have similar efficacy, although individual responsiveness to specific NSAIDs is well known. Second, generic NSAIDs are available and should be tried first because of their reduced cost. Third, several classes of NSAIDs, such as drugs of the propionic acid class—ibuprofen (Motrin), naproxen (Naprosyn), and oxaprozin (Daypro)—are popular because of their overall efficacy and gastrointestinal safety. Newer NSAIDs have emphasized low gastrointestinal side-effect profiles. For RA these include nabumetone (Relafen) and diclofenac (Voltaren). Fourth, once-a-day NSAID therapies dramatically increase compliance but may increase the side effect rates, especially with respect to the stomach and kidney. Fifth, the total dose of NSAIDs for RA has traditionally been in the highest range used for any chronic arthritis. In summary, NSAIDs are used in almost every patient with RA. The clinician must be aware of the somewhat unpredictable and frequently silent gastrointestinal bleeding, renal insufficiency, hepatotoxicity, fluid retention, and central nervous system alterations caused by NSAIDs.

SELECTED COMPLICATIONS OF CHRONIC RA

Chronic diseases such as RA can be complicated by osteoporosis, atherosclerotic heart disease, and medication reactions. A review of RA, with respect to those problems, emphasizes the complex interactions of disability, systemic disease, and exposure to potentially toxic medications over several decades. Potential risk factors for osteoporosis include female sex, menopause status, immobility, corticosteroid therapy (even low dose), and cytokine production that augments bone resorption. Exercise programs, estrogen replacement at the earliest signs of menopause, adequate calcium intake in the 1000-mg-daily range with concomitant vitamin D 400 IU per day, and the use of the lowest dose of corticosteroid, i.e., prednisone 5 mg in a single morning dose, may reduce the risk of fracture. There is currently a renewed interest in concomitant coronary vascular disease in the autoimmune diseases. In SLE, premature coronary artery disease appears linked to the combination of the corticosteroid with the vasculitis itself. In RA, the data that relate corticosteroid use to coronary artery disease are much less clear, but close scrutiny for this problem is advised. For the clinician, it means that even casual reference to chest discomfort by a patient with long-standing RA on corticosteroid therapy should be investigated further.

Patients with RA discontinue medications because of either a lack of continued efficacy or adverse reactions. When side effects appear in any therapeutic regimens for a chronic disease, the "old" drugs that have been useful for many months are as likely as the recently started medication to be the cause. For instance, the use of NSAIDs in RA can result in upper gastrointestinal bleeding, and the presentation of this problem can occur anytime from 1 month to several years after the therapy is begun. On the other hand, the renal function abnormalities related to the prostaglandin blockade by NSAIDs usually occur during the first several months after initiation. Surprisingly, it is the NSAIDs rather than the DMARDs that more often result in life-threatening complications. In part, it relates to the close monitoring for adverse effects in patients taking DMARDs such as MTX and azathioprine. On the other hand, surveillance for side effects from NSAIDs, which are used so frequently for a wide variety of musculoskeletal problems and have an overall very satisfactory safety record, is less intense. A cost-effective therapeutic approach to RA should have four overall guiding principles. First, early treatment may prevent long-term disability. Second, laboratory tests, especially for the monitoring of toxicity and disease activity, are a prominent component of the therapeutic cost. Several examples illustrate this point. MTX therapy requires the serial evaluation of blood for liver function and cytopenias. However, as the experience with this drug for RA has expanded over the last decade, it is clear that severe liver and blood problems are distinctly rare. Therefore, the original recommendation for monthly testing has been increased to 6-week intervals, and some rheumatologists obtain liver function tests and a CBC on an every-other-month schedule. Hydroxychloroquine therapy requires no blood test monitoring, but ophthalmic examinations should be performed every 6 to 12 months.

In a similar fashion, disease activity can be evaluated by a directed history of ADL rather than a primary reliance on blood tests such as the ESR. This test should be done as an additive evaluation when the ADL history is not clear. One test, the titer rheumatoid factor (RF), does not correlate with disease activity and should not be used serially. In fact, once the RF is positive in a patient with RA, there is virtually no reason to repeat it for the primary care physician.

Third, generic drugs, especially of the propionic acid class of NSAIDs, which includes ibuprofen and naproxen, are now available. Similarly, MTX and soon-to-go-generic hydroxychloroquine give the primary care physician full access to the DMARD class of medicines. When efficacy or compliance is the major factor, the rationale for continuation of the brand name can be justified, but this should be the exception.

Fourth, the clinician should be continually assessing how much of a patient's symptoms are related to ongoing inflammation, which require DMARDs, as opposed to the structural and mechanical sequelae of chronic arthritis, which may warrant orthopedic intervention.

Managed care insurance plans are developing or have developed algorithms for the care of RA; these need to be reviewed and evaluated for the inclusion of sound therapeutic principles rather than just arbitrary cost-cutting measures. The very nature of the waxing and waning course of chronic diseases often means that the effects of a therapeutic intervention done today may not be known for years or even decades. Based on the most appropriate scientific facts available, physicians who care for patients with RA need to be aware of the most cost-effective therapeutics.

In summary, the therapy of RA has been influenced by both the epidemiologic and the basic science research in this disease. Although the future may include monoclonal antibodies and cytokine alteration, the current cost-driven environment would suggest that early intervention with DMARDs, together with minimizing the risk of NSAID use, will be the central components of an integrated therapeutic plan that will result in the best outcomes.

JUVENILE RHEUMATOID ARTHRITIS

method of
CAROL B. LINDSLEY, M.D.
University of Kansas Medical Center
Kansas City, Kansas

Of the more than 100 different types of arthritis in children, the most common is juvenile rheumatoid arthritis (JRA). JRA is a disease characterized by arthritis of variable patterns and may be associated with nonarticular manifestations. It is estimated to affect up to 200,000 children in the United States. The disease onset can be from infancy to adulthood, but the peak incidence occurs between 1 and 4 and 9 and 14 years of age. The cause of JRA remains unknown. The onset frequently follows an upper respiratory tract infection or sometimes trauma, but no causative relationship between these events and the subsequent disease has been identified. Current areas of research with regard to etiology focus on an as-yet-unidentified viral agent, an exaggerated or abnormal immune response, a genetic predisposition, or a combination of these factors. In JRA in general, there is a 2:1 to 3:1 female/male ratio, although the sex ratio varies with different subtypes. There are three onset subtypes of JRA defined by the clinical manifestations present during the first 6 months of illness: systemic onset, polyarticular onset (many joints), and pauciarticular onset (few joints). The onset may be insidious or fulminant, and any joint can be involved initially.

Systemic-onset JRA affects 10 to 15% of the children with JRA, has a male predominance, and is characterized by persistent, intermittent fever with elevations to 103° to 106° F and an evanescent rash. Between the fever spikes, there is typically a drop to normal or subnormal levels. Usually, the spikes are in the late afternoon or early evening and are associated with periods of joint discomfort. In the majority of patients with systemic-onset JRA, a rash is associated with the high fever. Occasionally, a child has a rash alone. The evanescent rash is characterized by small salmon-pink lesions, generally 3 to 4 mm in diameter and often with central clearing. The rash is usually present over the anterior chest, axillae, and buttocks, and, to a lessor extent, on the extremities. It is generally nonpruritic. Fever and rash are often accompanied by hepatosplenomegaly, lymphadenopathy, and pericarditis. As the fever and rash subside over a period of weeks or months, the joint symptoms become more prominent. Over half these children develop polyarticular involvement, with about 25% progressing to severe deforming arthritis.

Polyarticular-onset JRA is characterized by involvement of five or more joints during the first 6 months of disease. It is more common in females and is characterized by symmetrical small joint involvement of the hands and feet. This subtype represents from 30 to 40% of all patients with JRA. Children may show mild systemic symptoms, such as low-grade fever and malaise, and morning stiffness is often present. The younger child may also have involvement of the tendon sheath (tenosynovitis), which causes diffuse swelling of the involved area, usually the hand or the foot. Frequently, there is early involvement of the cervical spine, wrists, and hips. A subgroup of polyarticular JRA involves children who are seropositive for rheumatoid factor. They tend to have an older age of onset, a high incidence of rheumatoid subcutaneous nodules, and progressive arthritis manifested by articular erosions and joint deformity. Except for the age of onset, this small subgroup (5 to 10% of all those with JRA) have a disease course similar to that of adult rheumatoid arthritis (RA).

Pauciarticular-onset JRA involves four or fewer joints during the first 6 months of disease. As in the polyarticular type, there is a female predominance. The most commonly affected joints are weight-bearing joints, most frequently knees and ankles. Pauciarticular JRA represents 40 to 50% of children with this disease and is divided into two subgroups. One subgroup includes boys with peripheral arthritis and the HLA-B27 histocompatibility antigen. Children with JRA in this subgroup are at increased risk for the ultimate development of spondylitis. The other subgroup of pauciarticular JRA involves young girls (less than 6 years of age) with an increased risk of chronic iridocyclitis. Chronic iridocyclitis is a prime cause of morbidity in this group and involves inflammation of the anterior uveal tract of the eye. If untreated, it may result in blindness. At least 80% of the chronic iridocyclitis that occurs in JRA occurs in this relatively small group and is often associated with the presence of antinuclear antibodies (ANAs). Thus, the ANA test is a marker for an increased risk of eye disease. As eye disease in young children may be entirely asymptomatic, regular examinations for the early detection of inflammation are critical (see the section "Eye Disease").

DIAGNOSIS

The diagnosis of JRA is dependent on the objective demonstration of chronic inflammation in one or more joints for a minimum of 6 weeks in a person younger than 16 years of age. Inflammation is characterized by swelling or limitation of motion associated with pain, tenderness, or increased warmth. Pain alone (arthralgia) is not adequate for the diagnosis. Other disease must be excluded. The specific exclusions considered in an individual patient depend on the type of onset and general clinical presentation, but should include viral and bacterial infections, malignancy, osteonecrosis, and other rheumatic diseases (e.g., systemic lupus erythematosus, psoriatic arthritis, Lyme disease, vasculitis). There is no specific diagnostic laboratory test for JRA. The majority of patients with active disease have an elevated erythrocyte sedimentation rate (ESR). However, it may be normal or mildly elevated in pauciarticular disease. The white blood cell count may be normal or elevated. Marked leukocytosis is often present in children with systemic disease (40,000 to 80,000 cells per μL) and is usually accompanied by thrombocytosis. A positive ANA test occurs in 30 to 40% of patients. The rheumatoid factor is found in only 5 to 10% and denotes a high-risk subgroup described earlier. By far, the majority of patients with JRA are seronegative for rheumatoid factor, and thus the absence of rheumatoid factor is not helpful in excluding the diagnosis of JRA. Synovial fluid analysis is particularly helpful in monoarticular arthritis to rule out bacterial infection and to document the presence of inflammatory fluid.

Characteristic radiographic changes in patients with JRA often occur late. Initially, only periarticular swelling and juxta-articular osteoporosis are present. These are followed at variable intervals by joint space narrowing, erosive changes, and finally joint fusion. The earliest radiographic changes often occur in the wrist.

TREATMENT

The goal of treatment is to relieve pain and stiffness, to preserve joint function, and to minimize the extra-articular manifestations including psychosocial and school problems. The four main components of long-term treatment are drug therapy, physical and occupational therapy, education of the patient and the family about the disease, and the use of appropriate community services. To monitor disease activity and its response to therapy, parameters such as morning stiffness, active joint count (those with swelling or limitations of motion and pain or tenderness) and selected laboratory tests such as the ESR and complete blood count (CBC) are the most helpful.

Drug Therapy

First-Line Agents

The first-line agents provide anti-inflammatory, antipyretic, and analgesic effects and include aspirin and more than 20 nonsteroidal anti-inflammatory drugs (NSAIDs). Traditionally, aspirin has been the drug of choice in the treatment of JRA, but in most pediatric rheumatology centers it has been replaced by naproxen or ibuprofen. Aspirin is readily available and the least expensive of all NSAIDs. If used, the dosage is 75 to 90 mg per kg (weight <25 kg) per 24 hours (maximum 4 grams per day). The initial dosage and aggressiveness of treatment obviously depend on the severity of the child's symptoms. High-dose salicylate therapy must be closely monitored with serum salicylate levels (therapeutic range 15 to 30 mg per dL) 3 to 7 days after the initiation of therapy and then periodically. In an individual patient, a small increment in the blood level may make a significant difference in the control of symptoms. Moreover, a small increment in oral dosage can result in a relatively large increase in the serum level. Children should be carefully monitored for signs of salicylism (lethargy, lability, tinnitus, or hyperpnea). As the serum level increases, the risk of hepatotoxicity increases, and liver function tests, aspartate aminotransferase (AST) and alanine aminotransferase (ALT) levels should be monitored closely. The salicylate therapy should be discontinued or the dosage reduced if the AST and ALT values consistently

TABLE 1. **Nonsteroidal Anti-Inflammatory Drugs**

Drug	Dosage (mg/kg/day)	Doses per Day
Tolmetin sodium (Tolectin)	20–50	3–4
Naproxen (Naprosyn, Aleve)	10–20	2
Ibuprofen (Advil, Motrin, Nuprin, Rufen)	30–40	3–4

exceed 100 IU. A variety of salicylates is available, including enteric-coated aspirin (Ecotrin), slow-release aspirin (ZORprin), choline magnesium trisalicylate (Trilisate), and salsalate (Disalcid), which are generally well tolerated. Because of the high incidence of gastrointestinal (GI) side effects, salicylates should be taken with food to minimize irritation. Antacids or sucralfate (Carafate)* may also be helpful. Because of the possible risk of Reye's syndrome, salicylates should be discontinued during serious viral illness, especially influenza, and on exposure to chickenpox.

The U.S. Food and Drug Administration (FDA) has approved other NSAIDs for use in children younger than 14 years of age, including tolmetin sodium (Tolectin), naproxen (Naprosyn, Aleve), and ibuprofen (Advil, Motrin, Nuprin, Rufen) (Table 1). Naproxen, choline magnesium trisalicylate, and ibuprofen are available in liquid preparation (see Table 1).

Other NSAIDs that are used in the treatment of children and especially adolescents with JRA include sulindac (Clinoril), 5 to 7 mg per kg per day, and indomethacin (Indocin), 1.5 to 3 mg per kg per day (maximum 150 mg daily†). Other NSAIDs with twice or single daily dosing include nabumetone (Relafen) and oxaprozin (Daypro). There is some evidence that sulindac may have fewer renal side effects, and indomethacin is often particularly effective in treating HLA-B27–positive pauciarticular JRA. Six to 12 weeks may be required for optimal response to NSAID therapy. Thereafter, a different NSAID is usually tried.

The most common side effect of the NSAIDs is gastrointestinal toxicity, including abdominal pain, dyspepsia, peptic ulcer disease, and gastrointestinal bleeding. Hepatic and renal toxicity can also occur. Urinalysis should be obtained every 3 to 4 months, and, if abnormalities are noted, further evaluation should be done. Central nervous system effects are rare but necessitate discontinuation of NSAIDs. Photosensitivity reactions have been reported with most NSAIDs but are common with naproxen, especially facial scars (pseudoporphyria). Long-term multiple NSAID therapy should be avoided.

Second-Line Agents (Slow-Acting Antirheumatic Drugs)

Those patients (40 to 50% of those with JRA) who have persistent polyarticular involvement unresponsive or only partially responsive to NSAID therapy

for 3 to 6 months or steroid dependence or toxicity are candidates for therapy with second-line agents. Unresponsiveness is judged by persistence of a patient's symptoms, particularly joint stiffness or swelling, or fever, and usually radiographic evidence of progressive joint disease. Approximately 50% of patients respond to treatment with gold, hydroxychloroquine, or penicillamine. Response often requires a minimum of 8 to 12 weeks, and treatment is associated with a significant risk of toxicity. Thus, treatment should not be initiated without clear indications. Gold treatment can be in the form of either oral medication, auranofin (Ridaura); or parenteral gold salts, aurothioglucose (Solganal) or gold sodium thiomalate (Myochrysine). Auranofin is usually well tolerated in the dosage of 0.1 to 0.2 mg per kg per day but may be less effective than a parenteral preparation and is not currently approved by the FDA for use in young children. Parenteral gold salts should be given by weekly intramuscular injections. After test injections of 0.25 mg per kg, then 0.5 mg per kg, 0.75 mg per kg per week initially is given to a weekly maximum of 50 mg and continued for 20 weeks. If good response occurs, the injections are maintained at less frequent intervals (every 2 to 3 weeks) for at least 1 year or longer if clinical response is continued and toxicity is avoided. Both oral and parenteral gold require baseline hematologic, hepatic, and renal studies followed by weekly (parenteral gold salts) or biweekly (auranofin) CBCs, urinalysis, and clinical examination for toxicity (rash, mouth ulcers). Patients with systemic JRA may be at increased risk for toxicity. Hydroxychloroquine (Plaquenil),* 5 to 7 mg per kg per day, is well tolerated and is effective in about 50% of the patients. Regular ophthalmic monitoring for retinal toxicity must be done initially and then every 3 to 6 months. Penicillamine (Cuprimine, Depen)* has had limited testing in children but appears to be effective about 50% of the time. It is initiated in a dosage of 5 mg per kg per day and is increased gradually to a maximum of 10 mg per kg per day. Close monitoring for renal toxicity, dermatitis, or a lupus-like syndrome must be done.

Sulfasalazine (Azulfidine)* has received limited experience in children, although it has been shown to be effective in adults with RA. The initial course is 40 to 60 mg per kg per day in divided doses with meals for 6 to 12 weeks, followed by a gradual reduction of dosage to approximately 25 to 30 mg per kg per day. Sulfasalazine appears to be most useful in those with persistent polyarthritis or spondyloarthritis unresponsive to other regimens but is associated with bone marrow toxicity, dermatitis, and gastrointestinal irritation and is contraindicated in patients with prior salicylate or sulfa toxicity or glucose-6-phosphate dehydrogenase deficiency.

Methotrexate

Studies of methotrexate (Rheumatrex) following morning oral dose in children with JRA show efficacy

---

*Not FDA-approved for this indication.
†Exceeds dosage recommended by the manufacturer.

---

*Manufacturer's warning: Efficacy in the treatment of JRA has not been established.

in the treatment of polyarthritis unresponsive to conservative regimens and slow-acting antirheumatic agents. Efficacy has been shown at dosages below those known to be associated with toxicity, and safety for long-term oncogenesis and sterility has been demonstrated. However, methotrexate can be associated with increased susceptibility to infection, bone marrow suppression, GI ulceration, hepatitis and cirrhosis, pulmonary insufficiency, and pneumonitis. Therefore, baseline hematologic, hepatic, and renal studies should be done before the institution of therapy. The regular dosage is 10 mg per m² orally once a week in the morning with water or clear liquids. The initial dose should be low (one-quarter to one-half of the regular dose) with a gradual increase to full dosage. Periodic CBC, urinalysis, and AST and ALT determinations should be performed every 2 weeks initially, then every 1 to 2 months. Periodic testing for serum levels of methotrexate may be helpful if the response is poor. One-hour levels should be approximately 6 $\times$ 10^{-7} mol/L, followed by a 24-hour level of less than 2.2×10^{-8} mol/L.

The major concern with long-term methotrexate usage is potential liver damage. Acute hepatitis as well as chronic damage with fibrosis and cirrhosis may occur. If AST levels exceed 200 IU, the drug should be withheld and only restarted when a return to normal levels occurs. Once the total cumulative dose of 2.5 grams has been reached, the therapy should be reviewed.

Therapy with an NSAID is usually continued during the use of any of the second-line drugs. Caution and careful monitoring should be used when an NSAID is used in combination with methotrexate, as toxicity of the latter may be increased.

Other Agents

Immunosuppressive agents, including cyclophosphamide (Cytoxan), azathioprine (Imuran), and chlorambucil (Leukeran), are not approved for the treatment of JRA. However, azathioprine has been used in adult RA and selected cases of JRA. Weekly intravenous methylprednisolone, intravenous gamma globulin, and cyclosporin therapy are also used selectively, but the use of these agents remains experimental.

Corticosteroids

Oral corticosteroids may be required for severe systemic disease or progressive chronic uveitis. As low a daily dosage as possible (usually <1 mg per kg per day) should be used initially, with slow tapering to alternate-day treatment as symptoms permit. Significant toxicity, including growth retardation, increased susceptibility to infection, and iatrogenic Cushing's syndrome, is associated with prolonged daily therapy. Intravenous steroid pulse therapy may be used to control life-threatening systemic disease or a serious flare of polyarticular disease. Methylprednisolone sodium succinate (Solu-Medrol), 10 to 30 mg per kg per dose in a single pulse given over 60 minutes every day for 3 days, or every other day for 3 doses, has been used. Close monitoring of fluid balance, electrolyte levels, and cardiovascular functions should be done during infusion in a hospital setting. Potential toxicities of such therapy include acute fluid and electrolyte imbalances, sudden death from arrhythmia, hypertensive crisis, GI hemorrhage, seizure disorder, osteonecrosis, hyperglycemia, ketosis, and increased risk of infection.

Selective use of intra-articular corticosteroids (triamcinolone hexacetonide [Aristospan], 20 mg per mL, 25 mg for large joints, and 10 mg for small joints) can be beneficial. Particular caution is needed with regard to serial injections (more than three) and hip joint injections. Close follow-up regarding overuse of the injected joint and infection is needed.

Physical and Occupational Therapy

Each child needs a balanced rest and activity program tailored to current disease activity. Physical and occupational therapy are an important component of JRA treatment. Almost all children with JRA require an exercise program at one time or another. Painful joints are held in flexion and used with decreased frequency, often leading to flexion contractures within a short time. The longer the duration of symptoms without adequate therapy, the more difficult it is to reverse these changes. Inflamed joints should receive range-of-motion exercise at least once daily. With active inflammation, the exercise program consists initially of passive range-of-motion exercise and thereafter a progressive program should be instituted under the direction of a physical or occupational therapist. As disease activity diminishes, passive exercises can be replaced by active ones and ultimately by progressive strengthening exercises. Emphasis is almost always on joint extension rather than flexion, as flexion contractures are common problems. In addition to prescribed exercises, swimming and bicycle or tricycle riding are excellent all-around activities. Many children have shoulder and hip girdle involvement and particularly benefit from swimming. Normal play or sport activities, however, do not take the place of prescribed exercises. Many small aids, such as doorframe pulleys, tilt tables, writing spacers, and self-help devices, are helpful in selected patients. Heat is good for relieving morning stiffness and muscle spasm and can be accomplished with an early morning shower, the use of an electric blanket or sleeping bag, or the use of a heated water bed. Adequate rest is important, but prolonged bed rest is contraindicated.

Splinting is helpful in maintaining functional position, particularly of wrists and knees. Splints can be made from either plaster or plastic material; appropriate fit is important. Splints are most beneficial when worn at night to rest the joints. Dynamic splints and serial casting are helpful in selected patients. Elastic joint supports help protect knees or ankles during vigorous activity. Fitted soft cervical collars may relieve cervical spine discomfort and help maintain good posture. Firm collars may be required in the child with C1–2 subluxation. Crutches or a cane temporarily reduce the load on a painful hip or knee to permit continued mobility. Orthotic devices such as metatarsal bars, heel cushions, and medial arch supports are often useful.

Surgery

A small number of children ultimately require artificial joint replacement. Hip and knee replacements are the most common and the most successful. Other surgical procedures, such as soft tissue release of contractures, correction of micrognathia, synovectomy, and cervical spine stabilization, may be helpful in selected patients.

Eye Disease

Periodic eye examination by an ophthalmologist, including slit-lamp examination, is required every 4 to 6 months to prevent injury from chronic iridocyclitis, which is often asymptomatic in the young child and is associated with JRA in 10 to 15% of patients.* Known risk factors for iridocyclitis include young age (less than 6 years), arthritis pattern (pauciarticular onset), and a positive ANA. Activity of eye disease does not correlate with arthritis activity. If detected early, iridocyclitis usually responds to topical corticosteroids and mydriatic agents. Progressive eye disease may require oral corticosteroid therapy. Adjunctive NSAID therapy may reduce the eye disease activity. Complications of chronic iridocyclitis include cataracts, glaucoma, and blindness.

GENERAL ISSUES OF CHRONIC DISEASE

JRA is a chronic disease, and there are several generic issues important to optimal management. Compliance with the medical regimen, including medication, an exercise program, and splinting, is a problem. Most children respond to simple behavior management strategies, particularly if instituted early. Parents should be encouraged to treat their children with JRA as normally as possible. Extremes should be avoided, such as being insensitive to the child's needs or being overindulgent. Depression and low self-esteem may require specific psychosocial intervention, especially in the teenager. Family counseling may be indicated.

The nutritional aspects of chronic disease are best addressed with careful monitoring of the child's growth parameters and periodic dietary surveillance. Children may require iron, calcium, or caloric supplementation. No special diet is needed, but a well-balanced one with adequate calories to account for any increased metabolic need is appropriate.

Education is an ongoing need for both the parent and the child. The child needs to have information regarding the disease and its treatment, and the goals of the treatment should be reiterated and modified as age-appropriate. The child should attend school regularly and particpate in a regular or alternative physical education program if at all possible. Federal law requires that schools provide adequate programs for children with special needs (Public Law 94-142). Communication between the family and the school is of major importance to optimize the child's educational experience. Individual education programs (IEPs) or privileges such as an elevator pass, two sets of books (home and school), the use of a tape recorder, or assistance at lunch may be needed. Educational materials are available from the Arthritis Foundation and American Juvenile Arthritis Organization.

The multiple aspects of care of the child with JRA are best dealt with by close cooperation between the primary physician and a health care team with expertise in the care of the child with arthritis including a nurse specialist, occupational and physical therapist, dietician, psychologist, dentist, ophthalmologist, and orthopedist.

The overall prognosis for a child with JRA is good. Ten to 15 years after disease onset, up to 75% of the children are in remission. Most of these children have a polycyclic course with periods of disease remissions and exacerbations. The highest risk for long-term deformity is in patients with seropositive polyarticular disease or persistent polyarticular disease after systemic onset. Deformity involving wrists and hips is of particular concern and may progress in spite of relatively good disease control.

Other complications include growth disturbances, particularly leg length discrepancy, micrognathia, and scoliosis. The mortality from JRA in the United States is less than 1%, usually secondary to systemic infection associated with immune suppressive therapy or rarely amyloidosis.

ANKYLOSING SPONDYLITIS

method of
GLEN T. D. THOMSON, M.D.,
SAMUEL MARK STEINFIELD, B.Sc.,
  B.M.R.(P.T.), and
RON MATTHEW GALL, B.M.R.(P.T.)
*University of Manitoba Pan Am Sports Medicine
  Center*
Winnipeg, Manitoba, Canada

Ankylosing spondylitis (AS) is an inflammatory systemic disease that affects predominantly the spine and sacroiliac joints. AS is a member of a larger family of disorders

---

*See American Academy of Pediatrics Section on Rheumatology and Section on Ophthalmology: Guidelines for ophthalmologic examinations in children with juvenile rheumatoid arthritis. Pediatrics *92*:295–296, 1993.

The support of the Arthritis Society of Canada is gratefully acknowledged.

TABLE 1. **Spondyloarthropathy Family**

Predominant axial joint arthritis
  AS
  AS associated with ulcerative colitis or Crohn's disease
  AS associated with psoriasis
Predominant peripheral joint arthritis
  Reactive arthritis following dysentery (*Salmonella, Shigella, Yersinia, Campylobacter*)
  Reactive arthritis following venereal infection (*Chlamydia, Ureaplasma*)
  BASE (*B*27, *a*rthritis, *s*acroiliitis, *e*nthesitis) (same clinical disease as reactive arthritis but no antecedent clinical infection)

Abbreviation: AS = ankylosing spondylitis.

known as the spondyloarthropathies (SpA), which include both postinfectious "reactive arthritis" and arthropathies associated with inflammatory bowel disease and psoriasis (Table 1). Many clinical and laboratory features overlap the specific disease designations in the SpA (Table 2). HLA-B27 transgenic rat research has demonstrated this interaction of host genetic type, microbial infection, and gut inflammation in the etiopathogenesis of SpA.

AS affects between 0.1 and 0.2% of the white population and is recognized more frequently in men (3:1). The incidence of AS follows the frequency of HLA-B27 in the population. Even though more than 90% of AS patients have the HLA-B27 phenotype, only 1 or 2% of those with HLA-B27 develop AS. This increases tenfold if a first-degree relative has AS.

CLINICAL FEATURES AND COURSE

AS usually begins insidiously in the individual's late teens or early twenties as alternating or bilateral buttock pain or thoracolumbar pain. The patient awakes at night because of back pain. The morning stiffness improves with exercise and with nonsteroidal anti-inflammatory drugs (NSAIDs) but not with analgesics alone. It is unusual for peripheral joint arthritis to be present at the onset except in adolescent patients. The presence of extra-articular features of SpA or a positive family history of SpA may raise the index of suspicion of AS (see Table 2).

There is a spectrum of severity in AS from asymptomatic radiologic sacroiliitis to complete ankylosis of the axial skeleton (bamboo spine). Peripheral joint arthritis complicates 10% of cases of AS and is usually confined to girdle joints (hips and shoulders). Individuals in whom there is an early age of onset, hip arthritis, and failure to respond to medication have a worse long-term prognosis.

Arthritis of the costotransverse and costospinal joints may lead to restriction of chest expansion, although there is minimal impairment of breathing in nonsmokers. Arthritis of the costosternal, manubriosternal, sternoclavicular, and acromioclavicular joints is also frequent.

Iritis can occur in up to 30% of AS patients at some point in their lives. The iritis is primarily associated with the HLA-B27 phenotype, not the AS.

Among the less frequent manifestations of AS are aortic insufficiency and cardiac conduction defects. Upper lobe pulmonary fibrosis may occur and may be complicated by infections such as aspergillosis. Cauda equina syndrome with saddle anesthesia and characteristic diverticula on myelography is a late manifestation of AS, as is secondary amyloidosis.

Many patients remain functional and continue to work despite chronic pain and physical limitations. Prolonged inflammatory back pain and consequent inactivity result in additional mechanical back pain. The typical alteration of posture results in muscle imbalances, such as lengthening of antigravity muscles and shortening of their antagonists, resulting in joint contracture.

The longevity of patients with AS is reduced by systemic complications such as amyloidosis. Fractures of the cervical spine due to minor trauma may lead to spinal cord damage, quadriplegia, and death.

INVESTIGATIONS

Laboratory tests are nonspecific. The erythrocyte sedimentation rate (ESR) is elevated in 75% of patients, especially those with peripheral joint arthritis. Other acute phase reactants, such as C-reactive protein, are elevated, and the serum IgA may be mildly to moderately elevated. The rheumatoid factor and antinuclear antibody test are negative. HLA-B27 typing is costly and is seldom helpful because of the high frequency (10%) of well individuals with HLA-B27 in typical white populations.

Plain radiographs of the sacroiliac joints or other spinal joints are usually normal for several years after the onset of symptoms. Nuclear medicine scans are more sensitive to early change but are not specific. Computed tomography (CT) and magnetic resonance imaging (MRI) may demonstrate early erosive changes of the sacroiliac joints and are the most definitive (albeit costly) early investigations.

MANAGEMENT

The goals of therapy are (1) to reduce pain and stiffness and (2) to maintain good posture and range of motion. The physiotherapy program (Table 3) is facilitated by NSAID therapy (Table 4). Phenylbuta-

TABLE 2. **Features of Spondyloarthropathy Family**

Clinical Features

Axial arthritis or sacroiliitis: low back, alternating buttock, or thoracolumbar junction pain lasting more than 3 months
Oligoarthritis: high frequency of lower limb, asymmetrical involvement (but not exclusively)
Enthesitis: plantar fasciitis, Achilles enthesitis
Dactylitis: "sausage" digit
Ocular inflammation: iritis, conjunctivitis (in reactive arthritis)
Mucocutaneous inflammation: psoriasis, balanitis, keratoderma, blennorrhagia
Bowel inflammation: Crohn's disease, ulcerative colitis, or subclinical inflammation on ileocolonoscopy
Urologic inflammation: sterile urethritis, sterile prostatitis
Family history: AS, reactive arthritis or Reiter's syndrome, psoriasis, Crohn's disease, or ulcerative colitis
Infectious history: antecedent nongonococcal venereal infection or dysenteric infection within previous 6 weeks

Laboratory Features

Seronegative: negative tests for rheumatoid factor and antinuclear antibody
HLA-B27: present in more than 90% of cases of idiopathic AS but in only 50 to 75% of patients in whom antecedent infection or associated disease (psoriasis, Crohn's disease, ulcerative colitis) is present
Radiologic sacroiliitis: spectrum of changes from joint line erosions (earliest) to joint space "pseudo-widening" and reactive sclerosis, culminating in complete joint ankylosis

Abbreviation: AS = ankylosing spondylitis.

TABLE 3. **Physiotherapy Programs**

1. Education*
   The disease
   Posture, body mechanics, resting and sleeping positions
   Modification of activity and exercise during exacerbation
   Appropriate sporting activities (e.g., swimming)
   Proper use of heat and ice
2. Prevention of contractures
   Specific stretching and strengthening exercises
3. Reduction of pain and inflammation
   Ultrasound, electrical stimulation, acupuncture
4. Maintenance or improvement of range of motion
   Manual therapy techniques (e.g. passive joint mobilization
   and muscle stretching)

*Additional educational materials available from the Arthritis Foundation, the Ankylosing Spondylitis Association, and the Arthritis Society (Canada).

zone was commonly used in the past but has been abandoned because of rare but life-threatening hematologic side effects. Salicylates are not of much therapeutic benefit in AS or other SpA.

Use of second-line drugs in refractory cases should be considered with the help of a rheumatologist (Table 5). Sulfasalazine (Azulfidine) 1 gram orally twice daily for 3 months may improve symptoms. Increasing the dose to 3 grams per day for an additional 3 months may be necessary if the response is suboptimal. The dose at which the patient becomes asymptomatic should be maintained for an additional 3 to 4 months. If the patient remains asymptomatic, tapering the dose by 500 mg every 4 months to a dose of 1 gram per day may be desirable.

Methotrexate (Rheumatrex) in oral doses of 7.5 to 15 mg per week may also be helpful in treating patients with refractory AS. Gold therapy (Myochrysine, Ridaura) or hydroxychloroquine (Plaquenil) has been used in patients with refractory peripheral joint arthritis.

Refractory peripheral joint monarthritis, sacroiliitis, and enthesitis may respond to corticosteroid injection. When no bony changes are evident on radiographs, cervical spine restriction of range of motion may be improved by aggressive physiotherapy

TABLE 4. **NSAID Therapy**

Choose a nonsalicylate NSAID: indomethacin (Indocin), naproxen (Naprosyn), diclofenac (Voltaren), tenoxicam (Mobiflex),* piroxicam (Feldene), ketoprofen (Orudis), sulindac (Clinoril), tolmetin (Tolectin), flurbiprofen (Ansaid), ibuprofen (Motrin, Advil), fenoprofen (Nalfon)
Prescribe full dose
Do *not* use combinations of NSAIDs
Use time-release formulations or suppository to treat night pain and morning stiffness
Trial period for an NSAID is 2–3 weeks minimum
Switch to another NSAID if previous response is suboptimal
Add cytoprotective agent if there is a high risk for ulcer
Allow reduction or cessation of therapy after several months to determine efficacy of current NSAID
Educate patient about the benefits and potential risks of NSAIDs

*Not available in the United States.
Abbreviation: NSAID = nonsteroidal anti-inflammatory drug.

TABLE 5. **Indications for Second-Line Therapy in AS**

1. Failure to achieve control of peripheral joint arthritis
2. Failure to achieve control of axial symptoms with NSAIDs
   IF
   a. Early disease is present (within 5 years of onset) *or*
   b. Increased ESR, C-reactive protein, or serum IgA is present *or*
   c. Axial symptoms with minimal or no radiologic ankylosis and/or positive bone scan

Abbreviations: AS = ankylosing spondylitis; ESR = erythrocyte sedimentation rate; NSAID = nonsteroidal anti-inflammatory drug.

and a short course of systemic corticosteroids: prednisone 0.5 mg per kg per day given orally for a week followed by a rapid taper during the following week, or intramuscular methylprednisolone acetate (Depo-Medrol) 2 mg per kg. Pulsed intravenous corticosteroids (methylprednisolone sodium succinate [Solu-Medrol] 1 gram intravenously daily for one to three doses) may provide short-term benefit to patients with refractory systemic AS. Systemic daily oral corticosteroids should not be used as long-term therapy for AS.

Analgesics and muscle relaxants can be used as adjunctive therapy for AS, particularly in patients who are disturbed by night pain. Amitriptyline (Elavil) 10 to 50 mg orally at bedtime may also be helpful in encouraging sleep and relieving pain.

COMPLICATIONS

Iritis

Immediate referral to an ophthalmologist is warranted to confirm the diagnosis and begin therapy with topical corticosteroids and mydriatic or cycloplegic eye drops. Refractory cases may require systemic corticosteroids.

Suspected Spinal Fracture

Plain radiographs may not immediately reveal a fracture. Tomography, CT, MRI, or bone scan may be necessary to rule out a fracture. Referral to a spinal trauma specialist is advisable.

Total Hip Replacement

There is an increased risk of heterotopic ossification in AS patients. Postoperative radiation should be considered as prophylaxis.

ASSOCIATED DISEASES

Inflammatory Bowel Disease

Treatment of the bowel disease medically or surgically will not influence the course of AS. NSAIDs may exacerbate bowel inflammation, but NSAIDs absorbed in the proximal gut may be better tolerated than slow-release or enteric preparations.

An acute self-limited peripheral joint arthritis is

seen in 5% of Crohn's disease patients. NSAIDs or intra-articular injections are sufficient to relieve the symptoms. Successful treatment of the underlying bowel disease terminates the acute arthritis.

Psoriasis

The activity of the skin disease does not influence the course of AS. Sulfasalazine (Azulfidine) therapy sometimes results in significant skin improvement.

Psoriatic arthritis of the peripheral joints can be initially treated with NSAIDs. In refractory cases, methotrexate may cause improvement in both the joint and the skin diseases.

Reactive Arthritis

Postdysenteric and postvenereal reactive arthritis may be a self-limited disease of less than 6 months' duration or may become a chronic arthritis characterized by a waxing and waning course. The presence of Reiter's triad (conjunctivitis, urethritis, and arthritis) at onset is more frequent in postvenereal reactive arthritis. Acute flares usually respond to the same NSAIDs used for AS. A 3-month course of tetracycline 250 mg orally four times per day or minocycline (Minocin) 100 mg orally twice a day may be successful in treating refractory cases of postvenereal reactive arthritis. Sulfasalazine in the same doses used for AS may be helpful in patients with chronic reactive arthritis.

TEMPOROMANDIBULAR DISORDERS

method of
H. T. PERRY, D.D.S., Ph.D.
Northwestern University Dental School
Chicago, Illinois

The temporomandibular joints (TMJs) are located at each end of the mandible and are actively involved in speech, mastication, deglutition, and facial expression, as well as other lower facial movements and functions. As in all other joints in the body, the movements of the TMJs depend on muscle contraction with capsular and ligament guidance and limitation. The combination of the jaws, jaw joints, teeth, tongue, and associated musculature is referred to as the "stomatognathic system." Disturbances in the normal or accepted function of this system have accumulated a series of terms or classifications over the years: Costen's syndrome, myofascial pain dysfunction syndrome, TMJ pain dysfunction syndrome, oromandibular pain dysfunction syndrome, and craniomandibular dysfunction syndrome. Today, the most common and generally accepted term is "temporomandibular disorders" (TMD).

ANATOMY

The TMJs are classified as ginglymoarthrodial—a combination of a hinge and a sliding joint. The extensive function range may well contribute to some of the components of TMD. The articular surfaces are lined with fibrocartilage as opposed to the hyaline cartilage of most other joints. The articular portion of the mandible, the condyle, is seated in the glenoid fossa with an interposed fibrous disk. This disk has a biconcave shape in the anteroposterior plane. The disk comprises three zones: (1) the anterior band, which is fused to the capsule of the TMJ; (2) the intermediate zone, the thinnest portion of the disk; and (3) the posterior zone, the thickest portion of the disk, which is attached in a bilaminar fashion, the posterosuperior attachment of which is fibroelastic and attaches to the posterior articular lip, the postglenoid process, and the tympanosquamosal fissure. The posteroinferior portion is more fibrous and vascular. It attaches to the posterior portion of the condylar neck, just inferior to the articular tissues.

The articular capsule and ligaments are important in normal functional support of the TMJ. The fibrous portion of the capsule is attached to the squamous temporal bone along the lines of the articular surface of the articular eminence and fossa. The articular capsule is quite thin medially, posteriorly, and anteromedially but thicker laterally and anterolaterally. The heavier lateral portion of the capsule is termed the "temporomandibular ligament."

The synovial system of this joint lines all structures of the articulation that are not subject to compression. The greatest concentration of synovium is found in the upper and lower surfaces of the bilaminar zone and the connective tissue at the posterior attachment of the disk to the capsule.

The blood supply to the disk and capsule is primarily via the superficial temporal artery. The proprioceptive and nociceptive nerves of the capsule and periphery of the disk are supplied by the auriculotemporal, deep temporal, and masseteric branches of the trigeminal nerve.

Four primary muscle pairs are responsible for the majority of mandibular movement: (1) the masseter muscles, (2) the temporalis muscles, (3) the medial pterygoids, and (4) the lateral pterygoids. They are innervated by the third division of the trigeminal nerve.

SIGNS AND SYMPTOMS

A simple evaluation triad summarizes the signs and symptoms of this disorder:

1. Joint sounds with jaw movement (past or present)
   a. Clicking, snapping, popping
   b. Crepitus, crepitation
2. Mandibular movement alteration
   a. Deviation in opening or closing
   b. Limitation in opening or closing
   c. Irregular movement patterns in function
3. Pain with jaw movement
   a. Arthrogenous
   b. Myogenous

Some professionals consider excessive tooth wear as another diagnostic sign. It is believed that such tooth wear is possible evidence of parafunctional jaw use, such as gnashing of the teeth (bruxism), clenching of the teeth, or other oral habits that involve lip, cheek, or tongue biting.

PREVALENCE

General population studies in the United States and abroad have concluded that nearly 70% of the population will experience some of the signs and symptoms of this triad during their lifetime. However, the percentage having symptoms severe enough to warrant treatment has been shown to be as low as 6%. The greatest frequency of occurrence appears to be in the age group from 20 to 40 years. In most studies reported, the majority of patients are female, outnumbering males by a ratio of 8 : 1. Since such a general prevalence of signs and symptoms exists, the present rationale is to avoid treatment for symptoms other than pain. Many clinicians believe that patients with TMD signs and symptoms should be evaluated and monitored inasmuch as some may develop pain associated with a progression of other symptoms.

The significance of various signs in conjunction with pain provides an indication to the clinician for possible therapy. The two principal sources of pain are those of the masticatory muscles (myogenous) and those of the joint, intracapsular and extracapsular (arthrogenous). Frequently the two pain types will overlap and thus create a third, less distinct, nociceptive pattern.

Tenderness to palpation of the elevator muscles of the mandible, as well as other cranial and cervical muscles, is the most commonly noted muscle pain, subjectively described by the patient as a dull ache to sharp, shooting pain. When the temporalis is involved, it is reported as a "headache."

It should be stressed that many of the muscle symptoms are self-limiting and transient; they may fluctuate with general health changes or with periods of stress.

Arthrogenous pain is often the result of intracapsular disk displacement. This is the most common arthropathy of the TMJ. Frequently, the patient will exhibit a click on mouth opening and a subtle soft click on closure. This is classified as a reciprocal displacement with reduction, as the disk returns to its more normal condyle-fossa position. That position, as determined with magnetic resonance imaging (MRI) and arthrographic studies, would place the disk on top of the condyle, with its thickest posterior band at the superior surface of the condyle. This has been called the "12 o'clock position." Other studies have noted slight normal variations to anterior, posterior, medial, or lateral of this "ideal" location. Longitudinal epidemiologic studies have indicated that there may be a progressive pattern with disk displacement. The first stage is characterized by the reciprocal click. Later there is disk displacement without reduction and possible locking. Then there is a period of articular and muscle pain with movement restriction. The terminal stage is characterized by crepitation and mandibular movement restriction, which in most instances is later accompanied by a slow resolution of symptoms. This typical sequence emphasizes that initial extensive therapy should be avoided and the therapist should direct treatment efforts toward the relief of pain with supportive efforts to provide range-of-motion improvement and jaw stability.

CAUSE

Many theories of cause have evolved over the years. Several of the proposals have been discarded with research and clinical experience. At present, there is consensus among those who treat TMD patients that a spectrum of factors may exist that have a bearing over time on the occurrence and continuance of the TMD signs and symptoms. In the broader scope of TMD, just as for any other bodily affliction, causative factors relate to the patient's physical status, including that of the dentition; the patient's behavioral responses to life's events; and the patient's psychosocial status.

Most clinicians cite predisposing factors in considering cause; this includes any processes that could initiate un-

usual masticatory function and create the possibility of TMD. There are often precipitating factors that in association with the predisposing element will initiate TMD. Most common of these is immediate trauma to the face or jaws. This may occur in many forms, from the macrotrauma of a direct blow to the mandible or side of the face to the microtrauma related to abnormal joint/muscle loading in mastication, yawning and stretching, extended mouthpiece use in diving or contact sports, long dental appointments with an open mouth, excessive mandibular opening stretch (as in cheerleaders and singers), unusual or abnormal masticatory loading (as in extended periods of gum chewing), and the parafunctional/nonmasticatory jaw movements associated with grinding or clenching of the teeth and other oral habits. These are but some of the major precipitating factors that have been cited. Undoubtedly, there are others.

Once the patient experiences the TMD problem, acknowledged perpetuating factors, if continued, will adversely affect the therapist's efforts to resolve the patient's problem. Inclusive in this category are any of the precipitating factors as well as the patient's stress or emotional response to the disturbance. Thus, exacerbation of the symptoms can result in the patient's noncompliance with the therapist's instructions.

In addition to these suspected causative factors, other local or systemic disturbances may create symptom/sign overlap or mimic the basic TMD symptoms. The possibility of their occurrence emphasizes the need for a clear differential diagnosis to positively identify the patient's problems as TMD prior to initiation of therapy. Some of the factors that may contribute to, mimic, or exacerbate the TMD symptoms are outlined in Table 1.

TABLE 1. **Local and Systemic Disturbances That May Complicate Diagnosis of Temporomandibular Disorders**

I. Arthritis
  A. Traumatic
  B. Infectious
  C. Inflammatory
    1. Rheumatoid
    2. Still's disease (juvenile rheumatoid arthritis)
    3. Ankylosing spondylitis
    4. Psoriatic
    5. Reiter's syndrome
  D. Autoimmune disorders and mixed connective tissue disease
    1. Scleroderma
    2. Sjögren's syndrome
    3. Lupus erythematosus
  E. Degenerative
  F. Metabolic crystal–induced
    1. Gout
    2. Hyperuricemia
II. Neural (components)
  A. Odontogenic—toothache
  B. Phantom tooth pain—atypical odontalgia
  C. Vascular—temporal arteritis
  D. Sinus disease
  E. Oral dysesthesia—burning mouth syndrome
  F. Aural pain
  G. Ophthalmic pain
  H. Intracranial lesions
  I. Cluster headaches
  J. Migraine headaches
  K. Hormonal headaches
  L. Salivary gland disturbances

PATIENT EVALUATION

The physician can often utilize the patient's subjective assessment of symptoms to objectively evaluate the nature of the complaint. A simple questionnaire is given to the patient to fill out (Table 2).

A brief examination of the patient's stomatognathic function is easily conducted by the physician. The patient is asked to slowly open the mouth as far as possible without pain. The normal range of such a movement in the adult is from 47 to 52 mm (approximately the width of the three middle fingers). If there is deviation from one side to another or a restriction in opening, it should be noted and evaluated for pain. Joint sounds can often be evaluated by light finger pressure over the temporomandibular ligament just anterior to the external auditory meatus. Frequently, a more accurate evaluation may be made with a stethoscope or by placing the little finger gently in the auditory meatus when the jaw is moved.

Palpation of the temporal and masseter muscles often provides the examiner with evidence of taut, sore muscle areas or of a subjective response of muscle pain to pressure.

It is important to evaluate the patient's dental health as well as current and past dental experiences with the pain and dysfunction symptoms. A thorough knowledge of some of the significant disturbances that mimic TMD (see Table 1) is essential in making an accurate diagnosis.

Imaging of the jaw and TMJs may be indicated when a degenerative disturbance is suspected or gross facial asymmetries exist. The occurrence of disk displacement with self-reduction can accurately be determined by physical examination and jaw movement patterns. This would not appear on radiographs, but would be noted by an arthrogram or MRI scan. The latter is most often reserved for presurgical diagnosis. The existence of crepitus frequently suggests arthropathy, and if the bone destruction or bone alterations are significant, radiographs would confirm it.

Many practitioners and clinics utilize the diagnostic skills and tests of a behaviorist to thoroughly evaluate and examine the chronic TMD patient. Specific personality evaluation tests are available, and their value in the total diagnosis has been confirmed in both research and the literature.

MANAGEMENT

Pain is the most consistent complaint of patients seeking treatment. The many possible facial/cranial causes of pain necessitate a gradual and conservative treatment approach. An improper diagnosis with aggressive procedures may exacerbate the patient's problem. The primary goals of the physician are to properly recognize the problem, to prevent those factors that aggravate the problem, to provide proper maintenance and support to the patient and the patient's jaw structure, and to manage and control those features of function or health that have created the problem.

Home care instruction should include the application of moist heat to the area of the muscle pain; elimination of hard or chewy foods; and voluntary restriction of jaw movement in yawning, singing, and chewing. The health professional may find it necessary to prescribe mild medications such as nonsteroidal anti-inflammatories, muscle relaxants, and/or aspirin.

In the patient examination, evidence indicating the need for a dental orthotic is often found. This intraoral appliance is fabricated to fit either the upper or the lower teeth of the patient. The purpose is to provide stability to the bite when the teeth are closed together in occlusion. The most frequently recommended and utilized orthotic fits the maxillary teeth. Some practitioners use a soft vinyl orthotic for patients when tooth clenching is suspected as the cause of the muscle or joint pain. These appliances are custom designed by the dentist for the patient. They are usually worn full-time with removal only at mealtime. Their purpose is to reduce imbalance or abnormal loading on the joints and to provide some balance of the occlusion for muscle relief. These appliances are not designed for long-term wear. If worn for several months without constant monitoring by the dentist, they can cause irreversible changes to the patient's dentition, which adds to the patient's jaw problems.

The management of more severe intracapsular disk problems has been addressed recently with the orthopedic procedures of arthrocentesis and arthroscopic surgery. Arthroplastic surgery has been utilized for the most severe degenerative joint problems. However, the success of these measures has been reported as minimal.

The majority of patients with a true TMD problem respond satisfactorily to conservative therapy, home care, and time. The small percentage of those diagnosed with TMD that involves intracapsular changes with disk breakdown, fibrocartilage destruction, and bony condylar lesions and change should be managed in a true orthopedic manner by qualified and competent oral/maxillofacial surgeons.

Many patients diagnosed with TMD who fail to respond to the conservative therapy described may fit the chronic pain patient category. These patients may need the total commitment of a chronic pain clinic, with the possible use of physical therapy, biofeedback, pharmacologic therapy, and psychological counseling.

TABLE 2. **Brief Patient Temporomandibular Disorders Questionnaire**

1. Do you have difficulty or pain while chewing or talking?
2. Does your jaw hurt when you yawn?
3. Do you have difficulty in closing your teeth together?
4. Do you have pain in the jaw when you awaken?
5. Do you have difficulty in getting the jaw to move in the morning?
6. Do you now or did you ever hear sounds in the joint with jaw movement?
7. Do you have jaw muscle (cheek) pain?
8. Do you have temporal pain, headaches?
9. Do you have pain, soreness in the teeth?
10. Do you clench your teeth during the day?
11. Have you been made aware of tooth grinding during sleep?
12. Do you recall a blow or trauma to your face or jaw prior to your present complaints?

BURSITIS, TENDINITIS, MYOFASCIAL PAIN, AND FIBROMYALGIA

method of
LAWRENCE F. LAYFER, M.D., and
CALVIN R. BROWN, JR., M.D.
Rush Medical College
Chicago, Illinois

Soft tissue pain, rather than true arthritis, is the most common musculoskeletal reason for a patient to see a physician. Our lifestyles frequently lead to minor traumas or repetitive stress, which may precipitate such injuries. These are divided into tendinitis, bursitis, myofascial pain syndromes, or fibromyalgia, classified more on the basis of anatomic considerations and associated symptoms than on laboratory testing. Therefore, a knowledge of the location of bursae and tendons commonly involved with these inflammations, as well as the common sites of "trigger points" in myofascitis, is crucial to appropriate diagnosis. These syndromes have similar treatment plans, and once learned for a single site they can be extended to other sites easily. Systemic symptoms associated with widespread tenderness suggest the fibromyalgia syndrome rather than a regional disorder. The illness has its own special treatments.

BURSITIS AND TENDINITIS

Bursitis and tendinitis are often secondary to acute or chronic, repetitive trauma. They sometimes result from abnormal body mechanics during work or recreation. Tendinitis or tenosynovitis often results from prolonged or repetitive tasks. Failure to condition properly before a sport or activity can lead to soft tissue injury, particularly for the older recreational athlete. These conditions are commonly described and frequently observed, yet there is little objective scientific study of them. Therefore, much of what follows is based on clinical observation rather than controlled trial.

A careful history is essential to establish the diagnosis, with emphasis on work habits, leisure activities, and body mechanics. Physical examination must include attention to factors such as body habitus, posture, and maneuvers that reproduce or accentuate pain. Most of these disorders cannot be diagnosed by radiology or laboratory tests. When a diagnosis of bursitis or tendinitis is considered, the physician must carefully palpate the involved area for localized tenderness. When pain overlies a joint, synovitis or an internal derangement must be considered.

Some general concepts of therapy apply to this group of disorders as a whole. Most respond to rest, local protection, and so-called counterirritants such as ice. The mnemonic "RICE," for *r*est, *i*ce, *c*ompression, and *e*levation, is particularly useful to recall for acute treatment. Ice, in particular, when applied promptly may prevent excessive bleeding or soft tissue swelling. Nonsteroidal anti-inflammatory drugs (NSAIDs) and salicylates may be useful, but drug therapy should not be the only method of treatment.

Local injections of corticosteroid combined with 1 to 5 mL of procaine or lidocaine often quickly reduce symptoms. The crystalline preparations triamcinolone acetonide (Kenalog) or methylprednisolone acetate (Depo-Medrol) are preferred, and never more than 40 mg should be administered to one site. When used judiciously and infrequently, and never when there is sepsis, this form of therapy has proved safe and effective in controlled clinical trials as well as in extensive clinical use. Measures to relieve pain and inflammation must be followed by therapeutic exercise and correction of causative biomechanical factors. Individualized exercises are an integral part of management and are often overlooked or underutilized by treating physicians. The clinician can direct the patient in the performance of simple exercise with adequate instruction, or the services of a physical therapist can be utilized, particularly because the excercise program must be modified as it continues. The patient must be educated to understand that pain relief may depend upon a conscientious program of therapy and exercise over an adequate period of time, often several weeks or months. It should be emphasized to patients that routine day-to-day activities are not an adequate substitute for prescribed exercise.

Tendinitis

Tendons may tear or be partially ruptured but are not truly inflamed. Thus, the term *tendinitis* actually refers to inflammation of the peritendinous tissues or the synovial sheaths surrounding them, properly referred to as tenosynovitis. This distinction is important because corticosteroid should be injected into the surrounding tissues or synovial sheath and not the tendon itself. Injection directly into the tendon, particularly if repeated, can lead to weakening and rupture of the tendon. Most instances of tendinitis result from overuse or unaccustomed activity; thus rest, splinting, or both are important therapeutic modalities.

Bursitis

Bursae lie either superficially, where their swelling and inflammation can be felt, or deep, where involvement must be inferred from pain referral patterns and exacerbation by movement of associated structures. Bursitis is rarely visualized on imaging studies, including radiography and magnetic resonance imaging. When possible, aspiration of fluid can be helpful for diagnosis; if the fluid is not clear, it should be sent to the laboratory for culture. For noninfective bursitis, rest combined with use of an NSAID for at least 1 week after symptoms have abated is effective. If more rapid relief of symptoms is sought, injection of a mixture of 1 mL of a long-acting steroid such as triamcinolone (Aristospan), betamethasone (Celestone), or methylprednisolone (Depo-Medrol), combined with 1 to 3 mL of 1% lidocaine, can be given. Septic bursitis is usually due to *Staphylococcus aureus*, particularly in immunocompromised hosts. Systemic treatment with oral dicloxacillin may be effective in mild cases; in more severe cases or in immunocompromised patients, intravenous antibiotics for 7 to 10 days, combined with needle or open surgical drainage, are required.

Regional Syndromes

Shoulder

Rotator cuff tendinitis is perhaps the most common cause of shoulder pain. Because the subacromial bursa and rotator cuff tendons are so close, often the two structures are involved, which is referred to as the "impingement syndrome," and specific differentiation is clinically impossible. This tendinitis is believed to result from repetitive trauma and compression of the bursa and tendons between the humeral head below and the inferior surface of the acromion above the impingement. With impingement syndrome, the patient complains of a painful arc of from 60 to 120 degrees of abduction. Pain is also reproduced or exacerbated by simultaneous forward flexion and internal rotation of the shoulder. Treatment consists of rest and physical therapy modalities, followed by range-of-motion exercises as soon as tolerated. NSAIDs may be beneficial; however, an injection of corticosteroid and anesthetic into the subacromial space is the most frequently effective treatment.

Bicipital tendinitis is manifested by pain in the anterior region of the shoulder and often more diffusely as well. Palpation over the bicipital groove reveals localized tenderness, although both involved and uninvolved sides should be compared because normal tendons can be somewhat tender. Pain can also be reproduced by supination of the forearm against resistance (Yergason's sign) or shoulder flexion against resistance (Speed's test). Bicipital tendinitis and impingement syndrome may coexist. Occasionally the tendon may sublux out of the groove with a sensation of "snapping," particularly when an abducted shoulder is rotated internally and externally. Treatment consists of locally applied ice, rest, and range-of-motion exercises. NSAIDs are useful, and a small amount of corticosteroid injected into the tendon sheath can be helpful.

Elbow Region

The olecranon bursa is frequently involved with bursitis. This can arise secondary to trauma or as an idiopathic condition. Frequently the swelling is great but there is little pain. It is important to note that the elbow range of motion is not lost; if a decrease has occurred, intra-articular involvement must be suspected. The bursa generally should be aspirated if the diagnosis is uncertain. Inflammatory bursitis can occur secondary to gout, pseudogout, or rheumatoid arthritis. Trauma yields a bloody fluid. With septic olecranon bursitis, pain is more frequent, and culture is positive. Aspiration and protection alone

are often effective treatment, but a small amount of corticosteroid can be injected in nonseptic conditions. Septic bursitis requires aspiration, to maintain drainage, and appropriate antibiotics.

Lateral epicondylitis, known as "tennis elbow," is a common occurrence in individuals who use their arms repetitively. Tennis actually accounts for only a small percentage of affected individuals; occupational or other recreational activities are the usual cause. Pain is exacerbated with hand grip, such as a handshake or carrying a briefcase. Localized tenderness over and anterior to the lateral epicondyle is the hallmark. Treatment consists of altering the inciting activity, along with local application of ice and antiinflammatories. A forearm brace can be worn that does not interfere with activities. Ultimately, a steroid injection using a fine-gauge needle may be needed for relief, and surgical excision of the bursa can be considered in the most refractory cases.

Medial epicondylitis, or golfer's elbow, is less common than lateral epicondylitis. Resistance to wrist flexion reproduces the pain, which is felt in the area of the medial epicondyle. In all other respects, the condition is managed similarly to lateral epicondylitis.

Wrist and Hand

De Quervain's tenosynovitis results from repetitive thumb pinches combined with wrist movement. Symptoms include pain, tenderness, and occasional swelling over the radial styloid. Pain can be reproduced by folding the thumb and then deviating the wrist to the ulnar side, known as "Finkelstein's test." Treatment involves local application of ice, splinting, and NSAIDs. Local corticosteroid injection in the abductor pollicis tendon sheath has been shown to be effective in controlled trials.

Tenosynovitis can occur in other flexor or extensor tendons of the wrist in addition to those involved in De Quervain's tenosynovitis. The findings vary depending upon which tendon or group of tendons is involved, usually on either the flexor or extensor side. Pain on resisted movement helps define the involved tendons. Treatment is similar to that for other forms of tendinitis.

Inflammation of the volar flexor tendons of the fingers, the flexor digitorum superficialis and profundus, is extremely common. Pain in the palm is felt with finger flexion and palpation of localized tenderness and swelling of the flexor tendon sheaths. Sometimes a nodule of fibrous tissue develops that can interfere with normal gliding of the tendon within the sheath, producing locking or triggering of a digit. The middle and index fingers are most often involved. This tenosynovitis is seen in conjunction with overuse, osteoarthritis, and rheumatoid arthritis. Injection of long-acting corticosteroid into the tendon sheath is usually effective, although surgery is occasionally necessary.

Hip Region

Trochanteric bursitis is common, but it is often not appreciated and is underdiagnosed. The main symptom is aching pain over the greater trochanter of the hip, but it also can have a radiating quality down the lateral thigh, mimicking radiculopathy. It is important to recognize that true hip joint pathology usually produces pain in the groin, thus helping differentiate these two conditions. The onset is usually gradual, and walking or lying on the hip may intensify the pain. Physical examination reveals point tenderness over the trochanteric area on palpation. External rotation may exacerbate the pain as well, again felt laterally over the trochanter. Calcification of the bursa has been noted occasionally.

Injection with long-acting corticosteroid via a fine-gauge needle of adequate length to fully penetrate the bursal space (up to 3.5 inches of needle length in large patients) is effective. Nonsteroidal drugs, weight loss, and gluteus-strengthening exercises help in management as well.

Iliopsoas bursitis provides an exception to many of the common themes of bursitis elsewhere. This bursa lies deep to the iliopsoas muscle, just anterior to the hip joint and adjacent to the femoral vessels. Thus groin and thigh pain suggestive of true hip joint pathology may be suggested. A limp, and holding of the hip joint in flexion to minimize pain, may be seen. Occasionally, the swelling may be so extensive that a femoral mass can be palpated; otherwise, contrast injection and plain radiography, or magnetic resonance imaging may be necessary to visualize this deep structure. With recurrent involvement, excision may be necessary.

Knee

Anserine bursitis produces pain and tenderness over the medial aspect of the knee just below the joint line. The bursa extends between tendons of the quadriceps muscles that insert below the knee and tibial collateral ligament. It occurs commonly in middle-aged and older women who are overweight and have osteoarthritis of the knee. Rest, stretching of the quadriceps muscles, and corticosteroid injection are effective treatments.

Similar to the olecranon bursa in its superficial location, the prepatellar bursa causes swelling superficial to the kneecap. Thus trauma, either acute or cumulative from kneeling, is a common causative factor. Pain is usually minimal, even in cases of significant swelling. Protection plays an important role in treatment in addition to the other modalities typically used in bursitis. Septic bursitis can result if penetration occurs; as with septic bursitis in the olecranon, aspiration, culture, and appropriate antibiotics should be given.

Patellar tendinitis, also known as jumper's knee, occurs predominantly in athletes who run and jump. Pain and tenderness are localized over the patellar tendon. Rest, ice, and anti-inflammatories are effective; corticosteroid injection is contraindicated, as it has been associated with tendon rupture.

Ankle and Foot

Achilles' tendinitis results from athletic overuse or trauma. It is also associated with systemic inflammatory conditions such as Reiter's syndrome and anklyosing spondylitis. Pain and tenderness, sometimes with associated swelling, occur around the tendon and particularly at its insertion at the calcaneus. In addition to typical management, shoe heel cushions and gentle stretching are helpful. The Achilles tendon is prone to rupture, so caution needs to be emphasized in cases of prolonged or intense inflammation; again, steroid injection is strictly avoided. This tendinitis is frequently associated with plantar fasciitis.

Plantar fasciitis refers to a condition of pain and tenderness on the plantar surface of the heel. The calcaneal bursa also lies in direct contact with the plantar fascia at its insertion on the posterior calcaneus; thus the two conditions are usually inseparable. Trauma from athletic activity, and particularly activity associated with heel striking, is recognized as a precipitating factor. Heel cup cushions, NSAIDs, arch supports, and Achilles' tendon–stretching exercises are useful. Corticosteroid injection is indicated in more severe cases and does not seem to be associated with increased risk for rupture here.

Posterior tibial tendinitis produces pain just posterior to the medial malleolus in the ankle. Eversion, especially against resistance, reproduces pain. Chronic tendon inflammation or systemic inflammation such as rheumatoid arthritis can result in rupture, causing progressive flatfoot. With rupture, the patient will be unable to rise on the ball of the affected foot. Reconstruction can be considered if appropriate.

Fibromyalgia

Fibromyalgia (FM) (fibrositis) is a syndrome of chronic, often disabling, diffuse musculoskeletal aches and pains associated with soft tissue tenderness. A strong female predominance is noted, and any age group is affected (including children), but it most often occurs in young to middle-aged adults. FM is common, being responsible for 20% of rheumatology and 5% of general medical visits. The pains are wide-ranging, and by diagnostic criteria must be in the upper and/or lower bilateral extremities, as well as in the axial skeleton. Tenderness to palpation of at least 11 of 18 "tender points" (symmetrical occiput, upper costochondral, trapezius, lower cervical, supraspinatus, gluteal, lateral epicondyle, greater trochanter, and medial knee fat pad) is needed for diagnosis. Tender points are not pathologic areas, and pain is not limited to these sites. Control points (forehead, anterior thigh, nail bed) may help distinguish malingering. Joint, neural, and muscle examinations are normal except for findings due to incidental concomitant illness. Associated symptoms, such as irritable bowel, headaches, nonrestorative sleep and sleep disturbance, fatigue (similar to chronic fatigue syndrome), paresthesias, and a sense of distal extremity swelling, are common. Laboratory tests are normal.

The differential diagnosis includes systemic illnesses (polymyalgia rheumatica, polymyositis, hypo-thyroid condition, rheumatoid arthritis, Lyme disease, sleep apnea, and so on), as well as local conditions (osteoarthritis, lumbar or cervical radiculopathy). Although most now believe psychologic factors do not cause FM, concomitant depression must be looked for. The etiology remains unknown. Spontaneous and secondary (trauma, infectious) onsets are noted. No histologic abnormalities have been noted, and metabolic muscle abnormalities as the cause of symptoms remain speculative. Abnormalities of stage 4 non–rapid eye movement (REM) sleep are noted, but whether these are a primary cause is unclear. It is currently thought that abnormalities of neurotransmitters, such as substance P and serotonin, point to neurologic abnormalities as the cause.

The treatment approach is multifocused. Tricyclic antidepressants such as amitriptyline (Elavil),* 10 to 50 mg, and muscle relaxers such as cyclobenzaprine (Flexeril), 10 to 20 mg at night, have been shown to be useful in short-term studies, perhaps because of their neurotransmitter-altering abilities. Fluoxetine (Prozac)* may be useful for the same reasons and is frequently used but as yet untested. NSAIDs such as ibuprofen (Motrin) or naproxen (Naprosyn) may be used for pain (not their anti-inflammatory effects), but these have variable efficacy. Long-term side effects, such as ulcer and platelet and renal dysfunction, limit their use in a chronic illness. Acetaminophen (Tylenol), 650 to 1000 mg two to four times a day, can be tried. Narcotics (Darvon or Tylenol No. 3) should be reserved for those unable to tolerate symptoms on other regimens and then in a restricted and controlled manner. Full-dose antidepressants should be used for those with concomitant depression. Psychological therapy for stress management and depression in those patients willing to accept this type of therapy is appropriate. Local injections of 2 to 5 ml of lidocaine (Xylocaine 1%) (with or without a small amount of injectable steroid such as triamcinolone hexacetonide [Aristospan]) into tender or trigger points may be useful. Physical therapy with heat, range-of-motion exercises, and muscle stretching should be tried.

Low-impact aerobics has been found in at least one study to lower pain and is useful for cardiovascular fitness. Sleep evaluations should be attempted. Other modalities, such as biofeedback, transcutaneous electrical nerve stimulators (TENS), and acupuncture may be of value in selected patients. Treatment of local conditions (osteoarthritis, radiculopathy) is important. Since symptoms are chronic, often with poor response to multiple treatment plans, and may be debilitating and disruptive, attention to patient education is important. The nondeforming, noncrippling nature of the illness should be emphasized. Goals should be set for function in daily schedules. Family and coworkers should be talked to. Above all, patients need to feel that they have a trusted and nonjudgmental friend in the physician.

---

*Not FDA-approved for this indication.

Myofascial Pain Syndrome

The myofascial pain syndrome is similar to fibromyalgia in that soft tissues are tender to touch. Both are commonly seen in a primary care setting. However, the pain in myofascial pain syndrome is usually not generalized but regional, and systemic symptoms such as fatigue are not present. The pain on palpation of soft tissue, so typical of fibromyalgia, is present in myofascial illness but tends to be local.

Palpation of the area reveals a contracted muscle with spasm, with an increase in symptoms upon stretching of the muscle. Pain may radiate to a referred area distal to the tender area upon palpation, leading to the designation of these points as trigger points, as opposed to the tender points of fibromyalgia. Common sites of involvement include the trapezius or occipital muscles, leading to referred headaches, and the gluteal area, leading to referred sciatica-like pain, especially when the pain is located near the piriformis muscle.

Treatment includes local injections of Xylocaine, which may be diagnostic as well as therapeutic, followed by stretching of muscle. Local spray coolants such as ethyl chloride before stretching may be useful. Local measures as outlined in other areas of this review may also be used. A search for precipitant causes in the lifestyle of the patient is worthwhile, as avoidance of recurrences may hinge on such discovery.

OSTEOARTHRITIS

method of
ARTHUR L. WEAVER, M.D.
Arthritis Center of Nebraska
Lincoln, Nebraska

Osteoarthritis (OA) is characterized by progressive loss of articular cartilage (narrowing of the joint space), new subchondral bone formation (sclerosis), and formation of new bone at the joint margins (osteophytes). Early clinical features include joint pain aggravated by activity, stiffness after inactivity (gelling), bony enlargement (Heberden's and Bouchard's nodes in the distal and proximal interphalangeal joints, respectively), and occasional low-grade synovitis (perimenopausal females, erosive OA). Late clinical features include instability of the joint, low-grade synovitis owing to degeneration of cartilage and bone, limitation of motion, and functional impairment.

OA is the most prevalent of joint diseases with an economic impact 30-fold greater than that of rheumatoid arthritis. It is the major cause of disability and limitation of activity in our elderly population. The most common joints affected by OA are the distal and proximal interphalangeal joints and the first carpometacarpal joint of the hands, the first metatarsophalangeal joints of the feet, and the hips, knees, and spine. Secondary forms of OA may occur with inflammatory joint disease, physical factors (obesity, trauma, avascular necrosis), and endocrine and metabolic disorders (diabetes, hemochromatosis, gout, and pseudogout).

TREATMENT

The principal objectives in the management of patients with OA are to reassure and educate the patient, to relieve the symptoms of pain and stiffness with minimal risk, to preserve function or minimize functional loss, and to delay progression of the disease.

Patient Education

Patient education and reassurance are of vital importance to the successful management of all rheumatic diseases. It is imperative for patients to understand clearly the chronic nature of OA and to know that the symptoms are generally mild, that the pain can usually be managed effectively, and that the progression of the disease is slow. Patients should be reassured that they do not have an inflammatory condition such as rheumatoid arthritis, and that OA infrequently causes crippling or fatal complications. The Arthritis Foundation publishes a useful educational booklet entitled *Osteoarthritis* and, in addition, can provide the names of nearby rheumatologists, the location of dry land and water exercise programs, and if necessary, a reference to appropriate support groups.

Obese patients should be advised to reduce their weight, thereby reducing the stress on weight-bearing joints. Other than weight reduction, there is no evidence that dietary manipulation has a role in the management of OA.

Prolonged and repeated overuse of involved joints can be detrimental. Thus the need for rest and protection of these joints must be emphasized as one of the most effective ways of alleviating pain and slowing the progression of OA. Periods of daily joint rest should be prescribed in accordance with the location and the extent of joint involvement. The misconception that vigorous exercise is beneficial for an involved joint must be dispelled at the time of initial evaluation. Patients must be advised to modify or avoid stressful activities such as participation in certain sports and recreational activities. Occupational activities must be assessed and, if necessary, modified to prevent disease progression in those patients with significant joint involvement.

Physical and Occupational Therapy

Patients with OA should be involved in an exercise program designed to improve general fitness as well as a program of graduated exercise for involved joints. Such a program has the potential to enhance their general well-being, help maintain cartilage integrity, help prevent muscle atrophy and osteoporosis, decrease muscle spasm, and help maintain a full range of joint motion. Active rather than passive and isometric rather than isotonic exercises are preferred. Joint pain persisting for longer than 45 to 60 minutes after completing a given exercise necessitates that that activity should be modified or discontinued. Moist heat (moist packs, soaks, hydrotherapy, paraffin baths) provides excellent muscle relaxant effects and facilitates an exercise program. Conversely, the use of ice massage to an affected area may relieve the pain in some patients.

Physical and occupational therapists can provide instruction in joint protection, work simplification and modification, energy conservation, postural training, back care, and positions of rest in addition to instruction in exercise programs and methods of heat and cold application. Specific aids (canes, crutches, splints, walkers, cervical collars, braces, corsets, prescription shoes, and orthotics) and assistive devices (grab bars, hand railings, extended and built-up handles, and elevated chairs and toilet seats) can reduce weight-bearing and stress on involved lower extremity joints, reduce pain and stiffness, provide stability, and promote continued independence. Transcutaneous electrical nerve stimulation has been proved to be beneficial in some cases of painful OA of the spine.

Pharmaceutical Agents

The use of pharmaceutical agents in the management of OA is currently controversial. Most of the medications are prescribed for the relief of pain and stiffness and low-grade inflammation. No data exist to suggest that any of the available agents are chondroprotective and in view of the potential toxicity of many of the medications used, a conservative approach seems prudent.

Simple analgesics such as acetaminophen administered on a regular basis are frequently effective in the management of pain in OA. Other analgesics such as tramadol hydrochloride (Ultram), propoxyphene hydrochloride (Darvon), and low-dose codeine may be useful for acute flares, but narcotic preparations should be used cautiously and infrequently.

Nonsteroidal anti-inflammatory drugs (NSAIDs), including aspirin, have been the mainstay of the medical management of OA for several years. The rationale for using NSAIDs has been that they are capable of reducing the inflammation that accompanies the pain and stiffness in this disease.

Salicylates are tolerated by many patients, especially the newer (buffered, delayed-release, enteric-coated, and nonacetylated) forms. The continued search for aspirin substitutes with fewer side effects has resulted in the development of several new NSAIDs. Improved patient compliance has been demonstrated with the newer agents administered only once or twice daily.

Caution is advised with the use of salicylates and NSAIDs in OA. Monitoring for potential side effects is imperative, and the physician must be alert to the risk factors involved in potential gastrointestinal toxicity (elderly, tobacco use, concurrent steroid therapy, previous ulcer disease and treatment, chronic disease states, previous NSAID side effects) and renal toxicity (elderly, hypertensive, diseases associated with decreased circulating blood volume, pre-existing renal dysfunction, and concurrent use of other medication).

A variety of other pharmaceutical agents have been used in OA. Muscle relaxants must be dispensed cautiously but can be used to reduce the muscle spasm adjacent to involved joints. Amitriptyline* may be useful in helping reduce the pain, anxiety, and sleep disturbance often present in these patients. Topical capsaicin (Zostrix) has been reported to provide pain relief in some patients with OA when applied to individual joints.

Intra-Articular Corticosteroids

Systemic corticosteroid therapy clearly has no place in the treatment of OA. However, intra-articular corticosteroid therapy can provide quick and sometimes long-lasting relief when used judiciously in selected patients. Such therapy is adjunctive and most effectively used in patients who have one or two persistently painful and inflamed joints or in those patients with associated crystal deposition disease. Utilizing aseptic technique, larger joints should be aspirated and then injected with a longer-acting steroid preparation such as triamcinolone hexacetonide. In smaller joints, the use of a more soluble preparation such as triamcinolone acetonide reduces the risk of atrophy in the overlying skin. Primary capsular and ligamentous injections in tender areas around involved joints can also be a useful adjunctive therapy. Patients should be advised to rest the injected joint for several days, and a given joint should not be injected more often than once every 4 to 6 months. If no benefit occurs following injection, further steroid injections are best avoided.

Surgery

Surgical intervention in OA is indicated for patients with intractable pain unrelieved by medical measures, significant loss of function, and marked joint instability. Wash-out of the joint can be accomplished by arthroscopy and tidal irrigation. Débridement of cartilage and spurs and removal of loose bodies can be accomplished by arthroscopy and arthrotomy. Bony decompression is occasionally useful in early osteonecrosis and to relieve severe pain. Osteotomy of the knees (if the disease is localized to the medial or lateral compartment) may be an effective temporizing procedure. Total joint arthroplasty is reserved for patients with severe disease of the hip, knee, and occasionally other joints and results in excellent pain relief and near-normal motion in most instances. Total joint replacement should not be utilized to return the patient to a vigorous lifestyle. The patients should be informed prior to surgery of possible complications including thrombophlebitis and pulmonary emboli, nerve injury, infection, and loosening with prosthetic failure. Arthrodesis is of value in patients whose weight or physical activity is too demanding for total joint re-

*Not FDA-approved for this indication.

placement and as a salvage procedure for failed total joint replacement.

Rheumatology Consultation

The primary care physician should be able to provide appropriate care for the majority of patients with OA. The rheumatologist can provide expert assistance in instances of questionable diagnosis, cases of secondary OA, erosive OA, unusual sites of joint involvement (shoulders, elbows, ankles), uncontrolled symptoms, determination of appropriate surgical referral, joint injection therapy, and the possible use of investigational agents that may provide a more direct therapeutic approach in the management of OA.

POLYMYALGIA RHEUMATICA AND GIANT CELL ARTERITIS

method of
JOSEPH G. RENNEY, D.O., and
RICHARD M. SILVER, M.D.
Medical University of South Carolina
Charleston, South Carolina

Two closely associated rheumatic diseases, polymyalgia rheumatica (PMR) and giant cell arteritis (GCA), rarely occur before the sixth decade of life, with peak incidences in the eighth and ninth decades. Women are affected about twice as often as men. The etiology of these two diseases is not understood. There appears to be an association of the HLA-DR4 histocompatibility antigen with both PMR and GCA. Both the cellular and humoral immune systems have been implicated, but not proved to be involved, in the pathogenesis of PMR and GCA. In GCA, there is inflammation in the walls of medium and large arteries, often in association with granulomas consisting of multinucleated histiocytic and foreign body giant cells, collections of lymphocytes, plasma cells, and/or fibroblasts. Granulomas, along with demonstrable immune globulin and complement deposition intracellularly or near the elastic tissue of the arterial wall, suggest a cell-mediated immune reaction to arterial wall antigens. Elevated serum levels of interleukin-6 that decrease with treatment have been found in both PMR and GCA patients. Giant cells are not always apparent on microscopic examination. Pathologic findings in PMR are rare, but muscle biopsy may show a nonspecific Type II muscle atrophy. A transient lymphocytic synovitis involving the knee, sternoclavicular, shoulder, and sacroiliac joints has been described in patients with PMR.

CLINICAL FEATURES

Nonspecific systemic symptoms of PMR and GCA such as fatigue, low-grade fever, and anorexia and weight loss may be abrupt or insidious in onset. Fever in GCA frequently has high spikes that follow no specific pattern. Common clinical features of GCA include a throbbing headache with or without scalp tenderness; visual disturbances such as diplopia, ptosis, and transient (amaurosis fugax) or permanent blindness; and muscle claudication (especially those used in mastication). Jaw claudication is usually asymmetrical and worsens with continued chewing. Neurologic manifestations of GCA are typical of those seen in transient ischemic attacks (TIAs) and cranial neuropathies. Cough (productive or nonproductive), sore throat, hoarseness, angina pectoris, and congestive heart failure are less frequent clinical presentations of GCA. In PMR, high spiking fevers are generally absent. Common features of PMR include arthralgias, myalgias, morning stiffness or "gelling phenomenon," and the aforementioned synovitis. Achiness and nocturnal pain of the proximal limb and axial muscles (shoulder girdle, neck, and/or hips) are classically reported in PMR. Muscle strength is usually preserved, although the pain associated with movement may render muscle testing inaccurate. Muscle atrophy and impaired range of motion may develop later in the disease.

LABORATORY STUDIES

The erythrocyte sedimentation rate (ESR) is usually markedly elevated. Acute phase reactant proteins (fibrinogen, alpha$_2$ globulins), platelets, gamma globulins, and complement components may be increased, and the negative acute phase protein, albumin, may be decreased. A mild to moderate normochromic anemia is commonly present. Leukocyte count and differential, blood urea nitrogen, creatinine, urinalysis, creatine kinase, aldolase, rheumatoid factor, and antinuclear antibodies are either normal or negative. Alkaline phosphatase and aspartate aminotransferase (AST) may be mildly elevated. Electromyograms and muscle biopsy are normal.

DIAGNOSIS

In any patient over the age of 50 years with an elevated ESR, the differential diagnosis should include PMR or GCA. A careful history for any of the clinical features, recent or remote, will help guide the clinician. In those patients with headache, jaw claudication, amaurosis fugax or blindness, TIAs, cranial neuropathies, or angina pectoris, a superficial temporal arterial biopsy should be considered the test of choice to rule out GCA. Even after 7 days of treatment with steroids, the temporal artery histopathology may show features consistent with GCA. Bilateral temporal artery biopsy reduces the rate of false-negative results.

TREATMENT

Nonsteroidal anti-inflammatory drugs or salicylates may be tried as initial treatment in PMR, but in most cases, corticosteroids are required. Treatment with prednisone 5 to 15 mg per day is usually sufficient to suppress the musculoskeletal achiness and stiffness. This dose is not adequate to treat underlying GCA. In patients with suspected or documented GCA, treatment consists of prednisone 0.5 to 1.0 mg per kg per day in divided doses. After 4 to 6 weeks, the dose of prednisone may be reduced slowly if the patient has responded. Steroids should be tapered and discontinued after 1 to 2 years, with treatment resuming at the first clinical sign of disease activity. The prognosis for both diseases, once treated, is generally good. In cases refractory to steroids, treatment with methotrexate or azathioprine may be considered.

OSTEOMYELITIS

method of
RICHARD N. GREENBERG, M.D.
University of Kentucky Medical Center
Lexington, Kentucky

and

JOSE H. SALGADO, M.D., M.P.H.
Newburgh, Indiana

The treatment of osteomyelitis should be scientific (not empirical). Treatment should be based on several important criteria: the age of the patient, adequate circulation at the site of infection, presence of necrotic tissue, presence of a foreign body at the site of infection, allergies to medication, and the results of cultures. In addition, treatment is influenced by the patient's signs and symptoms and by whether the infection is acute or chronic. Recent advances have dramatically improved the therapy of osteomyelitis for some patients.

PATHOPHYSIOLOGY

The bones of neonates and infants up to 18 months of age contain numerous transphyseal vessels. In this type of circulation, infection can occur on both sides of the metaphysis and can lead to destruction of the epiphysis and the metaphysis. Neonatal osteomyelitis can be subtle but very destructive, involving numerous bones. The most common pathogens at this time are *Staphylococcus aureus*, *Haemophilus influenzae* type B, Enterobacteriaceae, and streptococci (groups A and B, and pneumococci).

In children, infection caused by hematogenous spread of organisms most often involves rapidly growing bone (long bones) and tends to start just beneath the metaphysis, where the nutrient arterioles bend. Infection tends to spread through the cortex and may collect under a sturdy periosteum, where it is confined by a fibrous capsule (Brodie's abscess). Any significant collection of purulent material can eventually lead to an ineffective blood supply and avascular bone. Hence, early treatment of children with osteomyelitis provides better long-term results than treatment after the development of purulent material in the periosteum, with subsequent sequestrum (devitalized bone) or involucrum (new periosteal bone). *Staphylococcus aureus* causes osteomyelitis in children of all ages. *Pseudomonas aeruginosa* is generally the cause of osteomyelitis in children older than 9 years.

In adults, because the periosteum is firmly attached to bone, subperiosteal abscesses form infrequently; instead, adults develop chronic suppurative and necrotic lesions with sequestrum and avascular bone. Patients older than 50 years of age may develop osteomyelitis as a result of a contiguous focus of infection (infected surgical wound or a soft tissue infection) or vascular insufficiency.

Osteomyelitis can be classified on the basis of pathogenesis as hematogenous, secondary to contiguous focus of infection, or secondary to peripheral vascular disease. In addition, osteomyelitis can be considered acute or chronic. The symptoms of acute osteomyelitis are typically fever and bone pain; on the other hand, chronic osteomyelitis is often indolent, with periodic exacerbations characterized by sinus tract drainage and associated bony sequestra. A distinction between the two categories of osteomyelitis is sometimes difficult to establish. A classification based on anatomic staging and host factors has been proposed by Mader and Cierney and is found in the 1993 edition of *Conn's Current Therapy*.

SPECIAL CONSIDERATIONS

In addition to age, other important predispositions to osteomyelitis include the presence of diabetes mellitus, sickle cell disease, or severe peripheral vascular disease; the presence of a prosthesis or metal device; immunologic status, a long illness, and a history of fracture, surgery, or trauma; the specific location (e.g., spine, hip, foot); and hematogenous or nonhematogenous origin.

Diabetics often develop foot infections that require a combination of antibiotics because of the presence of multiple organisms: *S. aureus*, Enterobacteriaceae (i.e., aerobic gram-negative rods), *Corynebacterium*, and anaerobic bacteria. These infections heal with adequate débridement and appropriate antibiotics as long as there is adequate circulation. Amputation rather than antimicrobial treatment is indicated when circulation to the infected bone is compromised and inadequate. Circulation to the infected site must be verified either by physical examination or by special vascular studies. Diabetics also often "hide" infection because they have an increased threshold for pain. Hence, not only a detailed examination (especially in paraplegics) but also a scanning procedure (discussed later) may be required to find occult osteomyelitis. Any cellulitis or draining skin lesions in a diabetic patient should be considered to involve the underlying bone until proved otherwise.

Osteomyelitis in a patient with sickle cell disease is frequently associated with hematogenous spread of the organisms. The infection usually occurs in the diaphysis of long bones and is caused by *Salmonella* species, other aerobic gram-negative rods, or *S. aureus*. An important problem in treating these patients is distinguishing between infection and infarction. A negative bone scan suggests the presence of infarction. Osteomyelitis is more likely to cause elevations in temperature, white blood cell count, and erythrocyte sedimentation rate; in addition, the results of a bone scan will be positive. Blood, stool, and bone cultures should be taken and may reveal *Salmonella* species infection. Once cultures have been taken, presumptive treatment should include coverage for *Salmonella* species (e.g., ampicillin, trimethoprim-sulfamethoxazole, ciprofloxacin, or another effective quinolone antibiotic).

The clinical picture of patients with significant peripheral vascular disease can suggest osteomyelitis, even though in actuality these patients have bone infarction caused by significant vascular trauma and interruption of the arterial blood supply. This condition occurs especially often after vascular surgery. Cultures of affected bone (and bone biopsy whenever possible) are needed to rule out infection. Patients with osteomyelitis must be evaluated for adequate circulation to the infected bone.

Patients with a metal apparatus or prosthesis at the infection site cannot be considered curable unless treatment eventually includes removal of the foreign object and sterilization of the site (proved by culture) before the prosthesis is reintroduced. Often the condition of these patients is too severe to permit removal of the foreign object; treatment is then directed toward suppression of the infection. Suppressive treatment is often achieved with oral antibiotics rather than parenteral antibiotics. Regardless of whether treatment is given for cure or suppression, cultures identifying the pathogen are necessary for successful therapy. Suppressive treatment always includes the inher-

ent risk of bacteremia, and patients should be instructed to seek attention if symptoms such as fever, dizziness, and nausea occur. Bacteremia in the presence of an infected appliance demands removal of the foreign object.

Immunologically compromised patients can harbor unusual pathogens. Culturing must be extensive, and consideration must be given to the possibility of finding unusual bacterial and fungal species. One such fungal pathogen, *Sporothrix schenckii*, often infects joints or may appear as a cellulitis but actually has invaded the underlying bone. Sporotrichosis is associated with contamination of wounds through gardening or other contact with the soil. Other fungal pathogens include *Blastomyces dermatitidis*, *Histoplasma capsulatum*, *Cryptococcus neoformans*, *Candida* species, *Mucor* species, and *Coccidioides immitis*.

Location of the lesion often suggests a pathogen and influences the presumptive treatment. Osteomyelitis of the spine is occasionally seen after hematogenous dissemination of uropathogens (*Escherichia coli*, *Klebsiella* species), *S. aureus*, group B streptococci, or *Mycobacterium tuberculosis*. The spine is the most frequent site of tuberculous osteomyelitis in adults, whereas the metaphysis of long bones is the most frequent site in children (followed by the hip and the knee). *Mycobacterium tuberculosis* is the most common pathogen involving the ribs. Rarely, other mycobacteria are bone pathogens. Infection of the foot after a nail puncture is frequently caused by *Pseudomonas aeruginosa*, presumably introduced from the host's own skin flora. Anaerobic osteomyelitis (especially *Bacteroides* species) may occur in the long bones and in the skull and facial bones in association with previous fractures, diabetes, sinusitis, or human bites.

Bone infections related to trauma (open fractures) may be caused by pathogens from the host's own flora or by those introduced by the contaminating elements. Human bites can lead to osteomyelitis involving mouth flora, including anaerobic organisms. Cat bites can introduce *Pasteurella multocida* (a common organism in the oral secretions of cats), *Rochalimaea* species or *Bartonella* species. *Bartonella* infection is most often found in patients with acquired immune deficiency syndrome (AIDS). Dog bites may introduce aerobic gram-negative rods, including *Capnocytophaga* (DF-2 organisms or dysgonic fermenters: slow-growing, gram-negative rods commonly found in the oral secretions of dogs) as well as anaerobic organisms.

Hematogenous osteomyelitis in children is nearly always caused by *S. aureus*. This organism also is common in bone infections related to indwelling catheters (e.g., in hemodialysis patients) or intravenous infections (e.g., drug addicts). Drug addicts sometimes develop osteomyelitis caused by gram-negative rods (especially *P. aeruginosa*) and *Candida* species.

Nonhematogenous osteomyelitis either is a result of contiguous spread of pathogens from nearby infected soft tissue (e.g., decubital ulcers) or is related to trauma. These patients may not exhibit systemic signs unless the infection becomes bacteremic as well. Surgical wound infection after midsternotomy may lead to sternal osteomyelitis; the bacteria most frequently found are *S. aureus*, *Staphylococcus epidermidis*, and *P. aeruginosa*.

Vertebral osteomyelitis is generally acquired after bacteremia originating from infections of the skin, intravenous drug abuse, urinary tract infections, and endocarditis. The patient complains of dull back pain and progressive paraplegia caused by an epidural abscess. The etiologic diagnosis is made by blood cultures or isolation of pathogens from a needle biopsy of the vertebral body or disk space. *S. aureus* and Enterobacteriaceae are more frequently isolated, but tuberculosis, salmonellosis, brucellosis, candidiasis, or other fungi can also involve the spine. Magnetic nuclear resonance imaging (MRI) is extremely helpful in evaluating the extent of infection in vertebral osteomyelitis. MRI is more precise than computed tomography (CT) scans and may preclude a myelogram.

PATIENT EVALUATION

The patient's history may provide clues about the types of pathogens present. These clues include nail puncture *(P. aeruginosa)*; exposure to plants *(S. schenckii)* or sea water (atypical mycobacteria, *Vibrio* species, and *Aeromonas* species); recent skin infection *(S. aureus)*; human bite (anaerobes); hemodialysis *(S. aureus)*; drug addiction *(Staphylococcus* species, *Pseudomonas* species); dental work or periodontal disease (mouth flora); animal bite or exposure *(Pasteurella multocida*, DF-2 organisms, *Rochalimaea* species and *Brucella* species); and exposure to tuberculosis.

The duration of the infection is particularly important in children. It seems that if acute osteomyelitis is treated early (within 1 week of the onset of symptoms), shorter courses of antibiotics (3 to 4 weeks instead of 6 weeks) without surgical débridement may be effective. Thus, the duration of chills, sweating, fever, malaise, and pain; inability to flex or move the involved area; joint pain; redness or erythema of skin; swelling of soft tissue; or muscle spasms should be assessed.

Chronic infections are often characterized by drainage or open sinus tracts, and prior pathogens tend to be the current ones. A foul odor from sinus tract drainage is highly suggestive of the presence of anaerobes. Unusual pathogens may be present in immunologically compromised patients or in those who have recently traveled to tropical areas. Any metal or prosthetic devices should be identified.

Identification of a history of drug allergies is essential. Any recent surgery or joint aspirations (or injections) should be noted.

It is important to realize that neonates may have no signs or symptoms except for fever, vomiting, diarrhea, or all three.

Physical examination should identify the area involved (e.g., tenderness to palpation, swelling, redness, and warmth over the infected bone). A draining sinus with a feculent odor indicates the presence of anaerobic pathogens. In children especially there may be only an inability to move the adjacent joint. Systemic signs include not only fever, chills, and malaise but also evidence of an underlying disease (periodontal disease, sinusitis, signs of diabetes mellitus, or signs of decreased peripheral circulation such as decreased pulses and lack of nail bed filling).

LABORATORY EVALUATION

Laboratory evaluation includes a white blood cell count with differential count and a Westergren eythrocyte sedimentation rate. These test results are followed during treatment and should return to normal or preinfection values if the osteomyelitis is cured or suppressed. Some individuals prefer serum C-reactive protein rather than erythrocyte sedimentation rate. In studies involving acute hematogenous osteomyelitis in children, the C-reactive protein increased and decreased faster than the sedimentation rate, reflecting the effectiveness of therapy.

Other blood tests used for particular patients may include a sickle cell preparation or determination of blood glucose level. A skin test for tuberculosis is indicated in any patient with spine or rib osteomyelitis or an infection that does not appear to have an easily identified bacterial pathogen as a cause.

IMAGING

Radiographic films, radionuclide scans, computed tomography, and magnetic resonance imaging are used to locate the infection and to observe for spread of infection. Because these procedures can be expensive (Table 1), judgment and restraint are required to order only the tests that are indicated. Radiographic films should be obtained of the area or areas in which osteomyelitis is suspected based on the history or physical examination. The first radiographic sign of osteomyelitis is soft tissue swelling (there may be no such evidence for up to 14 days). Later, bone destruction and periosteal elevation occur.

A ^{99m}Tc bone scan is specific for increased osteoblastic activity or bone formation (it is not diagnostic for infected bone because it can be positive in areas of trauma, tumor, synovitis, arthritis, or noninfected inflammatory processes). It is positive as early as 3 days after the onset of symptoms and is helpful in locating the osteomyelitis when the radiograph appears normal. The scan can miss infected avascular areas. This test is unnecessary if the involved area is known. Our review of 30 studies evaluating ^{99m}Tc three-phase bone scans in 1460 patients with suspected bone infections found a combined sensitivity of 547/591 (93%) but a low specificity of 553/869 (64%).

Although the ^{67}Ga citrate scan may be more specific for infection, it is less sensitive than the ^{99m}Tc scan, and its resolution is not as good in small bones. A large amount of purulent material and active phagocytosis at the infected site are required to produce a positive scan. A review of 15 papers evaluating ^{67}Ga citrate scans in the diagnosis of osteomyelitis found an overall sensitivity of 209/257 (81%) and a specificity of 188/272 (69%). This scan is unnecessary if the involved area has been identified.

The ^{111}In-labeled leukocyte scan uses the labeling of the host's own leukocytes, which are then reinjected into the patient and accumulate in areas of infection. The scan is specific for osteomyelitis when the infection occurs in areas of increased bone remodeling. We reviewed 22 published studies evaluating ^{111}In-labeled leukocyte scans in a total of 1199 patients with suspected osteomyelitis and found a sensitivity of 498/586 (85%) and a specificity of 549/613 (85%). The false-positive results were primarily caused by the presence of rheumatoid arthritis, healing fractures, noninfected prostheses, and metastatic carcinoma.

TABLE 1. **Cost of Radiographic and Scanning Procedures***

Procedure	Cost (US $)
X-ray (foot)	57
X-ray (spine)	73
Total body scan	375
Three-phase bone scan	313
Total body gallium scan	650
^{111}In leukocyte scan—total body	639
CT scan of lumbar spine (with contrast)	517
MRI scan of lumbar spine (with contrast)	800
Erythrocyte sedimentation rate	14

*1995, University of Kentucky Medical Center, does not include physician charge.

Abbreviations: CT = computed tomography; MRI = magnetic resonance imaging.

When infection is extensive or near vital organs, CT scan or MRI is helpful. These expensive studies are of special value in following vertebral osteomyelitis and infection involving the skull, pelvic area, or hips. Both modalities can delineate the depth and extent of bone involvement. MRI has the best resolution. We reviewed 14 studies in which MRI was used in the diagnosis of possible osteomyelitis; the overall sensitivity was 245/261 (94%) and the specificity was 154/174 (89%).

Two experimental imaging modalities appear promising: the ^{99}Tc-HMPAO-labeled leukocyte scan has a reported sensitivity of 91/103 (88%) and a specificity of 71/86 (83%), and labeled antigranulocyte antibodies have a reported sensitivity of 172/193 (89%) and a specificity of 118/136 (87%). At this time prospective studies with high-resolution ultrasonography do not support the use of this modality. One recent study examining nine patients had a sensitivity of 63% and a diagnostic accuracy of 58%.

When radiographic results are normal and bone infection is still a consideration, the current practice is to obtain a whole-body three-phase bone scan or gallium scan in neonates and children and a ^{99m}Tc bone scan, an MRI, or a CT scan in adults.

It is not possible at this time to claim with certainty that positive scans indicate a need for continued treatment of an infection. Treatment should end at 6 weeks if the clinical condition has completely healed, or when the patient's condition has returned to baseline with no further radiographic evidence of bony destruction. Scans at this time can be misleading and are unnecessary. It is preferable to follow the patient clinically and to re-treat him or her if symptoms recur or to continue treatment if the infection has not totally healed.

ISOLATION OF THE PATHOGEN

Blood cultures (up to three sets, each drawn at a different time) show the pathogen in most cases of acute hematogenous osteomyelitis but rarely in cases of chronic osteomyelitis (less than 5%). Bone cultures identify the pathogen in nearly all cases of acute osteomyelitis and in at least 60% of chronic infections.

Treatment should never start until after at least one set of blood cultures (aerobic and anaerobic) has been taken. Furthermore, an aspirated sample from the infected bone should be obtained with a 16- or 18-gauge needle (with an inner stylet if possible) before treatment is begun. Because acute hematogenous osteomyelitis can be associated with potential life-threatening complications, every effort should be made to obtain blood and bone material for culture quickly so that presumptive treatment with antibiotics can begin. In contrast, patients with chronic osteomyelitis need not be treated until surgical débridement and gathering of material for bone cultures has been performed. Treatment for these patients can begin in the operating room once material for cultures has been obtained.

If bone aspiration is attempted, the needle should enter through an uninvolved area of skin that has been prepared with an iodine-containing disinfectant (iodine disinfectants work quickly, whereas alcohol requires several minutes to sterilize). Lidocaine can be used only to anesthetize the skin; it should not be injected along the periosteum because it can retard bacterial growth in culture. Specimens from infected bone should be analyzed for Gram's stain and for aerobic, anaerobic, mycobacterial, and fungal cultures. Even if only a few drops of serosanguineous material are obtained, they should be sent to the pathology laboratory

for, at least, culture and Gram's stain. When patients are immunocompromised (including those with human immunodeficiency virus infection) or are suspected of harboring fungal pathogens, bone should also be stained for fungal pathogens. In addition, these stains must include a silver stain if *Bartonella* species are suspected.

Transport of the material to the laboratory is critical, and one should consult the laboratory personnel for the best transport method available in the hospital. If transport medium is not available, one should leave the material in the syringe and send it to the laboratory as quickly as possible.

Deep wound cultures or cultures taken from sinus tracts are misleading and a waste of money. Skin-colonizing organisms may mislead the physician, and the true pathogens may not be recovered.

Stool and urine cultures for *Salmonella* species are indicated for patients with sickle cell disease.

TREATMENT

Basic Concepts

Treatment of osteomyelitis requires removal of necrotic, avascular, infected bone and relatively long-term antibiotic treatment. Amputation may be necessary if an inadequate blood supply cannot be improved. Surgery is not necessary for every patient because children and neonates treated early for acute hematogenous osteomyelitis are often cured with appropriate antibiotic treatment alone.

Chronic osteomyelitis requires surgical débridement for cure. The type of surgery is determined by the extent of the infection and may include removing a metal appliance or prosthesis or immobilizing bone. For infected knee arthroplasties, resection arthroplasty is much more efficient than débridement alone in controlling the infection. If a foreign object must remain in place to stabilize a fracture or maintain a joint, antimicrobial treatment should be designed to suppress the infection and allow the patient to be discharged from the hospital. Suppressive treatment is usually provided by an oral antibiotic given for several months and is restarted if symptoms recur. An occasional patient may require nearly lifelong daily administration of antibiotics to suppress infection in a prosthetic joint. If all foreign objects can be removed from the bone, a cure is attempted. For patients with large or multiloculated cavities in long bones or with long bone infections for which bone grafting can be used, the Ilizarov procedure should be considered. This radical and relatively painful procedure has succeeded in eradicating debilitating chronic osteomyelitis that is refractory to all other treatments.

Initial Treatment

Choice of antibiotic depends on which pathogen is present. Empirical treatment does not exist. Once cultures have been taken, it is important to select the appropriate treatment on the basis of the patient's evaluation. If the patient is acutely ill (possibly bacteremic), an initial combination of antimicrobials such as vancomycin, an aminoglycoside (e.g., gentamicin, tobramycin, or amikacin), and metronidazole in an adult or cefotaxime and an aminoglycoside in a child can be used. This coverage is extensive (and potentially toxic) but may be necessary in a severely ill individual with acute hematogenous osteomyelitis. The regimen is changed to appropriate (cost-effective) and safer drugs as soon as the culture reports are available.

Treatment Guidelines

Parenteral or oral antibiotics, or both, are preferable to local application of antibiotics alone. One can determine whether the choice (a parenteral or oral antibiotic) is appropriate by obtaining serum bactericidal levels against isolated pathogens. Serum bactericidal activity is the only true laboratory measure of an antibiotic's effectiveness in osteomyelitis. In adults, trough (just before the next dose) serum bactericidal (i.e., not serum bacteriostatic) levels should exist at 1:2 dilutions or higher of serum in patients with acute bone disease and at 1:4 dilutions or higher of serum in patients with chronic bone disease. In children, peak (30 minutes after dosing) serum bactericidal levels should exist at 1:8 dilutions or higher except for streptococci, which should be at 1:32 dilutions or higher.

Children who respond after only 2 weeks of intravenous treatment may be switched to an effective oral antibiotic for an additional 3 to 4 weeks. Treatment for cure requires a total of 6 or more weeks of antibiotic therapy except in cases of vertebral osteomyelitis, mycobacterial disease, or fungal disease. Vertebral osteomyelitis therapy continues for up to 6 months and is stopped only when radiographs and computed tomography or MRI show no further disease and the Westergren erythrocyte sedimentation rate has returned to baseline. Mycobacterial disease is usually treated initially with four drugs: isoniazid (isoniazid use requires pyridoxine as well), rifampin, pyrazinamide, and ethambutol. Treatment should continue until the possibility of multidrug-resistant tuberculosis is ruled out. If *M. tuberculosis* is not drug resistant, isoniazid, rifampin, and pyrazinamide are continued for 2 months, followed by isoniazid and rifampin for an additional 4 months. If the patient is unable to take both isoniazid and rifampin, alternative drugs must be used and continued for up to 18 months. Two effective drugs should always be used to treat active tuberculosis. Fungal therapy requires amphotericin B or perhaps a new imidazole derivative (ketoconazole, fluconazole, or itraconazole); the treatment plan should be discussed with an infectious disease specialist.

Antibiotics for Specific Organisms

For osteomyelitis caused by *Staphylococcus* species, an appropriate initial choice is oxacillin or nafcillin (vancomycin for methicillin-resistant staphylococci or for the patient with penicillin allergy) (Table 2). No oral agent can be relied on to provide consistently adequate serum bactericidal levels against staphylococci. Once the patient has shown clinical improvement and has been treated with parenteral antimicrobials for several weeks, oral regimens may be tried. Patients treated with oral agents must be carefully observed for signs of treatment failure and must have adequate serum bactericidal levels. Oral agents with antistaphylococcal activity include cloxacillin, dicloxacillin, and clindamycin. These agents could be combined with rifampin, which has been shown to enhance nafcillin activity in chronic staphylococcal osteomyelitis. Rifampin should not be used alone because patients rapidly develop resistance to it. Currently available quinolone antibiotics are rarely effective treatment for staphylococcal osteomyelitis. We use them only as a last resort because we have found them frequently ineffective. When quinolone antibiotics are used, great care must be taken to observe and evaluate the patient frequently.

Osteomyelitis caused by *Streptococcus* species is treated with penicillin; penicillin-allergic patients may receive vancomycin, a first-generation cephalosporin, a long-acting cephalosporin (ceftriaxone, cefonicid), or clindamycin. Currently available quinolones are ineffective.

Osteomyelitis caused by *Haemophilus* species (a consideration in children) is treated with ampicillin, cefotaxime, trimethoprim-sulfamethoxazole (co-trimoxazole), a quinolone, cefuroxime, or ceftriaxone.

Bone infections caused by Enterobacteriaceae (e.g., *E. coli, Klebsiella* species, *Proteus* species) are treated with ampicillin (if the pathogen is sensitive), a third-generation cephalosporin (cefotaxime), a monobactam (aztreonam), an aminoglycoside (gentamicin), or a quinolone. *Pseudomonas* infections of bone require an aminoglycoside (gentamicin) and a beta-lactam antibiotic such as ceftazidime or aztreonam. Ciprofloxacin is always ineffective if the minimal inhibitory concentration of the *Pseudomonas* species is equal to or greater than 1 μg per mL. We have not found the current quinolone antibiotics effective in the treatment of *Pseudomonas* osteomyelitis.

Anaerobic osteomyelitis is treated with metronidazole; this agent can be given orally (over 80% absorption). Other choices include intravenous clindamycin, piperacillin, cefoxitin, cefotetan, or other agents with adequate anaerobic coverage.

Overall, the best antibiotic is the least toxic agent with adequate serum bactericidal activity.

Treatment with Oral Agents

A combination of the oral agents ciprofloxacin and metronidazole should be excellent for osteomyelitis caused by Enterobacteriaceae and anaerobes. After adequate débridement, these drugs may be reasonable for treatment of osteomyelitis of the foot. However, such coverage is *inadequate* for elimination of *Pseudomonas* species, *S. aureus*, or *Streptococcus* species. At this time, oral therapy is possible if the patient can receive oral medication, is able to absorb

TABLE 2. **Antibiotic Preferences for Osteomyelitis***

Organism	Drug	Daily Dose Children (mg/kg)	Daily Dose Adults	Hours Between Doses	Route of Administration	Wholesale Daily Price (US $)†
Methicillin-sensitive *Staphylococcus aureus*	Nafcillin (oxacillin)	50–100	8 gm	6	IV	68.06
	Cefazolin	40–100	6 gm	8	IV	20.35
	Clindamycin	20–40	2.7 gm	8	IV	18.60
Methicillin-resistant *S. aureus* and other staphylococci	Vancomycin	15–40	2 gm	12	IV	22.34
Streptococcus species	Penicillin	100,000–200,000 U 100–300	15–20 million U	4–6	IV	15.02
Enterobacteriaceae (*Escherichia coli, Proteus* species, *Klebsiella* species)	Ampicillin	100–300	8 gm	6	IV	18.72
	Aztreonam	50–200	6 gm	8	IV	85.98
	Cefotaxime	—	6 gm	8	IV	57.70
	Aminoglycoside‡					
	Ciprofloxacin		1.5 gm	12	PO	10.32
Pseudomonas species	Aminoglycoside with aztreonam§ or	—	8 gm (aztreonam)	6	IV	114.80
	Aminoglycoside with ceftazidime or	30–100	6 gm (ceftazidime)	8	IV	90.06
	Aminoglycoside with piperacillin	—	16–18 gm (piperacillin)	4	IV	82.00
Salmonella species (ampicillin-sensitive, ampicillin-resistant)	Ampicillin	100–300	8 gm	6	IV	18.72
	Trimethoprim-sulfamethoxazole	10/50	480/2400–640/3200 mg	6–12	IV	50.00
	Ciprofloxacin	—	1.5 gm	12	PO	10.32
Haemophilus species (ampicillin-sensitive, ampicillin-resistant)	Ampicillin	100–300	8 gm	6	IV	18.72
	Cefotaxime	50–200	6 gm	8	IV	57.70
	Trimethoprim-sulfamethoxazole	10/50	480/2400–640/3200 mg	8–12	IV	50.00
	Aztreonam	—	6 gm	8	IV	85.98
Anaerobes	Metronidazole‖	15–35	1.5–2 gm	8–6	PO or IV	0.30 or 23.43
	Clindamycin	25–40¶	2.7 gm	8	IV	18.60
	Ampicillin/sulbactam	110/55	12/4 gm	6	IV	52.25

*The drug listed is the first choice. Other drugs are options if reason exists to choose an alternative agent. Daily dose assumes normal renal function.

†Wholesale prices according to the Red Book, 1994.

‡The most cost-effective aminoglycoside is gentamicin, followed by netilmicin. Tobramycin and amikacin are least cost effective. Aminoglycosides could be used initially until sensitivities are available but should be discontinued if the Enterobacteriaceae species are sensitive to less toxic agents.

§In severe *Pseudomonas* infections (potential for bacteremia is present), the combination of an aminoglycoside and a beta-lactam agent should be used. Aztreonam, the most specific beta-lactam for *Pseudomonas* species, is preferred.

‖Safety and efficacy in children have not been established.

¶May exceed manufacturer's recommended dose.

drugs via the gastrointestinal tract, and has an anaerobic pathogen (metronidazole) and/or an Enterobacteriaceae organism (ciprofloxacin or a comparable quinolone). Oral treatment is also indicated for suppressive therapy for an infected prosthesis. The combination of rifampin and ofloxacin was successful in 74% of patients with *Staphylococcus*-infected orthopedic implants when given for up to 9 months.

Local Treatment with Beads, Cement, and Flaps

Local administration of antibiotics to bone is currently being studied. Antibiotic-impregnated poly-methyl methacrylate beads placed in open bone cavities after débridement have yielded good results in animal models. In vitro studies also suggest that local delivery of an appropriate antibiotic is possible. If beads are to be used, the antibiotic must remain active against the pathogen once the bone has been prepared with the polymethyl methacrylate. The use of aminoglycosides in impregnated beads has been studied most thoroughly; these agents are stable and active against sensitive aerobic, gram-negative rods and staphylococci. Aminoglycosides cannot be used for streptococci or anaerobic infections. Beads need to be removed or replaced after 2 to 3 weeks because a dense fibrous tissue starts to surround them. There is also a real concern that these beads could act as foreign bodies and could harbor pathogens (resistant to antibiotics in the beads), thus prolonging the infection. Not enough data are available to recommend treatment with beads alone; however, beads plus systemic antibiotics help to deliver antibiotic to both vascular and avascular areas of infection.

Use of antibiotic-impregnated cement cannot be recommended if its purpose is to deliver antibiotic to an infected area. In theory, the cement could be used as prophylaxis in sterile areas. The use of such cement to prevent infection (rather than systemic antibiotic prophylaxis) is debatable. In uncontrolled trials, the use of antibiotic-impregnated cement has been reported to contribute to successful revision of infected arthroplasties. The primary advantage of antibiotic-impregnated beads and cement is that high local concentrations of antibiotics in bone can be achieved for a short period; serum levels remain nearly negligible, and systemic toxicity is unusual.

Local administration to bone of appropriate antibiotics by means of a drug pump is investigational.

For certain patients (e.g., those with long bone infections), antibiotic beads and microvascular muscle grafting may assist in clearing the infection before bone grafting can be performed. Bone grafts may form the nidus for sequestered bacteria if the wound is not sterile. It is not clear whether hyperbaric oxygen treatment assists in the resolution of osteomyelitis. Hyperbaric oxygen treatment does speed soft tissue healing in areas with vascular compromise.

COMMON SPORTS INJURIES

method of
JAMES C. PUFFER, M.D.
University of California at Los Angeles School of Medicine
Los Angeles, California

Sports injuries occur as a result of two basic mechanisms. The first of these is the result of acute trauma, when an extrinsic force that is applied to bone, ligament, or a musculotendinous unit exceeds the inherent tensile strength of that structure, resulting in its failure. These *macrotraumatic* injuries result commonly in fracture or ligamentous or musculotendinous disruption. More commonly, however, injuries occur as the result of accumulated microtrauma—microscopic, subclinical injury that occurs as a result of repetitive forces placed on anatomic structures over time. The accumulation of repeated microtrauma can lead to a prostaglandin-mediated inflammatory response and the subsequent development of pain when the inflammation occurs in soft tissue. This phenomenon is known as an *overuse syndrome*. Overuse syndromes constitute the largest group of sports injuries seen by primary care physicians. Overuse syndromes of the shoulder and knee are seen most frequently. The appropriate diagnosis and management of these conditions are essential in promoting prompt recovery and guaranteeing timely return to play.

TREATMENT OF OVERUSE SYNDROMES OF THE SHOULDER

The athlete with a painful shoulder usually presents with a history of participation in a sport that requires the overhead use of the upper extremity. These sports include all throwing sports, volleyball, tennis, racquetball, and swimming. Repeated microtrauma occurs as a result of repeated tensile overload of the rotator cuff and "wringing out" of the cuff over the head of the humerus during adduction and extension of the shoulder. Impingement of the cuff and subacromial bursa can result in microtrauma as well and can occur secondary to degenerative disease of the acromioclavicular (AC) joint or acromion (primary impingement) or to instability of the glenohumeral joint (secondary impingement). Physical examination usually elicits tenderness over the supraspinatus tendon, the subacromial bursa, the long head of the biceps, or any of these structures in combination. A positive impingement sign may be present, and the patient may demonstrate clinical signs of glenohumeral instability. X-ray examination is usually unremarkable, although occasionally calcifications can be appreciated in the subacromial bursa or the rotator cuff just proximal to its insertion in the greater tuberosity of the humerus; in older patients, a subacromial spur or degenerative disease in the AC joint may be present to explain impingement. Essential in the treatment of this disorder is an assessment of the underlying mechanism responsible for producing microtrauma and the degree to which pain compromises athletic performance. After the mechanism responsible for repetitive injury has been identified, functional classification of pain into four distinct types is critical in providing a stepwise approach to the management of this disorder, as well as all other overuse syndromes (Table 1).

Type I pain is best managed by relative rest with a 25% reduction in workload (e.g., number of pitches thrown, number of meters swum, etc.). Additionally, the athlete is begun on a stretching program that is designed to restore normal resting muscle length as well as promote the mobilization of the inflammatory by-products of exercise. The athlete is instructed to perform these exercises both before and after activity. The importance of ice massage in reducing the inflammatory response after completion of physical activity is also stressed. Approximately 15 minutes should be spent icing the shoulder after exercise. Therapeutic ultrasound can serve as effective adjunctive therapy, and all athletes should begin a shoulder rehabilitation program directed at correcting specific deficiencies noted during the physical examination. This usually concentrates on strength-

TABLE 1. **Functional Classification of Pain**

Type I	Pain after activity only
Type II	Pain during activity, not restricting performance
Type III	Pain during activity, restricting performance
Type IV	Chronic, unremitting pain

ening muscles of the shoulder girdle through proprioceptive neuromuscular facilitation and progressive resistance exercises as tolerated.

Type II pain should also be treated with enforcement of relative rest. The workload should be reduced by approximately 50%. In addition to the use of ultrasound, ice, stretching exercises, and rehabilitation, athletes whose pain falls into this category are most effectively managed with the initiation of nonsteroidal anti-inflammatory therapy. Many effective nonsteroidal agents are currently available, and the choice of a specific agent should be predicated on physician preference and patient tolerance. Naproxen 375 mg orally twice daily and ibuprofen 600 mg orally four times daily are effective agents that can be used for these purposes.

Type III pain is by definition pain that precludes competitive athletic performance, and for these reasons the athlete should be encouraged to rest the shoulder completely. Oral anti-inflammatory agents and physical therapy should be used in these individuals, and it is usually this group of patients who benefit from an injection of corticosteroid into the subacromial bursa. From 20 to 30 mg of triamcinolone acetonide suspension mixed with two mL of 1% lidocaine (Xylocaine) can be used for this purpose depending on the estimated size of the bursa. The injection should never be placed into the rotator cuff since it has been demonstrated that this can result in local atrophy and increased risk for subsequent rupture. An anterior or posterior approach may be used, and unimpeded flow occurs if the needle is correctly positioned within the bursa. Resistance to flow indicates that the needle is in the rotator cuff thereby necessitating repositioning.

Type IV pain is pain that is chronic, is unremitting, and has not been amenable to conservative therapy. In these patients special consideration should be given to surgical intervention with the ultimate goal of relieving pain and restoring function. This usually requires correction of underlying instability in younger athletes or subacromial decompression in older athletes.

OVERUSE SYNDROMES OF THE KNEE

Knee pain is commonly encountered in athletes who participate in running and jumping sports. Specific diagnosis is dependent on the elicitation of pain over specific anatomic structures. The differential diagnosis of knee pain by anatomic location is described in Table 2. Patellofemoral arthralgia is seen most frequently in the patient who reports a history of pain on walking up and down stairs, stiffness after

TABLE 2. **Differential Diagnosis of Knee Pain by Anatomic Location**

Medial	Lateral
Synovial plica syndrome	Iliotibial band syndrome
Anserine bursitis	Popliteus tendinitis
Voschel's bursitis	Biceps femoris tendinitis
Torn medial meniscus	Lateral retinaculitis
Medial retinaculitis	Torn lateral meniscus
Stress fracture proximal tibia	
	Inferior
Intra-articular	Infrapatellar tendinitis
Chondromalacia patella	Infrapatellar bursitis
Osteochondral fracture	Osgood-Schlatter disease
Degenerative joint disease	Stress fracture of proximal
Torn meniscus	tibia
Cystic, discoid, or	Fat pad syndrome
degenerating meniscus	
Loose bodies	Superior
	Suprapatellar tendinitis
	Suprapatellar bursitis

sitting for long periods of time (positive movie house sign), and pain during or after activity. Physical examination usually elicits tenderness over the medial facet, and a positive compression test can be demonstrated. The seated Q angle is usually in excess of 5 degrees, and passive patellar tilt and/or excessive lateral or restricted medial patellar glide may be demonstrated. Genu varum, external tibial torsion, and "squinting" patellas can be observed. X-ray examination may demonstrate signs of early degenerative change but most commonly is unremarkable. Athletes with this malady should be treated in a stepwise fashion as described earlier based on functional classification of their pain. However, paramount in minimizing the recurrence of this disorder is the careful evaluation of lower extremity biomechanics with correction of lower-extremity-to-hindfoot and hindfoot-to-forefoot malalignment, which can lead to hyperpronation and abnormal tracking of the patella within the patellofemoral groove. The use of flexible or rigid orthotics can be useful in this regard. In those instances in which this disorder can be specifically linked to abnormal tracking of the patella, quadricep setting exercises that concentrate on enhancing the strength and tone of the vastus medialis muscle are important in attempting to restore normal alignment of the patella, thereby minimizing recurrence. This can be enhanced by McConnell's taping of the patella. There is little, if any, role for the use of injectable steroid in and around the knee. Only in those instances in which an inflammatory bursitis can be elicited should injectable steroids be used, and then these should be injected only into the specific bursal structures that are affected.

Section 15

Obstetrics and Gynecology

ANTEPARTUM CARE

method of
KATHRYN M. ANDOLSEK, M.D., M.P.H.
Duke University Medical Center
Durham, North Carolina

The infant mortality rate in the United States is markedly worse than in other industrialized countries despite greater expenditures on health care. The causes are multifactorial. They include poverty, substance abuse, domestic violence, tobacco use, and inadequate nutrition. Perinatal technology has made brilliant advances, but access to primary obstetric care often remains limited because of factors related to geography, health insurance, transportation, education, and social support.

The majority of adverse birth outcomes are related to prematurity and other conditions that may be prevented, or at least ameliorated by appropriate obstetric management. Unfortunately, waiting until pregnancy is recognized and the woman seeks obstetric care generally means that care occurs too late to affect the most critical period in fetal development—17 to 56 days after conception. Most women during this crucial early period of pregnancy are unaware that they are pregnant.

For this reason, all health care providers, even those who do not specifically provide obstetric services, need to recognize and accept their critical role in affecting birth outcomes. They play an important role by identifying potential risk factors and developing management strategies when caring for any woman in the reproductive age group. This process has been referred to as "preconception care."

PRECONCEPTION CARE

Preconception care includes risk assessment, education and health promotion, and management or referral for medical or psychosocial conditions that affect the morbidity and outcome of a potential pregnancy. At least 60% of primary health care providers should provide age-appropriate preconception care and counseling. Such care and counseling need to be available in many settings. A public health strategy targets schools, youth centers, and correctional and other institutions. It also is a natural part of an individual health care encounter for a woman in the reproductive age group. It is perhaps most effectively provided as part of general preventive care or during primary care visits for other medical conditions. Preconception assessment is similar to the medical history, physical examination, and laboratory evaluation commonly addressed at the first prenatal visit. However, the timing of this assessment *before* conception (1) allows the visit to include an emphasis on family planning to perhaps modify when, or even if, conception will take place and (2) provides an opportunity to modify factors that affect birth outcome before conception, or at least at a very early time in fetal development.

Men should also be encouraged to seek assessment and counseling either alone or, optimally, with their partners. Male factors are increasingly understood as directly or indirectly associated with pregnancy outcome.

There is considerable overlap in the medical assessment of a patient before conception and early in her prenatal care. These common factors are discussed first.

Poverty. The incidence of low income is directly correlated with the rates of infant mortality, very low birthweight, low birthweight, and prematurity. Women who seek medical care and are discovered to be socioeconomically disadvantaged should be offered referral that can address eligibility for social service programs including nutrition, education, housing, and vocational assistance.

Congenital Anomalies. Preconception assessment identifies potential parents at risk and provides them with knowledge in order to facilitate informed decisions about their reproductive options. As advances are made in preventing and managing many genetic or other congenital conditions, this information needs to be systematically disseminated to families on whose lives it impacts. For example, women who have had an infant with a neural tube defect can markedly decrease their risk of recurrence in a subsequent pregnancy by using a dietary supplement of 4 mg of folic acid the month before and 3 months after conception.

Common inherited disorders include Tay-Sachs disease in Jews of Ashkenazic background; beta-thalassemia in Greeks and Italians; alpha-thalassemia in individuals from Southeast Asia, the Philippines, and North Africa; hemoglobinopathies such as sickle cell anemia in African Americans or other black patients; and cystic fibrosis in whites.

The issues are frequently complex. Cleft lip with or without cleft palate is one of the most common congenital malformations, occurring in about 1 in 1000 births. At the present time, the precise risk of inheritance cannot be calculated. Risk can only be estimated from the frequency of transmission observed in similar families. If a father has cleft lip, the risk to the baby is approximately 3.5%. The risk is higher if the mother has the cleft condition. Surgery often results in excellent functional and cosmetic outcomes. Counseling needs to provide parents with all pertinent and current information.

The preconception assessment approach gives parents information and counseling to decide whether to conceive (or perhaps adopt) and the available technology to diagnose, and increasingly treat, medical conditions in their children, once conceived. The ethical imperatives inherent in this counseling have recently been addressed by the Council on Ethical and Judicial Affairs of the American Medical Association. The council stresses that counseling should "include discussion of the reasons for and against testing, as well as discussion of the inappropriate uses of genetic testing. . . . Physicians should inform women or couples without an elevated risk of the reasons why prenatal diagnosis may not be desirable in their case."

Unintended Pregnancies. Unintended pregnancies are associated with delayed prenatal care and poorer birth outcomes. Often the best outcome of a preconception assessment may be the recognition that a woman does not desire a pregnancy at the current time. Contraceptive counseling can then be initiated.

Lifestyle Risks. Many of the lifestyle risks that contribute to adverse birth outcome constitute risks to a woman's general health status. These include poor nutrition; alcohol abuse; tobacco use; prescription or illegal drug use; lack of exercise; environmental exposure to heavy metals, organic solvents, other chemicals, and radiation through the work place or hobbies; and unprotected sexual activity.

Nutrition. Maternal folic acid supplementation has been shown to reduce the incidence of fetal neural tube defects. All women who may become pregnant should supplement their diet with 0.4 mg of folic acid daily. Women in the reproductive age group need information on the value of this supplementation. Nutritional assessment should also include other common conditions such as overweight, underweight, eating disorders, pica, megavitamin supplementation, and dietary practices likely to be inadequate in basic nutrients.

Alcohol. Excessive alcohol intake in early pregnancy may result in fetal alcohol syndrome, the leading preventable known cause of mental retardation and birth defects. The prevalence of fetal alcohol syndrome exceeds that of Down's syndrome or neural tube defects. Eleven percent of women who consume between 1 and 2% of absolute alcohol a day will have infants who develop this syndrome. Surveys consistently reveal women's lack of knowledge regarding pregnancy and alcohol use. Reliable tools, such as the CAGE instrument, are available to screen for alcohol abuse in the office setting. The CAGE involves four questions:

Have you ever felt the need to *c*ut down on your drinking?

Have you ever felt *a*nnoyed by another's criticism of your drinking?

Have you ever felt *g*uilty about your drinking?

Have you ever felt the need for an *e*ye opener (early morning drink)?

A woman with any positive response should be further evaluated. The physician should evaluate high-risk women even more carefully. At particular risk are women who are older, are heavy tobacco users, and present late for prenatal care. Alcohol use or abuse in significant others, family, and friends should be scrutinized. Management of the addicted woman generally involves a multidisciplinary effort. Benzodiazepines and psychotropic medications are generally contraindicated for withdrawal symptoms in pregnant women. Local and state resources are catalogued by the National Council on Alcoholism, 511 K Street N.W., Washington, D.C. 20005.

Tobacco Use. At some point during their pregnancy, 25% of pregnant women smoke. Even more are exposed through passive smoke at home or in the work place. Smoking is associated with adverse pregnancy outcomes such as infertility, low birthweight, perinatal death, placenta previa, abruptio placentae, and spontaneous abortion.

If the woman is motivated to stop smoking, a management strategy can be initiated. Identifying problem tobacco use during the preconception period allows the use of nicotine substances such as gum or the transdermal release system if it is felt to be beneficial. Unfortunately these are contraindicated during pregnancy. A quit date can be established and documented in the chart. The woman should be seen in follow-up shortly after the quit date. There are many community programs affiliated with the American Cancer Society, the American Heart Association, the American Lung Association, and local hospitals.

Other Substances of Abuse. As many as 10 to 15% of women use cocaine, heroin, methadone, amphetamines, phencyclidine, or marijuana during pregnancy. The use of cocaine in the first trimester and before pregnancy can be associated with congenital defects and placental abruption, even if the woman later discontinues such use. Heroin withdrawal during pregnancy may be life-threatening for the fetus. Withdrawal is more safely undertaken preconception.

Physical, Chemical, and Radiologic Agents and Work Conditions. Preconception assessment allows modifications to decrease or eliminate risks of exposure. In some cases, job reassignment or even a change of occupations may be indicated.

Unprotected Sexual Activity. Unprotected sexual activity and risky sexual behavior place women at risk of human immunodeficiency virus (HIV) infection and other sexually transmitted diseases. The Centers for Disease Control and Prevention (CDC) released a draft of their recommendations in February 1995 for HIV screening in pregnant women and their subsequent care throughout pregnancy. They recommend that screening be offered to all patients since there is now sufficient evidence that treatment decreases vertical transmission to the infant. In addition, recommendations regarding breast-feeding are altered in HIV-positive women. Treatment of tuberculosis in an HIV-positive pregnant woman also varies. Copies of this document can be obtained through the CDC National AIDS Clearinghouse, Box 6003 Rockville, MD 20849-6003 or by calling 1-800-458-5231. Women need frank, honest discussions on how to modify their risk of acquiring HIV infection through abstinence, selection of sexual partners, and the use of condoms.

Medication Use. The average woman uses 4 to 11 drugs during pregnancy; 40% of these drugs are taken in the first trimester, often before she is aware of the pregnancy. Some commonly prescribed drugs affect fetal development. These include isotretinoin; folic acid antagonists such as co-trimoxazole; warfarin; valproic acid; lithium; and gold. Women using these medications need to be aware of their reproductive consequences, offered effective contraception, and given the opportunity to discontinue the drug or substitute a less toxic substance when pregnancy is contemplated.

Chronic Medical Conditions. Women with chronic medical conditions may be at particular risk for an adverse birth outcome. The underlying condition itself may pose adverse reproductive consequences. Medication or other therapeutic modalities used to manage the condition may pose independent yet additive risks.

PHENYLKETONURIA. Women with phenylketonuria need to resume a phenylalanine-restricted diet before conception and throughout pregnancy to reduce the fetal risk of mental retardation, microcephaly, and low birthweight.

DIABETES. Women with poorly controlled diabetes at the time of conception deliver infants with higher rates of congenital anomalies as well as infants with macrosomia. The most common congenital malformations in these infants develop before the seventh week of gestation. These rates can be decreased by improved glycemic control before conception.

HYPERTENSION. The control of hypertension may worsen during pregnancy. Women with hypertension are at increased risk for preeclampsia. Some antihypertensive medications compromise fetal development. A woman with hypertension who is treated with medication may need to adjust her dose of medication or substitute another medication to one felt to be safer in pregnancy. Angiotensin-converting enzyme medications, for example, have been associated with fetal demise when used in the second or third trimesters of pregnancy. Diuretics are generally avoided.

EPILEPSY. Women with epilepsy are at risk of adverse birth outcomes because of their disease, hypoxia if they seize, and the medications prescribed to control seizures. Women who have been seizure-free for at least 2 years and have a normal electroencephalogram may be offered a trial of medication before contemplating pregnancy. Trimethadione (Tridione), paramethadione (Paradione), and valproate (Depakene) are contraindicated during pregnancy. The least toxic medication that controls seizures should be prescribed. Serum levels can be monitored to keep the patient at the lowest therapeutic level that controls the seizures.

CERVICAL ABNORMALITIES. The cervix should be assessed cytologically before pregnancy. Abnormalities should be treated before conception.

Infectious Disease. Rubella immunity should be assessed. Fifteen percent of women are not immune to rubella. Increasing numbers of congenital rubella syndrome cases have been reported since 1988. Women without a history of vaccination and no contraindication to immunization can be vaccinated without serologic testing. Women previously vaccinated or with a history compatible with the disease can be tested to ensure immunity. Once immunity has been demonstrated in an adult, no further testing is necessary.

If maternal rubella infection occurs in a woman without immunity before 11 weeks of gestation, there is a fetal anomaly rate of 90%. The risk is 33% when the infection occurs during Weeks 11 to 12. Although the risk of congenital rubella secondary to vaccination is low, it is recommended that conception be postponed for 3 months after rubella immunization. Women who are inadvertently vaccinated, however, should be reassured that the fetal risk is negligible, and this should not be a reason to consider pregnancy termination. If a woman is already pregnant, rubella vaccination should be postponed until after delivery. Approximately 25% of women develop arthralgias and transient arthritis after vaccination.

TETANUS. The tetanus status can be ascertained. Tetanus toxoid should be given if there has been no previous administration during the preceding 10 years. This vaccine can be given even if the woman is already pregnant.

HEPATITIS B. A woman's hepatitis B status should be determined in the preconception period. Hepatitis B infection is common: one in 20 persons in the United States become infected with hepatitis B virus (HBV). Vertical transmission to infants is highly likely. Of those women who are hepatitis B surface antigen (HBsAg) positive, 70% transmit the infection to their newborn; 90% of babies without treatment become carriers; and 25% of the babies die of liver complications. If a woman is HBsAg-negative and at risk of HBV infection because of lifestyle or occupational factors, the hepatitis B vaccine should be recommended along with counseling on ways to diminish risk (abstinence or safer sexual practices, eliminating intravenous drug use, and not sharing needles). Hepatitis B vaccine can be given during pregnancy. Screening of sexual partners is recommended, with counseling and vaccination offered to those at risk.

HUMAN IMMUNODEFICIENCY VIRUS. High-risk women and their sexual partners should be offered HIV testing. Perinatal transmission can be decreased from 27 to 8% in women who are taking antiretroviral medication during pregnancy and delivery. The CDC has published a draft of recommendations calling for HIV testing of all pregnant women and outlining issues in their care.

VARICELLA. With the recent availability of the varicella vaccine, women without previous varicella infection may be candidates for vaccination.

Other Laboratory Testing. A Pap smear should be obtained to screen for cervical abnormalities. Many of these, if present, are more easily treated before conception than during pregnancy. Mammography may also be indicated depending upon the woman's age and risk of breast cancer.

Some authors recommend a hemoglobin or hematocrit test to detect iron deficiency and a urine dipstick test for protein and sugar levels, although these have not been demonstrated to be clearly efficacious. Women in high-risk groups, and their sexual partners, can be offered screening for gonorrhea, syphilis, chlamydia infection, and tuberculosis. Any identified infection can be treated before conception.

Toxoplasmosis screening remains controversial. Pregnant women in the United States are less likely to have had previous infection and immunity than women in France, where a more aggressive screening program has been undertaken. In the United States it is felt that the proportion of seronegative women who would require serial testing would be much higher, and screening is not currently felt to be cost effective.

Genetic Consultation. Genetic consultation should be considered for women

1. Older than 35 years of age at the time of a pregnancy (although most congenital malformations occur in infants of women less than 35 years of age)
2. With a family history of congenital anomalies or inherited disorders
3. With a previous child with abnormal development or mental retardation
4. From an ethnic background associated with a high prevalence of inheritable diseases
5. With a history of chemical use due to industrial exposure or exposure to teratogens
6. With a previous history of three or more consecutive spontaneous abortions

Genetic tools include serum markers, amniocentesis, and chorionic villus sampling. Amniocentesis is usually performed at 16 weeks of gestation. The risk of fetal loss is 0.5 to 1%. Amniocentesis can cause leakage of amniotic fluid into the vagina, puncture of the fetus, or induction of amniotic fluid bands. Chorionic villus sampling is generally performed between 9 and 11 weeks of gestation, and testing can be completed in hours to days, rather than the weeks necessary for amniocentesis. Since no amniotic fluid is obtained, it does not assess alpha-fetoprotein levels. The risk of fetal loss is estimated to be 1 to 2%. Compared with amniocentesis, chorionic villus sampling has a slightly higher risk of procedure failure and fetal loss, and approximately 3 to 10% of women subsequently require amniocentesis for adequate genetic diagnosis.

Domestic Violence. Each year, 4 million women are victims of physical assault. Domestic violence against women occurs more frequently than burglary, mugging, or other physical crimes combined. Although 35% of women cared for in a hospital emergency room experience ongoing abuse, only 5% of the victims are identified. Abuse is a significant factor in miscarriage and abortion, in addition to rape, attempted suicide, alcohol and drug abuse, psychiatric disease, and child abuse. The incidence of domestic violence increases during pregnancy; 4 to 7% of pregnant women are abused. At particular risk are women who have completed fewer than 12 years of education, of nonwhite races, younger than 19 years of age, unmarried, living in crowded conditions, with an unwanted pregnancy, and with delayed or no prenatal care. However, abused women are from every socioeconomic background, occupation, and educational level.

Higher rates of violence can be detected when women are specifically questioned:

"Within the past year have you been hit, slapped, kicked, or otherwise physically hurt by someone?
"Since you have become pregnant have you been hit, slapped, kicked, or otherwise physically hurt by someone? If yes, by whom?
"Within the last year has anyone forced you to have sexual activities? If yes, whom?"

Abuse during pregnancy characteristically recurs and often escalates. Head trauma is the most frequent form of abuse. In addition to maternal morbidity, domestic violence is associated with preterm labor and chorioamnionitis.

Since the best predictor of abuse during pregnancy is a history of prior abuse, attempts should be made to assess all women as a part of preconception health appraisal with referral to appropriate community resources once an abused patient is identified.

Diagnosis of Pregnancy. A presumptive diagnosis of pregnancy can be made by clinical signs and symptoms in over 90% of patients. Amenorrhea and common physical complaints such as fatigue, breast tenderness, urinary frequency, and morning sickness are usually the first signs. Laboratory testing can be confirmatory. The latex agglutination inhibition tests are the most widely available and least expensive. They are not specific and produce many false-negative results. Radioimmunoassay of the beta subunit of human chorionic gonadotropin (hCG) is the most sensitive and most reliable test as well as the most expensive. In its quantitative or qualitative form, it becomes positive within a few days after conception. The monoclonal antibody test provides a good compromise with regard to cost, availability, and reliability. It may use either urine or serum, and common drugs do not commonly cause test interference.

Transabdominal ultrasonographic identification of a gestational sac is frequently possible 5 weeks after the patient's last menstrual period (LMP). A sac can be demonstrated even earlier with transvaginal probes.

Early obstetric ultrasound examination is usually necessary only when the patient is being evaluated for consideration of an ectopic pregnancy or when

TABLE 1. Historical Features Assessed at First Prenatal Visit

Menstrual and contraceptive history
Gynecologic and obstetric history
Details of past pregnancies
Medical and surgical history—especially gynecologic and obstetric
Prior hospitalizations
Environmental exposures
Medications
Allergic reactions and drug reactions
Diethylstilbestrol (DES) exposure
Family history of hereditary diseases, multiple gestation
Social factors
Tobacco, alcohol, substance abuse
Domestic violence and social support
Review of systems for pregnancy-related symptoms such as nausea, vomiting, abdominal pain, constipation, headaches, syncopal episodes, vaginal bleeding or discharge, dysuria or urinary frequency, swelling, varicosities, hemorrhoids

clinical gestational dating is uncertain. Fetal heart tones can be detected by Doppler ultrasound examination as early as 9 to 12 weeks from the LMP. The DeLee fetoscope detects fetal heart tones at 18 to 20 weeks from the LMP. Fetal activity, or quickening, is generally perceived between 16 and 20 weeks of pregnancy. As soon as pregnancy is recognized, the woman should be enrolled in prenatal care.

PRENATAL CARE

Prenatal care reduces the incidence of low birthweight and improves perinatal outcome. Figure 1 presents a flow diagram of suggested care for the prenatal patient.

First Prenatal Visit. At the first prenatal visit

TABLE 2. Physical Examination at First Prenatal Visit

Height
Weight
Fundi
Thyroid
Breast
Lungs
Heart
Abdomen
Presence of fetal heart tones
Extremities
Reflexes
Pelvic examination
External genitalia
Vagina
Cervix ("erosion" is common)
Uterus (At 12 weeks the uterus fills the pelvis and the fundus is palpable at the symphysis pubis. By 16 weeks the fundus is midway between the symphysis pubis and the umbilicus. At 20 weeks it reaches the umbilicus. Between 20 and 32 weeks the number of weeks of pregnancy correlates roughly with the number of centimeters from the top of the symphysis pubis to the top of the uterine fundus.)
Adnexa
Evidence for any infections such as condylomata, herpes simplex, or *Neisseria.*

TABLE 3. Routine First Trimester Laboratory Evaluation

Complete blood count
ABO blood typing
Rh factor test
Antibody screen
Urinalysis
Urine culture (able to diagnose group B streptococcal bacteriuria)
Serologic test for syphilis
Rubella titer (if previously unknown)
Pap smear
Hepatitis B soluble antigen test
HIV test

the physician should complete a risk assessment, patient history, and physical examination. Unfortunately, formal risk assessment scoring systems correlate poorly with birth outcomes. Half the adverse outcomes occur in patients who are felt to have low-risk pregnancies. Most formal risk assessment systems currently in use target specific populations. A great deal of judgment is necessary to decide which assessments benefit individual patients. Assessment can identify some high-risk patients with treatable risk factors. Some of these factors have been discussed in the context of a preconception evaluation and will not be repeated in this section.

It is important to try to establish an accurate estimated date of confinement. This date is the cornerstone for much of the subsequent care during pregnancy. For the woman with a reliable menstrual pattern, the mean duration of pregnancy as calculated from the LMP is 280 days, or 40 weeks. Many use Nägele's rule:

$$EDC = LMP - 3 \text{ months} + 7 \text{ days}$$

Physical examination may demonstrate uterine enlargement, isthmus softening (Hegar's sign), and vaginal or cervical cyanosis (Chadwick's sign). Uterine length, rather than width or volume, most accurately reflects gestational age and correlates well with ultrasonographic measurements from 6 to 14 weeks. Table 1 outlines the historical features important to assess at the first prenatal visit. Table 2 outlines the physical examination that should be completed at the first prenatal visit. Table 3 provides routine first trimester laboratory evaluation. Table 4 highlights laboratory evaluation that can be used for groups specifically at risk. Table 5 outlines laboratory evaluations and their recommended timing during pregnancy. This information should be collected and orga-

TABLE 4. Laboratory Evaluation for Patients "At Risk"

Gonorrhea test
Tuberculosis skin testing
Cervical culture for chlamydia
Hemoglobin electrophoresis
Tay-Sachs screening
Urine or blood toxicologic analysis

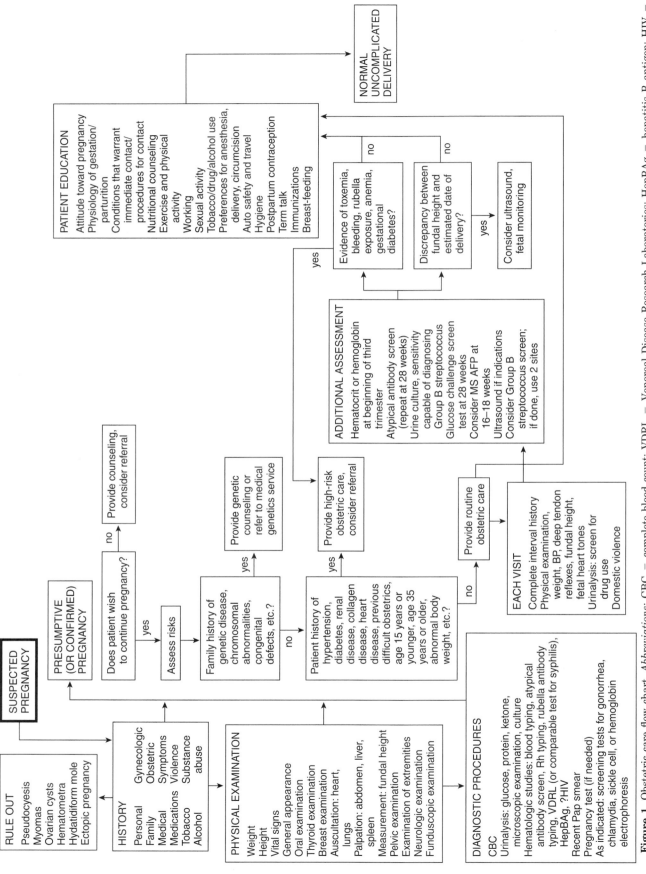

Figure 1. Obstetric care flow chart. *Abbreviations:* CBC = complete blood count; VDRL = Venereal Disease Research Laboratories; HepBAg = hepatitis B antigen; HIV = human immunodeficiency virus; BP = blood pressure; MS AFP = alpha-fetoprotein. (Adapted from Normal Pregnancy Reference Guide #17, 2nd ed. Lexington, KY, American Board of Family Practice, 1985, pp IV–V.)

TABLE 5. **Routine Prenatal Care**

Routine Prenatal Care	Risk Assessment						
	All Visits	First Visit	Each Trimester	16–18 Weeks	24–28 Weeks	26–28 Weeks	First Visit & 36 Weeks
Weight	x						
Blood pressure	x						
Blood type		x					
Antibody titer		x			x if Rh −		
Complete blood count		x	x				
Rubella titer		x					
Pap smear		x					
Urine dipstick	x						
Urine culture				x			
Hepatitis B antigen		x					
HIV		x					
VDRL		x					
Gonorrhea culture							x*
Chlamydia							x*
Group B streptococci						†	
Alpha-fetoprotein				x†			
Glucose					x		
Substance abuse	x						
Violence	x						
Others (if indicated)							
Tuberculosis							
Amniocentesis							
Sickle cell or hemoglobin electrophoresis							
Uric acid							
Not routinely indicated							
Ultrasound							
Home uterine monitoring							

*For women at high risk.
†Suggested by some; not proved to be cost effective.

nized into an easily accessible obstetric database. The format of the obstetric record should allow quick and easy identification of basic information, the most common risk factors, pertinent prenatal issues organized by trimester, and psychosocial and medical issues pertinent to each visit or trimester and should facilitate documentation and communication among other health providers or sources of care. Ongoing parameters such as dates of health encounters; fundal height; fetal heart tones; blood pressure; weight; urine protein and glucose levels; and pertinent laboratory values, as well as information about consultation (such as nutritional or genetic) and patient education should be easily displayed as well as documented by the use of flow sheets.

Many examples of this type of charting are commercially available. Computerized medical records have the advantage of allowing the availability of these data "on line" among geographically different sites, including the hospital or birthing center. The information collected, recorded, and analyzed allows risk assessment as well as ongoing management of the pregnancy. Situations that increase risk include pre-existing medical illness; previous pregnancy complications such as perinatal mortality, prematurity, fetal growth retardation, malformations, placental accidents, and maternal hemorrhage; substance abuse; and evidence of poor maternal nutrition. Identification of some categories of risk, such as risk

of preterm labor, may require adaptation of routine prenatal care, such as more frequent visits and additional methods of evaluation such as ultrasound. Other risks that are identified may lead to consultation or referral with a secondary or tertiary source of obstetric care, such as a perinatal center. Table 6 lists common items in the obstetric database, their significance, and implications for management.

Subsequent Prenatal Care. For low-risk pregnancies the recommended frequency of prenatal visits is every 4 weeks to 28 weeks, every 2 weeks from 28 to 36 weeks, and weekly until delivery. For women who benefit from additional education or develop complications, more frequent evaluation is recommended. At each visit, weight, blood pressure, uterine size, auscultation of fetal heart tones, the presence of edema or proteinuria, and any new symptoms or new issues should be recorded. Educational materials should supplement extensive anticipatory guidance. Childbirth preparation classes are recommended.

Nutrition. Prepregnancy weight for height is correlated with gestational weight gain and newborn birthweight. The effect of any given amount of weight gain is greater in thin women and least in obese women. For any given amount of weight gain, young adolescents give birth to smaller infants than older women. They should be instructed to gain on the higher side of the recommendations. Recommenda-

Text continued on page 977

TABLE 6. **Obstetric Database***

Data Collected	Significance	Management or Additional Screening
Medical History		
GENERAL		
Maternal age <18 years	Increased incidence of preeclampsia, low birthweight of child, associated low socioeconomic status.	Frequent visits. Refer to adolescent pregnancy program.
Maternal age >35 years	Increased incidence of chromosomal abnormalities (especially Down's syndrome), hypertension, placenta previa, abruptio placentae, hydatidiform mole, pregnancy-induced hypertension, diabetes, infants >4000 gm or <2500 gm, cesarean section, maternal mortality, spontaneous abortions, and stillbirths.	Consider chorionic villi sampling, amniocentesis at 14 to 16 weeks, closer prenatal surveillance.
Paternal age >42 years	Incidence of chromosomal abnormalities.	Consider amniocentesis.
Diabetes mellitus	Incidence of stillbirth, macrosomia, hydramnios, fetal anomalies.	Glucola screening
Hypertension	Incidence of preeclampsia, eclampsia, intrauterine growth retardation, size and date discrepancies.	Frequent blood pressure checks; alter medications if necessary to reduce fetal toxicity.
Allergies and adverse reactions (especially to drugs).	Possibly used in pregnancy: narcotics, antibiotics.	Have patient avoid allergic reactions.
Maternal DES exposure	Increased incidence of uterine abnormality, spontaneous abortion, prematurity, incompetent cervix. Most exposed women can carry pregnancy to term.	Frequent cervical checks beginning mid-second trimester to rule out effacement or dilatation.
Herpes simplex Type II	Risk of neonatal infection if active lesions present at birth. Small risk of primary infection produces congenital abnormality.	No need for third-trimester screening with viral cultures. Instead, examine all women in labor for active lesions.
Congenital heart lesions including mitral valve prolapse	Consider need for subacute bacterial endocarditis prophylaxis at delivery. No need for prophylaxis for mitral valve prolapse in routine vaginal delivery.	Assess classification of cardiac disease; consider consultation for anything except mitral valve prolapse.
Urinary tract infection or pyelonephritis	Pyelonephritis leads to increased incidence of premature labor.	Frequent laboratory evaluation to rule out urinary tract infection.
Thromboembolic disease	Risk of pulmonary embolus.	Regular checks for phlebitis; prescribe support stockings.
Seizure disorder	Antiseizure medications teratogenic; drug levels affected by pregnancy.	Consider consultation, preconception trial off medication; if seizure free >2 years and normal EEGs, change to less teratogenic drug or lower dose.
Activity	Not associated with adverse birth outcome except in rare occupations.	See section on activity.
Nutrition	Assess eating disorders, pica, adequacy of calcium, protein, calories.	Consider nutritionist referral.
SURGICAL		
Pelvic trauma or surgery	? adequacy of pelvis secondary to surgery or trauma, previous uterine surgery, or cesarean section.	Type of uterine surgery or cesarean section determines if attempt at vaginal delivery is possible; obtain previous operative notes; consultation for cesarean section if vaginal delivery is to be attempted.
Major surgery (heart, kidneys)	Depends on surgery and subsequent functional status.	Consider consultation.
Obstetric-Gynecologic		
Parity	Primigravida, increased incidence of preeclampsia. Parity >5, increased incidence of hypertension, uterine inertia, postpartum bleeding.	Monitor frequently for symptoms and signs of preeclampsia.
Spontaneous abortions	>3 increases incidence of fetal loss. As many as half of pregnancies may end in miscarriage, usually before implantation. Only one spontaneous abortion does not carry poor prognosis for future fertility.	Consider consultation ? cerclage.

TABLE 6. **Obstetric Database*** *Continued*

Data Collected	Significance	Management or Additional Screening
Therapeutic abortions	CONTROVERSIAL—>2 increases fetal loss to two to three times normal up to 28 weeks.	Consider consultation ? cerclage.
Premature labor	Increased incidence of subsequent premature labor.	? bed rest; frequent cervical checks in third trimester, consider group B streptococcal screening from urine, cervix, and rectum and treatment in labor; consider consultation. Screen for other cervical or vaginal infections.
Prior complications in labor	Depends on complication.	Consider consultation.
Cesarean section		Consider consultation; consider trial of vaginal labor or VBAC.
Preeclampsia	Increased risk of preeclampsia but less than that of primigravid patients.	Rule out underlying chronic hypertension; add uric acid and coagulation studies to laboratory studies.
Gestational diabetes mellitus	High risk of gestational diabetes mellitus (50%) in subsequent pregnancies.	Consider glucose screening at 12 weeks. If negative, repeat at 24–28 weeks.
Rh status	Risk of erythroblastosis fetalis if mother Rh-negative and baby Rh-positive.	Rh screen in entry at 28 weeks. $Rh_o(D)$ immune globulin for bleeding, at 28 weeks, and postpartum.
Prior fetal anomalies	Depends on anomaly.	May benefit from genetic counseling, amniocentesis, ultrasonography.
Birthweight of prior babies	Infant >4500 gm, high incidence of gestational diabetes mellitus; infant <2500 gm, depends on reason for low birthweight.	Management depends on cause.
Length of previous labors	Look for history of precipitous labors.	Low tolerance for checking patient in labor and delivery near term.
Previous abnormal Pap smear	Cervical trauma with treatment (conization, cryosurgery) or current abnormal Pap smear.	Check past and current Pap tests.
Interval from last pregnancy	<1 year, greater maternal morbidity (anemia and malnutrition).	Nutrition consultation.
Drug Use		
Alcohol	High incidence of fetal alcohol syndrome, low birthweight, spontaneous abortions, fetal and/or maternal withdrawal (esp. >2 drinks/day or periodic binge drinking).	All patients should be screened for use; if positive, refer for multidisciplinary treatment program. Cutting down even in third trimester benefits baby!
Tobacco (10 cigarettes/day or more)	High incidence of spontaneous abortions, low birthweight.	Support smoking cessation "cold turkey"; refer to area programs; avoid transdermal nicotine.
Marijuana	? Increased SAB, placental dysfunction; decreased birthweight, prematurity, ? chromosomal abnormalities.	Most users also use other psychoactive substances.
Caffeine	>2 cups/day may affect incidence of low birthweight, spontaneous abortions; may be a teratogen.	Encourage patient to decrease amount consumed.
Cocaine	Woman at greater risk if cocaine is sole drug of abuse; crack increases incidence of preterm labor, low birthweight, hemorrhage.	
Opiates	Affected infants born addicted. Methadone still problematic, though delayed infant withdrawal.	
Prescription and over-the-counter drugs	Depends on medication.	Check on association with pregnancy outcome; consider folic acid supplementation if on oral contraceptives within 1 year of pregnancy.
Family History		
Sickle cell trait	Screen for sickle cell trait. Pregnant women with trait more prone to urinary tract infections. If trait positive, child at risk, and father should be screened.	If mother has sickle cell trait, screen her for urinary tract infection with monthly urine cultures, and screen father for sickle cell trait. If father is positive, screen child at appropriate age. If mother has sickle cell disease, refer.

Table continued on following page

TABLE 6. **Obstetric Database*** *Continued*

Data Collected	Significance	Management or Additional Screening
Diabetes	Increased congenital defects if hyperglycemic before conception; this risk can be decreased with euglycemia.	Normalized blood sugar before conception.
Congenital abnormalities		Consider obstetric consultation, amniocentesis ultrasonography, genetic counseling.
Neural tube defects	Higher incidence of neural tube defects.	Alpha-fetoprotein, amniocentesis, and/or ultrasonography; ? preconception vitamins.
Multiple gestations	Higher incidence of multiple gestations.	Watch for size-date discrepancy; ? ultrasonography.
Trisomy, dislocations, translocation	Higher incidence of subsequent genetic abnormality.	Genetic counseling, chorionic villus sampling, amniocentesis.
Tay-Sachs disease	Hexosaminidase A activity.	Screen Ashkenazic Jews, individuals of Mediterranean origin; check blood smear or hemoglobin electrophoresis.
Other genetic conditions, inborn errors of metabolism		Genetic counseling.
Social History		
Partner's involvement	If no involvement, mother at risk for being single parent; establish source of emotional and financial support.	Consider scheduling partner for appointment; invite to prenatal visits, classes.
Economic status	Low economic status associated with high fetal morbidity.	Seek appropriate social services.
Pregnancy: planned or unplanned; wanted or unwanted	If pregnancy unplanned or unwanted, increased incidence of poor prenatal care and child abuse.	Increase visits as indicated.
Education level	No relationship to prenatal outcome, may influence infant care.	Providers need to pay attention to work choice, literacy, and reading level of any printed material.
Social support of family and community	Affects economic, emotional support.	Increase visits as indicated.
Work plans	Usually no effect on outcome except in certain occupations.	
Pets	Cats, risk of toxoplasmosis.	Have patients avoid cats, especially changing litter. TORCH titer not useful screen.
Domestic violence	Occurs in all educational and socioeconomic groups. 4–7% affected. Pregnancy may precipitate increase in violence.	Providers need to specifically ask at early visit.
Exercise	May affect fertility; little study in pregnancy. Joint laxity may predispose to injury.	Patient should use comfort as a guide, avoid hypertension and dehydration, overheating, hot tubs and saunas in the first trimester; limit heart rate to ≤140 beats per minute. Additional calories needed. Abdominal trauma should be avoided.
Physician Examination		
Pregnant weight (weight at entry)	≤80% ideal body weight (IBW), risk of poor nutrition, cephalopelvic disproportion; ≥120% IBW, risk of gestational diabetes, large-for-gestational-age infant, hypertension, cephalopelvic disproportion.	Consider nutrition consultant, weight gain should be based on BMI (see text).
Blood pressure	Blood pressure 140/90 or blood pressure rise: >30 systolic, >15 diastolic.	High incidence of chronic hypertension, preeclampsia.
Pelvic lesions	Herpes, risk of neonatal infection at delivery, low risk of primary infection to baby; HPV infection, risk of neonatal infection and maternal bleeding at delivery.	Examine for herpetic lesions in all women in labor; consider consultation, treat lesions carefully during pregnancy (use trichloroacetic acid instead of podophyllin).
Uterine size and shape	If fibroids or uterine abnormalities, high incidence of premature labor; fibroids may degenerate.	Consider consultation.

TABLE 6. **Obstetric Database*** *Continued*

Data Collected	Significance	Management or Additional Screening
Previous cesarean scar	See "Medical History"; pelvic surgery, low incidence of dehiscence or uterine rupture.	Consultation; obtain previous operative notes to ascertain location of uterine scar.
Clinical pelvimetry	Pelvic adequacy.	Check for tight pelvis, but essentially all patients are given trial of labor.
Extremities, phlebitis edema	Risk of pulmonary embolus; rule out underlying causes, especially preeclampsia.	Avoid warfarin or aspirin therapy; patient should elevate feet, use support stockings; treat preeclampsia if present.

Laboratory Data
URINALYSIS

Data Collected	Significance	Management or Additional Screening
Proteinuria	Rule out underlying renal disease, urinary tract infection, preeclampsia.	Follow-up as indicated by evaluation.
Glycosuria	Rule out diabetes mellitus. This is poor screen, as it usually reflects recent meals.	Check blood sugar.
Urine culture (Uricult)	Rule out urinary tract infections. Asymptomatic bacteriuria during pregnancy associated with high risk of overt urinary tract infection; however, magnitude of risk, effectiveness of antibiotics in reducing it, and the value of screening still controversial. Screen with culture medium able to diagnose group B streptococcal bacteria.	Treat infection, then test for cure. If two infections, do monthly urine cultures and/or suppression.
VDRL/RPR	Rule out syphilis with its risk for fetal anomalies.	If positive, rule out false-positive in pregnancy (need FTA and titer).
Hematocrit	<30 = anemia. Consider empirical treatment with oral iron. If no response, dilution, iron deficiency, hemoglobinopathy. Only severe anemia correlates with poor pregnancy outcome.	Prescribe $FeSO_4$. Use other iron preparations if GI intolerance. Avoid iron dextron (Imferon). Check hematocrit each trimester.
Platelet count	If decreased, may represent ITP or precursor to preeclampsia/HELLP syndrome.	
Glucose screening after 50 gram of carbohydrate load	If ≤140 mg after 50-gm carbohydrate load, (can be nonfasting), full 3-hour GTT, GTT and if either 2 abnormal values and abnormal FBS (see table below), diagnose as diabetes.	

Criteria for Evaluating Results of Glucose Tolerance Test

Time (h)	O'Sullivan Criteria Plasma Glucose (mg/dL)	Whole Blood (mg/dL)	Plasma Glucose Oxidase Method (mg/dL)
Fasting	105	90	95
1	190	165	180
2	165	145	155
3	145	125	140

Data Collected	Significance	Management or Additional Screening
Blood type	Rh-negative associated with risk of erythroblastosis fetalis; ABO abnormality associated with high incidence of fetal jaundice.	If titer negative, give $Rh_o(D)$ immune globulin (RhoGAM) at 28 weeks and every 12 weeks until delivery. Repeat ideally within 72 h postpartum (but up to 4 weeks). Also need to give same immune globulin for amniocentesis, bleeding in second and third trimester, external version, after ectopic, SAB, or TAB.
Antibody screen	If positive, check titer.	Streptomycin can cause OTO toxicity in the infant and should be avoided; pyrazinamide ? safety. Isoniazid, rifampin, ethambutol are safe (with Isoniazid need vitamin B_6).

Table continued on following page

TABLE 6. **Obstetric Database*** *Continued*

Data Collected	Significance	Management or Additional Screening
Rubella titer	15% of women are not immune; infants are susceptible to congenital rubella.	Though risk of congenital rubella secondary to vaccination is low, wait until after birth to immunize mother. If exposure occurs, check rubella titer every 2 weeks if first titer is <1:8. Fourfold increase indicates recent infection; options need to be discussed, including therapeutic abortion. Inadvertent vaccination of pregnant women should not lead to therapeutic abortion in absence of other conditions and evidence.
Sickle cell trait	Occurs in blacks and Southeast Asians; mothers with trait are more prone to urinary tract infections.	Hemoglobin electrophoresis. If sickle trait, screen monthly for urinary tract infection. If mother positive, screen father to see if infant at risk for sickle cell disease.
Pap test	Screen for dysplasia.	Consider obstetric referral for colposcopy and possible biopsy if not available.
Gonorrhea culture	Possible neonatal infection.	Treat infection, test for cure. Treat sexual partner(s). Screen for gonorrhea last trimester, depending on prevalence of gonorrhea in population. Value of routine gonorrhea culture in low-risk patients may be overstated.
Tetanus immunization status	Risk of maternal, perinatal tetanus.	Give tetanus toxoid during pregnancy if mother has not had one in 10 years.
Alpha-fetoprotein	Associated with neural tube defects; increase in incidence of fetal demise; other associations under investigation; need careful laboratory evaluation and thorough counseling.	Offer to all with full discussion. Document patient with. If screening, perform at 7–18 weeks. Correlate with race, weight.
Hepatitis B soluble antigen (HBsAg)	Vertical transmission highly likely; 70% transmit infection to newborn, 90% of babies become carriers, 25% of babies die of liver complications	Universal screening for HBsAg recommended. Immunize if HBsAg negative but at risk.
TORCH screen (see rubella and herpes)	Toxoplasmosis in 1.1/1000 live births, 8% of babies are infected; 90% of women have no clinical illness; cytomegalovirus, 3–5% of women shed virus at term; 1–25% of newborns excrete virus.	Routine screening not recommended; toxoplasmosis screen only if clinical suspicion; good hygiene emphasized; patients should cook raw meat thoroughly, wash hands after handling raw meat, avoid cat litter, wear gloves while in contact with soil. Cytomegalovirus, no treatment at present. Female health personnel or day care personnel without antibodies may be at risk. CMV is the most common congenital viral infection. Screen women at high risk with PPD, with recent multidrug resistance check. Most recent recommendations are that infant needs INH too.
Chlamydia tests	Infection may cause diseases in newborn; increase in premature labor, decrease in postpartum endometritis.	Screen high-risk women at first visit and 36 weeks; if positive, treat with 1.5 gm of erythromycin for 7 days. Treat sexual partners.
Amniocentesis		Offer to women >35 years (or when fathers are >42 years) or with previous child with chromosomal anomaly. May be used to determine fetal sex if couple is at risk for X-linked disorder. It may also be part of management plan for Rh or abnormal alpha-fetoprotein.
Group B streptococcal infection	Can cause preterm labor: bacteria, puerperal infection of mother, vertical transmission in labor most common cause of neonatal sepsis. Early disease within 48 hours. Respiratory distress and sepsis. Late disease within 4 weeks most typically meningitis.	CONTROVERSIAL as routine screen; however, patients with previously infected infant or with premature rupture of membranes with or without labor, preterm labor prolonged for 18 hours, need treatment.

TABLE 6. **Obstetric Database*** *Continued*

Data Collected	Significance	Management or Additional Screening
Tuberculosis		No screening except in high-prevalence settings.
AIDS testing	Consider for all women. About one-third of infants will develop AIDS; rate decreases with AZT treatment of mother.	Informed consent for testing necessary. If positive, should be managed with multidisciplinary input.
Parvovirus B_{19}	< one-third of maternal infections result in fetal infection; infection increases SAB stillbirth, nonimmune hydrops.	No known antiviral treatment; gamma globulin not effective if exposed. If exposed, check IgM. If positive, monitor with MS-AFP and ultrasound.
Varicella	5–10% of adult women susceptible; infection increases preterm labor, maternal encephalitis, and pneumonia. Congenital varicella syndrome affects 10% of babies exposed in first trimester. If mother infected, 5–21 days before delivery generally mild infection in infant. If mother infected, 4 days before or 2 days after delivery, baby is at risk for infection.	Consider immunizing non-pregnant women who have not had varicella infection. Consider VZIG within 72 h of birth. Pregnant patient exposed to chickenpox or shingles: consider IgG titer if no personal history of chickenpox. If nonimmune, ? effect of VZIG within 96 h of exposure.

*Revised from Andolsek KM: Obstetric standards of prenatal, intrapartum and postpartum management. Philadelphia, Lea & Febiger, 1990, pp. 30–36.
Abbreviations: DES = diethylstilbestrol; EEG = electroencephalogram; VDRL = Venereal Disease Research Laboratories; RPR = rapid plasma reagin; SAB = spontaneous abortion; HPV = human papilloma virus; ITP = idiopathic thrombocytopenic purpura; HELLP = hemolysis (intravascular), elevated liver enzymes, low platelets; GTT = glucose tolerance test; FBS = fasting blood sugar; TORCH = change to toxoplasmosis titer; AZT = zidovudine; VZIG = varicella zoster immune globulin; VBAC = vaginal birth after cesarean section; FTA = fluorescent treponemal antibody; GI = gastrointestinal; TAB = therapeutic abortion; OTO = otic; PPD = purified protein derivative; INH = isoniazid; MS–AFP = maternal serum alpha fetoprotein.

tions are based on weight-for-height categories, or a body mass index (BMI = weight/height)

	Recommended Pregnancy Weight
BMI	Gain (Pounds)
Low	28 to 40
Normal	25 to 35
High	15 to 25

For most women, this degree of weight gain requires an additional 300 kcal per day (35 kcal per kg of pregnant body weight). Caloric requirements for pregnant adolescents are higher. Women 11 to 14 years of age need 2200 kcal per day just for their own growth; additional calories are needed to meet pregnancy requirements. Most women who consume an adequate diet do not need to increase their protein intake. Sodium restriction has not been found to be beneficial. Iron supplementation is controversial. There is little evidence to suggest that routine iron supplementation during pregnancy improves clinical outcomes for the mother, fetus, or newborn. Pregnant women with a hemoglobin level less than 10 mg per dL are at an increased risk for having preterm or low-birthweight newborns and other adverse outcomes. However, it is not clear whether the anemia is responsible for these outcomes or whether they can be prevented through iron supplementation. Iron improves maternal hematologic indexes but has not been shown to improve outcomes. Many providers limit additional iron to women with hemoglobin levels of less than 10 mg per dL. If it is prescribed, it can be given as ferrous sulfate, ferrous gluconate, or ferrous fumarate.

Additional folic acid is recommended daily for all women; 4 mg if they have a history of a previous baby with a neural tube defect; at least 0.4 mg if they have no such previous history. Specific folic acid supplementation is generally necessary. If a women tries to get this amount by simply increasing quantities of over-the-counter multivitamin supplements, she may receive toxic doses of other vitamins. Folic acid needs are greater in women with multiple gestations, those who have previously used oral contraceptives, those who were pregnant within the previous 2 years, or those who are dependent on (or are abusers of) alcohol.

Most pregnant women do not require additional calcium supplementation unless they have a diet extremely low in calcium or are adolescent. Milk servings should be increased to three or four per day.

Consultation with a nutritionist is recommended. This is particularly important in managing patients with nonstandard weight-gain patterns; diabetic patients; adolescents; individuals with lactose intolerance or hyperemesis; vegetarians; patients with multiple gestations; women who have had three or more pregnancies within 2 years; and those with excessive vitamin intake or with symptoms of pica (compulsive eating of non-nutritive substances like starch or ice), citta (excessive unusual food cravings), or edema.

Mid-Trimester Screening Tests. Any first-trimester tests, like tests for HIV, that, if positive, would affect management should be repeated in the mid-trimester if risk factors continue.

Screening for gestational diabetes is currently recommended by most authorities at 26 to 28 weeks. The standard test is the 50-gram glucose load followed an hour later by a serum glucose determination. The patient does not need to be fasting. Values greater than 140 mg per dL should result in a 3-hour oral glucose tolerance test. Criteria for the interpretation of this test are presented in Table 6 with the "Glucola" entry.

Ultrasonography. Four major randomized controlled clinical trials involving 15,935 pregnant women demonstrated an identical rate of live births and proportion of newborns with Apgar scores below 7 with or without routine ultrasonography. The only difference that could be demonstrated in perinatal mortality was that screened fetuses with major malformations were aborted. In the nonscreened group these babies were born and frequently died at birth. On the other hand, there was a 2.4 per 1000 rate of false-positive findings suggesting malformations where there were none. This is about the same rate as for "real" malformations.

Compared with the use of indicated ultrasonography, routine ultrasound examinations have not been shown to have any effect on perinatal morbidity or mortality for either mothers or infants, nor does routine ultrasonography reduce unnecessary intervention that may occur from an erroneous perception that a pregnancy is postdated.

The American College of Obstetricians and Gynecologists (ACOG) has reconfirmed its recommendation against routine ultrasound screening. Some concerns regarding long-term safety to the fetus remain.

Although ultrasonography has not been found to be beneficial as a routine screen, it is an extremely valuable tool when used in the diagnosis and management of suspected abnormal conditions. Some of these indications include estimating gestational age (when clinical dating is not possible); excluding an ectopic pregnancy; localizing the placenta before amniocentesis; locating the placenta to exclude placenta previa; following fetal growth in the fetus with suspected intrauterine growth retardation; detailing placental abnormalities; detecting fetal death in a patient with a missed abortion or threatened abortion; assisting in the prenatal diagnosis of infants with congenital abnormalities, choriocarcinoma, or hydatid mole; providing adjunct information to other procedures; evaluating pregnant women with a pelvic mass; documenting fetal position; and assessing fetal well-being through fetal movements or amniotic fluid volume. Parental bonding may be enhanced by viewing the infant with real-time ultrasonography.

Home Uterine Activity Monitoring. Home uterine activity monitoring (HUAM) has not been shown in randomized clinical trials to improve birth outcomes. It does document the presence of contractions, many of which are not perceived by the patient. The ACOG in 1989 and again in 1992 stated that HUAM was investigational and not for routine clinical use. The Agency for Health Care Policy and Research in 1992 reported that data did not support the widespread use of HUAM, nor was it felt to be any more effective than other methods for reducing the incidence of preterm labor.

Herpes Cultures. In the past, women with a history of herpes simplex virus (HSV) infection had samples cultured weekly beginning at 36 weeks. If the culture was negative at the time of delivery, they were allowed to attempt a vaginal delivery. If the culture was positive or uncertain, cesarean section was recommended. These weekly surveillance cultures are no longer recommended. Most women who shed HSV at the time of delivery have no past history of the illness. Current management recommendations for pregnant patients are as follows:

1. The use of weekly prenatal cultures should be abandoned (if this has been the standard).
2. There is no role for amniocentesis in assessing infection.
3. At the time of labor the genital area of all women in labor should be inspected. If there are no genital herpetic lesions, vaginal delivery is acceptable.
4. If lesions are present, no scalp electrodes should be used.
5. If there are herpetic lesions when labor or rupture of membrane occurs, a cesarean section should be performed in 4 to 6 hours. These infants should be closely watched, as they have an approximately 6% chance of illness.
6. If remote lesions are present, vaginal delivery is acceptable, but lesions should be excluded from the field by draping.
7. Isolation is not necessary for the mother, who can hold her baby and breast-feed. She needs to use strict handwashing measures and prevent contact between the baby and infected lesions or their secretions.
8. Since 70% of HSV-infected babies are delivered by mothers without a past clinical history of HSV, or signs or symptoms of disease at delivery, HSV should be suspected in all ill infants.

Controversial Screening Methods. Screening for group B streptococcal (GBS) infection in pregnancy remains controversial. GBS infection is the leading cause of life-threatening perinatal infection in the United States. From 15 to 40% of pregnant women are asymptomatic carriers, and 8% are colonized at the time of labor. In mothers, GBS infection causes maternal chorioamnionitis, endomyometritis, cystitis, and pyelonephritis and increases the incidence of premature rupture of membranes (PROM) and preterm delivery. Furthermore, 75% of babies born to colonized mothers are colonized. From 1 to 3 per 1000 live births have an early onset of the disease. This risk increases to 10 per 1000 live births if the mother is colonized and 40 per 1000 if other risk factors are present. Early onset of the disease generally occurs within 7 days of birth; two-thirds of babies develop symptoms within 6 hours. These babies have a 15% mortality rate due to bacteremia, pneumonia, and meningitis. In late onset of the disease (0.5 to 1.0 per 1000 live births), meningitis is more common.

Screening has been problematic for several reasons. No one site is exclusively predictive of perinatal infection. Over the course of pregnancy a positive site frequently spontaneously becomes negative. Negative culture sites become positive. Even among infants of colonized mothers, the overall attack rate is low. If culture-positive women receive oral antibiotics, over two-thirds relapse by term if treatment is discontinued.

Antepartum chemoprophylaxis has been successful when directed at urinary tract colonization. Antepartum treatment of GBS bacteriuria reduces the incidence of PROM and preterm labor.

Intrapartum intravenous antibiotic therapy decreases mother-to-baby colonization, decreases the early onset of neonatal sepsis, and decreases postcesarean endometritis. There is no effect on the late onset of neonatal disease.

Some authorities recommend screening all pregnant women at 28 weeks of gestation.

If samples from women are cultured, both rectal and lower vaginal sites should be used concurrently. Culturing samples from only one of these sites misses 25% of GBS carriers. Women with positive cultures and one or more of the risk factors listed in Table 7 should be treated intrapartum.

If the maternal colonization status is not known, women should be treated if one of these clinical risk factors is present.

Some authorities advocate treating all women in labor. Unfortunately the degree of risk reduction obtained is about the same as that of significant adverse reactions to parenteral antibiotics among patients not previously known to be allergic. The ACOG does not recommend routine rectal and vaginal screening. Women with preterm labor and PROM are screened and treated with antepartum antibiotics if positive for GBS. Women are screened for GBS bacteriuria and treated antepartum if culture is positive.

The ACOG recommends that all women be treated intrapartum regardless of their colonization status if any of the clinical risk factors listed in Table 7 are present. Intrapartum chemoprophylaxis regimens are listed in Table 8.

Immunizations. Pregnancy may be a time to update a woman's immunization status. Table 9 lists the immunizations considered safe in pregnancy. Some would defer immunization until the second trimester in case the woman develops fever with the theoretical impact of hyperthermia on early development. Indications remain the same as for nonpregnant patients.

In general, live-virus vaccines are contraindicated in pregnant women. These include measles, mumps, varicella, oral poliomyelitis, and rubella. Some are contraindicated unless exposure is unavoidable,

there is close continued exposure, or the patient travels to areas in which diseases such as yellow fever and typhoid are endemic.

If polio vaccination is necessary, inactivated polio vaccine (IPV) should be considered rather than oral polio vaccine (OPV).

Exercise. Benefits of exercise to the pregnant woman include enhanced well-being, fitness, weight control, improved sleep, less constipation, and less water retention. Risks include joint laxity, especially in the second and third trimesters. Joint laxity increases instability and predisposes to injury. Potential risks include an increase in the maternal core temperature, producing hyperthermia in the fetus. Women who have been physically active before pregnancy are usually able to continue their activity, making necessary adjustments for coordination and balance. They should avoid high-impact sports or those with potential abdominal blunt trauma. Inactive women should be encouraged to start a program of graduated aerobic exercise.

Sports considered unsafe at any point in pregnancy include scuba diving, boxing, hockey, soccer, and tackle football. If weight lifting, the woman should avoid the supine position and the Valsalva maneuver.

Many authorities recommend restricting the mother's maximum heart rate to 140 beats per minute. Alternatively, a target heart rate for the woman can be calculated:

60 to 70% of (220 − patient age)   For most patients
80 to 85% of (220 − patient age)   For well-trained athletes

TABLE 8. **Intrapartum Chemoprophylaxis Regimens for Group B Streptococcal Infection**

Intrapartum ampicillin
500 mg IV q 6 h
2 gm IV then 1 gm q 4 h (+ treating newborn with ampicillin 50 mg/kg q 12 h for 4 doses)
2 gm IV q 6 h (if no delivery 500 mg q 6 h PO for 14 days)
1 gm IV q 6 h until delivery
Intrapartum penicillin
Penicillin G 5 million U IV q 6 h; if no delivery after 18 h, Penicillin V 1 million U q 8 h till active labor
Erythromycin or clindamycin can be used in penicillin-allergic women.

TABLE 7. **Risk Factors for Intrapartum Chemoprophylaxis Against Group B Streptococcus**

Preterm labor at less than 37 weeks of gestation
PROM at less than 37 weeks of gestation
Fever during labor
Multiple birth
Rupture of membranes beyond 18 h
Sibling of baby had GBS infection

Abbreviations: PROM = premature rupture of membranes; GBS = group B streptococcal.

TABLE 9. **Immunizations Considered Safe in Pregnancy**

Tetanus toxoid
Tetanus-diphtheria
Rabies
Hepatitis B
Pneumococcus
Cholera
Plague
Influenza
Immune globulins (e.g., hepatitis B, rabies, tetanus, varicella, hepatitis A, measles)

If her heart rate exceeds 140 or her recovery rate is 110 at 5 minutes or 100 or more at 10 minutes, the intensity of her workout should be decreased. An additional 200 to 300 calories for each 20- to 30-minute session of low-intensity aerobic workout is recommended. A 10-minute warm-up and 5-minute cool-down are suggested. The high-intensity part of a workout should be limited to 10 to 15 minutes. Exercising in hot, humid weather should be avoided when possible.

Role of the Father. Fathers often have been excluded from the process of prenatal care. However their inclusion in this process offers many advantages. Common acute care needs of fathers can be addressed. As many as 10 to 25% of prospective fathers develop the couvade syndrome during the first trimester of their partner's pregnancy. Paternal anxiety is expressed as somatic symptoms similar to what their partners may be experiencing including nausea, cramps, changes in appetite, diarrhea, increased blood pressure, abdominal bloating, or toothache. This syndrome can occur for the first time or recur during the ninth month.

Health maintenance can be addressed in individuals who characteristically do not present for wellness care.

Sometimes addressing the father's health issue is part of a strategy for the mother as well. For example, tobacco or other substance use in either parent may be better managed by involvement, and ideally abstinence, by their partner.

Special concerns for the father may include change in sexual drive and activity; his impending role change and its impact on his relationship with the mother and the work place; financial concerns; and often the increase in contact with other relatives that pregnancy frequently precipitates.

Involving the father also allows him and the mother the opportunity to address important developmental tasks for themselves as a couple. These tasks, common responses, and recommendations for physicians have been detailed.

The role of the support person, often the father, cannot be underestimated. Meta-analysis of 10 randomized trials evaluating the effect of a labor companion reveals lower rates of cesarean section and operative vaginal delivery as well as improved fetal outcomes.

Psychosocial Issues. Pregnancy is an opportunity to address the psychological and mental health issues of women. Some of these are well managed by systematic attention to education and anticipatory guidance. The woman should be included in as much of the management plan as possible, increasing her overall participation and sense of control. For some women this involves writing their own birth plan of hoped-for circumstances.

Family issues need to be addressed. The father, or other support individuals, needs to be included. Siblings require attention. Some psychosocial issues are an integral part of managing a "medical" condition, for example, domestic violence or substance abuse, in which a multidisciplinary approach is generally necessary. A common psychological issue is the perinatal experience of grief. More women experience perinatal death than have a pregnancy complicated by chronic diseases. Miscarriages are common and affect perhaps 25% of pregnancies. Strategies for facilitating grieving have been reviewed.

Assessment of Fetal Well-being. Fetal well-being is generally assessed inferentially from clinical parameters obtained during routine prenatal visits. These include symptom review, weight gain, blood pressure, fundal height measurement, report of fetal movements, and periodic auscultation of fetal heart tones. When there is concern regarding fetal compromise, additional testing is necessary. Some of these concerns include pregnancy prolonged beyond 41 to 42 weeks; suspicion of intrauterine growth retardation; maternal diabetes or hypertension; previously unexplained stillbirth; or the mother's report of decreased fetal movement.

BIOCHEMICAL ASSESSMENT. In the past, serial serum estriol and human placental lactogen levels have been used. They are not currently recommended to assess fetal health, growth, or development.

FETAL MOVEMENT (KICK COUNTS). Quickening has long been recognized as a significant clinical correlate of gestational age. A woman who notes fetal movements for 25 weeks has a 90% or greater chance of having a baby who is at least 38 weeks of gestation. If daily fetal movements are recorded by mothers, women report 90% of the fetal movements detectable electronically.

Maximum fetal movement occurs between 29 and 38 weeks of gestation. Later in pregnancy, babies move more between 10 P.M. and 2 A.M. Movements are affected by diurnal variation, cord compression, congenital abnormalities, hydramnios, sound, and food or glucose intake of the mother.

One common method to systematically assess movement is to ask pregnant women to determine the period of time needed to record 10 fetal movements. The provider should be called if they do not feel 10 movements within 12 hours. Another method is to ask the mother to choose an hour each morning to lie on her side and concentrate on the baby's movements. If the baby moves four times she may stop counting and resume her daily activities. If the baby moves less than four times during the hour she should continue counting for another hour. If there are still fewer than four movements per hour she should be instructed to call or come in for assessment. To date, fetal kick counts are the only antenatal testing method that has been demonstrated to improve obstetric outcome in a randomized clinical trial. However, there is a high false-positive rate.

NONSTRESS TEST. If a fetus is suspected of compromise, the first assessment of well-being is usually the nonstress test. A healthy fetus accelerates its heart rate in response to its movement. If these accelerations occur, the baby is generally safe in its intrauterine environment for another week. The test is conducted by asking the mother to lie in the lateral supine position. A continuous fetal heart rate tracing is obtained from external Doppler equipment. The mother should report each fetal movement. She can record these on her own, or an observer can make a notation on the tracing. The effect of fetal movements on the fetal heart rate is recorded. A normal fetus has a variable baseline heart rate. The fetus responds to movement with an acceleration in fetal heart rate of at least 15 beats or more per minute above its baseline. A reactive nonstress test is defined as one that demonstrates at least two accelerations from an established baseline in a 20-minute interval. These accelerations consist of a rise from the baseline of at least 15 beats per minute with a return back to the baseline lasting at least 15 seconds. Poor baseline beat-to-beat variability, the presence of decelerations, or a lack of acceleration with fetal movement constitutes a nonreactive, or positive, nonstress test. Further evaluation is necessary for these patients even though the test has a poor predictive value and only a small percentage of nonreactive tests do in fact indicate a compromised fetus.

CONTRACTION STRESS TEST. The contraction stress test uses intravenous oxytocin, or breast nipple stimulation, to produce contractions. It evaluates fetal heart rate activity electronically in response to contractions.

This test has been the "gold standard" of uteroplacental well-being. It was used whenever a nonstress test was nonreactive or suspicious. Contraindications include ruptured chorioamnion, previous premature labor, previous classic cesarean section, known or suspected placenta previa, hydramnios, or multiple gestation. The test requires an in-hospital stay. A fairly standard protocol administers oxytocin at 0.5 mU per minute, doubling the dose every 10 to 15 minutes until three contractions occur. Each contraction needs to last 40 to 60 seconds. Three contractions need to occur within 10 minutes. An alternative method uses nipple stimulation of a breast for 2 minutes; this is stopped for 5 minutes and the cycle is repeated until three contractions, each 40 to 60 seconds in duration, occur within 10 minutes. A test is considered positive if decelerations follow at least half the contractions or three or more consecutive contractions. For those patients delivery should be considered.

This test has been replaced in many centers by the biophysical profile, or modified biophysical profile. These tests do not require hospitalization or placement of intravenous lines, or risk precipitation of labor.

BIOPHYSICAL PROFILE. The biophysical profile combines the nonstress test with ultrasound measurements of normal fetal reflex activities and amniotic fluid measurements. It has a lower false-positive and false-negative rate than the nonstress test and contraction stimulation test. It is an outpatient procedure. A score of 2 (normal) or 0 (abnormal) is assigned to each of five variables for a maximum possible score of 10. The variables are

Gross body movements
Fetal tone
Fetal breathing patterns
Assessment of amniotic fluid volume
Nonstress testing

The best correlates of fetal well-being are with the quantitative assessment of amniotic fluid volume and the nonstress test. Some providers have therefore "modified" this test to include just these two measurements. However, whether this modified test actually identifies a group of patients at increased risk for perinatal outcome or, if so, does it better than a weekly nonstress test or no monitoring remains controversial.

ECTOPIC PREGNANCY

method of
MARIAN L. McCORD, M.D., and
FRANK W. LING, M.D.
University of Tennessee College of Medicine
Memphis, Tennessee

The incidence of ectopic pregnancy has quadrupled over the past 20 years. The most recent statistics suggest a rate of 16.0 ectopic pregnancies per 1000 reported pregnancies, with the highest rates in women ages 35 to 44 years (27.2 per 1000 reported pregnancies). Ectopic pregnancy remains a major cause of morbidity and mortality, accounting for 5 to 6% of all maternal deaths in the United States.

RISK FACTORS

Independent risk factors consistently shown to increase the risk of tubal pregnancy include previous laparoscopically proven pelvic inflammatory disease, previous tubal pregnancy, current intrauterine device use, and previous tubal surgery for infertility. Other factors that have been shown to modify risk include contraceptive choice, prior abdominal surgery, previous pregnancies, and fertility status.

INITIAL ASSESSMENT

Diagnosing ectopic pregnancy is difficult because of the wide spectrum of clinical presentations, from asymptomatic to acute abdomen and hemodynamic shock. The physician must maintain a high degree of suspicion for ectopic pregnancy.

Pertinent information includes menstrual history, previous pregnancy outcome, history of infertility, current contraceptive status, risk factor assessment, and current symptoms. The classic triad of pain, amenorrhea, and vaginal bleeding is present in only about 50% of patients. Abdominal pain is the most common presenting complaint, but the severity and nature of the pain vary widely. It may be unilateral or bilateral; dull, sharp, or crampy in nature; and either continuous or intermittent. Shoulder and back pain, which is thought to result from hemoperitoneal irritation of the diaphragm, is a worrisome symptom.

On examination, the abdomen may be nontender or mildly tender, with or without rebound. Cervical motion tenderness may or may not be present. The uterus may be slightly enlarged, with findings similar to those of a normal pregnancy. An adnexal mass, palpable in up to 50% of cases, varies in size, consistency, and tenderness and may be a corpus luteum rather than an ectopic pregnancy. Rupture of a tubal pregnancy may result in significant intra-abdominal hemorrhage. The patient may present with tachycardia followed by hypotension, diminished (or absent) bowel sounds, abdominal distention, and rebound tenderness. Frequently, the pelvic examination is inadequate due to pain and guarding.

A urinary human chorionic gonadotropin (hCG) test should be obtained in all patients suspected of being pregnant, with a positive result not establishing the location of the pregnancy. Current urinary pregnancy tests using monoclonal antibody technology are sensitive enough to detect pregnancy by the first day of a missed menstrual cycle. If the test is negative, a pregnancy in any location is unlikely. A complete blood count (CBC) to determine the patient's hematologic status is essential. Serial hematocrits should be obtained when rupture is suspected to monitor the patient's status preoperatively. Blood typing and antibody status are required. Rh_O (D) immune globulin (RhoGAM) is indicated for all pregnant, Rh-negative, unsensitized women.

DIAGNOSTIC TESTS

Taken together, the accuracy of the history and physical examination is less than 50%. Additional tests are frequently required to differentiate ectopic pregnancy from early viable or abnormal intrauterine pregnancy. In our institution, a screening algorithm (Figure 1) helps make a definitive diagnosis of unruptured ectopic pregnancy, in many cases without laparoscopy. The tests used in this algorithm include single serum progesterone, serial quantitative βhCG, vaginal ultrasonography, and curettage with identification of villi.

A single serum progesterone level may determine the viability of a first-trimester pregnancy. Only 1.5% of ectopic pregnancies are associated with a level of 25 ng per mL or greater. A progesterone level less than 5 ng per mL is highly suggestive of, but not diagnostic of, nonviability. The chance of viability with a progesterone level less than 5 ng per mL is 0.15%.

Measurements of βhCG are used in three ways. First, serial titers can identify an abnormal pregnancy, without regard to location. A 66% rise in hCG titer over 48 hours represents the lower limit of normal for viable intrauterine pregnancies (15% of women with viable intrauterine pregnancies will have a less than 66% rise in the hCG titer over 48 hours, and 15% of those with ectopic pregnancies will have a greater than 66% rise in the hCG titer over 48 hours). In our experience, no viable gestation is associated with an βhCG rise of less than 50% over 48 hours. Second, correlation of βhCG levels helps with the accurate interpretation of ultrasound findings. Third, βhCG measurements obtained 12 to 24 hours after evacuation of the uterus by curettage pinpoints the location of the pregnancy: an expected drop in hCG is diagnostic of nonviable intrauterine gestation. Plateaued or rising levels are diagnostic of ectopic pregnancy.

Two assay standards of βhCG measurement are widely used: the Second International Standard (2nd IS) and the Third International Standard (3rd IS), which was formerly known as the First International Reference Preparation (1st IRP). As a general rule of thumb, the 2nd IS is approximately half of the 3rd IS—for example, if a level is reported as 500 mIU per mL (2nd IS), it is equivalent to a level of 1000 mIU per mL (3rd IS). One must know the standard employed to interpret the results accurately.

With transvaginal sonography, diagnosis of an intrauterine pregnancy is possible 1 week earlier than with transabdominal sonography. When βhCG exceeds 2000 mIU per mL (3rd IS), virtually all intrauterine gestations are identified. Nonvisualization of an intrauterine gestation indicates ectopic pregnancy or recently completed abortion. When βhCG is below this discriminatory zone, the differential diagnosis includes normal intrauterine pregnancy, too early for visualization; abnormal intrauterine gestation; recent abortion; and ectopic pregnancy. Detection of ectopic cardiac activity and measurement of mass size guide therapy.

Endometrial suction curettage is used in patients with abnormal hCG titers (i.e., <50% rise in hCG titer over 48 hours) to differentiate ectopic from nonviable intrauterine gestations. A nonviable intrauterine gestation can be verified by identification of chorionic villi or rapid decline in hCG titers over 12 to 24 hours. Absence of villi with plateaued or rising hCG titers is diagnostic of ectopic pregnancy.

MANAGEMENT

Diagnosis at the earliest possible time maximizes the therapeutic options available. Treatment prior to rupture prevents catastrophic outcomes, minimizes pelvic organ damage, and decreases cost and recuperation time. If an ectopic pregnancy can be identified prior to rupture or irreparable tubal damage, consideration may be given to optimization of future fertility and nonsurgical treatment.

Operative management is currently the most widely used treatment for ectopic pregnancy. Linear salpingostomy is the procedure of choice when the patient wishes to retain her potential for future fertility. The products of conception are removed through an incision made into the tube on its antimesenteric border. Wedge resection may be necessary, particularly for isthmic gestations. Reconstruction is usually performed at a later date. Salpingectomy is performed if the patient does not desire future fertility or the tube is irreparably damaged. Laparoscopy is replacing laparotomy as the surgical approach of choice. However, the surgical approach ultimately depends on the hemodynamic stability of the patient, the size and location of the ectopic mass, and the surgeon's expertise.

As 60 to 70% of all ectopic pregnancies occur in histologically normal tubes, resolution without surgery may spare the tube from additional trauma and improve fertility potential. Medical therapy primarily revolves around the use of methotrexate,* although other agents have been studied, including potassium chloride, hyperosmolar glucose, prostaglandins, and RU-486 (mifepristone).†

Methotrexate is a folic acid analogue that inhibits dehydrofolate reductase and thereby prevents synthesis of DNA. High doses of methotrexate can cause leukopenia, thrombocytopenia, bone marrow aplasia,

---

*Not FDA-approved for this indication.
†Investigational drug in the United States.

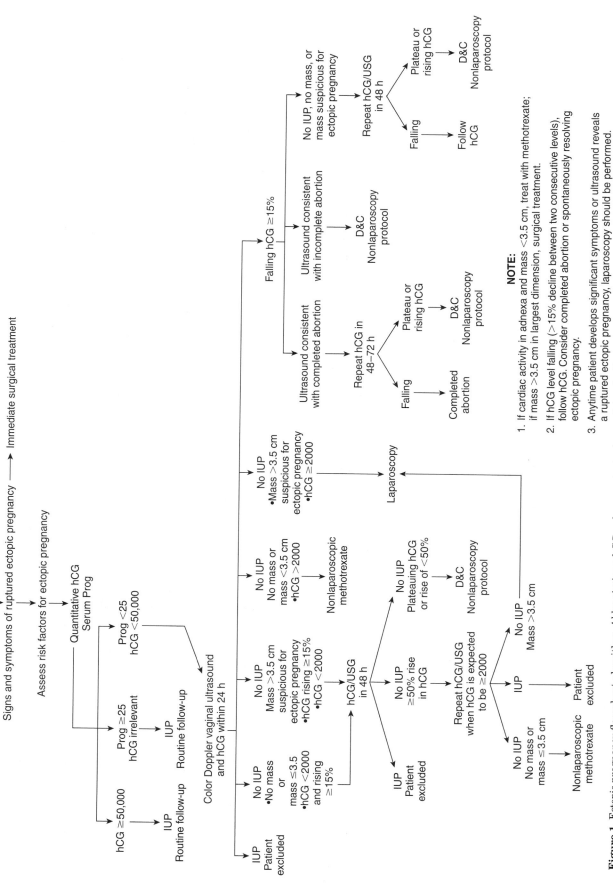

Figure 1. Ectopic pregnancy flow chart algorithm. *Abbreviations:* hCG = human chorionic gonadotropin; Prog = progesterone; IUP = intrauterine pregnancy; USG = ultrasound; D&C = dilatation and curettage. (Redrawn from Stovall TG, Ling FW: Ectopic pregnancy: Diagnostic and therapeutic algorithms minimizing surgical intervention. *J Reprod Med* 38:808, 1993.)

The following text appears within the figure:

Positive urine pregnancy test → Signs and symptoms of ruptured ectopic pregnancy → Immediate surgical treatment

Assess risk factors for ectopic pregnancy

Quantitative hCG
Serum Prog

hCG ≥50,000
IUP
Routine follow-up

Prog ≥25
hCG irrelevant
IUP
Routine follow-up

Prog <25
hCG <50,000
IUP
Routine follow-up

Color Doppler vaginal ultrasound and hCG within 24 h

IUP
Patient excluded

No IUP
•No mass or mass ≤3.5
•hCG <2000 and rising ≥15%

No IUP
Mass >3.5 cm suspicious for ectopic pregnancy
•hCG rising ≥15%
•hCG <2000

No IUP
No mass or mass <3.5 cm
•hCG >2000

No IUP
•Mass >3.5 cm suspicious for ectopic pregnancy
•hCG ≥2000

hCG/USG in 48 h

Nonlaparoscopic methotrexate

Laparoscopy

IUP
Patient excluded

No IUP
≥50% rise in hCG

No IUP
Plateauing hCG or rise of <50%

D&C
Nonlaparoscopy protocol

Repeat hCG/USG when hCG is expected to be ≥2000

IUP
Patient excluded

No IUP
No mass or mass ≤3.5 cm
Nonlaparoscopic methotrexate

No IUP
Mass >3.5 cm

IUP
Patient excluded

Falling hCG ≥15%

Ultrasound consistent with completed abortion

Ultrasound consistent with incomplete abortion
D&C
Nonlaparoscopy protocol

Repeat hCG in 48–72 h

Falling
Completed abortion

Plateau or rising hCG
D&C
Nonlaparoscopy protocol

No IUP, no mass, or mass suspicious for ectopic pregnancy

Repeat hCG/USG in 48 h

Falling
Follow hCG

Plateau or rising hCG
D&C
Nonlaparoscopy protocol

NOTE:

1. If cardiac activity in adnexa and mass <3.5 cm, treat with methotrexate; if mass >3.5 cm in largest dimension, surgical treatment.

2. If hCG level falling (>15% decline between two consecutive levels), follow hCG. Consider completed abortion or spontaneously resolving ectopic pregnancy.

3. Anytime patient develops significant symptoms or ultrasound reveals a ruptured ectopic pregnancy, laparoscopy should be performed.

TABLE 1. **Single-Dose Methotrexate Protocol for Ectopic Pregnancy Treatment**

Day	Therapy
0*	hCG, D & C, CBC, SGOT, BUN, creatinine, blood type + Rh
1	MTX, hCG
4	hCG
7†	hCG

*In those patients not requiring D & C prior to MTX initiation (hCG >2000 mIU/mL [3rd IS] and no gestational sac on transvaginal ultrasound), day 0 and day 1 are combined.

†If <15% decline in hCG titer between days 4 and 7, give second dose of MTX 50 mg/m² on day 7. If ≥15% decline in hCG titer between days 4 and 7, follow weekly until hCG is <15 mIU/mL.

Abbreviations: hCG = quantitative human chorionic gonadotropin-beta, mIU/mL; D & C = dilatation and curettage; CBC = complete blood count; SGOT = serum glutamic-oxaloacetic transaminase, units/L; BUN = blood urea nitrogen; MTX = intramuscular methotrexate, 50 mg/m².

From Stovall TG, Ling FW: Single-dose methotrexate: An expanded clinical trial. Am J Obstet Gynecol *168*:1760, 1993.

ulcerative stomatitis, diarrhea, hemorrhagic enteritis, alopecia, dermatitis, elevated liver enzymes, and pneumonitis. Side effects are infrequent at the low doses used for ectopic pregnancy treatment. Citrovorum factor reduces the incidence of these side effects and is generally used when multiple doses are required. Importantly, long-term follow-up of women treated with methotrexate for gestational trophoblastic disease shows no increase in congenital malformation, spontaneous abortion, or secondary tumors after chemotherapy.

Medical treatment with methotrexate is appropriate for a patient with an unruptured ectopic pregnancy less than 3.5 cm in size who desires future fertility and is capable of complying with an outpatient regimen of treatment and follow-up. Presence of cardiac activity is a relative contraindication. Many dosing regimens have been described. In the most commonly utilized protocol (Table 1), a single 50 mg per square meter, body surface area, intramuscular dose is given. During treatment, patients must refrain from alcohol, multivitamins (containing folic acid), and sexual intercourse. Pelvic examination is to be avoided. Patients should be informed that they will experience some pelvic discomfort during resolution. Nonsteroidal analgesics may be taken. Patients with persistent pain should be assessed with a hematocrit, ultrasonography, and observation to exclude rupture.

REPRODUCTIVE FUNCTION

The potential for reproductive function has generally involved the study of treatment efficacy, tubal patency, and pregnancy outcome. A woman's chance of achieving a subsequent intrauterine pregnancy or a recurrent ectopic pregnancy is a result of many factors, including her fertility status, previous childbearing, the underlying cause of the ectopic pregnancy, and the status of the involved and contralateral tubes. Salpingostomy, whether by laparoscopy or laparotomy, and methotrexate treatment appear to be equivalent in efficacy. Each has an efficacy of 95%, with the remaining 5% of patients requiring further treatment (because of rupture during methotrexate treatment or persistent trophoblastic tissue following salpingostomy). Outcomes for salpingostomy and methotrexate treatment, respectively, are similar: tubal patency, 86% versus 77%; pregnancy rate, 78% versus 63%; and recurrent ectopic rate, 21% versus 11%. Multicenter, randomized, prospective analysis of the treatment modalities is required before definitive conclusions can be drawn.

VAGINAL BLEEDING IN LATE PREGNANCY

method of
JON M. KATZ, M.D.
Columbia Hospital for Women Medical Center
Washington, D.C.

Vaginal bleeding in late pregnancy is a rare but potentially serious event to both the mother and the fetus. Bleeding may indicate an event as innocuous as term labor or may signal the ultimate consequence of abruptio placentae—stillbirth of the fetus and maternal consumptive coagulopathy.

The complaint of vaginal bleeding may be elicited at the time of routine prenatal care but more likely will be via a telephone call. From studies done to correlate patient descriptions of bleeding with actual blood loss, it is apparent that it is difficult for patients to quantify the amount of blood lost. If a patient describes scant bleeding after an internal examination or coitus, she can be reassured. If the patient is at term and describes a "bloody show," the consequence of dilatation of the cervix, with tearing of small veins, she can be reassured and instructed that the latent phase of labor may be starting. Otherwise, the complaint of vaginal bleeding should be evaluated in a labor and delivery setting. The patient's vital signs should be obtained, and a fetal heart monitor should be utilized to evaluate both fetal well-being and maternal contractions. If the vital signs are stable, the bleeding is not excessive, and there is no evidence of fetal compromise, a conservative approach is recommended. If records indicate that the patient has had a sonogram noting the absence of placenta previa, a sterile speculum examination is done to exclude rupture of the membranes, cervical neoplasm, or infection. If the amniotic sac is intact, a sterile vaginal examination is performed to exclude or confirm the diagnosis of labor. If the patient's vital signs are unstable, the patient is bleeding profusely, or there is fetal distress, the evaluation must be performed expeditiously to minimize maternal and fetal morbidity.

The differential diagnosis includes symptomatic placenta previa, bleeding as a consequence of separation of the placenta implanted in the immediate vicinity of the cervical canal; abruptio placentae, bleeding from the placenta located elsewhere in the uterine cavity; or vasa praevia, velamentous insertion of the umbilical cord with rupture of a fetal vessel at the time of rupture of the membranes, associated with fetal hemorrhage. The classic teaching that a patient with a symptomatic placenta previa presents with painless vaginal bleeding and a patient with abruptio placentae presents with painful uterine contractions should be abandoned. A bleeding placenta previa may elicit painful uterine contractions suggestive of abruptio placentae, and abruptio placentae may mimic normal labor or present with the sequela of a concealed abruptio—a stillbirth without obvious vaginal bleeding.

Irrespective of the actual diagnosis, it is critical that a large-bore intravenous line be established, fluid resuscitation be initiated, and blood studies be obtained for evaluation of anemia and consumptive coagulopathy and to serve as baseline values if the bleeding continues. Blood for typing and screening for potential transfusion should be sent to the laboratory. If there is fetal distress or life-threatening maternal hemorrhage, an operating room should be opened in preparation for possible cesarean section, and nursery and anesthesia personnel should be notified accordingly.

PLACENTA PREVIA

The incidence of placenta previa ranges from 0.3 to 0.5% of all deliveries. Risk factors include multiparity, advanced maternal age, prior cesarean section, history of induced abortion, and cigarette smoking. If a placenta previa is diagnosed on routine second-trimester sonography, there is an approximately 97% chance for migration to a normally implanted site (lateral, posterior, anterior, or fundal) as the uterus grows and the lower uterine segment develops. If a previa is diagnosed in the third trimester, the chance of placental migration is markedly decreased, especially if the previa is associated with vaginal bleeding.

Most frequently, bleeding from a patient with placenta previa starts without warning and is rarely so profuse as to result in significant maternal hemodynamic instability or fetal distress. Most often, but not always, the bleeding ceases spontaneously and recurs, with episodes of intermittent bleeding. Management of a patient with bleeding as a consequence of placenta previa should be based on the degree of maternal hemorrhage and on fetal well-being. If there is evidence of fetal distress, life-threatening maternal hemorrhage, or any hemorrhage in a patient with a term gestation, prompt cesarean section is the treatment of choice. If the mother is stable and fetal well-being is confirmed, evaluation with sonography is indicated.

A confirmatory diagnosis can be made with great accuracy by transabdominal sonography. The location of the placenta in relationship to the internal cervical os is determined. Various types of previa may be identified. A total previa entirely covers the internal os, a partial previa is eccentrically located and partially covers the os, a marginal previa is defined as one in which the edge of the placenta appears adjacent to the cervical os, and a low-lying placenta is located in the less vascular lower uterine segment such that the edge is in close proximity to but does not reach the os. Irrespective of the type of previa, extensive bleeding may occur. A false-positive diagnosis of previa may be made in a patient with a distended bladder as the bladder compresses the anterior lower uterine segment, making an anteriorly located placenta appear as a previa. Confirmation of a placenta previa should be done after the bladder is nearly empty. A fetal body part may obscure the location of the internal os, and endovaginal sonography may provide better visualization of landmarks to confirm the diagnosis. Translabial sonography has also been utilized to visualize crucial landmarks without the need to insert the vaginal probe.

Once the diagnosis is confirmed and there is no evidence of fetal compromise, labor, or maternal coagulopathy, a conservative approach can be instituted. Bleeding placenta previa is a relative contraindication to tocolytic therapy; however, uterine relaxation may shorten the time the patient continues to bleed and arrest preterm labor. Systemic corticosteroid therapy to promote fetal lung maturation is given weekly until the achievement of 34 weeks' gestation. Hospitalization is continued until term unless the patient is stable, lives within 15 minutes of the hospital, and is compliant with bed rest. If a patient is chronically hospitalized due to recurrent bleeding and has completed 34 weeks' gestation, an amniocentesis is performed to determine fetal lung maturity. If the lung profile is mature, cesarean section is promptly performed.

A patient with placenta previa is more likely than a patient with a normally implanted placenta to have a placenta accreta, increta, or percreta, three forms of invasive growth of the placenta through the maternal myometrium. Whenever a cesarean section is performed for placenta previa, 2 to 4 U of crossmatched blood must be readily available, as well as the instruments and personnel to perform uterine or hypogastric artery ligation or hysterectomy.

ABRUPTIO PLACENTAE

In contrast to patients with placenta previa, patients with abruptio placentae have bleeding from a normally implanted placenta. The incidence has been reported from 0.44 to 1.3% of all deliveries, with a perinatal mortality rate from 20 to 35%. The etiology of abruptio placentae is unknown. Risk factors include multiparity, hypertensive disorders (both chronic hypertension and pregnancy-induced hypertension), maternal blunt trauma, cigarette smoking, cocaine use, preterm premature rupture of the membranes, and retroplacentally located uterine leiomyoma. The initial event is hemorrhage into the basal decidua, which may dissect to the margin of the placenta and ultimately to the level of the cervix or may be concealed within the margins of the placenta. A decidual hematoma forms, with compression and destruction of adjacent placenta, reducing the overall area for diffusion of nutrients and removal of waste products.

The extent of vaginal bleeding varies considerably. There may be profuse bleeding with minimal placental separation that does not compromise the fetus, or there can be total placental separation leading to stillbirth and maternal coagulopathy with little or no bleeding. Vaginal bleeding is the most common symptom, occurring in 78% of cases, and patients may also complain of uterine tenderness and backache. Signs such as fetal distress, uterine hypertonus, idiopathic preterm labor, and fetal demise are also diagnosed in association with abruptio placentae.

The initial management of patients with abruptio placentae is similar to the care of those with bleeding placenta previa. Maternal vital signs should be obtained and a physical examination done to evaluate hemodynamic instability, uterine resting tone, contractions, and fetal viability. After an ultrasound is done to exclude a placenta previa, a vaginal examination is performed to determine the presence and stage of labor. Blood studies are performed to exclude anemia and disseminated coagulopathy, and blood is sent for type and crossmatch. A normal blood pressure reading, or even hypertension, does not exclude the possibility of hypovolemia. Hemorrhagic shock is usually in proportion to the extent of vaginal bleeding. If the patient is stable and there is no evidence of labor or fetal distress, sonography is employed to evaluate the nature of the bleeding. Initially, retroplacental bleeding may appear hypoechoic, but as the clot organizes, it may appear indistinct from normal placental tissue. Negative ultrasound findings do not exclude potentially life-threatening abruptio placentae.

Consumption of clotting factors such as platelets and fibrinogen, with the production of fibrin degradation products, is one serious sequela of abruptio placentae. Also known as disseminated intravascular coagulation, this occurs in up to 30% of women with abruptio placentae severe enough to kill the fetus and is much less common in situations without fetal compromise. The induction of the clotting cascade occurs both intravascularly and retroplacentally. This creates a bleeding tendency and may complicate surgery to deliver a fetus by cesarean section. In addition, fibrin may be deposited in small vessels of various organ systems, leading to ischemic tissue damage such as renal tubular necrosis and adult respiratory distress syndrome.

Treatment of a patient with abruptio placentae depends on the mother's medical condition, the fetus's gestational age, and fetal well-being. If there is fetal distress in a potentially viable fetus or excessive maternal hemorrhage, prompt cesarean section with simultaneous blood and electrolyte replacement therapy is indicated. If there is no evidence of fetal distress or maternal hemorrhage creating hypovolemia or anemia, conservative therapy, especially in the case of a markedly immature fetus, is indicated. Because the etiology of abruptio placentae is often not determined, the patient should be hospitalized for observation. Exacerbation of maternal chronic hypertension should be controlled, and cigarette smoking and illicit cocaine use eliminated. If preterm labor is confirmed, tocolytic therapy with magnesium sulfate is instituted. Betamethasone therapy is given to all patients at risk for delivery at less than 34 weeks' gestation and repeated on a weekly basis. Anemia is corrected with transfusion of packed red blood cells to keep the hematocrit greater than 30%. Platelets are transfused if the platelet count drops below 20,000 per μl when a vaginal delivery is anticipated, and below 50,000 per μl when a cesarean section is anticipated. Fresh frozen plasma, cryoprecipitate, or both are utilized if there is clinically active bleeding, the fibrinogen is less than 100 mg per dL, and cesarean section is anticipated.

The route of delivery is dependent on fetal viability, fetal distress, degree of maternal hemorrhage, and presence of consumption coagulopathy. If the fetus is dead and hemorrhage is managed by intravenous fluid and blood replacement, vaginal delivery is preferable. Vaginal delivery with removal of the placenta will initiate myometrial contraction and constriction of bleeding vessels and thus control hemorrhage. Unless there is continued bleeding, the coagulopathy will correct in 24 to 48 hours without the need for replacement of coagulation factors. Labor may occur with contractions of normal frequency, duration, and intensity, or the uterus may be hypertonic. Internal monitoring with a scalp electrode and intrauterine pressure catheter may provide more accurate information to ensure fetal well-being. Oxytocin is not contraindicated in a hypotonic uterus or a first-stage arrest when fetal distress and cephalopelvic disproportion are excluded. Cesarean section is indicated in the presence of fetal distress, uncontrollable maternal hemorrhage, and failed induction of labor. At the time of laparotomy, extravasation of blood into the uterine musculature and beneath the serosa—called Couvelaire uterus—may be encountered. These myometrial hematomas are not an indication for cesarean hysterectomy because they seldom interfere with uterine contractions sufficiently to produce postpartum hemorrhage. Postoperatively, patients are followed with frequent hematocrits, platelet counts, and clotting studies and are supported with blood, platelets, fresh frozen plasma, and cryoprecipitate as clinically indicated. Urine output is monitored hourly to assess renal perfusion.

RECURRENCE RISK AND MANAGEMENT IN A SUBSEQUENT PREGNANCY

The risk of recurrence of abruptio placentae reportedly ranges from 4 to 16%. Management strategies vary, owing to the fact that the etiology of abruptio placentae is often undetermined and separation may occur suddenly, without warning, any time late in gestation. Methods of fetal surveillance, such as weekly non–stress tests, serial ultrasound evaluation of fetal growth and biophysical assessment, and Doppler flow analysis, are readily available but may not be effective in anticipating the problem. Some studies suggest that in subsequent pregnancies, low-dose aspirin therapy, 81 mg per day, should be instituted from the time the pregnancy is confirmed with sonography until delivery. Weekly nonstress tests are initiated, starting several weeks before the gestational age at which the abruptio occurred in the previous pregnancy and continuing until delivery. Sonography is indicated to evaluate fetal growth and well-being if clinical measurements or nonstress testing indicates a potential problem. Labor is induced when the patient's cervical Bishop score is greater than 6 or she has reached her estimated date of confinement, assuming there is no other contraindication to vaginal delivery.

HYPERTENSIVE DISORDERS OF PREGNANCY

method of
PHYLLIS AUGUST, M.D.
Cornell University Medical College
New York, New York

The hypertensive disorders complicating pregnancy are among the most challenging medical problems in prenatal care. High blood pressure complicates approximately 10% of all pregnancies and is responsible for considerable maternal and fetal morbidity. Most important, the therapeutic goals of treating hypertension in pregnancy differ from those in nonpregnant individuals. When managing hypertensive gravidas, the major objective is delivery of a healthy, mature fetus without compromising maternal well-being, whereas in nonpregnant populations, the primary focus is on long-term prevention of cardiovascular disease. This is best accomplished by close maternal and fetal surveillance, nonpharmacologic therapy, judicious use of antihypertensive medication, and timely delivery of the fetus.

An overall appreciation of the unique physiologic adaptations to normal pregnancy is necessary for appropriate management of hypertensive gravidas. Although this subject is outside the scope of this article, the more significant changes are worth mentioning. Normal pregnancy is associated with increased cardiac output, vasodilatation, lower blood pressure, and hypervolemia. There are increases in both glomerular filtration rate and renal blood flow. Dramatic endocrine adaptations include changes in hormonal systems that may influence volume regulation and vascular reactivity. These include large increases in estradiol, estriol, and progesterone, as well as marked stimulation of all components of the renin-angiotensin-aldosterone system. Most of the aforementioned changes are apparent by the end of the first trimester, reaching a peak in midpregnancy, then leveling off toward term.

The Importance of Accurate Diagnosis. The important diagnostic issue in pregnancy hypertension is the identification of preeclampsia, as this disorder is associated with the greatest maternal and fetal morbidity and mortality. Important interventions, such as a decision to deliver, are often based on clinical impressions of the disease responsible for the hypertension. Thus the appropriate diagnosis may have significant implications for the future of the fetus.

Terminology. Although there are many proposed classification schemes for the hypertensive disorders of pregnancy, we use the 1972 report of the Committee on Terminology of the American College of Obstetricians and Gynecologists, believing it the most practical of all those proposed. In this nosology, women with hypertension in pregnancy are classified into four groups: (1) preeclampsia-eclampsia; (2) chronic hypertension; (3) chronic hypertension with superimposed preeclampsia; or (4) transient hypertension.

PREECLAMPSIA: DIAGNOSIS, PATHOPHYSIOLOGY, TREATMENT

Diagnosis

Preeclampsia, the disorder unique to pregnancy, occurs primarily in primigravidas after the 20th week of gestation and is characterized by elevated blood pressure, proteinuria, generalized edema, and at times coagulation and/or liver function abnormalities. Preeclampsia complicates about 6% of first pregnancies. Other risk factors include family history, multiple gestation, chronic hypertension, diabetes, hydatidiform mole, nonimmune hydrops fetalis, and extremes of reproductive age.

The clinical course of preeclampsia is marked by its potentially explosive nature. Women with mildly elevated blood pressure and even minimal proteinuria can rapidly progress to eclampsia, the convulsive form of the disorder. Thus, even when the disorder is considered mild, close scrutiny and even hospitalization are warranted. Another complication in seemingly stable patients is a variant that goes by the acronym HELLP syndrome (*h*emolysis, *el*evated *l*iver enzymes, *l*ow *p*latelet counts). Such patients often present with right upper quadrant and epigastric pain and a peripheral blood smear consistent with a microangiopathic hemolytic anemia. This is a life-threatening emergency that requires prompt termination of the pregnancy.

Elevations in blood pressure after midpregnancy in previously normotensive women are often the initial clue to the development of preeclampsia. The standard criteria for diagnosing hypertension in pregnancy are (1) systolic blood pressure increases of 30 mm Hg or greater; and (2) diastolic blood pressure (Korotkoff 5) increases of 15 mm Hg or greater compared with the average of values prior to 20 weeks' gestation. When prior blood pressures values are not known, a reading of 140/90 mm Hg is considered abnormal. Thus, a level of 120/80 mm Hg may represent substantial hypertension in a woman whose previously recorded value was 90/50 mm Hg.

Controversy exists on how to measure blood pressure in pregnant women. The National High Blood Pressure Education Program (NHBPEP) Working Group on Hypertension in Pregnancy of the United States recommends that Korotkoff 5 (disappearance) be used to designate diastolic pressure, whereas a World Health Organization task force suggests Korotkoff 4 (muffling). We recommend using the disappearance of sound because it is the value used in nonpregnant populations, and the fourth sound may overestimate diastolic pressure by 5 to 10 mm Hg.

The definition of abnormal proteinuria in pregnancy is 300 mg or more per 24 hours. Dipstick determinations of proteinuria may be erroneous or misleading, and it is advisable to confirm qualitative evidence of proteinuria with a timed urine collection. The diagnosis of preeclampsia in the absence of proteinuria is uncertain; however, it is important to recognize that proteinuria may be a late manifestation of this disorder. Therefore, it may be necessary to treat women as preeclamptic before proteinuria develops.

Edema frequently occurs during normal gestation, and its presence alone is not a useful diagnostic criterion for preeclampsia—nor does its absence make preeclampsia an unlikely diagnosis. Sudden and rapid weight gain is more likely in women who develop preeclampsia.

The standard laboratory evaluation for a woman suspected of having preeclampsia includes urinalysis, hematocrit, platelet count, serum creatinine, urea nitrogen, uric acid, and albumin levels, as well as liver function tests.

Pathophysiology

Preeclampsia is characterized by vasospasm and reduced perfusion of multiple organs, including uterus, placenta, kidney, brain, and liver. Many believe that early abnormalities in the development of placental blood vessels initiate the disease in the early second trimester. This then results in decreased placental perfusion. Systemic illness in the mother appears later in gestation and is characterized by generalized endothelial cell dysfunction, vasospasm, and reduced organ flow.

Features of maternal disease include hypertension, which is characterized by marked lability of blood pressure, and increased sensitivity to vasoconstrictors, particularly angiotensin II. Plasma volume is reduced compared with normal pregnancy, as are glomerular filtration rate and renal blood flow. Liver and brain involvement are features of severe disease. Eclampsia, the convulsive phase, is a major cause of death in women with this disease. The mechanism of the convulsions is not known, but they may be due to cerebral edema, vasospasm, and ischemia, as well as hypertensive encephalopathy.

PREVENTION AND TREATMENT OF PREECLAMPSIA

Prevention

At the present time there are no proven preventive strategies for preeclampsia. Two current approaches, however, are still under investigation as of early 1995. These are low-dose aspirin and calcium supplementation. Data from several small clinical trials conducted in the mid-1980s suggest that low-dose aspirin (50 to 150 mg daily) administered early in gestation may prevent preeclampsia. The hypothesized mechanism was the reversal of the imbalance between prostacyclin and thromboxane that has been observed to be present in women with preeclampsia. More recently, larger trials have not substantiated the earlier positive results. The largest clinical trial performed to date included more than 9000 women, and in the study group as a whole, there were no apparent benefits in the aspirin-treated group. There are still several large trials in progress, focusing on "high-risk" women. We do not recommend routine use of prophylactic aspirin to prevent preeclampsia. In certain extremely high-risk patients who have had severe preeclampsia at an early gestational age, with poor fetal outcome, it may be appropriate to recommend this approach until the results of larger trials are published.

The rationale for the use of calcium supplementation to prevent preeclampsia stems from the observation that a high dietary intake of calcium in certain South American populations is associated with a lower incidence of preeclampsia. Furthermore, calcium supplementation lowers blood pressure in normotensive pregnant women and some nonpregnant essential hypertensive patients. Results of published trials are promising and currently larger multicenter trials are in progress. The dosage of calcium carbonate that has been shown to be beneficial is 1 to 2 grams per day.

Treatment

The development of hypertension in late pregnancy, especially when the diagnosis of preeclampsia appears certain, is a clear indication for hospitalization. This approach is advisable even when preeclampsia is only suspected, given the explosive nature of the disease. Once the diagnosis is made, the patient usually remains hospitalized until delivery. Occasionally, if after careful evaluation a woman appears to have very mild disease (i.e., minimally elevated blood pressure, normal renal function, minimal proteinuria, normal fetal testing), or if signs and symptoms ameliorate, she can be discharged and her clinical course closely followed at home.

Delivery is the only cure for preeclampsia, although occasionally the disease appears to develop in the first postpartum week, or transiently worsen in the immediate puerperium. The decision to deliver is extremely important for the future health and well-being of the fetus and is made by the obstetrician, but internists involved in the care of pregnant women must be cognizant of the issues involved in such decisions.

When preeclampsia develops close to term, and fetal maturity is certain, then delivery is advisable. Difficulties arise if the disease manifests when the fetus is still quite immature and its survival in doubt; then one must decide whether it is safe for the mother to postpone delivery. Most physicians would terminate the pregnancy in the presence of persistent severe hypertension (diastolic blood pressure greater than 110 mm Hg), abnormal liver function tests, low platelet count (less than 100,000 per mm^3), deteriorating renal function, significant headache or visual disturbances, and right upper quadrant discomfort. Conservative management in such cases may not be associated with improved fetal outcome and may in fact result in serious maternal morbidity. On the other hand, when a woman remote from term has but mild-to-moderate hypertension and no signs of deteriorating renal or hepatic function or coagulopathy, temporization should be attempted, though it may be necessary to administer antihypertensive therapy to maintain blood pressure in a safe range (e.g., less than 110 mm Hg diastolic, see later). Such women should be treated in the hospital, where it is easier to monitor progression of the disease and intercede rapidly when complications arise. Also, hospitalization permits frequent antepartum testing, including nonstress testing, sonography, and biophysical profiling, which are the tests that help predict fetal jeopardy, and the decision to continue temporization can be made on a day-to-day basis. It must be stressed, however, that conservative treatment of early preeclampsia entails risks and is appropriate only at a tertiary care center, where aggressive monitoring of maternal and fetal status is possible.

If a decision to postpone delivery is made, then the most important therapeutic intervention is enforcing modified bed rest. This is obviously best accomplished in a hospital setting, as most women are unable to get sufficient rest at home, especially if they have small children.

The role of antihypertensive therapy in the management of preeclampsia is controversial, largely because of the concern that lowering maternal blood pressure might further compromise placental perfusion, whereas there is no evidence to suggest that lowering maternal blood pressure cures or reverses preeclampsia. At best it may help avoid premature delivery when the level of blood pressure is the most worrisome manifestation of disease. Thus, reduction of pressure is performed primarily for maternal safety.

There is disagreement regarding what level of blood pressure should be treated. In the peripartum period, many authorities would begin therapy when diastolic pressure is 105 mm Hg or greater. Excessive reduction of blood pressure (e.g., below 90 mm Hg) should be avoided since it may compromise placental function. If temporization is planned, then it is advisable to start treatment when diastolic levels approach 100 mm Hg. Therapy should be individualized, however, taking into consideration the woman's early pregnancy blood pressures, the rate of rise, and the symptoms. If clinicians are unable to control blood pressure satisfactorily with two antihypertensive agents within 24 to 48 hours, the advisability of continuing the pregnancy is questionable. The recommended antihypertensive agents for acute hypertension in the peripartum period are shown in Table 1.

The treatment and/or prevention of eclamptic convulsions is controversial. In the United States, parenteral magnesium sulfate is routinely administered in the peripartum period to prevent convulsions. Outside the United States, either the drugs phenytoin, phenobarbital, or diazepam or nothing is used as an alternative to magnesium sulfate. A large multicenter trial comparing magnesium sulfate, diazepam, and phenytoin in patients with eclampsia is underway, and reports have appeared that calcium channel blockers with central actions might be alternative ways to prevent and treat eclampsia.

In very severe or extremely complicated cases, invasive hemodynamic monitoring may be useful, particularly when respiratory difficulties or bleeding arises. We find the need for Swan-Ganz catheterization relatively uncommon, as most cases can be managed using clinical acumen alone.

CHRONIC HYPERTENSION: DIAGNOSIS AND TREATMENT

Chronic hypertension refers to hypertension that precedes conception and is usually due to essential hypertension. In many patients blood pressure decreases substantially during gestation, and pregnancies proceed uneventfully in about 85% of women. However, such women are at increased risk for the development of *superimposed preeclampsia*, which is

TABLE 1. **Drug Therapy of Acute, Severe Hypertension in Pregnancy**

Drug	Dose/Route	Onset of Action	Adverse Effects	Comments
Hydralazine (Apresoline)	5 mg IV/IM, then 5–10 mg q 20–40 min; or constant infusion 0.5–10 mg/h	IV: 10 min IM: 10–30 min	Headache, flushing, tachycardia, nausea, vomiting; possible increase in ventricular arrhythmia	Possible limited availability but is familiar to all OB staff
Labetalol (Normodyne, Trandate)	20 mg IV then 20–80 mg q 20–30 min, up to 300 mg; or 1–2 mg/min constant infusion until desired effect	5–10 min	Flushing, nausea, vomiting, tingling of scalp	Experience limited, compared with hydralazine
Nifedipine (Procardia)	10 mg PO; repeat in 30 min if necessary, then 10–30 mg PO 4–6 h	15–20 min	Flushing, headache, tachycardia, nausea, inhibition of labor	Synergistic interaction with MgSO$_4$; limited pregnancy experience
Diazoxide (Hyperstat)	30–50 mg IV q 5–15 min	2–5 min	Inhibition of labor; hyperglycemia, fluid retention with repeated doses	Doses of 150–300 mg may cause severe hypotension

Abbreviation: MgSO$_4$ = magnesium sulfate.

diagnosed when blood pressure suddenly increases in late pregnancy, often associated with the onset of proteinuria and/or hyperuricemia, thrombocytopenia, and liver function abnormalities. The prevalence of chronic hypertension in pregnancy is not known and differs widely in different geographic areas, but it is probably between 3 and 10% of all pregnancies. Some women with chronic hypertension manifest proteinuria early in pregnancy owing to the presence of intrinsic renal disease. Most other forms of chronic hypertension are rare in gestation, but, when they occur, they can be deceptive. These include collagen diseases such as periarteritis and scleroderma, and pheochromocytoma in which life-threatening hypertensive crises can occur. Cushing's syndrome may exacerbate in pregnancy and is associated with poor fetal outcome. Primary aldosteronism, on the other hand, may ameliorate during pregnancy because of the increased levels of progesterone that may decrease kaliuresis and lower blood pressure.

Hypertensive women contemplating pregnancy should be evaluated prior to conceiving. It is important to exclude secondary forms of hypertension, particularly those that may be curable (renovascular, primary aldosteronism, pheochromocytoma). Patients with intrinsic renal disease or with renal transplants should be advised about the risks of pregnancy, especially if azotemia (creatinine level greater than 1.4 mg/dL) and hypertension are present. Preconception counseling permits for adjustments in lifestyle that may be necessary during pregnancy if elevated blood pressure resists control— specifically, the possibility that restricted activity (including job furlough), bed rest, or even hospitalization may be advisable. Furthermore, certain antihypertensive agents that are either contraindicated in pregnancy (e.g., angiotensin-converting inhibitors) or that have not been used extensively and thus whose teratogenic potential is virtually unknown (most antihypertensives) can be discontinued and, if necessary, other medications believed safer for pregnancy prescribed. Finally, one should counsel women with a history of severe hypertension, especially those who require multidrug therapy, against conceiving, and such a scenario is an indication for therapeutic abortion in early pregnancy.

Close medical supervision is the mainstay of management of pregnant women with chronic hypertension. Frequently, blood pressure drops during the first and second trimesters, and it may be possible to reduce or discontinue medication, provided patients are evaluated on a regular basis. If blood pressure does not decrease in midpregnancy, then it may be prudent to recommend limitation of activity. Weight reduction and exercise are not advised during gestation. On the other hand, pregnancy is the ideal time to abandon smoking, given the motivational incentives that accompany this condition. Although sodium restriction is generally not recommended during pregnancy, if a pregnant woman with hypertension has been satisfactorily treated with a low-salt diet before conception, it is not necessary to modify this approach during pregnancy.

The majority of women with chronic hypertension in pregnancy will have mild-to-moderate elevations in blood pressure, and thus the risk of acute cardiac or cerebrovascular complications is extremely low. In the small percentage of women who have severe hypertension (and who decline to terminate), the increased risk of cerebral hemorrhage, heart failure, and myocardial infarction necessitates close monitoring and aggressive treatment at all stages of gestation.

As noted, objectives of treatment in pregnant women are to minimize the short-term risks to the mother of elevated blood pressure, while maintaining fetal well-being. When maternal hypertension is severe (diastolic blood pressure 110 or more mm Hg), treatment should be instituted to avoid hypertensive vascular damage.

The indications for treatment of mild-to-moderate hypertension during pregnancy are less clear, owing to concerns regarding exposure of the fetus to antihypertensives of unproved safety. Excessive blood pressure reduction is to be avoided, and a conservative approach is recommended. If diastolic blood pressure early in the first trimester is between 90 and 100 mm Hg, it is reasonable to anticipate the expected physiologic decrease in blood pressure before prescribing antihypertensives. If in the initial trimester the diastolic blood pressure is below 90 mm Hg and the patient is ingesting antihypertensive drugs, reduction of dose or discontinuance of the medication can be considered. The NHBPEP Working Group has recommended treatment when diastolic blood pressures are consistently 100 mm Hg (Korotkoff 5) or greater. Methyldopa (Aldomet) is the drug of choice, because of its long record of safe use in pregnancy (Table 2).

The diagnosis of superimposed preeclampsia is made when a woman with known or suspected chronic hypertension develops acute elevations in blood pressure, in association with significant proteinuria and/or other laboratory manifestations of preeclampsia (e.g., hyperuricemia, low platelet count, elevation in platelet count). The same principles of treatment apply, with respect to timing of delivery and management of hypertension outlined in the preceding discussion of treatment of preeclampsia and chronic hypertension. Women with preexisting hypertension who develop preeclampsia are more prone to both maternal and fetal complications; thus, any increase in blood pressure in the second half of pregnancy should be given careful attention.

Transient Hypertension

In late pregnancy or the immediate puerperium, some women experience mild or moderate elevations of blood pressure that normalize rapidly postpartum. This entity, designated transient hypertension, usually has a benign course and probably affects women destined to develop essential hypertension later in

TABLE 2. **Drug Therapy of Chronic Hypertension in Pregnancy**

Drug	Daily Dose	Adverse Effects and Comments
Agent of Choice		
Methyldopa (Aldomet)	500–3000 mg in 2–4 divided doses	Safety for mother and fetus (after first trimester) is well documented
Second-Line Agents		
Hydralazine (Apresoline)	50–300 mg in 2–4 divided doses	Few controlled trials, but extensive experience; usually causes fluid retention when used alone
Labetalol (Normodyne, Trandate)	200–1200 in 2–3 divided doses	Less experience than with methyldopa, but compares favorably with methyldopa. Fatal hepatotoxicity reported in nonpregnant patients
Beta-adrenergic inhibitors	Depends on specific agent used	Might cause fetal bradycardia and impair fetal responses to hypoxia. Risk of intrauterine growth retardation when begun in first or second trimester
Calcium channel blockers	Depends on specific agent used	Relatively limited data; may inhibit labor; may be used as single agents without causing sodium retention
Clonidine (Catapres)	0.1–0.8 mg in divided doses	Limited data; useful if above agents unsuccessful or not tolerated
Prazosin (Minipress), other alpha blockers	Depends on agent used	Limited information
Diuretics	Depends on agent used	May cause volume depletion, electrolyte imbalance, pancreatitis, and thrombocytopenia. May be used in individuals successfully treated with diuretics when not pregnant, if other agents not successful. Reduction of dose should be attempted
Contraindicated		
Angiotensin-converting enzyme inhibitors		Fetal loss reported in animals. Oligohydramnios, neonatal anuric renal failure reported after second and third trimester exposure

life. However, this diagnosis is often made retrospectively, after delivery, when it is certain that the features of preeclampsia have not developed. Thus, because of the potential hazards of not recognizing preeclampsia, women with transient hypertension are often managed in the hospital, using the same principles already outlined.

OBSTETRIC ANESTHESIA

method of
BRADLEY E. SMITH, M.D.
Vanderbilt University Medical Center
Nashville, Tennessee

The "consumer movement," which has encouraged a healthy new emphasis on full participation by the parents in the birth process, has also accelerated acceptance of regional obstetric anesthesia and has led to the long-awaited demise of the routine use of heavy medication and general anesthesia in obstetrics in the United States. Nonetheless, anesthesia still probably accounts for 7% of maternal mortality in obstetric patients in the United States. Aspiration of vomitus may still cause one-fourth of obstetric anesthesia deaths. Obstructed airway, inability to intubate the trachea, laryngospasm, anoxia, overdose of anesthetic, and chronic hypoventilation all result in maternal and fetal mortality and morbidity. Regional anesthesia also presents the possibility of serious complications; these include convulsions, "total spinal block," and hypotension with epidural block. "Spinal" anesthesia, although effective and safer than epidural anesthesia, is fast losing popularity, largely because it has not been possible to maintain it

for long periods during labor and because of fear of "spinal headache." The decision about which pain relief method to use should be based not only on the obstetric situation but also on the abilities of the anesthetist. Poorly qualified or inexperienced anesthesia personnel must not be asked to perform difficult and potentially hazardous types of anesthesia, thus exposing two lives to serious complications.

CHOICE OF ANESTHESIA AND ANALGESIA IN NORMAL PREGNANCIES

Psychological Techniques

The numerous psychological techniques can be divided into "natural childbirth," "psychoprophylaxis," and "medical hypnosis." Psychological preparation for labor benefits most patients, but its unpredictability and the great amount of time necessary to implement it often make it impractical for routine use. However, these techniques, along with regional anesthesia, have the important advantage of preserving the mother's ability to respond to and with the baby immediately after birth and to receive the psychological benefits of participation in the birth process.

Sedative and Narcotic Management of Labor Pain

Use of excessive analgesics and sedatives may extend the latent and active phases of labor. However, when labor is well established, only certain general inhalational anesthetics will completely inhibit uterine contractions. (Spinal, peridural, and thiopental anesthesia uncomplicated by hypotension does not influence the force of uterine contractions but may reduce the effectiveness of conscious muscular expulsive efforts.) Doses of sedatives and narcotics sufficient to reduce labor pain significantly without blocks or other adjuncts almost universally cause depression of breathing, cardiovascular function, and alertness in the newborn baby. Recently, however, fentanyl (Sublimaze), in doses of 25 µg given intravenously by patient-controlled analgesia (PCA) pump with a 10-minute lockout, has been used by some to decrease the pain of labor.

Pudendal Block

Pudendal block is still a useful option to establish surgical anesthesia of the perineum with no effect on the course of labor, and it can be administered by the obstetrician. This block provides adequate anesthesia for simple spontaneous delivery, with episiotomy, and is even sufficient to allow some motivated women to experience vacuum extraction or minor outlet forceps procedures. Approximately 10 mL of 1% lidocaine (Xylocaine) deposited on each pudendal nerve at the origin of the sacrosciatic ligament is usually sufficient and rarely causes complications.

Paracervical Block Anesthesia for Vaginal Delivery

This block has regrettably fallen from favor because of a fear of fetal bradycardia and possible cardiac depression. It provides excellent relief of labor pains in both the first and second stages of labor but should be combined with pudendal block for the delivery itself. It is established by infiltration of approximately 10 mL of 1% lidocaine (many centers forbid the use of bupivacaine [Marcaine] for this block) at positions corresponding to four and eight o'clock around the cervix during careful fetal heart monitoring. The anesthetist should wait between injections and observe the fetal heart rate while administering the drug. Bradycardia or fetal death can occur when paracervical block is administered in a high dosage, too rapidly, or without monitoring, but the incidence is low.

Continuous Lumbar Peridural Analgesia for Vaginal Delivery

Continuous lumbar peridural analgesia allows the use of smaller doses of local anesthetic drugs than does a caudal block. Complete anesthesia of the perineum is somewhat delayed with this method compared with a caudal block, but hypotension and toxic reactions are less frequent because of the smaller dose and the lesser vascularity at the site of injection. Minor slowing of total labor may occur because of the reduced reflex urge to push down vigorously in second-stage labor and because of unnecessary degrees of muscle block. These inconveniences can be minimized by limiting the concentration of local anes-

thetic and the spread of block and by maintaining good coaching during the second stage to encourage pushing. Several large clinical studies show that *acceleration* of labor by minimizing the effects of pain and fear actually occurs as frequently as inhibition of labor by epidural anesthesia.

Epidural Technique for Vaginal Delivery

Establishment of the epidural block before the cervix is dilated 3 to 4 cm may slow the latent phase of labor. After the sterile preparation and drape, a special needle (a 17-gauge Weiss needle serves well) is placed in the epidural space, and a plastic catheter is inserted. A test dose given to detect intravascular or subarachnoid placement is very important. One common test protocol includes 3 mL of 1.5% lidocaine with 1:100,000 epinephrine given through the plastic catheter. If no excitement, convulsions, respiratory impairment, tachycardia, or other signs of intravascular or subarachnoid injection are apparent after 3 minutes, a therapeutic dose of 8 mL of 0.25% bupivacaine with 40 µg of fentanyl is given through the epidural catheter. Analgesia usually develops within 20 minutes with little loss of muscle tone. Analgesia for labor can be maintained with an infusion by pump of 10 to 14 mL per hour of a mixture of 0.125% bupivacaine with 5 µg per mL of fentanyl at a rate of 10 to 14 mL per hour into the same catheter. Bolus doses of up to 4 mL can be given if the analgesia level is inadequate. An additional dose just before delivery is sometimes needed to improve perineal anesthesia; some prefer 0.25% bupivacaine without fentanyl for this final dose.

Spinal Anesthesia ("Saddle Block") for Vaginal Delivery

Spinal anesthesia is usually administered in primiparous patients when the head is at about the +2 to +3 station late in second stage, but it may be established earlier in multiparous patients. Hypotension occurs in approximately 18% of patients receiving saddle block anesthetics, so blood pressure should be monitored carefully, especially immediately after the block and after delivery of the infant.

Spinal Block Technique for Vaginal Delivery

After arachnoid puncture with the smallest possible needle (many now prefer the Sprotte design to avoid "spinal headaches"), a dose of 25 to 40 mg of lidocaine, or 0.5 mL of 0.75% bupivacaine in dextrose diluted to 1.5 to 2 mL with 5% dextrose should produce anesthesia to T10 if the patient sits erect for 30 seconds after the injection before lying down. Anesthesia will be complete during forceps manipulations and episiotomy.

Inhalation Analgesia

The use of a potent inhalational anesthetic agent in exceedingly low concentrations (subanesthesia) is a safe and simple analgesic technique that has fallen into disuse because of the expressed desire of many women to be entirely alert at the time of birth. However, this technique can allow the mother to remain conversant, cooperative, and self-controlled without danger to the baby. Constant inhalation of 40 to 50% nitrous oxide and oxygen, 0.5 to 0.8% enflurane (Ethrane), or 0.3 to 0.5% isoflurane (Forane) is effective in producing demonstrable analgesia and degrees of amnesia in approximately 90% of cases. All these agents have essentially no effect on the fetus at these low concentrations.

General Anesthesia

When general anesthesia is necessary, the dose or depth and the duration of anesthesia prior to delivery must be minimized. Mixing of all intravenous and inhalational anesthetics with the fetal blood begins almost immediately after administration. The use of unconscious general anesthesia usually calls for endotracheal intubation because of the possibility of aspiration of gastric contents or loss of patency of the airway. This technique usually requires two persons, one of whom presses the cricoid cartilage directly against the vertebrae, thereby "pinching" the esophagus closed (Sellick's maneuver).

Inhalational Anesthetic Agents

Inhalational anesthetics pass the placenta immediately, and in anesthetic concentrations, all produce significant depression in the newborn in anesthetic concentrations. All but nitrous oxide can lead to postpartum uterine bleeding. Although they are of great help in certain obstetric complications (e.g., tetanic uterine contractions), their routine obstetric use is not recommended because their effects make the baby "sleepy." However, in subanesthetic concentrations (i.e., 0.5 to 0.8% enflurane or 0.3 to 0.5% isoflurane), they produce amnesia and some analgesia and reduce stress responses during light general endotracheal anesthesia, along with nitrous oxide at 40 to 50%.

Thiopental

Thiopental (Pentothal) induction of maternal general anesthesia may cause some depression of breathing in the newborn. In full-term infants, the danger is real but of small magnitude, and a dose of 3.5 mg per kg given intravenously is commonly used. It was mistakenly thought in the past that a long period between the injection and delivery allows "redistribution" of the drug in the baby, but it is clear now that the shortest interval practical between induction of anesthesia and delivery of the baby is safest. Greater caution should be used with thiopental when dealing with "high-risk" or premature babies.

Ketamine

Although slower in achieving induction, ketamine (Ketalar) in small doses (up to 0.75 mg per kg) is recognized as a safe alternative to thiopental as an induction agent in obstetrics. In small doses, both immediate and delayed newborn alertness appears to be better than with thiopental, and the blood pressures of both mother and newborn are better supported. Neurologic complications and respiratory depression may be caused by larger ketamine doses. Rarely, hallucinations by mothers during emergence from ketamine anesthesia occur, but at these low doses, they are very infrequent and are usually prevented by postpartum doses of diazepam (Valium).

CHOICE OF ANESTHESIA AND ANALGESIA IN COMPLICATED PREGNANCIES

Forceps

Forceps are rarely used in modern obstetrics but still have indications. During the use of forceps or vacuum extraction devices, a relaxed perineum and a quiet patient aid in preventing maternal vaginal lacerations and extension of the episiotomy and help minimize trauma to the baby's head. These conditions are provided by spinal and peridural blocks, which also allow the mother to participate in the birth.

Breech Presentation

Vaginal delivery of babies presenting by breech became infrequent because of evidence that both neonatal mortality and intellectual development were more favorable after cesarean birth of breech babies. However, the incidence of vaginal breech births is now increasing again as the risk/benefit ratio is becoming better understood. Today, many experts advocate epidural analgesia for breech births. An alternative choice for pain management in vaginal breech birth consists of good psychic support supplemented by minimal narcotics and tranquilizers, a paracervical block in the first stage, and a quick induction of general endotracheal anesthesia, including succinylcholine (Anectine), when the infant's umbilicus becomes visible. This sequence, combined with the "following hand" pressure on the mother's abdomen just above the pubis, may obviate forceps and minimize the transfer of anesthetic to the baby.

Multiple Births

Useful methods of pain management for the vaginal delivery of the first baby of twins may include the use of limited doses of systemic analgesia (i.e., narcotics and tranquilizers) during the first and early second stage, occasionally supplemented by light inhalational or continuous epidural analgesia. Anesthesia for delivery of the first baby can also be provided by pudendal block and inhalational analgesia or by regional block. The second baby may be delivered under pudendal or local anesthesia in some cases. A significant increase in neonatal mortality is associated with multiple births if intrauterine manipulation (e.g., version and breech extraction) is attempted while the mother is under local or regional anesthesia. If the second infant is to be delivered by means of version and breech extraction, endotracheal halothane anesthesia may be used to relax the uterus, but preparations for active resuscitation of the baby should be made in advance.

Tetanic Contractions

The older standard method of rapid relaxation of the uterus during tetanic contractions used inhalation anesthesia. Endotracheal halothane at concentrations of only 1 to 2% is effective within 2 to 4 minutes, but hypotension is frequent, and endotracheal intubation using prophylactic cricoid pressure is recommended to guard against aspiration of vomitus. Intravenous "beta stimulator" catecholamines do not work as completely or as rapidly. Regional anesthesia does not relax the uterus. Intravenous nitroglycerin (in 100- to 300-μg boluses) may relax the uterus but often causes dangerous maternal hypotension.

Fetal Distress

When fetal distress exists, further depression of the newborn by potent anesthetics given to the mother should be minimized. Although some doctors have advocated spinal anesthesia at this time, no time should be wasted, nor should hypotension be tolerated. If local anesthesia is not sufficient, general anesthesia may be produced rapidly and obstetric delivery expedited.

Antepartum Hemorrhage

Sudden antepartum bleeding leading to hypotensive maternal blood pressure is detrimental to the fetus. Hypovolemia is an added danger to the mother with anesthesia of any type. All forms of major regional anesthesia are frequently contraindicated in this emergency because the resulting sudden sympathetic blockade paralyzes the compensatory mechanisms ordinarily required to maintain the mother's blood pressure during hemorrhage. Management by local anesthesia, pudendal block, or subanesthetic inhalational analgesia is recommended when applicable, but maternal vascular volume should be restored as rapidly as possible with the appropriate fluid. Vasopressors should *not* be used in place of adequate volume replacement. Ketamine 0.75 mg per kg, succinylcholine (1.5 mg/kg), oxygen, endotracheal intubation (by Sellick's technique), and 50% oxygen with 50% nitrous oxide is a popular method of obtaining general anesthesia in this emergency. Potent inhalational anesthetics may accentuate the hypotension caused by hypovolemia.

Pregnancy-Induced Hypertension (Toxemia of Pregnancy)

In a toxemic pregnancy, maternal liver and kidney function may be poor, convulsions are frequently en-

countered, severe maternal hypertension and increased sensitivity to vasopressors occur frequently, and the infant is often born prematurely and is undernourished. Most obstetric anesthesiologists favor continuous regional analgesia because of its antihypertensive quality and because of the minimal concomitant drug depression in the infant. However, some obstetricians still worry that hypotension develops more easily in response to regional block. Current worldwide experience does not validate this concern. Of course, care should be taken to evaluate and correct the hypovolemia frequently seen in toxemia before the regional blocks are placed. In managing general anesthesia, efforts to attenuate the hypertensive response to endotracheal intubation are important. Intravenous magnesium sulfate, which is frequently used by obstetricians, synergizes with anesthetic muscle relaxants and may contribute to newborn drug depression. Nitroglycerin 100 to 300 μg by intravenous bolus is sometimes used for this purpose.

Prematurity

Respiratory and cardiovascular depression is extremely common after the use of analgesic and anesthetic agents in premature infants. Continuous regional block is the analgesic method of choice during the first and second stages of labor. "Saddle block" is excellent for delivery but is not suitable for labor. Pudendal block is not dangerous but does not relax the birth canal sufficiently to minimize head trauma to the premature baby.

Diabetes

Anesthesia should be directed toward reducing stress. Although hypotension and other complications must be avoided, major regional analgesia is desirable when practical. Insulin and glucose control should be meticulous and should be frequently monitored during labor and the induction of anesthesia. Intravenous glucose intake must be carefully controlled because maternal hyperglycemia may stimulate excessive insulin release by the baby, leading to postpartum hypoglycemia.

Cardiac Disease

Fewer than 2% of pregnant patients suffer from severe heart disease, less than half the incidence noted 40 years ago. Although valvular sequelae of rheumatic fever still predominate, an increasing proportion of pregnant cardiac patients today suffer from complicated congenital heart defects. Continuous regional analgesia is very popular for patients with a wide variety of acquired or congenital heart lesions. Great caution should be exercised in regard to the potential of regional anesthesia to precipitate heart failure by a sudden decrease in peripheral resistance. In addition, the potential for reversal of abnormal shunts because of changing vascular resistance should be borne in mind. Indications for invasive monitoring should be neither more nor less stringent than those used in patients with similar cardiac conditions about to undergo major surgical interventions. Certainly all pregnant cardiac patients should be continuously monitored with electrocardiography, and there should be continuing consultation with the physician caring for the cardiac condition.

Sickle Cell Disease

Sickle cell disease remains a grave threat to women with the SS configuration and their babies. Although some centers report excellent results with exchange transfusion in pregnant sickle cell patients, others disagree. Anesthesia for these patients also remains controversial. However, it should be noted that general anesthesia has not been followed by complications in a large reported series of surgical patients, and inhalational anesthetics have even been reported to be protective against sickling for several hours after anesthesia. Although stasis in the peripheral vascular bed and possible coagulation problems at the needle site have theoretically been objections to major regional analgesia in sickle cell disease, no objective evidence has ever been offered to support these objections.

ANESTHETIC TECHNIQUES FOR CESAREAN SECTION

Major regional analgesia is favored for cesarean section today in most large institutions because of its favorable effects on both mother and infant, provided the anesthesiologist is aware of and alert to the potential dangers. Prophylactic and therapeutic means of avoiding or treating common complications should be used. Such measures include preanesthetic intravenous volume expansion fluids, slight Trendelenburg position, prevention and correction of aortocaval compression by displacement of the uterus to the left, and preparation for administration of ephedrine, either prophylactically or therapeutically. Intravenous doses of 12.5 mg as needed are more controllable than intramuscular doses for either use.

Epidural Block Technique

When the patient is transferred to the operating table, she is placed in the left lateral position. An intravenous line is started with a 16- to 18-gauge plastic catheter, and 800 to 1500 mL of intravenous lactated Ringer's solution without dextrose is administered (to avoid rebound neonatal hypoglycemia). The epidural catheter is placed and tested for safety as outlined in the section on vaginal delivery. After the test dose, medication for cesarean section under epidural block could include 15 to 22 mL of bupivacaine 0.5% mixed with 100 µg of fentanyl or 4 mg of morphine and administered in three divided doses.

Pain following extraction of the infant is treated by reinforcing the block routinely with 75% of the original dose of local anesthetic and fentanyl or morphine every hour, provided that a pinprick test verifies safe block level. During both epidural and spinal anesthesia, unpleasant sensations may be a problem for the mother, even with high block levels. In such an event, intravenous analgesics and tranquilizers may be used in reduced doses. However, narcotics and benzodiazepines synergize their respiratory depressant effects when used together, particularly during high regional block analgesia. Extreme alertness for respiratory depression should always be exercised. Fentanyl 25 µg per intravenous bolus and midazolam (Versed) 0.5 mg per bolus are common combinations. If analgesia remains inadequate, general endotracheal anesthesia with Sellick's technique can be instituted rather than continuing to reinforce intravenous sedation.

Spinal Anesthesia Technique

Bupivacaine 0.75% in doses of 8 to 13 mg, with 20 µg of fentanyl or 0.2 mg of "spinal morphine" (Duramorph) mixed with 0.2 mL of 1:1000 fresh epinephrine, is adequate for subarachnoid block for cesarean section. After blocking, the patient is placed supine in a slight (10 degrees) Trendelenburg position, head on a pillow, and table tilted 15 degrees to the left. A pillow, balloon, or wedge is placed under the right hip to displace the uterus from the vena cava and aorta.

Arterial blood pressure is monitored at least every 60 seconds. If the systolic pressure falls 30% below the preanesthesia level or below 100 mmHg, the left uterine displacement is increased, the Trendelenburg position is steepened, the rate of intravenous infusion is increased, and oxygen by face mask is administered; ephedrine 12.5 mg intravenously—in increments, if necessary—can be given. Phenylephrine is not accepted by many anesthesiologists in this circumstance.

General Anesthesia

Premedication is usually omitted because of its effect on the baby. An intravenous infusion is started using a 16- or 18-gauge needle. Neutralization of acid stomach contents and suppression of further secretion of acid gastric content is desirable, when possible, by giving 30 mL of sodium bicitrate (Bicitra) orally. The patient is placed on the operating table in the left lateral recumbent position until the start of the skin preparation. The dangers of aortocaval compression are also present during general anesthesia, so the mother's right hip should be elevated on a pillow or the uterus deflected during cesarean section under general as well as regional anesthesia. During preparations, the patient is preoxygenated for 3 minutes. When the surgeon is ready, 0.6 mg of scopolamine and 0.3 mg of pancuronium are given about 3 minutes before induction.

Thiopental 3.5 mg per kg intravenously may depress even full-term infants slightly, even in this small dose; however, the degree of "sleepiness" is not important in most full-term healthy babies. Ketamine in small doses (0.75 mg per kg intravenously) seems to be well tolerated but in higher doses may cause *profound* neurologic and respiratory problems in the baby. Many obstetric anesthesiologists still prefer muscle paralysis induced by succinylcholine 2 mg per kg intravenously, followed by a variable intravenous infusion. However, others use 0.1 mg per kg of pancuronium (Pavulon) given intravenously, followed by smaller increments as needed.

Either thiopental 3.5 mg per kg, up to a maximum of 250 mg, or ketamine 0.75 mg per kg, up to 60 mg, is given as a bolus intravenously, followed by succinylcholine 2 mg per kg, followed by a continuous drip of 0.2% succinylcholine. *Cricoid pressure should be instituted and maintained by someone other than the anesthetist as soon as consciousness is impaired.* Intubate the trachea and check ventilation in both lungs with a stethoscope before permitting the incision.

After tracheal intubation, many elect to administer only nitrous oxide 4 liters per minute and oxygen 4 liters per minute until the cord is clamped. In this case, the level of anesthesia can be deepened with thiopental, narcotics, or potent inhalational agents as soon as the cord is clamped. The continuing use of succinylcholine drip (or pancuronium) should be monitored with a nerve block stimulator. Some experts advocate adding a small dose of fentanyl, sufentanil (Sufenta), or alfentanil (Alfenta) or approximately one-half the minimal alveolar concentration of a potent inhalational agent before the birth to reduce the maternal stress response and the possibility of memory. However, the possibility of respiratory depression in the baby after these drugs are administered should not be disregarded.

POSTPARTUM ANALGESIA

Pain After Vaginal Delivery

The intensity of pain in the period following vaginal delivery is rarely as severe as that following cesarean section. Therefore, a variety of oral analgesic agents is commonly employed for this purpose. Rarely, a few doses of common parenteral opioid agents are used. In recent years, a wide variety of antiprostaglandins has been employed with increasing success, sometimes without the need for other analgesics. In a patient with a large episiotomy or perineal lacerations, it may be anticipated that the pain will be severe enough to warrant the use of techniques described later in conjunction with cesarean section.

Pain After Cesarean Section

A variety of methods of treatment of pain after cesarean section may be suitable. Oral and parenteral opioids or even milder oral analgesics such as oxycodone 5 mg and acetaminophen 325 mg (Percocet) orally every 6 hours, often in conjunction with antiprostaglandins (e.g., ibuprofen [Motrin] 400 mg orally every 6 hours), have become standard in treating this type of pain. Recent research shows that many deficiencies exist in this method, including "peaks and valleys" in the intensity of pain due to the varying blood levels achieved by intermittent intramuscular injection. However, this method is by far the least costly of all those described in this section, and it may be expedient and sufficient in many patients.

Patient-Controlled Analgesia (PCA)

Although the concept of PCA is well over 25 years old, its popularity has surged in the past few years. This method has been shown to result in a less variable blood concentration of the analgesic agent. In addition, numerous studies verify that eliminating the peaks and valleys of analgesia, along with the undefinable psychological comfort of the patient's knowing that she can instantly obtain relief from pain, clearly results in overall administration of a lesser total dose of analgesic agent during any given period. Unexpected apnea from the respiratory depressant effects of opioids has been reported but is not as frequent as that reported after intrathecal or epidural use of opioids. However, because of the need for specialized electronic gear and the preparation by the pharmacy of large volumes of analgesic agent to be placed in the reservoir, this method of analgesia entails significant additional expense.

COMPLICATIONS OF GENERAL ANESTHESIA

Airway Obstruction

Eleven obstetric patients were reported to have died in New York City in one 2-year period due to failure to achieve and maintain control of the patients' access to air (the "airway") and ventilation of the lungs during induction of general anesthesia for obstetric delivery. Therefore, it is essential that before induction of general anesthesia, the obstetrician and the anesthetist agree on the steps to be taken should intubation of the trachea prove impossible. These will vary according to the condition of the mother and the baby. This "failed intubation" protocol should be instituted quickly and skillfully.

Aspiration of Gastric Contents

Aspiration of stomach contents is a major hazard during heavy sedation or general anesthesia and occurs even under major regional anesthesia. Gastric emptying may be slowed because of the pain of labor or by the administration of narcotic pain relievers. In addition, the patient frequently has eaten a meal just before the onset of labor. Emptying the stomach artificially by administering apomorphine or performing gastric lavage is very unpleasant, dangerous, and unreliable. Aspiration of gastric contents is now reported to be fatal in fewer than 10% of aspirations by obstetric patients in reporting university hospitals. Until very recently, however, careful reports from Great Britain demonstrated that 35% of all anesthetic-related obstetric deaths were directly caused by inhalation of stomach contents. Although the majority of these deaths occurred during attempted tracheal intubation under general anesthesia, only half of them occurred in patients with "difficult" intubation conditions. Forty percent of those who died received prophylactic antacids orally to prevent acid damage to the lungs, and half were receiving attempted prophylactic external cricoid pressure (Sellick's maneuver). Nonetheless, both measures are firmly indicated in obstetrics.

Treatment of aspiration pneumonia should be based on the principles of immediate establishment of unimpeded ventilation, suppression of transudation by positive end-expiratory intratracheal pressure, and careful monitoring for inadequate ventilation or the delayed development of bacterial pneumonia. Although steroid therapy after aspiration into the trachea has been advocated by many, evidence from animal research indicates that it is ineffective. So-called prophylactic antibiotics are almost universally avoided by experts because of the tendency to favor the growth of opportunistic organisms. The combination of ranitidine (Zantac) 150 mg and metoclopramide (Reglan) 10 mg given orally 90 minutes before surgery as prophylaxis against acid aspiration has been reported to be effective in nearly eliminating these risk factors but has not yet been recommended by the U.S. Food and Drug Administration in obstetric patients.

COMPLICATIONS OF BLOCK ANESTHESIA

Hypotension and Circulatory Failure

Hypotension and circulatory failure may account for 34% of all maternal deaths due to anesthesia and are also a hazard to the fetus. The most frequent cause of maternal death is the aortocaval compression syndrome complicated by blockade of the sympathetic nervous system incidental to spinal or epidural anesthesia. This syndrome can be diagnosed by the presence of hypotension, dyspnea, and acute apprehension, often with tachycardia. It is treated by lifting the uterus to the left or placing the patient on her left side or tilting the patient to the left with a pillow. Further treatment of hypotension includes position change, vigorous fluid infusion, and, if necessary, intravenous ephedrine in 12.5-mg bolus doses. Large doses of alpha-agonist vasoconstrictors such as phenylephrine are NEVER used because they further depress uterine blood flow despite restoring maternal blood pressure, although some experts occasionally use 2 μg/kg of phenylephrine in refractory hypotension.

Seizures Due to Local Anesthetics

Convulsions may constitute about 11% of all disastrous complications of regional anesthesia. Frequently incorrectly attributed to previously undiagnosed eclamptic seizure, unexpected neurologic events ranging from disorientation and bizarre behavior to tonic-clonic convulsions following the injection of a local anesthetic drug should be assumed to be due to the local anesthetic until proved otherwise, even in pregnant patients. Local anesthetic–induced convulsions are rarely due to "allergy" but most often result from elevated blood concentrations of the local anesthetic. Subarachnoid ("spinal") anesthesia almost never results in convulsions due to the very small dose of local anesthetic, which is usually injected to produce subarachnoid block. Although lidocaine-induced convulsions have relatively benign neurologic and cardiovascular sequelae after prompt therapy, convulsions due to bupivacaine are much more serious and have been associated with conduction defects in the human myocardium that are very difficult to reverse once established. Emergency treatment of local anesthetic convulsions consists of skillful support of ventilation and monitoring and support, when necessary, of cardiovascular function. The injection of a small dose of rapid-acting barbiturate, such as 100 mg of thiopental sodium or a small dose of diazepam—for example, 5 mg given intravenously along with succinylcholine 40 to 80 mg—followed by intermittent positive-pressure breathing, is very useful. Generally, the baby should not be delivered at this time because the fetal blood level of anesthetic will be high until it has had time to be redistributed. Blood pressure should be monitored and supported with 12.5-mg boluses of ephedrine if necessary.

Massive Subarachnoid Instillation of Local Anesthetic ("Total Spinal")

Unintended total spinal anesthesia is still a frequent problem during attempted epidural anesthesia and may occur in as many as 1 per 1000 attempted epidural blocks. The epidural catheter can "migrate" into the subdural space from the epidural space some hours after original institution of the block, leading to a "total spinal" after a reinjection. The resulting duration of the respiratory and cardiovascular embarrassment can be expected to be relatively shorter than the planned duration of the intended subarachnoid block. But total spinal anesthesia resulting from subarachnoid instillation of local anesthetic that was intended for the epidural space is a life-threatening emergency because the quantity of local anesthetic injected is frequently 4 to 10 times greater than is used for intentional subarachnoid anesthesia. Patients experiencing this unfortunate situation should be adequately sedated immediately until the return of spontaneous vital functions is complete. Skillful application of intermittent positive-pressure breathing and monitoring and support of cardiovascular activity usually prevent the otherwise fatal outcome of this complication.

Unilateral or Uneven Peridural Block

Some desired segments are not blocked in as many as 10% of patients undergoing peridural blocks. The cause may be a laterally placed catheter, use of volumes that are too small, insufficiently strong concentrations of local anesthetic agent, or perhaps lateral positioning of the patient during injection. The remedy may be to pull back the catheter and inject more anesthetic volume, place the patient on the unblocked side, or inject a larger volume of a more concentrated solution.

Inadvertent Dural Puncture During Attempted Peridural Block

Even a skilled anesthetist may puncture the dura in up to 2% of attempts. A second attempt at an epidural in an adjacent interspace is routine in this event, but extreme care should be taken to administer and observe test doses at every subsequent injection into the epidural catheter. Because postpartum headaches occur in 25 to 75% of patients who have experienced inadvertent dural puncture by the epidural needle, immediate precautions against headache may be desirable. Immediate postpartum instillation of large volumes (up to 60 mL) of "normal" saline has been very successful. Bed rest, hydration, use of intravenous caffeine sodium benzoate or intravenous theophylline, or other conservative measures are often successful in treating these headaches once they are established. Persistent "spinal headaches" are usually eliminated by injections of autologous blood (10 mL) in the epidural space no sooner than the third postpartum day.

HAZARDS TO THE NEWBORN FROM OBSTETRIC ANESTHESIA

Three main factors may contribute to anesthesia-related morbidity in newborns: (1) sedatives, analgesics, and anesthetics administered to the mother during labor; (2) trauma of labor and delivery; and (3) asphyxia due to impaired exchange of respiratory gases during labor and delivery. Obstetric factors such as toxins from amnionitis, muscular depression due to magnesium sulfate, and other factors cannot be disregarded. A newborn is more susceptible to anesthetic overdose than an adult because the undeveloped brain is more susceptible to these drugs. Modern practice attempts to minimize the use of prepartum sedatives by encouraging the use of psychological techniques such as prepared childbirth, regional analgesia techniques, and the concurrent use of synergistic but less depressant drugs. Phenothiazines, for example, add to the analgesia of narcotics, diminish nausea and vomiting, and cause little direct respiratory depression, although some may cause hypotension. Propiomazine (Largon) in incre-

mental doses of 5 mg intravenously or promethazine (Phenergan) in increments of 12.5 mg intravenously can often be used with good effect. Benzodiazepines such as midazolam (Versed) and diazepam (Valium) are sometimes used in laboring women but may be more dangerous to their subsequent newborn baby than are the aforementioned medications.

POSTPARTUM CARE

method of
BERNARD GONIK, M.D., and
WALTER CHAIM, M.D.
Wayne State University School of Medicine
Detroit, Michigan

The terms "postpartum" and "puerperium" are used interchangeably, although by strict definition the first implies after *labor* and the latter begins after *delivery*. From an operational perspective, the two terms are synonymous, with this time period ending when physiologic and anatomic adaptations of pregnancy return to their nonpregnant states. During the postpartum period, usually lasting 6 weeks after delivery, uterine involution occurs and ovulation is re-established; the physiologic hydronephrosis of pregnancy resolves; and hematologic, immunologic, and biochemical parameters return to baseline values.

IMMEDIATE POSTPARTUM PERIOD

The immediate postpartum period is arbitrarily defined as the first several hours to days after delivery and is singled out because of specific events or complications that may require attention. During the immediate postpartum period, vital signs should be frequently monitored, and uterine contractility and the degree of vaginal bleeding should be assessed.

Postpartum Hemorrhage

Postpartum hemorrhage is traditionally defined as an estimated blood loss in excess of 500 mL in the first 24 hours after delivery. However, quantitative measurements are rarely undertaken, and in all likelihood, this amount of blood loss occurs commonly in association with both vaginal and cesarean deliveries. Overall, postpartum hemorrhage has been reported to occur in approximately 5% of deliveries and is still a leading cause of maternal mortality. Causes of postpartum hemorrhage include

Uterine atony   50%
Lower genital tract injury   20%
Uterine or placental anomalies   20%
Subinvolution or retained products or
     coagulopathies   10%

The management of postpartum hemorrhage includes early recognition, large-bore intravenous access, crystalloid (and, as soon as available, blood product) replacement, and identification and correction of the causative factors. The birth canal should be carefully inspected, with special attention to the episiotomy site and cervix. Determining the general source of bleeding (upper vs. lower tract) is essential. Under normal conditions, the uterus should be firm and well contracted below the umbilicus when palpated abdominally. If atony is suspected, the bladder should be emptied and the uterus elevated out of the pelvis and manually massaged. The following pharmacologic agents are available to increase uterine tone in an attempt to reduce bleeding due to atony:

Oxytocin (Pitocin)   20 U in 1000 mL intravenously (10 mL per min)
Methylergonovine (Methergine)   0.2 mg intramuscularly
Prostaglandin (carboprost tromethamine) (Hemabate)   250 μg intramuscularly

Surgical intervention may be required to correct an anatomic defect (e.g., uterine rupture) or if atony cannot be medically controlled. In this latter case a variety of approaches have been considered including radiographic embolization of the affected vessels, uterine or hypogastric artery ligation, and hysterectomy. Coagulation abnormalities associated with blood product replacement should be monitored and corrected as indicated.

Infection

Puerperal febrile morbidity can be defined in a number of different ways. Our preference is a temperature of 38° C or greater on two occasions at least 4 hours apart, within any 24-hour period, usually excluding the first 24 hours after delivery. A careful physical examination, with selective laboratory testing, is needed to determine the cause of the febrile morbidity. Several of the more common reasons for *non*infectious febrile morbidity are breast engorgement (discussed later), atelectasis after surgery, wound seroma formation, and peripheral intravenous line–related thrombophlebitis. Infectious causes include urinary tract infection, pneumonia, and paraendometritis. This latter cause is the usual reason patients receive therapeutic parenteral antibiotics in the postpartum period. Pelvic cellulitis, infected hematoma formation, wound infection, and septic pelvic thrombophlebitis are infectious disease complications usually identified later during the hospitalization. All these infectious disease complications are more commonly found after cesarean (vs. vaginal) delivery.

Uterine infections are typically polymicrobial, including both gram-positive and gram-negative aerobes and anaerobes. The diagnosis of paraendometritis is based on the presence of fever, inappropriate uterine tenderness, foul-smelling lochial drainage, and no other identifiable cause. Laboratory studies are of limited value, in that leukocytosis is commonly associated with parturition and blood cultures are usually negative. Some clinicians recommend a transcervical culture of the endometrial cavity, looking for resistant organisms in the event the patient does not respond to the initial empirical therapy. Antimicrobial therapy should be broad spectrum to cover the wide array of potential pathogens. A common regimen would include ampicillin 2 grams every 6 hours, and gentamicin 80 to 100 mg every 8 hours, titrated to peak and trough levels. Because of the concern for adequate anaerobic coverage, especially after cesarean delivery, clindamycin (Cleocin) is frequently added at a dose of 900 mg every 8 hours. Numerous studies have demonstrated that in the mild to moderately infected patient, equivalent efficacy can be achieved using any of a variety of newer-generation, broad-spectrum penicillin-like (or cephalosporin-like) monotherapies. Parenteral therapy is usually continued until the patient is afebrile for at least 24 to 48 hours. In the otherwise uncomplicated postpartum patient, further outpatient antibiotic therapy is not needed.

Failure of initial treatment is uncommon but may be related to inadequate antibiotic therapy, abscess formation, or the development of septic pelvic thrombophlebitis. One should be cautious not to equate persistent fever with antibiotic failure since other diagnoses such as drug fever or an underlying unrelated cause (e.g., collagen vascular disease) must be entertained. Computed tomography (CT) scanning may be useful in localizing a pocket of pus within the abdomen or pelvis, or to identify clot within the ovarian vein. If suspicious, the wound or episiotomy site must be explored and opened for drainage and debridement if necessary. If pelvic thrombosis is suspected, full heparinization is recommended until lysis of the fever and should probably be continued for a total of 7 to 10 days.

Bladder Function

Intravenous fluids are usually infused overzealously in most labor and delivery units. Additionally, routine oxytocin administration, with its antidiuretic effect, may result in bladder distention and impairment of function. Therefore, postpartum bladder function should be carefully monitored, and bladder emptying should not be delayed over 4 hours after delivery. Patients at particularly high risk are those using conduction anesthesia and those with periurethral trauma at delivery. If unable to spontaneously void, the postpartum patient should be straight-catheterized, with the volume recorded. If serial catheterizations are anticipated, a Foley catheter should be left in place for 24 to 48 hours. With early ambulation, bladder complications, as well as other common problems such as constipation, peripheral venous thrombosis, and pulmonary embolism, are less frequent.

Breast Engorgement and Feeding

Within 48 to 72 hours after delivery, engorgement of the breasts is noticed by most women and may cause varying degrees of discomfort. A well-managed breast-feeding program (for example, every 3 hours alternating each breast) resolves the engorgement.

At the same time a well-fitted brassiere is recommended for support. Oxytocin (Syntocinon) sniffing (5 IU poured onto a gauze) 15 minutes before breast-feeding is also very helpful. If engorgement increases and fever appears in association with local redness and induration, it may be due to mastitis. In addition to scheduled emptying of the breast milk, antibiotics (e.g., an antistaphylococcal penicillin or cephalosporin) should be administered for this latter condition. For women who choose not to breast-feed, minimizing breast stimulation and a firm-fitting breast binder should result in a decrease in engorgement over several days. Bromocriptine is no longer recommended by the manufacturer for lactation suppression.

Episiotomy Site Care

If delivery is associated with the suturing of an episiotomy or a vulvar tear, special attention must be given to postpartum vulvar hygiene. The parturient should be taught to perform "front to back" vulvar cleansing, and the use of sitz baths. An ice pack applied to the perineum helps reduce edema and discomfort during the first 24 hours after episiotomy repair. The topical application of an anesthetic spray also brings some relief. Stool softeners are commonly prescribed, especially if the repaired perineal defect extended into the rectal sphincter or mucosa.

After Birth Pains

Most women notice discomfort and crampy pains associated with uterine contractions after birth and early on with breast feeding. Good relief can be achieved with common analgesics such as acetaminophen, codeine, or any of the nonsteroidal anti-inflammatory agents. These drugs should not be withheld because of concerns over their accumulation in breast milk.

EXTENDED POSTPARTUM PERIOD

The extended postpartum period can be defined as the time between the patient's discharge from the hospital and the "6 week" postpartum visit. Aside from the physical changes that are occurring, one must be cognizant of, and sensitive to, the significant psychosocial adaptations that are also present.

Late Hemorrhage

Vaginal bleeding after delivery becomes scantier after the first 24 hours and progresses from lochia rubra to lochia serosa and finally to lochia alba when leukocytes replace erythrocytes in the vaginal drainage. The two most common pathologic causes of serious bleeding late in the puerperium are retention of placental fragments and subinvolution at the placental site. These two entities must of course first be differentiated from the return of menses, which also can occur in this same time frame (particularly in

the non-breast-feeding woman using a nonhormonal form of contraception). Initial attempts at controlling the bleeding in the hemodynamically stable individual should be medically directed, using either methylergonovine or prostaglandins, as previously specified. If the bleeding does not subside, surgical curettage is needed but may iatrogenically induce more vigorous hemorrhage if subinvolution is the underlying cause. On rare occasion, more aggressive surgical intervention must be entertained, including radiographic embolization, hypogastric artery ligation, or hysterectomy.

Immunization

During the first 72 hours after delivery, women with an Rh-negative blood group type whose newborns are Rh-positive must receive anti-D immune globulin (RhoGAM) 300 µg to reduce the risk of sensitization. On occasion, additional amounts of immune globulin are needed because of concerns for excessive fetomaternal hemorrhage. This can be quantified by performing a Kleihauer-Betke stain on a postpartum maternal blood sample and calculating the extrapolated volume of fetal red cells in the maternal circulation. In some institutions, the postpartum period is chosen to begin an immunization program for the mother, including vaccination against rubella and hepatitis B, and to receive diphtheria–tetanus toxoid booster, when indicated.

Breast Care

Breast-feeding should be encouraged in most circumstances for promotion of mother-child bonding and to satisfy most of the infant's immediate nutritional needs. Breast-feeding can be continued for variable periods of time, with the child usually weaned when solid foods are a stable component of the diet. Nipples require cleaning of the areola with water and mild soap; attention should be paid to the presence of fissures, so that local infection does not develop. At times, the temporary use of a nipple shield is necessary. For breast-feeding women, a protein-rich diet is recommended, and women are frequently encouraged to maintain adequate hydration.

Depression

Postpartum depression is a well-recognized complication of pregnancy, yet few clinicians focus on this diagnostic evaluation during the routine care of their patients. Most often, depression is associated with the birth of the first child and can present insidiously. Postpartum "blues" can be identified in up to 80% of parturients, usually beginning several days after delivery, and spontaneously remitting within a few weeks. Symptoms can include insomnia, irritability, anxiety, loss of appetite, and fatigue. Encouraging family emotional and physical support, rest, and occasional counseling are usually adequate interventions. Major postpartum depression is identified in approximately 10 to 12% of women, occurring in the first several weeks to months after delivery. Treatment may include psychiatric counseling, hospitalization, and antidepressant or antipsychotic medications. Recurrences in subsequent pregnancies are common for this more serious type of depression.

Weight Regulation

Uterine evacuation at term produces a loss of 5 to 6 kg of weight. A further decrease of 2 to 3 kg is achieved by diuresis during the first postpartum week. As suggested earlier, for breast-feeding women a protein-rich diet is recomended, but nonlactating women need no different diet than healthy nonpregnant women. Prenatal vitamins are continued for variable periods of time after delivery, but the benefit of this practice is doubtful if nutrition is otherwise adequate. Conversely, many women are identified to have iron-deficiency anemia during or after their pregnancy, and iron supplementation is probably of some value. Most women approach their prepregnancy weight 6 months after delivery, but still retain on average a surplus of 1.4 kg. A weight-reduction program can be instituted any time after delivery and should have both caloric and exercise components.

Contraception

Contraception counseling is one of the most important tasks of the attending clinician during the early puerperium, considering that ovulation will reestablish itself approximately 4 weeks after delivery in nonlactating women. Combination oral contraceptive pills may be started as early as 2 to 3 weeks after delivery for both lactating and nonlactating women. In some of our patients, we begin contraceptive management before discharge from the hospital using injectable medroxyprogesterone acetate. Intrauterine contraceptive device (IUD) placement is usually attempted in the appropriately selected patient at the examination 4 to 6 weeks postpartum or with completion of the first menses. Breast-feeding affords some protection from pregnancy because of a delay in the onset of ovulation but is a poor contraceptive choice in those absolutely unwilling to be pregnant. Barrier method contraception should always be discussed, because of its ease of use and the added advantage of reducing the risk of sexually transmitted diseases.

Activity

Normal physical activity after routine vaginal delivery can be resumed after a couple of days, including bathing, driving, and some household or work-related functions. Reinitiation of sexual activity should be determined according to the woman's level of comfort. The episiotomy site is usually healed by 2 weeks after repair but can maintain some degree of induration and tenderness for an additional 6 weeks.

Most women regain their usual level of energy by 6 weeks postpartum.

RESUSCITATION OF THE NEWBORN

method of
SCOTT A. JOHNSON, M.D., and
ALFRED L. GEST, M.D.
Baylor College of Medicine
Houston, Texas

At birth, the newborn must make rapid cardiopulmonary adaptations to make the transition from intrauterine to extrauterine life. An effective neonatal resuscitation protocol ensures the accomplishment of a successful transition to postnatal life.

In utero the placenta is the organ of respiration, and the lungs are filled with fluid. Because the lung does not function to oxygenate the blood in utero, oxygenated blood from the placenta through the umbilical vein traverses the ductus venosus, enters the inferior vena cava, and empties into the right atrium. This blood is then shunted through the foramen ovale into the left side of the heart, which in turn distributes oxygenated blood to the brain and peripheral circulation. The right side of the heart primarily receives blood with a lower oxygen content that is ejected into the pulmonary artery but is then diverted to the aorta rather than to the high-resistance lungs through the ductus arteriosus. This blood is then distributed to the placenta through the aorta and umbilical arteries to receive oxygen and nutrients and to release carbon dioxide and waste products.

As the newborn is delivered and takes the first few breaths, several changes occur that allow the lungs to become responsible for respiration: First, the lungs expand as they are filled with gas, and fetal lung fluid gradually leaves the alveoli by moving into the extra-alveolar interstitium, which is eventually cleared by lung lymphatics. At the same time, the pulmonary vascular resistance decreases precipitously while pulmonary blood flow correspondingly increases. With occlusion of the umbilical cord, systemic vascular resistance increases. Even though the foramen ovale and ductus arteriosus remain anatomically open, the decrease in pulmonary vascular resistance and the increase in systemic vascular resistance effectively reverse the direction of blood flow through them. Elevated pulmonary vascular resistance caused by hypoxia, acidosis, and hypothermia leads to right-to-left shunting through the foramen ovale and ductus arteriosus, thus prolonging the fetal circulatory pathways and impairing oxygen delivery. It is apparent that minimization of hypoxia, acidosis, and hypothermia at birth helps to ensure a smooth transition to a normal postnatal circulation.

Fortunately, the first few breaths of most newborn infants are effective and allow the cardiopulmonary adaptations previously discussed to take place. However, some infants are asphyxiated in utero and are born with ineffective respirations or apnea, which leads to hypoxia and acidosis, making these adaptations difficult.

In animal studies, total asphyxia initially causes a short period of increased respiratory effort, which is followed by apnea. This condition is known as "primary apnea," and during this time spontaneous respirations can be restored by tactile stimulation. However, if asphyxia continues, the infant develops gasping respirations, the heart rate continues to decrease, and the blood pressure begins to fall. The infant then takes a last gasping breath (the "last gasp") and enters a period known as "secondary apnea." Now the infant is unresponsive to stimulation, and only positive-pressure ventilation restores spontaneous respiration. The longer the delay in resuscitation, the longer it takes for spontaneous respirations to occur. Because the fetus may experience asphyxia in utero, he or she may undergo primary and secondary apnea in utero. Therefore, when the infant is born apneic, one cannot differentiate between primary and secondary apnea, and one must assume that the infant is in secondary apnea and initiate positive-pressure ventilation.

PREPARATION

Preparation is the essential first step in effective neonatal resuscitation. According to *The Textbook of Neonatal Resuscitation*, published by the American Heart Association and the American Academy of Pediatrics, 90% of hospitals where deliveries occur have only Level 1 nurseries. Therefore, it is essential to ensure that personnel who are adequately skilled in neonatal resuscitation are present at every delivery, whether or not perinatal problems are anticipated. In deliveries at which a normal, healthy infant is expected, one person (e.g., physician, nurse, respiratory therapist) who has the skills to perform a complete neonatal resuscitation must be present. If this person is also caring for the mother, another person who is capable of initiating and assisting with neonatal resuscitation must be present. It is inappropriate to have someone "on call" to provide neonatal resuscitation because this may cause unnecessary delay. During high-risk deliveries at which neonatal asphyxia is likely, two persons not involved in the care of the mother must be readily available, and one of these two must be skilled in endotracheal intubation and the administration of medications.

Equipment needed for a complete resuscitation is listed in Table 1. This equipment should be present in every delivery area and should be routinely checked to ensure that it is working properly. When the antepartum or intrapartum history suggests that an asphyxiated infant may be born, all equipment needed should be taken out of the packages and prepared for use. One should quickly check to ensure that the radiant warmer is heating, that oxygen is flowing through the tubing, that suction is functioning properly, that the resuscitation bag and mask can provide an adequate seal and generate pressure, and that the laryngoscope light source is functional. Several minutes into the resuscitation of a cyanotic infant is not the time to realize that the valve to the oxygen source was never opened. For multiple gestations, a full complement of equipment and personnel is needed for each infant.

INITIAL STEPS OF RESUSCITATION

Although there are certain aspects of neonatal resuscitation that make it unique, it should be noted that the basic ABCs of resuscitation in any age group

TABLE 1. **Requirements for Resuscitation**

Environment

    Radiant warmer
    Blankets, towels (warm)
    Wall clock with sweep second hand

Suction

    Bulb syringe
    Suction catheters (No. 6, 8, 10 French)
    Regulated wall suction
    Meconium aspirators

Airway Management

    Stethoscope
    Oxygen
    Flow meter
    Oxygen tubing
    Infant resuscitation bag with manometer and pressure relief valve
    Masks (premature and infant sizes)
    Laryngoscope
    Size 0 and 1 laryngoscope blades
    Endotracheal tubes (2.5-, 3.0-, 4.0-mm diameters)
    Stylets

Vascular Access

    Umbilical catheters (No. 3.5 and 5.0 French)
    Umbilical catheterization tray
    Syringes (1-, 3-, 5-, 10-, 20-, and 60-mL)
    Needles
    Stopcocks
    Suture
    Sterile saline (10 mL)
    IV catheters
    IV tubing
    Umbilical tape

Medications

    Epinephrine (1:10,000)
    Naloxone hydrochloride (Narcan) (1 mg/mL or 0.4 mg/mL)
    IV solutions (normal saline, 10% dextrose)
    Sodium bicarbonate (4.2%, 0.5 mEq/mL)
    Albumin (5%)
    Sterile water

Miscellaneous

    Gloves
    Masks, with eye shield
    Quick reference card for ages and weights

still apply (*a*irway, *b*reathing, *c*irculation). Most infants respond to airway management and the initiation of positive-pressure ventilation if needed. Chest compressions and, in particular, medications are rarely necessary. This also applies to infants with medical complications such as those in whom prenatal diagnosis has detected complex congenital heart disease or hydrops fetalis. The basic rules of neonatal resuscitation still apply, and one should not forget the ABCs in the excitement that sometimes accompanies delivery of an infant with a complex prenatally detected condition. As we begin to discuss the individual steps of neonatal resuscitation, the importance of continuous evaluation of the patient to assist in the necessary decision-making process involved in neonatal resuscitation cannot be overemphasized.

One very important and unique aspect of newborn resuscitation is temperature control. Simply keeping the newborn warm decreases morbidity more than any other component of resuscitation. In fact, paying attention to temperature should come before the "A" in the ABCs. Cold stress in the newborn leads to increased oxygen consumption and increased metabolic demand, which further complicates the resuscitation of the asphyxiated newborn. This is especially true in the very-low-birthweight infant (less than 1.0 kg). The large surface area of the newborn relative to body mass and the newborn's poor insulating ability (decreased body fat, particularly in preterm infants) accelerate heat loss.

Heat can be lost by four different mechanisms: evaporation, convection, radiation, and conduction. Evaporative heat loss is increased by failure to dry off amniotic fluid. This evaporative heat loss is exacerbated in very-low-birthweight infants whose skin is thin and less keratinized. Convective heat loss occurs when ambient air temperature is less than the infant's skin temperature. Heat loss by radiation to cold objects in a delivery room is a major cause of thermal stress in newborns, and if the baby is placed on cool blankets or towels for resuscitation, heat loss by conduction can occur. It is easy to see how quickly a newborn can lose heat and how important it is for the first steps of resuscitation to include ways to minimize this heat loss. This is easily accomplished by placing the newborn under a prewarmed radiant heat source and quickly drying the infant with a prewarmed towel or blanket. Remember to remove the wet blanket or towel from the infant or evaporative heat loss will continue. Drying of the infant also has the added benefit of providing gentle stimulation, which may aid in the onset of spontaneous respirations.

Establishment of an open airway is accomplished by placing the neonate on his or her back with the neck in a neutral to slightly extended position on a flat radiant warmer bed. The neck should not be hyperextended or underextended, and the warmer bed should not be in the Trendelenburg position as was once recommended. If needed, a rolled blanket or towel may be placed under the shoulders, elevating them approximately 1 inch off the mattress. The newborn should now be in the best position to maintain an open airway.

When the infant has been correctly positioned, the mouth and nose should be suctioned quickly. The material in the mouth should be suctioned first to decrease the risk of aspiration should the infant gasp. A bulb syringe or mechanical suction device may be used. Deep suctioning of the esophagus and stomach or prolonged suctioning is contraindicated because it can produce a vagal response leading to apnea and bradycardia. According to the update to the *Interim Training Guidelines for Neonatal Resuscitation*, published by the American Heart Association and the American Academy of Pediatrics, suctioning should be limited to 3 to 5 seconds. This time limit in addition to avoidance of deep suctioning should lessen the risk of vagal-induced apnea or bradycardia.

The next step is to provide tactile stimulation. The infant has already been dried and suctioned, which in many cases will initiate respirations. If not, there are two (and only two) safe and appropriate ways of providing additional tactile stimulation: (1) slapping or flicking the soles of the feet and (2) rubbing the infant's back. Other actions such as slapping the baby's back or buttocks or blowing cool oxygen or air into the baby's face can result in unnecessary bruising and hypothermia, respectively. If there is no response to one or two flicks of the feet, it is not appropriate to then try to rub the infant's back. The time elapsed from placing the baby under the warmer to positioning, suctioning, and providing additional tactile stimulation should be 15 to 20 seconds. During this time period, the adequacy of respirations should be assessed. Because one must assume that apnea noted at birth may be secondary apnea, it is now time to proceed to positive-pressure ventilation.

The initial steps of warming, positioning, suctioning, and applying tactile stimulation are applied in every newborn delivery. The remaining guidelines to resuscitation depend on the evaluation of the infant while those initial steps are being performed. Apgar scores are of little value to the pediatrician or neonatologist at the delivery. Continued need for resuscitation depends on three clinical signs: (1) respiratory effort, (2) heart rate, and (3) color. If the infant has a regular breathing pattern after tactile stimulation, proceed to check the heart rate. If the infant is gasping or apneic, positive-pressure ventilation should be given. When respiratory effort has been evaluated and the appropriate action taken, the heart rate is monitored. If the heart rate is more than 100 beats per minute, proceed to evaluate the infant's color. If the heart rate is less than 100, even if the infant has spontaneous respirations, proceed to positive-pressure ventilation. The heart rate can be monitored by auscultation or palpation of the pulse in the umbilical cord, although it is generally more prudent to auscultate, especially for the less experienced caregiver. Constant monitoring of the heart rate determines the extent of resuscitation, as is discussed later.

The infant's color should be evaluated next. Peripheral cyanosis (acrocyanosis) is common in the newborn, but central cyanosis is abnormal. Central cyanosis involves the entire body, including the mucous membranes. If central cyanosis is present in a newborn with adequate respirations and a heart rate of more than 100, free-flowing oxygen should be administered. In this instance, positive-pressure ventilation is not indicated. Oxygen should be delivered at a flow rate of 5 liters per minute via an oxygen hose and held steadily (not waved back and forth) ½ inch from the infant's nares. This will deliver approximately 80% inspired oxygen to the infant. The infant should receive a high concentration of oxygen until he or she turns pink, then oxygen should be gradually withdrawn to the degree that the newborn can maintain a pink color.

MECONIUM–STAINED AMNIOTIC FLUID

Another situation unique to resuscitation of the newborn is that of meconium-stained amniotic fluid.

Thin, watery meconium-stained fluid has not been proved to contribute to increased perinatal morbidity, and specific management of these infants is probably unnecessary. However, thick and particulate meconium-stained amniotic fluid can lead to meconium aspiration syndrome, with or without persistent pulmonary hypertension. To minimize this risk, the baby's mouth, pharynx, and nose should be suctioned with a No. 10 French catheter by the obstetrician as the baby's head is delivered but before the shoulders are delivered. After delivery, the baby should be placed under a radiant warmer, and before drying, any remaining meconium should be suctioned from the hypopharynx. The trachea should then be suctioned under direct vision. This is best accomplished by intubating the infant with an endotracheal tube and applying suction (no more than 100 mmHg) as the endotracheal tube is withdrawn. Passing a suction catheter through the endotracheal tube is inappropriate because it may be too small to suction particulate meconium. Reintubation followed by repeat suctioning should be performed until all meconium is removed, provided the infant remains stable. Free-flowing oxygen should be provided with all intubation attempts to minimize the risk of hypoxia. It is important to monitor the heart rate continuously because positive-pressure ventilation may have to be initiated in the asphyxiated infant before all the meconium can be removed from the trachea. If positive-pressure ventilation has to be initiated prior to removal of all meconium in the trachea, complete resuscitation (including chest compressions and medications if needed) should be performed until the heart rate is over 100, at which time repeat tracheal suctioning can then be performed. Gastric contents should be suctioned for meconium to prevent the possibility of later regurgitation and aspiration. However, this should be done only after resuscitation is completed and the infant is stable.

POSITIVE–PRESSURE VENTILATION

Positive-pressure ventilation is sometimes needed during the course of neonatal resuscitation. This can be provided by bag-and-mask ventilation or by bag-and-endotracheal tube. Although an anesthesia bag may be used, it is a more difficult technique to master, and in our opinion it is not nearly as effective at delivering the higher pressures sometimes required to resuscitate a sick newborn. A self-inflating resuscitation bag is preferable, and it should be equipped with a face mask and an oxygen reservoir, which enables the bag to deliver a higher concentration of oxygen (90 to 100%). Without the oxygen reservoir, the self-inflating bag is unable to deliver a high concentration of oxygen. The flow of oxygen through the tubing should be increased to 8 to 10 liters per minute and should be connected to the oxygen inlet on the resuscitation bag. The self-inflating bags have a pressure-release valve, commonly called a "pop-off valve," that usually releases at 25 to 35 cmH$_2$O pressure. It is often necessary to occlude this pop-off

valve to generate a sufficient amount of pressure to ventilate a newborn's nonaerated lungs effectively, especially with the first few breaths. With the pop-off valve occluded, care should be taken not to overventilate the newborn because this may cause a pneumothorax. A pressure manometer should always be used in conjunction with the bag to prevent overdistention of the lung.

Masks come in different shapes and sizes, with or without cushioned rims. The mask rim should be cushioned and should cover the chin, mouth, and nose but not the eyes. It is recommended that masks be available for full-term and premature infants. The bag-and-mask apparatus should already have been tested for adequacy by forming an airtight seal against the palm of one's hand and generating pressure. At the time of need for bag-and-mask ventilation, the baby should already be in the correct position for an open airway with the neck in a neutral to slightly extended position. The newborn has already been suctioned and tactilely stimulated not more than twice. If respirations remain inadequate, bag-and-mask ventilation should be initiated.

The ventilator should stand in a position that does not obstruct the view of the newborn's chest. The mask is placed over the baby's face, and light downward pressure is applied with one hand. Constant reevaluation is necessary to ensure that the seal is adequate and that chest expansion is occurring with each assisted ventilation. If chest expansion is inadequate, the most common problem is an inadequate seal. Second, the infant's airway could be blocked by improper positioning or occluded by secretions. It may be necessary to reposition the infant or suction the infant's mouth and nose. If a good seal is obtained and an airway is maintained, increasing the pressure may be necessary to move the chest. Pressures of 20 to 40 cmH$_2$O are often required in infants with respiratory conditions that decrease lung compliance. The infant should be ventilated at a rate of 40 to 60 times per minute.

After 15 to 30 seconds of bag-and-mask ventilation, the heart rate determines the next step of resuscitation. If the heart rate is more than 100 and spontaneous respirations have begun, bag-and-mask ventilation is gradually decreased, free-flowing oxygen is provided, and one observes the infant for continuation of effective respirations. If the heart rate is 60 to 100 and increasing, bag-and-mask ventilation is continued. If the heart rate is 60 to 100 and not increasing, the adequacy of ventilation is reassessed, and if the heart rate remains less than 80, chest compressions are begun. If the heart rate is less than 60, the adequacy of ventilation is again assessed, and chest compressions are begun immediately. The adequacy of the seal between the mask and the baby's face cannot be overemphasized.

CHEST COMPRESSIONS

Chest compressions are performed on the lower third of the sternum, located between an imaginary line drawn between the nipples and the xyphoid process. Care must be taken to avoid applying pressure directly over the xyphoid. The thumb technique may be used by encircling the infant's body with both hands and placing the thumbs on the sternum and the fingers under the infant. The thumbs are used to compress the sternum. The two-finger method uses the tips of the first two fingers or the middle and ring finger placed in a perpendicular position over the lower sternum. Only the fingertips should rest on the chest and pressure should be applied directly downward to decrease the risk of fractured ribs or a pneumothorax. The amount of pressure used should be the amount sufficient to depress the sternum ½ to ¾ of an inch. According to the new *Interim Training Guidelines for Neonatal Resuscitation*, published by the American Heart Association and the American Academy of Pediatrics in April 1993, chest compressions should be interposed with ventilation in a ratio of 3:1. This amounts to 90 compressions and 30 breaths per minute. Therefore, the ventilation rate used during chest compressions is lower than the 40- to 60-range recommended when chest compressions are not being performed. The heart rate should be evaluated every 30 seconds and compressions continued until the heart rate is over 80.

ENDOTRACHEAL INTUBATION

Endotracheal intubation is indicated when prolonged positive-pressure ventilation is required or bag-and-mask ventilation is deemed ineffective. It is also indicated in such special circumstances as infants born with thick or particulate meconium in the amniotic fluid or infants with congenital diaphragmatic hernia. Intubation is a skill that takes practice and that becomes better with experience. In preparation for intubation, the laryngoscope should be equipped with a No. 0 blade for premature infants and a No. 1 blade for full-term infants, although many skilled intubators find that a No. 0 blade is sufficient for full-term infants also. Double-check to see that the light source is functional. Select the proper size of endotracheal tube based on the baby's weight. A 2.5-mm (internal diameter) tube is appropriate for an infant weighing less than 1.0 kg, 3.0 mm is best for infants weighing 1.0 to 2.0 kg, and 3.5 mm is appropriate for infants weighing more than 2.0 kg. Use of a stylet is optional but is usually unnecessary because the stiffness of the endotracheal tube is adequate for manipulation during intubation. Mechanical suction (not to exceed 100 mmHg) should be available as well as free-flow oxygen to provide a high concentration of oxygen during the procedure to minimize hypoxia. The resuscitation bag and mask remain at the bedside for use between intubation attempts; the bag will be connected to the endotracheal tube after intubation is completed.

When intubation is needed, the infant should already be in the proper position, that is, with the head in a midline position and the neck in a neutral to slightly extended position. The laryngoscope handle is held in the left hand and the blade is inserted between the tongue and the palate until the tip of the blade rests in the vallecula. Once inserted, the glottis is visualized by lifting the entire blade in an "up and outward" motion. With this motion, the intubator's entire arm should move in the desired direction. The laryngoscope should never be rotated in a "prying" or "can opener" type of maneuver. At least two people are required for endotracheal intubation. The second person prepares the tape for securing the tube in place, administers free-flow oxygen during the attempt, monitors the heart rate, limits the time of the attempt to no more than 20 seconds, assesses whether the attempt is successful, helps determine the appropriateness of the position of the tube, and helps secure the tube in place. The intubation attempt should not last more than 20 seconds. Bag-and-mask ventilation should be performed between attempts. Suctioning is sometimes necessary to provide adequate visualization of the glottis. Once the glottis is in view, the endotracheal tube is inserted with the right hand until the vocal cord guideline (the heavy black line near the tip of the tube) is at the level of the vocal cords. A guideline for estimating that the endotracheal tube is in a good location is to add 6 to the infant's weight in kilograms. This provides the centimeter mark at which the endotracheal tube should be taped at the lip. It is important for the intubator to hold the endotracheal tube securely until it is taped into position and to always listen for equal breath sounds bilaterally in the axillae of the infant. One should be sure to record the position at which the tube is taped because this is useful for repositioning later and for determining whether the tube has inadvertently shifted in position.

Often one is so elated at passing the tube successfully that he or she fails to pay attention to the distance that it is inserted. Much harm can come from inserting an endotracheal tube too far. If it is inserted too far, it can rest in the right main stem bronchus, causing poor oxygen and carbon dioxide exchange and overdistention of that lung segment, possibly leading to pulmonary interstitial emphysema and pneumothorax. In the premature infant, extra care should be taken to ensure good endotracheal tube placement because the "6 plus weight in kilograms" rule may be less reliable; the tube may need to be inserted less far. To ensure against esophageal intubation, listen for air entering the stomach and observe for gastric distention. This usually becomes apparent because secretions enter the endotracheal tube and the patient does not respond clinically. Always obtain a chest radiograph to confirm the position of the endotracheal tube.

MEDICATIONS

Resuscitation medications are rarely needed in the newborn. However, in the newborn whose heart rate remains less than 80 despite adequate ventilation with 100% oxygen and effective chest compressions for more than 30 seconds, or in the newborn with a heart rate of 0, medications should be administered. The initial medication in such a situation is epinephrine. Epinephrine increases cardiac output by increasing the heart rate and myocardial contractility and increases blood pressure by causing peripheral vasoconstriction. It should be given rapidly and can be given intravenously or via an endotracheal tube in a dose of 0.1 to 0.3 mL per kg of 1:10,000 solution. The intravenous route is preferable because plasma concentrations with the endotracheal route are sometimes low. However, intravenous access has usually not been established when the first dose of epinephrine is required, so it may be preferable to give the higher recommended dose when the drug is administered by the endotracheal route. Epinephrine may be repeated every 5 minutes if the heart rate remains less than 100. If there is no response to epinephrine, one should suspect metabolic acidosis in the asphyxiated infant. In this case, or in the case of documented metabolic acidosis, sodium bicarbonate is indicated in a dose of 2 mEq per kg. It can only be given intravenously. Intracranial hemorrhage has been associated with the use of bicarbonate in animal studies. To reduce that risk, sodium bicarbonate in the commercially available 4.2% solution (0.5 mEq per mL) should be given slowly over a minimum of 2 minutes, not to exceed a rate of 1 mEq per minute. Hypovolemia may be present in the newborn and is usually a known event (e.g., umbilical cord accidents) and is indicated by pallor, poor perfusion despite a normal pH and PO_2, and weak pulses despite a good heart rate. Hypovolemia must also be considered if there is no response to the administration of epinephrine and bicarbonate. A dose of 10 mL per kg of volume expander should be given slowly intravenously. In the premature infant, this volume should always be given over at least 30 minutes to decrease the risk of intraventricular hemorrhage. However, in the hypovolemic asphyxiated full-term infant it may be necessary to administer the volume over 5 to 10 minutes. It is essential to monitor the heart rate and discontinue medications once the heart rate is over 100.

In the special instance of a baby born with respiratory depression to a mother who received narcotics within 4 hours of delivery, naloxone hydrochloride (Narcan) in a dose of 0.1 mg per kg given rapidly is indicated. In our experience this is a rare occurrence, and we find that naloxone is often given when it is unwarranted. Remember that apnea can always be effectively controlled with bag-and-mask ventilation while the narcotic administration history is checked. When needed, naloxone may be given by endotracheal tube, intravenously, intramuscularly, or subcutaneously. The intravenous route is preferable. Naloxone should not be given if the mother had a narcotic addiction, because this may precipitate withdrawal in the infant. The infant who receives naloxone should be observed, because the narcotic causing the respiratory depression may have a longer duration of action than the naloxone, which has a dura-

tion of action of 1 to 4 hours. Therefore, the dose of naloxone may need to be repeated.

Successful neonatal resuscitation requires communication between the resuscitation team and the obstetric staff, advanced preparation, and skilled and knowledgeable personnel. This expertise should be available at all hospitals for every newborn delivery regardless of the presence of highly specialized perinatal services. We encourage all hospitals delivering babies to have skilled personnel available for all deliveries. Preferably, these personnel will have completed The Neonatal Resuscitation Program offered by the American Academy of Pediatrics and the American Heart Association.

CARE OF THE HIGH-RISK NEONATE

method of
GLEN A. GREEN, M.D., and
JAMIL H. KHAN, M.D.
Eastern Virginia Medical School
Norfolk, Virginia

In the United States, approximately 2 to 4% of the estimated 4 million infants born annually require some type of special care shortly after birth. Resuscitation is required in an estimated 80% of the infants born weighing 1500 grams or less and in an additional significant but undetermined number of infants over 1500 grams. Anticipation of and preparation for potential problems or special care in the delivery room begin with good communication between the obstetric and pediatric care providers.

Approximately 10% of all pregnancies are considered to be high risk. Although many of the infants requiring special care come from this high-risk population, a significant number have a benign prenatal history.

EXTRAUTERINE ADAPTATION

At the time of delivery, the infant has to make many physiologic adjustments in order to adapt to the extrauterine environment. A successful transition depends on the transfer from a placental cardiorespiratory support to the effective utilization of the newborn's lungs in coordination with changes in the cardiovascular system.

Physiology

Before birth, the placenta provides the nutrients and exchange of gases for the fetus. In utero, the lungs are filled with fluid and receive approximately 7% of the cardiac output. The flow of oxygenated blood comes from the umbilical vein into the inferior vena cava, through the ductus venosus, and across the foramen ovale to more directly enter the systemic circulation. The less oxygenated blood returns from the body to the right atrium via the superior vena cava, is pumped out the pulmonary artery, bypasses the lungs through the ductus arteriosus, and enters the placenta via the two umbilical arteries (Figure 1).

The fluid in the lungs is removed by a sequence of events beginning with partial reabsorption with the initiation of labor, then physical expression during passage through the vaginal canal, and finally, gradual reabsorption with breathing. The successful expansion of the lungs with effective gas exchange is critical for survival. The circulation must also change to ensure adequate pulmonary blood flow. The clamping of the umbilical cord causes an increased systemic resistance, with subsequent closure of the foramen ovale and increased blood flow to the lungs. The ductus arteriosus and ductus venosus close shortly after birth, and the "normal" circulation is established.

Thermoregulation

Temperature regulation is very important in providing optimal neonatal care. The delivery room temperature should be a comfortable 24° to 27° C. After birth, the infant is immediately dried with a warm towel and placed in a warm environment. Constant attention is given to avoid the mechanisms of heat loss, including evaporation, convection, conduction, and radiation. Hypothermia will impair the newborn's adaptation to extrauterine life and may cause peripheral vasoconstriction, leading to a metabolic acidosis.

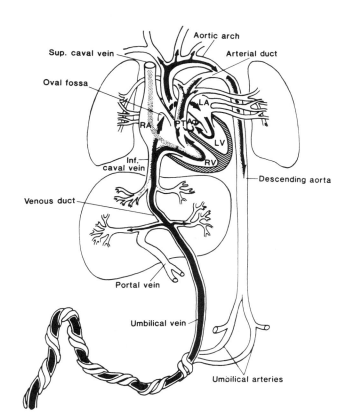

Figure 1. Diagram of the course of the fetal circulation. (From Long WA: Fetal and Neonatal Cardiology. Philadelphia, WB Saunders, 1990, p 4.)

Thus, careful attention must be given to ensure proper thermoregulation even during a complicated and intense resuscitation.

In the nursery, thermal control continues to be a priority. Maintaining a neutral thermal environment—the environmental temperature at which caloric loss (as measured by oxygen consumption) is minimized—helps promote growth and stability.

Assessment of Adaptation

The infant's response to labor and delivery and subsequent extrauterine adaptation are generally measured by the Apgar score. However, the need for resuscitation is best determined by assessing the infant's respiration, heart rate, and color. The American Heart Association and the American Academy of Pediatrics Neonatal Resuscitation Program have established standardized guidelines for neonatal resuscitation. All facilities with a delivery service should require the presence of someone specifically qualified in neonatal resuscitation at each delivery. Additional information is provided in the section on neonatal resuscitation.

A brief physical examination should be done in the delivery room to ensure that the infant is not compromised and has no major anomalies. This physical examination in combination with the history of the pregnancy, labor, and delivery will determine whether the infant should go to the term nursery, the intermediate nursery, or the newborn intensive care unit. In all cases, the infant will need close observation to ensure a successful adaptation to extrauterine life.

NEWBORN INFANT ASSESSMENT

History

The history of the pregnancy, labor, and delivery and the medical history of the parents and their families are critical in formulating a differential diagnosis and in determining an appropriate diagnostic and therapeutic plan. A copy of the pertinent obstetric records and prenatal laboratory results should be sent to the nursery. The newborn record should include:

1. Social demographics (parents' names, ages, and marital status).

2. Mother's obstetric history, including the number of pregnancies, any problems with the pregnancies, and their outcomes.

3. The estimated date of confinement based on the last menstrual period.

4. Results of any fetal testing (e.g., ultrasonography, amniocentesis).

5. Maternal systemic diseases.

6. Maternal drug history, including medications (prescription and nonprescription), alcohol, tobacco, and any substance abuse.

7. Recent infections or exposures.

8. Maternal blood type and serologic tests.

9. Family history of inherited diseases.

10. Current pregnancy problems, such as pre-eclampsia, polyhydramnios, oligohydramnios, surgery, or trauma.

11. Labor and delivery information, including duration of ruptured membranes; fetal monitoring abnormalities; fever; analgesics or anesthesia; mode of delivery; complications, such as abruptio placentae, meconium, or nuchal cord; initial assessment, including resuscitation requirements; Apgar scores; and placental examination, if indicated.

The history should be complete and may require further questioning of the parents, family, and/or obstetric physician.

Gestational Age Assessment

An integral part of the newborn assessment is an estimation of the gestational maturation. Prenatal estimates of gestational age are routinely calculated using the mother's last menstrual period. The most accurate ultrasonic gestational age assessment is obtained from the crown-rump length at 5 to 12 weeks' gestation. The New Ballard Score (Figure 2) is used in the author's nursery and provides a valid estimation of postnatal maturation for infants with gestational ages greater than 20 weeks. An infant whose birth occurs between 38 weeks 0 days (260th day) and 42 weeks 6 days (294th day) from the onset of the last menstrual period is classically defined as term. Therefore, a preterm birth occurs before 38 weeks and a post-term birth occurs after 43 weeks from the onset of the last menstrual period.

Optimal preparation for preterm deliveries requires an understanding of the etiologies of preterm delivery and anticipation of special needs. The etiology for a preterm delivery is usually not known but may be associated with fetal abnormalities (e.g., fetal distress), obstetric conditions (e.g., abruptio placentae, incompetent cervix, uterine malformations), multiple gestations, acute or chronic maternal illness (e.g., preeclampsia, chorioamnionitis, diabetes, urinary tract infections), malnutrition, maternal age younger than 16 or older than 35 years, or inaccurate gestational assessment.

Post-term infants usually have a normal head circumference and length. However, they generally lose weight after 42 weeks of gestation owing to nutritional deprivation. Mortality is increased with postmaturity, so careful gestational age assessment and close monitoring of fetal well-being are vital. Complications of postmaturity include meconium aspiration, persistent pulmonary hypertension, hypoglycemia, polycythemia, hypocalcemia, and perinatal depression.

Birthweight Classification

The generally accepted definitions for birthweight classifications are as follows:

Normal birthweight (NBW): 2500 grams or more

Low birthweight (LBW): less than 2500 grams

Very low birthweight (VLBW): less than 1500 grams

Small for gestational age (SGA): weight less than two standard deviations below the mean for gestational age or less than the tenth percentile

Large for gestational age (LGA): weight greater than two standard deviations above the mean for gestational age or more than the ninetieth percentile

The most common cause of SGA infants in the United States is uteroplacental insufficiency, which can be due to preeclampsia, smoking, hypertension, or cardiopulmonary disease. Other associations with SGA infants include malnutrition, congenital infections (e.g., rubella, cytomegalovirus), chromosomal abnormalities, multiple gestations, and a constitutionally small size.

LGA infants may have hyperinsulinism and need close blood sugar monitoring (e.g., those with Beckwith's syndrome or infants of diabetic mothers). Further risks associated with being LGA include birth trauma (e.g., brachial plexus injuries), polycythemia, and perinatal depression.

Fetal growth and maturation are individualized and depend on a combination of factors that include genetic predisposition, nutrition, obstetric conditions, and maternal illnesses and stress. Therefore, a newborn infant may exhibit clinical behavior that is either advanced or delayed for his or her gestational age. An individualized care plan must then be created based on the history, physical examination, and clinical course.

Physical Examination

A thorough physical examination should be performed on each newborn. The weight, length, and head circumference should always be recorded. A general appraisal of a naked infant under a warming unit allows a quick assessment for cardiorespiratory difficulties, major anomalies, jaundice or meconium staining, and overall activity level. It is usually better to examine the infant in the following order: inspection, auscultation, palpation, and manipulation.

Head. Inspection of the head reveals the shape and any scalp deformities or lesions such as bruises, puncture marks, or lacerations. A caput succedaneum is a subcutaneous collection of blood and edema, whereas a cephalohematoma is a subperiosteal collection of blood. Therefore, a cephalohematoma does not cross cranial sutures. The anterior and posterior fontanelles and the sagittal, coronal, lambdoid, and frontal sutures should all be palpated. Widening of the sutures and large fontanelles indicate possible intracranial pathology or hypothyroidism.

Eyes. Ophthalmic evaluation for the light reflex helps identify possible cataracts, glaucoma, retinoblastoma, and other abnormalities. Gentle inspection is required to avoid trauma to the eye and eyelid.

Neuromuscular Maturity

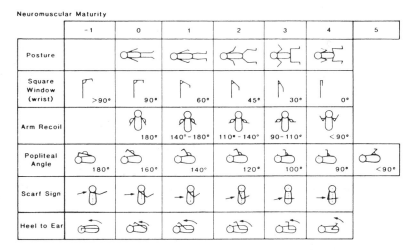

Physical Maturity

Maturity Rating

score	weeks
-10	20
-5	22
0	24
5	26
10	28
15	30
20	32
25	34
30	36
35	38
40	40
45	42
50	44

Figure 2. Expanded New Ballard Score includes extremely premature infants and has been refined to improve accuracy in more mature infants. (From Ballard JL, Khoury JC, Wedig K, et al: New Ballard Score, expanded to include extremely premature infants. J Pediatr *119*:417–423, 1991.)

Ears. The shape, size, and position of the ears may indicate possible chromosomal abnormalities or syndromes. The ear is considered "low-set" if the helix is below the horizontal plane at the level of the corner of the orbit.

Mouth. Evaluation of the mouth may detect a cleft palate, the presence of teeth, or other anomalies. Asymmetry of movement of the lips, tongue, and face indicates possible underlying neurologic impairments.

Nose. Flaring of the nasal alae may indicate respiratory distress. Patency of the nasal passage can be ensured by passage of a catheter through the nares into the nasopharynx.

Neck. The trachea should be midline, and no clefts, sinuses, or masses should be present. The thyroid gland is not normally palpable at any gestational age.

Heart. The normal newborn heart rate is usually between 120 and 160 beats per minute but may range from 80 to 180 beats per minute. The rate may vary with respirations and activity. Auscultation of the heart should be performed while the infant is quiet to determine heart position. Normal position on the left may occur, or dextrocardia may be present. The presence of a murmur may or may not indicate underlying pathology. When the ductus arteriosus is closing, a transient murmur may be heard; yet a serious heart anomaly may present with no murmur at all. Femoral pulses should be palpated to help assess for coarctation of the aorta. When further evaluation of cardiac structure and function is required, four extremity blood pressures, chest radiograph, electrocardiogram, and cardiology consultation should be considered.

Lungs. The respiratory rate is generally between 40 and 60 breaths per minute. Regular respirations may be interrupted by 5 to 10 seconds of not breathing. However, apnea of more than 20 seconds, associated with oxygen desaturation or bradycardia or requiring stimulation to recover, is abnormal. Symmetrical breath sounds should be present upon auscultation. In general, the infant should have good color and be in no distress.

Abdomen. The abdomen should appear symmetrical and be neither distended nor scaphoid. The umbilical cord should have two arteries and one vein. The liver may be palpated approximately 2 to 3 cm below the right costal margin along the midclavicular line. The spleen is not generally palpable. If the liver and spleen are enlarged, suspect a hemolytic or infectious disease. The kidneys may be felt with deep palpation in the first few days of life, since little abdominal muscle is present. However, if the kidneys are easily palpable, they may be enlarged and warrant further evaluation.

Genitalia. The uncircumcised male always has a significant degree of phimosis. The term male's penis should be greater than 2.5 cm in length; the urethral meatus should be visualized and any degree of hypospadias documented. The testes should be palpated by running a finger down from the internal ring on either side to the base of the penis. The testes are trapped in the scrotum and should be of equal size bilaterally. The female genitalia at birth are notable for an enlarged labia majora. The labia should be spread and any anomalies such as an imperforate hymen documented. A benign mucosal tag may be present from the vaginal wall, and a creamy white discharge is commonly noted from the vagina. After a few days, this discharge may become bloody (pseudomenses).

Anus. Patency, position, and size (approximately 10 mm in diameter) of the anus should be assessed. Digital examination is generally not indicated and may be traumatic.

Spine. The back, especially the lumbar, sacral, and cervical areas, should be carefully inspected for evidence of a pilonidal sinus tract, meningocele, or other anomalies.

Extremities. Anomalies of the digits (syndactyly, abnormal number or placement), club feet, and hip dislocation are common abnormalities. Checking the passive range of motion of all extremities is recommended. When examining the hips, a "clicking" sensation may be felt due to possible movement of the ligamentum teres in the acetabulum. This should not be confused with the "clunk" felt with dislocation and relocation of the femoral head in the acetabulum. Fetal positioning frequently causes mild deformities of the extremities such as tibial torsion and forefoot adduction. If the forefoot adduction can be corrected with passive motion, it will generally resolve spontaneously. Mild tibial torsion and bowing will also resolve spontaneously.

Neurologic Function. Observation of the infant before and during the physical examination is the most valuable part of the neurologic evaluation. The behavioral state, level of alertness, and gestational age of the infant, along with any external environmental stimulation, all have a significant influence on the examination. Primitive reflexes such as the Moro reflex, the palmar grasp reflex, and the rooting reflex help determine equal and symmetrical movement and strength. Tone and posture are readily assessed during manipulation of the infant. Deep tendon reflexes help demonstrate functional sensory, motor, and proprioceptive nerve function. The Babinski response and unsustained ankle clonus may be elicited in the newborn and are normal.

Laboratory Assessment

Routine laboratory assessment usually includes a hematocrit and blood glucose. A central venous hematocrit of less than 40% in a newborn indicates significant anemia. The etiology of the anemia must be investigated and may include hemolysis or acute or chronic blood loss, as is seen with ABO blood group incompatibility, abruptio placentae, and fetal-maternal hemorrhage, respectively. A central hematocrit of more than 65% indicates polycythemia and is associated with potential hyperviscosity. Anemia and polycythemia are discussed later in the "Hematologic" section.

Serum glucose concentrations decrease after birth owing to the loss of the placental glucose supply and the stresses of birth. Hypoglycemia is functionally defined as a blood glucose level less than 40 mg per dL. We therefore recommend the evaluation of any infant with a blood glucose level of less than 40 mg per dL. The blood glucose concentration should be assessed for every infant admitted to the nursery. A rapid approximation of the blood glucose may be obtained using reagent strips and following the test instructions. The accuracy of the results is dependent on proper skin preparation, appropriate storage of the reagent strips, and effective use of the reagent strips and/or glucose meter. If a low blood glucose value is determined, a blood sample may be sent to the laboratory for confirmation of hypoglycemia. Treatment should begin immediately while confirmatory results are pending. We recommend an initial intravenous infusion of 2 mL per kg of 10% glucose water followed by maintenance glucose administration as outlined in the "Fluid and Electrolytes" section. Asymptomatic term infants who are at risk for hypoglycemia (e.g., intrauterine malnutrition) or who have "borderline" low blood sugar may be given early oral feedings and followed closely.

FLUID AND ELECTROLYTES

If an infant is not expected to receive enteral nutrition in the immediate newborn period, intravenous dextrose and water is begun. Initial fluids consist of 10% glucose water unless the infant weighs less than 1000 grams, in which case 5% glucose water is used. If glucose concentrations higher than 12% are required, a central venous line must be used to avoid peripheral vein injury. The recommended rates of administration are outlined in Table 1.

Glucose administration should be considered in terms of the total glucose per kilogram per minute. The glucose requirements for a term infant, preterm infant over 1000 grams, and preterm infant less than

TABLE 1. **Initial Intravenous Fluid Infusion Rates***

Weight (gm)	Rate
500–750	150 mL/kg/day
750–1000	120–150 mL/kg/day
1000–1500	100–120 mL/kg/day
>1500	80 mL/kg/day

*Fluid should be restricted to 60 mL/kg/day if renal impairment is suspected.

1000 grams are 8 to 9 mg per kg per minute, 5 to 7 mg per kg per minute, and 4 to 6 mg per kg per minute, respectively.

Increased fluid needs may be anticipated in certain clinical situations, such as extreme immaturity secondary to excessive insensible water loss and inability to concentrate urine, sepsis with third spacing, excessive gastrointestinal losses (diarrhea, emesis, increased gastric tube output), or the use of a radiant heater or phototherapy. Placing the infant in a warm, humidified environment with a plastic shield or isolette and using a humidified ventilator or oxyhood help minimize fluid losses. Signs of dehydration include excessive weight loss, hypernatremia, hypotension, tachycardia, and decreased urine output. Excess free water may present with excessive weight gain, hyponatremia, body edema, and increased respiratory needs, with a radiograph demonstrating an increased hazy appearance. An infant's fluid status is best assessed by monitoring the infant's weight, serum sodium, and urine output closely. In an immature infant, however, the urine specific gravity and urine output may not be reliable indicators of the fluid status owing to the kidneys' impaired ability to concentrate and dilute the urine. In general, normal urine output is 1 to 4 mL per kg per hour.

In the first several hours of life, the infant's serum electrolytes generally reflect those levels present in the mother. We generally do not recommend measuring the infant's serum electrolytes before 12 hours of age unless the mother has electrolyte imbalances. Maintenance sodium and potassium are begun at 2 to 3 mEq per kg per day and 1 to 2 mEq per kg per day, respectively. Potassium is added only after renal function is ensured, as evidenced by urine output. The serum electrolyte levels are monitored at least daily and more frequently if they are unstable or the infant's clinical condition is changing. Normal sodium levels are between 130 and 150 mEq per dL; normal potassium levels are between 3.5 and 5.5 mEq per dL. Hypernatremia may be caused by dehydration, iatrogenic factors, or renal disease. Hyponatremia may be caused by iatrogenic factors such as the use of diuretics or excess free water administration; syndrome of inappropriate antidiuretic hormone; congestive heart failure; or renal disease. Hyperkalemia may be associated with renal disease, severe acidosis, or iatrogenic causes. Hypokalemia may result from iatrogenic causes such as diuretic therapy or nasogastric suctioning, emesis, or metabolic alkalosis. Treatment of the electrolyte imbalance should be based on identifying and correcting the underlying cause.

Hypocalcemia is commonly seen in infants of diabetic mothers, preterm infants, and asphyxiated infants. Hypocalcemia is generally defined as a total serum calcium less than 7.0 mg per dL or an ionized serum calcium less than 4.0 mg per dL. Signs of hypocalcemia include tremulousness, cardiac arrhythmias, and seizures. Treatment is with 100 to 200 mg per kg of calcium gluconate. We recommend infusing the calcium intravenously over 20 to 30 minutes unless an emergency exists, in which case cautious, slow intravenous push may be indicated. The heart rate should be monitored closely during rapid intravenous administration of calcium, since profound bradycardia may be a complication.

NUTRITION

Parenteral nutrition should be initiated if the infant is not going to receive adequate enteral nutrition within 3 to 5 days. Parenteral nutrition generally consists of amino acids, glucose, electrolytes, vitamins, minerals, and lipids. We start amino acids at 0.5 to 1 gram per kg per day and incrementally increase by approximately 0.5 gram per kg per day to a maximum of 3 grams per kg per day. Glucose is initially infused at 5 to 8 mg per kg per minute and incrementally increased by 0.5 to 2 mg per kg per minute per day, depending on the glucose tolerance of the infant. The serum glucose may be maintained between 150 and 180 mg per dL if no glycosuria is present and increased calories are necessary. The desirable glucose infusion rate should range from a minimum of 5 mg per kg per minute to a maximum of 14 mg per kg per minute. Lipids are begun at 0.5 to 1 gram per kg per day and incrementally increased by 0.5 gram per kg per day to a maximum of 3 grams per kg per day. In general, the lipid calories delivered should not be greater than 50% of the total parenteral calories. The infant's parenteral caloric goal is estimated to be 90 to 110 kcal per kg per day.

Many feeding schedules have been devised for infants of various sizes and gestations and with many different conditions. In general, small feedings at slow rates are recommended initially for all high-risk infants. The initiation of enteral nutrition may be delayed in infants with a history of possible asphyxia or compromised intestinal perfusion. Enteral feeding is begun once the infant's clinical condition is stable and the schedule is tailored to the individual patient. The complex coordinated mechanism of sucking and swallowing is not present in preterm infants until approximately 32 to 34 weeks postconceptional age. Therefore, nasogastric feedings are recommended prior to this age. An enteral caloric goal of 120 calories per kg per day is desired. Proprietary formulas are available for preterm infants that provide an increased amount of protein, vitamins, and minerals and have a high caloric concentration (24 kcal per ounce). Further advantages of preterm proprietary formulas include a ratio of whey to casein of 60:40 and an osmolarity of less than 300 mOsm per liter; medium chain triglycerides are 40 to 50% of the fat composition, and the carbohydrates used take into account the limited lactase present in preterm infants.

SPECIAL PROBLEMS

Neurologic

Hypoxic-Ischemic Encephalopathy

Hypoxic-ischemic encephalopathy may result in a spectrum of manifestations from severe to mild. The effects of hypoxia and ischemia are difficult to separate clinically, and both contribute to the resulting injury. The degree of asphyxia necessary to cause permanent neurologic damage is only slightly less than would be lethal. Asphyxia this severe generally results in impairment of many organ systems, especially neurologic, renal, metabolic, cardiovascular, and pulmonary. Severely affected infants may present in the initial hours of life with stupor or coma, have irregular respirations, and lack complex reflexes such as the Moro and sucking reflexes. Seizures may develop, generally between 6 and 24 hours after the insult has occurred. With time, the infant may worsen and develop brain stem dysfunction. Ultrasonography of the brain may reveal edema or hemorrhages. A computed tomography (CT) scan is more useful in determining the extent of neurologic injury after approximately 2 to 4 weeks. An electroencephalogram (EEG) may be used in conjunction with clinical evaluation to help indicate the severity of the damage. Poor prognosis may be present if the EEG demonstrates a burst suppression pattern. However, medications such as phenobarbital may also depress the EEG. In general, asphyxia should be suspected and the infant observed closely if the Apgar score at 5 minutes or later is less than 3; a metabolic or mixed acidosis (pH < 7.00) is determined on an umbilical cord arterial blood sample; neurologic sequelae are evident, including hypotonia, stupor, coma, or seizures, particularly in the first 24 to 48 hours; prolonged resuscitation is required; or multiorgan system impairment is noted.

Management may be broken down into three periods of time: prenatal, delivery room, and postnatal. Prenatal management is performed by the obstetrician and includes close monitoring for fetal distress or placental compromise and optimizing the management of any maternal condition that would add to a hypoxic-ischemic insult. Delivery room management involves effective resuscitation and treatment of any conditions such as meconium aspiration or shock that would worsen the hypoxia or ischemia. A high Apgar score (> 6 at 5 minutes) generally indicates no significant peripartum asphyxia. A low Apgar score (< 3 at 5 minutes) may result from asphyxia, but other factors such as maternal anesthesia and neuromuscular disorders could also result in low Apgar scores. Note that Apgar scores alone do not indicate the presence of asphyxia. In postnatal management, it is critical that attention be paid to restoring adequate perfusion and oxygenation. This may include providing oxygen or assisted ventilation, in addition to restoring blood volume with packed red blood cells, 5% albumin, Plasmanate, or fresh-frozen plasma.

Seizures

The incidence of neonatal seizures cannot be accurately delineated, since many of the subtle manifestations of a seizure go undetected in newborns. The clinical presentation of a tonic-clonic seizure pattern is rare in neonates. More commonly, buccal and oral movements (lip smacking, chewing), apnea, gaze abnormalities, and tonic posturing of a limb are present, indicating subtle seizures. Other patterns include focal clonic seizures, multifocal clonic seizures, myoclonic seizures, and tonic seizures. The etiology of the seizure should be actively sought and any underlying condition identified. Neonatal encephalopathy, cerebral contusion, and intracranial hemorrhage account for up to 40% of all neonatal seizures. Metabolic problems, infections, developmental brain anomalies, focal infarcts, and drug withdrawal are included in the differential diagnosis of neonatal seizures. An EEG may be a helpful adjunct in the clinical determination of seizures, but a normal EEG at one time does not mean that seizures have not occurred or that they will not reappear in the future. Treatment is directed at correcting any underlying condition, providing supportive care, and, if indicated, initiating anticonvulsant therapy. We recommend phenobarbital (Luminal) at a loading dose of 20 mg per kg as the anticonvulsant of choice. Phenytoin (Dilantin), diazepam (Valium), and lorazepam (Ativan) may also be of benefit in certain situations. The overall prognosis in neonatal seizures is primarily dependent on the etiology of the seizure. In general, the more premature the infant, the more abnormal the background EEG (such as burst suppression pattern), and the more serious the disorder that provokes the seizure, the poorer the prognosis.

Subependymal Hemorrhage–Intraventricular Hemorrhage

Subependymal hemorrhage–intraventricular hemorrhage (SEH–IVH) involves bleeding from the subependymal germinal matrix with or without rupture into the ventricle. The incidence of SEH–IVH in infants younger than 34 weeks' gestation is approximately 20 to 30% and is inversely related to gestational age. Most hemorrhages occur in the first few days of life, and by 5 days after delivery, more than 90% of the hemorrhages and any progression of the lesions have occurred. The clinical presentation depends on the severity, site, and rapidity of the hemorrhage. The signs and symptoms are nonspecific, and in up to 50% of cases, the hemorrhages are asymptomatic. Real-time gray-scale portable sector ultrasonography is the most reliable and accurate method to evaluate infants for the presence of SEH–IVH. Management is directed at prevention of the hemorrhage by avoiding rapid intravenous administration of osmotically active agents such as sodium bicarbonate, minimizing manipulations of the infant, and attempting to maintain physiologic homeostasis. Once an SEH–IVH has occurred, the treatment is primarily supportive and is aimed at avoiding extension of the hemorrhage. Complications of SEH–IVH include hyperbilirubinemia, seizures, and posthemorrhagic hydrocephalus. The prognosis is dependent on many variables, and in general, the more extensive the hemorrhage, the more likely there will be motor or cognitive impairment. When parenchymal damage is present, some form of motor impairment is common.

Cardiac

Cardiac Disease

Congenital heart disease occurs in about 8 in every 1000 live births. Approximately 60% of babies with congenital heart disease present in the first month of life, and two-thirds of these in the first week. In patients with significant mixing of oxygenated and deoxygenated blood in the heart, some degree of cyanosis may be apparent even in the delivery room.

The most common congenital heart disease is a ventricular septal defect (VSD). VSDs are usually asymptomatic in the first week of life, although a murmur may be heard. As the pulmonary vascular resistance drops over the first 2 months of life, increased pulmonary blood flow develops, and right-sided heart failure with respiratory symptoms may develop. Small VSDs often close spontaneously, so an expectant management strategy—with medical treatment using diuretics and digoxin, if needed—is used when possible. Atrial septal defects are almost always asymptomatic in the newborn period and can be followed clinically. In either case, surgical intervention should be employed if necessary to avoid the development of pulmonary hypertension in childhood.

Cyanotic congenital heart disease is usually apparent in the newborn period. The most common cyanotic lesions are transposition of the great vessels and tetralogy of Fallot (VSD, pulmonary stenosis or atresia, right ventricular hypertrophy, and the aorta "overriding" the VSD). Less common cyanotic lesions include endocardial cushion defects, total anomalous pulmonary venous return (to the right side of the heart), tricuspid atresia, and truncus arteriosus. In addition, hypoplastic left heart syndrome, with severe underdevelopment of the left atrium, ventricle, and ascending aorta, may also present with cyanosis. Congenital heart defects in which either the pulmonary or the systemic circulation is dependent on flow of blood through the ductus arteriosus are often referred to as ductal-dependent lesions. In addition to structural heart lesions, severe coarctation of the aorta is ductal dependent. The ductus arteriosus does not close immediately after delivery but starts to constrict during the first few days of life. If there is a strong suspicion of ductal-dependent heart disease, we begin a continuous intravenous infusion of prostaglandin E_1 (alprostadil [Prostin VR Pediatric]) 0.05

to 0.1 μg per kg per minute to maintain the patency of the ductus arteriosus.

Crucial to the appropriate treatment of congenital heart disease, and to its differentiation from other conditions, is a definitive determination of the cardiac anatomy and physiology. A careful physical examination, measurement of four-extremity blood pressures, and chest radiographs are part of the initial evaluation. In addition, real-time ultrasound scanning to visualize the intracardiac structures and pulsed Doppler technology to ascertain the direction of flow and to estimate pressures have provided a dramatic advancement in neonatal diagnostic cardiology. Invasive cardiac catheterization is now reserved for more complex anomalies, some preoperative studies, and situations in which a therapeutic procedure may be needed emergently, such as a balloon atrial septostomy to allow adequate mixing of pulmonary and systemic circulations in transposition of the great vessels.

Palliative or definitive repair is possible for most defects. For others, such as hypoplastic left heart syndrome, cardiac transplantation is often used. For some patients with multiple, complex lesions, no therapy may be beneficial, and death may occur in the neonatal period.

Complete congenital heart block is a total failure of atrial impulses to be conducted to the ventricles and is due to either a structural interruption in or a degeneration of the cardiac conduction tissue. It occurs in about 1 in 15,000 pregnancies. Heart rates are usually 50 to 80, and the condition is amenable to prenatal diagnosis; if not diagnosed, it may lead to emergent delivery for bradycardia. Congestive failure may develop either in utero (possibly leading to hydrops fetalis) or after birth, especially with lower (<60) heart rates. Many of these infants are born to mothers with connective tissue diseases or serologic markers for these diseases without symptoms. However, approximately 40% of these patients have structural heart disease. If this diagnosis is established and the neonate is in no distress, only careful observation is needed. Acute symptomatic bradycardia can be treated with chronotropic agents such as isoproterenol (Isuprel) and/or with epicardial pacing if needed. Prognosis depends on the underlying heart disease but is generally good.

Patent Ductus Arteriosus

A patent ductus arteriosus (PDA) is physiologically appropriate in utero and usually closes in term infants shortly after birth. However, a PDA becomes hemodynamically significant in approximately 20% of preterm infants weighing less than 1750 grams. The clinical signs of a PDA may include a systolic ejection murmur, increased pulse pressure greater than 25 mmHg, a hyperdynamic precordium, cardiomegaly, and/or a worsening respiratory status. Not every infant with a PDA manifests all these findings, making the diagnosis difficult at times. A two-dimensional echocardiogram confirms the diagnosis. Treatment is generally pharmacologic with intravenous indomethacin (Indocin) at varying doses, depending on the age of the infant. Surgical treatment may be necessary if medical treatment is unsuccessful in closing the PDA. Supportive care and close monitoring should be provided.

Hypotension

Hypotension is a common problem in the special care nursery. Supportive measures should be initiated while the underlying etiology is investigated. The initial therapy is intravascular volume expansion with 10 mL per kg of 5% albumin, Plasmanate solution, or normal saline. If, after intravenous infusion of 20 to 30 mL per kg of volume expanders, the blood pressure remains low, inotropic therapy should be considered. We recommend beginning with dopamine (Intropin) 2 to 10 μg per kg per minute and adding dobutamine (Dobutrex) 5 to 20 μg per kg per minute if necessary.

Respiratory

Respiratory Distress Syndrome

Respiratory distress syndrome (RDS), also known as hyaline membrane disease (HMD), is a pulmonary process characterized by an inadequate amount or function of pulmonary surfactant. Without surfactant, the lungs are stiff and noncompliant; atelectasis, unequal gas distribution, increased work of breathing, and hypoxia develop, leading to respiratory failure. The incidence of RDS is inversely correlated with gestational age; it is uncommon after 34 weeks of gestation, and it is seen in the majority of patients born at 30 weeks or less. RDS affects about 40,000 babies annually in the United States, and over 2000 die from it.

Modern obstetric care can lessen the occurrence of RDS through aggressive management and tocolysis of preterm labor and through the administration of glucocorticoids, such as betamethasone (Celestone Soluspan), to the mother more than 24 hours before delivery to enhance fetal lung maturity. Analysis of amniotic fluid for markers of lung maturity, such as a lecithin/sphingomyelin ratio of greater than 2.0 and the presence of phosphatidyl glycerol, can help in determining the optimal time of delivery for a preterm baby.

Treatment of RDS is directed at maintaining adequate oxygenation and ventilation, using the least amount of support needed. Overaggressive support may predispose to acute complications such as air leaks (e.g., pneumothorax, pulmonary interstitial emphysema) and chronic lung disease (bronchopulmonary dysplasia). In mild cases, provision of oxygen by hood may be sufficient. Use of continuous positive airway pressure (CPAP) through nasal prongs helps prevent atelectasis while allowing the patient to do all of his or her own breathing. If support of ventilation is needed to avoid significant acidosis or the oxygen requirement is high, endotracheal intubation and institution of mechanical ventilation are indi-

cated. Once the patient is intubated, if the oxygen requirement is 30% or greater, we treat with replacement surfactant (Survanta or Exosurf).

Surfactant replacement therapy has dramatically impacted the care of VLBW babies and is credited with a significant fall in infant mortality. Surfactant is given through the endotracheal tube directly into the trachea. For patients with a high risk of having RDS, many physicians employ surfactant prophylactically, giving it soon after intubation, often in the delivery room. This approach may be especially useful in patients weighing less than 1000 grams. Alternatively, treatment with surfactant only after RDS is diagnosed avoids unnecessary administration of the drug and allows for more careful monitoring during treatment. If this approach is used, we recommend prompt treatment once significant RDS is diagnosed. Surfactant treatment may be repeated as frequently as every 6 hours for up to as many as four doses, depending on the product. For especially severe disease or in the presence of air leaks, high-frequency ventilation, particularly oscillatory ventilation, employing tiny tidal volumes and rates of 600 to 900 cycles per minute may be beneficial.

Persistent Pulmonary Hypertension and Meconium Aspiration

As noted in the section on physiology, only about 7% of cardiac output passes through the pulmonary circulation. Large amounts of blood are shunted from the right atrium to the left atrium at the foramen ovale, and from the pulmonary artery to the aorta through the ductus arteriosus. Elevated pulmonary vascular resistance, caused by constriction of vascular smooth muscle in small pulmonary arterioles and by the fluid-filled, atelectatic state of the in utero lung, leads to this small amount of pulmonary blood flow. If the normal transition in circulation and expansion of the lungs fails, pulmonary resistance and pressure may remain high, leading to persistent pulmonary hypertension of the newborn (PPHN), formerly known as persistent fetal circulation (PFC). PPHN may occur in term or near-term babies with sepsis, meconium aspiration, RDS, and pulmonary hypoplasia.

In PPHN, blood continues to be shunted away from the lung at both the foramen ovale and ductus arteriosus, resulting in hypoxia and hypercarbia, which then worsen the PPHN. Pulmonary vascular resistance decreases with lung inflation, increased oxygen levels, and alkalosis. Treatment of PPHN is directed at maintaining an adequate systemic blood pressure, a normal or above-normal arterial P_{O_2}, and a normal or above-normal pH. Controversy exists about aggressive hyperventilation versus "gentle" ventilation. We suggest mild hyperventilation, adequate lung expansion as evidenced on x-rays and by examination, and use of vasopressors to maintain blood pressure.

Other methods that may be useful for severe disease include inhaled nitric oxide, an experimental drug that is given as a gas and causes pulmonary vasodilatation but is inactivated before any systemic effect, and extracorporeal membrane oxygenation (ECMO), in which a patient is connected to a cardiopulmonary bypass machine that includes a membrane oxygenator, which can support gas exchange only (veno-venous ECMO) or, more commonly, can support both pulmonary and cardiac function (venoarterial ECMO).

Meconium is present in the amniotic fluid in 10% of all pregnancies and in 30 to 40% of post-term babies at delivery. Meconium consists of sloughed intestinal epithelial cells, secretions of the gastrointestinal tract, and swallowed debris present in the amniotic fluid. It is unclear whether meconium-stained amniotic fluid always indicates asphyxia; however, in the presence of other signs of fetal compromise, meconium is a marker for fetal distress. With distress, deep gasping respirations occur in utero, and meconium in amniotic fluid may be carried far down the fetal bronchial tree. If not well suctioned, babies with meconium-stained fluid have a high chance of developing meconium aspiration syndrome (MAS), characterized by a chemical pneumonitis, airway occlusion and air trapping from the tenacious thick meconium, and PPHN. MAS may be fatal and often requires aggressive neonatal care, including treatment with ECMO.

All infants with meconium should have careful and complete suctioning (by the delivering clinician) of the oro- and nasopharynx using a No. 10 French or larger catheter to remove any meconium present *immediately*, preferably after delivery of the baby's head and before delivery of the shoulders. Personnel trained in neonatal resuscitation should be present at the time of delivery, and the newborn should be moved to an infant warmer for further care without delay.

When thick meconium is present, if the baby is depressed or there has been inadequate obstetric suctioning, the neonate should be intubated by someone trained in neonatal resuscitation, ideally before the first breath, to clear the airway of meconium. Since 9% of babies who have no meconium visible in the pharynx after obstetric suctioning may have meconium present below the vocal cords, visualization of the cords without intubation is insufficient. If meconium is obtained from below the vocal cords, intubation and suctioning should be repeated until no further meconium is obtained. Usually, after 2 to 5 minutes of intubation and suctioning, one should consider standard resuscitative measures. We use clinical judgment and the presence of bradycardia to help guide the timing of initiation of manual ventilation.

For a vigorous, pink, nondistressed baby with thin or terminal meconium, the risk of depression and trauma from intubation may be greater than any potential benefit.

Congenital Diaphragmatic Hernia

Congenital diaphragmatic hernia (CDH) is caused by failure of the Bochdalek foramen to close at 8 to 10 weeks' gestation, leading to the presence of bowel and sometimes other intra-abdominal organs in the thoracic cavity. This results in pulmonary hypoplasia and compression of the lungs that worsens with bag-and-mask ventilation. CDH is seen in 1 in 2500 to 4000 live births. Approximately 90% of CDHs occur on the left side, and about two-thirds of affected infants are male. A scaphoid abdomen, shift in heart sounds to the right, unequal breath sounds, and respiratory distress should arouse suspicion of this defect, but there may be no findings other than respiratory distress. If CDH is suspected, we recommend immediate intubation and manual ventilation as well as placement of a gastric sump to keep the bowel decompressed. The patient should be stabilized prior to operative repair. PPHN is expected in these patients and many require treatment with ECMO. Infants with CDH have a 30 to 50% mortality, due mostly to pulmonary failure.

Gastrointestinal

Hyperbilirubinemia

Virtually all newborns develop serum bilirubin concentrations in excess of normal adult values of 1.5 mg per dL, and most manifest at least mild jaundice. A current challenge for practitioners is to know when to evaluate, when to treat, and when to follow clinically and avoid unnecessary intervention.

Bilirubin is produced as a metabolite from the breakdown of heme-containing proteins. Newborns are predisposed to hyperbilirubinemia because they have increased bilirubin production due to shortened fetal red blood cell (RBC) life span (70 to 80 days versus 120 days for an adult RBC), increased hematocrit, frequent bruising due to the delivery process, and a higher rate of ineffective hematopoiesis, resulting in bilirubin production from RBC precursors. Also, hepatic metabolism of bilirubin is decreased in neonates, including uptake into the hepatocyte, conjugation, and export into the biliary system. Finally, there is an increased enterohepatic circulation of bilirubin in newborns due to decreased breakdown by intestinal bacteria, increased beta-glucuronidase activity in the intestinal mucosa, and slow feeding initially.

Hyperbilirubinemia is a concern because very high levels of unconjugated (or indirect) bilirubin, in the presence of hemolytic diseases, have been associated with severe bilirubin encephalopathy, also called kernicterus. Kernicterus literally describes a yellow staining of the basal ganglia. Accompanying clinical features may include seizures, feeding intolerance, changes in alertness, apnea, and death. Sequelae include hearing loss, choreoathetoid cerebral palsy, and sometimes mental retardation. Administration of anti-Rh antibodies (RhoGAM) to Rh-negative mothers has dramatically diminished Rh hemolytic disease. Hemolytic disease due to ABO incompatibility is usually less severe. Documented kernicterus in the absence of hemolytic disease is extraordinarily rare and occurs only at extremely high bilirubin levels.

We recommend a cautious clinical approach to jaundice, consistent with recommendations from the American Academy of Pediatrics. The blood type of every mother should be ascertained. If the mother is Rh-negative, the baby should be given careful attention. In healthy term babies, jaundice (indicating a bilirubin >5 mg per dL) noted within the first 24 hours of life is usually abnormal and may indicate hemolytic disease. The evaluation should include at least a total bilirubin level and a determination of the baby's blood type, and possibly measurement of hematocrit and hemoglobin.

After 24 hours, most normal newborns exhibit jaundice; levels tend to have a cephalocaudal distribution, so that jaundice of only the face may indicate low bilirubin levels, but jaundice of the feet indicates higher levels. Since the goal of treatment is to prevent disease (kernicterus), treatment decisions need to be based on the clinical situation rather than strictly on the bilirubin level. Phototherapy, which acts by a photoisomerization of bilirubin, resulting in exposure of polar groups and increased water solubility, is the first therapy employed. However, the importance of maintaining good enteral feeding (breast milk if the mother is nursing, formula otherwise) must not be overlooked. If it appears that the bilirubin level is nearing a danger zone for developing kernicterus despite phototherapy, then a double-volume exchange transfusion with fresh whole blood or hematocrit-specific (50%) blood from components (packed red cells and fresh-frozen plasma) should be carried out. Briefly, this involves replacement of the infant's blood with donor blood that is compatible with both the infant's and the mother's blood. This is carried out using one or two central umbilical catheters and is done slowly over 1 to 2 hours, with small amounts being removed, and replaced with an equal volume of donor blood, so as to maintain hemodynamic stability.

Premature infants and babies with hemolytic disease are at much higher risk for kernicterus. Therefore, treatment in both these groups is indicated at lower bilirubin levels than in patients with no underlying pathology. Breast-feeding infants, if feeding adequately during the first few days, probably have bilirubin levels similar to those of formula-fed babies. However, hospital practices such as separation of mothers and babies, adherence to rigid schedules, and forced supplementation, particularly with glucose water, can all interfere with the establishment of normal feeding and thus worsen jaundice. After the first few days, breast-feeding babies do have higher bilirubin levels than formula-fed babies. Only if bilirubin levels become markedly elevated in an otherwise well baby should interruption of breast-feeding be considered, and then only temporarily.

Abdominal Wall Defects

Abdominal wall defects result in intra-abdominal organs being present outside of the abdomen. An omphalocele is a congenital defect in the formation of the umbilical and supraumbilical portions of the abdominal wall due to failure of the defect in the abdominal wall to close by week 10 of gestation. Usually, the examination shows an intestine-filled sac with a large base and the umbilical cord implanting on the sac. The incidence of omphalocele is 1 in 6000 to 10,000 live births. Up to two-thirds of these patients have associated anomalies, including trisomies (30%), cardiac lesions (20%), other gastrointestinal anomalies, and other midline defects such as bladder exstrophy. The prognosis depends on the associated anomalies. Survival is 70% or greater without associated anomalies, but mortality with serious cardiac disease approaches 80%.

Gastroschisis is the herniation of abdominal contents through an abdominal wall defect, usually just to the right of the umbilicus. Although the abdominal defect may be fairly small, there may be a large amount of abdominal contents present outside of the peritoneal cavity, with the potential for vascular occlusion. There is no sac covering the organs, and they are often matted together with fibrinous, exudative tissue. Approximately 50% of these patients are born prematurely, and 15 to 20% have intestinal atresias. Gastroschisis occurs in about 1 in 20,000 live births. This condition has a 10 to 30% mortality, and establishment of enteral feedings is usually a slow process.

For either lesion, the patient should immediately be placed on a radiant warmer and the defect gently wrapped in warm saline–soaked sterile gauze, with attention to preserving organ perfusion. Gastric suction with a properly placed sump catheter to keep the bowels decompressed should also be initiated. We recommend that the entire lower half of the baby be placed in a sterile "bowel bag" to minimize heat and water loss from the lesion and to protect the exposed abdominal organs. Emergent pediatric surgical repair consists of returning the protruding organs to the peritoneal cavity and closure of the defect. If a large volume of organs is present and the abdominal cavity is small, a staged repair is done, wherein a "silo" of synthetic material (Dacron or other) is created to hold the intestines. The organs are then gradually reduced into the abdominal cavity, with definitive closure occurring as a second procedure at about 1 week of life.

Acute Renal Failure

Acute renal failure is used to describe a severe, rapid decrease in glomerular filtration rate. Acute renal failure may be subdivided into prerenal failure, or renal failure due to insufficient systemic and/or renal circulation; intrinsic renal failure, or renal failure due to parenchymal damage to the kidneys; and obstructive renal failure, or renal failure due to mechanical obstruction in the urinary collecting system.

The diagnosis of the etiology and type of acute renal failure is of great importance. With prompt diagnosis, prerenal failure may be reversible if fluids and diuretics are given early. Early diagnosis of obstruction of the urinary tract may aid in correcting the problem and lead to an improved outcome. Finally, early recognition of acute renal failure helps avoid excess intravascular fluids and the accumulation of electrolytes and medications.

Evaluation includes a careful history consisting of family history of renal malformations, presence of oligohydramnios in the pregnancy, prenatal ultrasonography revealing abnormalities of the urinary tract or kidney, and history of severe perinatal asphyxia. The physical examination includes evaluation of the external genitalia and palpation of the abdomen to assess for abdominal masses, kidney and bladder size, and abdominal wall musculature. Laboratory evaluation includes daily serum creatinine assessment of infants who are at risk for acute renal failure. If oliguria (defined as urine output less than 1 mL per kg per hour over 8 to 12 hours) is present, placement of a catheter in the bladder helps rule out lower urinary tract obstruction and can determine if urine is being made. If urine is present, this allows for more careful assessment of urinary output and allows collection of urine for analysis.

If there is no evidence of congestive heart failure, a fluid challenge of an isotonic solution such as 0.9% saline at approximately 10 to 20 mL per kg may be given over 1 to 2 hours. If the oliguria continues, furosemide (Lasix) 2 mg per kg should be given intravenously. If urine output remains less than 1 mL per kg per hour, intrinsic renal failure should be suspected and intravenous fluids restricted (approximately 60 mL per kg per day in a 1-day-old term infant). Ultrasound evaluation of the kidney and renal tract is helpful. When obstruction of the urinary tract is suspected, a voiding cystourethrogram is also recommended.

Specific concerns in infants with acute renal failure include fluid overload, hyponatremia, hypertension, hyperkalemia, hyperphosphatemia, hypocalcemia, and metabolic acidosis. Management of intrinsic renal failure is primarily supportive care until the kidney recovers and renal function improves.

Hematologic

Polycythemia

Polycythemia in neonates is defined by a venous hematocrit greater than 65% and has an incidence of approximately 1 to 5%. The diagnosis should be suspected with a screening capillary hematocrit of greater than 69%. Capillary hematocrits may be 5 to 15% higher than venous hematocrits owing to decreased skin perfusion. Neonatal polycythemia may result from placental red cell transfusions such as with twin-to-twin transfusion, maternal-fetal transfusion, delayed cord clamping, or cord stripping. Another etiology is increased fetal erythropoiesis resulting from intrauterine hypoxia that may be related to placental insufficiency. Others who are predisposed to polycythemia include infants of diabetic mothers and infants with Beckwith-Wiedemann syndrome; trisomy 21, 13, or 18; or congenital hypothyroidism. The problems associated with polycythemia are related to the increase in whole blood viscosity.

Clinical findings of hyperviscosity include feeding problems, lethargy, jitteriness, tachypnea, plethora, and, rarely, seizures. However, many polycythemic infants are asymptomatic. Polycythemia is very uncommon in preterm infants.

Symptomatic polycythemia is treated with a partial exchange transfusion to reduce the red cell mass by replacing whole blood with either a plasma substitute (5% albumin, Plasmanate) or an isotonic crystalloid (normal saline) of equal volume. The amount of blood to be exchanged can be calculated using a target hematocrit (Hct) of 55% and an infant blood volume (BV) of 80 mL per kg:

Volume of exchange (mL) =

$$\frac{\text{BV (80 mL per kg)} \times \text{wt (kg)} \times (\text{observed Hct} - \text{desired Hct})}{\text{Observed Hct}}$$

The isovolemic exchange is usually performed utilizing 10- to 20-mL aliquots of blood drawn from umbilical or peripheral arterial or venous catheters.

The long-term outcome is dependent on the individual situation, taking into account the severity of clinical symptoms, any underlying condition, and the potential complications of the partial exchange transfusion, if performed. The neurologic prognosis for asymptomatic polycythemic infants, treated or untreated, is controversial. Some experts do not recommend a partial exchange transfusion in asymptomatic infants unless the hematocrit exceeds 70%. Others perform the exchange at 65%. Any polycythemic infant should undergo a partial exchange transfusion if symptoms of hyperviscosity are present.

Anemia

The evaluation of anemia must consider the normal developmental changes in the red cell mass that occur in the first few months of life. The hemoglobin nadir in a term infant is approximately 6 to 12 weeks of life, whereas a preterm infant's nadir is a few weeks earlier. In general, neonatal anemia at term is defined as a venous hemoglobin of less than 13 mg per dL or a hematocrit of less than 39%. The causes and laboratory manifestations of anemia in the first week of life are listed in Table 2. The diagnostic approach to neonatal anemia must include a thorough family and obstetric history, a careful physical examination, and selected laboratory studies. The laboratory evaluation may include a Coombs' test, which, if positive, is supportive of an immune hemolytic anemia. If a fetal-maternal hemorrhage is suspected, a Kleihauer-Betke preparation of the mother's blood should be performed. Other specific tests may be helpful, depending on the clinical history and presentation.

The decision to transfuse RBCs, the method of transfusion (10 to 15 mL per kg or a partial exchange transfusion), and the type of blood product to be used (packed RBCs, whole blood, or irradiated RBCs) all depend on the infant's clinical condition and physiologic needs.

TABLE 2. **Etiologies and Laboratory Findings of Neonatal Anemia**

Symptom	Cause	Hematocrit	Reticulocyte Count	Bilirubin
Blood loss	Fetal-maternal or twin-twin transfusions; obstetric accidents (abruptio placentae or placenta previa)	Normal or decreased	Increased or normal	Normal
Hemolysis	Immune hemolytic anemia; infection; red blood cell membrane disorders; red blood cell enzyme deficiencies	Decreased	Increased	Increased
Decreased red blood cell production	Infection (cytomegalovirus); congenital leukemia	Decreased	Decreased	Normal

Infectious Disease

The overall incidence of bacterial sepsis is approximately 0.1 to 1% in live births. Multiple risk factors for perinatal infections have been identified. Maternal risk factors include premature onset of labor, prolonged rupture of membranes (>24 hours), maternal sepsis, chorioamnionitis, and cervical or vaginal bacterial colonization. The most important neonatal risk factor is prematurity. Other neonatal risk factors include instrumentation, low Apgar score (<5 at 1 minute), twin pregnancy, and underlying disease processes or anomalies.

A newborn infant's granulocyte function (chemotaxis, phagocytosis, and bactericidal activity) is deficient compared with that of an adult. The neonate also has relatively low concentrations of specific antibody, complement, and opsonins. The more immature the infant, the less the amount of transplacental IgG acquired. IgA and IgM are not transplacentally transported, and fetal synthesis does not begin until around the thirtieth week of gestation. Thus, specific and nonspecific defense mechanisms are underdeveloped in neonates, predisposing them to infections by a wide variety of pathogens.

An infection in a newborn can present with subtle, nonspecific clinical findings. These may include respiratory distress, hypotension, hypoglycemia, temperature instability, metabolic acidosis, decreased activity, poor feeding, mottling or pallor, apnea, and jaundice. Laboratory evaluation generally includes a complete blood count. A leukocyte count of less than 5000, a total neutrophil count of less than 1500, and an immature (band) to total neutrophil ratio of greater than 0.2 have been associated with an increased risk of bacterial infection.

Cultures are crucial in determining the diagnosis and course of treatment of bacterial infections. Before antibiotic therapy is instituted, blood cultures should be obtained by sterile technique from a peripheral site or from a fresh, sterilely placed catheter. If a nosocomial infection is suspected, two blood cultures obtained from separate sites within 6 hours of each other are recommended. Urine cultures are generally not necessary in the first 24 hours of life unless there is evidence of urinary tract anomaly. A suprapubic aspiration or sterile catheterization is the method of choice in obtaining a urine specimen. Cerebrospinal fluid cultures are also necessary but may not be obtainable if significant cardiovascular or respiratory instability is present. A chest x-ray is essential in evaluating an infant with respiratory distress. The x-ray helps limit the differential diagnosis but is never diagnostic for infection. Localized infiltrates are unusual in congenital pneumonia, and the x-ray pattern is typically indistinguishable from that of RDS. If the neonate has abdominal symptoms, an evaluation should be done for signs of obstruction, perforation, or necrotizing enterocolitis (pneumatosis intestinalis).

Clinical judgment must always be used in conjunction with a careful history and physical examination to determine the extent of the laboratory and radiographic evaluation. In all patients with known risk factors, close observation is necessary, and medical management may need to be modified, depending on the infant's clinical course.

Infections in neonates are caused by a large variety of organisms and are acquired in several ways. In utero infections may occasionally result from transplacental passage of organisms such as viral infections, tuberculosis, and syphilis. More commonly, the fetal environment becomes contaminated by an ascending infection that occurs after the membranes have ruptured. Infants may also acquire an infectious organism when passing through the birth canal. Other infants may become infected after losing their skin integrity, as with punctures and instrumentation, or through the mucous membranes.

This wide spectrum of virulent organisms commonly includes those listed in Table 3. Other pathogens frequently identified include herpes simplex virus, *Chlamydia trachomatis, Neisseria gonorrhoeae,* and syphilis. Nosocomial infections frequently include those in Table 3 as well as possible *Candida* species, anaerobic organisms, and many other bacteria too numerous to list.

The initial antibiotic therapy depends on an assessment of which organisms are most likely to be involved. In general, the antibiotics should include coverage for gram-positive and gram-negative organisms. Therefore, we recommend initiating a combination of ampicillin (Omnipen) and an aminoglycoside such as gentamicin (Garamycin). If renal function is in question (e.g., with severe asphyxia or renal anomalies), ampicillin and cefotaxime (Claforan) are recommended. Nosocomial infections frequently in-

TABLE 3. **Selected Intrauterine and Perinatally Acquired Bacterial Infections in the Neonate**

Organism	Microbiology	Clinical Manifestations	Suggested Treatment*
Group B beta-hemolytic streptococci	Gram-positive cocci in pairs	Pneumonia, sepsis, meningitis	Penicillin G
Escherichia coli	Gram-negative bacilli	Sepsis, meningitis, urinary tract infection	Ampicillin and aminoglycoside
Listeria monocytogenes	Gram-positive bacilli	Intrauterine—abortion Perinatal—sepsis, meningitis	Ampicillin
Nosocomial Infections			
Staphylococcus epidermidis	Gram-positive cocci in clusters	Sepsis, meningitis	Vancomycin
Staphylococcus aureus	Gram-positive cocci in clusters	Skin infection, sepsis	Penicillinase-resistant penicillin
Pseudomonas aeruginosa	Gram-negative bacilli	Pneumonia, sepsis, urinary tract infection	Ticarcillin or mezlocillin and aminoglycoside

*Sensitivities to antibiotics must be assessed to ensure proper treatment owing to the possible presence of resistant organisms.

volve resistant organisms; therefore, a combination of a penicillinase-resistant penicillin and an aminoglycoside or vancomycin (Vancocin) and cefotaxime may be indicated. Clindamycin (Cleocin) may be added if anaerobic organisms are probable, such as with bowel perforation and/or peritonitis. If a fungal or herpesvirus infection is strongly suspected, amphotericin B (Fungizone) or acyclovir (Zovirax), respectively, should be initiated.

Once a specific organism is isolated from a culture, the therapy should be adjusted to the antimicrobial sensitivities identified. The postconceptional age and postnatal age must be considered when determining the dose of antibiotic and the interval of administration. Selected antibiotic doses and administration intervals for term infants are recommended in Table 4. The duration of therapy is dependent on the diagnostic findings, the organism involved, and the infant's clinical response. The duration is best measured from the time repeat cultures become negative. We recommend 7 to 10 days for sepsis and pneumonia with no evidence of focal infection, 14 days for meningitis caused by group B streptococci or *Listeria monocytogenes*, and a minimum of 21 days for meningitis caused by gram-negative bacilli. If the cultures are negative or unreliable owing to previous antibiotic therapy in the mother or infant but the infant is strongly suspected of having an infection and improves with therapy, antibiotics should be continued for approximately 7 days. In our nursery, if reliable cultures are negative for longer than 72 hours and the infant is healthy and doing well, antibiotics are discontinued.

SPECIAL CONSIDERATIONS

Surgical Emergencies

Surgical problems constitute a significant portion of special care nursery admissions, and many need to be recognized and managed expeditiously in order to optimize the outcome. Pediatric surgery consultation is strongly recommended if any infant has a condition that may require major surgery.

Several key management principles should be considered when addressing a potential neonatal surgical problem. If a bowel obstruction or diaphragmatic hernia is suspected, gastric suction with a properly placed sump catheter is indicated. Shock, electrolyte imbalances, and dehydration should always be corrected or steps taken to help prevent these problems from developing. Antibiotics may be indicated, as in the case when bowel integrity is in question. A warm, sterile saline cover should be applied to any exposed viscera, with careful attention to preserving organ perfusion. Emergent invasive procedures may be necessary to stabilize the infant, such as thoracentesis or chest tube insertion in the case of a pneumothorax or chylothorax. In general, the evaluation and management of neonates with surgical problems should be conducted in close consultation with a pediatric surgeon.

Infants of Diabetic Mothers

Infants of diabetic mothers are a select population that shares special concerns. Good prenatal care with

TABLE 4. **Selected Antibiotic Doses and Administration Intervals for Term Infants***

Antibiotic (Route)	Dosage (mg/kg)	Postnatal Age (Days)	Interval (Hours)
Ampicillin (IV, IM)	100	0–7	12
		>7	8
Gentamicin† (IV, IM)	2.5	0–7	12
		>7	8
Cefotaxime (Claforan) (IV, IM)	50	0–7	12
		>7	8
Oxacillin (Prostaphlin) (IV, IM)	25	0–7	12
		>7	8
Vancomycin† (IV)	15	All	8

*Term infants are those 37 to 44 weeks postconceptional age. Preterm infants or infants with renal or hepatic dysfunction need dosage and administration interval adjustments.

†The dose and administration interval may need adjustment based on serum drug concentrations.

Adapted from Young TE, Mangum OB: NeoFax™ '94: A Manual of Drugs Used in Neonatal Care, 7th ed. Columbus, OH: Ross Products Division, Abbott Laboratories, USA, 1994, pp 8, 10, 26, 37, 44.

close attention to glucose control is important for the well-being of the fetus. Communication between obstetric and pediatric personnel is critical in preparing for the infant's delivery and arranging appropriate nursery care. Hypoglycemia is commonly present in infants of diabetic mothers as a result of the hyperinsulinemia that has occurred in response to the mother's hyperglycemia. The infant's serum glucose should be followed closely in the first few hours of life. Management of hypoglycemia is the same as that outlined earlier.

Specific problems frequently observed in infants of diabetic mothers include hypocalcemia, RDS, polycythemia, poor feeding, hyperbilirubinemia, macrosomia, transient cardiac ventricular septal hypertrophy, sepsis, and an increased incidence of congenital abnormalities, especially involving the central nervous system and heart.

Infants Exposed to Maternal Substance Abuse

Substance abuse continues to be a problem and affects many pregnant women. Physicians caring for newborn infants should inquire whether the mother has any history of substance abuse. If narcotic abuse is present, naloxone (Narcan) is contraindicated, since it may precipitate a severe withdrawal reaction. Fetal alcohol syndrome may be difficult to diagnose but should be considered if the mother has consumed significant amounts of alcohol during her pregnancy.

Fortunately, most newborn infants exposed to alcohol, nicotine, cocaine, or other drugs in utero are asymptomatic and do not require specialized nursery care. They do, however, require a supportive, educated nursery staff and social service system to help provide optimal care for the infant and family.

Multiple Births

In the United States, it is estimated that 12 per 1000 naturally occurring pregnancies result in a twin delivery. A higher incidence of multiple births is present in mothers who received treatment for infertility or had in vitro fertilization. Monozygotic or identical twinning accounts for one-third of twin pregnancies; dizygotic or fraternal twinning accounts for the other two-thirds. Early detection of pregnancy with twins is important because of increased maternal and fetal complications. Perinatal mortality in twin births is 4 to 11 times greater than that in single births. This increased mortality is primarily due to the increased frequency of premature delivery, with an average twin delivery occurring at approximately 37 weeks' gestation. Placental vascular interconnections, twin transfusion syndrome, and more frequent congenital anomalies also contribute to the increased morbidity and mortality of twins. Management for multiple gestational delivery begins with appropriate preparation for each infant. Separate resuscitation teams should be available if problems are anticipated. The infants should be carefully examined for congenital anomalies, growth retardation, and prematurity. Blood pressure and hematocrit should be measured to determine if twin transfusion syndrome is present. Support for the family, including possible home assistance and financial assistance, should also be discussed prior to discharge.

Neonatal Death and Parental Bereavement

Good communication is critical to the development of trust and understanding between parents and health care providers. Patient care conferences offer an opportunity for the primary care team (attending physician, primary nurse, and social worker) to share information with the parents and for the parents to ask questions. Each family has individual needs and may cope with stress and difficult news differently.

Death is an unfortunate event that is encountered in every special care nursery. Anticipation of the death may help prepare the family and enable support services to be available. Adequate time and a private place for the family to hold the infant should be provided, if possible. The child's dignity should always be preserved and the process of bereavement discussed with the family. At the time of death, any technical aspects of the infant's death can be explained in a clear, simple manner. An autopsy may be recommended, and its importance and limitations are also explained. Information about community resources and bereavement support services may be offered. Finally, a follow-up appointment with the family in approximately 2 months affords the opportunity to discuss any unresolved questions or feelings, review the results of the autopsy, and explore the psychological effects of grieving on the family.

The news of the infant's death should also be communicated to the referring obstetrician, pediatrician, and/or family physician.

Extreme Prematurity and the Limit of Viability

The question "What is the limit of viability?" has ethical and social as well as medical dimensions and remains difficult to answer. Should eventual quality of life and potential disability be factored into the decision? What input should parents have in the decision? Clearly, the limit of viability has changed over time; survival of extremely premature babies has increased dramatically in the last decade. Current experience suggests that at 25 weeks, aggressive resuscitation is indicated; these babies have 70 to 80% total survival, the majority without severe abnormalities on cranial ultrasound. At 24 weeks, survival is about 50%. However, about half of these infants have significant cranial ultrasound abnormalities. At 23 weeks, survival is 10 to 20%, with most survivors having significant cranial ultrasound abnormalities. At 22 weeks, resuscitation seems inappropriate, as there are virtually no survivors.

Changes in technology and legal requirements in some areas may influence the approach to this group of patients.

We believe that it is crucial to explain one's approach to the family and to clearly state that the baby is too immature to survive if resuscitation is not carried out. One must be ready at delivery to quickly assess the maturity of the infant, particularly if the dates are unsure. Resuscitation is then begun if the patient is more mature than expected; only warmth, comfort, and a chance for the mother to hold the baby are provided if the infant is clearly previable. If significant uncertainty about viability exists, we advocate beginning resuscitation and intensive care, but it should be stated overtly to the family that if it becomes clear that survival is very unlikely, intensive care should be withdrawn.

OUTCOME AND FOLLOW-UP

Critically ill term infants and all VLBW (≤1500 grams) infants are at increased risk for long-term medical and developmental morbidity, compared with healthy term infants. However, the vast majority of them will be normal. Specific factors that may increase the chances of abnormal outcome include severe intracranial hemorrhage (Grades 3 and 4), periventricular leukomalacia, prolonged mechanical ventilation and bronchopulmonary dysplasia, and intrauterine growth retardation. The more premature the infant, especially at less than 28 weeks, the greater the rate of disability. The baby's home environment, measured by such variables as socioeconomic status and highest level of maternal education, exerts a strong effect on outcome. Up to 25% of VLBW babies may have some degree of impairment, such as cerebral palsy or mental retardation. Hearing or visual impairment and seizures are less common. A later hidden morbidity may be seen in the school-age years, with possible increases in learning and behavioral problems. VLBW babies are more likely to develop chronic medical problems (usually respiratory) and to require hospitalization during the first few years of life.

Sick newborns are at higher risk for developmental problems, making careful follow-up essential. We believe that these babies need a primary care provider (a "medical home") who can coordinate care needs and handle routine well baby care. In addition, higher-risk babies benefit from participation in a neonatal follow-up clinic. Such a clinic is usually multidisciplinary, with participation by speech, physical, and occupational therapists; neonatology and developmental pediatricians; nurses; and social workers. Developmental assessment, usually every 4 to 6 months, allows early identification of problems and referral to early intervention programs and institution of specific therapies. If outcome appears normal after 2 years of age, the parents can usually be reassured that development most likely will continue to progress normally. If abnormalities are detected, the family can be so informed in a sensitive manner by people who have had an ongoing relationship with the patient and family. Action can then be taken to help each child develop and function to the best of his or her ability.

NORMAL INFANT FEEDING

method of
WILLIAM J. KLISH, M.D.
Baylor College of Medicine
Houston, Texas

BREAST–FEEDING

Breast-feeding remains the optimal choice of infant feeding by all major societies and agencies, including the American Academy of Pediatrics and the World Health Organization. These groups base their recommendations on the strong scientific evidence of decreased infant mortality in developing countries and decreased morbidity in developed countries seen in exclusively breast-fed infants compared with those fed human milk substitutes. No commercially processed infant formula has been developed that reproduces the immunologic properties, nutrient bioavailability, digestibility, and trophic effects of human milk.

Breast-feeding also offers psychological and behavioral benefits to both mother and infant. The postpartum status of the mother is improved by hormones released during breast-feeding. Infant sucking induces the release of oxytocin, thereby accelerating the involution of the uterus. Exclusive breast-feeding resulting in frequent nipple stimulation can suppress ovulation. However, in developed countries, where more "structured" feeding schedules are practiced, suppression may not be sustaining and therefore not used as a form of birth control. Animal studies have demonstrated an increased threshold for maternal stress, presumably due to the hormones released during breast-feeding.

The Physician's Role in Infant Feeding Decision-Making

Prenatal visits should include discussion on infant feeding issues. This provides the parents an opportunity to make an informed choice by gaining information. Allowing for an open discussion of the facts about infant feeding helps diffuse guilt that results from lack of knowledge or of support of breast-feeding from a physician. Studies have demonstrated that prenatal education and breast-feeding support from family, especially the infant's father, and friends are associated with a mother's choice of breast-feeding regardless of maternal age, ethnic group, educational level, or marital status. Prenatally, mothers are intensely focused on the birth experience, therefore breast-feeding instruction and information will need to be reviewed following delivery. The office or clinic environment can send a strong message to parents about the priorities of the clinician. An office complete with formula advertisements in the form of posters, pads, and pencils gives a subtle message that may undermine any verbal "lip service" to breast-feeding.

A thorough history should be obtained and a breast examination performed during the prenatal period. Histories of breast surgery and breast-feeding experiences should be obtained. Previous breast surgery is not a contraindication to breast-feeding; however, the type of surgery (augmentation vs. reduction) and surgical technique utilized (periareolar vs. submammary) might affect lactation performance and must be considered during progression of lactation.

An assessment of nipple type will allow for early intervention when appropriate. Flat and inverted nipples are not always of concern since the infant latches onto the areola and not the nipple. Breast care beyond normal daily hygiene is not necessary. Practices such as "toughening of the nipples" are not recommended and can occasionally damage breast tissue.

Initiation of Breast-Feeding

Breast-feeding is enhanced by early initiation. It is ideal to place the infant at the breast immediately following birth. Test feedings of water are not necessary to assess suck and swallow. Subsequent feedings are usually sporadic, depending on the use of maternal medication during labor and delivery, but they should not be more than 3 to 4 hours apart. Frequent feedings provide the necessary hormonal stimulation needed for establishment of an adequate maternal milk volume. To allow for adequate milk transfer to the infant, proper positioning and latch-on at the breast are important. This is facilitated with "hands-on" instruction provided by knowledgeable nursing or medical staff. Breast-feeding books and videos are helpful but should not be used as a replacement for supportive assistance. Hospital policies that support rooming-in options and avoid water and glucose feedings for the infant after breast-feeding send a clear affirmative message to breast-feeding mothers. Controlled studies have demonstrated clearly that infants who are given water, glucose water, or formula instead of human milk in the first week of breast-feeding lose more weight, regain it more slowly, and have higher bilirubin levels and fewer stools.

Early feedings should not be timed to some predetermined duration. Each infant is individual in feeding behavior and, especially in the first few days, may be too sleepy to nurse for long durations. Feeding durations may range from 3 to 20 minutes at each breast. Improper positioning and latch-on at the breast rather than length of feeding is associated with the degree of nipple soreness. Both breasts are usually offered at each feed; however, some infants may fall asleep before taking the second breast. An understanding that the fat content in the milk increases as the breast is emptied further validates the importance of not limiting feeding duration. This change in milk fat content also explains why an infant can get an adequate volume and caloric intake by nursing one breast at a feed.

Frequent feedings that allow time for complete breast emptying are associated with adequate maternal lactogenic hormone levels and increased milk volume. Most infants will drive their mothers milk volume by waking for 10 to 12 feeds in a 24-hour period. Some infants may sleep for one extended duration of 4 hours in a 24-hour period and as a result cluster those ten or so feedings in a tighter period. Given these variations in infant behavior and the move to shorter hospital stays, instruction regarding breast-feeding should be kept simple and as uncomplicated as possible. Discharge information should be simple and emphasize what to expect in terms of breast changes with the increase in milk flow, the frequency and duration of feedings, and signs of adequate milk intake, including stooling and urination patterns.

Early Breast-Feeding Management and Follow-Up

With the change to shorter hospital stays following delivery, breast-feeding mothers are discharged with little instruction prior to the transition from colostrum to transitional and subsequent mature milk. Most mothers will experience increased breast fullness during the first few days following delivery. However, a distinction should be made between breast fullness and engorgement. Breast fullness is a normal transitory state during which the breast tissue remains compressible, allowing the infant to suck efficiently and comfortably. Engorgement is caused by improper positioning as well as delay or restriction of feeding frequency and duration. It presents as generalized, swollen, rigid tissue resulting in a taut, shiny appearance to the breast. Given this tightness, the infant finds it difficult to grasp the breast, causing increased milk stasis and maternal discomfort. Prompt intervention is needed to promote milk flow and reduce swelling. An electric *intermittent* minimum pressure breast pump along with warm compresses may be needed to facilitate milk flow. Providing the primiparous mother with information on these breast changes, emphasizing the importance of frequent feedings, will significantly reduce the chances of severe engorgement.

Another result of early hospital discharge is loss of the physician's opportunity to observe the establishment of successful breast-feeding. To compensate for this, a mechanism for early postpartum follow-up is essential to assure breast-feeding success. A visit to the office on the third day postpartum will allow the physician to assess the infant's positioning at the breast, passing of meconium stool, urination patterns, and maternal breast changes. On postpartum day 6, a follow-up phone call is helpful to document feeding frequency and duration, to check urine and stool frequency, and to offer support and information.

This should be followed by a clinic (or home) visit at 2 weeks to check the infant's weight gain. Follow-up allows monitoring of the mother's and infant's progress and early intervention when necessary. Exclusively breast-fed infants receiving adequate milk intake usually follow the pattern described in Table 1.

Inadequate infant weight gain may be due to infant or maternal factors. An assessment of the breast-feeding mother-infant dyad is necessary to make a thorough assessment. Treating only one member of this dyad is not sufficient if breast-feeding is to be preserved. The most common cause of inadequate milk supply is improper instruction to the mother. Maternal stress and fatigue can result in a faulty milk ejection (let-down) reflex. When supplemental feeding is necessary, the mother should continue breast stimulation via mechanical breast pumping to maintain milk volume. If milk volume is maintained, exclusive breast-feeding can again resume once the infant's weight gain improves.

When mothers complain of sore nipples, the first step is to observe the infant latching to the breast. Infants should latch on the soft tissue of the areola, not at the base of the nipple. Mothers with flat or inverted nipples may not experience a problem breast-feeding since the infant sucks the areola and not the nipple. If the physician is not experienced in observing breast-feeding, an *experienced* individual should be consulted.

Breast-Feeding and Maternal Employment

Many women return to work outside the home following delivery. Continuation of breast-feeding is possible during work but requires some planning and support. Mothers have reported that maintenance of lactation is easier if return to work is delayed for a few months postpartum. When that is not possible, a gradual return to full-time employment may facilitate the development of feeding and pumping schedules. The mother will need to express her milk during the work day in order to maintain hormonal levels and milk volume. A variety of electrical and battery-operated breast pumps are available for purchase or rent. Expressed breast milk should be refrigerated and fed to the infant within 48 hours. Glass or hard plastic is ideal for milk storage. When using soft plastic bags, it is best to use two layers of bags to prevent leakage during storage. Mothers should be informed that it is normal to see a decrease in ex-pressed milk volume during a 5-day work week. Breast-feeding exclusively on the weekend will restore the lowered volume.

Many companies have seen a decrease in employee absenteeism caused by infant illness when mothers can continue breast-feeding. Some companies provide facilities to allow privacy while pumping. Enabling a mother to continue this breast-feeding relationship following her return to work makes the transition from full-time mother to working mother less stressful.

Pros and Cons in Breast-Feeding

Maternal Fever

Maternal fever *is not* a contraindication to breast-feeding. The maternal ability to manufacture secretory IgA specific to the infection her infant is exposed to and excrete it in her milk provides her infant with a unique and potent protection from infection. Cessation of breast-feeding during this time will prevent this elegant protective cycle from occurring.

Some Maternal Medications

Breast-feeding is contraindicated during maternal use of drugs of abuse (e.g., heroin, cocaine). Few other drugs are contraindicated during breast-feeding. Up-to-date references are important to keep current with recommendations. The Physicians' Desk Reference is a poor resource for information on excretion of drugs in breast milk.

Breast Cancer

A mother with breast cancer should not nurse her infant, to allow her to receive immediate definitive treatment. Prolactin levels remain very high during lactation, and prolactin may advance some mammary cancers.

HIV-Positive Mother

The Centers for Disease Control and Prevention and the U.S. Public Health Service recommend that women who test positive for human immunodeficiency virus (HIV) should be counseled to avoid breast-feeding.

FORMULA–FEEDING

Since not all mothers are able or willing to breast-feed their infants, substitute methods of infant feeding have always been available. The history of modern infant formulas began in 1849 when Baron Justus von Leibig recognized that all living tissue, including food, was composed of different proportions of carbohydrate, fat and protein. This resulted in the first commercially available human milk substitute, Baron von Leibig's Soluble Food, which was available in the United States by 1869. The composition of infant formulas has evolved greatly during the past century as our understanding of nutrient requirements, absorptive physiology, and metabolic distur-

---

TABLE 1. **Signs of Adequate Milk Intake in the Exclusively Breast-Fed Infant**

Nurses approximately 8–10 times/24 h; may cluster the feeds
Has the least 6 (paper) to 8 (cloth) wet (pale yellow urine) diapers/24 h
Transition from meconium (tarry) to milk stool (yellow, seedy) by day 7 postpartum; may have as many as 5–10 stools/day during the first month, less often after 4 weeks
Initial weight loss not exceeding 10% of birthweight
Regains birthweight by the second week of life, with an average weight gain of 30 gm/day thereafter

bances has advanced. A large array of routine and special-purpose infant formulas is currently available. To select the proper formulas for particular circumstances, it is necessary to understand the significance of the various nutrients composing them.

Energy Content of Infant Formulas

Infant formulas contain energy in the form of carbohydrate and fat, as well as protein, minerals, vitamins, and water in amounts sufficient to meet all the nutritional requirements of a healthy, growing infant. The energy content of a routine infant formula is 20 kcal per ounce. This caloric density was chosen because human milk contains an average of 20 kcal per ounce, although there are significant variations in the energy content of human milk depending on the stage of lactation. Formulas for premature infants usually contain 24 kcal per ounce because premature infants frequently have difficulty ingesting an adequate volume of formula. Occasionally, formula for premature infants is mixed to provide 27 to 30 kcal per ounce.

Carbohydrates in Infant Formulas

Lactose

Lactose is the most common sugar in infant formula. Since lactose is the disaccharide found in almost all mammalian milks, including human milk, it is the logical choice for the carbohydrate for routine infant feeding. Human milk contains approximately 7 grams of lactose per dL (7%). Most infant formulas also contain 7% lactose.

Lactose is hydrolyzed on the brush border of the intestine by lactase, a disaccharidase enzyme, releasing the monosaccharides glucose and galactose, which are then absorbed. The enzyme lactase is present in a relatively small amount compared with the other disaccharidases. For every unit of lactase activity present on the intestinal brush border, there are 2 units of sucrase activity and approximately 6 to 8 units of maltase activity. It is for this reason that lactose intolerance can occur after acute gastroenteritis. Nonspecific injury to the intestinal mucosa will affect lactase activity more significantly than the other, more plentiful, disaccharidases.

Because lactose is absorbed less efficiently than other sugars such as sucrose or starch, some is allowed to enter the distal bowel. There it is fermented by intestinal bacteria, resulting in a slightly lower pH in the intestinal lumen. This change in the intestinal milieu appears to favor the growth of acidophilic bacteria, such as lactobacillus, at the expense of less favorable, pathogenic bacteria. The lower pH also appears to enhance the absorption of calcium and phosphorus from the distal small intestine.

Premature infants are born with less lactase than full-term infants have. Infants born at 30 to 34 weeks' gestation have intestinal lactase levels approximately 50% of the level in a full-term infant.

Lactose is still an important component of the diet of the premature infant because of the aforementioned benefits. However, because of this limited lactose tolerance, formulas for premature infants contain lactose combined with other carbohydrates to decrease the lactose load.

Even though lactose intolerance is a well-recognized complication of acute gastroenteritis, it does not occur as often as one might expect. In a study of infants admitted to the hospital with acute diarrhea, only 13% developed significant clinical symptoms of lactose intolerance and required a change in formula. Almost all the infants who developed lactose intolerance recovered their ability to absorb lactose within 30 days. Most infants, therefore, do not have to be lactose-restricted simply because they develop acute gastroenteritis. Infants who do develop secondary lactose intolerance and are switched to a lactose-free formula should be rechallenged with lactose within a month to determine recovery.

Sucrose

Sucrose-based formulas are indicated for the feeding of infants with lactose intolerance. These formulas should be used only when indicated, because sucrose has a less favorable influence on intestinal pH in the normal infant. Occasionally, infants are born with sucrase-isomaltase deficiency and cannot tolerate sucrose. These infants, however, should be able to tolerate lactose-containing formulas. Infants with significant generalized small bowel disease may malabsorb sucrose. For these infants, formulas are available with starches, such as modified corn syrup solids or glucose polymers, as the carbohydrate source.

Modified Starch and Emulsifiers

Under normal circumstances, starch is digested in the intestinal lumen by alpha-amylase secreted by the pancreas and salivary glands. This results in a mixture of maltose, isomaltose, and alpha-limit dextrans, which are low-molecular-weight starches (3 to 5 glucose units). These products are then further hydrolyzed to glucose by maltase enzymes present on the intestinal brush border. The glucose formed is either absorbed directly or spilled back into the lumen of the intestine for distal absorption. An alternate pathway for the digestion of starch is through hydrolysis by glucomylase, which is a brush border enzyme. Pancreatic amylase secretion is low in the neonate, so starch is digested largely by intestinal glucoamylase. Very few clinical situations have been documented, however, in which starch is not tolerated by the normal newborn infant.

Most infant formulas contain starch in one form or another. It may be present as an emulsifier, such as tapioca or corn starch, or added to a formula for calories. Several products are available commercially for use as a calorie additive to formulas that are derived from the hydrolysis of cornstarch.

An advantage of adding modified or partially hydrolyzed starch or glucose polymers to formulas as a source of calories is that they have little effect on osmolality because of their relatively large molecular weights. They are readily absorbed because they can be hydrolyzed by maltase, the most abundant disaccharidase. They are colorless, impart little sweetness, and have low viscosity, so they can be added in significant amounts without changing the physical characteristics of a formula. Care must be taken whenever additives are put in formulas that they do not dilute the other ingredients and result in nutrient imbalances. For example, a standard 20 cal per ounce formula normally contains about 10% of its calories as protein. If this formula is fortified to 30 cal per ounce by adding carbohydrate, the protein content drops to about 6.5% of the calories, which represents a marginal protein intake in a normal child.

Fat

Long Chain Triglycerides

Fat provides the major source of energy for growing infants. In human milk, about 50% of the energy is from fat, and in commercial formulas fat provides 40% to 50% of the energy. Most routine infant formulas contain vegetable oil as the source of fat. Cow milk contains less essential fatty acid (linoleic acid) than does human milk. This initially led manufacturers of infant formulas to add vegetable oil to the skimmed cow milk base of their preparations. These oils continue to be used not only because of their essential fatty acid content but also because they are better absorbed from the infant gut than is butter fat.

Fatty acids essential for humans are the derivatives of 18:2 6 (ω 6) fatty acid, or linoleic acid. This acid cannot be made in mammalian tissue. Linoleic acid and its derivative 20:4 6 arachidonic acid are components of cell membranes, but more importantly they serve as precursors for prostaglandins. Essential fatty acid should provide at least 3% of the total caloric intake of an individual. Human milk contains about 7% of the calories as linoleic acid, depending on the maternal diet. Unmodified cow milk has only about 1%. Most commercial infant formulas contain more than 10%.

Fat is the most difficult component of food to digest and absorb because of its hydrophobic nature. A normal adult can absorb only about 95% of ingested fat. Infants are less efficient and sometimes absorb as little as 85% of the ingested fat. A very sophisticated system for the absorption of long chain triglycerides exists. Ingested triglycerides are emulsified by bile salts. The small emulsion particles, or micelles, provide a large surface area for the action of pancreatic and human milk lipase. Lipase removes the two outer fatty acids from the glycerol backbone of the triglyceride, leaving the easily absorbed monoglyceride and the fatty acids. These pass into the mucosal cells of the small intestine where they are reassembled into triglycerides, coated with a protein, and extruded as chylomicrons into the lymphatics of the small bowel. The longer the chain length of the fatty acid, the slower the absorption. The introduction of double bonds into a fatty acid enhances absorption.

Medium Chain Triglycerides

Medium chain triglycerides are absorbed more efficiently than are long chain triglycerides in normal infants. The addition of medium chain triglycerides to formula for premature infants enhances not only the absorption of fat but also the absorption of calcium and magnesium.

Most of the uniqueness associated with medium chain triglycerides is due to one physical property. Medium chain fatty acids are partially soluble in water. At 20° C, 69 mg of octanoic acid (C_8) will dissolve in 100 ml of H_2O, compared with 0.7 mg of palmitic acid (C_{16}). Pancreatic lipase hydrolyzes medium chain triglycerides more effectively than long chain triglycerides, resulting in more efficient digestion when lipase is decreased in the intestinal lumen. Once octanoic acid is released, it is so hydrophilic that it will enhance the solubility of other triglycerides. Because of this property, medium chain triglycerides can bypass the need for emulsification by bile acids. About half the absorbed medium chain triglycerides is transported directly into the portal venous system rather than the lymphatics. Medical indications for the use of medium chain triglycerides are pancreatic insufficiency, hepatic insufficiency, and those diseases that affect the lymphatics of the intestinal tract, such as lymphangiectasia and perhaps severe congestive heart failure.

Medium chain triglycerides do have side effects, however. If they are malabsorbed, either because of overfeeding or intestinal mucosal disease, they enhance secretion in the distal small bowel, resulting in diarrhea. Some studies have implied that feeding medium chain triglycerides alters the postprandial metabolic rate, resulting in an increase in the caloric requirements for an individual. The advantage of the increased absorption of this fat could be offset by this increase in calorie requirements.

Casein

Casein is a group of milk-specific proteins characterized by their low solubility at an acidic pH, resulting in curd formation, and by their ability to form complex micelles with calcium and phosphorus salts. There are four electrophoretic groups of casein, which are represented in cow milk in the following proportion: alpha (50 to 55%), beta (30 to 35%), kappa (15%), and gamma (5%). Genetic and species variations are present in each group. Human casein is more heterogeneous than cow casein, and beta-casein is predominant. Differences exist in the amino acid composition between human and bovine casein even within the electrophoretic groups, accounting for slight differences in the biologic value and antigenicity of these proteins.

Whey

Whey represents the protein that remains in solution after casein has been precipitated by acid. It is a mixture of proteins that has important biologic functions. The predominant whey protein in human milk is alpha-lactalbumin, which is involved in lactose synthesis. Lactoferrin is the second most abundant whey protein in human milk and is thought to play a role in iron absorption as well as in local host defense. Lysozyme, another whey protein, has antibacterial properties; because it is resistant to digestive enzymes, it can pass intact through the infant's intestinal tract. Immunoglobulins composed principally of secretory immunoglobulin A are present and impart local intestinal immunity to the infant fed human milk. Beta-lactoglobulin is the predominant protein found in whey of bovine milk. Its function is unknown.

Whey-predominant formulas tend to mimic human milk more closely, making these formulas more popular, particularly for the feeding of the premature infant. These have the advantage of being rapidly emptied from the stomach because of little curd formation. They appear to have virtually eliminated lactobezoars, which were occasionally seen in preterm infants in the past. They may help minimize gastroesophageal reflux because they are emptied more rapidly from the stomach.

Soy Proteins

Because they are lactose-free, soy-based protein formulas are primarily indicated for use in infants with lactose intolerance. They also can be fed to infants of strict vegetarians if the parents refuse to use products based on cow milk. Most soy formulas, however, are used for infants who are suspected of having cow milk protein intolerance. Infants known to be sensitive to cow milk protein should have soy protein introduced cautiously, because these infants may also be intolerant to soy.

A potential problem that could arise from the prolonged feeding of soy formula is bone demineralization. Phytic acid is a contaminant in the processing of soy protein and can form a complex with certain minerals like calcium and zinc. This results in the decreased absorption of these minerals. The absence of lactose in soy formula is an additional factor that can interfere with calcium absorption. Most soy protein–based formulas have additional calcium added to offset any calcium malabsorption.

Hydrolyzed Protein

Hydrolyzed cow milk protein formulas are designed for use in infants who are intolerant of intact cow milk protein. They are also helpful in infants who have a limited ability to absorb nutrients because of either a short gut or intestinal mucosal disease. The protein is hydrolyzed enzymatically and broken down to free amino acids and small peptides. However, some products contain larger-molecular-weight peptides that are capable of antigenic expression. In infants with known protein hypersensitivity, it is important to select a product that contains little antigenic potential.

Formulas based on hydrolyzed protein do have several disadvantages. They tend to taste bad because of the presence of sulfated amino acids, which tend to impart a sulfur-like flavor. The more complete the hydrolysis, the worse the flavor. The osmolality of formulas prepared with hydrolyzed protein tends to be high, and they may cause osmotic diarrhea if used improperly. They are also expensive.

Infant Formula Classification

Commercially available infant formulas fall into several categories. Examples of each category are listed in Tables 2 through 5.

Formulas for premature infants differ from regular infant formulas in that they contain more calories and greater amounts of all nutrients, including minerals such as sodium, potassium, calcium, and phosphorus. Most formulas for premature infants are whey predominant, the fat is a blend of medium chain and long chain triglycerides, and the formula contains a low concentration of lactose. These formulas are recommended for feeding low-birthweight newborns until they achieve a body weight of approximately 1.8 kg. The composition of these formulas differs markedly from that of human milk. When the very-low-birthweight infant is fed human milk exclusively, the infant's needs for growth may not be met, and certain nutrient deficiencies may develop. However, since human milk may provide immunologic protection, the use of a human milk fortifier will supplement the nutrients deficient in human milk.

INTRODUCTION TO SOLID FOODS

Solid foods can be introduced to infants at 4 to 6 months of age, depending upon development as well as social, cultural, and economic considerations. The feeding of solids prior to 4 months of age offers no nutritional or developmental benefits and may result in excessive weight gain. Up until about 4 months of age the feeding of solids by spoon is difficult because of the presence of the extrusion reflex. When food is placed on the anterior half of the tongue, this protective reflex causes the tongue to move forward, pushing food from the mouth. Mothers attempt to cope with this reflex by scraping the food from the chin and pushing it back in. There is no need to feed with a spoon until this reflex spontaneously disappears at 4 to 5 months of age. At 6 months of age, an infant's iron stores may be diminished, so the introduction of solids to supplement this nutrient is desirable.

When solid foods are introduced, single-ingredient foods should be selected and introduced one at a time at no less than 3-day intervals to permit the identification of food intolerances if present. Infant cereal is the optimal first supplemental food since it contains not only additional energy but is fortified with iron. Cereal should be fed by spoon and not

TABLE 2. **Formulas Designed for the Normal Newborn Infant; Standard Milk-Based Formulas**

Formula	Gm/dL			Mg/dL			Source		Osmolality (mOsm/kg of H₂O) and General Comments
	Pro	Fat	CHO	$\frac{Na}{K}$	$\frac{Ca}{P}$	Fe	CHO	Fat	
Similac (Ross) (20 kcal/ 30 mL)	1.45	3.6	7.2	$\frac{18}{71}$	$\frac{49}{38}$	0.15	Lactose	Coconut oil, soy oil	(300) Whey:casein ratio is 18:82
					(w/iron, 1.2)				
Similac (24 kcal/30 mL)	2.2	4.3	8.5	$\frac{28}{107}$	$\frac{73}{57}$	0.18	Lactose	Coconut oil, soy oil	(380) Whey:casein ratio is 18:82; available for hospital use only
					(w/iron, 1.5)				
Similac Concentrate, mixed to 24 kcal/oz	2.6	4.3	8.6	$\frac{22}{84}$	$\frac{58}{45}$	1.4	Lactose	Coconut oil, soy oil	Prepared from standard Similac concentrate. Patient requires formula instruction prior to discharge
Similac (27 kcal/30 mL)	2.5	4.8	9.5	$\frac{31}{121}$	$\frac{82}{64}$	0.2	Lactose	Coconut oil, soy oil	(410) Whey:casein ratio is 18:82
Enfamil (Mead Johnson) (20 kcal/30 mL)	1.5	3.8	6.9	$\frac{18}{72}$	$\frac{52}{35}$	0.1	Lactose	Palm olein; soy oil, coconut oil, sunflower oil	(300) Whey:casein ratio is 60:40
					(w/iron, 1.3)				
SMA (Wyeth) (20 kcal/30 mL)	1.5	3.6	7.2	$\frac{15}{56}$	$\frac{42}{28}$	1.2	Lactose	Coconut oil, safflower oil, oleo, soy oil	(300) Milk-based formula with a low renal solute load; whey:casein ratio is 60:40
Gerber	1.5	3.6	7.1	$\frac{22}{72}$	$\frac{50}{39}$	0.3	Lactose	Palm oil, soy oil, coconut oil, sunflower oil	(320) Whey:casein ratio is 18:82
					(w/iron, 1.2)				
Good Start	1.6	3.4	7.3	$\frac{16}{65}$	$\frac{43}{24}$	1.0	Lactose, malto-dextrins	Palm oil, oleic, safflower oil, corn oil	(260) Hydrolyzed whey protein formula

Abbreviations: Pro = protein; CHO = carbohydrate; Na = sodium; Ca = calcium; Fe = iron; K = potassium; P = phosphorus.

TABLE 3. **Formulas Designed for the Infant with Simple Formula Intolerance; Soy-Based Formulas**

Formula	Gm/dL			Mg/dL			Source		Osmolality (mOsm/kg of H₂O) and General Comments
	Pro	Fat	CHO	$\frac{Na}{K}$	$\frac{Ca}{P}$	Fe	CHO	Fat	
Isomil (Ross) (20 kcal/ 30 mL)	1.8	3.7	6.8	$\frac{30}{73}$	$\frac{71}{51}$	1.2	Corn syrup solids, sucrose	Soy oil, coconut oil	(240) Soy protein isolate formula; lactose-free formula
Isomil SF (Ross) (20 kcal/30 mL)	1.8	3.7	6.8	$\frac{30}{73}$	$\frac{71}{51}$	1.2	Hydrolyzed cornstarch	Soy oil, coconut oil	(180) Soy protein isolate formula; lactose- and sucrose-free
Prosobee (Mead Johnson) (20 kcal/ 30 mL)	2.0	3.5	6.7	$\frac{24}{81}$	$\frac{63}{49}$	1.3	Corn syrup solids	Palm olein, coconut oil, soy oil, sunflower oil	(200) Soy protein isolate formula; lactose- and sucrose-free
Nursoy (Wyeth) (20 kcal/30 mL)	1.8	3.6	6.9	$\frac{20}{70}$	$\frac{60}{42}$	1.2	Sucrose	Oleo, coconut oil, safflower oil, soy oil	(244) Soy protein isolate formula; lactose-free; no corn syrup solids
I-Soyalac (Loma Linda) (20 kcal/30 mL)	2.1	3.7	6.7	$\frac{28}{78}$	$\frac{68}{47}$	1.3	Sucrose, tapioca starch	Soy oil	(206) Soy protein isolate formula; corn-free; lactose-free; Fe-fortified
Soyalac (Loma Linda) (20 kcal/30 mL)	2.1	3.7	6.7	$\frac{29}{78}$	$\frac{63}{37}$	1.3	Corn syrup solids, soy, sucrose	Soy oil	(273) Soy protein isolate formula; lactose-free; Fe-fortified

Abbreviations: Pro = protein; CHO = carbohydrate; Na = sodium; Ca = calcium; Fe = iron; K = potassium; P = phosphorus.

TABLE 4. **Special Formulas for Infants with Complex Absorptive Disorders**

| Formula | Gm/dL | | | Mg/dL | | | Source | | Osmolality (mOsm/kg of H_2O) and General Comments |
	Pro	Fat	CHO	$\dfrac{Na}{K}$	$\dfrac{Ca}{P}$	Fe	CHO	Fat	
Alimentum (Ross) (20 kcal/30 mL)	1.9	3.8	6.8	$\dfrac{29}{79}$	$\dfrac{70}{50}$	1.2	Sucrose, modified tapioca starch	MCT oil, safflower oil, soy oil	(370) For malabsorption problems; protein is casein hydrolysate with added amino acids; 50% fat from MCT oil
Nutramigen (Mead Johnson) (20 kcal/30 mL)	1.9	2.6	8.9	$\dfrac{31}{73}$	$\dfrac{63}{42}$	1.3	Corn syrup solids, modified corn starch	Corn oil, soy oil	(320) For malabsorption problems; protein is casein hydrolysate with added amino acids
Pregestimil (Mead Johnson) (20 kcal/30 mL)	1.9	3.7	6.9	$\dfrac{26}{73}$	$\dfrac{62}{42}$	1.3	Corn syrup solids, modified corn starch, dextrose	MCT oil, corn oil, soy oil, safflower oil	(300) For malabsorption problems; protein is casein hydrolysate with added amino acids; 55% fat from MCT oil
Pregestimil (24 kcal/30 mL)	2.3	4.4	8.3	$\dfrac{31}{88}$	$\dfrac{74}{50}$	1.6	Same as Pregestimil 20	Same as Pregestimil 20	(360) For malabsorption problems; patient needs formula instruction prior to discharge
Portagen (Mead Johnson) (20 kcal/30 mL)	2.3	3.2	7.7	$\dfrac{37}{83}$	$\dfrac{63}{47}$	1.3	Corn syrup solids, sucrose	MCT oil, corn oil	(220) Medium chain triglyceride formula for lactose intolerance; protein is sodium caseinate; 87% MCT oil
Lofenalac (Mead Johnson) (20 kcal/30 mL)	2.2	2.6	8.7	$\dfrac{31}{68}$	$\dfrac{63}{47}$	1.3	Corn syrup solids, modified tapioca starch	Corn oil	(360) Low phenylalanine formula used in treatment of phenylketonuria; protein is specially processed casein hydrolysate reduced in phenylalanine with other added amino acids
Phenyl-Free (Mead Johnson) (25 kcal/30 mL)	3.3	1.1	10.7	$\dfrac{66}{223}$	$\dfrac{83}{83}$	1.9	Sucrose, corn syrup solids, modified tapioca starch	Corn oil, coconut oil	(790) Protein provided as amino acids without phenylalanine
Lacto-Free (Mead Johnson) (20 kcal/30 mL)	1.5	3.7	6.9	$\dfrac{20}{73}$	$\dfrac{55}{37}$	1.1	Corn syrup	Palm oil, soy oil, coconut oil, sunflower oil	(200) For lactose intolerance, lactose-free, milk protein isolate; whey:casein ratio is 20:80
Similac PM 60/40 (Ross) (20 kcal/30 mL)	1.5	3.8	6.9	$\dfrac{16}{58}$	$\dfrac{38}{19}$	0.15	Lactose	Soy oil, coconut oil	(280) Low renal solute load; minerals comparable to human milk. Lactalbumin:casein and calcium:phosphorus ratios comparable to those of human milk; low iron formula
S-29 (Wyeth) (20 kcal/30 mL)	1.7	2.2	9.8	$\dfrac{1.0}{32}$	$\dfrac{16}{19}$	1.3	Lactose	Oleo, coconut oil, safflower oil, soybean oil	(360) Very low renal solute load; whey protein
Calcilo XD (Ross) (20 kcal/30 mL)	1.6	4.1	7.5	$\dfrac{16}{60}$	$\dfrac{7}{18}$	1.3	Lactose	Corn oil, coconut oil	(277) Whey protein; low calcium formula

Abbreviations: Pro = protein; CHO = carbohydrate; Na = sodium; Ca = calcium; Fe = iron; K = potassium; P = phosphorus.

added to the nursing bottle except for medically indicated reasons such as gastroesophageal reflux.

The order in which solid foods have traditionally been introduced has been cereal, fruit, yellow vegetables, green vegetables, meats and desserts. There is no physiologic reason for this order of introduction. After cereals, the food introduced can be at the discretion of the mother.

Commercially prepared strained foods or those prepared at home are both acceptable. If infant foods are prepared at home, precaution should be taken to avoid highly seasoned food or food salted to adult taste. The salt content of commercially prepared American baby food is low. Honey should not be fed to infants younger than 12 months of age, because of its association with infant botulism.

The amount of water needed by infants to replace their losses and provide for growth is available in both human milk and infant formula during the nursing period. Healthy infants require little or no supplemental water except in hot weather. When solid foods are introduced, additional water is required because the renal solute load is high in solid foods from their higher protein and salt content. Infants should be offered water to allow an opportunity to fulfill fluid needs without an obligatory intake of extra calories. Fruit juices are not good choices as a water substitute, since they may introduce poor eating habits by emphasizing the sweet flavor. If placed in a bottle that an infant is allowed to drink from over prolonged periods, fruit juice increases the risk of nursing bottle caries.

TABLE 5. **Formulas for Low-Birthweight Infant**

Formula	Gm/dL			Mg/dL			Source		Osmolality (mOsm/kg of H₂O) and General Comments
	Pro	Fat	CHO	Na/K	Ca/P	Fe	CHO	Fat	
Enfamil Premature, Iron-Fortified (Mead Johnson) (24 kcal/30 mL)	2.4	4.0	8.8	31/82	131/66	1.5† (Low Fe, 0.2)	Corn syrup solids, lactose	Soy oil, MCT oil, coconut oil	(310) For low-birthweight infants; available for hospital use only; whey:casein ratio is 60:40; 40% fat from MCT oil
Similac Special Care, Iron-Fortified (Ross) (24 kcal/30 mL)	2.2	4.4	8.6	35/105	146/73	1.5† (low Fe, 0.3)	Lactose, hydrolyzed cornstarch	MCT oil, soy oil, coconut oil	(280) For low-birthweight infants; available for hospital use only; whey:casein ratio 60:40; 50% fat from MCT oil; recommended vitamin D supplement 400 IU/day
Similac Special Care (Ross) (20 kcal/30 mL)	1.8	3.6	7.1	29/87	122/61	0.2	Lactose, hydrolyzed cornstarch	MCT oil, soy oil, coconut oil	(235) Available for hospital use only
Similac Natural Care (Ross) (24 kcal/30 mL)	2.2	4.4	8.6	35/104	170/85	—	Lactose, hydrolyzed cornstarch	MCT oil, soy oil, coconut oil	Designed to be mixed with human milk or to be fed alternately with human milk to low-birthweight infants
Enfamil Human Milk Fortifier with EBM* (Mead Johnson) @ 4 pkt/100 mL	1.7	3.5	9.7	27/68.6	116/59	0.2	Glucose polymers, lactose	—	(380) For low-birthweight infants, or infants with volume restriction on expressed breast milk; available for hospital use only; whey:casein ratio 60:40. Recommended mixture is 2 pkt of fortifier/100 mL human milk for 24 h, afterwards increased to 4 pkt/100 mL for full fortification; does not contain iron

*Expressed breast milk.
†Also available as low iron formula.
Abbreviations: Pro = protein; CHO = carbohydrate; Na = sodium; Ca = calcium; Fe = iron; K = potassium; P = phosphorus.

Vitamin Supplements

Vitamin K is effective in preventing hemorrhagic disease of the newborn because it prevents or minimizes the postnatal decline of the vitamin K–dependent coagulation factors II, VII, IX, and X. Vitamin K is given as a single intramuscular dose of 0.5 to 1 mg or an oral dose of 1.0 to 2.0 mg. Large doses of water-soluble vitamin K analogues can produce hyperbilirubinemia.

Questions still exist about whether breast-fed infants require any vitamin or mineral supplements before the introduction of solid foods at 6 months of age. The vitamin D content of human milk is low, and rickets can occur in breast-fed infants who are deeply pigmented and have an inadequate exposure to sunlight. Therefore, vitamin D supplementation is recommended for these breast-fed infants at a dose of 400 IU per day. There is no evidence that vitamins A or E are needed for healthy breast-fed term infants. Bottle-fed infants receive adequate vitamins in formula. Supplementation is not necessary.

Fluoride supplementation is not recommended until after the first 6 months of age.

DISEASES OF THE BREAST

method of
HELENA R. CHANG, M.D., PH.D., and
KIRBY I. BLAND, M.D.
Brown University School of Medicine
Providence, Rhode Island

BENIGN BREAST DISEASE

Fibrocystic Disease (Proliferative and Nonproliferative)

"Fibrocystic disease of the breast" is a nonprecise pathologic term that refers to the spectrum of proliferative and nonproliferative lesions of the organ. Fibrocystic disease may be an asymptomatic condition, or it may present as pain, as a lump that fluctuates with the menstrual cycle, or as nipple discharge. Fibrocystic disease may be of either a proliferative or a nonproliferative type.

The pain that is associated with fibrocystic disease frequently affects premenopausal women, but seldom does pain affect postmenopausal women. When postmenopausal women are symptomatic, they are usually on estrogen replacement therapy. The pain is frequently cyclic and not well localized and may be associated with gross cysts. The management is conservative if malignancy is not suspected. Mild pain may resolve spontaneously. Elimination of methylxanthine derivatives from the diet, avoiding excessive salt during premenstrual times, wearing supportive but not compressive brassieres, and the occasional use of analgesics may be sufficient to control moderate pain. In severe cases, danazol (Danocrine) 200 to 400 mg daily for 4 to 6 months may relieve pain in 70% of treated women. The side effects of danazol include weight gain, irregular menstruation, headache, and gastrointestinal symptoms. When the pain is localized and persistent, surgical biopsy may be necessary to rule out the possibility of breast cancer.

The lumps associated with fibrocystic disease are frequently found at biopsy. If the lumps are cystic, needle aspiration for a complete resolution is sufficient. Persistent and solid lumps may require surgical removal, even when fine-needle cytologic examination reveals a nonmalignant condition. The pathologic examination may show the nonproliferative or proliferative hyperplasia, with or without atypia. The nonproliferative fibrocystic disease carries no risk of subsequent breast cancer. A finding of proliferative lesions without atypia carries a slightly higher risk for cancer development. Although atypia is an infrequent finding, it is associated with a risk of breast cancer that is four times that of the general population. The risk rises to eight times if there is a family history of breast cancer.

Nipple discharge can be another clinical manifestation of fibrocystic disease. When the discharge is spontaneous, unilateral, single-duct, with or without palpable mass, and with or without blood, ductal exploration and excision may be necessary to determine the diagnosis. A mammogram and cytologic examination are important parts of the work-up, but a negative finding does not change or replace the surgery if discharge persists. The other differential diagnoses are papilloma and cancer of the breast.

Benign Breast Tumors

Fibroadenoma. Fibroadenoma usually affects young women. Most fibroadenomas are nontender, mobile, spherical, or lobulated solid masses. Most fibroadenomas are the adult type. The other variants are juvenile fibroadenomas and giant fibroadenomas. The former type is characterized by florid glandular hyperplasia and stromal cellularity. The latter type is pathologically similar but is larger. Rarely, breast cancer may coincide with the fibroadenoma. When the malignancy is confined to the fibroadenoma, the prognosis is excellent. When the surrounding breast tissues are involved by the breast cancer, the outcome is the same as that of breast cancer without fibroadenoma.

Intraductal Papillomas. Intraductal papillomas are breast lesions with papillary configurations. These can be solitary intraductal papillomas, peripheral papillomas, or papillomatosis.

The solitary intraductal papillomas are a disease of the major lactiferous ducts and present with spontaneous bloody nipple discharge from a single duct. The complaint is usually restricted to one breast. It may or may not have a palpable mass. Treatment is surgical excision of the duct and draining of the segment of breast tissue. Permanent sections of the tumor are required to evaluate papillary lesions of the breast. Intraductal papillomas are benign conditions.

Peripheral intraductal papillomas are multiple and frequently bilateral. Peripheral intraductal papillomas tend to affect younger women and carry an increased risk of developing breast cancer. The papillomas present with a nondiscrete mass on palpation, with or without nipple discharge. Mammography may show an ill-defined density with a dilated duct. Surgical excision is the treatment of choice. Patients should be followed up.

Papillomatosis is a disease predominantly affecting young women. It may present as a mobile, nontender mass, similar to that of a fibroadenoma. This condition is a known marker for increased chances of breast cancer development. The treatment is surgical removal and an appropriate follow-up program.

Inflammatory Lesions

Various metabolic and cellular events stimulate the breast parenchyma and ducts to produce inflammatory lesions. These benign disorders are categorized as follows.

Fatty Necrosis. Fatty necrosis, which may be caused by trauma to the breast, presents as a nontender hard mass. Mammography may show a density with or without calcification. Without a known causative surgical event, the mass should be surgically removed to rule out malignancy.

Silicone Injection Reactions. Reactions to silicone injection frequently appear as multiple hard nodules that may be tender. A history of foreign body reaction may clarify the diagnosis.

Mondor's Disease. Mondor's disease is a thrombophlebitis of the thoracoepigastric vein with a cordlike band and superficial skin retraction. This is accompanied by pain in the breast. Mondor's disease is usually caused by breast surgery or radiation. It is a self-limited disease and is frequently resolved within 2 months.

Mammary Ductal Ectasia. Mammary ductal ectasia may be caused by duct obstruction secondary to squamous metaplasia and can lead to periductal mastitis at the terminal subareolar ducts. The manifestations are nipple inversion, a subareolar painful mass, and a nipple discharge. Bacterial infection may be present, with abscess formation. When an abscess is present, drainage with antibiotics coverage is the treatment of choice. The abscess cavity should be biopsied to rule out breast cancer. Recurrence of ductal ectasia after incision and drainage of focal abscesses is common. After the acute infection and inflammation subside, the major ducts beneath the areola should be excised together with the skin at the previous drain site. This is known as the "Hadfield procedure." Fewer recurrences develop after the use of this technique. Occasionally, the nipple and areola are removed for a refractory condition.

Lactational Mastitis. Lactational mastitis is a cellulitis of the breast. Women may present with redness, tenderness, and warmth at the involved segment as well as chills and fever. This should be differentiated from a duct obstruction, which also presents with swelling and pain but with no redness and fever. Lactational mastitis should be treated with warm compresses, promoting milk drainage from the involved segment, and antibiotics. This condition, if ignored, may evolve into abscess.

BREAST CANCER SCREENING

The incidence of breast cancer has been increasing in the United States in the past 2 decades. This increase may partially be explained because breast cancer is diagnosed earlier. The remaining difference is likely to be due to a real rise in the incidence of breast cancer. Many possible causes have been suggested, such as a high-fat diet, alcohol consumption, pesticide exposure, and hormonal treatment. A clear policy for cancer prevention is not available at the present time. Early breast cancer detection remains the most effective program to reduce breast cancer mortality. The recommended guidelines for breast cancer screening are as follows:

1. Women of 20 to 39 years of age with no particular risk factors are advised to perform breast self-examination (BSE) monthly and to have a clinical breast examination (CBE) every 2 to 3 years. The baseline mammographic examination is recommended at age 35.

2. Women aged 40 to 49 years should have a monthly BSE and a yearly CBE and mammographic examination. Recently, the National Cancer Institute (NCI) recommended that annual mammography be postponed until the age of 50 years. The NCI claims that there is no evidence that breast cancer mortality is reduced by screening asymptomatic women in their forties. In making this recommendation, the NCI ignores the trend of various studies to favor a screening program. In addition, there were not enough participants in the studies used by the NCI to make their recommendation valid. The American Cancer Society and the American College of Surgeons are not changing their guidelines for women in this age group.

3. Women aged 50 to 75 should continue to follow the recommendations made for women in their forties. The need for routine mammographic screening for women older than 75 depends on each woman's overall health, and a yearly mammogram may not be necessary.

4. Women at excessive risk, such as a family history of premenopausal breast cancer in first-degree relatives or a previous personal biopsy showing atypia or lobular carcinoma in situ, should receive a CBE twice a year and yearly mammography beginning at the age of 35 years.

DIAGNOSIS AND TREATMENT OF MALIGNANT NEOPLASMS

The diagnosis of cancer in a palpable breast mass can be made by either fine-needle aspiration cytologic examination or an open biopsy. Occasionally, the incisional biopsy may be more appropriate if the suspicious tumor is locally advanced or if the tumor involves the nipple areolar complex. When the lesion is not palpable and is detectable only by mammography, it can be surgically removed with needle localization placed under radiographic guidance.

During the open biopsy, the placement of incisions, orientation of the specimen, and pathologic examination for freezing specimens to determine the amount of estrogen receptor (ER) and progesterone receptor (PR) are all important considerations during the process of making a diagnosis.

Once the diagnosis is made, preoperative staging is critical in planning optimal treatment. The preoperative staging consists of a thorough history and physical examination, a blood laboratory study, and radiographic images. A chest x-ray (CXR) film is part of the staging study. Bone scan is indicated for patients with symptoms: abnormal alkaline phosphatase or serum calcium levels; palpable lymph nodes; a big primary tumor; and aggressive histopathologic features. CT scan of the abdomen is indicated only when liver function is abnormal or an abdominal physical examination suggests organomegaly.

If metastasis is not found, the local-regional treatment is the choice for treating patients with Stages I and II breast cancer. Preoperative chemotherapy is recommended for Stage III breast cancer. For metastatic disease, chemotherapy is the treatment of choice and any local treatment is limited to palliation.

Local Regional Treatment

Both modified radical mastectomy and breast conservation are effective treatments for local regional involvement by breast cancer. The modified radical mastectomy consists of the removal of the breast and axillary lymph nodes with the preservation of pectoralis major muscle and frequently the pectoralis minor muscle as well. The breast conservation treatment consists of partial mastectomy, axillary lymph node removal, and postoperative irradiation of the breast. The latter treatment is the preferred treatment for women with a tumor size less than 4 or 5 cm. The surgical goal is to achieve a tumor-free margin after partial mastectomy and to achieve a good cosmetic result. The axillary lymph node removal is for staging and regional control of the disease. Radiation reduces the local recurrence from 40 to 10% in women with partial mastectomy and with adequate margin. Women who are pregnant or who have had previous breast radiation are not candidates for breast conservation treatment. Other factors such as those responsible for increasing local recurrence, those resulting in poor cosmetic outcomes, and those affecting the early detectability of subsequent recurrences may influence a choice of modified radical mastectomy over breast conservation treatment.

A local recurrence in the breast after breast conservation therapy behaves like a primary tumor. In approximately 85% of cases, a local recurrence can be treated by salvage mastectomy, and approximately 65% survive for 5 years after salvage mastectomy. Chest wall recurrence after mastectomy, on the other hand, represents a local sign of an advanced disease. Very few patients survive without additional systemic treatments. The goal of local treatment is to keep the patient free of complications of local disease.

In treating ductal carcinoma in situ (DCIS), the conventional treatment is total mastectomy, which provides a cure rate of 99%. Recent reports of patients with DCIS treated by breast conservation suggest that most women can be treated by a combination of excision and radiation. Patients with large or palpable DCIS, particularly the comedo type, and those whose DCIS is multicentric, are best treated by mastectomy. When breast conservation is chosen for treating DCIS, one must understand that even with clear margins and radiation, a recurrence may occur and a certain percentage will return with an invasive cancer.

The finding of lobular carcinoma in situ (LCIS) is now being viewed as a marker for high risk of developing breast cancer in both breasts. The condition itself does not require treatment; however, patients should be informed of the associated risks and closely monitored. Although mammography is not very sensitive to detect LCIS, cancers that develop in these women tend to be the invasive lobular and ductal cancers, which are readily detectable by mammography. It is reasonable to include mammography in the follow-up program in addition to the twice-a-year CBE.

Systemic Adjuvant Treatment

Histopathologic features and the nodal status are the most powerful predictors of the outcome of the initial treatment. The presence of histologically documented nodal metastasis and the absolute number of nodes that are involved by metastases correlate directly with the rate of recurrence and survival. The size of the invasive breast cancer, the mitotic index,

the DNA ploidy, and the levels of ERs and PRs in the tumor provide additional prognostic and management information. The positivity of ERs and PRs indicates a better prognosis and a likely responsiveness to the tamoxifen treatment. Other molecular prognosticators such as HER-2-*neu* oncogene and cathepsin D are nonstandardized parameters and have limited usefulness at the present time.

It has been shown that adjuvant systemic therapy can reduce recurrence and improve survival. Benefits are shown in both young and postmenopausal women, in women with positive node(s), and in women with negative nodes but with other high-risk features. Young women and postmenopausal women in good health who have nodal metastases should receive systemic adjuvant chemotherapy. The commonly used cytotoxic chemotherapy regimens are CMF (cyclophosphamide [Cytoxan], methotrexate, 5-fluorouracil [5-FU], CAF (cyclophosphamide, doxorubicin [Adriamycin], 5-FU), and CMF plus VP-16 (etoposide [VePesid]). In postmenopausal women, the less toxic chemotherapy is selected with the addition of a subsequent tamoxifen treatment. In women of 70 years of age or older, or between 50 and 70 years in marginal health, tamoxifen (Nolvadex) alone is a reasonable adjuvant agent to reduce tumor recurrence.

Although most adjuvant treatment is given after the local-regional treatment, the neoadjuvant therapy is recommended for patients with a large tumor size or those who have skin or chest wall involvement. Local-regional treatment in these patients is mainly to evaluate the response of the tumor to the drug treatment and to prevent complications resulting from local tumor invasion.

A subset of cancer patients, i.e., those with inflammatory breast cancer or with 10 or more positive nodes, may benefit from dose-intensified chemotherapy and autologous bone marrow or peripheral blood stem cell transplantation. A higher cure rate may be expected from this new approach. Although patients with metastatic disease who respond dramatically to the initial chemotherapy may have a sustained remission by adding a bone marrow transplantation protocol to the treatment, this approach is nonstandard and requires further investigation before recommendation.

Treatment for Metastatic Breast Cancer

The common sites of breast cancer metastases are bone, liver, lung, brain, chest wall, adrenal, and ovaries. Local treatments such as surgical resections and radiation are largely palliative and do not change the overall outcome. Surgical resection of an isolated metastasis should be practiced with extreme caution, particularly when the resection is expected to be associated with significant morbidity and mortality. Systemic treatment is the choice in treating metastatic disease. Hormonal treatment such as tamoxifen or progestational agents is preferred in postmenopausal women with tumors that are either positive or of unknown status. Chemotherapy is more appropriate in those who became refractory to the hormonal treatment, although most chemotherapy-induced responses are not long-lasting. The response rate of patients with metastases is generally much higher to the first-line than to the second-line chemotherapy regimens. Cytotoxic agents such as cyclophosphamide, doxorubicin, 5-FU, methotrexate, paclitaxel (Taxol), cisplatin (Platinol), and VP-16 are among the first-line agents.

Oncologic emergencies such as hypercalcemia, central nervous system metastases, spinal cord compression, unstable bony metastases, intestinal obstruction or perforation, or massive pleural effusion should be dealt with promptly and specifically.

Patients having hypercalcemia of greater than 12 mg per dL should be admitted to the hospital for treatment. The initial appropriate treatment includes hydration and diuresis. For life-threatening hypercalcemia, a short course of high-dose calcitonin (Calcimar) (8 IU per kg, intramuscularly every 6 to 8 hours) may result in an immediate response. After hydration, etidronate (Didronel) and gallium nitrate (Ganite) may be added as part of the short-term treatment.

Metastases of breast cancer to the brain may be associated with signs and symptoms such as headache, mental change, seizures, nausea or vomiting, dizziness, difficulty in walking, visual or hearing changes, vertigo, and facial numbness. Spinal symptoms include lower motor neuron weakness, paresthesias, radicular pain, incontinence, and stiff neck. Immediate corticosteroid (dexamethasone) therapy minimizes future edema. Prompt radiographic examinations and neurosurgical and radiation consultations are required.

Suspected intestinal obstruction or perforation should be treated with proximal decompression of the gastrointestinal tract after surgical evaluation on an urgent or emergent basis.

Nonstable bony metastasis should be treated with rest and immobilization. Patients should be promptly evaluated by radiographic examinations. The orthopedic surgeon as well as radiation oncologist should be consulted promptly to prevent or to correct pathologic fracture.

Respiratory distress from massive pleural effusion can be treated with chest tube drainage and subsequent administration of a sclerosing agent to prevent subsequent recurrence.

ENDOMETRIOSIS

method of
TONY G. ZREIK, M.D.,
JILL S. FISCHER, and
DAVID L. OLIVE, M.D.
Yale University School of Medicine
New Haven, Connecticut

Endometriosis is one of the most commonly encountered gynecologic diseases in reproductive-age females, yet it is among the most engimatic of conditions. The literature on endometriosis is extensive and often contradictory, reflecting the wide range of symptoms, signs, and physical appearances of the lesions. Recent studies, however, have produced new insights into this complex disorder.

Endometriosis is classically defined as the presence, in locations other than the endometrial cavity or musculature, of tissues that are biologically and morphologically similar to normal endometrium. Traditionally, pathologists have required the presence of both endometrial glands and stroma to firmly establish the diagnosis, but the pathologic effect of one or the other of these tissue components, when present alone, has not been adequately assessed.

PATHOGENESIS

Although many theories of histogenesis and etiology have been advanced, three main theories still dominate current thinking. The original theory of coelomic metaplasia stated that peritoneal mesothelium cells, under certain unspecified stimuli, may undergo a metaplastic transformation that changes their physiologic function and appearance into that of endometrium. However, despite the fact that both endometrial and peritoneal cells derive from the same surface (coelomic wall epithelium), it has never been shown that peritoneal cells can differentiate further.

A second theory of histogenesis speculated that during menstruation, viable endometrial tissue is transported through the fallopian tubes to ectopic locations, where it implants and grows. In support of this theory of retrograde menstruation proposed by Sampson are the findings of viable endometrial cells in the menstrual effluent in the fallopian tubes and the fact that experimentally implanted endometrium can grow within the peritoneal cavity.

The third theory, known as the induction theory of endometriosis, is in fact a combination of the two previously mentioned theories. It states that the shed endometrium releases unknown substances that induce undifferentiated mesenchymal tissue to form endometriosis.

The latter two theories are most supported by epidemiologic, surgical, and experimental data; thus, it appears that retrograde menstruation is a necessary first step for a significant portion of resultant endometriosis. Regardless of which theory of histogenesis is correct, however, it is important to realize that since retrograde menstruation is a near universal phenomenon, additional factors must be responsible for the expression of the disease. Such additional factors might include the degree of retrograde flow or an impaired immune response, resulting in the inability to remove refluxed menstrual debris. Several studies have shown that women with a greater amount of retrograde menstruation, such as those with menorrhagia or outflow tract obstruction, are at greater risk of developing endometriosis. In addition, subtle alterations in the immune system may modify a woman's risk of developing endometriosis. It has further been suggested that growth factors in the peritoneal fluid of women with endometriosis may enhance the likelihood of transplantation. However, the role of factors that determine the degree of retrograde menstruation and the immunologic factors that may affect a woman's susceptibility to the implantation of refluxed endometrial cells remains to be fully elucidated.

Clinical and epidemiologic studies have suggested a familial predisposition toward endometriosis. A sevenfold increased risk of endometriosis among the first-degree relatives of patients with the disease compared with their husband's first-degree relatives was noted, and although data from large twin studies are unavailable, small studies showed endometriosis in 75% of monozygotic twin pairs. These studies suggest that genetic transmission is highly likely, with the suspected mode of inheritance being polygenic or autosomal dominant with variable penetrance.

PRESENTATION

Endometriosis may present with a wide variety of symptoms but is not always symptomatic. Although some symptoms are strongly suggestive of endometriosis, there are no pathognomonic symptoms. Pelvic pain is the most common symptom of endometriosis, presenting as primary or secondary dysmenorrhea, dyspareunia, or nonspecific lower abdominal pain. It most frequently occurs as dysmenorrhea, starting 1 to 2 days before the menstrual flow and lasting for the duration of the flow. Some women, however, experience the most intense pain around the time of ovulation.

Infertility is commonly associated with endometriosis. Although it is clear that adhesion formation resulting from endometriosis can lead to infertility when reproductive organs are involved, it is unclear whether any causal relationship exists between simple endometriosis implants and infertility. In addition, the symptoms of endometriosis may be quite variable and are mostly determined by the areas of involvement. For example, pain in the flank and iliac fossa may indicate involvement of the ureter, and rectal bleeding may be an indication of bowel involvement.

Although most frequently seen in the pelvis, endometriosis has been found in most areas of the body, including the umbilicus, abdominal scars, diaphragm, stomach, kidneys, and lungs.

DIAGNOSIS

Laparoscopy is considered the "gold standard" for the diagnosis of endometriosis. Unfortunately, the lesions of endometriosis do not necessarily have a single characteristic appearance. Thus, the precision of laparoscopic diagnosis is wholly dependent on the skill of the surgeon responsible for recognizing the disease.

Thorough systematic visualization of the pelvis is essential, with particular attention to the ovaries, the anterior and posterior peritoneum, and the uterosacral ligaments. Typical endometriosis lesions appear as stellate-scarred lesions surrounded by reddish-blue powder-burn implants on the peritoneal surfaces of the pelvis. Atypically appearing implants include clear vesicles, white fibrotic scarring, and red polypoid lesions. Recently, a pattern of evolution of these lesions has been suggested, their appearance being subtle in the teenage years and more obvious a decade later.

Considerable interest in a laboratory method for the diagnosis of endometriosis has been expressed in recent years. Present studies on serum markers for the disease focus on two areas: the CA 125 antigen and antiendometrial antibodies. An elevated CA 125 level in the peripheral blood has been repeatedly described in women with endometriosis. However, the sensitivity and specificity of this test for screening are suboptimal, making the test of questionable value for diagnostic screening but possibly useful in monitoring responses to treatment. In addition, although endometrial antibodies are detected in the serum in a high percentage of patients with endometriosis, these levels do not appear to correlate with the severity of the disease.

Imaging techniques have traditionally been of limited value in the diagnosis of endometriosis. However, of the currently available modalities, magnetic resonance imaging (MRI) seems to have the most potential. Endometriomas can be differentiated from other adnexal masses quite consistently, with an overall accuracy greater than 90%. Fat-saturation technique appears to be superior to conventional MRI and may be useful as a noninvasive monitoring technique to follow the response of endometrial implants to various therapies.

PATHOLOGIC FEATURES

Endometriotic implants have traditionally been described as bluish-gray "powder burns." The color is attributed to menstrual cyclicity of the ectopic endometrium, with hemolysis and encapsulation of the debris by scarring. The ectopic endometrium may also appear as nonpigmented clear vesicles, white plaques, and reddish petechiae or flamelike areas. These implants may range in size from several millimeters to centimeters and may be superficial or deeply invasive. When endometriotic cysts occur in the ovary, they are termed endometriomas.

Microscopically, endometrial implants show a varied histology, which corresponds roughly to gross appearance. The red polypoid lesions are closest to ectopic endometrial tissue, and the white lesions contain sparse glands and stroma with increased fibrous tissue. The black powder-burn lesions are fibrotic and probably inactive. Similarly, endometriomas are quite nondescript, with simple cuboidal epithelium surrounded by fibrous tissue.

PATHOPHYSIOLOGY

Pain

Although many mechanisms explaining pain in endometriosis have been proposed, all remain speculative. Recent investigations revealed that the deeper the lesion, the greater the likelihood of pain. The mechanism for this may be the induction of fibrosis in surrounding tissues or the inflammation of nerve fibers around implants. Endometrial implants produce prostaglandins, and prostaglandin synthetase inhibitors have been shown to decrease the pain symptoms that accompany endometriosis. In addition, visceral pain may result from invasion of the gastrointestinal or genitourinary tract.

Supporting the relationship between endometriosis and pelvic pain is the apparent effectiveness of medical treatment in relieving pain. Virtually all hormonal therapies directed at suppressive endometriotic implants have proved effective in relieving pain associated with endometriosis. Thus, it is likely that a cause-and-effect relationship exists.

Infertility

Three separate factors may play a role in infertility associated with endometriosis: implants, ovarian endometriomas, and adhesions. When adhesions causing anatomic distortion of the pelvis or obstruction of the fallopian tubes are present, the result is often infertility. However, the mechanisms of infertility associated with endometriosis without obvious pelvic adhesive disease are poorly understood. Many possibilities have been suggested, including altered prostaglandin secretion and metabolism, impaired immunity, increased macrophage activity with sperm phagocytosis, ovulatory dysfunction with altered folliculogenesis, luteal phase defect, luteinized unruptured follicles, impaired fertilization, defective implantation, and embryo toxicity against early embryonic development.

Despite the apparent association between infertility and mild endometriosis, there is a paucity of evidence identifying the specific mechanisms of such resultant infertility. Furthermore, human data strongly dispute such a causal relationship. Indeed, mild endometriosis is not infrequent in fertile women, and expectant management or no treatment of endometriosis yields pregnancy rates that are similar to those in treatment groups. Accordingly, mild or minimal endometriosis may be an incidental finding and of no importance in the pathogenesis of infertility.

TREATMENT

Medical strategies to combat endometriosis are focused on hormonal alteration of the menstrual cycle, creating states of pseudopregnancy, pseudomenopause, or chronic anovulation.

Danazol (Danocrine), a synthetic derivative of testosterone, causes anovulation by attenuating the midcycle surge of luteinizing hormone secretion, thus preventing further reflux of endometrial tissue into the peritoneal cavity. Direct inhibition of several enzymatic steps in the steroidogenic pathway may also serve to inhibit estrogen-induced growth and maintenance of the disease. A number of side effects have been attributed to danazol, most resulting from the androgenic effects of the drug; some, such as deepening of the voice, are irreversible. Good results have generally been obtained when danazol is used to treat the anatomic manifestation of endometriosis, although the duration of this physical improvement is unknown. Similarly, pain relief has been noted in 84 to 92% of treated patients at the conclusion of numerous uncontrolled trials. However, there is no evidence that danazol enhances pregnancy rates for women with endometriosis-associated infertility.

Progestogens cause deciduation of endometrial tissue with eventual atrophy. They work against endometriosis by creating an unfavorable steroid environment and by decreasing cyclic bleeding and subsequent reflux of menstrual fluid into the peritoneal cavity. Side effects are reversible and may include breast tenderness, abnormal uterine bleeding, nausea, fluid retention, and depression. One progestogen, medroxyprogesterone (Provera), has been demonstrated to be as effective as danazol in decreasing the physical manifestations of the disease and in providing pain relief. Like danazol, however, progestogens have not been shown to be an effective treatment for infertility.

Gestrinone is an antiprogestational steroid with additional androgenic and antiestrogenic effects. It is believed to enhance lysosomal degradation of the cell via a progesterone withdrawal effect. Side effects are mostly mild and transient and include voice changes, hirsutism, and clitoral hypertrophy. Improvement in pelvic pain has been shown in over 90% of patients while they were taking medication; however, within 1 year following discontinuation of the drug, recurrence of pain was observed in up to 30%. Similar to the previously mentioned medications, gestrinone treatment results in no improvement in fertility.

More recently, the use of gonadotropin-releasing hormone (GnRH) analogues to produce a medical oophorectomy has become popular in the treatment of endometriosis. Continuous administration of these drugs leads to desensitization of pituitary receptors and down-regulation of the pituitary-ovarian axis. Side effects are secondary to hypoestrogenism and may include hot flushes, vaginal dryness and subsequent dyspareunia, amenorrhea, headache, depression, and osteoporosis. GnRH analogues are comparable to danazol and superior to placebo in relieving endometriosis-associated pain. Studies reporting pregnancy rates following GnRH agonist therapy have suffered from small sample size, inconsistent staging, and variable length of follow-up; they have failed to show an enhanced fertility in patients with endometriosis.

Oral contraceptives are the most common drug regimen in the treatment of endometriosis, used in over 40% of patients with the disease. Despite their widespread use, no data are available regarding their effect on disease manifestations. Similarly, no data have been published on the effect of oral contraceptives on fertility. Oral contraceptives have been shown to be as efficacious as GnRH analogues for the treatment of endometriosis-associated pain, however.

All the aforementioned drugs appear to be roughly equivalent in diminishing the anatomic extent of the disease and in reducing pain. However, there is no evidence that medical treatment is beneficial in women with endometriosis-associated infertility.

Unlike medical treatment, surgical treatment of endometriosis may be effective against both infertility and pelvic pain. Surgical procedures for endometriosis are often labeled either "radical" or "conservative." Conservative surgery does not imply the use of any particular technique or procedure but merely indicates that the surgery is designed to preserve or improve fertility. Radical surgery, consisting of removal of the uterus and ovaries and resection of all endometriotic lesions, should be reserved for patients with severe symptoms who have no further desire for pregnancy.

Although laparotomy has long been the standard surgical therapy for endometriosis, laparoscopy is becoming increasingly important in the treatment of most, perhaps all, cases of endometriosis. Laparoscopy offers several advantages over laparotomy. Along with the ability to treat at the time of initial diagnosis, laparoscopy is associated with a shortened hospital stay, a reduced morbidity, and a decreased postoperative adhesion rate. Several methods for endometriosis removal or destruction through the laparoscope are currently available:

1. Electrosurgical energy, in the form of unipolar or bipolar instrumentation, is widely used in operative laparoscopy. This modality has distinct therapeutic effects on tissues, such as fulguration, desiccation, or vaporization.

2. Thermocoagulation differs from electrosurgery in that no electricity comes into contact with the tissues. Instead, the electrical current is converted to

heat within the electrode itself, and this heat is then transmitted to tissues by convection.

3. Laser energy sources are presently available for use through the laparoscope, including carbon dioxide, argon, Nd:YAG, and KTP crystals. The advantage of lasers involves their ability to localize the generated energy source, producing a well-defined limit of tissue damage.

Small peritoneal implants of endometriosis can be effectively treated with coagulation or vaporization once biopsies are obtained for diagnostic purposes. With larger lesions, excision to the level of healthy tissue becomes increasingly important and may be accomplished with lasers, electrosurgery, or scissors. It is also important to excise rather than merely separate adhesions, which may leave endometriotic implants that are capable of causing adhesion reformation postoperatively.

Conservative surgery has been used extensively in an attempt to enhance fertility. When compared with expectant management, conservative surgery produced significantly better results for severe endometriosis, and both modalities were equally effective for mild or moderate disease.

In addition to treatments directed at the disease itself, many treatments are directed merely at the symptoms and should be tailored to the individual patient's needs. Accordingly, an infertile woman with minimal endometriosis may be treated similarly to a patient with unexplained infertility—with gonadotropins for ovulation induction, coupled with intrauterine inseminations or in vitro fertilization and embryo transfer (IVF/ET). In general, however, a major intervention such as IVF/ET should not be considered in the initial management of endometriosis-associated infertility, except in an older patient or in patients with severe tuboperitoneal adhesive disease.

Although extensive research has been generated on the different aspects of endometriosis, many questions regarding the pathogenesis, pathophysiology, and clinical management of the disease remain unanswered. Thus, basic research must be supplemented by well-constructed clinical trials to improve on the current diagnostic and treatment options.

DYSFUNCTIONAL UTERINE BLEEDING

method of
STEVEN R. BAYER, M.D.
Boston Regional Center for Reproductive Medicine
Stoneham, Massachusetts

and

ALAN H. DeCHERNEY, M.D.
Tufts University School of Medicine
Boston, Massachusetts

Abnormal uterine bleeding is one of the most common problems that challenge the gynecologist on a routine ba-

sis. The abnormal bleeding can be secondary to a benign physiologic process or can be a sign of underlying pathology within the reproductive tract. Dysfunctional uterine bleeding (DUB) is defined as the abnormal bleeding that occurs in the absence of pelvic pathology or a systemic disorder. In the majority of cases anovulation is the cause of DUB. During the pubertal and perimenopausal periods, anovulatory bleeding is a common occurrence and is transitory. The unopposed estrogen associated with chronic anovulation or polycystic ovarian disease can also result in abnormal bleeding. The diagnosis of DUB is one of exclusion, and the clinician must complete a thorough evaluation to rule out all other causes before the diagnosis can be established and the appropriate therapy instituted.

DIAGNOSING ABNORMAL UTERINE BLEEDING

The average menstrual cycle is 29 days in length, with a range of 23 to 39 days. The normal duration of the menstrual period is 2 to 7 days, and the average blood loss is 40 mL. Among women, the length of the menstrual cycle and the duration and amount of bleeding can vary; however, for an individual woman these parameters remain relatively consistent from cycle to cycle. Only when a woman perceives a deviation from her norm does she have reason to seek medical advice.

Once a patient presents with abnormal bleeding, the clinician must first determine whether an evaluation is even indicated (Figure 1). This decision is easy to make when a woman presents with heavy, active bleeding. But others present only with a history of abnormal bleeding. For these patients the clinician must initially rely on the menstrual history. The regularity of the menstrual cycles and duration of the menses, in the past and present, are important pieces of information. It is also important to know whether the abnormal bleeding is an isolated event or a chronic occurrence. For those patients complaining of menorrhagia, the clinician can try to estimate the amount of blood loss by the number of tampons or pads used. However, this approach has been shown to be notoriously inaccurate. Nevertheless, a menstrual period that lasts longer than 7 days or is accompanied by clotting is very suggestive of excessive bleeding. In addition, laboratory evidence of anemia provides objective evidence that the bleeding has been excessive. When the clinician determines that the frequency of the menstrual periods or the amount of blood loss is abnormal, further evaluation is indicated.

The next step is to determine whether the bleeding is ovulatory or anovulatory in nature. Bleeding that occurs at regular intervals and is preceded by premenstrual symptoms is ovulatory. Prolonged bleeding that occurs at irregular intervals is probably anovulatory in nature. However, the bleeding pattern of many patients is between these extremes, and the patient's ovulatory status may be uncertain. A simple and inexpensive test to determine a patient's ovulatory status is charting the basal body temperature. A biphasic temperature chart demonstrating an increase in temperature of 0.5 to 1.0° F is compatible with an ovulatory cycle. For those patients who are not compliant with the temperature charting, a serum progesterone level that is greater than 3.0 ng per mL or an endometrial biopsy that shows secretory changes is diagnostic of previous ovulation.

Abnormal uterine bleeding that is ovulatory in nature has a number of causes. The pelvic examination may identify pathology within the reproductive tract that may explain the bleeding. An enlarged uterus can suggest preg-

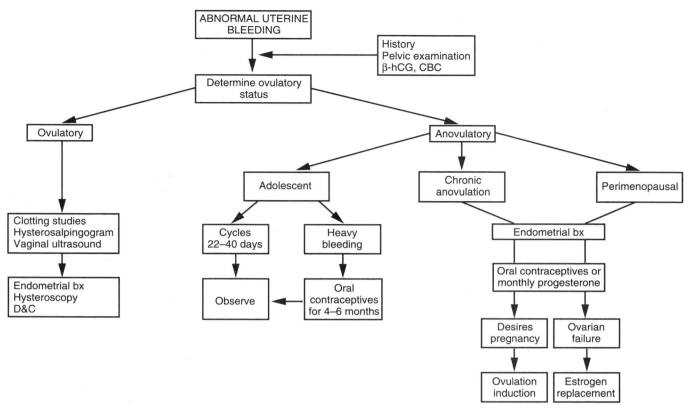

Figure 1. Evaluation and treatment of abnormal uterine bleeding. *Abbreviations*: β-hCG = beta-human chorionic gonadotropin; CBC = complete blood count; bx = biopsy; D&C = dilatation and curettage.

nancy, adenomyosis, or uterine fibroids (the submucous variety is commonly associated with abnormal bleeding). To determine the number, size, and location of uterine fibroids, vaginal sonography and hysterosalpingography can be useful. Coagulation disorders can also be a cause of the abnormal bleeding. When no cause is evident, hysteroscopic examination of the uterine cavity with endometrial sampling is indicated.

The pubertal and perimenopausal periods represent states of transition, during which anovulation is common. In the pubertal woman, there is a delay in the maturation of the positive feedback that is necessary for the luteinizing hormone (LH) surge. Therefore, many of the initial cycles after menarche are anovulatory. The bleeding that results is from an estrogen withdrawal, occurs at 22- to 45-day intervals, and is light to moderate in amount. In these cases, simple observation is warranted. However, when the bleeding is protracted or occurs at longer intervals, chronic anovulation should be suspected.

During the perimenopause, estradiol levels of the follicular phase are lower and may not be sufficient to initiate an LH surge; as a result, ovulation will not occur. Withdrawal bleeding occurs when the estradiol levels decline. This transition can last from months to years before all ovarian follicles are exhausted and menopause ensues.

Pathologic causes of anovulation can result from dysfunction at any level of the hypothalamic-pituitary-ovarian axis. Ovarian failure can be the result of increasing age, a sex chromosomal abnormality, or an autoimmune disorder. Hypothalamic dysfunction can be secondary to weight loss, anxiety, or chronic illness. Both hypothalamic dysfunction and ovarian failure can produce amenorrhea, but in transition DUB can occur. Chronic anovulation or polycystic ovarian disease can be secondary to hyperprolactinemia, obesity, hyperandrogenism, or insulin resistance. Any patient with anovulation should have assessment of serum prolactin, thyroid-stimulating hormone (TSH), and gonadotropin levels.

Regardless of the cause, chronic anovulation is associated with menstrual irregularity. A patient with chronic anovulation can present with a wide range of abnormal menstrual patterns, including amenorrhea, light bleeding occurring at irregular intervals, or profuse bleeding following a period of amenorrhea. The sustained, unopposed estrogen associated with chronic anovulation can also place a patient at risk for endometrial cancer.

TREATMENT OF DYSFUNCTIONAL UTERINE BLEEDING

The three main goals of treatment are to stop acute bleeding, to avert future bleeding episodes, and to prevent long-term complications, i.e., endometrial cancer. In cases of severe bleeding, initial stabilization is followed by dilatation and curettage to evacuate clots and remove hypertrophic endometrial tissue. In less severe cases, drug therapy with progestational or estrogenic agents can be effective (Table 1).

Natural Progesterone

The main advantage of using natural progesterone is that the endogenous hormone is being replaced

TABLE 1. **Progestational Treatment in Dysfunctional Uterine Bleeding**

	Acute	Chronic
Intramuscular Route		
Progesterone-in-oil	100–200 mg	—
Depo-medroxyprogesterone acetate (Depo-Provera)	150 mg	150 mg q 3 mon
Oral Preparations		
Medroxyprogesterone acetate (Provera)	20–40 mg q day	10 mg q day × 12
Megestrol acetate (Megace)	40–120 mg q day	—
Norethindrone (Norlutin)	1–5 mg q day	1 mg q day × 12
Norethindrone acetate (Norlutate, Aygestin)	1–5 mg q day	1 mg q day × 12
Oral contraceptives	1–4 tabs q day	1 tab q day

and it does not have the deleterious effects on the lipoprotein system that are associated with the synthetic progesterone preparations. The recent development of the micronization process allows the oral administration of natural progesterone. However, the major disadvantage of the medication is that it has a short half-life and must be taken several times a day to achieve therapeutic serum levels. Natural progesterone can also be administered by intramuscular injection, and a dose of 100 to 200 mg should be adequate in controlling an acute bleeding episode. It can be used on a monthly basis as well.

Synthetic Progesterone

Orally potent synthetic progestational agents have been the mainstay of medical treatment for DUB. These include 17-OH-progesterone derivatives (medroxyprogesterone acetate [Provera] and megestrol acetate [Megace]) and 19-nortestosterone derivatives (norethindrone [Norlutin], norethindrone acetate [Aygestin], norethynodrel, ethynodiol diacetate, norgestrel, and norgestimate). The latter are common progestational agents in oral contraceptives. The administration of depo-medroxyprogesterone acetate intramuscularly has a sustained progestational effect that can last for up to 6 months. This long-acting preparation can be useful in patients with DUB who are poorly compliant or mentally incompetent. When progestational treatment does not produce improvement or resolution of the bleeding in 24 to 48 hours, dilatation and curettage with a hysteroscopy should be performed to rule out other causes.

Estrogen

Estrogen therapy has a role in the treatment of DUB. Long-term treatment with oral contraceptives or progestational therapy can result in atrophic changes in the endometrium that can lead to breakthrough bleeding. Resolution of the bleeding can be achieved with 10 to 20 μg of ethinyl estradiol (Estinyl) or 1.25 to 2.5 mg of conjugated estrogens (Premarin) for 10 days. Estrogen therapy may also be useful in the patient who undergoes a curettage for heavy bleeding but has only minimal tissue removed. In these patients chronic bleeding can denude the endometrial lining, and intravenous conjugated estrogens administered at a dose of 25 mg every 4 hours (for a maximum of 3 doses) are effective therapy. When bleeding stops, oral progestational therapy should be started to stabilize the endometrium.

Individualizing Treatment

1. For the adolescent with heavy bleeding, treatment with an oral contraceptive should be initiated and continued for 3 to 6 months, followed by observation. Some patients may resume a normal menstrual pattern, whereas others go on to develop chronic anovulation and require continued treatment with a progestational agent.

2. For the adult woman who presents with an acute episode of abnormal bleeding that was preceded by normal menses, a pregnancy test should be checked. If negative, the patient can be started on a short course of a progestational agent, such as medroxyprogesterone acetate (10 mg for 5 to 10 days). If the bleeding does not resolve, other causes of the bleeding should be sought.

3. In women with chronic anovulation, monthly administration of a progestational agent will prevent irregular bleeding and provide protection against the development of endometrial cancer. The duration of treatment, not the dose, is important. A study showed that a 12-day course is needed to provide optimal protection. Monthly progesterone will achieve this goal. Another good alternative is the use of oral contraceptives, which will also help improve hyperandrogenic symptoms.

4. The perimenopausal patient with anovulatory bleeding should be treated with a 12-day course of progesterone each month. Once withdrawal bleeding ceases, estrogen replacement should be started. Some perimenopausal patients fluctuate between ovulatory and anovulatory cycles, which can create some difficulty with management. In selected patients, the use of low-dose contraceptive agents up to the time of menopause can prove efficacious. Once ovarian failure is documented (by an elevated follicle-stimulating hormone [FSH] test performed on day 7 of the placebo pills), the patient's regimen can be changed to a standard hormonal replacement.

AMENORRHEA

method of
LORI-LINELL H. HALL, M.D., and
DAVID S. GUZICK, M.D., PH.D.
University of Pittsburgh School of Medicine
Pittsburgh, Pennsylvania

Amenorrhea, the absence of menstrual bleeding, is a common condition and a frequent reason that women of reproductive age seek health care. Many diverse conditions, such as congenital anatomic disorders of the female reproductive tract, endocrinopathies including hypothalamic, thyroid, or adrenal disease, and chronic systemic illness may present with amenorrhea. Although definitions of amenorrhea are not uniform, women who fail to menstruate by the age of 16 years in the presence of normal secondary sexual characteristics or by the age of 14 years in the absence of normal secondary sexual characteristics should be investigated. Furthermore, in a woman who has previously been menstruating, 3 months of amenorrhea is considered abnormal and should be evaluated.

Traditionally, amenorrhea is classified as either primary (women who have never menstruated) or secondary (women who have previously menstruated for a variable time before the cessation of menses). However, some causes most commonly associated with primary amenorrhea (e.g., gonadal dysgenesis) may present as secondary amenorrhea, while others most commonly associated with secondary amenorrhea (e.g., hyperandrogenic anovulation) may present as incomplete puberty with primary amenorrhea. This article focuses on the diagnosis of patients with amenorrhea based on clinical presentation and the judicious use of laboratory testing. We attempt to provide a conceptual approach to the evaluation of amenorrhea that emphasizes clinical assessment. A careful history and physical examination alone will guide the clinician to the appropriate major diagnostic categories; a judicious use of a small number of laboratory tests will then lead to definitive diagnosis.

PRIMARY AMENORRHEA

It is common for reviews of the diagnostic assessment of primary amenorrhea to make heuristic use of flow charts. We do some of that here, but emphasize the initial categorization of individuals with primary amenorrhea according to four types of clinical presentation: sexual infantilism, congenital genital ambiguity, acquired virilization, or incomplete puberty. This categorization follows an approach developed by Dr. Paul MacDonald* in his teachings to house staff and fellows at the University of Texas, Southwestern Medical School. Using this classification system forces the clinician to think about the key features of a patient's clinical presentation; furthermore, once the patient is assigned to one of the four major categories, there is then a laboratory test or clinical finding that distinguishes between one or another of the major diagnoses. In this manner, the combination of clinical assessment and limited laboratory testing almost always guides the clinician to the likely diagnosis. If several options remain in a particular diagnostic grouping, additional laboratory tests can determine the possibilities.

We emphasize the clinical approach to the four broad categories of primary amenorrhea based on history, physical examination, and one or two diagnostic tests within each category. This completes the diagnostic evaluation for the vast majority of women presenting with primary amenorrhea. Less common causes are not reviewed in detail.

*One of the authors (DSG) learned this approach as a fellow of Dr. MacDonald. However, responsibility for any errors of omission or commission remains with the authors.

Sexual Infantilism

Sexual infantilism is characterized by the absence of secondary sexual development, corresponding to Tanner Stage 1. This can be most readily assessed clinically by the absence of breast budding. However, breast development may have been induced by exogenous estrogen administration, as it is common for patients in this category to have been placed on oral contraceptives to induce cyclic withdrawal bleeding. In such cases the clinician must, by history, ascertain the status of secondary sex characteristics at the time of initial presentation for primary amenorrhea before exogenous estrogen therapy.

As indicated in Figure 1, the absence of secondary sex characteristics is caused by the lack of endogenous estrogen production due either to an inability of the ovaries to produce estrogen even when stimulated by gonadotropins or to a lack of adequate gonadotropin stimulation of normally responsive ovaries. Discrimination between these two possibilities can be readily accomplished by testing the serum follicle-stimulating hormone (FSH) level. An elevated FSH level (>30 mIU per mL) implies ovarian unresponsiveness, whereas a normal or low level of FSH implies a lack of ovarian stimulation. If the FSH level is elevated, the patient should be examined for the presence or absence of a uterus. The presence of a uterus is good (but not perfect) office-based evidence for the absence of a Y chromosome; a karyotype should be obtained for confirmation. If a uterus is present, by far the most common cause of sexual infantilism is gonadal dysgenesis, which is also the most common cause of primary amenorrhea generally. Gonadal dysgenesis is characterized by "streak" gonads that do not contain any germinal elements. Patients with the classic form of gonadal dysgenesis, Turner's syndrome or 45,XO gonadal dysgenesis (O designates the absence of the second sex chromosome), generally present with short stature (<58 inches) and can display a variety of other characteristics such as a webbed neck, a shieldlike chest with side-set nipples, and shortening of the fourth or fifth digits. Other karyotypic variants include mosaicism, structural abnormalities of the second sex chromosome, and pure gonadal dysgenesis (i.e., XX or XY). In patients with pure XY gonadal dysgenesis or mosaics with a Y chromosome, there is a risk of gonadal malignancies, i.e., dysgerminomas or gonadoblastomas; thus, it is generally recommended that the gonads be removed. Malignancy is a more common problem in congenital genital ambiguity or acquired virilization; however, such neoplasms in an XY individual presenting with sexual infantilism are rare.

Initiation of low-dose estrogen therapy (0.3 mg of conjugated equine estrogens [Premarin]) at 12 to 13 years of age in conjunction with a progestin (5 mg of medroxyprogesterone acetate [Provera]) promotes the development of secondary sex characteristics and is associated with a growth spurt without an acceleration of bone age or a reduction in the final height. The estrogen can be given each day with the proges-

- Characterized by no endogenous estrogen production
- Two possible defects:
  1) Inability of gonads to produce estrogen
  2) Failure of pituitary to secrete gonadotropin
- Evaluation: draw FSH; if elevated, examine patient for presence of uterus and obtain karyotype.

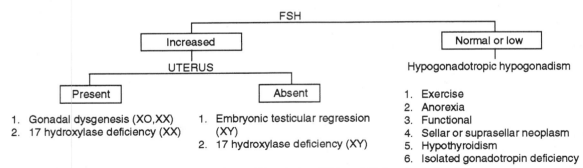

Figure 1. Sexual infantilism. *Abbreviation*: FSH = follicle-stimulating hormone.

tin added on the first through the twelfth calendar day of each month. This regimen induces regular withdrawal bleeding, thus simulating normal menstrual cycles. Once the final height is achieved, an estrogen-progestin oral contraceptive can be used to prevent the long-term sequelae of hypoestrogenism without increasing the risk of endometrial hyperplasia or cancer.

Karyotypic females with 17-alpha-hydroxylase deficiency present with sexual infantilism and primary amenorrhea due to negligible estrogen production from deficiency of C_{21} and C_{19} steroids. Progesterone, 11-deoxycorticosterone, and corticosterone levels are elevated. Hypertension and hypokalemic alkalosis may be present. Treatment is aimed at providing the missing steroids. Sex steroids must be given to effect sexual development. In patients with an absent uterus and elevated FSH level, 17-alpha-hydroxylase deficiency with an XY karyotype or embryonic testicular regression may be the cause. Karyotypic males may present with disorders ranging from normal-appearing female external genitalia and a blind vaginal pouch to ambiguous genitalia or a small phallus with hypospadias (see next section).

Patients with primary amenorrhea, sexual infantilism, and a normal or low FSH level have hypogonadotropic hypogonadism by exclusion. Idiopathic and genetic forms of multiple pituitary hormone deficiency are also included in this group. Deficiency of pulsatile gonadotropin-releasing hormone (GnRH) may be caused by a congenital defect that is undetected until puberty as well as by trauma, tumors, vascular lesions, or inflammatory processes. Psychiatric and functional conditions can also suppress GnRH. Gonadotropin-deficient patients are usually of normal height for age when seen during adolescence when compared with patients with constitutional delay in growth and puberty.

Craniopharyngioma, originating from the pituitary stalk, is the most common tumor associated with sexual infantilism. The peak incidence is between 6 and 14 years. Patients often present with headache,

visual changes, short stature, diabetes insipidus, and hypothyroidism. In addition to gonadotropin deficiency, there may be deficiency in thyroid-stimulating hormone (TSH), adrenocorticotropic hormone (ACTH), growth hormone (GH), and vasopressin. Computed tomography (CT) or magnetic resonance imaging (MRI) is useful for diagnosis. Surgical excision is typically required, and postoperative radiation therapy is often needed due to incomplete tumor resection. Other rare central nervous system tumors associated with sexual infantilism and primary amenorrhea include germinomas, astrocytomas, and hypothalamic or optic gliomas occurring independently or in conjunction with neurofibromatosis.

Functional gonadotropin deficiency, typically associated with secondary amenorrhea, may be associated with primary amenorrhea when there is severe systemic or chronic disease, malnutrition, hypothyroidism, anorexia nervosa, and extreme exercise or psychogenic stress. Weight loss to less than 85% of ideal weight for height due to chronic disease or dieting is associated with gonadotropin deficiency. Chronic renal disease in childhood may be associated with sexual infantilism, although normal gonadotropin secretion ensues after kidney transplant. A delay in puberty and subsequent menarche may be noted in patients with hypothyroidism; treatment with thyroxine can initiate puberty. Patients with anorexia nervosa may present with primary amenorrhea and sexual infantilism or delayed puberty in association with suppressed GnRH pulsatility and other neuroendocrine derangements. Psychotherapy, behavioral modification, and dietary modification are the mainstays of therapy. Exercise, particularly vigorous training starting before puberty, such as gymnastics and ballet dancing, may also be associated with low gonadotropin levels and primary amenorrhea or delayed sexual development. The underlying cause is unclear but may involve body composition and changes in neuroendocrine signals from the brain that promote fuel mobilization, redistribution, and utilization. Counseling concerning the risks of excessive exercise and assurance of adequate caloric intake is advisable.

Congenital Genital Ambiguity

The patient with congenital genital ambiguity often attracts medical attention at the time of birth. However, if the ambiguity is subtle, he or she may not be seen until a later age when parental concern, signs of an enzyme deficiency, if present, or amenorrhea brings the patient to a physician. Thus, a careful history of events surrounding delivery and subsequent pediatric examinations, as well as a detailed genital examination, is important. If a patient with primary amenorrhea is placed in the category of congenital genital ambiguity, a disorder of fetal endocrinology is likely: either incomplete masculinization of a male fetus or virilization of a female fetus in utero (Figure 2). If a uterus is present the karyotype differentiates between an XX individual with a probable enzyme deficiency and some variant of gonadal dysgenesis or true hermaphroditism (coexistence of ovarian and testicular tissue). Patients with an XX karyotype may be further categorized according to 17-hydroxyprogesterone levels. An elevated 17-hydroxyprogesterone level indicates congenital adrenal hyperplasia, most commonly due to 21-hydroxylase deficiency. In patients with a normal 17-hydroxyprogesterone level, genital ambiguity may be due to in utero exposure to maternal androgens or a variant of gonadal dysgenesis. In patients with an absent uterus and an XY karyotype, incomplete virilization due to androgen resistance such as testicular feminization is a possible cause. Testosterone enzyme defects and embryonic testicular regression are also possibilities.

Acquired Hirsutism and Virilization

Primary amenorrhea associated with acquired hirsutism or virilization, various degrees of genital and breast maturation, but no genital ambiguity is an infrequent yet important presentation of primary amenorrhea as it raises the possibility of a dysgenetic gonadal tumor. The karyotype differentiates between women with a likely dysgenetic gonadal tumor and those with either Cushing's syndrome or an ovarian or adrenal cause (Figure 3).

Incomplete Puberty

Patients with incomplete puberty are characterized by primary amenorrhea in a setting of normal secondary sexual characteristics (Figure 4). These patients can be divided into two categories: those with a müllerian abnormality (i.e., the absence of a normal female reproductive tract) and those with a normal uterus and vagina. In patients with an abnormal female reproductive tract, disorders of vertical fusion resulting in vaginal abnormalities but a normal uterus give rise to a transverse vaginal septum. If the septum is at the introitus, it is called an imperforate hymen. These are obstructive lesions due to a lack of normal vertical fusion of the downgrowing

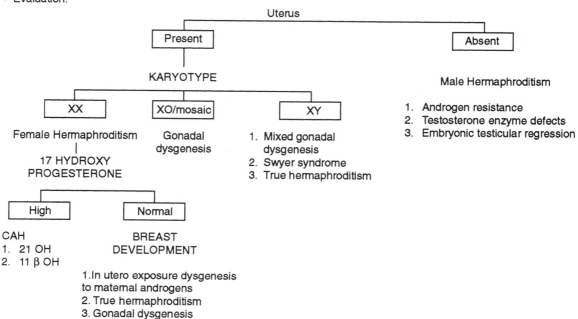

- Characterized by abnormal androgen representation in utero
- Two possible problems:
  1) Incomplete masculinization of male fetus
  2) Virilization of female fetus
- Evaluation:

Figure 2. Congenital genital ambiguity. *Abbreviation*: CAH = congenital adrenal hyperplasia.

- Characterized by primary amenorrhea in a setting of varying degrees of genital and breast maturation, no genital ambiguity, but acquired hirsutism or virilization.
- Evaluation:

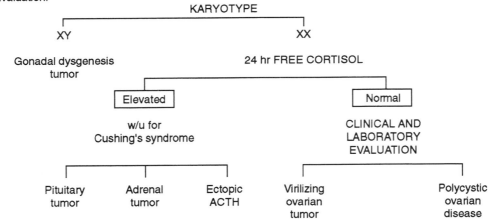

Figure 3. Acquired hirsutism or virilization. *Abbreviations*: w/u = work-up; ACTH = adrenocorticotropic hormone.

müllerian duct and upgrowing urogenital sinus during embryogenesis. Clinical presentation of these patients includes primary amenorrhea, cyclic lower abdominal pain, and often a vaginal mass due to hematocolpos. Defects in vertical fusion may occur anywhere along the vagina. Correction of the problem involves excision of the septum.

In patients with an absent uterus, müllerian agenesis (Mayer-Rokitansky-Kuster-Hauser syndrome) or testicular feminization syndrome may be the cause of primary amenorrhea. Müllerian agenesis is the second most common cause of primary amenorrhea.

These patients have a normal 46,XX karyotype but lack a uterus and vagina. Ultrasound or MRI may be used to confirm the diagnosis. An intravenous urogram is indicated for evaluation because of the high incidence of renal anomalies (15 to 40%). Ovarian function is normal in these women, but they are unable to carry a pregnancy because of the absence of a uterus. Ovarian stimulation, oocyte retrieval, fertilization in vitro, and transfer of embryos to a volunteer surrogate with a uterus are possible means of having a genetic offspring. A vagina can be created surgically or through progressive dilation of

- Characterized by primary amenorrhea in a setting of genital and breast maturation and no genital ambiguity
- Can be conveniently divided into two categories: those with an associated abnormality of the uterus and /or vagina and those with a normal uterus and vagina.
- Evaluation:

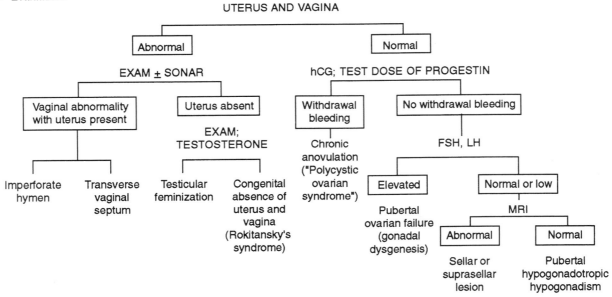

Figure 4. Incomplete puberty. *Abbreviations*: hCG = human chorionic gonadotropin; FSH = follicle-stimulating hormone; LH = luteinizing hormone; MRI = magnetic resonance imaging.

the blind-ending vaginal pouch or dimple on the perineum. Patients often require extensive teaching and training concerning sexual functioning and their inability to carry a pregnancy.

Testicular feminization, or androgen resistance syndrome, is also characterized by primary amenorrhea, an absent uterus, a blind-ending vaginal pouch, and a 46,XY karyotype. Although these patients have normal breast development, pubic and axillary hair are scant. This disorder, either X-linked recessive or X-linked dominant, is due to a defect in the androgen receptor. In patients who present with an inguinal hernia and primary amenorrhea, complete androgen resistance should be suspected. These patients may be differentiated clinically from those with müllerian agenesis because of their paucity of pubic and axillary hair. An elevated serum testosterone level confirms the diagnosis. Breast development in these women probably results from a lack of suppression of breast tissue anlage by testosterone during fetal life, stimulation of breast tissue by estrogens derived from direct testicular secretion, and peripheral aromatization of testosterone to estrogens. Bilateral gonadectomy is essential after breast development because of the increased risk of malignancy in inguinal and abdominal testes.

Evaluation of women with a normal reproductive tract and primary amenorrhea is similar to the evaluation of those with secondary amenorrhea. Once pregnancy has been eliminated as an explanation, a progestin (e.g., 10 mg of medroxyprogesterone acetate for 5 to 10 days) may be given as a clinically useful (though not perfect) test to differentiate those with normal estrogen levels from those with hypoestrogenism. Estrogen priming of the endometrium is required before progestin-induced withdrawal bleeding. In general, if withdrawal bleeding ensues, chronic anovulation or polycystic ovarian syndrome is the most likely cause of the amenorrhea. Clinical presentation includes primary amenorrhea or perimenarchal oligoamenorrhea, and commonly hirsutism as well as obesity. In adolescent patients, low-dose oral contraceptives containing 30 to 35 µg of ethinyl estradiol may be prescribed to initiate and maintain cyclic menses. When fertility becomes desirable, ovulation can usually be induced with clomiphene citrate.

In patients with no withdrawal bleeding in response to a progestin challenge, the serum FSH level should be measured. An elevated FSH level indicates pubertal ovarian failure or gonadal dysgenesis. Patients with gonadal dysgenesis who have some secondary sexual development are usually mosaics, i.e., 45 XO/XX. Treatment is as outlined above, i.e., estrogen-progestin therapy. If gonadotropin levels are normal or low, an MRI is indicated to investigate the possibility of a sellar or suprasellar lesion such as craniopharyngioma or germinoma. A normal MRI suggests pubertal hypogonadotropic hypogonadism. Further evaluation and management follow guidelines as previously outlined under sexual infantilism.

SECONDARY AMENORRHEA

Women with secondary amenorrhea (Figure 5) should be evaluated for physiologic causes including pregnancy, lactation, and premature menopause. Once these causes have been excluded, the possibility of hyperprolactinemia should be assessed. A progestin challenge test is sometimes used in women with secondary amenorrhea to differentiate between those with normal and those with low estrogen levels, although a clinical history and physical examination can generally accomplish the same goal.

Acquired abnormalities of the outflow tract associated with normal estrogen levels and secondary amenorrhea, assessed by the lack of withdrawal bleeding and/or physical examination, include Asherman's syndrome and rarely cervical stenosis. Women with Asherman's syndrome or intrauterine adhesions have either amenorrhea or hypomenorrhea. Most patients give a history of dilation and curettage, or of previous uterine surgery such as metroplasty, myomectomy, or cesarean section. Se-

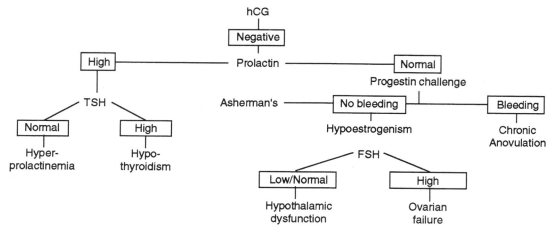

Figure 5. Secondary amenorrhea. *Abbreviations*: hCG = human chorionic gonadotropin; TSH = thyroid-stimulating hormone; FSH = follicle-stimulating hormone.

vere pelvic infections such as tuberculosis or schistosomiasis are rare causes of Asherman's syndrome. Diagnosis by hysterosalpingogram reveals multiple filling defects or, less commonly, obliteration of the uterine cavity. Hysteroscopic lysis of intrauterine adhesions is the preferred method of treatment, after which 90% of patients resuming normal menses. Cervical stenosis can be a cause of secondary amenorrhea due to a surgical procedure such as conization for cervical neoplasia.

Prolactin, the primary hormone controlling lactation, is secreted by the lactotrophs of the anterior pituitary and is under inhibition by dopaminergic neurons in the hypothalamus. An elevated prolactin level in nonpregnant women is a common cause of secondary amenorrhea. Many conditions are associated with abnormal prolactin secretion, including breast examination; stress; decreased oral intake; a host of medications such as estrogens, antidopaminergic drugs, and opioids; prolactinomas; and destructive lesions of the hypothalamus. Hyperprolactinemia may also be associated with chronic renal failure, hypothyroidism and ectopic production by bronchogenic tumors.

Women presenting with secondary amenorrhea should have an assessment of the serum prolactin concentration regardless of the presence or absence of galactorrhea, as about one-third of women with hyperprolactinemia do not have galactorrhea. Because of the myriad causes of an elevated prolactin level (>20 ng per mL), a second blood test should be done to confirm the diagnosis, preferably midmorning in the fasting state. The TSH level should be measured to investigate the possibility of primary hypothyroidism as a cause of amenorrhea and galactorrhea due to stimulation of the lactotrophs by excess thyrotropin-releasing hormone (TRH) secretion. Hyperprolactinemia in the face of a normal TSH level might prompt evaluation of the pituitary by MRI or CT. Even mild elevations of prolactin levels may be associated with pituitary adenomas, although the natural history of microadenomas (i.e., <1 cm) is typically benign. With or without an adenoma, the amenorrhea should be treated, as hypoestrogenism increases the risk of osteoporosis. A dopamine agonist, such as bromocriptine (Parlodel), 2.5 mg per day with increasing increments of 2.5 mg at 2-week intervals if necessary, should normalize the prolactin level with the resumption of regular cyclic menses. Bromocriptine treatment should be initiated at night to avoid postural hypotension. Patients unable to tolerate oral bromocriptine because of gastrointestinal side effects may take it intravaginally. Women who become pregnant during bromocriptine treatment may discontinue its use once pregnancy is diagnosed although it is not associated with an increased risk of fetal malformations. Patients in whom medical management fails, particularly those with macroadenomas, may require surgical intervention or rarely radiation therapy.

Women who respond to a progestin challenge with withdrawal bleeding may be classified as having chronic anovulation with estrogen present. Polycystic ovarian syndrome is the most common cause of secondary amenorrhea in this setting. Women frequently present with chronic anovulation beginning at menarche, with evidence of androgen excess. Hyperinsulinemia is common. Obesity is stereotypic but is not a necessary characteristic. Treatment depends on the reproductive goals of the patient. If pregnancy is not desired, low-dose oral contraceptives may be prescribed. Patients desiring fertility usually ovulate in response to clomiphene citrate (Clomid, Serophene) 50 mg administered daily from days 3 to 7 or 5 to 9 of the menstrual cycle. Dosage may be increased by increments of 50 mg up to 200 mg per day; approximately 75 to 80% of patients ovulate. In those who do not respond to clomiphene, gonadotropins or laparoscopic ovarian drilling may be used.

Other rare causes of secondary amenorrhea with normal estrogen levels are thyroid disorders, adult-onset adrenal hyperplasia, Cushing's disease, and ovarian and adrenal tumors.

Women with a normal outflow tract who do not respond with withdrawal bleeding after a progestin challenge are hypoestrogenic. Determining gonadotropin levels allows further subclassification. Those with FSH levels greater than 30 mIU per mL have hypergonadotropic hypogonadism or gonadal failure, whereas those with low or normal values have hypothalamic-pituitary dysfunction secondary to weight loss, stress, exercise, anorexia nervosa, hypothalamic or pituitary tumors, and isolated gonadotropin deficiency. As noted above, these causes may also be associated with primary amenorrhea. In hypothalamic amenorrhea, suppression of GnRH secretion is responsible for low or decreased gonadotropin levels and resultant hypoestrogenism. Counseling often corrects the disorder, with the resumption of menstrual cyclicity. However, in those with persistent amenorrhea, the administration of pulsatile GnRH or of gonadotropins may be utilized for ovulation induction if pregnancy is desired. Oral contraceptives or estrogen-progestin treatment is indicated to maintain normal bone density in women not interested in fertility. Exercise amenorrhea is similarly the result of reduced GnRH pulse frequency. Reduction in the amount of exercise often corrects the amenorrhea. However, pulsatile GnRH or gonadotropin therapy may also be necessary for ovulation induction. Hormone replacement therapy to prevent bone loss is indicated if the patient declines to alter her exercise program. Simple weight loss in anorexia nervosa does not explain the amenorrhea in these patients. An absent or diminished luteinizing hormone (LH) response to GnRH has been a consistent finding. Psychiatric counseling is necessary because of the potential life-threatening nature of this disorder. Hormone replacement therapy should be administered until sufficient weight gain allows a return of cyclic menses.

Women with hypergonadotropic hypergonadism include some patients with gonadal dysgenesis who may menstruate for a variable amount of time before ovarian failure. A woman who presents with secondary amenorrhea before the age of 30 years should have a karyotype obtained to rule out the presence of a Y chromosome because of the risk of gonadal malignancy. Treatment should be aimed at correcting the hypoestrogenism with hormone replacement or oral contraceptives. Most women with gonadal dysgenesis are infertile, although pregnancies have been reported in women with 46,XX/45,XO karyotype. Normal pregnancy and delivery may be accomplished with donor eggs, in vitro fertilization, endometrial synchronization, and early support of the pregnancy with exogenous estrogen and progesterone.

Amenorrhea and elevated gonadotropin levels in a woman before the age of 40 years are considered premature ovarian failure. Causes include ovarian failure secondary to chemotherapy, pelvic irradiation, and ovarian surgery as well as genetic or autoimmune causes. In the transition to ovarian failure, follicular depletion may not be complete, and spontaneous ovulation and pregnancy may occasionally occur. A karyotype and thyroid and adrenal evaluation including specific endocrine antibody testing should be performed. Complications of estrogen deficiency may be prevented by hormone replacement therapy. In those desiring pregnancy, donor oocytes with synchronization of the endometrium have resulted in pregnancy rates of 30 to 50%.

DYSMENORRHEA

method of
SAMANTHA M. PFEIFER, M.D.
University of Pennsylvania
Philadelphia, Pennsylvania

"Dysmenorrhea" refers to painful menstruation and can be classified as primary or secondary, based on the cause. In primary dysmenorrhea, there is no detectable pelvic pathology, whereas secondary dysmenorrhea is caused by other disease processes or conditions. Primary dysmenorrhea occurs more frequently in women in their late teens and early twenties. The initial onset occurs at least 6 months to 1 year after menarche, coinciding with the onset of ovulation. The symptoms tend to improve with age and parity. Smoking has been associated with more severe symptoms. The incidence of primary dysmenorrhea is difficult to quantify but is in the range of 50 to 70%. In the United States, the incidence reported among adolescents is 60%. As many as 5 to 14% of women regularly miss work or school because of this condition.

The predominant symptom of primary dysmenorrhea is recurrent, sharp, crampy, and spasmodic lower abdominal pain. It usually begins within hours of the onset of menstrual flow and may last 1 to 3 days. The pain is located in the suprapubic area and may radiate to the lower back, sacrum, or upper thigh. Nausea, vomiting, diarrhea, or a combination of these symptoms may also be present. The pain is similar during each menstrual cycle, and the patient is able to predict the course. Primary dysmenorrhea is not associated with prodromal symptoms, as can occur with premenstrual syndrome or some causes of secondary dysmenorrhea. The diagnosis of primary dysmenorrhea is made by careful history and physical examination. The history reveals predictable pain symptoms that began shortly after menarche. Primary dysmenorrhea is rarely seen in a woman who has had years of relatively painless menses. The physical examination should be completely normal. Specifically, a normal mobile uterus, normal-sized adnexa, and normal cervix and vagina should be visualized and/or palpated on pelvic examination. A rectovaginal examination is an important part of this assessment. At the time of symptoms, the abdomen should be nontender.

In obtaining the history and performing the physical examination, it is important to keep in mind and exclude the multiple causes of secondary dysmenorrhea to ensure the correct diagnosis. Important causes of secondary dysmenorrhea include mullerian anomalies such as imperforate hymen, vaginal septum, and blind uterine horn (communicating or noncommunicating). These patients usually present at a similar time as patients with primary dysmenorrhea but should be distinguished by an abnormal pelvic examination. Endometriosis can present as progressive dysmenorrhea and infertility. Although the examination may be normal, associated physical findings typically include a fixed uterus and adnexa, focal persistent tenderness, and uterosacral nodularity detected on rectovaginal examination. Adenomyosis typically affects older patients and is associated with menorrhagia and a "boggy" uterus. Uterine myomas may be associated with menorrhagia, and an enlarged, irregular uterus is usually present. Intrauterine (submucous) myomas or polyps are more often associated with menorrhagia than dysmenorrhea and are often present with a normal-sized uterus. Cervical stenosis can present as dysmenorrhea but is also associated with absent or scant menses. Pelvic inflammatory disease can also be associated with dysmenorrhea but is usually associated with other symptoms.

Imaging studies are not beneficial in diagnosing primary dysmenorrhea but can exclude other pelvic pathology that may cause secondary dysmenorrhea. Pelvic ultrasonography is useful in the detection of uterine myomas and adnexal pathology, and magnetic resonance imaging (MRI) is excellent for distinguishing mullerian anomalies. Computed tomography (CT) is usually not helpful in defining pelvic pathology. If the pelvic examination is inadequate due to body habitus or patient compliance or if an abnormality is detected, an ultrasound or possibly an MRI may be indicated. In patients believed to have primary dysmenorrhea, laparoscopy should be reserved for only those who fail an adequate trial of medical therapy and is indicated to exclude the presence of pathology causing secondary dysmenorrhea.

PATHOPHYSIOLOGY

Prostaglandins are responsible for the severe uterine contractions observed in patients with dysmenorrhea. Prostaglandins are synthesized in the endometrium in response to the fall in progesterone that takes place at the end of a nonpregnant ovulatory cycle. The mechanism is as follows: Phospholipids from the sloughing endometrium are converted to arachidonic acid by the enzyme phospholipase A_2. Arachidonic acid can then be metabolized by two different pathways: (1) by cyclooxygenase to ultimately produce prostaglandins PGE_2, PGF_{2a}, PGD_2, and prostacyclin, or (2) by lipoxygenase to produce leukotrienes. All these end products are thought to be involved in producing dysmenorrhea, but the prostaglandins are the most important.

Patients with dysmenorrhea have been shown to have significantly higher levels of prostaglandins in the endometrium and menstrual fluid compared with patients without dysmenorrhea. This suggests that overproduction of prostaglandins, rather than an increased sensitivity, is responsible for the observed symptoms. Further evidence supporting prostaglandins as the mediators of dysmenorrhea is the success of prostaglandin synthetase inhibitors in relieving symptoms in these patients.

Excessive uterine contractions induced by prostaglandins, predominantly $PGF_{2\alpha}$, are widely recognized as being responsible for dysmenorrhea. By placing a pressure sensor within the uterus, asymptomatic menstruating women have been shown to have contractions of 50 to 80 mmHg lasting 15 seconds. In contrast, patients with dysmenorrhea experience contractions in excess of 400 mmHg lasting greater than 90 seconds. These excessive contractions may lead to decreased uterine perfusion, with resulting hypoxia, ischemia, and pain. Other proposed factors include prostaglandin-induced hypersensitivity of pain receptors, direct vasoconstriction caused by elevated levels of leukotrienes (known potent vasoconstrictors), and additional stimulation of uterine contractions by vasopressin.

TREATMENT

The most common treatment for primary dysmenorrhea consists of nonsteroidal anti-inflammatory drugs (NSAIDs) and oral contraceptives. The NSAIDs work by inhibiting the synthesis of prostaglandins. The most effective NSAIDs for the treatment of dysmenorrhea are those that inhibit the breakdown of arachidonic acid by the enzyme cyclooxygenase. These are the propionic acid derivatives (naproxen, naproxen sodium, ketoprofen, flurbiprofen), the acetic acid derivatives (indomethacin, ketorolac, diclofenac), and the fenamates. The commonly used agents are listed in Table 1.

Many studies have evaluated the success of nonsteroidal drugs in treating primary dysmenorrhea and

have found significant relief of symptoms in 80% of patients. All the drugs appear to be equally effective compared with placebo, but no clear advantage of one drug over the others has consistently been found. An individual's response to one particular drug may be variable. Therefore, it is important to try two or three different agents, preferably from different classes, before concluding that the therapy is ineffective.

The drugs are most effective when started at the onset of symptoms and taken continuously for the expected duration of symptoms. Taking the drugs on an "as needed" basis or prophylactically has not been found to be as effective. The drugs should not be taken for longer than 5 days to avoid side effects. Since no drug is superior to another, the first drug tried is a matter of patient or physician preference or convenience.

Oral contraceptives are also very effective in the treatment of primary dysmenorrhea and are the treatment of choice for those patients who also desire contraception. These agents work by inhibiting ovulation and decreasing the amount of endometrial tissue produced in a given cycle. In this way, fewer prostaglandins are produced and the amount of menstrual bleeding is decreased, thereby reducing the factors responsible for dysmenorrhea.

The combined oral contraceptive is effective in the treatment of primary dysmenorrhea in 90% of patients. Monophasic pills may be more effective than triphasic pills. Relief of symptoms is usually noted within the first few cycles. If symptoms persist, a nonsteroidal agent should be added. These drugs work by different mechanisms and complement each other. There are no adverse interactions.

Progestin-only contraceptives may be useful in relieving symptoms of primary dysmenorrhea in patients who are unable to tolerate combined oral contraceptives. Medroxyprogesterone acetate (Depo-Provera) and the progestin-only pill are effective because, in addition to producing an atrophic endometrium, these agents successfully inhibit ovulation. Implantable progestins, such as levonorgestrel (Norplant), do not reliably inhibit ovulation and therefore are not as effective.

In general, a 6-month trial of nonsteroidal drugs and/or oral contraceptives is recommended. If there is little or no response, the diagnosis of primary dysmenorrhea should be questioned, even in light of a normal history and examination. Causes of secondary dysmenorrhea should be investigated. A laparoscopy at this point should be considered to investigate causes of secondary dysmenorrhea, such as endometriosis, even in women in their late teens or early twenties. In this way, the appropriate therapy can be instituted.

Treatment of women with proven primary dysmenorrhea that is resistant to traditional therapy has included the use of beta agonists and calcium channel blockers to decrease uterine activity. Transcutaneous electric nerve stimulation (TENS) in combination with nonsteroidal drugs has also been reported to be effective. Surgical ablation of uterosacral or

TABLE 1. **Prostaglandin Synthetase Inhibitors**

Drug	Brand Name	Dosage
Phenylpropionic acid derivatives		
Ibuprofen	Motrin, Advil, Nuprin, Rufen	400–600 mg q 6 h
Naproxen	Naprosyn	250–500 mg q 6 h
Naproxen sodium	Anaprox	275–550 mg q 6 h
Ketoprofen	Orudis	50 mg q 8 h
Flurbiprofen*	Ansaid	50 mg q 6 h
Acetic acid derivatives		
Indomethacin	Indocin	25–50 mg q 6 h
Ketorolac tromethamine	Toradol	10 mg q 6 h
Diclofenac potassium	Cataflam	50 mg q 8 h
Fenamates		
Mefenamic acid	Ponstel	250–500 mg q 6 h
Meclofenamate sodium*	Meclomen	50–100 mg q 6 h
Oxicams		
Piroxicam*	Feldene	20–40 mg/day

*Commonly used but not specifically labeled by the FDA for treatment of dysmenorrhea.

presacral nerves should be considered only in those women with incapacitating symptoms refractory to all other treatments. These nontraditional therapies should be undertaken only in extreme cases and only after careful consideration.

PREMENSTRUAL SYNDROME

method of
JOSEPH F. MORTOLA, M.D.
Harvard Medical School
Boston, Massachusetts

Recent advances in elucidating the pathophysiology of premenstrual syndrome (PMS) have permitted the development of sound pharmacologic interventions for this previously treatment-resistant disorder. The earlier high failure rates of medical therapy for PMS can largely be attributed to improper diagnosis of the syndrome, overinclusion of patients with poorly characterized symptoms in controlled clinical trials, and underutilization of rigorous experimental methodology in studies of the efficacy of various therapies. Although there are presently no medications approved by the U.S. Food and Drug Administration (FDA) for the treatment of PMS, extensive well-designed studies have been conducted that can guide the clinician's treatment of the disorder. As a result, less proven nonpharmacologic modalities such as dietary modification, exercise regimens and psychotherapy are more quickly supplanted by the use of medication. Prior to initiation of treatment, however, accurate diagnosis is required, particularly since PMS often mimics other disorders, including depression, anxiety disorders, and thyroid disease.

DIAGNOSIS

The prevalence of PMS is estimated to be 2.5% of women of reproductive age. Although prevalence rates of up to 80% have been reported, this is attributable to the inclusion of a large number of women with normal premenstrual symptoms, referred to as molimina, in the PMS population. Currently, diagnostic criteria are available that permit a more accurate assessment of women in need of medical intervention because of disabling disruption of social, vocational, and avocational performance (Table 1). Even with such strict diagnostic criteria, however, PMS is among the most common disorders in reproductive-age women.

Although more than 150 symptoms have been ascribed to PMS, careful statistical analysis in well-selected populations reveals the symptom constellation to be much more specific and well defined. Only a select group of symptoms occurs selectively in the luteal phase of the menstrual cycle with sufficient frequency to merit inclusion in the syndrome. The most common of these symptoms are fatigue (92% of women with PMS), irritability (91%), depression (85%), breast tenderness, and bloated sensations in the abdomen or extremities. Appetite disturbance restricted to the luteal phase of the cycle is seen in 75% of women with PMS and is usually experienced as increased food cravings, particularly for carbohydrates. The other frequently noted behavioral symptoms include mood lability with alternating sadness and anger (81%), oversensitivity to trivial environmental events (69%), crying spells (65%), social withdrawal (65%), and difficulty concentrat-

TABLE 1. Diagnostic Criteria for Premenstrual Syndrome

1. Presence of self-report of at least one of the following somatic *and* affective symptoms during the 5 days prior to menses in each of the three prior menstrual cycles:

Affective	**Somatic**
Depression	Breast tenderness
Angry outbursts	Abdominal bloating
Irritability	Headache
Anxiety	Swelling
Confusion	
Social withdrawal	

2. Relief of the above symptoms within 4 days of the onset of menses, without recurrence until at least cycle day 12.
3. Presence of the symptoms in the absence of any pharmacologic therapy, hormone ingestion, or drug or alcohol use.
4. Reproducibility of the symptoms during two cycles of prospective recording.
5. Presence of identifiable dysfunction in social or economic performance by one of the following criteria:
   Marital or relationship discord confirmed by partner
   Difficulties in parenting
   Poor work or school performance; poor attendance or tardiness
   Increased social isolation
   Legal difficulties
   Suicidal ideation
   Seeking medical attention for somatic symptoms

From Mortola JF, Girton L, Beck L, et al: Depressive episodes in premenstrual syndrome. Am J Obstet Gynecol *161*:1682, 1984.

ing (47%). Common physical symptoms also include acne (71%) and gastrointestinal upset (48%). Although less often observed, vasomotor flushes (18%), heart palpitations (13%), and dizziness (13%) occur more frequently in women with PMS than in women who do not suffer from the syndrome.

None of the symptoms of PMS is unique to the disorder, and even presentation of the entire constellation of symptoms is less important in establishing the diagnosis than is the timing of the symptoms' occurrence with respect to the menstrual cycle. From the fourth day of menses until at least cycle day 12, symptoms, if they occur at all, are sporadic and no more common than would be expected in the general population. This criterion for the relatively symptom-free interval is applicable to most reproductive-age women, although women with menstrual cycles that are typically shorter than 26 days may have the onset of symptoms slightly earlier than day 12. The importance of prospectively documenting symptoms in establishing the diagnosis of PMS has been demonstrated in numerous studies. Validated symptom inventories such as the Calendar of Premenstrual Experiences (University of California, San Diego) are the most reliable methods of establishing the diagnosis (Figure 1). Prospective recording over the course of two menstrual cycles is optimal in order to assure reproducibility in the timing of symptoms. Scores on such inventories should reveal at least a twofold increase in total symptom severity during the last week of the menstrual cycle as compared with the second week.

In addition to the type of symptoms and their timing, several other criteria should be fulfilled in order to accurately diagnose PMS. These include the identifiable presence of socioeconomic difficulties and the absence of pharmacologic therapy with hormonal agents such as oral contraceptives.

Name _____ Month/Year _____ Age _____ Unit # _____

Begin your calendar on the *first* day of your menstrual cycle. Enter the calendar date below the cycle day. Day **1** is your *first* day of bleeding. Shade the box above the cycle day if you have bleeding. ■ Put an **X** for spotting. ☒

If more than one symptom is listed in a category, i.e., nausea, diarrhea, constipation, you do not need to experience all of these. Rate the most disturbing of the symptoms on the 1-3 scale.

Weight: Weigh yourself before breakfast. Record weight in the box below date.
Symptoms: Indicate the severity of your symptoms by using the scale below. Rate each symptom at about the same time each evening.

     0 = **None** (symptom not present)   2 = **Moderate** (interferes with normal activities)

     1 = **Mild** (noticeable but not troublesome)   3 = **Severe** (intolerable, unable to perform normal activities)

Other Symptoms: If there are other symptoms you experience, list and indicate severity.
Medications: List any medications taken. Put an **X** on the corresponding day(s).

	Cycle Day	1	2	3	4	5	6	7	8	9	10	11	12	13	14	15	16	17	18	19	20	21	22	23	24	25	26	27	28	29	30	31	32	33	34	35	36	37	38	39	40
Bleeding																																									
Date																																									
Weight																																									
SYMPTOMS																																									
Acne																																									
Bloatedness																																									
Breast tenderness																																									
Dizziness																																									
Fatigue																																									
Headache																																									
Hot flashes																																									
Nausea, diarrhea, constipation																																									
Palpitations																																									
Swelling (hands, ankles, breast)																																									
Angry outbursts, arguments, violent tendencies																																									
Anxiety, tension, nervousness																																									
Confusion, difficulty concentrating																																									
Crying easily																																									
Depression																																									
Food cravings (sweets, salts)																																									
Forgetfulness																																									
Irritability																																									
Increased appetite																																									
Mood swings																																									
Overly sensitive																																									
Wish to be alone																																									
Other Symptoms 1. ____																																									
2. ____																																									
Medications 1. ____																																									
2. ____																																									

Figure 1. Calendar of Premenstrual Experiences (COPE). (© University of California, San Diego; Department of Reproductive Medicine, Division of Reproductive Endocrinology.)

DIFFERENTIAL DIAGNOSIS

The differential diagnosis of PMS includes a rather large number of medical and psychiatric disorders. Fortunately, the majority of these can be easily excluded by use of a prospective symptom calendar, history and physical examination, and simple laboratory investigation. In a study of 263 women presenting with the complaint of PMS, the use of oral contraceptives was found to confound the diagnosis in 10.6%. Early menopause was found in 10.2%. The most common disorders were depression and anxiety disorders, which were observed in 30.5%. These were easily identified by the absence of a symptom-free interval by either self-reporting or on prospective recording. Eating disorders were observed in 5.3%, and substance abuse disorders in 3.8%. Medical conditions, the most common of which were diabetes and thyroid disease, were found in 8.6%. Menstrual cycle irregularities were obtained by history in 16.6%. Because of the medical conditions and perimenopausal conditions that may present as PMS, laboratory evaluation should include serum glucose, thyroid-stimulating hormone, and follicle-stimulating hormone.

PATHOPHYSIOLOGY

PMS is a psychoneuroendocrine disorder that has recently been the subject of considerable scientific investigation. There is extensive evidence that the pathophysiologic basis of PMS is primarily the result of changes in central nervous system neurotransmitter economy that are induced by cyclical fluctuations in ovarian steroid (estrogen and progesterone) levels. There is currently a basis for implicating adrenergic, opioid, gamma-aminobutyric acid (GABA), and serotonin systems in the behavioral manifestations as well as the physical manifestations of PMS. Each of these neurotransmitter systems has been demonstrated to be influenced by estrogen and/or progesterone. The reason that women show different degrees of sensitivity to these ovarian steroid–induced neurotransmitter alterations, however, remains unknown. It is more likely that these differences in susceptibility are biologically endowed than that they are the result of environmental contingencies.

TREATMENT

Selective Serotonin Reuptake Inhibitors

Selective serotonin reuptake inhibitors (SSRIs)* are the first-line pharmacologic intervention for PMS. SSRIs are a novel class of antidepressants that act with relative specificity on the serotonergic system and hence differ from the majority of antidepressants, which have simultaneous effects on several neurotransmitter systems. Unlike SSRIs, classic antidepressants are remarkably ineffective in the treatment of PMS; in fact, they show even less efficacy in some studies than placebo. This is consistent with data that PMS and depression have distinct neuroendocrine manifestations.

Fluoxetine (Prozac) is the SSRI that has been most studied in PMS. It has been demonstrated in independent, double-blind, placebo-controlled studies to have a success rate of 90% in the 85% of patients who can tolerate the medication. This yields an overall

---

*Not FDA-approved for this indication.

response rate of 75%. The clinical demonstration of the efficacy of SSRIs in PMS is supported by the finding of differences in serotonin markers in women with PMS and fluctuations of serotonin levels during the menstrual cycle. The effective dose of fluoxetine is 20 mg daily. It is best taken in the morning, as it is generally an activating drug. In a minority of patients, it is sedating, and these individuals are best treated with an evening or bedtime regimen. Although it is safe to prescribe 60 to 80 mg per day in single or divided doses, the vast majority of patients respond to a 20-mg dose. Widely publicized reports of an increased risk of suicidal or homicidal behavior in patients who are on fluoxetine have been refuted in careful studies. Nonetheless, patient acceptance of the drug continues to be a problem. Reassurance that the earlier reports are unsubstantiated is often required. Recently, a small study suggested that fluoxetine administration in patients with PMS may be limited to the luteal phase. In clinical practice, the medication is started on day 14 of the menstrual cycle and continued until day 2 of the following cycle. This is a desirable method of initiating therapy, since smaller total monthly doses are required. Not infrequently, patients are unable to tolerate a full 20-mg dose of fluoxetine with either luteal-phase-only administration or full-cycle administration. In these patients, doses as small as 5 mg per day should be prescribed initially. Fluoxetine is available in a convenient elixir form for this purpose. In addition to fluoxetine, clinical trials have demonstrated the efficacy of other SSRIs, including sertraline and paroxetine. These are normally used as second-line interventions because of the more extensive clinical information available on fluoxetine.

Approximately 15% of patients taking SSRIs experience side effects of sufficient severity or discomfort to warrant discontinuation of the drug. The most commonly reported side effects are agitation or insomnia, gastrointestinal disturbance and headache, and sexual dysfunction, which may include loss of libido, impotence, and anorgasmia. Each of these occurs with sufficient severity to require discontinuation of treatment in approximately 5% of patients. A larger percentage of patients experiences these symptoms to lesser degrees.

The most commonly observed side effect of SSRIs is headache. This occurs in up to 20% of patients. Often the headaches resolve during the first 2 weeks of therapy. A variety of gastrointestinal complaints have been noted in up to 15% of patients on fluoxetine. These most commonly include nausea and diarrhea. Approximately 9% of patients on fluoxetine report marked anorexia. In patients with PMS, this has not been noted to a degree that warrants discontinuation of the drug. Rarely, hematologic disturbances, including anemia and thrombocytopenia, as well as alterations in liver enzymes have been observed in patients on SSRIs. These do not occur with sufficient frequency to mandate routine monitoring of asymptomatic patients.

The incidence of a decline in libido during treatment with SSRIs is reported to be approximately 2% in studies of depressed patients. However, this may be falsely low due to the already decreased libido that usually accompanies depression. In nondepressed patients, it appears that decreased libido is more commonly noted, particularly in women with PMS.

Although large doses of SSRIs given to animals have not been associated with birth defects, human studies are lacking. The use of fluoxetine in pregnant or breast-feeding patients should therefore be discouraged. Contraception is recommended for patients with PMS treated with SSRIs.

Benzodiazepines

At least two double-blind studies have demonstrated the efficacy of alprazolam (Xanax)* in the treatment of PMS. The usual dose is 0.25 mg four times a day during the luteal phase of the cycle. Occasionally, higher doses of 0.5 mg up to four times a day are required. Although efficacy has been demonstrated at these doses, clinically, many patients report significant improvement when the medication is taken during the luteal phase on an as-needed basis.

The side effect of greatest concern is alprazolam's addictive potential. This has prompted a number of clinicians to substitute other benzodiazepines for alprazolam in the treatment of PMS. Although there is a sound theoretical rationale to posit that other benzodiazepines may have an efficacy similar to that of alprazolam based on their biochemical similarity, this has not been demonstrated in controlled studies. Moreover, although alprazolam may be more addictive than some other benzodiazepines, all agents in this class carry a substantial risk of addiction. For this reason, the use of benzodiazepines in PMS should be carefully restricted to luteal-phase administration in reliable patients. Addiction to alprazolam has not been reported when restricted to use during this prescribed interval.

Withdrawal symptoms similar to those observed with barbiturates have been noted on discontinuation of alprazolam prescribed on a daily basis. These can range from mild anxiety, dysphoria, and/or insomnia to more severe manifestations of muscle cramps, nausea, perspiration, and tremor. Withdrawal seizures have also been reported. Patients with underlying seizure disorders are not candidates for alprazolam because of the repeated alteration in the seizure threshold induced by the cyclical initiation and discontinuation of the drug.

In addition to addiction, three other side effects of alprazolam are frequently observed. Drowsiness occurs in up to 40% of patients. This symptom sometimes resolves after a period of weeks on the medication. Lowering the dose and using a more frequent dosing schedule are often successful in relieving this side effect. Approximately 5% of individuals on alpra-

zolam have hypotension. Lightheadedness has also been reported in a similar number of individuals. Discontinuation of therapy is less commonly required in individuals experiencing the latter two side effects. A number of more idiosyncratic symptoms have been reported in patients on alprazolam. Among the most disturbing of these is paradoxic agitation. This usually resolves only by stopping the drug.

Administration of alprazolam has not been demonstrated to be safe in pregnancy and has been reported to cause lethargy in the infants of nursing mothers. Women on this agent for PMS should be instructed to use reliable methods of birth control.

GnRH Agonists*

In 1984, Muse and colleagues published the first results demonstrating a dramatic reduction of symptoms in women with PMS using daily injections of a gonadotropin-releasing hormone (GnRH) agonist. Since that time, several other reports using different GnRH agonists have confirmed these results. GnRH agonists cause pituitary desensitization to native GnRH, which is thought to be the result of internalization of the GnRH receptor. Depending on the potency of the agonist, the desensitization phase (termed down-regulation) requires 7 to 21 days. Once down-regulation has been established, it persists for as long as the agonist is administered. During down-regulation, luteinizing hormone (LH) and follicle-stimulating hormone (FSH) secretion by the pituitary is substantially reduced. As a result, there is insufficient stimulation of the ovary for normal sex steroid production. Circulating estrogen levels are therefore in the postmenopausal range, and progesterone levels are similarly low.

The daily subcutaneous injection form of GnRH agonists is cumbersome for the patient. Administration of GnRH analogues may be associated with localized pain and irritation at the injection site. More recently, depot formulations of the compounds have become available. These are administered as monthly intramuscular injections. A nasal spray has also been formulated that is available for two- or three-times-a-day use. Although the nasal spray is less uncomfortable than subcutaneous administration, absorption may be somewhat more erratic, and patient reliability becomes a greater concern.

In women, the side effect profile of GnRH agonists is largely the result of hypoestrogenism. Most women on the medication experience significant hot flashes. These are generally classic postmenopausal hot flashes that last for minutes and tend to be more pronounced on the upper torso and face. The hot flashes tend to be most bothersome at the initiation of the down-regulation phase. In some women, they continue to be highly disturbing, but in others, their perceived severity decreases over weeks to months.

The acute menopausal syndrome includes emotional lability and insomnia in addition to hot

---

*Not FDA-approved for this indication.

*Not FDA-approved for this indication.

flashes. In general, these symptoms tend to be less disturbing than the symptoms of severe PMS.

The long-term use of GnRH analogues is limited by the effects of chronic hypoestrogenism. The most pronounced of these is osteoporosis. As a result, use of GnRH analogues is limited to a period of 6 months unless accompanied by serial bone densitometry to demonstrate maintenance of bone integrity. There is also concern regarding the long-term consequences of negating the putative protective effect of estrogen on cardiovascular disease in women. Large epidemiologic studies are required to quantify this risk. Other symptoms of menopause, although not posing health risks, are also of concern when prescribing GnRH analogues. These include vaginal dryness, an increase in urinary tract symptoms, and a decrease in skin collagen content.

Given the association between breast and gynecologic cancers and ovarian function, there is a potential protective effect of long-term GnRH agonist administration on breast, ovarian, and endometrial carcinoma risk. Proof of this association also awaits large-scale epidemiologic studies.

In order to reverse the potential side effects of GnRH agonist administration, low-dose estrogen and progestin replacement therapy, similar to that used in postmenopausal women, has been advocated. Since almost all the short- and long-term side effects of the therapy are the result of this hypoestrogenism, this approach is based on a sound rationale. There is substantial evidence to suggest that this "add-back" therapy may maintain the majority of the beneficial effects of GnRH agonists on the symptoms of PMS.

TREATMENTS OF UNPROVEN EFFICACY

Progesterone*

Until recently, progesterone given in the form of vaginal or rectal suppositories was widely prescribed for PMS. This was based on uncontrolled studies. Progesterone has now been shown to be no more effective than placebo in treating PMS symptoms. Moreover, there is evidence that both the physical and the emotional symptoms of PMS may be progesterone induced. Thus, administration of progesterone commonly results in increased breast tenderness, bloating of the abdomen and extremities, and emotional lability. The use of progesterone in the treatment of PMS cannot be advocated.

Oral Contraceptives*

The success of treating PMS with oral contraceptive agents has not been consistent. For the most part, the side effects of oral contraceptive agents, including mood effects (particularly depression), water retention, and appetite changes, are precisely those that women with PMS experience. There appears to be a small percentage of women for whom oral contraceptives provide a preferable hormonal milieu to their endogenous estrogen and progesterone. In general, however, these agents are not effective in the treatment of PMS.

Vitamin B₆*

At least one placebo-controlled study of vitamin B_6 in PMS showed efficacy, although other studies failed to replicate these results. The efficacy of vitamin B_6 therapy in the syndrome is therefore controversial. At high doses (>600 mg per day), vitamin B_6 therapy has been associated with peripheral neuropathy. If this therapy is tried in PMS, patients must be cautioned against excess dosages.

Diet and Dietary Supplements

Multiple dietary supplements have been attempted in PMS, including magnesium, linoleic acid in the form of evening primrose oil, and multiple vitamin regimens. None of these has proved effective in treating PMS. Dietary restriction, such as the elimination of caffeine and chocolate, has not been demonstrated to be effective in PMS either.

DRUGS USED FOR SPECIFIC INDICATIONS

Premenstrual Migraines and Danazol

Although several reports have indicated the efficacy of danazol (Danocrine)* in PMS, since the advent of GnRH analogues, its use has been largely restricted to the treatment of premenstrual migraines. Danazol is a derivative of the synthetic androgen 17-alpha-ethinyl testosterone. As such, it possesses significant androgenic properties. Administration of danazol results in amenorrhea in a majority of women. The objective of therapy is to obtain the beneficial effects that occur secondary to this amenorrhea. The usual dose is 600 to 800 mg per day in divided doses. The side effect profile of danazol is considerable and is the result of both its androgenic activity and its antiestrogen properties. Acne and weight gain are commonly reported. Decreased breast size is a particularly disturbing complaint for many women. More rarely, overtly masculinizing side effects are noted, including deepening of the voice and clitoromegaly. Fluid retention on danazol therapy is particularly disturbing to women with PMS.

The antiestrogenic side effects, although better tolerated by most women than the androgen effects, can be quite bothersome. These are the same side effects observed with GnRH analogues and include hot flashes, vaginal dryness, and emotional lability. Although the osteoporosis that accompanies GnRH agonist therapy is less of a concern with danazol, the effects on lipid profiles are more worrisome. This is due to the combined adverse effects of hypoestrogenism and hyperandrogenism. For this reason, the use of danazol should be accompanied by monitoring of lipid profiles.

Danazol is contraindicated during pregnancy because of in utero female pseudohermaphroditism. There have also been reports of hepatotoxicity, manifested by increased liver function tests, while on danazol. Therefore, liver function studies should be monitored periodically in patients taking this drug. Taken together, approximately 80% of women on danazol experience side effects.

Based on the risk/benefit ratio, danazol is a poor choice for most patients with PMS. Overall, it is less efficacious and has many more side effects than GnRH analogues. Danazol may be somewhat more effective, however, in treating premenstrual migraines than are GnRH analogues. But because there are conventional, effective antimigraine medications with fewer side effects than danazol, danazol should not be considered a first-line agent even in premenstrual migraines.

Water Retention and Diuretics

Of the diuretics that have been used in PMS, spironolactone (Aldactone) has achieved the greatest popularity. This is largely the result of specific properties of this agent that are uniquely suited to hormonally based disorders. Spironolactone is an aldosterone inhibitor. As such, it shares considerable structural similarity with steroid hormones. Because of its steroidal properties and diuretic effects, spironolactone showed promise as an effective agent in the treatment of PMS. It was hypothesized that the inhibition of steroidogenesis seen with this agent might also improve hormonally related mood changes as well as the physical symptoms of breast tenderness, water retention, and weight gain that accompany PMS. Overall, the results achieved with spironolactone have been disappointing, and it appears to be a mildly helpful agent at best. Nonetheless, because of its antisteroidal properties, it remains the diuretic most often chosen in the treatment of the water-retention symptoms of PMS.

Because of its aldosterone antagonist activity, spironolactone is a potassium-sparing diuretic. Patients should therefore be warned against taking potassium supplements while using this medication. Hypotensive effects are rarely observed in healthy young women.

Spironolactone has been associated with a number of side effects in women. They occur rarely, but when they do occur, gastrointestinal symptoms are the most common. Central nervous system side effects also occasionally occur, including drowsiness, lethargy, headache, and mental confusion. Because of its inhibition of steroid synthesis, irregular menses are not uncommon in patients taking spironolactone daily.

Many of the side effects of spironolactone have been noted with long-term daily administration. In general, adverse reactions are fewer when use is limited to the luteal phase of the cycle. Because spironolactone is now used primarily to treat the water-retention symptoms of PMS, therapy can be limited to short-term administration—usually for 7 to 10 days in the luteal phase of the cycle. Many of the agents that are most effective in treating overall PMS symptoms, particularly the mood and appetite disturbances, are less effective in relieving the water-retention symptoms of bloating and breast tenderness. In these cases, spironolactone provides a relatively safe adjunctive therapy.

Other diuretics have also been tried in PMS, with variable success in alleviating the water-retention symptoms. For the most part, these are reserved for spironolactone failures or those individuals with significant side effects from spironolactone. The most commonly used class of diuretics after spironolactone is the thiazides. Thiazide diuretics are often combined with an antikaliuretic agent such as triamterene. Even with these preparations, however, hypokalemia remains the major concern. Not uncommonly, diuretics are abused by women who become highly concerned about their weight. Particularly in women with PMS who are concerned about bloating, cautions about the overuse of diuretics should be stressed.

In addition to hypokalemia, thiazide diuretics are occasionally associated with anaphylactic responses, hematologic and central nervous system disturbances, and serious cardiac arrhythmias. Fortunately, these are rare events.

Overall, the side effect profile is better and the dosage tolerance range is higher with spironolactone than with thiazide diuretics. For this reason, as well as the potential for some beneficial effects exerted by its antisteroid properties, spironolactone remains the diuretic of choice for PMS. The use of more potent diuretics or low-dose thiazides in patients with PMS should be discouraged.

MENOPAUSE

method of
WULF H. UTIAN, M.D., PH.D.
University Hospitals of Cleveland
Cleveland, Ohio

In the United States, there were 47 million women over the age of 45 years in 1995. The number of women aged 40 to 54 years will increase 52% by 2010. The current median age of menopause is 51.3 years. However, approximately 8% of women undergo premature menopause before the age of 40 years.

Menopause represents the final cessation of menses. During the time of the climacteric (the phase in the aging of women that marks the transition from the reproductive to the nonreproductive stage of life), deficiency of follicular inhibin and estrogen leads to decreased negative feedback, which results in an increase in levels of follicle-stimulating hormone (FSH) and luteinizing hormone (LH). Thus, chronic elevated plasma FSH levels are the best diagnostic test for menopause.

The tissue or organs directly affected by this relative estrogen deficiency are those with specific estrogen receptors, such as the ovaries, endometrium, vaginal epithelium, hypothalamus, urinary tract, bone, circulatory system, and skin. The resultant symptoms or problems that may occur when these various tissues and organs become estrogen-deficient are summarized in Table 1.

The gradual decline of total circulating estrogen may be associated with an alteration in menstruation, usually manifesting as irregular cycles with a lighter menstrual flow, less frequent menses, and finally, a total absence of menstruation (menopause). If anovulatory cycles occur, the absence of progesterone can result in irregular, heavy menstrual periods.

The most frequent symptom bringing a woman to a physician's office is the hot flash. Hot flashes, which can begin several years before the actual menopause, occur in up to 80% of women. The equivalent problem of night sweats can impair sleep and result in secondary symptoms of fatigue, irritability, memory impairment, and poor concentration. The mechanism for hot flashes may be that of estrogen deprivation for central neurotransmitters required to stabilize the thermoregulatory center in the hypothalamus.

During the perimenopausal period, the risk of cardiovascular disease in women begins to increase to a rate similar to that in men. The decrease in estrogen production is thought to be one factor responsible for this acceleration of risk. Estrogen probably has an impact on cardiovascular disease through a positive effect on lipid metabolism as well as direct vasomotor effects enhancing blood flow and perfusion.

After cardiovascular disease, the most significant problem related to estrogen deficiency is osteoporosis. By the age of 80 years, about 25% of all women have sustained one or more fractures of the proximal femur, vertebrae,

or distal radius. Hip fractures are associated with high morbidity and mortality rates.

CONFIRMING MENOPAUSE

An interval of 6 months or more of secondary amenorrhea in a woman older than 50 years of age is usually diagnostic of menopause, especially if accompanied by the development of hot flashes or a low estrogen profile on physical examination (e.g., atrophic vaginal smear, absence of cervical mucus, atrophic endometrium on biopsy). In younger women, the menses should be absent for at least 1 year for menopause to be diagnosed with the same degree of confidence.

A negative response (no menstruation) to a progestogen challenge test (e.g., medroxyprogesterone acetate [Provera] one 10-mg tablet a day orally for 7 days) is confirmatory of low estrogen production and is usually the only special test necessary. If some doubt exists and urgent diagnostic confirmation is requested, measurement of the plasma FSH level is an adequate adjunct.

MENOPAUSE MANAGEMENT

Menopause should be considered as an excellent event to initiate a formal primary preventive health care program for women in their middle years and beyond. Selective cost-effective screening should therefore be utilized for menopause-related and age-related problems. Particularly if hormone replacement therapy (HRT) is being considered, the observation of a few basic precautions suffices to eliminate avoidable problems. The general state of health of every patient must be fully evaluated by currently accepted methods, including full history and physical examination. In particular, these points are of importance:

1. An indication for treatment must exist.
2. There should be no contraindications to estrogen.
3. Menopause should be confirmed, preferably by amenorrhea for a minimum of 3 months and the presence of specific estrogen-deficiency symptoms, or elevated plasma FSH and low estrogen levels.
4. A full general examination, including determination of blood pressure, breast examination, and pelvic examination with cervical and vaginal cytologic smears, is essential.
5. An attempt should be made to evaluate the degree of estrogen deficiency. These are adjuncts to diagnosis:
   a. Severity of hot flashes.
   b. Hormonal cytology.
   c. Plasma FSH level (usually necessary).
   d. Plasma estradiol or estrone level (usually unnecessary).
   e. Fasting urinary calcium/creatinine ratio or bone markers (rarely indicated).
6. The patient should be fully informed and must agree to regular check-ups.
7. Special and more frequent attention must be given to the patient considered at risk.
8. A mammogram should be completed.

TABLE 1. **Potential Problems of the Untreated Climacteric**

Target Organ	Possible Symptom or Problem
Vulva	Atrophy, dystrophy, pruritus vulvae
Vagina	Dyspareunia, blood-stained discharge, vaginitis
Bladder and urethra	Cystourethritis, ectropion, frequency or urgency, stress incontinence
Uterus and pelvic floor	Uterovaginal prolapse
Skin and mucous membranes	Atrophy, dryness, or pruritus; patient easily traumatized; loss of resilience and pliability; dry hair or loss of hair; minor hirsutism of face; dry mouth
Vocal cords	Voice changes (reduction in upper register)
Cardiovascular system	Atherosclerosis, angina, coronary heart disease
Skeleton	Osteoporosis with related fractures, backache
Breasts	Reduced size, softer consistency, drooping
Neuroendocrine system	Hot flashes, psychological disturbances

Modified from Utian WH: Menopause in Modern Perspective. New York, Appleton-Century-Crofts, 1980, p 111.

9. Bone densitometry should be considered.
10. Cholesterol screening is indicated.

Minimal Follow-Up Requirements

The patient must be seen at least every 12 months to assess general health, clinical response, and adequacy of dosage. Follow-up visits should include, minimally, breast and pelvic examinations with cytology and blood pressure check-up.

An annual endometrial biopsy is not recommended for the patient on cycled progestin. When indicated, various methods exist for obtaining endometrial specimens for cytologic or histologic diagnosis of the endometrial state. Most have not been widely used as screening tests because they are expensive, complicated, and unreliable.

Treatment

The modern therapeutic armamentarium is broad but in some respects superficial. Diet and nutrition, exercise, and hormonal medications receive the most attention, and the latter the most debate.

Hormone Replacement Therapy

HRT of varying types, formulations, doses, and routes of administration produces certain benefits and entails certain side effects and risks. The benefits include alleviation of hot flashes, urogenital atrophy, osteoporosis, and possibly, coronary heart disease, as well as improvement in sexual response, mood, sleep, and memory. In addition, HRT may promote longevity. Negative responses to HRT include nausea, mastalgia, menstrual bleeding, increased necessity for surgery, uterine and breast cancer, thromboembolic disease, hypertension, and gallstones.

The objective of modern prescribing habits is to enhance benefits and reduce risks. Already, the outcome of therapy has been reflected in lower mortality rates in users than in nonusers and enhanced feeling of well-being and quality of life.

Clearly, the most widely recognized reason for prescribing estrogen for menopausal women is to control symptoms. Estrogen effectively reduces the vasomotor, somatic, and associated psychological components of the menopausal syndrome. Recently, however, the role of estrogen in the prevention of disease, particularly osteoporosis, urogenital atrophy, and atherosclerotic cardiovascular disease, has prompted consideration of this treatment for a more long-term goal. Bone loss occurring after menopause can be prevented by the use of estrogen. This significantly reduces the morbidity and mortality of associated fractures. Atrophic changes, which can occur earlier in the menopause than previously recognized, also respond to estrogen treatment.

The incidence of angina or myocardial infarction is lower in estrogen users than in nonusers, and overall mortality rates from cardiovascular disease appear to be reduced as well.

Unopposed estrogen replacement is a known risk factor for endometrial carcinoma, but the effects on ovarian and breast tissue remain uncertain. The increased risk of endometrial carcinoma seems to be related to both the dosage and the duration of unopposed estrogen treatment. Progestins are known to protect against endometrial hyperstimulation, but the optimal duration of therapy each month and the maximally protective agent and dose remain to be determined.

The enhancement of liver function by orally administered estrogens is thought to contribute to some of the negative effects of HRT. Avoidance of this so-called first-pass metabolism by nonoral administration of estrogen through a skin patch or cream seems a logical way of minimizing hepatic effects while retaining the benefits of hormone therapy. However, studies of vaginal administration of ethinyl estradiol and conjugated equine estrogens have shown that enhanced liver action is still present. Apparently, the first-pass effect is not the sole mechanism by which estrogens affect the liver.

Contraindications to estrogen replacement are few. These include a history of breast cancer, a recent history of endometrial cancer, active liver disease, or the presence of thrombophlebitis.

BLEEDING RELATED TO HORMONE THERAPY

Any form of abnormal bleeding, be it unpredictable, prolonged, or excessive, requires histologic evaluation of the endometrium. This principle applies whether bleeding occurs on therapy (breakthrough bleeding) or during the pill-free days (withdrawal bleeding).

Once a histologic diagnosis has been made and cancer excluded, there are two ways to treat abnormal bleeding responses to hormonal therapy. The first is to cease therapy and observe. The second is to adjust the type and dose of hormone being administered. In this respect, progestogens, alone or in combination with estrogen therapy, are drugs of considerable value. Progestogen therapy for longer than 7 days seems to induce unpleasant minor side effects (fluid retention, tender breasts, reversal of mental tonic effect).

SELECTION OF DRUG AND REGIMEN

It is currently recommended that estrogen be prescribed continuously. Progestin is recommended for all women with an intact uterus, but not for those without. Protocols and drug preparations, combinations, and permutations are innumerable, being based on the fact that no right combination is yet the most preferable.

The current recommended protocol is continuous estrogen, either oral or transdermal, for all patients, with cycled progestin added on calendar days 1 to 12 for those with an intact uterus. Although the latter has the disadvantage of inducing monthly cycles, the use of combined-continuous estrogen and progestin has not yet proved to be as effective and safe as sequential therapy, particularly in relation to potential prevention of coronary disease (Table 2).

TABLE 2. **Current Protocols for Hormone Replacement Therapy**

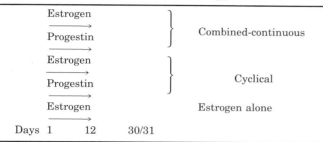

Estrogen is usually prescribed as conjugated equine estrogen (Premarin) 0.625 mg per day, micronized 17-beta-estradiol (Estrace) 1 mg, or transdermal estradiol patch (Estraderm) 0.05 mg. Frequently prescribed progestins are medroxyprogesterone acetate (Provera) 5 to 10 mg and norethindrone acetate (Micronor, Norlutate, Aygestin) 0.35 to 2.5 mg for days 1 to 12. Lower doses of progestin are used for the combined-continuous regimen—for example, Micronor 0.35 mg and Provera 2.5 mg.

TREATING ADVERSE EFFECTS

The incidence of estrogen-induced side effects is usually low, provided that the drugs are correctly selected and prescribed. The type and severity of adverse effects are influenced by individual patient idiosyncrasy, general health, selection of drug and dose, mode of administration, and so on.

Nausea occurs in up to 20% of patients during the first 2 to 3 months of therapy. Treatment may require reduction in estrogen dose but is usually successfully achieved by reassurance, advice to take tablets with the evening meal, and prescription of antiemetic preparations. Alternatively, conversion to nonoral administration (i.e., the transdermal estrogen skin patch) is usually effective.

Retention of excessive amounts of fluid may manifest as breast tenderness or weight gain. Reassurance, once again, is usually of value. Occasionally, the dosage of estrogen or progestin needs reduction, or a change of preparation may be required. The use of diuretics is not recommended.

Nonhormonal Medications

Alternative therapeutic regimens should be considered for specific indications.

Hot Flashes. Clonidine (Catapres), a centrally acting alpha-adrenergic agonist in doses of 0.1 to 0.2 mg twice daily, is effective in about 30% of patients. Vitamin E has not been tested in randomized studies. For women with treated breast cancer, megestrol acetate (Megace) 40 to 80 mg per day may be effective.

Osteoporosis. Calcium supplementation is essential to reduce bone loss, but it is not an estrogen substitute. Calcitonin may be indicated. Various diphosphonates are currently in clinical trial.

Vaginal Dryness. Local water-soluble lubricants (K-Y Jelly, Surgilube, Astroglide) and synthetic mucopolysaccharide moisturizers (Replens) may relieve dyspareunia.

Adjuncts to Drug Therapy

It is often gratifying to note the extent to which additional counseling can further enhance the quality of life of women seeking perimenopausal medical advice. These are but a few areas in which judicious counseling can be of value:

1. Correct diet, particularly use of weight-reducing diets where indicated.
2. Total body care, including advice about oral and dental hygiene, cosmetics, and care of skin and nails.
3. Physical fitness programs. Selective exercise programs, both home plans and health studio plans, can be recommended after a satisfactory physical examination.
4. Marital counseling.
5. Psychosexual counseling.
6. Smoking cessation programs.

Useful exercise programs and diet styles for the perimenopausal woman are described in *Managing Your Menopause.**

---

*Utian WH: Managing Your Menopause. Englewood Cliffs, NJ: Simon and Schuster Fireside Press, 1990.

VULVOVAGINITIS

method of
BARBARA D. REED, M.D., M.S.P.H.
University of Michigan
Ann Arbor, Michigan

Vulvovaginitis is one of the most common complaints of women at the physician's office. A majority of women are affected at some time in their lifetimes, many several times, resulting in considerable morbidity, inconvenience, discomfort, and disruption of usual activities. Furthermore, elucidating the cause of vaginal symptoms is often difficult, and the treatment is not always successful in alleviating either symptoms or the causative agent.

CAUSES

The most common causes of vaginal symptoms are listed in Table 1. Although bacterial vaginosis, candidal vulvovaginitis (CVV), and trichomonal vaginitis make up the majority of diagnoses for women with vaginal symptoms, clarifying the diagnosis and identifying women who have

TABLE 1. **Common Causes of Vaginal Symptoms**

Bacterial vaginosis	Vulvodynia
Candidal vulvovaginitis	Vestibulitis
Trichomonal vaginitis	Lichen sclerosis
Atrophic vaginitis	Seborrheic dermatitis
Allergic reaction	Unknown cause
Foreign body	

been previously misdiagnosed (by themselves or by medical providers), as well as those who have poorly understood vaginal symptoms are important to maximize outcome.

DIAGNOSIS

The common types of vaginal problems differ in presenting symptoms, physical examination findings, office laboratory findings, and treatment. Patients typically present with complaints of increased or discolored vaginal discharge, altered vaginal odor, or genital itching or irritation. The examination may be totally unremarkable despite the presence of infection, or it may reveal vulvar or vaginal erythema, edema, or excoriations; an abnormal discharge; or a fishy odor. The office laboratory examination may similarly be helpful in differentiating the cause, or it may be normal. The major differences in clinical presentation and evaluation of the common diagnoses associated with vaginal symptoms are depicted in Table 2.

However, such a table may lead to the erroneous conclusion that the diagnosis of vaginitis is so straightforward that it can be made over the telephone or can be inferred despite conflicting findings from symptoms, signs, and laboratory data. In contrast, the symptoms, signs, and risk factors for vaginal problems are inexact and only suggest probable diagnoses—they cannot accurately indicate the diagnosis. Only with identification of the organism (for CVV and trichomonal vaginitis), or close adherence to clinical criteria for the diagnosis (for bacterial vaginosis), can diagnostic accuracy be optimal for these infections. Consideration of other maladies (e.g., vulvodynia, vestibulitis, and allergic vaginitis) is needed to avoid repeatedly treating

women for infections they do not have, and to direct therapy appropriately.

OFFICE AND CENTRAL LABORATORY ASSESSMENT

Because the symptoms and signs of vaginitis are not diagnostic, careful attention to the in-office laboratory procedures is important. As shown in Table 2, the diagnosis of CVV requires identification of the organism, either microscopically, normally using a potassium hydroxide (KOH) preparation, or by culture. Similarly, *Trichomonas vaginalis* identification microscopically or by culture is required to make that diagnosis (the normal saline [NS] preparation method is described later). The diagnosis for bacterial vaginosis (previously referred to by numerous other names, such as *Gardnerella* vaginitis and nonspecific vaginitis), can be made using the Amsel criteria (Table 2).

Specimen collection for vaginal discharge should include placing vaginal discharge from the midportion of the vagina into approximately 0.5 mL of saline solution that can be applied to a slide immediately prior to microscopic examination. This enhances the probability of detecting *Trichomonas vaginalis*, an organism that requires a fluid medium for motility. A microscopic slide with a shallow depression in it can be used for the hanging-drop test to maximize the probability that motile *Trichomonas* will be observed.

The normal findings of an examination of vaginal fluid include a pH of less than 4.8, a negative whiff test when potassium hydroxide is applied, microscopic evidence of vaginal squamous cells surrounded by a moderate number

TABLE 2. **Findings Associated with Bacterial Vaginosis, Candidal Vulvovaginitis, Trichomonal Vaginitis, Vulvodynia, and Vestibulitis**

	Symptoms	Signs	In-Office Laboratory Data	Diagnostic Criteria
Bacterial Vaginosis	Increased discharge; vaginal odor, often increased after intercourse	Creamy, homogeneous discharge (may be discolored); vaginal odor	Clue cells;* amine odor after KOH applied to discharge; high pH of discharge (≥4.8); decreased lactobacilli; presence of curved or short rods on NS prep	Amsel criteria: 3 of the following: 1. Homogeneous discharge 2. pH ≥4.8 3. Clue cells 4. Amine odor
Candidal Vulvovaginitis	Vaginal or vulvar itching (may be severe); with or without discharge; discharge may be curdlike	Vulvar/vaginal erythema, edema, excoriations; thick, curdlike discharge; satellite lesions	Budding yeast or hyphae on KOH prep; WBCs common on NS prep	Positive KOH prep (budding yeast forms or hyphae) *or* Positive culture
Trichomonal Vaginitis	Increased discharge—often thin or creamy, may be discolored; may also have vaginal odor; irritation may be present	Thin, sometimes bubbly discharge, may be discolored; strawberry cervix (uncommon)	May have amine odor with KOH; motile *Trichomonas* on fresh, moist NS prep or hanging-drop prep	Positive NS prep with motile *Trichomonas* seen *or* Positive culture
Vulvodynia	Chronic, idiopathic burning pain at introitus, often following acute onset	Minimal vulvar findings; local tenderness with occasional erythema, edema, or fissures	None diagnostic; rule out co-infection	None definitive; practical diagnosis made by the presence of classic symptoms without co-infection present
Vestibulitis	Tenderness in the vulvar vestibule; dyspareunia common	Point tenderness at gland openings; vulvar erythema of varying degree	None diagnostic; rule out co-infection	None definitive; compatible history and physical examination without evidence of co-infection

*Clue cells are vaginal epithelial cells covered with bacteria, with the smooth epithelial cell borders obscured.
Abbreviations: KOH = 10% potassium hydroxide solution; NS = normal saline; WBC = white blood cell; prep = preparation.

of long rods, few or no white blood cells, and lack of clue cells or motile *Trichomonas vaginalis*. The presence of parabasal cells (vaginal epithelial cells that have a rounder appearance than normal, which suggests estrogen deficiency) can also be assessed.

Also at the time of the vaginal examination, vaginal discharge should be smeared, undiluted, directly onto a microscopic slide as a visible thick layer for the KOH preparation. The addition of a drop of KOH may then be made at any time prior to microscopic examination, with the amine odor assessed at that time by smelling the slide for a "fishy" fragrance.

A third vaginal specimen may be collected for culture if desired in the case of an unclear etiology, and a cervical specimen should be collected and sent to the laboratory for evaluation for *Chlamydia trachomatis* or *Neisseria gonorrhoeae* if cervical discharge or risk factors are present. The value of culturing for any other vaginal organisms is controversial. Few data exist substantiating a role for Group B streptococcus or *Escherichia coli* in symptomatic vaginitis, and knowledge of the presence of these organisms is not currently considered useful to guide therapy.

Although women with symptoms of vaginitis are more likely to harbor human papillomavirus infection than are controls, no reports prove that vaginal symptoms are caused by this virus. Assuring that the cervical cytology screening is current in symptomatic women is reasonable.

Data from the cytology smear are rarely useful in making the diagnosis of the cause of vaginal symptoms. Although the positive predictive value of the presence of *Candida* species on the cytology report is good, the sensitivity of this finding is low. The diagnosis of *Trichomonas vaginalis* or *Chlamydia trachomatis* on cytology smear reports is not accurate, and these data should prompt repeat evaluation—not diagnosis and treatment.

Accuracy of the Office Diagnosis of Vaginitis

The accuracy of symptoms, signs, and office laboratory tests for vaginitis differs greatly by the diagnosis. For bacterial vaginosis, the office evaluation is sufficient by itself—if the Amsel criteria are met, treatment can be initiated, with approximately 90% accuracy in the diagnosis. The predictive value of individual factors associated with bacterial vaginosis is less accurate, with a 30 to 60% false-positive rate for isolated findings of amine odor, high pH, or clue cells. The clinical diagnosis of CVV and trichomonal vaginitis are more commonly inaccurate. Only approximately 50% of women with a thick, white vaginal discharge have CVV. In addition, the false-negative rate of not seeing hyphae or budding yeast in vaginal discharge from women with CVV is 37 to 81% and that for not seeing *Trichomonas vaginalis* in infected women is 23 to 58%.

If the diagnosis remains unclear following the in-office laboratory assessment, further testing may be required, including culturing for *Candida* species, culturing for *Trichomonas vaginalis*, evaluating the woman's hormonal status, and reevaluating over time. Cultures for *Candida* can be performed using selective media (such as Sabauraud CG agar), or the specimens can be transported to the central laboratory using standard transport tubes or media for culture there. Culture for *Trichomonas vaginalis* requires special media that should be inoculated in the office. Modified Diamond's Media (available from Remel Pharmaceuticals, Lenexa, Kansas) is a liquid medium for *Trichomonas* culture that also allows diagnosis of *Candida* infection simultaneously. This culture is positive in 1 to 2 days for *Candida* but takes as long as 9 days for *Trichomonas*

growth. Vulvodynia, vestibulitis, and allergic vaginitis are diagnoses suggested by the history, the absence of co-infections, and the physical findings. The accuracy of these diagnoses is not well studied, partially due to the lack of a "gold standard," and needs further evaluation.

TREATMENT

Treatment for vaginal symptoms is specific to the etiology of the disorder. The recommended treatment modalities for acute, recurrent, and resistant bacterial vaginosis, CVV, and trichomonal vaginitis are shown in Table 3.

The number of effective treatments for bacterial vaginosis has recently increased. Previous recommendations included the use of oral metronidazole or clindamycin, with amoxicillin, erythromycin, and tetracycline being much less effective. Side effects of oral metronidazole include gastrointestinal symptoms (nausea, heartburn, and a metallic taste), hypersensitivity, an Antabuse-like reaction if alcohol is ingested, and rare peripheral neuropathy or seizures. Metronidazole is contraindicated in the first trimester of pregnancy. The availability of vaginal clindamycin and metronidazole has increased the options for local therapy for bacterial vaginosis. The efficacies of these vaginal preparations are similar to the oral medications. These preparations are usually well tolerated, with side effects being primarily local irritation or hypersensitivity and subsequent CVV. Gastrointestinal side effects may occur in patients using vaginal metronidazole. Both vaginal drugs are minimally absorbed (less than 5%) in the systemic circulation, and the Antabuse-like reaction is less common with topical than with oral metronidazole therapy.

Treatment of sexual partners of women with bacterial vaginosis is controversial, with only isolated studies showing benefit. At this time treatment of partners should be reserved for couples in whom bacterial vaginosis is recurrent or persistent.

Topical therapy for CVV remains the recommendation for intermittent episodes, with imidazole (miconazole, clotrimazole, butoconazole) and triazole (terconazole) preparations showing superior clinical efficacy (85% cure rate) compared with the older polyene preparations such as nystatin. Several topical antifungals are now available over the counter, and prescription-only formulations may also be used. Treatment with boric acid suppositories has not been well studied but appears to be very effective in eradicating *Candida* species; however, these are not commercially available and require pharmacist preparation. The options for oral therapy for CVV have expanded with the availability of newer antifungals with lower rates of liver toxicity and high *Candida* eradication rates compared with those achieved with ketoconazole: these include fluconazole and itraconazole.* Oral ketoconazole has a 5 to 10% risk of reversible hepatitis, and a 1 in 15,000 chance of potentially serious hepatitis, with the side effects of fluconazole

---

*Not FDA-approved for this indication.

TABLE 3. **Treatment Protocols for Bacterial Vaginosis, Candidal Vulvovaginitis, and Trichomonal Vaginitis**

Etiology	Treatment	Dose	Cost ($)
Bacterial Vaginosis	Metronidazole (Flagyl, Protostat)	500 mg PO twice daily for 7 days	$4.98
	Clindamycin (Cleocin) 2% vaginal cream	5 gm (100 mg clindamycin) intravaginally, once daily for 7 days	$39.98
	Metronidazole vaginal gel (Metro-Gel)	5 gm (37.5 mg metronidazole) intravaginally, twice daily for 5 days	$33.98
For resistant cases	Clindamycin (Cleocin)	300 mg PO twice daily for 7 days	$25.55
	Povidone-iodine (Betadine)	Gel or suppositories intravaginally, bid for 14–28 days	No longer available
During pregnancy (need for treatment during pregnancy is controversial)	Clindamycin (Cleocin)	300 mg PO twice daily for 7 days	$25.55
Candidal Vulvovaginitis	Miconazole (Monistat 3)	200-mg suppository intravaginally, 1 each night for 3 nights	$34.98
		or	
	(Monistat 7) (OTC)	2% vaginal cream, one application intravaginally each night for 7 nights	$16.99
		or	
	(Monistat) (OTC)	100-mg vaginal tablet, intravaginally each night for 7 nights	$16.99
	Clotrimazole (recommended, but not commercially available in this dose)	200-mg vaginal tablet, intravaginally, each night for 3 nights	Not available
	(Gyne-Lotrimin, Mycelex-7, Femcare) (all OTC)	100-mg vaginal tablet intravaginally each night for 7 nights	$20.98
	(Gyne-Lotrimin, Mycelex-7, Femcare) (all OTC)	1% vaginal cream, one application intravaginally each night for 7 nights	$20.98
	(Mycelex-G)	500-mg vaginal tablet intravaginally, once	$21.98
	Butoconazole (Femstat)	2% cream, one application intravaginally each night for 3 nights	$29.98
	Terconazole (Terazol 3)	80-mg suppository or 0.8% vaginal cream, one application each night for 3 nights	$29.98
		or	
	(Terazol 7)	0.4% vaginal cream intravaginally, each night for 7 nights	$29.98
	Tioconazole (Vagistat-1)	6.5% ointment intravaginally once	$12.98
Resistant or recurrent cases	Any of the above drugs	Dose used for 7-day regimens, but extended to a 14- to 21-day course	$33.98 to $89.94
	Fluconazole (Diflucan)	150 mg PO once	$18.98
	Ketoconazole (Nizoral)	200 mg orally twice daily for 5 to 14 days	$38.98 for 5 days
	Itraconazole (Sporanox)*	200 mg orally once daily for 3 days	$26.98
	Gentian violet vaginal staining	Once or twice in one week	Office charge
	Boric acid	600-mg capsule twice daily intravaginally for 14 days (formulated by pharmacist)	$14.00 approximately
Prophylactic regimens	Clotrimazole	One 500-mg vaginal tablet monthly	$21.98
	Ketoconazole	200 mg PO twice daily for 5 days each month	$38.98
	Fluconazole	150 mg orally each month	$18.98
	Miconazole	100-mg vaginal tablet twice weekly	$16.99 for 7 doses
Trichomonal Vaginitis	Metronidazole (Flagyl, Protostat)	2 gm PO in a single dose, or 500 mg PO twice daily for 7 days for both patient and partner(s)	$4.98
Persistent or recurrent cases	Metronidazole	500 mg PO twice daily for 14 days or 2 gm PO for 3 days plus one of the following	$4.98
	Metronidazole gel (MetroGel-Vaginal)	5 gm intravaginally twice daily for 5 days	$33.98
	Povidone-iodine suppositories (Betadine)	One suppository intravaginally twice daily for 14 to 28 days	No longer available
	Clotrimazole (Gyne-Lotrimin, Mycelex-G)	100-mg vaginal tablet intravaginally at bedtime for 7 nights	$20.98
Pregnancy	Metronidazole	2 gm PO one time only after first trimester	$4.98
	Clotrimazole	100 mg intravaginally at bedtime for 7 nights	$20.98
Lactation	Metronidazole	2 gm PO one time, with discontinuation of breast-feeding for 24 h	$4.98

*Not FDA-approved for this indication.

and itraconazole being primarily nausea and diarrhea (2 to 6% of patients), occasional headache, and rare hypersensitivity. Oral treatment for CVV is recommended for women with persistent infection or in those with frequent recurrence. Suppressive therapy with periodic doses of vaginal or oral antifungals has been suggested for women with very frequent or predictable infection, such as in women with perimenstrual infections. Withdrawal of suppression may be attempted approximately every 6 months to reevaluate continued need. For pregnant women with CVV, data are primarily available for miconazole and clotrimazole. These can be used in the second and third trimester in women with CVV if symptoms warrant therapy. There is no recommendation for treatment of the male partners of women with CVV, and this should be avoided unless the partner shows signs of infection or infection is documented. Topical treatment of men does not alter the course in the female partner.

Oral metronidazole remains the recommended treatment for trichomonal vaginitis, and all sexual partners should also be treated. In patients with persistent infection, the possibility of reinfection, co-infection with other genital pathogens, noncompliance with the treatment regimen, and metronidazole resistance should be considered. Resistant cases can be treated with prolonged courses and higher doses of metronidazole, and the addition of vaginal preparations of metronidazole, povidone-iodine, or clotrimazole should be considered. Because of the lack of effective alternatives for treatment of this infection, desensitization and in-hospital treatment of women with symptomatic trichomonal vaginitis who have a hypersensitivity to metronidazole should be considered. Treatment in pregnancy is controversial, with studies suggesting that infection with *Trichomonas vaginalis* during pregnancy is associated with premature delivery, low birthweight, and postpartum endometritis. Whether these complications are due to the *Trichomonas* infection is unclear. If considered, metronidazole should be used after the first trimester of pregnancy.

Treatments for vulvodynia and vestibulitis are less well studied and defined. Treatment options for vulvodynia include medication for chronic *Candida* infection when appropriate (used over a prolonged course, often 4 to 6 months), local therapy as effective (including ice packs, bland emollients), localized topical 2 to 5% lidocaine in an emollient base (for vestibulitis or dysesthetic vulvodynia), or tricyclic antidepressants for chronic pain—especially in women with dysesthetic vulvodynia or pudendal vulvodynia (saddle distribution from the mons pubis to the groin, and upper inner thighs). Topical or systemic estrogen replacement may be tried in elderly women with dysesthetic vulvodynia. Potent topical steroids should be avoided unless hypertrophic lichen sclerosis is present. Surgical remedies for vestibulitis, such as vestibulectomy with vaginal advancement, have had some success in recalcitrant cases and should be reserved for women unresponsive to other therapies

in whom the potential benefit outweighs the risk of continued pain. Laser therapy for vulvodynia and vestibulitis may be associated with short-term improvement, but long-term results are poor, and hence this is not recommended.

Follow-Up

Women with symptoms that fail to resolve in 1 to 2 weeks, and those with recurrence within 1 month, should be reevaluated in the office. Occasionally, treatment of one infection will allow diagnosis of unrecognized co-infections that were obscured in the original evaluation (such as cervicitis or trichomonal vaginitis). Confirming the diagnosis and using additional laboratory methods if the diagnosis is unclear are crucial in these cases. The treatment strategies for resistant or recurrent cases (shown in Table 3) can then be used if indicated.

TOXIC SHOCK SYNDROME

method of
P. JOAN CHESNEY, M.D.
University of Tennessee College of Medicine
Memphis, Tennessee

Toxic shock syndrome (TSS) is fatal in 3 to 5% of cases, usually as a result of irreversible respiratory failure, refractory cardiac arrhythmias, or severe bleeding. Such deaths could potentially be prevented by early recognition, early and intensive monitoring, and treatment of each of the well-described multisystem components of this disease. Most of the sequelae are probably toxin-mediated, but some appear to be related to the degree and duration of hypotension and are therefore potentially preventable.

PATHOGENESIS

TSS appears to be mediated by a toxin produced by certain strains of *Staphylococcus aureus*. As with other bacterial toxin–mediated diseases, the bacteria themselves are usually present in only a single focus and often only in relatively small numbers. With few exceptions, blood, urine, and cerebrospinal fluid cultures are negative. Positive cultures are obtained from the focus of infection. Around surgical wounds or a site of infection there is often minimal or no inflammatory reaction that would suggest the presence of a staphylococcal infection. Thus, numerous case reports suggest that in a patient with TSS, all recent surgical wounds and any suspected sites should be opened, irrigated, and cultured even when no clinical evidence of inflammation is apparent.

The toxins that mediate this syndrome and their mechanism of action are not yet defined with certainty. Toxic shock syndrome toxin–1 (TSST-1), a protein of molecular weight 24,000, is a valuable marker for the *S. aureus* strains isolated from 95% of menstrually associated cases of TSS. In nonmenstrual TSS, as few as 63% of *S. aureus* isolates produce TSST-1, suggesting the likely involvement of other unidentified toxins, particularly in nonmenstrual cases.

TSST-1 has been shown to be a potent inducer of monokines and lymphokines in vitro. Incubation of TSST-1 with macrophages and lymphocytes results in the rapid production of interleukin-1, tumor necrosis factor (TNF), interferon-gamma, and lymphotoxin. The specific roles of these mediators and TSST-1 in the pathophysiology of TSS is unclear. Monoclonal antibodies to both TSST-1 and TNF have provided protection in animal models of TSS.

The two most important pathophysiologic effects of the toxin(s) and mediators in this syndrome are inducing a decrease in peripheral venous tone and extensive capillary leakage of intravascular fluid into the interstitial spaces, resulting in a rapidly progressive hypovolemia. In addition to the ensuing poor tissue perfusion, the toxin or mediators appear to have direct toxic effects on the myocardium, kidneys, lungs, liver, muscles, lymphoid tissue, and, possibly, the central and peripheral nervous systems. Hence, the three most important, immediate principles of management are rapid restoration of the intravascular volume, inactivation and/or elimination of the toxin, and drainage and treatment of the focus of infection.

TREATMENT

As noted in Table 1, immediate and appropriate monitoring for the early signs of the well-described acute complications secondary to multisystem organ damage should be established in all hospitalized patients.

Although antimicrobials have not been proved to modify the outcome of the acute illness in menses-associated cases, their use is clearly indicated in all cases to eradicate organisms from the infected site. In all cases, they should be used to treat the rare patient with positive blood or urine cultures, and to prevent recurrences in menstrually associated cases.

TSS-associated strains of *S. aureus* are usually resistant to penicillin and ampicillin but uniformly sensitive to the beta-lactamase–resistant (BLR) penicillins. For patients allergic to penicillin, vancomycin hydrochloride (Vancocin) or clindamycin hydrochloride (Cleocin) are the drugs of first choice. A BLR

TABLE 1. **Monitoring of Toxic Shock Syndrome Patients**

Initial

Clinical	*Laboratory*
Blood pressure	Electrolyte and acid-base status
Urine output	Serum calcium and phosphorus
Respiratory rate	levels
Heart rate	Chest x-ray examination
Heart sounds	Electrocardiogram
Pulmonary sounds	Coagulation status
Temperature	Blood urea nitrogen and
Weight	creatinine levels
Level of consciousness	Liver function tests
	Stool guaiac test
	Cultures of infected focus, blood, and urine

Prolonged Hypotension (>2 h)

Central venous pressure
Pulmonary artery wedge pressure
Mean arterial pressure
Cardiac index
Arterial blood gas levels
M-mode and two-dimensional echocardiograms

penicillin is administered at a maximal intravenous dose appropriate for the patient's age until the patient is afebrile and has not required pressor agents for 2 to 3 days. At that time an oral BLR penicillin is administered, 100 mg per kg per day every 6 hours not to exceed 4 grams per day. Clindamycin hydrochloride may be used at 25 mg per kg per day not to exceed 1.2 grams per day. Combined intravenous and oral therapy should total 10 to 14 days. In bacteremic patients, the possibility of additional therapy for endocarditis or other complications should be considered.

In vitro, concentrations of clindamycin below the minimal inhibitory concentration of *S. aureus* have been shown to "turn off" the production of TSST-1 despite continued growth of the organism. This phenomenon is not seen with other antibiotics such as ampicillin. The significance of this phenomenon has yet to be studied in humans.

Of equal importance to antimicrobial selection is identification of the infected focus, removal of all foreign bodies (tampons, gauze packing, sutures, prostheses, etc.), and drainage, irrigation, and culture of the suspected focus. The correct techniques for removing and/or eradicating any toxins are not known, as the tissue distribution, sites, and mechanisms for inactivation of TSST-1 and other unidentified toxins are not yet known.

One patient with TSS due to *S. aureus* infection of a herniorrhaphy incision did not recover for 5 days despite aggressive resuscitation and intravenous nafcillin (Nafcil) administration until povidone-iodine (Betadine) irrigation and soaks of a well-drained, normal appearing but still infected wound were instituted. Saline irrigations and povidone-iodine irrigations and soaks of infected foci including the vagina should be considered as additional means of eradicating the source of toxin. Povidone-iodine is readily absorbed from the vagina after only a 2-minute application, leading to fivefold to 15-fold increases in serum total iodine and inorganic iodide concentrations within 15 minutes. This finding should be noted when this form of therapy is considered.

Aggressive management of hypovolemic TSS patients as outlined in Table 2 is crucial. The most important aspect of the nonspecific symptomatic therapy is fluid replacement. The rapid restoration of intravascular volume to achieve adequate tissue perfusion should be accomplished immediately. The fluid replacement required to maintain organ perfusion may far exceed the amount of fluid calculated to be necessary, based on normal replacement and fluid deficit volumes, because of the ongoing capillary leak syndrome. Thus, some adults have required 12 liters of fluid in the first 24 hours in addition to vasopressors in order to stabilize the circulating blood pressure. Edema is inevitable as a result of the continued vascular capillary fluid leak. Close monitoring in an intensive care unit determines when the correct intravascular volume has been achieved. Peripheral edema and pleural and pericardial effusions can sequester massive volumes of fluid. Once the patient's

TABLE 2. **Supportive and Symptomatic Therapy**

Hypovolemia and Hypotension	**Adult Respiratory Distress Syndrome**
Initial therapy:	Anticipate.
Oxygen, intubation, PEEP	**Electrolyte and Acid-Base Status**
1. Large-bore intravascular catheter	Correct initial hyponatremia and acidosis.
2. Rapid administration of crystalloid 20–40 mL/kg over 1 h to stabilize BP and achieve urine output of ≥2 mL/kg/h	**Hypocalcemia**
	Anticipate hypocalcemia and tetany. Maintain physiologic levels.
3. Methylprednisolone sodium succinate (Solu-Medrol), 30 mg/kg q 6 h for 2 doses	**Acute Renal Failure**
	Avoid nephrotoxic drugs. Monitor and dialyze if necessary.
If no response after 1 h:	**Thrombocytopenia and DIC**
1. Transfer to ICU.	Use fresh-frozen plasma and platelets if needed.
2. Continue crystalloid at 20 mL/kg/h; may require many times maintenance to restore BP.	**Edema, Pericardial and Pleural Effusion**
3. Establish CVP line.	Maintain adequate intravascular volume before using diuretic to mobilize extravascular fluid.
4. Correct electrolyte, calcium, and acid-base status.	**Hypoferremia and Anemia**
If no response after 2–4 h:	No treatment unless blood loss.
1. Place pulmonary artery Swan-Ganz and arterial catheters.	**Hepatic Dysfunction**
2. Establish status of myocardium and lungs.	Avoid drugs conjugated in liver.
3. Consider use of dopamine hydrochloride or dobutamine hydrochloride (Dobutrex) for myocardial dysfunction.	**Central Nervous System Dysfunction**
	Anticipate irrational behavior, seizures.
4. Use appropriate therapy for myocardial dysfunction if needed.	
5. Look for sources of bleeding.	
If BP remains unstable after 12–24 h:	
1. Look for continued source of toxin production.	
2. Consider other techniques for toxin removal (see text).	

Abbreviations: BP = blood pressure; CVP = central venous pressure; DIC = disseminated intravascular coagulation; ICU = intensive care unit; PEEP = positive end-expiratory pressure.

blood pressure is stable, the judicious use of diuretics helps to mobilize fluid.

Numerous reports have documented the initial hemodynamic changes to be markedly decreased system vascular resistance, decreased mean arterial pressure, and increased cardiac output (CO). In some patients, however, after an initial phase of increased CO, myocardial contractility decreases, presumably owing to a toxin-mediated cardiomyopathy. This results in a decreased CO, increased pulmonary artery wedge pressure (PAWP), and increased central venous pressure (CVP). This stage of myocardial dysfunction may not be readily apparent from the nonspecific electrocardiogram findings but is quickly recognized from increased CVP and PAWP readings, a decreased cardiac index, and an abnormal echocardiogram. Early recognition of myocardial failure and potential arrhythmias should lead to changes in management such as decreasing the amount of fluid volume administered and considering afterload reduction, a subject beyond the scope of this discussion. Whereas dopamine may be effective in the early stages before myocardial dysfunction develops, dobutamine or a combination of both is preferable when myocardial damage has been demonstrated.

A retrospective study demonstrated that a short course of methylprednisolone (Solu-Medrol) or dexamethasone (Decadron) was associated with a reduction in the duration of fever and severity of disease if given early enough. As well, steroids appeared beneficial in an animal model. Steroids should probably be reserved for the severely ill patient unresponsive to fluid resuscitation.

Severely ill patients need to be cared for in an intensive care setting so that, if present, myocardial dysfunction, hemodynamic derangements, pulmonary edema, adult respiratory distress syndrome, acute renal failure, encephalopathy, and disseminated intravascular coagulation can be appropriately monitored and treated.

No recommendation can be made concerning the use of antitoxin for the treatment of this presumably toxin-mediated disease, as the roles of TSST-1, other toxins, and mediators have not yet been clarified. Absent or low titers of antibody to TSST-1 are found in almost all patients at the onset of menstrual TSS. The acquisition of antibody to TSST-1 in control populations is age-related, with more than 88% of individuals aged 20 years or more having high titers of antibody. The failure to develop antibody after menstrual TSS appears to correlate with an ongoing risk of recurrent disease.

High levels of antibody to TSST-1 have been found in both intramuscular and intravenous immune globulin (IVIG) preparations. In the rabbit subcutaneous whiffle ball or tampon model of TSS, human IVIG given at the time of administration of toxin or organism prevented TSS. When IVIG was given 8 hours later, it decreased the mortality from 90 (in control animals) to 16% (p < .001). When IVIG was given 29 hours after TSST-1 administration, the increase in survival among the IVIG-treated animals was still significant. No adverse reactions were noted in the IVIG-treated animals, and there was no evidence of disease mediated by the formation of antigen-antibody complexes.

Thus, for a number of reasons, consideration might be given to the administration of IVIG to patients severely ill with TSS. IVIG has been given to several patients with sepsis and septic shock in an intensive care setting with no adverse effect. As TSS is now a relatively rare disease, a controlled study of the effect of IVIG on outcome may be difficult to implement. It is also possible that early administration of IVIG would blunt the immune response to TSST-1 and/or other toxins, increasing the possibility of a recurrent episode. The potential risks and benefits of this form of therapy will have to be weighed for each patient.

If an unstable blood pressure persists despite aggressive management and if an unsuspected site of infection with continued toxin production cannot be found, anecdotal case reports suggest that techniques that might remove toxins from the blood such as plasmapheresis or hemodialysis might be useful. These forms of therapy have not been studied and should be considered investigational.

Other multisystem manifestations commonly present in hospitalized patients with TSS are listed in Table 2. Each complication should be managed using standard guidelines. The anticipation and early recognition of these complications is of great importance. Although hypocalcemic tetany is uncommon, hypocalcemia that appears to be mediated by a toxin-induced calcitonin-like molecule is common. Close attention to maintaining physiologic calcium concentrations may be important.

Hypoferremia, most often incidentally detected on routine chemistry panels, is a physiologic response to acute inflammation and need not be treated.

PREVENTION

Adequate therapy of the initial episode of TSS is the cornerstone to prevention of recurrence in menstrually associated TSS. Without therapy, up to 65% of women who develop their initial episode of TSS during menses experience at least one more episode during subsequent menses. Subsequent episodes may be mild or severe. Recurrence is rare in patients who have developed nonmenstrually associated TSS. Women who develop TSS with menses take many months to develop antibody to TSST-1. Patients with

nonmenstrual TSS develop antibody soon after their illness.

Administering a BLR penicillin during the acute illness and discontinuing tampon use decreases the recurrence rate to less than 5% in menses-associated cases. Such women may remain susceptible to TSS until they have developed anti-TSST-1 antibody. Serum antibody levels to TSST-1 could be monitored and tampon use cautiously resumed once a significant titer had been achieved. Such individuals may also continue to be at risk as long as they are colonized with TSST-1–producing strains of *S. aureus* and have no antibody to TSST-1. Thus, repeat vaginal cultures several months after the initial episode may be of help in identifying persistent carriers. Aside from encouraging patients to continue to avoid tampon use, optimal management of such carriers is not known but might include a course of an oral antibiotic such as rifampin to eliminate cervicovaginal *S. aureus* carriage.

The patterns of tampon use that minimize the risk of TSS are unclear. The use of superabsorbent tampons clearly increases the risk of TSS, and such tampons can now be identified by the consumer-based manufacturer's absorbency labels. The use of pads at night and tampon removal when symptoms suggestive of TSS develop are two recommendations with which most investigators would concur. The optimal frequency for changing tampons to minimize risk is not clear.

For women who have had TSS, with menses, postpartum, or with a vaginal infection or contraceptive use, tampon use should be discontinued until antibody to TSST-1 is present. Certain precautions may prevent the initial episode of TSS. Physicians should instruct their patients to use tampons judiciously.

Prevention of TSS associated with nasal surgery has been attempted using single-dose cefazolin (Kefzol) with inconsistent results.

CHLAMYDIA TRACHOMATIS INFECTION

method of
KIMBERLY A. WORKOWSKI, M.D.
Emory University
Atlanta, Georgia

Chlamydia trachomatis is the most common sexually transmitted bacterial pathogen in the United States, accounting for an estimated 4 million infections annually. In most instances, the initial lower genital tract infection is asymptomatic and hence difficult to recognize clinically. Undetected infections can cause serious sequelae, including pelvic inflammatory disease, infertility, and ectopic pregnancy. Thus, as a leading cause of pelvic inflammatory disease and infertility, chlamydial infections are an important threat to women's reproductive health.

EPIDEMIOLOGY

Although the prevalence of genital chlamydial infection has ranged from 2 to 20% in various settings, precise

TABLE 1. Demographic Risk Factors

Age <19 years
Nonwhite race
Multiple sexual partners
Single marital status
Nonbarrier contraceptive use

epidemiologic data are not currently available owing to the lack of uniform reporting nationwide. Demographic factors associated with an increased risk of chlamydial infection include young age, nonwhite race, multiple sexual partners, single marital status, concurrent gonorrhea, and nonbarrier contraceptive methods (Table 1). Transmission rates vary, depending on the presence of symptoms in the index case and whether the sexual encounter is casual or continuous. Recent studies using DNA amplification techniques indicate that approximately 50 to 75% of male partners and 55 to 60% of female partners are infected.

BIOLOGY

Chlamydia are distinguished from all other microorganisms on the basis of their unique life cycle, involving an alteration between two highly specialized morphologic forms adapted to either intracellular or extracellular environments. *C. trachomatis* is one of the three species within the genus *Chlamydia*. *C. trachomatis* can be differentiated into 18 serovars or strains based on monoclonal antibody–based typing assays. Serovars A, B, Ba, and C are associated with endemic trachoma, serovars D to L with genital tract disease, and L1 to L3 with lymphogranuloma venereum. Chlamydia are obligate intracellular parasites that infect squamocolumnar epithelial cells, causing damage from replication of the organism as well as from the resultant inflammatory response.

CLINICAL MANIFESTATIONS

Cervicitis

Clinical recognition of chlamydial cervicitis depends on a high index of suspicion and careful examination, because the majority of women are asymptomatic (Table 2). Findings suggestive of chlamydial infection include easily induced endocervical bleeding, mucopurulent endocervical discharge, and hypertrophic ectopy. Gram's stain of endocervical secretions from women with chlamydial cervicitis usually shows more than 30 polymorphonuclear leukocytes per 1000× field.

Urethritis

Although urethral symptoms may develop in women with chlamydial infection, the majority of women with urethral infection do not have dysuria or urinary frequency. However, chlamydial urethritis should be suspected in young women with dysuria lasting more than 7 to 10 days, lack of hematuria, presence of suprapubic tenderness, use of birth control pills, and sterile pyuria.

Endometritis and Salpingitis

Histologic evidence of endometritis is present in approximately 50% of women with mucopurulent cervicitis and almost all of those with salpingitis. The presence of endometritis in women with chlamydial cervicitis correlates with a history of intermenstrual bleeding. The proportion of women with cervical chlamydial infection who develop upper genital tract infection (endometritis, salpingitis, pelvic peritonitis) is thought to be significant. One study showed that 30% of women with both gonococcal and chlamydial infections treated only for gonorrhea subsequently developed salpingitis. Studies of the long-term complications of salpingitis underscore the impact of so-called silent infection. Infertility due to obstructed fallopian tubes and ectopic pregnancy have been correlated with serologic evidence of chlamydial infection.

Perihepatitis

Recent studies suggest that chlamydia is more commonly associated with perihepatitis than is gonococcal infection. Perihepatitis should be suspected in women with right upper quadrant pain, fever, nausea and vomiting, and salpingitis.

Neonatal Infection

The attack rate of chlamydial conjunctivitis in infants varies from 18 to 50%, and that of chlamydial pneumonitis from 3 to 18%. Chlamydial pneumonitis is clinically indistinguishable from pneumonitis caused by other pathogens. Other infant infections thought to be caused by *C. trachomatis* include otitis media, bronchiolitis, and vulvovaginitis.

TABLE 2. Spectrum of *Chlamydia trachomatis* Infections in Women

| Diagnosis | Clinical Criteria | Laboratory Criteria | |
		Presumptive	*Confirmatory*
Mucopurulent cervicitis	Mucopurulent cervical discharge, cervical ectopy and edema, easily induced endocervical bleeding	Cervical Gram's stain ≥30 polymorphonuclear leukocytes/1000X (nonmenstruating women)	Culture, direct antigen test (cervix), polymerase chain reaction
Acute urethral syndrome	Dysuria—frequency >7 days; new sexual partner	Pyuria, no bacteriuria	Culture or direct antigen test (cervix, urethra)
Pelvic inflammatory disease	Lower abdominal pain, adnexal tenderness, mucopurulent cervical discharge	Cervical mucopus	Culture or direct antigen test (cervix, endometrium, tube)
Perihepatitis	Right upper quadrant pain, nausea, vomiting, fever, salpingitis	Cervical mucopus	*C. trachomatis* serology

DIAGNOSTIC TESTING

Isolation of *C. trachomatis* by cell culture is the most sensitive and specific test available for detection. However, isolation rates depend on strict sample handling and culture procedures. Therefore, specimens should be immediately placed in specific transport media and frozen at $-70°$ C if specimens cannot be inoculated into tissue culture within 24 hours of acquisition. Additionally, the use of cell culture is beyond the capability of most laboratories owing to its technical demands, labor intensity, and high cost. As a result, nonculture methods of detecting chlamydia in genital specimens based primarily on antigen detection or nucleic acid hybridization methods offer reasonable alternatives. At present, there are three nonculture-based assays used for the detection of *C. trachomatis* antigens: a fluorescent monoclonal antibody for direct visualization of the organism, enzyme immunoassays for antigen detection, and a nucleic acid hybridization test. Compared with cell culture, these tests have a reported sensitivity of 70 to 90% in populations in which the prevalence of chlamydial infection exceeds 8%. However, in populations in which the prevalence of chlamydial infection is below 5%, the positive predictive value of a nonculture test may be less than 50%. Confirmatory testing can be performed using blocking antibodies, competitive probes, or a different nonculture test to confirm the initial result. The recent commercial development of nucleic acid amplification methods using the polymerase chain reaction offers more sensitive assays and may soon provide extremely accurate noninvasive methods (urine testing) for screening asymptomatic patients.

TREATMENT

The recommended treatment regimen for uncomplicated chlamydial urethral, endocervical, and rectal infections is doxycycline (Vibramycin) 100 mg twice daily for 7 days or azithromycin (Zithromax) in a single 1-gram dose (Table 3). Azithromycin offers the advantage of single-dose therapy with proven efficacy in recent comparative trials with doxycycline in the treatment of uncomplicated chlamydial infections. Alternative regimens include a 7-day regimen of ofloxacin (Floxin) 300 mg twice daily; erythromycin base 500 mg four times daily; or erythromycin ethylsuccinate 800 mg four times daily.

TABLE 3. **Treatment Regimens for Uncomplicated Urethral, Endocervical, or Rectal Chlamydial Infections**

Recommended Regimens
Doxycycline (Vibramycin) 100 mg PO twice daily for 7 days
or
Azithromycin (Zithromax) 1 gm PO in single dose

Alternative Regimens
Ofloxacin (Floxin) 300 mg PO twice daily for 7 days
or
Erythromycin base 500 mg PO four times daily for 7 days
or
Erythromycin ethylsuccinate 800 mg PO four times daily for 7 days

In Pregnancy
Erythromycin base 500 mg PO four times daily for 7 days
Amoxicillin 500 mg PO three times daily for 10 days

Pregnant women with chlamydial infection should not be treated with doxycycline, ofloxacin, or erythromycin estolate. Azithromycin has not yet been evaluated in pregnancy. Recommendations for treatment in pregnancy include a 7-day regimen of either erythromycin base 500 mg four times daily or erythromycin ethylsuccinate 800 mg four times daily. An alternative regimen for pregnant patients intolerant to erythromycin is amoxicillin 500 mg three times daily for 10 days.

Although a routine test of cure during the immediate post-treatment period is not recommended for the standard treatment regimens, retesting should be considered after using the alternative regimens. However, a nonculture test for confirming organism eradication should be performed at least 3 to 4 weeks after antimicrobial therapy owing to the possibility of prolonged antigen shedding, resulting in a false-positive test.

Additionally, screening for other sexually transmitted diseases should be considered, along with referral of the sexual partner for evaluation and treatment.

PELVIC INFLAMMATORY DISEASE

method of
MARIAN E. WULF, M.D.
University of Texas Medical School at Houston
Houston, Texas

Pelvic inflammatory disease (PID) is an ascending infection of the uterus, the fallopian tubes, and adjacent structures. PID is the most frequent serious infection of women in the United States, affecting over 1 million women per year. The acute manifestations of PID include acute salpingo-oophoritis, endometritis, the development of a tubo-ovarian complex or a tubo-ovarian abscess, and pelvic peritonitis. The chronic sequelae of PID are equally devastating and include infertility, ectopic pregnancy, chronic pelvic pain, and the risk of recurrent PID. Each episode of PID increases a woman's chance of developing infertility from tubal damage. Because PID can present in myriad forms and can have such profound effects, it is important to have a low threshold for diagnosing and treating it when evaluating women with gynecologic complaints.

PID ascends from the cervix and vagina into the upper genital tract most frequently during the first 7 days after menstruation. The polymicrobial nature of this disease has been clearly established. The two most common pathogens are *Neisseria gonorrhoeae* and *Chlamydia trachomatis*. Other pathogens involved in PID include *Escherichia coli*, anaerobic cocci, *Bacteroides* species, and possibly the genital mycoplasmas. Cultures from a tubo-ovarian abscess are usually positive for anaerobic bacteria, not *N. gonorrhoeae* or *C. trachomatis*.

RISK FACTORS

Many predisposing factors for PID have been identified. Women between the ages of 15 and 25 years account for the majority of cases of PID. Women with a history of multiple sexual partners, a previous history of PID, and a history of a sexually transmitted disease are also at increased risk. A history of vaginal douching has been implicated in increasing the risk of acquiring PID.

The type of contraception used can also affect the risk of acquiring PID. Barrier methods of contraception and oral contraception have a protective effect against PID. Insertion of an intrauterine contraceptive device within the previous month is associated with an increased incidence of PID. History of a tubal sterilization dramatically decreases but does not eliminate the risk of PID.

CLINICAL PRESENTATION

The term "PID" is used to describe a broad spectrum of disease, ranging from mild or subclinical symptoms (atypical PID) to rupture of a tubo-ovarian abscess with acute purulent peritonitis. Consequently, there is a wide variation in the clinical presentation. The most common presenting symptom is lower abdominal pain, usually bilateral. More subtle presenting complaints may include a change in vaginal discharge, abnormal uterine bleeding, genitourinary and gastrointestinal symptoms, and dyspareunia. Systemic complaints such as fever, chills, nausea, and vomiting may also be present. Apparently, many women with PID have silent disease, as evidenced by the presence of hydrosalpinges and pelvic adhesions in women with infertility and no history of PID.

Physical examination usually reveals lower abdominal tenderness, adnexal tenderness, and pain with cervical motion. The adnexal tenderness may be unilateral in a significant number of cases. Rebound tenderness and the presence of an adnexal mass may help clarify the diagnosis. Perihepatitis (Fitz-Hugh-Curtis syndrome) may be present with right upper quadrant pain and tenderness to palpation. Perihepatitis is more commonly associated with *C. trachomatis* salpingitis. Fever, leukocytosis, an elevated erythrocyte sedimentation rate, and an elevated C-reactive protein may also be present.

Laboratory evaluation of endocervical specimens for *N. gonorrhoeae* and *C. trachomatis* should be performed using either culture or nonculture techniques. A urine pregnancy test helps rule out ectopic pregnancy, which often mimics PID in the clinical presentation. A culdocentesis may reveal purulent fluid that can be cultured. Ultrasonography can be useful in diagnosing adnexal masses, especially when severe tenderness prevents an adequate pelvic examination. Diagnostic laparoscopy can be useful in clarifying the diagnosis and in ruling out ectopic pregnancy and appendicitis. Screening for other sexually transmitted diseases such as HIV or syphilis is often appropriate.

TREATMENT

The goal of treatment for PID is to prevent the chronic sequelae such as ectopic pregnancy and tubal infertility by early diagnosis and prompt initiation of antibiotic therapy. Because of the wide variety of organisms implicated in the pathogenesis of PID, appropriate regimens must provide empirical broad-spectrum coverage. There is no single agent currently available that covers *C. trachomatis* and all the aerobic and anaerobic species involved in PID.

Table 1 lists the 1993 Centers for Disease Control and Prevention (CDC) recommendations for the outpatient treatment of PID. This regimen consists of cefoxitin (Mefoxin) 2 grams intramuscularly with probenecid (Benemid) 1 gram orally, followed by a

TABLE 1. 1993 CDC Guidelines for the Ambulatory Management of Acute PID

Regimen A
Cefoxitin (Mefoxin) 2 gm IM *plus* probenecid (Benemid) 1 gm PO
or
Ceftriaxone (Rocephin) 250 mg IM
or
Ceftizoxime (Cefizox) 1 gm IM
or
Cefotaxime (Claforan) 1 gm IM
plus
Doxycycline (Vibramycin) 100 mg PO bid for 14 days
Regimen B
Ofloxacin (Floxin) 400 mg PO bid for 14 days
plus
Clindamycin (Cleocin) 450 mg PO bid for 14 days
or
Metronidazole (Flagyl) 500 mg PO bid for 14 days

From Centers for Disease Control and Prevention: 1993 sexually transmitted diseases treatment guidelines. MMWR *42*(RR-14):78–80, 1993.

14-day course of doxycycline (Vibramycin) 100 mg twice daily. Alternatively, ceftriaxone (Rocephin), ceftizoxime (Cefizox), or cefotaxime (Claforan) can be used in place of cefoxitin as a single injection, with antichlamydial activity provided by a 14-day course of doxycycline. A second ambulatory regimen involves the patient taking two medications orally for 14 days: ofloxacin (Floxin) with either clindamycin (Cleocin) or metronidazole (Flagyl). Patients with PID who are treated as outpatients need to be re-evaluated within 72 hours. If there is no response to treatment, the patient needs to be hospitalized for confirmation of the diagnosis and parenteral antibiotic therapy.

The CDC recommends hospitalization of patients with PID in the following situations: There is an uncertain diagnosis, and surgical emergencies such as ectopic pregnancy or appendicitis need to be excluded; a pelvic abscess is suspected; the patient is pregnant; the patient is an adolescent; the patient has human immunodeficiency virus (HIV) infection; the patient cannot follow or tolerate an outpatient regimen; the patient has failed to respond to outpa-

TABLE 2. 1993 CDC Guidelines for the Inpatient Treatment of Acute PID

Regimen A
Cefoxitin (Mefoxin) 2 gm IV q 6 h
or
Cefotetan (Cefotan) 2 gm IV q 12 h
plus
Doxycycline (Vibramycin) 100 mg bid IV or PO q 12 h
Regimen B
Clindamycin (Cleocin) 900 mg IV q 8 h
plus
Gentamicin (Garamycin) loading dose (2 mg/kg of body weight) IV or IM followed by maintenance dose of 1.5 mg/kg q 8 h

From Centers for Disease Control and Prevention: 1993 sexually transmitted diseases treatment guidelines. MMWR *42*(RR-14):78–80, 1993.

tient therapy; or clinical follow-up within 72 hours of the initiation of therapy cannot be arranged.

Table 2 lists the 1993 CDC recommendations for parenteral treatment of PID. Regimen A consists of cefoxitin or cefotetan and doxycycline. Regimen B consists of clindamycin and gentamicin. Many clinicians prefer regimen B when a tubo-ovarian abscess is present because of clindamycin's more effective anaerobic coverage. Parenteral antibiotics should be continued for at least 48 hours after the patient has shown significant improvement, and then oral antibiotics should be used to complete a 14-day course of treatment. The CDC recommends either doxycycline 100 mg twice daily or clindamycin 450 mg four times daily as the oral antibiotic.

Evaluation and treatment of the patient's sexual partner are essential to preventing reinfection, regardless of the regimen used to treat PID.

UTERINE LEIOMYOMA

method of
SANFORD M. MARKHAM, M.D.
Georgetown University Medical Center
Washington, District of Columbia

Uterine leiomyomas are not only the most common pelvic neoplasm in women, but they are also the most common uterine neoplasm. The incidence of uterine leiomyoma is reported to be approximately 20% in women over the age of 30 years; however, postmortem examinations of women suggest a somewhat higher incidence, as do diagnostic laparoscopies for the assessment of infertility, pregnancy wastage, and pelvic pain. Because of their incidence and their impact on women's health and quality of life, these uterine tumors are of great importance. Abnormal uterine bleeding, abdominal pelvic pain, abdominal pelvic organ dysfunction (urinary frequency, constipation), and altered reproductive capacity (infertility, pregnancy wastage, premature delivery) have all been related to uterine leiomyoma.

PATHOPHYSIOLOGY

Recent studies have demonstrated that many uterine leiomyomas are cytogenetically abnormal. Chromosomes 7, 12, and 14 have been found to be most frequently involved in leiomyoma and include both translocations and deletions. Many other chromosomes, including the X chromosome, have also been implicated. The concept that most human tumors, including uterine leiomyoma, are cytogenetically abnormal clones is rapidly gaining acceptance. This theory suggests that uterine leiomyomas are composed of genetically abnormal clones of cells derived from a single progenitor that has undergone mutation. The mutation results in cells that respond abnormally to one or more growth factors resulting in tumor cell growth, whereas adjacent normal myometrial cells, without mutation, replicate in a conditioned and normal fashion. Other studies indicate that a number of growth factors, including insulin-like growth factors and their binding proteins, play a modulating role in uterine leiomyoma growth. It is also possible that epidermal growth factor as well as others also modulates leiomyoma growth, with some growth factors stimulated by estrogen and others by progestins. This variable modulation concept may explain why some uterine leiomyomas respond more dramatically than others to gonadotropin-releasing hormone agonist (GnRHa).

Uterine leiomyomas generally occur in one of three anatomic locations: (1) intramural (occurring in the midportion of the myometrium), (2) subserosal (projecting outwardly into the pelvic cavity), or (3) submucosal (projecting into the uterine cavity). Subserosal leiomyomas may grow into the broad ligament or other adjacent structures. Both subserosal and submucosal leiomyomas may also become pedunculated. Some subserosal leiomyomas have become detached from their uterine surface and reattached to other tissues and/or organs in the abdominal cavity. These migratory tumors are referred to as parasitic leiomyomas.

Approximately 80% of uterine leiomyomas are multiple. The most common histologic changes of uterine leiomyomas are degeneration, hemorrhage, and ulceration. These changes may occur in up to two thirds of all uterine leiomyomas. Degenerative changes include (1) hyaline degeneration, (2) hydropic (edema) degeneration, (3) red (infarction) degeneration, (4) calcific degeneration, (5) myxomatous degeneration, and (6) fatty degeneration. Whether myomas also degenerate into leiomyosarcomas (LMS) or whether LMS develop spontaneously remains controversial. Most data favor a malignant degeneration process. Such a malignant degeneration of uterine leiomyoma to LMS occurs in approximately 0.5% of all leiomyomas. In either case, uterine LMS accounts for only 1.3% of all uterine malignancies. The histologic difference between leiomyomas and LMS is based on the numbers of mitoses per high-power field (HPF) and the presence of atypia seen on histologic examination. Tumors with fewer than five mitoses per ten HPF examinations and no atypia are considered to be benign.

Adenomyosis is sometimes confused with uterine leiomyoma because of similar presenting symptoms and physical findings. Differentiation of the two pathologies has historically been based on histologic examination. However, magnetic resonance imaging (MRI) appears to have the ability to make a presurgical differentiation. Such a distinction is important, since conservative management of adenomyosis generally is of little benefit.

SYMPTOMS

Though a majority of leiomyomas are asymptomatic, approximately 33% do present with symptoms. These symptoms include abnormal uterine bleeding, pelvic pain and/or pressure, and reproductive abnormalities (infertility, pregnancy wastage, and preterm labor).

DIAGNOSIS

The diagnosis of uterine leiomyoma is made primarily by physical examination. However, the patient's history and imaging techniques may be supportive as well as diagnostic. Leiomyomas are suspected when, on bimanual examination, the uterus is found to be enlarged, irregular in outline, firm, and nontender. Imaging techniques useful when the physical examination fails to provide a clear diagnosis include pelvic ultrasonography (US), MRI, and/or computed tomography (CT) scanning. Of these imaging techniques, pelvic ultrasonography is both effective and least expensive and therefore preferred. If adenomyosis must also be ruled out, MRI has recently proved to be effective. The diagnosis of uterine leiomyoma is also frequently made in asymptomatic patients undergoing laparoscopy or laparotomy for other pelvic pathology.

The evaluation of a patient with uterine leiomyoma should attempt to determine accurately the number, location, and size of each uterine tumor. Traditionally, the total uterine leiomyoma size has been estimated on the basis of equivalent gestational size. Imaging techniques now allow the assessment of uterine volume, which may prove to be far more accurate in following patients.

Additional studies of importance in assessing uterine leiomyoma include (1) hematocrit or hemoglobin and (2) coagulation studies (fibrinogen, prothrombin time, bleeding time), in patients with abnormal uterine bleeding; and/or (3) endometrial biopsy, in patients at risk for endometrial hyperplasia. Occasionally surgical diagnostic procedures (laparoscopy, hysteroscopy) are required to assess accurately the location, number, and size of the uterine tumor. Generally, however, imaging techniques such as ultrasonography provide this information, obviating the need for surgical procedures (Table 1).

MANAGEMENT

Management of uterine leiomyoma depends on (1) symptoms resulting from the tumor, (2) size and number of tumors, (3) the patient's desire to maintain reproductive function, and (4) the patient's age. Active management (medical or surgical) is not generally recommended for uterine leiomyoma under the equivalent of a 12 weeks' gestational size with minimal or no symptoms. As the composite uterine volume increases above this size or if rapid growth occurs or if symptoms of abnormal uterine bleeding, significant pelvic pain, or reproductive function disorders occur that are likely related to the tumors, then active management should be considered.

Treatment for uterine leiomyoma may be divided into two general options: expectant management or

active management. Active management may include medical or surgical options (Table 2).

Expectant management is the treatment of choice in patients with minimal or controllable symptoms (menorrhagia/metrorrhagia) whose tumors are stable in size or are noted to be only slow growing after 2 years of observation. Interval examinations should be every 6 months for 2 years, and then yearly thereafter unless significant changes occur during this period. The abnormal uterine bleeding may be controlled with nonsteroidal anti-inflammatory drugs, progestins, or low-dose oral contraceptives (Table 3).

Medical management of uterine leiomyoma is based on the finding that estrogens generally stimulate uterine growth. GnRHa suppresses pituitary gonadotropin release, which in turn suppresses ovarian estrogen production. The resulting hypoestrogenemia

---

TABLE 1. **Evaluation of Uterine Leiomyoma**

Abdominal-pelvic examination

Imaging procedures (when physical examination is inconclusive):
  Ultrasonography
  Magnetic resonance imaging
  Computed tomography scanning

Hematologic studies (with abnormal bleeding):
  Hemoglobin or hematocrit
  Coagulation/bleeding studies:
    Prothrombin time
    Bleeding time
    Fibrinogen
    Platelets

Histologic studies (with abnormal bleeding):
  Endometrial biopsy
  Curettage

Adjuvant procedures (when tumor size affects other pelvic organ function):
  Intravenous pyelogram
  Barium enema

Adjuvant procedures (when diagnosis is unclear with above testing):
  Hysteroscopy
  Laparoscopy

TABLE 2. **Management Options for Treating Uterine Leiomyoma**

Expectant management
  Uterine size under the equivalent of 12 weeks' gestation
  Minimal or controllable symptoms

Medical management
  Gonadotropin-releasing hormone agonist (GnRHa) suppression
  GnRHa suppression with estrogen/progestin "add-back"

Surgical management
  Hysteroscopic excision of submucous/pedunculated leiomyoma
  Laparoscopic excision/destruction of subserous leiomyoma
  Laparotomy with myomectomy
  Hysterectomy (abdominal/vaginal)

Combined medical/surgical management
  Preoperative GnRHa suppression
  Conservative/definitive surgery

TABLE 3. **Expectant Management of Leiomyoma**

Initial abdominal/pelvic examination followed by repeat examinations every 6 months for 2 years, then yearly

Symptom control
  Abnormal uterine bleeding
    Nonsteroidal anti-inflammatory drugs (NSAIDs)
      1. Ibuprofen (Motrin), 400 mg PO q 4 h beginning with earliest onset of bleeding
      2. Naproxen sodium (Anaprox), 550 mg PO initially, then 275 mg PO q 6 h beginning with earliest onset of bleeding
      3. Mefenamic acid (Ponstel), 500 mg PO initially, then 250 mg PO q 6 h beginning with earliest onset of bleeding
    Progestins
      1. Medroxyprogesterone acetate (Provera), 10 mg PO daily × 14 days each month, starting cycle day 12
      2. Norethindrone (Micronor) 0.35 mg PO daily × 14 days each month, starting cycle day 12
      3. Norgestrel (Ovrette), 0.075 mg PO daily × 14 days each month, starting cycle day 12 or daily without break
    Oral contraceptive agents
      1. Norgestrel and ethinyl estradiol (Ovral), 1 tablet daily for 21 of 28 days
      2. Desogestrel and ethinyl estradiol (Ortho-Cept), 1 tablet daily for 21 of 28 days
      3. Norethindrone and mestranol (Norinyl 1 + 50), 1 tablet daily for 21 of 28 days
  Abdominal/pelvic pain:
    NSAIDs as listed above

TABLE 4. **Medical Management of Leiomyoma**

Uterine leiomyoma size reduction through ovarian/estrogen
    suppression
    Submucous leiomyoma >2 cm
    Subserous leiomyoma greater than equivalent 12 weeks'
      gestation size

Gonadotropin-releasing hormone agonist (GnRHa) ovarian/
    estrogen suppression*
    Leuprolide acetate (Lupron Depot), 3.75 mg IM monthly × 3
      months
    Nafarelin acetate (Synarel), 200 µg intranasally bid × 3
      months
    Goserelin acetate (Zoladex), 3.6 mg SC monthly × 3 months

GnRHa ovarian/estrogen suppression* with estrogen/progestin
    "add-back"
    3 months of one of the above GnRHa followed by
    Continued GnRHa, plus
      (1) Conjugated estrogens (Premarin), 0.625 mg PO qd
      (2) Medroxyprogesterone acetate (Provera), 2.5 mg PO qd

*GnRHa does not have FDA approval for medical management of uterine leiomyoma; however, sufficient research and clinical data support its merit in leiomyoma management.

is associated with a reduction in uterine volume of approximately 40%. This reduction is usually more prominent in leiomyomas in which the uterine composite size is greater than 12 weeks' gestation. The effect of GnRHa is maximal at approximately 3 months of therapy, with little or no additional size reduction beyond this time. Following cessation of GnRHa therapy, rapid re-growth of tumors back to pretreatment size is most commonly observed. Therefore, this management option is generally only recommended as a presurgical adjuvant or in patients with pending menopause. Longer management with

TABLE 5. **Surgical Management of Leiomyoma**

Hysteroscopic excision of submucous/pedunculated leiomyoma
    <2 cm without GnRHa ovarian/estrogen suppression
    >2 cm with GnRHa ovarian/estrogen suppression
    20% of cases require additional management at a later date

Laparoscopic excision/destruction of subserous/pedunculated
    leiomyoma
    Excision limited by size of leiomyoma
    Destruction of leiomyoma by laser or bipolar electrocautery
    Because of potential complications, this procedure is still
      considered investigational

Laparotomy with myomectomy
    For patients who fail to conceive or who experience recurrent
      pregnancy wastage in whom the leiomyoma would appear to
      be a contributing cause
    For patients who wish to preserve reproductive capacity (see
      Table 6)

Hysterectomy (abdominal/vaginal)
    For patients with
      >12 weeks' gestation equivalent size uterus
      Rapidly growing leiomyoma
      Excessive abnormal uterine bleeding unresponsive to
        conservative management
      Abdominal/pelvic pain unresponsive to conservative
        management
    Abdominal hysterectomy the preferred route except in smaller
      symptomatic leiomyoma
    Retention of ovaries in premenopausal patients (see Table 7)

GnRHa is reported to be beneficial with utilization of "add-back" therapy following the first 12 weeks of GnRHa administration (Table 4).

Surgical management includes four separate operative options: (1) laparoscopic excision/destruction of leiomyoma, (2) hysteroscopic resection of pedunculated or broad-based submucous leiomyoma, (3) laparotomy with myomectomy, and (4) hysterectomy (Table 5). The decision to utilize a surgical approach should be based on the adverse effects that the leiomyomas have on the patient's quality of life. Symptomatic patients (abnormal uterine bleeding/abdominal pelvic pain/reproductive disorders) are candidates for surgical intervention if the symptoms can be reasonably related to the leiomyoma. Laparoscopic excision of pedunculated leiomyoma or coagulation of the leiomyoma by laser or electrical current has enjoyed some success; however, these approaches are applicable only to the small, subserous leiomyoma and at this time are not recommended for the larger tumors that warrant major surgical intervention. Hysteroscopic resection of submucous leiomyoma offers a less extensive surgical approach to uterine cavitary lesions when the tumors are felt to be related to abnormal uterine bleeding or reproductive disorders. It is recommended that these surgical procedures be preceded by GnRHa suppression for a 3-month period to reduce the size of the tumor (particularly with tumors over 2 cm) as well as to reduce blood loss during the procedure. It should be noted, however, that approximately 20% of patients require additional surgery after hysteroscopic resection of leiomyoma.

Laparotomy with myomectomy may be considered for the patient who meets the American College of Obstetricians and Gynecologists (ACOG) criteria for myomectomy (Table 6) or who is desirous of main-

TABLE 6. **ACOG Criteria for Myomectomy***

Indication: Leiomyomas in infertility patients, as a probable
          factor in failure to conceive or in recurrent pregnancy
          loss

Confirmation of indication: In the presence of failure to conceive
                  or recurrent pregnancy loss:
  1. Presence of leiomyomas of sufficient size or specific location
    to be a probable factor
  2. No more likely explanation exists for the failure to conceive
    or recurrent pregnancy loss

Actions prior to procedure:
  1. Evaluate other causes of male and female infertility or
    recurrent pregnancy loss
  2. Evaluate the endometrial cavity and fallopian tubes, e.g.,
    hysterosalpingogram
  3. Document discussion that complexity of disease process may
    require hysterectomy
    (Unless otherwise stated, each numbered item must be
    present)

*Evaluation of the quality of care provided with this procedure, when performed for the indication listed, will be possible through assessment of ongoing or repetitive patterns of care ("trending").

Modified from The American College of Obstetricians and Gynecologists: Uterine Leiomyomata. Technical Bulletin No. 192. Washington, DC, ACOG, © 1994.

TABLE 7. ACOG Criteria for Hysterectomy for Leiomyomas

Procedure: Hysterectomy, abdominal or vaginal*

Indication: Leiomyomas

Confirmation of indication: Presence of 1 or 2 or 3
1. Asymptomatic leiomyomas of such size that they are palpable abdominally and are a concern to the patient
2. Excessive uterine bleeding evidenced by *either* of the following:
    a. Profuse bleeding with flooding or clots or repetitive periods lasting for more than 8 days
    b. Anemia due to acute or chronic blood loss
3. Pelvic discomfort caused by myomas (a or b or c)
    a. Acute and severe
    b. Chronic lower abdominal or low back pressure
    c. Bladder pressure with urinary frequency not due to urinary tract infection

Actions prior to procedure:
1. Confirm the absence of cervical malignancy
2. Eliminate anovulation and other causes of abnormal bleeding
3. When abnormal bleeding is present, confirm the absence of endometrial malignancy
4. Assess surgical risk from anemia and need for treatment
5. Consider patient's medical and psychological risks concerning hysterectomy

Contraindication:
1. Desire to maintain fertility, in which case myomectomy should be considered
2. Asymptomatic leiomyomas of size less than 12 weeks' gestation determined by physical examination or ultrasound examination

(Unless otherwise stated, each numbered and lettered item [except contraindications] must be present)

*Evaluation of the quality of care provided with this procedure, when performed for indications 2 and 3, will be possible through assessment of ongoing or repetitive patterns of care ("trending").

Modified from The American College of Obstetricians and Gynecologists: Uterine Leiomyomata. Technical Bulletin No. 192. Washington, DC, ACOG, © 1994.

taining her reproductive capacity, presents with symptoms requiring surgical intervention, or is unresponsive to expectant management. GnRHa suppression for a 3-month period has proved to be beneficial in reducing tumor volume and operative bleeding in patients whose leiomyomas have a composite size of greater than 12 weeks' gestation. It should be kept in mind that approximately 25% of patients who have undergone a myomectomy will later require another surgical procedure, as the recurrence rate is approximately 50% in patients with multiple leiomyomas.

Hysterectomy may be considered in symptomatic patients who are uninterested in further reproductive function provided the ACOG criteria for hysterectomy for leiomyoma are met (Table 7).

ENDOMETRIAL CANCER

method of
JOHN P. CURTIN, M.D.
Memorial Sloan-Kettering Cancer Center
New York, New York

EPIDEMIOLOGY

Adenocarcinoma of the endometrium is the most common malignancy of the female genital tract, and it was estimated that there would be 33,000 new cases diagnosed in the United States in 1995. The disease is generally diagnosed in an early stage, and the prognosis for most patients is good. Treatment is primarily surgical, and radiotherapy is reserved for the patient unable to tolerate a surgical procedure or as adjuvant therapy after hysterectomy.

The overall lifetime risk of an American white woman's developing adenocarcinoma of the endometrium is 2.7%; the risk in African American women is one-half that of white women, and the incidence is lowest in Asian women. The incidence of endometrial cancer has remained relatively stable over the past several decades with the exception of a statistical increase in incidence in the mid-1970s. This increase in the number of new cases of endometrial cancer was the result of the widespread practice of prescribing unopposed estrogen therapy to postmenopausal women. Once this association was noticed and physician prescription practices changed, the incidence returned to the same level as previously recorded. The increased incidence noted in the 1970s was not accompanied by an increase in the rate of death due to endometrial cancer, probably reflecting the relatively indolent nature of endometrial cancer associated with estrogen replacement therapy.

Endometrial adenocarcinoma is primarily a disease of Western society, with the highest incidence rates noted in the United States and European countries. The median age at diagnosis is approximately 59 years, and the diagnosis is uncommon in women younger than 40 years of age (less than 5 to 10% of all cases). The prime risk factors associated with endometrial cancer include obesity, a high-fat diet, low parity, hormonal replacement therapy, and increasing age. Less commonly, patients are at risk for endometrial cancer because of a genetic predisposition (i.e., Lynch II syndrome) or an estrogen-producing neoplasm of the ovary, such as a granulosa cell tumor. The known risk factors and the relative risk associated with these factors are presented in Table 1. Several factors are known to decrease the overall incidence of endometrial cancer, including oral contraceptives, high parity, and smoking (probably related to a decrease in weight).

The presumed common mechanism of these risk factors is increased estrogen stimulation of the endometrium. Pro-

TABLE 1. Risk Factors Associated with Endometrial Cancer

Risk Factor	Relative Risk
Obesity (>50 lb)	2–11
Nulliparity	2
Late menopause	2
Estrogen (unopposed)	2–5
Estrogen and progesterone	1.6
Diabetes	1.5–2.0
Hypertension	1.5–2.0

longed stimulation of the endometrium by estrogen results in a progression from simple hyperplasia to hyperplasia with atypia to invasive cancer; endometrial hyperplasia is theoretically a reversible condition and often responds to progesterone therapy. More recently, there have been reports of an increased risk of endometrial neoplasia associated with the use of tamoxifen (Nolvadex), which is prescribed as adjuvant therapy after a diagnosis of breast cancer. Tamoxifen competes for the estrogen-binding sites located in the nuclear region of the breast cancer cell, which is presumed to explain in part the mechanism of action in the decreasing rate of recurrences and second primaries in breast cancer patients. It appears, however, that in endometrial cells, tamoxifen acts as a weak estrogenic agent. There is continued debate about whether there is a true increased rate of endometrial cancer in women receiving tamoxifen as adjuvant therapy for breast cancer, since these women are already at risk because of their diagnosis of breast cancer. The value of routine screening of women taking tamoxifen is undetermined.

DIAGNOSIS AND INITIAL EVALUATION

The classic symptom of endometrial cancer is postmenopausal bleeding. The recognition by both the patient and the physician of the significance of postmenopausal bleeding accounts for the large percentage of patients diagnosed with early-stage disease. The rate of endometrial cancer diagnosis in patients with postmenopausal bleeding ranges between 5 and 20%. Less commonly, the diagnosis is prompted by the finding of an abnormal Pap smear demonstrating either normal or abnormal endometrial cells in a postmenopausal woman not on hormonal replacement. In younger women irregular bleeding is common. Patients with advanced disease often present with symptoms similar to those of advanced ovarian cancer, with increasing abdominal girth due to ascites and/or intra-abdominal metastasis.

The standard diagnostic test for the patient suspected of having endometrial neoplasia is dilatation and curettage (D & C) of the endometrial cavity. In the past several years, there has been a shift toward the use of endometrial biopsy and ultrasound in the initial management of the patient who presents with postmenopausal bleeding. Endometrial biopsy has the advantage of ease of use, with an acceptable degree of sensitivity and specificity. Endometrial biopsy can be successfully done on the majority of postmenopausal women and avoids the need for a surgical procedure, with the associated higher costs. Recent reports have introduced the ultrasonic measurement of endometrial thickness as another method to evaluate the postmenopausal woman with bleeding; when the endometrial stripe is less than 5 to 10 mm thick, the likelihood of endometrial neoplasia is small. Hysteroscopy is now commonly added to the D & C procedure to ensure a more accurate evaluation of the endometrium. Some concern has been raised regarding the potential for transtubal implantation of the hysteroscopic fluid contaminated with endometrial cancer cells during the hysteroscopic procedure. To date, there is no clinical evidence to support this concern, and the suspicion of an endometrial neoplasm is not a contraindication to hysteroscopy.

Once the histologic diagnosis is confirmed by a sampling of the endometrium, the standard therapy is hysterectomy with bilateral salpingo-oophorectomy (BSO). The preparation of the patient for surgery does not involve any special tests other than those required for preoperative studies. Since this disease is predominantly a disease of older women, a medical consultation is often appropriate. The only routine medical imaging study ordered is a two-view chest radiograph. Patients with early endometrial cancer do not benefit from routine imaging studies, including computed tomography (CT) scans, pelvic ultrasound, or magnetic resonance imaging (MRI) studies. Before the surgical procedure, the patient should also have undergone the screening studies for the two most common malignancies among women in this age group, namely, breast cancer and colon cancer. Finally, most patients are candidates for autologous blood donation, and patients are given the opportunity to bank 1 to 2 U of blood before the surgical procedure.

SURGICAL TREATMENT AND STAGING

Standard surgical therapy for endometrial cancer is a total abdominal hysterectomy (TAH) and BSO. A midline incision is preferred to allow a more thorough inspection and exploration of the abdominal cavity. The surgeon should aspirate the pelvic fluid for cytologic examination at the beginning of the procedure; saline can be instilled in the cul-de-sac and aspirated if there is no obvious fluid present. After cytologic sampling, the pelvis and abdominal cavity are carefully explored. Important areas of concern in the pelvis include the size and consistency of the uterus, evidence of peritoneal implants, and/or suspicious enlargement of the ovaries. The pelvic lymph nodes are palpated. Exploration of the abdomen includes the omentum, large bowel and appendix, small bowel, stomach and pancreas, pericolic peritoneum, diaphragms, gallbladder, and liver. As is true for ovarian cancer, the exploration is both a visual and a tactile examination; suspicious nodules or roughened areas of peritoneum should be excised for histologic examination.

The hysterectomy is performed as a simple hysterectomy and BSO; rarely, a modified or radical hysterectomy is indicated for the patient who presents with gross cervical involvement. In the very young patient with an endometrial cancer, consideration can be given to ovarian preservation if the endometrial cancer is not thought to represent a genetic syndrome (i.e., endometrial cancer in a patient with polycystic ovarian disease). The vaginal cuff is closed and drains are not required.

Although endometrial cancer staging is now based on surgical staging, not all patients should be subjected to an extended surgical staging procedure. Based on the large surgical staging study conducted by the Gynecologic Oncology Group (GOG), patients with clinical early-stage endometrial cancer can be assigned to low-risk and high-risk groups, according to the pathologic features of the tumor (grade and histologic subtype) and the depth of myometrial invasion. The grade and histologic subtype are known preoperatively, and the depth of myometrial invasion can be determined by gross inspection of the opened uterus in the operating room; if there is no obvious deep invasion (>50%) of the myometrium, the uterus is then sent for frozen section analysis to rule out deep invasion.

When the patient is at high risk for possible lymphatic spread (Table 2), the pelvic and aortic lymph nodes are sampled. This procedure differs from a therapeutic lymph node dissection as performed for early cervical cancer. To sample the pelvic lymph nodes, the lymph-bearing tissue over the external iliac vessels is removed and the dissection is carried down to the obturator space. The aortic lymph nodes are sampled on both the right and the left sides. In the GOG study of over 600 patients with endometrial adenocarcinoma, 48 women (7%) were found to have metastasis to the aortic lymph nodes. An important observation is that in 47 of the 48 cases the patients had one or more of the following high-risk factors: Grade 3 histologic type, deep myometrial invasion, and/or clinical evidence of adnexal or pelvic lymph node involvement.

Although TAH is considered the standard treatment of endometrial cancer, vaginal hysterectomy is another option that has been used for the patient who may not be able to tolerate an abdominal incision. More recently, laparoscopic-assisted vaginal hysterectomy (LAVH) has been reported in limited series of patients. The LAVH technique has the advantage of allowing a complete inspection of the peritoneal cavity and collection of a cytologic specimen. Depending on the level of experience of the laparoscopic surgeon, pelvic and aortic lymph node sampling is also possible via the laparoscope. The theoretical advantage of this approach is shorter hospitalization and a faster return to normal activities after the surgical procedure, although this has not been proved in a prospective clinical trial.

PROGNOSTIC FACTORS

The most important prognostic factor for patients with adenocarcinoma of the endometrium is the stage at the time of diagnosis. The current surgical staging guidelines are presented in Table 3 and represent a shift from the clinical staging of endometrial cancer that was employed before 1988. Since the revised staging system was derived from clinicopathologic studies of prognostic factors, the current staging takes into account many of the factors indicating a poor prognosis, such as the depth of myometrial invasion, cervical invasion, adnexal metastasis, and lymph node metastasis. One area of controversy is whether positive peritoneal cytologic findings alone are associated with a poorer prognosis; positive cytologic findings are equated with other known poor prognostic factors (high grade, deep myometrial inva-

TABLE 3. International Federation of Gynecology and Obstetrics (FIGO) Staging of Endometrial Cancer

Stage	Characteristics
IA G123	Tumor limited to endometrium
IB G123	Invasion to less than one-half of the myometrium
IC G123	Invasion to more than one-half of the myometrium
IIA G123	Endocervical glandular involvement only
IIB G123	Cervical stromal invasion
IIIA G123	Tumor invasion of serosa or adnexa, or positive peritoneal cytologic finding
IIIB G123	Vaginal metastases
IIIC G123	Metastases to pelvic or para-aortic lymph nodes
IVA G123	Tumor invasion of bladder or bowel mucosa
IVB	Distant metastases, including intra-abdominal and inguinal lymph nodes

Degree of histopathologic differentiation: Cases of carcinoma of corpus should be classified (or graded) according to degree of histologic differentiation, as follows: G1 = 5% or less of a nonsquamous or nonmorular solid growth pattern; G2 = 6–50% of a nonsquamous or nonmorular solid growth pattern; G3 = more than 50% of a nonsquamous or nonmorular solid growth pattern.

sion, adnexal metastasis, and serosal invasion) in the subgroup of patients classified as Stage IIIA. Age is also an important determinant of prognosis in women with adenocarcinoma of the endometrium, with younger patients having an improved prognosis compared with older patients. This overall good prognosis is especially apparent in women younger than 40 years of age at the time of diagnosis; in one series there were no deaths due to endometrial cancer in this population of young women.

The histologic subtype of adenocarcinoma is also an important prognostic factor. Simple adenocarcinoma is the most common type of uterine cancer and accounts for approximately 80% of all endometrial cancers. Prognosis is dependent on the grade of the tumor. Stage I adenocarcinoma of the endometrium confined to the uterus has an expected 5-year survival ranging between 80 and 98%, depending on grade and depth of invasion. Aortic lymph node metastases are associated with a significant drop in survival, estimated to be approximately 40% by 5 years. Patients with advanced, unresectable intra-abdominal disease or distant metastases at diagnosis have a poor prognosis, with fewer than 5 to 10% alive at 5 years after diagnosis.

Other historic subtypes include clear cell, papillary, and papillary serous cancers. Although relatively uncommon, these histologic variants are important because of the poor prognosis associated with these types. Patients with papillary serous cancers of the endometrium are more likely to have advanced disease at the time of diagnosis. The pattern of spread for papillary serous tumors is like that of ovarian cancer, and intraperitoneal dissemination is common; surgical staging for patients known to have papillary serous cancers should include multiple peritoneal biopsies and an omental biopsy. When patients with papillary serous tumors have disease confined to the uterus at the time of diagnosis, they are at higher risk of recurrence. Patients with advanced

TABLE 2. Indications for Extended Surgical Staging in Endometrial Cancer

Suspicious pelvic or aortic nodes
Deep myometrial invasion
Grade 2 or 3
Adnexal metastasis
High-risk histologic findings (papillary, papillary serous)
Cervical involvement

or recurrent disease respond poorly to either chemotherapy or radiation and often die of their disease. Patients with clear cell or papillary tumors have a poorer prognosis that is comparable to that of patients with poorly differentiated adenocarcinoma.

As would be expected, endometrial adenocarcinomas often contain hormonal receptors, and the levels of receptors as measured either by the cytosol protein method or by immunohistochemical staining are another predictor of prognosis. Patients with high levels of nuclear hormonal receptors, especially high progesterone receptor levels, have a significant survival advantage over those patients with low levels of hormonal receptors. In a multivariate analysis of women with early-stage endometrial cancer, only the age of the patient, the grade of the tumor, and the progesterone receptor status were significant predictors of overall survival. Estrogen and progesterone receptor studies can be obtained at the time of hysterectomy for patients with endometrial cancer. This information not only provides some information regarding prognosis, but may also determine therapy if the patient subsequently develops a recurrence, since patients with progesterone receptor–rich tumors are more likely to respond to hormonal therapy.

ADJUVANT THERAPY

Postoperative adjuvant radiation therapy is prescribed for patients at higher risk of recurrence after hysterectomy and BSO. Determination of risk is similar to the decision process that identifies patients who should have lymph node sampling. If the patient has had surgery and has no evidence of disease spread beyond the uterus, a combination of whole pelvic radiation therapy and intracavitary therapy is usually reserved for patients with deep myometrial invasion and/or high-grade tumors; less than 50% of all patients with endometrial cancer require both external and internal radiotherapy after hysterectomy. The radiation therapy is begun after recovery from surgery (approximately 6 to 8 weeks), and the dose of pelvic radiation prescribed is 4500 cGy. Intracavitary radiation is delivered via a high-dose-rate machine in our institution, and the usual total dose to the vaginal mucosa is 2100 cGy, given in three applications. Patients with minimal myometrial invasion who do not meet the criteria for external beam radiation therapy receive the intracavitary radiation therapy alone. Only patients with no myometrial invasion (Stage IA) receive no postoperative radiation therapy.

Patients with evidence of lymphatic metastasis should receive extended-field radiation in addition to pelvic radiation therapy; the extent of additional treatment depends on the location of the documented lymph node metastasis. If there is pelvic lymph node metastasis only, then the treatment field should be extended to include the lower aortic lymph nodes. If aortic nodal metastases are found, the radiation field should include a full aortic "chimney." Patients with completed resection of peritoneal metastases are candidates for whole abdominal radiation therapy with a pelvic boost. For patients with positive peritoneal cytologic findings alone, there is considerable debate on the role of adjuvant therapy. Various authors have suggested that patients with malignant cells in the peritoneum are candidates for intraperitoneal ^{32}P therapy. Another recommendation is to treat these patients with progestins. Our bias has been to use intraperitoneal ^{32}P therapy for those patients with strongly positive peritoneal cytologic findings and other high-risk factors.

THERAPY OF ADVANCED OR RECURRENT DISEASE

Patients who present with either advanced unresectable disease or recurrent disease are candidates for hormonal therapy or chemotherapy. The choice of therapy is based on the histologic subtype, the grade of the original tumor, and, if available, the estrogen and progesterone receptor levels. Patients with well-differentiated adenocarcinomas should receive a progestin as an initial therapy. The two most commonly prescribed agents are megestrol acetate (Megace) (160 mg per day) and medroxyprogesterone (Provera) (10 to 20 mg per day). These agents are well tolerated with minimal side effects. Response rates range from 15 to 40%, and in some instances, the response can be long-lasting. If the patient progresses on hormonal therapy, then chemotherapy is indicated.

The most active agent for advanced endometrial adenocarcinoma is doxorubicin (Adriamycin). A recent study reported that there was a survival advantage when cisplatin was combined with doxorubicin, compared with doxorubicin alone. Since doxorubicin is contraindicated in patients with cardiac disease, which is relatively common in women with endometrial cancer, an alternative would be cisplatin alone. Other chemotherapeutic agents reported to be active against endometrial cancer include ifosfamide (Ifex) and paclitaxel (Taxol).

ROUTINE FOLLOW-UP

Women who have completed initial treatment of endometrial cancer are followed on a close basis for the first 2 years after therapy, since most recurrences are diagnosed within that time frame. Surveillance for recurrent disease includes a complete physical examination, including a vaginal cytologic examination and an internal rectovaginal examination. It is equally important for the clinician to ensure that the patient has been screened for other common cancers by following the recommendations for yearly mammograms and screening sigmoidoscopy.

Regular chest x-ray films or a CT scan of the abdomen and pelvis is not indicated in the absence of symptoms. A diagnosis of endometrial cancer is listed as a contraindication to estrogen replacement therapy. Several retrospective reports have prescribed estrogen replacement therapy to long-term survivors of endometrial cancer who were free of disease several years after treatment. The safety of this approach has not been proved in a prospective clinical trial.

CARCINOMA OF THE UTERINE CERVIX

method of
MITCHELL MORRIS, M.D.
The University of Texas M. D. Anderson Cancer
Center
Houston, Texas

Despite the use of large-scale cervical cancer screening programs in industrialized nations, invasive cervical cancer continues to be a significant problem around the world. Although screening programs have decreased mortality from cervical cancer in the past 4 decades in the United States, there continue to be approximately 14,000 new cases of cervical cancer annually. Nearly half of these women will die of their disease, making the early detection of cervical cancer even more important.

EPIDEMIOLOGY AND ETIOLOGY

A number of epidemiologic factors have been associated with cervical cancer, including early age at first intercourse, multiple sexual partners, lower socioeconomic status, cigarette smoking, and a male sexual partner in a high-risk group. The most important thing about these variables is that they all reflect a high risk of acquiring a sexually transmitted disease, an association that has been noted for a number of years. In the past 15 years, investigators have turned their attention to the human papillomavirus (HPV) as a causative agent of cervical carcinoma. Using molecular techniques, they have found that the overwhelming majority of women with invasive or preinvasive surgical lesions have HPV DNA fragments incorporated into the host genome, strongly suggesting a causative relationship. Research investigating methods of combating HPV is under way, and a vaccine may be developed in the next decade.

PATHOLOGY

The classification of malignant lesions of the cervix is summarized in Table 1.

Abnormalities of the cervix progress through a series of stages, beginning with preinvasive changes that are confined to the intraepithelial area. Squamous intraepithelial lesions (SILs) can be detected either by histologic technique through a biopsy or by a Pap smear. It is believed that dysplastic lesions progress first to in situ carcinoma and then to invasive disease. When an in situ lesion progresses beyond the basement membrane of the epithelium, it is considered to be invasive with the potential for further growth and the formation of metastatic lesions. The earliest phase of cervical invasion has been termed "microinvasive carcinoma." This is defined in the United States as lesions that involve 3 mm or less in depth from the basement membrane of the epithelium. The risk of metastatic disease of these lesions is close to zero. Lesions that invade more than 3 mm or those that have lymph-vascular space involvement are considered frankly invasive and must be treated with more radical therapies.

Squamous carcinoma makes up between 85 and 90% of invasive cervical cancers. Adenocarcinoma of the cervix makes up between 10 and 15% of these lesions. There are some who believe that adenocarcinoma has a worse prognosis and a greater propensity toward early spread. This has been difficult to prove.

Clear cell carcinoma is a variant of cervical cancer that has been associated with intrauterine exposure to diethylstilbestrol (DES) but is not limited to those with such exposure. Clear cell carcinoma is treated in the same fashion as the other variants.

DETECTION AND STAGING

Preinvasive Lesions

Cervical screening programs with Pap smears are the best method of detecting preinvasive lesions. The Pap smear is best performed on a patient who has not had intercourse or douched for 24 hours. A sampling from both the exocervix, obtained with a plastic or wooden spatula, and from the endocervix, preferably obtained with an endocervical brush, should be smeared on a glass slide and promptly fixed. Before the smear is obtained, the cervix should be well visualized. No lubricants other than a small amount of water should be used as this may induce artifact. If the cells are allowed to dry before fixation, artifact will result. The interval for performing a Pap smear has been controversial. Most recommend that once a woman becomes sexually active or reaches the age of 18, annual cervical screenings should be performed. After three consecutive normal smears, if the patient is in a low-risk group, this interval may be lengthened at the discretion of the physician.

When confronted with the abnormal Pap smear, the clinician is obligated to perform further investigation before any therapy. It should be kept in mind that the Pap smear is a screening test and is not a diagnostic test.

Colposcopy is the routine method of further investigating the abnormal smear. With the use of the colposcope, abnormal areas of the cervix can be properly identified and biopsied. The results of these biopsies and the observations using the colposcope guide further therapy. Those patients in whom the entire lesion is visualized and whose biopsy does not show invasive cancer may be treated by conservative means. Cryotherapy is perhaps the most widely employed method of treating cervical dysplasia (SIL). Most

TABLE 1. **Histologic Classification of Invasive Cancers of Uterine Cervix**

Squamous carcinoma
  Microinvasive carcinoma
  Clinically invasive carcinoma
  Verrucous carcinoma
Adenocarcinoma
  Endocervical adenocarcinoma
  Endometrioid adenocarcinoma
  Clear cell carcinoma
  Papillary adenocarcinoma
  Mucinous adenocarcinoma
  Medullary adenocarcinoma
Variants of adenocarcinoma
  Adenoma malignum (minimal deviation adenocarcinoma)
  Adenoid cystic carcinoma
  Mesonephric carcinoma
Mixed epithelial carcinoma
  Adenosquamous carcinoma
  Glassy cell carcinoma
  Mucoepidermoid carcinoma
Neuroendocrine carcinoma
  Carcinoid
  Small cell carcinoma
Undifferentiated carcinoma
Melanoma
Metastatic lesions

cryosurgical units use a liquefied gas, usually nitrogen, nitrous oxide, or carbon dioxide, to cool a silver alloy probe that is applied to the cervix. The procedure lasts several minutes until an ice ball completely covers the affected area of the cervix along with a margin of normal tissue. The amount of time required to produce such an effect is variable and depends on the size of the lesion, the configuration of the cervix, and the timing of the freeze. With this technique for cervical dysplasia 85 to 95% of patients are cured.

An alternative to the use of cryotherapy has been the loop electrosurgical excision procedure (LEEP). In this procedure an electrical current applied to a wire loop is used to excise a cone-shaped portion of the cervix. In addition to its being an outpatient therapeutic procedure, a tissue sample is obtained for pathologic analysis to definitively rule out cervical cancer.

Invasive Disease

Invasive disease may be detected on a Pap smear but is also often detected by the signs and symptoms with which patients present. In its early stages cervical carcinoma tends to be asymptomatic. Early symptoms may include vaginal discharge, odor, and abnormal vaginal bleeding. The vaginal bleeding may take on any pattern of menometrorrhagia or postmenopausal bleeding. Postcoital bleeding may be seen from disruption of a friable cervical lesion.

Early lesions may be diagnosed during a routine pelvic examination. Any time a gross cervical lesion is visible, a biopsy is indicated, regardless of the results of a Pap smear. Because of the associated inflammation and necrosis, a cytologic smear of an invasive cancer is occasionally reported as inflammation. *Every* visible cervical lesion should be biopsied to enable a definitive histologic diagnosis.

More advanced lesions may be characterized by pelvic pain, heavy bleeding, or unilateral leg edema. This indicates that there is infiltration of surrounding tissues.

Cervical cancers are often characterized by their appearance as either exophytic or endophytic. An exophytic lesion protrudes from the cervix and can be easily visualized and measured. Endophytic lesions, on the other hand, can be more difficult to detect; they may not be easily visible and may expand the endocervix before detection. Adenocarcinoma is more commonly endophytic.

Cervical cancer spreads in two predominant patterns: direct extension and lymphatic dissemination. Cervical cancer spreads from the cervix to the adjacent upper vagina, parametrial tissues, and, in later stages, the bladder or rectum. This is best assessed through a careful rectal and vaginal examination. Direct extension into the uterine cavity is difficult to detect and probably does not affect the prognosis. Occasionally, patients with advanced cancers present with an asymptomatic hydroureter from involvement of the collecting system on one side or the other. Very occasionally, patients with advanced cancer present in renal failure due to bilateral ureteral obstruction.

The lymphatic spread pattern of cervical cancer is fairly predictable and proceeds in a stepwise fashion. Initially, tumor spreads through paracervical lymphatic channels to the pelvic node chains in the obturator, internal iliac, and external iliac vessels. This then spreads cephalad to the common iliac chain and paraortic lymph nodes. More advanced cases can have more widespread nodal dissemination.

Metastatic disease resulting from hematogenous dissemination is unusual but can be seen in women with recurrent disease.

STAGING

Staging Procedures

Cervical cancer is staged by clinical evaluation that allows comparison between treatment results from radiation therapy and those from surgery. The majority of cervical cancer patients are treated with radiation therapy. The rules for staging of cervical carcinoma have been established by the International Federation of Gynecology and Obstetrics (FIGO), and the staging system used today is presented in Table 2. It should be noted that several important prognostic variables are not included in FIGO staging.

Pretreatment evaluation of a patient with cervical cancer depends on the extent of disease at the time of initial presentation (Table 3). A thorough history and physical examination should be performed with complete evaluation of peripheral lymph node chains. Pelvic examination, particularly the rectovaginal examination, is important in determining the size of the lesion and the presence of vaginal or parametrial spread.

All patients should undergo a chest radiograph. An intravenous pyleogram is also a useful modality to identify ureteral obstruction. Cystoscopy and flexible sigmoidoscopy are often a useful method for evaluating the bladder and rectum to rule out invasion before initiation of ther-

TABLE 2. **International Federation of Gynecology and Obstetrics Staging of Cervical Carcinoma**

Preinvasive Carcinoma	
Stage O:	Carcinoma in situ; intraepithelial carcinoma.
Invasive Carcinoma	
Stage I:	Carcinoma confined to cervix (extension to corpus should be disregarded).
IA:	Preclinical carcinoma.
	IA1: Minimal microscopically evident stromal invasion (early stromal invasion).
	IA2: Lesions detected microscopically that can be measured. Upper limits of measurement should not be deeper than 5 mm from base of epithelium (surface or glandular). Second dimension, horizontal spread, must not exceed 7 mm. Larger lesions are staged as IB.
IB:	All other Stage I lesions.
Stage II:	Carcinoma extends beyond cervix onto either vagina or parametrium but not to lower third of vagina and not to pelvic wall.
IIA:	No obvious parametrial involvement.
IIB:	Obvious parametrial involvement.
Stage III:	Carcinoma extends to either lower third of vagina or to pelvic wall. Hydronephrosis or nonfunctioning kidney, unless they are known to be due to another cause, necessitates allocation to stage IIIB.
IIIA:	Involvement of lower third of vagina. No extension to pelvic wall.
IIIB:	Extension to pelvic wall or hydronephrosis or nonfunctioning kidney.
Stage IV:	Carcinoma extends beyond true pelvis or involves mucosa of bladder or rectum. Bullous edema does not permit assignment to Stage IV.
IVA:	Spread to bladder or rectum.
IVB:	Spread to distant organs.

TABLE 3. **Pretreatment Evaluation of Cervical Cancer**

Studies Permitted for Staging

Physical examination
Routine blood examination
Chest radiography
Intravenous pyelography
Barium enema examination
Cystoscopy
Sigmoidoscopy

Optional Studies That May Not Be Used for Staging

Computed tomography
Magnetic resonance imaging
Lymphangiography
Surgical staging

apy. This should be reserved for patients with more advanced lesions. A barium enema can also be performed.

Although not used in staging, other radiologic tests may be useful to evaluate the para-aortic nodes. Computed tomography (CT), magnetic resonance imaging (MRI), and lymphangiography are all useful modalities for defining the spread of cervical cancer. A lymphangiogram is probably the most accurate and cost effective but has limited availability. A pelvic and abdominal CT scan can be performed to rule out the presence of para-aortic nodal metastases.

Surgical staging is a controversial concept in the treatment of cervical cancer. In this procedure a retroperitoneal approach to the para-aortic and pelvic lymph nodes is taken. The rationale is to help define the optimal radiation field for patients with advanced disease. In reality, very few patients have treatment decisions based on surgical staging, and it should be considered an investigational modality. There is no useful tumor marker for cervical carcinoma on a routine basis. The squamous carcinoma antigen level is elevated in the majority of patients; however, it does not affect treatment planning and should be considered investigational.

Prognostic Factors

The two most important prognostic factors for determining outcome in patients with cervical carcinoma are the size of the tumor and the FIGO stage. Other prognostic factors include the presence of nodal metastases, lymph-vascular invasion, variant histologic findings, and grade.

MICROINVASIVE CERVICAL CARCINOMA

Treatment of microinvasive cervical carcinoma has excellent results. These lesions should be documented with either a conization or a hysterectomy specimen. After hysterectomy or conization with negative margins the cure rate is approximately 99%. Because there is very little risk of lymph node metastases, it is not necessary to address these nodes with treatment. Conization alone permits younger patients to maintain fertility.

TREATMENT

Careful choice of a primary therapy for cervical carcinoma is critical since recurrent disease is usu-

ally not curable. Primary approaches are radical hysterectomy, radiation therapy, and multimodality therapy.

Radical Hysterectomy

For FIGO Stage IB and IIA lesions, radical hysterectomy has long been the standard therapy. This procedure involves the removal of not only the uterus but also the cardinal and uterosacral ligaments, the pubocervical ligaments, and the upper one-third of the vagina. Also performed as part of this procedure is a complete pelvic lymphadenectomy, removing the lymph nodes from the obturator and the internal iliac, external iliac, and lower common iliac chains. Many surgeons also sample the upper common iliac and lower para-aortic lymph nodes.

The procedure begins with an abdominal exploration, with careful inspection of the peritoneal surfaces, liver, bowel, ovaries, and other pelvic organs. Pelvic and para-aortic nodes should be carefully palpated for clinically evident metastatic disease. If extrauterine disease is present, most surgeons discontinue the procedure and treat the patient with radiation therapy. If only one or two pelvic lymph nodes are positive, some surgeons excise them and continue with the radical hysterectomy.

The ideal candidate for radical hysterectomy is a younger woman who is in good health and preferably not obese. The cancer should be confined to the cervix, although some patients with upper vaginal involvement may be adequately treated with radical hysterectomy. Larger lesions, even though they may be Stage IB, are probably best treated by radiation therapy.

One of the major advantages of radical hysterectomy is ovarian preservation. Since ovarian metastases from early cervical cancer are exceedingly rare, the ovaries may remain in situ if further ovarian function is desired. After surgery, further prognostic information can be obtained through pathologic analysis of the specimen. If there are lymph node metastases, positive surgical margins, or parametrial spread, most women receive postoperative pelvic radiation therapy. The results for patients treated with radical hysterectomy are excellent, with 5-year survival rates ranging from 75 to 95%.

Radical hysterectomy has the potential for complications. In addition to blood loss and infection, there is a loss of innervation to the bladder, occasionally resulting in serious urinary retention. Likewise, many women complain of chronic constipation after the procedure. Vaginal shortening is usually not a significant problem since this organ is distensible and elastic enough to accommodate partial resection.

Radiation Therapy

Ionizing radiation is the expected therapy for the majority of women who present with cervical carcinoma. There are two phases to treatment with radiation therapy. Initially, external beam radiation therapy is given to the pelvic area. The standard treatment field measures 15 by 15 cm and treatment is usually given by a four-field technique. The lower border of the field is generally placed at the midpubis or 4 cm below the lowest level of vaginal disease. The upper border is placed at L4–5. The lateral borders are placed at least 1 cm lateral to the pelvic margins. These borders can be tailored to the distribution of tumor and the patient's anatomy. Occasionally extended-field radiation is employed when disease is suspected in the para-aortic area. Extended-field radiation does have additional complications due to the greater volume of irradiated normal tissue.

External therapy both eradicates microscopic disease in the pelvic lymph nodes and shrinks the central tumor in the cervix and paracervical tissues to provide superior geometry for the appropriate placement of a radiation implant. External therapy is given in a series of small fractions, most commonly 1.8 to 2.0 Gray daily, lasting for 4 to 5 weeks for a total of 40 to 50 Gray. After external radiation, patients usually receive two radiation implants. Intracavitary therapy, also referred to as "brachytherapy," uses a variety of applicator devices designed to give an intense dose of radiation to the central pelvis while sparing surrounding tissues. The first system is usually inserted approximately 1 week after the conclusion of the external beam therapy, and the second system a week later. Once inserted the system is loaded with cesium and left in place for approximately 48 hours.

Multimodality Therapy

The effectiveness of radiation therapy is related to the size and oxygenation of the tumor. Larger tumors tend to be hypoxic and therefore radioresistant, while those with a rich blood supply are more radiosensitive. Larger tumors have been prone to treatment failure, and a variety of therapies have been designed to try to overcome this relative radioresistance.

Radiation sensitizers potentiate the effect of radiation on tumors. The most commonly used radiation sensitizer for cervical cancer has been hydroxyurea. Some investigators have shown that the combination of hydroxyurea and radiation therapy produces superior results compared with radiation alone. Chemotherapeutic agents, including 5-fluorouracil and cisplatin (Platinol), have also been used in a similar fashion as radiosensitizers. Whether radiosensitizers truly improve survival is unknown.

An alternative to radiosensitizers has been neoadjuvant chemotherapy. In this setting, chemotherapy is used to shrink the tumor before radiation. Again, data are conflicting as to whether this improves survival or not.

Radiation therapy also has a set of complications. In the acute setting most patients experience diarrhea and occasionally urinary frequency. Long-term complications occur in very few patients but may be serious. These include stricture of the intestine with obstruction or perforation, chronic diarrhea, short bowel syndrome, and fistula formation.

POST-TREATMENT SURVEILLANCE

Seventy-five percent of cervical cancer recurrences occur within 2 years of therapy. By the end of 5 years, 95% of patients destined to have recurrent disease have relapsed. These figures help us plan our follow-up. Patients should be seen every 3 to 4 months during the first 2 years after therapy, and every 6 months for 3 years after that. Follow-up examination should include assessment of lymph node areas, examination of the chest and abdomen, and thorough pelvic examination including the rectovaginal examination. A Pap smear should also be obtained. These examinations can be particularly difficult in women who have received radiation therapy since fibrosis can often mimic recurrent disease. Distinguishing between these two may be difficult even for the experienced clinician. Bimanual and rectovaginal examination often shows fibrosis to be smooth, while recurrent disease is tender and nodular. Follow-up radiologic studies probably have little value in surveillance since any patient with distant disease is incurable.

MANAGEMENT OF RECURRENT CERVICAL CANCER

The great majority of women with recurrent disease are incurable. Recurrent cervical cancer may occur in the central pelvis, on the side wall of the pelvis, or at distant sites. The most common distant sites include the para-aortic or other distant lymph nodes, the lung, or bone (most commonly vertebral bodies). The importance of surveillance is to detect the few patients who will have a central pelvic recurrence. This group of patients are candidates for curative therapy through radical surgery.

Treatment of recurrent disease is based on a type of primary therapy delivery. Those with pelvic recurrence after radical hysterectomy may be treated with radiation therapy, and this may be successful in some cases. Central recurrence may be treated through a whole pelvic field with an implant. Patients who have already received pelvic radiation are usually not candidates for additional radiation.

Pelvic Exenteration

Pelvic exenteration is a very radical procedure that includes the removal of the pelvic reproductive organs including the uterus, tubes, ovaries, and vagina; the bladder and distal ureters; the rectum and anus; and the pelvic floor, including the pelvic peritoneum and levator muscles and usually the pelvic lymph nodes as well. Occasionally, a more limited procedure may be performed. Extensive reconstructive procedures including a myocutaneous gracilis flap for vaginal reconstruction, continent urinary conduit for bladder reconstruction, and colostomy are performed on these women so that they may return to a normal lifestyle after surgery. Approximately 50% of patients with recurrent cervical cancer confined to the center of the pelvis who undergo pelvic exenteration can be cured by this procedure.

Chemotherapy for Recurrent Cervical Cancer

Chemotherapy for recurrent cervical carcinoma should be regarded as a palliative intervention. The opportunity for cure is very small, and even the best regimens have low response rates. The most active chemotherapeutic agent in the treatment of recurrent cervical cancer is cisplatin. The response rate is approximately 30%, but even responders tend to relapse quickly. The overall median survival after recurrence that cannot be treated with surgery is on the order of 7 months.

Palliative Therapy

Perhaps one of the most important roles of a physician treating a woman with recurrent cervical cancer is delivering proper palliative care. The management of pelvic pain, renal failure, and infection is an important aspect of the total care of the patient.

Advanced cervical cancer often results in severe pelvic pain. A lesion on the pelvic side wall or involving sacral nerve endings or bone can make pain intolerable. Physicians should understand the cause of this pain and be ready to provide aggressive narcotic analgesia. Occasionally, when systemic analgesics fail, it is necessary to place a semipermanent indwelling epidural catheter or perform a nerve block.

Many women suffer from lymphatic and venous outflow obstruction from the lower extremity and have a painful leg. This should not be treated the same way as deep vein thrombosis since the risk of pulmonary embolism is small. Heparin sometimes does alleviate the symptoms.

Women with progressive cervical cancer often die from renal failure secondary to ureteral obstruction. When such renal failure occurs, the obstruction may be bypassed through percutaneous nephrostomy tubes. Before this procedure is performed, the physician and patient in conjunction with the family should have a serious discussion about the overall prognosis and whether such a procedure is desirable. With no effective second-line therapy, saving a patient from death by uremia only to have her suffer with progressive pelvic pain may not be helpful.

NEOPLASMS OF THE VULVA

method of
KEVIN O. EASLEY, J.D., M.D., and
DAVID G. MUTCH, M.D.
Washington University School of Medicine
St. Louis, Missouri

A wide variety of pathologic processes can affect the vulva. Over the years, there have been various terminologies and classification schemes used to describe these diseases. The present classification system is that proposed in 1989 by the International Society for the Study of Vulvar Disease (Table 1).

NON-NEOPLASTIC EPITHELIAL DISORDERS OF SKIN AND MUCOSA

Non-neoplastic disorders that may involve the vulva include lesions that were previously described by a number of terms, including lichen sclerosus, lichen sclerosus et atrophicus, leukoplakia, and kraurosis vulvae. The older terminology included lesions with both benign and malignant potential. The new classification system better categorizes vulvar lesions and clearly sets apart those with malignant potential. The gross appearance of these lesions is often quite similar, yet treatments can vary significantly, depending on the diagnosis. In addition, although it is believed that these lesions do not have malignant potential, it is known that non-neoplastic vulvar lesions can coexist with a neoplastic lesion. Consequently, biopsy must be utilized liberally with persistent or suspicious lesions to ensure accurate diagnosis and exclude a neoplastic process.

Lichen Sclerosus

Lichen sclerosus of the vulva may present at any age. The patient typically complains of a persistent, severe pruritus and often shows marked excoriations of the perineum secondary to persistent scratching. The affected skin generally appears thin, hypopig-

TABLE 1. **Nomenclature of Vulvar Diseases**

Non-Neoplastic Epithelial Disorders of Skin and Mucosa*
Lichen sclerosus
Squamous hyperplasia, not otherwise specified (formerly hyperplastic dystrophy without atypia)
Other dermatoses
Classification of Vulvar Intraepithelial Neoplasia (VIN)
Squamous intraepithelial neoplasia (formerly dystrophy with atypia)
VIN I: mild dysplasia (formerly mild atypia)
VIN II: moderate dysplasia (formerly moderate atypia)
VIN III: severe dysplasia (formerly severe atypia)
VIN III: carcinoma in situ

*Mixed non-neoplastic epithelial disorders may occur, and in such cases, both components should be reported. When a non-neoplastic disorder occurs with a neoplastic one, it should be diagnosed as VIN.

mented, and parchment-like. In long-standing cases there may also be a finding of agglutination and stenosis of the labia and vaginal introitus. The pathophysiologic abnormality in these patients is not clear, but there is evidence to suggest an autoimmune etiology. It has also been shown that these patients demonstrate lower activity levels of 5-alpha-reductase and androgenic hormone levels.

Microscopically, one finds loss of rete ridges and thinning of the epithelium. Subcutaneous edema and chronic inflammation are generally present. Hyperkeratosis is a variable finding. Hyperplasia of the epithelium may or may not be present. If present, however, the abnormality should be classified as lichen sclerosus with associated squamous hyperplasia.

Treatment consists of topical 2 to 3% testosterone propionate, prepared in a petrolatum or stearin-lanolin base. Depending on the severity of the disease, application frequency varies. It is prescribed in a tapering fashion: twice daily until symptomatic control is achieved, then gradually reduced to applications once or twice per week. Patients should be counseled that it takes months for noticeable improvement, and lifelong treatment is generally required. They should also be made aware of possible androgenic side effects, including clitorimegaly and hirsutism. These may necessitate discontinuation or a decrease in dosage. If phimosis is present, testosterone may result in pain if clitorimegaly occurs below the agglutinated tissues. The bothersome pruritus may continue well into treatment and is usually worse at night. Soaks, followed by air drying of the vulva, and/or the use of topical fluorinated corticosteroids or systemic antipruritics may be necessary to help break this itch-scratch cycle. Hygienic measures should also be encouraged. In severe refractory cases, steroid or alcohol subdermal injection of the involved areas may rarely be necessary. Skinning vulvectomy has also been utilized in such cases. Table 2 outlines various treatment options.

In prepubertal females, in patients who cannot tolerate the side effects experienced with testosterone, or in patients who show no improvement with testosterone therapy, a 1 to 2% preparation of topical progesterone may be of benefit.

Squamous Hyperplasia

Squamous cell hyperplasia clinically appears as a thickened, irregular pale epithelium, often described as plaquelike. Pruritus is usually the presenting complaint. Histopathology reveals acanthosis, with elongation and widening of the rete ridges, and marked hyperplasia of the squamous epithelium. The etiology of squamous hyperplasia is uncertain but it is often precipitated by local irritants. Removal of possible culprits, such as soaps, deodorized tissues or sanitary products, laundry detergents, or other agents that may be in contact with the affected area, often alleviates the problem and prevents recur-

TABLE 2. Treatment of Vulvar Dystrophy

Lichen Sclerosus

1–2% testosterone propionate mixed in a petrolatum or stearin-lanolin cream base
or
1–2% progesterone ointment mixed in a petrolatum or stearin-lanolin cream base
Massage affected areas twice daily until symptomatic improvement is obtained, then gradually taper dosage to once or twice per week

Hyperplastic Dystrophy

0.025 or 0.01% fluocinolone acetonide (Fluonid, Synalar, Synemol) applied as a thin film 2–4 times daily

Antipruritic Therapies

Hygienic measures, including soaks and thorough drying of the vulva
Avoidance of occlusive clothing
Cool Burow's solution (Domeboro tabs) topically if the vulva is inflamed
or
Crotamiton lotion (Eurax) massaged into affected areas twice daily
For more severe cases, use of oral antipruritics at night to prevent inadvertent scratching while sleeping (the following are adult dosages):
    Diphenhydramine hydrochloride (Benadryl) 25–50 mg q 6–8 h
    Hydroxyzine hydrochloride (Atarax) 25–50 mg q 6–8 h
In severe, refractory cases, use of alcohol or steroid injection or skinning vulvectomy

rences. If atypia is present in the epithelium, it is classified and treated as vulvar intraepithelial neoplasia (VIN). Treatment of squamous hyperplasia consists of controlling the pruritus. Use of topical fluorinated corticosteroids for no more than 4 to 6 weeks is generally successful.

Other Dermatoses

Lichen planus is less common than the previously described disorders, and its etiology is poorly understood, although it is believed that autoimmunity plays a role. These patients usually present with complaints of vulvar burning, irritation, and pruritus but are occasionally asymptomatic. Grossly, this abnormality appears similar to lichen sclerosus secondary to the thinning of the epithelium and can present with atrophy and agglutination of vulvar structures. Biopsy is necessary for diagnosis; microscopically, there is a lymphocytic infiltrate with liquefaction necrosis of the basal epithelial cells. Acanthosis and hyperkeratosis may also be seen. Treatment with topical fluorinated corticosteroids may initially be used for control of symptoms, followed by the use of other oral or topical agents, including antibiotics, immune suppressive agents, and retinoids.

There are a number of other benign dermatologic abnormalities that may affect the vulva, including yeast vulvitis, atopic dermatitis, psoriasis, vulvar vestibulitis, hidradenitis suppurativa, and Behçet's syndrome. Indicated diagnostic tests should be undertaken, with a low threshold for consultation or biopsy in atypical, persistent, or uncertain cases.

This serves to rule out a neoplasm and allows accurate diagnosis and appropriate treatment.

TUMORS OF THE VULVA

Cystic tumors occur fairly frequently on the vulva. Commonly encountered lesions include Bartholin gland cysts and epidermal cysts. Bartholin gland cysts occur when the duct dilates secondary to occlusion. It presents as a palpable mass. It may be asymptomatic or exquisitely tender, depending on the degree of dilatation and whether or not infection is present. Treatment is indicated if the patient is symptomatic. Placement of a Word catheter for 4 to 5 weeks allows epithelialization of a new tract for drainage of the gland and is a procedure easily done in the office with the patient under local anesthesia. If the cyst recurs or presents in a female older than 40 years of age, consideration should be given to excision of the gland, which can be done as an outpatient surgical procedure. The excised specimen should be sent for pathologic examination to rule out malignancy. Epidermal cysts, inclusion cysts, and sebaceous cysts refer to a number of small, usually asymptomatic cystic inclusions found just below the epidermis, usually within the labia majora. Their etiologies are thought to be the result of trauma or obstruction of sebaceous gland ducts. Removal is usually not necessary.

Benign solid tumors of the vulva can arise from epithelial tissues or underlying glandular, adipose, connective, muscular, or neural tissues. Fibromas commonly occur on the vulva and are generally small and asymptomatic, but they may become large enough to warrant removal for reasons of comfort or cosmesis. Acrochordons or fibroepithelial polyps are rare benign vulvar tumors. They may arise in hair-bearing areas of the vulva and can vary significantly in presentation, ranging from a small papillomatous growth to a large polypoid lesion. Again, removal is dictated by patient desire. Papillomas of the vestibule are frequently seen. They are of no clinical significance but may be mistaken for human papillomavirus (HPV) and occasionally needlessly treated. Colposcopy with 3% acetic acid can result in mistakenly identifying normal vaginal mucosa as being HPV-infected because of acetowhite changes normally seen in this glycogen-rich mucosa. Biopsy can distinguish these lesions from HPV by their lack of nuclear changes. Endometriosis can present on the vulva, often appearing as a nodule near a previous episiotomy site. Patients may give a history of cyclical swelling and/or tenderness. Lipomas arise from underlying adipose tissues, are usually slow growing, and present as painless firm masses. Vascular hemangiomas may be of several varieties, with the majority presenting as capillary hemangiomas in children that usually regress spontaneously. Senile hemangiomas occur in adults and are of no clinical significance. Leiomyomas, hidradenomas, and neuro-

mas are other benign tumors that may be infrequently encountered as vulvar tumors.

HUMAN PAPILLOMAVIRUS

HPV is the most frequently encountered sexually transmitted disease today. It is an epitheliotropic virus and affects epithelial surfaces of the skin and mucous membranes. Although it more commonly affects the cervix, vulvar infection is also frequently encountered. HPV infections are classified as latent, subclinical, or clinical. Clinical infections cause local epithelial proliferation, typically resulting in a cauliflower-like growth called "condyloma acuminatum." It less frequently results in a small plaquelike wart or a keratotic-type growth that is visible using colposcopy after application of 3% acetic acid.

More than 60 different subtypes of HPV have been identified, and of these, more than 20 subtypes have been shown to be involved in anogenital tract infections. Further, these subtypes have been categorized based on their oncogenic potential. Table 3 lists some of the more commonly encountered subtypes by category. It should be noted that this classification scheme may vary, depending on the study. Subtypes 6 and 11 are those most often responsible for vulvar HPV infections, but they are in the low-risk category for malignant predisposition.

VIN is associated with HPV in 80 to 90% of patients, with subtype 16 found most often. HPV is associated with invasive vulvar cancers as well. This association more often occurs in a younger subset of patients. Because of this association and the tendency for HPV to involve multiple genital tract sites, it is important that a thorough evaluation of the vulva, vagina, cervix, and perianal areas be done. Under magnification, following application of 3% acetic acid, atypical acetowhite areas may become apparent that are not typical for HPV and warrant biopsy. A cervical Pap smear should also be taken if one has not been done recently. DNA probes are available to aid in detecting specific HPV DNA subtypes, but the role of this diagnostic technique in clinical management is uncertain.

Therapy of genital HPV infections varies significantly, with excision, cryotherapy, laser ablation, interferon injections, and topical agents as available treatment alternatives (Table 4). Although removal of all symptomatic and/or visible lesions may be the goal of therapy, it is often difficult to attain. Even after all visible lesions have been successfully treated, permanent cure is unlikely. Recurrences are common, as latent disease generally persists in nor-

TABLE 3. **Oncogenic Potential of HPV Subtypes**

Low Risk	Moderate Risk	High Risk
6, 11	30, 33, 35, 39, 51, 52, 56, 63	16, 18, 31, 45

TABLE 4. **Treatment of Vulvar HPV Infection**

Topical Therapy

Concentrated trichloroacetic acid (50–85% solution)
Podophyllum resin 25% in tincture of benzoin (Pod-Ben-25)
Podofilox (Condylox)
Fluorouracil (Efudex cream)

Surgical Therapy

Cryotherapy
Simple local excision
Electrosurgical excision
CO_2 laser ablation

mal-appearing adjacent tissues and may subsequently progress to clinically obvious disease. Changes in the immune status of the patient also affect the frequency and degree of clinically detectable HPV recurrences.

The majority of vulvar condylomas can be treated with topical caustic agents that cause sloughing of the HPV-infected epithelium. Trichloroacetic acid (TCA) as a 50 to 85% solution is frequently used. Visible lesions are coated at weekly intervals. TCA is a strong desiccant, and efforts should be made to confine application to the lesion and avoid contact with surrounding normal tissues. Podophyllin is also available as topical therapy but is generally not as effective. In addition, its use is contraindicated in pregnancy. Both TCA and podophyllin require an office visit for careful application. Podofilox (Condylox) is a topical agent that can be easily applied by the patient. After the diagnosis of HPV has been made, this agent allows safe and early treatment of new lesions and avoids the expense and inconvenience of frequent office visits.

Ablative therapy is usually reserved for lesions unresponsive to topical agents or for extensive lesions not amenable to topical treatment. Interferon injections have met with mixed results and are not commonly used. Topical fluorouracil (Efudex) is a cytotoxic agent that was occasionally used in the past, but because of extreme discomfort and low patient compliance, it is infrequently used today. In patients with impaired immune status, such as renal transplant recipients, who suffer from persistent condylomas, fluorouracil has been used intermittently in low doses and shown to be successful in controlling recurrences in cases in which other agents have failed. It should be avoided in pregnancy, however, because of its teratogenic potential.

Management of the sexual partners of patients with documented HPV infection is somewhat controversial, but studies to date have shown no difference in treatment failure rates in women whose male partners were treated compared with women whose partners were not treated.

The finding of HPV genital tract infection in a child should alert one to the possibility of sexual abuse. It should be noted, however, that although the overwhelming majority of HPV infections are the result of sexual transmission, latent or subclinical

virus has been detected in women who have never had vaginal intercourse. This points out that the natural history and clinical significance of latent and subclinical disease are poorly understood, making it difficult to counsel patients who have this virus.

VULVAR INTRAEPITHELIAL NEOPLASIA

VINs are classified using terminology similar to that used for cervical intraepithelial neoplasia (see Table 1). The gross appearance of VIN varies, with discoloration common. The lesions often appear as nodules or plaques. It can present as a single lesion or as multifocal disease, the latter occurring more often in younger patients. VIN often affects the hairless areas of the vulva, especially the posterior fourchette and labia. Symptoms are also quite varied, ranging from none to pruritus or vulvar irritation. It is important to stress that the gross appearance varies considerably, and diagnosis is dependent on biopsy. In addition, because of the occasional multifocal presentation of VIN, a thorough colposcopic inspection of the entire vulva, vagina, and cervix is indicated, following treatment with 3% acetic acid. Liberal use of biopsy is encouraged and it can easily be done as an office procedure with a Keyes punch biopsy after local injection. Placement of silver nitrate or a plug of Gelfoam generally ensures hemostasis, and sutures are rarely necessary.

VIN is associated with other sexually transmitted diseases, especially HPV, as discussed earlier.

Although invasive vulvar cancers are often found to have adjacent areas of VIN, the potential for malignant transformation is still not clear. Malignant transformation of VIN is believed to be more likely to occur in elderly or immunocompromised patients.

Treatment of VIN is dependent on the degree of neoplasia present and patient symptoms. VIN I can generally be followed with examinations every 3 to 6 months. Vulvar inspection grossly or with colposcopy, using acetic acid or toluidine blue in combination with acetic acid, is generally sufficient to allow detection of a progressive lesion. Instructing the patient in self-examination to aid in detecting early vulvar changes is also recommended.

VIN III should be treated, but there is no consensus on a best method of treatment, and opinions vary considerably. The reported incidence of associated invasive vulvar cancer is 5 to 10%; consequently, some discourage the use of ablative therapy, such as CO_2 laser, for fear of missing this diagnosis. Treatment with wide local excision or skinning vulvectomy has been recommended. However, as the majority of these invasive cancers are minimally invasive (<1 mm), most believe that a thorough examination by a qualified physician, combined with the liberal use of biopsy, will exclude invasive disease; in such qualified hands, ablative therapy is appropriate.

Treatment of VIN II is controversial, with some

authorities proposing only observation and others recommending treatment.

INVASIVE VULVAR CANCER

Vulvar cancer, although the fourth most common female genital tract malignancy, is relatively rare, accounting for only approximately 5% of gynecologic malignancies, with an incidence of 1.6 per 100,000. Over 90% of these lesions are squamous cell carcinoma. Melanoma is the next most common pathologic type, accounting for 5% of vulvar carcinomas. The remaining 5% include adenosquamous carcinomas, sarcomas, and Bartholin gland carcinomas. Extramammary Paget's disease of the vulva is quite rare. It involves the vulvar skin and microscopically appears similar to Paget's disease of the breast, with large pale cells that appear to be infiltrating the epithelium from below.

Squamous Cell Carcinoma

Although the median age group affected with squamous cell carcinoma of the vulva is reported to be those in their sixties, the age of onset appears to be decreasing. Berek and Hacker, in their textbook *Practical Gynecologic Oncology* (2nd edition), state that this disease may in fact have two presentations. The more common variety is seen in postmenopausal women and is often preceded only by vulvar pruritus. A less commonly encountered second type is that seen in younger women, who present with risk factors also seen in cervical dysplasia, including a history of multiple sexual partners, smoking, and the presence of HPV. A coexisting second primary malignancy or preinvasive lesion is found in 15 to 20% of patients with vulvar squamous cell carcinoma, most often of the cervix or vagina. Consequently, it is imperative that a careful and thorough evaluation be done to look for a coexisting neoplasm; at the very least, this mandates colposcopy of the cervix and vagina.

Although older studies reported associated risk factors, including nulliparity, diabetes, hypertension, and obesity, more recent reports, using newer epidemiologic techniques, have not confirmed these findings.

Etiology

HPV has been reported to be present in approximately 25% of cases of vulvar cancer, predominantly types 6 and 16, but it has not been proved to be a causative factor. There is also controversy regarding the malignant potential of preinvasive VIN. In general, however, VIN is not thought to have significant malignant potential, except in medically compromised or elderly patients. The fact that vulvar cancer is more common in lower socioeconomic groups and in an older population has resulted in the proposal that it is the result of poor personal hygiene. Vulvar dystrophies have also been suggested as pre-existing lesions that can result in vulvar carcinoma. To date, however, none of these theories is supported by the available data.

Clinical Presentation

The lesion may occur anywhere on the vulva. It may begin as a small bump or nodule that subsequently ulcerates and does not heal. Other presentations may include a wartlike growth that appears similar to, and is often confused with, condyloma acuminatum.

The majority of lesions arise on the labia majora but they can occur on the labia minora, clitoris, or other areas of the perineum. Symptoms vary, but vulvar pruritus is the most common presenting complaint and is present in about 50% of patients. Other less common symptoms, secondary to a more advanced vulvar lesion, may include a bulge or mass, pain, bleeding or discharge, a nonhealing ulcer, and urinary symptoms of dysuria or frequency.

Diagnosis is dependent on a tissue diagnosis, and biopsy of any persistent vulvar lesion is mandatory. An adequate biopsy should contain surrounding normal skin as well as underlying dermis to allow complete pathologic evaluation. For well-demarcated lesions, a wedge biopsy, with surrounding normal tissue and underlying dermis, should be obtained. When possible, the entire lesion should be completely removed, obtaining a 1-cm margin of surrounding normal tissue. Failure to perform a biopsy of a vulvar lesion is a common cause of delay in diagnosing this disease. In spite of this delay, the majority of vulvar lesions are diagnosed at a relatively early stage because of vulvar cancer's characteristic slow progression.

Spread

Vulvar squamous cell cancers spread most often by contiguous growth to the surrounding tissues of the urethra, vagina, and anus. Lymphatic drainage is initially to the inguinal nodes—first to the superficial group, then to the deeper femoral nodes, and from there to the pelvic nodes. As a rule, lymphatic spread is only to the ipsilateral group of inguinal nodes. Involvement of the contralateral inguinal nodes is unlikely, except in three situations: when the ipsilateral nodes are positive; when the vulvar lesion crosses or occurs in the midline, such as on the clitoris; and when the vulvar lesion occurs on the anterior labia minora. Hematogenous spread to distant sites may also occur, including the expected sites of bone, lung, and liver.

Staging

One of the purposes of staging is to allow one to determine a prognosis and tailor treatment based on that prediction. Staging of vulvar cancers was previously based only on a clinical examination. This was changed to a surgical staging system in 1988 (Table 5). In general, the stage of disease in vulvar cancer is dependent on the size of the lesion, the

TABLE 5. **FIGO Staging of Vulvar Carcinoma**

Stage	TNM System	Description
O	Tis	Carcinoma in situ, intraepithelial carcinoma
I	T1, N0, M0	Tumor confined to the vulva and/or perineum, 2 cm or less in greatest dimension, nodes are not palpable
II	T2, N0, M0	Tumor confined to the vulva and/or perineum, more than 2 cm in greatest dimension, nodes are not palpable
III	T3, N0, M0 T3, N1, M0 T1, N1, M0 T2, N1, M0	Tumor of any size with (1) adjacent spread to the lower urethra and/or the vagina, or the anus, and/or (2) unilateral regional lymph node metastasis
IVA	T1, N2, M0 T2, N2, M0 T3, N2, M0 T4, any N, M0	Tumor invades any of the following: upper urethra, bladder mucosa, rectal mucosa, pelvic bone, and/or with bilateral regional node metastasis
IVB	Any T, any N, M1	Any distant metastasis, including pelvic lymph nodes

presence or absence of inguinal lymph node involvement, and the degree of local spread of disease. A 1991 Gynecologic Oncology Group study looked at the present staging system and identified two factors that this system fails to consider adequately: that patients will do well, regardless of the stage of disease, if lymph nodes are negative; and that the prognosis in patients with lymph node involvement is highly dependent on the number of lymph nodes involved.

Prognostic Factors

In addition to stage and lymph node status, other prognostic factors include size of the lesion, depth of invasion, and tumor grade. Lesions less than 2 cm in size carry a better prognosis, and lesions greater than 4 cm have a higher risk for local recurrence. Depth of invasion is highly correlated with risk of lymph node involvement and, consequently, overall prognosis. Depth of invasion is measured from the most superficial dermal papilla adjacent to the tumor to the deepest focus of invasion.

As previously noted, outcome is highly dependent not only on whether there is lymphatic spread of disease but also on the extent of that spread. Inguinal lymph nodes are reportedly involved in approximately 10% of vulvar cancers, and pelvic lymph node involvement occurs in 5%. Overall, 5-year survival is 90% if lymph nodes are negative. Survival drops to 50% if inguinal nodes are positive. With pelvic nodal metastasis, survival is only 10%. The number of lymph nodes involved is the single most important prognostic variable. Overall 5-year survival is shown in Table 6, which is based on the most recent staging system. Five-year survival based on the number of lymph nodes involved is shown in Table 7.

Treatment

Historically, vulvar cancer was treated with radical surgery, which included an en bloc vulvar resection and bilateral groin dissection of inguinal lymph nodes. Following this radical approach, survival was noted to improve, but there was an associated high morbidity, with an 85% incidence of wound breakdown. Severe psychosexual sequelae were also noted to occur as a result of this rather disfiguring surgery. Treatment of vulvar cancer has changed significantly over the years owing to these factors as well as to evidence that survival is not negatively affected with a less radical approach. Today, the key to treatment is individualization based on the stage and location of the lesion and on the age, health, and desires of the patient.

With early Stage I lesions (<2 cm, no suspicious nodes), a radical local excision can be done. This consists of removing the entire lesion, with at least

TABLE 6. **Five-Year Survival Based on Stage**

Stage	5-Year Survival (%)
I	98
II	85
III	74
IV	31

From Homesley HD, Bundy BN, Sedlis A, et al: Assessment of current International Federation of Gynecology and Obstetrics staging of vulvar carcinoma relative to prognostic factors for survival (a Gynecologic Oncology Group study). Am J Obstet Gynecol *164*:997, 1991.

TABLE 7. **Five-Year Survival Based on Lymph Node Involvement**

Number of Positive Groin Nodes	5-Year Survival (%)
1–2	75.2
3–4	36.2
5–6	24
≥7	0

From Homesley HD, Bundy BN, Sedlis A, et al: Assessment of current International Federation of Gynecology and Obstetrics staging of vulvar carcinoma relative to prognostic factors for survival (a Gynecologic Oncology Group study). Am J Obstet Gynecol *164*:997, 1991.

a 1-cm tumor-free margin, and taking the underlying tissue down to the level of the inferior fascia of the urogenital diaphragm. If the depth of invasion is 1 mm or less, omission of groin dissection may be considered, as nodal metastasis is extremely unlikely. If adequate margins cannot be obtained, postoperative radiation therapy should be given.

If depth of invasion is found to be greater than 1 mm, ipsilateral inguinal dissection should be undertaken. If there are one or no positive nodes, no further therapy is necessary. The presence of two or more positive nodes requires additional treatment with groin and pelvic node irradiation. Some also recommend groin dissection of the contralateral nodes if the ipsilateral nodes are determined to be positive intraoperatively. Historically, a pelvic lymph nodes dissection was recommended when two or more positive groin nodes were found. A 1977 Gynecologic Oncology Group study, however, showed that pelvic lymph node dissection offered no survival advantage over radiation therapy. As lymph node dissection also results in comparatively greater morbidity, pelvic and groin irradiation is now the preferred adjuvant therapy when inguinal nodes are found to contain disease.

Inguinal dissection carries significant morbidity, including infection, wound breakdown, cellulitis, and lymphedema. In addition, these complications are made significantly worse with radiation therapy. As a result, a more conservative approach has recently been proposed that entails performing only a superficial inguinal node dissection and omitting the dissection of the deeper femoral nodes if the nodes are otherwise not suspicious. A 1992 Gynecologic Oncology Group study reported on a series of 121 patients who had undergone such a superficial inguinal node dissection, with 6 patients suffering a recurrence in a previously negative, superficially dissected groin. Although it is not clear that these recurrences occurred in the undissected femoral nodes, because of the known mortality of 90% if recurrence occurs in an undissected groin, some continue to undertake a complete inguinal dissection when dissection is indicated, in spite of the significant associated morbidity.

If the lesion is greater than 2 cm and/or involves minimal spread to the urethra, vagina, or anus, and there are no suspicious groin nodes, treatment may consist of radical vulvectomy or radical local excision, with bilateral groin node dissection of both inguinal and possibly femoral nodes. The need for additional postoperative radiation therapy depends on the status of the dissected nodes, with further therapy indicated if two or more nodes are positive. If it is a relatively large lesion, preoperative radiation therapy may be given in an effort to shrink the tumor and allow a less radical and less disfiguring subsequent surgery.

If more extensive local spread, infiltration of bladder or rectal mucosa, or bulky positive groin nodes are present, it is considered advanced disease. In the past, these patients were treated with exenteration, with survival at 5 years reported to be approximately 50%. Today, recommended treatment consists of preoperative radiation therapy, with or without neoadjuvant chemotherapy, followed by resection of the tumor bed and groin dissection to remove bulky nodes.

In patients with bulky positive groin nodes, radiation therapy has not been as successful in preventing pelvic recurrences as it has been in patients with palpably normal but positive groin nodes. It is hypothesized that the size of these nodes prevents adequate sterilization by irradiation. It is therefore recommended that these patients undergo preoperative pelvic computed tomography (CT) scan. If bulky pelvic nodes are present and, following groin dissection, frozen section confirms metastatic disease, removal of the enlarged pelvic lymph nodes should be considered. Postoperative groin and pelvic irradiation should also be given.

Recurrence

The risk of recurrence correlates closely with the number of positive groin nodes. There is little risk of recurrence if there are fewer than three positive groin nodes. If three or more groin nodes are positive, there is a high risk of recurrence, both locally and at regional and distant sites.

Local recurrences can usually be treated with local excision. When there is a regional or distant recurrence, management is difficult, and long-term survival is unlikely. Treatment options include palliative surgery and/or radiation therapy. Chemotherapy for distant disease has generally not been effective, having a dismal response rate.

Melanoma

Melanoma is responsible for approximately 5% of vulvar cancers. It most often occurs on the anterior labia minora and clitoris. Staging is based on Clark's levels, as the prognosis in this malignancy is mainly dependent on depth of invasion. With less than 1 mm of invasion, treatment consists of radical local excision only. If invasion is greater than 1 mm, bilateral groin dissection is also undertaken. Pelvic nodal dissection has not been shown to affect survival. The overall prognosis for vulvar melanoma is poor, with a mean 5-year survival of approximately 30%.

Bartholin Gland Carcinoma

Bartholin gland carcinoma is a rare malignancy. Diagnostic criteria, as proposed by Honan, are strict, which may result in some degree of underreporting of this entity. The carcinoma must be located deep in the labia majora, have overlying intact skin, and have some recognizable normal glandular tissue present. Treatment is essentially the same as for squamous cell cancer of the vulva. Prognosis is also similar, stage for stage, to squamous cell carcinoma of the vulva. Diagnosis of Bartholin gland carcinoma generally occurs at a later stage, however, because of its deeper location. Overall survival is consequently lower.

Other Cell Types

Basal cell carcinoma is treated by radical local excision. Lymph node involvement is rare.

Extramammary Paget's disease, named after its counterpart in the breast, typically presents as a weeping, erythematous lesion on the vulva. Pruritus is common. An underlying adenocarcinoma is present in about 15 to 20% of patients. A second primary malignancy reportedly occurs in about one-third of patients, commonly involving the breast, cervix, or gastrointestinal tract, and should be excluded. Treatment involves wide local excision, with removal of the underlying dermis because of the risk of a coexisting underlying adenocarcinoma. Multiple frozen sections may be indicated intraoperatively to ensure negative surgical margins, as the disease usually extends beyond the borders of the grossly visible lesion. Recurrences can be treated with laser ablation, as underlying adenocarcinomas are unlikely.

Verrucous carcinoma is grossly and histologically similar in appearance to condyloma acuminatum but differs in that it is locally invasive. It is generally a disease of postmenopausal women. Treatment consists of radical local excision. Radiation therapy is contraindicated, as it may result in malignant transformation with distant metastatic spread. Recurrences are treated with additional surgery, and long-term survival is excellent.

There are a number of other vulvar neoplasms that are extremely rare, including sarcomas, adenocarcinomas of ectopic breast tissue, neuroendocrine tumors of the skin, adenosquamous carcinomas, and metastatic tumors. This re-emphasizes the need for adequate biopsy of any persistent vulvar abnormality.

VENOUS THROMBOEMBOLISM IN OBSTETRICS AND GYNECOLOGY

method of
A. KONETI RAO, M.D., and
SUNITA B. SHETH, M.D.
Temple University School of Medicine
Philadelphia, Pennsylvania

PATHOGENESIS

Venous thrombi are intravascular deposits composed predominantly of fibrin and red cells, with a variable platelet and leukocyte component. Although the term "thrombophlebitis" has been used, inflammation plays only a limited role in the pathogenesis of deep vein thrombosis (DVT) and pulmonary embolism (PE). Venous thromboembolism is, therefore, a more appropriate term. Pathogenetic factors for the development of venous thrombosis were defined by Virchow in 1856 to be stasis, endothelial injury, and hypercoagulability. In pregnancy, these factors are routinely observed. Compression of the inferior vena cava by the gravid uterus reduces blood return from the lower extremities and results in stasis. During pregnancy there is an increase in several of the plasma-clotting factors, and post partum, tissue injury becomes a contributing factor as well. Despite this, the risk of venous thromboembolism in the antepartum period is not significantly increased over that of the nonpregnant female of childbearing age. In contrast, the relative risk in the postpartum period is increased 5- to 20-fold, with the risk being higher after cesarean section than after vaginal delivery. Thus, although venous thromboembolism is uncommon during pregnancy, it is a major cause of postpartum maternal mortality and morbidity.

A number of other factors may contribute to venous thromboembolism in obstetric patients, including immobilization, obesity, varicose veins, and infection during the immediate puerperium. In addition, the presence of underlying inherited deficiencies of plasma proteins, such as antithrombin III, protein C, and protein S, and the recently described hereditary resistance to activated protein C, constitutes an important predisposing factor. Patients with antiphospholipid antibodies have a high risk of venous thromboembolism. Despite the more frequent occurrence of leg swelling and pain in the third trimester, recent studies indicate that the frequency of DVT documented by objective testing is spread equally in all three trimesters. There is a very striking propensity for DVT to occur in the left leg, possibly due to compression of the left iliac vein by the right iliac artery.

Patients undergoing gynecologic surgery are also considered at increased risk for the development of DVT and PE in the postoperative period. The incidence of DVT following hysterectomy ranges from 7 to 27%, depending on the procedure used. The thrombosis may originate during the operative procedure or 3 to 5 days after the surgery. Most thrombi originate in the calf, and about 20% of these may propagate proximally, making the risk of PE a reality. Factors contributing to this risk include age over 40 years, obesity, malignancy, and the use of oral contraceptives at the time of surgery.

DIAGNOSIS

Clinical examination is both insensitive and nonspecific and cannot be relied on in making the diagnosis of DVT. The classic syndrome of swelling, pain, venous distention, and pain on abrupt dorsiflexion of the foot (Homan's sign) is present in less than a third of patients with a documented DVT. In the presence of suggestive clinical findings, objective tests corroborate the diagnosis less than half the time. Pregnancy can confound the clinical presentation, because lower extremity edema and pain are frequently seen in the third trimester. Thus, the diagnosis of DVT must be established by objective tests.

The standard diagnostic test for DVT is ascending venography, which can detect both distal calf vein thrombi and proximal thrombi in the popliteal, femoral, and iliac veins. Disadvantages of this invasive procedure include patient discomfort, contrast medium–induced thrombosis, difficulty in identifying old from new clots, technical difficulty in cannulating pedal veins, and cost. During pregnancy, exposure of the fetus to ionizing radiation constitutes another drawback.

Noninvasive tests include impedance plethysmography (IPG), B-mode ultrasonography, and duplex Doppler ultrasonography, all of which are more sensitive for detection of proximal than distal thrombosis. By measuring changes in electrical resistance, IPG measures the decrease in venous outflow following a proximal obstruction. IPG is highly specific and sensitive for proximal DVT in symptomatic patients; however, in a recent study it was found to be less sensitive than in earlier reports. IPG is insensitive to nonocclusive proximal thrombi, and any process that causes venous obstruction, such as pregnancy, may lead to a false-positive test.

Real-time B-mode ultrasonography has a sensitivity of over 95% in symptomatic patients with proximal DVT and allows visualization of the thrombus. Failure of the vein to collapse with compression (compression ultrasonography) is the most sensitive finding. Duplex imaging combines B-mode ultrasonography with Doppler flow-detection ultrasonic imaging and has a sensitivity of 93% and a specificity of 98% in the symptomatic nonpregnant patient with proximal DVT. This technique can detect occlusive and nonocclusive thrombi. Disadvantages include the inability to visualize the iliac veins uniformly and the inadequate sensitivity in asymptomatic patients with proximal DVT, which limits its role as a screening test in patients at high risk for developing DVT. Other diagnostic techniques available include computer-assisted tomography and magnetic resonance venography, both of which can detect thrombosed proximal lower extremity, pelvic, and abdominal veins. Their role in routine diagnosis of DVT is limited by high cost and availability.

In the pregnant patient, a diagnosis of DVT may be made using duplex ultrasonographic imaging or IPG. In many centers, duplex imaging has become the noninvasive diagnostic method of choice for acute DVT. A diagnosis of proximal DVT may be reliably made based on an abnormal IPG study during the first two trimesters, but a positive test in the third trimester should be confirmed either with duplex imaging or contrast venography. A normal duplex imaging or IPG does not exclude a distal or calf vein thrombosis. The test in this case should be repeated on day 2 after referral and again on days 3, 5, 7, 10, and 14 to detect proximal extension of distal thrombosis. In the absence of evidence of a proximal DVT on serial testing, anticoagulation may be safely withheld.

If noninvasive testing for DVT is not available, then a limited contrast venogram should be performed, shielding the abdomen. A complete venogram should be done if the former is negative. Unilateral venogram without shielding will expose the fetus to a total absorbed dose of about 305 mrads, and a limited venogram with shielding of the abdomen is associated with an exposure of well under 50 mrads.

Pulmonary embolism, a potentially fatal complication of DVT, must be suspected in any patient who presents with a sudden onset of dyspnea that may be associated with fever, tachycardia, pleuritic chest pain, and hemoptysis. Massive PE may also present with cardiovascular collapse and acute cor pulmonale. The true incidence of PE is unknown, and silent, clinically unrecognized PE occurs far more frequently than is currently considered, underscoring the need for a high index of clinical suspicion. The importance of objective testing to establish the diagnosis of PE cannot be overemphasized. The general approach remains the same as in nonpregnant patients. A ventilation-perfusion lung scan is the first test to obtain to establish diagnosis. Ventilation scintigraphy involves administration of radiolabeled xenon gas, and the perfusion scan employs the injection of radiocolloid particles into the circulation. A normal perfusion scan excludes the diagnosis of PE, and a high-probability scan, defined by a segmental or larger perfusion defect with normal ventilation, can make the diagnosis with certainty. A low-probability scan makes the probability of PE low if combined with a strong clinical impression that PE is unlikely. However, in the presence of a clinical likelihood and a nondiagnostic scan, pulmonary angiography, the "gold standard" for the diagnosis of PE, should be performed. The amount of radiation exposure can be minimized by performing the pulmonary angiography via the brachial route (instead of the femoral route) and with abdominal shielding. An alternative approach in patients with nondiagnostic ventilation-perfusion scans is to obtain noninvasive studies of the lower extremities. A substantial number of PEs originate in the lower extremities, and therefore evidence for a proximal DVT would define an indication for anticoagulation and may obviate the need for a pulmonary angiogram.

TREATMENT

Management of the pregnant patient with venous thromboembolism entails special considerations, and they are discussed here. In general, the guidelines for treatment of DVT and PE in nonpregnant patients with gynecologic disorders remain the same as for all other patients, and they are presented elsewhere in this book.

Use of Antithrombotic Agents During Pregnancy

Anticoagulant therapy is used during pregnancy for the treatment or prophylaxis of venous thromboembolic disease, for the prevention and treatment of systemic embolism associated with valvular heart disease (including prosthetic valves), and in the management of patients with antiphospholipid antibody syndrome. The use of anticoagulants during pregnancy brings up special considerations with respect to their effects on the fetus and the mother. Heparin does not cross the placenta, but oral anticoagulants do and may cause adverse effects on the fetus. Recent studies suggest that heparin is relatively safe, with no increased risks to the fetus. Warfarin (Coumadin) induces an embryopathy consisting of nasal hypoplasia or stippled epiphyses after exposure in utero during the first trimester. This has been reported to occur in 28% of infants after exposure between 7 and 12 weeks. Central nervous system abnormalities have also been described with warfarin use in pregnancy.

Two potential maternal complications of anticoagulation that assume special importance in the pregnant patient are hemorrhage and heparin-induced osteoporosis, the latter being related to prolonged heparin administration. During pregnancy, the rate of bleeding in patients treated with heparin appears no different from that in nonpregnant patients. However, anticoagulation may contribute to excessive bleeding during delivery. It has been recently observed that the anticoagulant effect of heparin may persist for a prolonged period (up to 28 hours) after subcutaneous injection; this effect has been associated with an increased risk of hemorrhage during the delivery. Therefore, heparin therapy should be discontinued 24 hours prior to elective induction of labor, and careful administration of protamine sulfate may be appropriate in patients with marked anticoagulant effect at delivery. Warfarin therapy should be avoided in the weeks before delivery. Long-term heparin therapy has been reported to cause osteoporosis in about 17% of pregnant patients treated with subcutaneous heparin, and this may be associated with a small risk of symptomatic fractures. The risk of osteoporosis may be dependent on dose and duration of heparin therapy; bone changes may be reversible following discontinuation of heparin.

Use of anticoagulants in the nursing mother assumes importance in view of the increased risk of venous thromboembolism in the postpartum period. Heparin can be safely administered to nursing mothers and is not secreted into breast milk. Warfarin administration to the mother does not alter plasma levels of vitamin K–dependent factors or induce an anticoagulant effect in the breast-fed infant.

Therapy of Venous Thromboembolism During Pregnancy

Patients who develop either a DVT or PE during pregnancy should be treated with a continuous intravenous infusion of heparin for 5 to 10 days followed by subcutaneous injections every 12 hours in full doses. The activated partial thromboplastin time (aPTT) should be prolonged to 1.5 to 2.5 times control, and therapy should be continued until delivery. Initiation of intravenous therapy is best achieved with a bolus of 5000 to 10,000 U of heparin. During therapy with subcutaneous heparin, the dose should be adjusted to achieve an aPTT of 1.5 times control at 6 hours post injection. Heparin should be discontinued immediately before delivery. Anticoagulation should be reinstituted post partum with heparin and warfarin. Heparin should be discontinued once therapeutic anticoagulation with warfarin is achieved (International Normalized Ratio of 2 to 3). Warfarin should be administered for at least 2 weeks thereafter. All patients receiving heparin should be carefully followed with platelet counts obtained at least three times a week. Heparin-induced thrombocytopenia and thrombosis are infrequent complications but result in major sequelae.

Low-molecular-weight heparins (LMWH) constitute a new class of anticoagulants that are likely to have a major impact on management of patients with venous thromboembolism. LMWH have a longer plasma half-life and a more predictable anticoagulant response compared with standard heparin; these features permit administration once daily and without the laboratory monitoring routinely used for conventional heparin therapy. LMWH do not cross the placental barrier, and their role in management of pregnant patients needs to be defined.

Patients with massive PE, especially with shock, and extensive proximal DVT are candidates for thrombolytic therapy with streptokinase, tissue plasminogen activator, or urokinase. An alternative is emergency embolectomy for life-threatening PE. Despite numerous case reports of successful use of thrombolytic agents for treatment of PE during pregnancy, more information is needed to develop firm guidelines for their use during pregnancy. Apart from the risks of excessive hemorrhage, particularly during delivery and post partum, there is not enough clinical experience available to exclude the possibility of a teratogenic effect when administered in the first trimester.

Surgical treatment for acute DVT (thrombectomy) is based on the rationale that removal of the clot should rapidly restore venous patency and protect venous valvular function. Surgical thrombectomy has been recommended for the treatment of extensive iliofemoral deep vein thrombosis and for phlegmasia cerulea dolens, in which extensive venous occlusion results in a compromised arterial circulation and viability of the limb is threatened. Further clinical trials are needed to establish the potential benefits of venous thrombectomy. Patients with PE who have a contraindication to anticoagulation or who sustain a PE despite adequate anticoagulation are candidates for vena caval interruption techniques. Vena caval filters are effective in preventing recurrent PE.

Deep calf vein thrombosis has the potential for proximal propagation and subsequent embolization. One approach is to treat patients with symptomatic calf vein thrombosis with analgesics and follow them carefully with serial noninvasive tests for 10 to 14 days to detect evidence of proximal propagation, which would be an indication for anticoagulation. An alternative approach is to treat them with anticoagulation at initial detection.

Pregnant patients with a history of previous DVT or PE should be treated with 5000 U of heparin every 12 hours subcutaneously; the risk of recurrence in such patients is 4 to 12%. Because of the risks of warfarin embryopathy, women on long-term oral anticoagulation should be carefully counseled regarding the risks of pregnancy. In the event of unexpected pregnancy, warfarin should be replaced with subcutaneous heparin injections. In the context of planned pregnancy, two options can be considered: to replace warfarin with heparin prior to conception or to perform frequent pregnancy tests and substitute heparin when pregnancy is achieved.

A special scenario pertains to pregnant patients who have circulating antiphospholipid antibodies, deficiency of plasma AT-III, protein C, or protein S, or other states (e.g., resistance to activated protein C) that are considered to be associated with an enhanced risk of thromboembolism. Such patients with a previous history of DVT or PE should be treated with subcutaneous heparin, with the dose adjusted to achieve an aPTT of 1.5 to 2.5 times control. Patients without a previous history of venous thromboembolism should be treated with low-dose subcutaneous heparin during pregnancy.

Prevention of Venous Thromboembolism

Venous thromboembolism is a major cause of morbidity and mortality in hospitalized patients, accounting for over 100,000 deaths in patients each year in the United States. Fatal PE has been considered the most common preventable cause of hospital death. Moreover, of the patients who eventually die of PE, two thirds survive less than 30 minutes after the event. These facts emphasize the pressing need to prevent DVT and PE in patients at risk. This is relevant to patients hospitalized with gynecologic disease and for surgery. In these patients the approaches to preventing DVT are based on the potential risks of venous thromboembolism, benefits of the various interventions, and the possible complications related to their use. The risk of thromboembolic events is increased by factors such as older age (more than 40 years), obesity, prolonged bed rest, varicose veins, estrogen treatment, malignancy, duration of surgery, and a history of previous thromboembolic events. In low-risk patients (less than 40 years of age), without any clinical risk factors, and undergoing minor operations, no specific prophylaxis, other than early ambulation and graduated compression stockings, is recommended. In moderate-risk patients over the age of 40 years undergoing major operations (more than 60 minutes in duration) but without any additional risk factors, therapy with low-dose subcutaneous heparin (5000 U twice daily) is recommended. An alternative approach is the use of external pneumatic compression in patients prone to wound complications such as hematomas and infections. Because of the increased risk of venous thromboembolism in the postpartum period, there is a strong rationale to administer low-dose subcutaneous heparin to these patients. In high-risk patients over the age of 40 years undergoing major surgery and having additional risk factors, it is recommended that heparin (5000 U subcutaneously every 8 hours) be administered. In patients with multiple risk factors, this can be combined with other approaches, such as intermittent pneumatic compression.

Important new agents currently in extensive clinical trials are the low-molecular-weight heparins that have not yet been licensed in the United States for use in patients undergoing general or gynecologic surgery. In several trials in general surgery patients, LMWH have been found to be superior to therapy with standard low-dose subcutaneous heparin in preventing DVT without a corresponding increase in major bleeding complications. LMWH have the potential of becoming major therapeutic agents in this context in the near future.

Septic Pelvic Vein Thrombosis

Prior to the antibiotic era, puerperal infection with resultant pelvic venous system thrombophlebitis was a major cause of maternal morbidity but now is a rather uncommon complication of pelvic surgery or delivery. Risk factors include puerperal sepsis, infected abortion, or postoperative infection. Clinical findings may include high-spiking fevers and chills, nausea, vomiting, tender indurated cords on pelvic examination, a tender abdominal mass just beyond the uterine cornu, abdominal guarding and an ileus. Alternatively, the diagnosis may be less obvious, with a presentation of enigmatic fever or persistent fever spikes with occasional accompanying chills and the absence of other clinical findings. Except for the fever, the patient may not appear ill. Since the presentation can be variable, one must have a high index of suspicion. In addition to obtaining cultures, the diagnosis may be confirmed by a noninvasive test such as computed tomography or magnetic resonance imaging. Therapy consists of therapeutic anticoagulation and appropriate antibiotics. Patients whose course is complicated by septic pulmonary emboli resulting in pleural effusions, pulmonary infarctions, or abscesses may require a vena caval filter.

CONTRACEPTION

method of
CATHERINE L. DEAN, M.D., M.P.H.
Washington University School of Medicine
St. Louis, Missouri

Two-thirds of American women have at least one unintended pregnancy by the time they reach menopause. Despite readily available contraceptives, more than one-half of the nearly 6 million pregnancies annually in the United States are unintended. Fifty percent of women presenting with unintended pregnancy report they were using contraception at the time they conceived. Thus, it is essential that health care providers understand the reasons contributing to the surprisingly high lifetime failure rate of contraception in order to reduce the number of unintended pregnancies.

DETERMINANTS OF CONTRACEPTIVE CHOICE

A woman's choice of a contraceptive method is key in determining her risk for future unintended pregnancy. The health care provider's role in counseling women is critical in providing all the necessary information needed to make the best choice. The ideal contraceptive is a balance between effectiveness, ease of compliance, safety (real or perceived), reversibility (or permanence), and personal acceptability. Moreover, the woman must understand that all contraceptive methods, even when used correctly, can fail and result in pregnancy.

The health care provider can further assist the woman with her choice by informing her of any non-contraceptive health benefits (Table 1). Protection against sexually transmitted diseases (STDs) is a critical noncontraceptive benefit for women at risk. The simultaneous use of two contraceptive methods can add protection against STDs and lower the risk of contraceptive failure.

Effectiveness

Many women are not aware of the differing levels of effectiveness between various contraceptive methods. One needs to remember that just as contraceptives fail women, women sometimes fail to use contraceptives correctly each time. Thus, the failure rate of any given contraceptive applies to women in general, not to any one individual. For example, the diaphragm has an 18% first-year failure rate. That failure rate would be lower with a 40-year-old woman with biologically declining fertility who rarely has intercourse, compared with a 20-year-old woman in her reproductive prime who has frequent intercourse.

Ease of Compliance

Contraceptive methods that are compliance-independent are permanent sterilization, implants, long-acting injectables, and intrauterine devices (IUDs). These methods require differing amounts of medical intervention, from one-time implementation, as with sterilization, to relatively infrequent maintenance (varying between 3 months and 10 years). Because of their ease of use, failure rates are low and are rarely due to user error.

Contraceptive methods that are compliance-dependent are pills, all barrier methods, spermicides, withdrawal, periodic abstinence, and the lactational amenorrhea method (LAM). The pill is intercourse-independent and requires strict compliance: A woman must take the pill at the same time every day. The woman has to honestly assess whether she can remember to take her pill correctly because inconsistent use is associated with high failure rates. All the barrier and spermicide methods are intercourse-dependent. The woman has to consider her sexual lifestyle, and whether she will have the needed method at hand each time intercourse occurs. Withdrawal requires trust in the partner and complete ejaculatory control. Periodic abstinence and LAM both require the woman to monitor her reproductive cycle and abstain or use another method during potentially fertile times.

Safety

Generally, contraception is safe for most women. However, certain women should not use specific contraceptive methods, particularly in the presence of certain medical conditions. Specific safety considerations are discussed in the sections on methods.

More important is to differentiate between real safety considerations and misconceptions. A woman will not use a method that she fears. If the health care provider cannot educate her and her support system as to the safety of a given method *to their satisfaction*, another method should be chosen.

Personal Acceptability

Only the woman can decide, for her own specific set of reasons, what methods are most acceptable for her. These reasons generally change over time. Partner acceptance is important as well. She may prefer a barrier method that her partner does not like. She may want a method that is quickly reversible under her control. It is important that she understands it is acceptable to change her mind and try a different method. The cost of the method may limit her choice. Many women use one method while saving money for another method. Finally, the desire for future fertility, if any, is an important consideration in choosing a contraceptive method.

TABLE 1. **Noncontraceptive Benefits of Major Methods of Contraception**

Contraceptive Method	Noncontraceptive Benefits
Sterilization	None known.
Levonorgestrel implant (Norplant), medroxyprogesterone acetate (Depo-Provera), progestin-only pills	May protect against PID; decreased anemia; reduced menstrual pain and blood loss; lactation not affected; decreased risk of endometrial and ovarian cancer.
IUD	Copper IUD, none known; progestin IUD may decrease menstrual blood loss and pain.
Combined oral contraceptive pill	*Decreases* ovarian cancer, endometrial cancer, PID, benign breast disease, dysmenorrhea, ectopic pregnancies; *increases* menstrual regularity, bone density.
Male condom	Protects against STDs; delays premature ejaculation.
Female condom	Protects against STDs.
Diaphragm, cervical cap	Protects somewhat against STDs.
Spermicide	Protects against STDs.
Periodic abstinence, withdrawal	None known.
Lactational amenorrhea method	Provides excellent nutrition for infant during first 6 months.

Abbreviations: PID = pelvic inflammatory disease; STD = sexually transmitted disease; IUD = intrauterine device.

SURGICAL STERILIZATION

One-third of reproductive-age women in the United States rely on sterilization as their contraceptive method, making this the most popular method. Twenty-five percent of women have had a tubal ligation, and 11% of women depend on their partner's vasectomy. These methods are highly effective, with failure rates of less than 1%. Both male and female sterilization are low-risk surgical procedures, making sterilization much safer than pregnancy, in terms of morbidity and mortality. Couples must be carefully counseled as to the intended permanence of these methods, since reversal procedures are expensive and unreliable. The first-year failure rate for tubal ligation is 0.4%, and for vasectomy, 0.15%.

COMPLIANCE-*INDEPENDENT* REVERSIBLE METHODS

Levonorgestrel Implant

Levonorgestrel implant (Norplant) is the first contraceptive in this new drug delivery system approved by the Food and Drug Administration (FDA). This implant system consists of six Silastic rods containing the progestin levonorgestrel; they are placed just under the skin in the upper inner arm. The implants slowly release the hormone, which then inhibits ovulation, suppresses the endometrium, and thickens cervical mucus. Norplant is effective for 5 years, with failure rates equal to sterilization in the first 2 years of use. The overall failure rate is 3 per 1000. When the implant is removed, fertility returns almost immediately.

Contraindications to this implant system are pregnancy, undiagnosed abnormal vaginal bleeding, most antiseizure medications, active pulmonary emboli or thrombophlebitis, and breast cancer. The most significant side effect is menstrual disturbances, which all women should be counseled to expect. Most women like the method, with 85% of women continuing to use it after 1 year.

Medroxyprogesterone Acetate Injectable

Medroxyprogesterone acetate (Depo-Provera) (DMPA) 150 mg intramuscularly provides 12 weeks of contraception with a 2-week grace period. DMPA inhibits ovulation, thickens cervical mucus, and suppresses the endometrium. The effectiveness is similar to that of the levonorgestrel implant, and contraindications to its use are generally the same. DMPA also causes menstrual disturbances but is more likely to cause amenorrhea after 6 months of use. Of key significance, a return of fertility could be delayed up to 18 months after cessation.

Intrauterine Devices

The copper IUD (ParaGard T 380A) is FDA-approved for 8 years of use, and Progestasert, the progesterone IUD, is FDA-approved for 1 year of use. Studies from the Centers for Disease Control and Prevention have confirmed that IUDs are very safe in the appropriately screened patient, that is, a woman who is in a mutually monogamous relationship. Although there is a slightly increased risk of infection related to insertion for the first few months, there is no additional risk of infection from the IUD itself. However, if the woman should contract an STD, the STD infection is likely to be severe when an IUD is in place, often leading to tubal damage and subsequent infertility. This is why patient selection is crucial. Unfortunately, IUDs remain underutilized in the United States. The highly publicized Dalkon Shield litigation has created many negative perceptions concerning the IUD. With public health education, women in the United States are now gradually choosing the IUD as their contraceptive method. IUDs are highly effective and have a "typical use" first-year failure rate of 0.8% for the copper IUD (ParaGard T 380A) and 2% for the Progestasert System.

COMPLIANCE-*DEPENDENT* REVERSIBLE METHODS

Oral Contraceptives

Oral contraceptives remain the number one reversible contraceptive choice of women in the United States. The most commonly used pill is the combined estrogen and progestin pill used for 21 days, with a 7-day pill-free interval. The "mini-pill," progestin only, is used much less frequently and must be taken daily.

Although the new lower-dose pills are much safer than the original formulations, there are still some women who should not use the pill. Fortunately, this list continues to decrease with increased knowledge about the current pill formulations. Major contraindications include thrombophlebitis or thromboembolism (current or past), stroke, coronary heart disease, breast cancer, other estrogen-dependent cancer, current impaired liver function, benign hepatic adenoma or liver cancer, smoking past the age of 35, and pregnancy. Women with the following conditions may be able to use the pill with extreme caution and close follow-up: hypertension (medication-controlled), controlled diabetes mellitus, migraine headaches that start after pill use, sickle cell disease (SS) or sickle C (SC) disease, active gallbladder disease, Gilbert's disease (congenital hyperbilirubinemia), age over 50 years, and lactation.

The reduced hormonal content of current pills has also decreased undesirable side effects. The most common side effects are breakthrough bleeding and amenorrhea. Both can generally be corrected by changing pill formulations. Women need to be warned of these side effects so they do not stop using the pill before seeking medical care.

The oral contraceptive pill has many noncontraceptive benefits summarized in Table 1. Oral contraceptives are highly effective when used correctly and have a "typical use" first-year failure rate of 3%.

Barrier or Spermicide Methods

Male Condom

Condoms are the second most popular reversible contraceptive method in the United States. Latex condoms have been shown to protect against STDs and are now widely promoted for use in addition to most other contraceptive methods for safer sexual practices. Condoms are available in various sizes, lubricated or nonlubricated, with or without spermicide, with or without a reservoir tip, and in a variety of textures and colors. Lambskin condoms are available for those with latex allergies but are not as effective at infection prevention. Condoms have a "typical use" first-year failure rate of 12% when used alone. Efficacy is increased when they are used with a vaginal spermicide.

Female Condom

The Reality female condom consists of a polyurethane sheath containing two flexible rings. One ring is inside and serves as an insertion guide and internal anchor. The second larger ring serves as an external anchor. The interior sheath is prelubricated with a silicone-based lubricant. It does not contain spermicide and cannot be used with a male condom. The female condom is available over the counter, is disposable, and is intended for only one use. The female condom protects against STDs and pregnancy. The "typical use" first-year failure rate of the female condom used alone is 21%.

Diaphragm

The diaphragm is the first female contraceptive method ever used in the United States. The diaphragm must be fitted by a health care provider, and the woman must be taught proper placement. Spermicide is placed in the cap and around the rim at the time of insertion, and the diaphragm may be inserted up to 6 hours before intercourse. The diaphragm must remain in place for at least 6 hours after intercourse. Repeated intercourse needs to be preceded with additional spermicide placed by an applicator. The diaphragm should not be left in place for more than 24 hours because of the possible risk of toxic shock syndrome. Some women cannot be properly fitted with a diaphragm, particularly in the presence of a cystocele. The "typical use" first-year failure rate is 18%.

Cervical Cap

The Prentif cavity rim cervical cap fits snugly on the cervix and is held in place by suction. It must be fitted by a health care provider, and the woman must be taught proper placement. All the previous caveats regarding the diaphragm also apply to the cervical cap, except the cap may be worn for up to 48 hours, and additional spermicide with repeated intercourse is not needed. Some women cannot be fitted with the cap. The "typical use" first-year failure rate is 18% in nulliparous women and 36% in parous women.

Sponge

The manufacturer of the Today sponge has stopped producing the contraceptive because of excessive costs of FDA-required manufacturing plant upgrades that have made the product unprofitable. The polyurethane sponge was impregnated with nonoxynol 9 and lasted 24 hours. The sponge was available over the counter, came in one size, and did not require any special training or fitting. The "typical use" first-year failure rate in nulliparous women is 18%, and in parous women, 36%.

Foam, Suppositories, Jellies, Film

Vaginal spermicides are available in a variety of formats. They have been shown to reduce the transmission of STDs such as gonorrhea and chlamydial infection. The effect of spermicide on human immunodeficiency virus (HIV) infection without a condom is unclear. Nonoxynol 9 is the active agent in most spermicidal products. Octoxynol is also available in the United States. Spermicides are necessary with vaginal barrier methods such as the diaphragm and cervical cap. Spermicides are much more effective when used with a condom than when used alone. When used alone, the "typical use" first-year failure rate of spermicides is 21%.

Behavioral Methods

Withdrawal

Withdrawal and condoms are the only two male reversible contraceptive methods. Withdrawal depends on trust and absolute ejaculatory control. Withdrawal can be used with other methods to further improve contraceptive efficacy. When no other contraceptive method is available, withdrawal can significantly reduce conception rates. When used alone, the "typical use" first-year failure rate is 18%.

Periodic Abstinence

Fertility awareness methods are used to prospectively predict ovulation and thereby allow the couple to abstain from intercourse during the "unsafe" time of the cycle. Highly motivated women with regular cycles can achieve low failure rates. Women with irregular cycles are poor candidates for these methods. The "typical use" first-year failure rate is 20%.

Lactational Amenorrhea Method

Women who are exclusively breast-feeding generally do not ovulate for the first 6 months. However, if during the first 6 months weaning begins, if the infant's diet is supplemented, or if menses return, other forms of contraception should be initiated. Clinical studies estimate a "perfect use" 6-month failure rate of 0.7%.

Emergency Contraception

Emergency contraception can dramatically reduce unintended pregnancy from unprotected intercourse. Condoms can break, diaphragms can be dislodged or forgotten, and rape continues to occur.

Hormonal Method

The use of higher-dose combined oral contraceptive pills within 72 hours of a single episode of unprotected intercourse during the midcycle is highly effective at preventing pregnancy. The best-known regimen is 100 micrograms of ethinyl estradiol and 1.0 mg of norgestrel (two Ovral tablets) taken immediately and two more tablets taken in 12 hours. Transient nausea and vomiting is a common side effect with this method. Clinical studies indicate emergency contraceptive pill treatment reduces the risk of pregnancy by 75%.

Postcoital Intrauterine Device Insertion

Insertion of the ParaGard copper IUD within 5 to 7 days after unprotected midcycle intercourse is also a highly effective contraceptive method, with the resulting pregnancy rate less than 1%.

Section 16

Psychiatric Disorders

THE MANAGEMENT OF ALCOHOLISM

method of
AIDAN FOY, M.B., M.Sc.
Newcastle Mater Misericordiae Hospital
Newcastle, New South Wales, Australia

Alcohol-related problems are common in all areas of medical practice, from trauma surgery to psychiatry. Although there is some evidence that a modest alcohol intake is protective, it is generally agreed that daily consumption of more than 30 grams for a man and more than 20 grams for a woman approximately doubles age-adjusted mortality. Consumption of over 80 and over 60 grams, respectively, for men and women produces one of the traditional diseases due directly to alcohol.

Therefore, all treatment of alcoholism is essentially intended to prevent the alcohol-related diseases, their complications, or the financial, social, emotional, and family problems caused by alcohol dependence. In terms of community health, alcohol-associated conditions affect many more people and are more important than the classic "alcoholic" diseases, and the greatest effort in primary and secondary prevention should be directed at them. Tertiary prevention of alcohol-related disability is more concerned with the treatment of alcohol dependence.

PRIMARY PREVENTION

It is now well established that the overall level of alcohol consumption by a society as a whole is directly related to the level of alcohol-related problems, so primary prevention consists of measures to reduce consumption either overall or in certain situations. Primary prevention measures can be directed at nations, small communities, minority groups, or people in specified high-risk situations.

A full discussion of primary prevention is beyond the scope of this book, but there are essentially two approaches, legislative and educational. Legislation can take the form of licensing laws governing the sale and consumption of liquor, localized prohibition (a community choosing to forbid the sale and/or consumption of alcohol), or drunk driving laws. The random breath testing policy used in Australia has been credited with achieving a 30% reduction in mortality from motor vehicle accidents and is, in effect, a form of targeted prohibition. Educational initiatives usually consist of campaigns aimed at specific target groups, such as youth, and more general campaigns aimed at publicizing the "safe drinking rules" (Table 1). They can be used in addition to a legislative approach.

SECONDARY PREVENTION

In the context of alcohol-related disease, secondary prevention refers to the prevention of such disease by recognizing the association between drinking and individual medical conditions, drawing this to patients' attention, and assisting them to change. This is the area that impacts most on medical practice and where doctors can make their greatest contribution in dialogue with individual patients. There are six simple steps to follow:

1. Be aware of the common diseases that are associated with alcohol consumption. These are not the traditional "alcoholic" conditions but rather those that alcohol increases the risk for and in which alcohol is associated with complications or is likely to interfere with therapy (Table 2).

2. Take a quantitative alcohol history. How many days a week does the patient drink alcohol? How much in grams? (A standard drink equals 10 grams absolute alcohol.) For how long (in months or years) has this pattern continued?

3. Explain the association between the disease in question and alcohol consumption.

4. Make a brief assessment of alcohol dependence. There are now at least three simple questionnaires—CAGE (*c*ut down, *a*nger, *g*uilt, *e*ye-opener), TWEAK (*t*olerance, *w*orry, *e*arly morning, *a*mnesia, *c*ut down), and the Trauma Scale (Table 3)—that can be used as screening tests. These have been criticized for being obvious in their intent, but if they are introduced at an appropriate moment and used tactfully, they are useful. For hospitalized patients, with more serious conditions and more available time, the Canterbury Alcoholism Screening Test (CAST) (Fig-

TABLE 1. **The Rules of "Safe" Drinking for Men (Women)**

Average three (two) standard drinks per day or fewer
No more than six (four) drinks in any one day
Maximal rate of drinking is three (two) drinks in the first hour, then one per hour thereafter
No drinking on inappropriate occasions* or against advice

*Circumstances vary with the individual.

TABLE 2. **Alcohol-Related Conditions**

Alcohol Increases the Risk
Hypertension
Trauma—motor vehicles, other accidents, assaults, self-harm
Chronic anxiety
Depression
Gastrointestinal upset—gastritis, esophagitis, Mallory-Weiss lesion
Complications of pregnancy
Alcohol Is Associated with Complications
Diabetes
Chronic airway limitation
Alcohol Interferes with Therapy
Diabetes
Hyperlipoproteinemia
Psoriasis
Plus most of the other above-mentioned conditions
Traditional "Alcoholic" Diseases
Cirrhosis
Pancreatitis
Brain damage

ure 1) or AUDIT (*a*lcohol *u*se *d*isorders *i*dentification *t*est) questionnaires can be useful.

5. If the patient does not appear to be alcohol dependent, negotiate an agreement to follow the rules of safe drinking, appropriately modified for the individual situation.

6. If the patient appears dependent or simple measures are not effective, refer the patient for formal treatment of alcohol dependence.

TERTIARY PREVENTION

The aim of tertiary prevention is to limit disability from alcohol dependence or alcohol-related disease. This phase incorporates formal treatment of alcoholism and alcohol dependence.

As the treatment program is put together, each patient proceeds through three separate stages: crisis/entry, consolidation/induction, and maintenance. Different techniques are aimed at different outcomes in each stage.

Crisis/Entry

This phase refers to management of a specific alcohol-related problem that has brought the patient to notice. In medical practice, this is usually an alcohol-related illness or an urgent request for detoxification, but there are other signs, such as distress following a marital breakup or arrest for an alcohol-related offense. This immediate crisis needs attention in its own right, but the patient must be encouraged to make the connection with alcohol use and progress to the next stage.

It is essential to appreciate that the first presentation of an alcohol problem that is causing family dysfunction may be seen in a child or spouse of the drinker.

In the crisis phase, medical treatment, detoxification, and family support are used. The goals are defined by the immediate problem plus an appreciation by the patient that things need not be this way.

Induction/Consolidation

Having dealt with the crisis, the patient moves in the second phase to change from a drinking lifestyle to a sober lifestyle. This is not "treatment" in the traditional sense. The patient is not a passive recipient but an active partner in management, and his or her personal autonomy must be preserved. All successful forms of therapy work in some way to regain or extend patients' power over their own lives.

TABLE 3. **Questionnaires**

CAGE
Over the past 12 months, have you felt
1. That you should cut down on your drinking?
2. Annoyed by anyone commenting on your drinking?
3. Guilty about your drinking?
4. That you needed an early morning drink to get going?
Two or more positive responses suggest dependence.

Trauma Scale
Since your eighteenth birthday, have you
1. Broken a bone or dislocated a joint?
2. Been injured in an automobile accident?
3. Suffered a head injury?
4. Been injured in a fight or assaulted (excluding sporting injuries)?
5. Been injured while or after drinking alcohol?
Two or more positive responses suggest dependence.

TWEAK
1. Do you need three or more drinks to feel the effect? (If yes, score 2.)
2. Can you "hold" five or more drinks without getting drunk? (If yes, score 2.)
3. Do you worry about your drinking? (If yes, score 2.)
4. Do you need an early morning drink to get going? (If yes, score 1.)
5. Do you sometimes forget what happened the night before? (If yes, score 1.)
6. Have you tried to cut down on your drinking? (If yes, score 1.)
A score of ≥ 3 suggests dependence.

Please Tick: YES/NO

Q1.   When did you last drink? (Discontinue if response is "never"). . . . . □□

Q2.   Have you been admitted to hospital more than once because of accidents?

(By accidents, we mean all types) . . . . □□

Q3.   Have any close family members such as a parent, brother, spouse, or sister,

had drinking problems?. . . . . □□

Thinking over THE LAST THREE MONTHS-

Q4.   Do you drink before lunch fairly often?. . . . . □□

Q5.   After the first glass or two of alcohol do you ever feel a craving for more?. □□

Q6.   Do you find you are thinking a lot about alcohol?. . . . . □□

Q7.   Do you sometimes drink alcohol against your doctor's advice?. . . . . □□

Q8.   When you drink a lot of alcohol, do you tend to eat less?. . . . . □□

Q9.   In the morning do you sometimes feel that you might be sick (vomit)?. . . . . □□

Q10.   Have you found that your hands have been trembling a lot?. . . . . □□

Q11.   Have you ever used alcohol to get rid of trembling or the feeling that

you might be sick?. . . . . □□

Q12.   Have you ever been criticised at work because of your drinking?. . . . . □□

Q13.   Do you prefer to drink alone?. . . . . □□

Q14.   Do you think you're in worse shape because of your drinking?. . . . . □□

Q15.   Do you ever have a guilty conscience about drinking?. . . . . □□

Q16.   In order to cut down your drinking, have you ever felt it necessary

to limit it to certain occasions or to certain times of the day?. . . . . □□

Q17.   Do you feel you should drink less?. . . . . □□

Q18.   Do you think that without alcohol you would have fewer problems?. . . . . □□

Q19.   When you're upset do you drink alcohol to calm down?. . . . . □□

Q20.   Are there times when you'd like to stop drinking?. . . . . □□

Q21.   Would you get along better with your spouse/partner/the people

you're closest to if you didn't drink?. . . . . □□

Q22.   Have you ever deliberately tried to do without any alcohol at all?. . . . . □□

Q23.   Have you often been told that your breath smells of alcohol?. . . . . □□

5 POSITIVE RESPONSES TO Q'S 2-23 IS POSITIVE

Q24.   On the average, write in the number you would normally drink in a week:

Spirits/Liqueurs   Nip □   Bottle (sm) □   Bottle (lrg) □

Beer   Glass □   Can □

Wine   Glass □   Bottle □

Sherry   Glass □   Bottle □

Cocktails   Glass □

Figure 1. Canterbury Alcoholism Screening Test. (From Elvy GA, Wells JE: The Canterbury alcoholism screening test (CAST): A detection instrument for use with hospitalized patients. NZ Med J 97:111–115, 1984.)

TABLE 4. **Criteria for Alcohol Dependence (DSM–IV)**

Tolerance
Episodes of withdrawal
Drinking more or for longer than intended
An inability and/or a persistent desire to cut down
Excessive time used in obtaining/using/recovering from alcohol
Important activities given up in favor of drinking
Drinking in spite of alcohol-related physical or psychological problems
The presence of three or more criteria defines alcohol dependence.

Adapted from American Psychiatric Association: Diagnostic and Statistical Manual of Mental Disorders, Fourth Edition. Washington, DC, American Psychiatric Association, 1994.

The approach chosen should always follow a careful assessment of the patient. The scale and extent of problems, the degree of dependence based on the standard criteria (Table 4), the degree of brain damage, and psychological characteristics are the main components of this assessment. An individual program can then be developed by making a series of choices. Should abstinence or controlled drinking be the goal? Is group or individual treatment best? Should the program be highly structured or loose? Is inpatient treatment necessary? Is detoxification required? Are any additional services such as relaxation training or conjoint counseling with the partner necessary? Is a psychiatric assessment required?

The precise approach varies with each patient but consists of a core program with "add-ons" of additional services, as mentioned earlier. The most commonly available core programs are inpatient treatment, drug therapy, and counseling.

Inpatient Rehabilitation. These highly structured programs usually last about 6 weeks. They are useful for highly dependent people with an abstinence goal who have lost the capacity to respond to normal social and family obligations and need to relearn this as an essential part of recovery.

Disulfiram (Antabuse). Disulfiram inhibits acetaldehyde dehydrogenase, causing acetaldehyde accumulation and the disulfiram-ethanol reaction (DER) when alcohol is consumed. Therefore, the patient must avoid alcohol consumption in order to avoid the reaction. In traditional approaches, the drug has been used in a highly structured way, including administration under supervision. A more recent approach is to use the drug with self-monitoring in intelligent, well-motivated people whose decision making is relatively internally located.

Other drugs are currently undergoing trials, including fluoxetine (Prozac),* naltrexone (Trexan), and calcium antagonists. All show some promise when allied with a contingency management type of counseling approach.

Individual Counseling. At some stage, most patients require or will accept individual counseling. There are five main modalities:

1. Twelve-step/introduction to Alcoholics Anonymous (AA). The counseling sessions are directed at encouraging greater knowledge of AA and assisting the patient to make optimal use of the fellowship.

2. Cognitive/behavioral. Insight-oriented therapy based on goal setting, testing goals against achievement, and encouraging active, informed decision making.

3. Motivational interviewing. Usually used early on, at the boundary of the crisis and induction phases, this approach is designed to make the connection between drinking and problems and to explore alternatives.

4. Medical counseling. Essentially a form of motivational interviewing centered around a particular medical problem.

5. Controlled drinking. Approaches that are designed to help patients to control their drinking are appropriate only for those who have neither serious medical problems nor established dependence. Most programs use cognitive-behavioral techniques and require 2 to 6 months of abstinence first.

Other Approaches. There are a variety of group educational and therapeutic programs. Some disulfiram programs use group techniques, and there is AA, which is undoubtedly one of the best approaches available for alcohol-dependent individuals committed to recovery.

Maintenance Phase

This is the phase of recovery that occupies the rest of the patient's life. AA, with its ready-made social network and supportive philosophy, is often crucial, as is continuing medical care for any lingering alcohol-related illnesses. Other networks based on church, social, or sporting activities are also helpful.

WITHDRAWAL

The alcohol withdrawal syndrome is characterized by a state of autonomic hyperactivity that is usually self-limited and corresponds to the period of readaptation of the central nervous system from alcohol-induced neuroadaptation. During this period, the patient is vulnerable to stress and at risk of developing the more serious complications of seizures, hallucinations, or delirium. Careful monitoring of the level of vulnerability, minimizing stress, and damping down the hyperexcitable state are cornerstones of therapy, regardless of the setting.

Identification of Patients at Risk

Some patients present to an alcoholism unit or their family doctors requesting detoxification. In a general hospital, characteristics indicating that a patient is at risk are:

A blood alcohol of 0.2 grams per dL or above without impairment of consciousness.
An alcohol intake of 100 grams (10 standard drinks) daily.

*Not FDA-approved for this indication.

Admission with an alcohol-related diagnosis.
A recent history of alcohol withdrawal.

The risk is increased if the medical condition is also a cause of stress—for example, shock, hypoxia, sepsis, or pain.

Objective Monitoring

Monitoring is reassuring to the patient and gives early warning if a reaction is not responding to simple measures. A validated clinical scale such as the Clinical Institute Withdrawal Assessment—Alcohol (CIWA-A) should be used. This collates observations of autonomic hyperactivity, level of arousal, and sensory changes to provide a numerical score. Scores are calculated every 4 hours routinely, every 2 hours if the score is 15 or more, and hourly if it is 20 or more. There is a modified short version, CIWA-Ar, which is more suitable for use outside a general hospital.

Reduction of Stress

Stress can be emotional, physiologic, or pharmacologically induced. Good nursing care by confident and supportive attendants in a comfortable, well-lit environment is essential, accompanied by reassurance and gentle reality orientation. Good medical care is crucial, particularly the avoidance of shock, hypoxia, sepsis, or other physical stressors. Finally, drugs that add to adrenergic activity, such as the tricyclic antidepressants or amine uptake inhibitors, should be suspended.

Drug Therapy

Choosing the right patients and the right time for treatment is far more important than the choice of drug. Seizures, hallucinations, or delirium can be prevented if sedation is given when scores continue to rise or symptoms do not settle.

Diazepam (Valium) is the drug of choice because of its cross-reactivity with alcohol at the GABA receptor, its long half-life, and its safety. Haloperidol (Haldol) is a dopamine antagonist that is effective against hallucinations. Phenytoin (Dilantin) is occasionally necessary for seizures. The following drugs are not recommended: Chlormethiazole* is effective but produces marked respiratory depression, increased bronchial secretion, and disturbances of thermoregulation. Alcohol should never be used, because to prevent withdrawal reliably, blood levels of 0.08 grams per dL are needed, and the drug is then rapidly excreted, increasing the risk of a secondary withdrawal. Phenothiazines lower the seizure threshold.

Management of Particular Situations

Uncomplicated, Mild, Self-Limited Reaction. The primary symptoms of autonomic hyperactivity,

_____
*Not available in the United States.

nausea, anxiety, and sleep disturbances usually occur while the blood alcohol level is still above zero and remit within 48 hours. Usually firm reassurance and simple measures suffice, but if symptoms persist or there are two scores of 15 or one of 20, load with diazepam by giving 20 mg at 2-hour intervals until scores are below 10. The patient should be examined before each dose, and care should be taken if the patient is elderly, hypoxic, or has liver disease. The situation should be reviewed after 60 mg, and no more than 120 mg should be given.

Concurrent Serious Illness. No seriously ill patient should ever be sedated without careful assessment and the advice of appropriate specialists. The signs of hypoxia are often identical to those of alcohol withdrawal, and sedation is hazardous in patients with respiratory failure. Therefore, it is best to decide in advance whether sedation will be used and whether assisted ventilation will be offered. In liver disease, a lower dose of sedative can be used. Alternatively, oxazepam, which is eliminated by conjugation rather than oxidation, can be substituted. Advice of a specialist should be sought.

Seizures. Not all seizures that occur during withdrawal are due to withdrawal. If the seizures are focal, they must be investigated. If a patient is already on anticonvulsants, these should be continued through the detoxification and reviewed afterwards. Otherwise, one or two seizures should be treated by initiating diazepam. If more than two seizures occur, load with phenytoin 12 to 15 mg per kg and continue the drug at 200 to 400 mg daily for 5 days.

Hallucinations. Hallucinations usually develop within 48 hours, are poorly formed, involve one or more senses, and are accompanied by hyperactivity. Treatment consists of 2.5 to 10 mg of haloperidol, depending on the patient's size, age, and general condition; it can be repeated in an hour, if necessary. All such patients also need diazepam. In a small number of patients with chronic hallucinosis who are calm and have preserved insight, no treatment is needed.

Delirium. In spite of our best efforts, some patients develop an excited delirium with hallucinosis and autonomic hyperactivity at 48 to 72 hours after the last drink. They should be handled in as reassuring a way as possible; given simple, clear instructions; and reoriented in time, place, and person at every opportunity. Medical management requires attention to fluids and electrolytes, including zinc and magnesium; sedation with diazepam and haloperidol; and investigation for underlying causes. Most reactions remit spontaneously in 3 to 7 days. Mortality is less than 1%.

Unexpected Deterioration. If a reaction occurs late, is unduly severe, is unduly prolonged, or appears to recur after adequate treatment, there is usually an underlying cause such as shock, sepsis, hypoxia, myocardial infarction, or undiagnosed pain. These patients should always be investigated.

DRUGS OF ABUSE

method of
DAVID M. COSENTINO, M.D.,
JAVIER I. ESCOBAR II, M.D., and
MARC J. BAYER, M.D.
*University of Connecticut Health Center
Farmington, Connecticut*

More than 20,000 different pharmaceutical agents are now available in the United States. Of these, fewer than 20 are involved in greater than 90% of toxic ingestions. These include prescription drugs such as narcotics, barbiturates, benzodiazepines, and analgesics, as well as illicitly manufactured agents such as cocaine, amphetamines, designer drugs, and hallucinogens. A growing number of intoxications also result from ingestion and inhalation of solvents and plants. This article focuses on the presentation and treatment of the acutely intoxicated patient. In addition, we review the wide array of medical complications resulting from drug abuse and the management of withdrawal from these substances.

GENERAL MANAGEMENT PRINCIPLES

The clinician is often forced to manage the poisoned patient, without either specific knowledge of the poison or the benefit of a clinically specific toxidrome. In this event, the physician should rely on a guideline of general management principles.

The initial evaluation should always begin with a thorough assessment and proper management of the patient's airway, breathing, and circulation. Serial vital signs should be assessed, as they can frequently give helpful clues to the clinical status of the patient, as well as to the nature of the offending drug. Once the patient has been stabilized, the administration of oxygen, 50% dextrose, naloxone, thiamine, and flumazenil must be considered.

Oxygen is useful in all drug overdoses and should be administered routinely. Traditionally, dextrose, naloxone, and thiamine have been given empirically. However, this method has recently been challenged, and these agents are now administered based on clinical and laboratory evaluation.

Prior to administration of dextrose, the clinician should obtain a glucose level because it has been shown that patients with cerebral ischemia have a worse neurologic outcome after dextrose therapy. A bedside determination of glucose can now be made very rapidly and accurately with reagent test strips if the sample is obtained from the antecubital fossa. This is preferred over fingerstick samples, which may vary widely if the patient is hypotensive. If the glucose level is less than 80 mg per dL in the face of altered mental status, then 50 mL of 50% dextrose should be administered.

Thiamine 100 mg should be given intravenously to all patients presenting with altered mental status. Administration may prevent the development of peripheral neuropathy and/or Wernicke-Korsakoff syndrome. Because thiamine is necessary for glucose metabolism, it should be given prior to dextrose in order to prevent a potential exacerbation of thiamine deficiency.

Naloxone (Narcan), a pure opioid antagonist, should be given to those patients presenting with an altered mental status and one or more of these clinical signs: respirations less than or equal to 12 per minute, miosis, or circumstantial evidence of opioid abuse. Although naloxone is usually not harmful, it should be withheld if the clinical scenario is not consistent with acute opioid overdose. The physician should, however, keep in mind that some patients may initially present with agitation that may progress to a state consistent with opioid intoxication, as may be seen after use of a speedball (a combination of heroin and cocaine). In this scenario, naloxone therapy should be reconsidered as the patient begins to show signs consistent with opioid overdose. Dosing is the same as with definitive acute opioid intoxication.

Flumazenil (Romazicon) is a relatively new drug that works as a competitive antagonist of benzodiazepines at central nervous system (CNS) receptor sites. It reverses the respiratory depressant, sedative/hypnotic, ataxic, amnestic, anxiolytic, and muscle relaxant effects of all benzodiazepines. However, it has been associated with significant toxicity under certain conditions, and therefore must be used with caution. The contraindications for flumazenil use are listed in Table 1.

Life-threatening seizures, particularly after co-ingestion of tricyclic antidepressants and/or proconvulsants, have been reported following flumazenil use. Acute benzodiazepine withdrawal may occur in the habituated patient, and dysrhythmias have been noted in approximately 1% of patients. Because resedation occurs in greater than 60% of cases, the patient must be monitored closely after being given flumazenil. Dosing is further discussed later under specific management of sedative-hypnotic overdose.

PRINCIPLES OF RESTRAINTS

The clinician may need to restrain the acutely agitated patient. In this situation, one must first decide between physical and chemical restraints. Chemical restraints are often preferred because physical restraints in a thrashing patient may lead to rhabdomyolysis. With phencyclidine (PCP) intoxication,

TABLE 1. **Contraindications to Flumazenil (Romazicon)**

Use of benzodiazepines for seizure control
Recent or present use of benzodiazepines for seizure control, long-term sedation, or maintenance
Known or suspected co-ingestion of tricyclic antidepressant and/or other proconvulsant
Severe head trauma (use cautiously)

TABLE 2. **Various Routes of Administration of Cocaine and Their Differing Effects**

Route	Onset	Peak Action	Duration of Euphoria	Half-Life
Inhalation	7 s	1–5 min	20 min	40–60 min
Intravenous	15 s	3–5 min	20–30 min	40–60 min
Nasal	3 min	15 min	45–90 min	60–90 min
Oral	10 min	60 min	60 min	60–60 min

however, both types of restraints may be necessary if the patient is extremely agitated.

Chemical restraint is best accomplished by administration of the neuroleptic haloperidol (Haldol), a butyrophenone, 5 to 10 mg intravenously or intramuscularly. This drug has a better safety profile than barbiturates and phenothiazines, and its effectiveness is well documented in the literature. This agent produces sedation in addition to a sense of indifference to environmental stimulation. After haloperidol has been given, however, the physician should monitor the patient closely because of its potential to lower seizure thresholds. For patients who remain agitated or when prolonged sedation is necessary, an excellent protocol is to combine haloperidol 5 mg with lorazepam (Ativan) 2 mg, both being given either intravenously or intramuscularly. If necessary, the dose can be repeated in 30 minutes. If dystonic reactions occur (rare), these can be controlled by diphenhydramine (Benadryl) 25 to 50 mg intravenously or benztropine (Cogentin) 1 to 2 mg intravenously.

Phenothiazines are not recommended for use as chemical restraints, as they have been shown to cause paradoxical hyperthermia, lower the seizure threshold, and increase the serum half-life of amphetamines.

SYMPATHOMIMETICS

The most commonly abused stimulant drugs are cocaine and amphetamines. However, caffeine, phenylpropanolamine, nicotine, ephedrine, and pseudoephedrine, which can be easily obtained from over-the-counter preparations and diet pills, are also widely abused. These drugs activate the sympathetic nervous system, causing release of neurotransmitters such as norepinephrine and epinephrine. Less frequently, they cause increased release or decreased reuptake of dopamine and serotonin.

Amphetamines can be taken orally, topically, intravenously, or by inhalation. Oral and intravenous use had been the most popular routes of administration until the advent of "ice," a form of methamphetamine that can be smoked. Effects of "ice" can last up to 36 hours, whereas orally ingested amphetamines usually produce effects lasting only 4 to 8 hours. These drugs are metabolized primarily in the liver with small amounts being metabolized by renal mechanisms.

Cocaine, which is made from the leaves of *Erythroxylon coca*, can be administered by numerous routes including nasal insufflation, smoking, intravenously, orally, or through placement in various body orifices. Cocaine may be ingested as the crystalline salt, cocaine hydrochloride, or as the free cocaine base, of which one common form is "crack." Onset, intensity, and duration of effects are listed in Table 2. Cocaine is metabolized primarily by the liver, where it is hydrolyzed to benzoylecgonine, which can then be detected in the urine.

Most of the clinical manifestations of stimulant drug intoxication are a result of excessive central and peripheral sympathetic overdrive. The use of lower doses of stimulants generally does not lead to acute medical complications. These patients often show signs of euphoria, stimulation, fatigue, diminished appetite, restlessness, and anxiety and rarely present to the Emergency Department.

A specific constellation of signs and symptoms (toxidromes) is associated with sympathomimetic use, as shown in Table 3. Initial stimulation may be followed by abrupt generalized CNS depression.

Malignant hyperthermia, cardiac vasospasm, car-

TABLE 3. **Signs and Symptoms of Sympathomimetic Toxidrome**

Central Nervous System	Respiratory System
Agitation	Tachypnea
Anxiety	Respiratory depression/failure
Confusion	Pneumomediastinum
Delirium	Pneumothorax
Dizziness	Crack lung
Headache	Pulmonary edema
Tremors	**Gastrointestinal System**
Delusions	
Hallucinations	Nausea
Paranoia	Vomiting
Seizure	Diarrhea
Ischemic/hemorrhagic stroke	Abdominal cramping
Toxic encephalopathy	Constipation
Focal neurologic deficits	**Metabolic and Other Systems**
Coma	
Cardiovascular System	Hyperthermia
	Rhabdomyolysis
Hypertension	Reactive mydriasis
Sinus tachycardia	Tremor
Bradycardia	Muscle rigidity
Electrocardiographic repolarization abnormalities	Pale, diaphoretic skin
Tachydysrhythmias	Dehydration
Cardiac ischemia/infarction	
End-organ ischemia	
Cardiomyopathy	
Subendocardial fibrosis	
High-output congestive heart failure	
Myocardial necrosis	
Myocarditis	
Aortic dissection	
Shock	

diac ischemia, dysrhythmia, and seizures are particularly dangerous presentations of cocaine abuse. Any young, otherwise healthy adult who presents with symptoms suggestive with these, should be suspected of cocaine and/or amphetamine abuse, and appropriate symptomatic treatment should be implemented. If cocaine use is suspected, an electrocardiogram should be obtained and the patient should be placed on a cardiac monitor, regardless of age. Drug abuse should not be ruled out simply on the basis of denial by the patient, as fear of legal or parental consequences may often contribute to a falsified history.

Both amphetamines and cocaine are easily detected in the urine up to 2 to 3 days after their use. However, treatment should never be withheld pending a drug test. If diagnosis is unclear, complete blood count, electrolytes, glucose, urinalysis, renal function tests, and thyroid testing may be helpful. If there is a focal neurologic deficit or altered mental status, a lumbar puncture may be beneficial after a mass lesion has been ruled out by computed tomography scan.

Prehospital care should focus on frequent vital signs, intravenous line placement, and cardiac monitoring, if possible. Once in the Emergency Department, care should be symptom-directed. Patients with altered mental status and/or who are acutely agitated should be managed according to the general guidelines discussed previously.

Dysrhythmias range from mild sinus tachycardia to life-threatening ventricular arrhythmias. Ventricular ectopy or tachycardia may be initially treated with esmolol (Brevibloc), a beta$_1$ specific blocker, an intravenous loading bolus of 500 µg per kg over 1 minute followed by 50 to 100 µg per kg per minute intravenously for 4 minutes, if the patient is not hypertensive. Lidocaine (Xylocaine) 1 mg per kg intravenous push followed by 2 to 4 mg per minute intravenously should be reserved for second-line use as it can lower the seizure threshold. Supraventricular tachycardias should not be treated unless hemodynamically significant. Sinus tachycardia is usually self-limited and may be treated with a short-acting benzodiazepine if deemed necessary. Hemodynamically significant paroxysmal supraventricular tachycardia (PSVT) may be treated with esmolol as described earlier or verapamil (Calan, Isoptin), a calcium channel blocker, 0.075 to 0.15 mg per kg intravenous push over 2 to 5 minutes. Verapamil can be repeated after 30 minutes if necessary. If the PSVT is associated with hypertension, labetalol (Normodyne), an alpha and beta blocker, 10 to 20 mg intravenously, or verapamil, may be used. In this situation, esmolol can be combined with an alpha blocker such as phentolamine.

Hypertension is a frequent occurrence after stimulant drug overdose and should be managed aggressively. Phentolamine (Regitine) 5 mg intravenously in an adult (1 mg in a child), is the drug of choice to control blood pressure in this situation. A rise in heart rate may be seen following administration, and this can be controlled with esmolol. If the increase in blood pressure is significant, nitroprusside (Nipride) 0.5 to 5 µg per kg per minute intravenously can also be used. If intravenous access is unattainable, nifedipine (Procardia) 10 mg orally should be administered. Beta blockers are not a good choice in these patients because of the risk of unopposed alpha stimulation.

Benzodiazepines, in sufficient doses, are the treatment of choice for agitation and tremors. Likewise, seizures should be treated with diazepam (Valium) 5 mg intravenously over several minutes. If the patient continues to seize, the dose should be repeated until seizures are controlled or a dose of 40 mg has been given. Unresponsive seizures should then be managed by loading with phenytoin (Dilantin) intravenously up to a total dose of 15 to 18 mg per kg. Alternatively, phenobarbital (Luminal) 15 mg per kg intravenously may be used. After phenobarbital administration, it is important to monitor the patient closely because of the risk of subsequent respiratory depression and/or hypotension developing. Because hyperthermia may contribute to life-threatening seizure activity, temperatures greater than 105° F should be treated with external cooling until the temperature is less than 102° F.

Rhabdomyolysis can be readily tested for with a urine dipstick. A heme-positive result is suggestive of rhabdomyolysis, and treatment should be initiated. A high urine flow rate (>300 mL per hour) should be maintained with intravenous fluids, and urine alkalization with intravenous sodium bicarbonate will protect the renal tubules from myoglobin toxicity.

If oral overdose is suspected, gastric lavage followed by activated charcoal along with a cathartic should be administered. Ipecac-induced emesis should be avoided because of the high possibility of seizures resulting in airway compromise and aspiration. For those patients who have ingested packets of cocaine, activated charcoal should be given and whole-bowel irrigation considered. Induced emesis and/or endoscopy should not be performed because of the life-threatening risk of packet rupture. These patients should be monitored very closely for signs and symptoms of cocaine intoxication, which merit surgical intervention.

Withdrawal symptoms from stimulant drug abuse are rarely physiologically life-threatening. However, because of the relative depletion of dopamine and norepinephrine in the withdrawal period, depressive symptoms along with increased craving are common. This leads to an increased risk of suicide, and these patients may require antidepressants.

NARCOTICS

Narcotics are a group of drugs, naturally occurring or synthetic, used principally as analgesics. Substances are included in this group because of their clinical similarity to opium. Unlike the sympathomimetics, these drugs are commonly prescribed by practicing physicians, and this serves as a major source of abuse. The most frequently abused agents are

TABLE 4. **Commonly Abused Narcotics**

Natural	Semisynthetic	Synthetic
Morphine	Heroin	Methadone (Dolophine)
Opium	Hydromorphone (Dilaudid)	Fentanyl (Sublimaze)
Codeine	Hydrocodone (Lorcet, Vicodin)	Diphenoxylate (Lomotil)
	Oxycodone (Roxicodone)	Propoxyphene (Darvon)

listed in Table 4. Approximately 5% of drug intoxications involve narcotics; however, one in every four deaths reported from poisoning in the United States and Canada involve these agents.

Narcotic agents interact with various opiate receptors in the CNS causing analgesia, euphoria, miosis, sedation, respiratory depression, dysphoria, and psychiatric symptoms such as delusions and hallucinations. These agents are used illicitly, through oral, inhalational, subcutaneous, and intravenous routes. Parenteral use of narcotics is of greatest concern because of the high incidence of potentially lethal infections, including endocarditis, hepatitis, human immunodeficiency virus (HIV), septic emboli, pneumonia, subcutaneous abscesses, cellulitis, and tetanus. The majority of opioids have their onset of action within 1 hour of administration, although several, such as methadone, produce more latent effects.

Patients abusing narcotics typically present with the triad of CNS depression, respiratory depression, and miosis. A detailed listing of the most frequent signs and symptoms of opioid toxicity is given in Table 5. Some important exceptions to this clinical picture should be noted. First, convulsions may be seen after use of meperidine (Demerol), codeine, or propoxyphene (Darvon). Second, mydriasis or normal pupils may be seen after ingestion of meperidine or diphenoxylate (Lomotil).

Since narcotic overdoses often present with CNS and respiratory depression, the clinician must first support and maintain the patient's airway, breathing, and circulation. The general management principles described previously should then be followed. Naloxone should initially be given intravenously as a 2-mg bolus. A response should be seen in seconds to minutes. If there is no initial response, repeat doses can be given at 2- to 3-minute intervals until a total dose of 10 mg. At this point, if there is no response, it is unlikely that narcotic toxicity is the sole cause of CNS depression. Severe cases of narcotic overdose, however, may require up to 24 mg of naloxone for reversal of symptoms. Naloxone therapy may precipitate narcotic withdrawal. This, however, is not life-threatening and usually subsides in 20 to 30 minutes. The clinician should, though, be prepared to restrain a suddenly agitated patient. Because of the short half-life of naloxone, a continuous infusion may be required to maintain alertness. This should be administered intravenously at an hourly dose of two-thirds of the dose required to arouse the patient. A patient should never be released soon after receiving naloxone because the ingested narcotic may have a longer half-life than naloxone, and its toxic effects may break through. As with stimulant overdoses, emesis should not be induced if the patient has an altered level of consciousness. If oral intake is suspected, a gastric lavage followed by activated charcoal may be administered.

The withdrawal syndrome from narcotics typically begins 6 to 12 hours after the last dose of the offending agent. Symptoms peak from 36 to 48 hours and usually subside in 5 to 10 days. Initially, one sees restlessness, insomnia, lacrimation, rhinorrhea, and diaphoresis. Eventually, the patient develops mydriasis, piloerection, myalgias, arthralgias, and abdominal cramping. In severe cases, patients may complain of nausea, vomiting, and diarrhea. Sinus tachycardia and hypertension may also be seen. Treatment is aimed at managing the symptoms as well as preventing or minimizing the withdrawal component. Methadone (Dolophine) 5 to 10 mg, given orally or intramuscularly, seems to be adequate in mitigating withdrawal symptoms, regardless of the amount of drug abused.

SEDATIVE–HYPNOTICS

This group of CNS depressants is composed of a wide variety of drugs including benzodiazepines, barbiturates, carbamates, alcohols, and over-the-counter preparations. Like some of the narcotic agents, these drugs are frequently prescribed by physicians. They are used mainly for their anxiolytic and sedative properties. Benzodiazepines and barbiturates are the most commonly abused drugs in this class. These agents exert their effects by binding to the gamma-aminobutyric acid (GABA) receptor and enhancing its inhibitory function in the CNS. Sedative-hypnotics are usually taken orally. They are metabolized primarily in the liver and excreted in the urine, where they are readily detectable.

Patients who are acutely intoxicated may present with different degrees of CNS depression ranging from ataxia and drowsiness to coma. Respiratory depression and hypotension can result from an acute overdose. High doses of barbiturates may also cause hypothermia, pulmonary edema, temporary paralysis, and bullous lesions on the fingers, buttocks, or knees. Benzodiazepines rarely cause respiratory depression if taken alone. However, these agents are often taken with other sedative drugs, thus potentiating the respiratory depressant effect of these other

TABLE 5. **Characteristics of Narcotic Toxicity**

Central nervous system depression—coma
Respiratory depression—cyanosis
Miosis
Hypothermia
Bradycardia
Pulmonary edema
Orthostatic hypotension
Urinary retention
Decreased gastrointestinal motility

agents. Over-the-counter antihistamines and glu-thetimide (Doriden) in overdose produce anticholinergic actions in addition to CNS depression. Methaqualone overdose may also present with myoclonus, hyperreflexia, and hypertonicity, which can progress to seizures. Chloral hydrate overdose may produce cardiovascular collapse or dysrhythmias in addition to CNS and respiratory depression.

Ipecac-induced emesis must be avoided as the risk for onset of vomiting following CNS sedation from the abused agent exists. In the patient with an altered level of consciousness, gastric lavage with multiple doses of activated charcoal and a cathartic should be administered.

Fewer than 1 out of every 50 people who overdose with sedative-hypnotics die. These patients usually present with an altered level of consciousness; therefore, initial management should follow the general management principles outlined previously. If flumazenil is administered, it should initially be given as 0.2 mg intravenously. If there is no response after 1 to 2 minutes, 0.3 mg should be administered. Subsequent doses of 0.5 mg can be given until a positive response is noted or a total dose of 3 mg has been given. These patients then need to be monitored closely for seizures, dysrhythmias, and resedation. Renal clearance of long-acting barbiturates can be greatly enhanced by alkalization of the urine with 1 to 2 mEq per kg of sodium bicarbonate, given by intravenous push. It should then be subsequently administered to maintain a urinary pH of 7 to 8. Diuresis should also be accomplished by administration of intravenous normal saline. These treatments, however, are ineffective for all other sedative-hypnotic drug poisonings and therefore should be performed only when the offending agent is known. Peritoneal dialysis is no longer recommended in CNS depressant overdoses. Hemodialysis has been shown to be variably effective, and hemoperfusion to be effective in removing significant amounts of phenobarbital. These treatment modalities, however, should be reserved for lethal ingestions only.

Withdrawal from sedative-hypnotics is generally considered to be more dangerous than that from other substances. Initial withdrawal symptoms may develop anywhere from 24 hours to 2 weeks after termination of drug use. These symptoms include insomnia, anxiety, and irritability, which may progress to tremors, diaphoresis, nausea, vomiting, agitation, and frank hallucinations. The seizures and/or hyperthermia that may subsequently develop places these patients at extreme risk for death. These patients, therefore, should undergo detoxification while hospitalized. An appropriate dose of a barbiturate or another cross-tolerant sedative-hypnotic should be administered to control clinical symptoms of withdrawal. The dose should remain unchanged for 2 to 3 days, and then tapered by approximately 10% each subsequent day. Both phenobarbital and diazepam have been proved effective because their long half-lives allow for a slow decline in serum drug concentration.

PLANTS AND HALLUCINOGENS

Hallucinogens are drugs that produce alterations in perception, thought, and mood. This is a heterogeneous group of substances, some of which are derived from natural products, such as plants, and others that are chemically synthesized. Some commonly abused drugs are listed in Table 6.

PCP ("angel dust")-intoxicated patients may present with a wide range of clinical signs including cholinergic, anticholinergic, adrenergic, and CNS effects. In addition, mood changes, including extremely violent behavior, disoriented thoughts, and visual/tactile hallucinations are commonly seen. Physical examination may reveal vertical and horizontal nystagmus, depressed pupillary light reflex, ataxia, tremors, muscle weakness, and slurred speech. Severe medical complications may include rhabdomyolysis and its sequelae, seizures, hypertension, hyperthermia, and respiratory depression/apnea.

Intoxication from other hallucinogens and plants is much less likely to present for medical attention. Lysergic acid diethylamide (LSD) primarily affects the CNS causing alterations in mood and behavior, as well as visual hallucinations. The designer drugs, including MDA, MDMA ("Ectasy"), and MDEA ("Eve"), are a class of drugs created for the purpose of avoiding legal consequences. Many of these drugs are amphetamine derivatives and therefore produce sympathomimetic activity in addition to hallucinogenic effects. Psilocybin and psilocin are potent hallucinogenic compounds contained within *Psilocybe* mushrooms. These mushrooms are commonly referred to as "magic mushrooms," "blue legs," or "liberty cap." In addition to hallucinations, these drugs can produce mild sympathomimetic effects. Few adverse reactions occur and fatality is unusual, but has been reported, most often in children. Mescaline is the principal active ingredient of the peyote cactus (*Lophophora williamsii*). Effects are similar to those seen with LSD; however, more intense visual hallucinations can be seen. Jimsonweed (*Datura stramonium*) is most commonly abused by adolescents and children. Clinically, it produces both central and peripheral anticholinergic effects, as well as auditory and visual hallucinations.

Marijuana, the most commonly abused illicit substance in the United States, is the dried form of either *Cannabis sativa* or *C. indica,* and hashish is the resin produced from their flowers. The psychoactive agent found in these plants is tetrahydrocannab-

TABLE 6. **Commonly Abused Plants and Hallucinogens**

Plants	Hallucinogens
Peyote	Lysergic acid diethylamide (LSD)
Mushrooms (psilocybin, psilocin)	Phencyclidine (PCP)
	Mescaline
Peyote	Designer drugs (MDA, MDMA, MDEA)
Jimsonweed	
Marijuana and hashish	

inol (THC). Although not usually hallucinogenic, marijuana can produce a variety of mood-altering effects. The most common adverse reactions are panic and dysphoria.

Treatment of hallucinogen and plant intoxication is centered on supportive care. Many patients can be reassured in a calm, quiet environment or "talked down" from an agitated or hallucinatory state. More severe cases may require sedation with benzodiazepines and a butyrophenone, which should be administered as previously discussed. Gastric lavage is usually not indicated unless the patient is seen within 30 minutes of oral ingestion.

SOLVENTS

Volatile substance abuse refers to the intentional inhalation of chemical vapors. These compounds are generally hydrocarbon derivatives and can be divided into six major structural classes (Table 7). The potential for danger is increased because these agents are readily available at home and in industry. Although prevalent in the adult population, solvents are most commonly abused by adolescents.

Inhalation is most commonly achieved by "sniffing," but "bagging" and "huffing" are other commonly used routes. "Sniffing" refers to directly inhaling the agent from an open container, whereas "huffing" involves inhalation of the agent from a rag dampened with the solvent. "Bagging" involves inhaling the substance directly from a closed container or plastic bag. This is the most dangerous method of inhalation because of the potential for asphyxia. An alteration in mental status is the most commonly seen presentation of acute solvent intoxication. In addition to CNS disturbances, gastrointestinal complaints, cyanosis, respiratory symptoms, syncope, or cardiac arrest may be seen. Sudden death, which typically occurs after physical exertion, has been reported to be secondary to the development of a cardiac dysrhythmia. A wide array of medical complications can also occur secondary to chronic abuse of solvents.

Symptomatic management is the norm for cases of acute solvent intoxication. Cardiac monitoring is initially helpful for the detection of dysrhythmias. If necessary, antiarrhythmics should be administered. Other complications, such as respiratory distress, seizures, and coma, may be managed by standard emergency medical modalities. Neuropathic abnormalities, which are sometimes seen with nitrous oxide abuse, may be corrected with vitamin B_{12} and thiamine supplements. Acute methemoglobinemia may also be seen and can be treated with methylene blue.

Substance abuse continues to be a major medical problem in the United States. Although drug therapy may be necessary to manage the acutely intoxicated patient, education is most essential in curtailing continuing abuse. Keep in mind that your region most likely has a Poison Control Center that is staffed by physician toxicologists 24 hours a day. These experts can supply useful immediate advice on the management of patients intoxicated with substances of abuse.

ANXIETY DISORDERS

method of
MICHAEL R. WARE, M.D., and
JAMES C. BALLENGER, M.D.
Medical University of South Carolina
Charleston, South Carolina

Anxiety is a universal human emotion. It may be experienced on a continuum ranging from mild uneasiness and slight apprehension to terrifying panic. Anxiety in small doses may be beneficial, serving to help an individual cope with a difficult or dangerous situation. Conversely, intense anxiety is associated with significant social and occupational impairment.

Often unappreciated by many physicians, anxiety generally produces several significant symptoms in more than one organ system. Most frequently patients relate disturbances in the nervous, cardiovascular, and gastrointestinal organ systems. The manifestations of anxiety vary among patients but generally involve symptoms in cognitive, affective, behavioral, and somatic areas. Cognitively, patients may report thoughts of impending doom, impaired attention and concentration, and preoccupation with physical health or other worries. Tenseness, nervousness, apprehension, and fear are common affective symptoms. Behaviorally, patients often exhibit hand wringing, hyperventilation, pacing, and tremor. The most common presentation of anxiety, however, is somatic. Somatic symptoms frequently reported to physicians include light-headedness and headache, tightness of or a lump in the throat, shortness of breath, palpitations or chest tightness, gastrointestinal disturbances, and paresthesias in the extremities.

The differential diagnosis of anxiety involves a range of medical and psychiatric conditions. Briefly, anxiety may present as a complication of substance abuse. Intoxication from sympathomimetic agents such as caffeine, cocaine, or amphetamines, or use of hallucinogens such as lysergic acid diethylamide (LSD), may result in anxiety. Further, withdrawal from sedative-hypnotic drugs and alcohol commonly involves anxiety complaints. Prescription medica-

TABLE 7. **Classification and Sources of Commonly Abused Solvents**

Aliphatic Hydrocarbons	**Ketones**
Gasoline	Nail polish remover
Petroleum ether	
Kerosene	**Aromatic Hydrocarbons**
Lighter fluid	Model glue or cement
Hair styling mousse	Adhesives
Ethers	**Alkyl Nitrates**
Gasoline engine primer	Aphrodisiacs
Alkyl Halides	
Aerosol cans	
Freon	
Typewriter correction fluid	
Dry cleaning fluid	
Spot removers	
Paints, varnishes, and lacquers	

tions, including insulin, theophylline, and steroids, also need to be considered culprits in the differential diagnosis. Finally, the practitioner must exclude a variety of medical illnesses that may masquerade as an anxiety disorder. These include endocrinopathies such as hyperthyroidism and Cushing's syndrome, pulmonary diseases resulting in hypoxia for any reason, cardiovascular etiologies such as arrhythmia and angina, and neurologic illnesses such as seizure disorders. A careful history and physical examination plus screening laboratory tests will assist the physician in eliminating most of these organic etiologies.

Once both the substance-precipitated and the medically induced causes of anxiety are ruled out, the potential psychiatric causes need to be explored. Anxiety may be a complication of another primary psychiatric illness. Major depression, dissociative disorders, and acute psychosis in a schizophrenic patient are frequently associated with anxiety. The most effective therapy for these secondary anxiety complaints is the adequate treatment of the underlying primary psychiatric condition.

The *Diagnostic and Statistical Manual of Mental Disorders, 4th Edition* (DSM–IV) outlines the American Psychiatric Association's criteria for the diagnosis of the primary anxiety disorders. We briefly review the diagnosis and presentation of these disorders and describe the acute management of each illness. Because of the chronicity and comorbidity associated with the anxiety disorders, we strongly encourage ongoing consultation with a psychiatrist experienced in the management of these disorders.

PANIC DISORDER

Patients with panic disorder (PD) suffer from recurrent, unexpected, discrete episodes of intense fear or discomfort, termed "panic attacks." The attack has a sudden onset, generally builds to peak intensity within 10 minutes, and dissipates within 30 minutes. It is often associated with a sense of imminent danger or impending doom and a strong urge to escape. The somatic and cognitive symptoms of an attack include palpitations, sweating, trembling or shaking, shortness of breath, feelings of choking, chest pain or discomfort, nausea or abdominal distress, dizziness or light-headedness, derealization or depersonalization, a fear of losing control or going crazy, a fear of dying, paresthesias, and hot flashes or chills. The frequency and severity of the attacks vary across and within individuals. Some patients experience as few as one to two attacks per month, whereas others may have their attacks daily. A subgroup of patients with PD may experience only the somatic symptoms of an attack and report no apprehension, fear, or anxiety. These nonfearful panic attacks have been described principally in patients being treated in primary care, cardiology, and neurology practices.

Epidemiologic surveys show that about 1.6% of urban adults suffer from PD. The community lifetime prevalence is higher (about 3.5%), and many of these patients are found in primary care settings. PD has its peak onset in patients in their early twenties but may begin as early as childhood. About two-thirds to three-fourths of panic patients are female. Research has demonstrated that most patients with PD are co-morbid for other psychiatric problems. Typically, panic patients often develop major depressive epi-

sodes, have high rates of substance abuse and suicidal ideation, and experience other anxiety disorders, particularly generalized anxiety disorder and agoraphobia. Agoraphobia is defined as anxiety about being in places or situations from which escape might be difficult (elevators) or embarrassing (classrooms), or in which help may not be available in the event of suffering a panic attack (airplanes). At least half of all patients presenting for treatment generally have PD complicated by agoraphobia. This phobic avoidance substantially limits the social and occupational lives of many panic patients.

The successful treatment of PD and phobic avoidance often requires a multimodal strategy combining cognitive, behavioral, and pharmacologic therapies. Cognitively, patients should be reassured that their symptoms have a biologic basis that is amenable to therapy. Catastrophic appraisals ("I will die from this attack") need to be challenged, and patients need to be educated to avoid substances that are likely to exacerbate their anxiety such as alcohol, recreational substances, caffeine, and sympathomimetic agents. Exposing patients gradually to their feared agoraphobic situations or unpleasant interoceptive physical sensations further diminishes panic attack frequency, generalized anxiety, and phobic avoidance. Recently, studies have demonstrated promising results with these combined cognitive/behavioral treatments.

Pharmacologic trials document that at least 75% of panic patients will have a good response to any of three classes of medication: the tricyclic antidepressants (TCAs), monoamine oxidase inhibitors (MAOIs), and benzodiazepines (BZs). Of the TCAs, imipramine (Tofranil)* has been convincingly demonstrated to be effective at reducing panic attack frequency, avoidance behavior, and anticipatory anxiety (the fear of another panic attack). The drug is best initiated at a dose of 10 mg per day and increased by 10 mg every day or two until a dose of 50 mg daily is reached. The dose may then be gradually raised in 25-mg increments every 3 to 4 days to reach a final dose of 100 to 250 mg per day. This slow titration minimizes the hypersensitive reactions many panic patients have to medications and reduces the patient's fear of losing control. Generally, a delayed onset of action is seen with TCAs, taking 6 to 12 weeks to reach maximal effectiveness. Other TCAs demonstrating efficacy in the treatment of PD include nortriptyline (Pamelor),* desipramine (Norpramin),* and clomipramine (Anafranil).*

Phenelzine (Nardil),* a MAOI, is highly effective at reducing panic attacks and avoidance behavior. However, the side effect profile of orthostatic hypotension, weight gain, and sexual dysfunctions, plus the necessity of remaining on a tyramine-free diet, discourages many physicians and patients from utilizing this compound. Doses should start at 15 mg per day at breakfast and increase by 15 mg every 3 to 4 days to achieve a therapeutic level of 60 to 90

---

*Not FDA-approved for this indication.

mg daily, splitting the dose between breakfast and lunch. Like the TCAs, the MAOIs have a delayed onset of action, taking 6 to 12 weeks to reach maximal efficacy.

Alprazolam (Xanax) is a high-potency BZ and is the only drug approved by the Food and Drug Administration (FDA) for the treatment of PD. Alprazolam also demonstrates marked efficacy at reducing anticipatory anxiety and phobic avoidance. It is generally well tolerated by patients and produces beneficial effects within the first week of use, a significant advantage compared with the antidepressants. Disadvantages of alprazolam include initial sedation and ataxia and impairment of complex motor skills (such as driving a car). Fortunately, tolerance develops to these side effects within 7 to 10 days. The greatest disadvantage of the BZs is the potential for a withdrawal syndrome on discontinuation of the drug. However, slow, gradual, and flexible tapering over 2 to 4 months minimizes transient recurrence of anxiety symptoms. Alprazolam is best initiated at a dose of 0.25 to 0.5 mg three times daily. The average maintenance dose is 2 to 6 mg daily, although some patients require higher doses (6 to 10 mg per day). Clonazepam (Klonopin), another high-potency BZ, has also been found effective in the treatment of PD, generally in doses of 1 to 3 mg daily. Because of its long half-life, clonazepam can be given twice daily. Less extensive data suggest that other BZs are effective in the treatment of PD and include lorazepam (Ativan) and diazepam (Valium).

The newer serotonin-reuptake inhibitors, highly efficacious and popular as antidepressants, are currently being tested in PD patients. Several open studies already support fluoxetine (Prozac)* as being effective at reducing panic attack frequency and avoidance behavior. Many panic patients cannot tolerate standard fluoxetine doses, and the practitioner is advised to start at low doses of 2.5 to 5.0 mg daily at breakfast. Most patients respond at doses ranging from 5 to 20 mg daily. Common adverse events include agitation, insomnia, restlessness, and jitteriness. Sertraline (Zoloft)* and paroxetine (Paxil)* are currently undergoing double-blind trials and appear to be effective.

GENERALIZED ANXIETY DISORDER

Generalized anxiety disorder (GAD) is characterized by excessive anxiety and worry (apprehensive expectation) that occurs more days than not for a period of at least 6 months. The patient often worries about everyday routine life circumstances, such as finances, health of family members, job responsibilities, or household chores, but finds it difficult to control the worry. The anxiety and worry are associated with physical symptoms including restlessness, easy fatigability, difficulty in concentrating, irritability, muscle tension, and sleep disturbances. Overall, the intensity, frequency, or duration of the anxiety and worry are clearly out of proportion to the likely occurrence or impact of the feared event. The age of onset of GAD is typically in the late teens or early twenties, but it may occur much later. The onset is gradual, with the course of illness fluctuating over a patient's lifetime. Stressful life events commonly exacerbate the illness. The lifetime prevalence of GAD is about 5%, making it one of the most common anxiety disorders. Co-morbidity is typical in GAD, with most patients suffering from coexisting major or minor depressions, substance abuse, and a variety of other anxiety disorders, particularly social phobia (SP) and PD.

The successful treatment of GAD incorporates both psychotherapeutic management and pharmacotherapy. At a minimum, supportive therapy aims to support and educate the patient and teach cognitive and behavioral techniques to improve coping skills and minimize the effects of daily life stress. Pharmacotherapy options include BZs, the azapirone anxiolytic buspirone (BuSpar), and sedating antidepressants. For years, the BZs have been the mainstay of pharmacologic treatment. Since no one BZ has shown superiority in the treatment of GAD, the physician is encouraged to select an agent familiar to him or her. Marked advantages of the BZs include a high safety margin, rapid onset of anxiolytic action, and intermittent dosing options. These agents are best avoided in patients who abuse alcohol or other substances. Patients should be warned about the sedation, ataxia, and impaired psychomotor activity that result from early BZ use. These adverse effects resolve over a period of 7 to 10 days. During an acute episode of GAD, the BZ is usually prescribed for a period of 6 to 8 weeks before an attempt is made to taper and discontinue the drug. If relapse occurs, try intermittent dosing with therapy directed at the fluctuating anxiety symptoms.

Buspirone (BuSpar) offers anxiolytic efficacy without the aforementioned adverse effects of the BZs. Also, it is devoid of the withdrawal syndrome typical of BZs. Drawbacks to the use of buspirone include the requirement of regular dosing for several weeks for the drug to become effective, and lower rates of acceptability by patients compared with the BZs. Buspirone is initiated at a dose of 5 mg three times daily and increased to its effective range of 30 to 60 mg daily over a period of several weeks.

Sedating antidepressants, including imipramine (Tofranil),* clomipramine (Anafranil),* and trazodone (Desyrel),* have been prescribed successfully in the treatment of GAD. Sedation, weight gain, and potential lethality in overdose situations are disadvantages of their use. However, these agents can be dosed once per day at night to minimize patient complaints, and they are devoid of the abuse liability associated with BZs. Imipramine is the most studied drug of the group and is best initiated at a low dose of 10 mg at night and increased gradually to produce

*Not FDA-approved for this indication.

*Not FDA-approved for this indication.

symptom resolution. Efficacious doses for imipramine range from 50 to 200 mg daily.

OBSESSIVE-COMPULSIVE DISORDER

The essential diagnostic features of obsessive-compulsive disorder (OCD) are recurrent obsessions or compulsions that are severe enough to consume at least 1 hour of time per day or cause the patient marked distress or impairment. At some point during the course of the illness, the individual recognizes that the obsessions or compulsions are excessive or unreasonable. Obsessions are persistent ideas, thoughts, impulses, or images that are intrusive and inappropriate and cause the patient marked anxiety. The obsessions are not simply excessive worries about real-life problems but usually involve themes of danger or harm. The most common obsessions are fears of contamination (acquiring the human immunodeficiency virus [HIV] by shaking hands), repeated doubts (left stove on), aggressive impulses (harming one's child), and a marked need for symmetry or orderliness (socks in a drawer). Compulsions are repetitive behaviors (handwashing, checking, ordering) or mental acts (counting, repeating words or phrases) performed in response to obsessional thoughts. The goal of the compulsion is to prevent a dreaded event (becoming HIV-positive) or to reduce anxiety or distress. Resisting the compulsions enhances anxiety or tension for the patient.

The lifetime prevalence of OCD is 2.5%. It has a bimodal age of onset, with about one-third of patients developing symptoms by age 15 years. The average onset for adults who suffer from OCD is about age 23 years. A little over half of all patients are female, and patients generally have a chronic waxing and waning course once OCD develops. The majority of OCD patients are co-morbid for other psychiatric disorders. About one-third demonstrate another anxiety disorder, particularly PD, SP, or specific phobia, and at least half will suffer from major depression. Substance abuse of alcohol and sedative-hypnotic drugs is common as patients attempt to self-medicate their anxiety.

Despite its severity and chronicity, OCD is a treatable disorder. A form of behavior therapy, involving in vivo exposure with response prevention and antidepressants that substantially enhance serotonergic neurotransmission, dramatically reduces OCD symptoms. The behavior treatment is best instituted by a skilled therapist who works in conjunction with the treating physician. Briefly, the therapist gradually exposes the patient to the specific fears but prevents practice of the rituals. At least half of all patients treated with this form of behavioral therapy respond with about a 75% reduction in both obsessions and compulsions. Research demonstrates that the therapeutic effect is long-lasting. Behavior treatment may be initially preferred by a patient phobic about taking medications.

The TCA clomipramine (Anafranil) and the serotonin-specific reuptake inhibitor fluoxetine (Prozac) are both FDA-approved for the treatment of OCD. Because of delayed response to pharmacotherapy, both agents should be given for at least 10 weeks in adequate doses before deciding that a patient is refractory. Clomipramine is generally effective at doses from 150 to 250 mg daily. To minimize the anticholinergic and adrenergic side effects, clomipramine should be started at 25 mg nightly and increased by 25 mg every 2 to 4 days. Exceeding a dose of 250 mg daily will greatly increase the risk of seizure activity from clomipramine. Fluoxetine (Prozac) has demonstrated efficacy in doses ranging from 20 to 80 mg daily. The practitioner is advised to start the drug at 20 mg every morning and to delay further dose increases for several weeks. This allows the physician to determine which patient may respond at lower fluoxetine doses, thereby minimizing side effects (insomnia, anorexia, nausea, sexual dysfunctions) and reducing costs. Unfortunately, no clinical predictors exist to suggest which drug to try first; if patients fail one drug, they should receive a trial with the other. Pharmacotherapy of OCD usually results in a 35 to 60% reduction in both obsessions and compulsions in approximately 70% of patients. This substantial clinical improvement can be further enhanced by the addition of in vivo exposure with response prevention. On the horizon, three serotonin-specific reuptake inhibitors either are awaiting FDA approval (fluvoxamine [Luvox]) for use in OCD or are currently being tested for efficacy (sertraline [Zoloft], paroxetine [Paxil]).

POST-TRAUMATIC STRESS DISORDER

The onset of post-traumatic stress disorder (PTSD) follows exposure to extreme traumatic events in which the patient experienced, witnessed, or was confronted with an event that involved actual or threatened death, serious injury, or threat to physical integrity. Traumatic events that produce intense fear, helplessness, or horror in the PTSD patient include military combat, personal assaults (rape or mugging), natural disasters, severe automobile accidents, or being diagnosed with a life-threatening illness. The characteristic symptoms of PTSD resulting from exposure to extreme trauma include persistent re-experiencing of the event through dreams or recollections; persistent autonomic arousal as demonstrated by exaggerated startle responses, hypervigilance, and insomnia; and persistent avoidance of stimuli associated with the trauma, along with numbing of general responsiveness. The likelihood of developing PTSD is enhanced as the intensity of, and physical proximity to, the trauma increases. Stressors of human design (torture, rape) appear more traumatizing than acts of God (earthquake).

PTSD may begin at any age, including childhood. Symptoms usually develop within the first 90 days after the trauma, but onset may be delayed months or years. The community lifetime prevalence is 1% but for at-risk groups (combat veterans), the prevalence is much higher. A history of behavior difficulties as a child predisposes an adult to develop PTSD. Psychiatric co-morbidity in PTSD is very common, with the patient at increased risk for substance abuse (alcohol, sedative-hypnotics), major and minor depression, or another anxiety disorder, especially OCD, PD, and generalized anxiety disorder.

There is a paucity of well-controlled trials evaluating the efficacy of either psychotherapeutic management or pharmacotherapy of PTSD. Supportive psychotherapy goals include patient education, activation of social supports, and assessment and treatment of co-morbidity. One study has demonstrated that both cognitive behavioral therapy and prolonged exposure in imagination were superior to counseling in the treatment of rape victims.

Pharmacotherapy trials to date have mostly utilized combat veterans, and the generalizability of these results to community trauma patients is unclear. No medication has FDA approval for the treatment of PTSD, but trials of antidepressants, BZs, anticonvulsants, lithium, and clonidine have been conducted. Medications are generally more effective against the positive symptoms of PTSD, including the autonomic arousal, dreams, nightmares, and recollections related to the trauma. The avoidance behavior and withdrawal associated with PTSD are less responsive to pharmacotherapy. Phenelzine (Nardil) has been the most frequently researched drug, and studies indicate that doses from 60 to 90 mg daily are effective. The drug is best started at 15 mg every morning and increased by 15 mg every 3 to 4 days, dividing doses between breakfast and lunch. The use of MAOIs requires a tyramine-free diet for the patient and predisposes the individual to weight gain, postural hypotension, and sexual dysfunctions. The TCAs imipramine (Tofranil)* and amitriptyline (Elavil)* both demonstrate at least modest efficacy in PTSD, especially when used in doses ranging up to 300 mg daily. To minimize the anticholinergic and adrenergic side effects, begin both drugs at 25 mg at night and increase the dose by 25 mg every 2 to 4 days to achieve a therapeutic effect. Several uncontrolled trials have investigated the efficacy of fluoxetine (Prozac)* in PTSD. Doses found effective have ranged from 20 to 80 mg daily. Few data are available to support the use of either BZs or lithium in the pharmacotherapy of PTSD at this time. In addition, BZs should be used with caution because of the frequency of co-morbid substance abuse found in patients with PTSD.

SOCIAL PHOBIA

The essential feature that characterizes social phobia (SP) is a marked and persistent fear of social or performance situations that may result in embarrassment. The patient recognizes that the fear is excessive or unreasonable but will either avoid a potentially humiliating situation or endure it with great distress. Consequently, social or performance situations markedly constrict a patient's daily routine. Patients are convinced that others can detect their social anxiety (trembling hands, quaking voice) and thus may avoid public speaking, eating, drinking, or writing in public. Palpitations, tremors, sweating, and blushing are common autonomic symptoms when the individual is confronted with the phobic situation. Generalized SP, with fears of most social situations (dating, parties, classrooms), accounts for well over half of all cases of this anxiety disorder. Limited SP implies that the patient is restricted in only one or possibly several situations, and this form of SP is associated with much less disability than the generalized type.

Community epidemiologic studies in adults have determined a lifetime prevalence of SP ranging from 2.8 to 13.3%. In most clinical samples, both sexes are equally represented or the majority are male. The mean age of onset is 15 years, but most cases begin in childhood. Onset after age 25 years is uncommon. Once present, the illness is chronic and unremitting and is associated with substantial psychiatric co-morbidity. Over half of patients report coexisting specific phobias, and about one-third develop major or minor depressions. OCD, agoraphobia, and alcohol abuse also frequently coexist with SP.

Both nonpharmacologic and pharmacologic therapies have demonstrated efficacy in the treatment of SP. Studies have identified cognitive behavioral treatment as particularly beneficial, with long-lasting results. In this form of nonpharmacologic treatment, the therapist carefully delineates the patient's specific feared situations, provides instruction in anxiety management techniques, develops cognitive reframing strategies, and initiates a behavioral exposure program. In general, this form of treatment is well accepted by patients and can be performed in groups.

The pharmacotherapy of SP is still in its infancy, and no medication has been FDA-approved for SP. A variety of medications, including MAOIs, BZs, beta blockers, and the newer serotonin-specific reuptake inhibitors, have been tested to date. Limited SP (performance anxiety in a musician) is probably best treated with intermittent doses of beta blockers or BZs. For instance, 20 to 80 mg of propranolol (Inderal)* or 25 to 100 mg of atenolol (Tenormin)* taken 1 to 2 hours before a performance will suppress autonomic symptoms of SP. Small doses of alprazolam (Xanax), 0.5 to 1.0 mg, or clonazepam (Klonopin), 0.25 to 0.5 mg, can accomplish similar results. Intermittent use of medication minimizes cost and adverse effects and eliminates the fear of dependency from taking medications regularly. We suggest a "test dose" of the beta blocker or BZ on a trial run ahead of time to avoid unexpected reactions in the midst of a performance.

For patients with the more severe generalized SP, phenelzine (Nardil) appears to be the most efficacious medication. Starting at 15 mg every morning, the

---

*Not FDA-approved for this indication.

*Not FDA-approved for this indication.

drug may be increased by 15 mg every 3 to 4 days to obtain a range of 60 to 90 mg daily, divided between breakfast and lunch. Again, phenelzine use requires a tyramine-free diet for safe use, and patients are likely to complain about weight gain, orthostatic hypotension, and sexual dysfunctions. Fluoxetine (Prozac),* starting at 20 mg every morning and increased as needed up to 80 mg daily, has been shown in several uncontrolled trials to be very effective against both limited and generalized SP. Because fluoxetine has a more benign side effect profile and requires no dietary restrictions, many practitioners prefer starting with fluoxetine before trying phenelzine. However, at least 5 weeks must elapse between stopping fluoxetine and starting phenelzine, to prevent the potentially lethal serotonin syndrome. Alprazolam (Xanax), when used at between 2 to 6 mg daily, and clonazepam (Klonopin), prescribed 1 to 3 mg daily, have shown significant therapeutic benefits in the treatment of SP. Many practitioners are reluctant to use BZs regularly in this population because of concerns about coexisting substance abuse, particularly alcohol ingestion. Other medications are currently being tested in SP.

SPECIFIC PHOBIA

The essential diagnostic feature of specific phobia is substantial and persistent fear of a circumscribed object or situation that significantly interferes with a patient's social and occupational performance. Despite knowing that the fear is excessive or unreasonable, the patient continues to avoid the feared situation or endures it only with great distress or anxiety. The level of anxiety usually varies as a function of both the degree of proximity to the feared stimulus and the extent to which escape from the stimulus is limited. Specific phobia is subtyped by class of feared object or situation. Patients with animal subtypes fear animals and insects (dog, snake, roach), whereas natural environment subtype patients fear storms, heights, or water. Blood injection–injury subtype patients fear blood and invasive medical and dental procedures, whereas situational subtypes fear being trapped in tunnels, elevators, airplanes, and enclosed places or on bridges.

Specific phobia is the most common primary anxiety disorder, with a lifetime prevalence of 11.3%. Most specific phobias begin in childhood, although the situational subtype may begin in adulthood. At least one-half to two-thirds of all patients are female. Specific phobias are commonly co-morbid with other anxiety disorders, with PD with agoraphobia being the most common coexisting illness.

Although specific phobia is the most common anxiety disorder, it is the one with the least morbidity and therefore the one least frequently treated. Many patients simply avoid the feared stimulus when possible or endure it with anxiety when necessary. The most effective treatment for specific phobia is exposure to the feared object or situation. Usually, the patient is exposed in vivo in small progressive steps to the stimulus. With repeated exposure, the patient's fear gradually diminishes, and avoidance is minimized or eliminated. The effect of this behavior therapy is rapid and durable, with positive results lasting years.

Pharmacotherapy is limited to treating patients with specific phobias who have failed to respond to behavior therapy, or who cannot encounter their feared situation often enough to adequately desensitize to their fear. For instance, a patient with fear of flying may benefit from small doses of a BZ prior to the flight. Alprazolam (Xanax), 0.5 mg taken 1 to 2 hours before departure, minimizes anticipatory anxiety and autonomic symptoms during the flight and facilitates patient comfort during exposure to the feared situation.

BULIMIA NERVOSA

method of
JAMES E. MITCHELL, M.D., and
SCOTT CROW, M.D.
University of Minnesota
Minneapolis, Minnesota

Bulimia nervosa is an eating disorder that was first described as a discrete and common diagnostic entity by Gerald Russell in 1979. The disorder is characterized by binge-eating episodes, during which the individual consumes large amounts of food in a short period of time, frequently followed by self-induced vomiting or other compensatory behaviors, such as laxative abuse.

In the latest revision of the psychiatric nomenclature (Diagnostic and Statistical Manual of Mental Disorders, fourth edition [DSM-IV]) the criteria for bulimia nervosa have been altered, and bulimia nervosa has now been subdivided into purging and nonpurging types.

Most patients with bulimia nervosa who have been described in the literature, and in particular those who have been the focus of treatment research, have been of the purging subtype; very little is known about nonpurging patients who engage in other types of compensatory behaviors, such as excessive exercise or fasting, although these patients are occasionally seen in clinical practice. Therefore, most of our discussion focuses on purging bulimia nervosa.

In addition to the abnormal eating and compensatory behaviors, most of these patients can also be characterized by certain distinct psychological symptoms. In particular, most of them are very preoccupied with body weight and shape concerns, and most fear that they will become overweight, despite the fact that most are of normal or low weight. These psychopathologic symptoms are also seen in anorexia nervosa.

The disorder has been described in all socioeconomic groups. It does appear, however, to be seen most commonly among women in industrialized societies in which a high positive value is placed on slimness as a model of attractiveness for young women, and where food is freely available to the general population. Prevalence studies suggest that 1 to 2% of women in such societies may develop this

---

*Not FDA-approved for this indication.

disorder, while prevalence studies in preindustrial countries suggest that bulimia nervosa occurs very rarely in such settings. Therefore, cultural factors are extremely important in understanding this disorder.

The median age of onset of bulimia nervosa is around 18 years, but it can occur anytime during adolescence or young adulthood; it is rare for patients to report an age of onset beyond 40 years. It is interesting that the age of onset clusters around the age of 18, this being the time when many young women are leaving home and going into the work force or to college. This crucial period of role transition seems to be a high-risk time for the development of this disorder, although it usually develops in an individual who has been weight-preoccupied and dieting intermittently during much of adolescence.

DIAGNOSTIC CRITERIA

As summarized in Table 1 the hallmark of the disorder is the binge-eating episode. Although at times these appear to be precipitated by discrete cues such as stressful events or unpleasant emotions, often the binge-eating episodes become almost a scheduled or institutionalized activity, occurring usually late in the day when the individual returns home from work or school.

The caloric content of binge-eating episodes can vary dramatically, but commonly as many as 3000 to 5000 calories are consumed. The most commonly ingested binge-eating foods include those that are easily prepared and that tend to be high in fat and carbohydrates, ice cream being the most common binge food. These same foods tend to be avoided at times when the individual is not binge-eating.

Many individuals describe feeling "out of control" and having an altered sense of reality while binge-eating. After binge-eating they then usually engage in some compensatory behaviors; this is most often self-induced vomiting, but at other times they may ingest drugs as a way of attempting to precipitate weight loss, for example, large amounts of laxatives or diuretics, both of which result in a decrease in body weight through the loss of fluid rather than ingested calories. Rarely patients with bulimia nervosa use ipecac to induce vomiting, which is particularly dangerous given the dose-dependent cardiomyopathy that this agent can cause.

CO-MORBIDITY

Although some individuals with bulimia nervosa are relatively free of other problems, it is not uncommon to encounter co-morbid psychopathologic conditions in these patients. Most commonly seen are affective disorders, particularly recurrent depression, and the lifetime risk for a co-morbid affective disorder is surprisingly high, often 70 to 80% in many studies. The prevalence of anxiety disorders has also been carefully examined, and appears relatively common. Co-morbid substance abuse problems also have received considerable attention, since they markedly complicate the treatment of these patients. These patients appear to be at increased risk for the abuse of both typical substances of abuse (such as alcohol) and atypical substances of abuse, such as laxatives, diuretics, diet pills, and ipecac. Screening for both types of problems should be part of a routine evaluation.

Bulimia nervosa has also been associated with certain personality disorders, particularly so-called Cluster B, Axis II disorders, which generally are characterized by poor insight, problems with affect regulation and impulsivity, and difficulties with interpersonal relationships.

MEDICAL COMPLICATIONS AND MEDICAL MANAGEMENT

Most patients with bulimia nervosa are at a relatively normal body weight, and one does not usually see the marked physical changes associated with starvation that one encounters with anorexia nervosa patients. However, despite a grossly normal body weight, many patients with bulimia nervosa evidence subtle changes suggestive of malnutrition, including, on screening laboratory examination, elevations in beta-hydroxybutyric acid and free fatty acid levels, and fasting hypoglycemia. Interestingly, brain imaging studies using computed tomography (CT) or magnetic resonance imaging (MRI) have demonstrated "pseudoatrophy" in some patients with bulimia nervosa, again suggesting problems with malnutrition, although the degree of atrophy is usually less severe than in anorexia nervosa.

On physical examination there are a few clues that

TABLE 1. **Diagnostic Criteria for Bulimia Nervosa**

A. Recurrent episodes of binge-eating. An episode of binge-eating is characterized by both of the following:
  1. Eating, in a discrete period of time (e.g., within any 2-hour period), an amount of food that is definitely larger than most people would eat during a similar period of time and under similar circumstances
  2. A sense of lack of control over eating during the episode (e.g., a feeling that one cannot stop eating or control what or how much one is eating)
B. Recurrent inappropriate compensatory behavior in order to prevent weight gain, such as self-induced vomiting; misuse of laxatives, diuretics, enemas, or other medications; fasting; or excessive exercise.
C. The binge-eating and inappropriate compensatory behaviors both occur, on average, at least twice a week for 3 months.
D. Self-evaluation is unduly influenced by body shape and weight.
E. The disturbance does not occur exclusively during episodes of anorexia nervosa.

Specify type:
Purging type: During the current episode of bulimia nervosa, the person has regularly engaged in self-induced vomiting or the misuse of laxatives, diuretics, or enemas.
Nonpurging type: During the current episode of bulimia nervosa, the person has used other inappropriate compensatory behaviors, such as fasting or excessive exercise, but has not regularly engaged in self-induced vomiting or the misuse of laxatives, diuretics, or enemas.

From American Psychiatric Association: Diagnostic and Statistical Manual of Mental Disorders, fourth edition. Washington, DC: American Psychiatric Association, 1994, pp 549–550.

are useful when one makes this diagnosis. The best area of focus is the teeth. Recurrent episodes of vomiting are associated with decalcification of the dental surfaces that are exposed to the vomitus, and the majority of patients who have been actively binge-eating and vomiting for over 4 years have obvious evidence of enamel erosion. Interestingly, the amalgams or fillings are relatively resistant to the acid and therefore often project above the surface of the teeth.

Some patients with bulimia nervosa evidence salivary gland hypertrophy, often involving the parotid glands, which at times can be dramatic and which may persist intermittently for several months during recovery. Some patients with bulimia nervosa also show callus or scar formation on the dorsum of the hand or knuckles, apparently resulting from trauma to these areas when using the hand to stimulate the gag reflex to induce vomiting.

On laboratory testing, patients with bulimia nervosa not uncommonly evidence fluid and electrolyte abnormalities. Most commonly metabolic alkalosis, hypochloremia, and occasionally hypokalemia are seen. Edema generally is suggestive of laxative or diuretic abuse, both of which result in reflex fluid retention. Chronic hypokalemia and fluid depletion can result in cardiac abnormalities and in kaliopenic nephropathy, both of which are fortunately rare. The use of ipecac can lead to the development of myopathy and, of particular concern, cardiomyopathy, which requires careful assessment.

Many patients with bulimia nervosa have a variety of gastrointestinal complaints including constipation, diarrhea, bloating after eating, abdominal pain, and dyspepsia. Gastric dilatation and ruptures have also been reported and may be the leading cause of death in these patients. Various subtle endocrine abnormalities have been described in bulimic patients including reduced levels of triiodothyronine (T_3), hypersecretion of cortisol, and failure to suppress cortisol activity after dexamethasone administration, although there is evidence that this latter finding may be at least partially attributable to dexamethasone malabsorption.

ETIOLOGY

There are three variables that correlate highly with the development of the disorder:

1. Female sex: bulimia nervosa is rare in males, who account for only 2 to 8% of the cases.
2. Age of onset in teen to early adult years: bulimia nervosa seems to develop in the context of dieting during adolescence or early adulthood, and rarely outside of this context.
3. Cultural variables: bulimia nervosa and other similar eating disorders appear to exist almost exclusively in societies in which a high positive value is placed on slimness as a model of attractiveness, and where obesity is disparaged.

However, all three of these variables identify a very large group of girls and women, most of whom do not develop full-blown eating disorders or bulimia nervosa, although many of whom experiment with some bulimic behaviors. The reason why some move from experimentation to the ongoing problem is unclear, although some early genetic studies suggest that there may be genetic diathesis for the development of this disorder, with a high concordance rate for monozygotic twins.

Bulimia nervosa tends to cluster in families in which other psychopathologic conditions are present, particularly affective disorders and alcohol abuse. Therefore, there is some suggestion that families with these other sorts of problems and impulse-control disorders may be at increased risk for having children who develop eating disorders. A core family pattern that predisposes to the development of eating disorders has really not been described, although many families with eating disorders are markedly disrupted by the course of the disorder even if problems were not present before the onset of the disorder.

Other risk factors may also be operative, and it is possible that certain physiologic changes that develop in the course of the eating disorder may perpetuate the behavior. For example, recent biologic studies suggest that serotonin, a neurotransmitter involved in appetite regulation and impulse regulation, may be abnormal in patients with bulimia nervosa. Also, elevated levels of a peptide known to increase appetite, the pancreatic polypeptide PYY, have been found in bulimic patients after a period of eating stability. Some bulimic patients may have impaired satiety responses, including impaired peripheral release of certain satiety hormones such as cholecystokinin. Also, recently it has been demonstrated that nociceptive (pain) thresholds may be altered in patients with bulimia nervosa. These changes suggest that some underlying abnormalities in biologic processes controlling mood, appetite, and satiety may predispose to the development of this disorder or develop in the context of the disorder and tend to maintain it.

DIAGNOSIS AND TREATMENT

The most important ingredient in the diagnosis of eating disorders is a high index of suspicion. Disorders of mood and eating are common enough in adolescent girls and young adult women that questions about such problems should be included in the routine evaluation of such patients. The physician should routinely inquire about the presence of binge-eating, protracted fasting, and compensatory behaviors such as self-induced vomiting. Also, it is useful to inquire about body image. Although some bulimics will deny such symptoms, a straightforward, nonjudgmental approach will increase the likelihood of a valid response.

Most patients with bulimia nervosa can be successfully treated out of hospital. However, they tend to be somewhat difficult to work with for many health professionals, and the available treatment studies suggest that they do best in structured programs that use techniques designed specially to treat this group. Hospitalization may be considered in patients who fail to respond to outpatient treatment, who are co-morbidly depressed to the point where suicide is of concern, or in whom mental instability is a problem.

The treatment literature on bulimia nervosa has centered on the parallel development of two strategies: pharmacologic strategies, primarily using antidepressant drugs, and psychotherapy or counseling approaches. We discuss each in turn.

Pharmacotherapies

More than a dozen placebo-controlled double-blind antidepressant trials of bulimia nervosa have been published, and the results are fairly consistent in showing that traditional antidepressant drugs do have a potent and significant suppressant effect on binge-eating and purging behavior. Also, if co-morbid mood problems are present, not uncommonly such symptoms improve as well. The available studies suggest that individuals who are not depressed at baseline may respond equally well to antidepressant treatments, suggesting that the mechanism of action may be other than the antidepressant effect. Many tricyclic antidepressant compounds and monoamine oxidase (MAO) inhibitors have been used experimentally. However, in recent years, the serotonin re-uptake inhibitors have become the agents of choice, mainly because they appear to be as equally efficacious as the older agents, but better tolerated, with lower drug discontinuation rates secondary to side effects. The agent that has been studied in the most subjects, in two large multicenter trials, is fluoxetine hydrochloride (Prozac)*; this drug appears to work optimally in these patients at dosages higher than those usually employed in the treatment of depression, typically 60 mg a day for bulimia nervosa.

Although there are dramatic and significant reductions in the frequency of target eating behaviors with antidepressant treatment, and at times impressive improvement in symptoms of mood, many patients with bulimia nervosa remain symptomatic despite antidepressant treatment. This raises questions as to whether or not antidepressants are a sufficient treatment for these patients. Also, although antidepressants can be quite useful, the available research suggests high rates of relapse when the drugs are discontinued; thus, although there may be short-term advantages in terms of cost and symptom management, over time these benefits may be outweighed by prophylactic effects obtained with psychotherapy approaches.

Several studies have examined the combined use of antidepressants and psychotherapy, and these studies suggest that for eating disorder symptoms, psychotherapy approaches are probably superior; however, there is some evidence that on certain variables, such as depression and anxiety, the combination may be superior, although this has yet to be adequately tested with the newer serotonin re-uptake inhibitors.

Psychotherapy

Paralleling the interest in antidepressant treatment, a fairly large treatment literature on psychotherapy approaches has developed. Initial studies compared active treatments with waiting list control groups or minimal interventions, but more recently psychotherapy studies have progressed to the point at which active treatments are being compared and dismantling studies are being undertaken. The results of these studies are quite consistent in showing that cognitive behavioral therapy (CBT) techniques, delivered in either group or individual formats, appear to be as effective as or more effective than the comparison treatments that have been used. These have become accepted as the most commonly recommended type of treatment in the field. There are a number of common elements among these CBT treatments:

1. There is strong emphasis on nutritional counseling. In many of the programs patients are given a structured meal-planning system at the beginning of treatment and strongly encouraged to eat regular, balanced meals, while treatment focuses on the problem of dietary restraint as a precipitant to binge-eating.
2. Other behavioral techniques are employed, such as examining cues associated with binge-eating and the consequences of the behavior (both positive and negative). Many of these programs also focus on cognitive restructuring techniques around weight and shape concerns and irrational beliefs about food and dieting. For example, it is very common for patients with bulimia nervosa to believe that they should eat as little fat as possible, or no fat at all, and that if they eat a "regular" amount of food they will become obese. These sorts of beliefs can be challenged using a Socratic dialogue.
3. Self-monitoring is also very useful. Research has shown that simply having patients record when and how much they are binge-eating can be very helpful in teaching them to gain control of the behavior.
4. Psychoeducational principles regarding the illness are also quite useful.
5. Alternative ways of dealing with uncomfortable affective states, such as anger, can be developed.
6. Family involvement may be useful, particularly for younger patients who are living at home. The relative advantages of group versus individual therapy have not been adequately tested.

COURSE AND OUTCOME

Unfortunately, many patients with bulimia nervosa go untreated and have the illness chronically

*Not FDA-approved for this indication.

or in a chronic relapsing fashion over many years. Carefully designed research studies have shown that using structured techniques, 60 to 80% of patients with bulimia nervosa can learn to control their eating behavior during the course of a relatively short-term therapy, such as 3 to 4 months. However, there is a risk that 20 to 25% of these patients will relapse, usually within 6 months after treatment, and follow-up care and further treatment are indicated in an attempt to prevent or minimize this relapse.

DELIRIUM

method of
LARRY E. TUNE, M.D.
Emory University
Atlanta, Georgia

Delirium is a common, serious, often unrecognized neuropsychiatric syndrome defined by the presence of global cognitive decline and altered level of consciousness. The incidence is approximately 10 to 15% in medical and surgical patients, but it can be much higher in selected patient populations (e.g., up to 30% in geriatric patients). The syndrome is of considerable clinical importance because it can be associated with increased morbidity and mortality. Early detection is critical, as treatment of the underlying cause is the cornerstone of management. Clinical management requires skilled psychopharmacologic and psychosocial management.

Diagnostic criteria include (1) disturbance of consciousness, with associated impairments in attention; (2) significant changes in cognitive functioning (e.g., recent onset of impairments in memory, orientation, language) that cannot be explained by a pre-existing condition; (3) clinical features that develop acutely or subacutely (usually hours to days) and tend to fluctuate over time; and (4) evidence from clinical examination that a specific cause is responsible for the disturbance (Table 1). Because these symptoms are often subtle, clinical assessment can be facilitated by the use of a standardized mental status examination of cognitive performance. The most widely used is the Mini-Mental State Examination (MMSE). It has the advantage of providing a brief, reproducible assessment of a range of cognitive domains. Clinicians should have a high index of suspicion for delirium in patients who perform poorly on this examination. Unfortunately, disturbances of consciousness are not so readily operationalized. Generally, this is manifested by changes in the patient's level of alertness and responsiveness and accessibility to questioning on clinical examination. Typically, the delirious patient is drowsy or inaccessible to questioning, although some delirious states are characterized by hyperalertness. Delirium is distinguished from dementia, and indeed from other psychiatric disturbances, principally by the accurate assessment of the patient's level of consciousness. There are a number of associated symptoms that should alert the clinician to the possibility of acute delirium. These symptoms incude perceptual disturbances (e.g., hallucinations, delusions, illusions); disturbed sleep-wake cycle, including worsening of symptoms as the evening progresses (sundowning); fluctuations in level of activity; and agitation through the day.

The most frequently identified risk factors for delirium

TABEL 1. Common Causes of Delirium

Metabolic or Endocrine

Electrolyte abnormality (especially Na^+, K^+, Ca^{2+}, and Mg^{2+})
Hyperglycemia or hypoglycemia
Hypoxia or hypercarbia
Liver or kidney failure
Thyroid disorder
Fever

Infection

Sepsis
Pneumonia
Urinary tract infection or upper respiratory infection
(especially in elderly patients)

Drug Toxicity

Anticholinergics, including most psychoactive medications
Lithium
Steroids
Digoxin
Theophylline

Drug or Alcohol Withdrawal

Central Nervous System Lesion

Acute stroke
Subdural hematoma
Postictal state
Raised intracranial pressure
Head trauma
Encephalitis or meningitis
Vasculitis

Multifactorial

are age, pre-existing cognitive impairment (especially pre-existing dementia), and polypharmacy. Table 1 lists the most common causes of delirium. The first step in approaching a delirious patient is a careful clinical examination. It is critical that this examination include a review of all medications taken by the patient, since the most common cause of delirium is medication intoxication. A large number of prescription medications are associated with delirium. In many instances, blood levels are available to assist in the clinical assessment and should be determined when a delirious patient is on these medications (e.g., digoxin, theophylline, lithium). One possible mechanism of toxicity is through the anticholinergic effects of multiple prescription medications. This has been shown in elderly patients, who are likely to be on multiple medications with cumulative anticholinergic effects. Table 2 lists the 24 most commonly prescribed medications in the elderly and their potential for anticholinergic effects. Under normal circumstances, these medications taken alone rarely cause delirium. However, when administered in combination, especially in vulnerable individuals, the risk of delirium increases. Drug withdrawal from alcohol and benzodiazepines should also be considered, especially in patients showing signs of autonomic instability (tachycardia, sweating, orthostasis). At times, a test dose of the suspected agent may assist in the diagnosis, although such interventions lack diagnostic specificity. Should a routine clinical examination fail to yield the etiology, a computed tomography (CT) or magnetic resonance imaging (MRI) scan of the head (to rule out stroke, masses, or subdural hematoma), followed by a lumbar puncture, is important to the clinical assessment. Finally, electroencephalography (EEG) may be useful in identifying delirious patients. Typically, the EEG shows generalized slowing, which may improve as the patient improves. However, the EEG cannot reliably distinguish delirium from dementia.

TABLE 2. **Presence or Absence of Anticholinergic Effects in 24 Medications Commonly Prescribed for the Elderly**

Medication	Anticholinergic Effects*
Furosemide (Lasix)	+
Digoxin	+
Hydrochlorothiazide and triamterene (Dyazide)	+
Hydrochlorothiazide	−
Propranolol (Inderal)	−
Salicylic acid	−
Dipyridamole (Persantine)	+
Theophylline anhydrous	+
Nitroglycerin	−
Insulin	−
Warfarin (Coumadin)	+
Prednisolone	+
Methyldopa (Aldomet)	−
Nifedipine (Procardia)	+
Isosorbide dinitrate	+
Ibuprofen	−
Codeine	+
Cimetidine (Tagamet)	+
Diltiazem hydrochloride (Cardizem)	−
Captopril (Capoten)	+/−
Atenolol (Tenormin)	−
Metoprolol (Lopressor)	−
Timolol (Blocadren)	−
Ranitidine (Zantac)	+

*+ = present; − = absent.

MANAGEMENT OF DELIRIUM

The management of behavioral symptoms of delirium, including agitation resulting from perceptual disturbances, usually requires combined pharmacologic and psychosocial intervention. The most widely used medication is haloperidol (Haldol) in doses of 0.5 to 2.0 mg per day. This is generally well tolerated, even when administered intravenously. Newer atypical antipsychotic medications, which are associated with fewer extrapyramidal side effects (e.g., risperidone [Risperdal] 0.5 to 1.0 mg per day), are gaining popularity. Less commonly used, primarily because of the sedative effects, are low doses of benzodiazepines. Benzodiazepines have been successfully used in delirious patients who experience side effects from haloperidol, including paradoxic agitation due to akathisia. It is critical that medications be reviewed daily, since the behavioral symptoms of delirium are often short-lived. Psychosocial interventions focus on providing a predictable, reassuring environment. These include avoiding excessive stimulation, frequently orienting the patient to time and location, providing frequent interactions between the patient and staff or family, and explaining the syndrome to both the patient and the family (i.e., explaining that the confusion and agitation have a medical cause). The syndrome is very frightening, and some cautious explanation can allay anxiety.

MOOD DISORDERS

method of
DAVID A. SOLOMON, M.D., and
MARTIN B. KELLER, M.D.
Brown University
Providence, Rhode Island

Although psychiatrists as well as primary care physicians have become increasingly aware that mood disorders are chronic and recurrent illnesses, posing a public health problem and affecting lifetime productivity, they remain underdiagnosed and undertreated. It is important for the medical field to adjust to the conceptual shift that mood disorders are medical disorders analogous to diabetes or hypertension. The consequences of these disorders can be very serious, ranging from social and physical disability to suicide. The physical, social, and role functioning of patients with a depressive disorder, for example, is often significantly worse than that associated with hypertension, angina, diabetes, advanced coronary artery disease, arthritis, back problems, lung problems, and gastrointestinal disorders. Patients with depression tend to have significantly more days in bed, worse perceived current health, and more bodily pain than do patients with major chronic medical conditions.

PREVALENCE

Mood disorders have a high lifetime prevalence: 5% for major depression; 3% for dysthymia; and 1% for bipolar disorder. Each year depression alone affects 10 to 14 million people in the United States. The median age at onset for major depression is 25 years; the corresponding age for bipolar disorder is 19 years. Half of all patients who recover from an episode of major depression at a tertiary care center will have a recurrence within 2 years. The natural history of bipolar disorders is marked by even higher rates of recurrence.

Co-morbidity is frequently seen in mood disorders. Although anxiety and depression are two separate disorders, research shows that approximately 60% of patients with depression have some anxiety symptoms, and 25% of those patients have panic attacks. Other co-morbid conditions include substance abuse, chronic medical conditions, and personality disorders.

LOW LEVEL OF TREATMENT

Many patients suffering from depression for as long as 2 years or more still receive minimal, insufficient, or no treatment at all. Research demonstrates that half of the patients who recover from a major depression receive no preventive treatment prior to their next episode. There are several explanations for low levels of somatic treatment. Patients may not seek evaluation, or clinicians may miss the initial diagnosis. Patients may refuse treatment or not comply with it. Some physicians prefer psychosocial treatment, and others may be concerned with medical contraindications or the issue of overdose attempts by patients with suicidal ideation. When medication is prescribed, the dose may be inadequate or side effects may arise and necessitate discontinuation.

Based on treatment research gathered for over a decade, it is clear that low levels of treatment alone do not cause the high rate of chronicity, relapse, and recurrence found in patients suffering from mood disorders. It is, however, clinically important to note that most of the available data reflect that the majority of patients do not receive adequate treatment for their mood disorders.

Further, there is a tendency for patients receiving the lowest levels of somatotherapy to remain ill for the longest period of time. This suggests that some severely ill patients who previously may have been thought to be resistant to treatment may in fact have received either inadequate levels of treatment or treatment for too short a period of time. Some researchers have concentrated on whether early intervention shortens the length of an episode, whereas others have focused on assessing the prospective pattern of recurrence following short-term treatment and recovery. Both areas of research are still being investigated. There is concurrence, however, that prophylactic drug treatment can reduce the risk of recurrence.

COSTS

The low levels of treatment for mood disorders disrupt social and physical functioning and create a heavy economic burden on patients and society. The direct costs of these illnesses include hospitalization and medication. Some of the more subtle but equally precarious economic strains come from repeated hospital stays, nursing home care, and the support costs of outpatient care including medical doctors, psychologists, and social workers.

Also troublesome are the indirect costs that influence the economic burden of mood disorders. The high morbidity of these illnesses reduces the productivity and therefore the income of both the patient and the employer. Other productivity losses are incurred by absenteeism, safety risks, high employee turnover, decreased quality of life, increased strain on relationships, and overall value of time spent by caregivers. Mortality is the ultimate loss in productivity.

Additional expenses are incurred by the social welfare administration and criminal justice system, which assist in treating, maintaining, and tracking those patients who make their way into those systems. Although current figures estimate that depressive disorders alone pose a $50 billion burden nationally, it is hard to quantify the effect of welfare dependence, disability, human loss and suffering, lost income and homelessness, and unreported or unrecognized illness, especially in primary care. It is crucial to recognize the significance of the costs of untreated mood disorders.

CLINICAL DESCRIPTIONS

Mood disorders are diagnosed by the clinical history and mental status examination. Criteria for each diagnosis are specified in the *Diagnostic and Statistical Manual of Mental Disorders*, 4th edition* (DSM-IV). The primary disorders described subsequently are major depression, dysthymia, and bipolar disorder. Descriptions of other mood syndromes such as hypomania and cyclothymia as well as modifiers of mood disorders, such as psychotic, catatonic, melancholic, atypical, postpartum, single episode, recurrent, rapid cycling, and seasonal pattern, can be found in DSM-IV.

Major Depression

According to the DSM-IV criteria, to diagnose an episode of major depression, at least five of the following symptoms must be present during the same 2-week period, and they must represent a change from the patient's previous level of functioning. Further, at least one of the symptoms must be either (1) depressed mood or (2) loss of interest or pleasure.

1. Depressed mood most of the day, nearly every day, as indicated by either subjective report (i.e., feels sad or empty) or observation made by others (i.e., appears tearful) Note: In children and adolescents, this can be an irritable mood.
2. Markedly diminished interest or pleasure in all, or almost all, activities most of the day, nearly every day (as indicated either by subjective account or observation made by others).
3. Significant weight loss when not dieting or weight gain (i.e., more than 5% of body weight in a month), or a decrease or increase in appetite nearly every day. Note: In children, consider failure to make expected weight gains.
4. Insomnia or hypersomnia nearly every day.
5. Psychomotor agitation or retardation nearly every day (observable by others, not merely subjective feelings of restlessness or being slowed down).
6. Fatigue or loss of energy nearly every day.
7. Feelings of worthlessness or excessive or inappropriate guilt (which may be delusional) nearly every day (not merely self-reproach or guilt about being sick).
8. Diminished ability to think or concentrate, or indecisiveness, nearly every day (either by subjective account or as observed by others).
9. Recurrent thoughts of death (not just fear of dying), recurrent suicidal ideation without a specific plan, or a suicide attempt or a specific plan for committing suicide.

The definition also states that these symptoms cause clinically significant distress or impairment in social, occupational, or other important areas of functioning and are not due to the direct effects of a substance (i.e., drugs of abuse, medication) or a general medical condition (e.g., hypothyroidism). Major depression should not be diagnosed in the context of

---

*From American Psychiatric Association: *Diagnostic and Statistical Manual of Mental Disorders*, 4th ed. Washington, D.C., American Psychiatric Association, 1994.

bereavement (i.e., after the loss of a loved one) unless the symptoms persist for longer than 2 months or are characterized by marked functional impairment, morbid preoccupation with worthlessness, suicidal ideation, psychotic symptoms, or psychomotor retardation.

Dysthymia

Dysthymic disorder is defined by
A. Depressed mood for most of the day, for more days than not, as indicated by subjective account or observation made by others, for at least 2 years. In children and adolescents, mood can be irritable, and duration must be at least 1 year.
B. In addition, criteria include the presence, while depressed, of at least two of the following:
  1. poor appetite or overeating
  2. insomnia or hypersomnia
  3. low energy or fatigue
  4. low self-esteem
  5. poor concentration or difficulty in making decisions
  6. feelings of hopelessness.
C. During the 2-year period (1 year for children and adolescents) of the disturbance, the person has never been without the symptoms in A and B for more than 2 months at a time.
D. No major depressive episode has existed during the first 2 years of the disturbance (1 year for children and adolescents)—i.e., the episode is not better accounted for by chronic major depressive disorder, or major depressive disorder in partial remission.
  Note: There may have been a previous major depressive episode provided there was a full remission (no significant signs or symptoms for 2 months) before the dysthymic disorder developed. In addition, after these 2 years (1 year for children and adolescents) of dysthymic disorder, there may be superimposed episodes of major depressive disorder, in which case both diagnoses may be given.
E. Patient has never had a manic episode or an unequivocal hypomanic episode.
F. The disorder does not occur exclusively during the course of a chronic psychotic disorder such as schizophrenia or delusional disorder.
G. The disorder is not due to the direct effects of a substance (e.g., drugs of abuse, medication) or a general medical condition (e.g., hypothyroidism).

Bipolar Disorder

Bipolar disorder is characterized by recurrent episodes of mania and major depression. Between episodes, patients may experience full remission but are just as likely to suffer significant morbidity that falls short of meeting the full criteria for a mood episode. Such subsyndromal symptoms increase the risk of relapse. Within the DSM-IV diagnosis of bipolar disorder there are many categories of distinction including hypomanic, single episode, depressed, cyclothy-

mic, and due to a medical condition, and there are even examples of bipolar disorder not otherwise specified. For the purposes of common use and brevity, this article outlines the criteria for manic episode as follows:
A. A distinct period of abnormally and persistently elevated, expansive, or irritable mood lasting at least 1 week (or any duration if hospitalization is necessary).
B. During the period of mood disturbance, at least three of the following symptoms persist (four if the mood is irritable) and are present to a significant degree:
  1. inflated self-esteem or grandiosity
  2. decreased need for sleep (e.g., feels rested after only 3 hours of sleep)
  3. more talkative than usual or feels pressure to keep talking
  4. flight of ideas or subjective experience that thoughts are racing
  5. distractibility (i.e., attention too easily drawn to unimportant or irrelevant external stimuli)
  6. increase in goal-directed activity (either socially, at work or school, or sexually) or psychomotor agitation
  7. excessive involvement in pleasurable activities that have a high potential for painful consequences (e.g., unrestrained buying sprees, sexual indiscretions, or foolish business investments).
C. Mood disturbance is sufficiently severe to cause marked impairment in occupational functioning or in the usual social activities or relationships with others or necessitates hospitalization to prevent harm to self or others.
D. The disorder is not due to direct effects of a substance (e.g., drugs of abuse or medication) or a general medical condition (e.g., hyperthyroidism).
  Note: Manic episodes that are clearly precipitated by somatic antidepressant treatment (e.g., medication, electroconvulsive therapy, light therapy) should not count toward a diagnosis of bipolar disorder.

GENETICS

Evidence of the heritability of mood disorders comes from genetic-epidemiologic studies, using three different methods. Twin, family, and adoption studies indicate that major depression and bipolar disorder are at least partially caused by genetic transmission. In family studies, for example, relatives of patients are two to three times more likely to incur a mood disorder than are relatives of case controls. Twin studies, conducted over a span of 50 years, reveal an average concordance rate of 65% for monozygotic twins and 14% for dizygotic twins. There appears to be at least a partial overlap in the genetic transmission of major depression and bipolar disorder. Furthermore, the heritability of these disorders, as shown by twin studies, is comparable to that of illnesses such as diabetes and hypertension.

More recent findings have made use of the techniques of molecular genetics. These genetic mapping studies have reported a linkage of bipolar disorder to markers on the X chromosome (color blindness, glucose-6-phosphate dehydrogenase deficiency, Factor IX, and the Xg blood group), and a linkage of bipolar illness and major depression to markers on chromosome 11 (insulin-*ras* oncogene) and chromosome 6 (human leukocyte antigen). None of these findings has been consistently replicated, meaning either that these specific linkages do not exist or that genetic heterogeneity is present in the population.

When counseling patients and their families about childbearing and the risk of a child's incurring the illness, the following figures may be useful. If one parent has a mood disorder and the other is not ill, there is roughly a 30% risk of having a child with a mood disorder. If one parent has bipolar disorder and the other parent has a mood disorder, the risk is 50 to 75%. Finally, first-degree relatives of patients with a bipolar disorder have at least a 25% chance of developing a mood disorder.

COURSE AND OUTCOME

Clinical research has consistently provided evidence that mood disorders are chronic and recurrent conditions. Despite the previously held clinical belief that depressed patients tend to make complete recoveries from acute depressive episodes, a significant percentage of patients suffering from mood disorders remain chronically ill. More than 20% of patients remain ill with major depression for 2 years, 12% fail to recover after 5 years, and the risk of remaining ill for 10 years is 7%. Patients spend as much as 20% of their lifetime in depressive episodes. Up to 20% may commit suicide.

Factors found to predict a slower time to recovery are longer duration and increased severity of the initial episode, prior history of a nonaffective psychiatric disorder (suggesting that the depression in these subjects was secondary to a disorder such as alcoholism), lower family income, and being married. Research data confirm that a significant percentage of depressed patients experience multiple episodes or lengthy episodes without returning to the "pre-depression" state of well-being. This differs from earlier theories that depression consisted of discrete episodes of illness alternating with clearly defined well periods.

Probabilities of recovery calculated for intervals ranging from 1 week to 5 years show that the chances of recovery from major depression are highest within the first 6 months following accurate diagnosis and treatment. The longer patients remain ill, the less likely recovery becomes, as suggested by the fact that only 28% of patients observed recovered during the second 6 months, whereas 54% recovered during the first 6 months after enrollment in the study. The majority of patients who do not recover during the 5 years experience subsyndromal symptoms of depression most of the time. Their illness resembles chronic minor depression or dysthymia with episodes of major depression rather than major depression alone.

Among patients who do recover from acute episodes of major depression, relapse is frequent, although the risk of relapse tends to decrease the longer the patients remain well. Among patients who relapse, the probability of remaining ill for 1 year or more is 22%.

DIFFERENTIAL DIAGNOSIS

Clinicians, particularly in the primary care setting, may encounter patients with mixed anxiety and depressive symptoms that do not meet the full criteria for either an anxiety or mood disorder. It appears that a significant number of patients in the community, as many as 10% of patients with depressive symptoms, fall into this subclinical population. This is an area that is receiving extensive attention; in DSM-IV, this problem is discussed in an appendix on the mixed anxiety-depression syndrome.

The differential diagnosis of major depression includes organic mood syndrome with depression, primary degenerative dementia of the Alzheimer type, multi-infarct dementia, schizoaffective disorder of the depressive type, adjustment disorder with depressed mood, and uncomplicated bereavement. The differential diagnosis of mania includes organic mood syndrome with mania, schizophrenia, schizoaffective disorder of the bipolar type, cyclothymia, attention-deficit hyperactivity disorder, and borderline personality disorder.

TREATMENT

Three types of treatment are currently used for severe depression: pharmacotherapy, psychotherapy, and electroconvulsive therapy. Antidepressant medications are usually the first approach in treatment because of their demonstrated efficacy and rapid effect. Three classes of antidepressants are generally used for treating major depression: tricyclic antidepressants (TCAs) such as imipramine, monoamine oxidase inhibitors (MAOIs) such as phenelzine, and selective serotonin re-uptake inhibitors (SSRIs) such as fluoxetine. In addition, there are several atypical compounds. Prescriptions for antidepressant medications require close monitoring of the patient because of the risk of overdose or suicide.

TCAs are effective and widely used, and have historically been the first-line antidepressant. They are rapidly absorbed and metabolized in the liver. Their mechanism of action is a function of their ability to block re-uptake of the neurotransmitters norepinephrine and serotonin. These medications interact with many other pharmacologic agents including MAOIs, alcohol, oral contraceptives, antihistamines, beta-adrenergic blockers, clonidine, diuretics, class II antiarrhythmics, and anticholinergic drugs. Even when used within the therapeutic range, they cause significant and sometimes unacceptable side effects: sedation, increased heart rate, cardiac rhythm disturbances, postural hypotension, dry mouth, blurred vision, constipation, urinary retention, sexual dysfunction, and weight gain. The elimination half-life is such that the TCAs can be given once a day and, because of their hypnotic effect, are usually administered at bedtime (Table 1).

The MAOIs inhibit the enzyme that degrades biogenic amines, including catecholamines. The MAOIs are effective antidepressants but are less widely used than TCAs because they produce severe adverse interactions with sympathomimetic drugs and food products containing amines such as tyramine. They are, however, more effective than TCAs in treating depression characterized by symptoms of anxiety, phobic features, panic attacks, hysterical features, or reversed vegetative symptoms (e.g., increased sleep, increased appetite). Patients taking MAOIs must be educated about the importance of avoiding medications, foods, and beverages that contain vasoactive amines and the hypertensive crisis that can ensue. MAOIs are prescribed on a twice-a-day or three-times-a-day basis (Table 2).

The recent introduction of a new class of antidepressant medications, the SSRIs, has had a profound impact on depression pharmacotherapy. As denoted

TABLE 1. Tricyclic Antidepressants: Preparations and Doses

Generic Name	Brand Name	Dosage Forms	Usual Dosage Range (mg/day)*
Amitriptyline	Elavil, Endep	10, 25, 50, 75, 100, 150 mg	100–300
Clomipramine	Anafranil	25, 50, 75 mg	100–250
Desipramine	Norpramin	10, 25, 50, 75, 100, 150 mg	100–300
	Pertofrane	25, 50 mg	
Doxepin	Sinequan Adapin	10, 25, 50, 75, 100, 150 mg	100–300
Imipramine	Tofranil Janimine Sk-Pramine	10, 25, 50, 75, 100, 125, 150 mg	100–300
Imipramine pamoate	Tofranil PM (sustained release)	5, 100, 125, 150 mg	150–300
Maprotiline	Ludiomil	25, 50, 75 mg	100–150
Nortriptyline	Pamelor Aventyl	10, 25, 50, 75 mg	50–150
Protriptyline	Vivactil	5, 10 mg	15–60
Trimipramine	Surmontil	25, 50, 100 mg	150–300

Common or Troublesome Side Effects

Anticholinergic	Dry mouth and nasal passages, constipation, urinary hesitance, esophageal reflux
Autonomic	Orthostatic hypotension, palpitations, intracardiac conduction slowing, increased sweating, increased blood pressure, tremors
Allergic	Skin rashes
Central nervous system	Stimulation, sedation, delirium, myoclonic twitches (generally at high dosages), nausea, speech blockage, seizures and extrapyramidal symptoms
Other	Weight gain and impotence

*Dosage ranges are approximate.

TABLE 2. Monoamine Oxidase Inhibitors: Preparations and Doses

Generic Name	Brand Name	Dosage Forms	Usual Dosage Range (mg/day)*
Isocarboxazid	Marplan	10 mg	20–50
Phenelzine	Nardil	15 mg	45–90
Selegiline†	Eldepryl	5 mg	20–50
Tranylcypromine	Parnate	10 mg	30–50

Common or Troublesome Side Effects

Anticholinergic	Dry mouth, constipation, urinary hesitance
Autonomic	Orthostatic hypotension, hypertensive crisis (interactions with food or medications), hyperpyrexic reactions, myoclonic twitches, muscle cramps and myositis-like reactions
Central nervous system	Stimulation during the day, sedation (particularly daytime and due to insomnia during the night), insomnia during the night
Other	Weight gain, anorgasmia, sexual impotence

*Dosage ranges are approximate.
†Not FDA-approved for this indication.

by their name, the SSRIs are highly selective in blocking the re-uptake of serotonin and have little direct effect on norepinephrine. The SSRIs have a relatively mild side effect profile and are usually better tolerated than TCAs and MAOIs. The elimination half-life is such that the SSRIs can be given once a day and, because of their stimulating effect, are usually administered in the morning (Table 3).

The atypical compounds are a heterogeneous group of drugs with novel structures and mechanisms of action. Venlafaxine was approved quite recently and is given in three divided doses. Bupropion is also prescribed on a three-times-a-day basis. Both amoxapine, which has some properties of a neuroleptic, and trazodone should be considered second-line drugs. Amoxapine is given once a day, usually at bedtime, whereas trazodone is prescribed in two or three divided doses. This past year, the Food and Drug Administration (FDA) approved the use of nefazodone (Serzone), a compound structurally related to trazodone. Nefazodone is also administered in two or three divided doses (Table 4).

TABLE 3. Selective Serotonin Re-uptake Inhibitors: Preparations and Doses

Generic Name	Brand Name	Dosage Forms	Usual Dosage Range (mg/day)*
Fluoxetine	Prozac	10, 20 mg	20–40
Fluvoxamine†	Luvox	50, 100 mg	50–300
Paroxetine	Paxil	20, 30 mg	20–50
Sertraline	Zoloft	50, 100 mg	50–200

Common or Troublesome Side Effects

Anticholinergic	Nausea, diarrhea, vomiting
Autonomic	Restlessness, nervousness, tremulousness
Central nervous system	Insomnia and daytime drowsiness
Other	Sexual dysfunction and headaches

*Dosage ranges are approximate.
†Not FDA-approved for this indication.

TABLE 4. **Atypical Compounds: Preparations and Doses**

Generic Name	Brand Name	Dosage Forms	Usual Dosage Range (mg/day)*
Amoxapine	Asendin	25, 50, 100, 150 mg	200–300
Bupropion	Wellbutrin	75, 100 mg	200–450
Nefazodone	Serzone	100, 150, 200, 250 mg	300–600
Trazodone	Desyrel	50, 100, 150, 300 mg	150–400
Venlafaxine	Effexor	37.5, 50, 75, 100 mg	75–375

Common or Troublesome Side Effects

Amoxapine	Sedation, dry mouth, constipation, nausea, blurred vision, anxiety, restlessness. In addition, neuroleptic side effects may occur, including akathisia, tremor, tardive dyskinesia, and neuroleptic malignant syndrome
Bupropion	Agitation, restlessness, insomnia. Risk of seizures may be higher than for other antidepressants, and the total daily dose should not exceed 450 mg
Nefazodone	Dizziness, headache, nausea, drowsiness, asthenia
Trazodone	Sedation (trazodone is often used as a hypnotic), orthostatic hypotension, nausea, vomiting, priapism
Venlafaxine	Anorexia, nausea, sedation, dizziness. Less commonly, palpitations, fatigue, headache, constipation, anxiety, dry mouth, sexual dysfunction, diaphoresis, increased blood pressure and increased heart rate

*Dosage ranges are approximate.

Somatic treatments are the most effective for severe depression, but psychotherapy has been proved to be effective either as an alternative or in combination with medication. Candidates for psychotherapy as an alternative to medication include those who refuse medication, those for whom antidepressant pharmacotherapy is contraindicated, those who cannot tolerate the side effects, and those whose depressive symptoms are refractory to pharmacotherapy. Psychotherapy is most useful as an adjunct to pharmacotherapy.

Three psychotherapeutic approaches have been modified or developed specifically for the treatment of depression: cognitive therapy, behavioral therapy, and interpersonal therapy. Cognitive therapy is based on the premise that depression results from faulty cognition, which leads to an unrealistic outlook and set of expectations. Therapy aims to identify the specific distorted cognitions and replace them with corrected patterns of thinking. Behavioral psychotherapy views depression as a result of the loss of positive reinforcement. Therapy seeks to create specific systems of self-reinforcement that will improve the balance of positive versus negative interactions. Interpersonal psychotherapy (IPT) is based on the premise that difficulties in interpersonal relationships are the cause or result of depression, and it focuses on the resolution of current conflicts. IPT was developed especially for the treatment of depression.

Each of these are short-term interventions, usually involving 12 to 20 sessions over 12 to 16 weeks.

It had been thought that because psychotherapeutic techniques help patients develop more effective coping strategies, these techniques would produce more lasting benefits in the long-term treatment of depression. In the few studies available, IPT and a combination of cognitive and behavioral therapies have been effective in preventing relapse. Nevertheless, somatic therapy appears to provide even better results.

The treatment of bipolar disorder and acute mania requires the use of specific antimanic medications (Table 5). This past year, the FDA approved the use of valproic acid for treatment of bipolar disorder. The only other approved medication is lithium. Carbamazepine is not FDA approved for this indication, but it is frequently used as a second-line agent for patients not responsive to lithium. Often, an antipsychotic medication such as haloperidol or chlorpromazine is also required to manage acute symptoms. It should be noted that several drugs can induce mania, including tricyclic antidepressants, amphetamines, and steroids. Caffeine and over-the-counter stimulants may have the same effect.

Electroconvulsive therapy (ECT) is usually reserved for severely depressed or manic patients who have not responded to pharmacotherapy, for whom medication is contraindicated, or for whom immediate effective intervention is essential (e.g., suicidal patients). It has been debated whether ECT is more rapidly effective than medication. ECT is not considered to have lasting effects, and maintenance medication must be administered following a course of

TABLE 5. **Specific Antimanic Medications**

Generic Name	Brand Name	Dosage Forms	Therapeutic Plasma Levels
Lithium carbonate	Eskalith	300 mg	0.8–1.0 mM/L
	Lithane	300 mg	
	Lithonate	300 mg	
	Lithotabs	300 mg	
	Eskalith CR (sustained release)	450 mg	
Lithium citrate syrup	Cibalith-S	8 mEq/5 mL (480-mL bottle)	0.8–1.0 mM/L
Valproic acid	Depakote Depakene	125, 250, 500 mg	50–125 μg/mL
Carbamazepine*	Tegretol	200 mg (chewable: 100 mg)	4–12 μg/mL

Common or Troublesome Side Effects

Lithium	Gastrointestinal distress (nausea, vomiting, diarrhea), impaired renal function (polyuria), tremor, hypothyroidism, electrocardiographic changes, acne, psoriasis
Valproic acid	Sedation, gastrointestinal distress, tremor, hepatotoxicity, alopecia
Carbamazepine	Sedation, gastrointestinal distress, tremor, leukopenia, hepatotoxicity

*Not FDA-approved for this indication.

ECT. Maintenance ECT, given once a month or once every 2 months, is also an option.

The results of most studies point to a combination of pharmacologic and psychotherapeutic treatments as being most effective in the management of mood disorders. A three-phase plan for pharmacologic treatment of depression has been proposed that includes acute, continuation, and maintenance stages as the best means of preventing recurrence.

CONTINUATION AND MAINTENANCE

A number of investigators have recently explored the role played by maintenance treatment in the outcome of major depressive disorder. They uniformly note that surprisingly few studies have attempted to address the questions of whether and how early intervention influences the subsequent course of patients' illness, whether somatotherapy shortens episodes and decreases their likelihood, and how the discontinuation of medication impacts the course of the illness.

Research shows that it takes a median of 25 weeks for patients to achieve stabilization from an initial episode of major depression. Continuation therapy is the uninterrupted extension of pharmacotherapy after the acute episode has resolved. Medication is thus continued to consolidate the remission and forestall relapse of the acute episode. When therapy is extended for longer periods for the purpose of preventing recurrence of a new episode, this prophylaxis is referred to as maintenance therapy. Maintenance treatment is particularly important for patients at high risk of repeated episodes. Risk factors for recurrent episodes include history of frequent or multiple episodes, double depression (major depression plus pre-existing dysthymia), onset after age 60, long duration of individual episodes, family history of affective disorder, co-morbid anxiety disorder, or substance abuse.

Studies of maintenance pharmacotherapy suggest that such treatment results in a 30 to 40% reduction in relapses (i.e., a 50% relapse rate in patients on maintenance treatment as opposed to an 80% relapse rate in patients not receiving maintenance therapy). However, the costs and benefits of such treatment must be carefully weighed on a case-by-case basis because long-term somatotherapy entails both economic expense and the risk of side effects. For patients with repeated episodes, severe symptoms, or inter-episode dysthymia, the benefits of treatment frequently outweigh the costs.

Contrary to long-held clinical wisdom, patients with mood disorders experience a significant risk of chronicity, relapse, and recurrence. For example, patients with double depression may never return to a pre-illness healthy personality because the underlying dysthymia frequently persists even after acute episodes of major depression have ended.

Given these facts, and given the high levels of morbidity and mortality associated with mood disorders, it is especially disturbing that these illnesses are underdiagnosed and undertreated. Only 20% of patients with depression are treated in the mental health sector. It is imperative that clinicians who treat major depression remain aware of its pernicious nature and of the many effective options available for its treatment. Primary care physicians should seek psychiatric consultation or referral for patients who fail to respond to acute therapy, deteriorate during maintenance treatment, develop new co-morbidity, or desire to discontinue prophylactic treatment.

Given the complexity of treatment decisions, no single report to date fully describes or explains the reason for the gap between the availability of treatments demonstrated by controlled clinical trials to be effective for depression, and the treatment actually received by individual patients in clinical practice. However, the accumulation of concordant findings from different investigators with complementary strengths and weaknesses provides strong evidence that such a gap exists.

Research has demonstrated that there is a need for a conceptual shift in the understanding of major depression. It is a chronic medical disorder, analogous to diabetes or hypertension, and requires long-term maintenance treatment. The approach to treatment should include early recognition, treatment of the acute episode, stabilization to avoid relapse, and maintenance to prevent recurrence. The need for continuation and maintenance treatment is an issue that now deserves increased attention, especially with the availability of new classes of antidepressant drugs that have excellent efficacy and more favorable side effect profiles.

SCHIZOPHRENIA

method of
DANIEL E. CASEY, M.D.
Oregon Health Sciences University School of Medicine
Portland, Oregon

Schizophrenia is the most severe and disabling of all mental illnesses. The prevalence is approximately 1%, with the onset usually occurring in the late teens to midtwenties. Men and women are effected equally. Until the advent of neuroleptic drugs in the 1950s, there were no consistently effective medical approaches to schizophrenia. These agents have now become the mainstay of managing both the acute and the chronic phases of schizophrenia. Secondary therapeutic approaches include supportive counseling, patient and family education, and vocational training tailored to each patient's abilities.

The large majority of patients have both positive and negative psychotic symptoms. Positive symptoms include delusions, hallucinations (usually auditory), and disorganized thinking patterns that are marked by incomprehensible or illogical statements. Negative symptoms, such as anergia, emotional blunting or flatness, avolition-apathy, and anhedonia, constitute the loss of personality characteristics that are normally present. During acute exacerbations, positive symptoms often dominate, whereas negative symptoms may be more apparent in the chronic phases of illness. The initial episodes and exacerbations usually have a gradual onset over several days, weeks, or months and are accompanied by a steadily deteriorating level of function. The differential diagnosis includes schizoaffective disorder (major depressive or manic symptoms are also present), delusional disorder (nonbizarre delusions that focus on an aspect of daily life), brief reactive psychosis (symptoms similar to schizophrenia that are present for at least 1 day but less than 4 weeks with eventual return to full functioning), psychosis due to other medical conditions, and substance-induced psychotic disorders (psychosis within 1 month of substance intoxication or withdrawal).

The etiology of schizophrenia is unknown. However, the preponderance of evidence supports a biologic basis of this disorder, which includes contributions from genetic, perinatal, neurodevelopmental, neuroanatomic, and neuropharmacologic factors. The relative contributions of each of these factors has yet to be determined.

ANTIPSYCHOTIC DRUG CHARACTERISTICS

Mechanism of Action

Although there are numerous dopamine receptor subtypes, the mechanism of action that is common to all efficacious antipsychotic drugs is the blockade of central nervous system dopamine D_2 receptors. There is a high correlation between the affinity of neuroleptics for D_2 receptors and effective antipsychotic daily dosage. The effects of drugs on other receptor subtypes of dopamine, serotonin, or noradrenaline have been proposed as mechanisms for their antipsychotic efficacy. To date these hypotheses are unproved, though indirect supportive data have been used to explain the possible mechanism of action of the two newest antipsychotic compounds, clozapine (Clozaril) and risperidone (Risperdal).

Receptor-binding profiles of neuroleptics also strongly correlate with side effects. High-milligram, low-potency compounds such as chlorpromazine (Thorazine), thioridazine (Mellaril), or clozapine have high anticholinergic, antihistaminic, and anti–alpha-adrenergic receptor antagonistic properties that correlate with high rates of sedation, dry mouth, blurred vision, constipation, hypotension, and increased pulse rates, and low rates of extrapyramidal syndrome (EPS) side effects. At the opposite end of the continuum, low-milligram, high-potency compounds such as haloperidol (Haldol) and fluphenazine (Prolixin) have minimal activities on these receptors and have much lower rates of these troublesome side effects, but do have high rates of acute EPS. Risperidone is somewhat of an exception to this rule. At efficacious antipsychotic doses (2 to 6 mg per day) it has low EPS rates, but at higher doses it has EPS rates that are similar to those of other high-potency drugs (Table 1).

Drug Choice

Neuroleptic drugs have equal antipsychotic efficacy (see Table 1). Most patients who do poorly with one medicine also do poorly with another, though this is not always the case, and trials with drugs from different chemical classes are warranted when the first treatment regimen is unsuccessful. Clozapine is an exception to this generalization because it has superior efficacy in treatment-resistant schizophrenia.

TABLE 1. **Estimated Equivalent Oral Doses of Neuroleptic Drugs Commonly Used to Treat Schizophrenia and Other Psychoses**

Generic Name	Brand Name	Estimated Equivalent Dose (mg)*	Common Dose Range (mg)[†,‡]	Relative Potency	Extrapyramidal Syndromes
Phenothiazines					
Chlorpromazine	Thorazine	100	200–900	Low	Low
Thioridazine	Mellaril	100	200–800	Low	Low
Perphenazine	Trilafon	8	16–64	Intermediate	Intermediate
Trifluoperazine	Stelazine	5	5–40	High	High
Fluphenazine	Prolixin	2	5–20	High	High
Butyrophenones					
Haloperidol	Haldol	2	5–20	High	High
Thioxanthenes					
Thiothixene	Navane	5	5–60	High	High
Dibenzazepines					
Clozapine	Clozaril	50	125–900	Low	Minimal
Loxapine	Loxitane	15	25–250	Intermediate	Intermediate
Indoles					
Molindone	Moban	10	50–225	Intermediate	Intermediate
Benzisoxazole					
Risperidone	Risperdal	1	2–16	High	Low-High

*Equivalents are derived from clinical trials that span a range of study designs that do not routinely compare one neuroleptic against the other.
†Common daily dose ranges are derived from clinical experience. These do not necessarily correlate in a 1:1 ratio with the estimated dose equivalents.
‡Doses below and above the common dose range are occasionally used in special circumstances.
Adapted from Casey DE: Schizophrenia: Psychopharmacology. *In* Jefferson JW, Greist JH (eds): The Psychiatric Clinics of North America: Annual of Drug Therapy. Philadelphia, WB Saunders Co, 1994, pp 81–99.

Sedating high-milligram, low-potency compounds are often used for agitated patients, whereas nonsedating low-milligram, high-potency neuroleptic drugs are frequently selected for the withdrawn psychotic patient. Though this is common practice, either the high- or low-potency compounds appear to be equally effective in treating both these subgroups of patients. It is not possible to predict from the clinical symptoms which drug will have the better acute, intermediate, and long-term outcomes. If additional sedation is needed during the initial phases of treatment, adjunctive therapy with benzodiazepines, such as lorazepam (Ativan) (0.5 to 3.0 mg per day) may be used.

Several drug-delivery choices are available with the neuroleptics. Many of the compounds are available as oral concentrates, tablets, short-acting injectable, and long-acting injectable depot decanoate (lasting 2 to 4 weeks) formulations like haloperidol and fluphenazine. During the acute-treatment phase it is necessary to start planning for chronic maintenance treatment. Serious consideration should be given to the long-acting depot neuroleptics for patients who would prefer or benefit from biweekly or monthly injections. This consideration is particularly important for patients with histories of noncompliance and exacerbations of psychosis when medicines are discontinued.

Low to moderate doses of neuroleptics are equally efficacious to high daily doses for most patients (see Table 1). Side effects are dose-related, so that escalating doses are associated with increasing side effect frequency and severity. However, some patients are poor absorbers or rapid drug metabolizers and may require higher doses.

Blood Levels

Drug blood levels are usually not beneficial in treating schizophrenia. Because of individual differences in absorption and metabolism, blood levels from the same daily dose vary widely among patients. Clinical outcome correlates poorly with blood levels, in part because of the wide variation in clinical response. In contrast, side effects, particularly EPSs, do show a positive dose and blood-level relationship. Clozapine is an exception: clozapine blood levels should approximate 350 ng per mL or more before it can be concluded that the patient has had an adequate therapeutic trial. Clozapine blood levels over 600 ng per mL are associated with higher rates of seizures.

ACUTE TREATMENT

Initial or recurring acute psychotic episodes require drug therapy. If relapse is associated with noncompliance it is important to address the underlying issues of noncompliance. This is particularly so if drug side effects were the cause of drug discontinuation. Changes in the drug type, dose, and method of administration are parameters to consider when revising treatment. Neuroleptic drugs should be initiated at the lower end of the dose range and gradually titrated upward to the desired level over a period of a few to several days.

The range of response varies greatly among patients. A minority have an excellent response that allows them to return to their prior level of function. Most patients have partial benefit but remain somewhat symptomatic and do not return to prior functioning levels. Approximately 10 to 30% of patients are described as treatment-resistant, or are nonresponders. Both positive and negative symptoms usually improve during drug therapy, but positive symptoms often improve more in the acute-treatment phases.

The therapeutic time course is gradual. Most patients begin to show improvement within a few days, but 2 to 4 weeks are frequently needed before the patient shows substantial clinical gains. Several months of treatment are required before maximal benefit is obtained.

Unfortunately, it is not possible to predict at the outset of treatment who will benefit. The best predictor of current response is the response to prior therapy. Education of the patient, the family, and friends is valuable to aid in early recognition of symptom recurrence. Reinstituting treatment in early relapse is usually associated with shorter symptomatic episodes and decreased morbidity.

MAINTENANCE THERAPY

Most acute psychotic episodes should continue to be treated with maintenance neuroleptic therapy for up to 1 year. If this is the initial psychotic episode, gradual downward titration of the neuroleptic after the patient has done well for 6 to 12 months is appropriate. However, if there have been many episodes of relapse associated with drug dose decrease or discontinuation, extended, open-ended maintenance is recommended. The dose required to initially treat the psychosis may be decreased by 25 to 50% in the extended maintenance phase for many patients. This strategy should be carefully considered as many patients are now receiving lower doses than were previously used in the acute-treatment phases, so that there may be a narrower dose range to work with for dose decreases in maintenance therapy.

Although maintenance therapy is usually with oral medicines, long-acting depot neuroleptics given at 2- to 4-week intervals are an underutilized alternative treatment strategy. This depot approach ensures delivery of medicine on a daily basis and provides relatively low stable blood levels with manageable side effects. On the other hand some patients dislike regular injections and are noncompliant with treatment appointments.

TREATMENT RESISTANCE

Although the majority of patients benefit from neuroleptic treatment, a sizable minority (10 to 30%) have minimal or no benefit. Treatment resistance has been operationally (though arbitrarily) defined as being ill for 2 or more years and failing to benefit substantially from at least two different pharmacologic classes of antipsychotic drugs given at clinically relevant doses for at least 1 month each. If a patient fails to improve substantially after 4 to 6 weeks of continuous treatment at effective doses, several treatment options are available. These include (1) raising the current drug dose substantially, (2) adding another psychotropic drug such as lithium or carbamazepine (Tegretol) (combining clozapine and carbamazepine should be avoided because of concern about additive risks of agranulocytosis), (3) switching to another traditional neuroleptic drug, (4) reducing the drug dosage, (5) continuing the current treatment for an additional 4 to 6 weeks, (6) switching to clozapine or risperidone. Substantially increasing the dose may help a few patients, but it is usually not helpful to the majority of patients, and increased side effects are a predictable disadvantage. Adding other psychotropic drugs may help some patients but not others. Switching drugs to another chemical class of agents appears to provide little benefit, unless the other drug is clozapine, or perhaps risperidone. Decreasing the drug dosage may be helpful in those patients whose improvement has been substantially impaired by side effects. Waiting for time to bring additional benefits is a therapeutic principle in all of medicine.

If none of the above alternatives work or if there is well-established treatment resistance, switching to clozapine is the next logical step. Approximately 30 to 65% of those who are resistant to standard neuroleptic therapy show clinically relevant improvement with clozapine. It is not possible to predict in advance who will benefit from clozapine. Usual daily doses are in the 300 to 450 mg per day range but may go up to 900 mg per day. Between 3 and 6 months of clozapine treatment is needed before treatment failure can be determined. If clozapine fails, risperidone may be useful, but it has not been extensively studied in treatment-resistant patients.

Clozapine has substantial side effects. The most serious problem is agranulocytosis in 1 to 2% of patients. The main risk period is between 6 weeks and 6 months, but a few cases have occurred later. If the total white blood cell count drops below 3000 per mm^3 and the granulocytes drop below 1500 per mm^3, clozapine therapy should be discontinued. Weekly blood tests are required as part of a clozapine monitoring system that is linked with weekly prescriptions. Leukocytopenia and agranulocytosis are usually reversible when detected early. Fevers and infections should be carefully monitored as indicators of impairment to the granulocyte system. Another troublesome side effect is seizures: there is an approximate 5% incidence rate with 1 year of clozapine therapy. Adding phenytoin (Dilantin) or reducing the clozapine dose is usually effective. Sedation can be a dose-limiting factor, although partial to full tolerance develops over many weeks. Hypersalivation is also a problem for some patients. Hypotension and or moderate increases in the pulse rate (10 to 20 beats per minute) may be clinically relevant side effects. On the positive side, clozapine has a minimal risk of acute EPS and is likely to have a very low liability for tardive dyskinesia (TD).

SIDE EFFECTS

Neuroleptic drugs have many side effects because they affect many neurotransmitter subtypes. The major problems are the neurologic motor symptoms of acute EPSs and TD (Table 2). Acute EPSs usually develop early in therapy, whereas TD develops after many months or years of chronic treatment. EPSs, which include akathisia, dystonia, and parkinsonism, occur in 50 to 75% of patients and are described in Table 2. Acute dystonic reactions occur more often in younger patients, particularly males, whereas drug-induced parkinsonism occurs more often in older patients. Akathisia occurs equally in all age groups. These symptoms cause both motor and mental impairments and are frequent reasons for drug noncompliance. TD occurs in approximately 20% of patients and is usually mild, but may be irreversible. TD develops in 50 to 70% of elderly persons receiving chronic neuroleptic treatment. It also occurs significantly more often in females and patients with non-insulin-dependent diabetes receiving neuroleptic drugs.

Managing acute EPSs is usually successful with the addition of anti-EPS drugs or reducing neuroleptic dose (Table 3; also see Table 2). Most of the anti-EPS medicines are highly anticholinergic or antihistaminic. Thus, they have many of their own undesirable side effects on the autonomic nervous system.

Thermoregulatory dysfunction is also a consequence of neuroleptic treatment in a small minority of patients (0.01 to 1%). It occurs with all neuroleptic treatment including clozapine and risperidone. Symptoms are hyperthermia, rigidity, and autonomic nervous system instability. Elevations of creatine phosphokinase (CPK) levels are commonly but not always part of the clinical picture. This disorder usually develops during the initial phases of treatment, but it may occur at any time. Treatment approaches include (1) stopping all neuroleptic and other psychotropic drugs, (2) providing supportive treatment for temperature control and electrolyte imbalances as well as maintaining cardiovascular and renal functions, and (3) effective drug treatment with dopamine agonists such as bromocriptine (Parlodel) or other drugs such as dantrolene (Dantrium) or benzodiazepines.

All commercially available neuroleptic drugs, with the exception of clozapine, raise prolactin levels by antagonizing dopamine receptors in the pituitary. This can be associated with mild galactorrhea in 2 to 5% of patients and improves by decreasing neuroleptic doses. Irregular menses can also be associated with neuroleptics, but the exact extent and clinical impact of this problem are unknown.

TABLE 2. **Acute Extrapyramidal Syndromes and Tardive Dyskinesia**

Syndrome	Symptoms	Distinguish from Psychiatric Symptoms	Period of Symptom Onset (Days)	Treatment
Acute EPSs				
Acute dystonia	Briefly sustained or fixed abnormal postures of the limbs, trunk, neck, face, eyes, tongue	Manipulation, hysteria, seizures, catatonia	1–5	Benztropine (1–2 mg) or diphenhydramine (25–50 mg) IM or IV is diagnostic and curative.
Parkinsonism	Tremor, rigidity, bradykinesia (akinesia), mask face, decreased arm swing	Depression, negative symptoms of psychosis	5–30	Reduce neuroleptic dose. Use anti-EPS agents.
Akathisia	Subjective complaints or motor restlessness, pacing, rocking, shifting foot to foot	Severe agitation, psychotic decompensation	1–30	Reduce neuroleptic dose. Use lipophilic beta-adrenergic blockers; propranolol. Use anti-EPS agents.
Tardive Dyskinesia Syndromes				
Tardive dyskinesia	Orofacial-lingual dyskinesia, choreoathetosis in limbs and trunk	Stereotypy or mannerisms of psychosis	Months to years	No consistently effective treatment. Use lower neuroleptic dose.
Tardive dystonia	Persisting abnormal postures in the limbs, trunk, neck, face, eyes, tongue	Acute dystonia, idiopathic dystonia	Months to years	No consistently effective treatment. High-dose anticholinergics or clozapine may help.
Tardive akathisia	Persisting subjective and objective restlessness	Acute akathisia, psychotic agitation	Months to years	No consistently effective treatment. Propranolol or anti-EPS agents may help.

Abbreviation: EPS = extrapyramidal syndrome.
Adapted from Casey DE: Schizophrenia: Psychopharmacology. *In* Jefferson JW, Greist JH (eds): The Psychiatric Clinics of North America: Annual of Drug Therapy. Philadelphia, WB Saunders Co, 1994, pp 81–99.

PSYCHOSOCIAL TREATMENT

Neuroleptic drugs reduce psychotic symptoms in the majority of patients. However, schizophrenia is a pervasive disorder that affects all aspects of daily life. Therefore, psychosocial interventions are necessary. Counseling to assist patients and their families in adjusting to the demands and limitations of the illness is appropriate. Additionally, vocational rehabilitation according to the patient's abilities is often necessary. Neuroleptic drugs help patients become more able to benefit from these additional multidisciplinary approaches.

TABLE 3. **Estimated Equivalent Oral Doses of Anti–Extrapyramidal Syndrome Agents**

Generic Name	Brand Name	Usual Daily Dose (mg)
Anticholinergic or Antihistaminic Agents		
Benztropine	Cogentin	1–6
Biperiden	Akineton	2–10
Diphenhydramine	Benadryl	25–150
Orphenadrine	Norflex	50–300
Procyclidine	Kemadrin	5–30
Trihexyphenidyl	Artane	5–15
Dopamine Agonist		
Amantadine	Symmetrel	100–300
Beta Blocker		
Propranolol	Inderal	20–120

Adapted from Casey DE: Schizophrenia: Psychopharmacology. *In* Jefferson JW, Greist JH (eds): The Psychiatric Clinics of North America: Annual of Drug Therapy. Philadelphia, WB Saunders Co, 1994, pp 81–99.

PANIC DISORDER

method of
MURRAY B. STEIN, M.D.
University of California, San Diego
La Jolla, California

"Panic disorder" is a common condition (affecting 1 to 2% of the general population) wherein the sufferer experiences recurrent panic attacks. "Panic attacks" are acute paroxysms of physical and emotional symptoms that occur unexpectedly, especially in the early phases of the illness. Panic attacks typically begin suddenly, reach their peak within seconds or minutes, and vary widely in their duration. The panic attacks themselves consist of anxious feelings and somatic symptoms such as tachycardia and shortness of breath (Table 1), in addition to "cognitive" symptoms such as the fear of doing something uncontrolled, the fear of going crazy, or the fear of dying. The latter fear leads people with panic attacks to seek help in the emergency room, where they often present with the conviction that they are having heart attacks, strokes, or some other acute medical emergency. Patients with panic disorder are also known to present to cardiologists, neurologists, and primary care physicians with physical complaints (e.g., chest pain, dizziness) that are ultimately proved to be attributable to panic disorder. This fact makes it essential that medical clinicians be familiar with this disorder and its treatment.

DIAGNOSTIC ISSUES

Panic disorder should be strongly considered whenever the clinical presentation includes a constellation of episodic physical symptoms that occur suddenly and are associated with fearfulness or anxiety. In particular, the occurrence of such symptoms in young persons should raise the clinician's level of suspicion, as should a family history of panic disorder. Panic disorder usually has its onset in the late teens or early twenties, with a predilection for females over males (2:1 ratio). It is also known to run in families. Even though panic disorder may figure prominently in the differential diagnosis, it is almost always necessary to rule out other common physical conditions before concluding that the diagnosis is panic disorder. This medical evaluation should be thorough and sufficient to reassure both the patient and the physician that an occult medical disorder is not being missed, but it need not initially include extensive tests to rule out exotic disorders such as pheochromocytoma. A suggested approach to medical evaluation is presented in Table 2. The clinician is reminded that drug abuse should always be strongly considered; this includes the excessive use of caffeine.

Other psychiatric disorders also enter into the differential diagnosis of panic disorder. First among these is major depression, which, in truth, is not so much a *differential* diagnosis as an *additional* diagnosis. Approximately 35% of patients who present with panic disorder are also clinically depressed at the time, but this is often missed because the dramatic nature of the panic attacks overshadows the depressive symptoms. It is therefore mandatory that the presence of depression be systematically evaluated in any patient who presents with panic attacks. In particular, the presence of suicidal ideation should be ascertained,

TABLE 1. **Symptoms of Panic Attacks (DSM–IV)**

A panic attack is a discrete period of intense fear or discomfort in which four (or more) of the following symptoms develop abruptly and reach a peak within 10 minutes:

Palpitations, pounding heart, heart racing
Sweating
Trembling or shaking
Shortness of breath or smothering sensations
Choking sensations
Chest pain or discomfort
Nausea or abdominal distress
Dizziness, lightheadedness
Derealization (feelings of unreality) or depersonalization (being detached from oneself)
Fear of losing control
Fear of going crazy
Fear of dying

TABLE 2. **Medical Evaluation in Panic Disorder**

Routine Work-Up

Complete physical examination, including neurologic assessment
Complete blood count, electrolytes, liver function tests, serum calcium and phosphate
Routine electrocardiogram with rhythm strip
Thyroid function screening (thyroxine and thyroid-stimulating hormone)

Special Situations

Prominent palpitations or chest pain: consider Holter monitor, echocardiogram, exercise stress test
Loss of consciousness or prominent headaches: consider electroencephalogram or computed tomography or magnetic resonance imaging of the head
Intermittent or chronic hypertension: consider urinary catecholamines and vanillylmandelic acid to rule out pheochromocytoma

Other Suggestions

If patient fails to respond to standard treatments, re-evaluate for possible medical illness that may have been missed initially

as this necessitates immediate intervention to ensure the patient's safety. The co-morbid presence of major depression also influences the choice of treatment, in that an antidepressant would be strongly recommended.

Panic attacks can also occur in syndromes other than panic disorder, and this sometimes presents a diagnostic dilemma. For example, persons who experience panic attacks whenever they have to give a speech or whenever they have to perform in front of a crowd probably suffer from a condition known as "social phobia." Social phobia involves the fear of situations wherein the individual is subject to the scrutiny of others. In such situations, the individual fears that he or she will say or do something embarrassing or that his or her anxiety will be evident to other people. What differentiates social phobia from panic disorder is the fact that in social phobia, panic attacks are restricted to social situations (i.e., they do not occur out of the blue), and the person with social phobia knows *why* he or she is afraid (e.g., "because I'm going to look like an idiot"). The differential diagnosis of panic disorder and social phobia can be difficult, and there are occasions when both disorders are present simultaneously. Fortunately, many of the treatments for panic disorder (e.g., high-potency benzodiazepines, monoamine oxidase inhibitors, serotonin transport inhibitors) are also helpful for social phobia, so there is some cause for consolation when the differential diagnosis of these disorders remains unresolved.

Some persons with "post-traumatic stress disorder" can experience panic attacks. Post-traumatic stress disorder was classically described in Vietnam-era war veterans who experienced panic attacks, excessive irritability, chronic nervousness, and flashbacks (vivid recollections of traumatic events). However, it has recently been recognized that post-traumatic stress disorder may also afflict persons who have been either recently (e.g., rape victims, victims of other violent crimes or natural disasters) or remotely (e.g., child abuse victims) traumatized. In most cases, the diagnosis of post-traumatic stress disorder should occasion referral to a mental health provider for specialized counseling. In some cases, however, the primary care physician should be prepared to provide pharmacotherapeutic support, which might involve the use of antidepressants.

When anxiety is more of a chronic, unremitting condition

seen in association with excessive worry, then the diagnosis of "generalized anxiety disorder" should be considered.

COMPLICATIONS

The main complication of panic disorder is agoraphobia. The Greek translation for "agoraphobia" is "fear of the marketplace," and this has colloquially been interpreted as a fear of wide-open spaces. Persons with agoraphobia, however, do not fear wide-open spaces; they fear and avoid situations in which they believe that they might have a panic attack. Usually, the person begins to avoid places where a panic attack has actually occurred (e.g., the supermarket), but this soon generalizes to include many places with lots of people (e.g., church, school) or other places where escape might be difficult if a panic attack were to occur (e.g., movie theater, driving in traffic, lines at the bank). The extent of the individual's phobic avoidance (i.e., the severity of the agoraphobia) can fluctuate over time and can range from very limited avoidance (e.g., avoiding driving during rush hour) to severe avoidance (e.g., being unable to walk more than two blocks from home unless accompanied by a companion). Some patients with panic disorder—more men than women—for reasons that are not apparent, develop little or no phobic avoidance. But in persons who do develop agoraphobia, this can be a major source of disability that can lead to emotional and/or financial dependence (e.g., job loss).

Another potential complication of panic disorder is substance abuse, particularly alcoholism. In what may be an attempt to self-medicate, some persons with panic disorder resort to alcohol or unprescribed benzodiazepines to reduce the frequency and intensity of their anxiety. It is thus incumbent on physicians to determine the extent of alcohol and other substance abuse in their patients before prescribing medications for their condition. In patients with a history of alcohol or minor tranquilizer abuse, the prescription of benzodiazepines for panic disorder should be undertaken judiciously, and usually only in consultation with a psychiatrist. For some patients, the specific treatment of substance abuse should be the primary focus of treatment, with the panic disorder treatment deferred until the substance abuse is under control. In some cases, however, the simultaneous management of the substance abuse and panic disorder becomes necessary in order to effect improvement in either condition.

The concomitant presence of major depression, which in some cases may be considered a complication of panic disorder, was described earlier.

TREATMENT

The treatment of panic disorder can be among the most satisfying professional events in clinical medical practice. The majority of patients with panic disorder get much better, they get better quickly, and their level of functioning improves dramatically. For physicians who are apathetic or nihilistic about the treatment of psychiatric disorders, the treatment of patients with panic disorder provides an exciting revelation. This said, it must also be recognized that the treatment of panic disorder requires the application of the full range of the physician's skills: as a diagnostician, an educator, a motivator, and a pharmacotherapist.

Education and Counseling

Patient Education

Patients with panic disorder benefit enormously from education about the nature of their illness. As mentioned earlier, the physician must ascertain that an underlying physical condition is not the proximate cause of the panic attacks, and the patient must be made aware of the reasons behind any diagnostic tests that are ordered. Once it is clear that the diagnosis is panic disorder, the clinician can proceed to discuss the ramifications of this diagnosis with the patient. When the physician can give a name to the patient's seemingly inexplicable constellation of frightening symptoms and inform the patient that treatments are available, the patient's condition almost always improves immediately. It is important to let patients know that they are not the only ones in the world suffering from this condition, that it is a disorder well recognized by the medical community, and that they are neither losing their minds nor suffering from a gravely mysterious, undiagnosed condition.

Patients with panic disorder should be advised to avoid caffeinated substances (which need to be reduced gradually, by the equivalent of one cup of coffee per day, lest caffeine withdrawal headaches and somnolence supervene) and to avoid sleep deprivation, both of which have been shown to make panic attacks worse. Regular aerobic exercise can be recommended for its anxiolytic effects in patients in whom this is not contraindicated. In many communities, anxiety disorder self-help groups are available, and patients should be made aware of these valuable sources of support and educational materials.

Counseling

When the physician is fortunate enough to see patients in the early stages of the illness, it is critical to let them know that they should attempt to continue their usual routines and to force themselves to continue doing things, even if it makes them anxious. This will prevent extensive agoraphobic complications, which are much more difficult to treat once they have been established. Patients who present at the point where they already have phobic limitations should be encouraged to gradually put themselves into anxiety-provoking situations and to stay in them for progressively longer periods of time. A hierarchy can be established in which a patient is encouraged to confront the least frightening situations first (e.g., driving the car a block from home when there is no traffic) and then to build on this to attack more difficult situations (e.g., driving a mile from home during rush hour). Usually these suggestions for in vivo exposure, as it is called, should be made when it is apparent that medications, if used, are beginning to work and that panic attacks have lessened.

For patients with agoraphobia, it is critical that they begin to tackle situations and places that they previously avoided. Without this, they may remain stuck at home—granted, without panic attacks, but still stuck at home. For patients whose agoraphobia is particularly severe, it may be helpful to enlist the help of a significant other (e.g., spouse or friend) who can act as a facilitator and monitor of the patient's exposure therapy.

Most patients also benefit from some explanation about how their thinking can exacerbate their symptoms and contribute to the maintenance of the disorder. Patients with panic disorder often "somatize" and "catastrophize," meaning that they assume that the symptoms they experience are indicative of serious bodily dysfunction and, moreover, that the worst (e.g., a heart attack) is inevitably going to occur. When it can be pointed out to them that these assumptions are not necessarily true, some patients are able to see their symptoms and their reaction to them in a different light.

Pharmacologic Treatment

Not all patients with panic disorder require pharmacotherapy. Approximately one in three patients does well merely with appropriate education, reassurance, and counseling about the disorder. But for the remaining patients, formal cognitive-behavioral therapy (which is usually provided by a psychologist or psychiatrist with special training), pharmacotherapy, or a combination of the two will probably be required. In the medical setting, it is important to realize that many patients are presenting at that particular time because they are in imminent danger of becoming disabled by their panic disorder (e.g., losing a job or having to quit school). For this reason, instituting prompt treatment can be of paramount importance.

Antidepressants

The pillar of the pharmacologic treatment of panic disorder is the use of antidepressants. So-called antidepressants have been shown over the past decade to be efficacious in blocking the occurrence of panic attacks, even in patients who are not depressed. Given that many patients with panic disorder are also clinically depressed, however, antidepressants offer the capacity to treat both the anxiety and the depressive symptoms with a single agent. With treatment with benzodiazepines alone, depressive symptoms are unlikely to improve. For this reason, and because benzodiazepines are associated with some risk of abuse and physical dependence, antidepressants are the initial medication of choice for panic disorder.

A list of antidepressants that are useful in the treatment of panic disorder, along with suggested dosages, is included in Table 3. This list is not exhaustive. In fact, most antidepressants are probably useful for treating panic disorder, with a few possible exceptions such as bupropion (Wellbutrin), trazodone (Desyrel), and amoxapine (Asendin). Also, medications with prominent anticholinergic effects, such as

TABLE 3. **Commonly Used Antidepressants for Panic Disorder**

Medication	Starting Dose	Therapeutic Dose
Tricyclic and Heterocyclics		
Imipramine (Tofranil)	10–25 mg at bedtime	100–300 mg/day
Desipramine (Norpramin)	10–25 mg at bedtime	100–300 mg/day
Selective Serotonin Re-uptake Inhibitors		
Fluvoxamine (Luvox)	25 mg at bedtime	100–300 mg/day
Paroxetine (Paxil)	10 mg at bedtime	20–40 mg/day
Sertraline (Zoloft)	50 mg once daily	100–200 mg/day

amitriptyline (Elavil), should probably be avoided, as patients with panic disorder tolerate these side effects poorly. The selective serotonin re-uptake inhibitors (SSRIs) as a group are particularly well tolerated by patients with panic disorder.

When prescribing antidepressants for patients with panic disorder, it is critical that the initial dosage be very low (e.g., 10 to 25 mg of imipramine [Tofranil]* per day or 10 mg of paroxetine [Paxil]* per day) and that subsequent increments in dosage be made slowly. Ultimately, most patients with panic disorder do need full antidepressant doses (e.g., 150 mg imipramine per day or 20 to 40 mg of paroxetine per day), but these doses must be reached more slowly than would be the case in the treatment of patients with major depression. If the initial doses are too high, patients tend to experience a plethora of adverse effects, including the temporary exacerbation of their anxiety. By using small initial doses, by warning patients that they may experience a transient worsening of their symptoms, and by being readily available to answer questions about side effects, physicians can help patients get through this often difficult initial treatment phase.

Included in the category of antidepressants are the monoamine oxidase inhibitors (MAOIs). These drugs, which include phenelzine (Nardil)* and tranylcypromine (Parnate),* are arguably the most effective of the antipanic agents. However, because of the low-monoamine diet that must be prescribed in order to prevent a hypertensive crisis, the MAOIs are usually reserved for refractory cases. Clinicians should be aware of their existence, however, so that patients who do not respond to standard treatments can be referred for treatment with these agents.

Benzodiazepines

High-potency benzodiazepines such as alprazolam (Xanax),* clonazepam (Klonopin),* and lorazepam (Ativan)* are all of proven efficacy in the treatment of panic disorder. They have several advantages over the antidepressants: they work quicker (often within the first few doses or days, whereas antidepressants

---

*Not FDA-approved for this indication.

typically require weeks to work), and they tend to have fewer side effects (sedation is the main side effect with these agents). For these reasons, they have been favored by many American physicians in the treatment of panic disorder. Concerns about "addiction" to these agents are certainly overdone; in fact, most patients with panic disorder take less medication than prescribed and are eager to stop taking it as soon as possible. Nonetheless, patients do become physically dependent on benzodiazepines, and patients must be advised that these drugs cannot be stopped abruptly, lest they experience a rebound of their anxiety, insomnia, or, at the extreme, seizures. A disadvantage of the benzodiazepines is that some patients find it inordinately difficult to stop using them; when they do, their anxiety recurs with a vengeance. Very slow tapering of the benzodiazepine and psychological support can ameliorate these symptoms, but for some patients, this remains a definite problem.

When prescribed, benzodiazepines are best used on a regular dosing schedule rather than on an as-needed basis. Suggestions for benzodiazepine dosages in panic disorder are included in Table 4.

TABLE 4. **Benzodiazepine Dosages for Panic Disorder**

Medication*	Starting Dose	Therapeutic Dose
Alprazolam (Xanax)	0.25 mg tid–qid	2.0–4.0 mg total per day
Clonazepam (Klonopin)	0.25 mg every morning and at bedtime	1.0–2.0 mg total per day
Lorazepam (Ativan)	0.5 mg tid–qid	3.0–8.0 mg total per day

*Approximate order of potency: clonazepam $2\times$ > alprazolam $2\times$ > lorazepam.

Duration of Treatment

Most patients who are treated with medications for panic disorder should continue taking them for 9 to 12 months before any attempt is made at dosage reduction or discontinuation. If medications are discontinued earlier than this, relapse rates are unacceptably high. If possible, patients should be referred for specialized cognitive-behavioral therapy, as there is evidence that this may facilitate their eventual discontinuation of medication and, more important, may reduce their rate of relapse in the future.

Section **17**

Physical and Chemical Injuries

BURNS

method of
JOHN A. GRISWOLD, M.D.
Texas Tech University Health Sciences Center
Lubbock, Texas

The skin is the largest organ of the body and is made up of two layers. The more superficial is the epidermis or cellular layer, whereas the deeper is the dermis, a relatively acellular layer containing mostly collagen. The lowest layer of the epidermal portion contains the basal layer of replicating epithelial cells, which provides the major source for new cells as more superficial cells slough. The dermis contains skin appendages such as hair follicles and glands, which are also lined by replicating epithelial cells. The dermis also contains the vast majority of pain-related nerve endings.

The skin's function is to act as a protective barrier against injury and invading organisms. It plays a significant role in the control of body core temperature. It helps control insensible fluid loss through evaporation and serves as a primary sensory organ, providing constant information related to the environment. Damage to an organ system this large and with such wide-ranging activities can have catastrophic effects on the person as a whole. This damage not only causes a loss of function in the areas mentioned but also stimulates the release of inflammatory mediators such as eicosanoids, vasoactive peptides, and cytokines. On a local level, such substances may be protective, but once they are released in large amounts systemically, they can have additional detrimental effects. Therefore, burn injury is not simply a mechanical damage to a protective organ system but a stimulus causing a hormonal or chemical response that has a wide array of effects supplementing the disruption of homeostasis.

There are approximately 2.5 million burn injuries suffered in the United States each year of sufficient magnitude to require medical help. Of these, 100,000 require hospitalization, and 10,000 to 12,000 patients die each year from their burns. Although only a small number of burns result in trauma they have a major impact on overall cost to society due to the chronicity and intensity of rehabilitation and subsequent disability. The direct cost of burn care exceeds $1 billion annually, but the indirect cost for vocational and physical rehabilitation is estimated to be between $3 billion and $4 billion each year.

DESCRIPTION OF BURN TEAM AND BURN CENTERS

Burn centers arose out of the need for a comprehensive, coordinated approach to the care of patients with burn injuries. Organized therapy of burn care became one of the first and strongest examples of the true team approach in medicine involved in a specific type of disease or injury. A burn center is made up of a group of dedicated professionals who come together, each with his or her own expertise in a specific area, each providing a part in the care and recovery of burn patients.

This team begins with the firefighters and paramedics responsible for the rescue, stabilization, and transport of burn victims to a health care facility. Their role as part of the team cannot be overstated, and they are all too often forgotten as an important element in the care of burn patients.

Nursing care far outreaches that of traditional nursing activities, not only in the intensity of critical care support but also in the in-depth understanding of wounds, wound management, and wound healing, along with a solid grasp of all aspects of pain management.

Wound technicians are intimately involved in the daily débridement of wounds and are like magicians, applying dressings that are protective and comfortable yet still allow freedom of movement for therapy.

The role of physical therapists has always been strong in burn centers and has long been emphasized as a crucial element in burn care. From the time of the incident, physical therapists begin therapeutic maneuvers to prevent loss of function and strength. The physical therapist is one of the few members of the team who has continuous interaction with individual burn patients, caring for them from the very beginning of their injuries through the long, drawn-out process of their recovery.

Occupational therapists are experiencing growing activity in support of burn patients. Besides splinting joints and newly grafted areas to prevent loss of function and protect healing wounds, they have become experts in upper extremity rehabilitative therapy, especially where burns of the hand are concerned. They also play an intense role in educating both the family and the patient, initiating and continuing activities of daily living, and complementing the physical therapist from the time of the injury through the end of recovery.

One of the newer members of the burn team is the speech therapist. The speech therapist's involvement is vital not only to aid in communication with patients who are mechanically ventilated due to severe burn injuries and/or smoke inhalation, but also to initiate facial muscle exercise and massage, along with techniques for voice preservation.

Nutritionists and pharmacists often make up the nutrition support team and are helpful in constructing enteral and parenteral approaches to calorie intake in a patient population that has the highest metabolic demands of any disease or injury known. The pharmacist is also helpful in providing antimicrobial protection and pain management.

The respiratory therapist is crucial in the management of patients with lung injury, which is currently a major cause of mortality in burn centers.

All members to this point have specific expertise in dealing with the physical damage that occurs after burn injury. Equally important is the psychological impact of such injuries, which is felt not only by the patients but also by their families. For this reason, a team of experienced psychiatrists and psychologists is necessary to guide patients and their families through the prolonged recovery period. This includes not only therapeutic sessions with individual patients and families but also support groups where patients and families in similar circumstances can meet and vocalize their thoughts, concerns, and fears in a constructive manner.

The physician is the last member of the burn team. Although the physician may be the coordinator or director of the burn center, he or she plays an equal role in the care of burn patients. It would be impossible for burn surgeons to obtain successful functional and cosmetic outcomes for these patients without the support of all the other members of the team.

INITIAL MANAGEMENT

At the scene, the initial concern of rescue personnel approaching an area where a burn injury has occurred should be safety. Firefighting and emergency personnel attempting to rescue burn patients constitute 1% of all burn victims. They are often required to work in areas that pose significant threats to their own safety. Once the scene is determined to be safe—electrical current shut off, protective clothing donned in situations of possible chemical contact, appropriate equipment used in situations of fire—emergency personnel can then focus on rescue and stabilization of burn victims prior to transporting them to a health care facility.

Rescue personnel should begin a rapid initial assessment once the scene is safe for themselves and the victim. This includes a quick evaluation of the size of the burns using the rule of nines, which divides the body surface into areas of 9% in order to estimate the size of the injury. In an adult, these areas are 9% for the head and neck, 18% for the anterior trunk, 18% for the posterior trunk, 9% for each arm, and 18% for each leg, with 1% remaining for the perineum. The body surface of a child differs from that of an adult; the head is much larger, and the lower extremities are smaller. Therefore, 14% is applied to each leg and 18% to the head and neck in children under the age of 6 years. Another simple way to determine body surface area is to use the palm of the patient's hand, which should equal approximately 1% of total body surface area. This method is useful in splattered scald burns or chemical burns with multiple small wounds, which make the use of the rule of nines somewhat difficult. The patient should be exposed well enough for the rescue personnel to determine the extent of burns as well as to look for associated injuries. Because this exposure may pose a risk to body temperature, it might best be done within the transport vehicle. The ABCs (airway, breathing, circulation) play a major role in

the evaluation of these patients; airway and breathing should be optimal and circulation supported. This may require beginning resuscitation using two large-bore intravenous lines, which can be placed through burned skin if necessary. Many of these patients may also have suffered blunt trauma and should therefore be treated appropriately with cervical collars and backboard stabilization.

CARE IN THE EMERGENCY CENTER

The most important point is that the initial evaluation of a burn victim after arrival in the emergency center should ignore the burned skin and look for more subtle and more life-threatening injuries. Burn patients, like all other trauma patients, should be approached in the standard way, beginning with a primary survey directed at investigation for and initial treatment of potentially life-threatening and rapidly fatal injuries. The burned skin does not fall into this category. Although a burn patient may have suffered only thermal injury, many situations involving a fire expose such individuals to other types of trauma such as blunt or penetrating wounds. Evaluation of the airway, breathing, and circulation is the first step, and the cervical spine must be stabilized until an injury is ruled out by x-rays. Evaluation of the burn wound and determination of its severity should probably be done as the last part of the secondary survey once life-threatening injuries and associated injuries have been evaluated.

One aspect of a burn injury that may be immediately life-threatening is the consequences of smoke inhalation. During the primary survey involving airway and breathing, the possibility of severe smoke inhalation must be ascertained and dealt with appropriately. Steps should already have been taken during transport in the form of oxygen administered by face mask. There are three components to smoke inhalation that produce a respiratory injury. First, the heat can damage the upper aerodigestive tract above the glottis, resulting in progressive edema and possible upper airway obstruction. The lungs have an incredible ability to warm or cool inhaled air below the vocal cords but are not as efficient in the supraglottic area. Since this aspect of smoke inhalation injury produces a progressive obstruction, the key to therapy is to maintain a patent airway and approach patients in a preventive or prophylactic manner. Therefore, we must be able to identify those who are at risk by their presenting signs and symptoms. Subtle evidence may include skin burns of the head and neck, soot around or in the mouth and nose, and erythema of the oral pharynx. Certainly, concern should arise for patients who have hoarseness, stridor, wheezing, or the acute development of coughing. The primary indicator from the history is an injury that occurred in an enclosed space where the patient was forced to breathe the heated smoke. Probably the most important physical finding is carbonaceous sputum. If the patient has a productive cough and carbon particles within the sputum, this individual is at significant risk for developing progressive airway obstruction. In patients who are at risk for developing heat-related edema of the upper airway, endotracheal intubation is the treatment of choice before airway compromise occurs. The endotracheal tube is kept in place until the edema resolves. This can be easily evaluated by deflating the endotracheal cuff and checking to see whether the patient can breathe around the endotracheal tube.

The second component of smoke inhalation injury is carbon monoxide poisoning. Carbon monoxide has an affinity for hemoglobin 280 times that of oxygen and therefore reduces the oxygen delivery to tissue, resulting in hypoxia. The half-life of carbon monoxide in individuals breathing room air (21% oxygen) is approximately 3½ to 4 hours. However, the half-life in those breathing 100% oxygen is 30 to 45 minutes. It is therefore crucial that prehospital emergency care providers administer oxygen immediately upon rescuing the patient from the scene of injury. There is also some subtle evidence that carbon monoxide alters cytochrome C systems, important energy pathways for cellular activity. This seems to occur in addition to the hypoxia, and carbon monoxide should therefore be considered a cytotoxin. The treatment of choice for carbon monoxide inhalation is oxygen.

The third component of injury from smoke inhalation is a pulmonary parenchymal poisoning due to the toxic fumes and chemicals that are produced. This begins to be subtly evident as airway irritation and increased mucus production develops. This progresses to loss of ciliary activity, mucosal sloughing, and eventual damage of the alveolocapillary membrane, ultimately leading to the development of adult respiratory distress syndrome (ARDS).

Once life-threatening injuries have been evaluated and the possibility of smoke inhalation determined, attention can then be directed toward the burn wound. In addition to determining the body surface area, as mentioned earlier, the depth of the wound needs to be evaluated as well.

First-degree burns involve only the cellular or epidermal layer. They heal quickly—within several days—usually by peeling, and rarely cause any systemic response. Burns into the dermis are second-degree burns and have recently been divided into superficial and deep partial-thickness injuries because the depth of the dermis is not consistent throughout. In the upper one-third, known as the papillary dermis, there are more structures containing replicating epithelial cells (skin appendages such as hair follicles) to provide for a rapid closure of the wound. In addition, there is loosely packed collagen, which helps reduce the possibility of scar formation. Burns in this upper one-third are usually uniform in color, pink to red. They are usually moist and painful and often heal within 3 weeks, rarely leaving much of a cosmetic or functional deficit. Burns in the deeper two-thirds of the dermis are known as deep partial-thickness wounds and involve the reticular dermis, where there are fewer structures containing new replicating cells and more densely packed collagen. These burns tend to be of multiple colors, less moist, and less painful because pain nerve endings have been destroyed. These burns take longer than 3 weeks to heal and often result in a hyperpigmented, hypertrophic scar. Burns of this depth may best be treated by excision and grafting, since today's techniques produce results that are much better than what the body can produce itself. Third-degree burns extend below both layers of the skin. They are dry and leathery, can be depressed or contracted, and are often painless. These wounds require some type of surgical procedure to heal, usually excision and grafting.

Once the initial assessment of the burn victim has been completed and the severity of the burn injury has been evaluated by body surface area and depth, preparations are made to begin stabilization treatment of the burn wound. If the patient is being prepared for transport to a burn center, initial care for the burn wound should consist of simple covering with a clean sheet or blanket. This is important for several reasons. First, covering the burn wound with creams, ointments, or solutions will reduce body temperature, especially since one of the major ways to control body temperature has now been destroyed. Hypothermia can have significant negative effects in a burn patient, increasing metabolic rate and requiring an increase in resuscitation needs. Second, application of creams and ointments will necessitate additional wound cleansing once the patient arrives at the burn center in order to evaluate the burn wound. Finally, the application of ointments and creams may eliminate the possibility of using biologic dressings as a means of wound support to speed healing.

RESUSCITATION

Resuscitation begins at the same time as the initial assessment of the injured patient and possibly even during prehospital transport. The first step is starting two large-bore intravenous lines, with lactated Ringer's as the solution of choice at a rate determined by the patient's initial needs, which can be anywhere from an estimated maintenance rate to wide-open infusion. Once in the emergency center, however, a more specific approach can be undertaken after the severity of the burn injury has been determined. Although there are many formulas available for resuscitation of burn patients, probably the most commonly used formula is the Parkland or Baxter formula, which uses 2 to 4 mL of lactated Ringer's multiplied by the patient's weight in kilograms and then by the percentage of body surface involved (2 to 4 mL × body weight (kg) × burned body surface (%). In other words, a patient who weighs 80 kg with a 50% burn using the 4-mL level would require 16 liters of lactated Ringer's over the first 24 hours. The first half is equally divided over the first 8 hours, starting from the time of the injury. This is important to remember, especially if a patient has gone several hours without resuscitation prior to arrival in the emergency center. In this situation, the hourly rate may need to be increased in order to complete half of the infusion within the first 8 hours from the time of the injury. The second half is delivered equally over the remaining 16 hours. The best means of evaluating adequate resuscitation and maintenance of perfusion to vital organs is urine output, with a goal of 30 to 50 mL per hour in adults or 1 to 2 mL per kg per hour in children under the age of 6 years or weighing less than 30 kg. In young children, an additional maintenance volume of intravenous fluid containing glucose is necessary due to their low glycogen stores, rapid release and utilization, and subsequent possibility of hypoglycemia. It is our practice to use D5 ¼ to ⅓ normal saline as the maintenance fluid for several reasons. More hypertonic fluid such as D5W can aggravate hyponatremia, which is often seen within the first 24 to 48 hours after resuscitation. In addition, the use of D5LR can sometimes be mistakenly increased as a resuscitation fluid and result in hyperglycemia.

The need for such resuscitation in burn patients is due to a shock state that develops from the injury. This shock is a form of hypovolemic shock. In contrast to other types of trauma patients, however, this is not a volume lost outside the body but rather a loss of intravascular volume to the extravascular-extracellular and intracellular spaces due to an alteration in capillary integrity caused by the massive amounts of injury-related hormones and enzymes released after a burn. This volume loss begins immediately after the injury and progresses in severity over the first 8 to 12 hours. Over the second 12 hours after injury, the loss plateaus and begins to reduce by the end of 24 hours as the capillary integrity returns toward normal. With a stabilization in capillary permeability over the second 24 hours, resuscitation approaches tend to change toward mobilization of extravascular fluid back to the intravascular space. This is often done with the use of large-molecule or colloid-like solutions such as albumin or Plasmanate. There is a lack of agreement about the approach to the second 24 hours of resuscitation. Several formulas are available to calculate the colloid needs during the second postinjury day.

There are those who believe that hypertonic saline solutions have an advantage over isotonic crystalloid solutions during the first 24 hours of resuscitation. These solutions are used in an attempt to reduce the volume of resuscitation required and therefore reduce the edema that develops after a burn injury. The high salt concentration of these fluids increases the salt volume in the extracellular space, causing an osmotic pull of fluid from the intracellular to extracellular compartments. Theoretically, this should improve cellular function, since most cells tend to swell slightly after a burn injury due to alterations in cell membrane potential and damage to the sodium-potassium pump. The intracellular space becomes a reservoir for additional resuscitation fluid for the intravascular space. It is hoped that the amount of resuscitation volume can be reduced,

therefore minimizing skeletal edema as well as edema in vital organs. Unfortunately, in most situations, hypertonic saline solutions perform no better compared with isotonic solutions and may cause additional morbidity. Several recent studies, including our own experience, have shown an increased risk of renal failure in patients treated with hypertonic saline solutions. Another problem with hypertonic saline solutions is that patients require close, continuous monitoring by both nurses and physicians while the fluid is infusing. This alone is a disadvantage in comparison with a simple-to-use, readily available, inexpensive fluid such as lactated Ringer's.

BURN WOUND MANAGEMENT

Treatment of damaged skin from a burn injury is usually centered around the application of an ointment or cream with antimicrobial capabilities. It is definitely true that wounds heal more rapidly in a moist environment. If the burned skin is allowed to dry and desiccate, healing comes to a halt. However, a wound that is kept too moist may macerate, which also retards healing.

Reduction of bacterial colonization and risk of infection is accomplished by dressing changes, cleansing of the wound, and the application of topical antimicrobial ointments and creams. By far the most effective means of reducing bacterial colonization is wound cleansing, which is done by showering the injured area and sponging or wiping with a mild soap. The antimicrobial effects of creams and ointments may help slightly, but they are not as important as débriding the wound during dressing changes.

Antimicrobial ointments and creams are also known to delay wound healing. Their toxic effect on replicating epithelial cells can range from mild to severe, and even the most gentle antibiotic cream can delay epithelial cell replication to some degree. There is also some evidence that these antimicrobial creams and ointments hinder the production and deposition of ground substance, such as chondroitin sulfate, which acts as the glue that allows keratinocytes, fibroblasts, and myofibroblasts to migrate and stick to the open wound. The faster the damaged skin can be placed in a cream or ointment that provides an appropriate moist environment without the healing retardation of antimicrobial creams and ointments, the quicker the wound will heal. For this reason, once we are sure that the wound is well débrided and the risk of infection minimal, we use a water-soluble petrolatum ointment.

Biologic dressings are quite useful and effective in burns that are of uniform depth and of superficial partial thickness. A biologic dressing should be applied to the wound as soon after the injury as possible and should adhere to the wound while healing occurs underneath. The characteristics of a biologic dressing should be similar to skin, in that it reduces pain, reduces temperature and fluid loss, protects against invading bacteria, and speeds healing. Probably the most frequently used biologic dressing in the past was pigskin, which is easily applied, covered for 24 hours, and reinspected to ensure adherence to the wound. Once adherence has occurred, the pigskin and wound can be left open and can be treated like the patient's own skin. Clothes can be worn over the area, and the patient can bathe without difficulty. There are now many synthetic and semisynthetic substances, such as Biobrane (Dow B. Hickam, Inc.) or SkinTemp (BioCore, Inc.), that work similarly to pigskin.

All small third-degree burns and many deep partial-thickness burns are treated with excision and grafting. The most common approach is a tangential or sequential excision of the burn wound down to healthy tissue, usually deep dermis or subcutaneous fat. A split-thickness piece of skin, usually 0.0012 to 0.0015 inch thick, is applied once hemostasis is obtained. This can be meshed to allow the donor skin to expand and prevent fluid accumulation. However, burns of less than 5 to 10% body surface area might best be covered with a sheet graft for improved cosmetic outcome. A dressing is then applied and affixed to the wound to apply moderate pressure, which improves graft take and prevents any shearing forces that may cause graft loss. It is the job of the surgeon to protect the graft with a dressing that allows the patient's rapid return to therapy activities postoperatively, even while graft adherence is taking place. A dressing should be constructed that allows even patients with lower extremity wounds to mobilize quickly.

A recent advance in the care of deep burn wounds is the use of cultured keratinocytes. Within the first 24 to 48 hours after admission, a 1- to 2-cm^2 area of full-thickness skin is excised, usually from the groin or axilla, and the remaining wound is closed primarily. The full-thickness piece of skin can be then digested in the tissue culture laboratory, collecting and saving the viable replicating keratinocytes. Over a 15- to 17-day period, approximately 15 to 20% of body surface area can be grown from each 1 cm^2 of skin. In addition, it is now possible to develop cultured keratinocytes anchored to a dermal base. This improves its durability and makes handling easier at the time of application. It may also improve graft take.

REHABILITATION THERAPY

The rehabilitation phase in the care of a burn patient differs somewhat from that in other types of injuries, in which rehabilitation is usually a second step after the acute trauma has healed. In burn patients, rehabilitation or therapy begins from the time of the injury. This is crucial to maintain strength and mobility in order to shorten an already long road to recovery. The physical and occupational therapists are vital in this phase, as mentioned earlier. It is important that they play a role in the assessment of the burn patient and develop a therapy program within the first 24 hours after injury. The addition of vigorous therapy to appropriate wound care can produce an outcome that is quite satisfactory for both the patient and the individuals caring for him or her.

DISTURBANCES DUE TO COLD

method of
JEFFRY P. McKINZIE, M.D., and
KEITH D. WRENN, M.D.
Vanderbilt University Medical Center
Nashville, Tennessee

Exposure to cold may cause illness in several ways. Cold injury may be limited predominantly to local tissue effects (as seen in frostbite, immersion foot, or chilblains) or may result in manifestations of systemic hypothermia. Patients frequently present with a combination of local and systemic signs and symptoms. Although cold injury is often anticipated in persons with a known exposure to a cold environment, it may also occur in surprisingly temperate climatic conditions. A careful history and physical examination coupled with a high index of suspicion will help the clinician avoid misdiagnosis, especially when exposure to a cold environment is not obviously apparent.

Many predisposing factors have been identified for the development of cold injury. Important environmental factors include low ambient temperature, prolonged duration of exposure, high humidity, and high wind chill factor. Predisposing patient characteristics include altered mental status of any cause (including intoxicants, head injury, or psychiatric disorders), hypovolemia, malnutrition, fatigue, lack of acclimatization, and lack of adequate shelter and protective clothing. Persons at the extremes of age are also predisposed because of impaired thermoregulatory mechanisms. Societal factors such as the increased prevalence of homelessness and the increased interest in cold weather recreational activities also come into play. Predisposing conditions that contribute mainly to local tissue injury include diabetes mellitus, arteriosclerosis, prior cold injury, and other causes of peripheral vascular disease or peripheral neuropathy.

LOCAL COLD INJURY

Local cold injury may be divided into two categories based on the degree of local tissue hypothermia: freezing injuries and nonfreezing injuries. Freezing injuries include the various stages of frostbite. Nonfreezing injuries include immersion foot and chilblains.

Frostbite

Frostbite is caused by the cooling of body tissues to the point of ice crystal formation. Such tissue freezing generally results from exposure to extremely cold environmental temperatures for a period of several hours. Historically, frostbite has been a significant cause of morbidity and mortality during cold weather military campaigns. Vivid descriptions of frostbite and hypothermia were recorded by Baron de Larrey, the surgeon-in-chief of Napoleon's Grand

Army, during the retreat from Moscow in the winter of 1812 to 1813. More recently, over 1 million cases of frostbite injury were recorded during the two World Wars and the Korean War. Today, frostbite remains a significant medical problem for both military and civilian populations, especially in cold climate regions. A 12-year review of frostbite in the civilian population of Saskatchewan, Canada, demonstrated that the "typical" frostbite patient is a male aged 20 to 50 years. The most common body parts affected, in decreasing order of incidence, are lower extremities only (47%), combined lower and upper extremities (31%), upper extremities only (19%), and face or trunk only (3%).

Pathophysiology

Extensive laboratory and clinical observations have clarified the pathophysiologic events leading to frostbite injury. Initially, a cold-induced vasoconstriction occurs followed by vasodilatation, that is, the "hunting response." Arteriovenous anastomoses in the cooled extremity allow shunting of blood around capillary beds back to the central circulation, as the body attempts to preserve core temperature and perfusion of vital organs. This results in more rapid cooling and ischemia in peripheral tissues. As cooling continues, ice crystal formation occurs in the extracellular fluid space, causing increased extracellular osmotic pressure, diffusion of water across cell membranes, and cellular dehydration. Enlarging extracellular ice crystals also cause direct structural cellular damage. As freezing continues, protein denaturation and destruction of essential enzymes occur. Cell membrane damage and increased cell wall permeability result in critical endothelial cell injury and impaired microvascular function.

When the frozen part is thawed, vasodilatation and capillary leakage occur, resulting in tissue edema. Erythrocyte sludging and platelet aggregation cause microvascular stasis that may progress to vessel thrombosis and tissue ischemia. Concurrently, the arachadonic acid inflammatory cascade is activated with release of thromboxane and prostaglandins. These and other inflammatory mediators, such as oxygen free radicals, produce further tissue injury. The combined injurious effects of tissue freezing, inflammation, and ischemia may ultimately result in tissue necrosis and gangrene.

Clinical Manifestations

In the past, the classification of frostbite was similar to that of thermal burns, based on the extent and depth of tissue injury, that is, first-, second-, third-, and fourth-degree frostbite. This classification scheme was problematic since it is generally difficult or impossible for the clinician to accurately assess the full extent of tissue injury at the time of initial evaluation. Therefore, a simpler classification is now in use that allows the clinician in the acute setting to more easily divide frostbite injury into one of two types: superficial or deep.

The precursor to frostbite is frostnip. The onset of frostnip is signaled by the sudden loss of cold sensation in the affected part, which instead feels numb and painful. The skin is cold, may be blanched or flushed, and remains pliable. Frostnip is completely reversible with immediate treatment by removing the affected part from the cold environment and rewarming it. Rewarming results in tingling, pain, and redness that quickly resolve.

Superficial frostbite involves freezing of the skin and subcutaneous tissues. The skin is cold and waxy-white and does not blanch. The frozen part is usually anesthetic. With thawing, the area becomes painful and flushed as reperfusion occurs. Edema develops rapidly and is often accompanied within the first 24 hours by the development of clear bullae filled with serous fluid. If these bullae are left undisturbed, they are gradually reabsorbed, leaving a dark, dry eschar. The presence of the eschar may give the impression of deep underlying gangrene. After several weeks, however, the eschar begins to spontaneously separate, revealing shiny red epithelial tissue beneath it. This "new" skin is delicate and very sensitive to heat and cold and may perspire excessively.

Deep frostbite involves not only the skin and subcutaneous tissues but also muscle, tendons, neurovascular structures, and bone. The frozen part is anesthetic and has a hard woodlike consistency. The area is typically ashen-gray, cyanotic, or mottled in appearance and may remain this way even after rewarming. Edema develops but bullae may be absent or may develop in a delayed fashion. Unlike the clear bullae seen with superficial frostbite, these bullae are filled with hemorrhagic exudate, denoting a more severe injury to the subdermal vascular plexus. The bullae gradually dry, forming a hard, black eschar. Over a period of weeks to months, nonviable tissue becomes mummified and a line of demarcation develops between healthy and necrotic tissue.

The true extent of tissue loss is often not apparent until several weeks after the frostbite injury. Two factors that may accelerate this process, however, are (1) freeze-thaw-refreeze injury, and (2) infection. Extensive clinical experience has shown that thawing of a frostbitten part with subsequent refreezing results in more tissue destruction. Patients with this injury pattern rapidly develop gangrene. Likewise, infection superimposed on frostbite injury accelerates the development of gangrene.

Diagnosis

Frostbite is a clinical diagnosis that may be challenging at times, particularly if a history of cold exposure is not readily apparent. Less than 20% of frostbite victims present for medical care with the involved body parts still frozen. Thawing may occur spontaneously or through active intervention by the victim prior to arrival. An accurate history may be difficult to obtain due to concurrent altered mental status, peripheral neuropathy, or other coexisting conditions. Such conditions may make the patient unaware of the extent of cold exposure or unable to relate such an exposure to medical personnel. Thus, a high index of suspicion is required.

Treatment

The first priority in the treatment of frostbite is preservation of life. Patients with frostbite often have coexisting systemic hypothermia and may have other potentially life-threatening injuries or conditions. Therefore, initial assessment and resuscitation must be directed at supporting the ABCs (airway, breathing, and circulation) and treating immediate threats to life. The victim should be removed from the cold environment as soon as possible and the frozen part should be protected to avoid further injury. Due to the disastrous effects of freeze-thaw-refreeze injury, rewarming of the frozen part should be delayed until there is no risk of refreezing. It is far better for a hiker to finish a hike with frostbite and then seek definitive care than to thaw the frozen extremities on the trail and experience refreezing during completion of the journey.

If the body part is still frozen, it should be thawed in a circulating warm water bath carefully maintained at a temperature between 38° and 42° C (100.4° and 108° F). A whirlpool or Hubbard tank is ideal if available. Temperatures exceeding 42° C may cause secondary thermal injury and should be avoided. The affected part should not be rubbed or massaged during rewarming since this may exacerbate tissue injury. Rapid rewarming by the described method usually requires 10 to 30 minutes for complete thawing. Narcotic analgesics may be required since patients often experience throbbing, burning pain during and after thawing. Thawing is complete when the distal tip of the affected part flushes, signaling reperfusion. Rapid rewarming in warm water is superior to other rewarming methods and results in greater tissue preservation. Potentially harmful techniques include ice water massage, snow massage, and use of excessive dry heat (e.g., campfire, motor exhaust). All these techniques have been popular in the past and are still occasionally used by frostbite victims attempting self-treatment.

Complications that may be encountered during rewarming include exacerbation of systemic hypothermia and disturbances of electrolyte or acid-base balance. These may develop due to the rush of cold acidemic blood from the injured part back into the central circulation during thawing. Core temperature, acid-base status, and electrolytes should be carefully monitored in anticipation of these problems.

After thawing, patients should be admitted for further care in all but the mildest cases of frostbite. The injured extremities should be kept elevated to minimize edema. Whirlpool baths are used twice daily for 20 minutes at temperatures of 32° to 35° C (90° to 95° F) to gently clean and débride the area. Surgical soaps, such as povidone-iodine, hexachlorophene, or chlorhexidine gluconate, can be added to the whirlpool solution to prevent superficial bacterial overgrowth. Gentle range of motion of involved joints is facilitated during hydrotherapy and helps to prevent contractures. Following whirlpool therapy, the area is gently blotted dry, elevated, and left open to the air. Injured digits should be separated with sterile gauze, cotton, or lamb's wool to prevent maceration. The use of ointments or moist dressings is generally not recommended.

Some experts advocate leaving blisters intact since they provide a sterile biologic dressing for the underlying injured tissues. Using this approach, blisters are only débrided if they rupture or become infected. Others favor routine blister débridement or aspiration since blister fluid contains thromboxane and other inflammatory mediators that may exacerbate tissue injury. Some advocate use of topical aloe vera, a thromboxane inhibitor. Systemic thromboxane inhibitors, such as ibuprofen or aspirin, may also be used. Tetanus prophylaxis should be administered when appropriate. Systemic antibiotics are generally unnecessary in the absence of infection. Vasoconstrictive agents, including nicotine, should be avoided.

Surgical treatment of frostbite should initially be conservative. Escharotomy may be required when hardened eschar prevents adequate range of motion of involved joints. In addition, fasciotomy is occasionally necessary due to the development of compartment syndrome. Surgical débridement and amputation, however, should be delayed until the demarcation between viable and nonviable tissue is clear. This may require as long as 30 to 90 days. Angiography or technetium-99m scintigraphy may be helpful in assessing perfusion of the injured area. Early amputation is performed only in the presence of obvious septic gangrene.

Numerous experimental therapies have been suggested for the treatment of frostbite. Various drug regimens have included antithrombotic agents such as heparin and low-molecular-weight dextran, thrombolytic agents, and vasodilators such as phenoxybenzamine (Dibenzyline) or calcium channel blockers. Other experimental treatments include sympathectomy (medical or surgical) and hyperbaric oxygen therapy. None of these therapies has been shown to consistently enhance tissue salvage.

Immersion Foot

Immersion foot is a clinical syndrome caused by prolonged exposure of the feet to a wet and usually occlusive environment. This poorly understood disorder is plagued by a confusing nomenclature containing many colorful pseudonyms such as "trench foot," "jungle rot," "swamp foot," "paddy foot," and "sea boot." Historically, immersion foot accounted for huge numbers of military casualties in both World Wars, the Korean War, and the Vietnam conflict. More recently, the disorder has become increasingly common among the homeless civilian population.

Immersion foot is a spectrum of disease, the presentation of which depends mainly on the duration of exposure, the temperature of the medium, and the susceptibility of the victim. As originally described, "immersion foot" refers to the injury pattern seen with exposure to cold but nonfreezing water. Subsequently, clinical variants related to warm water exposure have been described. "Warm water immersion foot" refers to injury to the soles of the feet that occurs with immersion in relatively warm water, 15° to 32° C (59° to 90° F) for up to 72 hours. The term "tropical immersion foot" is used to denote longer periods of warm water immersion with resultant injury to not only the soles but also the dorsum of the feet.

Pathophysiology

The pathologic hallmark of immersion foot is waterlogging of the thick stratum corneum of the soles of the feet. As much as 1 to 2 grams of water may be absorbed per hour by the foot, with greater absorption occurring in freshwater than in salt water. The permeability coefficient of the thicker plantar skin is ten times greater than that of the thinner dorsal skin. In addition, the thinner dorsal skin is able to more efficiently shunt water to the circulation and the thick plantar skin retains more water within the stratum corneum. Therefore, injury to the plantar skin develops more rapidly and is usually more extensive than injury to the dorsal skin. Biopsies of affected skin reveal thickening and fragmentation of the stratum corneum, capillary narrowing, edema, and lymphocytic vasculitis within the dermis. In classic immersion foot, exposure to cold water results in local tissue hypothermia that further increases tissue injury. Intense cold-induced vasoconstriction results in tissue ischemia. In severe cases, intravascular thrombosis, fat necrosis, wallerian degeneration of peripheral nerves, and even gangrene may result.

Clinical Manifestations

The threshold for development of signs and symptoms depends to some extent on the temperature of the water. In warmer water, symptoms usually develop after approximately 48 hours of exposure, whereas in colder water injury generally occurs earlier. The soles of the feet are usually involved within 72 hours and the dorsal skin may withstand injury for over 72 hours in warm water.

Itching is one of the earliest symptoms of immersion foot and may precede visible signs of injury. As the syndrome progresses, the patient usually presents with cool, swollen, painful feet. The soles are white, wrinkled, and very tender to palpation. Ambulation may be difficult or impossible due to pain. Erythema and abrasions may be seen over pressure points from shoes or socks. Femoral adenopathy and fever are common. Involvement of the dorsum of the foot usually takes the form of discrete erythematous papules with associated edema and a sharp line of demarcation relative to the level of submersion. This is the sine qua non of "tropical immersion foot," which generally denotes exposure in warm water for greater than 72 hours.

Although the initial appearance of the foot is similar, significant differences exist between "warm water immersion foot" and "classic immersion foot" seen with colder exposures. Four distinct phases are described with cold exposure. The first phase is the exposure, followed by the prehyperemic phase in which the foot is cold, numb, cyanotic, and pulseless. This stage usually lasts for a few hours and is followed by the hyperemic stage in which the feet are warm with bounding pulses and increasing swelling. Pain and blister formation occur during this stage. Gangrene is not uncommon. The hyperemic phase may last for up to 10 weeks. Finally, there is the posthyperemic stage during which cold sensitivity and hyperhidrosis are seen despite a normal appearance of the feet. This stage may last many years. With colder exposures, the extent of initial injury and the incidence of long-term sequelae increase.

The role of infection in the pathogenesis of immersion foot is controversial. The systemic febrile response with associated femoral lymphadenopathy suggests a possible infectious component. Bacterial colonization with various gram-negative organisms such as *Pseudomonas* and *Klebsiella* has been noted. These organisms generally reflect the flora of the water in which the feet were immersed. The prompt response of most cases to conservative management without antibiotics, however, implies that bacterial infection is a minor component of the syndrome. Cases of secondary bacterial infections, such as streptococcal cellulitis, have been reported. Fungal pathogens do not appear to play a role in the syndrome.

Treatment

The treatment of uncomplicated immersion foot is conservative. The cornerstones of therapy are bed rest, elevation of the legs, and air-drying at room temperature. Nonsteroidal anti-inflammatory agents may be used for pain control. Most cases respond rapidly to these measures with noticeable improvement within 24 to 48 hours and complete resolution within 1 to 2 weeks. Antibiotics appear to play little role in the treatment of immersion foot unless secondary cellulitis or gangrene is present.

The key to preventing immersion foot is good foot care with adequate time for air-drying. Keeping the feet dry at least 8 hours out of every day is optimal. Boots are better than tennis shoes in preventing the syndrome. However, footwear with thermal insulation or waterproof material may make the situation worse by causing excessive perspiration and maceration of the feet. In situations where prolonged exposure to moisture is unavoidable (e.g., military maneuvers), daily application of silicone grease to the soles of the feet has been shown to be helpful.

Chilblains (Pernio)

Chilblains, or pernio, is a cold-induced inflammatory vasculitis caused by prolonged exposure to a nonfreezing cold environment. The condition is most common in women and children but can be seen in all ages, both sexes, and all races. The incidence of chilblains is highest in areas with cold, damp climates, including certain coastal areas of the United

States. Because many physicians are unfamiliar with the disorder, misdiagnosis is common and may give rise to unnecessary diagnostic testing or inappropriate therapies.

The patient with chilblains typically presents during late fall or winter with bluish-purple maculopapular lesions on acral skin areas, such as the hands, feet, and face. Occasionally, overlying blisters, erosions, or ulcers may be seen. Histologic examination of biopsy specimens reveals lymphocytic perivascular cuffing with endothelial edema. Pruritus or burning pain at the site of the lesions is often reported. The lesions usually resolve spontaneously in 1 to 3 weeks but recurrent episodes are common in susceptible individuals. The differential diagnosis includes Raynaud's syndrome, Kaposi's sarcoma, lupus erythematosus, septic emboli, atheromatous emboli, and polycythemia vera. These conditions can usually be excluded by history and clinical findings with occasional selected laboratory tests.

Treatment is generally conservative and supportive. Adequate protective clothing and avoidance of cold exposure will speed recovery as well as prevent future attacks. Judicious use of local heat, gentle massage, and application of lubricants to keep the skin supple may also be helpful. A recent study supports the use of nifedipine (Procardia)* 20 mg three times daily as an adjunctive therapy. Nifedipine appears to reduce the pain associated with chilblains and to speed resolution of the lesions.

Systemic Hypothermia

Hypothermia is defined as the lowering of core body temperature to 35° C (95° F) or less. Although hypothermia is a preventable condition, approximately 780 persons die from exposure to cold each year in the United States. Death rates from hypothermia vary significantly by age, sex, and race. Nearly half of all hypothermia-related deaths occur among persons over 65 years of age. The male/female ratio of hypothermia deaths is almost 3 : 1. Differences in hypothermia mortality by race probably reflect socioeconomic factors, such as nutrition and access to adequate shelter. The death rate for nonwhite persons is almost four times higher than that for whites.

Hypothermia can be classified etiologically into two categories: primary and secondary. Primary or accidental hypothermia occurs when the body's normal thermoregulatory mechanisms of heat conservation are overwhelmed by environmental cold stress. Primary hypothermia includes immersion and nonimmersion exposures. Examples include the inadequately clothed hiker caught in a blizzard, the cold water near-drowning victim, and the homeless person without access to adequate shelter. Secondary hypothermia occurs when the body's thermoregulatory mechanisms are impaired because of some preexisting condition and are unable to respond adequately to cold stress. Disorders that predispose to hypothermia include endocrine diseases (diabetes mellitus, hypothyroidism, hypoadrenalism, hypopituitarism), malnutrition, cardiovascular diseases (myocardial infarction, vascular insufficiency), erythrodermas (burns, psoriasis, exfoliative dermatitis), neurologic diseases (head injury, stroke, tumor, spinal cord injury), drugs or toxins (alcohol, phenothiazines, antidepressants, barbiturates), and multiple trauma. Iatrogenic hypothermia may also be seen in postoperative patients, following massive infusions of cold crystalloid or blood or due to overzealous treatment of heat stroke.

Thermoregulation

Heat loss occurs through a combination of four mechanisms: radiation, conduction, convection, and evaporation. Normally, 55 to 65% of the body's heat loss occurs through radiation to the surrounding environment. Radiative heat losses are increased when a large temperature gradient exists between the body and the surrounding environment or when a large body surface area is exposed. Evaporation normally accounts for about 30% of heat loss, with about 25% occurring via the skin and 5% via the airway. Conduction is the transfer of heat by direct contact. Because air possesses poor thermal conductivity, conduction accounts for only about 15% of heat loss in a dry environment. Conductive heat loss increases dramatically, however, with wet clothing or cold water immersion since there is a 20- to 30-fold increase in the thermal conductivity of water over that of air. Convection, caused by cooling air currents, is normally a minor component of heat loss but can increase greatly in a windy environment. The "wind chill factor" is a quantitative measure reflecting the potential magnitude of convective heat loss.

Thermoregulation is controlled by nuclei in the preoptic anterior hypothalamus that act as the body's "thermostat." When exposure to a cold environment occurs, impulses from cutaneous thermoreceptors are transmitted to the hypothalamus via the spinothalamic tract. Temperature receptors in the hypothalamus also react directly to blood temperature. In response to the cold stimulus, the hypothalamus activates the sympathetic nervous system causing release of norepinephrine, increased heart rate, and peripheral vasoconstriction. Stimulation of the extrapyramidal tract causes shivering, which can increase the basal metabolic rate two to five times. Stimulation of the anterior pituitary gland by the hypothalamus indirectly causes increased release of thyroxine and adrenal steroids, which further increases metabolic rate and thermogenesis. Adaptive behavioral responses also occur that cause the individual to seek a warmer environment. The overall physiologic effect is an increase in heat production and a decrease in heat loss.

Pathophysiology

Hypothermia may be classified as mild, moderate, or severe based on the magnitude of decline in the

---

*Not FDA-approved for this indication.

patient's core body temperature and the associated physiologic effects. In mild hypothermia, body temperature ranges from 32° to 35° C (90° to 95° F). At this stage, an initial increase in metabolic rate occurs with tachycardia, tachypnea, increased muscle tone, vasoconstriction, and maximal shivering thermogenesis. Subsequently, a progressive slowing of bodily functions results in bradycardia, hypoventilation, depressed cerebral metabolism, and decreased oxygen utilization. Cold-induced diuresis causes decreased circulating blood volume and progressive hemoconcentration.

Moderate hypothermia, from 28° to 32° C (82° to 90° F), causes a further decline in basal metabolic rate and bodily functions. Hyporeflexia, dilated pupils, depressed level of consciousness, and associated electroencephalographic changes are seen. Cardiac output falls and cardiac arrhythmias become increasingly common. Shivering typically ceases at 31° C (88° F) and the patient becomes essentially poikilothermic.

In severe hypothermia, below 28° C (82° F), cardiopulmonary and neurologic functions are further depressed. Coma, peripheral arreflexia, and loss of ocular reflexes are seen. Cardiac output declines by more than 50% and susceptibility to ventricular fibrillation is increased. Major acid-base disturbances are generally present. At 19° C (66° F) the electroencephalogram becomes flat and at 18° C (64° F) asystole develops.

Clinical Manifestations

Early findings in mild hypothermia may be subtle. Vague symptoms such as dizziness, fatigue, joint stiffness, nausea, and pruritus are common. Shivering is usually present except in elderly patients. Initial increases in heart rate and respiratory rate are replaced by bradycardia and bradypnea. Bronchorrhea and bronchospasm may be seen. The skin is pale and cool due to intense peripheral vasoconstriction. Early mental status changes include lethargy, flat affect, impaired judgment, and mild confusion. As neurologic function progressively deteriorates, the victim exhibits loss of fine motor coordination, ataxia, slurred speech, and maladaptive behavior such as paradoxical undressing.

In moderate hypothermia, further depression of the level of consciousness produces hallucinations and stupor. A common electrocardiographic finding is the Osborn (J) wave, an upward deflection occurring at the junction of the QRS complex and the ST segment (Figure 1). J waves may be seen at any temperature below 32° C (90° F) and become more pronounced as body temperature declines further. Atrial fibrillation and other dysrhythmias are also common. Hyporeflexia, pupillary dilatation, and loss of protective airway reflexes may occur.

In severe hypothermia, peripheral pulses and blood pressure may become imperceptible due to the combined effects of hypotension and vasoconstriction. The patient is usually comatose and may appear clinically dead with fixed and dilated pupils, loss of ocular reflexes, no response to noxious stimuli, and stiff extremities ("pseudo–rigor mortis").

Evaluation

Appropriate treatment of the hypothermic patient requires the ability to accurately determine core body temperature. Low-reading rectal probe and infrared tympanic thermometers are widely available and easy to use. Rectal temperature may lag behind true core temperature and is influenced by lower extremity temperature and probe placement. Insertion of the probe in cold feces or to a depth less than 15 cm may yield inaccurate results. Tympanic temperature correlates well with hypothalamic temperature and changes most rapidly with variations in core temperature. An esophageal probe may be used in the intubated patient. Bladder probes attached to a urinary catheter are also available.

Laboratory evaluation should include arterial blood gases to assess the adequacy of oxygenation and ventilation and determine acid-base status. Hypothermia shifts the oxyhemoglobin-dissociation curve to the left, causing decreased availability of oxygen to the body's tissues. A combined respiratory and metabolic acidosis is commonly seen due to hypoventilation, decreased tissue perfusion, and increased lactate production. Arterial blood gas values do not need to be corrected for the patient's lower body temperature since blood gas analyzers automatically warm the sample to 37° C (98.6° F). Additional routine laboratory studies should include a complete blood count, electrolytes, glucose, blood urea nitrogen, creatinine, prothrombin and partial thromboplastin times, amylase, liver function tests, toxicologic screen, and urinalysis. An electrocardiogram and chest radiograph should also be obtained. These studies will establish a baseline and will assist the clinician in detecting and treating the various complications of hypothermia.

Treatment

Initial treatment of the hypothermic patient should include a careful assessment of the ABCs (airway, breathing, circulation) with appropriate interventions as needed. Despite prior concerns regarding precipitation of cardiac arrhythmias, gentle endotracheal intubation after preoxygenation has been shown to be safe and should be performed when necessary. Slow, faint pulses may be difficult to detect but should be carefully sought, and cardiac monitoring should be initiated as soon as possible. Unnecessary initiation of cardiopulmonary resuscitation in the patient with spontaneous circulation, however faint, may be detrimental since the hypothermic myocardium is extremely irritable and susceptible to ventricular fibrillation.

Supplemental oxygen, an intravenous line, and continuous core body temperature monitoring should be initiated. An empirical intravenous fluid challenge of 250 to 500 mL of crystalloid may be beneficial since many patients are hypovolemic due to cold-induced diuresis and other factors. Intravenous flu-

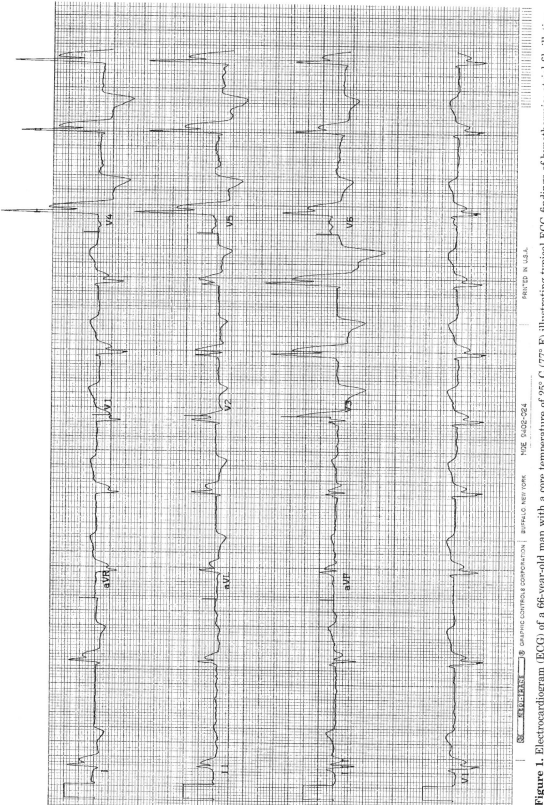

Figure 1. Electrocardiogram (ECG) of a 66-year-old man with a core temperature of 25° C (77° F) illustrating typical ECG findings of hypothermia: atrial fibrillation with slow ventricular response, prolonged QT interval, and Osborn (J) waves.

ids should be heated to 40° to 42° C (104° to 107.6° F) prior to administration. A 1-liter plastic bag of crystalloid typically requires 2 minutes on high power in a microwave oven to reach the proper temperature range. Warmed intravenous fluids help prevent further iatrogenic heat loss but do not provide sufficient heat to contribute significantly to rewarming. A nasogastric tube (following endotracheal intubation) and indwelling bladder catheter should be placed in moderate or severe cases. Measures to prevent further heat loss, including the removal of wet clothing, should be instituted in all patients. Gentle handling and minimal patient movement are important to avoid precipitation of arrhythmias. A careful history, when possible, and thorough examination should be performed to determine the presence of any precipitating factors or coexisting conditions that require specific treatment (e.g., traumatic injuries, hypothyroidism, or addisonian crisis).

As core temperature falls, the body becomes progressively less responsive to the pharmacologic actions of various medications (e.g., insulin, digoxin, pressors). In addition, decreased hepatic metabolism and increased protein binding can contribute to the accumulation of excessive medication levels that may produce toxicity when rewarming occurs. Therefore, excessive pharmacologic manipulation should be avoided and nonessential medications should be delayed until after rewarming.

Multiple rewarming modalities are available and can be divided into three categories: passive rewarming, active external rewarming, and active core rewarming. The choice of rewarming techniques to be used for a particular patient may vary depending on the severity of hypothermia, the presence of cardiovascular instability, the experience of the clinician, and the availability of specialized resources. Several rewarming methods may be used simultaneously to hasten the rewarming process.

Passive rewarming allows the patient to spontaneously rewarm utilizing the body's intrinsic heat production without the application of additional heat. The patient is kept dry and insulated with blankets to prevent further heat loss. Gradual rewarming occurs primarily due to shivering thermogenesis at a rate of about 0.5° C (0.9° F) per hour. Passive rewarming is suitable for the hemodynamically stable patient with mild hypothermia who is metabolically capable of heat generation. Passive rewarming may also be used as an adjunct to active rewarming methods in moderate and severe hypothermia.

Active external rewarming consists of the application of exogenous heat to the surface of the body—including the use of warm packs, heating blankets, radiant heat, and warm water immersion. Active external rewarming is noninvasive and most techniques are easy to perform. Disadvantages include the risk of thermal burns due to excessive heat application, the difficulty of monitoring the patient with certain techniques (e.g., warm water immersion), and core temperature afterdrop. Afterdrop is the continuing decrease in core body temperature that occasionally occurs after rewarming is initiated. The postulated cause of this phenomenon is peripheral vasodilatation that occurs with external rewarming, allowing the return of cooled blood from the periphery to the body's core. Because afterdrop may cause clinically significant deterioration of the hypothermic patient, this phenomenon should be anticipated and prevented whenever possible. Thus, active external rewarming should be used as the primary rewarming method only in patients with mild hypothermia who are hemodynamically stable. In more severe cases, application of external heat to the thorax only (while allowing the extremities to rewarm passively) may lessen the incidence of core temperature afterdrop, particularly when used in conjunction with core rewarming techniques.

Active core rewarming techniques produce the most rapid rewarming times but tend to be more invasive and carry various risks that must be considered. Core rewarming carries the advantage of preferentially rewarming the heart and other vital organs prior to rewarming the extremities. Active core rewarming should be used in hypothermic patients who are hemodynamically unstable, who have a core body temperature lower than 32° C (90° F), or who fail to respond to more conservative rewarming methods. One simple and safe method is the use of heated humidified air via face mask or endotracheal tube. A heating nebulizer or ventilator should be adjusted to heat inspired gases to 40° to 45° C (104° to 113° F) at the mouth. This approach prevents further evaporative heat loss via the airway and raises body temperature an average of 1° to 2° C per hour. In moderate-to-severe hypothermia, airway rewarming may be used as an adjunct to other more rapid rewarming techniques. Peritoneal lavage with warmed potassium-free dialysate (40° to 45° C) is a more invasive but effective approach, producing rewarming rates ranging from 2° to 4° C per hour. This technique is facilitated by the insertion of two catheters allowing continuous infusion and withdrawal of dialysate at a rate of about 6 liters per hour. Continuous pleural irrigation with warmed saline via two large-bore thoracostomy tubes is another method that has been used with success. Some experts advise inserting chest tubes on the right side only to reduce the chance of precipitating ventricular fibrillation. Continuous irrigation of the stomach, colon, or bladder with warmed fluids has limited rewarming benefit due to the small surface areas available for heat exchange.

Extracorporeal rewarming provides the most rapid and efficient means of rewarming. A standard cardiopulmonary bypass circuit can achieve rewarming rates of 1° to 2° C every 3 to 5 minutes. Successful resuscitation with complete clinical recovery has been reported using cardiopulmonary bypass even after prolonged cardiac arrest unresponsive to standard resuscitative and rewarming measures. Hemodialysis is another option that has been used with success, although rewarming is slower because flow rates are lower than that achieved with cardiopulmonary bypass. The use of countercurrent fluid warmers to provide continuous arteriovenous rewarming is also being investigated. Depending on the technique, extracorporeal rewarming can provide not only rapid rewarming rates but also varying amounts of hemodynamic and electrolyte control. Disadvantages of extracorporeal rewarming include the need for specialized equipment and personnel and the need for heparinization with its associated complications (particularly in the patient with traumatic injury).

Resuscitation of the hypothermic patient in cardiac arrest deserves a special note since it varies from the standard resuscitation protocols. At core temperatures below 30° C (<86° F), the heart is usually unresponsive to cardioactive drugs, pacemaker stimulation, and defibrillation. In the presence of ventricular fibrillation, if standard defibrillation (up to three shocks at 200, 300, and 360 joules) is unsuccessful, a single dose of 10 mg per kg of bretylium (Bretylol) should be administered and defibrillation repeated. If still unsuccessful, further intravenous medications and defibrillation attempts should be withheld until the patient is rewarmed above 30° C. Cardiopulmonary resuscitation should be continued while aggressive core rewarming techniques are initiated. Left thoracotomy or median sternotomy with direct mediastinal lavage using warmed saline should be considered. Cardiopulmonary bypass is another alternative with proven efficacy. The commonly repeated maxim, "No one is dead until they are warm and dead," is generally appropriate but cannot be literally applied in every case. Fixed dilated pupils, dependent lividity, and an apparent rigor mortis–like state are not always reliable criteria for withholding or discontinuing cardiopulmonary resuscitation in the hypothermic patient. In most cases, resuscitation should be continued until the core body temperature is raised above 32° C and the patient remains unresponsive to resuscitative efforts. However, the decision to terminate resuscitation must be individualized by the physician in charge based on the unique circumstances of each incident. A potassium level greater than 10 mEq per liter in a nonhemolyzed specimen has been advocated by some as an indicator for the futility of further resuscitative efforts.

DISTURBANCES DUE TO HEAT

method of
JAMES E. HAYES, M.D.,
KATHLEEN A. DELANEY, M.D., and
RON J. ANDERSON, M.D.
*The University of Texas Southwestern Medical
Center at Dallas*
Dallas, Texas

Physical disturbances due to heat encompass two types of clinical problems: disturbances caused by an excess of environmental heat that are not associated with life-threatening increase in body temperature and physical injury caused by severe elevations of body temperature that may or may not occur in an unusually hot environment. The first group includes non–life-threatening manifestations of heat illness such as heat exhaustion and heat syncope. The second group encompasses those patients with life-threatening elevations in body temperature (heat stroke) primarily associated with environmental exposure to heat, as well as patients without environmental heat exposure who develop severe hyperthermia in association with toxic, metabolic, or structural impairment of thermoregulation.

The epidemiologic literature on environmental heat injury describes two distinct groups of patients. Classic heat stroke occurs in populations affected by heat waves. It most commonly affects the elderly, whose risk of death due to all causes is increased during prolonged heat exposure. Patients with classic heat stroke have an indolent onset of illness, generally presenting after several days of heat exposure. Exertional heat stroke affects persons exercising vigorously in a hot environment. The largest case series come from studies of military recruits in basic training, athletes, and workers laboring in adverse environments such as mines. The term "nonseasonal heat stroke" describes those patients who develop severe hyperthermia in any season. These include psychotic, delirious, or seizing patients who may be taking drugs that affect thermoregulation and patients with neuromotor disturbances such as delirium tremens, parkinsonism, or neuromuscular rigidity.

Both the clinical manifestations of heat illness and its causes are best illuminated by examining the normal physiologic responses to heat. The human body maintains a remarkably constant temperature despite exposure to a wide range of environmental temperatures. Increases in body temperature occur during exposure to exogenous heat or endogenous heat from muscle activity or increased metabolic activity. The body responds to an increase in body temperature through finely tuned mechanisms mediated by the hypothalamus. Perfusion of the hypothalamus with warmed blood leads to peripheral vasodilatation and sweating. Cutaneous vasodilatation increases blood flow to the skin, requiring an increase in the cardiac output. This increased cutaneous circulation facilitates heat transfer to the environment, primarily through evaporation and convection. High ambient temperatures impair the body's ability to transfer heat to the environment by convection, and high humidity prevents evaporative heat loss.

Clinical experience shows that many patients who develop heat stroke have identifiable risk factors that impede heat loss. In healthy individuals, poor physical conditioning, use of drugs that impair thermoregulation, volume depletion, obesity, the use of protective clothing (firefighters, football players), and a recent move from a cool climate to a hot one have been cited as risk factors.

When the physiologic requirements for elimination of heat are considered, disease processes and drug effects that put patients at risk for hyperthermia are predictable. Alpha agonist drugs such as cocaine or ephedrine impair vasodilatation, and drugs with anticholinergic effects impair sweating. Beta blockers, calcium channel blockers, and diuretics limit the cardiac output. Neuroleptic medications decrease heat tolerance even when anticholinergic effects are limited, probably through direct effects on hypothalamic function. In addition, neuroleptic agents may precipitate severe muscular rigidity, resulting in increased heat production. The clinical significance and spectrum of these effects are very broad. A marathon runner taking an antihistamine or pseudoephedrine for seasonal allergies has a higher risk of heat stroke than the runner who does not use such medication. A military recruit who is volume depleted by the effects of alcohol consumption, a diarrheal illness, or inadequate fluid intake is at greater risk than his or her colleagues. A patient on large doses of chlorpromazine or haloperidol may develop heat stroke despite minimal activity during a heat wave, as might an elderly patient on a tricyclic antidepressant. The deadly combination of severe muscular exertion with the vasoconstrictive effects of cocaine is well known.

Patients with cardiac disease of any cause who cannot tolerate an increased cardiac output are at greater risk for heat illness, as are those with peripheral vascular disease or autonomic dysfunction. Extensive disruption of normal skin function caused by burns or dermatologic disorders impairs vasodilatation and sweating. Patients with structural abnormalities of the central nervous system or spinal cord may lack the neurologic capability to respond to increased body temperature.

Intense muscular activity, whether due to exercise, labor, agitation, or seizures, causes excess heat production and results in hyperthermia when heat production exceeds heat loss. Neuromuscular disturbances resulting in severe rigidity, myoclonus, choreoathetosis, or tremor may also precipitate severe hyperthermia. Rigidity associated with hyperthermia has been described in severe dystonic reactions (the so-called neuroleptic malignant syndrome), abrupt withdrawal of antiparkinsonian medications, and overdose of monoamine oxidase inhibitors. Malignant hyperthermia is an extremely rare disorder characterized by the sudden onset of muscular rigidity in patients with a congenital disturbance of calcium regulation in the sarcoplasmic reticulum. It is most commonly precipitated by inhalational anesthetics.

HEAT STROKE

The clinical effects of heat stroke are the result of injury to organ tissues by high body temperatures and are the same regardless of the precipitating factors. A temperature of 107.8° F (42° C) results in the denaturation of protein and the break down of phospholipid membranes. The extent of damage done to cells depends on the absolute tissue temperature and the length of time that the temperature is elevated. Many patients with heat stroke have lower recorded temperatures, especially when axillary or oral recordings are used. In addition, core temperatures from the rectum do not indicate the temperature of the brain or liver, which may be much higher. Frequently, patients who arrive in the emergency department with signs of heat stroke have been cooled in the field, so that their temperature does not reflect their risk of injury. By definition, all patients with heat stroke have altered mental states, ranging from confusion to coma. This is due to the direct effects of heat on the brain. Patients with heat stroke may be comatose for up to 4 hours and still have a good prognosis for recovery.

The hemodynamic effects of heat stroke depend on the volume state and cardiac function of the patient. Healthy athletes or military recruits who suffer heat stroke during exercise most commonly manifest tachycardia and a wide pulse pressure that reflects vasodilatation and increased cardiac output. Approx-

imately 50% are hypotensive. Significant volume depletion is not common in these patients, and vital sign abnormalities respond to modest fluid replacement and cooling. Elderly patients with classic heat stroke frequently have decreased cardiac output, vasoconstriction, and hypotension. They are more significantly volume depleted than the patient with exertional hyperthermia. Fragile elderly patients with heat stroke may require invasive monitoring for optimal volume resuscitation.

Heat damage affects many organs and physiologic functions. Renal failure is most often a consequence of rhabdomyolysis and myoglobin injury to the renal tubules. It occurs more often in patients with heat stroke associated with increased muscular exertion or rigidity. Coagulation disturbances have multiple causes. Early coagulopathy results from direct heat injury to clotting factors. Diffuse intravascular coagulation is associated with extensive heat injury to vascular endothelium and occurs in the most severe cases. Early thrombocytopenia is most often attributed to increased clearance of heat-injured platelets and, less often, to diffuse intravascular coagulation. Late coagulopathy is a consequence of hepatic failure and should be anticipated in patients with heat stroke. Elevation of hepatic enzymes occurs very early; however, other pathologic and clinical manifestations of hepatic injury are not seen for 2 to 3 days. Injury to the myocardium is diffuse, with nonspecific electrocardiographic changes and elevation of myocardial enzymes. Subendothelial petechiae and hemorrhages are noted at autopsy. Noncardiogenic pulmonary edema has been reported in more than 50% of autopsied heat stroke cases.

Laboratory abnormalities reflect heat injury to cells and metabolic processes. The lactate dehydrogenase is always elevated. Coagulation disturbances and thrombocytopenia should be sought. Concomitant respiratory alkalosis and lactic acidosis are common acid-base disturbances. Creatine phosphokinase elevation primarily reflects rhabdomyolysis. Potassium may be elevated as a result of tissue injury and renal failure or low because of aldosterone effect, which occurs during the process of acclimatization to heat. Hyperglycemia or hypoglycemia may be present. Hypophosphatemia is caused by heat injury to renal tubules and hyperventilation. Hyperphosphatemia is seen when rhabdomyolysis is extensive and is frequently associated with hypocalcemia, which is postulated to be secondary to binding of calcium by injured tissue. Spontaneous rebound hypercalcemia occurs during recovery. Calcium should not be used therapeutically in these patients. Because of the frequent elevation of phosphate when calcium is low, administration of calcium may precipitate soft tissue calcification. In addition, calcium acts as an intracellular toxin in injured cells whose membranes have lost the capacity to maintain normal electrolyte gradients. Administration of exogenous calcium may increase tissue injury. Judicious calcium administration should be considered only when severe tetany is present or when hyperkalemia does not respond to the administration of glucose, insulin, and sodium bicarbonate. In our experience, most patients with hyperkalemia as a result of skeletal muscle injury can be successfully managed without the use of calcium.

Along with the ABCs (airway, breathing, circulation) of basic resuscitation, cooling must be a major priority. The longer the patient is hyperthermic, the more injury occurs. Serious errors in the management of these patients occur in three ways: failure to detect the temperature elevation; failure to stop heat production by adequate control of agitation, rigidity, or seizures; and use of inadequate cooling techniques. Flexible rectal temperature probes that record temperatures above 106° F (41° C) and allow continuous monitoring of temperatures should be available.

The risk of the development of heat stroke in agitated patients should always be considered and core temperatures monitored closely. Agitation should be managed by titration with an intravenous benzodiazepine. The benzodiazepines may also effectively control rigidity and prevent shivering during cooling. Many older papers recommend the use of intravenous chlorpromazine to control shivering during cooling. Chlorpromazine (Thorazine) has anticholinergic effects that impair sweating and alpha-blocking effects that may precipitate shock in these unstable patients. In addition, chlorpromazine lowers the seizure threshold. The availability of benzodiazepines, which are effective for control of both shivering and agitation, makes the use of chlorpromazine an outmoded and dangerous intervention.

Dantrolene (Dantrium), an agent that blocks calcium influx into the sarcoplasmic reticulum, has been used with anecdotal success in the management of severe rigidity in patients with malignant hyperthermia precipitated by the induction of anesthesia. Without well-done controlled studies with dantrolene, we recommend that the clinician focus on aggressive cooling and use of intravenous benzodiazepines followed by neuromuscular blockade for initial treatment of muscular rigidity in severely hyperthermic patients, reserving trials of dantrolene for when these interventions fail in the critically ill patient. In less critically hyperthermic patients with suspected neuroleptic malignant syndrome who do not respond to benzodiazepines or dopamine receptor blockers such as bromocriptine, a trial of dantrolene may be reasonable.

Aggressive external cooling is rapidly effective in almost all cases of heat stroke. Although theoretical arguments have been raised against the use of ice water immersion because of the precipitation of vasoconstriction and shivering, this technique is readily available, does not require special equipment, and has been used widely with repeatedly demonstrated success. A modification of the immersion technique involves covering the patient with ice and wet sheets, with special attention to icing those areas where large vessels are near the surface, such as the neck, axillae, and groin, and using fans. The use of large fans and tepid water mists to achieve evaporative cooling minimizes vasoconstriction and is highly effective. This technique requires special equipment and is readily available only in settings where heat stroke is commonly managed. Cooling blankets are not adequate to cool a patient with life-threatening hyperthermia. Antipyretic agents such as salicylate and acetaminophen are not effective because, unlike in the patient with fever, the hypothalamic temperature "set point" is normal in patients with heat stroke. Occasionally, invasive cooling techniques such as iced gastric, rectal, or bladder lavage may be needed when cooling does not progress rapidly or temperature is extremely elevated. It should not take more than 30 minutes to bring the temperature down to 101° to 102° F (38° to 39° C). Cooling is usually stopped when the temperature reaches 102° F (39° C) to prevent progression to hypothermia.

Volume requirements vary depending on the cause of heat stroke. As noted previously, patients with exertional heat stroke usually respond to modest volume replacement (1 to 2 liters of normal saline or lactated Ringer's solution over 2 hours) and rapid cooling. A Foley catheter should be placed to monitor urine output. Fluid needs will be increased when significant rhabdomyolysis and myoglobinuria are present. This will be indicated by urine that is strongly positive for heme on routine dip but has few red cells, by elevation of the creatine phosphokinase (usually in the tens of thousands), and by early elevation of the serum creatinine. The most effective therapeutic intervention to protect the kidneys from injury due to the renal tubular deposition of myoglobin is the establishment of a brisk urine output. In most cases, volume expansion with intravenous fluids is effective and no further pharmacologic intervention is needed. In other cases, the addition of mannitol (12.5 grams per liter of intravenous fluid) or use of a loop diuretic may be necessary to establish urine flow. Animal studies have demonstrated that myoglobin precipitates more readily in an acid urine; hence, urinary alkalinization has long been recommended as adjunctive therapy in treatment of patients with rhabdomyolysis. Although it may be useful, no well-controlled studies have proved the efficacy of bicarbonate administration in the clinical setting. It is often difficult to alkalinize the urine effectively, and administration of bicarbonate causes electrolyte shifts that may further lower serum calcium and precipitate tetany.

Vasopressors should be avoided during the early process of rapid cooling, as their vasoconstrictive effects are deleterious to the cooling process. For patients with hypotension unresponsive to cooling and fluid infusion, pressors may be necessary, as well as Swan-Ganz monitoring to guide further resuscitation.

ACCLIMATIZATION

Physical acclimatization occurs over several weeks to months in persons who regularly exercise in the heat. Initially, the intravascular volume is increased with elevation of serum aldosterone and decrease in the concentration of sodium in the sweat and in the urine. Serum potassium is also decreased owing to the persistent aldosterone effect. Over time the kidney "escapes" from the renal aldosterone effects and a new state of sodium balance is reached. Hypokalemia may persist for several months. Sweat sodium content remains significantly decreased in the acclimatized person. The acclimatized person has earlier onset of sweating and a slower pulse rate and lower rectal temperature for a given degree of exercise.

HEAT EXHAUSTION

Heat exhaustion occurs during exercise in the heat and results in collapse or inability to continue the activity. It is differentiated from heat stroke by the presence of a normal mental status and by lower body temperatures, rarely exceeding 105° F (40.5° C). Patients with heat exhaustion are occasionally hypothermic. These patients generally demonstrate adequate thermoregulatory responses, with tachycardia, wide pulse pressure, and sweating. They may manifest hyponatremic dehydration when fluid intake has been adequate but salt intake inadequate. Hypernatremic dehydration occurs when fluid intake is inadequate. Patients with hypernatremia appear more dehydrated and have more prominent orthostatic hypotension. Lactic acidosis and respiratory alkalosis are common. The military experience suggests that heat exhaustion occurs in acclimatized trainees, whereas heat stroke occurs more commonly in unacclimatized trainees. Treatment is rest, cooling, and administration of saline-containing fluids, either orally or intravenously.

HEAT SYNCOPE

Heat syncope most commonly occurs early during exposure to a hot environment in persons who stand for long periods in the heat. It is due to the combined effects of venous pooling resulting from vasodilatation, decrease in venous return caused by inactivity, volume depletion, and orthostatic stress. Alcohol use may also contribute to the vasodilatation and volume depletion. These patients do not demonstrate an elevated temperature and recover quickly with simple rest and oral fluid replacement. Consciousness and a normal mental status should return rapidly once the patient is supine. Heat syncope should of course be diagnosed with caution in the elderly patient whose response to the cardiovascular stress of heat exposure may result in an exacerbation of underlying cardiac disease.

PREVENTION

Many interventions can result in the prevention of heat stroke. Patients with obvious risk factors should be cautioned and medications adjusted during the summer. Patients on psychiatric medications need close observation during the summer months. Pa-

tients hospitalized with behavioral or neuromotor disturbances that place them at risk should be closely observed. Adequate hydration and appropriate sedation need to be assured and temperatures closely monitored. Persons engaging in vigorous physical activity should have frequent cooling off periods, should drink fluids beyond their thirst, and should be closely observed for behavioral abnormalities that suggest the onset of hyperthermia. Adequate supplies of fluid and ready means for rapid cooling should be available at all sites where vigorous physical activity occurs. Careful attention to these simple measures has significantly decreased both the frequency and the mortality of heat stroke in the military and the athletic experiences.

SPIDER BITES AND SCORPION STINGS

method of
LUCINDA S. BUESCHER, M.D.
Southern Illinois University School of Medicine
Springfield, Illinois

More than 30,000 species of spiders exist; most are venomous, but few are considered a hazard to humans. When an individual encounters a spider with chelicerae (jaws) long enough to penetrate the skin, the envenomation may be painful but is rarely dangerous. The site of the bite is usually erythematous, edematous, and tender. Minor spider bites are sufficiently treated with gentle wound cleansing, resting and elevating the affected body part, applying cold compresses, using non-steroidal anti-inflammatory agents for pain and swelling, tetanus prophylaxis (if indicated), and antibiotics if secondary infection is suspected. It is crucial for the patient to bring in the spider for identification whenever possible because significant morbidity can result from bites by species of *Loxosceles* (fiddleback or violin spiders) and *Latrodectus* (widow spiders).

LOXOSCELES ENVENOMATION

Although the brown recluse, *Loxosceles reclusa,* is the most notable and widespread of this genus, four other species in the United States are known to cause cutaneous necrosis (necrotic arachnidism). These spiders are most prevalent in the south-central United States but have been reported in most states. They prefer a warm, dry habitat outdoors in a protected niche, but as they migrate north they move indoors. They spin inconspicuous matted webs. As its name implies, the spider is reclusive and a nocturnal feeder. Encounters with humans are rare, and bites usually result when the spider is trapped against the skin (often after occupying clothing left on the floor overnight).

Loxosceles spiders are tan or gray and demonstrate a distinctive dark brown, violin-shaped marking on the dorsal cephalothorax (*L. unicolor* has a very subtle marking). Another distinguishing feature is the presence of six eyes, rather than the usual eight found in most arachnids. The body measures 10 to 15 mm in length, and its leg span may be greater than 25 mm.

The actual *Loxosceles* bite usually goes unnoticed and often occurs on the lower abdomen or thigh or under the arm. Six to 12 hours after the bite, local signs and symptoms appear, including pruritus, pain, edema, erythema, and induration. A pustule or vesicle may appear at the bite site. If necrotic arachnidism is imminent, the center of the lesion becomes mottled dark blue or purple, surrounded by a white halo and finally a large area of reactive erythema, which is somewhat irregular in configuration due to gravitational effects. Over the ensuing 2 or 3 days this progresses to frank cutaneous necrosis, with stellate ulceration and eschar formation, requiring months to heal.

Systemic signs and symptoms such as headache, malaise, arthralgias, myalgias, fever, and a generalized, faintly papular eruption may accompany many bites, but viscerocutaneous loxoscelism is rare. This syndrome affects primarily children, who present with massive hemolysis. This can eventuate in renal failure, which may not appear until 2 to 3 days after the bite. Other findings include leukocytosis, leukopenia, thrombocytopenia, disseminated intravascular coagulation, convulsions, and coma.

Venom isolated from *Loxosceles reclusa* contains a number of enzymes, but the fraction responsible for cutaneous necrosis and hemolysis is sphingomyelinase D. This enzyme binds to target cell membranes and causes structural alterations that presumably initiate an inflammatory reaction. Neutrophil activation is essential for the development of cutaneous inflammation and necrosis following envenomation; complement, arachidonic acid metabolites, and lymphokines are likely participants as well.

Treatment

Since most *Loxosceles* bites are trivial, the same initial care noted earlier will suffice (i.e., cleanse, rest, elevate, cool compresses), and this should be employed until the lesion resolves. These measures should greatly diminish pain, but analgesics are often required. Administration of tetanus toxoid may be indicated, and antibiotics are necessary if cellulitis is suspected.

If an ulcer develops, dapsone,* 100 mg twice daily, should be initiated if the patient is not glucose-6-phosphate dehydrogenase (G6PD)–deficient. Regardless of G6PD status, some degree of hemolysis will occur (usually 1 to 2 grams per dL). Methemoglobinemia and leukopenia may occur as well but is rarely clinically significant. Dapsone should be continued until the wound has healed. Dapsone is a potent inhibitor of neutrophil function, and this is the presumed mechanism responsible for limiting tissue necrosis.

Surgical excision and grafting are rarely necessary and contraindicated in early stages of necrosis when graft failure is likely. Surgical intervention should be reserved for late eschars that fail to heal by secondary intention.

Cases of suspected systemic loxoscelism may show hemolysis and renal compromise. Systemic steroids in doses of 1 mg per kg per day should be initiated, along with appropriate fluid management.

Antivenin* is not widely available at this time. Its therapeutic significance is questionable because most bites are not symptomatic until many hours after envenomation, when tissue necrosis is already underway.

LATRODECTUS ENVENOMATION

Five widow spiders inhabit the United States. *Latrodectus mactans* is the most common species and can be found throughout the country, especially in the southern states. *Latrodectus variolus* is the northern black widow, and *L. hesperus* is the western black widow. These three species are all similar in appearance. The brown widow (*L. geometricus)* may be found in Florida and California, whereas the red widow (*L. bishopi)* is limited to Florida. They establish webs in dark, protected spaces indoors and out.

Female black widow spiders are shiny, with the characteristic, but variable, red or orange hourglass marking on the abdomen. Mature arachnids have a 3- to 4-cm leg span. Males are approximately half this size; thus their bites rarely result in significant symptoms.

The actual bite by a mature female widow is mild. A blue or red macule surrounded by a white halo and a faint urticarial eruption may ensue. Other local signs include piloerection, focal perspiration and lymphangitis.

Neurotoxic signs and symptoms begin within an hour, peak by 6 hours, and usually remit after 24 hours. Severe cramps and muscle contractions gradually spread from the inoculation site to involve the entire body. Abdominal rigidity mimics an acute abdomen, but distention and tenderness are lacking. Some authorities suggest that burning of the volar feet is a characteristic symptom of latrodectism. Additional findings are headache, anxiety, dizziness, diaphoresis, nausea, vomiting, salivation, lacrimation, respiratory distress, fever, priapism, hyperactive deep tendon reflexes, urinary retention, tachycardia, tremors, hypertension, paresthesias, and coma. Death occurs in less than 1% of bites.

Alpha-latrotoxin, a neurotoxin, is the venom released by black widow spiders. It induces a massive, calcium-dependent release of acetylcholine and catecholamines from synaptic terminals and blocks transmitter reuptake as well.

Treatment

Early application of ice packs to the blister site should slow absorption of venom. Tetanus immuniza-

---

*Not FDA-approved for this indication.

*Investigational drug in the United States.

tion status should be assessed and the patient monitored for signs of shock. Quick relief of cramping and pain may be achieved by intravenous calcium gluconate 10% solution (5 to 10 mL per dose maximum). Repeat dosing will be necessary every 1 to 4 hours as the effects on cramping are temporary. Additionally, pain relievers (including narcotics) and muscle relaxants are beneficial. The pain peaks at 2 to 3 hours, but may last for 48 hours. Suspected cellulitis at the bite site requires systemic antibiotics.

Antivenin (produced in horses) is available and is not species-specific. This is reserved for those patients with potential for severe complications (e.g., infants, young children, the elderly, patients with hypertensive heart disease or respiratory distress). Patients at risk for complications should be hospitalized and monitored for renal failure, convulsions, cardiac and respiratory failure, cerebral hemorrhage, and local cellulitis.

CENTRUROIDES STINGS

Scorpions have a crab-like appearance, with pincers on the front appendages, a segmented body and tail with a bulbous terminal segment, and a distal curved stinger. They vary in size from 2 to 10 cm. *Centruroides sculpturatus* is the only deadly species in the United States. It is yellowish-brown and less than 6 cm in length. This arthropod resides in southern Arizona, western New Mexico, and Mexico. The common striped scorpion *C. vittatus* is the most commonly encountered scorpion in southwestern states and has an extremely painful, nonfatal sting.

Scorpions are known to burrow into small crevices only to emerge at night to feed on insects and spiders. They may enter homes, especially attics, that provide cool, dark niches. They may appear around sinks, bathtubs, and toilets in their quest for water.

Most scorpion stings cause immediate sharp pain and local edema and erythema, but unless the patient has an allergy to the venom, stings are rarely of medical importance. Regional lymph node enlargement, local itching, paresthesias, fever, nausea, and vomiting may follow. The more deadly species inject a venom with greater neurotoxic and hemolytic activity. Systemic effects may not appear until 2 to 20 hours after envenomation. The patient may experience drowsiness, partial paralysis, muscle twitching, sialorrhea, perspiration, hypertension, tachycardia, and convulsions. Death may result from respiratory paralysis, peripheral vascular failure, or myocarditis.

Treatment

To minimize the absorption of venom, patients should remain calm and apply ice and pressure to the sting site. Antivenin (produced at Arizona State University by inoculation of goats with *C. sculpturatus* venom) is species-specific and should be administered in cases of severe envenomation and in young children. There is a high incidence of allergic hypersensitivity to the antivenin.

Supportive measures and careful monitoring for relapse and deterioration are mandatory. A parasympatholytic agent such as atropine sulfate (0.5 to 2.0 mg intravenously) may be beneficial. Muscle twitching will diminish with intravenous calcium gluconate 10% (10 mL per dose, or 0.1 mg per kg in children). Oxygen and positive-pressure breathing may be necessary for patients with impending respiratory failure. Tachycardia and severe hypertension may require temporary treatment with beta blockers and alpha blockers, respectively. Antiepileptic drugs are indicated to control seizures. Opiates and other narcotics are contraindicated as they have a synergistic effect with the venom.

SNAKE VENOM POISONING

method of
CHARLES H. WATT, JR., M.D., and
EDWARD L. HALL, M.D.
John D. Archbold Memorial Hospital
Thomasville, Georgia

Venomous snakebite in the United States is infrequent enough that many practitioners treat few, if any, snakebites over a lifetime of practice. There remains much confusion and controversy in the literature over the appropriate treatment of snakebite. This stems in part from the regional variation in snake species and in large degree from the complexity of the venoms themselves.

Worldwide there are approximately 32,000 deaths per year from venomous snakebite. In the United States there are approximately 8000 snakebites with envenomation per year, resulting in 12 to 16 deaths.

Crotalidae (rattlesnakes, cottonmouths, copperheads) and Elapidae (coral snakes) are the two poisonous snake families in the United States. Their venoms, symptoms, and treatment are different enough that they are addressed separately.

TREATMENT OF PIT VIPER (CROTALIDAE) ENVENOMATION

Pit vipers (Crotalidae) account for 99% of the venomous snakebites in the United States. They include the rattlesnakes, cottonmouths, and copperheads and are distinguished by their triangular head, retractable forward fangs, elliptical pupils, and the sensory "pit" found between the eye and nostril.

One should become familiar with the species in one's locale, but the identification of the exact species involved is not necessary to provide appropriate treatment.

Table 1 lists the dos and don'ts of the field treatment of snakebites. Safe, rapid transport to an appropriate medical facility is the first and foremost priority. Incision and suction are not recommended. The Extractor device (Sawyer Products) has been shown to remove a significant amount of venom if applied within a few minutes after the bite, and its use is recommended. The lymphatic constricting band, if

TABLE 1. **Field Treatment of Snakebite**

Do	Do Not
Get away from snake	Risk multiple bites trying to kill snake
Reassure and put victim at rest if possible	Exert unnecessarily
Immobilize bitten extremity and maintain at heart level	Elevate bitten extremity above heart
Remove constricting jewelry or clothing	Apply a tight "tourniquet"
Use Extractor if available	Use incisions or mouth suction
Apply lymphatic constricting band	Use electroshock
Secure safe, rapid transport to medical facility	Use ice or any form of cooling

used, should not occlude venous or arterial flow and should be placed 5 to 10 cm proximal to the bite so that it only mildly indents the skin. If a patient presents with a true tourniquet or constricting band in place, it should not be removed until you have intravenous access and have begun treatment. If the band is removed prematurely, immediate circulatory collapse can ensue because of the sudden systemic release of venom.

The use of ice or any method of cooling the bite site or extremity exacerbates the local tissue effects of the venom and can lead to severe tissue loss necessitating amputation. Cryotherapy is thus contraindicated. Electroshock has been advocated in the lay press but has no scientific merit, can produce burns or cardiac arrest, and should not be used.

Pit viper venom is a complex mixture of enzymes, bioactive enzymatic peptides, and other toxins that produce wide-ranging local physiologic derangements. Signs and symptoms are highly variable and dependent on the species, the amount of venom injected, the host response, and so forth. The symptoms are progressive over a highly variable period of time (minutes to hours). Fang marks must be present for envenomation to have occurred. These may not always be the "classic" two small puncture wounds but may be single or multiple punctures, scratches, or lacerations. They usually bleed easily. Swelling is very frequent and is usually present in 5 to 10 minutes. It can spread rapidly, or over several hours, to involve an entire extremity. It may be absent or minimal in deep bites that penetrate the fascia. Pain at the site is often immediate and severe but varies with the species. Vesicles, hemorrhagic blebs, and ecchymoses usually take several hours to form and can progress to necrosis.

Common systemic symptoms include weakness, numbness, tingling, dizziness, sweating, nausea, vomiting, fasciculations, and abdominal pain. The occurrence of a minty, rubbery, or metallic taste in the mouth is very specific for systemic rattlesnake envenomation. Laboratory findings indicating systemic envenomation include evidence of coagulopathy, bleeding, thrombocytopenia, fibrin degradation, and hypofibrinogenemia. When death occurs, it is generally secondary to shock and pulmonary edema resulting from coagulopathy and extreme capillary permeability.

The initial priority is to obtain a rapid pertinent history and physical examination. Up to 20% of pit viper bites result in no envenomation. There may be fang marks and a clear history, but if no further symptoms develop after several hours of observation, these patients can be discharged with no treatment other than local wound care and tetanus coverage.

Patients with signs and symptoms of envenomation should have immediate laboratory work to include a complete blood cell count (CBC); prothrombin time (PT) and partial thromboplastin time (PTT) measurement; tests for levels of fibrinogen and fibrin degradation products; a platelet count; a urinalysis; and tests for creatinine, blood urea nitrogen (BUN), and blood glucose levels. The levels of creatine phosphokinase (CPK) and/or lactate dehydrogenase (LD), if measured immediately and again 1 hour later, may help determine if envenomation has occurred. One should type and crossmatch blood and obtain arterial blood gas levels if hypotension, overt bleeding, or respiratory distress is present. Two large-bore intravenous lines should be initiated, and an electrocardiogram (ECG) obtained. If present, shock should be treated initially with volume resuscitation and judicious use of vasopressors.

The intravenous administration of polyvalent (Crotalidae) antivenin of equine origin (Wyeth) is the cornerstone of definitive management. This product is quite antigenic and thus should be given only when necessary to prevent disability, deformity, tissue loss, or systemic complications from envenomation. We use the following grading system to determine whether antivenin should be given and, if so, how much. Note that the grading of a bite should be determined by the most severe symptom or sign (e.g., the bite of a patient with no local reaction but with severe systemic signs is graded "severe").

Minimal Envenomation. Minimal envenomation means that there is a local reaction (edema, pain, ecchymosis) limited to the immediate area of the bite with no systemic manifestations. No antivenin should be given.

Moderate Envenomation. Moderate envenomation means that there is a local reaction involving less than one extremity but beyond the immediate area of the bite and/or non–life-threatening systemic manifestations (nausea, vomiting, oral paresthesias, unusual taste, minor alterations of laboratory values). The patient should be given 5 to 10 vials of antivenin.

Severe Envenomation. Severe envenomation means that there is a local reaction involving an entire extremity and/or severe systemic manifestations (hypotension, respiratory insufficiency, alteration of consciousness, pronounced tachycardia or tachypnea, overt bleeding, severe alteration of laboratory values). The patient should be given 15 to 30 vials of antivenin.

The species and size of pit viper involved can alter this schema (Mojave and some canebrake bites may require >30 vials). If the severity of the bite is in doubt, overtreatment is generally better than undertreatment. A common error is to underclassify a patient soon after the bite and not recognize the progressive nature of envenomation, which can worsen over several hours.

Antivenin is occasionally indicated for patients with severe local reaction alone, especially on the fingers or hand. The dosage is based entirely on the degree of envenomation and not patient size. Indeed, children usually need more antivenin than adults for an equivalent amount of envenomation. These guidelines for dosage are a starting point only. The dosage should be titrated to the patient's response. Good indicators for this titration are progression of swelling, pain, and the patient's general feeling of well-being. As neutralization of the venom occurs, vital signs return toward normal, the progression of edema slows, pain diminishes, and the patient "feels better." Continued monitoring of all parameters is essential.

Once the decision is made to give antivenin, one should not delay. Skin testing for allergy to horse serum should be done as outlined in the antivenin package insert. As anaphylaxis can be precipitated by skin testing, epinephrine premixed in a syringe and resuscitative equipment should be immediately available. If the skin test is negative, you should rapidly prepare at least five vials of antivenin and dilute with 500 mL of normal saline. Epinephrine should be ready and 5% dextrose in normal saline should be running intravenously. Then you should cautiously give 1 to 2 mL of the antivenin mixture, and if there are no signs of anaphylaxis, increase the rate of administration gradually over several minutes. You should try to administer the total estimated dose as rapidly as is tolerated. This should be accomplished in 1 to 4 hours maximum.

In skin test–positive patients or patients with known allergy to horse serum, antivenin can be cautiously given if life or limb is at stake. You should refer to the package insert and/or seek consultation. Pretreatment with diphenhydramine (Benadryl) 50 mg intravenously, ranitidine (Zantac) 50 mg intravenously, and aqueous epinephrine (1:1000) 0.01 mL per kg subcutaneously is imperative. Indeed, we advocate this pretreatment for all patients receiving antivenin. If anaphylaxis occurs, you should treat conventionally and stop the antivenin infusion.

Patients receiving antivenin must be monitored in a critical care setting for at least 24 hours. Coagulopathy responds well to antivenin if given rapidly and early enough. Blood and blood products are transfused only as indicated for bleeding or profound alterations of coagulation parameters.

Pulmonary edema responds well to antivenin but, when severe, may require intubation and ventilation with positive end-expiratory pressure. Antibiotics are needed only if there is advanced tissue necrosis. Once treatment is established, constricting bands should be removed, as these tighten rapidly with the progression of swelling.

Surgical incision or excision of the bite site is not indicated. Fasciotomy is indicated only for the rare patient with true compartment syndrome secondary to a subfascial bite or inadequate or delayed treatment, or for patients mistakenly treated with cryotherapy. The exception to this is digit dermotomy. This consists of a longitudinal incision through the medial or lateral skin of the envenomated finger to prevent necrosis and disability. It should be done for any significant bite to the finger and is a local procedure that should not delay other treatment. Surgical débridement is needed only for significant necrosis 3 to 10 days after the bite.

Most patients receiving antivenin develop some degree of serum sickness. This rarely requires rehospitalization. The symptoms of serum sickness should be described and patients told to expect and report them immediately. Steroids are of no use in the early treatment of snakebite but are the mainstay of treatment for serum sickness. The protocol for treatment of serum sickness is described elsewhere in this book.

A multicenter trial is currently in progress testing a new polyvalent Crotalidae Fab antivenin of ovine origin (CroTab,* Therapeutic Antibodies, Inc.). This antivenin shows promise to minimize the incidence of allergic reactions and thus greatly simplify the treatment of pit viper envenomation.

TREATMENT OF CORAL SNAKE ENVENOMATION

Envenomation by the eastern coral snake (Micrurus fulvius) represents 1% or less of the venomous bites in the United States. The coral snake's venom is neurotoxic, and symptoms of envenomation may be delayed up to 18 hours. They include weakness, paresthesias, headache, diplopia, dysphagia, dysphonia, and respiratory paralysis. In contrast to pit viper envenomation, there are few, if any, local symptoms. The treatment consists of the administration of 3 to 10 vials of antivenin (Micrurus fulvius) of equine origin (Wyeth). This antivenin neutralizes the venom but will not reverse established paralysis. Therefore, any patient determined to have been bitten by an eastern coral snake should be treated. If paralysis develops it can be quite prolonged, requiring intubation and mechanical ventilation. Muscular paralysis generally resolves very slowly over several weeks. Skin testing, antivenin administration, and general supportive care are the same as for pit viper envenomation.

Bites by imported exotic snake species should be handled by immediate consultation with your regional zoo or poison control center. They can access the Antivenin Index, which lists available antivenins and consultants.

---

*Investigational drug in the United States.

MARINE ANIMAL INJURIES

method of
BRUCE W. HALSTEAD, M.D.
World Life Research Institute
Colton, California

With the explosive increase in jet travel and underwater activities worldwide, there has been a corresponding increased exposure to hazardous marine animals in both tropical and temperate zones. Dangerous marine animals can be grouped into four major categories: those that inflict serious bites, venomous invertebrates and vertebrates, those that are poisonous to eat, and the electric fishes.

TRAUMATOGENIC FISHES AND REPTILES

Among the fishes, sharks head the list of the feared denizens of marine waters. It is estimated that there are about 350 species of sharks worldwide, but only 32 species have definitely been incriminated in human attacks. The great white shark (*Carcharodon carcharias*) is the largest and the heaviest of the predatory sharks dangerous to humans. It attains a length upward of 16 feet and a weight in excess of 3000 pounds. Another large shark that is probably more aggressive than the great white is the tiger shark, which attains a length of about 18 feet. Its weight is much less than that of the great white. Both sharks are found in tropical and temperate seas, and both may be found in inshore shallow waters. The bite of a large shark may attain a force of 18 tons.

Other sharks that can inflict fatal bites include the mako (*Isurus oxyrinchus*), length up to 12 feet; the Zambesi shark or bull shark (*Carcharhinus leucas*), length 12 feet; and the gray reef shark (*Carcharhinus amblyrhynchos*), length 7 feet. All are found in the Indo-Pacific region. The gray reef shark has a nasty temperament, is sometimes found in large schools, may go into a feeding frenzy, and can inflict bad bites. Any shark with adequate dentition is capable of producing a fatality under suitable circumstances.

Other biting fishes include the great barracuda, moray eel, and giant grouper. Most of their bites are relatively minor. One of the most dangerous of all the biting marine organisms is the saltwater crocodile (*Crocodylus porosus*), found in the western Indo-Pacific and Indian Oceans. Attacks by this crocodile are usually fatal.

Most shark and crocodile bites result in massive tissue and blood loss. The victim should be removed from the water as soon as possible and administered first aid on the beach immediately. The victim should be kept warm but out of the sun, and bleeding should be controlled by manual compression. The victim should be moved to a trauma center. Bleeding must be controlled to prevent hypovolemic shock; large blood vessels can be ligated or compressed manually. Pain should be controlled with a suitable narcotic.

Marine animal wounds are usually contaminated and should be surgically irrigated. Débridement is essential. The wound should be closed loosely, with drains inserted. Wounds are frequently contaminated with virulent bacteria of the genera *Vibrio, Pseudomonas, Erysipelothrix, Staphylococcus, Streptococcus*, and *Clostridium*, necessitating the use of appropriate antibiotics. Bacterial cultures of the wound are recommended. Tetanus prophylaxis is essential. All serious wounds should be treated with hyperbaric oxygen (HBO) therapy—1 hour at 2 atmospheres of pressure absolute (ATA) in the morning and again in the afternoon—for 1 to 3 weeks, depending on the extent of the wound. This treatment is important, since it will help speed healing and reduce scarring.

MARINE ENVENOMATIONS

Marine animals that possess venom glands are divided into stinging invertebrates—animals without backbones—and vertebrate fishes. All the stinging animals have one thing in common: they are equipped with a venom gland of some type. The venomous invertebrates range from sponges, which secrete irritating agents, to coelenterates such as hydroids, jellyfishes, corals, sea anemones, cone shells, octopuses, bristle worms, glycerid worms, and a variety of sea urchins.

Sponge dermatitis may be helped by sponging the area with vinegar. Anti-inflammatory agents and emollients such as aloe vera cream are helpful.

Hydroid, fire coral, Portuguese man-of-war, and most jellyfish stings can be very painful but usually subside when treated symptomatically. Special note should be taken of coral cuts, which can begin as minor cuts but become seriously infected with secondary bacterial invaders. Topical application of vinegar, hydrogen peroxide, antibacterial agents, emollients, and anti-inflammatory agents is helpful. If a cellulitis ensues, systemic antibiotics may be required. The most dangerous jellyfish is the sea wasp, *Chironex fleckeri*. Stings can be fatal, and treatment must be immediate. Pouring vinegar or isopropyl alcohol over the affected area inactivates any nematocysts in the adhering tentacles, which must not be touched with the bare hands. Commonwealth Serum Laboratories, Melbourne, produces an effective antivenin* against *Chironex*. Anyone traveling and diving along the northeast coast of Australia should avail themselves of this antivenin. The remainder of the treatment is symptomatic.

Some sea anemone stings, such as those of the hell's fire anemone (*Actinodendron*) and the Red Sea anemone (*Triactis*), are very painful and can ulcerate and produce a necrotic base. These anemone stings can result in a severe cellulitis and may take several months to heal. In addition to the usual treatment for coelenterate stings, HBO therapy may be necessary, using 2 ATA for 1 hour twice a day. The length of time HBO therapy is required varies with the

---

*Not available in the United States.

severity of the ulcer, but it speeds healing and reduces scarring.

Cone shell envenomations may be fatal. There is no antivenin available. Treatment is symptomatic. Live cone shells should be handled with extreme care to avoid the mouth parts and the venomous teeth.

The blue-spotted octopus (*Octopus maculosus*) possesses an extremely potent venom, and its bite may be fatal. There is no antivenin available. Treatment is symptomatic.

Bristle worms can cause a very irritating dermatitis with their setae, or bristles, which are situated on the side of each segment of the body. Some of the polychaete worms have powerful jaws and can inflict nasty bites. Glycerid worms can inflict painful bites with their venomous jaws. Visible setae in wounds should be removed with forceps. The smaller setae may be removed with the application of adhesive tape. Treatment is symptomatic.

Sea urchins can inflict painful wounds with their spines. *Diadema* is equipped with long spines that are venomous. Most of the spines that are embedded in a wound are almost impossible to remove because of the retrorse spinules covering the spines. It is generally best to leave the spines alone; after a few days, they will be absorbed into the subcutaneous tissues. Warm water soaks help. Spines embedded in a joint region may have to be surgically removed to avoid ankylosis. A granulomatous foreign tissue reaction may ultimately develop. Secondary bacterial invaders may be present, requiring antibiotic therapy. Tetanus prophylaxis is recommended. Some sea urchins such as *Toxopneustes* are equipped with venomous globiferous pedicellariae, which may appear to cover the outside of the sea urchin as though they were tiny flower-like rosettes. These are the venomous jaws, and some species have been known to produce fatalities. There is no known antivenin. Treatment is symptomatic.

There are numerous species of venomous fishes, including stingrays, horned sharks, ratfishes, catfishes, weeverfishes, scorpion fishes, lionfishes, stonefishes, toadfishes, surgeonfishes, and stargazers. Stingray and stonefish stings have produced fatalities. Treatment is aimed at alleviating pain, combating the effects of the venom, and preventing secondary infections. Stonefish antivenin* is available through Commonwealth Serum Laboratories in Australia. Otherwise, treatment is symptomatic. Fish stings should be immediately immersed in hot water, about 120° F, for 20 minutes. This will help attenuate the venom and the pain. Localized anesthetics may be needed. Stingray wounds generally need to be irrigated with normal saline. The integumentary sheath of the fish spine may have to be removed from the wound with the use of forceps or by irrigating the wound. Larger wounds may require a drain until the wound heals.

Sea snake envenomations can be serious and may result in fatalities. Sea snakes are equipped with a

---

*Not available in the United States.

flat paddle-like tail and are found only in the tropical Pacific westward to the Persian Gulf. Sea snake bites do not necessarily mean that the victim has been envenomated. Sea snake fangs are short and easily dislodged. There are about 51 species of sea snake, but only about 14 of them are known to have inflicted serious envenomations. Symptoms usually appear within 6 hours after the bite. The bite is usually painless. The presence of fang marks should be determined prior to therapy. The venom is a myotoxin and produces a flaccid paralysis. Initial symptoms of sea snake envenomation include painful muscle movements, paralysis of the legs, trismus, and ptosis. Once symptoms begin to appear, treatment should be instituted. If no symptoms appear after 6 hours, there is probably no envenomation, and treatment is unnecessary. If an envenomation has occurred, treatment with sea snake hydrophiid antivenin or elapid antivenin should be started as soon as possible. The complete instructions for use of the antivenin are given in the package insert.

ORAL INTOXICATIONS

Marine organisms that are poisonous to eat are divided into two major groups—the invertebrates and the vertebrates. The invertebrates include a variety of mollusks that transvector poisonous dinoflagellates, causing paralytic shellfish poisoning. Geographically, paralytic shellfish poisoning appears to be spreading throughout the world. Most public health agencies maintain close surveillance of poisonous shellfish in endemic areas. There is no known antidote for paralytic shellfish poisoning. Fatalities are usually caused by eating shellfish that have been feeding on toxic dinoflagellates, which may discolor the ocean and cause red tide. The victim dies of respiratory paralysis. Treatment is symptomatic. Contaminated shellfish may also spread a number of viral diseases such as polio, hepatitis, and coxsackievirus infection and bacterial diseases such as typhoid fever and cholera.

The sea anemone *Rhodactis* is poisonous when eaten raw but is safe to eat when cooked. It is found in Polynesia. Treatment is symptomatic.

Poisonings from the echinoderms—sea urchins and sea cucumbers—are rare but may be serious. The nature of the poisons is unknown. Treatment is symptomatic.

Poisonings from the Asiatic horseshoe crab, coconut crab, spiny lobster, and a variety of reef crabs may result in fatalities. The toxicity of these arthropods is generally unpredictable. It is suspected that in some cases the poison involved may be one of the members of the ciguatera complex; in other instances, tetrodotoxin may be involved. Treatment is symptomatic. There are no specific antidotes available.

Poisonings from marine vertebrates are not uncommon. Intoxications from some of the tropical sharks, such as *Carcharhinus amboensis*, may be serious and cause fatalities. The Greenland shark

(Somniosus) may be toxic when fresh but is edible when cooked.

There are about 400 species of tropical insular reef fishes that have been incriminated in ciguatera poisoning. Ciguatera involves a complex of poisons, some of which are among the most deadly marine biotoxins known. The poisons originate in the environment from the food chain, beginning with toxic dinoflagellates, which are ingested by herbivorous fishes and subsequently involve carnivorous fishes. Ciguatera is characterized by a spectrum of neurologic disturbances, including paresthesias, motor weakness, and gastrointestinal upset. Some of the worst offenders include moray eels, barracuda, and jack and red snappers. The treatment is to induce vomiting. Vitamin B complex and intravenous sodium ascorbate 25 grams three times a week in a slow drip in 250-mg normal saline solution during the acute phase may be helpful. Infusions of mannitol have been reported to be useful in relieving some of the acute symptoms. Calcium gluconate 1 to 3 grams intravenously over 24 hours has been reported to be useful.

Scombroid poisoning involves the scombroid fishes such as tuna, mackerel, skipjack, and related species. Poisonings are the result of ingesting fresh scombroids that have been inadequately refrigerated. A variety of bacteria are known to decarboxylate histidine to histamine in these dark-meated fishes. Scombroid poisoning is not an ordinary form of bacterial food poisoning. Scombroid fishes having a sharp peppery taste should be discarded. This is the most common form of fish poisoning worldwide. Treatment consists of antihistamines and inducing vomiting.

Puffer or fugu poisoning is caused by ingesting fishes of the suborder Tetraodontoidea. These fishes are also known as globefish, swellfish, swelltoads, mahi mahi, deadly death puffer, toados, and balloon fish. These fishes contain the deadly tetrodotoxin, which is a fast-acting poison with a high mortality rate. The treatment is to induce vomiting as soon as possible. There is no known antidote.

Marine turtles may become poisonous as a result of feeding on toxic algae. Ingestion of poisonous turtles can be fatal. There is no known antidote. Treatment is to induce vomiting.

Polar bear liver and kidneys may contain extremely high levels of vitamin A. Fatalities have occurred from eating polar bear viscera.

ELECTRIC FISH SHOCKS

There are about 250 species of electric fishes. Some of them are marine and others are freshwater inhabitants. The Amazonian electric eel discharges the greatest shock, which varies from 370 to 550 volts, sufficient to stun a human or a horse. These shocks may be painful but are generally not fatal. No treatment is required.

ACUTE POISONINGS

method of
HOWARD C. MOFENSON, M.D.,
THOMAS R. CARACCIO, Pharm.D., and
JOSEPH GREENSHER, M.D.
Long Island Regional Poison Control Center
East Meadow, New York

BASIC MANAGEMENT OF POISONINGS

The severity of the manifestations of acute poisoning exposures varies greatly with the age and intent of the victim. Accidental poisoning exposures make up 80 to 85% of all poisoning episodes and are most frequent in children under 5 years of age. Many of these episodes are actually ingestions of relatively nontoxic substances that require minimal medical care. Intentional poisonings constitute 10 to 15% of poisonings, and often these patients require the highest standards of medical and nursing care and the occasional use of sophisticated equipment for recovery. Suicide attempts represent a significant number of these poisonings, and the use of toxic substances is often involved. The majority of the drug-related suicide attempts involve a central nervous system (CNS) depressant, and "coma management" is vital to the treatment.

Sixty percent of patients who take a drug overdose do so with their own prescribed medication and 15% with drugs prescribed for relatives. The top poisoning categories for all ages are over-the-counter analgesics, sedative-hypnotics, benzodiazepines, cleaning agents and petroleum products, alcohol and substance abuse, pesticides, tricyclic antidepressants, plants, carbon monoxide, and opioids.

ASSESSMENT AND MAINTENANCE OF VITAL FUNCTIONS

Upper airway obstruction is the most common cause of death in intoxicated patients outside the hospital. Any patient who is comatose and has absent protective airway reflexes is able to tolerate an endotracheal tube (cuffed for those over the age of 7 to 9 years) and should have it inserted as soon as possible.

Ventilation is required if the respiratory rate and depth are inadequate.

The circulatory status is best assessed by the blood pressure and heart rate and rhythm. The circulatory clinical status and tissue perfusion may be inferred from the skin temperature, the return of color after pressure blanching (capillary filling), and the urine output. Intra-arterial blood pressure measurements are essential for adequate monitoring.

If the circulation fails to improve after adequate ventilation and oxygenation, a 15- to 20-cm elevation of the foot of the bed may aid by increasing the venous return to the heart. A fluid challenge also may improve the circulatory status if hypovolemia is the cause. If these measures fail, plasma expanders and similar products may be required. As a last resort, vasopressors may be needed. If these measures fail to produce a response, a central venous pressure or pulmonary artery wedge pressure (PAWP) line should be inserted to monitor for heart failure and fluid overload.

The level of consciousness of all intoxicated patients should be assessed and the time of assessment recorded. The Glasgow Coma Score used in head trauma is not useful in intoxications because alcohol, depressant drugs, and hypotension may give falsely lowered scores. The Reed Coma Scale is preferred (Table 1).

PREVENTION OF ABSORPTION AND REDUCTION OF LOCAL DAMAGE

Ocular exposure should be immediately treated with water or saline irrigation for 20 minutes with eyelids fully retracted. Neutralizing chemicals should not be used. All caustic and corrosive injuries should be evaluated by an ophthalmologist.

Dermal exposure is treated immediately with rinsing, not a forceful flushing in a shower, which might result in deeper penetration of the toxic substance. The skin should be rinsed with copious amounts of water for at least 30 minutes. Shampooing of the hair, cleansing of the fingernails and navel, and irrigation of the eyes are necessary in an extensive exposure. The clothes may have to be discarded. Leather goods are irreversibly contaminated and must be abandoned. Caustic (alkali) exposures often require hours of irrigation until the "soapy" feeling of the burn is gone. Dermal absorption may occur with pesticides, hydrocarbons, and cyanide.

Injected exposures to drugs and toxins or those introduced by envenomation may require a lymphatic restricting band and early suction. (See Antidotes 4 through 6 in Table 4.)

Inhalation exposure to toxic substances is treated by immediately removing the victim from the contaminated environment.

Gastrointestinal exposure is the most common route of poisoning, and an estimate of what, when, and how much of the toxic substance was ingested must be made. If there is a possibility of potential intoxication, gastrointestinal decontamination is performed rather than waiting for symptoms to develop.

Gastrointestinal Decontamination

To decrease gastrointestinal absorption, emesis should be induced or gastric aspiration and lavage performed. Neither of these methods is completely effective; each removes only 30 to 50% of the ingested substance. They are recommended up to 1 hour post-ingestion; however, there are few indications for induced emesis in the emergency department in an adult because it delays the administration of activated charcoal, which is more effective.

Emesis

Contraindications

Relative contraindications to the induction of emesis are (1) petroleum distillate ingestion of high-viscosity agents, (2) ingestions of agents that are likely to rapidly produce coma (short-acting barbiturates) or convulsions (propoxyphene, camphor, isoniazid, strychnine, tricyclic antidepressants) in less than 30 minutes and therefore may predispose to aspiration during emesis, and (3) prior significant vomiting.

Absolute contraindications to the induction of emesis are (1) caustic (alkali) or corrosive (acid) ingestions, (2) convulsions, because of the danger of aspiration and possible induction of laryngospasm, (3) coma, because of the possibility of aspiration with the loss of protective airway reflexes, (4) the absence of a cough reflex—an absence of the gag reflex is not a reliable indication of a lack of airway protection because a number of healthy people lack gag reflexes, (5) hematemesis, in which vomiting may produce additional damage, (6) age under 6 months, because of immature protective airway reflexes, (7) foreign bodies—emesis is ineffective and risks obstruction or aspiration, and (8) the absence of bowel sounds (when no bowel sounds are present, gastric lavage is preferred).

Inducing Emesis

Syrup of ipecac is the preferred agent but never fluid extract of ipecac, which is too potent, or salt water, which has produced fatal hypernatremia. It is not recommended that emesis be induced at home in children younger than 1 year of age; however, emesis can be performed in a medical facility under supervision when indicated. The dose of syrup of ipecac in the 6- to 9-month-old infant is 5 mL; in the 9- to 12-month-old, 10 mL; and in the 1- to 12-year-old, 15 mL. In children over 12 years and in adults, the dose is 30 mL. The dose may be repeated *once* if the child does not vomit in 15 to 20 minutes. The vomitus should be inspected for remnants of pills or toxic substances, and the appearance and odor should be noted.

TABLE 1. **Level of Consciousness (Reed Coma Scale)**

Stage	Conscious Level	Pain Response	Reflexes	Respiration	Circulation
0	Asleep	Normal	Normal	Normal	Normal
1	Coma	Decreased	Normal	Normal	Normal
2	Coma	None	Normal	Normal	Normal
3*	Coma	None	None	Normal	Normal
4†	Coma	None	None	Abnormal	Abnormal

*Patients in Stages 3 and 4 require intubation and placement in an intensive care unit.
†Patients in Stage 4 need intervention to sustain life.

Apomorphine is a parenteral emetic that must be freshly prepared. Its use is fraught with complications, although it produces more rapid onset of emesis than syrup of ipecac. We do not recommend its use in the cooperative patient. Naloxone (Narcan) should be available to reverse CNS depression.

Gastric aspiration and lavage may be preferable to the induction of emesis in cooperative adolescents or adults because a large tube can be introduced through the oral cavity. Contraindications to gastric aspiration and lavage in intoxicated patients are (1) caustic (alkali) and corrosive (acid) ingestions, because of the risk of esophageal perforation, (2) uncontrolled convulsions, because of the danger of aspiration and injury during the procedure, (3) ingestions of petroleum distillate products, (4) coma or absent protective airway reflexes, which require the insertion of an endotracheal tube to protect against aspiration, (5) significant cardiac dysrhythmias, which should be controlled first, and (6) hematemesis, which may be a relative contraindication.

The best results with gastric aspiration and lavage are obtained with the largest possible orogastric tube that can be reasonably passed (nasogastric tubes are not large enough for this purpose). In adults, a large-bore orogastric Lavacuator hose or a No. 42 French Ewald tube should be used; in children, a No. 22–28 French orogastric-type tube.

The amount of fluid used varies with the patient's age and size, but in general, aliquots of 150 to 200 mL per lavage are used in adolescents or adults and 5 mL per kg or 50 to 100 mL per lavage in children younger than 5 years of age.

Continuous gastric suction has been used for substances that have an enterohepatic recirculation or are actively secreted into the gastrointestinal tract, such as tricyclic antidepressants (imipramine [Tofranil]) and local anesthetics such as mepivacaine (Carbocaine) (Table 2).

Activated charcoal is produced by combustion of organic material in the absence of air until the carbon particle is formed. There are few relative contraindications to the use of activated charcoal: (1) it should not be administered before, concomitantly with, or shortly after syrup of ipecac because it may adsorb the ipecac and interfere with its emetic prop-

TABLE 2. Substances with Enterohepatic Recirculation

Chloral hydrate
Colchicine
Digitalis preparations (digoxin, digitoxin)
Glutethimide
Halogenated hydrocarbons (DDT derivatives)
Isoniazid
Methaqualone
Nonsteroidal anti-inflammatory drugs
Phencyclidine
Phenothiazines
Phenytoin
Salicylates
Tricyclic antidepressants

TABLE 3. Substances Poorly Adsorbed by Activated Charcoal

C—caustics and corrosives
H—heavy metals (arsenic, iron, lead, lithium, mercury)
A—alcohols (ethanol, methanol) and glycols (ethylene glycols)
R—Rapid onset or absorption (cyanide and strychnine)
C—chlorine and iodine
O—other substances insoluble in water
A—aliphatic and poorly adsorbed hydrocarbons
L—laxatives (sodium, magnesium, sorbitol)

erties, (2) it should not be given before, concomitantly with, or shortly after oral antidotes unless it has been proved not to interfere significantly with their absorption, (3) it does not effectively adsorb caustics and corrosives and may produce vomiting or cling to the esophageal or gastric mucosa and falsely appear as a burn on endoscopy, (4) it should not be given if there are no bowel sounds, and (5) it should not be given if the location of nasogastric tube cannot be confirmed (because of the potential for charcoal lung). Activated charcoal has no absolute contraindications, but it does not effectively adsorb alcohols, boric acid, caustics, corrosives, cyanide, metals, and drugs insoluble in aqueous acid solution (Table 3). Activated charcoal is a stool marker, indicating that the toxin has passed through the gastrointestinal tract and that no further significant absorption from the original ingestion will occur.

The dose of activated charcoal is 1 gram per kg per dose orally, with a minimum of 15 grams. The usual adolescent and adult dose is 60 to 100 grams. It is administered as a slurry mixed with water or by orogastric tube. A continuous nasogastric drip of activated charcoal, 0.25 gram per kg per hour, is an alternative in children. It should not be mixed with milk, marmalade, or starch because these interfere with charcoal's adsorptive action. Charcoal is administered with a cathartic initially. Subsequently, cathartics should be given every 24 hours.

Activated charcoal may be administered orally every 4 hours as long as bowel sounds are present, and it may be especially beneficial in intoxications that have an enterohepatic recirculation (see Table 2). Repeated dosing with oral activated charcoal has been shown to increase the clearance of many drugs without allowing enterohepatic recirculation (see later discussion of individual poisonings).

Catharsis is used to hasten the elimination of any remaining toxin in the gastrointestinal tract. Cathartics are relatively contraindicated (1) when ileus is indicated by an absence of bowel sounds, (2) in intestinal obstruction or evidence of intestinal perforation, and (3) in cases with a pre-existing electrolyte disturbance. Magnesium sulfate (Epsom salts) is contraindicated in renal failure; sodium sulfate (Glauber's salts), in heart failure or diseases requiring sodium restriction. Magnesium sulfate or sodium sulfate is administered in doses of 250 mg per kg per dose as 20% solutions. The adolescent and adult dose is 30 grams. In adults, sorbitol is given at 2.8 mL per kg to a maximum of 214 mL of a 70% solution. The cathartic should be given with the initial dose of activated charcoal. Sorbitol should be used with caution in children younger than 3 years of age and is not recommended in children under 1 year of age.

Dilutional treatment is indicated for the immediate management of caustic and corrosive poisonings but is otherwise not useful. Contraindications to dilution are (1) an inability of the patient to swallow, resulting in aspiration of the diluting fluid and (2) signs of upper airway obstruction, esophageal perforation, and shock. The administration of large quantities of diluting fluid—above 30 mL in children and 250 mL in adults—may produce vomiting, re-exposing the vital tissues to the effects of local damage and possible aspiration.

Neutralization has not been proved to be scientifically effective.

In whole-bowel irrigation, bowel-cleansing solutions of polyethylene glycol with electrolytes are used. It may be indicated with ingestions of substances that are poorly adsorbed by activated charcoal, such as iron, lithium, or sustained-release preparations. The procedure has been used successfully with iron overdose when abdominal radiographs reveal incomplete emptying of excess ingested iron. There are additional implications in other ingestions, e.g., body packing of illicit drugs, such as cocaine and heroin. The procedure is to administer, orally or by nasogastric tube, the solution (GoLYTELY or Colyte), 0.5 liter per hour in children younger than 5 years of age and 2 liters per hour in adolescents and adults. The end point is reached when the rectal effluent is clear. This takes approximately 2 to 4 hours. These measures should not be used if there is extensive hematemesis, ileus, or signs of bowel obstruction, perforation, or peritonitis.

USE OF ANTIDOTES

Antidotes are available for only a relatively small number of poisons. An available antidote should be administered only after the vital functions have been established. Table 4 summarizes the commonly used antidotes and their indications and methods of administration. Most informational, so-called first aid measures and antidotes on commercial product labels are notorious for their inaccuracy; it is preferable to contact the Regional Poison Control Center rather than follow the recommendations on these labels.

ENHANCEMENT OF ELIMINATION

The medical methods of the elimination of absorbed toxic substances are diuresis, dialysis, hemoperfusion, exchange transfusion, plasmapheresis, enzyme induction, and inhibition. Methods of increasing urinary excretion of toxic chemicals and drugs are being studied extensively, but the other modalities have not been well evaluated.

In general, these methods are needed in only a minority of instances and should be reserved for life-threatening circumstances or when a definite benefit is anticipated.

Diuresis

Diuresis increases the renal clearance of compounds that are partially reabsorbed in the renal tubules. Forced-fluid diuresis is based on the principle that it will shorten exposure to reabsorption at the distal renal tubules. The risks of diuresis are fluid overload, with cerebral and pulmonary edema, and disturbances in acid-base and electrolyte balance. Failure to produce a diuresis may imply prerenal or renal failure. If renal failure is present, dialysis should be considered.

Osmotic diuresis is meant to increase the osmotic gradient and prevent reabsorption from the proximal loop and distal tubules. Mannitol is used to initiate this type of diuresis, and then fluids are added in sufficient amounts to produce a diuresis similar to forced-fluid diuresis.

Acid and alkaline diuresis is based on the principle that inhibition of reabsorption of certain toxic agents can be encouraged by adjusting the urinary pH so the substance is maintained in its ionized form, which interferes with its passage back into the blood. Electrolyte and acid-base monitoring are necessary. Hypokalemia and hypocalcemia are frequent complications. Acid diuresis is accomplished by using ammonium chloride (Antidote 2, Table 4). Although it may enhance the elimination of weak bases, such as amphetamines and fenfluramine (Pondimin), it is not recommended. Ammonium chloride is contraindicated if rhabdomyolysis is present. Alkaline diuresis with sodium bicarbonate can be used in the therapy of weak acids, such as salicylates, and long-acting barbiturates, such as phenobarbital (Antidote 39, Table 4).

Dialysis

Dialysis is the extrarenal means of removing certain toxins from the body and can substitute for the kidney when renal failure occurs. Dialysis is never the first measure instituted; however, it may be lifesaving later in the course of a severe intoxication. It is needed in only a small minority of intoxicated patients (Table 5). Peritoneal dialysis is only one-twentieth as effective as hemodialysis. It is easier to use and less hazardous to the patient but also less reliable in removing the toxin; thus it is seldom used. Hemodialysis is the most effective means of dialysis but requires experience with sophisticated equipment. The patient-related criteria for dialysis are anticipated prolonged coma and the likelihood of complications, renal impairment, and deterioration despite careful medical management. Most dialyzable substances have a volume of distribution (Vd) of less than 1 liter per kg and protein binding of less than 50%.

Text continued on page 1160

TABLE 4. **Antidotes***

Medication	Indications	Comments
1. *N*-Acetylcysteine (NAC, Mucomyst, Mead Johnson). Glutathione precursor that prevents accumulation and helps detoxify acetaminophen metabolites. **Dose:** *Adult,* 140 mg/kg PO of 5% solution as loading dose, then 70 mg/kg PO q 4 h for 17 doses as maintenance dose. *Child,* same as for adult. **Packaged:** 10 and 20% solution in 4-, 10-, and 30-mL vials.	Acetaminophen toxicity. Most effective within first 8 h (to make more palatable, administer through a straw inserted into closed container of citrus juice). **AR:** Stomatitis, nausea, vomiting. See Acetaminophen in text. The full course of therapy is required in any patient whose level falls in the toxic range.	IV preparation experimental.‡ The dose of NAC should be repeated if the patient vomits within 1 h after administration. Methods to stop vomiting of the NAC are: (a) placement of a tube in the duodenum, (b) slow administration over 1 h, (c) ½ h before NAC dose use metoclopramide (Reglan), 1 mg/kg IV over 15 min (max dose 10 mg) q 6 h; infants 0.1 mg/kg/dose IM, IV. Droperidol (Inapsine), 1.25 mg IV; for extrapyramidal reactions, use diphenhydramine (see 19).
2. **Ammonium chloride.**	Not recommended.	
3. **Amyl nitrate.**	See 14, Cyanide antidote kit.	
4. **Antivenin,** black widow spider *(Latrodectus mactans).* **Dose:** 1–2 vials infused over 1 h. **Packaged:** 6000 U/vial with 2.5 mL of sterile water and 1 mL of horse serum 1:10 dilution.	Envenomation by black widow spider or by any *Latrodectus* spp producing severe symptoms. Most healthy adults survive with supportive care. Antivenin is used in elderly or infants or if there is underlying medical condition causing hemodynamic instability **AR:** Same as for 5, Antivenin Polyvalent because derived from horse serum.	Preliminary sensitivity test. Supportive care alone is standard management.
5. **Antivenin polyvalent** for Crotalidae (pit vipers), Wyeth, IV only. **Dose:** Depends on degree of envenomation: minimal: 5–8 vials; moderate: 8–12 vials; severe: 13–30 vials. Dilute in 500–2000 mL of crystalloid solution and start IV at slow rate, increasing after first 20 min, if no reaction occurs. **Packaged:** 1 vial (10 mL) of lyophilized serum, 1 vial of (10 mL) bacteriostatic water for injection, 1 vial (1 mL) of normal horse serum.	Venoms of crotalids (pit vipers) of North and South America. **AR:** Anaphylactic shock reaction occurs within 30 min. Serum sickness usually occurs 5–44 days after administration. It may occur in <5 days, especially in those who have received horse serum products in past. Signs and symptoms include fever, edema, arthralgia, nausea, and vomiting, as well as pain and muscle weakness.	Consider consulting with Regional Poison Control Center and herpetologist. Administer IV. Preliminary sensitivity test. Never inject in fingers, toes, or bite site.
6. **Antivenin,** North American coral snake, Wyeth, IV only. **Dose:** 3–5 vials (30–50 mL) by slow IV injection. First 1–2 mL should be injected over 3–5 min. **Packaged:** 1 vial of antivenin, 10 mL. 1 vial of bacteriostatic water (10 mL) for injection.	*Micrurus fulvius* (Eastern coral snake); *Micrurus tenere* (Texas coral snake). **AR:** Anaphylaxis (sensitivity reaction). Usually 30 min after administration. Signs and symptoms: Flushing, itching, edema of face, cough, dyspnea, cyanosis. Neurologic manifestations—usually involve the shoulders and arms. Pain and muscle weakness are frequently present, and permanent atrophy may develop.	Same as for Antivenin Polyvalent for Crotalidae. Will not neutralize the venom of *Micrurus euryxanthus* (Arizona or Sonoran coral snake).
7. **Atropine** (various manufacturers). Antagonizes cholinergic stimuli at muscarinic receptors. **Dose:** *Adult,* initial dose 2–4 mg IV. Dose every 10–15 min as necessary until cessation of secretions. Severe poisoning may require doses up to 2000 mg. *Child,* initial dose of 0.02 mg/kg to a max of 2 mg every 10–15 min as necessary until cessation of secretions. Use preservative-free atropine if infusion. **Packaged:** 0.3 mg/mL; 0.4 mg/mL in 0.5-, 1-, 20-, and 30-ml vials; 1 mg/mL in 1- and 10-mL vials.	Carbamate and organophosphate insecticide poisonings. Rarely needed in cholinergic mushroom intoxication (*Amanita muscaria, Clitocybe, Inocybe* spp). Lack of signs of atropinization confirms diagnosis of cholinesterase inhibition. **AR:** Flushing and dryness of skin, blurred vision, rapid and irregular pulse, fever, and loss of neuromuscular coordination. **Diagnostic Test:** *Child:* 0.01 mg/kg IV. *Adult:* 1 mg total.	If cyanosis, establish respiration first because atropine in cyanotic patients may cause ventricular fibrillation. If severe signs of atropinization, may correct with physostigmine in doses equal to one-half dose of atropine. If symptomatic, administer until the end point of drying secretions and clearing of lungs. Hallucinations, flushing of the skin, dilated pupils, tachycardia, and elevation of the body temperature are not end points and do not preclude atropine administration. Maintain atropinization for 12–24 hr, then taper dose and observe for relapse.

*This is for information purposes and is not intended to substitute for independent judgment. It is always advisable to review the package insert for the most up-to-date information. Contact Regional Poison Control Center for additional details on use.

†This dose may exceed the manufacturer's recommended dose.

‡Investigational drug in the United States.

§Not FDA-approved for this indication.

Abbreviations: AR = adverse reaction to antidotes; MP = monitoring parameters; FDA = US Food and Drug Administration; Conc = concentration; ECG = electrocardiogram; TIBC = total iron-binding capacity; G6PD = glucose-6-phosphate dehydrogenase; CNS = central nervous system; GI = gastrointestinal; AV = atrioventricular; EEG = electroencephalogram; RBC = red blood count; CBC = complete blood count.

Table continued on following page

TABLE 4. **Antidotes*** *Continued*

Medication	Indications	Comments
		Atropine has been administered successfully by IV infusion, although this method has not received FDA approval. **Dose:** Place 8 mg of atropine in 100 mL D5W or saline. Conc = 0.08 mg/mL. Dose range = 0.02–0.08 mg/kg/h or 0.25–1 mL/kg/h. Severe poisoning may require supplemental doses of IV atropine intermittently in doses of 2–4 mg until drying of secretions occurs.
8. **BAL** (British antilewisite; dimercaprol).	See 17, Dimercaprol.	
9. **Bicarbonate.**	See 39, Sodium bicarbonate.	
10. **Botulism antitoxin,** Connaught Medical Research Labs. **Dose:** *Adult,* 1 vial IV stat, then 1 vial IM, repeat in 2–4 h if symptoms appear in 12–24 h. *Child,* check with state health department.	Prevention or treatment of botulism.	Contact local or state health department for full management guidelines.
11. **Calcium disodium edetate** (EDTA, Disodium versenate, Riker). **Dose:** *Adult,* max 4 gm. *Child,* max 1 gm. Moderate toxicity: IM or IV, 50 mg/kg/day for 3–5 days. Severe toxicity: IV or IM, 75 mg/kg/day for 4–5 days. Dose divided into 3–6 doses daily. Dilute 1 gm in 250–500 mL saline or D5W, infuse over 4 h bid for 5–7 days. For lead levels over 69 µg/dL or if symptoms of lead poisoning or encephalopathy: Add BAL alone initially, 4 mg/kg, then combination BAL and EDTA at different sites. EDTA dose: 12.5 mg/kg IM. (See "Lead" in text for latest recommendations.) Modify dose in renal failure. **Packaged:** 200 mg/mL ampules.	For chelation of cadmium, chromium, cobalt, copper, lead, magnesium, nickel, selenium, tellurium, tungsten, uranium, vanadium, and zinc poisoning. **AR:** 1. Thrombophlebitis. 2. Nausea, vomiting. 3. Hypotension. 4. Transient bone marrow suppression. 5. Nephrotoxicity, reversible tubular necrosis (particularly in acid urine). 6. Fever 4–8 h after infusion. 7. Increased prothrombin time.	Hydrate first and establish renal flow. Avoid plain sodium EDTA because hypocalcemia may result. Procaine 0.25–1 mL of 0.5% for each mL of IM EDTA to reduce pain. Do not use EDTA orally. Limit use to 7 days (otherwise loss of other ions and cardiac dysrhythmias may occur). **MP:** Calcium levels, urinalysis, renal profile, erythrocyte protoporphyrin, blood lead, and liver profile. Contraindicated in iron intoxication, hepatic impairment, and renal failure.
12. (A) **Calcium gluconate** 10%. **Dose:** IV 0.2–0.5 mL/kg of elemental calcium up to max 20 mL (2 gm) over 10–15 min with continuous ECG monitoring. Titrate to adequate response. **Packaged:** 10% solution in 10-mL vial.	Calcium channel blocker poisoning, e.g., nifedipine (Procardia), verapamil (Calan), diltiazem (Cardizem). It improves blood pressure but does not affect dysrhythmias. Hypocalcemia as result of poisonings. Black widow spider envenomation.	Repeat dose as needed. Monitor calcium levels. Contraindicated with digitalis poisoning.
(B) **Calcium chloride.** **Dose:** IV 0.2 mL/kg up to max 10 mL (1 gm) with continuous IV monitoring. Titrate to adequate response. Rate should not exceed 2 mL/min. (C) **Infiltration of calcium gluconate.** **Dose:** Infiltrate each cm² of affected dermis and subcutaneous tissue with about 0.5 mL of 10% calcium gluconate using a 30-gauge needle. Repeat as needed to control pain. **Packaged:** 10% solution in 10-mL vial.	Hydrofluoric acid (HF) exposure (if irrigation with cool water fails to control pain). **AR:** IV bradycardia, asystole, necrosis with extravasation.	Infiltration with calcium gluconate should be considered if HF exposure results in immediate tissue damage and erythema and pain persist after adequate irrigation.
(D) **Calcium gel:** 3.5 gm USP calcium gluconate powder added to 5 oz of water-soluble lubricating jelly.	Dermal exposure of HF less than 20%.	Gel must have direct access to burn area; if pain persists, calcium gluconate injection may be needed. Placing loose-fitting surgical glove over gel when fingers are involved helps to keep preparation in contact with burn area.

*This is for information purposes and is not intended to substitute for independent judgment. It is always advisable to review the package insert for the most up-to-date information. Contact Regional Poison Control Center for additional details on use.
†This dose may exceed the manufacturer's recommended dose.
‡Investigational drug in the United States.
§Not FDA-approved for this indication.
Abbreviations: AR = adverse reaction to antidotes; MP = monitoring parameters; FDA = US Food and Drug Administration; Conc = concentration; ECG = electrocardiogram; TIBC = total iron-binding capacity; G6PD = glucose-6-phosphate dehydrogenase; CNS = central nervous system; GI = gastrointestinal; AV = atrioventricular; EEG = electroencephalogram; RBC = red blood count; CBC = complete blood count.

TABLE 4. **Antidotes*** *Continued*

Medication	Indications	Comments
13. **Chemet.**	See 42, Succimer.	
14. **Cyanide antidote kit,** Lilly. Nitrite-induced methemoglobin attracts cyanide off cytochrome oxidase, and thiosulfate forms nontoxic thiocyanate. **Doses:** *Adult,* amyl nitrite. Have patient inhale for 30 sec of every min. Use new ampule every 3 min. Reapply until sodium nitrite can be given. Then inject IV 300 mg (10 ml of 3% solution of sodium nitrite) over 20 min. Alternative: IV infusion, 300 mg in 50–100 mL of 0.9% saline over 20 min. Then inject 12.5 gm (50 mL of 25% solution) of sodium thiosulfate over 20 min. *Child,* use following chart for children's dosage. **Packaged:** 2- to 10-mL ampules sodium nitrite injection; 2- to 50-mL ampules sodium thiosulfate injection; 0.3-mL amyl nitrite inhalant.	Cyanide poisoning. **AR:** Hypotension, methemoglobinemia.	*Note:* If child is given adult dose of sodium nitrite, fatal methemoglobinemia may result. Do not use methylene blue for methemoglobinemia in cyanide therapy. Observe for hypotension and have epinephrine available. Cyanide kits should have amyl nitrite changed annually. Administer oxygen 100% between inhalations of amyl nitrite. Monitor hemoglobin, arterial blood gases, methemoglobin concentration (nitrite given to obtain methemoglobin level of 25%). Some add nitrite ampule to resuscitation bag.

Chart should be used to determine dose of sodium nitrite and sodium thiosulfate in children on basis of hemoglobin concentration on left. Average child with normal hemoglobin requires 0.33–0.39 mL/kg of sodium nitrite up to 10 mL over 20 min.

Hemoglobin (gm)	Initial Child Dose of Sodium Nitrite 3% (mL/kg) (do not exceed 10 mL)	Initial Child Dose of Sodium Thiosulfate (mL/kg) (do not exceed 12.5 gm)
8	0.22 (6.6 mg/kg)	1.10
10	0.27 (8.7 mg/kg)	1.35
12	0.33 (10 mg/kg)	1.65
14	0.39 (11.6 mg/kg)	1.95

If signs of poisoning reappear, repeat above procedure at one-half above doses. Each agent should be given at rate of over 20 min.

Medication	Indications	Comments
15. **Deferoxamine mesylate** (DFOM, Desferal, Ciba). Has remarkable affinity for ferric iron and chelates it. **Therapeutic dose:** *Adult,* 90 mg/kg† IM or IV q 8 h to maximum of 1 gm per injection; may repeat to maximum of 6 gm in 24 h. *Child,* same as adult. IV administration can be given by slow infusion at rate not exceeding 15 mg/kg/h. **Packaged:** 500 mg/ampule (powder).	DFOM is useful in treatment of symptomatic iron poisoning or cases where serum iron is greater than 500 μg/dL. If DFOM challenge test is positive, it is not definite indication that therapy is necessary in asymptomatic patient. Oral DFOM is not recommended. Iron intoxication. Therapeutic—see dose in left column. *Diagnostic trial:* Give deferoxamine, 50 mg/kg IM (up to 1 gm). If serum iron exceeds TIBC, unbound iron is excreted in urine, producing "vin rosé" color of chelated iron complex in the urine (pink-orange). However, may be negative with high serum iron exceeding TIBC. **AR:** Flushing of skin, generalized erythema, urticaria, hypotension, and shock may occur. Blindness has occurred rarely in patients receiving long-term, high-dose DFOM therapy. Continuous infusions of DFOM over 24 h have produced severe pulmonary manifestations such as adult respiratory distress syndrome. Contraindicated in patients with renal disease or anuria.	Therapy is usually continued until serum iron <100 μg/dL, or when positive "vin rosé" urine turns clear, or when patient is asymptomatic. Therapy is rarely required over 24 h. Establish good renal flow. To be effective, DFOM should be administered in first 12–16 h. In mild to moderate iron intoxication or shock, IV route only. Monitor serum iron levels, urine output, and urine color.
16. **Diazepam** (Valium, Roche). **Dose:** *Adult,* 5–10 mg IV (max 20 mg) at rate of 5 mg/min until seizure is controlled. May be repeated 2 or 3 times. *Child,* 0.1–0.3 mg/kg up to 10 mg IV slowly over 2 min. **Packaged:** 5 mg/mL; 2- and 10-mL vials.	Any intoxication that provokes seizures when specific therapy is not available, e.g., amphetamines, phencyclidine (PCP) use, barbiturate and alcohol withdrawal. Chloroquine poisoning. **AR:** Confusion, somnolence, coma, hypotension.	Intramuscular absorption is erratic. Establish airway and administer 100% oxygen and glucose.

*This is for information purposes and is not intended to substitute for independent judgment. It is always advisable to review the package insert for the most up-to-date information. Contact Regional Poison Control Center for additional details on use.

†This dose may exceed the manufacturer's recommended dose.

‡Investigational drug in the United States.

§Not FDA-approved for this indication.

Abbreviations: AR = adverse reaction to antidotes; MP = monitoring parameters; FDA = US Food and Drug Administration; Conc = concentration; ECG = electrocardiogram; TIBC = total iron-binding capacity; G6PD = glucose-6-phosphate dehydrogenase; CNS = central nervous system; GI = gastrointestinal; AV = atrioventricular; EEG = electroencephalogram; RBC = red blood count; CBC = complete blood count.

Table continued on following page

TABLE 4. **Antidotes*** *Continued*

Medication	Indications	Comments
17. **Dimercaprol** (Bal, Hynson, Westcott, & Dunning). **Dose:** Recommendations vary; contact Regional Poison Control Center. Prevents inhibition of sulfhydryl enzymes. Given deep IM only. *For severe lead poisoning*—see 11, Calcium disodium edetate. *For mild arsenic or gold poisoning*—2.5 mg/kg q 6 h for 2 days, then q 12 h on third day, and once daily thereafter for 10 days. *For severe arsenic or gold poisoning*—3–5 mg/kg q 6 h for 3 days, then q 12 h thereafter for 10 days.† *For mercury poisoning*—5 mg/kg initially, followed by 2.5 mg/kg 1 or 2 times daily for 10 days. **Packaged:** 100 mg/mL 10% in oil in 3-mL ampules.	For chelation of antimony, arsenic, bismuth, chromates, copper, gold, lead, mercury, and nickel. **AR:** 30% of patients have reactions: fever (30% of children), hypertension, tachycardia, may cause hemolysis in G6PD deficiency patients. Doses greater than recommended may cause various adverse effects: nausea, vomiting, headache, chest pain, tachycardia, and hypertension.	Contraindicated in instances of hepatic insufficiency, with exception of postarsenic jaundice. Should be discontinued or used only with extreme caution if acute renal insufficiency is present. Monitor blood pressure and heart rate (both may increase), urinalysis, qualitative urine excretion of heavy metal. Contraindicated in iron, silver, uranium, selenium, and cadmium poisoning.
18. **Dimercaptosuccinic acid** (DMSA).	See 42, Succimer.	
19. **Diphenhydramine** (Benadryl, Parke-Davis). Antiparkinsonian action. **Dose:** Adult, 10–50 mg IV over 2 min. *Child,* 1–2 mg/kg IV up to 50 mg over 2 min. Max in 24 h: 400 mg. **Packaged:** 10 mg/mL in 10- and 30-mL vials. 50 mg/mL in 1-, 5-, 10-, and 30-mL vials. Capsules, tablets 25 and 50 mg. Elixir, syrup 12.5 mg/5 mL.	Used to treat extrapyramidal symptoms and dystonia induced by pheno-thiazines and related drugs. **AR:** Fatal dose, 20–40 mg/kg. Dry mouth, drowsiness.	Continue with oral diphenhydramine, 5 mg/kg/day to 25 mg 3 times a day for 72 h, to avoid recurrence.
20. **EDTA.**	See 11, Calcium disodium edetate.	
21. **Ethanol** (ETOH). Competitively inhibits alcohol dehydrogenase. **Dose:** *Loading*—administer 7.6–10.0 mL/kg of 10% ETOH in D5W over 30 min IV or 0.8–1.0 mL/kg 95% ETOH PO in 6 oz of orange juice over 30 min. While administering loading dose, start maintenance. *Maintenance:* Volume of 10% ETOH needed IV or 95% oral solution (not in dialysis). See chart on maintenance dose, below. If patient is on dialysis, add 91 mL/h in addition to regular maintenance dose. See comments to prepare 10% solution if not commercially available. **Packaged:** 10% ethanol in D5W 1000 mL; 95% ethanol. May be given as 50% solution orally. *Maintenance Dose:*	Methanol, ethylene glycol poisoning. Ethanol infusion therapy may be started in cases of suspected methanol and ethylene glycol poisoning presenting with increased anion gap and osmolal gap, or if urine shows crystalluria of ethylene glycol poisoning or hyperemia of optic disk of methanol intoxication. **AR:** CNS depression, hypoglycemia.	Monitor blood ethanol 1 h after starting infusion and q 4–6 h. Maintain blood ethanol concentration of 100–200 mg/dL. Monitor blood glucose, electrolytes, blood gases, urinalysis, and renal profile at least daily. Continue infusion until safe concentration of ethylene glycol or methanol is reached. Ethanol-induced hypoglycemia may occur. Dialysis, preferably hemodialysis, should be considered in severe intoxication not controlled by ethanol alone. To prepare 10% ethanol for infusion therapy: Remove 100 mL from 1 L of D5W and replace with 100 mL of tax-free bulk absolute alcohol after passing through 0.22-µm filter; 50-mL vials of pyrogen-free absolute ethanol for injection are available from Aper Alcohol Company, Shelbyville, KY, telephone 800-456-1017, or American Reagent, Shirley, NY, telephone 800-645-1706.

Patient Category	mL/kg/h using 10% IV	mL/kg/h using 50% oral
Nondrinker	0.83	0.17
Occasional drinker	1.40	0.28
Alcoholic	1.96	0.39

Medication	Indications	Comments
22. **Fab** (antibody fragment, Digibind). **Dose:** Average dose used during clinical testing was 10 vials. Dosage details are specified by manufacturer. It should be administered by IV route over 30 min. Calculate on basis of body burden either by known amount ingested or by serum digoxin concentration.	Toxicity due to digoxin, digitoxin, oleander tea, with following: 1. Imminent cardiac arrest or shock. 2. Hyperkalemia > 5.5 mEq/L. 3. Serum digoxin >10 ng/mL at 6–12 h postingestion in adults. 4. Life-threatening dysrhythmias. 5. Ingestion over 10 mg in adults or 4 mg in child (0.3 mg/kg).	Contact Regional Poison Control Center. Preliminary sensitivity test. Administer through a 0.22-µm filter. Fab causes a rise in measured bound digoxin but a fall in free digoxin.

*This is for information purposes and is not intended to substitute for independent judgment. It is always advisable to review the package insert for the most up-to-date information. Contact Regional Poison Control Center for additional details on use.

†This dose may exceed the manufacturer's recommended dose.

‡Investigational drug in the United States.

§Not FDA-approved for this indication.

Abbreviations: AR = adverse reaction to antidotes; MP = monitoring parameters; FDA = US Food and Drug Administration; Conc = concentration; ECG = electrocardiogram; TIBC = total iron-binding capacity; G6PD = glucose-6-phosphate dehydrogenase; CNS = central nervous system; GI = gastrointestinal; AV = atrioventricular; EEG = electroencephalogram; RBC = red blood count; CBC = complete blood count.

TABLE 4. **Antidotes*** *Continued*

Medication	Indications	Comments
Calculation of Dose of Fab: 1. Known amount ingested multiplied by bioavailability (0.8) = body burden. Body burden divided by 0.6 = number of vials. 2. Known serum digoxin (obtained 6 h postingestion) multiplied by Vd (5.6 L/kg) and weight in kg divided by 1000 = body burden. Body burden divided by 0.6 = number of vials.	6. Bradycardia or second- or third-degree heart block unresponsive to atropine.	40 mg binds 0.6 mg of digoxin.
23. **Flumazenil** (Mazicon, Roche Labs), Benzodiazepine (BZP) receptor antagonist. **Dose:** 1. *Management of BZP overdose:* (Caution) 0.2 mg (2 mL) IV over 30 sec; may repeat after 30 sec with 0.3 mg (3 ML). Further doses of 0.5 mg over 30 sec. If no response in 5 min and max of 5 mg, cause of sedation is unlikely to be BZP. 2. *Reversal of conscious sedation or in general anesthesia:* 0.2 mg (2 mL) IV over 15 sec; may repeat in 45 sec. Doses may be repeated at 60-sec intervals to max dose of 1 mg (10 mL). If resedation, repeated doses may be administered at 20-min intervals to max 1 mg (0.2 mg/min). Max 3 mg should be given in any 1 h. **Packaged:** 0.1 mg/mL in 5- and 10-mL multiple-use vials.	1. Reversal of sedative effects of BZP general anesthesia. 2. Sedation with BZP for procedures. 3. Caution in management of overdose. **AR:** Convulsions, dizziness, injection site pain, increased sweating, headache, and abnormal or blurred vision (3–9%).	Not treatment for hypoventilation. Caution with overdose. Flumazenil is not recommended for cyclic antidepressant poisoning, or if patient has seizures or increased intracranial pressure. Flumazenil has been associated with seizures in long-term benzodiazepine use or dependency.
24. **Folic acid.**	See 28, Leucovorin.	
25. **Folinic acid.**	See 28, Leucovorin.	
26. **Glucagon.** Works by stimulating production of cyclic adenyl monophosphate. **Dose:** 50–150 µg/kg over 1 min IV followed by a continuous infusion of 1–5 mg/h in dextrose. Then taper over 5–12 h. 2 mg of phenol per 1 mg of glucagon. 50 mg is the maximum amount of phenol recommended; therefore, toxicity may result when high doses of glucagon are used. **Packaged:** 1-mg (1 U) vial with 1-mL diluent with glycerin and phenol; also in 10-mL size.	Beta blocker, quinidine, and calcium channel blocker intoxication. **AR:** Glucagon is generally well tolerated—most frequent reactions are nausea, vomiting.	Do not dissolve the lyophilized glucagon in the solvent packaged with it when administering IV infusion because of possible phenol toxicity. Use D5W, not 0.9% saline. Effects of single dose observed in 5–10 min and last for 15–30 min. A constant infusion may be necessary to sustain desired effects.
27. **Labetalol hydrochloride** (Normodyne, Schering; Trandate, Glaxo). Nonselective beta and mild alpha blocker. **Dose:** IV 20 mg over 2 min. Additional injections of 40 or 80 mg can be given at 10-min intervals until desired supine blood pressure is achieved. Max dose 300 mg. Alternative: Slow IV infusion: 200 mg (40 mL) is added to 160 or 250 mL of D5W and given at 2 mg/min. Titrate infusion according to response. **Packaged:** Solution 5 mg/mL in 20 mL.	Hypertensive crises secondary to cocaine. **AR:** GI disturbances, orthostatic hypotension, bronchospasm, congestive heart failure, AV conduction disturbances, and peripheral vascular reactions.	Concomitant diuretic enhances therapeutic response. Patient should be kept in supine position during infusion. **MP:** Monitor blood pressure during and after administration.
28. **Leucovorin.** **Dose:** For methanol poisoning: 1 mg/kg up to 50 mg IV q 4 h for 6 doses. For methotrexate overdose, see comments. **Packaged:** 3 mg/mL (1 mL), 5 mg/mL (1 and 5 mL), 50 mg/vial.	1. **Methanol poisoning§:** Active form of folic acid used to enhance metabolism of formic acid in animals to carbon dioxide and water. 2. **Methotrexate (MTX) overdose:** Supplies tetrahydrofolate cofactor, which is blocked by methotrexate. **AR:** Allergic sensitization.	For MTX overdose, initial dose can be given IV or IM in MTX equivalent dose up to 75 mg. If MTX blood level is measured 6 h postingestion and is above 10^{-8} molar or is unavailable, give 12 mg q6h after MTX level is below 10^{-8} molar. Alternatively, if GI function is adequate, may give orally 10 mg/m² q6h until MTX levels are lowered to less than 10^{-8} molar. Leucovorin in doses of 5–15 mg/day PO has also been recommended to counteract hematologic toxicity from folic acid antagonists such as trimethoprim and pyrimethamine.

*This is for information purposes and is not intended to substitute for independent judgment. It is always advisable to review the package insert for the most up-to-date information. Contact Regional Poison Control Center for additional details on use.
†This dose may exceed the manufacturer's recommended dose.
‡Investigational drug in the United States.
§Not FDA-approved for this indication.
Abbreviations: AR = adverse reaction to antidotes; MP = monitoring parameters; FDA = US Food and Drug Administration; Conc = concentration; ECG = electrocardiogram; TIBC = total iron-binding capacity; G6PD = glucose-6-phosphate dehydrogenase; CNS = central nervous system; GI = gastrointestinal; AV = atrioventricular; EEG = electroencephalogram; RBC = red blood count; CBC = complete blood count.

Table continued on following page

TABLE 4. **Antidotes*** *Continued*

Medication	Indications	Comments
29. **Methylene blue.** Methylene blue reduces ferric ion of methemoglobin to ferrous ion of hemoglobin. **Dose:** *Adult,* 0.1–0.2 mL/kg of 1% solution (1–2 mg/kg) over 5 min IV. Max adults 7 mg/kg. *Child,* same as adults. Max infants 4 mg/kg. May repeat in 1 h if necessary. Repeat only once. **Packaged:** 1% 10-mL ampules.	Methemoglobinemia. **AR:** GI (nausea, vomiting), headache, hypertension, dizziness, mental confusion, restlessness, dyspnea, hemolysis, blue skin, blue urine, burning sensation in vein when IV dose exceeds 7 mg/kg. Treatment is unnecessary unless methemoglobin is over 30% or respiratory distress is present.	Saliva, urine, and other body fluids may turn blue. Contraindications: Renal insufficiency, cyanide poisonings when sodium nitrite is used to induce methemoglobinemia; in G6PD-deficiency patients. Monitor hemolysis, methemoglobin level, and arterial blood gases. Avoid extravasation because of local necrosis.
30. **Naloxone** (Narcan). Pure opioid antagonist. **Dose:** *Adult,* 0.4–2.0 mg IV and repeat at 3-min intervals until respiratory function is stable. Before excluding opioid intoxication on basis of lack of naloxone response, minimum of 2 mg in child or 10 mg in adult should be administered. *Child,* initial dose is 0.1 mg/kg IV. **Packaged:** 0.02 mg/mL, 0.4 mg/mL ampule, 10-mL multidose vial.	1. Comatose (not just lethargic) patient. 2. Ineffective ventilation or adult respiratory rate <12. 3. Pinpoint pupils. 4. Circumstantial evidence of opioid intoxication, e.g., known drug abuser, track marks, opioid paraphernalia. **AR:** Relatively free of adverse reactions. Rare reports of pulmonary edema. Should be administered with caution in pregnancy.	Naloxone infusion therapy should be used if large initial dose was required, repeated boluses are necessary, or long-acting opiate is involved. In infusion therapy initial response dose is administered every hour and may need to be boostered in half-hour after starting. Infusion may be tapered after 12 h of therapy. Naloxone infusion: calculate daily fluid requirements, add initial response dose of naloxone multiplied by 24 to solution. Divide fluid by 24 h for naloxone infusion rate/h. Does not cause CNS depression. Routes: IV and endotracheal are preferred routes. Pentazocine (Talwin), dextramethorphan, propoxyphene (Darvon), and codeine may require larger doses.
31. **Nicotinamide,** various manufacturers. **Dose:** *Adult,* 500 mg IM or IV slowly, then 200–400 mg q 4 h. If symptoms develop, the frequency of injections should be increased to q 2 h (max 3 gm/day). *Child,* One-half suggested adult dose. **Packaged:** 100 mg/mL: 2-, 5-, 10-, and 30-mL vials; 25- and 50-mg tablets.	Vacor poisoning: phenylurea pesticide intoxication. *Note:* Vacor 2% is now available only to professional exterminators. 0.5% Vacor is available to general public and can be toxic to children if swallowed. **AR:** Large doses—flushing, pruritus, sensation of burning, nausea, vomiting, anaphylactic shock.	Nicotinamide is most effective when given within 1 h of ingestion. Do not use niacin or nicotinic acid in place of nicotinamide. Monitor liver profile.
32. **Oxygen** 100%. **Dose:** *Adult,* 100% oxygen by inhalation or 100% oxygen in hyperbaric chamber at 2–3 atm. *Child,* Same as adult.	Carbon monoxide or cyanide exposure, methemoglobinemia. Any inhalation intoxication.	The t½ of carboxyhemoglobin is 240 min in room air 21% oxygen; if patient is hyperventilated with 100% oxygen, t½ of carboxyhemoglobin is 90 min; in chamber at 2 atm, t½ is 25–30 min.
33. **Pancuronium bromide** (Pavulon, Organon). Nondepolarizing (competitive) blocking agent. **Dose:** *Adults and children,* initially, 0.1 mg/kg IV; for intubation, 0.1 mg/kg IV, repeated as required (generally every 40–60 min).† **Packaged:** Solution 1 mg/mL in 10 mL. 2 mg/mL in 2- and 5-mL containers.	Neuromuscular blocking agent. Used for intubation and seizure control, acts in 2 min, lasts 40–60 min. **AR:** Main hazard is inadequate postoperative ventilation. Tachycardia and slight increase in arterial pressure may occur due to vagolytic action.	Required dose varies greatly, and a peripheral nerve stimulator aids in determining appropriate amount. Should monitor EEG, because motor effect may be abolished without decreasing electric discharge from brain.
34. **D-Penicillamine** (Cuprimine, Merck; Depen, Wallace Labs). Effective chelator and promotes excretion in urine. **Dose:** *Adults,* 250 mg 4 times daily PO for up to 5 days for long-term (20–40 days) therapy; 30–40 mg/kg/day in children. Max 1 gm/day. For chronic therapy, 25 mg/kg/day in 4 doses. **Packaged:** 125- and 250-mg capsules.	For chelation of heavy metals: arsenic, cadmium, chromates, cobalt, copper, lead, mercury, nickel, and zinc. **MP:** Routine urinalysis, white blood count differential, hemoglobin determination, direct platelet count, renal and hepatic profiles. Collect 24-h urine, quantify for heavy metal. **AR:** Leukopenia (2%); thrombocytopenia (4%); GI—nausea, vomiting, diarrhea (17%); anaphylactic shock, fever, rash, lupus syndrome, renal and hepatic injury.	This is not considered standard therapy for lead poisoning after chelation therapy. May produce ampicillin-like rash, allergic reactions, neutropenia, and nephropathy. Contraindication: hypersensitivity to penicillin.

*This is for information purposes and is not intended to substitute for independent judgment. It is always advisable to review the package insert for the most up-to-date information. Contact Regional Poison Control Center for additional details on use.

†This dose may exceed the manufacturer's recommended dose.

‡Investigational drug in the United States.

§Not FDA-approved for this indication.

Abbreviations: AR = adverse reaction to antidotes; MP = monitoring parameters; FDA = US Food and Drug Administration; Conc = concentration; ECG = electrocardiogram; TIBC = total iron-binding capacity; G6PD = glucose-6-phosphate dehydrogenase; CNS = central nervous system; GI = gastrointestinal; AV = atrioventricular; EEG = electroencephalogram; RBC = red blood count; CBC = complete blood count.

TABLE 4. **Antidotes*** *Continued*

Medication	Indications	Comments
35. **Physostigmine salicylate** (Antilirium, O'Neil). Cholinesterase inhibitor; a diagnostic trial is not recommended. **Dose:** *Adult,* 1–2 mg IV over 2 min; may repeat every 5 min to max dose of 6 mg. *Child,* IV, 0.5 mg (0.02 mg/kg) over paralysis, 2 min to max of 2 mg q 30–60 min if symptoms recur.† Once effect is accomplished, give lowest effective dose. **Packaged:** 1 mg/mL in 2-mL ampule.	Not advised for use in diagnostic testing or for routine use in treating anticholinergic effects. Reserve for life-threatening complications. **AR:** Death may result from respiratory paralysis, hypertension or hypotension, bradycardia or tachycardia or asystole, hypersalivation, respiratory difficulties or convulsions (cholinergic crisis).	Do not consider for toxicities due to the following: antidepressants, amoxapine, maprotiline, nomifensine, bupropion, trazodone, imipramine. IV administration should be at a slow controlled rate, not more than 1 mg/min. Rapid administration can cause adverse reactions.
36. **Pralidoxime chloride** (2-PAM, Protopam, Ayerst). Cholinesterase reactivator; acts by removing phosphate. **Dose:** *Adult,* 1–2 gm IV infused in 100–250 mL saline IV over 15–30 min. Repeat in 1 h if needed. Repeat q 8–12 h when needed; if toxicity is severe, can give 0.5 gm/h infusion. *Child,* 25–50 mg/kg IV over 30 min. No faster than 10 mg/kg/min. Max 12 gm/24 h. **Packaged:** 1 gm/20-mL vials.	Organophosphate insecticide (OPI) poisoning. Not usually needed in carbamate insecticide poisoning. Most effective if started in first 24 h before bonding of phosphate. **AR:** Rapid IV injection has produced tachycardia, muscle rigidity, transient neuromuscular blockade. IM: conjunctival hyperemia, subconjunctival hemorrhage, especially if concentrations exceed 5%. Oral: nausea, vomiting, diarrhea, malaise.	Should be used only after initial treatment with atropine. Draw blood for RBC cholinesterase level before giving 2-PAM. Use of 2-PAM may require reduction in dose of atropine. End point is absence of fasciculations and return of muscle strength. **MP:** Monitor renal profile and reduce dose accordingly. t½: 1–2 h. Reversal of OPI effects at 4 µg/mL of 2-PAM. Start early because "aging" of PO_4 on acetylcholinesterase makes it more difficult to reverse.
37. **Protamine sulfate.** **Dose:** 1 mg neutralizes 90–115 U of heparin, max dose 50 mg IV over 5 min at 10 mg/mL. **Packaged:** 5 mL (50 mg); 25 mL (250 mg).	Heparin overdose. **AR:** Rapid administration causes anaphylactoid reactions.	**MP:** Monitor thromboplastin times. Doses of up to 200 mg have been tolerated over 2 h in adult.
38. **Pyridoxine** (Vitamin B₆). Gamma–amino acid agonist. **Dose:** *Unknown amount ingested:* 5 gm over 5 min IV. *Known amount:* add 1 gm of pyridoxine for each gram of INH ingested IV over 5 min. **Packaged:** 50 and 100 mg/mL; 10 and 30 mL.	Isoniazid (INH), monomethyl hydrazine mushrooms. **AR:** Unlikely owing to the fact that vitamin B₆ is water-soluble. However, nausea, vomiting, somnolence, and paresthesia have been reported from chronic high doses; up to 52 gm IV and up to 357 mg/kg have been tolerated.	Pyridoxine is given as 5–10% solution IV mixed with water. It may be repeated every 5–20 min until seizures cease. Some administer pyridoxine over 30–60 min. **MP:** Correct acidosis, monitor liver profile, acid-base parameters. Lethal dose of pyridoxine in animals is 1 gm/kg.
39. **Sodium bicarbonate.** **Dose:** IV 1–3 mEq/kg as needed to keep pH 7.5 (generally 2 mEq/kg q 6 h). When alkalinization is desired to correct acidosis to pH of 7.3, use 2 mEq/kg to raise pH 0.1 unit. **Packaged:** 50 mL and 50-mEq ampule.	To promote urinary alkalinization for salicylates, phenobarbital (weak acids with low volume of distribution and excreted in urine unchanged). To correct severe acidosis. To promote protein binding and supply sodium ions into Purkinje cells in cyclic antidepressant intoxication. **AR:** Large doses in patients with renal insufficiency may cause metabolic alkalosis. In patients with ketoacidosis, rapid alkalinization with sodium bicarbonate may result in clouding of consciousness, cerebral dysfunction, seizures, hypoxia, and lactic acidosis.	Alkaline diuresis. Assessment of need for bicarbonate should be based on both blood and urine pH. Maintain blood pH at 7.5. Keep urinary output at 3–6 mL/kg/h. May use diuretic to enhance diuresis. Potassium is necessary to produce alkaline diuresis. Monitor electrolytes, calcium, pH of both urine and blood, arterial blood gases.
40. **Sodium nitrite.**	See 14, Cyanide antidote kit.	
41. **Sodium thiosulfate.**	See 14, Cyanide antidote kit.	
42. **Succimer** (DMSA, Chemet, McNeil Consumer Products). **Dose:** 10 mg/kg or 350 mg/m² q 8 h for 5 days, then 10 mg/kg or 350 mg/m² q 12 h for 14 more days (see following chart). Therapy course lasts 19 days. **Packaged:** 100-mg capsule.	For chelation in children only when blood lead is >45 µg/dL. **AR:** Rashes, nausea, vomiting, an elevation of serum transaminases occur in 6–10% of patients.	Minimum of 2 weeks between courses is recommended unless venous lead indicates need for more prompt therapy. Patients who have received Ca-EDTA or BAL may use succimer after an interval of 4 weeks. In young children capsule can be opened and sprinkled on soft food. Monitor venous lead before therapy, on Day 7, and weekly for rebound. Monitor following tests: CBC, platelets, ferritin, liver.

*This is for information purposes and is not intended to substitute for independent judgment. It is always advisable to review the package insert for the most up-to-date information. Contact Regional Poison Control Center for additional details on use.

†This dose may exceed the manufacturer's recommended dose.

‡Investigational drug in the United States.

§Not FDA-approved for this indication.

Abbreviations: AR = adverse reaction to antidotes; MP = monitoring parameters; FDA = US Food and Drug Administration; Conc = concentration; ECG = electrocardiogram; TIBC = total iron-binding capacity; G6PD = glucose-6-phosphate dehydrogenase; CNS = central nervous system; GI = gastrointestinal; AV = atrioventricular; EEG = electroencephalogram; RBC = red blood count; CBC = complete blood count.

Table continued on following page

TABLE 4. **Antidotes*** *Continued*

Medication	Indications	Comments

Pediatric Dosing Chart

Weight (lb)	Weight (kg)	Dose (mg)	No. of Capsules
18–35	8–15	100	1
36–55	16–23	200	2
56–75	24–34	300	3
76–100	35–44	400	4
>100	>45	500	5

43. **Vitamin K** (AquaMEPHYTON, Merck). Promotes hepatic biosynthesis of prothrombin and other coagulation factors. Competitive antagonist of warfarin. It may be administered orally in absence of vomiting.

Dose: *Adult,* 2.5–10 mg IV, depending on potential for hemorrhage. Oral dose is 15–25 mg/day. Severe bleeding, 5–25 mg slow IV push. Rate 1 mg/min. Repeat q 4–8 h depending on prothrombin time. *Child,* 1–5 mg IV may be given orally when vomiting ceases at dose of 5–10 mg/day.

Packaged: 2 mg/mL in 0.5 mL ampules. 2.5- or 5-mL vials. Child oral dose 5–10 mg.

Indications: Overdose of warfarin (Coumadin) or superwarfarins, salicylate intoxication.

Comments: Fatalities from anaphylactic reaction have been reported after IV route. It takes 24 h for vitamin K to be effective. Need for further vitamin K is determined by prothrombin time. If bleeding is severe, fresh blood or plasma transfusion may be needed.

*This is for information purposes and is not intended to substitute for independent judgment. It is always advisable to review the package insert for the most up-to-date information. Contact Regional Poison Control Center for additional details on use.

†This dose may exceed the manufacturer's recommended dose.

‡Investigational drug in the United States.

§Not FDA-approved for this indication.

Abbreviations: AR = adverse reaction to antidotes; MP = monitoring parameters; FDA = US Food and Drug Administration; Conc = concentration; ECG = electrocardiogram; TIBC = total iron-binding capacity; G6PD = glucose-6-phosphate dehydrogenase; CNS = central nervous system; GI = gastrointestinal; AV = atrioventricular; EEG = electroencephalogram; RBC = red blood count; CBC = complete blood count.

Hemoperfusion

Hemoperfusion is the extracorporeal exposure of the patient's blood to an adsorbing surface (charcoal or resin). This procedure has extended extracorporeal removal to a large range of substances that were formerly either poorly dialyzable or nondialyzable. Hemoperfusion may be used for agents that have high protein binding, low aqueous solubility, and poor distribution in the plasma water. In these cases, hemodialysis is relatively ineffective. Hemoperfusion has proved useful in glutethimide intoxication, barbiturate overdose even with short-acting barbiturates, and intoxication with theophylline, tricyclic antidepressants, or chlorophenothane (DDT). Activated charcoal cartridges are the primary type of hemoperfusion that is currently available. In general, supportive care is all that is required. Analysis of studies with hemodialysis and hemoperfusion does not indicate that they reduce morbidity or mortality substantially except in certain cases (Table 6).

SUPPORTIVE CARE, OBSERVATION, AND THERAPY OF COMPLICATIONS

The comatose patient is on the threshold of death and must be stabilized initially by establishing an airway. Intubation should be accomplished in any comatose patient.

An intravenous line should be inserted in all comatose patients, and blood should be collected for appropriate tests, including toxicologic analysis (10 mL of clotted blood, initial gastric aspirate, 100 mL of urine). The initial management of the comatose patient should include the administration of 100% oxygen, 100 mg of thiamine intravenously, 50% glucose as an intravenous bolus, and 2 to 10 mg of naloxone (Narcan) intravenously. Other causes associated with coma and mimicking intoxications should be eliminated by examination and laboratory tests (trauma, infection, cerebrovascular accident, hypoxia, and endocrine-metabolic causes).

Pulmonary edema complicating poisoning may be cardiac or noncardiac in origin. Fluid overload during forced diuresis may cause the cardiac variety, particularly if the drugs used have an antidiuretic effect (opioids, barbiturates, and salicylates). Some toxic agents produce increased pulmonary capillary permeability, and other agents may cause a massive sympathetic discharge resulting in neurogenic pulmonary edema (opioids and salicylates). Management consists of minimizing fluid administration and administering diuretics and oxygen. If renal failure is present, dialysis may be necessary. The noncardiac type of pulmonary edema occurs with inhaled toxins, such as ammonia, chlorine, and oxides of nitrogen, or with drugs, such as salicylates, opioids, paraquat, and intravenous ethchlorvynol (Placidyl). This type does not respond to cardiac measures, and oxygen with intensive respiratory management using me-

TABLE 5. Dialysis: Indications and Contraindications

Immediate Consideration of Dialysis: Life-Threatening Toxicities

Ethylene glycol with refractory acidosis
Methanol with refractory acidosis and levels consistently over 50 mg/dL
Lithium levels consistently elevated over 4 mEq/L
Amanita phalloides

Severe Toxicities Due to Dialyzable Drugs (Stage 3 or Higher on Reed Coma Scale)

Alcohol*	Iodides
Ammonia	Isoniazid*
Amphetamines	Meprobamate
Anilines	Paraldehyde
Antibiotics	Potassium*
Barbiturates* (long-acting)	Quinidine
Boric acid	Quinine
Bromides*	Salicylates*
Calcium	Strychnine
Chloral hydrate*	Thiocyanates
Fluorides	(Certain other drugs also dialyzable)

Conditions Requiring Dialysis for General Supportive Therapy

Uncontrollable metabolic acidosis or alkalosis
Uncontrollable electrolyte disturbance, particularly sodium or potassium
Overhydration
Renal failure
Hyperosmolality not responding to conservative therapy
Marked hypothermia
Stage 3 or higher on Reed Coma Scale

Dialysis Contraindicated on Pharmacologic Basis Except for Supportive Care: Nondialyzable Drug Toxicities

Antidepressants (tricyclic and monoamine oxidase inhibitors)
Antihistamines
Barbiturates (short-acting)
Belladonna alkaloids
Benzodiazepines (Valium, Librium)
Digitalis and derivatives
Hallucinogens
Meprobamate (Equanil, Miltown)
Methyprylon (Noludar)
Opioids (heroin, Lomotil)
Phenothiazines (Thorazine, Compazine)
Phenytoin (Dilantin)

*Most useful.

chanical ventilation with positive end-expiratory pressure (PEEP) is necessary.

Hypotension and circulatory shock may be caused by heart failure due to myocardial depression, hypovolemia (fluid loss or venous pooling), a decrease in peripheral vasculature resistance (adrenergic blockage), or a loss of vasomotor tone caused by CNS depression.

Renal failure may be due to tubular necrosis as a result of hypotension, hypoxia, or a direct effect of the poison (e.g., salicylate, paraquat, acetaminophen, carbon tetrachloride) on the tubular cells. With hemoglobinuria or myoglobinuria, hemoglobin or myoglobin may precipitate in the renal tubules and produce renal failure.

Cerebral edema in intoxicated patients is produced by hypoxia, hypercapnia, hypotension, hypoglycemia,

and drug-impaired capillary integrity. Computed tomography (CT) may aid in diagnosis. Therapy consists of correction of the arterial blood gas and metabolic abnormalities and the hypotension. Reduction of the increased intracranial pressure may be accomplished by giving 20% mannitol, 0.5 gram per kg, infused over a 30-minute period, and hyperventilation to reduce the Pa_{CO_2} to 25 mmHg. The head should be elevated, and intracranial pressure monitoring should be considered. Fluid administration should be minimized.

Seizures are caused by many substances, such as amphetamines, camphor, chlorinated hydrocarbon insecticides, cocaine, isoniazid, lithium, phencyclidine, phenothiazines, propoxyphene, strychnine, and tricyclic antidepressants, and by drug withdrawal from ethanol and sedative hypnotics. Recurring or protracted seizures require intravenous diazepam (Valium) and phenytoin and, if seizure persists, a neuromuscular blocking agent and assisted ventilation.

Cardiac dysrhythmias occur with poisoning. A wide QT interval occurs with phenothiazines, and a wide QRS complex occurs with tricyclic antidepressants, quinine, or quinidine overdose. Digitalis, cocaine, cyanide, propranolol, theophylline, and amphetamines are among the more frequent toxic causes of dysrhythmias. Correction of metabolic disturbances and adequate oxygenation correct some of the dysrhythmias; others may require antidysrhythmic drugs or a cardiac pacemaker or cardioversion.

Metabolic acidosis with an increased anion gap is seen with many agents in overdose. There is a mnemonic by which to remember these agents: MUD PILES (*m*ethanol, *u*remia, *d*iabetic ketoacidosis, *p*araldehyde and *p*henformin, *i*ron and *i*soniazid, *l*actic acidosis, *e*thylene glycol and *e*thanol, and *s*alicylate,

TABLE 6. Plasma Concentrations Above Which Removal by Extracorporeal Means May Be Indicated

Drug	Plasma Concentration (mg/dL)*	Method of Choice
Phenobarbital	10	HP>HD
Other barbiturates	5	HP
Glutethimide	4	HP
Methaqualone	4	HP
Salicylates	80	HD>HP
Ethchlorvynol	15	HP
Meprobamate	10	HP
Trichloroethanol	5	HP
Paraquat	0.1	HP>HD
Theophylline	6 (chronic)	HP
	10 (acute)	
Methanol	50	HD
Ethylene glycol	Unknown	HD
Lithium	4 mEq/L	HD
Ethanol	500	HD

*1 mg/dL = 10 μg/mL.
Abbreviations: HP = hemoperfusion; HD = hemodialysis.
Modified from Haddad L, Winchester JF (eds): Clinical Management of Poisoning and Drug Overdose. Philadelphia, WB Saunders Co, 1983, p 162.

starvation, and solvents such as toluene). Assessment of the arterial blood gases, serum electrolytes, and plasma osmolality may be a clue to the etiologic agent. Intravenous sodium bicarbonate may be needed when the pH is below 7.1 if there is adequate ventilation.

Hematemesis can be produced by caustics and corrosives, iron, lithium, mercury, phosphorus, arsenic, mushrooms, plant poisons, fluoride, and organophosphates. Therapy consists of fluid and blood replacement and iced saline lavage if there is no esophageal damage. Although controversial, antacids, H_2 blockers, sucralfate, or misoprostol may be used.

TOXICOKINETICS FOR THE PRACTICING PHYSICIAN

Toxicokinetics is clinical pharmacokinetics from the viewpoint of the toxicologist. Pharmacokinetics is a mathematic description of what the body does to a drug. Knowledge of the toxicokinetics of a specific toxic agent allows the physician to plan a rational approach to the definitive management of the intoxicated patient after the vital functions have been stabilized.

The LD_{50} (the lethal dose for 50% of experimental animals) and the MLD (the minimal lethal dose) are seldom relevant in human intoxications but indicate potential toxicity of the substance. Protein binding of toxic agents influences the volume distribution, elimination, and action of the drug. Diuresis and dialysis are usually reserved for drugs with less than 50% protein binding. The "therapeutic blood range" for a drug is the range of drug concentrations at which the majority of the treated population can be expected to receive therapeutic benefit. The "toxic blood range" is the range of drug concentrations at which this majority would be expected to have toxic manifestations. The drug range values are not absolute. Blood concentrations are a quantitative aid in determining whether more specific measures need to be instituted in correlation with the clinical manifestations. The "apparent Vd" is the percentage of body mass in which the drug is distributed. It is determined by dividing the amount absorbed by the blood concentration. When a substance has a large Vd (above 1 liter per kg), as do most lipid-soluble chemicals, and is concentrated in the body fat, it is not available for diuresis, dialysis, or exchange transfusion. Elimination routes of detoxification allow the physician to make therapeutic decisions, such as using ethanol to interfere with the metabolism of methanol and ethylene glycol into more toxic metabolites. Urine identification is usually qualitative and allows only the identification of an agent.

Never manage a poisoned patient solely by laboratory tests, and always treat according to the manifestations of poisoning, not the laboratory test results. The laboratory toxicology analyst should be given whatever historical information is available so that the agent can be sought and identified as rapidly as possible. Toxicologic analysis is like a mini research project, unlike most other laboratory tests. Specimens for toxicologic analysis require the patient's name, the date, the time of exposure, the time the specimen was drawn, any therapeutic drugs administered, the patient's manifestations, and other relevant data. The toxicologic specimens that should be obtained for analysis are (1) vomitus or initial gastric aspiration, (2) blood, 10 mL (ask the analyst about the type of container and anticoagulant), and (3) urine, 100 mL. Acetaminophen plasma concentrations should be assessed in all suicide attempts.

COMMON POISONS AND THERAPY

Abbreviations Used in the Following List of Common Poisons

t½	=	half-life (time required for blood level to drop by 50% of original value)
Vd	=	volume of distribution (liters per kg)
TLV	=	threshold limit value in air
TWA	=	time-weighted average
PPM	=	parts per million in air and water
ECG	=	electrocardiogram
CPK	=	creatine phosphokinase
PEEP	=	positive end-expiratory pressure
EEG	=	electroencephalogram
BUN	=	blood urea nitrogen
EDTA	=	ethylenediaminetetraacetic acid

Conversion Factors

1 gram	=	1000 milligrams (mg)
1 milligram (mg)	=	1000 micrograms (μg)
1 microgram (μg)	=	1000 nanograms (ng)

Standard International Units:

1 mole	=	mol wt in grams per liter
1 millimole	=	mol wt in mg per liter
1 micromole	=	mol wt in μg per liter

Blood levels:

1 microgram per milliliter (mL)	=	100 μg per dL
	=	1 mg per liter
	=	1000 ng per mL
100 milligrams per deciliter (dL)	=	0.1 gram per dL
	=	1000 mg (1 gram) per liter
	=	1 mg per mL

Acetaminophen (APAP, Tylenol). *Toxic dose:* Child, 3 grams or more; adult, 7.5 grams or more. Liver toxicity, 140 mg per kg. *Toxicokinetics:* Absorption time, 0.5 to 1 hour. Vd, 0.9 liter per kg. *Route of elimination:* Liver. Draw peak blood level after 4 hours in overdose. *Manifestations:* First 24 hours: malaise, nausea, vomiting, and drowsiness, followed by latent period of 24 hours to 5 days; then hepatic symptoms, disturbances in clotting mechanism, and renal damage. *Management:* (1) Activated charcoal may be given when N-acetylcysteine (NAC) therapy is contemplated. In these circumstances, separate activated charcoal from NAC administration by 1 to 2 hours. (2) Give NAC for a toxic overdose (Antidote 1, Table 4). Start and give a full course if a toxic dose has been ingested or if blood concentrations are above the toxic line on the nomogram shown in Figure 1. (3) In this instance, a saline sulfate cathartic

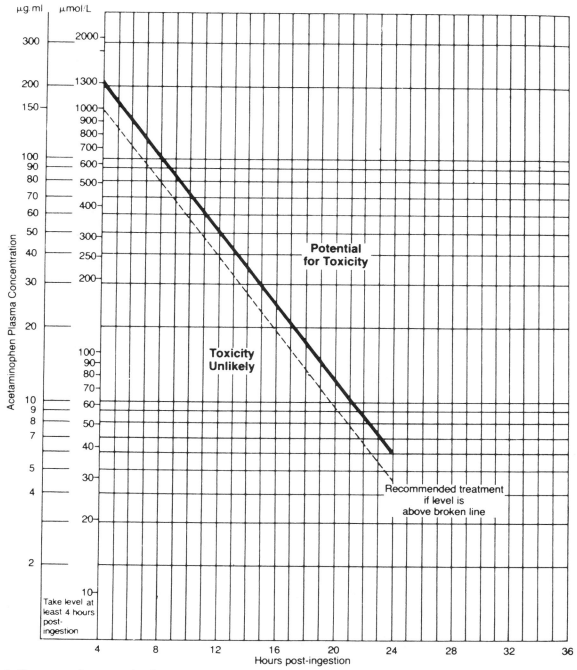

Figure 1. Nomogram for acetaminophen intoxication. Start *N*-acetylcysteine therapy if levels and time coordinates are above the lower line on the nomogram. Continue and complete therapy even if subsequent values fall below the toxic zone. The nomogram is useful only in acute, single ingestions. Serum levels drawn before 4 hours may not represent peak levels. (From Rumack BH, Matthew H: Acetaminophen poisoning and toxicity. Reproduced by permission of Pediatrics, Vol. 55, Page 871, Copyright 1975.)

is preferred to sorbitol. Treat at 50% APAP plasma levels of nomogram if the patient has a history of alcoholism or is taking enzyme inducer medication, i.e., anticonvulsants. *Laboratory aids*: APAP level, optimally at 4 to 6 hours. Plot levels on the nomogram in Figure 1 as a guide for treatment. Monitor liver and renal profiles daily.

Acids. See Caustics and Corrosives.

Alcohols

1. Ethanol (grain alcohol). *Manifestations*: Blood ethanol levels over 30 mg per dL produce euphoria; over 50, incoordination and intoxication; over 100, ataxia; over 300, stupor; and over 500, coma. Levels of 500 to 700 mg per dL may be fatal. Chronic alco-

holic patients tolerate higher levels, and the correlation may not be valid. *Management*: (1) Gastrointestinal decontamination. Caution: The rapid onset of CNS depression may preclude the induction of emesis. Activated charcoal and cathartics are not indicated. (2) Give 0.25 gram per kg of dextrose, 50%, intravenously if the blood glucose level is less than 60 mg per dL. (3) Thiamine, 100 mg intravenously, if chronic alcoholism is suspected, to prevent Wernicke-Korsakoff syndrome. (4) Hemodialysis is indicated in severe cases when conventional therapy is ineffective (rarely needed). (5) Treat seizures with diazepam (Valium) followed by phenytoin (Dilantin) if the patient is unresponsive. (6) Treat withdrawal with hydration and chlordiazepoxide (Librium) or diazepam. Large doses of sedatives may be required for delirium tremens. *Laboratory aids*: Arterial blood gases, electrolytes, blood ethanol levels, glucose; determine anion and osmolar gap and check for ketosis. Chest radiograph to determine whether aspiration pneumonia is present. Liver function tests and bilirubin levels.

2. ISOPROPANOL (rubbing alcohol). Normal propyl alcohol is related to isopropanol but is more toxic. *Manifestations*: Ethanol-like intoxication with acetone odor to breath, acetonuria, acetonemia without systemic acidosis, gastritis. With worsening acidosis, there is multiorgan failure, with death from complications of intractable acidosis. *Management*: (1) Gastrointestinal decontamination. Activated charcoal and cathartics are not indicated. (2) Hemodialysis in life-threatening overdose (rarely needed). *Laboratory aids*: Isopropyl alcohol levels, acetone, glucose, and arterial blood gases. The lack of excess acetone in the blood (normal 0.3 to 2 mg per dL) within 30 to 60 minutes or acetone in the urine within 3 hours excludes the possibility of significant isopropanol exposure.

3. METHANOL (wood alcohol). *Toxic dose*: One teaspoonful is potentially lethal for a 2-year-old child and can cause blindness in an adult. The toxic blood level of methanol is above 20 mg per dL, the potentially fatal level over 50 mg per dL. *Manifestations*: Metabolism may delay onset for 12 to 18 hours or longer if ethanol is ingested concomitantly. Hyperemia of optic disk, violent abdominal colic, blindness, and shock. With worsening acidosis, there is multiorgan failure, with death from complications of intractable acidosis. *Management*: (1) Gastrointestinal decontamination up to 1 hour after ingestion. Activated charcoal and cathartics are not indicated. (2) Treat acidosis vigorously with sodium bicarbonate intravenously. (3) If methanol is clinically suspected because of metabolic acidosis, with an anion gap if the methanol concentration is above 20 mg per dL, immediately initiate ethanol therapy intravenously or by mouth to produce a blood ethanol concentration of 100 to 150 mg per dL (Antidote 21, Table 4). (4) Folinic acid and folic acid have been used successfully in animal investigations. Administer leucovorin, 1 mg per kg up to 50 mg IV every 4 hours for six doses. (5) Consider hemodialysis if the blood methanol level is greater than 50 mg per dL or if significant metabolic acidosis or visual or mental symptoms are present. *Note*: The ethanol dose has to be increased during dialysis therapy. (6) Continue therapy (ethanol and hemodialysis) until the blood methanol level is preferably undetectable and there is no acidosis and no mental or visual disturbances. This often requires 2 to 5 days. (7) Ophthalmology consultation. *Laboratory aids*: Methanol and ethanol levels, electrolytes, glucose, and arterial blood gases.

Alkali. See Caustics and Corrosives.

Amitriptyline (Elavil). See Tricyclic Antidepressants.

Amphetamines (diet pills, various trade names). *Toxicity*: Child, 5 mg per kg; adult, 12 mg per kg has been reported as lethal. *Toxicokinetics*: Peak time of action is 2 to 4 hours. t½—8 to 10 hours in acid urine (pH less than 6.0) and 16 to 31 hours in alkaline urine (pH 7.5). *Route of elimination*: Liver, 60%; kidney, 30 to 40% at alkaline urine pH; at acid urine pH, 50 to 70%. *Manifestations*: Dysrhythmias, hyperpyrexia, convulsions, hypertension, paranoia, violence. *Management*: (1) Gastrointestinal decontamination. Avoid induced emesis because of rapid onset of action. (2) Control extreme agitation or convulsions with diazepam (Valium). Chlorpromazine (Thorazine) may be dangerous if ingestion is not pure amphetamine. (3) Treat hypertensive crisis with nitroprusside at 0.3 to 2 mg per kg per minute; maximum infusion rate 10 μg per kg per minute; should never last more than 10 minutes. (4) Acidification diuresis is not recommended. (5) Treat hyperpyrexia symptomatically. (6) If focal neurologic symptoms are present, consider cerebrovascular accident. Obtain a CT scan. (7) Observe for suicidal depression that may follow intoxication. (8) In life-threatening agitation, use haloperidol (Haldol). (9) Significant life-threatening tachydysrhythmia may respond to the alpha and beta blocker labetalol (Normodyne; Antidote 27, Table 4) or other appropriate antidysrhythmic agents. In a severely hemodynamically compromised patient, use immediate synchronized cardioversion. *Laboratory aids*: Monitor for rhabdomyolysis (CPK), myoglobinuria, hyperkalemia, and disseminated intravascular coagulation. Toxic blood level, 10 μg per dL.

Aniline. See Nitrites and Nitrates.

Anticholinergic Agents. Examples are antihistamines: hydroxyzine (Atarax), diphenhydramine (Benadryl); antipsychotics (neuroleptics): phenothiazines (Thorazine); antidepressant drugs (tricyclic antidepressants): imipramine (Tofranil); antiparkinsonian drugs: trihexyphenidyl (Artane), benztropine (Cogentin); over-the-counter sleep, cold, and hay fever medicines (methapyrilene); ophthalmic products (atropine); plants: jimsonweed *(Datura stramonium)*, deadly nightshade *(Atropa belladonna)*, henbane *(Hyoscyamus niger)*; and antispasmodic agents for the bowel (atropine). *Toxicokinetics*: See Table 7. *Manifestations*: Anticholinergic signs—hyperpyrexia, dilated pupils, flushing of skin, dry mucosa, tachycardia, delirium, hallucinations, coma, and convulsions. *Management*: (1) Gastrointestinal decontamination

TABLE 7. **Toxicokinetics of Anticholinergic Agents**

Drug	Potential Fatal Dose	Time to Peak Effect	Volume of Distribution (L/kg)	t½ (h)	Excretion Route
Atropine	Child: 10–20 mg; adult: 100 mg	1–2 h, may be prolonged in overdose	2.3	2–3	Renal (30–50%); hepatic (50–70%)
Diphenhydramine	Child: 25 mg/kg; adult: 2–8 gm	2 h, may be prolonged in overdose	3.3–6.8	3–10	98% hepatic

up to 12 hours postingestion. *Note*: Use caution with emesis if treating a diphenhydramine overdose because of rapid onset of action and seizures. (2) Control seizures with diazepam (Valium). (3) Control ventricular dysrhythmias with lidocaine (Xylocaine). (4) Physostigmine (Antidote 35, Table 4) for life-threatening anticholinergic effects refractory to conventional treatments. (5) Relieve urinary retention by catheterization to avoid reabsorption. (6) Treat cardiac dysrhythmias only if tissue perfusion is not adequate or if the patient is hypotensive. (7) Control hyperpyrexia by external cooling. No antipyretics.

Anticonvulsants. See Table 8. *Toxic dose*: Specific anticonvulsant blood levels and the clinical manifestations indicate toxicity. In general, the ingestion of five times the therapeutic dose is expected to have the potential for toxicity. *Management*: (1) Gastrointestinal decontamination up to 12 hours postingestion. Repeated doses of activated charcoal shorten t½ of carbamazepine, phenobarbital, primidone, phenytoin, and possibly others. Naloxone (Narcan) (Antidote 30, Table 4) may improve valproic acid–induced coma. (2) Monitor specific anticonvulsant blood lev-

els. (3) The effectiveness of hemoperfusion and dialysis has not been established.

Antidepressants. See Tricyclic Antidepressants.

Antifreeze. See Alcohols (Methanol) and Ethylene Glycol.

Antihistamines (H₁-Receptor Antagonists). See Anticholinergic Agents. Newer nonsedating long-acting preparations—terfenadine (Seldane) and astemizole—may produce prolonged QT intervals and torsades de pointes. In patients who have impaired hepatic function or are receiving cimetidine, ketoconazole, or macrolide antibiotics, the metabolism of terfenadine and astemizole may be inhibited. All children who ingest these newer nonsedating antihistamines or adults who ingest more than the therapeutic dose require close cardiac monitoring for 24 hours. Gastrointestinal decontamination is advised.

Arsenic and Arsine Gas. *Toxic dose*: In humans, the inorganic arsenic trioxide toxic dose is 5 to 50 mg; the potential fatal dose is 120 mg or 1 to 2 mg per kg. Sodium arsenite is nine times more toxic than arsenic trioxide. Organic arsenic is less toxic. The maximal allowable concentration for prolonged

TABLE 8. **Anticonvulsants**

Drug	Peak Time of Action (Steady State)	Volume of Distribution (L/kg)	t½ (h)	Route of Elimination (%)	Protein Binding (%)	Blood Level (µg/mL)	Comment*
Carbamazepine (Tegretol)	8–24 h (2–4 days)	1.0	18–54	Liver (98)	70	Therapeutic, 4–10	Related to tricyclic antidepressants, can cause dysrhythmias
Ethosuximide (Zarontin)	24–48 h (5–8 days)	0.8	36–55	Liver (80–90)	0	Therapeutic, 40–100	
Phenytoin (Dilantin)	PO, 6–12 h IV, 1 h (5–10 days)	1.0	24; varies in toxic doses: zero-order kinetics	Liver (95)	90	Therapeutic, 10–20; toxic, 20–30; nystagmus only, 30–40; ataxia, 40+; coma, convulsions	Dysrhythmias with parenteral use only
Primidone (Mysoline)	?3–4 days	0.6	Parent, 3–12; metabolites, 30–36	Liver	60	Therapeutic, 6–12 primidone and 15–40 phenobarbital (PB); toxic, over 50 primidone and over 40 PB (see Barbiturates)	Metabolized to active metabolites phenylethylmalonamide and PB; overdose gives white crystals in urine†
Valproic acid (Depakene)	?1–2 days	0.4	5–15	Liver (80–100)	84–96	Therapeutic, 50–100	Produces nausea and vomiting, changes in liver function
Clonazepam (Clonopin)	?		20–60	Liver (98)	90	Therapeutic, 20–70 ng/mL	
Phenobarbital (Luminal)	3–6 h	0.75	50–120	Liver	30	Therapeutic, 15–40	

*Manifestations: The major manifestations of these agents are depression of consciousness and respiratory depression. Other significant manifestations are mentioned in this column.

†Primidone produces whorls of shimmering white crystals in the urine from precipitation of intact primidone in massive overdose.

TABLE 9. **Comparative Acute Toxicities of Some Common Arsenicals**

Arsenic Compound	Lethal Dose
Arsenate	5–50 mg/kg
Arsenites	<5 mg/kg
Arsenic trioxide (insoluble)	120 mg total
Arsenic trioxide (soluble)*	13 mg total

*Nine times as toxic as insoluble form.

exposure is 0.05 PPM. See Table 9. Humans are more sensitive than rodents to arsenic. Acute poisoning results from accidental ingestion of arsenic-containing pesticides. (Ant traps sold in some states contain arsenic.) *Toxicokinetics*: Arsenates are water-soluble and arsenite is lipid-soluble. The soluble forms of arsenic are rapidly absorbed by inhalation and ingestion. Arsenic crosses the placenta and can cause fetal damage. Distributes into spleen, liver, kidneys. *Excretion*: In urine, 90%. After acute ingestion, it takes 10 days to clear a single dose; after chronic ingestion, up to 70 days. *Arsine gas*: Forms when active hydrogen comes in contact with arsenic. This may occur when zinc, antimony, lead, or iron is contaminated with arsenic and comes in contact with acid. This causes arsine inhalation intoxication characterized by a latent period of 2 to 48 hours and a triad of abdominal pain, jaundice (due to hemolysis), and hematuria. *Manifestations*: Arsenic intoxication produces gastroenteritis, neurologic and cardiac abnormalities, subsequent renal involvement. A garlic odor to the breath may be a clue. Smaller doses and prolonged low-level exposure produce subacute (stomatitis) and chronic (peripheral neuropathy) symptoms. *Management*: (1) Gastrointestinal decontamination. Activated charcoal is ineffective. Cathartics are not advised because of the potential for diarrhea. Follow with abdominal radiographs because arsenic is radiopaque. Consider whole-bowel washout if usual methods fail to remove arsenic. (2) Intravenous fluids to correct dehydration and electrolyte deficiencies. (3) Treat shock with oxygen, blood, and fluids as needed. (4) In severe cases, administer BAL (dimercaprol) (Antidote 17, Table 4). (5) In chronic poisoning, D-penicillamine (Antidote 34, Table 4) may be used to chelate arsenic. Therapy should be continued in 5-day cycles until the urine arsenic level is less than 50 μg per liter. (6) Treat liver and renal impairment. (7) Hemodialysis is effective in acute poisoning and can be used concurrently with chelation therapy in severe cases, especially if renal failure develops. (8) Arsine intoxication is treated by exchange transfusion and hemodialysis if renal failure occurs. BAL is ineffective. *Laboratory aids*: Blood arsenic and 24-hour urine arsenic levels. Excessive exposure is indicated by a level of 50 μg per liter of arsenic in urine, but persons whose diets are rich in seafood may excrete larger amounts. View values over 50 μg per day with suspicion. Monitor ECG and renal function. A blood arsenic level above 1.0 mg per liter is toxic, and one of 9 to 15 mg per liter is

potentially fatal (false values occur in inexperienced laboratories).

Aspirin. See Salicylates.

Atropine. See Anticholinergic Agents.

Barbiturates. See Table 10. *Management*: (1) Gastrointestinal decontamination. Avoid emesis in short-acting barbiturate intoxications. Activated charcoal and a cathartic in repeated doses have been shown to reduce the serum half-life of phenobarbital and increase the nonrenal clearance by over 50%. Give every 4 hours while the patient is comatose. (2) Supportive and symptomatic care is all that is necessary in the majority of cases. (3) Alkalinization with sodium bicarbonate, 2 mEq per kg intravenously during the first hour, followed by sufficient sodium bicarbonate (Antidote 39, Table 4) to keep the urinary pH at 7.5 to 8.0, enhances the excretion of long-acting barbiturates. Alkalinization is not useful for short-acting barbiturate intoxication. Forced diuresis should be used with caution because of fluid overload. At present, alkalinization without diuresis is advocated. (4) In severe cases that do not respond to conservative measures, consider hemodialysis and hemoperfusion. (5) Treat any bulla as a local second-degree skin burn. (6) Give intensive care monitoring to the comatose patient. *Treatment of withdrawal: In an emergency*, use thiopental (Pentothal) or diazepam (Valium) intravenously. If the patient is stable, pentobarbital is given orally and the patient examined after 1 hour for signs of intoxication (nystagmus, slurred speech, and ataxia). If none is present, the dose is repeated every 3 hours until these signs develop. This is the stabilizing dose; the patient is maintained on this dose for 72 hours and then changed to phenobarbital, 30 mg substituted for each 100 mg of pentobarbital. The phenobarbital is tapered, decreasing by 10% or 30 mg every 3 to 5 days. *Laboratory aids*: Emergency plasma barbiturate concentrations rarely alter management.

Benzene. See Hydrocarbons.

Benzodiazepines (BZPs). See Table 11. *Toxicity*: Low toxic potential. More than 500 mg has been ingested without respiratory depression. Benzodiazepines have an additive effect with sedatives, such as alcohol and barbiturates. Most patients intoxicated with benzodiazepines alone recover within 24 hours. Many of these agents have active metabolites with a long plasma t½, so performance in skilled tasks, such as driving, may be impaired. Withdrawal may be delayed. *Manifestations*: CNS depression. Deep coma leading to respiratory depression suggests the presence of other drugs. *Management*: (1) Gastrointestinal decontamination. (2) Supportive and symptomatic care. (3) Flumazenil (Romazicon) is a recently approved specific benzodiazepine antagonist. It is not a treatment for hypoventilation and should be used with caution in overdose cases because of dependency and seizures (Antidote 23, Table 4). (4) Withdrawal, if it occurs, is treated with a long-acting benzodiazepine on a tapering schedule. *Laboratory aids*: Document benzodiazepines in urine. Quantitative blood levels are not useful.

TABLE 10. **Features of Barbiturates***

Feature	Long-Acting (LAB)	Intermediate-Acting (IAB)	Short-Acting (SAB)
Duration (h)	>8	3–8	<3
Medical use	Anticonvulsants	Sedative hypnotics	
Half-life (h)	>50	<50	<50
DEA	Schedule IV	Schedule II	Schedule II

Feature	Barbital	Phenobarbital†	Amobarbital	Pentobarbital	Secobarbital
Trade name	Veronal	Luminal	Amytal	Nembutal	Seconal
Slang name	—	Purple hearts	Blues	Yellows	Red devils
pKa	7.8	7.24	7.9	7.96	7.9
Elimination route	Renal 20% Hepatic 80%	Renal 30% Hepatic 70%	Hepatic 98%	Hepatic >90%	Hepatic >90%
Onset IV (min)	22	12	—	0.1	0.1
Onset oral	1 h	20–60 min	13–30 min	15–30 min	10–30 min
Peak conc oral (h)	12–18	6–18	3–4	2–4	1–2
Protein-bound (%)	6	20–40	40–60	40–65	40–60
Oral Doses					
Fatal dose (gm)	10	8	5	3	3
(mg/kg)	75	65	40	50	30
Toxic dose (mg/kg)	>10	10	>6	>6	>6
Adult nontolerant (mg)	—	300	200–300	200–300	200
Therapeutic dose (mg/kg)	2–6	2–6	2–6	2–6	6
Adult dose (mg)	300–500	100–200	100–200	100–200	100–200
Blood Concentrations					
Therapeutic (µg/mL)	5–8	15–40	5–6	1–5	1–5
Toxic (µg/mL)	>30	>40	10–30	>10	>10
Lethal‡ (µg/mL)	>100	>100	>50	>35	>35
Duration (h)	16	6–8	6	6	6
Elimination t½ (h)	56–96	50–120	15–40	15–30	22–29
Volume of distribution (L/kg)	—	0.75	0.5	0.65	1.5
Available					
Capsule (mg)	—	16	65, 200	50, 100	50, 100
Tablet (mg)	—	16, 32, 65, 100	15, 30, 50, 100	—	100
Elixir (mg/5 mL)	—	15, 20	—	20	—
Suppository (mg)	—	—	—	30, 60, 120, 200	—

Manifestations

Low dose: Euphoria, ataxia, incoordination, nystagmus on lateral gaze

High dose: Flaccid coma, hypotension, respiratory depression, pulmonary edema (particularly with the short-acting barbiturates), subcutaneous bullae (6%), dermatographia

---

*Classification into long-acting, intermediate, and short-acting has no relationship to the duration of coma.

†The t½ in children is approximately 50% of adult.

‡These levels are not absolute, and tolerance occurs.

Abbreviations: DEA = Drug Enforcement Agency; conc = concentration; t½ = half-life.

Bleach. Household bleaches are 4 to 6% sodium hypochlorite. Commercial types are 10 to 20%. *Manifestations*: Difficulty in swallowing; pain in mouth, throat, chest, or abdomen. General household strength bleach does not produce burns; commercial strength bleach may. Inhalation of gases produced by mixing chlorine bleach with acids (toilet bowl cleaner and rust removers—chlorine gas) or with household ammonia (chloramine gas) causes irritation of mucous membranes, eyes, and upper respiratory tract. *Management*: (1) Ingestion—(a) Avoid gastrointestinal decontamination procedures. Dilute with small amounts of water or milk. Avoid acids. (b) Use esophagoscopy only if unusually large amounts have been ingested, the patient is symptomatic, or the product was stronger than the average household bleach. (2) Inhalation—remove from contaminated area. Observe for pulmonary edema. (3) Ocular exposure requires immediate gentle irrigation with water for at least 15 minutes, followed by fluorescein dye stain to detect any damage.

Botulism. See the article "Food-Borne Illness" in Section 2.

Brake Fluid. See Ethylene Glycol.

Calcium Channel Blockers. Used in treatment of effort angina, supraventricular tachycardia, and hypertension. See Table 12. *Manifestations*: Hypotension, bradycardia within 1 to 5 hours, CNS depression, and gastric distress. Manifestations are delayed after the ingestion of slow-release preparations. *Management*: (1) Gastrointestinal decontamination. If long-acting preparation, consider whole-bowel

TABLE 11. **Benzodiazepines (BZPs)**

Drug	Oral Dosage Range	Time to Peak Oral Plasma Levels (h)	$t\frac{1}{2}$ (h)	Major Active Metabolites ($t\frac{1}{2}$ in h)	Elimination Rate
Anxiolytics					
Diazepam (Valium)	6–40 mg/day	1–2	14–100	Desmethyldiazepam (50–100 h)	Slow
Chlordiazepoxide (Librium, Libritabs, various others)	15–100 mg/day	2–4	5–30	Desmethylchlordiazepoxide, demoxepam, desmethyldiazepam (50–100 h)	Slow
Clorazepate (Tranxene)	15–60 mg/day	1–2.5	1.1–2.9	Desmethyldiazepam (50–100 h)	Slow
Prazepam (Centrax)	20–60 mg/day	6	0.6–2	3-Hydroxyprazepam, desmethyldiazepam (50–100 h)	Slow
Halazepam (Paxipam)	60–160 mg/day	1–3	1.6–5.3	N-3-Hydroxyhalazepam, desmethyldiazepam (50–100 h)	Slow
Oxazepam (Serax)	30–120 mg/day	1–2	8–25	None	Rapid to intermediate
Lorazepam (Ativan)	2–6 mg/day	2–5	10–20	None	Intermediate
Alprazolam (Xanax)	0.75–4 mg/day	0.7–1.6	6–26	α-Hydroxyalprazolam	Intermediate
Hypnotics					
Flurazepam (Dalmane)	15–60 mg	0.5–2	50–100	Desalkylflurazepam ($t\frac{1}{2}$ = 50–100)	Slow
Midazolam (Versed)	5–30 mg/day IV	0.3–0.8	1.2–12.3	None	—
Flunitrazepam (Rohypnol— investigational, Roche)	1–2 mg	<1	0.5–2	7-Aminoflunitrazepam ($t\frac{1}{2}$ = 23), N-desmethylflunitrazepam ($t\frac{1}{2}$ = 31)	—
Temazepam (Restoril)	15–30 mg	2–3	10–20	None	Intermediate
Triazolam (Halcion)	0.125–0.5 mg	0.5–1.5	2–5	α-Hydroxytriazolam	Rapid
Quazepam (Doral)	7.5–15 mg	1–2	>39	2-Oxoquazepam N-desalkylflurazepam	Intermediate
Estazolam (ProSom)	1–2 mg	1–2	12–15	1-Oxo estazolam	Intermediate
Anticonvulsants					
Clonazepam (Klonopin)	1.5–20 mg/day	1–4	18–50	None	—
Zolpidem* (Ambien)	5–20 mg/day	2	1.5–2.5	None	Rapid

*Not a benzodiazepine chemically but an imidazopyridine that is a selective benzodiazepine-1 receptor agonist.

washout. If patient is symptomatic, obtain a cardiac consult. May need pacemaker. (2) Treat hypotension and bradycardia with positioning, fluids, and calcium gluconate or chloride (Antidote 12B, Table 4). Dopamine or norepinephrine may be used if necessary. If calcium fails, use sodium bicarbonate, glucagon, or both (Antidote 26, Table 4). (3) Heart block—may respond to intravenous calcium (Antidote 12B, Table 4) or atropine sulfate, 0.5 to 1 mg, if no response. (4) Ventricular pacing may be required in the severely intoxicated patient. (5) Patients receiving digitalis run the risk of toxicity and should be carefully monitored. (6) Extracorporeal washout measures are generally not considered to be useful. *Laboratory aids*: Specific drug levels, blood sugar and calcium, ECG.

Camphor (external analgesic rubs, Vicks VapoRub 4.8%, Campho-Phenique 11%). Many camphorated oil products were removed from the marketplace in September, 1982. Five milliliters of camphorated oil (20% camphor) equals 1 gram of camphor. *Toxicity*: More than 10 mg per kg by ingestion may cause seizures. Adult, 5 grams has been fatal; child, 1 gram. *Toxicokinetics*: Time to onset of manifestations, 5 to 90 minutes. Readily and rapidly absorbed

through the skin, mucous membranes, and gastrointestinal tract, and crosses the placenta. *Route of elimination*: Rapidly metabolized in liver to glucuronide form, which is excreted in urine. Pulmonary excretion causes a distinctive odor on the breath. *Manifestations*: Nausea, vomiting, and burning epigastric pain. Seizures may occur suddenly and without warning within 5 minutes of ingestion. Apnea and vision disturbances may occur. *Management*: Medical evaluation and admission should be considered for ingestion of over 50 mg per kg or over 3000 mg. (1) Induction of emesis is contraindicated because of early seizures. (2) Remove residual drug by gastric lavage. (3) Administer activated charcoal and a saline cathartic. Avoid giving oils or alcohol. (4) Treat seizures with intravenous diazepam (Valium). (5) Treat apnea with respiratory support.

Carbon Monoxide (CO). This is an odorless gas produced from incomplete combustion; it is found also as an in vivo metabolic breakdown product of methylene chloride (paint removers). Observe for the symptoms described in Table 13. Contrary to popular belief, the skin rarely shows a cherry-red color in the living patient. *Toxicokinetics*: CO is rapidly absorbed

TABLE 12. **Kinetics of the Calcium Channel Blockers**

Parameter	Nifedipine	Verapamil	Dilti-azem	Nicardipine	Nimodipine	Felodi-pine*	Amlodi-pine	Bepridil	Isradi-pine
Class	Dihydro-pyridine	Phenylal-kylamine	Benzothia-zepine	Dihydro-pyridine	Dihydro-pyridine	Dihydro-pyridine	Dihydro-pyridine	Dihydro-pyridine	Dihydro-pyridine
Trade name	Procardia	Calan, Isoptin	Cardizem	Cardene	Nimotop	Plendil	Norvasc	Vascor	DynaCirc
Preparations	10-, 20-mg cap	40-, 80-, 120-mg tab	30-, 60-, 90-, 120-mg tab	20-, 30-mg cap	30 mg cap	None	2.5-, 5-, 10-mg tab	200-, 300-, 400-mg tab	2.5-, 5-mg cap
Slow-release preparation	30-, 60-, 90-mg cap	120-, 180-, 240-mg tab	60-, 90-, 120-, 180-, 240-, 300-mg tab	30-, 45-, 60-mg cap	None	5, 10 mg tab	See above	None	None
Bioavail-ability (%)	65–70	20–30	40	35	3–30	20	60–65	60	17
Mean toxic dose	340 mg	3.2 gm	?rare toxicity	NA	NA	NA	—	—	—
Serious toxic amount	Lowest 200 mg	40 mg/kg child 2–3 gm adult	Up to 300 mg well tolerated by adults	NA	NA	NA	—	—	—
Dose range (mg/day)	30–120	120–480	90–360	60–120	60–360	5–30	2.5–10	200–400	2.5–15
Max daily dose (mg/day)	—	—	—	—	—	—	10	400	20
Onset of action (min)									
Oral	<20	30–120	<15	<20	<20	—	—	—	—
IV	<1	<3	<1	—	—	—	—	—	—
SL	3–5	—	—	—	—	—	—	—	—
Peak action									
Oral	30–90 min	60–90 min	30–60 min	60 min	60 min	2.6–6 h	6–9	2–3	2–3
SL	20 min	—	—	—	—	—	—	—	—
Sustained	—	4–8 h	3–4 h	—	—	—	—	—	—
Peak blood conc (min)	30–60	90–120	120–180	60	NA	NA	—	—	—
t½ (h)	3–6	6–12	4–9	8	1–8	24	35–50	33–42	5–10.7
Duration (h)	4–12	6–12	—	4–6	NA	—	24	24	12
Protein binding (%)	92–98	90–99	70–85	>95	>95	NA	98	99	97
Volume of distribution (L/kg)	1–5	4.5–7	3–5	NA	—	—	21	8	3
Elimination	Renal 50–70%	Hepatic 60–65%	Renal 70–80%	Hepatic	—	—	Hepatic	Hepatic	Hepatic
Metabolite	Inactive	Active mild norverapamil	Active 50% parent diacetyl-diltiazem	NA	NA	NA	Pyridine deriv. (not active)	17 metabo-lites (one active)	None active

*Anonymous: Felodipine—another calcium channel blocker for hypertension. Med Lett *33*:115–116, 1991.
Abbreviations: cap = capsules; tab = tablets; NA = no available information; SL = sublingual; conc = concentration.

TABLE 13. **Progression of Signs and Symptoms with Carbon Monoxide (CO) Exposure**

CO in Atmosphere (PPM)	Duration of Exposure (h)	Saturation of Blood (%)	Signs and Symptoms
Up to 0.01	Indefinite	1–10	None
0.01–0.02	Indefinite	10–20	Tightness across forehead, slight headache, dilatation of cutaneous vessels
0.02–0.03	5–6	20–30	Headache, throbbing temples
0.04–0.06	4–5	30–40	Severe headache, weakness and dizziness, nausea and vomiting, collapse, leukocytosis
0.07–0.10	3–4	40–50	Above, plus increased tendency to collapse and syncope, increased pulse and respiratory rate
0.11–0.15	1.5–3	50–60	Increased pulse and respiratory rate, syncope, Cheyne-Stokes respirations, coma with intermittent convulsions
0.16–0.30	1–1.5	60–70	Coma with intermittent convulsions, depressed heart action and respirations, death possible
0.50–1.00	1–2	70–80	Weak pulse, depressed respirations, respiratory failure, and death

through the lungs. The rate of absorption is directly related to alveolar ventilation. Elimination occurs through the lungs. The t½ in room air equals 5 to 6 hours; in 100% oxygen, 90 minutes; in hyperbaric oxygen, 20 minutes. The nomogram pictured in Figure 2 can be used to decide quickly whether serious CO intoxication is likely to have occurred and to select patients at high risk or who need early management in the intensive care unit or need hyperbaric oxygen. *Management*: (1) Remove the patient from contaminated area and expose to fresh air. Establish vital functions. (2) Give 100% oxygen to all patients until the carboxyhemoglobin level falls to

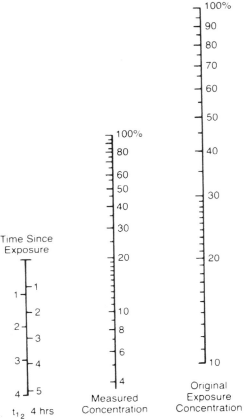

Figure 2. Nomogram for calculating carboxyhemoglobin concentration at time of exposure. The time since exposure is given on two scales to allow for the effects of previous oxygen administration on the half-life (t½) of carboxyhemoglobin (left-hand scale assumes a t½ of 3 hours). *Note*: The nomogram assumes a t½ of carboxyhemoglobin of 4 hours in a subject breathing room air. Most patients will not have received supplementary oxygen before admission, and at best this will have been administered via a face mask, giving a maximal fractional inspired oxygen concentration of 50 to 60% with little effect on carboxyhemoglobin elimination. The scale on the left side of the time column makes allowances for prior oxygen supplements by assuming a short t½ of 3 hours. The nomogram may help decide quickly whether serious carbon monoxide intoxication is likely to have occurred and may help select patients at high risk for early management in the intensive care unit. The nomogram may be an oversimplification because patients usually are not resuscitated with constant concentrations of oxygen, and many patients may hyperventilate, thus changing elimination characteristics. (Redrawn from Clark CJ, Campbell D, Reid WH: Blood carboxyhaemoglobin and cyanide levels in fire survivors. Lancet *1*[8234]:1332–1335, © by The Lancet Ltd, 1981.)

5% or less. Assisted ventilation may be necessary. The exposed pregnant woman should be kept in 100% oxygen for several hours after the carboxyhemoglobin level is zero because carboxyhemoglobin concentrates in the fetus and oxygen is needed five times longer to ensure elimination of CO from fetal circulation. CO or hypoxia may be teratogenic. (3) Monitor arterial blood gases and carboxyhemoglobin levels. Determine carboxyhemoglobin level at time of exposure by using nomogram. *Note*: A near-normal carboxyhemoglobin level does not rule out significant CO poisoning. (4) Only if pH is below 7.1 after correction of hypoxia and adequate ventilation, give sodium bicarbonate to correct acidosis. (5) Indications for 100% oxygen and, if possible, therapy with hyperbaric oxygen—(a) carboxyhemoglobin level higher than 25%, (b) carboxyhemoglobin level higher than 15% in a child or in a patient with cardiovascular disease, (c) carboxyhemoglobin level higher than 10% in a pregnant woman (and monitor fetus), (d) abnormal or ischemic chest pain or ECG abnormality, (e) abnormal chest radiograph, (f) presence of hypoxia, myoglobinuria, or abnormal renal function, or (g) history of unconsciousness, syncope, or neuropsychiatric symptoms. The most important indication for the hyperbaric chamber is a history of unconsciousness. A list of hyperbaric oxygen chambers can be obtained by contacting a Regional Poison Control Center. (6) Treat seizures with intravenous diazepam (Valium). (7) Monitor ECG, chest radiograph, and serum CPK and lactate dehydrogenase levels. (8) Treat cerebral edema with elevation of the patient's head, minimizing intravenous fluid and hyperventilation; if needed, give mannitol and monitor intracranial pressure. (9) Re-evaluate after recovery for neuropsychiatric sequelae. *Laboratory aids*: Arterial blood gases show metabolic acidosis and normal oxygen tension but reduced oxygen saturation, as measured by a co-oximeter.

Carbon Tetrachloride. See Hydrocarbons.

Caustics and Corrosives. Common acid substances are hydrochloric acid, sulfuric acid (battery acid), carbolic acid (phenol), nitric acid, oxalic acid, hydrofluoric acid, and aqua regia (mixture of hydrochloric and nitric acids). These are used as cleaning agents. Common alkaline substances are sodium or potassium hydroxide (lye), sodium hypochlorite (bleach [Chlorox]), sodium carbonate (nonphosphate detergents), potassium permanganate, ammonia, electric dishwasher agents, cement, and flat disk batteries. *Manifestations*: Dysphagia, drooling, pain in the throat or abdomen. Esophageal or gastric perforation, chest or abdominal pain, and peritoneal irritation may occur. *Toxicity*: Acids produce mucosal coagulation necrosis. They usually do not penetrate deeply (exception: hydrofluoric acid). The gastric mucosa is the primary site of injury. Alkalis produce liquefaction necrosis and saponification and penetrate deeply. Oropharyngeal and esophageal damage by solids is more frequent than that by liquids. Liquids are more likely to produce gastric damage. *Toxic dose*: Potential fatal dose of concentrated acid or alkali is 5 mL. The absence of oral burns does not exclude the possibility of esophageal burns (seen in 10 to 15% of patients). *Management*: (1) Dilute with milk or water immediately up to 30 mL in children or 250 mL in adults. Neutralization with acidic or alkaline agents is contraindicated. Dilute only if patient can swallow. Contraindications to dilution are an inability to swallow and signs of respiratory distress, shock, or esophageal perforation. (2) Gastrointestinal decontamination is contraindicated. In acid ingestions, however, some authorities advocate nasogastric intubation and aspiration in the early postingestion phase. The patient should receive only intravenous fluids after dilution until surgical consultation is obtained. Dermal and ocular decontamination should be carried out. (3) Endoscopy at 12 to 48 hours postingestion may be indicated to assess the severity of burn. (4) Steroids are controversial. (5) Antibiotics are not useful prophylactically. (6) Barium swallow may be necessary at 10 days to 3 weeks to assess the severity of damage. (7) Esophageal dilatation may need to be performed at 2- to 4-week intervals if evidence of stricture is found. (8) Interposition of the colon may be necessary if dilatation fails to provide an adequate-sized esophagus. (9) Inhalation management requires immediate removal from the environment, and clinical, radiographic, and arterial blood gas evaluation when appropriate. Oxygen and respiratory support may be required.

Chloral Hydrate. See Sedative Hypnotics.

Chlordane. See Organochlorine Insecticides.

Chlordiazepoxide (Librium). See Benzodiazepines.

Chlorine Gas. Chlorine gas is a yellow-greenish gas with an irritating odor, used in bleach, in the manufacture of plastics, and for water purification. Exposure usually results from transportation mishaps, industrial accidents, chemistry experiments, the mixing of household cleaners with bleach containing hypochlorite, and accidental release around swimming pools. Its density is greater than that of air, and an odor is detected at concentrations of less than 0.04 to 0.2 PPM. Chlorine acts as an oxidizing agent and also reacts with tissue water to form hypochlorous and hydrochloric acids and generate free oxygen radicals. *Toxic dose*: The threshold limit value is less than 1 PPM, but mild mucous irritation occurs in some patients; 30 PPM produces choking and chest pain; 60 PPM produces pulmonary edema; 400 PPM for 30 minutes is lethal; and 1000 PPM is fatal in a few minutes. *Management*: (1) Remove the patient from the contaminated environment and stabilize vital functions. Use decontamination procedures for dermal and ocular contamination as indicated. Protect rescue personnel with breathing apparatus. There are patients who have responded to nebulized 3.75% sodium bicarbonate (4 mL) (prepared by diluting 2 mL of 7.5% intravenous sodium bicarbonate with 2 mL of saline). *Classification*: If patient is symptomless or presents with a cough that clears up in less than 1 hour, advise rest for 12 hours and ask the patient to report if symptoms occur; no vigorous exercise for 24 hours. If symptoms persist beyond the period of exposure, admit to hospital and treat with bronchodilators (use aerosol beta agonists and theophylline, not epinephrine) and humidified oxygen. Noncardiac pulmonary edema is treated with PEEP; corticosteroids are controversial; furosemide (Lasix) may be used. For conjunctival irritation, use copious water irrigation and fluorescein stain for corneal damage. For dermal burns, use copious water irrigation and conventional treatment of burns. *Laboratory aids*: Chest radiograph (may not reflect damage for 24 hours), arterial blood gases, cardiac monitor for dysrhythmias.

Chlorpromazine (Thorazine). See Phenothiazines and Other Major Neuroleptics.

Clinitest Tablets. See Caustics and Corrosives.

Cocaine (benzoylmethylecgonine). *Toxic dose*: The potential fatal dose is 1200 mg, but death has occurred with 20 mg parenterally. *Toxicokinetics*: See Table 14. *Manifestations*: Hypertension, convulsions, hyperthermia, and cardiac dysrhythmias. *Management*: Supportive care. Avoid the induction of emesis or gastric lavage because of the rapid onset of action of cocaine. Blood pressure and thermal monitoring. Control anxiety, convulsions, and life-threatening dysrhythmias with diazepam (Valium). Lidocaine (Xylocaine) is controversial. Nitroprusside infusion, 0.5 to 10 μg per kg per minute, may be used for severe hypertension. Avoid propranolol (Inderal). Labetalol intravenously (Antidote 27, Table 4) has been used to control life-threatening hypertension and tachycardia but has been shown to increase the mortality in mice given cocaine. Most cases of hypertension and tachycardia are transient and can be managed without drugs or careful titration of benzodiazepines. A nonthreatening environment to reduce all sensory stimuli and protect the patient from

TABLE 14. **Pharmacotoxicokinetics of Cocaine**

Type	Route	Time to Onset of Action	Peak	t½	Possible Fatal Dose (Adult)
Hydrochloride	Insufflation	1–5 min	15–60 min	60–75 min	750–800 mg
	Ingested	Delayed	50–90 min	Sustained	1.4 gm
	IV	30–120 s	5–11 min	60–90 min	20–800 mg
Coca paste	Smoked	—	—	Not known	—
Crack and free base	Smoked	(Fastest) 5–10 s	5–11 s	Up to 20 min	Not known

injury is required. Apply precautions against suicide attempts and monitor the fetus if the patient is pregnant. The management of the "body packer" and "body stuffer" is to administer repeated doses of activated charcoal (except plastic vials), secure venous access, and have drugs readily available for treating life-threatening manifestations until contraband is passed in the stool. Surgical removal may be indicated if the material does not pass the pylorus. Endoscopy may be used to remove hard plastic vials, but not the bags, containing crack. Whole-body irrigation may be useful if plastic vials or bags were ingested.

Codeine. See Opioids.

Corrosives. See Caustics and Corrosives.

Cyanide. See Table 15. Hydrocyanic acid and sodium and potassium salts act rapidly and are extremely poisonous. The acid is extremely volatile, producing cyanide, which has a distinctive odor of bitter almonds and can produce death within minutes after inhalation. Cyanide interferes with the cytochrome oxidase system. *Classes of cyanides and derivatives*: (1) Hydrogen cyanide and simple salts in large doses produce death in 15 minutes. (2) Halogenated cyanides, such as cyanogen chloride, produce irritant and vesicant gases that may cause pulmonary edema. (3) Nitriles, such as acrylonitrile and acetonitrile (artificial-nail removers). (4) Residential fires. (5) Cyanides are used as fumigants (hydrogen cyanide), in synthetic rubber (acrylonitrile), in fertilizers (cyanamide), in metal refining (salts), and in the home in some silver and furniture polishes. (6) Cyanide in the seeds of fruit stones is harmful only if the capsule is broken. *Manifestations*: Seizures, stupor, cardiac dysrhythmias, pulmonary edema, lactic acidemia, decreased arterial venous oxygen difference. Bright red venous blood. *Management*: Attendants should not administer mouth-to-mouth resuscitation. (1) Immediately, 100% oxygen. If cyanide was inhaled, remove the patient from the contaminated atmosphere. (2) Cyanide antidote kit (Antidote 14, Table 4). Use antidote only if certain of diagnosis or residential fires involving plastics, urethane, or upholstery plus (a) significant toxicity (impairment of consciousness), (b) manifestations not corrected by oxygen and out of proportion to carboxyhemoglobin level, and (c) lactic acidosis and bright red venous blood with high or normal Pa_{O_2}. (3) Gastrointestinal decontamination by gastric lavage. *No* syrup of ipecac. Activated charcoal is used but is not very effective (1 gram binds only 35 mg of cyanide). (4) Treat seizures with intravenous diazepam (Valium). (5) Correct acidosis. (6) Other antidotes: In Europe, dicobalt edetate, 600 mg, is used intravenously, followed by 300 mg if the response is not satisfactory. Hydroxocobalamin (vitamin B_{12a}) is a useful antidote but must be given immediately after exposure in large doses. Dose: 1800 mg of vitamin B_{12} per dL of potassium cyanide (KCN) is usually required (forms cyanocobalamin [vitamin B_{12}]).

DDT and Derivatives. See Organochlorine Insecticides.

TABLE 15. **Sources of Cyanide and Their Toxicity**

Plants Containing Cyanide Glycosides		
Common Name	*Part of Plant**	*Botanical Name*
Apple	Seeds	*Malus* spp
Apricot	Seeds	*Prunus armeniaca*
Arrow grass		*Triglochin* spp
Bamboo	Sprouts, stems	Tribe Bambuseae
Bermuda grass		*Cynodon dactylon*
Bird's-foot trefoil		*Lotus corniculatus*
Bitter almond	Seeds	*Prunus amygdalus amara*
Blackthorn, sloe		*Prunus spinosa*
Calabash tree		*Crescentia cujete*
Cassava	Beans and roots	*Manihot esculenta*
Catclaw		*Acacia greggi*
Cherry laurel		*Prunus laurocerasus*
Chokecherry		*Prunus virginiana*
Cotoneaster		*Cotoneaster* spp
Cycad nut		*Zamia pumila*
Elderberry	Leaves and shoots	*Sambucus* spp
Eucalyptus		*Eucalyptus cladocalyx*
False sago palm		*Cycas circinalis*
Flax		*Linum usitatissimum*
Hyacinth bean	Bean	*Dolichos lablab*
Hydrangea	Leaves and bulb	*Hydrangea* spp
Jetbead		*Rhodotypos tetrapetala*
Johnson grass		*Sorghum halepense*
Lima bean		*Phaseolus lunatus* (not in United States)
Mountain mahogany		*Cercocarpus montanus*
Passionflower (African)		*Adenia volkensii*
Peach	Seed	*Prunus persica*
Pear	Seeds	*Pyrus communis*
Plains bahia		*Bahia oppositifolia*
Plum	Seed	*Prunus domestica*
Poison suckleya		*Suckleya suckleyana*
Queen's delight		*Stillingia sylvatica*
Sudan grass		*Sorghum* spp
Velvet grass		*Holcus lanatus*
Vetch	Seed	*Vicia sativa*

*In most cases, cyanide is distributed throughout the plant.

Hydrogen Cyanide Liberated from Samples of Carcinogenic Glycosides

Sample	*HCN (mg/gm or mL)*
Laetrile (amygdalin)*	
Sigma	55.9
Tablet yellow	400
Kemdalin	14.1
Apricot seeds	2.92
Peach seeds	2.60
Apple seeds	0.61

*Laetrile is 500-mg tablet for oral use, which is 6% cyanide by weight.

Forms of Cyanide and Their Toxicity

Product	*Toxicity (Potential Lethal Dose)*
Hydrocyanic acid	50 mg (1.0 mg/kg)
Potassium or sodium cyanide	150–300 mg (2 mg/kg)
Ferriferrocyanide (Prussian blue)	50 gm
Sodium nitroprusside	5 mg/kg causes toxicity
Bitter almonds	
Oil	2 oz
Almonds	50–60 (each contains 0.001 gm of cyanide)
Pulp	240 gm
Apricot seeds	
Wild	100 gm of moist seeds = 217 mg of cyanide
Cultivated	100 gm of seeds = 8.7 mg of cyanide

Desipramine (Norpramin, Pertofrane). See Tricyclic Antidepressants.

Diazepam (Valium). See Benzodiazepines.

Digitalis Preparations. See Table 16. *Manifestations*: Manifestations may be delayed 9 to 18 hours. Abdominal pain, nausea, vomiting, diarrhea, dysrhythmias, heart block, CNS depression, colored-halo vision. No dysrhythmia on ECG is characteristic of digitalis toxicity. *Management*: (1) Gastrointestinal decontamination. Avoid ipecac syrup; it may increase the vagal effect if the patient is symptomatic. Repeated doses of activated charcoal may interrupt enterohepatic recirculation. Gastric lavage may in- crease vagal effect. Pretreat with atropine 0.01 mg per kg if symptomatic. (2) Treat hemodynamically unstable ventricular dysrhythmias with Fab (antibody fragment [Digibind], Antidote 22, Table 4). Antidysrhythmic agents and a pacemaker should be used only when Fab therapy fails. Phenytoin (Dilantin) and lidocaine (Xylocaine) also may be administered for ventricular dysrhythmias. Magnesium sulfate, 20 mL of 20% intravenously given slowly over 20 minutes, has been useful for malignant ventricular dysrhythmias, such as torsades de pointes. (3) Treat bradycardia and second- and third-degree atrioventricular block with atropine or low-dose phe-

TABLE 16. **Toxicity and Kinetics of Common Digitalis Preparations**

Characteristics	Digoxin	Digitoxin
Trade name	Lanoxin	Crystodigin
Loading dose (LD) over 18–24 h	Varies with age	Varies with age
Premature infant (mg/kg)	0.005	—
Child <10 years (mg/kg)	0.020–0.060	<2 years 0.025–0.040
Child >10 years (mg/kg)	0.010–0.015	>2 years 0.020–0.040
Total adult (mg)	0.5–7.5	0.8–1.4
Maintenance dose (MD) (% of LD)	23–35	10
Total adult (mg)	0.125–0.50	0.05–0.20
Toxic dose		
Child (mg/kg)	0.3	NA
Normal adult (mg)	2	3–5
Adult fatal dose (mg)	10–20	3–10
Gastrointestinal absorption (%)	50–80	90–100
Tablet bioavailable (%)	60–75	—
Capsule bioavailable (%)	95	—
Elixir bioavailable (%)	85	—
Onset oral (min)	15–30	25–120
Peak IV (h)	1.5–6	4–12
Peak oral (h)	3–6	4–12
Duration of action	3–6 days	2–3 weeks
Protein bound (%)	25	>90
Volume of distribution (L/kg)		
In neonate	7.5–10	—
In infants and children	16	—
In adults	5–8	0.6
Fetal plasma concentrations equal maternal concentrations		
t½		
In premature infants (h)	37–170	—
In neonates (h)	35–69	—
In infants (h)	19–35	—
In adults	26–45 h (1½ days)	6–8 days or longer
Shorter t½ in overdose (h)	6–22	—
Elimination (%)	Renal 75	Liver 80
Active metabolite	None	8% converted digoxin
Plasma concentration should be measured 6–8 h after last dose		
Therapeutic plasma concentration (ng/mL)	0.5–2	15–30
Toxic plasma concentration	>4 ng/mL; varies	>35 ng/μg/mL
There is considerable overlap between therapeutic and toxic ranges		
Normal blood concentrations do not exclude toxicity		
Serious toxic concentration (ng/mL)	>10	—
Healthy children tolerate high concentrations better than adults		
Enterohepatic recirculation (%)	Up to 14	30
Availability		
Capsules (mg)	0.05, 0.1, 0.2	—
Tablets (mg)	0.125, 0.25, 0.50	0.05, 0.1, 0.15, 0.2
Elixir (mg/mL)	0.05	0.05

SI conversion factor: ng/ml $\times$ 1.281 = mmol/L.
Abbreviation: NA = not available.
From Clinical Data Handbook 1988, pp 472–474; AMA Drug Evaluations. Chicago, AMA, 1986, pp 425–427.

nytoin, 25 mg per dose intravenously in adults. If patient is unresponsive, use Fab (Table 4). Insertion of a pacemaker should be seriously considered. Avoid isoproterenol, which causes dysrhythmias. External pacing may be needed. (4) Treat hyperkalemia (above 5.5 mEq per liter) with Fab (antibody fragment; Table 4). Avoid calcium. Hemodialysis is the treatment of choice for severe or refractory hyperkalemia. (5) Direct current countershock may cause life-threatening dysrhythmias. (6) Specific Fab antibody fragments (Table 4) have been used if cardiac arrest or shock is imminent; the dose is 10 mg in an adult, 4 mg (or over 0.3 mg per kg) in a child, or lower (0.2 mg per kg) in an adolescent. Fab is also given for hyperkalemia (serum potassium >5.5 mEq per liter), or serum digoxin toxicity (>10 ng per mL in adults or >5 ng per mL in children) at 6 to 8 hours postingestion, or life-threatening dysrhythmias. Contact Poison Control Center for calculation of Fab or use package insert. *Laboratory aids*: Monitor ECG and potassium and digitalis levels. Draw blood for digoxin levels 6 to 8 hours postingestion, as well as when it is given by the intravenous route. An endogenous digoxin-like substance that cross-reacts with most common immune assay antibodies, with values as high as 4.1 ng per mL, has been reported in newborns, patients with chronic renal failure, and patients with abnormal immune globulin levels. The bound digoxin blood concentrations rise after the use of Fab, but the free (usually unmeasured) digoxin level falls.

Diphenhydramine (Benadryl). See Anticholinergic Agents.

Doxepin (Sinequan, Adapin). See Tricyclic Antidepressants.

Ethchlorvynol (Placidyl). See Sedative Hypnotics.

Ethyl Alcohol. See Alcohols.

Ethylene Glycol (solvent, antifreeze). *Toxic dose*: Death has occurred after a 60-mL ingestion of 95% ethylene glycol; fatal dose is 1.4 mL per kg of 100% solution. The TLV is 50 PPM. *Toxicokinetics*: Time of onset, 30 minutes to 12 hours for CNS and metabolic abnormalities to occur (Phase I). Twelve to 36 hours postingestion, cardiopulmonary depression (Phase II). In Phase III (2 to 3 days postingestion), renal failure occurs. The t½ is 3 hours (during ethanol therapy this is prolonged to 17 hours). Urine oxalate or monohydrate crystals may be seen 4 to 8 hours postingestion but are not always present. *Management*: (1) Gastrointestinal decontamination up to 30 minutes postingestion. Activated charcoal and cathartics are not indicated. (2) Treat seizures with intravenous diazepam (Valium). Exclude hypocalcemia and treat if necessary. (3) Correct acidosis with intravenous sodium bicarbonate. (4) Initiate ethanol therapy to block metabolism (Antidote 21, Table 4) if the blood ethylene glycol level is higher than 20 mg per dL, or if the patient is symptomatic or acidotic with an increased anion gap or osmolar gap. Ethanol should be administered intravenously or orally to produce a blood ethanol concentration of 100 to 150 mg per dL. (5) Early hemodialysis is indicated if the ingestion was large; if the blood ethylene glycol level is greater than 50 mg per dL; if severe acid-base or electrolyte abnormalities occur despite conventional therapy; or if renal failure occurs. (6) Thiamine (100 mg per day) and pyridoxine (50 mg four times daily) have been recommended for 48 hours but have not been extensively studied. (7) Continue therapy (ethanol and hemodialysis) until the plasma ethylene glycol level is below 10 mg per dL, the acidosis has cleared, the creatinine level is normal, and the urinary output is adequate. *Laboratory aids*: Complete blood count, electrolytes, urinalysis (look for oxalate ["envelope"] and monohydrate ["hemp seed"] crystals), and arterial blood gases. The oral mucosa and urine fluoresce if ethylene glycol is present. Obtain ethylene glycol and ethanol levels, plasma osmolarity (use freezing point depression method). Calcium, creatinine, and BUN studies. An ethylene glycol level of 20 mg per dL is usually toxic (levels are very difficult to obtain). The oral mucosa and urine will appear fluorescent under Wood's light if ethylene glycol is present. Propylene glycol, a vehicle in many liquid and intravenous medications (phenytoin, diazepam), may produce spurious ethylene glycol levels.

Flurazepam (Dalmane). See Benzodiazepines.

Fluoxetine (Prozac). *Toxic dose*: greater than 3.5 mg per kg in children. Over 1800 mg has produced seizures in adults. Adult fatal dose, 6 grams. *Manifestations*: Minimal risk of cardiovascular or neurologic complications. *Toxicokinetics*: See Table 31. *Management*: See Tricyclic Antidepressants.

Glutethimide (Doriden). See Sedative Hypnotics.

Hallucinogens

1. LSD (lysergic acid diethylamide). *Toxic dose*: equal to or greater than 35 μg. Street doses are typically 50 to 300 μg. *Toxicokinetics*: Peak effect, 1 to 2 hours. Duration, 12 to 24 hours. t½, 3 hours. Route of elimination, hepatic.

2. MORNING GLORY SEEDS *(Rivea corymbosa* or *Ipomoea)*. These have one-tenth the potency of LSD.

3. MESCALINE/PEYOTE (trimethoxyphenethylamine, or the toxic principle of *Lophophora williamsii)*. *Toxic dose*: equal to or greater than 5 mg per kg. Each button of mescaline contains 45 mg (4 to 12 produce symptoms). *Toxicokinetics*: Peak effect, 4 to 6 hours. Duration, 14 hours.

4. PSILOCYBIN. Similar in effect to LSD but short-acting. Peak effect, 90 minutes. Duration, 5 to 6 hours.

5. NUTMEG *(Myristica)*. *Toxic dose*: 5 to 15 grams (1 to 3 nutmegs). Peak effect, 3 to 6 hours. Duration, up to 60 hours.

6. MARIJUANA *(Cannabis sativa)* (Δ^9-tetrahydrocannabinol, THC). One joint equals 500 mg of marijuana; when the plant is smoked, 50% is destroyed. *Toxicokinetics*: Time of onset, 2 to 3 minutes (smoked). Duration, 2 to 3 hours. t½, 28 to 47 hours (shorter for chronic user). *Note*: 1% of the metabolite can be detected in urine up to 2 weeks after use. *Manifestations*: Visual illusions, sensory perceptual distortions, depersonalization, and derealization. *Management*: "Talk-down" technique.

7. INHALANTS. Nitrites (amyl and isobutyl nitrite) act immediately; aromatic hydrocarbon in airplane model glues, plastic cements (benzene, toluene, xylene)—see Hydrocarbons; Nitrous Oxide.

8. TRYPTAMINE DERIVATIVES (DMT, *N*-dimethyltryptamine; DET, diethyltryptamine; DPT, dipropyltryptamine). Rapid onset of action, but duration is only 1 to 2 hours.

9. STP OR DOM (2,5-dimethoxy-4-methylamphetamine). Acts like LSD but lasts 72 hours or longer.

10. MDA (3-methoxy-4,5-ethylenedioxyamphetamine). Related to amphetamine, produces a mild LSD-like reaction lasting 6 to 10 hours ("love pill").

See also Alcohols, Amphetamines, Anticholinergic Agents, Barbiturates, Cocaine, Opioids, Phencyclidine, Phenothiazines and Other Major Neuroleptics, and Tricyclic Antidepressants.

Haloperidol (Haldol). See Phenothiazines and Other Major Neuroleptics.

Heroin. See Opioids.

Hydrocarbons

1. PETROLEUM DISTILLATES. Gasoline (petroleum spirit), 2 to 5% benzene; kerosene (coal oil, kerosene, jet aviation fuel No. 1, charcoal lighter fluid); petroleum naphtha (cigarette lighter fluid, ligroin, racing fuel); petroleum ether (benzin); turpentine (pine oil, oil of turpentine); and mineral spirits (Stoddard solvent, white spirits, varsol, mineral turpentine, petroleum spirit). *Manifestations*: Materials aspirated during the process of ingestion may produce pneumonitis. Hypoxia associated with aspiration, not absorption, is the cause of CNS depression. It is *unlikely* that a child accidentally or an adult during siphoning of gasoline would ingest a sufficient quantity to warrant the induction of emesis.

2. AROMATIC HYDROCARBONS. *Benzene*, a solvent used in manufacturing dyes, phenol, and nitrobenzene, has a TLV of 10 PPM by inhalation according to the Occupational Safety and Health Administration (OSHA). The National Institute for Occupational Safety and Health (NIOSH) value is 1 PPM. The adult ingested toxic dose is 15 mL. Chronic exposure may cause leukemia. A level of 200 PPM is fatal in 5 minutes. *Toluene*, used in manufacturing TNT, has an OSHA TLV of 200 PPM by inhalation; the NIOSH figure is 100. The adult ingested toxic dose is 50 mL. *Styrene* has an OSHA TLV of 100 PPM by inhalation. *Xylene*, used in the manufacture of perfumes, has an OSHA TLV of 100 PPM by inhalation. The adult ingested toxic dose is 50 mL. *Manifestations*: Asphyxiation, CNS depression, defatting dermatitis, and aspiration pneumonitis. A bite into a tube of household plastic cement by a young child does not warrant the induction of emesis. Ingestion of hydrocarbon with a benzene fraction over 5% may warrant induction of emesis.

3. ALIPHATIC HALOGENATED HYDROCARBONS. See Table 17 for common examples. *Manifestations*: Myocardial sensitization and irritability, hepatorenal toxicity, and CNS depression. Dichloromethane may be converted into carbon monoxide in the body. Trichloroethylene concentrates in the fetus (pregnant

TABLE 17. **Common Examples of Aliphatic Halogenated Hydrocarbons**

	Estimated Toxic Dose (Ingested 100%)*	TLV-TWA (PPM ACGIH)	Synonym(s)
1,2-Dichloromethane†	0.3 mL/kg,† one swallow adult, lethal >0.5 mL/kg	1	Methylene chloride
1,2-Dichloroethylene	150–200 mL toxic in adults or large intentional ingestion	200	Acetylene dichloride
1,2-Dichloropropane	0.3 mL/kg toxic, one swallow	75	Propylene dichloride
Tetrabromoethane	1 mL/kg toxic, several swallows	—	Acetylene tetrabromide
Tetrachloroethane	0.3 mL/kg toxic, one swallow	1	Acetylene tetrachloride
Tetrachloroethylene	1 mL/kg toxic, several swallows	50	Perchloroethylene
Tetrachloromethane	0.3 mL/kg toxic, one swallow	5	
1,1,1-Trichloroethane	5.0 mL/kg fatal, 150–200 mL toxic in adults or large intestinal ingestion	350	Methyl chloroform, Triethane, Glamorene Spot Remover, Scotchgard Typewriter fluid
Trichlorethylene	0.3 mL/kg toxic, >one swallow	50	Vapor degreaser, typewriter correction fluid, fire retardant
Trichloromethane	0.3 mL/kg toxic, one swallow	10	Cleaning agent, fumigant, insecticide
1,1,2-Trichloro-1,2,2-fluoroethane	>200 mL? toxic adult		
1,1,2-Trichloroethane	0.5 mL/kg toxic, >2.0 mL/kg lethal	10	Vinyl trichloride
Carbon tetrachloride	3–5 mL total amount Lethal 4 mL total	2	

*Estimated fatal dose assumes pure 100% of the halogenated hydrocarbon in the ingested product. At this dose it is recommended that medical evaluation be sought. A *swallow* in 2-year-old is approximately 5 mL (0.3 mL/kg), in adult, 15–20 mL. *Large intentional amount* is 120–150 mL in adults. The decision for medical evaluation should be based on the most toxic substance present at concentrations exceeding 10 to 20%.

†Amount of methylene chloride in a single Christmas tree bubbling fluid light (0.5 mL) is nontoxic if ingested by small children.

Abbreviations: ACGIH = American Conference of Government Industrial Hygienists; PPM = parts per million; TLV = threshold limit value for 8-hour workday; TWA = time-weighted average concentration for normal workday and 40-hour workweek to which nearly all workers may be repeatedly exposed.

women should not be exposed) and causes a disulfiram (Antabuse) reaction ("degreaser's flush") when associated with the ingestion of ethanol. The decision to induce emesis must be based on the toxicity of the agent.

4. DANGEROUS ADDITIVES. Dangerous additives to the hydrocarbons, such as heavy metals, nitrobenzene, aniline dyes, insecticides, and demothing agents, may warrant the induction of emesis.

5. HEAVY HYDROCARBONS. These have high viscosity, low volatility, and minimal absorption, so emesis is unwarranted. Examples are asphalt (tar), machine oil, motor oil (lubricating oil, engine oil), diesel oil (engine fuel, home heating oil), petrolatum liquid (mineral oil, suntan oils), petrolatum jelly (Vaseline), paraffin wax, transmission oil, cutting oil, and greases and glues.

6. PRODUCTS TREATED AS PETROLEUM DISTILLATES. Essential oils (e.g., turpentine, pine oil) are treated as petroleum distillates. Mineral seal oil (signal oil), found in some furniture polishes, is a heavy, viscous oil that *never* warrants emesis; it can produce severe pneumonia if aspirated. It has minimal absorption. *Management*: Dermal decontamination. Removal from the environment in inhalation.

FIRST AID TREATMENT. See Table 18. *The use of activated charcoal, oils, and cathartics is not advised in petroleum distillate ingestions. General management*: (1) In the asymptomatic patient: observe several hours for the development of respiratory distress. (2) In the symptomatic patient: supportive respiratory care for respiratory distress. Bronchospasm may be treated with intravenous aminophylline. Avoid epinephrine. Monitor ECG; arterial blood gases; liver, pulmonary, and renal function; serum electrolytes; serial radiographs. Observe for signs of intravascular hemolysis and disseminated intravascular coagulation. If cyanosis that does not respond to oxygen is present or the arterial Pa_{O_2} is normal, suspect methemoglobinemia that may require therapy with methylene blue. Steroids have not been shown to be beneficial. Antimicrobial agents are not useful in prophylaxis. (Fever or leukocytosis may be produced by the chemical pneumonitis itself.) It is not necessary to treat pneumatoceles. Most infiltrations resolve spontaneously in 1 week except for lipoid pneumonia, which may last up to 6 weeks.

Imipramine (Tofranil). See Tricyclic Antidepressants.

Iron. The iron content of some preparations appears in Table 19. *Toxic dose*: Range, 20 to 60 mg per kg or greater of elemental iron. Dose requiring induction of emesis, equal to or greater than 20 mg per kg. The potential fatal dose is 180 mg per kg (600 mg of elemental iron). *Toxicokinetics*: Absorption occurs chiefly in the small intestine. For excretion there is no normal route except blood loss or gastrointestinal desquamation. *Manifestations*: Phase I—mucosal injury possibly with hematemesis (1 to 6 hours postingestion). Phase II—patient appears improved (2 to 24 hours). Phase III—cardiovascular collapse and severe metabolic acidosis (12 to 48 hours). Phase IV—hepatic injury associated with jaundice (2 to 4 days). Phase V—sequelae of intestinal stricture and obstruction or anemia (2 to 6 weeks). Patients asymptomatic for 6 hours rarely develop serious intoxication manifestations. *Management*: (1) Gastrointestinal decontamination. Emesis should be induced in ingestions of elemental iron that are over 20 mg per kg. Emesis should be followed by gastric lavage in an adult or in a child who has ingested a chewable or liquid preparation. The

TABLE 18. **Initial Management of Hydrocarbon Ingestions**

Symptoms	Contents	Amount	Initial Management
None	Petroleum distillate only	<5 mL/kg	None
None	Heavy hydrocarbon	Any amount	None*
	Mineral seal oil		None
None	Petroleum distillate with dangerous additive (heavy metals, pesticide)	Depends on toxicity of additive	Gastric lavage with small-bore tube
	Aromatic hydrocarbons	>1 mL/kg	
	Halogenated hydrocarbons†		
	A. Very toxic compounds	>0.3 mL/kg	Gastric lavage
	B. Moderately toxic compounds	>0.5 mL/kg	Gastric lavage
	C. Low-toxicity compounds	>1.0 mL/kg	Gastric lavage
	D. Christmas bubbling light		Gastric lavage‡
Loss of protective airway reflexes, coma, seizures	Petroleum distillate with dangerous additive, aromatic or halogenated hydrocarbons	Same as aromatic or halogenated hydrocarbons above	Endotracheal tube before gastric lavage

*Emesis may be necessary if machine oil contains triorthocresyl phosphate (TOCP), which causes weakness, sensory impairment, and "partially reversible damage to the spinal cord."

†Amounts of halogenated hydrocarbons ingested assume 100% of product.

‡See footnotes A to D and hydrocarbon amounts above.

  A. More than one swallow in adult or 0.3 mL/kg in a child of 100% of 1,2-dichloromethane (methylene chloride), 1,2-dichloropropane (propylene dichloride), tetrachloroethane (acetylene tetrachloride), tetrachloromethane, trichloroethylene, tetrachloroethylene, trichloromethane, or tetrabromoethane (acetylene tetrabromide).

  B. Several swallows in an adult or 0.5 mL/kg in a child of 100% 1,2-dichloroethane (ethylene dichloride), 1,2-dichloroethylene (acetylene dichloride), 1,1,2-trichloroethane (vinyl trichloride), tetrabromoethane, tetrachloroethylene (perchloroethylene), or 1,1,2,2-tetrachloroethylene.

  C. A large intentional ingestion in an adult (150–200 mL) or over 1 mL/kg in a child of 100% 1,2-dichloroethylene, tetrachloromethane, 1,1,1,-trichloroethane (methyl chloroform), or 1,1,2-trichloro-1,2,2,-fluoroethane.

  D. The amount of dichloromethane (methylene chloride) in a single Christmas tree bubbling fluid light (0.5 mL) is nontoxic if ingested by small children.

TABLE 19. **Iron Content of Some Preparations**

Iron Salt	Elemental Iron Content (%)	Average Tablet Strength (mg)	Elemental Iron/ Tablet (mg)	Average FeSO₄ Strength (mg)
Ferrous sulfate (hydrous)	20	300	60	Drp 75/0.6 mL
	20	SR 160	32	Syp 90/5 mL
	20	195	39	Solu 125/mL
	20	325	65	Elxr 220/5 mL
Ferrous sulfate (dried)	30	200	60	
	30	SR 160	48	
Ferrous gluconate	12	320	36	Elxr 320/5 mL
Ferrous fumarate	33	200	67	
	33	SR 324	107	Drp 45/0.6 mL
	33	Chewable 100	33	Susp 100/5 mL

Abbreviations: SR = slow release; Drp = dropper; Syp = syrup; Solu = solution; Elxr = elixir; Susp = suspension.

solution to be used for lavage is saline 0.9% or 1 to 1.5% sodium bicarbonate to form ferrous carbonate salts, which are poorly absorbed. One hundred milliliters of this solution should be left in the stomach (prepared by dilution of a sodium bicarbonate ampule with saline). The use of deferoxamine (Desferal Mesylate) in the gastrointestinal tract is not recommended. The use of diluted Fleet Enema (mono- and dibasic sodium phosphate) solution risks severe hypertonic phosphate poisoning. Activated charcoal is not recommended. (2) Postlavage abdominal radiograph—if significant amounts of residual radiopaque material are present, consider whole-bowel irrigation with polyethylene glycol solution first. Removal by endoscopy or surgery may also be required because coalesced tablets have produced hemorrhagic infarction and perforation peritonitis. (3) Diagnostic chelation test—deferoxamine not reliable. (4) Indications for chelation therapy with deferoxamine are serum iron levels over 500 mg per dL or systemic signs of intoxication independent of the serum iron level. Chelation should be performed within 12 to 18 hours to be effective (Antidote 15, Table 4). *Laboratory aids*: Serum iron levels correlate with the clinical course. Iron levels that are below 350 mg per dL when taken at 2 to 6 hours predict an asymptomatic course; levels of 350 to 500 are associated with mild gastrointestinal symptoms (rarely serious); and levels greater than 500 suggest the possibility of serious Phase III manifestations. Draw blood for serum iron (SI) before administering deferoxamine because it interferes with analysis. Total iron-binding capacity is not necessary. An SI at 8 to 12 hours is useful to exclude delayed absorption from a bezoar or sustained-release preparation. White blood cell counts greater than 15,000 per µL, blood glucose levels over 150 mg per dL, radiopaque material present on abdominal radiograph, vomiting, and diarrhea predict iron levels greater than 300 mg per dL. Monitor complete blood counts, blood glucose, serum iron, stools, and vomitus for occult blood; electrolytes; acid-base balance; urinalysis and urinary output; liver function tests; BUN; and creatinine. Obtain type and match of blood in severe cases. Abdominal radiographs. Follow-up is necessary for sequelae in significant intoxications—gastrointestinal series for in-

testinal strictures and anemia secondary to blood loss. Patients who develop fever or toxic symptoms after iron overdose should have blood and stool cultures checked for *Yersinia enterocolitica*.

Isoniazid (INH, Nydrazid). This is an antituberculosis drug frequently used in suicide attempts by Native Americans and Eskimos. *Mechanism of toxicity*: It produces pyridoxine deficiency (doubles excretion of pyridoxine). *Toxic dose*: 1.5 grams, 35 to 40 mg per kg, produces convulsions; severe toxicity is seen at 6 to 10 grams; at 200 mg per kg it is an obligatory convulsant. *Toxicokinetics*: Absorption is rapid, with a peak in 1 to 2 hours (clinical symptoms may start in 30 minutes). The Vd is 0.6 liter per kg. It passes the placenta and into breast milk at 50% of the maternal serum level. Not protein-bound. Elimination is by the liver, which produces a hepatotoxic metabolite, acetylisoniazid. t½—Slow acetylators (2 to 4 hours) (50% of blacks and whites) may develop peripheral neuropathy. Fast acetylators (0.7 to 2 hours) (90% of Asians and a majority of patients with diabetes) may develop hepatitis. Excreted unchanged, 10 to 40%. *Major toxic manifestations*: Visual disturbances, convulsions (≥90% with one or more seizures), coma, resistant severe acidosis (due to lactate secondary to hypoxia, convulsions, and metabolic blocks). *Management*: (1) Control seizures with large doses of pyridoxine, 1 gram for each gram of isoniazid ingested (Antidote 38, Table 4). If the dose ingested is unknown, give at least 5 grams of pyridoxine intravenously. Diazepam (Valium) is given and works synergistically to control seizures. (2) Correct acidosis with fluids and sodium bicarbonate (pyridoxine may spontaneously correct the acidosis). (3) After the patient is stabilized, or if asymptomatic, gastrointestinal decontamination procedures may be carried out, keeping in mind the rapid onset of convulsions. Asymptomatic patients should be observed for 4 hours. (4) Hemodialysis is rarely needed but may be used as an adjunct for uncontrollable acidosis and seizures. Hemoperfusion has not been adequately evaluated. Diuresis is ineffective. *Laboratory aids*: Isoniazid toxic levels are above 10 to 20 µg per mL. Monitor the blood glucose (often hyperglycemia), electrolytes (often hyperkalemia), bicarbonate, arterial blood gases, liver function tests, BUN, and creatinine. If convulsions persist obtain an EEG. Monitor the temperature closely (often hyperpyrexia).

Isopropyl Alcohol. See Alcohols.

Kerosene. See Hydrocarbons.

Lead. *Acute* lead poisoning is rare. *Acute toxic dose*: 0.5 gram in children. *Management*: (1) Gastrointestinal decontamination. (2) Supportive care, including measures to deal with the hepatic and renal failure and intravascular hemolysis. (3) EDTA in all severe cases if lead levels confirm absorption. *Chronic* lead poisoning occurs most often in children 6 months to 6 years of age who are exposed in their environment and in adults in certain occupations. *Chronic toxic dose*: Determined by blood lead level and clinical findings. A level of 10 μg per dL or over is the threshold of concern in children; 40 μg per dL or over in adult workers; 30 μg per dL or over for those planning pregnancy. Medical removal from work at 60 μg per dL. *Toxicokinetics*: Absorption—10 to 15% of the ingested dose is absorbed in adults; in children up to 40% is absorbed with iron deficiency anemia. Inhalation absorption is rapid and complete. Vd—95% present in bone. In blood, 95% is in red blood cells. t½—35 days; in bone, 10 years. The major elimination route for inorganic lead is renal. Organic lead is metabolized in the liver to inorganic lead; 9% is excreted in the urine per day. *Manifestations of acute symptoms of chronic lead poisoning* (ABCDE): Anorexia, apathy, anemia; behavior disturbances; clumsiness; developmental deterioration; and emesis. Manifestations of encephalopathy are remembered by the mnemonic PAINT: *P*, persistent forceful vomiting; *A*, ataxia; *I*, intermittent stupor and lucidity; *N*, neurologic coma and convulsions; *T*, tired and lethargic. In adults, one may see peripheral neuropathies and "lead gum lines." *Management*: (1) Gastrointestinal decontamination with enemas if radiopaque foreign bodies are noted. Do not delay therapy until clear. (2) Remove from exposure. For children, see Table 20. Dimercaptosuccinic acid, a derivative of dimercaprol (BAL), is an oral agent approved by the FDA for chelation only in children with venous blood lead levels of over 45 μg per dL. The recommended dose is 10 mg per kg every 8 hours for 5 days, then every 12 hours for 14 days (Antidote 42, Table 4). *Laboratory aids*: (1) Provocation mobilization test—500 mg of EDTA per m² of body surface area for one dose given deeply intramuscularly with 0.5% procaine diluted 1:1; collect the urine for 8 hours. If the ratio of micrograms excreted in the urine to milligrams of Ca-EDTA administered is greater than 0.6, there is an increased lead body burden, and chelation should be carried out. (2) Evaluate complete blood count, levels of serum iron, or ferritin; repeat blood lead levels and erythrocyte protoporphyrin. (3) Flat plate of the abdomen and long bone radiographs (knees usually). (4) Renal function tests. (5) Monitor electrolytes, serum calcium, phosphorus, blood glucose.

Lindane. See Organochlorine Insecticides.

Lithium (Eskalith, Lithane). Most cases of intoxication have occurred as therapeutic overdoses. The toxic dose is determined by serum levels, although intoxication has occurred with levels in the therapeutic range. *Toxicokinetics*: Absorption is rapid, with complete peaking in 1 to 4 hours. Vd is 0.5 to 0.9 liter per kg. It is not protein-bound. The t½ therapeutically is 18 to 24 hours. The kidney excretes 89 to 98% unchanged, one-third to two-thirds in 6 to 12 hours. Excretion is decreased in the presence of hyponatremia and dehydration. The cerebrospinal fluid concentration is one-half the plasma concentration. The breast milk level is 50% of the maternal serum level—toxic to the nursling. *Manifestations*: The first sign of toxicity may be diarrhea. Fine tremor of hands, lethargy, weakness, polyuria and polydipsia, goiter and hypothyroidism, and fasciculations are side effects. Severe toxicity is manifested by ataxia, impaired mental state, coma, and seizures (limbs held in hyperextension with eyes open in "coma vigil"). Cardiovascular manifestations are dysrhythmias, hypotension, flat T waves, and an increased QT interval. *Management*: (1) Gastrointestinal decontamination may not be useful after 2 hours because of rapid absorption. In slow-release preparations, decontamination may be useful up to 24 hours postingestion. Activated charcoal is not indicated. Sodium polystyrene sulfonate (Kayexalate), 60 mL orally four times a day, is useful in preventing absorption. Determine serum sodium level before administration because this agent may aggravate existing hypernatremia. (2) Hospitalize if intoxication is suspected because seizures may occur unexpectedly. (3) Restore normothermia and fluid and electrolyte balance, particularly sodium. If diabetes insipidus is present, an infusion of sodium may cause hypernatremia. Current evidence supports saline infusion as enhancing excretion of lithium. An infusion of 1 to 2 liters of 0.89% saline (adults) or 20 mL per kg (children) should be started to correct fluid and electrolyte deficits. When fluid deficits are corrected, administer 0.45% saline. (4) Hemodialysis is the treatment of choice for severe intoxication. Lithium is the most dialyzable toxin known. Long runs should be used until the lithium level is less than 1 mEq per liter because of extensive re-equilibration rebound. Monitor levels every 4 hours after dialysis. Dialysis may have to be repeated. Expect a time lag in neurologic recovery. If hemodialysis is not available or delayed, peritoneal dialysis can be used but is less effective. (5) Monitor ECG. Refractory dysrhythmias may be treated with magnesium sulfate and sodium bicarbonate. (6) Avoid thiazides and spironolactone diuretics, which increase lithium levels. *Laboratory aids*: Lithium level determinations should be performed every 2 to 4 hours. Although they do not always correlate with the manifestations at low levels, they are predictive in severe intoxications. Levels of 0.6 to 1.2 mEq per liter are usually therapeutic. Levels over 4.0 mEq per liter are usually severely toxic. Other tests to be monitored are complete blood count (lithium causes leukocytosis), renal function, thyroid, ECG, and electrolytes. Factors that predis-

TABLE 20. **Choice of Chelation Therapy Based on Symptoms and Blood Lead Concentration**

Clinical Presentation	Treatment	Comments
Symptomatic Children		
Acute encephalopathy	BAL,* 450 mg/m²/24 h CaNa₂-EDTA, 1500 mg/m²/24 h	BAL, 75/m² q 4 h After 4 h, start infusion of EDTA or use IM q 4 h† Duration, 5 days Interrupt therapy for 2 days If blood Pb > 70 μg/dL, BAL and EDTA for 5 more days; EDTA alone if blood Pb = 45–69 μg/dL Other cycles depend on blood Pb rebound
Blood Pb > 70 μg/dL	BAL, 300 mg/m²/24 h CaNa₂-EDTA, 1000 mg/m²/24 h Do not use CaNa₂-EDTA alone if symptomatic	BAL, 50 mg/m² q 4 h After 4 h, start infusion of EDTA or use IM q 4 h† Duration, 5 days Interrupt therapy for 2 days Discontinue BAL in 3 days if blood Pb < 50 μg/dL; BAL and EDTA for 5 more days if blood Pb > 50 μg/dL Other cycles depend on blood Pb rebound
Asymptomatic Children		
BEFORE TREATMENT, MEASURE VENOUS BLOOD LEAD		
Blood Pb > 70 μg/dL	BAL, 300 mg/m²/24 h CaNa₂-EDTA, 1000 mg/m²/24 h	BAL 50 mg/m² IM q 4 h After 4 h, start infusion of EDTA or use IM q 4 h Duration, 5 days Discontinue BAL in 3 days if blood Pb < 50 μg/dL Give second course of EDTA if blood Pb > 45 μg/dL within 5 days Other cycles depend on blood Pb rebound
Blood Pb = 45–69 μg/dL‡	CaNa₂-EDTA, 1000 mg/m²/24 h or DMSA	EDTA, IM q 4 h or IV Duration, 5 days Give second course of EDTA if blood Pb > 45 μg/dL within 7–14 days; wait 5–7 days before giving second course If lead exposure controlled, give single IV or IM dose on outpatient basis Other cycles depend on blood Pb rebound
Blood Pb = 25–44 μg/dL	CaNa₂-EDTA, 1000 mg/m²/24 h	Provocation, EDTA test Duration, 5 days IM or IV Provocation test periodically
Guidelines for Chelation of Excess Lead in Adults		
INORGANIC LEAD§		
Symptomatic Cases		
Acute encephalopathy	BAL-EDTA	Same as for children
Abdominal pain, weakness, and colic	BAL-EDTA	Course for 3–5 days followed by oral penicillamine until urine Pb < 500 μg/24 h or 2 months, whichever less
Painless peripheral neuropathy	D-Penicillamine	For 1–2 months If blood lead >100 μg/dL, BAL-EDTA first course 3–5 days, followed by oral penicillamine
Asymptomatic Cases		
Blood Lead Concentrations (μg/dL)		
100	BAL-EDTA	
80–100	Penicillamine alone	
40–79 and EP > 60	Provocation test	
ORGANIC LEAD	No chelation therapy	

Note: OSHA requires that workers be removed from the work environment when lead levels exceed 50 μg/dL and until they are below 40 μg/dL.

*Dimercaprol.

†Some physicians prefer to give EDTA IM to avoid large fluid volumes in high intracranial pressure.

‡DMSA may be used.

§Data from Rempel D: The lead exposed worker. JAMA 262:532–534, 1989. Copyright 1989, American Medical Association.

Abbreviations: BAL = British antilewisite; Blood Pb = venous blood lead concentration; CaNa₂ = calcium disodium; DMSA = 2,3 dimercaptosuccinic acid; EDTA = ethylenediaminetetraacetic acid; EP = erythrocyte protoporphyrin.

Modified from Piomelli S, Rosen JF, Chisolm JJ Jr, Graef JW: Management of childhood lead poisoning. J Pediatr 105(4):527, 1984, and CDC Prevention of Childhood Lead Poisoning. Atlanta, CDC, 1991.

pose to lithium toxicity are febrile illness, sodium depletion, concomitant drugs (thiazide and spironolactone diuretics), impaired renal function, advanced age, and fluid loss in vomiting and diarrheal illness.

Lomotil (Diphenoxylate and Atropine). See Opioids and Anticholinergic Agents.

LSD (Lysergic Acid Diethylamide). See Hallucinogens.

Marijuana. See Hallucinogens.

Meperidine (Demerol). See Opioids.

Meprobamate (Equanil, Miltown). See Sedative Hypnotics, Nonbarbiturate.

Mercury. *Management*: (1) Inhalation of elemental mercury—remove from exposure. (2) Ingestion of mercuric salt—gastrointestinal decontamination. Do not induce emesis. A protein solution such as egg white or 5% salt-poor albumin can be given to reduce salt to mercurous ion (less toxic). Activated charcoal does absorb mercuric chloride. (3) Chelating agents (do not use Ca-EDTA because of nephrotoxicity): dimercaprol (BAL) enhances mercury excretion through the bile as well as the urine and is the first choice if renal impairment from the mercury exists (Antidote 17, Table 4). Alternatives are penicillamine (Antidote 34, Table 4) and *N*-acetyl-DL-penicillamine (investigational use). Use of BAL in methyl mercury intoxication increases the brain mercury level and appears to be contraindicated; penicillamine and its analogue should be used (decreases mercury levels in brain). Another chelator, 2,3-dimercaptosuccinic acid, holds promise of less toxicity and more specific therapy.* (4) Monitor fluid and electrolyte levels, renal function, hemoglobin levels. Obtain blood and urine mercury levels (consult the laboratory for proper collection technique and containers). (5) Hemodialysis early in the symptomatic patient is useful. (6) Newer but not established approaches are use of polythiol resin to bind the methyl mercury excreted in the bile; heat and sauna treatment to increase mercury excretion through perspiration; and a regional dialyzer system using L-cysteine. (7) Surgical excision of *local injection sites*. *Laboratory aids*: (1) Blood levels are below 2 to 4 μg per dL and urine levels below 10 to 20 μg per liter in 90% of the adult population. Levels above 4 μg per dL in blood and 20 μg per liter in urine probably should be considered abnormal. Blood levels are not always reliable after the first few hours. Exposed industrial workers' urine levels are 150 to 200 μg per liter. (2) In asymptomatic patients with urine levels under 300 μg per liter, a chelating challenge with BAL or penicillamine may bring a significant increase that may aid in establishing the diagnosis. (3) Approximately 150 μg per liter of mercury in urine is equivalent to 3.5 μg per dL in blood. (4) Methyl mercury is excreted mainly through the feces, so urine mercury would not be a reliable measurement. (5) Mercury is also excreted in the sweat and saliva. The parotid fluid level is approximately two-thirds that of the blood. Because the hair is porous, it may absorb mercury from the atmosphere; however, hair concentrations of 400 to 500 μg per gram are likely to be associated with neurologic symptoms. Radiographs of the abdomen for ingestion and chest radiographs for injections may be helpful in showing radiopaque material.

Methadone. See Opioids.

Methanol. See Alcohols.

Methaqualone. See Sedative Hypnotics, Nonbarbiturate.

Methyprylon (Noludar). See Sedative Hypnotics, Nonbarbiturate.

Narcotic Analgesics. See Opioids.

Neuroleptics. See Phenothiazines and Other Major Neuroleptics.

Nitrites (NO$_2$) and Nitrates (NO$_3$). These are readily available in both inorganic and organic forms. Organic nitrates used for angina pectoris are listed in Table 21. Inorganic nitrates have more toxicologic importance in small infants in vegetables (carrots, spinach, beets) and preservatives used in meat products and contaminated well water. *Potential fatal doses*: Nitrite, 1 gram; nitrate, 10 grams; nitrobenzene, 2 mL; nitroglycerin, 0.2 gram; and aniline dye (pure), 5 to 30 grams. *Toxicokinetics*: Time to onset of action of nitroglycerin sublingually is 1 to 3 minutes, with a time to peak action of 3 to 15 minutes and a duration of 20 to 30 minutes. Other routes have a slower onset (2 to 5 minutes) and longer duration of action (1.5 to 6 hours). Nitrites are potent oxidizing agents converting ferrous to ferric iron in the hemoglobin molecule, which cannot carry oxygen. Normally humans have 0.7% methemoglobin, which is converted by methemoglobin reductase into oxygen-carrying hemoglobin. *Route of elimination*: Liver detoxification by dinitration. *Toxic manifestations* depend on the level of methemoglobinemia. At 10%, "chocolate cyanosis" occurs; at 10 to 20%, headache, dizziness, and tachypnea occur; and at 50%, mental alterations are present and coma and convulsions may occur. Headache, flushing, and sweating are due

---

*Not FDA-approved for this purpose.

TABLE 21. **Organic Nitrates for Angina Pectoris**

Drug and Route	Trade Name	Time to Onset of Action (min)	Duration (h)
Nitroglycerin			
Oral	Many	Varies	4–6
Sublingual	Many	1–3	¼–½
2% ointment	Nitro-Bid	15	3–6
Transdermal	Nitrol		
	Nitro-Dur	30	2–4
Isosorbide dinitrate	Isordil		
Sublingual		1–3	1.3–3
Oral		2–5	4–6
Chewable		2–5	2–3
Timed release		Varies	—
Isosorbide mononitrate	ISMO	1–2	6–12
Pentaerythritol tetranitrate, oral	Peritrate	2–5	3–5
Erythrityl tetranitrate, oral	Cardilate	2–5	4–6

to the vasodilatory effect; hypotension, tachycardia, and syncope may also occur. Severe hypoxia may produce pulmonary edema and encephalopathy. Levels above 50% produce metabolic acidosis and ECG changes; cardiovascular collapse occurs at levels of 70%. *Management*: (1) Dermal decontamination, if indicated. Aniline dyes may be removed with 5% acetic acid (vinegar). (2) Gastrointestinal decontamination if ingested. (3) Hypotension can be treated by the Trendelenburg position and fluid challenge. Vasoconstrictors (dopamine or norepinephrine) are rarely needed. (4) Methylene blue (Antidote 29, Table 4) is indicated for methemoglobin levels above 30%, dyspnea, metabolic acidosis (lactic acidosis), or an altered mental state. (5) Oxygen, 100%, or a hyperbaric chamber should be used in symptomatic patients if methylene blue fails or is not effective, e.g., as in chlorate intoxication or glucose-6-phosphate dehydrogenase deficiency. *Laboratory aids*: Methemoglobin levels, arterial blood gases. Blood has a chocolate-brown appearance and fails to turn red on exposure to oxygen. Methemoglobin levels and oxygen saturation should be measured by co-oximeter, not by pulse oximetry.

Nortriptyline (Aventyl, Pamelor). See Tricyclic Antidepressants.

Opioids (Narcotic Opiates). See Table 22. The major metabolic pathway differs for each opioid, but they are 90% metabolized in the liver. Patients should be observed for CNS and respiratory depression and hypotension. Pulmonary edema is a potentially lethal complication of mainlining (intravenous use). *Manifestations*: All opiate agonists produce miotic pupils (except meperidine [Demerol] and diphenoxylate-atropine [Lomotil] early), respiratory and CNS depression, physical dependence, and withdrawal symptoms. *Management*: (1) Supportive care, particularly an endotracheal tube and assisted ventilation. (2) Gastrointestinal decontamination up to 12 hours postingestion, because opiates delay gastric emptying time, but this is of no benefit if overdose is by injection. Convulsions occur rapidly with propoxyphene (Darvon) and codeine overdose, and this may be an indication not to use an emetic for gastrointestinal decontamination in this drug overdose. (3) Naloxone (Narcan) (Antidote 30, Table 4) may be given in bolus intravenous doses and by continuous drip. Naloxone must be titrated against the clinical response and precipitation of withdrawal in narcotic addicts. It should be repeated as often as necessary, because the effects of many opioids in overdose can last 24 to 48 hours, whereas the action of naloxone lasts only 2 to 3 hours. *Larger doses are needed for buprenorphine, codeine, designer drugs, dextromethorphan, diphenoxylate, methadone, pentazocine, and propoxyphene.* (4) Pulmonary edema does not respond to naloxone, and the patient needs respiratory supportive care. Fluids should be given cautiously in opioid overdose because these agents stimulate the antidiuretic hormone effect and pulmonary edema is frequent. (5) *If the patient is comatose, give 50% glucose* (3 to 4% of comatose narcotic overdose patients have hypoglycemia). (6) *If the patient is agitated*, consider hypoxia rather than withdrawal and treat as such. (7) *Observe for withdrawal* signs and symptoms (nausea, vomiting, cramps, diarrhea, dilated pupils, rhinorrhea, piloerection). If these occur, stop naloxone.

OPIOID ADDICT WITHDRAWAL SCORE. Signs and symptoms of withdrawal are diarrhea, dilated pupils,

TABLE 22. **Opioids (Narcotic Opiates)***

Drugs		Equivalent IM		Time to Peak Action (h)	t½ (h)	Duration of Action (h)	Potential Toxic Dose (mg)
Generic	*Trade*	*Dose† (mg)*	*Oral† (mg)*				
Alphaprodine‡	Nisentil	40–60	—	—	2	1–2	—
Butorphanol	Stadol	2	—	0.5–1.0	3	2.5–3.5	—
Camphorated tincture of opium	Paregoric	—	25 mL	—	—	4–5	—
Codeine	Various	120	200	—	3	4–6	800
Diacetylmorphine	Heroin	5	60	—	0.5	3–4	100
Diphenoxylate	Lomotil	—	10	Delayed by atropine	2.5	14	300
Fentanyl	Sublimaze	0.1–0.2	—	0.5	4–6	0.5–2	—
Hydrocodone	Hycodan	5–10	5–10	—	3.8	3–4	100
Hydromorphone	Dilaudid	1.5	6.0	0.5–1.5	2–3	2–4	100
Meperidine	Demerol	50–100	75–100	0.5–1	2–5	3–4	1000
Methadone	Dolophine	10.0	20	2–4	22–97	4–12	120
Morphine	Various	10.0	60	0.3–1.5	2–3	3–4	200
Nalbuphine	Nubain	10.0	—	0.5–1.0	3–4	3–4	—
Oxycodone	Percodan	—	15	—	—	3–4	—
Oxymorphone	Numorphan	1.0	—	1	2–3	4–5	—
Pentazocine	Talwin	—	30–60	1	2–6	3–4	—
Propoxyphene	Darvon	—	65–100	2–4	8–24	2–4	500

*"Ts and blues" are a combination of pentazocine (Talwin) and tripelennamine (Pyribenzamine) used intravenously. Pentazocine now has naloxone added to it to counter this abuse. Innovar is fentanyl plus droperidol, used as an IV anesthetic.
†Dose equivalent to 10 mg of morphine.
‡Not available in the United States.

gooseflesh, hyperactive bowel sounds, hypertension, insomnia, lacrimation, muscle cramps, restlessness, tachycardia, and yawning. Each sign or symptom is given 0, 1, or 2 points, depending on the severity. A score of 1 to 5 is mild; 6 to 10, moderate; and 11 to 15, severe. Seizures are unusual with withdrawal. They indicate severity regardless of the rest of the score. *Management*: Mild withdrawal is treated with diazepam (Valium) orally, 10 mg every 6 hours; moderate withdrawal, with intramuscular diazepam; and severe withdrawal, with diazepam and diphenoxylate-atropine for the diarrhea. Methadone orally may be used, 20 to 40 mg every 12 hours, decreased by 5 mg every 12 hours. When 10 mg is reached, add diphenoxylate-atropine. Clonidine (Catapres), 6 μg per kg every 6 hours, can be used with informed consent. (This is an unlisted use of clonidine; the manufacturer states that relief from withdrawal symptoms has been reported with 0.8 mg per day.) *Laboratory aids*: For acute overdose obtain levels of blood gases, blood glucose, and electrolytes; chest radiographs; and ECG. Blood opioid levels confirm the diagnosis but are not useful for making a therapeutic decision. For drug abusers, consider testing for hepatitis B, syphilis, and human immunodeficiency virus (HIV) antibody (HIV testing usually requires consent).

PROPOXYPHENE (Darvon). *Manifestations*: Onset may be as early as 30 minutes after ingestion. Convulsions occur early. Patients may develop diabetes insipidus, pulmonary edema, and hypoglycemia. *Elimination*: Metabolism is 90% by demethylation in the liver. Peak plasma level 1 to 2 hours after oral dose. The t½ is 1 to 5 hours. As little as 10 mg per kg has caused symptoms, and 35 mg per kg has

caused cardiopulmonary arrest. Therapeutic blood level is less than 200 μg per mL. *Treatment* (in addition to the general management): (1) Emesis can be dangerous because of the rapid onset of seizures. (2) Indications for naloxone are respiratory depression, seizure activity, coma, and miotic pupils. Signs of naloxone effect are dilation of pupils, increased rate and depth of respirations, reversal of hypotension, and improvement of obtunded or comatose state. Larger doses of naloxone are often required and can be continued as an infusion of the initial response dose every hour. (3) Naloxone and intravenous glucose should be tried first to control seizures. If these fail, diazepam may be tried.

Organochlorine Insecticides (DDT derivatives). See Table 23 for a listing of these agents. The *toxic dose* varies greatly. For chlorophenothane (DDT), 200 to 250 mg per kg is fatal; 16 mg per kg causes seizures. For methoxychlor, 500 to 600 mg per kg is fatal. For chlordane, 200 mg per kg is fatal (chlordane house air guidelines are below 5 μg per m³; the occupational TLV is 500 μg per m³). These insecticides interfere with axon transmission of nerve impulses. Metabolism varies; they resist degradation in human tissue and the environment. They accumulate in adipose tissue; the elimination route is via the liver. *Manifestations*: CNS stimulation, convulsions, late respiratory depression, and increased myocardial irritability usually develop within 1 to 2 hours and may last for 1 week or more. Endrin produces liver toxicity with a guarded prognosis. Chronic exposure causes liver and kidney damage. *Management*: (1) Dermal decontamination; discard contaminated leather goods. Protect personnel. Gastrointestinal decontamination, no oils. Emesis can be dangerous,

TABLE 23. **Organochlorine Pesticides (DDT Derivatives)**

Chemical Name	Trade Name	Toxicity Rating	Fatal Dose (Adult)	Elimination Time	Comment
Endrin	Hexadrin	Highest	NA	Hours–days	Banned
Lindane	1% in Kwell; Benesan; Isotox; Gamene	Moderate to high	10 gm	Hours–days	Scabicide; general garden insecticide
Endosulfan	Thiodan	Moderate	NA	Hours–days	
Benzene hexachloride	BHC, HCH	Moderate	NA	Weeks–months	Banned, produces porphyria (cutanea tarda)
Dieldrin	Dieldrite	High	3 gm	Weeks–months	Banned in 1974
Aldrin	Aldrite	High	3 gm	Weeks–months	Banned in 1974
Chlordane (10% is heptachlor)	Chlordan	High	3 gm	Weeks–months	Restricted in 1979; termiticide
Toxaphene	Toxakil Strobane-T	High	2 gm	Hours–days	
Heptachlor	—	Moderate	NA	Weeks–months	Malignancy in rats; banned in 1976
Chlorophenothane	DDT	Moderate	NA	Months–years	Banned in 1972
Mirex	—	Moderate	NA	Months–years	Banned; red anticide
Chlordecone	Kepone	Moderate	NA	Months–years	Tidewater, Virginia, contamination
Methoxychlor	Marlate	Low	600 mg/kg	Hours–days	
Ethylan	Perthane	Low	NA	Hours–days	
Dicofol	Kelthane	Low	NA	Hours–days	
Chlorbenzilat	Acaraben	Low	NA	Hours–days	Banned

Abbreviation: NA = not available.

owing to rapid onset of seizures. Many of these agents are dissolved in petroleum distillates, presenting an aspiration hazard. (2) No adrenergic stimulants (epinephrine) should be used because of myocardial irritability. (3) Cholestyramine, 4 grams every 8 hours, has been reported to increase the fecal excretion. (4) Anticonvulsants, if needed.

Organophosphate and Carbamate Insecticides (OPIs). These may cause (1) irreversible inhibition of cholinesterase, either direct (tetraethyl pyrophosphate [TEPP]) or delayed (parathion or malathion), or (2) reversible inhibition of cholinesterase (carbamates). Examples of OPIs are listed in Table 24. Absorption is by all routes. The onset of acute toxicity is usually before 12 hours and always before 24 hours, unless the agents are absorbed by the dermal route or are liquid-soluble (fenthion), which may delay onset for 24 hours. Inhalation produces intoxication within minutes. *Toxic manifestations:* Garlic odor of the breath or gastric contents or from the container that the OPI is stored in. Miosis and muscle twitching are helpful clues to acute OPI poisoning. Early, cholinergic crisis—cramps, diarrhea, excess secretion, bronchospasms, bradycardia. Later, sympathetic and nicotine effects occur—twitching, fasciculations, weakness, tachycardia and hypertension, and convulsions. CNS effects are anxiety, confusion, emotional lability, and coma. Delayed respira-

TABLE 24. **Examples of Common Organophosphate Insecticides**

Common Name	Trade Name(s)	EFD (gm/70 kg)	LD$_{50}$ (mg/kg)
Agricultural Products (25–50% formulations, highly toxic; LD$_{50}$ is 1–40 mg/kg)			
Azinphos-methyl	Guthion	0.2	10.0
Chlortriphos	Calathion		
Demeton*	Systox		1.5
Disulfoton*	Di-Syston	0.2	12.0
Ethyl-nitrophenyl-thiobenzene PO$_4$	EPN		
Fonofos	Dyfonate		
Methamidophos†	Monitor		
Mevinphos	Phosdrin	0.15	
Monocrotophos	Azodrin		21.0
Octamethyldiphosphoramide	OMPA, Schradan		
Parathion	Thiophos	0.10	2.5
Ethyl parathion	Parathion		
Methyl parathion	Dalf		
Phorate	Thimet		
Terbufos	Counter		
Tetraethyl pyrophosphate	TEPP, Tetron	0.05	1.5
Animal Insecticides (moderately toxic; LD$_{50}$ is 40–200 mg/kg)			
Chlorfenvinphos (tick dip)	Supona, Dermaton		
Coumaphos	Co-ral		
DEF	DeGreen		
Dichlorvos‡	DDVP, Vapona		46
Dimethoate§	Cygon, De-fend		>500
Fenthion‖	Baytex		40
Leptophos	Phosvel		
Phosmet	Imidan		
Ronnel	Korlan		
Trichlorfon	Dylox	10.0	
Household and Garden Pest Control (1–2% formulations, low toxicity; LD$_{50}$ is 200–1400 mg/kg)			
Acephate¶	Orthene		>1000
Bromophos**			>1000
Chlorpyrifos** (toxic dose is 300 mg/kg)	Lorsban, Dursban, Pyrinex		>500
Dimpylate*††	Spectracide, Diazinon	25.0	>400
Dichlorvos‡‡	DDVP, Vapona (plastic strip)		
Malathion (>92%, <24 h)	Cythion	60.0	1375
Merphos	Folex		>1000
Temephos	Abate		<2000

*Most OPIs degrade in the environment in a few days to nontoxic radicals. These may be taken up by plants and fruits.
†Delayed neuropathy.
‡Found in flea collars and No-Pest Strips.
§t½ is <24 h.
‖Long-acting.
¶t½ is 1–6 days.
**Some authors classify this as moderately toxic; t½ is 27 h.
††In rats, t½ is 12 h.
‡‡Some authors classify this as moderately toxic.
Abbreviations: EFD = estimated fatal dose, common lawn chemical has 14.3%; LD$_{50}$ = dose that is fatal in 50% of animals; OPI = organophosphate insecticide.

tory paralysis and neurologic disorders have been described. *Management*: (1) Basic life support and decontamination with careful protection of personnel. (2) Atropine (Antidote 7, Table 4), if patient is symptomatic, every 10 to 30 minutes until drying of secretions and clearing of lungs occur. Maintain for 12 to 24 hours, then taper the dose and observe for relapse. (3) Intravenous pralidoxime (2-PAM) is required after atropinization (Antidote 36, Table 4). It should be given early. Its use may require reduction in the dose of atropine. (4) Careful dermal and gastrointestinal decontamination when patient is stable. (5) Suction secretions until atropinization drying is achieved. Intubation and assisted ventilation may be needed. (6) *Do not* use morphine, aminophylline, phenothiazine, or reserpine-like drugs or succinylcholine. *Laboratory aids*: Draw blood for red blood cell cholinesterase determination before giving pralidoxime. Levels are usually more than 90% depressed for severe symptoms. A postexposure rise of 10 to 15% determined at least 10 to 14 days without exposure is important in the diagnosis. Monitor chest radiograph, blood glucose, arterial blood gases, ECG, blood coagulation status, liver function, and the urine for the metabolite alkyl phosphate *p*-nitrophenol. *Note*: If the diagnosis is probable, do not delay therapy until it is confirmed by laboratory tests. Atropine is both a diagnostic and a therapeutic agent. A test dose of 1 mg in adults and 0.01 mg per kg in children may be administered parenterally. In the presence of severe cholinesterase inhibition, the patient fails to develop signs of atropinization.

PROPHYLAXIS. It is not medically advisable to administer atropine or pralidoxime prophylactically to workers exposed to organophosphate pesticides.

CARBAMATES (esters of carbonic acid). Carbamates cause reversible carbamylation of acetylcholinesterase. Pralidoxime is usually not indicated in the management, but atropine may be required. The major differences from OPI are that (1) toxicity is less and of shorter duration, (2) they rarely produce overt CNS effects because of poor penetration, and (3) cholinesterase returns to normal rapidly, so blood values are not useful in confirming the diagnosis. Some common examples of carbamates are ziram, aldicarb (Temik) (taken up by plants and fruit), Matacil (aminocarb, carazol), Vydate (oxamyl), Isolan, carbofuran (Furadan), methomyl (Lannate; Nudrin), mexacarbate (Zectran), and methiocarb (Mesural). These agents are all highly toxic. Moderately toxic are propoxur (Baygon) and carbaryl (Sevin). Some of these agents may be formulated in wood alcohol and have the added toxicity of methyl alcohol.

Paradichlorobenzene. See Hydrocarbons.

Paraquat and Diquat. Paraquat is a quaternary ammonia herbicide rapidly inactivated in the soil by clay particles. Nonindustrial preparations of 0.2% are unlikely to cause serious intoxications. *Toxic dose*: Commercial preparations such as Gramoxone 20% are very toxic; one mouthful has produced death. Systemic absorption in the course of occupational use is apparently minimal. Paraquat on marijuana leaves is pyrolyzed to nontoxic dipyridyl. *Toxicokinetics*: "Hit and run" toxin. Less than 20% is absorbed. The peak is 1 hour postingestion. *Route of elimination*: Kidney. Most of the dose is eliminated in the first 40 hours; it is detected in urine for 15 days. The Vd is over 500 liters per kg. *Manifestations*: Local corrosive effect on skin and mucous membranes. Acute renal failure in 48 hours (often reversible). Pulmonary effects in 72 hours are progressive, and oxygen aggravates the pulmonary fibrosis. Diquat does not produce effects on the lungs but produces convulsions and gastrointestinal distention. Long-term exposure may cause cataracts. Chlormequat's target organ is the kidney. *Management*: (1) Gastrointestinal decontamination despite corrosive effects should be done cautiously with a nasogastric tube. Repeated doses of activated charcoal are recommended. Dermal and ocular decontamination as needed. (2) Hemodialysis and hemoperfusion may be carried out in tandem. Hemoperfusion with charcoal alone, if started within 2 hours after ingestion, may be effective; if started after 2 hours, however, the results are poor. Continue hemoperfusion until blood paraquat levels cannot be detected. (3) Diuresis may be of value but consider the risk of fluid overload. (4) Niacin and Vitamin E have not been effective. (5) Avoid oxygen unless absolutely necessary (Pa_{O_2} below 60 mmHg) because this aggravates fibrosis. Some use hypoxic air, FI_{O_2} 10 to 20%. (6) Corticosteroids may help prevent adrenocortical necrosis. (7) Sepsis often develops within 7 to 10 days and should be treated appropriately. *Laboratory aids*: Blood levels above 2 μg per mL at 4 hours or above 0.10 μg per mL at 24 hours are usually fatal. Blood level testing and advice may be obtained from ICI America, 1-800-327-8633. Monitor renal, liver, and pulmonary functions and chest radiographs. Urine test for paraquat exposure—alkalinization and sodium dithionite give an intense blue-green color in exposure.

Parathion. See Organophosphate Insecticides.

Pentazocine (Talwin). See Opioids.

Perphenazine. See Phenothiazines and Other Major Neuroleptics.

Petroleum Products. See Hydrocarbons.

Phencyclidine (angel dust, PCP, peace pill, hog). This is the "drug of deceit" because it is substituted for many other drugs, such as tetrahydrocannabinol (THC) and mescaline. There are now at least 38 analogues. Smoking may give cyanide poisoning. Improper mixing has caused explosions. *Toxic dose*: Two to 5 mg smoked or "snorted" produces drunken behavior, agitation, and excitement. Five to 10 mg produces stupor, coma, and myoclonus convulsions. Ten to 25 mg smoked, snorted, or taken orally results in prolonged coma and respiratory failure. It is usually fatal over 25 mg (250 ng per mL blood concentration). *Toxicokinetics*: Weak base. Rapidly absorbed when smoked, insufflated nasally, or ingested and secreted into stomach gastric juice. Absorbed in alkaline intestine, but ion trapping takes place in acid gastric media. t½ is 30 to 60 minutes. Lipophilic drug with extensive Vd. The onset of action if smoked is 2 to 5 minutes (peak in 15 to 30 minutes); orally, 30 to 60 minutes. The duration at low doses is 4 to 6 hours, and normality returns in 24 hours. At large overdoses, coma may last 6 to 10 days (waxes and wanes). An adverse reaction in overdose occurs in 1 to 2 hours. *Route of elimination*: By liver metabolism (50%). Urinary excretion of conjugates and free PCP. *Manifestations*: Sympathomimetic, cholinergic, cerebellar. Observe for violent behavior, paranoid schizophrenia, self-destructive behavior. Clues to diagnosis are bursts of horizontal, vertical, and rotary nystagmus, coma with eyes open. *Management* (avoid overtreatment of mild intoxications): (1) Gastrointestinal decontamination up to 4 hours postingestion, but this may not be effective because PCP is rapidly absorbed. Insert nasogastric tube into stomach for administration of activated charcoal every 6 hours because PCP is secreted into the stomach even if it is smoked or snorted. (2) Protect patient and others from harm. "Talk down" is usually ineffective. Low sensory environment. Diazepam (Valium) may be used orally or intramuscularly in the uncooperative patient. (3) For behavioral disorders and toxic psychosis—diazepam. (4) Seizures and muscle spasm—control with diazepam, 2.5 mg, up to 10 mg (Antidote 16, Table 4). (5) Dystonia reaction—diphenhydramine (Benadryl) intravenously (Antidote 19, Table 4). (6) Hyperthermia—external cooling. (7) Hypertensive crisis (dopaminergic)—use nitroprusside, 0.3 to 2 μg per kg per minute. Maximum infusion rate—10 μg per kg per minute; should never last more than 10 minutes. (8) Acid diuresis ion trapping (controversial). Ammonium chloride use is not recommended because of rhabdomyolysis and the danger of myoglobin precipitation in the renal tubules (Antidote 2, Table 4). (9) Avoid phenothiazines in the acute phase of intoxication because they lower the convulsive threshold. May be needed later for psychosis. *Laboratory aids*: (1) Elevation of the CPK level is a clue to the amount of rhabdomyolysis occurring and the chance of development of myoglobinuria. Values up to 20,000 U have been reported. (2) Test urine for myoglobin and pigmented casts. Test urine with orthotoluidine; a positive test without red blood cells on microscopic examination suggests myoglobinuria. (3) Monitor urine and blood pH and urinary output if acidifying patient. (4) Measure PCP level. (5) Evaluate BUN, ammonia, electrolytes, blood glucose levels (20% of patients have hypoglycemia). (6) Test for PCP in gastric juice; levels are 40 to 50 times higher than in blood. *Complications*: Rhabdomyolysis, myoglobinuria, and renal failure. Dopaminogenic hypertensive crisis, cerebrovascular accident, encephalopathy, and malignant hyperthermia. Schizophrenic paranoid psychosis (induced in chronic users or precipitated in acute users). Loss of memory for months. Delayed toxicity and "flashbacks" occur. Teratogenic cases have been reported. Children have been intoxicated from inhalation in a room where adults were smoking PCP. PCP-induced depression and suicide have been reported.

Phenobarbital. See Barbiturates.

Phenothiazines and Other Major Neuroleptics.

Phenothiazines are represented by aliphatic compounds: chlorpromazine (Thorazine), promethazine (Phenergan), promazine (Sparine), triflupromazine (Vesprin), methoxypromazine (Tentone)*; piperazine compounds (dimethylamine series): acetophenazine (Tindal), fluphenazine (Prolixin), prochlorperazine (Compazine), perphenazine (Trilafon), trifluoperazine (Stelazine); and piperidine compounds: mesoridazine (Serentil), thioridazine (Mellaril), pipamazine (Mornidine).* Nonphenothiazines are the thioxanthines: chlorprothixene (Taractan), thiothixene (Navane); butyrophenones: haloperidol (Haldol), droperidol (Inapsine); dibenzoxazepines: loxapine (Loxitane); and dihydroindolones: molindone (Moban). These have pharmacologic properties similar to those of the phenothiazines. See Table 25. *Manifestations*: If patient is asymptomatic, monitor vital signs and ECG for at least 6 to 12 hours. Clues to phenothiazine overdose are miosis, tremor, hypotension, hypothermia, respiratory depression, radiopaque pills on radiograph of abdomen, and increased QT waves on the ECG. Anticholinergic actions are also present. Major problems are respiratory depression, myocardial toxicity (quinidine-like), neurogenic hypotension (antidopaminogenic), and idiosyncratic reaction, which may occur at therapeutic levels. Idiosyncratic reaction consists of opisthotonos, torticollis, orolingual dyskinesis, and oculogyric crisis (painful upward gaze) and can be mistaken for a psychotic episode. Extrapyramidal crisis is frequent in children and women. Malignant neuroleptic syndrome may occur. It is characterized by hyperthermia, muscle rigidity, and autonomic dysfunction. Death is usually due to cardiac effects. Phenothiazines are metabolized by the liver into many metabolites. Some remain in the body longer than 6 months. *Management*: (1) Gastrointestinal decontamination. Avoid emesis. If symptoms are already present, many of these agents have antiemetic action, so lavage may be required. Always provide gastric lavage to comatose patients after the airway is protected regardless of the time of ingestion because of inhibition of gastric motility. (2) Extrapyramidal signs (idiosyncratic reaction) can be treated with diphenhydramine (Benadryl) (Antidote 19, Table 4), or benztropine (Cogentin), 1 to 2 mg intravenously slowly. Symptoms recur, and these drugs should be continued orally for 5 to 7 days. *This is not the treatment of overdose*, only of the idiosyncratic reaction. (3) Monitor ECG for dysrhythmias and treat with antidysrhythmic agents. Avoid quinidine, procainamide, or disopyramide (Norpace). Treat the membrane depressant effects with intravenous sodium bicarbonate. (4) Hypotension is treated with the Trendelenburg position or fluid challenge or both. Vasopressors are used only if these fail. Dopamine (Intropin) should *not* be used to treat the hypotension because these drugs are antidopaminogenic. If a pressor agent is needed, use norepinephrine (levarterenol, Levophed). (5) Treat

---

*Not available in the United States.

TABLE 25. **Pharmacokinetics of Phenothiazines and Related Compounds**

Medication	Metabolism	Dose Equivalent (mg)	Absorption	Volume of Distribution (L/kg)	t½ (h)	Therapy
Aliphatic Type						
Moderate cardiotoxic and hypotensive effects; low sedation; moderate extrapyramidal effects; moderate anticholinergic effects						
Chlorpromazine (Thorazine) (high sedation)	Hepatic	100	Rapid	10–20	16–30	PO: child, 2 mg/kg/24 h; max <12 years old, 75 mg/24 h; adult, 200-2000 mg/24 h
Promethazine (Phenergan)	Hepatic	25	Rapid	—	12	PO: child, 0.1–0.5 mg/kg/dose; adult, 12.5–25 mg/dose (25–200 mg/24 h)
Piperazine						
Least cardiotoxic and hypotensive effects; very high extrapyramidal effects; moderate anticholinergic effects						
Prochlorperazine (Compazine)	Hepatic	15	Slow	10–35	8–12	PO: child, 0.1 mg/kg/dose (not <2 years old); adult, 10 mg/dose
Fluphenazine HCl (Prolixin) (injectible decanoate salt)	Hepatic	2	Rapid	—	2–12 (6.8–9.6 days)	PO: adult, 2.5–10 mg/24 h
Piperidine						
Highest cardiotoxic and hypotensive effects; low extrapyramidal effects; high anticholinergic effects						
Thioridazine (Mellaril) (high sedation)	Hepatic	100	Slow	3.5	26–36	PO: child, 1 mg/kg/24 h (not <3 years old); adult, 150–300 mg/24 h
Butyrophenone						
Low cardiotoxic and hypotensive effects; low sedation; very high extrapyramidal effects; very low anticholinergic effects						
Haloperidol (Haldol)	Hepatic	2–15	Rapid	20–30	12–22	PO: child, 0.1 mg/kg/24 h; adult, 20–100 mg/24 h
Droperidol (Inapsine)	Hepatic	2.5–10	NA	Large	2.2	IM/IV: child, 0.1–1.5 mg/kg/dose; adult, 2.5–10 mg/dose
Thioxanthene						
Low cardiotoxic and hypotensive effects; low sedation; high extrapyramidal effects; low anticholinergic effects						
Thiothixene (Navane)	Hepatic	2	NA	Large	34	PO: child, 0.25 mg/kg/24 h; adult, 16–60 mg/24 h (max, 60 mg)
Dibenzoxazepine						
Low cardiotoxic and hypotensive effects; low sedation; high extrapyramidal effects; low anticholinergic effects						
Loxapine (Loxitane)	Hepatic	15	NA	Large	3–4	PO: adult, initially 10 mg bid to max of 50 mg
Dihydroindolones						
Molindone (Moban)	Hepatic	10	Rapid	Large	1.5	PO: adult, initially 50–75 mg/24 h increased up to 225 mg

Peak levels occur mainly 1–4 h postingestion, and these drugs have enterohepatic recirculation. The pharmacokinetics of most phenothiazines resemble those of chlorpromazine. See pharmacokinetics for details.
Abbreviation: NA = not available.

neuroleptic malignant syndrome by discontinuing the offending agent, reducing the patient's temperature with external cooling, and correcting any metabolic imbalance. Dantrolene and bromocriptine are agents that have been shown to be useful pharmacologic adjuncts for the management of this syndrome. (6) Treat hypothermia or hyperthermia with external physical measures (not drugs). (7) Physostigmine should be avoided because it can produce seizures and cardiac toxicity. *Laboratory aids:* A ferric chloride test of urine can confirm exposure to phenothiazines if there is a sufficient blood level. Blood levels are *not* useful in management. A radiograph of the abdomen is useful to detect undissolved tablets, which may be radiopaque. Monitor arterial blood gases, renal and hepatic function, and levels of electrolytes and blood glucose for creatine kinase and myoglobinemia in neuroleptic malignant syndrome.

Phenylpropanolamine (PPA). See Amphetamines.

Primidone. See Anticonvulsants.

Propoxyphene. See Opioids.

Propranolol and Beta Blockers. Some of these agents available in the United States at this time are listed in Table 26. Beta blockers generally act as negative cardiac inotropes and chronotropes, although some have partial agonist activity with the opposite effect. *Toxic dose:* Varies considerably. *Toxicokinetics:* Time to peak action is 1 to 2 hours orally; the effects last 24 to 48 hours. In drugs with long half-lives, e.g., nadolol, it may take many days to recover from overdose toxicity (Table 26). *Manifestations:* Observe for bradycardia and hypotension. Fat-soluble drugs have greater intensity of CNS effects. Partial agonists may initially produce tachycardia and hypertension (oxprenolol, pindolol). ECG changes include differing degrees of atrioventricular conduction delay or frank asystole. May cause hypoglycemia. *Management:* (1) Gastrointestinal decontamination with gastric lavage and activated charcoal and cathartic. Before gastric lavage, treatment with atropine, 0.01 mg per kg for a child and 0.5 mg for an adult, has been suggested to decrease the vagal effect in patients with bradycardia or significant intoxications. Avoid induced emesis because of early onset of seizures and vagal stimulation. Asymptomatic patients may be discharged after 12 to 24 hours of observation. (2) Treat hypoglycemia (frequent in children) and hyperkalemia. (3) Control convulsions. (4) Cardiovascular manifestations: Bradycardia—if patient is hemodynamically stable and asymptomatic, no therapy. If patient is unstable (hypotension or atriovenous block), use atropine, glucagon, isoproterenol, and pacemaker. Ventricular tachycardia or premature beats—use lidocaine (Xylocaine), phenytoin (Dilantin), or overdrive pacing. Myocardial depression and hypotension—correct dysrhythmias; institute Trendelenburg positioning and fluids. Monitor with a PAWP catheter. If low cardiac output with low PAWP, give more fluids. If low cardiac output with normal PAWP, use glucagon (Anti-

TABLE 26. **Pharmacokinetic Properties of Beta Blockers**

Drug Name	Solubility and Absorption (%)	Plasma t½ (h)	Elimination Route	Time to Peak Concentration	Protein Binding (%)	Volume of Distribution (L/kg)	Beta₁ Cardiac Selective
Acebutolol* (Sectral) Dose: 400–800 mg MDD: 800 mg TPC: 200–2000 ng/mL	Moderate, lipid (90)	3–4, metabolite diacetolol	Hepatic, active metabolite	—	26	1.2	+
Alprenolol* (Aptin,† Betapin; Betacard) Dose: 200–800 mg MDD: 800 mg TPC: 50–200 ng/mL	Lipid (10)	3.1	Hepatic	1–3	85	3.4	−
Atenolol (Tenormin) Dose: 50–100 mg MDD: 100 mg TPC: 200–500 ng/mL	Water (46–62)	6–9	Renal, 95%	2–4	3–10	0.7	+
Betaxolol (Betoptic) (Kerlone) Dose: 1 drop in eye twice daily MDD: Not available	Water (70–90)	12–22	Hepatic, 3–12%	—	50–60	4.9–13	+
Bisoprolol (Zebeta) Dose: 5–20 mg	Water (82–94)	9–12	Renal, 50%	3–4	30	2.9	+
Carteolol (Cartrol) Dose: 2.5–10 mg MDD: 40 mg	Lipid (84)	6–11	Renal, 60%	1–3	15	NA	−
Esmolol (Brevibloc) Dose: IV 50–500 µg/kg/min (loading dose) MDD: 300 µg/kg/min	Water	9 min	Hepatic, plasma esterases	—	55	3.4	+
Labetalol (Normodyne, Trandate) Dose: 400–800 mg MDD: 1–2 gm	Water (50)	6–8	Hepatic, 95% Blocks alpha (weakly) and beta activity	—	50	11	−
Levobunolol (Betagan) Dose: Ophthalmic: 1 drop twice daily, 0.5%, 1%	Water (100)	6.1	Hepatic	—	—	—	−
Metoprolol (Lopressor) Dose: 50–100 mg MDD: 450 mg TPC: 50–100 ng/mL	Lipid (>95)	3–4	Hepatic	1–2	10	5.6	+
Nadolol (Corgard) Dose: 40–320 mg MDD: 320 mg TPC: 20–400 ng/mL	Water (15–25)	14–23	Renal, 70%	3–4	25	2.1	−

Table continued on following page

TABLE 26. **Pharmacokinetic Properties of Beta Blockers** *Continued*

Drug Name	Solubility and Absorption (%)	Plasma t½ (h)	Elimination Route	Time to Peak Concentration	Protein Binding (%)	Volume of Distribution (L/kg)	Beta₁ Cardiac Selective
Oxprenolol (Trasicor)‡ Dose: 80–320 mg MDD: 480 mg TPC: 80–100 ng/mL	Lipid (70–95)	1.5–3	Hepatic	1–2	80	1.5	−
Penbutolol (Levatol) Dose: 20–80 mg MDD: 80 mg	Lipid (100)	4–8	Hepatic	1–1.5	80–90	0.5	−
Pindolol* (Visken) Dose: 20–60 mg MDD: 60 mg TPC: 50–150 ng/mL	Lipid (>90)	3–4	Hepatic, 60%; renal, 40%	1.25	57	2.0	−
Practolol* (Eraldin)‡ Dose: 25–600 mg MDD: 800 mg TPC: 1500–5000 ng/mL	No longer available in United States because of adverse reactions Water (100)	6–8	Renal	3	40	—	+
Propranolol (Inderal) Dose: 40–160 mg MDD: 480 mg TPC: 50–100 ng/mL	Lipid (100) (70% first pass)	2–3	Hepatic; renal (<1%), active hydroxy metabolite	1.5	90–95	3.6	−
Sotalol (Betapace) Dose: 80–320 mg MDD: 480 mg TPC: 500–4000 ng/mL	Prolongs QT and may produce torsades de pointes Water (70)	5–13	Renal	2–3	54	0.7	−
Timolol§‖ Dose: 20 mg (Blocadren); ophthalmic (Timoptic, 0.25%, 0.5%), 1 drop twice daily MDD: 60 mg TPC: 5–10 ng/mL	Lipid (>90)	3–5	Hepatic, 80%; renal, 20%	4–5	<10	5.5	−

*Partial agonists.
†Investigational drug in the United States.
‡Not available in the United States.
§Substantial first pass.
‖Mitochondrial calcium protection during ischemia.
Abbreviations: MDD = maximal daily dose; TPC = therapeutic plasma concentration.

dote 26, Table 4). Avoid quinidine, procainamide, and disopyramide (Norpace). Glucagon is probably the drug of choice because it works through an adenyl cyclase mechanism not affected by the beta blockers. It is given as a bolus and may be continued as an infusion (Antidote 26, Table 4). If bronchospasm is present, give aminophylline. Hemodialysis or hemoperfusion for low-volume distribution drugs that are low–protein binding and water-soluble (nadolol, atenolol, and sotalol) particularly with evidence of renal failure. If hypoglycemia is present, give intravenous glucose. *Laboratory aids:* Monitor blood glucose, potassium, ECG, PAWP. Toxic blood level of propranolol is over 2 μg per mL.

Quinidine and Quinine (antidysrhythmic and antimalarial agents). *Toxic dose:* Quinidine in child, 60 mg per kg; in adult, 2 to 8 grams. Quinine, 15 mg per kg in child; 1 gram in adult. *Toxicokinetics:* There is 95 to 100% absorption, with peak action in 2 to 6 hours. The t½ is 3 to 4 hours (quinidine gluconate, 8 to 12 hours). Large Vd. Metabolized predominantly by the liver. *Manifestations:* Cinchonism (headache, nausea, vomiting, tinnitus, deafness, diplopia, dilated pupils). Myocardial depression, dysrhythmias, ECG changes—widening of PR and QT intervals and QRS complexes. Rashes and flushing. Hemolysis in glucose-6-phosphate dehydrogenase deficiency. Dementia reported. Quinidine produces more cardiovascular damage, and quinine produces more ocular damage. *Management:* (1) Obtain an immediate cardiac consultation. Electrophysiologic support of the heart should be readily available. (2) Gastrointestinal decontamination. Avoid emesis because of rapid onset of seizures and coma. (3) Monitor ECG and liver function. (4) May need antidysrhythmic drugs (but avoid Class IA antidysrhythmics), and pacemaker and alkalinization. Treat torsades de pointes in adults with magnesium sulfate, 2 grams intravenously over 2 to 3 minutes. *Laboratory aids:* Quinidine—therapeutic level 2 to 6 μg per mL. Toxic greater than 8 μg per mL. Fatal greater than 16 μg per mL. Quinine—therapeutic level 7 μg per mL. Toxic greater than 10 μg per mL.

Salicylates. *Toxic dose:* 150 mg per kg or 7.5 to

TABLE 27. **Quantities of Aspirin Ingested: Deposition and Manifestations***

Category	Amount Ingested (mg/kg)	Toxicity Expected	Gastrointestinal Decontamination	Manifestations Anticipated
Nontoxic	<150	No	No	None
Mild intoxication	150–200	Yes	Yes (ECF)	Vomiting, tinnitus, mild hyperventilation
Moderate intoxication	200–300	Yes	Yes (ECF)	Hyperpnea, lethargy, or excitability
Severe intoxication	300–500	Yes	Yes (ECF)	Coma, convulsions, severe hyperpnea
Very severe intoxication	>500	Yes	Yes (ECF)	Potentially fatal

*See toxic dose section for gastrointestinal decontamination.
Abbreviation: ECF = emergency care facility.

10 grams. See Table 27. Methyl salicylate (oil of wintergreen)—1 mL equals 1.4 grams of salicylate. One teaspoonful equals 21 adult aspirins. *Toxicokinetics:* Plasma concentration is significant in 30 minutes and peaks in 1 to 2 hours but may be delayed 6 hours or more in overdose with enteric-coated, sustained-release preparations or concretions. The t½ is 3 to 6 hours (therapeutic) to 12 to 36 hours (toxic). Urine pH influences urine salicylate elimination. *Manifestations of acute ingestion* (see Table 27): The metabolic disturbance in adults and older children is usually respiratory alkalosis; in children younger than 5 years of age, the initial respiratory alkalosis usually changes to metabolic or mixed metabolic acidosis and respiratory alkalosis, with acidosis predominating within a few hours. *Management:* Do not wait for a 6-hour salicylate level to start treatment of symptomatic patients. If hemodialysis may be required, suggest an immediate consult with a nephrologist. (1) Gastrointestinal decontamination is useful up to 12 hours postingestion because some factors delay absorption (food, enteric-coated tablets, other drugs), pylorospasm may delay emptying, and concretions may form. Activated charcoal should be administered every 4 hours until stools are black. Concretions may be removed by lavage, whole-body irrigation, endoscopy, or gastrostomy. (2) Intravenous fluid should be given as recommended in Table 28. Alkalinization (Antidote 39, Table 4) enhances

salicylate excretion. Potassium is essential to produce adequate alkalinization. Monitor both the urine and blood pH. Do not use the urine pH alone to assess the need for alkalinization. (3) Fluid retention can be treated with mannitol (20%), 0.5 gram per kg over 30 minutes, or furosemide (Lasix), 1 mg per kg intravenously. (4) Hyperpyrexia should be treated with external cooling. (5) Patients with abnormal bleeding or hypoprothrombinemia need Vitamin K, 10 to 50 mg intravenously, and, if bleeding continues, fresh blood or platelet transfusion (Antidote 43, Table 4). (6) Hemodialysis is indicated if there is persistent acidosis (pH <7.0) and lack of response to fluid or alkali in 6 hours; if serum salicylate levels are initially greater than 160 mg per dL or greater than 100 to 120 mg per dL at 6 hours postingestion (do *not* use the salicylate level as the sole criterion for dialysis); or if the patient has coma and uncontrollable seizures, congestive heart failure, acute renal failure, progressive deterioration despite good management. Lower levels such as 30 to 60 μg per mL may be an indication for hemodialysis in chronic salicylism with altered mental status. (7) Chronic toxicity is usually a more severe intoxication because of the cumulative pharmacokinetics of salicylates. Management needs are outlined in Table 29. *Laboratory aids:* The metabolic acidosis of salicylism has a moderately elevated anion gap. Hyperglycemia or hypoglycemia may exist. Serum salicylate levels used

TABLE 28. **Recommendations for Fluid Management for Moderate or Severe Salcylism***

Purpose	Rate (mL/kg/h)	Duration (h)	Electrolyte Concentration (mEq/L)				Glucose (%)
			Na	K	Cl	HCO₃	
Volume expansion	20	0.5–1.0	100	0	77	23	5–10
Administered as 0.45% saline with 23 mEq/L NaHCO₃							
Hydration Ongoing losses Alkalinization	4–8	Until therapeutic blood serum concentration is 30 mg/dL	56	40	56	1–2 mEq/kg child; 50–100 mEq adult	5–10
Administered as 0.33% saline and NaHCO₃ to obtain urine pH 7.5–8.0, blood pH 7.5							
Maintenance	2–6	—	mEq/kg/day				
			3	2	4		

*For severe acidosis (pH < 7.15), may require 1–2 mEq/kg of sodium bicarbonate every 1–2 h. Usual fluid loss is 200–300 mL/kg, but carefully monitor for fluid overload. Potassium may be needed in excess of 40 mEq/L when alkalinizing.

TABLE 29. **Management of Chronic Salicylate Intoxication**

Classification	Urine pH	Blood pH	Hydration	NaHCO₃ (mEq/L)	Potassium (mEq/L)
Mild	Alkaline	Alkaline	Yes	Yes*	20
Moderate	Acid†	Alkaline	Yes	pH 7.5†	40
Severe	Acid	Acid	Yes	pH 7.5	40‡
					80§

*Bicarbonate administered to keep blood pH at 7.5 and urine pH at 7.5–8.0.
†Paradoxical acid urine and alkaline blood indicate potassium depletion.
‡Normal serum potassium and electrocardiogram (ECG).
§Low serum potassium and/or abnormal ECG indicate potassium deficiency.

in conjunction with the Done nomogram (Figure 3) are useful predictors of expected severity following *acute single ingestions*. The Done nomogram is *not* useful in chronic intoxications or in methyl salicylate, phenyl salicylate, or homomethyl salicylate ingestions. The salicylate level for use in the Done nomogram should be obtained 6 hours postingestion. Before 6 hours, levels in the toxic range should be treated, and patients with levels below the toxic range should be retested if a potentially toxic dose is ingested. Monitor urine output, urine pH, electrolytes, arterial blood gases, blood glucose, prothrombin time, renal function, serum salicylate level, and urine salicylate with the ferric chloride test. Arterial blood pH should be kept at 7.5. *Prognosis*: Persistent vigorous treatment of salicylate ingestion is essential because recovery has occurred despite decerebrate rigidity.

Sedative Hypnotics, Nonbarbiturate. See Table 30. *Management*: Primarily supportive (especially intubation and ventilator therapy with continuous positive airway pressure for adult respiratory distress syndrome) with the use of hemoperfusion or hemodialysis in patients who are severely intoxicated and fail to respond to good supportive care and whose intoxication is life-threatening. Avoid emesis because of rapid onset of convulsions, apnea, and coma. (1) *Chloral hydrate* management includes cautious gastrointestinal decontamination. Avoid the use of epinephrine and catecholamines that may produce dysrhythmias. Propranolol, 0.1 mg per kg in 1-mg increments, appears to be more effective than lidocaine (Xylocaine) for ventricular dysrhythmias. Charcoal hemoperfusion may effectively remove chloral hydrate and its metabolite in patients who fail to respond and have potentially fatal plasma levels (20 μg per mL or higher). Hemodialysis may be ineffective because of lipid solubility. (2) *Ethchlorvynol* management includes gastrointestinal decontamination up to several hours postingestion. Charcoal hemoperfusion is the best method of extracorporeal removal when other measures fail in a life-threatening situation (ingestion of over 10 grams or 100 mg per kg, with serum levels of over 100 μg per mL in the first 12 hours or 70 μg per mL after 12 hours in patients with prolonged life-threatening coma). External rewarming if temperature is below 32° C (89.6° F). (3) *Glutethimide* management includes gastrointestinal decontamination up to 24 hours postingestion. Concretions may form. Charcoal hemoperfusion appears to be the best method of extracorporeal removal in life-threatening protracted coma when the patient has ingested over 10 grams and has a serum level of over 30 μg per mL. Treat hyperthermia with external cooling. (4) *Meprobamate* management includes gastrointestinal decontamination up to several hours postingestion, with charcoal hemoperfusion in prolonged coma with life-threatening complications. Concretions may form in the stomach and may require whole-bowel irrigation, endoscopy, or surgical removal. (5) *Methaqualone* management includes gastrointestinal decontamination up to 12 hours postingestion. Forced diuresis, dialysis, and hemoperfusion are not indicated. Fatalities are rare.

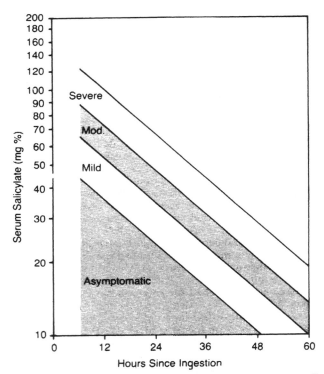

Figure 3. The Done nomogram for salicylate intoxication. For limitations of use, see *Laboratory aids*. (Redrawn from Done A: Salicylate intoxication: Significance of measurements of salicylate in blood in cases of acute ingestion. Reproduced by permission of Pediatrics, Vol. 26, Page 800, Copyright 1960.)

TABLE 30. **Nonbarbiturate Sedative Hypnotic Drugs**

Drug	Absorption and Toxic Dose	Time to Peak Effect (h)	Volume of Distribution (L/kg)	Protein Binding (%)	Elimination Route	Serum t½ (h)	Toxic Level (µg/mL)	Manifestations and Comment*
Chloral hydrate (Noctec)	Rapid TD, 2 gm FD, 4–10 gm	1–2	0.75–0.9	40	Hepatic 90% to active metabolite trichloro-ethanol (TCE)	4–8 min TCE: 8–12 h	100 (80 TCE—very toxic)	Pear-like odor, dysrhythmias (especially ventricular), hepatotoxicity, irritant to mucosa of GI tract, ARDS, radiopaque capsules
Ethchlorvynol (Placidyl)	Rapid TD, 2.5 gm FD, 10–25 gm	1–2	3–4	35–50	Hepatic 90%	10–25 in OD over 100	20–80	Prolonged coma up to 200 h, apnea, hypothermia, pulmonary edema, pink gastric aspirate, pungent odor
Glutethimide (Doriden) (highest mortality of all sedative hypnotics, 14%)	Slow, erratic TD, 5 gm FD, 10 gm	6	Large, 2–2.7	50	Hepatic 98% to toxic metabolite 4-hydroxy-glutarimide	10–40 in OD over 100	20–80	Prolonged, cyclic comas up to 120 h, anticholinergic signs, convulsions, recurrent apnea, hyperthermia
Meprobamate (Equanil, Miltown)	Rapid TD, 10–20 gm FD, 10–20 gm	4–8	10	20	Hepatic 90%	6–16	30–100	Coma, convulsions, pulmonary edema, apnea, concretions in stomach
Methaqualone (Quaalude, "love drugs")	Rapid TD, 800 mg FD 3–8 gm	1–3	2–6	80	Hepatic 90%	10–40	8–10	Hypertonia, hyper-reflexia, convulsions, apnea, acts "drunk," bleeding tendencies
Methyprylon (Noludar)	Rapid TD, 3 gm FD, 8–20 gm	2–4	1–2	—	Hepatic 97%	3–6 in OD over 50	30	Hyperactive, coma lasts 30 h, miosis, persistent hypotension, pulmonary edema, mortality rare

*Comment includes other features besides the typical manifestations of all these agents—coma, respiratory depression, psychological and physiologic withdrawal, hypotension, hypothermia (except glutethimide hyperthermia).
Abbreviations: TD = toxic dose; FD = fatal dose; OD = overdose; ARDS = adult respiratory distress syndrome; GI = gastrointestinal.

(6) *Methyprylon* management includes gastrointestinal decontamination and may require treatment of the hypotension with vasopressors of the alpha-adrenergic variety—e.g., levarterenol (norepinephrine, Levophed). The hypotension usually does not respond to position or fluids alone. This is a dialyzable drug, but dialysis usually is not necessary. Fatalities are rare.

Strychnine. Primarily available as a rodenticide and component of cathartics and "tonics." Adulterant of "street drugs," particularly marijuana and cocaine. *Toxic dose*: 5 to 10 mg; fatal in doses of 15 to 30 mg. *Toxicokinetics*: Rapid absorption. Manifestations may occur within 15 to 30 minutes. Low protein binding. Hepatic metabolism, which appears to be saturable. Twenty percent is excreted in urine. Has been found in the urine up to 48 hours after a 700-mg dose. *Manifestations*: Interferes with postsynaptic neurotransmitter inhibition by glycine. Hyperacusis is often the first sign. Mild cases—facial stiffness (trismus and risus sardonicus). Moderate cases—extensor muscle thrusts. Severe cases—tetanic convulsions with opisthotonos. Death occurs within 1 to 3 hours after ingestion. The prognosis for recovery improves if the patient survives beyond 5 hours. The complications of intoxication are lactic acidosis, hyperthermia, rhabdomyolysis and renal damage from precipitation of myoglobin in the renal tubules, and death from hypoxia. *Management*: (1) Emesis is contraindicated because of rapid absorption and the early onset of seizures. Gastric aspiration and lavage may be used after the seizures are controlled. Activated charcoal should be given and repeated. (2) Control convulsions with diazepam (Valium) or phenobarbital. (3) Supportive care for respiratory depression. (4) Acid diuresis and dialysis do not appear to be justified on the basis of available studies. (5) Paralysis with assisted ventilation is useful.

Tear Gas (lacrimators). CS (chlorobenzylidine), "riot control"; CN powder (chloroacetophenone, 1%); Mace (chloroacetophenone). *Management*: Dermal and ocular decontamination. Protect attendants from contamination. Ophthalmic evaluation. Oxygen therapy may be needed for dyspnea and respiratory distress.

Theophylline. *Toxic dose*: Acute, single dose greater than 10 mg per kg yields mild toxicity. Greater than 20 mg per kg, moderate manifestations. *Toxicokinetics*: Absorption is complete. Peak levels occur within 60 minutes after ingestion of liquid preparations; 1 to 3 hours after regular tablets; and 3 to 10 hours after slow-release preparations. Vd, 0.3 to 0.7 liter per kg. Protein binding, 15 to 40%. The t½ varies: 3.5 hours average in a child and 4.5 hours in an adult (range from 3 to 9 hours). In neonates and young infants the drug's half-life is much longer. Overdose increases the t½. *Elimination*: Hepatic metabolism, 90% (demethylation and oxidation); 8 to 10% is excreted unchanged in the urine. *Manifestations*: Acute toxicity generally correlates with blood levels; chronic toxicity does not. From 10 to 20 µg per mL is the therapeutic range, but mild gastrointestinal toxicity may occur in some. From 20 to 40 μg per mL is moderate toxicity, with gastrointestinal and CNS stimulation. Over 50 μg per mL, seizures and dysrhythmias may occur, but they may also occur at lower levels and without gastrointestinal symptoms. Children tolerate higher serum levels. Chronic intoxication is more serious and difficult to treat. Many factors increase theophylline concentration. *Management*: (1) Gastrointestinal decontamination in acute overdose, up to 4 hours with regular preparations and up to 8 to 12 hours with slow-release preparations. Test aspirate or vomitus for blood. Give activated charcoal every 4 hours until serum theophylline levels are less than 20 μg per mL. Do not induce emesis if hematemesis exists. If there is intractable vomiting, administer the antiemetic metoclopramide, 0.4 mg per kg per dose intravenously (maximum, 0.5 mg per kg per 24 hours) in infants and children, and 10 mg slowly over 15 minutes every 6 to 8 hours in adults. Alternative: droperidol, 2.5 mg intravenously or 0.05 to 0.1 mg per kg per dose every 6 to 8 hours if needed. Both drugs may cause extrapyramidal symptoms. Ondansetron is not recommended because it inhibits metabolism of theophylline. (2) Monitor ECG, obtain theophylline levels every 4 hours until they remain in the therapeutic range of 10 to 20 μg per mL. (3) Control seizures with diazepam (Valium). If coma, convulsions, or vomiting exists, intubate immediately. (4) Hypotension is treated with fluid challenge and, if this fails, vasopressors. (5) Hematemesis is managed with saline lavage and blood replacement if needed. (6) Charcoal hemoperfusion is the management of choice in life-threatening convulsions, dysrhythmias, hematemesis, or intractable vomiting refractory to conventional measures. It is recommended for acute intoxications with serum theophylline concentrations of 70 to 100 μg per mL, or with chronic overdoses with drug levels of 40 to 60 μg per mL, especially if the patient has risk factors that increase serum levels, e.g., age younger than 6 months or older than 60 years, liver disease, heart failure, viral infections, pneumonia, fever greater than 38.9° C (102° F); medications: macrolide antibiotics, oral contraceptives, cimetidine, beta blockers, carbamazepine, and caffeine. Differences in slow-release preparations from regular preparations: few or no gastrointestinal symptoms with high levels; peak concentration times may be 10 to 24 hours postingestion; and onset of seizures may occur 10 to 12 hours postingestion. *Laboratory aids*: Monitor theophylline levels, check for occult blood in vomitus and stools, monitor vital signs and hemoglobin and hematocrit (for hemorrhage). Monitor cardiac, renal, and hepatic function, electrolytes, blood glucose, arterial blood gases, and acid-base balance.

Toluene. See Hydrocarbons.

Tranquilizers. See Sedative Hypnotics.

Trichloroethylene. See Hydrocarbons.

Tricyclic Antidepressants (TCADs). See Table 31. These agents are generally rapidly absorbed from the gastrointestinal tract, but absorption may be prolonged in overdose owing to anticholinergic action. Their bioavailability has considerable variation among patients, and they are highly bound to plasma and tissue proteins. Protein binding decreases with decreasing pH. The Vd is large, usually 10 to 20 liters per kg. The TCADs are metabolized primarily in the liver. *N*-Demethylation of the tertiary amines yields the active secondary amine metabolites; hydroxylation gives rise to inactive metabolites. Forty percent is excreted in the feces and only 3% in the urine unchanged. The t½ varies from 9 to 198 hours. In an overdose, the t½ may be much longer. Tricyclic tertiary amines (metabolized to active metabolites) are amitriptyline (Elavil), imipramine (Tofranil), and doxepin (Sinequan, Adapin). Tricyclic secondary amines (metabolized to nonactive metabolites) are desipramine (Norpramin, Pertofrane), protriptyline (Vivactil), and nortriptyline (Pamelor). Tricyclic dibenzoxazepine (metabolized to a major metabolite) is amoxapine (Asendin). *Manifestations*: The onset of action varies from less than 1 hour to 12 hours after ingestion. The phases of intoxication are (1) consciousness with dry mouth, mydriasis, ataxia, increased deep tendon reflexes, and changes in the ST segment; (2) Stages I and II coma with hypertension, tachycardia above 160, mydriasis, and supraventricular tachycardia; and (3) Stages III and IV coma with hypotension, heart rate under 120, respiratory depression, tonic-clonic seizures, and ventricular dysrhythmias. The CNS effects occur early, and seizures are common. *Cardiovascular toxicity* is frequent in the serious poisonings and results from anticholinergic effects, sympathomimetic activity (by blocking reuptake of catecholamines), quinidine activity, catecholamine depletion, and alpha-adrenergic blockade. Cardiotoxic effects include cardiac dysrhythmias, hypertension, hypotension, and pulmonary edema.

Toxic dose: The TCADs have a narrow margin of safety. In a child a 375-mg dose and in adults as little as 500 to 750 mg have been fatal. The following dosages may serve as a guide to the degree of imipramine toxicity: Less than 10 mg per kg produces light coma, mydriasis, and tachycardia and has a good prognosis. At 20 mg per kg, Stage III manifestations are produced. At 30 mg per kg, fatalities may result. At 50 mg per kg, the mortality rate is increased. Over 70 mg per kg is rarely survived. Relative adult dosage equivalents may serve as a guide: amitriptyline, 100 mg; amoxapine, 125 mg; desipramine, 75 mg; doxepin, 100 mg; imipramine, 75 mg; maprotiline (Ludiomil), 75 mg; nortriptyline, 50 mg; and trazodone (Desyrel), 200 mg (see Table 31). Therapeutic blood levels are in the range of 50 to 170 ng per mL. If the QRS interval is less than 0.10 second for 6 hours, the prognosis is good. If it is greater than 0.10 second, seizures may occur, and if it is over 0.16 second, serious dysrhythmia may occur. In general, most antidepressants possess anticholinergic activity. The tricyclics produce dysrhythmias, hypotension, and seizures. The tetracyclics (amoxapine, maprotiline) produce convulsions that may result in rhabdomyolysis and renal dysfunction. The new

TABLE 31. **Kinetics of Cyclic Antidepressants**

Anti-depressant (Trade Name)	Absorption	Time to Peak Effect (h)	Volume of Distribution (L/kg)	t½ (h)	Protein Binding (1%)	Elimination	Toxic Level (ng/mL)	Availability	Therapeutic Plasma Level (Range) (ng/mL)	Adult (total daily dose) (mg)	Child (mg/kg/24 h)
TRICYCLIC TERTIARY AMINES (METABOLIZED TO ACTIVE METABOLITES)											
Amitriptyline (Elavil)	Slow	2–12	8–10	15–19	82–96	Hepatic	>500	Tab 10, 25, 75, 100, 150 mg	50–250	75–300	1.5–2.0
Imipramine (Tofranil)	Rapid (29–77%)	1–2	5–20	8–16	76–96	Hepatic	>500	Tab 10, 25, 50 mg; Cap 75, 100, 125, 150 mg	150–250	75–300	3–7
Doxepin (Sinequan, Adapin)	Rapid, complete	2–4	20	15–19	95	Hepatic	>150	Cap 25, 50, 75, 100, 150 mg	150–250	75–300	—
Trimipramine (Surmontil)	Rapid	2	NA	NA	Large	Renal		Cap 25, 50, 100 mg	100–200	75–300	—
TRICYCLIC SECONDARY AMINES (METABOLIZED TO NONACTIVE METABOLITES)											
Desipramine (Norpramin, Pertofrane)	Rapid, incomplete	4–6	28–60	18–28	73–92	Hepatic	>500	Tab 10, 25, 50, 100, 150 mg; Cap 10, 50 mg	125–300	75–300	—
Protriptyline (Vivactil)						Hepatic	NA	Tab 5, 10 mg	70–260	20–60	—
Nortriptyline (Aventyl)	Slow (46–77%)	7–8	21–57	50–150	93–95	Hepatic	>500	Cap 10, 25, 75 mg	50–150	75–200	1.5–2.0
TETRACYCLIC DIBENZOXAZEPINES (METABOLIZED TO MAJOR METABOLITES)											
Amoxapine (Asendin)	Rapid	1.5	Large	8–30	90	Renal and hepatic	NA	Tab 25, 50, 100, 150 mg	200–600	150–600	—
Maprotiline (Ludiomil)		8–24	22.6	27–58	88	Hepatic	>300	Tab 25, 50, 75 mg	200–600	75–300	—
TRIAZOLOPYRIDINES											
Trazodone (Desyrel)	Rapid	0.5–2	NA	4–13	89–95	Hepatic	NA	Tab 50, 100, 150 mg	800–1600	50–600	—
UNCLASSIFIED OR BICYCLICS (METABOLIZED TO ACTIVE METABOLITE)											
Fluoxetine (Prozac)	Rapid	4–6	14–102	24–96	94	Hepatic	>400	Cap 20 mg; syrup 20 mg/5 mL, 4-oz bottles	NA	20–80	—
Norfluoxetine (active metabolite) peak 76 h, half-life 5–7 days											
DIBENZAZEPINES											
Clomipramine* (Anafranil)	Rapid	3–5	12	21	98	Hepatic	500	Cap 25, 50, 75 mg	—	25–200	
Dimethylclomipramine (DM) (primary active metabolite) half-life 54–77 h											
AMINOKETONES											
Bupropion (Wellbutrin)	Rapid 5–20% bioavailability	2	NA	8–24	80	Hepatic	NA	Tab 75, 100 mg	—	200–450 tid	—
Several active metabolites relate to toxicity											

*Available to psychiatrists free of charge to treat patients: 1-800-842-2422 (Med Lett *30*:102–104, 1988).
Abbreviations: Toxic level = toxic serum concentration; NA = not available; Tab = tablets; Cap = capsules.

agents trazodone and fluoxetine (Prozac) appear to have mild sedative effects and cardiotoxicity, although orthostatic hypotension, vertigo, and priapism have been reported. Bupropion (Wellbutrin) is a phenylaminoketone antidepressant that produces dose-related seizures. Nomifensine (Merital) was withdrawn in 1986 because of reports of hemolytic anemia associated with it. *Management:* (1) Maintenance of vital functions. If the patient is asymptomatic, there should be vascular access, and cardiac monitoring should continue for at least 6 hours from admission or 8 to 12 hours postingestion. All children should be observed closely for 24 hours in an intensive care unit. If patient is symptomatic, obtain cardiac consultation and monitor in an intensive care unit until the patient is asymptomatic and shows no ECG abnormalities for at least 72 hours. (2) Gastrointestinal decontamination (omit emesis) if the patient is alert. Intact pills have been recovered by lavage up to 18 hours after ingestion. Suspected patients should have ECG monitoring. (3) Activated charcoal initially with a cathartic. No more than two doses of activated charcoal are advised. (4) Control seizures with intravenous diazepam (Valium). Intravenous phenytoin (Dilantin) may be added in patients with seizures not responding to diazepam alone. If not immediately successful, consider an aggressive approach to airway management and rapid-sequence intubation with paralysis by short nonpolarizing neuromuscular blockers such as vecuronium. (5) Cardiovascular complications of TCAD intoxication, including a QRS complex of over 0.14 second, ventricular tachycardia, severe conduction blocks, hypotension, or seizures, should *first* be treated by alkalinization of blood with sodium bicarbonate to a pH of 7.5 to 7.55 (Antidote 39, Table 4). Administer sodium bicarbonate 1 mEq per kg undiluted as a bolus and repeated twice a few minutes apart. If it does not affect cardiotoxicity, an infusion of sodium bicarbonate may follow to keep blood pH at 7.5 to 7.55 but not higher. Monitor serum sodium, potassium, and blood pH because fatal alkalemia and hypernatremia have been reported. Continuous infusion of bicarbonate by itself is of limited usefulness in TCAD intoxication because of its delayed onset. The combination of hyperventilation and sodium bicarbonate has produced fatal alkalemia. Alkalinization increases the protein binding of the TCAD. Serum potassium levels should be monitored because a sudden increase in blood pH can aggravate or precipitate hypokalemia. Specific cardiovascular complications should be treated as follows: *Hypotension*—norepinephrine (Levophed), a predominantly alpha-adrenergic drug, is preferred over dopamine. (Hypertension that occurs early rarely requires treatment.) *Serious conduction defects* are best managed with phenytoin, and patients may need a temporary transvenous pacemaker. *Sinus tachycardia* usually does not require treatment except for alkalinization. *Supraventricular tachycardia* with hemodynamic instability requires synchronized cardioversion, 0.25 to 1.0 watt-second per kg, after sedation. *Ventricular tachycardia*—after alkalinization and phenytoin, intravenous lidocaine (Xylocaine) (for one dose only) may be required for persistent ventricular tachycardia. Synchronized cardioversion may be needed if lidocaine fails. *Ventricular fibrillation* should be treated with direct current countershock. *Torsades de pointes* is treated with intravenous magnesium sulfate 20%, 2 grams over 2 to 3 minutes, followed by a continuous infusion of 5 to 10 mg per minute of isoproterenol, lidocaine, phenytoin, and bretylium and atrial or ventricular overdrive pacing to shorten the QT interval. *Laboratory aids*: Arterial blood gases with blood pH, ECG, serum electrolytes, BUN and creatinine, serum phenytoin level, urine output, and, in severe cases, central venous pressure, PAWP, or both should be monitored.

Turpentine. See Hydrocarbons.

Xylene. See Hydrocarbons.

Appendices and Index

REFERENCE INTERVALS FOR THE INTERPRETATION OF LABORATORY TESTS

method of
William Z. Borer, M.D.
Thomas Jefferson University Hospital
Philadelphia, Pennsylvania

Most of the tests performed in a clinical laboratory are quantitative in nature—that is, the amount of a substance present in blood or serum is measured and reported in terms of concentration, activity (e.g., enzyme activity) or counts (e.g., blood cell counts). The laboratory must provide reference values to assist the clinician in the interpretation of laboratory results. These reference ranges specify the physiologic quantities of substance (concentrations, activities, or counts) to be expected in healthy individuals. Deviation above or below the reference range may be associated with a disease process, and the severity of the disease process may be associated with the magnitude of the deviation. Unfortunately, a sharp demarcation between physiologic and pathologic values rarely exists, and the transition between these two is often gradual as the disease process progresses.

The terms "normal" and "abnormal" have been used to describe the laboratory values that fall inside or outside the reference range, respectively. Use of these terms is now discouraged because it is virtually impossible to define normality and because "normal" may be confused with the statistical term "gaussian." Reference ranges are established from statistical studies in groups of healthy volunteers. Although these study subjects must be free of disease, they may have lifestyles or habits that result in subtle variations in their laboratory values. Examples of these variables include diet, body mass, exercise, and geographic location. Age and gender may also affect reference values. When the data from a large cohort of healthy subjects fit a gaussian distribution, the usual statistical approach is to define the reference limits as two standard deviations above and below the mean. By definition, the reference range excludes the highest and the lowest 2.5% of the population. Nongaussian distributions are handled by different statistical methods, but the result is similar in that the reference range is defined by the central 95% of the population. In other words, the odds are 1 in 20

that a healthy individual will have a laboratory result that falls outside the reference range. If 12 laboratory tests are performed, the odds increase to about 1 in 2 that at least one of the results is outside the reference range. This means that all healthy individuals are likely to have a few laboratory results that are unexpected. The clinician must then integrate these data with other clinical information such as the history and physical examination to arrive at the appropriate clinical decision. The reference range for many tests (especially enzyme and immunochemical measurements) will vary with the method used. It is important that each laboratory establish reference ranges appropriate for the methods it employs.

SI UNITS

During the 1980s, a concerted effort was made to introduce SI units (le Système International d'Unités). The rationale for conversion to SI units is sound. Laboratory data are scientifically more informative when the units are based on molar concentration rather than mass concentration. For example, the conversion of glucose to lactate and pyruvate or the binding of a drug to albumin is more easily understood in units of molar concentration. Another example is illustrated as follows:

Conventional Units
1.0 gram of hemoglobin
Combines with 1.37 mL of oxygen
Contains 3.4 mg of iron
Forms 34.9 mg of bilirubin

SI Units
4.0 mmol of hemoglobin
Combines with 4.0 mmol of oxygen
Contains 4.0 mmol of iron
Forms 4.0 mmol of bilirubin

TABLE 1. **Base SI Units**

Property	Base Unit	Symbol
Length	meter	m
Mass	kilogram	kg
Amount of substance	mole	mol
Time	second	s
Thermodynamic temperature	kelvin	K
Electric current	ampere	A
Luminous intensity	candela	cd
Catalytic amount	katal	kat

TABLE 2. **Derived SI Units and Non-SI Units Retained for Use with the SI**

Property	Unit	Symbol
Area	square meter	m²
Volume	cubic meter	m³
	liter	L
Mass concentration	kilogram/cubic meter	kg/m³
	gram/liter	g/L
Substance concentration	mole/cubic meter	mol/m³
	mole/liter	mol/L
Temperature	degree Celsius	°C = °K − 273.15

TABLE 3. **Standard Prefixes**

Prefix	Multiplication Factor	Symbol
yocto	10^{-24}	y
zepto	10^{-21}	z
atto	10^{-18}	a
femto	10^{-15}	f
pico	10^{-12}	p
nano	10^{-9}	n
micro	10^{-6}	μ
milli	10^{-3}	m
centi	10^{-2}	c
deci	10^{-1}	d
deca	10^{1}	da
hecto	10^{2}	h
kilo	10^{3}	k
mega	10^{6}	M
giga	10^{9}	G
tera	10^{12}	T

The international use of SI units would also enhance the standardization of nomenclature to facilitate global communication of medical and scientific information. The units, symbols, and prefixes employed in the International System are shown in Tables 1, 2, and 3.

Unfortunately, problems have arisen with the implementation of SI units in the United States. Their introduction in 1987 prompted many medical journals to report laboratory values in both SI and conventional units in anticipation of complete conversion to SI units in the early 1990s. The lack of a coordinated effort toward this goal has forced a retrenchment on the issue. Physicians continue to think and practice using laboratory results expressed in conventional units and few, if any, American hospitals or clinical laboratories exclusively use SI units. It is not likely that complete conversion to SI units will occur in the foreseeable future, yet most medical journals will probably continue to publish both sets of units. For this reason the tables of reference ranges in this Appendix are given in both conventional units and SI units.

TABLES OF REFERENCE VALUES

Some of the values included in the tables have been established by the Clinical Laboratories at Thomas Jefferson University Hospital, Philadelphia, PA, and have not been published elsewhere. Other values have been compiled from the sources cited herein. These tables are provided for information and educational purposes only. They are intended to complement data derived from other sources including the medical history and physical examination. Users must exercise individual judgment when employing the information provided in this appendix.

Reference Values for Hematology

	Conventional Units	SI Units
Acid hemolysis (Ham test)	No hemolysis	No hemolysis
Alkaline phosphatase, leukocyte	Total score 14–100	Total score 14–100
Cell counts		
Erythrocytes		
Males	4.6–6.2 million/mm³	4.6–6.2 × 10^{12}/L
Females	4.2–5.4 million/mm³	4.2–5.4 × 10^{12}/L
Children (varies with age)	4.5–5.1 million/mm³	4.5–5.1 × 10^{12}/L
Leukocytes, total	4500–11,000/mm³	4.5–11.0 × 10^{9}/L
Leukocytes, differential counts*		
Myelocytes	0%	0/L
Band neutrophils	3–5%	150–400 × 10^{6}/L
Segmented neutrophils	54–62%	3000–5800 × 10^{6}/L
Lymphocytes	25–33%	1500–3000 × 10^{6}/L
Monocytes	3–7%	300–500 × 10^{6}/L
Eosinophils	1–3%	50–250 × 10^{6}/L
Basophils	0–1%	15–50 × 10^{6}/L
Platelets	150,000–400,000/mm³	150–400 × 10^{9}/L
Reticulocytes	25,000–75,000/mm³ (0.5–1.5% of erythrocytes)	25–75 × 10^{9}/L
Coagulation tests		
Bleeding time (template)	2.75–8.0 min	2.75–8.0 min
Coagulation time (glass tube)	5–15 min	5–15 min
D-dimer	<0.5 μg/mL	<0.5 mg/L

Reference Values for Hematology *Continued*

	Conventional Units	SI Units
Factor VIII and other coagulation factors	50–150% of normal	0.5–1.5 of normal
Fibrin split products (Thrombo-Welco test)	<10 µg/mL	<10 mg/L
Fibrinogen	200–400 mg/dL	2.0–4.0 g/L
Partial thromboplastin time (PTT)	20–35 s	20–35 s
Prothrombin time (PT)	12.0–14.0 s	12.0–14.0 s
Coombs' test		
Direct	Negative	Negative
Indirect	Negative	Negative
Corpuscular values of erythrocytes		
Mean corpuscular hemoglobin (MCH)	26–34 pg/cell	26–34 pg/cell
Mean corpuscular volume (MCV)	80–96 μm^3	80–96 fL
Mean corpuscular hemoglobin concentration (MCHC)	32–36 g/dL	320–360 g/L
Haptoglobin	20–165 mg/dL	0.20–1.65 g/L
Hematocrit		
Males	40–54 mL/dL	0.40–0.54
Females	37–47 mL/dL	0.37–0.47
Newborns	49–54 mL/dL	0.49–0.54
Children (varies with age)	35–49 mL/dL	0.35–0.49
Hemoglobin		
Males	13.0–18.0 g/dL	8.1–11.2 mmol/L
Females	12.0–16.0 g/dL	7.4–9.9 mmol/L
Newborn	16.5–19.5 g/dL	10.2–12.1 mmol/L
Children (varies with age)	11.2–16.5 g/dL	7.0–10.2 mmol/L
Hemoglobin, fetal	<1.0% of total	<0.01 of total
Hemoglobin A_{1C}	3–5% of total	0.03–0.05 of total
Hemoglobin A_2	1.5–3.0% of total	0.015–0.03 of total
Hemoglobin, plasma	0.0–5.0 mg/dL	0.0–3.2 µmol/L
Methemoglobin	30–130 mg/dL	19–80 µmol/L
Erythrocyte sedimentation rate (ESR)		
Wintrobe		
Males	0–5 mm/h	0–5 mm/h
Females	0–15 mm/h	0–15 mm/h
Westergren		
Males	0–15 mm/h	0–15 mm/h
Females	0–20 mm/h	0–20 mm/h

*Conventional units are percentages; SI units are absolute counts.

Reference Values* for Clinical Chemistry (Blood, Serum, and Plasma)

	Conventional Units	SI Units
Acetoacetate plus acetone		
Qualitative	Negative	Negative
Quantitative	0.3–2.0 mg/dL	30–200 µmol/L
Acid phosphatase, serum (Thymolphthalein monophosphate substrate)	0.1–0.6 U/L	0.1–0.6 U/L
ACTH (see Corticotropin)		
Alanine aminotransferase (ALT, SGPT), serum	1–45 U/L	1–45 U/L
Albumin, serum	3.3–5.2 g/dL	33–52 g/L
Aldolase, serum	0.0–7.0 U/L	0.0–7.0 U/L
Aldosterone, plasma		
Standing	5–30 ng/dL	140–830 pmol/L
Recumbent	3–10 ng/dL	80–275 pmol/L
Alkaline phosphatase (ALP), serum		
Adult	35–150 U/L	35–150 U/L
Adolescent	100–500 U/L	100–500 U/L
Child	100–350 U/L	100–350 U/L
Ammonia nitrogen, plasma	10–50 µmol/L	10–50 µmol/L
Amylase, serum	25–125 U/L	25–125 U/L
Anion gap, serum, calculated	8–16 mEq/L	8–16 mmol/L
Ascorbic acid, blood	0.4–1.5 mg/dL	23–85 µmol/L

Table continued on following page

Reference Values* for Clinical Chemistry (Blood, Serum, and Plasma) *Continued*

	Conventional Units	SI Units
Aspartate aminotransferase (AST, SGOT), serum	1–36 U/L	1–36 U/L
Base excess, arterial blood, calculated	0 ± 2 mEq/L	0 ± 2 mmol/L
β-carotene, serum	60–260 μg/dL	1.1–8.6 μmol/L
Bicarbonate		
Venous plasma	23–29 mEq/L	23–29 mmol/L
Arterial blood	21–27 mEq/L	21–27 mmol/L
Bile acids, serum	0.3–3.0 mg/dL	0.8–7.6 μmol/L
Bilirubin, serum		
Conjugated	0.1–0.4 mg/dL	1.7–6.8 μmol/L
Total	0.3–1.1 mg/dL	5.1–19.0 μmol/L
Calcium, serum	8.4–10.6 mg/dL	2.10–2.65 mmol/L
Calcium, ionized, serum	4.25–5.25 mg/dL	1.05–1.30 mmol/L
Carbon dioxide, total, serum or plasma	24–31 mEq/L	24–31 mmol/L
Carbon dioxide tension (Pco_2), blood	35–45 mmHg	35–45 mmHg
Ceruloplasmin, serum	23–44 mg/dL	230–440 mg/L
Chloride, serum or plasma	96–106 mEq/L	96–106 mmol/L
Cholesterol, serum or EDTA plasma		
Desirable range	<200 mg/dL	<5.20 mmol/L
LDL cholesterol	60–180 mg/dL	1.55–4.65 mmol/L
HDL cholesterol	30–80 mg/dL	0.80–2.05 mmol/L
Copper	70–140 μg/dL	11–22 μmol/L
Corticotropin (ACTH), plasma, 8 A.M.	10–80 pg/mL	2–18 pmol/L
Cortisol, plasma		
8:00 A.M.	6–23 μg/dL	170–630 nmol/L
4:00 P.M.	3–15 μg/dL	80–410 nmol/L
10:00 P.M.	<50% of 8:00 A.M. value	<50% of 8:00 A.M. value
Creatine, serum		
Males	0.2–0.5 mg/dL	15–40 μmol/L
Females	0.3–0.9 mg/dL	25–70 μmol/L
Creatine kinase (CK), serum		
Males	55–170 U/L	55–170 U/L
Females	30–135 U/L	30–135 U/L
Creatine kinase MB isoenzyme, serum	<5% of total CK activity	<5% of total CK activity
	<5% ng/mL by immunoassay	<5% ng/mL by immunoassay
Creatinine, serum	0.6–1.2 mg/dL	50–110 μmol/L
Estradiol-17β, adult		
Males	10–65 pg/mL	35–240 pmol/L
Females		
Follicular phase	30–100 pg/mL	110–370 pmol/L
Ovulatory phase	200–400 pg/mL	730–1470 pmol/L
Luteal phase	50–140 pg/mL	180–510 pmol/L
Ferritin, serum	20–200 ng/mL	20–200 μg/L
Fibrinogen, plasma	200–400 mg/dL	2.0–4.0 g/L
Folate, serum erythrocytes	2.0–9.0 ng/mL	4.5–20.4 nmol/L
	170–700 ng/mL	385–1590 nmol/L
Follicle-stimulating hormone (FSH), plasma		
Males	4–25 mU/mL	4–25 U/L
Females, premenopausal	4–30 mU/mL	4–30 U/L
Females, postmenopausal	40–250 mU/mL	40–250 U/L
γ-glutamyltransferase (GGT), serum	5–40 U/L	5–40 U/L
Gastrin, fasting, serum	0–110 pg/mL	0–110 mg/L
Glucose, fasting, plasma or serum	70–115 mg/dL	3.9–6.4 nmol/L
Growth hormone (hGH), plasma, adult, fasting	0–6 ng/mL	0–6 μg/L
Haptoglobin, serum	20–165 mg/dL	0.20–1.65 g/L
Immunoglobulins, serum (see Reference Values for Immunologic Procedures)		
Insulin, fasting, plasma	5–25 μU/mL	36–179 pmol/L
Iron, serum	75–175 μg/dL	13–31 μmol/L
Iron binding capacity, serum		
Total	250–410 μg/dL	45–73 μmol/L
Saturation	20–55%	0.20–0.55
Lactate		
Venous whole blood	5.0–20.0 mg/dL	0.6–2.2 mmol/L
Arterial whole blood	5.0–15.0 mg/dL	0.6–1.7 mmol/L
Lactate dehydrogenase (LD), serum	110–220 U/L	110–220 U/L
Lipase, serum	10–140 U/L	10–140 U/L
Lutropin (LH), serum		
Males	1–9 U/L	1–9 U/L
Females		
Follicular phase	2–10 U/L	2–10 U/L
Midcycle peak	15–65 U/L	15–65 U/L
Luteal phase	1–12 U/L	1–12 U/L
Postmenopausal	12–65 U/L	12–65 U/L

Reference Values* for Clinical Chemistry (Blood, Serum, and Plasma) *Continued*

	Conventional Units	SI Units
Magnesium, serum	1.3–2.1 mg/dL	0.65–1.05 mmol/L
Osmolality	275–295 mOsm/kg water	275–295 mOsm/kg water
Oxygen, blood, arterial, room air		
Partial pressure (Pa_{O_2})	80–100 mm Hg	80–100 mm Hg
Saturation (Sa_{O_2})	95–98%	95–98%
pH, arterial blood	7.35–7.45	7.35–7.45
Phosphate, inorganic, serum		
Adult	3.0–4.5 mg/dL	1.0–1.5 mmol/L
Child	4.0–7.0 mg/dL	1.3–2.3 mmol/L
Potassium		
Serum	3.5–5.0 mEq/L	3.5–5.0 mmol/L
Plasma	3.5–4.5 mEq/L	3.5–4.5 mmol/L
Progesterone, serum, adult		
Males	0.0–0.4 ng/mL	0.0–1.3 mmol/L
Females		
Follicular phase	0.1–1.5 ng/mL	0.3–4.8 mmol/L
Luteal phase	2.5–28.0 ng/mL	8.0–89.0 mmol/L
Prolactin, serum		
Males	1.0–15.0 ng/mL	1.0–15.0 μg/L
Females	1.0–20.0 ng/mL	1.0–20.0 μg/L
Protein, serum, electrophoresis		
Total	6.0–8.0 g/dL	60–80 g/L
Albumin	3.5–5.5 g/dL	35–55 g/L
Globulins		
Alpha$_1$	0.2–0.4 g/dL	2.0–4.0 g/L
Alpha$_2$	0.5–0.9 g/dL	5.0–9.0 g/L
Beta	0.6–1.1 g/dL	6.0–11.0 g/L
Gamma	0.7–1.7 g/dL	7.0–17.0 g/L
Pyruvate, blood	0.3–0.9 mg/dL	0.03–0.10 mmol/L
Rheumatoid factor	0.0–30.0 IU/mL	0.0–30.0 kIU/L
Sodium, serum or plasma	135–145 mEq/L	135–145 mmol/L
Testosterone, plasma		
Males, adult	300–1200 ng/dL	10.4–41.6 nmol/L
Females, adult	20–75 ng/dL	0.7–2.6 nmol/L
Pregnant females	40–200 ng/dL	1.4–6.9 nmol/L
Thyroglobulin	3–42 ng/mL	3–42 μg/L
Thyrotropin (hTSH), serum	0.4–4.8 μIU/mL	0.4–4.8 mIU/L
Thyrotropin-releasing hormone (TRH)	5–60 pg/mL	5–60 ng/L
Thyroxine (FT$_4$), free, serum	0.9–2.1 ng/dL	12–27 pmol/L
Thyroxine (T$_4$), serum	4.5–12.0 μg/dL	58–154 nmol/L
Thyroxine-binding globulin (TBG)	15.0–34.0 μg/mL	15.0–34.0 mg/L
Transferrin	250–430 mg/dL	2.5–4.3 g/L
Triglycerides, serum, after 12-hr fast	40–150 mg/dL	0.4–1.5 g/L
Triiodothyronine (T$_3$), serum	70–190 ng/dL	1.1–2.9 nmol/L
Triiodothyronine uptake, resin (T$_3$RU)	25–38%	0.25–0.38
Urate		
Males	2.5–8.0 mg/dL	150–480 μmol/L
Females	2.2–7.0 mg/dL	130–420 μmol/L
Urea, serum or plasma	24–49 mg/dL	4.0–8.2 nmol/L
Urea nitrogen, serum or plasma	11–23 mg/dL	8.0–16.4 nmol/L
Viscosity, serum	1.4–1.8 × water	1.4–1.8 × water
Vitamin A, serum	20–80 μg/dL	0.70–2.80 μmol/L
Vitamin B$_{12}$, serum	180–900 pg/mL	133–664 pmol/L

*Reference values may vary depending on the method and sample source used.

Reference Values for Therapeutic Drug Monitoring (Serum)

	Therapeutic Range	Toxic Concentrations	Proprietary Names
Analgesics			
Acetaminophen	10–20 μg/mL	>250 μg/mL	Tylenol
			Datril
Salicylate	100–250 μg/mL	>300 μg/mL	Aspirin
			Bufferin
Antibiotics			
Amikacin	25–30 μg/mL	Peak >35 μg/mL	Amikin
		Trough >10 μg/mL	

Table continued on following page

Reference Values for Therapeutic Drug Monitoring (Serum) *Continued*

	Therapeutic Range	Toxic Concentrations	Proprietary Names
Chloramphenicol	10–20 μg/mL	>25 μg/mL	Chloromycetin
		Peak >10 μg/mL	Garamycin
Gentamicin	5–10 μg/mL	Trough >2 μg/mL	
		Peak >10 μg/mL	Nebcin
Tobramycin	5–10 μg/mL	Trough >2 μg/mL	
		Peak >40 μg/mL	Vancocin
Vancomycin	5–10 μg/mL	Trough >10 μg/mL	
Anticonvulsants			
Carbamazepine	5–12 μg/mL	>15 μg/mL	Tegretol
Ethosuxamide	40–100 μg/mL	>150 μg/mL	Zarontin
		40–100 ng/mL	Luminal
Phenobarbital	15–40 μg/mL	(varies widely)	
Phenytoin	10–20 μg/mL	>20 μg/mL	Dilantin
Primidone	5–12 μg/mL	>15 μg/mL	Mysoline
Valproic acid	50–100 μg/mL	>100 μg/mL	Depakene
Antineoplastics and Immunosuppressives			
Cyclosporine	50–400 ng/mL	>400 ng/mL	Sandimmune
		>1 μmol/L 48 hr after	Mexate
Methotrexate, high dose, 48 hr	Variable	dose	Folex
Tacrolimus (FK-506), Whole blood	3–10 μg/L	>15 μg/L	Prograf
Bronchodilators and Respiratory Stimulants			
Caffeine	3–15 ng/mL	>30 ng/mL	
Theophylline (Aminophylline)	10–20 μg/mL	>20 μg/mL	Elixophyllin
			Quibron
Cardiovascular Drugs			
Amiodarone	1.0–2.0 μg/mL	>2.0 μg/mL	Cordarone
(Obtain specimen more than 8 hours after last dose)			
Digitoxin	15–25 ng/mL	>35 ng/mL	Crystodigin
(Obtain specimen 12–24 hours after last dose)			
Digoxin	0.8–2.0 ng/mL	>2.4 ng/mL	Lanoxin
(Obtain specimen more than 6 hours after last dose)			
Disopyramide	2–5 μg/mL	>7 μg/mL	Norpace
Flecainide	0.2–1.0 ng/mL	>1 ng/mL	Tambocor
Lidocaine	1.5–5.0 μg/mL	>6 μg/mL	Xylocaine
Mexiletine	0.7–2.0 ng/mL	>2 ng/mL	Mexitil
Procainamide	4–10 μg/mL	>12 μg/mL	Pronestyl
Procainamide plus NAPA	8–30 μg/mL	>30 μg/mL	
Propranolol	50–100 ng/mL	Variable	Inderal
			Cardioquin
Quinidine	2–5 μg/mL	>6 μg/mL	Quinaglute
			Tonocard
Tocainide	4–10 ng/mL	>10 ng/mL	
Psychopharmacologic Drugs			
			Elavil
Amitriptyline	120–150 ng/mL	>500 ng/mL	Triavil
Bupropion	25–100 ng/mL	Not applicable	Wellbutrin
			Norpramin
Desipramine	150–300 ng/mL	>500 ng/mL	Pertofrane
			Tofranil
Imipramine	125–250 ng/mL	>400 ng/mL	Janimine
Lithium	0.6–1.5 mEq/L	>1.5 mEq/L	Lithobid
(Obtain specimen 12 hours after last dose)			
Nortriptyline	50–150 ng/mL	>500 ng/mL	Aventyl
			Pamelor

Reference Values for Clinical Chemistry (Urine)

	Conventional Units	SI Units
Acetone and acetoacetate, qualitative	Negative	Negative
Albumin		
Qualitative	Negative	Negative
Quantitative	10–100 mg/24 hr	0.15–1.5 μmol/day
Aldosterone	3–20 μg/24 hr	8.3–55 nmol/day
δ-aminolevulinic acid (δ-ALA)	1.3–7.0 mg/24 hr	10–53 μmol/day
Amylase	<17 U/hr	<17 U/hr

Reference Values for Clinical Chemistry (Urine) *Continued*

	Conventional Units	SI Units
Amylase/creatinine clearance ratio	0.01–0.04	0.01–0.04
Bilirubin, qualitative	Negative	Negative
Calcium (regular diet)	<250 mg/24 hr	<6.3 nmol/day
Catecholamines		
Epinephrine	<10 µg/24 hr	<55 nmol/day
Norepinephrine	<100 µg/24 hr	<590 nmol/day
Total free catecholamines	4–126 µg/24 hr	24–745 nmol/day
Total metanephrines	0.1–1.6 mg/24 hr	0.5–8.1 µmol/day
Chloride (varies with intake)	110–250 mEq/24 hr	110–250 mmol/day
Copper	0–50 µg/24 hr	0.0–0.80 µmol/day
Cortisol, free	10–100 µg/24 hr	27.6–276 nmol/day
Creatine		
Males	0–40 mg/24 hr	0.0–0.30 mmol/day
Females	0–80 mg/24 hr	0.0–0.60 mmol/day
Creatinine	15–25 mg/kg/24 hr	0.13–0.22 mmol/kg/day
Creatinine clearance (endogenous)		
Males	110–150 mL/min/1.73m^2	110–150 mL/min/1.73m^2
Females	105–132 mL/min/1.73m^2	105–132 mL/min/1.73m^2
Cystine or Cysteine	Negative	Negative
Dehydroepiandrosterone		
Males	0.2–2.0 mg/24 hr	0.7–6.9 µmol/day
Females	0.2–1.8 mg/24 hr	0.7–6.2 µmol/day
Estrogens, total		
Males	4–25 µg/24 hr	14–90 nmol/day
Females	5–100 µg/24 hr	18–360 nmol/day
Glucose (as reducing substance)	<250 mg/24 hr	<250 mg/day
Hemoglobin and myoglobin, qualitative	Negative	Negative
Homogentisic acid, qualitative	Negative	Negative
17–Ketogenic steroids		
Males	5–23 mg/24 hr	17–80 µmol/day
Females	3–15 mg/24 hr	10–52 µmol/day
17–Hydroxycorticosteroids		
Males	3–9 mg/24 hr	8.3–25 µmol/day
Females	2–8 mg/24 hr	5.5–22 µmol/day
5–Hydroxyindoleacetic acid		
Qualitative	Negative	Negative
Quantitative	2–6 mg/24 hr	10–31 µmol/day
17–Ketosteroids		
Males	8–22 mg/24 hr	28–76 µmol/day
Females	6–15 mg/24 hr	21–52 µmol/day
Magnesium	6–10 mEq/24 hr	3–5 mmol/day
Metanephrines	0.05–1.2 ng/mg creatinine	0.03–0.70 mmol/mmol creatinine
Osmolality	38–1400 mOsm/kg water	38–1400 mOsm/kg water
pH	4.6–8.0	4.6–8.0
Phenylpyruvic acid, qualitative	Negative	Negative
Phosphate	0.4–1.3 g/24 hr	13–42 mmol/day
Prophobilinogen		
Qualitative	Negative	Negative
Quantitative	<2 mg/24 hr	<9 µmol/day
Porphyrins		
Coproporphyrin	50–250 µg/24 hr	77–380 nmol/day
Uroporphyrin	10–30 µg/24 hr	12–36 nmol/day
Potassium	25–125 mEq/24 hr	25–125 mmol/day
Pregnanediol		
Males	0.0–1.9 mg/24 hr	0.0–6.0 µmol/day
Females		
Proliferative phase	0.0–2.6 mg/24 hr	0.0–8.0 µmol/day
Luteal phase	2.6–10.6 mg/24 hr	8–33 µmol/day
Postmenopausal	0.2–1.0 mg/24 hr	0.6–3.1 µmol/day
Pregnanetriol	0.0–2.5 mg/24 hr	0.0–7.4 umol/day
Protein, total		
Qualitative	Negative	Negative
Quantitative	10–150 mg/24 hr	10–150 mg/day
Protein/creatinine ratio	<0.2	<0.2
Sodium (regular diet)	60–260 mEq/24 hr	60–260 mmol/day
Specific gravity		
Random specimen	1.003–1.030	1.003–1.030
24-hour collection	1.015–1.025	1.015–1.025
Urate (regular diet)	250–750 mg/24 hr	1.5–4.4 mmol/day
Urobilinogen	0.5–4.0 mg/24 hr	0.6–6.8 µmol/day
Vanillylmandelic acid (VMA)	1.0–8.0 mg/24 hr	5–40 µmol/day

Reference Values for Toxic Substances

	Conventional Units	SI Units
Arsenic, urine	<130 μg/24 hr	<1.7 μmol/day
Bromides, serum, inorganic	<100 mg/dL	<10 mmol/L
Toxic symptoms	140–1000 mg/dL	14–100 mmol/L
Carboxyhemoglobin, blood	*% Saturation*	*Saturation*
Urban environment	<5%	<0.05
Smokers	<12%	<0.12
Symptoms		
Headache	>15%	>0.15
Nausea and vomiting	>25%	>0.25
Potentially lethal	>50%	>0.50
Ethanol, blood	<0.05 mg/dL	<1.0 mmol/L
	<0.005%	
Intoxication	>100 mg/dL	>22 mmol/L
	>0.1%	
Marked intoxication	300–400 mg/dL	65–87 mmol/L
	0.3–0.4%	
Alcoholic stupor	400–500 mg/dL	87–109 mmol/L
	0.4–0.5%	
Coma	>500 mg/dL	>109 mmol/L
	>0.5%	
Lead, blood		
Adults	<25 μg/dL	<1.2 μmol/L
Children	<15 μg/dL	<0.7 μmol/L
Lead, urine	<80 μg/24 hr	<0.4 μmol/day
Mercury, urine	<30 μg/24 hr	<150 nmol/day

Reference Values for Cerebrospinal Fluid

	Conventional Units	SI Units
Cells	<5/mm³; all mononuclear	<5 × 10⁶/L, all mononuclear
Protein electrophoresis	Albumin predominant	Albumin predominant
Glucose	50–75 mg/dL (20 mg/dL less than in serum)	2.8–4.2 mmol/L (1.1 mmol less than in serum)
IgG		
Children under 14	<8% of total protein	<0.08% of total protein
Adults	<14% of total protein	<0.14 % of total protein
IgG index $\left(\dfrac{\text{CSF/serum IgG ratio}}{\text{CSF/ serum albumin ratio}}\right)$	0.3–0.6	0.3–0.6
Oligoclonal banding on electrophoresis	Absent	Absent
Pressure, opening	70–180 mmH$_2$O	70–180 mmH$_2$O
Protein, total	15–45 mg/dL	150–450 mg/L

Reference Values for Tests of Gastrointestinal Function

	Conventional Units		Conventional Units
Bentiromide	6-hr urinary arylamine excretion greater than 57% excludes pancreatic insufficiency	Maximum (after histamine or pentagastrin)	
β-carotene, serum	60–250 ng/dL	Males	9.0–48.0 mmol/hr
Fecal fat estimation		Females	6.0–31.0 mmol/hr
Qualitative	No fat globules seen by high-power microscope	Ratio: basal/maximum	
		Males	0.0–0.31
Quantitative	<6 g/24 h (>95% coefficient of fat absorption)	Females	0.0–0.29
		Secretin test, pancreatic fluid	
Gastric acid output			
Basal		Volume	>1.8 mL/kg/hr
Males	0.0–10.5 mmol/hr	Bicarbonate	>80 mEq/L
Females	0.0–5.6 mmol/hr		
		D-Xylose absorption test, urine	>20% of ingested dose excreted in 5 hr

Reference Values for Immunologic Procedures

	Conventional Units	SI Units
Complement, serum		
C3	85–175 mg/dL	0.85–1.75 g/L
C4	15–45 mg/dL	150–450 mg/L
Total hemolytic (CH⁵⁰)	150–250 U/mL	150–250 U/mL
Immunoglobulins, serum, adult		
IgG	640–1350 mg/dL	6.4–13.5 g/L
IgA	70–310 mg/dL	0.70–3.1 g/L
IgM	90–350 mg/dL	0.90–3.5 g/L
IgD	0.0–6.0 mg/dL	0.0–60 mg/L
IgE	0.0–430 ng/dL	0.0–430 µg/L

Lymphocyte Subsets, Whole Blood, Heparinized

Antigen	Cell Type	Percentage	Absolute
CD3	Total T cells	56–77	860–1880
CD19	Total B cells	7–17	140–370
CD3 and CD4	Helper-inducer cells	32–54	550–1190
CD3 and CD8	Suppressor-cytotoxic cells	24–37	430–1060
CD3 and DR	Activated T cells	5–14	70–310
CD2	E rosette T cells	73–87	1040–2160
CD16 and CD56	Natural killer (NK) cells	8–22	130–500

Helper/suppressor ratio: 0.8–1.8.

Reference Values for Semen Analysis

	Conventional Units	SI Units
Volume	2–5 mL	2–5 mL
Liquefaction	Complete in 15 min	Complete in 15 min
pH	7.2–8.0	7.2–8.0
Leukocytes	Occasional or absent	Occasional or absent
Spermatozoa		
Count	60–150 × 10⁶/mL	60–150 × 10⁶/mL
Motility	>80% motile	>0.80 motile
Morphology	80–90% normal forms	>0.80–0.90 normal forms
Fructose	>150 mg/dL	>8.33 mmol/L

REFERENCES

AMA Drug Evaluations, Annual. Chicago, American Medical Association, 1994.

Bick RL (ed): Hematology—Clinical and Laboratory Practice. St. Louis, Mosby–Year Book, 1993.

Borer WZ: Selection and use of laboratory tests. In Tietz NW, Conn RB, and Pruden EL (eds): Applied Laboratory Medicine. Philadelphia, WB Saunders Co, 1992 pp. 1–5.

Campion EW: A retreat from SI units. N Engl J Med 327:49, 1992.

Friedman RB, Young DS: Effects of Disease on Clinical Laboratory Tests, 2nd ed. Washington, DC, AACC Press, 1989.

Henry JB: Clinical Diagnosis and Management by Laboratory Methods, 18th ed. Philadelphia, WB Saunders Co, 1991.

Hicks JM, Young DS: DORA 1992–1993: Directory of Rare Analyses. Washington, DC, AACC Press, 1992.

Jacobs DS, Kasten BL, Demott WR, Wolfson WL: Laboratory Test Handbook, 2nd ed. Baltimore, Williams & Wilkins Co, 1990.

Kaplan LA, Pesce AJ: Clinical Chemistry—Theory, Analysis, and Correlation, 2nd ed. St. Louis, CV Mosby, 1989.

Kjeldsberg CR, Knight JA: Body Fluids—Laboratory Examination of Amniotic, Cerebrospinal, Seminal, Serous, and Synovial Fluids, 3rd ed. Chicago, ASCP Press, 1993.

Laposata M.: SI Unit Conversion Guide. Boston, New England Journal of Medicine Books, 1992.

Scully RE, McNeely WF, Mark EJ, McNeely BU: Normal reference laboratory values. N Engl J Med 327:718–724, 1992.

Speicher CE: The Right Test—A Physician's Guide to Laboratory Medicine, 2nd ed. Philadelphia, WB Saunders Co, 1993.

Tietz NW (ed): Clinical Guide to Laboratory Tests, 2nd ed. Philadelphia, W.B. Saunders Co., 1990.

Wallach J: Interpretation of Diagnostic Tests—A Synopsis of Laboratory Medicine, 5th ed. Boston, Little, Brown and Co, 1992.

Young DS: Determination and validation of reference intervals. Arch Pathol Lab Med 116:704–709, 1992.

Young DS: Effects of Drugs on Clinical Laboratory Tests, 3rd ed. Washington, DC, AACC Press, 1990.

Young DS: Implementation of SI units for clinical laboratory data. Ann Intern Med 106:114–129, 1987.

DRUGS APPROVED IN 1994

method of
DIRK S. LUCAS, PHARM.D.
University of Houston College of Pharmacy
Houston, Texas

Generic Name	Trade Name and (Manufacturer)	Dosage Form	Average Dosage Range	FDA Rating	Approved Use
Abcirximab	ReoPro (Centocor; Lilly)	2 mg/mL injection, 5-mL vials	0.25 mg/kg IV bolus 10–60 min before PTCA, followed by 10 µg/min IV infusion for 12 h	*	Platelet aggregation inhibition: adjunct to PTCA
Acrivastine; pseudoephedrine hydrochloride	Semprex-D (Adams; Burroughs Wellcome)	Capsules: 8 mg acrivastine, 60 mg pseudoephedrine HCl	1 capsule q 4–6 h, 4 times a day	1,4-S	Allergic rhinitis
Budesonide	Rhinocort (Astra)	Metered-dose inhaler for nasal administration, 32 µg/actuation, 200 actuations/canister	256 µg/day; 4 sprays in each nostril in the morning	1-S	Allergic rhinitis
Cysteamine bitartrate	Cystagon (Mylan)	50- and 150-mg capsules	Children through 12 years of age: 1.3 gm/m²/day; aged 12 years and older and more than 110 pounds: 2 gm/day	1-P,V	Nephropathic cystinosis
Dalteparin sodium	Fragmin (Pharmacia)	2500 IU/0.2-mL injection, prefilled syringes	2500 IU daily	1-S	DVT prophylaxis after abdominal surgery
Dorzolamide	Trusopt (Merck)	2% ophthalmic solution, 5- and 10-mL dropper bottles	One drop in affected eye 3 times daily	1-P	Glaucoma
Famciclovir	Famvir (SmithKline Beecham)	500-mg tablets	500 mg q 8 h	1-S	Acute herpes zoster
Fluvoxamine maleate	Luvox (Solvay; Upjohn)	50- and 100-mg tablets	50–300 mg/day	1-S	Obsessive-compulsive disorder
Imiglucerase	Cerezyme (Genzyme)	Powder for injection, 212 U/vial	2.5 U/kg 3 times a week to 60 U/kg once a week	1-P,V,E	Gaucher's disease
Lamotrigine	Lamictal (Burroughs Wellcome)	25-, 100-, 150-, and 200-mg tablets	300–500 mg/day	1-P	Epilepsy
Metformin hydrochloride	Glucophage (Bristol-Myers Squibb)	500- and 850-mg tablets	500–2550 mg/day	1-P	Type II diabetes mellitus
Nefazodone	Serzone (Bristol-Myers Squibb)	100- 150-, 200- and 250-mg tablets	200–600 mg/day	1-S	Depression
Pegaspargase	Oncaspar (Enzon; Rhone-Poulenc Rorer)	Injection, 3750 IU in 5-mL vials	2500 IU/m² q 14 days; if body surface area < 0.6 m²: 82.5 IU/kg q 14 days	*	Acute lymphoblastic leukemia
Rimexolone	Vexol (Alcon)	1% ophthalmic solution, 2.5-, 5-, and 10-mL dropper bottle	1–2 drops in conjuctival sac of affected eye 4 times daily	1-P	Postoperative inflammation after ocular surgery
Rocuronium bromide	Zemuron (Organon)	10 mg/mL injection, 5-mL vial	0.6–1.2 mg/kg	1-S	Adjunct to general anesthesia to provide skeletal muscle relaxation

Generic Name	Trade Name and (Manufacturer)	Dosage Form	Average Dosage Range	FDA Rating	Approved Use
Salmeterol xinafoate	Serevent (Allen & Hanburys)	25 μg/actuation, 60- and 120-actuation metered-dose inhalers	2 inhalations q 12 h	1-P	Asthma
Spirapril	Renormax (Sandoz)	3-, 6-, 12-, and 24-mg tablets	3–24 mg/day	1-S	Hypertension
Stavudine	Zerit (Bristol-Myers Squibb)	15-, 20-, 30-, and 40-mg capsules	30–80 mg/day	1-P,AA,E,H	HIV infection
Tacrolimus	Prograf (Fujisawa)	1- and 5-mg capsules 5 mg/mL injection, 1-mL ampules	0.05–0.1 mg/kg/day	1-P,E	Organ rejection prophylaxis
Vinorelbine tartrate	Navelbine (Burroughs Wellcome)	10 mg/mL injection, 1- and 5-mL vials	30 mg/m^2 weekly	1-P	Non–small cell lung cancer

Ratings: *   Biologic approval through an FDA procedure that does not assign a specific classification
      1   New molecular entity
      4   Combination product
      E   Treatment for a life-threatening or severely debilitating illness
      H   Accelerated approval
      P   Priority review, therapeutic gain
      S   Standard review, substantially equivalent
      V   Orphan drug
      AA   Treatment for acquired immune deficiency syndrome (AIDS) and/or its complications
Abbreviations: DVT = deep vein thrombosis; HIV = human immunodeficiency virus; PTCA = percutaneous transluminal coronary angioplasty.

TOP 200 DRUGS PRESCRIBED IN THE UNITED STATES

method of
DIRK S. LUCAS, PHARM.D.
University of Houston College of Pharmacy
Houston, Texas

Rank*	Generic Name	Brand Name (Manufacturer)	Cost Index†
1	Conjugated estrogens	Premarin (Wyeth-Ayerst)	$
2	Ranitidine	Zantac (Glaxo)	$$$
3	Amoxicillin	Amoxil (SmithKline Beecham)	$$
4	Levothyroxine	Synthroid (Boots)	$$
5	Digoxin	Lanoxin (Burroughs Wellcome)	$
6	Nifedipine	Procardia (Pratt)	$$$
7	Enalapril	Vasotec (Merck)	$$
8	Amoxicillin	Trimox (Apothecon)	$
9	Diltiazem	Cardizem (Marion Merrell Dow)	$$$
10	Fluoxetine	Prozac (Dista)	$$$$
11	Albuterol	Proventil inhaler (Schering)	$$
12	Amoxicillin	(Biocraft)	$
13	Amoxicillin; clavulanate	Augmentin (SmithKline Beecham)	$$$
14	Warfarin	Coumadin (DuPont)	$
15	Lovastatin	Mevacor (Merck)	$$$$
16	Ciprofloxacin	Cipro (Miles)	$$$
17	Medroxyprogesterone	Provera (Upjohn)	$$
18	Cefaclor	Ceclor (Lilly)	$$$
19	Albuterol	Ventolin inhaler (Allen & Hanburys)	$$
20	Sertraline	Zoloft (Roerig)	$$$$
21	Acetaminophen with codeine	(Purepac)	$
22	Captopril	Capoten (Bristol-Myers Squibb)	$$
23	Propoxyphene with acetaminophen	(Mylan)	$
24	Lisinopril	Zestril (Stuart)	$$
25	Ethinyl estradiol; norethindrone	Ortho-Novum 7/7/7 (Ortho)	$$$
26	Phenytoin	Dilantin (Parke-Davis)	$
27	Terfenadine	Seldane (Marion Merrell Dow)	$$$
28	Alprazolam	Xanax (Upjohn)	$$$
29	Clarithromycin	Biaxin (Abbott)	$$$$
30	Omeprazole	Prilosec (Merck)	$$$$
31	Famotidine	Pepcid (Merck)	$$$
32	Cephalexin	(Biocraft)	$
33	Hydrocodone with acetaminophen	(Watson Laboratories)	$
34	Alprazolam	(Geneva Generics)	$
35	Verapamil	Calan (Searle)	$$$
36	Loratadine	Claritin (Schering)	$$$
37	Cimetidine	Tagamet (SmithKline Beecham)	$$
38	Potassium chloride	K-Dur (Key)	$
39	Trimethoprim; sulfamethoxazole	TMP–SMZ (Biocraft)	$
40	Nabumetone	Relafen (SmithKline Beecham)	$$$$
41	Glyburide	Micronase (Upjohn)	$$$
42	Glipizide	Glucotrol (Pratt)	$$$
43	Terazosin	Hytrin (Abbott)	$$$
44	Triamterene with hydrochlorothiazide	(Geneva Generics)	$
45	Ethinyl estradiol; levonorgestrel	Triphasil (Wyeth-Ayerst)	$$$
46	Triamterene with hydrochlorothiazide	Dyazide (SmithKline Beecham)	$$
47	Penicillin V potassium	Veetids (Apothecon)	$
48	Glyburide	DiaBeta (Hoechst-Roussel)	$$$
49	Amlodipine	Norvasc (Pfizer)	$$$
50	Furosemide	(Mylan)	$
51	Acyclovir	Zovirax capsules (Burroughs Wellcome)	$$
52	Paroxetine	Paxil (SmithKline Beecham)	$$$$
53	Clonazepam	Klonopin (Roche)	$$$
54	Metoprolol tartrate	Lopressor (Geigy)	$$
55	Ibuprofen	IBU (Boots)	$
56	Estradiol	Estraderm (Ciba)	$$$
57	Acetaminophen with codeine	(Lemmon)	$
58	Naproxen	(Hamilton)	$
59	Furosemide	Lasix (Hoechst-Roussel)	$$
60	Cefuroxime axetil	Ceftin (Allen & Hanburys)	$$$$
61	Ketorolac tromethamine	Toradol (Syntex)	$$$
62	Diclofenac sodium	Voltaren (Geigy)	$$$
63	Ipratropium bromide	Atrovent (Boeringer Ingelheim)	$$$

Rank*	Generic Name	Brand Name (Manufacturer)	Cost Index†
64	Lisinopril	Prinivil (Merck)	$$
65	Hydrocodone with acetaminophen	Vicodin (Knoll)	$$
66	Erythromycin	Ery-Tab (Abbott)	$
67	Nizatidine	Axid (Lilly)	$$$
68	Amoxicillin	(Warner Chilcott)	$
69	Lorazepam	(Mylan)	$
70	Cefadroxil	Duricef (Mead Johnson)	$$$
71	Nitroglycerin	Nitrostat (Parke-Davis)	$
72	Etodolac	Lodine (Wyeth-Ayerst)	$$$
73	Timolol	Timoptic (Merck)	$$
74	Propoxyphene; acetaminophen	Propacet (Lemmon)	$
75	Pravastatin	Pravachol (Bristol-Myers Squibb)	$$$$
76	Cefprozil	Cefzil (Bristol Lab)	$$$
77	Propoxyphene; acetaminophen	Darvocet-N (Lilly)	$$
78	Beclomethasone	Beconase AQ (Allen & Hanburys)	$$$
79	Terfenadine; pseudoephedrine	Seldane-D (Marion Merrell Dow)	$$$$
80	Beclomethasone	Vancenase AQ (Schering)	$$$
81	Terconazole	Terazol (Ortho)	$$$
82	Estradiol	Estrace (Mead Johnson)	$
83	Verapamil	(Goldline)	$
84	Atenolol	Tenormin (Zeneca)	$$
85	Ethinyl estradiol; norgestrel	Lo/Ovral (Wyeth-Ayerst)	$$$
86	Prednisone	Deltasone (Upjohn)	$$
87	Ethinyl estradiol; norethindrone	Ortho-Novum (Ortho)	$$
88	Cefixime	Suprax (Lederle)	$$$$
89	Simvastatin	Zocor (Merck)	$$$$
90	Tretinoin	Retin-A (Ortho)	$$$$
91	Buspirone	BuSpar (Mead Johnson)	$$$$
92	Betamethasone; clotrimazole	Lotrisone (Schering)	$$
93	Oxycodone with acetaminophen	Roxicet (Roxane)	$
94	Pentoxifylline	Trental (Hoechst-Roussel)	$$$$
95	Furosemide	(Geneva Generics)	$
96	Triamterene with hydrochlorothiazide	(Rugby)	$
97	Triamcinolone acetonide	Azmacort (Rhone-Poulenc Rorer)	$$
98	Theophylline	Theo-Dur (Schering)	$
99	Ethinyl estradiol; desogestrel	Ortho-Cept (Ortho)	$$$
100	Acetaminophen with codeine	Tylenol with Codeine (McNeil)	$$
101	Carbamazepine	Tegretol (Basel)	$$
102	Amitriptyline	(Mylan)	$
103	Ketoconazole	Nizoral external (Janssen)	$$
104	Gemfibrozil	(Warner-Chilcott)	$
105	Potassium chloride	Micro-K (Wyeth-Ayerst)	$$
106	Potassium chloride	Klor-Con (Upsher-Smith)	$$
107	Penicillin V	(Mylan)	$
108	Propranolol	Inderal (Wyeth-Ayerst)	$$
109	Oxaprozin	Daypro (Searle)	$$$$
110	Mupirocin	Bactroban (SmithKline Beecham)	$$$$
111	Indapamide	Lozol (Rhone-Poulenc Rorer)	$$$
112	Cephalexin	(Zenith)	$
113	Hydrocodone with acetaminophen	(Warner-Chilcott)	$
114	Naproxen	Naprosyn (Syntex)	$$$
115	Cephalexin	(Apothecon)	$
116	Quinapril	Accupril (Parke-Davis)	$$
117	Triamterene with hydrochlorothiazide	Maxzide (Lederle)	$$
118	Nitroglycerin	Nitro-Dur (Key)	$$$
119	Atenolol	(Lederle)	$
120	Metoprolol tartrate	(Geneva Generics)	$
121	Hydrocodone with acetaminophen	Lortab (Whitby)	$$
122	Astemizole	Hismanal (Janssen)	$$$
123	Alprazolam	(Greenstone)	$
124	Ethinyl estradiol; levonorgestrel	Tri-Levlen (Berlex)	$$
125	Benazepril	Lotensin (Ciba)	$$
126	Levothyroxine	Levoxine (Daniels)	$
127	Verapamil	Verelan (Lederle)	$$
128	Erythromycin base	(Abbott)	$
129	Zolpidem	Ambien (Searle)	$$$$
130	Diazepam	Valium (Roche)	$$$
131	Nortriptyline	(Schein)	$
132	Naproxen sodium	(Hamilton)	$
133	Erythromycin ethylsuccinate	E.E.S. (Abbott)	$
134	Loracarbef	Lorabid (Lilly)	$$$$
135	Potassium chloride	(Ethex)	$
136	Cyclobenzaprine	(Mylan)	$

Table continued on following page

Rank*	Generic Name	Brand Name (Manufacturer)	Cost Index†
137	Cisapride	Propulsid (Janssen)	$$
138	Sucralfate	Carafate (Marion Merrell Dow)	$$$
139	Bumetanide	Bumex (Roche)	$$
140	Furosemide	(Rugby)	$
141	Ibuprofen	(Winsor)	$
142	Methylphenidate	Ritalin (Ciba)	$$$
143	Azithromycin	Zithromax (Pfizer)	$$$$
144	Glyburide	Glynase (Upjohn)	$$$
145	Tetracycline	Sumycin (Apothecon)	$
146	Erythromycin	PCE (Abbott)	$$
147	Nitrofurantoin	Macrobid (Procter & Gamble)	$$
148	Albuterol sulfate	(Lemmon)	$
149	Hydrocodone with acetaminophen	Lorcet Plus (UAD Labs)	$$
150	Sumatriptan	Imitrex (Cerenex)	$$$
151	Promethazine	Phenergan (Wyeth-Ayerst)	$$
152	Ethinyl estradiol; ethynodiol diacetate	Demulin (Searle)	$$$
153	Ibuprofen	Children's Motrin (McNeil)	$$
154	Isosorbide dinitrate	(Geneva Generics)	$
155	Erythromycin stearate	Erythrocin Stearate (Abbott)	$$
156	Furosemide	(Lederle)	$
157	Divalproex sodium	Depakote (Abbott)	$$$
158	Ethinyl estradiol; desogestrel	Desogen (Organon)	$$$
159	Ethinyl estradiol; norethindrone; ferrous fumarate	Loestrin Fe (Parke-Davis)	$$
160	Hydrocodone with acetaminophen	(Rugby)	$
161	Prochlorperazine	Compazine (SmithKline Beecham)	$$
162	Cromolyn sodium	Intal (Fisons)	$$$
163	Propoxyphene with acetaminophen	(Purepac)	$
164	Aspirin; caffeine; butalbital; codeine	Fiorinal with Codeine (Sandoz)	$$
165	Doxazosin	Cardura (Pfizer)	$$$
166	Beclomethasone	Vanceril (Schering)	$$$
167	Tamoxifen	Nolvadex (Zeneca)	$$$$
168	Atenolol	(Mylan)	$
169	Medroxyprogesterone	(Greenstone)	$
170	Triamcinolone acetonide	Nasacort (Rhone-Poulenc Rorer)	$$$$
171	Hydrochlorothiazide	(Geneva Generics)	$
172	Chlorhexidine gluconate	Peridex (Procter & Gamble)	$$
173	Ofloxacin	Floxin (Ortho)	$$$
174	Atenolol	(IPR Pharm)	$
175	Erythromycin	E-Mycin (Boots)	$
176	Amoxicillin	(Novopharm)	$
177	Nifedipine	Adalat (Miles)	$$
178	Thyroid	(Forest)	$
179	Ramipril	Altace (Hoechst-Roussel)	$$
180	Methylphenidate	(M.D. Pharm)	$
181	Mometasone furoate	Elocon (Schering)	$$
182	Hydrocodone with acetaminophen	(Qualitest)	$
183	Dicyclomine	(Rugby)	$
184	Amoxicillin	(Mylan)	$
185	Lorazepam	Ativan (Wyeth-Ayerst)	$$
186	Albuterol	Proventil nebulization (Schering)	$$
187	Ethinyl estradiol; norethindrone	Ovcon (Mead Johnson)	$$$
188	Guaifenesin; phenylpropanolamine	Entex LA (Procter & Gamble)	$$
189	Prednisone	Orasone (Solvay)	$
190	Lorazepam	(Purepac)	$
191	Theophylline	Slo-bid (Rhone-Poulenc Rorer)	$$
192	Diltiazem	Dilacor XR (Rhone-Poulenc Rorer)	$$
193	Levodopa; carbidopa	Sinemet (DuPont)	$$$
194	Isradipine	DynaCirc (Sandoz)	$$$
195	Trimethoprim; sulfamethoxazole	Cotrim (Lemmon)	$
196	Doxepin	(Mylan)	$
197	Estropipate	Ogen (Upjohn)	$$
198	Flurbiprofen	Ansaid (Upjohn)	$$$
199	Atenolol	(Geneva Generics)	$
200	Hydrochlorothiazide	(Purepac)	$

*The ranking is based on the total number of prescriptions for all preparations and strengths (unless noted) of drugs dispensed in U.S. community pharmacies.

†This is a comparison of the relative cost of drugs in a given therapeutic class. Less expensive drugs are noted by "$" and the more expensive drugs in the class as "$$$$." The relative cost is based on average wholesale price (AWP). The cost index is not an absolute indicator of cost; for example, drugs listed as "$$$$" are not exactly four times as expensive as drugs listed as "$."

NOMOGRAM FOR THE
DETERMINATION OF BODY SURFACE
AREA OF CHILDREN AND ADULTS

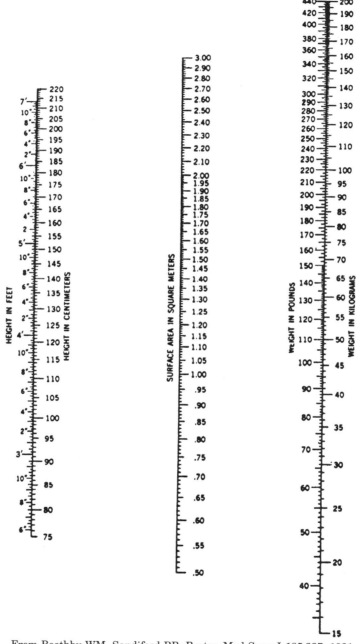

From Boothby WM, Sandiford RB: Boston Med Surg J *185*:337, 1921.

Index

Note: Page numbers followed by (t) refer to tables; page numbers in *italics* refer to illustrations.